Principles and Practice of Medical Genetics

Principles and Practice of Medical Genetics
Volume 2

Edited by

Alan E. H. Emery MD PhD (Johns Hopkins) DSc FRCP FLS FRS(E)
Emeritus Professor of Human Genetics and Honorary Fellow,
University of Edinburgh, Edinburgh, UK
Visiting Fellow, Green College, Oxford, UK
Research Director, European Alliance of Muscular Dystrophy
Associations, European Centre for Neuromuscular Diseases,
Baarn, The Netherlands

David L. Rimoin MD PhD
Steven Spielberg Chairman of Pediatrics; Director –
Ahmanson Pediatric Center, SHARE's Child
Disability Center and The Medical Genetics–Birth
Defects Center at Cedars Sinai Medical Center
Professor of Pediatrics and Medicine, University
of California at Los Angeles, Los Angeles, California, USA

Associate Editor
Jeffrey A. Sofaer BDS PhD DSc
Reader, Department of Oral Medicine,
University of Edinburgh, Edinburgh, UK

Editorial Assistant
Isobel Black RSA Cert

Foreword by
Victor A. McKusick MD
William Osler Professor of Medicine, The Johns Hopkins University
School of Medicine, Baltimore, Maryland, USA

SECOND EDITION

CHURCHILL LIVINGSTONE
EDINBURGH LONDON MELBOURNE AND NEW YORK 1990

CHURCHILL LIVINGSTONE
Medical Division of Longman Group UK Limited

Distributed in the United States of America by
Churchill Livingstone Inc., 1560 Broadway, New York,
NY 10036, and by associated companies, branches
and representatives throughout the world.

First edition 1983
Second edition 1990

ISBN 0 443 03583 0

British Library Cataloguing in Publication Data
Principles and practice of medical genetics. – 2nd. ed.
 Rimoin.
 1. Man. Diseases. Genetic factors
 I. Emery, Alan E. H.   II. Rimoin, David L.
 616.042

Library of Congress Cataloging in Publication Data
Principles and practice of medical genetics/edited by
 Alan E. H. Emery, David L. Rimoin; associate editor,
 Jeffrey A. Sofaer; editorial assistant, Isobel Black;
 foreword by Victor A. McKusick.
  – – 2nd ed.
       p.   cm.
  Includes bibliographical references.
  ISBN 0-443-03583-0
  1. Medical genetics.   I. Emery, Alan E. H.
  II. Rimoin, David L.,
 1936–
  [DNLM: 1. Genetics, Medical.   2. Hereditary
  Diseases.   QZ 50   P957]
 RB 155.P694   1990
 616'.042 – – dc20
 DNLM/DLC
 for Library of Congress   90-1784

Printed and bound in Great Britain by
William Clowes Limited, Beccles and London

Foreword

The six years since the first edition of *Principles and Practice of Medical Genetics* has seen the full-flowering of molecular clinical genetics. As discussed in my foreword for the first edition, medical genetics as a clinical speciality has been further strengthened by the new molecular diagnostic armamentarium.

It was in 1983, as the first edition was appearing, that the gene for Huntington disease was found to be linked to a DNA marker on the end of the short arm of chromosome 4. This was followed in relatively rapid succession by the linkage of other genetic disorders to markers at specific chromosome sites. The list now includes adenomatous polyposis of the colon (5q), childhood spinal muscular atrophy (5q), cystic fibrosis (7q), multiple endocrine neoplasia type II (10q), multiple endocrine neoplasia type I (11q), Wilson disease (13q), myotonic dystrophy (19q), polycystic kidney disease (16p), von Recklinghausen neurofibromatosis (17), bilateral acoustic neuroma (22q), Duchenne muscular dystrophy (Xp21), and many others. Each of these discoveries was welcomed with great enthusiasm by both the lay and the professional media and justly so: all of these conditions shared – at least at the time the linkage was determined – the characteristic that the nature of the fundamental defect was completely unknown, therefore no diagnostic test based thereon could be devised and rational management was hampered. Knowing the 'map location' of these disease genes meant that one could hope to test for the presence of the mutant gene by the linkage principle, i.e., by the company it keeps. It also meant that the basic gene defect might be elucidated by the approach of 'reverse genetics' – moving in on the segment of DNA altered in the mutation, determining how it differs from the normal, and most importantly, the nature and function of the normal gene that is changed. Definition of the precise genetic lesion makes it possible to do direct DNA diagnosis, by a process that might be called 'diagnostic biopsy of the genome'. Also, the improved understanding of pathogenesis is likely to enhance manage-ment by methods directed at the steps between gene and phene, i.e., without resort to gene therapy.

Remarkable indeed is the extent to which, since 1983, molecular methods have come into routine use in prenatal diagnosis, preclinical (premorbid or presymptomatic) diagnosis, and carrier detection of many of the above mentioned disorders as well as others. Cystic fibrosis and Duchenne muscular dystrophy are cardinal examples of diagnostic usefulness of molecular information, and in the case of DMD reverse genetics has been played out in full with identification of a muscle protein dubbed dystrophin as the site of the abnormality. The second edition of *Principles and Practice of Medical Genetics* is marked particularly by advances in this area of clinical molecular genetics.

A second area of remarkable advance since 1983 is that of somatic cell genetic disease. Traditionally, we employ the rather arbitrary but nonetheless useful three-way classification of diseases as to the role of genetic factors: monogenic (Mendelian) disorders, multifactorial disorders, and chromosomal disorders. Another large category of genetic disease is that caused by mutations in somatic cells. Cancers are prime examples. The chromosome theory of cancer, as advanced by Boveri in 1914 and others, has been massively corroborated in the last six years by the demonstration of many specific chromosomal aberrations in association with specific neoplasms, by the discovery of oncogenes, and by the correlation of the two approaches. Even cancers as intimately related to an environmental factor as small cell cancer of the lung is to cigarettes can be shown to have specific genetic changes that are responsible ultimately for the malignant change.

Obviously the new information on somatic cell mutation is valuable not only for understanding the malignant process but also for specific tumour diagnosis. Increasingly, we will depend on demonstration of specific DNA changes in the tumour rather than the relatively crude morphologic characteristics. Prognostication and management will be enhanced thereby. The

role of somatic cell mutations in congenital malformations and autoimmune disease is also under
exploration.

All these developments augur well for the future of
medical genetics, and are discussed in detail in this new
edition by contributors who are themselves internationally recognised authorities in their respective
fields. This new edition will therefore be welcomed by
all concerned in this rapidly advancing and exciting
subject.

Baltimore, Maryland, 1990   Victor A. McKusick

Preface to the second edition

Since the first edition of this book appeared in 1983 considerable changes have taken place in many aspects of medical genetics. These have been very largely due to the application of recombinant DNA techniques. This technology has helped our understanding of the fine structure of genes and is also beginning to unravel the molecular pathology of many inherited disorders. But perhaps of more immediate and practical importance, the technology has introduced novel and precise methods for detecting female carriers of X-linked disorders, pre-symptomatic cases of dominant disorders of late onset and in the prenatal diagnosis of genetic disease. These changes are reflected in most of the contributions to this new edition and their relevance will be apparent in almost all aspects of the subject.

As in the first edition we have enlisted the cooperation of internationally recognised experts to review developments in their respective fields. With no less than 116 chapters with 154 contributors there have been inevitable concerns about delays. But all have responded to our harassment and we believe that this new edition presents an up-to-date picture of the more important aspects of this rapidly growing subject.

Besides thanking our contributors we feel we must also acknowledge the invaluable help we have received from Mrs Isobel Black and the editorial team of Churchill Livingstone in Edinburgh, and Sheilah Levin and Susan Lane in Los Angeles. Finally we must also thank Dr Victor McKusick, in many ways the father of present-day medical genetics, for writing a Foreword to this new edition which we fervently hope will provide an important reference work for all those involved in this exciting field.

Edinburgh and Los Angeles, 1990   A.E.H.E.
D.L.R.

Preface to the first edition

Medical genetics has come of age as a unique speciality in medicine. All practitioners of medicine regardless of their individual speciality, encounter numerous patients with genetic disorders or conditions strongly influenced by hereditary factors and must be aware of their aetiology, pathogenesis, natural history and prognosis, as well as current approaches to their treatment and prevention. Unlike most other medical specialities, which are limited to a body system, age range or diagnostic modality, medical genetics has no such limits, involves all bodily systems and utilizes all manner of diagnostic and therapeutic modalities. In addition, the recent spectacular advances in cellular, biochemical and molecular genetics have been quickly translated into clinical applicability, and thus there are unique diagnostic tools available in modern genetics to which most practitioners of medicine have never been exposed.

There is a vast array of information available relating to genetic disease, which is found not only in genetics or general medical journals but appears throughout the many speciality and subspeciality medical journals and basic science journals as well. Although there are excellent textbooks and reference books dealing with the basic principles of medical genetics, or specific areas of medical genetics and broad catalogues of syndromes, inherited diseases and chromosomal diseases, there is no up-to-date reference source which attempts to cover all areas of medical genetics, from basic principles, to specific diseases, to therapy and prevention. Since most medical geneticists will encounter patients with a wide variety of genetic diseases and since most medical speciality textbooks do not pay a great deal of attention to the principles of genetics or genetic diseases, it was felt that a broad reference book in medical genetics, ranging from basic principles to applied genetics would be useful. The editors have undertaken the difficult task of trying to compile all of this information under one cover.

This task might have been easier 20 years ago when both of the editors were fellows and doctoral students at the Moore Clinic at Johns Hopkins Hospital with Dr Victor McKusick. At that time medical genetics was a relatively new speciality and the number of authors who could have contributed to this text was quite limited. The explosion of knowledge in genetics has been so great over the last two decades that complete coverage of all aspects of medical genetics is clearly impossible. Rather than ask relatively few individuals to contribute sections covering broad areas, such as the genetics of ophthalmology or the genetics of the endocrine glands, we have elected to conscript over 100 authors, each of whom has been asked to contribute to a relatively well defined area related to their own field of expertise. Thus each of the chapters is written by an individual who has had personal experience in the area in which he has been asked to write. The danger of this type of compilation is that there will be areas of medical genetics that have been excluded because they fell between the lines of the individual experts. We hope that our readers will bring these areas of omission to our attention so that they can be corrected in the next edition. We feel that we have included an outstanding group of international experts who have attempted to bring their current area of expertise to this readership in a relatively brief but complete form, with much of the information in useful tabular form and a fairly complete bibliography. We wish to thank these many individuals for their excellent contributions and apologize for the harassment they may have received from us.

In addition we would like to thank the individuals who contributed in a clerical and editorial fashion to this book including Margaret Fairbairn, Rita Anand, Dorothy Rivera, Toni Armstrong and Elena Hanson. We should also like to thank the publishers themselves especially Andrew Stevenson and Claire McLeod for their encouragement and much helpful advice. Finally, we should especially like to offer our gratitude to Dr Victor McKusick, who kindly agreed to write the foreword to this book. Dr McKusick's teaching, inspiration and encouragement were the prime factors in the development of both of our careers in medical genetics and thus we are doubly grateful to him.

Edinburgh and Los Angeles, 1983
A.E.H.E.
D.L.R.

Contributors

Dharam P. Agarwal PhD
Professor of Human Genetics, University of Hamburg, Hamburg, Federal Republic of Germany

Grace E. S. Aherne BSc MB BS DCH
Clinical Assistant, University Department of Ophthalmology, Royal Victoria Infirmary, Newcastle-upon-Tyne, UK

Chester A. Alper MD
Professor of Pediatrics, Harvard Medical School and The Center for Blood Research, Boston, Massachusetts, USA

Karl E. Anderson MD
Professor, Departments of Preventive Medicine and Community Health, Internal Medicine, and Pharmacology and Toxicology; Associate Director, Division of Human Nutrition; The University of Texas Medical Branch, Galveston, Texas, USA

Ingrun Anton-Lamprecht ScD
University Professor; Director of the Institute for Ultrastructure Research of the Skin, Department of Dermatology, Ruprecht-Karls University, Heidelberg, Federal Republic of Germany

Felicia B. Axelrod MD
Professor of Pediatrics, New York University Medical Center, New York, New York, USA

Howard P. Baden MD
Professor of Dermatology, Harvard Medical School, Boston, Massachusetts, USA

Gregory S. Barsh MD PhD
Assistant Professor, Department of Pediatrics, Stanford University School of Medicine, Howard Hughes Medical Institute, Stanford, California, USA

J. Bronwyn Bateman MD
Jules Stein Eye Institute for the Health Sciences, School of Medicine, University of California at Los Angeles, Los Angeles, California, USA

Peter Beighton MD PhD FRCP DCH
Director, MRC Research Unit for Inherited Skeletal Disorders; Professor of Human Genetics, University of Cape Town, South Africa

D. Timothy Bishop MSc PhD
Senior Scientist, Genetic Epidemiology Laboratory, IRCF, Leeds, West Yorkshire, UK

Gerry R. Boss MD
Associate Professor of Medicine, University of California at San Diego, San Diego, California, USA

Walter G. Bradley DM FRCP
Professor and Chairman, Department of Neurology, University of Vermont; Chief of Service, Medical Center Hospital of Vermont, Vermont, USA

Sarah Bundey MB FRCP
Lecturer in Clinical Genetics, University of Birmingham and Birmingham Maternity Hospital, Birmingham, UK

Peter H. Byers MD
Professor, Departments of Pathology and Medicine, University of Washington, Seattle, USA

Stephen D. Cederbaum MD
Professor of Psychiatry and Pediatrics, University of California at Los Angeles, Los Angeles, California, USA

Joel Charrow MD
Assistant Professor of Pediatrics, Northwestern University Medical School; Acting Head, Division of Genetics, Children's Memorial Hospital, Chicago, Illinois, USA

Ann C. Chandley DSc FRSE
Senior Scientist, MRC Human Genetics Unit, Western General Hospital, Edinburgh, UK

Albert de la Chapelle MD MScD
Professor and Chairman, Department of Medical Genetics, University of Helsinki, Helsinki, Finland

M. Michael Cohen, Jr DMD, PhD
Professor of Oral Pathology, Faculty of Dentistry;
Professor of Pediatrics, Faculty of Medicine,
Dalhousie University, Halifax, Nova Scotia, Canada

P. Michael Conneally PhD
Professor of Medical Genetics and Neurology, Indiana
University Medical Center, Indianapolis, Indiana, USA

C. Crawford MD
Academic Research Specialist, Department of
Pediatrics, Division of Endocrinology, Cornell
University Medical College, New York, New York, USA

David M. Danks MD BS FRACP
Director, Murdoch Institute for Research into Birth
Defects; Professor of Paediatric Research, Royal
Children's Hospital, Parkville, Australia

Robert J. Desnick MD PhD
Arthur J. and Nellie Z. Cohen Professor of Pediatrics
and Genetics; Chief, Division of Medical and
Molecular Genetics, Mount Sinai School of Medicine,
New York, New York, USA

John H. DiLiberti MD
Director of Pediatrics, St Francis Hospital and Medical
Center, Hartford; Associate Chairman, Department of
Pediatrics, University of Connecticut, Farmington,
Connecticut, USA

George N. Donnell MD
Professor of Pediatrics, University of Southern
California, Children's Hospital, Los Angeles,
California, USA

V. Dubowitz MD PhD FRCP DCH
Professor of Paediatrics and Neonatal Medicine, Royal
Postgraduate Medical School, Hammersmith Hospital,
London, UK

B. Dupont MD DSc
Member, Sloan-Kettering Institute for Cancer
Research, New York, New York, USA

Roswell Eldridge MD
Head, Clinical Neurogenetics, National Institute of
Neurological Disease and Stroke, NIH, Bethesda,
Maryland, USA

Richard Emanuel MA DM FRCP FACC
Senior Cardiologist, The Middlesex Hospital; Senior
Physician, National Heart Hospital; Lecturer, National
Heart and Lung Institute, London, UK

Alan E. H. Emery MD PhD (Johns Hopkins) DSc FRCP FLS
FRS(E)
Emeritus Professor of Human Genetics and Honorary

Fellow, University of Edinburgh, Edinburgh, UK;
Visiting Fellow, Green College, Oxford, UK; Research
Director, European Alliance of Muscular Dystrophy
Associations, European Centre for Neuromuscular
Diseases, Baarn, The Netherlands

Charles J. Epstein MD
Professor of Pediatrics and Biochemistry, University of
California at San Francisco, San Francisco, California,
USA

Richard W. Erbe MD
Chief, Division of Human Genetics; Professor of
Pediatrics and Medicine, The Children's Hospital of
Buffalo, Buffalo, New York, USA

Mark I. Evans MD
Director, Division of Reproductive Genetics, Hutzel
Hospital; Associate Professor, Department of
Obstetrics and Gynecology and Department of
Molecular Biology and Genetics, Wayne State
University, Detroit, Michigan, USA

Gerald M. Fenichel MD
Professor and Chairman, Department of Neurology,
Vanderbilt University, Nashville, Tennessee, USA

Delbert A. Fisher MD
Professor of Pediatrics and Medicine, University of
California at Los Angeles, Los Angeles, California,
USA

Uta Francke MD
Professor of Genetics and Pediatrics, Stanford
University Medical Center, Stanford, California, USA

F. Clarke Fraser OC MD PhD FRSC
Professor Emeritus of Human Genetics, McGill
Centre for Human Genetics, Montreal, Quebec,
Canada

Hans Galjaard MD PhD
Professor of Cell Biology and Human Genetics;
Chairman, Department of Clinical Genetics,
University Hospital, Erasmus University, Rotterdam,
The Netherlands

Ingrid Gamstorp MD
Professor of Child Neurology, Department of
Medicine, University Hospital, Uppsala, Sweden

Tobias Gedde-Dahl, Jr MD
Professor of Medical Genetics, Polar Institute of
Medical Genetics, Institute of Clinical Medicine,
University of Tromso, Norway

Bertil E. Glader MD PhD
Professor of Pediatrics, Stanford University School of

Medicine; Director, Hematology/Oncology Program, Children's Hospital at Stanford, California, USA

H. Werner Goedde PhD
Professor and Director, Institute of Human Genetics, University of Hamburg, Federal Republic of Germany

Lowell A. Goldsmith MD
James H. Sterner Professor of Dermatology and Chair, Department of Dermatology, School of Medicine and Dentistry, University of Rochester, Rochester, New York, USA

Richard M. Goodman MD (deceased)
Formerly Professor of Human Genetics, Sackler School of Medicine, Tel Aviv University; Formerly Professor of Human Genetics, Chaim Sheba Medical Center, Tel Hashomer, Israel

Stephen I. Goodman MD
Professor of Pediatrics, University of Colorado School of Medicine, Denver, Colorado, USA

Robert J. Gorlin DDS, MS
Professor of Oral Pathology, School of Dentistry; Professor of Pediatrics, Obstetrics and Gynecology, Dermatology, Pathology and Otolaryngology, School of Medicine, University of Minnesota, Minneapolis, Minnesota, USA

John M. Graham, Jr MD ScD
Director of Clinical Genetics and Dysmorphology, Medical Genetics Birth Defects Center, Ahmanson Pediatric Center, Cedars-Sinai Medical Center; Associate Professor of Pediatrics, School of Medicine, University of California at Los Angeles, Los Angeles, California, USA

Jean de Grouchy MD
Directeur de Recherche CNRS, Laboratoire de Cytogenetique Humaine et Comparée, Hôpital Necker-Enfants-Malades, Paris, France

Judith G. Hall MD
Director of Clinical Genetics Services and Professor of Medical Genetics, University of British Columbia, Vancouver, British Columbia, Canada

James W. Hanson MD
Professor of Pediatrics; Director, Division of Medical Genetics, University of Iowa, Iowa City, Iowa, USA

A. E. Harding MD FRCP
Reader in Clinical Neurology, Institute of Neurology; Consultant Neurologist, National Hospitals for Nervous Diseases, London, UK

P. S. Harper MA DM FRCP
Professor of Medical Genetics, University of Wales College of Medicine; Consultant in Medical Genetics, University Hospital of Wales, Cardiff, UK

Rodney Harris MSc MD FRCP FRCPath
Professor of Medical Genetics, St Mary's Hospital, Manchester, UK

John R. Heckenlively MD
Professor of Ophthalmology, Jules Stein Eye Institute for the Health Sciences, School of Medicine, University of California at Los Angeles, Los Angeles, California, USA

J. Z. Heckmatt MD MRCP
Senior Research Fellow and Honorary Consultant Paediatrician, Department of Paediatrics, Hammersmith Hospital, London, UK

Hugo S. A. Heymans MD PhD
Professor of Paediatrics, University of Groningen; Chairman, Department of Paediatrics, University Hospital, Groningen, The Netherlands

Harry R. Hill MD
Professor of Pediatrics and Pathology; Head, Division of Clinical Immunology and Allergy, University of Utah, Salt Lake City, Utah, USA

Richard E. Hillman MD
Professor of Child Health and Biochemistry; Director of Metabolic Genetics, University of Missouri-Columbia School of Medicine, Columbia, Missouri, USA

Kurt Hirschhorn MD
Herbert H. Lehman Professor and Chairman, Department of Pediatrics, Mount Sinai School of Medicine, New York, New York, USA

Rochelle Hirschhorn MD
Professor of Medicine and Chief, Division of Medical Genetics, New York University School of Medicine, New York, New York, USA

Susan Hodge DSc
Professor, Department of Psychiatry and Biostatics, New York State Psychiatric Institute, New York, New York, USA

Karen A. Holbrook BS MS PhD
Professor of Biological Structure, Adjunct Professor of Dermatology and Associate Dean for Scientific Affairs, University of Washington, Seattle, USA

P. Hooker MD PhD
Department of Dermatology, Harvard Medical School,

Massachusetts General Hospital, Boston,
Massachusetts, USA

William A. Horton MD
Professor, Pediatrics and Medicine; Director, Division
of Medical Genetics, University of Texas Health
Science Center at Houston, Houston, Texas, USA

Paul S. Ing PhD
Director of Cytogenetics, Boys Town National
Institute for Communication Disorders in Children,
Omaha, Nebraska, USA

Sherwin J. Isenberg MD
Professor and Vice Chairman, Department of
Ophthalmology, Jules Stein Eye Institute for the
Health Sciences, School of Medicine, University of
California at Los Angeles, Los Angeles, California,
USA

Charles E. Jackson MD
Chief, Clinical Genetics Division, Department of
Medicine, Henry Ford Hospital, Detroit; Clinical
Professor of Medicine, University of Michigan,
Detroit, Michigan, USA

Kenneth Lyon Jones MD
Professor of Pediatrics, School of Medicine, University
of California at San Diego, San Diego, California,
USA

Marilyn C. Jones MD
Associate Professor of Pediatrics, University of
California at San Diego; Children's Hospital at San
Diego, San Diego, California, USA

Stanley C. Jordan MD
Associate Professor, School of Medicine, University of
California at Los Angeles; Director, Pediatric
Nephrology and Transplant Immunology, Cedars-
Sinai Medical Center, Los Angeles, California, USA

Michael M. Kaback MD
Chairman, Department of Pediatrics, University of
California at San Diego, San Diego, California, USA

Hooshang Kangarloo MD
Professor of Radiological Sciences, University of
California at Los Angeles, Los Angeles, California,
USA

Haig H. Kazazian, Jr MD
Professor of Pediatrics and Director, Medical Genetics
Center, Johns Hopkins University, Baltimore,
Maryland, USA

John Kelemen MD
Clinical Assistant Professor of Neurology, Cornell

University Medical College; Assistant Attending,
Department of Neurology, North Shore University
Hospital, New York, New York, USA

Dennis K. Kinney PhD
Associate Psychologist and Acting Chief, Genetics
Laboratory, McLean Hospital, Belmont,
Massachusetts, and Department of Psychiatry,
Harvard Medical School, Boston, Massachusetts, USA

Hans-R. Koch MD
Professor of Ophthalmology, Department of
Microsurgery of the Eye, University of Bonn, Bonn,
Federal Republic of Germany

R. S. Lachman MD
Professor of Pediatrics and Radiology, Harbor—
UCLA Medical Center, University of California at Los
Angeles, Los Angeles, California, USA

Pulak Lahiri PhD
Reader, Department of Zoology, Calcutta University,
Calcutta, India

Jean-Marc Lalouel MD DSc
Professor of Human Genetics, Howard Hughes
Medical Institute, University of Utah, Salt Lake City,
Utah, USA

K. Michael Laurence MA DSc MB ChB FRCP(Ed)
FRCPath
Professor of Paediatric Research, Department of Child
Health; Consultant Clinical Geneticist and Co-
Director, Institute of Medical Genetics, University of
Wales College of Medicine and University Hospital of
Wales, Cardiff, UK

Claire O. Leonard MD
Associate Professor, Pediatric Department, University
of Utah, Salt Lake City, Utah, USA

Jules G. Leroy MD PhD
Professor and Chairman, Department of Pediatrics and
Medical Genetics, Ghent State University Medical
School, Ghent, Belgium

Jack Lieberman MD
Professor of Medicine, UCLA School of Medicine,
Los Angeles Veterans Administrations Medical
Center, Sepulveda, California, USA

H. A. Lubs MD
Professor of Pediatrics and Director, Genetics
Division, University of Miami, Miami, Florida, USA

C. A. Ludlam PhD FRCP FRCPath
Consultant Haematologist and Director, Haemophilia
Centre, Royal Infirmary, Edinburgh, UK

Stephen J. Marx MD
Chief, Mineral Metabolism Section, National Institute of Diabetes and Digestive and Kidney Disease, Bethesda, Maryland, USA

W. M. McCrae MB ChB FRCPE FRCP(G)
Consultant Physician, Royal Hospital for Sick Children; Senior Lecturer, Department of Child Life and Health, University of Edinburgh, Edinburgh, UK

V. V. Michels MD
Associate Professor, Department of Medical Genetics, Mayo Clinic, Rochester, Minnesota, USA

M. E. Miller MD (deceased)
Formerly Professor and Chairman, Department of Pediatrics, Children's Hospital, Pittsburg, Pennsylvania, USA

Orlando J. Miller BS MD
Professor and Chairman, Department of Molecular Biology and Genetics, School of Medicine, Wayne State University, Detroit, Michigan, USA

Hugo W. Moser MD
Professor of Neurology and Pediatrics, Johns Hopkins University; President, John F. Kennedy Institute for Handicapped Children, Baltimore, Maryland, USA

R. F. Mueller MB BS BSc MRCP
Consultant Clinical Geneticist, Department of Genetic Counselling, The General Infirmary, Leeds, UK

Henry L. Nadler MD
President, Michael Reese Hospital Medical Center, Chicago, Illinois, USA

M. I. New MD
Harold and Percy Uris Professor of Pediatric Endocrinology and Metabolism; Professor and Chairman, Department of Pediatrics, Cornell University Medical College, New York, New York, USA

W. G. Ng PhD
Professor of Pediatrics, School of Medicine, University of Southern California at Los Angeles, Los Angeles, California, USA

Reijo Norio MD
Professor of Clinical Genetics, University of Helsinki; Director, Department of Medical Genetics, Vaestoliitto, The Finnish Population and Family Welfare Federation, Helsinki, Finland

Eberhard Passarge MD
Professor of Human Genetics, Department of Human Genetics, University of Essen, Essen, Federal Republic of Germany

J. H. Pearn MD BSc PhD FRCP FRACP
Professor and Head, Department of Child Health, Royal Children's Hospital, Brisbane, Australia

Alan K. Percy MD
Professor of Pediatrics and Neurology, Baylor College of Medicine, Houston, Texas, USA

John A. Phillips III MD
Director, Division of Genetics; Professor of Pediatrics and Biochemistry, Vanderbilt University, Nashville, Tennessee, USA

David A. Price Evans MD DSc PhD FRCP
Honorary Professor of Medicine, King Saud University; Director of Medicine, Riyadh Armed Forces Hospital, Riyadh, Kingdom of Saudi Arabia

Reed E. Pyeritz MD PhD
Associate Professor of Medicine and Pediatrics, Johns Hopkins University School of Medicine; Director of Clinical Services, Division of Medical Genetics, Johns Hopkins Hospital, Baltimore, Maryland, USA

J. A. Raeburn TD MB ChB PhD FRCP(Ed)
Professor of Clinical Genetics, The Medical School, University of Nottingham, Nottingham, UK

C. T. Ramey MD
Professor, Frank Porter Graham Child Development Center, University of North Carolina, Chapel Hill, North Carolina, USA

Andrew P. Read MA PhD
Senior Lecturer in Medical Genetics, St Mary's Hospital, Manchester, UK

Vincent M. Riccardi MD
Professor of Medicine and Pediatrics, Baylor College of Medicine; Director, Baylor NF Program, Houston, Texas, USA

David L. Rimoin MD PhD
Steven Spielberg Chairman of Pediatrics; Director— Ahmanson Pediatric Center, SHARE's Child Disability Center and the Medical Genetics–Birth Defects Center at Cedars Sinai Medical Center; Professor of Pediatrics and Medicine, University of California at Los Angeles, Los Angeles, California, USA

Andrew G. Roberts PhD
Fellow in Molecular Genetics, Division of Medical and Molecular Genetics, Mount Sinai School of Medicine, New York, New York, USA

D. F. Roberts MD
Professor of Human Genetics, University of

Newcastle-upon-Tyne; Honorary Consultant in Genetics, Royal Victoria Infirmary, Newcastle-upon-Tyne, UK

T. F. Roe MD
Professor of Pediatrics, University of Southern California, Los Angeles, California, USA

Fred S. Rosen MD
President, The Center for Blood Research; James L. Gamble Professor of Pediatrics, Harvard Medical School, Boston, Massachusetts, USA

E. Roth MD
Department of Microsurgery of the Eye, University of Bonn, Bonn, Federal Republic of Germany

Jerome I. Rotter MD
Professor of Medicine and Pediatrics, School of Medicine, University of California at Los Angeles; Codirector, Cedars–Sinai Medical Center and The Medical Genetics–Birth Defects Center, Los Angeles, California, USA

Janet D. Rowley MD
Professor, Joint Section of Hematology and Oncology, University of Chicago, Illinois, USA; Part-time Senior Lecturer, Department of Medicine, University of Edinburgh, Edinburgh, UK

J. Roy Chowdhury MD MRCP
Professor of Medicine, Liver Research Center, Albert Einstein College of Medicine, New York, New York, USA

Namita Roy Chowdhury PhD
Associate Professor of Medicine, Albert Einstein College of Medicine, New York, New York, USA

R. Neil Schimke MD FACP
Professor of Medicine and Pediatrics, University of Kansas; Director, Division of Metabolism, Endocrinology and Genetics, Kansas University Medical School, Kansas City, Kansas, USA

R. B. H. Schutgens PhD
Head of Paediatric and Obstetric Clinical Chemistry Laboratory, University Hospital, Amsterdam, The Netherlands

C. Ronald Scott MD
Head, Division of Pediatric Genetics, Division of Genetics, Department of Pediatrics, School of Medicine, University of Washington, Seattle, Washington, USA

J. Edwin Seegmiller MD JD
Professor of Medicine, University of California at San Diego, La Jolla, California, USA

Margery Shaw MD JD
Professor Emeritus, Health Law, Health Law Program, University of Texas Health Science Center, Houston, Texas, USA

T. Shohat MD
Major, Epidemiology Branch, Israeli Defence Forces, Tel Aviv, Israel

Karol Sikora MA PhD FRCP FRCR
Professor of Clinical Oncology, Royal Postgraduate Medical School, London, UK

D. O. Sillence MB BS MD(Melb) FRACP FRCPA
Professor of Genetics, University of Sydney; Head, Medical Genetics and Dysmorphology Unit, Children's Hospital, Sydney, Australia

M. Simon MD (deceased)
Formerly Professor of Medicine, Hôpital Sud, Rennes, France

J. L. Simpson MD
Faculty Professor and Chairman, Department of Obstetrics and Gynecology, University of Tennessee, Memphis, Tennessee, USA

Rosalind Skinner MSc MD MFCM
Senior Medical Officer, Scottish Home and Health Department, Edinburgh, UK

J. A. Sofaer BDS PhD DSc
Reader, Department of Oral Medicine and Oral Pathology, University of Edinburgh, Edinburgh, UK

Robert S. Sparkes MD
Professor and Chief, Division of Medical Genetics, Department of Medicine, Health Sciences Center, University of California at Los Angeles, Los Angeles, California, USA

P. W. Speiser MD
Associate Professor of Pediatrics, Department of Pediatrics, Division of Pediatric Endocrinology, Cornell University Medical College, New York, New York, USA

M. Anne Spence PhD
Professor, Departments of Psychiatry and Biomathematics, University of California at Los Angeles, Los Angeles, California, USA

Jurgen Spranger MD
Professor of Pediatrics and Director, Children's Hospital, University of Mainz, Mainz, Federal Republic of Germany

Tom Strachan BSc PhD
Lecturer in Medical Genetics, St Mary's Hospital, Manchester, UK

Joel Sugar MD
Professor of Ophthalmology and Director of Cornea
Service, University of Illinois Hospital and Eye and
Ear Infirmary, Chicago, Illinois, USA

Graham C. Sutton PhD MFCM
Specialist in Community Medicine, Ackton Hospital,
Ackton, Pontefract, West Yorkshire, UK

P. K. Thomas DSc MD FRCP
Professor of Neurology, University of London and
Institute of Neurology, London, UK

Catherine Turleau MD
Directeur de Recherche CNRS, Laboratoire de
Cytogenetique Humaine et Comparée, Hôpital
Necker-Enfants-Malades, Paris, France

Gerd Utermann MD
Professor of Medical Biology and Genetics; Head,
Institute for Medical Biology and Genetics, University
of Innsbruck, Innsbruck, Austria

C. M. Vadheim PhD
Assistant Professor, Medicine and Pediatrics,
Department of Epidemiology, University of California
at Los Angeles, Los Angeles, California, USA

Demetris Vassilopoulos MD PhD
Reader in Neurology, University of Athens, Athens,
Greece

A. M. O. Veale MB ChB PhD FRACP MCCMNZ (deceased)
Formerly Professor of Human Genetics and
Community Health, Department of Community
Health and General Practice, University of Auckland,
Auckland, New Zealand

Friedrich Vogel Dr med Dr med hc
Professor of Human Genetics, University of
Heidelberg, Heidelberg, Federal Republic of Germany

R. J. A. Wanders PhD
Associate Professor, Department of Paediatrics,
University Hospital of Amsterdam, Amsterdam, The
Netherlands

Mette Warburg MD PhD
Consultant, Division of Pediatric Ophthalmology and
Handicaps, Gentofte Hospital, Gentofte, Denmark

James V. Watson MSc FRCR
Senior Clinical Scientist, Medical Research Council;
Honorary Consultant Oncologist, MRC Clinical
Oncology Unit, The Medical School, Cambridge, UK

A. Wegener DipBiol Dr rer nat
Department of Experimental Ophthalmology,
University of Bonn, Bonn, Federal Republic of
Germany

L. N. Went DSc
Emeritus Professor of Human Genetics, University of
Leiden, Leiden, The Netherlands

P. C. White MD
Associate Professor of Pediatrics, Department of
Pediatrics, Division of Pediatric Endocrinology,
Cornell University Medical College, New York, New
York, USA

Raymond L. White PhD
Investigator, Howard Hughes Medical Institute,
University of Utah, Salt Lake City, Utah, USA

Robert Williamson PhD FRCPath Hon MRCP Hon
MD(Turku)
Professor and Head of the Department of Molecular
Genetics, St Mary's Hospital, London, UK

Carl J. Witkop, Jr DDS MS
Professor of Oral Pathology and Genetics, University
of Minnesota, Minneapolis, Minnesota, USA

R. F. J. Withers PhD
Senior Lecturer in Human Genetics, The Medical
School, Middlesex Hospital, London, UK

J. Zonana MD
Professor of Medical Genetics, School of Medicine,
Oregon Health Sciences University, Portland, Oregon,
USA

Contents
Volume 2

Contents
Volume 1

56. The chondrodysplasias

D. L. Rimoin   R. S. Lachman

The skeletal dysplasias are a heterogeneous group of disorders associated with abnormalities in the size and shape of the limbs, trunk and/or skull which frequently result in disproportionate short stature. Until the 1960s, most disproportionate dwarfs were considered to have either achondroplasia (those with short limbs) or Morquio disease (those with a short trunk). It is now apparent that there are over 100 distinct skeletal dysplasias which have been classified primarily on the basis of their clinical or radiographic characteristics (see Appendix and General References).

CLASSIFICATION AND NOMENCLATURE

Current nomenclature for these disorders is most confusing and is based on the part of the skeleton that is affected radiographically (e.g. the epiphyseal dysplasias, the metaphyseal dysplasias); on a Greek term that describes the appearance of the bone or the course of the disease (e.g. diastrophic [twisted] dysplasia, thanatophoric [death-seeking] dysplasia; on an eponym (e.g. Kniest dysplasia, Ellis-van Creveld syndrome); or by a term that attempts to describe the pathogenesis of the condition (e.g. achondroplasia, osteogenesis imperfecta). The extent of the heterogeneity in these disorders and the variety of methods used for their classification have resulted in further confusion. Clinical classifications have divided the skeletal dysplasias into those with short-limbed dwarfism, and those with short-trunk dwarfism. The short-limbed varieties have been further subdivided on the basis of the segment of the long bones that is most severely involved. Other clinical classifications have been based on the age of onset of the disorder; those disorders that manifest themselves at birth (achondroplasia), versus those that first manifest in later life (e.g. pseudoachondroplasia). Associated clinical abnormalities have also been used to subdivide these disorders. Examples are the myopia of spondyloepiphyseal dysplasia congenita, the cleft palate of Kniest dysplasia, the fine hair of cartilage-hair hypoplasia, and the polydactyly and con-genital heart disease of the Ellis-van Creveld syndrome. Still other disorders have been classified on the basis of their apparent mode of inheritance; for example, the dominant and X-linked varieties of spondyloepiphyseal dysplasia.

The most widely used method of differentiating the skeletal dysplasias has been the detection of skeletal radiographic abnormalities. Radiographic classifications are based on the different parts of the long bones that are abnormal (epiphyses, metaphyses or diaphyses) (Figs 56.1 and 56.2). Thus there are epiphyseal and metaphyseal dysplasias which can be further divided depending on whether or not the spine is also involved (spondyloepiphyseal dysplasias, spondylometaphyseal dysplasias). Furthermore, each of these classes can be further divided into several distinct disorders based on a variety of other clinical and radiographic differences.

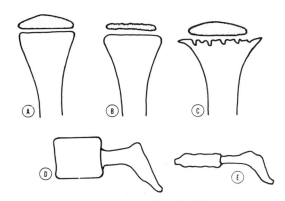

Fig. 56.1 Classification of chondrodysplasia based on radiographic involvement of long bones (A,B,C) and vertebrae (D,E).

Involvement	Disease category
A+D	Normal
B+D	Epiphyseal dysplasia
C+D	Metaphyseal dysplasia
B+E	Spondyloepiphyseal dysplasia
C+E	Spondylometaphyseal dysplasia
B+C+E	Spondyloepimetaphyseal dysplasia

895

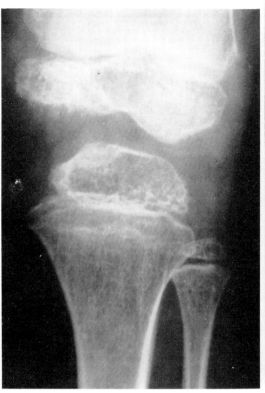

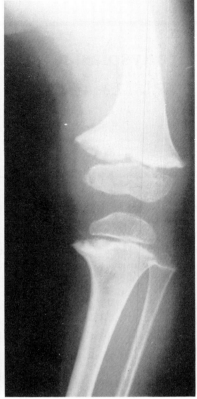

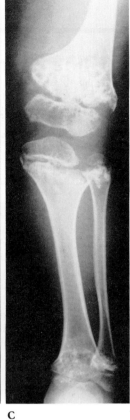

A   B   C

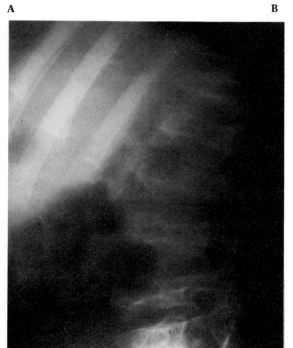

D

Fig. 56.2   Radiographs of knee (**A,B,C**) and spine (**D**) from patients with a variety of chondrodysplasias.

A   Epiphyseal dysplasia – note the small irregular epiphyses and normal metaphyses, from a patient with spondyloepiphyseal dysplasia congenita.

B   Metaphyseal dysplasia – note the irregular and widened metaphyses with normal epiphyses, from a patient with metaphyseal dysplasia, type Schmid.

C   Epimetaphyseal dysplasia – note the abnormal epiphyses and metaphyses from a patient with spondyloepimetaphyseal dysplasia – type Strudwick.

D   Platyspondyly – note the flat and irregular vertebrae from a patient with spondylometaphyseal dysplasia, type Kozlowski.

In an attempt to develop a uniform nomenclature for these syndromes, an International Nomenclature of Constitutional Diseases of Bone was proposed in 1970 and updated in 1977 and 1983 (see Appendix). This International Nomenclature divides the constitutional disorders of the skeleton into five major groups: the osteochondrodysplasias (abnormal growth or development of cartilage and/or bone); the dysostoses (malformations of individual bones, singly or in combination); the idiopathic osteolyses (a group of disorders associated with multifocal resorption of bone); the skeletal disorders associated with chromosomal aberrations; and primary metabolic disorders.

The osteochondrodysplasias are further divided into: (1) defects of growth of tubular bones and/or spine (e.g. achondroplasia), which are frequently referred to as chondrodysplasias (this chapter); (2) disorganized development of cartilage and fibrous components of the skeleton (e.g. multiple cartilaginous exostoses) and (3) abnormalities of density or cortical diaphyseal structure and/or metaphyseal modelling (e.g. osteogenesis imperfecta).

The chondrodysplasias are further subdivided into those disorders manifest at birth, as opposed to those that first become apparent in later life. This division may be purely artificial, since identical pathogenetic mechanisms of differing degrees of severity may occur in allelic disorders, resulting in differences in the age of manifestation. For example, both congenital and infantile presentations of osteogenesis imperfecta are seen within the same families manifesting dominant inheritance. On the other hand, many disorders which share common radiographic features and have thus been classified into one group, such as the metaphyseal dysplasias, almost certainly result from different pathogenetic mechanisms.

As short stature is a frequent finding in these disorders, the term 'dwarfism' has been historically used for them. However, 'dwarfism' is thought to result in stigmatization and is popularly unappealing, and for these and other reasons, the term 'dwarfism' has been dropped from the current nomenclature and replaced by the term 'dysplasia'. This latter term, which means 'disordered growth', reflects the probable pathogenesis of the majority of the chondrodysplasias. In contrast, malformations of single bones or groups of bones, which presumably do not reflect a generalized disorder of the skeleton, have been referred to as 'dysostoses'.

Although the International Nomenclature provides a uniform standard for referring to specific disorders, so that the same disease is called the same thing by all authors, many of the names are inaccurate. For example, achondroplasia and achondrogenesis are inaccurate terms in defining the pathogenesis of these conditions, but are so well entrenched in the literature that they persist. As the morphology, pathogenesis, and especially the basic biochemical defect in each of these disorders is unravelled, this nomenclature should be changed to refer to the specific pathogenetic or metabolic defect. The aetiological or pathogenetic nomenclature is now being used for certain skeletal dysplasias, such as the mucopolysaccharidoses, mucolipidoses and disorders of mineralization (e.g. β-glucuronidase deficiency, fucosidosis, hypophosphatasia).

CLINICAL EVALUATION

The osteochondrodysplasias are syndromes which represent generalized disorders of the skeleton and usually result in disproportionate short stature. Affected individuals usually present with the complaint of disproportionate short stature and the abnormality in stature must first be documented by the use of the appropriate growth curves with adjustment for ethnic background and parental heights (Rimoin & Horton 1978). In general, patients with disproportionate short stature have skeletal dysplasias, whereas those with relatively normal body proportions have endocrine, nutritional, prenatal or other nonskeletal defects. There are exceptions to these rules, as cretinism can lead to disproportionate short stature, and a variety of skeletal dysplasias, such as osteogenesis imperfecta and hypophosphatasia, may result in normal body proportions.

A disproportionate body habitus may not be readily apparent on casual physical examination. Thus anthropometric measurements, such as upper to lower segment ratio, sitting height and arm span must be obtained before the possibility of a mild skeletal dysplasia, such as hypochondroplasia or multiple epiphyseal dysplasia, can be excluded. Although sitting height is a more accurate measure of head and trunk length, it requires special equipment for consistent accuracy. Upper to lower segment ratios (U/L), on the other hand, provide a fairly accurate measure of body proportions and can be easily obtained. The lower segment measure is taken from the symphysis pubis to the floor at the inside of the heel, and the upper segment is obtained by subtracting the lower segment value from the total height. McKusick (1972), has published standard U/L curves for both Caucasian and Black Americans which are quite useful for rapid assessment of proportion. For example, a Caucasian infant has an upper/lower segment ratio of approximately 1.7; it reaches 1.0 at approximately 7–10 years, and then falls to an average U/L of 0.95 as an adult. Blacks, on the other hand, have relatively long limbs, and reach a U/L of approximately 0.85 as adults. Another index of limb versus trunk length is based on the arm span measurement, which usually falls within a few centimetres of total height. These measurements are

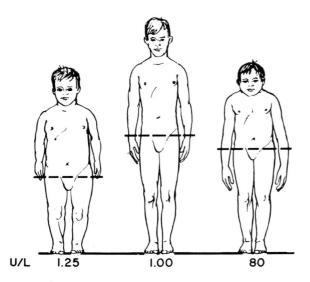

U/L   1.25   1.00   80

Fig. 56.3 Upper-Lower segment ratios in 8–10-year-old individuals with short limb dwarfism, proportionate stature and short trunk dwarfism, (from left to right respectively). The child on the left has short limbs and short stature with an elevated U/L, whereas the child on the right has a short trunk and short stature with a reduced U/L. U/L equals upper segment length/lower segment length.

most useful in determining whether or not an abnormally short individual is proportionate or not, and the type of disproportion present. For example, a short-limbed dwarf will have an abnormally high U/L ratio and an arm span which is considerably shorter than his height (Fig. 56.3).

As in the differential diagnosis of most other disorders, an accurate history, family history and physical examination may lead one to the correct diagnosis. As the International Nomenclature indicates, certain skeletal dysplasias have prenatal onset and manifest at birth, whereas others may not manifest until late infancy or early childhood. Thus a child who was normal until 2 years of age and then develops disproportionate short-limbed dwarfism is more likely to have pseudoachondroplasia or multiple epiphyseal dysplasia than achondroplasia or SED congenita. As has already been pointed out, classification on the basis of age of onset may not be totally accurate, as in certain disorders marked variability in expression is seen with both prenatal and postnatal onset of the disease in the same family (e.g. osteogenesis imperfecta type I). Furthermore, many parents may not notice short stature until 1 or 2 years of age, whereas, in reality, it existed from the time of birth.

A detailed physical examination may reveal the correct diagnosis or point to the likely diagnostic category (Table 56.1). First, one must establish whether the dispropor-

tionate shortening affects primarily the trunk or the limbs and, if the latter, whether it is proximal (rhizomelic), middle segment (mesomelic), or distal (acromelic), or a combination of these (Fig. 56.4). A disproportionately *large head* with frontal bossing and flattening of the bridge of the nose suggests achondroplasia or thanatophoric dysplasia. *Clover-leaf skull* is sometimes associated with thanatophoric dysplasia and rarely with campomelic dysplasia and a variety of malformation syndromes. *Congenital cataracts* suggest chondrodysplasia punctata. *Myopia* may be found associated with Kniest dysplasia or spondyloepiphyseal dysplasia congenita. Complete or partial *cleft palate*, bifid uvula or high-arched palate may be found in Kniest dysplasia, spondyloepiphyseal dysplasia congenita or diastrophic dysplasia. The *upper lip* is short and tethered in chondroectodermal dysplasia. Acute swelling of the *pinnae of the ears* in the newborn period, followed by cauliflower ears, is characteristic of diastrophic dysplasia.

Postaxial *polydactyly* is characteristic of chondroectodermal dysplasia and of the lethal short rib-polydactyly syndromes, and may also be seen in asphyxiating thoracic dysplasia (Fig. 56.5). Preaxial polydactyly is frequently observed in chondroectodermal dysplasia, short rib-polydactyly syndrome II (Majewski) and rarely in short rib-polydactyly syndrome I (Saldino-Noonan). In diastrophic dysplasia the *hands* are short and broad, the thumbs are hypermobile, proximally inserted and abducted leading to the 'hitch-hiker thumb' configuration, and flexion creases in the fingers are frequently absent (Fig. 56.5). In achondroplastic children, the hand has a trident appearance (Fig. 56.5). Hypoplastic *nails* are characteristic of chondroectodermal dysplasia, whereas the nails may be short and broad in the McKusick type of metaphyseal dysplasia (cartilage-hair hypoplasia). *Club feet* may be seen in infants with Kniest dysplasia, SED congenita, osteogenesis imperfecta, but are most characteristic of diastrophic dysplasia. Multiple *joint dislocations* suggest Larsen syndrome, Ehlers-Danlos syndrome type VII, or otopalatodigital syndrome; less severe degrees of joint laxity, particularly of the hands, may be seen in other types of skeletal dysplasia (e.g. cartilage-hair hypoplasia and pseudoachondroplasia). Bone *fractures*

Fig. 56.4 Different forms of disproportionate dwarfism.
A Short trunk dwarfism in a girl with Dyggve-Melchior-Clausen syndrome.
B Short limb dwarfism of the rhizomelic type in a boy with achondroplasia.
C Short limb dwarfism of the mesomelic type in a boy with mesomelic dysplasia, Langer type.
D Short limb dwarfism of the acromelic type in a girl with peripheral dysostosis.

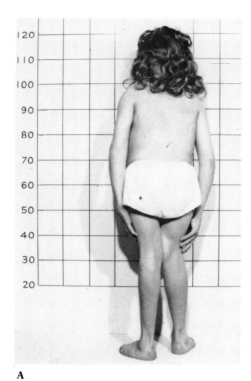

A

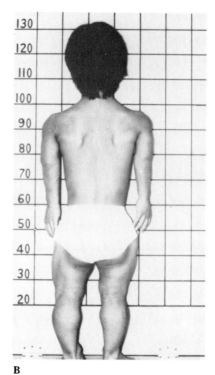

B

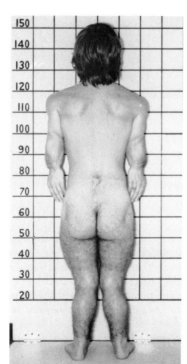

C

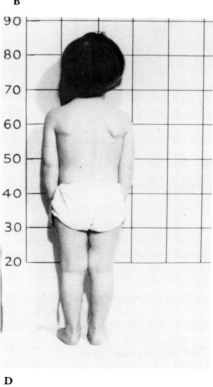

D

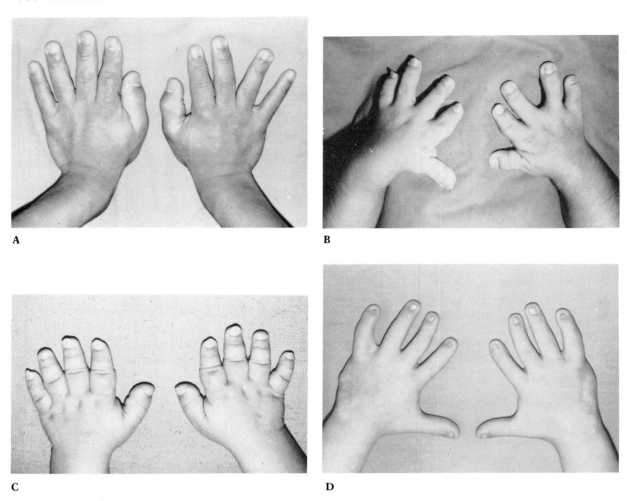

Fig. 56.5 Characteristic hand abnormalities in different types of chondrodysplasia.
A Achondroplasia – note the trident appearance of the hand and generalized brachydactyly.
B Diastrophic dysplasia – note the hitch-hiker thumb and symphalangism.
C Metaphyseal chondrodysplasia type McKusich – note the short hypermobile hands with squared off terminal phalanges.
D Chondroectodermal dysplasia – note the repaired postaxial polydactyly and the nail dysplasia.

may occur in all of the osteogenesis imperfecta syndromes and several types of hypophosphatasia, osteopetrosis, dysosteosclerosis and achondrogenesis type IA (Houston-Harris).

In the neonate or infant, a long, narrow *thorax* suggests asphyxiating thoracic dysplasia, chondroectodermal dysplasia or metatropic dysplasia. A very small thorax is also seen in thanatophoric dysplasia, the short rib-polydactyly syndromes and homozygous achondroplasia. In some neonates with spondyloepiphyseal dysplasia congenita,

the sternum and neck are short and the chest may be small with pectus carinatum producing early respiratory distress. In the child or adult, *scoliosis* is frequently seen in metatropic dysplasia, SMD and diastrophic dysplasia, whereas a short, broad thorax with Harrison's grooves is a frequent manifestation in various metaphyseal dysphasias.

Congenital *cardiac defects* are seen in several of the skeletal dysplasias. In chondroectodermal dysplasia the most common lesion is an atrial septal defect with a common atrium. In short rib-polydactyly syndrome I (Saldino-Noonan), a variety of very complex lesions involving the great vessels, transposition or double outlet right or left ventricle and ventricular septal defect have been reported, whereas in short rib-polydactyly syndrome II (Majewski), the most common cardiac defect is transposition of the great vessels.

Gastrointestinal manifestations are not common in the skeletal dysplasias, but congenital megacolon can be seen in cartilage-hair hypoplasia, malabsorption in the Schwachman-Diamond syndrome, and anorectal anomalies in short rib-polydactyly syndrome.

In the older child or adult, the complications associated with specific disorders may aid in the diagnosis. For example, *spinal stenosis* with symptoms of spinal cord claudication are characteristic of achondroplasia, whereas *odontoid hypoplasia* and C.1-C.2 subluxation are frequently seen in Morquio disease, metatropic dysplasia and spondyloepiphyseal dysplasia. *Genu varum* is seen in a number of skeletal dysplasias, but in achondroplasia it is associated with lateral curvature primarily of the middle segment of the limb with overgrowth of the fibula proximally, whereas in cartilage-hair hypoplasia, there is generalized bowing with marked overgrowth of the fibula distally (Fig. 56.6). In pseudoachondroplasia, genu varum, valgum or a windswept abnormality may be seen, but it is associated with severe instability and ligamentous laxity at the knees (Fig. 56.6). Thus, careful physical examination with delineation of all the skeletal and nonskeletal abnormalities can be quite helpful in arriving at a diagnosis.

A complete family history, details of stillborn children and parental consanguinity should be obtained. Parents should always be closely examined, looking for evidence of a dysplasia in a partially expressed form. This is especially important in dominantly inherited disorders with wide variability of expressivity, where a parent may be mildly affected without knowing it (e.g. osteogenesis imperfecta). The health of parental sibs, especially male sibs and male relatives of the mother, should be questioned, as some conditions are inherited in an X-linked fashion. Since each of the skeletal dysplasias most frequently presents as an isolated case in the family, an isolated instance of a skeletal dysplasia in a family cannot provide information as to the mode of inheritance of the particular disorder. However, the type of familial aggregation, when it occurs, can be most helpful. For example, affected sibs with normal parents suggests a recessive type of disease and argues against autosomal dominant disorders, such as achondroplasia and hypochondroplasia. However, germ cell mosaicism appears to account for this situation in osteogenesis imperfecta II

and may be much more common than previously appreciated. If two achondroplastic parents produce a severely affected offspring, it is most likely homozygous achondroplasia, rather than thanatophoric dysplasia. However, different modes of inheritance have been observed in disorders that cannot be distinguished clinically, such as the X-linked and certain autosomal forms of spondyloepiphyseal dysplasia.

RADIOLOGICAL EVALUATION

The next step in the evaluation of the disproportionately short patient is to obtain a full set of skeletal radiographs. A full series of skeletal views including anterior-posterior, lateral and Towne views of the skull, anterior-posterior and lateral views of the spine, anterior-posterior views of the pelvis and extremities, with separate views of the hands and feet is usually required. Lateral views of the foot are particularly helpful in identifying punctate calcification of the calcaneus which may be a clue to the diagnosis of the milder forms of chondrodysplasia punctata, confirming the absence of hypoplasia of calcaneus and talus in newborns with SED congenita, and in delineating the double ossification centres of the calcaneus in the Larsen syndrome. Skeletal radiographs alone will often be sufficient to make an accurate diagnosis, since the classification of skeletal dysplasias has been based primarily on radiographic criteria (Table 56.1). Attention should be paid to the specific parts of the skeleton which are involved (spine, limbs, pelvis, skull) and, within each bone, to the location of the lesion (epiphysis, metaphysis, diaphysis) (Figs 56.1 and 56.2). The skeletal radiographic features of many of these diseases change with age and it is usually beneficial to review radiographs taken at different ages when possible. In some disorders, the radiographic abnormalities following epiphyseal fusion are non-specific, so that the accurate diagnosis of an adult disproportionate dwarf may be impossible unless prepubertal films are available.

Radiological diagnosis is also based upon recognition of unique patterns of abnormal skeletal ossification, such as the total lack or marked reduction of ossification of the vertebral bodies in the achondrogenesis syndromes (Fig. 56.7). Some radiographic features characterize certain disorders. For example, in achondroplasia the acetabulae are flat with tiny sacrosciatic notches, rather square iliac wings with rounded corners, and an oval translucent area in the proximal femora and humeri in infants. In Kniest dysplasia and metatropic dysplasia, the long bones, and femora in particular, have a dumb-bell shaped appearance in the newborn period. Bowing of the limbs (campomelia) is observed in campomelic dysplasia, osteogenesis imperfecta, congenital hypophosphatasia,

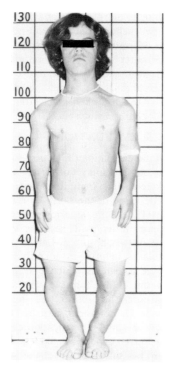

A

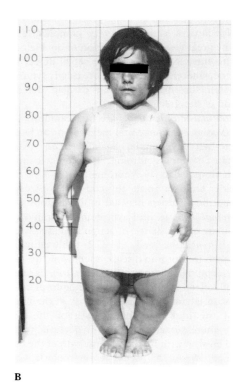

B

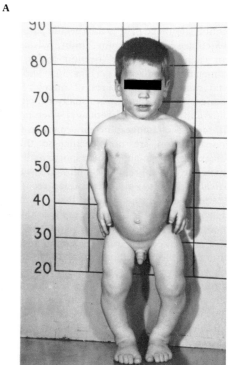

C

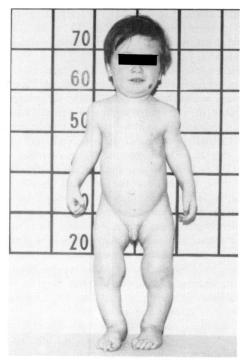

D

thanatophoric dysplasia and a heterogenous group of disorders with broad bent long bones.

There are calcified projections or spikes on the medial borders of the metaphyses of the femora in thanatophoric dysplasia; and medial and lateral borders in short rib-polydactyly syndrome I/III (Fig. 56.7). Cupping of the ends of the ribs and the long bones and metaphyseal flaring are features of a large number of dysplasias, including achondroplasia, the metaphyseal dysplasias, asphyxiating thoracic dysplasia and chondroectodermal dysplasia.

While fractures in the newborn suggest one of the osteogenesis imperfecta syndromes, fractures may also be seen in congenital osteopetrosis and severe hypophosphatasia. In achondrogenesis type IA (Houston-Harris), the ribs are thin and wavy with beading suggesting fractures, but the long bone and vertebral findings readily distinguish this from osteogenesis imperfecta. In the older individual, fractures may also be seen in a variety of osteopetrotic syndromes, including dysosteosclerosis and pycnodysostosis.

Retarded ossification manifest by absence of epiphyseal centres or marked delay in their ossification, is found in spondyloepiphyseal dysplasia congenita, Kniest dysplasia and other spondyloepimetaphyseal and multiple epiphyseal dysplasias. Stippling of the epiphyses is characteristic of the various forms of chondrodysplasia punctata, but may also be seen with cerebral-hepato-renal syndrome, Warfarin-related embryopathy and occasionally with chromosomal trisomy, lysosomal storage diseases, diphenylhydantoin-induced embryopathy, the Smith-Lemli-Opitz syndrome and congenital infections.

Rib shortening is most severe in the short rib-polydactyly syndromes and thanatophoric dysplasias, but may also be marked in patients with asphyxiating thoracic dysplasia, chondroectodermal dysplasia and metatropic dysplasia, and in some cases of metaphyseal dysplasia.

Marked decrease in or absence of ossification of the vertebral bodies suggests a diagnosis of achondrogenesis (Fig. 56.7). Marked reduction in ossification of the cervical, upper thoracic and lower lumbosacral vertebral bodies may also be seen in spondyloepiphyseal dysplasia congenita, Kniest dysplasia and other types of spondylo-epiphyseal dysplasias. Severe platyspondyly is characteristic of metatropic dysplasia, congenital lethal hypophosphatasia, lethal perinatal osteogenesis imperfecta type II, thanatophoric dysplasia, Morquio disease and spondylo-metaphyseal dysplasia (Kozlowski type), among others. In thanatophoric dysplasia, the vertebrae have a characteristic ossification defect so that they appear U-shaped in the thoracic spine, but with an inverted U-shaped in the lumbar spine (Fig. 56.7). In spondylometaphyseal dysplasia (Kozlowski type), the AP view of the spine is characteristic with a central core and widened platyspondylic bodies which overhang the pedicles, reminiscent of an open staircase. Coronal clefts of the vertebrae can be seen in Kniest dysplasia, Rolland-Desbuquois syndrome, Weisenbacher-Zweymuller syndrome, atelosteogenesis, short rib-polydactyly syndrome type I and various types of chondrodysplasia punctata.

These examples are representative of but a few of the many typical radiographic features seen in the skeletal dysplasia (Table 56.1). In many instances an accurate diagnosis can be made by simply examining the skeletal radiographs, but in other disorders only the general type of dysplasia, such as spondyloepiphyseal dysplasia, can be readily classified, and further information may be required to diagnose its exact form. Furthermore, only part of the heterogeneity of the skeletal dysplasias has been delineated to date and there are many disorders that will require morphological or biochemical studies for their exact delineation.

CHONDRO-OSSEOUS MORPHOLOGY

In recent years, morphological studies of chondro-osseous tissue have revealed specific abnormalities in many of the skeletal dysplasia (Rimoin 1975, Yang et al 1976, Stanescu et al 1977, Sillence et al 1979, Rimoin & Sillence 1981) (Table 56.1). In certain of these disorders, histological examination of chondro-osseous tissue may be useful in making an accurate diagnosis of the specific skeletal disorder. In other disorders, no histopathological alterations are present, or they are non-specific, and in these cases pathological examination is useful only in ruling out a diagnosis.

On morphological grounds, the chondrodysplasias can be broadly divided into: (1) those disorders which show no qualitative abnormality in endochondral ossification; (2) those in which there are abnormalities in cellular morphology; (3) those with abnormalities in matrix morphology; and (4) those in which the abnormality is primarily localized to the area of chondro-osseous

Fig. 56.6 Lower extremity abnormalities in different types of chondrodysplasia.
A Achondroplasia - note the genu varum with marked proximal overgrowth of fibula
B Metaphyseal chondrodysplasia, type McKusick - note the genu varum with marked distal overgrowth of the fibula.
C Pseudoachondroplastic dysplasia - note the marked genu varum involving the entire lower extremity.
D Metatropic dysplasia - note the genu varum with prominence of the knees and ankles.

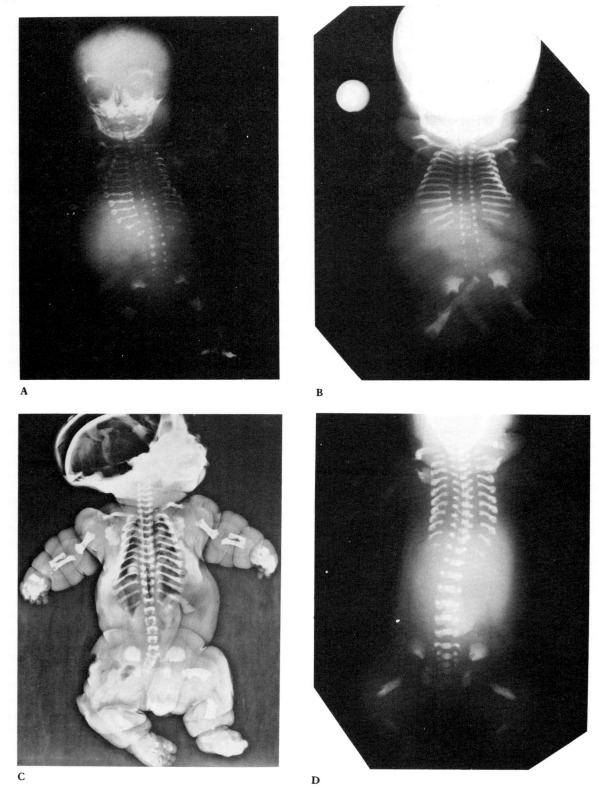

A

B

C

D

transformation. In certain disorders, abnormalities in two or more of these areas can be seen.

Conditions with minimal disturbance of endochondral ossification include achondroplasia and hypochondroplasia, where endochondral ossification is qualitatively normal, but where there are abnormalities in the height and arrangement of proliferative columns, particularly in the centre of the large growth plates. Ultrastructural studies show an increased number of dead chondrocytes and increased cytoplasmic glycogen. In asphyxiating thoracic dysplasia, where several workers have shown prominent lipid inclusions in chondrocytes, the growth plate organization is essentially normal.

In the achondrogenesis syndromes, defects in cellular morphology, matrix and/or chondro-osseous transformation can be seen. In achondrogenesis IA (Houston-Harris) the chondrocytes are large and contain prominent PAS-positive inclusions. Endochondral ossification is markedly disturbed with absence of columns of proliferative cells and lack of cellular hypertrophy. In achondrogenesis II (Langer-Saldino) there is complete disruption of endochondral ossification with large chondrocytic lacunae and little intervening matrix (Fig. 56.8). These changes suggest a metabolic defect leading to reduced synthesis of a matrix component.

In thanatophoric dysplasia (Fig. 56.8), and short rib-polydactyly type I and type II, there appears to be defective maturation of chondrocytes with reduced and disorganized columnization. Consequently, vascular invasion and chondro-osseous trabeculae are short and deformed with bridging between the trabeculae. Hypertrophic chondrocytes are irregularly arranged at the zone of chondro-osseous transformation and lack columnization. Bands of mesenchymal-like fibrous tissue extend from the perichondrial area into the growth plate.

Fig. 56.7 Radiographs of different forms of lethal neonatal dwarfism.

A Achondrogenesis, type IA (Houston-Harris) – note the irregular shortened ribs with anterior flare, abnormal iliac bones with some suggestion of ischial development, no ossification of vertebral bodies and the widened, extremely short femurs.

B Achondrogenesis type II (Langer-Saldino type) – note the almost entire lack of ossification of the vertebral bodies, the short ribs, the lack of ossification of the pubic and ischial bones, the characteristic ilia and shortened tubular femurs with cupped ends.

C Thanatophoric dysplasia – note the curved short long bones with metaphyseal spikes, short ribs, and inverted U-shaped vertebrae in the lumbar area.

D Short rib-polydactyly syndrome, type I (Saldino-Noonan type) – note the marked rib shortening and flaring, the apparently long trunk, characteristic femurs with pointed ends and a hypoplastic abnormal pelvis.

A group of conditions show dilatation of the chondrocyte rough endoplasmic reticulum, consistent with defective synthesis or abnormal processing of matrix proteins. These include pseudoachondroplasia, where the inclusions are prominent and in some cases show a highly regular RER inclusion (Fig. 56.8), consisting of alternating electron dense and electron lucent lamellae. Dilatation of the rough endoplasmic reticulum is seen also in spondylometaphyseal dysplasia (Kozlowski), autosomal recessive multiple epiphyseal dysplasia and Kniest dysplasia among others. Thus dilatation of the RER is not a diagnostic finding.

The matrix pathology in Kniest dysplasia is striking. Endochondral cartilage with paraffin processing shows dehiscence of matrix leading to the Swiss cheese cartilage appearance. With plastic embedding, these are areas of relatively acellular matrix surrounded by attenuated chondrocytes with a bubbly appearance to the perilacunar matrix.

Matrix abnormalities are also seen in diastrophic dysplasia, chondrodysplasia punctata (various types) and the Dyggve-Melchior-Clausen syndrome. In diastrophic dysplasia, the matrix of the reserve zone cartilage develops a particularly fibrillar appearance and shows areas of microscar formation (Fig. 56.8). Chondrocytes both by light microscopy and by electron microscopy are surrounded by dense corona of large collagen fibres. In Dyggve-Melchior-Clausen syndrome, chondrocytes by light microscopy appear to be arranged around a relatively large common lacuna with up to 10 chondrocytes clustered around each lacuna. In chondrodysplasia punctata of both the rhizomelic recessive and dominant Conradi-Hunermann varieties, there appears to be an alteration in epiphyseal and reserve zone cartilage matrix with areas of dystrophic (non-endochondral) ossification, fibrous dysplasia, and even areas of fat deposition.

New chondrodysplasias are constantly being reported. Morphological studies have often played an integral part in their investigation and nosology. For example, dyssegmental dysplasia, type Silverman-Handmaker and type Rolland-Desbuquois, appear to represent distinct syndromes showing large lateral vertebral clefts but differing in other radiographic features and morphology.

Syndromes with striking histopathological abnormalities have been reported by Stanescu et al (1977), (fibrochondrogenesis) and Greenberg et al (1988). Achondrogenesis IA (Houston-Harris) and IB (Fraccaro) have been distinguished one from the other by morphological as well as radiographic differences; whereas achondrogenesis type II (Langer-Saldino) and hypo-chondrogenesis have identical chondro-osseous morphology and appear to represent variability in a single disorder. Thus pathological analysis of chondro-osseous

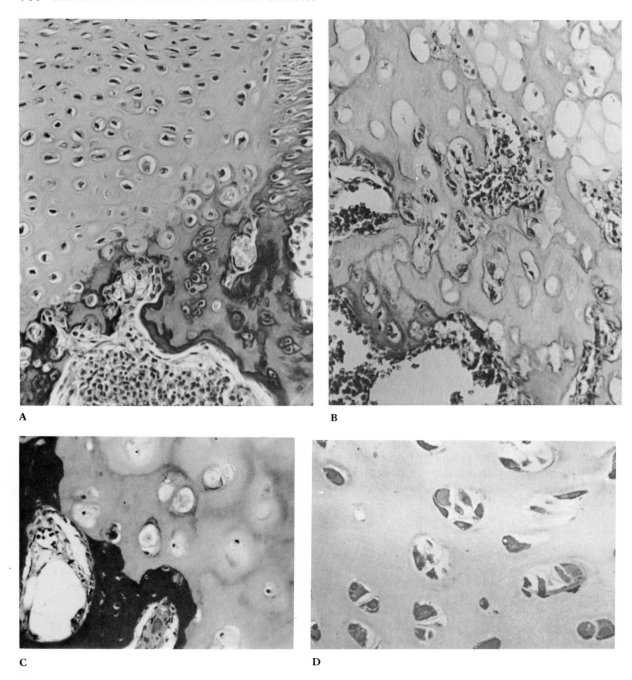

Fig. 56.8 Histological abnormalities in chondro-osseous tissue from various chondrodysplasia.
A Thanatophoric dysplasia – note the lack of cellular columns and the abnormal broad trabeculae in the lower right-hand corner.
B Achondrogenesis, type II (Langer-Saldino) – note the large chondrocytes with little intervening matrix and the incorporation of chondrocytes into the cartilaginous spicules.
C Diastrophic dysplasia – note the large chondrocytes surrounded by whorls of collagen and the intracartilaginous ossification (black).
D Pseudoachondroplasia – note the clusters of chondrocytes containing large greyish inclusion bodies.

tissue can be of great help in the diagnostic evaluation of the chondrodysplasias and can lead to the delineation of new syndromes.

BIOCHEMICAL STUDIES

In recent years, great progress has been made in our knowledge concerning the basic biology and technology of collagen and proteoglycan chemistry and a search for the biochemical defect in certain of the skeletal dysplasias has been performed. Nevertheless, except for the mucopolysaccharidoses and mucolipidoses and certain of the mineralization defects, such as hypophosphatasia, hypophosphataemic rickets and vitamin D dependency rickets, until recently the basic defect had not been uncovered in any of this large group of disorders.

Abnormalities in proteoglycan chemistry have been suggested in pseudoachondroplasia (Stanescu et al 1977). The cellular inclusion bodies which have been demonstrated in the chondrocytes in this disorder would also suggest an abnormality in proteoglycan chemistry and we have demonstrated immunohistochemical staining of these inclusion bodies with antibodies directed against the proteoglycan core protein. Specific abnormalities in cartilage proteoglycans have been demonstrated in several of the mouse chondrodysplasias, such as the sulphate donor defect in the brachymorphic mouse and an absence of proteoglycan core protein in the *cmd* mouse. Similar defects may well exist in certain of their human counterparts.

A specific defect in collagen chemistry has been suggested in numerous of the skeletal dysplasias (Rimoin & Sillence 1981). Cartilage collagen appears to be qualitatively and quantitatively normal, however, in human achondroplasia and the previously reported abnormalities in the type II collagen gene have not held up to further scrutiny. Likewise, the suggested abnormality in type II collagen in diastrophic dysplasia has been shown to be due to an artifact in the SLS collagen preparations. Type II collagen defects have now been demonstrated in achondrogenesis type II (Langer-Saldino), hypochondrogenesis, the spondyloepiphyseal dysplasias and Kniest dysplasia, and co-segregation of the Stickler syndrome with the type II collagen gene suggests that these disorders all represent a family of dysplasias caused by different mutations along the type II collagen gene (Byers 1989, Lee et al 1989, Murray et al 1989).

The rhizomelic form of chondrodysplasia punctata has been shown to be the result of a peroxisomal defect, as is the Zellweger syndrome, another disorder associated with stippled epiphyses.

In the other forms of chondrodysplasia punctata, however, peroxisomal metabolism has been found to be normal.

There are now numerous clues to possible biochemical defects in several of the other skeletal dysplasias. The rapid increase in the knowledge of the basic biology and technology of collagen and proteoglycan chemistry should pave the way for an exciting era in the detection of the basic defect in many of the skeletal dysplasias. However, the biochemical studies must take into account the known and potential heterogeneity in this group of disorders, if a single and consistent defect is to be found in any one disorder. Furthermore, the biochemist should take advantage of the numerous pathogenetic clues suggested by the morphological studies in deciding which disorders might be due to defects in collagen or proteoglycans chemistry, or to other defects in chondrocyte metabolism. The multiple defects in type I collagen in the osteogenesis imperfectas and in type II collagen in the spondyloepiphyseal dysplasias and achondrogenesis type II support Spranger's concept of families of bone dysplasias which have heterogeneous defects in a common metabolic pathway. Thus phenotypic heterogeneity may reflect intra- as well as inter-molecular heterogeneity.

SUMMARY

Thus clinical evaluation of the skeletal dysplasia requires a wide variety of clinical, radiographic and pathological tools. Diagnosis of the specific form of skeletal dysplasia can be of great importance in the prognosis, prevention and treatment of these disorders, and in the provision of accurate genetic counselling. Since space constraints prevent independent discussion of each of the many chondrodysplasias in this chapter, their salient clinical, radiographic, pathological and genetic characteristics are outlined in Table 56.1. The reader is referred to the classified bibliography for further details concerning each of these syndromes.

Table 56.1   Clinical, radiographic, morphological and genetic features in the chondrodysplasias (Associated with defects of growth of tubular bones and/or spine)

Dysplasia	Clinical features				Inheritance
	Head and neck	Chest and trunk	Limbs	Other	
A. Identifiable at birth *Usually lethal before or shortly after birth*					
Achondrogenesis IA (Houston-Harris)	round face, soft skull, short neck	short, round	very short	polyhydramnios common	AR
Achondrogenesis IB (Fraccaro)	round face, soft skull, short neck	short	very short	polyhydramnios common	AR
Achondrogenesis II/Hypochondrogenesis (Langer-Saldino)	round flat face, short neck	short, barrel-shaped	very short	distended abdomen, fetal hydrops	AR
Fibrochondrogenesis	+/− unusual facies with hypertelorism	narrow chest +/− omphalocele	short +/− contractures of hands & clubbed feet	+/− patent foramen ovale	AR
Thanatophoric dysplasia ± cloverleaf skull	large, bulging forehead, prominent eyes, depressed nasal bridge, wide fontanelles & sutures, ± cloverleaf skull	small, narrow, pear-shaped thorax	markedly short	± hydrocephalus, congenital heart & CNS defects	unknown
Atelosteogenesis Type 1	flat face, cleft palate, micrognathia	narrow, respiratory failure, scoliosis	severe rhizomelic shortening, finger deviation, joint dislocations, equinovarus deformity	premature birth, stillborn or neonatal death	unknown
Schneckenbecken dysplasia	large head, short neck, flat midface, +/− cleft palate	narrow chest, distended abdomen	very short long bones, hands & feet less severely affected	generalized oedema +/− cryptorchidism	AR
Short rib-polydactyly syndrome type I/III (Saldino-Noonan	round, flattened face	hydropic appearance, narrow thorax, protuberant abdomen	markedly short hands & feet, post-axial polydactyly	± defects of heart, kidneys, lungs, & GI tract	AR

	Radiological features				Chondro-osseous morphology
Skull	Ribs	Vertebrae	Pelvis	Limb bones	
poorly ossified	short, multiple fractured	unossified vertebral bodies	hypoplastic arch-like iliac bones, short vertical ischia	wedge-like femora with proximal metaphyseal spike, short broad tibiae and fibulae	hypervascular matrix, chondrocytes round with central nucleus and inclusion bodies, bone hypercellular & woven
poorly ossified	short, thin ribs, cupped ends, no fractures	unossified vertebral bodies	hypoplastic crenated iliae	short trapezoid femora, crenated tibiae, unossified fibulae	matrix devoid of collagen fibrils, dense collagenous ring around cells, lack of columns, fibrous zone between resting cartilage and woven bone
large calvarium, posterior ossification defect	short ribs	some vertebral ossificiation (thoraco-lumbar)	short ilia, flat acetabular roots; unossified pubic bones, ossified ischia	short broad, mild/moderate metaphyseal changes, long fibulae	large ballooned chondrocytes with ↓ matrix, growth plate hypercellular and irregular, sclerosed vascular channels
mid face hypoplasia	short, cupped 11 ribs	platyspondyly, coronal clefts	hypoplastic	short, dumb-bell shaped, metaphyseal flare, very short fibulae, ectopic ossification along long bones	densely fibrous collagenous matrix; growth plate markedly disorganized
large calvarium, short base, small foramen magnum	short, cupped and splayed anteriorly	hypoplastic, inverted U-shaped (AP), marked flattening with round anterior end (lateral)	small, short, flat spiculated acetabulum; small sacrosciatic notches	short, bowed, metaphyseal flaring (with medial spike-femora)	generalized disruption of growth plate, poor columns, fibrous bands and fibrous ossification
	short, 11 ribs	platyspondyly, coronal & sagittal clefting, scoliosis	small ilia, vertical block ischia, enlarged sacrosciatic notch	drumstick humeri, dysharmonic ossification short bones of hands, short metacarpals, dislocated knees	acellular areas of cartilage, areas containing cell clusters and large 'giant' cells
	short, splayed	platyspondyly, round anterior ossification	snail-shaped iliae	dumb-bell shaped, shortened, wide fibulae, precociously ossified tarsals	resting cartilage hypocellular, round chondrocytes with round central nucleus, growth plate short, peripheral spicules
	very short, horizontal	flat, wide intervertebral disc spaces	small ilia, flat acetabulum	very short, medial & lateral metaphyseal spurs, polydactyly	disorganized growth plate, broad short trabeculae

Table 56.1   Features in the chondrodysplasias (*contd.*)

Dysplasia	Clinical features				Inheritance
	Head and neck	Chest and trunk	Limbs	Other	
Short rib-polydactyly syndrome type II (Majewski)	short flat nose, low set ears, ± cleft lip or palate	hydropic appearance, narrow thorax, protuberant abdomen	moderately short, pre- or post-axial polydactyly	± PDA, dysplastic kidneys, respiratory tract anomalies	AR
Dyssegmental dysplasia, Rolland-Desbuquois type	short neck, micrognathia hypoplastic orbits, flat facies, cleft palate	narrow chest	short limbs, ↓joint mobility	± hirsutism ± hernia survival post newborn	AR
Dyssegmental dysplasia, Silverman-Handmaker type	short neck, micrognathia, hypoplastic orbits, flat facies, cleft palate	narrow chest	severe micromelia	encephalocele, ± hirsutism, ± patent ductus, stillborn or neonatal death	AR
Usually non-lethal dysplasias Chondrodysplasia punctata, rhizomelic type	flat face, depressed bridge & tip of nose		proximal shortening	cataracts, icthyosiform erythroderma, joint contractures	AR
Chondrodysplasia punctata, dominant type (Conradi-Hunermann) and X–linked dominant type	flat face, depressed bridge & tip of nose	± scoliosis	asymmetrical shortening	cataracts, icthyosiform erythroderma, alopecia, joint contractures	AD XD
Campomelic dysplasia, long-limbed type	large calvarium, small flat face, low set ears, micrognathia	small, narrow	bowed femora & tibiae with dimple at maximum convexity	respiratory distress, multiple anomalies, sex reversal	AR
Kyphomelic dysplasia (Campomelic dysplasia, short-limbed, normocephalic type)			all short & bowed		AR
Campomelic dysplasia, short-limbed, with craniosynostosis	large head, flat face		all short & bowed		unknown
Achondroplasia	large head, bulging forehead, low nasal bridge, prominent mandible	slight rib flaring	rhizomelic shortening, fatty folds of skin in infancy, genu varum	early otitis media, spinal stenosis	AD

Radiological features					Chondro-osseous morphology
Skull	Ribs	Vertebrae	Pelvis	Limb bones	
	very short, horizontal			short, ovoid tibiae, polydactyly, ± premature ossification of epiphyses	irregular columnization
midface-hypoplasia, mild micrognathia	short, flared	coronal clefting oversized vertebrae	wide, flared ilia, small sacrosciatic notches	short, broad tubular bones, dumb-bell femora; bowing, enlarged first metatarsals, accelerated ossification in newborn	resting cartilage contains patches of broad collagen fibres, growth plate normal
severe midface hypoplasia, micrognathia	very short flared ribs, malformed scapulae	anisospondyly with both coronal & sagittal clefting	small round dense, amorphous ilia	very short, broad angulated long bones, hypoplastic first metacarpals	mucoid degeneration of cartilage, disorganized growth plate, large, unfused calcospherites
		wide coronal clefts	trapezoid ilia, stippling of ischiopubis	stippled calcification in epiphyses, periarticular areas	↑vascularization of cartilage with dysplastic myxoid or fibrotic areas, irregular growth plate
flat facial bones		± coronal clefts, marked stippling of spinal processes & pedicles	stippling of ischiopubis	asymmetrical, mild shortening, stippled epiphyses, carpal & tarsal centres	cystic myxoid degeneration of cartilage, fibrous scarring at growth plate
enlarged, dolichocephalic, narrow, shallow orbits	narrow & wavy, often 11 pairs, hypoplastic scapulae	hypoplastic cervical bodies, others flattened, increased lumbar interpedicular distance	tall, narrow, increased acetabular angles, vertical ischia, hypoplastic ischiopubic rami	long, slender, bowed femora & tibiae	cartilage normal to slightly irregular, periosteal trabeculae converge at point of angulation
	11 pairs	mild flattening	mild narrowing	broad, angulated, widened metaphyses	periosteal trabeculae converge at point of angulation
cranio-synostosis ± clover-leaf deformity	slender		narrow ilia, hypoplastic ischiopubic rami	short, broad, angulated, epiphyseal delay	
large calvarium, short base, small foramen magnum	short, cupped anteriorly	decreased lumbosacral interpedicular distance, short pedicles	squared off ilia, small sacrosciatic notches	short, broad, oval radiolucency in proximal femora & humeri in infancy, relative overgrowth of fibulae	chondrocytes normal and growth plate regular-periosteal overgrowth

Table 56.1 Features in the chondrodysplasias (*contd.*)

Dysplasia	Clinical features				Inheritance
	Head and neck	Chest and trunk	Limbs	Other	
Diastrophic dysplasia	acute swelling of pinnae of ears in infancy – cauliflower ears	scoliosis	short with club feet, hitch-hiker thumbs, symphalangism	cleft palate	AR
Pseudodiastrophic dysplasia	large cranium, hypertelorism, flat nasal bridge, large malformed ear lobes, cleft palate	scoliosis	rhizomelic shortening, club feet, finger & elbow dislocations	± bluish sclerae	AR
Metatropic dysplasia		tail-like sacral appendage, trunk appears long & narrow at birth, develops severe scoliosis	short with prominent joints	long in length at birth, appears short limbed in infancy, short trunked later	AR & AD
Chondro-ectodermal dysplasia (Ellis-van Creveld)	± midline puckering of upper lip, ± natal teeth	long narrow chest	post-axial polydactyly of hands, ± of feet, acromesomelic shortening, nail dysplasia	congenital heart disease, epispadias	AR
Asphyxiating thoracic dysplasia (ATD) (Jeune)		long, narrow, prominent rosary, respiratory distress	variable shortening, short, broad hands & feet, ± post-axial polydactyly	respiratory insufficiency, progressive nephropathy	AR
Spondylo-epiphyseal dysplasia congenita, type Spranger-Wiedermann	± round flat face, short neck, prominent eyes, ± cleft palate	short barrel chest, ± pectus carinatum	mild rhizomelic shortening, normal hands ± club feet	± myopia, retinal detachment, hearing loss, subluxation of C1-C2	AD
Kniest dysplasia	flat face, prominent wide-set eyes, broad mouth ± cleft palate	short trunk	short, prominent knees, joint contractures	myopia, retinal detachment, hearing loss	AD
Mesomelic dysplasia, type Nievergelt			severe mesomelic shortening, equinovarus club-feet, brachydactyly, clinodactyly		AD
Mesomelic dysplasia, type Langer	micrognathia		severe mesomelic shortening		AR (probably homozygous for dyschond-rosteosis gene)

Radiological features					Chondro-osseous morphology
Skull	Ribs	Vertebrae	Pelvis	Limb bones	
ossified ear pinnae	precocious ossification of costal cartilages	± scoliosis & lumbar interpedicular narrowing		short with broad metaphyses, delayed epiphyseal ossification, short and/or oval 1st metacarpals	chondrocytes enlarged, clustered, degenerating, surrounded by dense collagen, cystic areas with fibrovascular tissue & intracartilaginous ossification
normal	slightly short, anterior flare	ovoid, platyspondyly, scoliosis	horizontal acetabular roofs	upper limb rhizomelia, elbow dislocations, multiple interphalangeal joint dislocations	resting cartilage normal, mild shortening of growth plate
	short, flared, cupped anteriorly	markedly flattened, wide intervertebral spaces (early) platyspondyly & scoliosis (late)	hypoplastic crescent-shaped ilia, low set anterior iliac spines	short, broad, club-like	chondrocytes vacuolated with inclusions, growth plate – irregular vascularization
	± short		squared ilia with hook-like spurs at acetabulae, similar to ATD	acromesomelic shortening with cone epiphyses, hamate-capitate fusion, slanting proximal tibial metaphyses	variable, ↑vascularity of cartilage, cartilage islands in metaphysis, irregular columns
	very short, cupped anteriorly		square, short ilia, flat acetabulae, spurs at margins of acetabulae	premature ossification capital femoral epiphyses, broad proximal femoral metaphyses	variable findings, lipid inclusions in chondroctyes, cartilage islands in metaphysis
	short	flattened, dorsal wedging (pear-shaped) ± odontoid hypoplasia	retarded ossification of pubic bones	retarded epiphyseal ossification & deformity – hips, knees, retarded ossification of carpal and tarsal centres, coxa vara	dilated RER in chondrocytes, microcysts in proliferative zone, columns short
frontal flattening, maxillary hypoplasia, shallow orbits	short	diffuse flattening, coronal clefts	small ilia, increased acetabular angles, irregular acetabular margins	club-like metaphyses, delayed ossification of femoral heads, cloud effect in epiphyseal plate regions	Swiss cheese cartilage with abnormal vacuolated matrix, perilacunar foaminess, dilated RER
				rhomboid-shaped radii, ulnae, tibiae, fibulae, radio-ulnar & tarsal synostoses	
mandibular hypoplasia				short & thick, hypoplastic fibulae & distal ulnae	

Table 56.1 Features in the chondrodysplasias (*contd.*)

Dysplasia	Clinical features				Inheritance
	Head and neck	Chest and trunk	Limbs	Other	
Mesomelic dysplasia, type Robinow	prominent forehead, hypoplastic mandible, hypertelorism, down-slanting palpebral fissures, short, flat nose		mesomelic shortening, hypoplastic nails	genital hypoplasia ± cryptorchidism	AD
Mesomelic dysplasia, type Rheinhardt			moderate mesomelic shortening, radial bowing, ulnar deviation of hands, lateral bowing of legs (cutaneous dimple)		AD
Acromesomelic dysplasia		small thorax, mild truncal shortening	meso- & acromelia with mild rhizomelia, square short hands, elbow deformities, upper extremities more severe than lower		AR
Cleido-cranial dysplasia	large, prominent forehead, wide persistent fontanelles & sutures	drooping shoulders & narrow chest, ± scoliosis	hyperextensible, ± coxa vara, fingers short & square	abnormal dentition	AD
Larsen syndrome	prominent forehead, flattened face, hypertelorism, ± cleft palate or uvula	soft, collapsing thorax	multiple dislocations	severe joint laxity, ± dysraphism of spine → neurological impairment	AD & AR
Oto-palato-digital syndrome I	prominent forehead & supraorbital ridges, hypertelorism, ± cleft palate, small jaw		short, broad thumbs & toes, broad phalanges	± hearing defect, ± mild mental retardation	XD
Oto-palato-digital syndrome II	prominent forehead, large fontanelle, midface hypoplasia, hypertelorism, micrognathia, cleft palate	narrow chest, scoliosis	rhizomelic shortening, dislocation of elbows & hips, camptodactyly, equinovarus deformity		XR
B. Identifiable in later life					
Hypochondroplasia	normal head to slight prominence of forehead	normal-mild lumbar lordosis	rhizomelic shortening of extremities, short broad hands, limited extension at elbow	mild short stature, muscular appearance	AD

		Radiological features			Chondro-osseous morphology
Skull	Ribs	Vertebrae	Pelvis	Limb bones	
		± posterior osseous fusion hemivertebrae		hypoplastic distal ulnae, ± radial head dislocations	
				short radii & ulnae, hypoplasia of distal ulnae & proximal fibulae	
		infancy & childhood oval shaped, adult-posterior wedging	hypoplasia of iliac base & irregular acetabulae	progressive shortening with metaphyseal flare, especially acro & mesomelia, mild epiphyseal delay, brachydactyly with cone epiphyses	
decreased ossification, multiple Wormian bones	absent or hypoplastic clavicles	± retarded ossification of bodies, posterior wedging	retarded ossification & hypoplastic pubis, hypoplasia of ilia	pseudoepiphyses of metacarpals & metatarsals, retarded ossification of carpals & tarsals	mild ↓ in growth plate height, ↓ periosteal ossification
craniofacial disproportion		± fusion defects of cervical spine		slender, multiple joint dislocations, duplication of calcanei	
small mandible with increased angle		narrow pedicles, wide lumbar interpedicular distance	small ilia ± dislocated hips	hypoplastic distal radii diffuse hand changes	
normal	thin, posteriorly pinched	early, slight cervical & thoracic platyspondyly	normal	early bowing of long bones, joint subluxations, carpal fusions, abnormal, hypoplastic metacarpals & metatarasals, round hypoplastic phalanges	no characteristic changes
	normal to slightly flared anteriorly	lumbosacral interpedicular narrowing, short pedicles, posterior scalloping	slightly short basilar segments of ilia	rhizomelia with short, wide bones, prominent deltoid tubercles, elongated fibulae	normal growth plate, with perhaps widened septa

Table 56.1 Features in the chondrodysplasias (*contd.*)

Dysplasia	Clinical features				Inheritance
	Head and neck	Chest and trunk	Limbs	Other	
Dyschondrosteosis			mesomelic shortening, dorsal subluxation distal end ulnae	mild short stature	AD
Metaphyseal dysplasia, type Jansen	prominent forehead		rhizomelic shortening, enlarged joints		AD
Metaphyseal dysplasia, type Schmid			waddling gait, bowed legs, generalized shortening of limbs		AD
Metaphyseal dysplasia, type McKusick (cartilage-hair hypoplasia)	fine sparse lightly pigmented hair, eyebrows		short, lax ligaments, short pudgy hands, telescoping fingers	± megacolon, immune defects, propensity to skin cancer	AR
Metaphyseal dysplasia with pancreatic insufficiency, neutropenia		± small narrow chest	± short	pancreatic insufficiency & malabsorption, neutropenia	AR
Spondylometaphyseal dysplasia, type Kozlowski		kyphoscoliosis pectus carinatum	waddling gait, knee & hip pain in childhood, limitation of large joints	short trunk, short stature	AD
Multiple epiphyseal dysplasia, type Fairbanks		thoracic kyphosis ± back pain	pain & stiffness in knees, hips & ankles, waddling gait		AD
Multiple epiphyseal dysplasia, type Ribbing			osteoarthropathy of hips	mild short stature	AD

Radiological features					Chondro-osseous morphology
Skull	Ribs	Vertebrae	Pelvis	Limb bones	
				radii & tibiae short in relation to ulnae and fibulae, Madelung-like deformity	
reticulate pattern in calvarium, sclerosis of base	splayed & cupped anteriorly		demineralized	metaphyses wide, splayed, frayed cortical erosion & sub-periosteal bone formation, abnormal phalanges	chondrocytes large, matrix fibrillar, cluster of hypertrophic cells at growth plate, irregular line of ossification with tongues of cartilage in metaphyses
				metaphyseal splaying & cupping in all long bones (especially hips), coxa vara	same as above
	splayed & cupped anteriorly			metaphyseal flaring & irregularity, especially knees, long distal fibulae	same as above
	± short, flared			mild generalized metaphyseal irregularity	same as above
		platyspondyly with open staircase appearance on AP view	narrow sacrosciatic notches. broad horizontal irregular acetabular roofs	metaphyseal irregularity, widened epiphyseal plate, coxa vara, marked retardation of carpal ossification	↓ proliferative zone, irregular columns, fibrous appearance to matrix, inclusions on EM
		end plate irregularity & Schmorl's nodes		small irregularly ossified epiphyses involving all areas, including small bones of the hands and feet	variable-normal to disturbed growth plate, inclusion bodies reported in chondrocytes, dilated RER
		normal but may have early onset of Schmorl's nodes		epiphyseal irregularity and delayed ossification, primarily involving the hips with other epiphyses less involved, non-mild involvement of hands and feet	

Table 56.1   Features in the chondrodysplasias (*contd.*)

Dysplasia	Clinical features				Inheritance
	Head and neck	Chest and trunk	Limbs	Other	
Arthro-ophthalmopathy (Stickler)	cleft palate, mandibular hypoplasia, midface hypoplasia		hypotonia, hyper-extension of joints, later joint pain and morning stiffness	marfanoid habitus, myopia, retinal detachment, conductive hearing loss	AD
Pseudoachon-droplastic dysplasia	normal skull and face	trunk appears disproportionately long	very short limbs with genu varum or valgum, hyper-mobility of joints, small broad hands	not manifested until at least 2 years of age	AD
Spondyloepiphyseal dysplasia tarda (X-linked)		sternal protrusion, back pain	osteoarthropathy of hips and knees	mild short trunk, short stature	XR
Brachyolmia (Hobaek type)		short trunk, back pain in adult, mild scoliosis		± punctate corneal opacities	AR
Brachyolmia (Maroteaux type)	± facial dysmorphism	short trunk, widely spaced nipples, pectus excavatum, back pain in adult, mild scoliosis	clinodactyly hyperlaxity of joints		AR
Dyggve-Melchior-Clausen dysplasia	short neck	thoracic kyphoscoliosis, lumbar lordosis, flared ribs, protruding sternum, short trunk	waddling gait, enlarged joints with restriction, small claw hands	mental retardation (most)	AR
Spondyloepi-metaphyseal dysplasia, type Strudwick	± cleft palate	pectus carinatum, scoliosis	genu valgum	resembles SED congenita at birth	?AR

Skull	Ribs	Radiological features				Chondro-osseous morphology
		Vertebrae	Pelvis	Limb bones		
		wedging of thoracic vertebrae & Schmorl's disease		mild epiphyseal dysplasia especially CFE & distal tibiae, irregular articular surfaces, degenerative arthrosis especially of hips		
		platyspondyly, anterior tongue-like protrusion, end plate irregularity	acetabular irregularity, hypoplastic ischium & pubis	epiphyseal & metaphyseal dysplasia, striking hand involvement with shortening of tubular bones with irregular metaphyses and small round epiphyses, marked CFE dysplasia		prominent inclusions in chondrocytes showing lamellar or granular RER dilatation on EM
		platyspondyly with hump-shaped centra	hypoplastic iliac wings	hypoplasia of large epiphyses and premature osteoarthrosis of hips		fairly normal with clustering of proliferative cells
	precocious costochondral calcification	platyspondyly, irregular vertebral end plates, lateral extended vertebral bodies, rectangular in shape				chondrocytes unevenly distributed, surrounded by dense staining material, growth plate short with clusters of hypertrophic cells
		platyspondyly, round anterior and posterior vertebral borders				
± microcephaly	mild flaring	anterior pointed platyspondyly, vertebral notching	lacy iliac crest, hypoplastic ilia pubae ischia and acetabular roof, small sacrosciatic notch	small epiphyses, especially CFE, brachydactyly, cone epiphyses, small carpal centres		foci of multiple degenerating chondrocytes surrounded by dense fibrous capsule
	splayed bulbous	platyspondyly, pear shaped vertebrae, end plate irregularity, scoliosis, C1-C2 subluxation	delayed ischial & pubic ossification	delayed epiphyseal ossification, clubbed shaped femora (1st year) metaphyseal and epiphyseal changes (after 3 years), dappling of metaphyses with fragmentation, greater involvement of fibula than tibia, ulna than radius		inclusion bodies in chondrocytes, hypocellular growth plates

Table 56.1 Features in the chondrodysplasias (*contd.*)

| Dysplasia | Clinical features | | | | Inheritance |
	Head and neck	Chest and trunk	Limbs	Other	
Oto-spondylo-mega-epiphyseal dysplasia (Weissenbacher-Zweymüller) OSMED	cleft palate, flat face	back pain	short limbs, large knees & elbows, decreased joint mobility in adults	normal stature, neurosensory deafness	?AR
Myotonic chondrodysplasia (Catel-Schwartz-Jampel)	characteristic pinched facial features (expressionless, immobile), narrow palpebral fissures, short neck	protuberant sternum	prominence & limited motion of large joints, coxa vara	microcornea, myopia, juvenile cataracts	AR
Parastremmatic dysplasia	short neck	stiffness of spine & kyphoscoliosis, increased AP diameter of thorax	abnormal gait, severe deformities of lower extremities, severe genu valgum, multiple joint contractures, short stubby hands	'twisted dwarfs'	AD or XD
Tricho-rhino phalangeal dysplasia, type I	pear-shaped bulbous nose, unusual philtrum, sparse, thin, slowly growing hair		brachydactyly, proximal interphalangeal swelling, thin nails		AD (? few AR)
Acrodysplasia with retinitis pigmentosa and nephropathy (Saldino-Mainzer)			brachydactyly	retinitis pigmentosa, interstitial nephritis, ± cerebellar ataxia	AR

AD – autosomal dominant
AR – autosomal recessive
XR – X–linked recessive
XD – X–linked dominant
CFE – capital femoral epiphysis
EM – electron microscopy
RER – rough endoplasmic reticulum

		Radiological features			Chondro-osseous morphology
Skull	Ribs	Vertebrae	Pelvis	Limb bones	
midface hypoplasia, mandibular hypoplasia	short	coronal clefts, platyspondyly	square iliac wings	short long bones, rhizomelia, especially femora, wide prominent metaphyses, late enlarged epiphyses	? normal
large skull with midface hypoplasia, platybasia	neuropathic thorax, downward tilted ribs	platyspondyly, irregular end plates	narrow ilia, acetabular hypoplasia	small epiphyses in proximal femora, humeri, radii, & short tubular bones, knee epiphyses enlarged, slight metaphyseal irregularity, usually coxa vara	
	slightly splayed 'woolly' changes in scapulae & clavicles	biconcave platyspondyly, 'flocky or woolly' end plates	large ischial & pubic bones with 'woolly' metaphyseal and apophyseal regions	marked woolly changes in carpal centres, and metaphyses with hypoplasia of epiphyses, especially CFE, twisted & shortened long bones	lack of columnization, ↓ osteoblasts and osteoclasts
				type 12 cone epiphyses of hands and feet, metaphyseal widening of femoral necks with sclerosis and hypoplastic appearing CFE associated with Legg Perthes like changes	
				cone epiphyses of hands and feet, metaphyseal widening of femoral necks with sclerosis and hypoplastic appearing CFE	

APPENDIX

INTERNATIONAL NOMENCLATURE OF CONSTITUTIONAL DISEASES OF BONE

Revision – May 1983

OSTEOCHONDRODYSPLASIAS

Abnormalities of cartilage and/or bone growth and development

Defects of growth of tubular bones and/or spine

Identifiable at birth   *Transmission*

Usually lethal before or shortly after birth

1. Achondrogenesis type I (Parenti-Fraccaro)   AR
2. Achondrogenesis type II (Langer-Saldino)
3. Hypochondrogenesis
4. Fibrochondrogenesis   AR
5. Thanatophoric dysplasia
6. Thanatophoric dysplasia with clover-leaf skull
7. Atelosteogenesis
8. Short rib syndrome (with or without polydactyly)
   a. type I (Saldino-Noonan)   AR
   b. type II (Majewski)   AR
   c. type III (lethal thoracic dysplasia)   AR

Usually non-lethal dysplasia

9. Chondrodysplasia punctata
   a. rhizomelic form, autosomal recessive   AR
   b. dominant X–linked form   XLD
                        lethal in male
   c. common mild form (Sheffield)
   Exclude: symptomatic stippling (Warfarin, chromosomal aberration. . .)
10. Campomelic dysplasia
11. Kyphomelic dysplasia   AR
12. Achondroplasia   AD
13. Diastrophic dysplasia   AR
14. Metatropic dysplasia (several forms)   AR,AD
15. Chondro-ectodermal dysplasia (Ellis-Van Creveld)   AR
16. Asphyxiating thoracic dysplasia (Jeune)   AR
17. Spondylo-epiphyseal dysplasia congenita
   a. autosomal dominant form   AD
   b. autosomal recessive form   AR
18. Kniest dysplasia   AD
19. Dyssegmental dysplasia   AR
20. Mesomelic dysplasia
   a. type Nievergelt   AD
   b. type Langer (probable homozygous dyschondrosteosis)   AR
   c. type Robinow
   d. type Rheinhardt   AD
   e. others
21. Acromesomelic dysplasia   AR
22. Cleido-cranial dysplasia   AD
23. Oto-palato-digital syndrome
   a. type I (Langer)   XLD
   b. type II (André)   XLR
24. Larsen syndrome   AR,AD
25. Other multiple dislocations syndromes (Desbuquois. . .)   AR

Identifiable in later life

1. Hypochondroplasia   AD
2. Dyschondrosteosis   AD
3. Metaphyseal chondrodysplasia type Jansen   AD
4. Metaphyseal chondrodysplasia type Schmid   AD
5. Metaphyseal chondrodysplasia type McKusick   AR
6. Metaphyseal chondrodysplasia with exocrine pancreatic insufficiency and cyclic neutropenia AR
7. Spondylo-metaphyseal dysplasia
   a. type Kozlowski   AD
   b. other forms
8. Multiple epiphyseal dysplasia
   a. type Fairbank   AD
   b. other forms
9. Multiple epiphyseal dysplasia with early diabetes (Wolcott-Rallisson)   AR
10. Arthro-ophthalmopathy (Stickler)   AR
11. Pseudo-achondroplasia
   a. dominant   AD
   b. recessive   AR
12. Spondylo-epiphyseal dysplasia tarda (X-linked recessive)   XLR
13. Progressive pseudo-rheumatoid chondrodysplasia   AR
14. Spondylo-epiphyseal dysplasia, other forms
15. Brachyolmia
   a. autosomal recessive   AR
   b. autosomal dominant   AD
16. Dyggve-Melchior-Clausen dysplasia   AR
17. Spondylo-epimetaphyseal dysplasia (several forms)
18. Spondylo-epimetaphyseal dysplasia with joint laxity   AR
19. Oto-spondylo-megaepiphyseal dysplasia (OSMED)   AR
20. Myotonic chondrodysplasia (Catel-Schwartz-Jampel)   AR
21. Parastremmatic dysplasia   AD
22. Tricho-rhino-phalangeal dysplasia   AD
23. Acrodysplasia with retinitis pigmentosa and nephropathy (Saldino-Mainzer)   AR

Disorganized development of cartilage and fibrous components of skeleton

1. Dysplasia epiphyseal hemimelica
2. Multiple cartilaginous exostoses   AD
3. Acrodysplasia with exostoses (Giedion-Langer)
4. Enchondromatosis (Ollier)
5. Enchondromatosis with haemangioma (Maffucci)
6. Metachondromatosis   AD
7. Spondyloenchondroplasia   AR
8. Osteoglophonic dysplasia
9. Fibrous dysplasia (Jaffe-Lichtenstein)
10. Fibrous dysplasia with skin pigmentation and precocious puberty (McCune-Albright)
11. Cherubism (familial fibrous dysplasia of the jaws)   AD

Abnormalities of density of cortical diaphyseal structure and/or metaphyseal modelling

1. Osteogenesis imperfecta (several forms)   AR,AD
2. Juvenile idiopathic osteoporosis
3. Osteoporosis with pseudo-glioma   AR
4. Osteopetrosis
    a. autosomal recessive lethal   AR
    b. intermediate recessive   AR
    c. autosomal dominant   AD
    d. recessive with tubular acidosis   AR
5. Pycnodysostosis   AR
6. Dominant osteosclerosis type Stanescu   AD
7. Osteomesopycnosis   AD
8. Osteopoikilosis   AD
9. Osteopathia striata   AD
10. Osteopathia striata with cranial sclerosis   AD
11. Melorheostosis
12. Diaphyseal dysplasia (Camurati-Engelmann)   AD
13. Cranio-diaphyseal dysplasia   AR
14. Endosteal hyperostosis
    a. autosomal dominant (Worth)   AD
    b. autosomal recessive (Van Buchem)   AR
    c. autosomal recessive (sclerosteosis)   AR
15. Tubular stenosis (Kenny-Caffey)   AD
16. Pachydermoperiostosis   AD
17. Osteodysplasty (Melnick-Needles)   AD
18. Fronto-metaphyseal dysplasia   XLR
19. Cranio-metaphyseal dysplasia (several forms)   AD
20. Metaphyseal dysplasia (Pyle)   AR or AD
21. Dysosteosclerosis   AR or XLR
22. Osteo-ectasia with hyperphosphatasia   AR
23. Oculo-dento-osseous dysplasia
    a. mild type   AD
    b. severe type   AR
24. Infantile cortical hyperostosis (Caffey disease, familial type)   AD

DYSOSTOSES

Malformation of individual bones, singly or in combination

Dysostoses with cranial and facial involvement

1. Craniosynostosis (several forms)
2. Cranio-facial dysostosis (Crouzon)
3. Acrocephalo-syndactyly
    a. type Apert   AD
    b. type Chotzen   AD
    c. type Pfeiffer   AD
    d. other types
4. Acrocephalo-polysyndactyly (Carpenter and others)   AR
5. Cephalo-polysyndactyly (Greig)   AD
6. First and second branchial arch syndromes
    a. mandibulo-facial dysostosis (Treacher Collins, Franceschetti)   AD
    b. acro-facial dysostosis (Nager)
    c. oculo-auriculo-vertebral dysostosis (Goldenhar)   AR
    d. hemifacial microsomia
    e. others
    (Probably parts of a large spectrum)
7. Oculo-mandibulo-facial syndrome (Hallermann-Streiff-Francois)

Dysostoses with predominant axial involvement

1. Vertebral segmentation defects (including Klippel-Feil)
2. Cervico-oculo-acoustic syndrome (Wildervanck)
3. Spregel anomaly
4. Spondylo-costal dysostosis
    a. dominant form   AD
    b. recessive forms   AR
5. Oculo-vertebral syndrome (Weyers)
6. Osteo-onychodysostosis   AD
7. Cerebro-costo-mandibular syndrome   AR

Dysostoses with predominant involvement of extremities

1. Acheiria
2. Apodia
3. Tetraphocomelia syndrome (Roberts) (SC pseudo thalidomide syndrome)   AR
4. Ectrodactyly
    a. isolated
    b. ectrodactyly-ectodermal dysplasia cleft palate-syndrome   AD
    c. ectrodactyly with scalp defects   AD
5. Oro-acral syndrome (aglossia syndrome, Hanhart syndrome)

6. Familial radio-ulnar synostosis
7. Brachydactyly, types A, B, C, D, E (Bell's classification) — AD
8. Symphalangism — AD
9. Polydactyly (several forms)
10. Syndactyly (several forms)
11. Poly-syndactyly (several forms)
12. Camptodactyly
13. Manzke syndrome
14. Poland syndrome
15. Rubinstein-Taybi syndrome
16. Coffin-Siris syndrome
17. Pancytopenia-dysmelia syndrome (Fanconi) — AR
18. Blackfan-Diamond anaemia with thumb anomalies (Aase-Syndrome) — AR
19. Thrombocytopenia-radial-aplasia syndrome — AR
20. Oro-digito-facial syndrome
    a. type Papillon-Leage — XLD lethal in male
    b. type Mohr — AR
21. Cardiomelic syndromes (Holt-Oram and others) AD
22. Femoral focal deficiency (with or without facial anomalies)
23. Multiple synostoses (includes some forms of symphalangism) — AD
24. Scapulo-iliac dysostosis (Kosenow-Sinios) — AD
25. Hand foot genital syndrome — AD
26. Focal dermal hypoplasia (Goltz) — XLD lethal in male

IDIOPATHIC OSTEOLYSES

1. Phalangeal (several forms)
2. Tarso-carpal
   a. including Francois form and others — AR
   b. with nephropathy — AD
3. Multicentric
   a. Hajdu-Cheney form — AD
   b. Winchester form — AR
   c. Torg form — AR
   d. other forms

MISCELLANEOUS DISORDERS WITH OSSEOUS INVOLVEMENT

1. Early acceleration of skeletal maturation
   a. Marshall-Smith syndrome
   b. Weaver syndrome
   c. other types
2. Marfan syndrome — AD
3. Congenital contractural arachnodactyly — AD
4. Cerebro-hepato-renal syndrome (Zellweger)
5. Coffin-Lowry syndrome — XLR

6. Cockayne syndrome — AR
7. Fibrodysplasia ossificans congenita — AD
8. Epidermal nevus syndrome (Solomon)
9. Nevoid basal cell carcinoma syndrome
10. Multiple congenital fibromatosis
11. Neurofibromatosis — AD

CHROMOSOMAL ABERRATIONS

PRIMARY METABOLIC ABNORMALITIES

Calcium and/or phosphorus

1. Hypophosphataemic rickets — XLD
2. Vitamin D dependency or pseudo-deficiency rickets
   a. type I with probable deficiency in 25 hydroxy vitamin D-1-alpha-hydroxylase — AR
   b. type II with target-organ resistance — AR
3. Late rickets (McCance)
4. Idiopathic hypercalciuria
5. Hypophosphatasia (several forms) — AR
6. Pseudo-hypoparathyroidism (normocalcaemic and hypocalcaemic forms, includes acrodysostosis) — AD

Complex carbohydrates

1. Mucopolysaccharidosis type I (alpha-L-iduronidase deficiency)
   a. Hurler form — AR
   b. Scheie form — AR
   c. other forms — AR
2. Mucopolysaccharidosis type II – Hunter (sulphoiduronate sulphatase deficiency) — XLR
3. Mucopolysaccharidosis type III – Sanfilippo
   a. type III A (heparin sulphamidase deficiency) — AR
   b. type III B (N-acetyl-alpha-glucosaminidase deficiency) — AR
   c. type III C (alpha-glucosaminide-N-acetyl transferase deficiency)
   d. type III D (N-actyl-glucosamine-6 sulphate sulphatase deficiency) — AR
4. Mucopolysaccharidosis type IV
   a. type IV A – Morquio (N-acetyl-galactosamine-6 sulphate-sulphatase deficiency) — AR
   b. type IV B (beta-galactosidase deficiency) — AR
5. Mucopolysaccharidosis type VI – Maroteaux-Lamy (aryl-sulphatase B deficiency) — AR
6. Mucopolysaccharidosis type VII (beta-glucuronidase deficiency) — AR
7. Aspartylglucosaminuria (Aspartyl-glucosaminidase deficiency) — AR

8. Mannosidosis (alpha-mannosidase deficiency)   AR
9. Fucosidosis (alpha-fucosidase deficiency)   AR
10. GM1-Gangliosidosis (beta-galactosidase deficiency) (several forms)   AR
11. Multiple sulphatase deficiency (Austin-Thieffry) AR
12. Isolated neuraminidase deficiency, several forms. Includes:
    a. mucolipidosis I   AR
    b. nephrosialidosis   AR
    c. cherry red spot myoclonus syndrome   AR
13. Phosphotransferase deficiency, several forms. Includes:
    a. mucolipidosis II (I cell disease)   AR
    b. mucolipidosis III (pseudo-polydystrophy)   AR
14. Combined neuraminidase beta-galactosidase deficiency   AR
15. Salla disease   AR

Lipids

1. Niemann-Pick disease (sphingomyelinase deficiency) (several forms)   AR

2. Gaucher disease (beta-glucosidase deficiency) (several types)   AR
3. Farber disease lipogranulomatosis (ceraminidase deficiency)   AR

Nucleic acids

1. Adenosine-deaminase deficiency and others   AR

Amino-acids

1. Homocystinuria and others   AR

Metals

1. Menkes syndrome (kinky hair syndrome and others)   AR

From: Annales De Radiologie 1983, vol. 26, p 457–462

GENERAL REFERENCES

Beighton P 1978 Inherited disorders of the skeleton. Churchill Livingstone, Edinburgh

Beighton P, Cremin B 1980 Sclerosing bone dysplasias. Springer-Verlag, Berlin

Byers P H 1989 Invited editorial: Molecular heterogeneity in chondrodysplasias. American Journal of Human Genetics 45: 1–4

Greenberg C R, Rimoin D L, Gruber H E, DeSa D, Reed M, Lachman R S 1988 A new autosomal recessive lethal chondrodystrophy with congenital hydrops. American Journal of Medical Genetics 29: 623–632

Horan F, Beighton P 1982 Orthopaedic problems in inherited skeletal disorders. Springer-Verlag, Berlin

Jones K L 1988 Smith's recognizable patterns of human malformation, 4th edn. Saunders, Philadelphia.

Kaufmann A J (ed) 1973 Intrinsic diseases of bones. Progress in Pediatric Radiology, vol 4, S Karger, Basel

Kozlowski K, Beighton P 1984 Gamut index of skeletal dysplasias. Springer-Verlag, Berlin

McKusick V A 1972 Heritable disorders of connective tissue, 4th edn. Mosby, St Louis

Martoteaux P 1974 Maladies osseuses de l'enfant. Flammarion, Paris

Maroteaux P 1979 Bone diseases of children. Lippincott, Philadelphia

Ornoy A, Borochowitz Z, Lachman R, Rimoin D 1988 Atlas of fetal skeletal radiology. Yearbook Medical Publishers, Chicago

Rimoin D L 1975 The chondrodystrophies. Advances in Human Genetics 5: 1–118

Rimoin D L (ed) 1976 Symposium on the skeletal dysplasias. Clinical Orthopaedics 114: 2

Rimoin D L, Horton W A 1978 Short Stature Part I and Part II. Journal of Pediatrics 92: 523–528, 697–704

Rimoin D L, Sillence D O 1981 Chondro-osseous morphology and biochemisty in the skeletal dysplasias. Birth Defects Original Article Series 17(1): 249–265

Sillence D, Rimoin D L, Lachman R 1978 Neonatal dwarfism. Pediatric Clinics of North America 25: 453

Sillence D O, Horton W A, Rimoin D L 1979 Morphologic studies in the skeletal dysplasias. American Journal of Pathology 96: 811

Spranger J 1985 Pattern recognition in bone dysplasia. In: Papadatos C J, Bartsocas C S (eds), Endocrine genetics and genetics of growth. Liss, New York, p 315–342

Spranger J W, Langer L O, Wiedemann H R 1974 Bone dysplasias. An atlas of constitutional disorders of skeletal development. Saunders, Philadelphia

Stanescu V, Stanescu R, Maroteaux P 1977 Morphological and biochemical studies of epiphyseal cartilage in dyschondroplasias. Archives Français de Pédiatrie (Suppl 3): 1

Taybi H, Lachman R 1990 Radiology of syndromes, skeletal dysplasias and metabolic disorders 3rd edn. Year Book Medical Publishers, Chicago

Wynne-Davies R, Hall C M, Appley A G 1985 Atlas of skeletal dysplasias. Churchill Livingstone, Edinburgh

Wynne-Davies R W, Hall C M, Young I D 1986 Pseudoachondroplasia: clinical diagnosis at different ages and comparison of autosomal dominant and recessive types: a review of 32 patients (26 kindreds). Journal of Medical Genetics 23: 425–434

Yang S S, Heidelberger K P, Brough P J, Corbett D P, Bernstein J 1976 Lethal short-limbed chondrodysplasia in early infancy. Perspectives of Pediatric Pathology 3:1

REFERENCES TO SPECIFIC SYNDROMES

OSTEOCHONDRODYSPLASIAS
Abnormalities of cartilage or bone growth and development,
or both
I. Defects of growth of tubular bones and/or spine

A. Identifiable at Birth

Achondrogenesis Type I

Beluffi G 1977 Achondrogenesis, type I. Fortschritte auf dem
Gebiete der Rontgenstrahten und der Nuklear Medizin 127:
341–344
Borochowitz Z et al 1988 Achondrogenesis type I: delineation
of further heterogeneity and identification of two distinct
subgroups. Journal of Pediatrics 112: 23–31
Houston C S, Awen C F, Kent H P 1972 Fatal neonatal
dwarfism. Journal of the Canadian Association of
Radiologists 23: 45–61
Maroteaux P, Stanescu V, Stanescu R 1976 The lethal
chondrodysplasias. Clinical Orthopaedics 114: 31
Sillence D O, Rimoin D L, Lachman R 1978 Neonatal
dwarfism. Pediatric Clinics of North America 25(3):
453–483
Yang Sheng-S, Brough A J, Garewal G S, Bernstein J 1974
Two types of heritable lethal achondrogenesis. Journal of
Pediatrics 85: 796–801

Achondrogenesis Type II (Langer-Saldino)

Borochowitz Z et al 1986 Achondrogenesis II –
Hypochondrogenesis: Variability vs. Heterogeneity.
American Journal of Medical Genetics 24: 273–288
Eyre D, Upton M, Shapiro F, Wilkinson R, Vautes G 1986
Non-expression of cartilage type II collagen in a case of
Langer-Saldino achondrogenesis. American Journal of
Human Genetics 39: 52–67
Godfrey M, Hollister D 1988 Type II achondrogenesis-hypo-
chondrogenesis. Identification of abnormal type II collagen.
American Journal of Human Genetics 43: 904–913
Horton W, Machado M, Chou I, Campbell D 1987
Achondrogenesis Type II, Abnormalities of extra-cellular
matrix. Pediatric Research 22: 324–329
Maroteaux P, Stanescu V, Stanescu R 1976 The lethal
chondrodysplasias. Clinical Orthopaedics 14: 31
Saldino R M 1971 Lethal short-limbed dwarfism:
achondrogenesis and thanatophoric dwarfism. American
Journal of Roentgenology 112: 185
Sillence D O, Rimoin D L, Lachman R 1978 Neonatal
dwarfism. Pediatrics Clinics of North America 25(3):
453–483
Yang Sheng-S, Brough A J, Garewal G S, Bernstein J 1974
Two types of heritable lethal achondrogenesis. Journal of
Pediatrics 85: 796–801

Fibrochondrogenesis

Eteson D J et al 1984 Fibrochondrogenesis: Radiologic and
Histologic studies. American Journal of Medical Genetics
19: 277–290
Whitley C B et al 1984 Fibrochondrogenesis. American
Journal of Medical Genetics 19: 265–275

Thanatophoric Dysplasia

Horton W A, Rimoin D L, Hollister D W, Lachman R S 1979
Further heterogeneity within lethal neonatal short-limbed
dwarfism: The platyspondylic types. Journal of Pediatrics
94: 736
Horton W, Hood O, Machado M, Ahmed S, Griffey E 1988
Abnormal ossification in thanatophoric dysplasia. Bone 9:
53–61
Langer L O, Spranger J W, Greinacher I, Herdman R C 1969
Thanatophoric dwarfism. Radiology 92: 285–294
Maroteaux P, Lamy M, Robert J M 1967 La nanisme
thanatophore. Presse Medicale 75: 2519
Ornoy A, Adomian G, Eteson D, Burgeson R, Rimoin D 1985
The role of mesenchymal-like tissue in the pathogenesis of
thanatophoric dysplasia. American Journal of Medical
Genetics 21: 613–630
Partington M W, Gonzales-Crussi F, Khakee S G, Wollin D G
1971 Cloverleaf skull and thanatophoric dwarfism. Report of
four cases, two in the same sibship. Archives of Disease in
Childhood 46: 656
Saldino R M 1971 Lethal Dwarfism: achondrogenesis and
thanatophoric dwarfism. American Journal of
Roentgenology 112: 185

Atelosteogenesis

Kozlowski K, Bateson E M 1984 Atelosteogenesis. Fortschr
Rontgenstr 140: 224–225
Maroteaux P et al 1982 Atelosteogenesis. American Journal of
Medical Genetics 13: 15–25
Sillence D O et al 1982 Spondylohumerofermoral hypoplasia
(Giant Cell Chondrodysplasia). American Journal of
Medical Genetics 13: 7–14
Sillence D O et al 1987 Atelosteogenesis. Pediatric Radiology
17: 112–118
Yang S S et al 1983 Two lethal chondrodysplasias with giant
chondrocytes. American Journal of Medical Genetics 15:
615–625

Schneckenbecken Dysplasia

Borochowitz Z et al 1986 A distinct lethal neonatal
chondrodysplasia with snail-like pelvis: Schneckenbecken
Dysplasia. American Journal of Medical Genetics 25: 47–59

Short Rib-polydactyly Syndrome Type I (Saldino-Noonan)
(perhaps several forms)

Bernstein R, Isdale J, Pinto M, Szaaigman J T, Jenkins T
1985 Short rib-polydactyly syndrome: A single or
heterogeneous entity? Journal of Medical Genetics 22:
46–53
Lowry R B, Wignall N 1975 Saldino-Noonan short rib-
polydactyly dwarfism syndrome. Pediatrics 56: 121–123
Saldino R M, Noonan C D 1972 Severe thoracic dystrophy
with striking micromelia, abnormal osseous development,
including the spine and multiple visceral anomalies.
American Journal of Roentgenology 114: 257–263
Sillence D O 1980 Non-Majewski short rib-polydactyly
syndrome. American Journal of Medical Genetics 7: 223
Spranger J, Grimm B, Weller M, Weissenbacher G, Herrmann
J, Gilbert E, Krepler R 1974 Short rib-polydactyly (SRP)
syndromes, type Majewski and Saldino-Noonan. Zeitschrift
fur Kinderheilkunde 116: 73

Short Rib-polydactyly Syndrome Type II (Majewski)

Bido-Lopez P, Ablow R C, Ogden J A, Mahoney M J 1978
A case of short rib-polydactyly. Pediatrics 61: 427–432

Chen H, Yang S, Gonzales E, Fowler M, Al Saadi A
    1980 Short rib-polydactyly syndrome. Majewski type.
    American Journal of Medical Genetics 7: 215
Majewski F, Pfeiffer R A, Lenz W et al 1971
    Polysyndaktylie, Verkurzte Gliedmassen und
    Genitalfehbildungen: Kennzeichen Eines Selbstandigen
    Syndromes. Zeitschrift fur Kinderheilkunde 111: 118–138
Silengo M C, Bell G L, Biagioli M, Franceschini P 1987
    Oral-facial-digital syndrome II: Transitional type between
    the Mohr and the Majewski syndromes: Report of two
    new cases. Clinical Genetics 31: 331–336
Spranger J, Grimm B, Weller M et al 1974 Short rib-
    polydactyly (SRP) syndromes, types Majewski and Saldino-
    Noonan. Zeitschrift fur Kinderheilkunde 116: 73–94

Dyssegmental Dysplasias

Aleck K A et al 1987 Dyssegmental Dysplasias. American
    Journal of Medical Genetics 27: 295–312
Stoss H 1985 Dyssegmental dysplasia. Pathologe 6: 88–95

Chondrodysplasia Punctata

Spranger J W, Opitz J M, Bidder U 1971 Heterogeneity of
    chondrodysplasia punctata. Humangenetik 11: 190–212

a. Rhizomelic Form

Schutgens R, Heymans H, Wanders R, Van Den Bosch H,
    Tager J 1986 Peroxisomal disorders: A newly recognized
    group of genetic diseases. European Journal of Pediatrics
    144: 430–440
Spranger J W, Bidder U, Voelz C 1971 Chondrodysplasia
    punctata (chondrodystrophia calcificans). II der Rhizomele
    typ. Fortschritte auf dem Gebiete der Rontgenstrahlen
    und der Nuklear Medizin 114: 327

b. Dominant Form

Afshani E, Girdany B R 1972 Atlanto-axial dislocation in
    chondrodysplasia punctata. Radiology 102: 399–401
Kaufman H J, Mahboubi S, Spackman T J, Capitanio M A,
    Kirkpatrick J 1976 Tracheal stenosis as a complication of
    chondrodysplasia punctata. Annals of Radiology 19:
    203–209
Silengo M C, Luzzatti L, Silverman F 1980 Clinical and
    genetic aspects of Conradi-Hunermann disease: A report of
    3 familial cases and review of the literature. Journal of
    Pediatrics 97: 911–917
Spranger J W, Bidder U, Voelz C 1970 Chondrodysplasia
    Punctata (chondrodystrophia calcificans) Type Conradi-
    Hunermann. Fortschritte auf dem Gebiete der
    Rontgenstrahlen und der Nuklear Medizin 113: 717–725
Theander G, Pettersson J 1978 Calcification in
    chondrodysplasia punctata. Acta Radiologica Diagnostica 1:
    205–221

*c. Other Forms. Exclude: Symptomatic stippling in other
    disorders (e.g. Zellweger syndrome, warfarin embryopathy)*

Curry C, Magenis R, Brown M et al 1984 Inherited
    chondrodysplasia punctata due to a deletion of the terminal
    short arm of an X chromosome. New England Journal of
    Medicine 311: 1010
Shaul W L, Emery H, Hall J G 1975 Chondrodysplasia
    punctata and maternal warfarin use during pregnancy.

American Journal of Diseases of Children 129: 360
Sheffield L J, Danks D M, Mayne V, Hutchinson L A 1976
    Chondrodysplasia punctata – 23 cases of a mild and
    relatively common variety. Journal of Pediatrics 89:
    916–923

Campomelic Dysplasia

Hoefnagel D, Wurster-Hill D H, Dupree W B, Benirschke
    K, Fuld G L 1978 Camptomelic dwarfism associated with
    XY-gonadal dysgenesis and chromosome anomalies.
    Clinical Genetics 13: 489–499
Khajavi A, Lachman R, Rimoin D et al 1976
    Heterogeneity in the campomelic syndromes. Radiology
    120: 641–647
Maroteaux P, Spranger J, Opitz J M, Kucera J, Lowry R B,
    Schimke R N, Kagan S M 1971 Le syndrome
    campomelique. Presse Medicale 79: 1157
Thurmon T F, DeFraites E B, Anderson E E 1973 Familial
    camptomelic dwarfism. Journal of Pediatrics 83: 841–843

**Other Dysplasias with Congenital Bowing of Long Bones
(several forms)**

Khajavi A, Lachman R, Rimoin D et al 1976
    Heterogeneity in the campomelic syndromes. Radiology
    120: 641–647
MacLean R, Prater W, Lozzio C 1983 Skeletal dysplasia with
    short angulated femora (kyphomelic dysplasia). American
    Journal of Medical Genetics 14: 373–380
Stuve A, Wiedemann H 1971 Congenital bowing of the
    long bones in two sisters. Lancet 2: 495

Achondroplasia

Langer L O Jr., Baumann P A, Gorlin R L 1967
    Achondroplasia. American Journal of Roentgenology,
    Radium Therapy and Nuclear Medicine 100: 12–26
Murdoch J L, Walker B A, Hall J G, Abbey II, Smith K K,
    McKusick V A 1970 Achondroplasia – a genetic and
    statistical survey. Annals of Human Genetics 33: 227–244
Pauli R, Scott C, Wassman E et al 1984 Apnea and sudden
    unexpected death in infants with achondroplasia. Journal of
    Pediatrics 104: 342–348
Pyeritz R, Sack G, Udvarhelyi G 1987 Thoracolumbosacral
    laminectomy in achondroplasia: Long term results in 22
    patients. American Journal of Medical Genetics 28:
    433–444
Rimoin D L, Hughes G N F, Kaufman R L, Rosenthal
    R E, McAlster W H, Silberberg R 1970 Endochondral
    ossification in achondroplastic dwarfism. New England
    Journal of Medicine 283: 728
Scott C I 1976 Achondroplastic and hypochondroplastic
    dwarfism. Clinical Orthopaedics 114: 18

Diastrophic Dysplasia

Gustavson K, Holmgren G, Jagells S, Jorulf H 1985 Lethal
    and non-lethal diastrophic dysplasia: A study of 14 Swedish
    cases. Clinical Genetics 28: 321–334
Hollister D W, Lachman R S 1976 Diastrophic dwarfism.
    Clinical Orthopaedics 114: 61–69
Horton W A, Rimoin D L, Lachman R S et al 1978 The
    phenotypic variability of diastrophic dysplasia. Journal of
    Pediatrics 93: 609–613

Lachman R S et al 1981 Diastrophic Dysplasia: The death of a variant. Radiology 140: 79–86

Lamy M, Maroteaux P 1960 La nanisme diastrophique. Presse Medicale 68: 1977–1980

Walker B A, Scott C I, Hall J G, Murdoch J L, McKusick V A 1972 Diastrophic dwarfism. Medicine 51: 1

Pseudodiastrophic Dysplasia

Eteson D J et al 1986 Pseudodiastrophic dysplasia: A distinct newborn skeletal dysplasia. Journal of Pediatrics 109: 635–641

Metatropic Dysplasia (several forms)

Beck M, Roubick M, Rogers J, Naumoff P, Spranger J 1983 Heterogeneity of metatropic dysplasia. European Journal of Pediatrics 140: 231–237

Boden S, Kaplan F, Fallon M et al 1987 Metatropic dwarfism: Uncoupling of endrochondral and perichondral growth. Journal of Bone and Joint Surgery 69A: 174–184

Gefferth K 1973 Metatropic dwarfism. Progress in Pediatric Radiology 4: 137–151

Jenkins P, Smith M D, McKinnell J S 1970 Metatropic dwarfism. British Journal of Radiology 43: 561–565

Maroteaux P, Spranger J, Wiedemann H R 1966 Der Metatropische Zwergwuchs. Archiv fur Kinderheilkunde 173: 211–226

Rimoin D L, Siggers D C, Lachman R S, Silberberg R 1976 Metatropic dwarfism, the Kniest syndrome and the pseudoachondroplastic dysplasias. Clinical Orthopaedics 114: 70

Chondroectodermal Dysplasia (Ellis-van Creveld)

Blackurn M G, Belliveau R E 1971 Ellis-van Creveld syndrome. American Journal of Diseases of Children 122: 267–270

Kozlowski K, Szmigiel C, Barylak A, Stropyrowa M 1972 Difficulties in differentiation between chondroectodermal dysplasia (Ellis-van Creveld syndrome) and asphyxiating thoracic dystrophy. Australasian Radiology 16: 401–410

McKusick V A, Egeland J A, Eldridge R, Krusen D R 1964 Dwarfism in the Amish. I. The Ellis-van Creveld syndrome. Bulletin of the Johns Hopkins Hospital 115: 306

Taylor G, Johansen C, Dorst S, Dorst J 1984 Polycarpaly and other abnormalities of the wrist in chondroectodermal dysplasia: The Ellis-van Creveld Syndrome. Radiology 151: 393–396

Asphyxiating Thoracic Dysplasia (Jeune)

Cortina J, Beltran J, Olague R, Ceres L, Alonson A, Lanuza A 1979 The wide spectrum of the asphyxiating thoracic dysplasia. Pediatric Radiology 8: 93–99

Herdman R C, Langer L O 1968 The thoracic asphyxiant dystrophy and renal disease. American Journal of Diseases in Children 116: 192–201

Kozlowski K, Szmigiel C, Barylak A, Stropyrowa M 1972 Difficulties in differentiation between chondroectodermal dysplasia (Ellis-van Creveld syndrome) and asphyxiating thoracic dystrophy. Australasian Radiology 16: 401–410

Langer L O Jr. 1968 Thoracic-pelvic-phalangeal dystrophy: asphyxiating thoracic dystrophy of the newborn, infantile thoracic dystrophy. Radiology 91: 447–546

Maroteaux P, Savart P 1964 La dystrophie thoracique asphyxiant; etude radiologique et rapports avec le syndrome d'Ellis et van Creveld. Annales Radiology 7: 332

Oberklaid F, Danks D M, Moyne V, Campbell B 1977 Asphyxiating thoracic dysplasia: clinical, radiological and pathological information on 10 patients. Archives of Disease in Childhood 52: 758

Spondyloepiphyseal Dysplasia Congenita

a. Type Spranger-Wiedemann

Bach C, Maroteaux P, Schaefer P, Bitan A, Crumiere C 1967 Dysplasia spondylo-epiphysaire congenitale avec anomalies multiples. Archives Françaises Pediatrie 24: 24–33

Hamidi-Toosi S, Maumenee I 1982 Vitreo-retinal degeneration in spondyloepiphyseal dysplasia congenita. Archives of Ophthalmology 100: 1104–1107

Harrod M, Friedman J, Currarino G, Pauli R, Langer L 1984 Genetic heterogeneity in spondyloepiphyseal dysplasia congenita. American Journal of Medical Genetics 18: 311–320

Kozlowski K, Bittel-Dobrzynska N, Budzynska A 1967 Spondyloepiphyseal dysplasia congenita. Annals of Radiology 11: 367–375

Lee B, Vissing H, Ramirez F, Rogers D, Rimoin D 1989 Identification of the molecular defect in a family with spondyloepiphyseal dysplasia. Science 244: 978–980

Murray L W, Bautista J, James P L, Rimoin D 1989 Type II collagen defects in the chondrodysplasias. I. Spondyloepiphyseal dysplasias. American Journal of Human Genetics 45: 5–15

Spranger J W, Langer L O Jr. 1970 Spondyloepiphyseal dysplasia congenita. Radiology 94: 313–322

Spranger J, Wiedemann H R 1966 Dysplasia spondyloepiphysaria congenita. Helvetica Pediatrica Acta 6: 598–611

b. Other Forms

Anderson C, Sillence D, Lachman R, Toomey K, Bull M, Dorst J, Rimoin D 1982 Spondylometaepiphyseal dysplasia, Strudwick type. American Journal of Medical Genetics 13: 243–256

Maroteaux P, Wiedemann H R, Spranger J, Kozlowski K, Lenzi L 1968 Essai de classification des dysplasies spondyloepiphysaires. Monographies de Genetique Medicale, Lyon, France

Spranger J, Langer L O 1974 Spondyloepiphyseal dysplasia. In: Skeletal Dysplasias. Birth Defects Original Articles Series X (9): 19

Kniest Dysplasia

Friede H, Matalon R, Harris V, Rosenthal I 1985 Craniofacial and mucopolysaccharide abormalities in Kniest dysplasia. Journal of Craniofacial Genetics 5: 267–276

Lachman R S, Rimoin D L, Hollister D W et al 1975 The Kniest syndrome. Radiology 123: 805

Maroteaux P, Spranger J 1973 La maladie de Kniest. Archives Francaises Pediatrie 30: 735

Poole A R, Pidoux I, Reiner A, Rosenberg L, Hollister D, Murray L, Rimoin D 1988 Kniest dysplasias characterized by an apparent abnormal processing of the C-propeptide of Type II collagen resulting in imperfect fibril assembly. Journal of Clinical Investigation 81: 579–589

Siggers D, Rimoin D L, Dorst J P et al 1974 The Kniest syndrome. In: Skeletal dysplasias. Birth Defects Original Article Series X(9): 193

Mesomelic Dysplasia

Kaitila II, Leisti J T, Rimoin D L 1976 Mesomelic skeletal dysplasias, Clinical Orthopaedics 114: 94–106

a. Type Nievergelt

Nievergelt K 1944 Positiver Vaterschaftorachivers auf Grund Erblicher Missbildungen der Extremitäten. Klaus-Stift Vererb Forsch 19: 157

Solonen K A, Sulamaa M 1958 Nievergelt syndrome and its treatment; a case report. Annales Chirurgiae et Gynaecologiae Fenniae 47: 142–147

b. Type Langer (probably Homozygous Dyschondrosteosis)

Espiritu C, Chen H, Wooley P V 1975 Mesomelic dwarfism as the homozygous expression of dyschondrosteosis. American Journal of Diseases of Children 129: 375

Goldblatt J, Wallis C, Vilgoen D, Beighton P 1987 Heterozygous manifestations of Langer mesomelic dysplasia. Clinical Genetics 31: 19–24

Langer L O Jr. 1967 Mesomelic dwarfism of the hypoplastic ulna, fibula mandible type. Radiology 89: 654–660

Silverman F N 1973 Mesomelic dwarfism. Progress in Pediatrics and Radiology 4: 546–562

c. Type Robinow

Butler M, Wadlington W 1987 Robinow syndrome: Report of two patients and review of literature. Clinical Genetics 31: 77–85

Kelly T E, Benson R, Temtamy S A, Plotnick L, Levin S 1975 The Robinow syndrome: an isolated case with a detailed study of the phenotype. American Journal of Diseases of Children 129: 383–386

Robinow M, Silverman F N, Smith H D 1969 A newly recognized dwarfing syndrome. American Journal of Diseases of Children 117: 645–651

d. Type Reinhardt

Reinhardt K, Pfeiffer R A 1967 Ulno-fibulare Dysplasie. Eine autosomal-dominant verebte Mikromesomelie ähnlich dem Nievergelts syndrom. Fortschritte auf dem Gebiete der Rontgenstrahlen und der Nuklear Medizin 107: 379

Acromesomelic Dysplasias

Campailla E, Martinelli B 1971 Deficit staturale con micromesomelia. Presentazione di due casi familiari. Minerva Ortopedica 22: 180

Langer L O, Garrett R T 1980 Acromesomelic dysplasia. Radiology 137: 349–355

Langer L O, Beals R K, Solomon I L et al 1977 Acromesomelic dwarfism: manifestations in childhood. American Journal of Medical Genetics 1: 87–100

Maroteaux P, Martinelli B, Campailla E 1971 Le nanisme acromesomelique. Presse Medicale 79: 1839

Cleidocranial Dysplasia

Faure C, Maroteaux P 1973 Cleidocranial dysplasia. Progress in Pediatrics and Radiology 4: 211

Forland M 1962 Cleidocranial dysostosis. A review of the syndrome. American Journal of Medicine 33: 792

Hawkins H B, Shapiro R, Petrillo C J 1975 The association of cleidocranial dysostosis with hearing loss. American Journal of Roentgenology, Radium Therapy and Nuclear Medicine 125: 944–947

Keats T E 1967 Cleidocranial dysostosis: some atypical roentgen manifestations. American Journal of Roentgenology, Radium Therapy and Nuclear Medicine 100: 71–74

Larsen Syndrome

Chen H, Chang C, Perrin E, Perrin J 1982 A lethal, Larsen-like multiple joint dislocation syndrome. American Journal of Medical Genetics 13: 149–161

Larsen L J, Schottstaedt E R, Bost R C 1950 Multiple congenital dislocations associated with characteristic facial abnormality. Journal of Pediatrics 37: 574

Latta R J, Graham B, Aase J, Scham S M, Smith D W 1971 Larsen's syndrome: a skeletal dysplasia with multiple joint dislocations and unusual facies. Journal of Pediatrics 78: 291

Micheli L J, Hall J E, Watts H G 1976 Spinal instability in Larsen's syndrome: Journal of Bone and Joint Surgery 58A: 562–565

Robertson F W, Kozlowski K, Middleton R W 1975 Larsen's syndrome. Clinical Pediatrics 14: 53–60

Steel H H, Kohl J 1972 Multiple congenital dislocations associated with other skeletal anomalies (Larsen's syndrome) in three siblings. Journal of Bone and Joint Surgery 54A: 75

Oto-palato-digital Syndrome I

Dudding B A, Gorlin R J, Langer L O 1967 The oto-palato-digital syndrome. American Journal of Diseases of Children 113: 214

Gall J C, Stern A M, Poznanski A K, Garn S M, Weinstein E D, Hayward J R 1972 Oto-palato-digital syndromes: comparison of clinical and radiographic manifestations in males and females. American Journal of Human Genetics 24: 24

Langer L O 1967 The roentgenographic features of the otopalato-digital (OPD) syndrome. American Journal of Roentgenology, Radium Therapy and Nuclear Medicine 100: 63

Kozlowski K, Turner G, Scougall J, Harrington J 1977 Oto-palato-digital syndrome with severe X-ray changes in two half brothers. Pediatric Radiology 6: 97–102

Pazzaglia U, Beluffi G 1986 Otopalatodigital syndrome in four generations of a large family Clinical Genetics 30: 338–344

Oto-palato-digital Syndrome II

Kaplan J, Maroteaux P 1984 Syndrome oto-palato-digital de Type II. Annales de Génétique 27: 79–82

Kozlowski K et al 1977 Oto-palato-digital syndrome with severe X-ray changes in two half brothers. Pediatric Radiology 6: 97–102

B. Identifiable in Later Life

Hypochondroplasia

Beals R K 1969 Hypochondroplasia. A report of five kindreds. Journal of Bone and Joint Surgery 51A: 728–739

Frydman M, Hertz M, Goodman R M 1974 The genetic entity of hypochondroplasia. Clinical Genetics 5: 223–229

Kozlowski K 1973 Hypochondroplasia. Progress in Pediatric Radiology 4: 238–249

Newman D E, Dunbar J S 1975 Hypochondroplasia. Journal of the Canadian Association of Radiologists 26: 95–103

Sommer A, Young-Wee T, Frye T 1987 Achondroplasia-hypochondroplasia complex. American Journal of Medical Genetics 26: 949–957

Walker B A, Murdock J L, McKusick V A, Langer L O, Beals R K 1971 Hypochondroplasia. American Journal of Diseases of Children 122: 95

Dyschondrosteosis

Carter A R, Currey H L 1974 Dyschondrosteosis (mesomelic dwarfism) – a family study. British Journal of Radiology 47: 634–640

Dawe C, Wynne-Davies R, Fulford G 1982 Clinical variation in dyschondrosteosis: a report on 13 individuals and 8 families. Journal of Bone and Joint Surgery 64B: 377–381

Espiritu C, Chen H, Wooley P V 1974 Mesomelic dwarfism as the homozygous expression of dyschondrosteosis. American Journal of Diseases of Children 129: 375–377

Felman A H, Kirkpatrick J A 1970 Dyschondrosteose. American Journal of Diseases of Children 120: 329–331

Kaitila II, Leisti J T, Rimoin D L 1976 Mesomelic skeletal dysplasias. Clinical Orthopaedics 114: 94–106

Langer L O Jr. 1965 Dyschondrosteosis: A hereditable bone dysplasia with characteristic roentgenographic features. American Journal of Roentgenology, Radium Therapy and Nuclear Medicine 95: 178–188

Maroteaux P, Lamy M 1959 La dyschondrosteose. Semaine des Hopiteaux de Paris 35: 3464–3470

Metaphyseal Chondrodysplasia Type Jansen

Charrow J, Poznanski A 1984 The Jansen type of metaphyseal chondrodysplasia: confirmation of dominant inheritance and review of radiographic manifestations in the newborn and adult. American Journal of Medical Genetics 18: 321–327

De Haas W H D, DeBoer W, Griffioen F 1969 Metaphyseal dysostosis. A late follow-up of the first reported case. Journal of Bone and Joint Surgery 51A: 290–299

Holt J F 1969 Discussion. In: Skeletal Dysplasias. Part IV, Birth Defects Original Article Series V (4): 73

Jansen M 1934 Über atypische Chondrodystrophie (Achondroplasie) und über eine noch nicht beschriebene angeborene Wachstrumstörung des Knochensystems. Metaphysäre Dysostose. Orthopedika Chirgica 61: 253–286

Metaphyseal Chondrodysplasia Type Schmid

Dent C E, Normand I C 1964 Metaphyseal dysostosis type Schmid. Archives of Disease in Childhood 39: 444

Kozlowski K 1964 Metaphyseal dysostosis. Report of five familial and two sporadic cases of a mild type. American Journal of Roentgenology, Radium Therapy and Nuclear Medicine 91: 601–608

Lachman R S et al 1988 Metaphyseal chondrodysplasia, Schmid type. Pediatric Radiology 18: 93–102

Stickler G R, Maher F R, Hunt J C, Burke E C, Rosevaer J W 1962 Familial bone disease resembling rickets (hereditary metaphyseal dysostosis). Pediatrics 29: 996

Wekselman R 1977 Familial metaphyseal dysostosis. American Journal of Roentgenology, Radium Therapy and Nuclear Medicine 59A: 690–691

Metaphyseal Chondrodysplasia Type McKusick

Lux S E, Johnston R B, August C S, Say B, Penchaszadeh V B, Rosen F S, McKusick V A 1970 Chronic neutropenia and abnormal cellular immunity in cartilage-hair hypoplasia. New England Journal of Medicine 282: 231–236

McKusick V A, Eldridge R, Hostetler J A, Ruangwit U, Egeland J A 1965 Dwarfism in the Amish II. Cartilage-hair hypoplasia. Bulletin of the Johns Hopkins Hospital 116: 285–326

Polmar S, Pierce G 1986 Cartilage-hair hypoplasia: Immunological aspects and their clinical implications. Clinical Immunology and Immunopathology 40: 87–93

Ray H C, Dorst J P 1973 Cartilage-hair hypoplasia. Progress in Pediatric Radiology 4: 270–298

Metaphyseal Chondrodysplasia with Exocrine Pancreatic Insufficiency and Cyclic Neutropenia

Schmerling D H, Prader A, Hitzig W H, Giedion A, Hadorn B, Kuhni M 1969 The syndrome of exocrine pancreatic insufficiency, neutropenia, metaphyseal dysostosis and dwarfism. Helvetica Paediatrica Acta 24: 547

Taybi H, Mitchell A D, Friedman G D 1969 Metaphyseal dysostosis and the associated syndrome of pancreatic insufficiency and blood disorders. Radiology 93: 563–571

Spondylometaphyseal Dysplasia

a. Type Kozlowski

Gustavson K H, Homgren G, Probst F 1978 Spondylometaphyseal dysplasia in two sibs of normal parents. Pediatric Radiology 7: 90–96

Kozlowski K 1976 Metaphyseal and spondylometaphyseal chondrodysplasias. Clinical Orthopaedics 114: 83

Kozlowski K, Maroteaux P, Spranger J 1967 La dysotose spondylometaphysaire. Presse Medicale 75: 2769

Riggs W, Summit R L 1971 Spondylometaphyseal dysplasia (Kozlowski). Radiology 101: 375

Thomas P S, Nevin N C 1977 Spondylometaphyseal dysplasia. American Journal of Roentgenology, Radium Therapy and Nuclear Medicine 128: 89–93 *b. Other forms*

Kozlowski K, Beemer F, Bens G et al 1982
Spondylometaphyseal dysplasia: report of 7 cases and essay of classification. In: Papadatos C, Bartsocas C (eds) Skeletal Dysplasia. Liss, New York p 89–101

Lachman R, Zonana J, Khajavi A et al 1978 The spondylometaphyseal dysplasias: clinical, radiologic and pathologic correlation. Annales de Radiologie 22: 125–135

Rimoin D L 1975 The chondrodystrophies. Advances in Human Genetics 5: 1

Schmidt B J, Becak W, Becak M L et al 1963 Metaphyseal dysostosis. Journal of Pediatrics 63: 106

Multiple Epiphyseal Dysplasia

Spranger J 1976 The epiphyseal dysplasias. Clinical Orthopaedics 114: 46

a. Type Fairbank

Fairbank H A T 1946 Dysplasia epiphysealis multiplex. Proceedings of the Royal Society of Medicine 39: 315–317

Jacobs J 1973 Multiple epiphyseal dysplasia. Progress in Pediatric Radiology 4: 309–324

Kozlowski K, Lipska E 1967 Hereditary dysplasia epiphysealis multiplex. Clinical Radiology 18: 330–336

Leed N E 1960 Epiphyseal Dysplasia mutliplex. American Journal of Roetgenology, Radium Therapy and Nuclear Medicine 84: 506–510

b. Other Forms

Hulvey J T, Keats T 1969 Multiple epiphyseal dysplasia. American Journal of Roentgenology, Radium Therapy and Nuclear Medicine CVI: 170–177

Juberg R C, Holt J F 1968 Inheritance of multiple epiphyseal dysplasia tarda. American Journal of Human Genetics 20: 549–563

Ribbing S 1937 Studien über Heredetaire, Multiple Epiphysenstorungen. Acta Radiologica 35(Suppl): 1–107

Arthro-ophthalmopathy

Francomano C, Liberfarb R, Hirose T et al 1987 The Stickler syndrome: evidence for close linkage to the structural gene of type II collagen. Genomics 1: 293–296

Opitz J M, Franc T, Hermann J 1972 The Stickler syndrome. New England Journal of Medicine 286: 546–547

Spallone A 1987 Stickler's syndrome: a study of 12 families. British Journal of Ophthalmology 71: 504–509

Stickler G B, Pugh D G 1967 Hereditary progressive arthro-ophthalmopathy II. additional observations on vertebral abnormalities, a hearing defect, and a report of a similar case. Mayo Clinic Proceedings 42: 495–500

Stickler G B, Belau P G, Farrell F J, Jones J D, Pugh D G, Steinberg A G, Ward L E 1965 Hereditary progressive arthro-ophthalmopathy. Mayo Clinic Proceedings 40: 433–455

Pseudoachondroplasia

a. Dominant

Ford N, Silverman R N, Kozlowski K 1961 Spondylo-epiphyseal dysplasia (pseudo-achondroplastic type). American Journal of Roentgenology, Radium Therapy and Nuclear Medicine 86: 462–472

Hall J G, Dorst J, Rotta J, McKusick V 1987 Gonadal mosaicism in pseudoachondroplasia. American Journal of Medical Genetics 28: 143–151

Maroteaux P, Lamy M 1959 Les formes pseudo-achondroplastiques des dysplasies spondylo-epiphysaires. Presse Medicale 67: 383–386

Phillips S J, Magsamen B F, Punnett H H, Kistenmacher M L, Campo R D 1974 Fine structure of skeletal dysplasia as seen in pseudoachondroplastic spondyloepiphyseal dysplasia and asphyxiating thoracic dystrophy. In: Skeletal Dysplasias. Birth Defects Original Article Series X(12) 314

b. Recessive

Hall J G 1975 Pseudoachondroplasia. In: Disorders of Connective Tissue. Birth Defects Original Article Series XI(6): 187

Spondyloepiphyseal Dysplasia Tarda

Bannerman R M, Ingall G B, Mohn J F 1971 X-linked spondylo-epiphyseal dysplasia tarda: clinical and linkage data. Journal of Medical Genetics 8: 291–301

Harper P S, Jenkins P, Laurence K M 1973 Spondylo-epiphyseal dysplasia tarda: a report of four cases in two families. British Journal of Radiology 46: 676–684

Iceton J, Horne G 1986 Spondyloepiphyseal dysplasia tarda: The X-linked variety in 3 brothers. Journal of Bone and Joint Surgery 68B: 616–619

Langer L O Jr. 1964 Spondyloepiphyseal dysplasia tarda. Hereditary chondrodysplasia with characteristic vertebral configuration in the adult. Radiology 82: 833–839

Maroteaux P, Lamy M, Bernard J 1957 La dysplasie spondyloepiphysaire tardive; description clinique et radiologique. Presse Medicale 65: 1205-1208

Brachyolmia

Fontaine G, Maroteaux P, Fariaux J P, Bosquet M 1975 Pure spondylar dysplasia or brachyolmy – appropos of a case. Archives Francaise Pediatrie 32: 695–708

Hobaek A 1961 Chondrodysplasia hereditaria infantalis. In: Hobaek A (ed): Problems of heredity chondrodysplasias: roentgenological, clinical and genetic study of 70 cases of hereditary chondrodysplasia in 42 Norwegian families. Oslo University Press, Oslo, p 82–95

Horton W A, Langer L O, Collins B C 1983 Brachyolmia Hobaek type: a clinical radiographic and histologic study. American Journal of Medical Genetics 16: 201–221

Shohat M, Lachman R, Gruber H E, Rimoin D L 1989 Brachyolmia: radiographic and genetic evidence of heterogeneity. American Journal of Medical Genetics 33: 209–219

Toledo S P, Mauro P A, Lamego C, Alves C A, Dietrich C P, Assisl M, Mattar E 1978 Recessively inherited, late-onset spondylar dysplasia and peripheral corneal opacity with anomalies in urinary mucopolysaccharides: a possible error of chondroitin-6 sulfate synthesis. American Journal of Medical Genetics 2: 385–395

Dyggve-Melchior-Clausen Dysplasia

Bonafede R P, Beighton P 1978 The Dyggve-Melchior-Clausen syndrome. Clinical Genetics 14: 24–30

Kaufman R L, Rimoin D L:, McAlister W H 1971 The Dyggve-Melchior-Clausen syndrome. Birth Defects Original Article Series VII: 144–149

Naffah J 1976 The Dyggve-Melchior-Clausen syndrome. American Journal of Human Genetics 28: 607

Schorr S, Legum C, Oschshorn M et al 1977 The Dyggve-Melchior-Clausen syndrome. American Journal of Roentgenology, Radium Therapy and Nuclear Medicine 128: 107–113

Spranger J W, Der Kaloustian J M 1975 The Dyggve-Melchior-Clausen syndrome. Radiology 114: 415

Spranger J W, Bierbaum B, Herrmann J 1976 Heterogeneity of Dyggve-Melchior-Clausen dwarfism. Human Genetics 33: 279

Spondyloepimetaphyseal Dysplasia (several forms)

Arias S, Mata M, Pinto-Cisternas J 1976 L'osteochondrodysplasie spondylo-metaphysaire type Irapa: nouveau nanisme over rachis et metatarscens courts. Nouvelle Presse Medicale 5: 319

Kozlowski K 1974 Micromelic type of spondylo-meta-epiphyseal dysplasia. Pediatric Radiology 2: 61

Kozlowski K, Budzinska A 1966 Combined metaphyseal and epiphyseal dysostosis. American Journal of Roentgenology, Radium Therapy and Nuclear Medicine 97: 21

Oto-spondylo-megaepiphyseal Dysplasias

Cortina H et al 1977 The Weissenbacher-Zwegenmuller Syndrome. Pediatric Radiology 6: 109–111

Giedion A et al 1982 Oto-spondylo-megaepiphyseal dysplasia (OSMED). Helvetica Paediatrica Acta 37: 361–380

Kelly T E et al 1982 The Weissenbacher-Zweggmuller syndrome: Possible neonatal expression of the Stickler syndrome. American Journal of Medical Genetics 11: 113–119

Myotonic Chondrodysplasia (Catel-Schwartz-Jampel)

Beighton P 1973 The Schwartz syndrome in Southern Africa. Clinical Genetics 4: 548–555

Edwards W, Rot A 1982 Chondrodystrophic myotonia (Schwartz-Jampel syndrome). American Journal of Medical Genetics 13: 51–56

Farrell S, Davidson R, Thorp P 1987 Neonatal manifestations of Schwartz-Jampel syndrome. American Journal of Medical Genetics 27: 799–805

Fowler W M, Loyzer R B, Taylor R G et al 1974 The Schwartz-Jampel syndrome. Its clinical, physiological and histological expression. Journal of the Neurological Sciences 22: 127

Kozlowski K, Wise G 1974 Spondylo-epi-metaphyseal dysplasia with myotonia. A radiographic study. Radiologia Diagnostica 6: 817

Van Huffelen A C, Gabrealo F J M, Van Luypen J S et al 1974 Chondrodystrophic myotonia. Neuropaediatri 5: 71

Parastremmatic Dysplasia

Horan F, Beighton P 1976 Parastremmatic dwarfism. Journal of Bone and Joint Surgery 58B: 343–346

Langer L O, Petersen D, Spranger J 1970 An unusual bone dysplasia: parastremmatic dwarfism. American Journal of Roentgenology, Radium Therapy and Nuclear Medicine 110: 550–560

Rask M R 1963 Morquio-Brailsford osteochondrodystrophy and osteogenesis imperfecta: report of a patient with both conditions. Journal of Bone and Joint Surgery 45A: 561–570

Trichorhinophalangeal Dysplasia

Bowen P, Piederman B, Hoo J 1985 The critical segment for the Langer-Giedion syndrome: 8q24.11-q24.12. Annales de Génétique 28: 224–227

Bühler E, Buhler U, Beuther C, Fessler R 1987 A final word on the trichorhinophalangeal syndromes. Clinical Genetics 31: 273–275

Felman A H, Frias J L 1977 Trichorhinophalangeal syndrome – study of 16 patients in one family. American Journal of Roentgenology, Radium Therapy and Nuclear Medicine 129: 631

Giedoin A, Burdea M, Fruchter Z et al 1973 Autosomal dominant transmission of the trichorhinophalangeal syndrome. Paediatrica Acta 28: 249

Kozlowski K, Blaim A, Malolepszy E 1972 Trichorhinophalangeal syndrome. Australasian Radiology XVI(4): 411–416

Pashayan H M, Solomon L M, Chan G 1974 The trichorhinophalangeal syndrome. American Journal of Diseases of Children 127: 257–261

Poznanski A K, Schmickel R D, Harper H A 1974 The hand in the trichorhinophalangeal syndrome. Birth Defects Original Article Series X(9): 209–219

Acrodysplasia with Retinitis Pigmentosa and Nephropathy (Saldino-Mainzer)

Ellis D, Heckenlively J, Martin C, Lachman D, Sakati N, Rimoin D 1984 Leber's congenital amouroses associated with familial juvenile nephronephthisis and cone-shaped epiphyses of the hands (The Saldino-Mainzer syndrome). American Journal of Ophthalmology 97: 233–239

Giedion A 1979 Phalangeal cone-shaped epiphyses of the hands (PhCSEH) and chronic renal disease – the conorenal syndromes. Pediatric Radiology 8: 32

Saldino R M, Mainzer F 1971 Cone-shaped epiphyses (CSE) in siblings with hereditary renal disease and retinitis pigmentosa. Radiology 98: 39

57. Disorders of bone density, volume and mineralisation

D. O. Sillence

This large group of genetic disorders of the skeleton consists of diseases characterised by abnormalities in the amount, density and remodelling of bone. It can be subdivided into the three following groups: disorders with a net decrease in skeletal tissue, disorders with a net increase of bone, and disorders of mineralisation and mineral metabolism.

DISORDERS WITH DECREASED BONE DENSITY

Decreased bone density may result from reduced production, defective mineralisation, increased breakdown of normal or defective bone, or a combination of these. Osteomalacia (i.e. undermineralised bone) characterises hereditary rickets and other disorders leading to defective mineralisation. Osteopenia (insufficient bone) characterises the hereditary osteoporoses and a number of other genetic and acquired diseases of childhood. Osteoporosis, i.e. the clinical syndromes resulting from osteopenia, is characterised by liability to fractures, particularly crush fractures of the vertebrae. The most important of the syndromes with osteoporosis numerically are the osteogenesis imperfecta syndromes.

Osteogenesis imperfecta

The term 'osteogenesis imperfecta' was advocated by Vrolik in 1840 to explain the origin of an hereditary skeletal condition leading to susceptibility to fracture and severe skeletal deformity. Also known as fragilitas ossium, osteopsathyrosis, Ekman-Lobstein and Vrolik disease, osteogenesis imperfecta is characterised by variable clinical severity.

The extreme variability in Osteogenesis Imperfecta (OI) results from genetic and biochemical heterogeneity. Four major syndrome groups, OI Types I–IV, are defined in the First International Nomenclature of Heritable Disorders of Connective Tissue (Beighton 1988). In each syndrome, further heterogeneity can be defined at the clinical, radiographic, collagen molecular or DNA level (Byers & Bonadio 1985, Cetta et al 1988). To these four syndrome groups must be added a number of essentially private syndromes (Sillence 1988).

Osteogenesis imperfecta Type I

This syndrome is characterised by osteoporosis leading to excessive bone fragility, distinctly blue sclerae and susceptibility to presenile conductive hearing loss in adolescents and adults with the disorder (Fig. 57.1).

Inheritance Inheritance in this syndrome is autosomal dominant with variable expressivity. Penetrance for fractures approximates 90% and for blue sclerae 100%. Hearing impairment is age related (Riedner et al 1980). Severity, measured by age of onset of fractures, fracture frequency in childhood and skeletal deformity, is correlated with a subgrouping based on the presence or absence of dentinogenesis imperfecta (DI) in the affected family (see below). Patients with OI Type I and DI have earlier and more marked manifestations than those with OI Type I and normal teeth (Paterson et al 1983).

Pathogenesis At the collagen biochemical level, these patients show approximately 50% reduction in synthesis of Type I procollagen. The mutations are heterozygous. Post-translational modification of Type I procollagen appears to be normal in contradistinction to OI Type II (see below). Linkage studies show segregation of the phenotype with pro alpha (1)I collagen gene (COLIA 1) restriction fragment length polymorphisms (RFLPs) demonstrating that mutations leading to OI Type I (at least the subgroup without DI) will be shown to be due to mutations affecting the synthesis of the pro alpha (1) collagen chain (Tsipouras et al 1984, Falk et al 1986).

Natural history This is the most common variety of osteogenesis imperfecta and has a birth frequency in the order of 1:30 000 live births and a population frequency similarly in the order of 1:30 000 (Sillence et al 1979a). The sclerae in these patients are generally of a deep blue-black hue. Fractures characteristically result from minimal trauma. Despite the tendency to bone fragility, accidental trauma does not always lead to fractures.

933

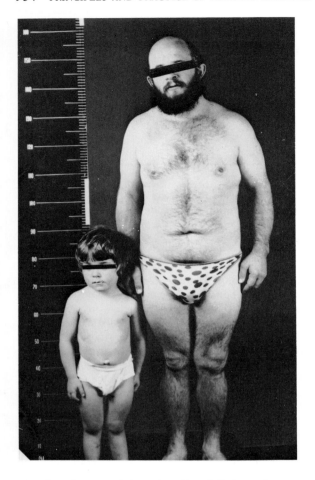

Fig. 57.1 Osteogenesis imperfecta Type I. Father and son showing mild shortening of stature. Both have intensely blue sclerae, numerous fractures and mild shortening of stature. Father wears a hearing aid.

Hereditary opalescent dentin (dentinogenesis imperfecta) is observed in some families with this trait and not others (Levin et al 1980, Paterson et al 1983). Opalescent dentin produces a distinctive yellowing and apparent transparency of the teeth which are often rapidly worn prematurely or broken. Some teeth with opalescent dentin may have a particularly greyish-blue hue. Radiological study of these teeth shows that they have short roots with constricted corono-radicular junctions.

Paterson and colleagues (1983) have shown that patients with OI Type I and normal teeth (OI 1) differ from patients with OI Type I with dentinogenesis imperfecta (OI 1.DI). The latter group are more likely to

have fractures at birth (25% versus 6%) and have a higher fracture frequency, more severe short stature, and skeletal deformity. Both groups have a similar frequency of joint hyperextensibility, bruising, deafness and joint dislocations.

When fractures occur at birth, generally there are only a few. Individuals with fractures at birth subsequently have no more deformity, handicap, or number of fractures than other individuals who have their first fracture after one year of age. Deformities of the limbs in this group are usually the result of fractures, but bowing, particularly of the lower limbs, is common. Other deformities such as genu valgum and flat feet with a metatarus varus deformity of the feet are common. Some adults have progressive kyphoscoliosis which may be of a severe degree. Kyphosis alone is common in older adults but rarely seen in children. There is usually excessive hyperlaxity of ligaments, particularly at the small joints of the hands, feet and knees, but this feature is less marked in adults.

Hearing impairment is a most troublesome complication. It is rarely present under 10 years of age. Approximately 100% of affected adults have recognisable hearing impairment by 50 years of age. Almost 40% of adults have severe hearing impairment. The hearing impairment is predominantly conductive but in some cases both conductive and sensorineural impairment is found (Riedner et al 1980).

There is a high frequency of premature arcus senilis in adults with OI Type I. No other visual abnormalities are associated with OI.

Radiographic studies in all patients in this group show generalised osteopenia, evidence of previous fractures and normal callus formation at the site of recent fractures. Deformities are usually the result of angulation at the site of previous fractures. However, bowing of the femora, tibiae and fibulae, and deformity in the bones of the feet, particularly metatarsus varus, are observed. Severe osteoporosis of the spine with codfish vertebrae is occasionally seen in these patients, but the majority have normally formed vertebral bodies with some wedging and flattening. Kyphoscoliosis is not usually diagnosed in childhood.

Spontaneous improvement is observed during adolescence with a marked reduction in the frequency of fractures.

Complications Complications include repeated fractures associated with minimal trauma. Ankle sprains and joint dislocation occur rarely.

Differential diagnosis 1. Juvenile idiopathic osteoporosis. The onset of fractures commonly commences in late childhood and the axial skeleton is more severely affected (Brenton & Dent 1976). Spontaneous improvement is the rule. The sclerae are not distinctly blue although the normal blueness of the sclerae in childhood must be distinguished from the distinct blueness of the sclerae in OI. Juvenile osteoporosis is sporadic.

2. Blue sclerae and keratoconus. In this autosomal recessive syndrome, blue sclerae are associated with keratoconus, middle ear bone conduction defect, joint hyperextensibility and spondylolisthesis without liability to fractures (Greenfield et al 1973).

3. Blue sclerae, familial nephrosis, thin skin and hydrocephalus. This autosomal recessive syndrome is not associated with skeletal fragility (Daentl et al 1978).

Therapy Comprehensive rehabilitation should be offered to improve mobility and muscle strength. Aggressive orthopaedic care with appropriate management of all fractures is necessary to avoid deformity and unnecessary immobilisation. Magnesium oxide, vitamin C, sodium fluoride, androgenic hormones and calcitonin have not shown consistent therapeutic efficacy.

Genetic counselling and prenatal diagnosis For an affected adult marrying a normal partner, there is a 50% chance of an affected child. Where two adults with OI Type I marry, there is a 25% chance for a severely affected infant homozygous for OI Type 1.

Ultrasound and radiographic studies prenatally will occasionally differentiate a normal from an affected fetus (Chervenak et al 1982). Prenatal prediction of OI Type 1 is feasible in some families where linkage to COLIA 1 (Collagen Type I, alpha-1 gene) or COLIA 2 (Collagen Type I, alpha-2 gene) polymorphisms can be demonstrated (Tsipouras et al 1987).

Osteogenesis imperfecta Type II

This syndrome group is characterised by extreme bone fragility leading to intrauterine or early infant death. The group is clinically and biochemically heterogeneous (Sillence et al 1984, Thompson et al 1987). Three subgroups which are useful for genetics and prognostic counselling are distinguished on a radiographic basis: (A) a subgroup with continuously beaded ribs and crumpled long bones (Fig. 57.2); (B) similar long bones but relatively normal ribs with few if any rib fractures; (C) long narrow dysplastic but beaded ribs with inadequately modelled long bones and multiple fractures. Collagen and DNA studies show that within each subgroup there is further biochemical and molecular heterogeneity.

Inheritance It is now clear from collagen biochemical and DNA studies that a majority of those instances of sibling recurrence where the proband has findings of subgroup A can be explained by parental gonadal mosaicism. True autosomal recessive inheritance may occur

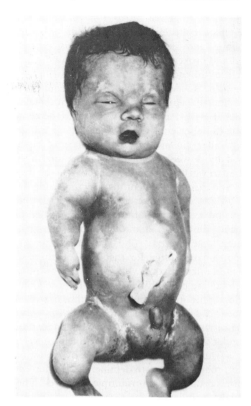

Fig. 57.2 Osteogenesis imperfecta Type II. Stillborn infant showing short deformed limbs with broad thighs fixed at right angles to trunk and relatively large head.

but, in the majority of cases examined biochemically, a heterozygous mutation is sufficient to produce the phenotype.

Where the proband has findings of subgroup B, the empiric recurrence risk is 7.7% (Thompson et al 1987). However, the frequent finding of sibling recurrence and parental consanguinity would suggest that a proportion of cases arise from autosomal recessive inheritance.

Subgroup C may represent an autosomal recessive disorder (Sillence et al 1984).

Pathogenesis A majority of cases with OI Type II studied at the biochemical or DNA level have been shown to have collagen defects. Diminished production of Type I collagen results from abnormal intracellular processing. Virtually all mutations have been heterozygous, either deletions or more commonly point mutations in the pro alpha (1) I or pro alpha (2) I chains. These disrupt triple helical folding of the two alpha (1) and one alpha (2) chains. Point mutations in glycine codons, such as glycine to cysteine which leads to disulphide bridging and glycine to arginine, disrupt helix formation (Byers &

Bonadio 1985, Bateman et al 1987, Tsipouras 1988). Severe tissue collagen deficiency leads to structurally weak bone and skin. The skeleton is progressively crushed and broken by muscle contraction during intra-uterine life (Sillence et al 1984).

Subgroup A Affected infants are commonly premature and, except where hydropic, with mean birth weight and birth length below the 50th percentile for gestation (Sillence et al 1984). One fifth are stillborn and the remainder die within hours or days of birth (90% deceased by 4 weeks of age, with maximum survival measured in weeks). General connective tissue fragility is present and dismemberment may occur during delivery.

The thighs are characteristically held in fixed abduction and external rotation (Fig. 57.2). The chest is small and limbs are markedly short and frequently angulated and bowed. The cranium often appears disproportionately large for the face and there is commonly mild micrognathia with a small narrow nose. Dark blue sclerae are present in virtually all those affected.

Radiographic study shows a small thorax with slightly shortened ribs which are thickened with continuous beading or wavy contours. The femora appear broad and rectangular with fine wavy margins (like a concertina) or are broad, undermodelled and very hypoplastic. Long and short tubular bones are demineralised, shortened and sometimes crumpled with multiple fractures. The tibiae are usually angulated. Vertebrae appear flattened and hypoplastic to a variable degree. The skull and face show diminished mineralisation and multiple ossification centres (Wormian bones). Pelves are hypoplastic with flattening of acetabular roofs and iliac crests.

Subgroup B These patients appear phenotypically similar to group A at birth but death from respiratory failure is not as likely. Survival for weeks to months and even several years is observed (Sillence et al 1984). Radiographically the ribs are shortened with few or no fractures. The long bones are broad and crumpled (accordion-like) as in group A. In those infants who survive the newborn period, a typical broad bone appearance develops in the first few weeks of life. The accumulation of rib fractures with callus formation produces an X–ray appearance indistinguishable from that of some babies with severe OI Type III.

Subgroup C This syndrome is extremely rare. All babies have been very small for gestational age and were stillborn or died in the newborn period (Sillence et al 1984, Thompson et al 1987).

Skeletal radiographs show slender, not so uniformly beaded ribs, slender long bones with fractures, twisting of the shafts of the femora and angulation deformities. There is extreme demineralisation of the skull and face.

Differential diagnosis 1. OI with microcephaly and cataracts. This autosomal recessive syndrome has clinical and radiographic features similar to OI Type II but all affected have had microcephaly and cataracts (Buyse & Bull 1978).

2. OI Type III. The distinction between these two syndromes is based on the clinical and radiographic findings at the time of birth. Infants with OI Type II, B subgroup, who survive to several months of age, will show skeletal radiographic findings indistinguishable from OI Type III.

Treatment Therapeutic intervention will not usually lead to survival. An occasional infant with milder subgroup B disease will survive and requires intensive management (see OI Type III).

Genetic counselling and prenatal diagnosis Where possible, collagen biochemical studies of cultured skin fibroblasts should be performed on all new cases to determine whether the mutation is heterozygous and whether collagen overmodification is present.

Byers et al (1988) have studied 65 complete families of OI Type II and found an empiric recurrence risk of approximately 6%. This is probably due to the rarer recessive form as well as germinal mosaicism for dominant mutations, although most cases of OI Type II are caused by fresh constitutional dominant mutations. Recurrence risks otherwise recommended for OI Type II are as follows; where the proband falls into subgroup A 1%; subgroup B 7%; and subgroup C 25% (Thompson et al 1987). On the other hand, parental consanguinity and recurrence in siblings, e.g. in some instances of subgroup B, is highly suggestive of autosomal recessive inheritance.

Serial ultrasound studies from the fourth to fifth gestational month are indicated in all future pregnancies, with a high likelihood of diagnosis of OI Type II based on limb shortening, fractures, or polyhydramnios (Shapiro et al 1982, Elejalde & Elejalde 1983).

In families with two or more previously affected offspring (gonadal mosaicism) and biochemically proven collagen over-modificiation, collagen synthesis can be studied in a chorion villus specimen taken at 10 weeks' gestation.

Osteogenesis imperfecta Type II

This syndrome is characterised by autosomal recessive inheritance of usually non-lethal OI with severe bone fragility leading to progressive deformity of the skeleton and usually light blue or normal sclerae (Sillence et al 1986) (Fig. 57.3).

Inheritance Recurrence in siblings and parental consanguinity point to autosomal recessive inheritance (Sillence et al 1986). The existence of families with

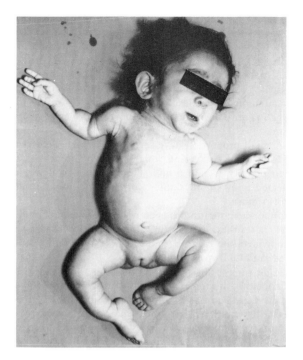

Fig. 57.3 Osteogenesis imperfecta Type III. Newborn with mild shortening and bowing deformities of the limbs.

childhood. While the sclerae may be blue at birth, observation of several patients with this syndrome suggests that the sclerae become progressively less blue with age. All patients have poor longitudinal growth and fall well below the third percentile in height for age and sex. Progressive kyphoscoliosis develops during childhood and progresses into adolescence. Hearing impairment has not been reported in children with this syndrome but it would not be surprising, in view of the severe osteopenia and liability to fractures, if there was significant involvement of the ossicular chain leading to hearing defect in some cases. The majority of patients do not have opalescent dentin.

At birth, there is usually over-modelling of the shafts of the long bones with widening of the femoral metaphyses and angulation of the tibiae. There is generalised osteopenia and multiple fractures. Within weeks to months, in the majority of infants, the shafts of the long bones show under-modelling producing a 'broad-bone' appearance. From several years of age, progressive disruption and repair of osseous trabeculae in the metaphyses may produce a 'popcorn' appearance similar to that seen in various forms of enchondromatosis. The ribs are thin, osteopenic and progressively crowded as platyspondyly increases. The skull shows multiple Wormian bones although these may not be evident until several weeks to months of age.

In the past approximately one third of the patients survived long term, reflecting not only the severity of the disorder but also the heterogeneity within the group. Death usually results from the complications of severe bone fragility, skeletal deformity including kyphoscoliosis, pulmonary hypertension and cardiac failure.

Differential diagnosis As these are severely affected infants, phenotypic features alone at birth do not allow distinction from other severely affected infants with OI Type I or Type IV. There is an overlap with infants with OI Type II. Family history, natural history of skeletal radiographic abnormalities and/or the demonstration of homozygosity for a biochemical defect are the features by which these patients may be distinguished from other cases with a progressively deforming phenotype with normal sclerae.

There are a number of rare private syndromes which may be distinguished from OI Type III (Sillence 1988).

Treatment Intensive rehabilitation and orthopaedic care should be instituted to prevent progressive deformity and provide for as normal a development as possible. Intramedullary rodding may improve mobility and prevent fractures and is also used to correct deformity. Various orthoses can be provided or designed by rehabilitation programmes. These improve mobility and normalize activities of daily living.

varying severity from newborn lethal OI (but distinct from OI Type II) to moderately severe OI compatible with childhood survival suggests that these cases may be genetically and biochemically heterogeneous.

Pathogenesis In one well documented case of OI Type III born to normal but consanguineous parents, the collagen gene mutation, a 4-nucleotide frameshift, alters the pro alpha (2) I chains which are not incorporated into the collagen triple helix. The collagen present in tissues such as bone and skin is composed of alpha (1) I trimers (Nicholls et al 1984). Studies with Type I collagen probes (COLIA 1 and COLIA 2) in several pedigrees of OI Type III exclude both the alpha (1) I and alpha (2) I collagen genes as the disease locus. Thus, there is a possibility that other loci concerned with collagen modification and secretion may be responsible for OI Type III in some families (Nicholls et al 1987).

Natural history These individuals have newborn or infant presentation with severe bone fragility and multiple fractures leading to progressive deformity of the skeleton. They are generally born at or near term and have normal birth weight and often normal birth length, although this may be reduced because of deformities of the lower limbs at birth. Fractures are present in the majority of cases at birth and occur frequently during

Osteogenesis imperfecta Type IV

This syndrome is characterized by osteoporosis leading to bone fragility without the characteristic features of the OI Type I syndrome (Sillence et al 1979a, Paterson et al 1983) (Fig. 57.4).

Inheritance Inheritance is autosomal dominant. As in OI Type I, families are observed with normal teeth (OI4) and with opalescent dentin (OI4.DI).

Pathogenesis Linkage studies with COLIA 1 and COLIA 2 probes have demonstrated that OI Type IV is linked to COLIA 2 and thus usually results from mutation affecting the pro alpha (2) I collagen chain. In one family a point mutation at the codon for the glycine position 1012 in the pro alpha (2) I chain changes the glycine to an arginine residue (Wenstrup et al 1987). This and similar mutations reduce collagen triple helix formation and stability and thus presumably reduce the amount of collagen available for bone formation.

Natural history The sclerae may be bluish at birth but become progressively less blue as the patient matures. All adolescents or adults have normal sclerae (Paterson et al 1983). These individuals have variable ages of onset of fractures which may be present at birth (approximately

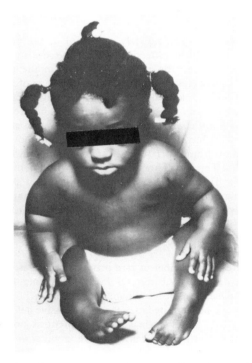

Fig. 57.4 Osteogenesis imperfecta Type IV. Patient aged 2 years (not walking) with mild bowing of the lower limbs and sclerae of normal hue; her father is similarly affected.

25%) or may not occur until adult life. Significant bowing of the lower limbs has been present at birth as the only feature of this syndrome. Some patients improve with age, in that bowing lessens. Just as in OI Type I, these patients appeared to show a spontaneous improvement at the time of puberty and very few fractures are encountered in adolescents and adults. However, the large majority of patients have short stature of postnatal onset.

A small proportion have severe progressive deformity of long bones and spine which is out of proportion to their severity as judged by fracture frequency. Those so affected show more skull deformity and more severe short stature.

Opalescent dentin has been observed in some families and not others, suggesting OI Type IV should be subdivided into two subgroups: OI Type IV with normal teeth and OI Type IV with DI.

Radiographically, this group is defined by generalised osteopenia. Although multiple fractures may be observed in the skeleton at birth and throughout life, as a group these patients have less osteopenia and fractures than infants with recessive varieties of osteogenesis imperfecta. The skull shows multiple Wormian bones.

Differential diagnosis 1. Juvenile idiopathic osteoporosis. This may be distinguished with difficulty from mildly affected cases of OI Type IV (with normal teeth) although in the former, the onset of fractures is usually late in the first decade and there is never a family history (Brenton & Dent 1976).

2. Osteoporosis with pseudogliomatous blindness (see below).

3. Other Mendelian disorders and inborn errors of metabolism characterised by osteopenia. Winchester, Cockayne and Rothmund-Thompson syndromes, and Fanconi pancytopenia are all autosomal recessive syndromes in which osteopenia may be found. Osteopenia is also a frequently recognised finding in homocystinuria, methylmalonic acidaemia, dibasic amino-aciduria, prolidase deficiency, glycogen storage disease type I, Menkes syndrome and Lowe oculo-cerebro-renal syndrome.

Treatment Treatment is as for OI Type I if mild, or OI Type III if severe.

Genetic counselling and prenatal diagnosis For the offspring of an affected parent by normal mating, there is a 50% chance of affected offspring. Ultrasound and radiographic prenatal diagnosis is unlikely to be definitive, although fractures and leg bowing may be detected in the third trimester.

Prenatal prediction of OI Type IV has been achieved by linkage analysis with COLIA 2 polymorphisms and could be offered in suitable families where linkage is demonstrated (Tsipouras et al 1987).

Osteoporosis – pseudoglioma syndrome

This rare syndrome is characterised by generalised osteoporosis leading to fractures and deformity of long bones and spine and various abnormalities of the anterior and middle segments of the eye (Saraux et al 1967, Frontali et al 1985).

The eye findings include microphthalmia, microcornea, corneal opacities, shallow anterior chamber, iris atrophy and lens opacity. The changes in the eye, initially characterised as pseudotumours, lead on towards phthisis bulbi in infancy. Mental retardation, hypotonia and joint hyperextensibility are variable manifestations.

DISORDERS WITH INCREASED BONE VOLUME OR DENSITY

Over 20 disorders are known with generalised or localised increase in the density or size of the skeleton or individual skeletal elements.

Osteopetrosis

Several forms have been described with an overlapping spectrum of clinical and radiographic features. Cases which present soon after birth often have a progressive course leading to death at an early age and are described as *osteopetrosis with precocious manifestations*. Cases with dominant inheritance or recessive inheritance of a usually milder disorder are designated *osteopetrosis with delayed manifestations*, sometimes known as osteopetrosis tarda or Albers-Schonberg disease.

Osteopetrosis with precocious manifestations

The precocious form of the disease is most frequently discovered during the first few months of life, but may present as failure to thrive, malignant hypocalcaemia, or anaemia with thrombocytopenia, or even because of severe, perhaps overwhelming infection. Rarely, fractures lead to medical attention.

Inheritance. Inheritance is generally autosomal recessive, although autosomal dominant inheritance of some cases with newborn presentation is possible.

Pathogenesis. While the exact defect is unknown, it is most likely that osteopetrosis results from either a defect in the maturation of osteoclasts from precursors or a metabolic defect in osteoclasts leading to impairment of bone resorption. Four osteopetrotic disorders have been described in the mouse: grey-lethal (gl), microphthalmic (mi), osteosclerotic (oc) and osteopetrotic (op). Three forms are known in the rat: incisor absent (ia), osteopetrotic (op) and toothless (tl). Which one, if any, is a model for human osteopetrosis is not known. However, the observation that mammalian osteopetrosis can be cured by parabiosis has led to successful cures with bone marrow transplantation in laboratory animals and in the human disorder (Marks & Walker 1976, Coccia et al 1980). Furthermore, some animal osteopetrosis, but not others, can be cured by infusion of monocyte (macrophage) precursors or immunocompetent cells. Milhaud and Labat (1978) have argued that the immunodeficiency observed in the 'op' rat is primary. This has certain parallels to human osteopetrosis, where Reeves et al (1979) have observed defective monocyte intracellular bacterial killing in human newborn osteopetrosis.

Natural history. Generalised hyperostosis may be recognised at birth but usually develops rapidly following birth and leads to crowding of the marrow cavity with anaemia and extramedullary haemopoiesis, hepatosplenomegaly and thrombocytopenia leading to purpura and ecchymosis. Anaemia appears to result not from inadequate erythropoiesis but rather from excessive extracorpuscular haemolysis. A defect in macrophage killing of bacteria may account for a tendency to severe and overwhelming infection. Progressive encroachment on the optic foramina may lead to optic atrophy and blindness. In some cases, evidence of optic nerve encroachment is present at birth. Hypocalcaemia is not an uncommon finding, and serum phosphorus may also be low. Elevated serum alkaline phosphatase is a constant finding. Radiologically, the diagnostic findings are a generalised increase in bone density combined with defective metaphyseal modelling and a 'bone-in-bone' appearance, most marked in the vertebral bodies. Diffuse hyperostosis leads to loss of demarcation of the cortex and medullary cavities. Irregular condensation of bone at the metaphyses may produce the appearance of parallel plates of dense bone at the ends of the long bones. The skull shows a dense base with normal to increased density of the vault and markedly increased density in the orbital margins.

Treatment. Treatment is aimed at decreasing or arresting progressive hyperostosis, correcting anaemia and thrombocytopenia, general supportive measures including prompt and vigorous treatment of infections and minimising neurological complications, particularly progressive optic atrophy due to encroachment of the optic foramina. A regimen of oral cellulose phosphate, prednisone and low calcium diet has been effective in some patients (Yu et al 1971). The prednisone arrests the progress of the anaemia. However, this regimen is rarely helpful in malignant osteopetrosis. Heparin therapy and parathormone to produce skeletal demineralisation have not produced a remission in patients with osteopetrosis. Neurosurgical unroofing of the optic foramina has been tried in some patients, but the results are difficult to interpret because of the complexities of such surgery and because optic atrophy is often established by the time the disorder is recognised and surgical intervention is attempted. Bone marrow transplantation of appropriately HLA-matched donor marrow has been reported to be curative in several patients, but the long-term success remains to be judged (Ballet et al 1977, Coccia et al 1980 Fischer et al 1986). Generally, the prognosis for survival is poor and death from complications such as anaemia, bleeding or overwhelming infection is not uncommon in the first few months or years.

Genetic counselling and prenatal diagnosis. For normal parents with one or more infants with congenital osteopetrosis, the risk approximates 25% for a subsequently affected infant.

Radiographic prenatal diagnosis has been generally unsuccessful in detecting increased bone density during the second trimester (Lachman & Hall 1979).

Osteopetrosis with later onset

Apart from cases with congenital or infantile presentation of osteopetrosis, there are a group of patients in whom the onset of the disease is recognised later (osteopetrosis tarda or Albers-Schonberg disease). The prevalence is 1/18 000 in Denmark (Bollerslev 1987).

Inheritance. In the majority of cases, this milder presentation of osteopetrosis is inherited as an autosomal dominant trait, although families with autosomal recessive inheritance have been reported.

Natural history. Patients may present in childhood, adolescence or young adult life because of fracture (10%), mild craniofacial disproportion, mild anaemia, complications arising from neurological involvement or osteitis with osteonecrosis, usually of the mandible. On the other hand, increased bone density may be discovered incidentally on routine radiological study for some non-skeletal problem (Graham et al 1973). Biochemically there is normal serum calcium, parathormone and calcitonin. Serum acid and alkaline phosphatases may be elevated, the latter with healing fractures.

Skeletal radiographs show generalised increased density of cortical bone with defective metaphyseal modelling of the long bones resulting in a club-shaped appearance. There is longitudinal and transverse osteodense striation at the ends of the long bones in over half the patients. The vertebral column shows alternating hyperlucent and very dense bands. The base of the skull is usually dense and thickened, but the face and vault are generally less severely involved.

Differential diagnosis

1. Pycnodysostosis. This is an autosomal recessive trait

characterised by generalised hyperostosis and short stature with onset at around 3 years of age. Distal acro-osteolysis and the radiographic pattern of involvement of the skeleton differ from osteopetrosis tarda (see below).

2. Dysosteosclerosis. In this disorder there is major involvement of the spine with flattening of the vertebrae (see below).

Treatment. Therapy should be directed at recognition and treatment of complications. Transfusion may be required for anaemia, and splenectomy may be useful in some patients. Frequent testing of visual field and acuity, and baseline radiographs of optic foramina, should be carried out. On the whole, treatment with low-calcium diet, parathormone, calcium chelating agents, corticosteroids and heparin therapy has not shown clear therapeutic advantages.

Pycnodysostosis

This is a rare generalised hyperostotic bone disease recognised from infancy by short limbs, short stature, characteristic facies and wide anterior fontanelle (Sugiura et al 1974) (Fig. 57.5).

Inheritance. This disorder is inherited as an autosomal recessive trait.

Natural history. The skull, which appears large, with frontal and occipital bossing and a wide anterior fontanelle, may bring the patient to attention. The hands and feet are short and broad and the nails may be deformed and brittle. The sclerae are often blue, and this, in combination with a tendency to fractures, may lead to confusion with osteogenesis imperfecta.

Radiographically, there is generalised increase in bone density without long bone or metaphyseal striation. The hands characteristically show hypoplasia or aplasia of the distal phalanges. The characteristic findings in the skull are wide sutures and Wormian bones, and in the face a small mandible with an obtuse mandibular angle.

Genetic counselling. For normal parents there is a 25% risk for further affected offspring. Ultrasound and radiographic prenatal diagnosis is not feasible.

Dysosteosclerosis

This is a rare autosomal recessive skeletal dysplasia characterised by generalised increase in bone density and short stature of postnatal onset. It is differentiated from osteopetrosis and pycnodysostosis by radiological evidence of platyspondyly with superior and inferior irregularity of vertebral ossification and clinical findings of a high incidence of developmental defects of the teeth with delayed eruption of primary dentition, severe hypodontia and early loss of the teeth (Houston et al 1978). Second-

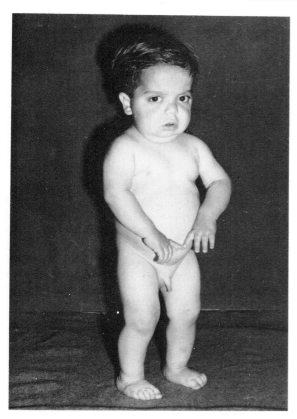

Fig. 57.5 Pycnodysostosis. Boy aged 2 years showing short limbs, short stature, large cranium and small chin (courtesy of Dr J S Yu, Royal Alexandra Hospital for Children, Camperdown, NSW, Australia).

ary dentition may fail to erupt. Otherwise, the complications, fractures, visual and hearing loss and recurrent infections of mandible and paranasal sinuses are very similar to those encountered in osteopetrosis.

Osteopoikilosis, osteopathia striata and melorheostosis

These three conditions are most commonly asymptomatic and are usually recognised during routine radiological study including skeletal films. Occasionally, patients are seen with both types of lesions.

In *osteopoikilosis*, numerous small osteo-dense round or oval foci are seen in the skeleton, most commonly in the epiphyses and carpal and tarsal centres. The disorder is inherited as an autosomal dominant trait and may be associated with joint pain in some 20% of cases and with skin lesions in an unknown proportion. These consist of slightly elevated whitish-yellow fibrocollagenous infiltra-

tions (dermatofibrosis lenticularis disseminata). There is an increased incidence of keloid formation.

In *osteopathia striata*, which is possibly also an autosomal dominant trait, linear regular bands of increased density are seen throughout the skeleton, radiating from metaphyses and with a fan-like array in the iliac wings. These should be distinguished from similar striations seen in osteopetrosis, which are associated with metaphyseal modelling defects, and transverse bands of osteodensity at the ends of the long bones. Typical changes of osteopathia striata are seen in the syndrome of focal dermal hypoplasia in which linear lesions consisting of dermal hypoplasia with herniation of the adipose tissue and skeletal defects of the limbs (hypoplasia, aplasia and syndactyly) occur.

In *melorheostosis*, irregular linear osteo-dense lesions are seen along the axis of the tubular bones. Single or multiple areas of skeleton maybe involved. No hereditary basis has been established but the pattern of lesions may be correlated with the sensory sclerotomes. It has been suggested that melorheostosis may be the late consequence of lesions of the sensory nerve supply to various skeletal elements (Murray & McCredie 1979). The lesions may be associated with shortening of certain bones leading to discrepancy in limb length, soft tissue contractures of the joints or palmar and plantar fasciae and intermittently painful swelling of affected joints. The radiological appearance of the osteo-dense lesions has been likened to candle wax flowing down the side of a candle. Management is directed at the orthopaedic complications.

CRANIOTUBULAR REMODELLING DISORDERS

This is a large group of disorders characterised by abnormal modelling as well as increased density of bone. A distinction has been drawn between the craniotubular dysplasias, e.g. craniodiaphyseal dysplasia, in which modelling abnormalities are prominent (Gorlin et al 1969) although there is also severe sclerosis of the skull, and the craniotubular hyperostoses, e.g. endosteal hyperostosis (Van Buchem), in which cranial and tubular bones are deformed by overgrowth of osseous tissue rather than by a defect in bone remodelling. This distinction is somewhat arbitrary as all these disorders result from excess bone deposition versus resorption with specifically different patterns of skeletal involvement. In essence, they are all disorders in which there is generally minimum involvement of the spine compared to osteopetrosis, pycnodysostosis and dysosteosclerosis, in which increased osteodensity is seen throughout the spine and the rest of the skeleton with minimal changes in the cranial vault.

In diaphyseal dysplasia (Camurati-Englemann), cranio-diaphyseal dysplasia, the craniometaphyseal dysplasias, frontometaphyseal dysplasia and pachydermoperiostosis, sclerosis in the region of optic foramina may lead to visual impairment, papilloedema and optic atrophy. Sclerotic narrowing of internal acoustic foramina and the middle ear may lead to various patterns of conductive or sensorineural hearing loss; encroachment on the facial foramina may lead to facial paresis and encroachment on the foramen magnum to long tract signs, hyperreflexia, weakness and even sudden death or paraplegia.

Diaphyseal dysplasia (Camurati-Englemann)

This is a rare craniotubular remodelling disorder (also known as progressive hereditary diaphyseal dysplasia) with significant neuromuscular involvement (Sparkes & Graham 1972).

Inheritance. Diaphyseal dysplasia is inherited as an autosomal dominant trait with variable penetrance and wide expressivity. There is considerable variation in the signs, symptoms and severity between affected individuals within the same family (Sparkes & Graham 1972).

Natural history. Symptoms usually begin between 4 and 10 years of age, but the onset of symptoms has been described as early as 3 months and as late as the sixth decade. Failure to thrive or gain weight, fatigability and abnormal gait are frequent presenting symptoms. Pain in the legs of progressively increasing severity may occur. The gait is characteristically wide-based and waddling, with reduced muscle mass and poor muscle tone. Flexion contractures may develop at the elbows and knees. Bow-leg or knock-knee deformity may be seen in the lower limbs, and the feet may be flat and pronated. Deep tendon reflexes in some cases have been hypoactive and in others hyperactive, with occasional ankle clonus. Increased lumbar lordosis and scoliosis may occur with variable degrees of back pain. Symptoms and signs of encroachment on cranial nerves may be present.

The radiographic features include symmetrical fusiform enlargement of the diaphyses of the long bones with normal epiphyses and metaphyses. In the diaphyses, there is enlargement of the cortex by endosteal and periosteal accretion of mottled new bone. The lesions are often first recognised centrally in the long bones and progress proximally and distally with gradual involvement of adjacent normal bone. In the skull there may be sclerosis of the frontal areas and base.

Serum calcium, phosphorus and serum alkaline phosphatase are characteristically normal. Muscle histology has been reported to show loss of individual muscle fibres with replacement by adipose tissue, atrophic muscle fibres, and slighly pyknotic sarcolemmal cell nuclei with hyalinisation and decrease in the prominence of cross-striations.

Treatment. Management of this condition should be aimed at maximising the mobility of the patient. Orthopaedic correction of deformity of lower limbs by appropriate osteotomy has been reported to help in the habilitation of these patients. There have been reports of good symptomatic response to low-dose steroid therapy (Allen et al 1970).

Craniodiaphyseal dysplasia

This is a rare craniotubular remodelling disorder characterised by massive hyperostosis and sclerosis of the skull and facial bones (Fig. 57.6) and hyperostosis and defective remodelling of the shafts of the tubular bones. The epiphyses and metaphyses are only mildly affected or spared. The early symptoms may be related to respiratory difficulty due to narrowing of the nasal passages (Gorlin et al 1969, Macpherson 1974).

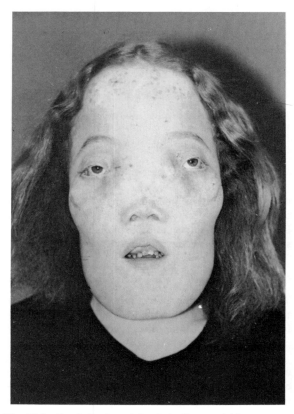

Fig. 57.6 Craniodiaphyseal dysplasia. Boy aged 13 years showing massive hyperostosis of cranium, facial bones and mandible (leontiasis ossea).

Inheritance. This disorder is inherited as an autosomal recessive trait.

Natural history. Flattening of the nasal root may be noted at birth, and symptoms may occur as early as 3 months of age. Hyperostosis of the cranial and facial bones is progressive in the first years of life, and frank prominence of nasal and adjacent maxillary bones is usually recognised by 1–2 years of age. Symptoms and signs produced by encroachment on cranial foramina are marked.

Skeletal radiographs show massive hyperostosis of the cranial bones developing rapidly during infancy and completely obscuring the detailed structures. The spine, ribs, clavicles and scapulae appear hypermineralised but normal in shape. The metaphyses of the long bones are poorly modelled and there is loss of normal funnelisation and tubulation so that the long bones appear broad and undermodelled. These patients are often of normal to tall stature.

Serum calcium and phosphorus appear to be normal, but serum alkaline phosphatase is markedly increased.

Treatment. There is no effective medical or surgical treatment to prevent the progressive craniofacial hyperostosis and sclerosis and its complications. Special attention should be given to amelioration of hearing and visual impairment and to psychosocial counselling for affected children and their families with this cosmetically disfiguring disorder.

Endosteal hyperostosis and sclereosteosis

This is a group of disorders characterised by marked accretion of osseous tissue at the endosteal (inner) surface of bone, leading to narrowing of the medullary canal or obliteration of the medullary space.

A rare dominantly inherited variety (Worth type) is frequently associated with the presence of a torus palatinus. The torus is a prominent midline ridge of the hard palate in the mouth and is noted in 5% of the population as a normal variant (Worth & Wollin 1966). Endosteal hyperostosis predominates in the long bones but marked hyperostosis of the cranium and lower jaw may occur. This disorder does not always run a benign course and neurological involvement may occur (Perez-Vincente et al 1987). Serum alkaline phosphatase may be markedly elevated.

A recessively inherited variety of endosteal hyperostosis (Van Buchem disease) is characterised by progressive mandibular enlargement from childhood, and in adult life by signs and symptoms resulting from sclerotic encroachment on optic and acoustic foramina. Serum alkaline phosphatase is markedly elevated. Radiographically, there is marked thickening of the skull starting in the base and extending to the vault, and increased density of the mandible after puberty. There is increased density of the cortices of tubular bones with narrowing of the marrow cavity.

Sclereosteosis, also an autosomal recessive trait, is clinically and radiologically almost indistinguishable from Van Buchem disease. Sclereosteosis has been differentiated by a high frequency of hyperostosis in the nasal and facial bones, producing a broad, flat nasal bridge and ocular hypertelorism with minor hand malformations. The latter consist of cutaneous syndactyly, radial deviation of the second and third fingers and absent or hypoplastic nails (Beighton et al 1976). Family studies from South Africa suggest that endosteal hyperostosis (Van Buchem disease) and sclereosteosis may be the same entity (Cremin 1979, Beighton et al 1984).

Tubular stenosis (Caffey-Kenny)

This disorder is characterised by narrowing of the medullary cavity and myopia. In some patients, tetanic seizures due to hypocalcaemia in infancy occur (Kenny & Linarelli 1966, Caffey 1967, Lee 1983).

Inheritance. Tubular stenosis is inherited as an autosomal dominant trait.

Natural history. Medullary stenosis may be recognised at an incidental radiographic study or as part of the investigation of the infant with clinical manifestations of hypocalcaemia. Other clinical features include delayed closure of the anterior fontanelle and early onset myopia.

Radiographically there is widening of the diaphyseal cortex in the long bones and short tubular bones of the hands and feet, without overall widening of the diaphyses leading to reduction of the medullary cavity. Rarely, vertebrae, pelvis, carpals, tarsals and skull may show increased density.

Pachydermoperiostosis

This is an unusual condition characterised by progressive thickening of the skin and clubbing of the fingers with onset in adolescence. Radiographic findings are similar to those observed in hypertrophic (pulmonary) osteoarthropathy without evidence of primary pulmonary neoplastic lesions (Rimoin 1965).

Inheritance. Pachydermoperiostosis is inherited as an autosomal dominant trait.

Natural history. Those affected develop a massive appearance of the limbs, which may be disproportionately long, and thickening of the facial skin with seborrhoeic hyperplasia. Complaints of easy fatigability, joint pain and blepharitis are frequent.

The skeletal changes include cortical thickening and

sclerosis of the tubular bones, thickening of the calvaria and base of the skull, which may lead to conductive and/or sensory hearing loss, and narrowing of other intervertebral foramina resulting in neurological symptoms.

Frontometaphyseal dysplasia

This produces a clinically striking facial appearance with a pronounced supraorbital ridge resulting from a torus-like bony overgrowth of the supraorbital ridges of the frontal bones (Fig. 57.7).

Inheritance. The disorder is inherited as an X-linked dominant trait (Gorlin & Winter 1980).

Natural history. The prominent supraorbital ridge which extends across the entire frontal bone may be recognised at birth, although in some cases not till later. It is associated radiographically with poor development of the frontal and other paranasal sinuses and with mandibular hypoplasia. The pelvis shows an unusually abrupt flare. The metaphyses of all the long and short tubular bones are undermodelled. Hirsutism, obstructive uropathy, congenital stridor and conductive deafness have

been observed. Scoliosis with various alterations of the modelling of the tubular bones may be present (Fitzsimmons et al 1982).

Craniometaphyseal dysplasias

This may also be a genetically heterogeneous group of disorders. Both autosomal dominant (Fig. 57.8) and recessive inheritance have been described with overlap in the clinical and radiographic findings between both groups of patients (Gorlin et al 1969, Carnevale et al 1983). The recessive variety is very rare.

Natural history. There is wide variability in the onset of symptoms and signs in families showing a dominant mode of inheritance, but some cases have been recognised in infancy. Clinically, both dominant and recessively inherited varieties show progressive facial dysmorphology with broad osseous prominence of the nasal root extending across the zygoma (Fig. 57.8). Difficulty with breathing and encroachment on the nasal passages may be recognised in the first 6 months of life. Signs and symptoms of sclerotic encroachment on cranial foramina vary in severity from patient to patient but may be unusually severe.

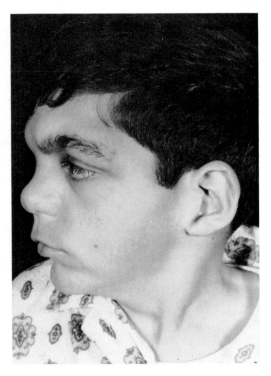

Fig. 57.7 Frontometaphyseal dysplasia. Boy aged 12 years showing torus-like hyperostosis of frontal bone extending across the cranium (from Danks et al, by permission of the publishers, American Journal of Diseases of Children 123: 254–258).

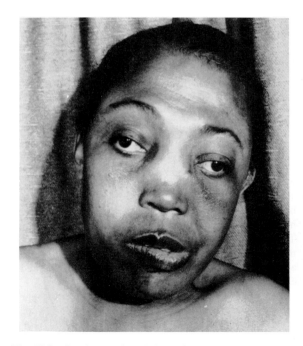

Fig. 57.8 Craniometaphyseal dysplasia (autosomal dominant) in a woman aged 42 showing hyperostosis of nasal process of frontal bone and adjacent maxilla and mandible (from Rimoin et al (1969) by permission of the publishers, Birth Defects Original Article Series 5(4): 96–104).

The essential radiological features are hyperostosis of the skull, nasal and maxillary bones extending bilaterally across the zygoma with failure of pneumatisation of the paranasal sinuses and mastoids, and hyperostosis of the mandible. The long bones show flaring and decreased density of the metaphyses (Ehrlenmeyer flask deformity) due to a failure of remodelling of the metaphyses during growth. Hyperostosis and sclerosis of the mandible develops but is less severe than in craniodiaphyseal dysplasia. Promising results have recently been reported in craniometaphyseal dysplasia with the use of high doses of calcitonin and calcitriol (Key et al 1988, Fanconi et al 1988, Cole & Cohen 1988).

Treatment. As in craniodiaphyseal dysplasia, the cosmetic and neurological problems in craniometaphyseal dysplasia may be considerable. Plastic surgery for the facial hyperostosis has been successfully performed.

Osteodysplasty (Melnick-Needles)

This disorder or group of disorders is characterised by 'abnormally shaped' bones.

Inheritance. Osteodysplasty is inherited as an autosomal dominant trait. Danks et al (1974) have described a severe 'precocious form' of osteodysplasty inherited as an autosomal recessive trait.

Natural history. The age at diagnosis is variable, and affected individuals usually present because of an abnormal gait with bowing of the extremities. Occasionally, dislocation of hips or delayed closure of the anterior fontanelle occurs. On the whole, these patients do not have short stature, and psychomotor development and adult height are normal. Facial appearance appears to be somewhat typical, with slight exophthalmos, protruding cheeks, a high, narrow forehead, prominent orbital rims, micrognathia and malaligned teeth. The lower thorax is narrow. There is incurving of the distal segments of the thumbs.

Radiographically, there is uneven thickening of the cortex of long bones, which have irregular contours and multiple constrictions producing a wavy border. The diaphyses are slightly curved and show metaphyseal modelling defects. Characteristically, there is coxa valga and dislocation of the hips is frequent. The ribs appear wavy, the pelvis is triangular and the iliac wings appear to be narrowed in the supra-acetabular portion.

DISORDERS OF MINERALISATION AND MINERAL METABOLISM

These disorders involve defective mineralisation, defective mineral metabolism or defective hormonal interactions with skeletal tissue during development.

Hyperphosphatasaemia with osteoectasia

In this disorder, progressive skeletal deformation is associated with marked elevation of alkaline phosphatase. As the clinical and radiological findings resemble Paget disease it has sometimes been known as juvenile Paget disease (Iancu et al 1978).

Inheritance. The disorder is inherited as an autosomal recessive trait.

Natural history. The disease usually has its onset between 2 and 3 years of age, when painful deformity of the extremities develops and leads to gait abnormalities and sometimes fractures. The clinical findings are similar to those of Paget disease in adults but are more generalised and symmetric in distribution. Short stature ultimately results. The skull is large, and radiographically the diploe is widened and there is loss of normal calvarial structure. Bony texture is variable with dense areas (showing a teased cotton-wool appearance) interspersed with lucent areas. Demineralisation is seen throughout the remainder of the skeleton. The long bones appear cylindrical, even fusiform, and deformed with the loss of normal metaphyseal modelling. Pseudocysts with a dense bony halo may be seen throughout the long bones.

Differential diagnosis

1. Marked elevation of serum alkaline phosphatase may be observed in a wide variety of disorders of density of cortical bones or metaphyseal remodelling. It is commonly observed with osteopetrosis, craniodiaphyseal dysplasia, and endosteal hyperostosis (Worth and Van Buchem types). However, the clinical and radiographic findings in osteoectasia are distinctive and unlike those in the foregoing conditions.

2. Infantile cortical hyperostosis (Caffey disease). This disorder is usually recognised in the first 3 months of life and is characterised by a febrile course with marked swelling of soft tissues over the face and jaws and progressive cortical thickening of the long and flat bones (Maroteaux 1979). The elevation of alkaline phosphatase is usually mild. Infantile cortical hyperostosis is characterised by repeated exacerbations with spontaneous regression after several years. Caffey disease is not familial. Corticosteroids have been demonstrated to be beneficial in relieving clinical symptoms during exacerbations.

Treatment: Clinical, radiographic and histopathologic amelioration of the skeletal lesions following treatment with human calcitonin has been reported (Woodhouse et al 1972, Whalen et al 1977).

Hypophosphatasia

This includes a number of conditions with overlapping phenotype but differing modes of inheritance characterised by bowing deformites of the skeleton of varying severity and a reduced serum alkaline phosphatase due to total absence of the bone/liver isozymes. There is also elevation of serum and urine phosphorylethanolamine (Rasmussen 1983).

Congenital lethal hypophosphatasia

Neonates with this disorder show disproportionately short limbs with bowing or angulation deformity. The skull vault is thin and membraneous. Radiographic studies show extremely poor ossification throughout the skeleton with thin ribs, hypoplastic vertebrae, demineralised facial bones and markedly reduced ossification of the skull vault. The metaphyses of the long bones are frayed and splayed, sometimes with a moth-eaten appearance (Currarino 1973).

Inheritance. The disorder is inherited as an autosomal recessive trait.

Pathogenesis. The alkaline phosphatase in chondroosseous tissue is important in the hydrolysis of phosphate esters to release phosphate ion for normal calcification. In congenital hypophosphatasia a deficiency in the production or stability of bone alkaline phosphatase enzyme leads to a deficiency in the availability of free phosphate necessary for calcification.

Natural history. In the most severe cases death occurs prenatally or in the newborn period due to respiratory distress. The serum alkaline phosphatase is low and the bone/liver isozyme measured in cultured fibroblasts is extemely low (Mulivor et al 1978).

Genetic counselling and prenatal diagnosis. There is a 25% recurrence risk for hypophosphatasia in sibs. Prenatal diagnosis can be achieved by measurement of the bone/liver isozyme in cultured amniotic cells (Mulivor et al 1978).

Hypophosphatasia tarda

Into this group fall patients with clinical, laboratory and radiographic evidence of hypophosphatasia which is of a milder degree (Rassmussen & Bartter 1978).

Inheritance. Both autosomal dominant and autosomal recessive modes of inheritance have been observed.

Natural history. Bowing of the legs may be recognised in early childhood. Premature craniosynostosis and premature loss of the teeth are also found. The serum alkaline phosphatase is reduced, and in both serum and urine there is elevation of phosphorylethanolamine.

Differential diagnosis. Pseudohypophosphatasia. This term was used by Scriver and Cameron (1969) to describe patients with clinical and radiographic findings of hypophosphatasia in the presence of a normal serum alkaline phosphatase but elevated urinary phosphorylethanolamine.

X-linked hypophosphataemic rickets

X-linked hypophosphataemic rickets (XLH) is recognised in infancy with bowing of the legs and radiographic evidence of rickets resistant to vitamin D therapy.

Inheritance. XLH is inherited as an X-linked dominant trait.

Pathogenesis. The discovery and investigation of the Hyp mouse, a rachitic mouse with vitamin D-resistant hypophosphataemia, has shed much light on the possible pathogenesis of human XLH rickets. Hyp is an X-linked trait in the mouse and therefore homology with human XLH follows (Ohno 1967). In the Hyp mouse it has been demonstrated that there is an intrinsic partial defect in the transport of phosphate across the renal brush border and epithelium of the small intestine (Tenenhouse et al 1978). Hypophosphataemia is the primary abnormality leading to the development of rickets. In human X-linked hypophosphataemic rickets, the renal phosphate handling is impaired, but opinions differ on whether there is impaired transport of phosphate at the intestinal level (Glorieux et al 1972). Some heterogeneity in phosphate transport would not be surprising, as there are at least four alleles in the mouse for the copper transport defect leading to mottled mice (Danks 1977).

Natural history. Abnormal vertical growth can be observed by 12 months and bow legs, leading to abnormal gait, are recognised in hemizygous males soon after. In heterozygous females the findings are much more variable. Some heterozygous females have only low serum phosphate while others demonstrate the full manifestations of the disease. While growth rate is consistently disturbed, the growth of children with XLH generally parallels the normal growth curves (Steendjik 1976). In some mildly affected individuals growth may accelerate at puberty and cross the third percentile. In others, the growth spurt of puberty may aggravate bowing of the legs.

Dentition may be late, and abnormal development of the maxillofacial region has been reported. The poor dental development may be associated with spontaneous dental abscesses. Deformities of the limbs are not limited to varus deformity. Valgus and sitting deformities may also develop.

In adults bowing of the legs and short stature may persist. In some patients evidence of active osteomalacia may be present. Overgrowth of bone at the site of muscle attachments may lead to joint limitation and various neurological compressive syndromes (Rasmussen & Anast 1983).

Differential diagnosis

1. Autosomal dominant hypophosphataemic bone disease (HBD). This can be distinguished from XLH by the absence of frank rachitic changes on skeletal X–ray in the presence of short stature with leg bowing and a low serum phosphorus (Scriver et al 1977). Clinical manifestations appear in late infancy. Leg bowing and short stature are less severe than in XLH, with comparable reduction of serum phosphorus. There is a similar selective impairment in renal tubular reabsorption of phosphorus but no abnormality in red cell membrane phosphorus transport (Scriver et al 1977).

2. Vitamin D-dependency rickets (VDD). This syndrome appears to be biochemically heterogeneous with two forms presently delineated

   a. Autosomal recessive VDD rickets. These patients have early infancy onset of hypocalcaemia, normal or low serum phosphorus, elevated serum alkaline phosphatase, generalised aminoaciduria and clinical and radiographic findings of severe rickets. Serum 25-hydroxy vitamin D is normal, but serum 1,25-dihydroxy vitamin D is below the limits of detection (Fraser et al 1973). The disorder presumably results from defective 1-α hydroxylation of 25-hydroxy vitamin D.

   b. Target organ resistance to 1,25-dihydroxy vitamin D. Brooke et al (1978) reported a 22-year-old Black patient with symptomatic osteomalacia, hypocalcaemia and hyperaminoaciduria from the age of 15 years. In this patient, plasma 25-hydroxy vitamin D was normal, but plasma 1,25-dihydroxy vitamin D was markedly increased. Osteomalacia in the face of elevated serum 1,25-dihydroxy vitamin D is thought to be due to impaired target organ responsiveness.

3. 'Steroid'-sensitive hypophosphataemic rickets. Dent (1976) has summarised the findings in a single patient with clinical and radiographic findings of hypophosphataemic rickets who appeared to respond to a small dose of cortisone and vitamin D.

4. Tumour rickets-delayed hypophosphataemic rickets of McCance. The onset of hypophosphataemia and rickets has been variable. McCance's (1947) patient had an unclassifiable tumour in the femur while Prader's case had a rib tumour identified as an osteoclastoma. Cure followed removal of the tumour. The cases have been reviewed by Salassa et al (1970).

Treatment. Oral supplementation with phosphate combined with vitamin D has demonstrated effectiveness in correcting hypophosphataemia, normalising growth and reducing bowing deformities of the lower limbs (Glorieux et al 1972). Scriver et al (1976) recommended an acidic oral phosphate supplement, as this is better tolerated. To be effective, phosphate must be given in five divided doses at 3–4 hours intervals throughout the day. Phosphate therapy alone leads to the development of secondary hyperparathyroidism (Glorieux et al 1972). Calcitriol (1,25-dihydroxy vitamin D_3) has been shown to be particularly effective in correcting the growth disorder in XLH (Chesney et al 1983) and is the vitamin D of choice in the management of XLH.

Genetic counselling. For XLH there is a 50% chance that a male child of an affected or carrier female will have hypophosphataemic rickets. Only a proportion of heterozygous females manifest the complete syndrome with short stature and leg deformities. All the daughters of affected males will be carriers or manifest the disorder.

Pseudohypoparathyroidism and related disorders

The clinical findings common to this group of disorders are disproportionate short stature with selective distal shortening of tubular bones, predominantly of metacarpals, but also of metatarsals and phalanges (Spiegel 1989). There is also a high frequency of mental retardation and ectopic, usually subcutaneous calcification (Nagant de Deuxchaisnes & Krane 1978).

In pseudohypoparathyroidism (PHP), the somatic abnormalities are associated with serum findings of hypoparathyroidism, i.e. low serum calcium and elevated serum phosphorus with resistance to the effects of circulating and exogeneous serum parathormone (PTH).

In pseudo-pseudohypoparathyroidism (Albright et al 1952) (PPHP), the somatic features of PHP occur in the presence of normal serum chemistries and normal end organ responsiveness to exogeneous PTH.

As PHP and PPHP are often both found in the same family, it is likely that they represent variability within the same dominant genetic disorder. Furthermore, physiological studies of parathormone-induced urinary cyclic AMP response suggest that this group of disorders is genetically heterogeneous (Nagant de Deuxchaisnes & Krane 1978).

Inheritance. While PHP appears to be genetically heterogeneous, the evidence suggests that in the majority the disorder is inherited as a dominant trait. In view of reported male-to-male transmission some forms of PHP and PPHP are likely to represent autosomal dominant inheritance, but many of these dominant cases may represent examples of type E brachydactyly (Mann et al 1962). The elevated female/male sex ratio of 2.1:1 observed in some studies (Spranger & Rohwedder 1965) must be explained by genetic heterogeneity with X–linked dominant inheritance, selection bias in favour of females or by the fact that the disease is more severe in females than males (Spranger & Rohwedder 1965). Mann et al (1962) have observed that males are not more severely affected than females, a fact which can be reconciled with autosomal rather than X–linked inheritance.

Cederbaum and Lippe (1973) have reported a family in which two sibs (a brother and sister) had classic PHP while both parents and grandparents appeared to be completely normal. This raises the possibility that there is an autosomal recessive form of PHP.

Drezner et al (1973) have described a patient who had normal serum phosphate and a subnormal phosphaturic response to exogeneous parathyroid extract but normal cyclic AMP response, presumably representing a further disorder, pseudohypoparathyroidism type II.

Pathogenesis. The demonstrable defect in serum and urinary cyclic AMP (c-AMP) generation by endogenous parathormone (PTH) suggest a defect in hormone binding at the PTH receptor in the pathway of generation of c-AMP (Spiegel 1989). Farfel et al (1980) have demonstrated, in five of 10 patients with PHP type I and in one patient with PHP type II, deficiency of a protein, the N protein which mediates between the PTH receptor and c-AMP generation. That five out of 10 patients representing one family did not show a defect in their assay system confirms the proposed genetic heterogeneity in pseudohypoparathyroidism.

Natural history. Symptomatic hypocalcaemia may be the presenting sign. Seizures, tetanic episodes and evidence of ectopic or intracranial calcification may also bring a child to attention. Mental retardation or a family history of short stature and mental retardation may be recorded. Affected individuals develop short stature with moderate obesity and dental anomalies. These consist of delayed eruption, enamel hypoplasia, dentin hypoplasia and teeth with short blunt roots.

Short digits arise from early closure of the epiphyses of the short tubular bones of the hands. The fourth and fifth digits are most often involved and the second least of all. The commonest phalanx affected is the distal first due to premature closure of its epiphysis. Cone-shaped epiphyses may be seen at the base of both first metacarpals.

Other skeletal anomalies are seen but less frequently. Radius curvus, cubitus valgus, coxa valga and vara and genu valgum and varum have been reported. Ectopic calcification usually appears in infancy and may be located in any site, but most commonly in the extremities around large joints.

Mental retardation is present in some 75% of cases with pseudohypoparathyroidism (PHP). The mean IQ is in the order of 60 (Smith 1982). Lenticular opacities have been reported in 44% of patients.

Complications

1. Diabetes mellitus. There are a number of reports of the coexistence of diabetes mellitus and PHP and of diabetes mellitus in the families of patients with PHP (Nagant de Deuxchaisnes & Krane 1978). Whether this is a true association or represents the segregation of a common trait (diabetes mellitus) in these cases is not established.
2. Hypothyroidism. This appears to have a real but rare association with PHP (Nagant de Deuxchaisnes & Krane 1978). The majority of cases with both features have primary hypothyroidism although secondary hypothyroidism with diminished TSH response to TRH has also been reported.

Differential diagnosis.

1. Causes of hypoparathyroidism and hypocalcaemia. These include both primary and secondary hypoparathyroid states and are excellently reviewed by Nagant de Deuxchaisnes and Krane (1978).
2. Syndromes of mental retardation, obesity, short stature and brachydactyly. These include Turner syndrome (XO gonadal dysgenesis), basal cell naevus syndrome, Gardner syndrome and type E brachydactyly (Halal et al 1986).

Treatment. The aim of treatment is to normalise serum calcium with supplementary dietary calcium and vitamin D. Treatment does not prevent the progression of lenticular opacities but may improve mental functioning. Additional calcium as lactate or gluconate can be added to achieve a blood calcium level of 2.12–2.37 mmol/l (8.5 to 9.5 mg/100ml). Calcitriol (1,25-dihydroxy vitamin D_3) is effective in the treatment of PHP with ready control of serum calcium.

REFERENCES

Albright F, Forbes A P, Henneman P H 1952 Pseudopseudohypoporathyroidism. Transactions of the Association of American Physicians 65: 337–350

Allen D I, Saunders A M, Northway W H, Williams G F, Schafer J A 1970 Corticosteroids in the treatment of Englemann's disease: progressive diaphyseal dysplasia. Pediatrics 46: 523

Ballet J J, Griscelli C, Coutris C, Milhaud G, Maroteaux P 1977 Bone-marrow transplantation in osteopetrosis. Lancet 2: 1137

Bateman J, Chan D, Walker I D, Rogers J G, Cole W G 1987 Lethal perinatal Osteogenesis Imperfecta due to the substitution of arginine for glycine at 391 of alpha I (1) chain of type I collagen. Journal of Biological Chemistry 262: 7021–7027

Beighton P 1988 International nomenclature of heritable

disorders of connective tissue. American Journal of Medical Genetics 29: 581–594

Beighton P, Durr L, Hamersma H 1976 The clinical features of sclerosteosis. A review of the manifestations in twenty-five affected individuals. Annals of Internal Medicine 84: 393–397

Beighton P, Barnard A, Hamersma H, van der Wouden A 1984 The syndromic status of sclerosteosis and van Buchem disease. Clinical Genetics 25: 175–181

Biering A, Iverson T 1955 Osteogenesis imperfecta associated with Ehlers-Danlos syndrome. Acta Paediatrica 44: 279–286

Bollerslev J 1987 Osteopetrosis. A genetic and epidemiologic study. Clinical Genetics 31: 86–90

Brenton D P, Dent C E 1976 Idiopathic juvenile osteoporosis. In: Bickel H, Stern J (eds) Inborn errors of calcium and bone metabolism. MTP Press, Lancaster, p 222–238

Brooke M H, Bell N H, Love L et al 1978 Vitamin D-dependent rickets type II: resistance of target organs to 1,25 dihydroxy vitamin D. New England Journal of Medicine 298: 996–999

Buyse M, Bull M 1978. A syndrome of osteogenesis imperfecta and cataracts. Birth Defects Original Article Series 14 (6B): 95–98

Byers P H, Bonadio J F 1985. The molecular basis of clinical heterogeneity in osteogenesis imperfecta. Mutations in type I collagen genes have different effects on collagen processing. In: Lloyd J K, Scriver C R (eds) Genetic and Metabolic Disease in Pediatrics Butterworths, London: p 56–90

Byers P H, Tsipouras P et al 1988. Perinatal lethal Osteogenesis Imperfecta (OI Type II): A biochemically heterogeneous disorder usually due to new mutations in the genes for Type I collagen. American Journal of Human Genetics 42(2): 237–248

Caffey J 1967 Congenital stenosis of medullary spaces in tubular bones and calvaria in two proportionate dwarfs, mother and son, coupled with transitory hypocalcemic tetany. American Journal of Roentgenology 100: 1–14

Carnevale A, Grether P, Del Castillo V, Takenaga Orzechowki A 1983 Autosomal dominant craniometaphyseal dysplasia. Clinical variability. Clinical Genetics 23: 17–22

Cederbaum S D, Lippe B M 1973 Probable autosomal inheritance in a family with Albright's hereditary osteodystrophy and an evaluation of the genetics of this disorder. American Journal of Human Genetics 25: 638–645

Cetta G, Ramirez F, Tsipouras P 1988 Third International Conference on Osteogenesis Imperfecta. Annals of the New York Academy of Sciences 543: 1–183

Chervenak F A et al 1982 Antenatal sonographic findings of Osteogenesis Imperfecta. American Journal of Obstetrics and Gynecology 143: 228–230

Chesney R W, Mazess R B, Rose P et al 1983 Long-term influence of calcitriol (1,25 dihydroxy vitamin D) and supplemental phosphate in X-linked hypophosphatemic rickets. Pediatrics 73: 559–567

Coccia P F, Krivitt W, Cervenka J et al 1980 Successful bone marrow transplantation for infantile malignant osteoporosis. New England Journal of Medicine 302: 701–708

Cole D E C, Cohen M M 1988. A new look at craniometaphyseal dysplasia. Journal of Pediatrics 112 (4): 577–578

Cremin B J 1979 Sclerosteosis in children. Pediatric Radiology 8: 173–177

Currarino G 1973 Hypophosphatasia. In: Kaufman H J (ed) Intrinsic Diseases of Bones S Karger, Basel p 469–494

Daentl D L, Townsend J L, Siegel R C et al 1978 Familial nephrosis, hydrocephalus, thin skin, blue sclerae syndrome: clinical structural and biochemical studies. Birth Defects Original Article Series 14(6B): 315–339

Danks D M 1977 Copper transport and utilisation in Menkes syndrome and in mottled mice. Inorganic Perspectives in Biology and Medicine 1: 73–100

Danks D M, Mayne V, Kozlowski K 1974 A precocious autosomal recessive type of osteodysplasty. Birth Defects Original Article Series 10(12): 124–127

Dent C 1976 Metabolic forms of rickets (and osteomalacia). In: Bickel H, Stern J (eds) Inborn Errors of Calcium and Bone Metabolism. MTP Press, St. Leonardsgate

Donnenfeld A E, Conradi K A, Roberts N S, Borns P F, Zackai E 1987 Melnick-Needles syndrome in males: a lethal multiple congenital anomalies syndrome. American Journal of Medical Genetics 27: 159–173

Drezner M, Neelon F A, Lebovitz H E 1973 Pseudohypoparathyroidism type II: a possible defect in the reception of the cyclic AMP signal. New England Journal of Medicine 289: 1056–1060

Eleialde B R, de Elejalde M M 1983 Prenatal diagnosis of perinatally lethal Osteogenesis Imperfecta. American Journal of Medical Genetics 14: 353–359

Falk C T, Schwartz R C, Ramirez F et al 1986 Use of the molecular haplotypes specific for the pro alpha 2(I) collagen gene in linkage analysis of the mild autosomal forms of Osteogenesis Imperfecta. American Journal of Human Genetics 38: 269–279

Fanconi S, Fischer J A et al 1988 Craniometaphyseal dysplasia with increased bone turnover and secondary hyperparathyroidism: Therapeutic effect of calcitonin. Journal of Pediatrics 112(4): 587–591

Farfel Z, Brickman A S, Kaslow H R, Brothers V M, Bourne H R 1980 Defect of receptor-cyclase coupling protein in pseudohypoparathyroidism. New England Journal of Medicine 303: 237–242

Fischer A, Griscelli G, Friedrich W et al 1986 Bone marrow transplantation for immunodeficiencies and osteoporosis. European Survey 1968–1985 Lancet 2 (2515): 1080–1084

Fitzsimmons J S, Fitzsimmons E M, Barrow M, Gilbert G B 1982 Fronto-metaphyseal dysplasia. Further delineation of the clinical syndrome. Clinical Genetics 22: 195–205

Fraser D, Kooh S W, Kind H P, Holick M F, Tanaka Y, De Luca H F 1973 Pathogenesis of hereditary vitamin D-dependent rickets. An inborn error of vitamin D metabolism involving defective conversion of 25-hydroxy vitamin D to 1α 25-dihydroxy vitamin D. New England Journal of Medicine 289: 817–822

Frontali M, Stomeo C, Dallapiccola B 1985 Osteoporosis — Pseudoglioma syndrome: report of three affected sibs and an overview. American Journal of Medical Genetics 22: 35–47

Glorieux F H, Scriver C R, Reade T M, Goldman H, Roseborough A 1972 Use of phosphate and vitamin D to prevent dwarfism and rickets in X-linked hypophosphatemia. New England Journal of Medicine 287: 481–487

Gorlin R J, Winter R B 1980 Fronto metaphyseal dysplasia - evidence for X-linked inheritance. American Journal of Medical Genetics 5: 81–84

Gorlin R J, Spranger J, Koszalka M F 1969 Genetic craniotubular bone dysplasias and hyperostoses, a critical analysis. Birth Defects Original Article Series 5: 79–95

Graham C B, Rudhe U, Eklof O 1973 Osteopetrosis. In: Kaufman H J (ed) Intrinsic Diseases of Bones Progress in Pediatric Radiology, vol 4. S Karger, Basel, p 375–402

Greenfield G, Romano A, Stein R, Goodman R M 1973 Blue sclerae and keratoconus: key features of a distinct heritable disorder of connective tissue. Clinical Genetics 4: 8–16

Halal F, Van Dup C, Lord J 1986 Differential diagnosis in young women with oligomenorrhoea and the pseudohypoparathyroidism variant of Albright's Hereditary Osteodystrophy. American Journal of Medical Genetics 21: 551–568

Houston C S, Gerrard J W, Ives E J 1978 Dysosteosclerosis. American Journal of Roentgenology 130: 988–991

Iancu T C, Almagor G, Friedman E, Hardoff R, Front D 1978 Chronic familial hyperphosphatasemia. Radiology 129: 669–676

Kenny F M, Linarelli L 1966 Dwarfism and cortical thickening of tubular bones. Transient hypocalcemia in a mother and son. American Journal of Diseases of Children 3: 201–207

Key L L, Volberg F, Baron R, Anast C S 1988 Treatment of craniometaphyseal dysplasia with calcitriol. Journal of Pediatrics 112(4): 583–587

Lachman R, Hall J G 1979 The radiographic prenatal diagnosis of the generalised bone dysplasias and other skeletal abnormalities. Birth Defects 15 (5A): 3–24

Lee W K, Vargas A, Barnes J, Root A W 1983 The Kenny-Caffey syndrome: growth retardation and hypocalcemia in a young boy. American Journal of Medical Genetics 14: 773–782

Levin L S, Brady J M, Melnick M 1980 Scanning electronmicroscopy of teeth in dominant osteogenesis imperfecta. Support for genetic heterogeneity. American Journal of Medical Genetics 5: 189–199

McCance R A 1947 Osteomalacia with Looser's nodes (Milkman's syndrome) due to a raised resistance to vitamin D acquired about the age of 15 years. Quarterly Journal of Medicine 16: 33–46

Macpherson R I 1974 Craniodiaphyseal dysplasia, a disease or group of diseases? Journal of the Canadian Association of Radiologists 25: 22–23

Mann J B, Alterman S, Hill A G 1962 Albright's hereditary osteodystrophy comprising pseudohypoparathyroidism and pseudo-pseudohypoparathyroidism, with a report of two cases representing the complete syndrome occurring in successive generations. Annals of Internal Medicine 56: 315–342

Marks S S, Walker D G 1976 Mammalian osteopetrosis - a model for studying cellular and humoral factors in bone resorption. In: Bourne G H (ed) The Biochemistry and Physiology of Bone, vol 4, 2nd edn. Academic Press, New York

Maroteaux P 1979 Bone diseases of children. J B Lippincott, Philadelphia

Melnick J C 1982 Osteodysplasty (Melnick and Needles syndrome). Progress in Clinical and Biological Research 104: 133–137

Milhaud G, Labat M L 1978 Thymus and osteoporosis. Clinical Orthopaedics 135: 260–271

Mulivor R A, Mennuti M, Zackai E H, Harris H 1978 Prenatal diagnosis of hypophosphatasia: genetic, biochemical and clinical studies. American Journal of Human Genetics 30: 271–282

Murray R O, McCredie J 1979 Melorheostosis and the sclerotomes: a radiological correlation. Skeletal Radiology 4: 57–71

Nagant de Deuxchaisnes C, Krane S M 1978 In: Avioli L V, Krane S M (eds) Metabolic Bone Disease, vol II. Academic Press, New York

Neuhauser G, Kaveggia E G, Opitz U M 1976 Autosomal recessive syndrome of pseudogliomatous blindness, osteoporosis and mild mental retardation. Clinical Genetics 9: 324–332

Nicholls A C, Osse G, Schloon H G et al 1984 The clinical features of homozygous $\alpha1(I)$ collagen deficient Osteogenesis Imperfecta. Journal of Medical Genetics 21: 257–262

Nicholls A C, Renouf D, Porter S, Pope F M 1987 Molecular abnormalities in Osteogenesis Imperfecta. Proceedings of IIIrd International Conference on Osteogenesis Imperfecta 15A

Ohno S 1967 Sex chromosomes and sex linked genes. Springer-Verlag, New York

Paterson C R, McAllion S, Miller R, 1983 Heterogeneity in Osteogenesis Imperfecta type I. Journal of Medical Genetics 20: 203–205

Paterson C, McAllion S, Miller R 1983 Osteogenesis Imperfecta with dominant inheritance and normal sclerae. Journal of Bone & Joint Surgery 65B: 35–39

Peres-Vincente J A, Rodrigues de Castro E, Lafuente J, Mateo M M, Gimenez-Roldan S 1987 Autosomal dominant endosteal hyperostosis. Report of a Spanish family with neurological involvement. Clinical Genetics 31: 161–169

Rasmussen H 1983 Hypophosphatasia. In: Stanbury J B, Wyngaarden J B, Frederickson D S, Goldstein J L, Brown M S (eds) The Metabolic Basis of Inherited Disease, 5th edn. McGraw-Hill, New York p 1497–1507

Rasmussen H, Anast C 1983 Familial hypophosphatemic rickets and Vitamin D-dependent rickets. In: Stanbury J B, Wyngaarden J B, Frederickson D S, Goldstein J L, Brown M S (eds) The Metabolic Basis of Inherited Disease, 5th edn. McGraw-Hill, New York, p 1743–1773

Rasmussen H, Bartter F C 1978 Hypophosphatasia. In: Stanbury J B, Wyngaarden J B, Frederickson DS (eds) The metabolic basis of inherited disease, 4th edn. McGraw Hill, New York, p 1340

Reeves J D, August C S, Humbert J R, Weston W L 1979 Host defences in infantile osteopetrosis. Pediatrics 64: 202–205

Riedner E D, Levin L S, Holiday M J 1980 Hearing patterns in dominant Osteogenesis Imperfecta. Archives of Otolaryngology 606: 737–740

Rimoin D L 1965 Pachydermoperiostosis (idiopathic clubbing and periostosis). Genetic and physiologic considerations. New England Journal of Medicine 272: 923–931

Saint-Martin J, Peborde J, Dupont H, Beguere A, Labes A 1979 Malformations osseuses complexes d'evolution lethale. Archives Francaises de Pediatrie 36: 188–193

Salassa R M, Jowsey J, Arnaud C D 1970 Hypophosphatemic osteomalacia associated with 'non-endocrine' tumours. New England Journal of Medicine 283: 65–70

Saraux H, Frezal J, Roy C, Avon J J, Hyat B, Lamy M 1967 Pseudo-gliome et fragilite osseuse hereditaire a transmission autosomal recessive. Annales d'oculaire (Paris) 200: 1241–1252

Scriver C R, Cameron P 1969 Pseudohypophosphatasia. New England Journal of Medicine 281: 604

Scriver C R, Glorieux F H, Reade T M, Tenenhouse H S 1976 X-linked hypophosphatemia and autosomal recessive Vitamin D dependency: models for the resolution of Vitamin D refractory rickets. In: Bickel H, Stern J (eds) Inborn errors of calcium and bone metabolism. MTP Press, St Leonardsgate

Scriver C R, MacDonald W, Reade I, Glorieux F H, Nogrady B 1977 Hypophosphatemic non-rachitic bone disease: an entity distinct from X-linked hypophosphatemia in the renal defect, bone involvement and inheritance. American Journal of Medical Genetics 1: 101–117

Shapiro J E, Phillips J A, Byers P H et al 1982 Prenatal diagnosis of lethal perinatal osteogenesis imperfecta (01 type II). Journal of Pediatrics 100: 127–134

Sillence D O 1988 Osteogenesis Imperfecta. Nosology and Genetics. Annals of the New York Academy of Sciences 543: 1–15

Sillence D O, Senn A S, Dank D M 1979a Genetic heterogeneity in Osteogenesis Imperfecta. Journal of Medical Genetics 16: 101–116

Sillence D O, Rimoin D L, Danks D M 1979b Clinical variability in Osteogenesis Imperfecta – Variable expressivity or genetic heterogeneity. Birth Defects Original Article Series 15 (5B): 113–129

Sillence D O, Barlow K K, Garber A P et al 1984 Osteogenesis Imperfecta type II. Delineation of the phenotype with reference to genetic heterogeneity, American Journal of Medical Genetics 17: 407–423

Sillence D O, Barlow K K, Cole W G 1986 Osteogenesis Imperfecta type III. Delineation of the phenotype with reference to genetic heterogeneity. American Journal of Medical Genetics 23: 821–832

Smith D 1982 Recognizable patterns of human malformation, 3rd edn. W B Saunders, Philadelphia

Sparkes R S, Graham C B 1972 Camurati-Engelmann disease. Journal of Medical Genetics 9: 73–85

Spiegel A 1989 Pseudohypoparathyroidism. In: Scriver C et al (eds) The metabolic basis of inherited disease. McGraw Hill, New York, p 2013–2027

Spranger J W, Rohwedder J 1965 Zur genetika der osteodystrophiahereditaria Albright. Medizinische Welt 41: 2308–2312

Steendjik R 1976 Aspects of growth and bone structure in hypophosphatemic rickets. In: Bickel H, Stern J (eds) Inborn Errors of Calcium and Bone Metabolism, MTP Press, St. Leonardsgate

Sugiura Y, Yamada Y, Koh J 1974 Pyknodysostosis in Japan: report of six cases and a review of Japanese literature. Birth Defects Original Article Series 10 (12): 78–98

Tenenhouse H S, Scriver C R, McInnes R R, Glorieux F H 1978 Renal handling of phosphate in vivo and in vitro by the X-linked hypophosphatemic male mouse (Hyp/X). Evidence for a defect in the brush border membrane. Kidney International 14: 236–244

Thompson E M, Young I D, Hall C M, Pembrey M E 1987 Recurrence risks and prognosis in severe sporadic Osteogenesis Imperfecta. Journal of Medical Genetics 24: 390–405

Tsipouras P, Borresen A L, Dickson L A et al 1984 Molecular heterogeneity of the mild autosomal dominant forms of Osteogenesis Imperfecta. American Journal of Human Genetics 36: 1172–1179

Tsipouras P, Schwartz R C, Goldberg I D et al 1987 Prenatal prediction of Osteogenesis Imperfecta (OI Type IV): exclusion of inheritance using a collagen gene probe. Journal of Medical Genetics 24: 406–409

Wenstrup R J, Cohn D H, Cohen T, Holbrook K A, Byers P H 1987 Heterozygosity for an arginine for glycine susbtitution in the triple helical domain of the alpha 2(I) collagen gene (COL 1 A2) produces the Osteogenesis Imperfecta type IV phenotype. Proceedings of the IIIrd International Conference on Osteogenesis Imperfecta 44A

Whalen J P, Horowith M, Krook L et al 1977 Calcitonin treatment in hereditary bone dysplasia with hyperphosphatasemia: a radiographic and histologic study of bone. American Journal of Roentgenology 129: 29–35

Woodhouse N J Y, Fisher M T, Sigurdsson et al 1972 Paget's disease in a five year old: acute response to human calcitonin. British Medical Journal 4: 267–269

Worth H M, Wollin D G 1966 Hyperostosis corticalis generalisata congenita. Journal of the Canadian Association of Radiology 17: 67–74

Yu J S, Oates K, Walsh K H, Stuckey S J 1971 Osteopetrosis. Archives of Disease in Childhood 46: 257–263

58. Abnormalities of bone structure

William A. Horton

INTRODUCTION

In the past few decades many disorders have been delineated which are characterized by abnormal skeletal development, collectively termed the skeletal dysplasias. A large number of these, designated the osteochondrodysplasias, are thought to result from disturbances in the normal ossification process. The osteochondrodysplasias have been subdivided into three categories: defects of growth of tubular bones and/or spine, disorganized development of cartilage and fibrous components of the skeleton, and abnormalities of density of cortical diaphyseal structure and/or metaphyseal modelling (Rimoin 1979). The disorders comprising the second category are the subject of this chapter. They can best be understood in the context of the normal ossification process.

The skeleton normally develops and grows through a combination of two distinct forms of ossification: endochondral and membranous (Rimoin & Horton 1978). In the latter form, bone develops directly from fibrous tissue. The calvarium, clavicles, body of the mandible, spinous processes of the vertebrae and part of the pelvis arise in this fashion. In addition, diaphyseal widening of individual bones occurs in this manner. The remainder of the skeleton develops through endochondral ossification, a more complex process in which a cartilage model for each bone is formed and is subsequently transformed into true bone. The cartilage anlagen arise early in embryonic development and, by mid pregnancy, ossification has spread throughout each bone leaving only the epiphyses as cartilaginous structures. Continued proliferation and hypertrophy of the cartilage bordering the ossification front (the endochondral growth plate) is responsible for linear growth of the bone. Highly organized zones of proliferative and hypertrophic cartilage can be identified within the growth plate. As the slowly progressing ossification front penetrates the cartilage at the cartilage-bone interface, true bone is laid down. Initially, it is immature or woven bone but, with modelling, this is replaced by mature or lamellar bone. (The

maturation process occurs in membraneous ossification as well.) Secondary centres of ossification which exhibit a similar sequence of events also develop in the epiphyses during late fetal life and throughout childhood. With completion of puberty, growth plate activity ceases and the structure is transformed into bone.

Certain generalizations can be made about the disorders discussed in this chapter. Several of them, such as hereditary multiple exostoses or enchondromatosis, are characterized by aberrant growth plate activity. The lesions in these disorders are restricted to bones which arise by endochondral ossification. The activity of these lesions tends to parallel that of the normal growth plate, i.e. growth during childhood, quiescence after puberty. In contrast, bone maturation is disturbed in some of the other disorders, such as fibrous dysplasia of bone. Puberty seems to have little effect on these lesions which may affect all bones. Thus, the clinical features in these disorders are often determined by the relationship of the specific abnormality to the normal ossification process.

DYSPLASIA EPIPHYSEALIS HEMIMELICA

Dysplasia epiphysealis hemimelica (DEH) is a developmental disorder of childhood characterized by asymmetrical growth of epiphyseal cartilage. Originally described as tarsomegalie in 1926, several designations have been used: tarsoepiphyseal aclasis, chondrodystrophy epiphysairi, benign epiphyseal osteochondroma, carpal osteochondroma, osteochondroma of the distal femoral epiphysis, epiphysealis hyperplasia, and intra-articular osteochondroma of the astragalus (Kettlecamp et al 1966, Barta et al 1973). The term DEH was introduced by Fairbank (1956) to distinguish this condition from multiple epiphyseal dysplasia and chondrodystrophica punctata. DEH has been extensively reviewed by several authors (Fairbank 1956, Kettlecamp et al 1966, Theodorou & Lantis 1968, Barta et al 1973).

Males are affected approximately three times as often as females. Symptoms usually arise between the ages of two and fourteen years but have been described as early as 18 months (Fasting & Bjerkreim 1976). In a few cases the diagnosis has been established during adulthood. Joint deformity, especially at the knee and ankle, restricted motion, and occasionally pain call attention to the condition. Bony hard swelling is found at the sites of the lesions which are usually confined to one side of a limb. The medial side is mainly affected in the leg, whereas in the arm, which is involved infrequently, the radial side predominates. The most common sites in order of decreasing frequency are: talus, distal femoral epiphysis, distal tibial epiphysis, proximal tibial epiphysis, tarsal navicular, median cuneiform and distal fibular epiphysis. The axial skeleton is rarely involved, but lesions of the pubis (Kettlecamp et al 1966) and scapula (Bigliani et al 1980) have been reported. Multiple lesions occur in about two thirds of the patients.

Skeletal radiographs reveal irregular enlargement of the affected epiphyses and tarsal and carpal bones. There is usually a lobulated multicentric mass adjacent to one side of the epiphysis or bone. In young children multiple ossification centres may be seen within this mass, but with time these fuse to form a single ossified mass which eventually becomes part of the adjacent bone. Mild widening of the metaphyses of affected bones may also be seen. When the talus is affected, the ossification centres may appear prematurely.

Histological examination of the lesions shows nests of proliferating and hypertrophic chondrocytes surrounding ossification centres. The appearance resembles that seen at secondary ossification centres; it is also indistinguishable from the pattern observed in osteocartilaginous exostoses.

The lesions and their secondary deformities tend to increase during the first few years of life, after which they become somewhat quiescent and enlarge only slightly as the child continues to grow. Both shortening and lengthening of the affected limbs compared to unaffected limbs has been described. New ossification centres may appear radiographically; however, as described earlier, these fuse with each other and the normal portion of the bone. Following puberty there is little change. Treatment must be individualized and usually involves excision of the lesions that contribute to deformities and interfere with normal function. Malignant degeneration of the lesions has not been described.

All cases of DEH reported to date have been sporadic. Moreover, in one instance, one of a pair of monozygotic twins was affected (Donaldson et al 1953). Hensinger et al (1974) however, reported the autosomal dominant transmission of DEH together with intracapsular chondromas, extraskeletal chondromas and osteochondromas.

HEREDITARY MULTIPLE EXOSTOSES

The formation of numerous cartilage-capped exostoses which give rise to deformities of the growing skeleton characterizes hereditary multiple exostoses. The syndrome has been recognized as a familial entity for well over a century. Many terms including diaphyseal aclasis, multiple osteochondromas, multiple osteocartilaginous exostoses, hereditary deforming osteochondrodysplasia and multiple exostoses have also been applied to it.

The clinical and radiographic features have been delineated by Solomon (1963, 1964) and Crandall et al (1984). The vast majority of patients are discovered during the first decade of life, often by the age of two years. Bony lumps of the scapula and tibia are usually noted first, probably because of the conspicuous nature of these areas. Skeletal radiographs at this time, however, usually show lesions in other bones. Palpable masses have been detected soon after birth in affected infants known to be at risk for the condition. The lesions characteristically appear and increase in size during childhood. After completion of puberty, no new lesions form, and the activity of existing lesions ceases. Asymptomatic ones may be detected by X-ray at any age. In addition, some lesions may actually disappear with time. The lesions are juxtaepiphyseal in origin and most frequently reside at the ends of tubular bones, vertebral borders of the scapula, iliac crest and ribs. Involvement of vertebral bodies, patella, carpal and tarsal bones is rare; however, the lesions can arise in any bone which develops by endochondral ossification. The radiographic appearance of the individual lesions varies considerably. In general, they appear as projections of the bone from which they come; the overlying cortex and inner marrow cavity are continuous with those of the parent bone.

The earliest lesion viewed radiographically is an asymmetrical overgrowth of the metaphyseal cortical bone which lies immediately adjacent to the growth plate. As the parent bone lengthens two patterns may evolve. Normal growth of the juxtaepiphyseal metaphyseal bone may resume, so that the exostosis appears to migrate toward the diaphysis as the bone elongates (Fig. 58.1). Alternatively, the exostosis may continue to expand at the metaphysis producing an irregular club- or sometimes cauliflower-shaped end of the bone (Fig. 58.2). Pedunculated lesions which point away from the joint may also be seen near the metaphysis. The behaviour of the lesions is unpredictable, varying from one bone to another within

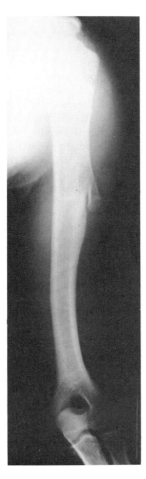

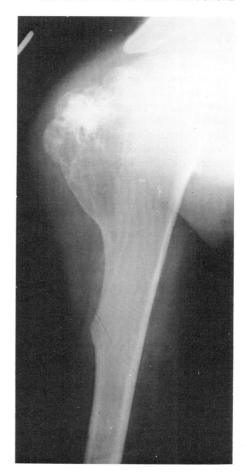

Fig. 58.1   Radiograph showing exostosis of the diaphysis of the humerus in a 16-year-old boy with hereditary multiple exostoses.

Fig. 58.2   Radiograph showing exostosis of the proximal humerus in 18-year-old female with hereditary multiple exostoses.

the same individual and even within the same bone (Solomon 1963).

In two thirds of patients the clinical picture is dominated by skeletal deformities distinct from the actual exostoses. They result from reduced linear growth of the affected long bones. In a study of 76 patients Solomon (1961) found that forearm deformities, including bowed radius, conical ulna and radiohumeral dislocations, were present in 50% of patients, while genu valgum, valgus deformities of the ankles, and deformities of the hands were present in 21, 45 and 17%, respectively. Except for the valgus deformities of the ankles, these deformities were asymmetrical. Scoliosis and pelvic and thoracic deformities were occasionally found as well. Short stature due to shortened extremities was common (41%) but was

rarely severe. Shapiro et al (1979) noted frequent limb length discrepancies. Crandall et al (1984) have estimated that half of affected persons are moderately or severely handicapped.

The most serious complication of this syndrome is malignant degeneration of the exostoses. Although development of chondrosarcoma has been reported in as many as 25% of patients (Jaffe 1943), the actual incidence is probably much lower, in the range of 5–10% of patients (Solomon 1974, Ochsner 1978). Some families may be more prone to malignant degeneration than others (Crandall et al 1984). The tumours tend to occur in the pelvic girdle, most commonly arising from the ilium or proximal femur and less often in the shoulder girdle. The diagnosis is most frequently made in the early thirties, and the first signs are usually swelling and, rarely, pain or neurological symptoms (Ochsner 1978). The tumours generally grow slowly and metastasize late. Since the exostoses do not normally enlarge after completion of puberty, any swelling or pain associated with the lesion, especially in the pelvic or shoulder region, should suggest malignant change. Other rare complications include large pelvic exostoses which cause urinary obstruction and renal failure, malposition of a pregnant uterus, intestinal obstruction and spinal cord compression (Solomon 1963, Vinstein & Franken 1971). Treatment depends upon the particular deformities and complications that occur, although most patients require surgery. The most common procedures include removal of exostoses which interfere with function, contribute to deformity, produce compression or are suspected of undergoing malignant degeneration; epiphysiodeses to compensate for reduced growth of affected bones; excision of the radial head in cases of humero-radial dislocation; and correctional osteotomies for specific deformities (Shapiro et al 1979).

Examination of an exostosis histologically shows a projection of trabecular bone covered by a cartilage cap. In children and adolescents columns of normally appearing proliferating and hypertrophic chondrocytes are found along the bony margin. The appearance is very similar to a normal growth plate except that the cartilage-bone interface is irregular and collections of hypertrophic chondrocytes are found in the bone (Spjut et al 1971). In the adult, the cartilage is reduced to a thin rim or is absent altogether.

Hereditary multiple exostoses is inherited as an autosomal dominant trait. When studied radiographically, there is essentially complete penetrance. Males and females are equally affected, but there is little tendency toward similarity in the distribution and type of lesions and deformities within families (Solomon 1964).

Several theories have been proposed to explain the pathogenesis of the cartilaginous tumours. Virchow originally postulated that a fragment of the growth plate becomes separated, is rotated 90 degress and proceeds to grow in the new direction (Spjut et al 1971). Others have suggested that collections of chondrocytes arising from the proliferative layer of the metaphyseal perichondrium give rise to the tumour, or that a defect in that perichondrial ring which normally surrounds the hypertrophic zone of the growth plate permits the aberrant cartilage growth (Solomon 1963). Langenskiold (1967) speculated that a layer of undifferentiated cells at the cartilage-bone interface fails to differentiate into osteoblasts, as normally occurs and instead retains its chondrogenic potential producing the abnormal cartilage growth. Ogden (1976)

has proposed that a biochemical defect exists which prevents synchronous cartilage growth at the growth plate. Cells at the periphery, which may be under less physical constraint, are permitted to expand multidirectionally producing the exostosis. Increased excretion of mucopolysaccharides in the urine was reported in 1960 by Lorincz. However, Solomon (1964), who performed more extensive studies, found that mucopolysaccharide excretion was normal in adults and only slightly increased in affected children; he felt that the abnormalities simply reflected the increased bulk of cartilage in these children.

Despite the lack of understanding regarding the origin of the exostoses, certain aspects of the disorder have been defined. The distribution of lesions is related to the growth rate of the individual bones; sites contributing the greatest to the overall skeletal growth show the highest frequency of exostoses. In addition, the normal process of bone remodelling affects the evolution of the individual lesions, explaining the phenomena of migration and disappearance of exostoses (Solomon 1963).

LANGER-GIEDION SYNDROME

In the Langer-Giedion syndrome, multiple exostoses occur as a component of a multisystem disorder. Also known as the tricho-rhino-phalangeal (TRP) syndrome type II and acrodysplasia with exostoses, this syndrome is rare. The first two cases were described independently by Langer (1968) and Giedion (1969). Hall, together with Langer, Giedion and others reported five additional patients and delineated the syndrome in 1974. Several more cases have been added to the literature (Kozlowski et al 1977, Stoltzfus et al 1977, Murachi et al 1979, Oorthuys & Beemer 1979, Wilson et al 1979, Buhler et al 1980, Brocas et al 1986, Fryns & Van den Berghe 1986, Zaletaev et al 1987). Heavy eyebrows, large bulbous nose with thickened alae and septum, prominent elongated philtrum, thin upper lip together with mild microcephaly, large poorly-developed protruding ears, and sparse scalp hair give rise to a characteristic craniofacial appearance. Other consistent features have included mental retardation, delay in the onset of speech, short stature, multiple exostoses, cone-shaped epiphyses and loose skin. The mental retardation is generally mild to moderate in degree. In one patient who was initially considered to be mentally retarded, intelligence was eventually determined to be normal after a profound hearing deficit was found (Oorthuys & Beemer 1979). A hearing loss has been detected in half the patients tested. The delay of speech development has been observed in at least two patients with normal audiograms, however, and it appears to be out of proportion to the degree of mental retardation.

The multiple exostoses are similar in clinical behaviour and radiographic appearance to those seen in hereditary multiple exostoses. Diminished linear growth of affected bones and secondary deformities occur as well. No cases of malignant degeneration have been reported but most of the patients described to date have been children.

Several types of cone-shaped epiphyses have been described by Giedion (1969). All patients with this syndrome have had the type 12 in which the distal epiphyses of the metacarpal and proximal epiphyses of the phalanges of the hand are affected. Small conical shaped epiphyses appear to invaginate into the adjacent metaphyses often with fusion and widening of the metaphyses (Hall et al 1974). These abnormalities are not visible radiographically before the age of 3–4 years, however, because ossification of the epiphyses in the hand bones is insufficient before this age. Epiphyseal irregularities have been found in other parts of the skeleton. In particular, Perthes-like changes in the capital femoral epiphyses have been seen in half the patients. This generalized epiphyseal disturbance is probably responsible for the short stature exhibited in all the cases.

The occurrence of multiple fractures has been mentioned as a component of the syndrome; however, it has been demonstrated in only three of the thirteen patients. Moreover, one patient had only a single traumatic fracture of the humerus (Gorlin et al 1969), and the two others were identical twins who showed generalized skeletal demineralization. In fact, Hall et al (1974) questioned whether this feature was a part of the syndrome or simply a second abnormality restricted to the twins.

Although most of the children have cutaneous involvement, it has varied with age. The loose skin seems to be most striking during early childhood and regresses or even disappears between the ages of 6 and 14 years. Small brown to black maculopapular nevi are found on the face, scalp, neck and upper trunk of the older children, but have not been seen prior to age 4 years.

Small deletions of the long arm of chromosome 8 (q24.11-q24.13) have been identified in most patients with the Langer-Giedion syndrome in whom high resolution banding has been done (Wilson et al 1979, Brocas et al 1986, Fukushima 1986, Zaletaev et al 1987). Such studies have confused the nosology of the TRP syndromes, however, because deletions typical of TRP type II have been detected in two patients with clinical and radiographic features of TRP type I (Fryns & Van den Berghe 1986, Parizel et al 1987).

ENCHONDROMATOSIS

Enchondromatosis is another rare disorder of the developing skeleton. It was originally described by Ollier who called it dyschondroplasia, but it has been variably referred to as Ollier disease, multiple enchondromatosis, multiple enchondromas and internal enchondromatosis (Fairbank 1948). It must be distinguished from a similar but yet distinct disorder, Maffucci syndrome, in which the combination of multiple enchondromas and cutaneous haemangiomas and other tumours is found.

The manifestations of the disorder result from the occurrence of cartilaginous tumours in the metaphyses of bones that are formed in cartilage. They have been best described by Fairbank (1948). Both long and short tubular bones are preferentially involved and the more rapidly growing ends of these bones are the most frequently affected sites. For example, lesions in the region of the knee joint and at the lower ends of the radius and ulna are particularly common sites, while the phalanges and the pelvis are somewhat less common. The scapula, ulna, ribs, sternum, base of the skull, and facial bones are rarely affected, and the cuboid bones, such as the vertebrae, carpal and tarsal bones, usually escape. Tumours do not occur in the calvarium. By definition, more than one lesion must be present; however, the involvement may vary considerably from enchondromas affecting a single limb to tumours throughout the skeleton. In the latter instance, the lesions are asymmetrical and bilateral in the majority of cases (Mainzer et al 1971).

The characteristic deformities result from direct expansion of the tumours and from reduced linear growth of the affected bones. The most common deformities include phalangeal enlargement, asymmetrical shortening of the limbs, bowing of the long bones, ulnar deviation of the wrist, dislocation of the radial head and genu valgum. In rare instances when the base of the skull is involved, facial asymmetry and cranial nerve compression may occur. Fractures of the affected bones are uncommon. Considerable variability has been noted regarding the severity of the deformities, ranging from asymptomatic lesions detected only by X-ray, to extensive disfigurement and disability, e.g. massive swelling of fingers and toes.

The disorder is usually detected during childhood but has been identified at birth in an infant who exhibited asymmetrical limb shortening (Mainzer et al 1971). The appearance of new lesions as well as tumour growth and progression of deformities occurs in an unpredictable fashion during childhood. The lesions often regress and deformities stabilize after puberty. Renewed growth during adulthood suggests sarcomatous degeneration. The occurrence of this complication is probably less than in the Maffucci syndrome (below), but actual figures are not known.

Radiographically the lesions vary from a minute foci of incompletely calcified epiphyseal cartilage extending linearly from the growth plate into the metaphysis of the bone to large tumorous masses of cartilage which produce extensive metaphyseal enlargement (Fig. 58.3) Irregular calcifications are often found within the tumour. Thinning and disruption of the cortex of the overlying bone may occur; and there may be abnormal metaphyseal modelling. In addition, radiolucent defects often extend into the shaft of the bone (Lachman & Horton 1979). The radiographic changes of enchondromatosis may be influenced by age (Mainzer et al 1971). For example, despite shortening of a bone, typical lesions may not be seen during infancy. Furthermore, there may be a gradual 'filling in' on the lesions with normal-appearing bone after puberty.

The tumour pathologically consists of lobulated masses of irregularly dispersed chondrocytes encased within bone. Proliferative and hypertrophic cells are found, and some areas resemble the normal endochondral growth plate. In tissue from older patients intracartilaginous ossification may be seen (Spjut et al 1971).

Enchondromatosis has occurred in a sporadic fashion in almost all cases reported to date. Both sexes are affected, but it is more common in males (Fairbank 1948). The source of the metaphyseal enchondromas is not known. They may represent unresorbed portions of growth plate tissue that become incorporated into the metaphysis as the bone lengthens, or may arise de novo within the metaphysis.

MAFFUCCI SYNDROME

In 1891 an Italian, Maffucci, described a patient with enchondromas and superficial haemangiomas. Today the syndrome in which this combination occurs bears his name; however, it is recognized that the manifestations are much more extensive. The skeletal manifestations are similar to those seen in isolated enchondromatosis. Expanding cartilaginous tumours in the metaphyses of tubular bones, primarily, develop during childhood. The metacarpals and phalanges of the hand are the most common sites, although lesions are frequently observed in the tibia, fibula, femur, radius, ulna and humerus as well (Lewis & Ketchum 1973). The tumours tend to be asymmetrical and bilateral, and cannot be distinguished radiographically or histologically from those found in patients with enchondromatosis. Likewise, tumour ex-

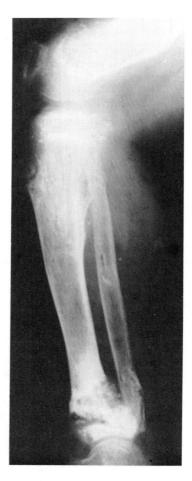

Fig. 58.3   Radiograph showing enchondromas in distal femur and proximal and distal tibia and fibula in a 12-year-old boy with enchondromatosis.

pansion and shortening of involved bones leads to a similar array of deformities. Spontaneous fractures through areas of advanced rarefaction have been reported in 26% of patients in one series (Anderson 1965). Cranial nerve palsies due to involvement of the base of the skull have also been described (Loewinger et al 1977).

The major nonskeletal manifestation of the disorder is the occurrence of simple or cavernous cutaneous haemangiomas (Anderson 1965). Usually located on the limbs, they lie in the deep layers of the skin and subcutaneous tissues. Their size varies from a few millimetres in diameter to many centimetres. They are not limited to the skin but may also be found throughout the viscera. There is a slight tendency for the haemangiomas and enchondromas to show a similar distribution with regard to laterality, but no direct relationship exists between the two. Phlebectasia is commonly observed, and thrombosis and subsequent calcification often occur within the vascular spaces. In fact, phleboliths seen on X-ray are found in nearly half the patients with this condition (Anderson 1965). In reporting a patient with enchondromas and fibromuscular dysplasia of cerebral arteries, Slagsvold et al (1977) speculated that this arterial lesion might represent another vascular manifestation of the disorder. Lymphangiomatosis has been described in a number of cases (Lewis & Ketchum 1973, Loewinger et al 1977). Other nonskeletal manifestations seen in the Maffucci syndrome include vitiligo, hyperpigmentation and nevi (Loewinger et al 1977). The majority of the soft tissue lesions are painless, although mild discomfort as well as increased skin temperature may accompany the haemangiomas (Lewis & Ketchum 1973).

The skeletal abnormalities do not usually present until early or mid childhood, but the haemangiomas are often detected at or shortly after birth. The clinical picture through puberty is dominated by the skeletal lesions; as with enchondromatosis, it is unpredictable. After the completion of puberty, however, the enchondromas do not usually progress, although this is not invariable (Anderson 1965). The predisposition to neoplasia during adulthood is well established. The greatest risk is for sarcomatous degeneration of the enchondromas which has been estimated to occur in 15–25% of patients (Anderson 1965, Lewis & Ketchum 1973, Sun et al 1985, Schwartz et al 1987). The risk does not correlate with the severity of involvement. Malignant degeneration of haemangiomas and lymphangiomas also occurs, and patients may develop multiple primary tumours. There are also reports of many other malignant and benign tumours occurring in patients with the Maffucci syndrome. These include osteosarcoma, fibrosarcoma, glioma, mesenchymal ovarian carcinoma, carcinoma of the pancreas, uterine polyps and fibroids, adrenal cortical adenomas, thecoma of the ovary and multiple fibromas (Braddock & Hadlow 1966, Lewis & Ketchum 1973, Sun et al 1985, Schwartz et al 1987). Chromophobe adenoma of the pituitary has been noted in 7 of 114 reported cases (Schnall & Genuth 1976). Because of the isolated nature of many of these reports, it is not clear if these associations are significant or simply coincidental. Sudden enlargement of either skeletal or non skeletal tumours during adulthood, however, should make one suspicious of malignant degeneration.

The treatment consists of orthopaedic and surgical intervention to minimize deformities and for cosmetic purposes. Careful surveillance for malignant degeneration of both skeletal and nonskeletal tumours, especially in the brain and abdomen, is essential.

The Maffucci syndrome occurs in all races with equal sex distribution. All cases have been sporadic and affected women have produced unaffected offspring (Lewis & Ketchum 1973). Normal karyotypes have been obtained in several instances (Lewis & Ketchum 1973). To explain the numerous mesenchymal tumours, it is generally thought that the syndrome results from a generalized defect in the mesodermal tissues (Anderson 1965, Lewis & Ketchum 1973, Loewinger et al 1977); however, the nature of this defect is unknown.

METACHONDROMATOSIS

Metachondromatosis is a distinct syndrome in which both exostoses and enchondromas are found. Only 14 cases have been reported. Thirteen were members of three families in which the trait showed autosomal dominant transmission (Maroteaux 1971, Giedion et al 1975, Hinkel et al 1984). The other was a sporadic case described by Lachman et al (1974). In addition, Cameron (1957) reported a patient (case no. 2) who may have had this syndrome. The patient exhibited multiple exostoses, enchondromas involving the metatarsal and tarsal bone of the left foot and a single haemangioma of the left big toe.

Clinically, patients may be short and usually present with exostoses, preferentially affecting the tubular bones of the hands and feet. In contrast to the lesions seen in hereditary multiple exostoses which point away from the epiphyses, the exostoses in this syndrome point toward the joint. In addition to the exostoses, irregularly calcified lesions which are sometimes separated from bone have been observed near the epiphyses (Giedion et al 1975). An unusual feature of the syndrome is the tendency for the tumours to regress and actually disappear in adulthood (Maroteaux 1971, Giedion et al 1975, Hinkel et al 1984).

The enchondromas are found in the metaphyses of long bones and in the iliac crest which is an unusual location for the tumours in enchondromatosis and the Maffucci syndrome (Fig. 58.4). Irregularity of the end plates of the vertebral bodies has also been seen. Presumably this defect together with the metaphyseal involvement by enchondromata is responsible for the short stature. Treatment consists of surgery when indicated. The risk of malignant degeneration of the cartilaginous tumours is not known.

FIBROUS DYSPLASIA OF BONE

Fibrous dysplasia of bone is characterized by the replacement of bone by dysplastic fibrous tissue. Although initially confused with osteitis fibrosa cystica of hyperparathyroidism, it was recognized as a separate entity in

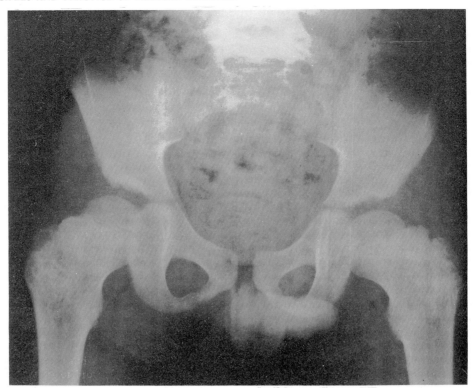

Fig. 58.4 AP radiograph of pelvis showing enchondromas in both iliac crest and exostoses of femoral necks in an 8-year-old with metachondromatosis. (Courtesy of R S Lachman, Los Angeles, C A.)

1937 by Albright et al, who described the skeletal lesions in association with increased skin pigmentation and endocrine disturbances. Five years later, Lichtenstein and Jaffe (1942) delineated the pathological features of the skeletal lesions which they termed fibrous dysplasia of bone, and observed that the extraskeletal abnormalities did not occur when only a single bone was involved. The disorder has since been defined further by several reviews in which the features of nearly 300 patients have been examined (Fries 1957, Harris et al 1962, Leeds & Seaman 1962, Stewart et al 1962, Reed 1963, Firat & Stutzman 1968, Henry 1969). Although there has been a tendency to classify fibrous dysplasia on the basis of whether or not extraskeletal features are found, it appears more appropriate to divide it on the basis of whether the lesions involve one or more than one bone, since the extraskeletal features occur only in the latter instance.

Monostotic fibrous dysplasia

Patients with monostotic disease are thought to be much more common than those with the polyostotic form. The most frequently affected sites in monostotic fibrous dysplasia are the craniofacial bones, including the skull, maxilla, and mandible; ribs; femur; tibia; and humerus. The pelvis, other long bones, vertebrae, and tarsal bones are occasionally involved (Harris et al 1962, Firat & Stutzman 1968, Henry 1969). The lesions in the extremities usually present during adolescence with pain, swelling, and pathological fractures. The craniofacial lesions are often heralded by swelling, asymmetrical growth of the skull or face and occasionally unilateral proptosis; they tend to occur in the second and third decade. Rib lesions are often asymptomatic and may be discovered at any age, often as an incidental finding on a chest X-ray (Henry 1969).

The earliest radiographic change consists of a loss of density at the site of the lesion. Later there is expansion of the bone with erosion and thinning of the cortex from within. The shaft may exhibit a 'ground glass' appearance, upon which prominent trabeculae are superimposed. In long bones the lesions appear to begin in the metaphysis and extend into the diaphysis (Stewart et al 1962). Sclerosis may be associated with involvement of the facial bones.

The lesions tend to grow slowly prior to adolescence, however, their activity is variable (Smith 1965, Gross & Montgomery 1967). After puberty, they usually become inactive; but Henry (1969) observed that several patients developed symptoms, often pathological fractures of long bones, beyond this age. He also noted fibrous dysplasia may become activated or reactivated during pregnancy. Malignant degeneration does occur, but rarely. Schwartz and Alpert (1964) calculated the incidence to be approximately 0.4% of patients. Osteogenic sarcoma was the predominant tumour and occurred at an average age of 32 years, following a mean lag time of 13.5 years after the initial presentation. Several of the patients in whom malignant degeneration has occurred have received previous radiation therapy (Harris et al 1962, Schwartz & Alpert 1964).

Although the radiographic appearance of fibrous dysplasia is characteristic, it is not pathognomonic. Therefore, in the monostotic form, a biopsy is necessary to confirm the diagnosis. Histologically, the lesions consist of poorly defined partially calcified trabeculae of bone embedded within dense, cellular fibrous tissue. The bone is immature (woven) in type; no lamellar (mature) bone is found. The trabeculae are rimmed by only a few osteoblasts, and there is a paucity of osteoclasts (Fries 1957, Harris et al 1962, Reed 1963, Spjut et al 1971). These changes seem to vary little with age. Cysts, dense fibrosis, islands of cartilage and lamellar transformation of woven bone, have also been described. Reed (1963) feels that these changes are nonspecific and reflect previous surgery, trauma, fractures and haemorrhage.

All cases of monostotic fibrous dysplasia have occurred on a sporadic basis. Males and females are equally affected. The pathogenesis of the condition is poorly understood. In 1942 Lichtenstein and Jaffe proposed that a defect in the bone forming mesenchyme results in the replacement of normal bone by dense fibrous tissue. This tissue then gives rise through metaplasia to woven bone which fails to mature into lamellar bone. Although the latter portion of this hypothesis, i.e. arrest of bone maturation, is still widely held (Fries 1957, Reed 1963, Spjut et al 1971), the nature of the primary defect remains unknown.

The treatment of monostotic fibrous dysplasia involves surgery to remove abnormal tissue. If this is not possible curettage of the lesion and packing it with bone chips is indicated. Treatment is successful when the lesion is completely removed. However, if not, recurrence is common.

Polyostotic fibrous dysplasia

In polyostotic fibrous dysplasia, the McCune-Albright or Albright syndrome, bone lesions which are identical to those found in the monostotic form of the disease occur in multiple bones, in association with abnormal skin pigmentation and a variety of endocrine disturbances. The bone lesions are the only invariable component of the syndrome. They are found throughout the skeleton, although the most frequent sites are the femur, tibia, pelvis, phalanges, ribs, humerus, and base of the skull (Harris et al 1962). The radiographic appearance of the extracranial lesions is essentially the same as seen in monostotic fibrous dysplasia (Fig. 58.5). Cranial involvement is usually characterized by diffuse sclerosis of the base of the skull, often involving the sphenoid, sella turcica and roof of the orbit, together with thickening of the occiput and obliteration of the paranasal sinuses. Radiolucent areas may be scattered through these areas of increased density.

The bone lesions are usually evident by the age of 10 years, and patients most often present with a limp, leg pain, or fracture (Harris et al 1962). Deformities are common; they include leg length discrepancy, coxa vara, shepherd's-crook deformity of the femur, bowing of the tibia, Harrison's groove and protrusio acetabuli. Most patients have at least one fracture and many have

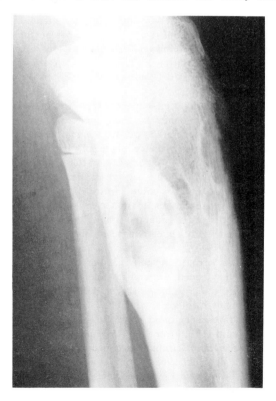

Fig. 58.5 Radiograph showing fibrous lesions in the proximal tibia in a 14-year-old female with polyostotic fibrous dysplasia.

repeated ones. Extensive craniofacial involvement may produce facial deformities as well as cranial nerve compression, hearing loss, sinusitis and lacrimal duct obstruction (Leeds & Seaman 1962). Spinal cord compression has been associated with vertebral involvement (Montoya et al 1968). The progression of the deformities is often associated with the extension of existing lesions. Puberty seems to have no effect on such extension or on the incidence of fractures. New lesions may appear, usually after puberty, and spontaneous improvement rarely occurs (Harris et al 1962). An elevation of serum alkaline phosphatase may be found.

Malignant degeneration has been reported more often in polyostotic than in monostotic fibrous dysplasia (Schwartz & Alpert 1964). It is thought that the higher incidence in the former is due to the greater number of lesions; the risk per lesion is the same in both (Gross & Montgomery 1967). The risk is relatively low, 0.4% of patients, and the complication occurs less often in the craniofacial region than in other parts of the skeleton (Leeds & Seaman 1962). Several of the patients with this complication have received prior radiation therapy (Gross & Montgomery 1967).

The extraskeletal manifestations of polyostotic fibrous dysplasia involve the skin and endocrine glands. The cutaneous lesions consist of brown flat patches of pigmentation. They follow an irregular contour and are frequently evident at birth. They may be extensive and may, but not necessarily, overlie the bone lesions (Rimoin & Hollister 1979).

Sexual precocity occurs in about one-third of patients, mostly females. In contrast to the sequence of events seen in normal girls undergoing puberty, and in most types of sexual precocity, vaginal bleeding usually occurs first and may precede breast development and the appearance of axillary and pubic hair by many years (Benedict 1962). It may appear as early as three months of age. The early bleeding is usually scant and irregular and normal menstrual periods begin at the time of expected puberty. Moreover, fertility appears to be unaffected (Rimoin & Hollister 1979). Accelerated skeletal maturation accompanies the sexual precocity. Laboratory findings in patients have been difficult to interpret. Girls with precocious puberty have larger than normal ovaries containing cysts (Foster et al 1986). Gonadal and adrenal steroids have been found to be elevated in the plasma (Danon et al 1975, Foster et al 1984); however, both low and high levels of circulating gonadotropins have been observed (Benedict 1962, Danon et al 1975, Lightner et al 1975, Foster et al 1984). Benedict (1962) noted that in three such cases in which ovarian tissue had been examined, no evidence of ovulation was found. However, active spermatogenesis was seen in a testicular biopsy

from a six-year-old boy with this condition (Hall & Warrick 1972).

Hyperthyroidism is a common feature, occurring in 30% of patients in one series (Benedict 1962). It may also contribute to the accelerated skeletal maturation. The thyroid abnormality is mild, and distinct from Graves disease in that ocular changes are lacking and histologically there is no lymphocytic infiltration in the thyroid tissue. Instead, diffuse hyperplasia is found (Hall & Warrick 1972). Thyroid stimulating hormone levels have been determined as being low on three occasions (DiGeorge 1975). Features of acromegaly and pituitary gigantism have been described several times, and an elevation of growth hormone has been detected at least once (Hall & Warrick 1972, Lightner et al 1975). Cushing syndrome due to bilateral adrenal hyperplasia has been documented at least three times (Aarskog & Tveterras 1968, Danon et al 1975). Hyperparathyroidism has been observed twice (Firat & Stutzman 1968, Sasaki et al 1985).

Two theories have evolved to explain the endocrine manifestations of the syndrome. The first states that hypersecretion of hypothalamic hormones leads to overactivity of various target endocrine glands (Hall & Warrick 1972, Lightner et al 1975). The other proposes autonomous hyperplasia of multiple endocrine glands (Danon et al 1975, Giovanelli et al 1978, Foster et al 1984, Lee et al 1986, Mauras & Blizzard 1986). The evidence to date gives the greatest support to the latter hypothesis; and it has been suggested that the regulation of cyclic adenosine monophosphate in endocrine organs is disturbed (Lee et al 1986). Further, Happle has proposed that the manifestations result from mosaicism of a lethal dominant gene that requires the presence of normal cells for survival (Happle 1986). The mosaicism hypothesis might explain the highly variable nature of the skeletal and endocrine abnormalities.

Other abnormalities have rarely been observed in patients with polyostotic fibrous dysplasia and may be components of the syndrome. Multiple intramuscular myxomas have been noted in 11 patients (Wirth et al 1971). They tend to develop in clusters, especially in the thigh region, and usually present during adulthood. Hyperplasia of reticuloendothelial tissue and both lymphoid and myeloid metaplasia have also been described (DiGeorge 1975).

Except in two instances, the reported cases of polyostotic fibrous dysplasia have all been sporadic. Hibbs and Rush (1952) reported a mother with skin pigmentation, possible precocious puberty and fibrous lesions of several bones. A biopsy of a bone lesion was consistent with fibrous dysplasia. Her daughter had cystic bone lesions of multiple bones but no skin or endocrine abnormalities. A

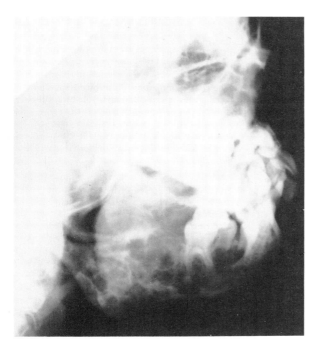

Fig. 58.6 Lateral radiograph of the jaw showing the multilocular lesions mandible in an 8-year-old girl with cherubism.

biopsy was also consistent with fibrous dysplasia. Firat and Stutzman (1968) described a mother and daughter both with documented hyperparathyroidism and cystic bone lesions (maxilla and mandible in the mother and mandible only in the daughter). Neither had skin or other endocrine manifestations. A bone biopsy in the mother showed dysplastic fibrous tissue consistent with fibrous dysplasia of bone, although osteitis fibrosa cystica was also considered.

CHERUBISM

In 1933 Jones reported four sibs with an unusual facial appearance; they appeared to be looking toward the heavens. He coined the term 'cherubism.' Despite the introduction of numerous descriptive designations, including familial multilocular cystic disease of the jaws, familial fibrous dysplasia of the jaws, familial fibrous swelling of the jaws, familial bilateral giant cell tumour of the jaw, familial intraosseus fibrous swelling of the jaw, disseminated juvenile fibrous dysplasia of the jaws and familial osseus dysplasia of the jaws, the term cherubism seems to be firmly established (Thompson 1959).

By 1970 over 70 cases had been described. The clinical features of cherubism vary considerably (Thompson 1959, Burland 1962, Khosla & Korobkin 1970). In general, the affected children present with painless symmetrical swelling of the jaws between the ages of 18 months and 7 years. The swelling progresses rapidly over the next 2–3 years after which it slows until puberty. Depending on the severity, the swelling can range from little more than broadening of the lower jaw to marked fullness of the lower face associated with thickening of the maxilla. In the most severe cases, maxillary expansion pushes the floor of the the the orbit upward. The cherubic look results from the combination of the displaced orbit and poorly supported lower eyelid; the altered facial contour permits the rim of sclerae to be exposed above the lower eyelid (Burland 1962). It is uncommon.

Maxillary involvement occurs only when mandibular involvement is severe. When present, it may be viewed intraorally. The aveolar processes may become thickened and the vault of the palate obliterated to the extent that speech is impaired. Dental abnormalities including delayed eruption, missing or displaced teeth, premature loss of deciduous teeth and absence of permanent molars have been observed. Enlargement of submandibular lymph nodes has also been described frequently. After puberty there is a gradual normalization of the facial appearance, although in most cases there is some degree of residual enlargement (Burland 1962). Treatment varies with the degree of involvement and may often not be needed because of the tendency toward spontaneous improvement.

Radiographs of the mandible taken during childhood reveal bilateral symmetrical well-defined multilocular radiolucent areas associated with expansion of bone and cortical thinning (Fig. 58.6) (Cornelius & McClendon 1969). The mandibular rami are always involved. The entire mandible may become involved except for the condyles which are always spared (Khosla & Korobkin 1970). Similar changes are seen in the maxilla when it is affected. The maxillary sinuses may be obliterated. In adults the radiolucent areas fill in with granular bone and become dense and sclerotic. The radiographic changes of the young are pathognomonic but those seen in adults are not.

Histologically, the bone is replaced by cellular fibrous tissue containing scattered trabeculae of woven bone and numerous collections of giant cells which resemble osteoclasts. Interestingly, the bone affected by the pathological process is derived from the first branchial arch. The basic abnormality is unknown.

Cherubism is an autosomal dominant trait. A review of 21 families showed that the penetrance is 100% in males and 50 to 70% in females (Anderson & McClendon 1962). There is considerable variability however and X-rays may be needed to detect mildly affected individuals, especially during adulthood.

REFERENCES

Aarskog D, Tveterras E 1968 McCune-Albright's syndrome following adrenalectomy for Cushing's syndrome in infancy. Journal of Pediatrics 73: 89–96

Albright F, Bulter A M, Hampton A O, Smith P 1937 Syndrome characterized by osteitis fibrosa disseminata, areas of pigmentation and endocrine dysfunction with precocious puberty in females. New England Journal of Medicine 216: 727–746

Anderson D E, McClendon J L 1962 Cherubism – hereditary fibrous dysplasia of the jaws. Oral Surgery, Oral Medicine and Oral Pathology 15 (Suppl 2): 5–16

Anderson I F 1965 Maffucci's syndrome, report of a case with a review of the literature. South African Medical Journal 39: 1066–1070

Barta O, Schanzl A, Szepesi J 1973 Dysplasia epiphysealis hemimelica. Acta Orthopaedica Scandinavica 44: 702–709

Benedict P H 1962 Endocrine features in Albright's syndrome (fibrous dysplasia of bone). Metabolism 11: 30–45

Bigliani L U, Neer C S, Parisien N, Johnson A D 1980 Dysplasia epiphysealis hemimelica of the scapula, a case report. Journal of Bone and Joint Surgery 62 A: 292–294

Braddock G T F, Hadlow V D 1966 Osteochondroma in endochondromatosis (Ollier's disease). Journal of Bone and Joint Surgery 48 B: 145–149

Brocas H, Buhler E M, Simon P, Malik N J, Vassart G 1986 Integrity of the thyroglobulin locus in tricho-rhino-phalangeal syndrome II. Human Genetics 74: 178–180

Buhler U K, Buhler E M, Stolder G R, Jani L, Jurik L P 1980 Chromosome deletion and multiple cartilaginous exostoses. European Journal of Pediatrics 133: 163–166

Burland J G 1962 Cherubism, familial bilateral osseous dysplasia of the jaws. Oral Surgery, Oral Medicine and Oral Pathology 15 (Suppl 2): 43–68

Cameron J M 1957 Maffucci syndrome. British Journal of Surgery 44: 596–598

Cornelius E A, McClendon J L 1969 Cherubism – hereditary fibrous dysplasia of the jaws. American Journal of Radiology 106: 136–143

Crandall B F, Field L L, Sparkes R S, Spence M A 1984 Hereditary multiple exostoses, report of a family. Clinical Orthopedics 190: 217–219

Danon M, Robboy S J, Kim S, Scully R, Crawford J D 1975 Cushing syndrome, sexual precocity, and polyostotic fibrous dysplasia (Albright syndrome) in infancy. Journal of Pediatrics 87: 917–921

DiGeorge A M 1975 Albright syndrome, is it coming of age? Journal of Pediatrics 87: 1018–1020

Donaldson J S, Sankey H H, Girdany B R, Donaldson W F 1953 Osteochondroma of distal femoral epiphysis. Journal of Pediatrics 43: 212–216

Fairbank H A T 1948 Dyschondroplasia, synonyms Ollier's disease, multiple enchondromata. Journal of Bone and Joint Surgery 30 B: 689–708

Fairbank T J 1956 Dysplasia epiphysealis hemimelica (tarsoepiphyseal aclasis). Journal of Bone and Joint Surgery 38 B: 237–257

Fasting O J, Bjerkreim I 1976 Dysplasia epiphysealis hemimelica. Acta Orthopaedica Scandinavica 47: 217–225

Firat D, Stutzman L 1968 Fibrous dysplasia of the bone, review of twenty-four cases. American Journal of Medicine 44: 421–429

Foster C M, Ross J L, Shawker T, Pescovitz O H, Loriaux D L, Cutler G B Jr 1984 Absence of pubertal gonadotropin secretion in girls with McCune-Albright syndrome. Journal of Clinical Endocrinology and Metabolism 58: 1161–1165

Foster C M, Feuillan P, Padmanabhan V et al 1986 Ovarian function in girls with McCune-Albright syndrome. Pediatric Research 20: 859–863

Foles J W 1957 The roentgen features of fibrous dysplasia of the skull and facial bones, a critical analysis of thirty-nine pathologically proved cases. American Journal of Roentgenology 77: 71–88

Fryns J P, Van den Berghe H 1986 8q24.12 interstitial deletion in trichorhinophalangeal syndrome type I. Human Genetics 74: 188–189

Fukushima Y 1986 A simple method for high-resolution banding of chromosomes and its application to diagnosis of birth defects. Hokkaido Igaku Zasshi 61: 935–946

Giedion Von A 1969 Die periphere dysostose (PD)-em sammelhegriff. Fortschr Roentgenstr 1 10: 507–524

Giedion A, Kesztler R, Muggiasca F 1975 The widened spectrum of multiple cartilageinous exostosis (MCE). Pediatric Radiology 3: 93–100

Giovannelli G, Bernasconi S, Banchini G 1978 McCune-Albright syndrome in a male child, a clinical and endocrinologic enigma. Journal of Pediatrics 92: 220–226

Gorlin R J, Cohen M M, Wolfsen J 1969 Tricho-rhino-phalangeal syndrome. American Journal of Diseases of Children 118: 595–599

Gross C W, Montgomery W W 1967 Fibrous dysplasia and malignant degeneration. Archives of Otolaryngology 85: 97–101

Hall B D, Janger L O, Giedion A, Smith D W, Cohen M M, Beals R K, Brandner M 1974 Langer-Giedion syndrome. Birth Defects Original Article Series 10: 147–164

Hall R, Warrick C 1972 Hypersecretion of hypothalamic releasing hormones, a possible explanation of the endocrine manifestations of polyostotic fibrous dysplasia (Albright's syndrome). Lancet 1: 1313–1316

Happle R 1986 The McCune-Albright syndrome, a lethal gene surviving by mosaicism. Clinical Genetics 29: 321–324

Harris W H, Dudley H R, Barry R J 1962 The natural history of fiberous dysplasia, an orthopaedic, pathologic, and roentgenographic study. Journal of Bone and Joint Surgery 44 A: 207–233

Henry A 1969 Monostotic fibrous dysplasia. Journal of Bone and Joint Surgery 51 B: 300–306

Hensinger R N, Cowell H R, Ramsey P L, Leopold R G 1974 Familial dysplasia epiphysealis hemimelica associated with chondromas and osteochondromas, a report of a kindred with variable expression. Journal of Bone and Joint Surgery 56 A: 1513–1516

Hibbs R E, Rush H P 1952 Albright's syndrome. Annals of Internal Medicine 37: 587–593

Hinkel G K, Rupprecht E, Harzer W 1984 Metachondromatosis, report of a family with 4 cases. Helvetica Paediatrica Acta 39: 481–489

Jaffe H L 1943 Hereditary multiple exostoses. Archives of Pathology 36: 335–357

Jones W A 1933 Familial multilocular cystic disease of the jaws. American Journal of Cancer 17: 946–950

Kettlekamp D B, Campbell G J, Bonfiglio M 1966 Dysplasia epiphysealis hemimelica, a report of fifteen cases and a review of the literature. Journal of Bone and Joint Surgery 48 A: 746–766

Khosla V M, Korobkin M 1970 Cherubism. American Journal

of Diseases of Children 120: 458–461

Kozlowski K, Harrington G, Barylak A, Bartoszewica B 1977 Multiple exostoses mental retardation syndrome (ale-calo or MEMR syndrome), description of two childhood cases. Clinical Pediatrics 16: 219–224

Lachman R S, Horton W A 1979 Endochondromatosis. In: Bergsma D (ed) Birth Defects Compendium, 2nd edn. Alan Liss, New York, p 392–393

Lachman R S, Cohen A, Hollister D, Rimoin D L 1974 Metachondromatosis. Birth Defects Original Article Series 10: 171–178

Langenskiold A 1967 The development of multiple cartilaginous exostoses. Acta Orthopaedica Scandinavica 38: 259–266

Langer L O 1968 The thoracic-pelvic-phalangeal dystrophy. Birth Defects Original Article Series 4: 55–64

Lee P A, Van Dop C, Migeon C J 1986 McCune-Albright syndrome, long-term follow-up. Journal of the American Medical Association 256: 2980–2984

Leeds N, Seaman W B 1962 Fibrous dysplasia of the skull and its differential diagnosis, a clinical and roentgenographic study of 46 cases. Radiology 78: 570–582

Lewis R J, Ketchum A S 1973 Maffucci's syndrome, functional and neoplastic significance, case report and review of the literature. Journal of Bone and Joint Surgery 55 A: 1465–1479

Lichtenstein L, Jaffe H L 1942 Fibrous dysplasia of bone, a condition affecting one, several or many bones, the graver cases of which may present abnormal pigmentation of the skin, premature sexual development, hyperparathyroidism or still other extraskeletal abnormalities. Archives of Pathology 33: 777–816

Lightner E S, Penny R, Frasier S D 1975 Growth hormone excess and sexual precocity in polyostotic fibrous dysplasia (McCune-Albright syndrome), evidence for abnormal hypothalamic function. Journal of Pediatrics 87: 922–927

Loewinger R J, Lichtenstein J R, Dodson W E, Eisen A Z 1977 Maffucci's syndrome, a mesenchymal dysplasia and multiple tumour syndrome. British Journal of Dermatology 96: 317–322

Lorincz A E 1960 Urinary acid mucopolysaccharides in hereditary deforming chondrodysplasia (diaphyseal aclasia) Federation Proceedings 19: 148

Mainzer F, Minagi H, Steinbach H L 1971 The variable manifestations of multiple enchondromatosis. Radiology 99: 377–388

Maroteaux P 1971 Metachondromatose. Zeitschrift fur Kinderheilkunde 109: 246–261

Mauras N, Blizzard R M 1986 The McCune-Albright syndrome. Acta Endocrinologica [Supplement] 279: 207–217

Montoya G, Evarts C M, Dohn D F 1968 Polyostotic fibrous dysplasia and spinal cord compression. Journal of Neurosurgery 29: 102–105

Murachi S, Itoh H, Sugiura Y 1979 Tricho-rhino-phalangeal syndrome type II, the Langer-Giedion syndrome. Japanese Journal of Human Genetics 24: 27–36

Ochsner P E 1978 Zum problem der neoplastischen entarung bei multiplen kartilagnaren exostosen. Zeitschrift fur Orthopadie 116: 369–378

Ogden J A 1976 Multiple hereditary osteochondromata, report of an early case. Clinical Orthopaedics and Related Research 116: 48–60

Oorthuys J W E, Beemer F A 1979 The Langer-Giedion-syndrome (tricho-rhino-phalangeal syndrome type II).

European Journal of Pediatrics 132: 55–59

Parizel P M, Dumon J, Vossen P, Rigaux A, De Schepper A M 1987 The tricho-rhino-phalangeal syndrome revisited. European Journal of Radiology 7: 154–156

Reed R J 1963 Fibrous dysplasia of bone, a review of 25 cases. Archives of Pathology 75: 480–495

Rimoin D L 1979 International nomenclature of constitutional diseases of bone with bibliography. Birth Defects, Original Article Series 15: 1–29

Rimoin D L, Hollister D W 1979 Fibrous dysplasia, polyostotic. In: Bergsma D (ed) Birth defects compendium. Alan Liss, New York, p 444–445

Rimoin D L, Horton W A 1978 Short stature, Part I. Journal of Pediatrics 92: 523–528

Sasaki H, Tsutsu N, Asano T, Yamamoto T, Kikuchi M, Okumura M 1985 Coexisting primary hyperparathyroidism and Albright's hereditary osteodystrophy, an unusual association. Postgraduate Medical Journal 61: 153–155

Schnall A M, Genuth S M 1976 Multiple endocrine adenomas in a patient with the Maffucci syndrome. American Journal of Medicine. 61: 952–956

Schwartz D T, Alpert M 1964 The malignant transformation of fibrous dysplasia. American Journal of Medical Science 247: 1–20

Schwartz H S, Zimmerman N B, Simon M A, Wroble R R, Millar E A, Bonfiglio M 1987 The malignant potential of enchondromatosis. Journal of Bone and Joint Surgery [AM] 69: 269–274

Shapiro F, Simon S, Glimcher M J 1979 Hereditary multiple exostoses; anthropometric, roentgenographic, and clinical aspects. Journal of Bone and Joint Surgery 61 A: 815–824

Slagsvold J E, Bergsholm P, Larsen J L 1977 Fibromuscular dysplasia of intracranial arteries in a patient with multiple enchondromas (Ollier's disease). Neurology 27: 1168–1171

Smith J F 1965 Fibrous dysplasia of the jaws. Archives of Otolaryngology 81: 592–603

Solomon L 1961 Bone growth in diaphyseal aclasis. Journal of Bone and Joint Surgery 43 B: 700–716

Solomon L 1963 Hereditary multiple exostosis. Journal of Bone and Joint Surgery 45 B: 292–304

Solomon L 1964 Hereditary multiple exostoses. American Journal of Human Genetics 16: 351–363

Solomon L 1974 Chondrosarcoma in hereditary multiple exostosis. South African Medical Journal 48: 671–676

Spjut H J, Dorfman H D, Fechner R E, Ackerman L V 1971 Tumors of bone and cartilage, Fascicle 5, Atlas of Tumor Pathology. Armed Forces Institute of Pathology, Washington DC

Stewart M J, Gilmer W S, Edmonson A S 1962 Fibrous dysplasia of bone. Journal of Bone and Joint Surgery 44 B: 302–318 E

Stoltzfus E, Ladda R L, Lloyd-Still J 1977 Langer-Giedion syndrome, type II tricho-rhino-phalangeal dysplasia. Journal of Pediatrics 91: 277–280

Sun T C, Swee R G, Shives T C, Unni K K 1985 Chondrosarcoma in Maffucci's syndrome. Journal of Bone and Joint Surgery [AM] 67: 1214–1219

Theodorou S, Lantis G 1968 Dysplasia epiphysialis hemimelica (epiphyseal osteochondromata), report of two cases and review of the literature. Helvetica Paediatrica Acta 2: 195–204

Thompson N 1959 Cherubism, familial fibrous dysplasia of the jaws. British Journal of Plastic Surgery 12: 89–103

Vinstein A L, Franken E A 1971 Hereditary multiple

exostoses, a report of a case with spinal cord compression. Radiology 112: 405–407

Wilson W G, Herrington R T, Aylsworth A S 1979 The Langer-Giedion syndrome: Report of a 22-year-old woman. Pediatrics 64: 542–545

Wirth W A, Leovitt D, Enzinger E M 1971 Multiple intramuscular myxoma, another extraskeletal manifestation of fibrous dysplasia. Cancer 27: 1167–1173

Yunis J J 1980 Nomenclature of high resolution human chromosomes. Cancer Genetics and Cytogenetics 2: 221–229

Zaletaev D V, Kuleshov N P, Lure I V, Marincheva G S 1987 Langer-Giedion syndrome and deletion in the long arm of chromosome 8. Genetika 23: 907–912

59. Dysostoses

J. G. Hall

INTRODUCTION

The dysostoses constitute that group of disorders in which the skeletal involvement is predominantly manifested in abnormalities of individual bones. These abnormalities can occur singly or in combinations. They may represent malformations, disruptions or deformations of bone or connective tissue (Spranger et al 1982). By comparison, the skeletal dysplasias have a generalized abnormality in cartilage or bone growth and development, or both. A discussion of the dysostoses becomes a discussion of the specific conditions in which abnormalities of individual bones are observed. In some ways it is only a listing of specific conditions, since at this time very little is known about the pathogenesis of the dysostoses or what the specific patterns of their involvement reflect about developmental processes. The revised International Nomenclature of Constitutional Diseases of Bones (Maroteaux 1983) will be followed in this discussion. In the International Nomenclature, the dysostoses are broken down into those primarily concerned with craniofacial involvement, those with predominantly axial involvement and those with predominant involvement of the extremities. These designations are arbitrary for the convenience of organization and categorization on clinical grounds, and in no way reflect basic mechanisms. In most cases, the other systems which may be involved will probably be the best clue to the basic mechanism of disease.

The dysostoses with craniofacial involvement are discussed in the chapter on craniofacial syndromes. Many of the dysostoses with predominantly axial involvement and with predominant involvement of the extremities will be included here, however only conditions which have been relatively well defined will be discussed. With the burgeoning of clinical genetics and dysmorphology, numerous syndromes have been and are being described. In many cases, abnormalities of individual bones are part of these newly defined syndromes. However, it is impossible to cover the variability and spectrum of many of the newly described or, as yet, poorly defined disorders

within the scope of this chapter. Numerous excellent books on syndromes include extensive discussion of the dysostoses (Warkany 1971, Poznanski 1974, Gorlin et al 1976, Beighton 1978, Temtamy & McKusick 1978, Bergsma 1979, Maroteaux 1979, Smith 1982, Wiedemann et al 1985, Goldberg 1987, McKusick 1988, Taybi & Lachman 1990) and in addition new computer programs have been developed by several centres aimed at identifying specific rare disorders and providing references (POSSUM 1987, Winter et al 1985).

The dysostoses include a number of conditions in which there is absence or partial absence of a bone or set of bones. Limb and skeletal development occur before the eighth week of gestation; consequently the predominant features of most dysostoses have been determined early in development. However, some (for instances the Poland anomaly/Poland sequence) are thought to be disruptions, and others (for instance camptodactyly) are thought to represent deformations, so some of the abnormalities may not be determined until much later. Those anomalies determined early would be readily apparent prenatally with ultrasonography; therefore, genetic counselling offering prenatal diagnosis is a consideration for many of these conditions.

DYSOSTOSES WITH PREDOMINANTLY AXIAL INVOLVEMENT

Vertebral segmentation defects including the Klippel-Feil anomaly (Klippel-Feil sequence)

Abnormal segmentation can involve any of the vertebral bodies (Fig. 59.1) but is most frequently seen in the cervical area (Fig. 59.2). Cervical vertebral segmentation anomalies are referred to as the Klippel-Feil anomaly (Klippel-Feil sequence) whether they involve fusion of two segments or the entire cervical spine, in spite of the fact that there are actually several distinct subcategories, as defined by Gunderson et al (1967). The mechanism which leads to the malformations seen in the Klippel-Feil anomaly appears to be a failure of the normal segmentation and fusion processes of the mesodermal somites, which would occur between the third and seventh weeks of gestation. Bouwes Bavinck and Weaver (1986) have proposed that this occurs on the basis of a vascular accident early in development.

Clinically, there is a classic triad of: (1) short neck (the head of patients with cervical involvement seems to sit directly on the thorax) often with the presence of pterygium colli; (2) the hairline usually seems low; and (3) there is painless limitation of head movement. The scapula is frequently high. If true neurological compromise is present, it may imply that the spinal cord has been compressed or even that there is a congenital structural anomaly of the spinal cord. The most severe form of cervical segmentation defect is discussed under spondylocostal dysplasia. Hemivertebrae, defective posterior elements (spina bifida occulta), clefting of the vertebral body anteriorly, reduction in the number of vertebrae and anomalies at the occipital-atlantal articulation may be seen (Goldberg 1987). Segmentation abnormalities in the C2–C3 region may lead to subluxation and secondary cord compression; thus, careful flexion and extension films of the neck should always be taken of patients with the Klippel-Feil anomaly. Abnormal segmentation in the thoracic and lumbar area can lead to scoliosis, either congenital, or developing during early childhood. Subluxation of the vertebrae can also occur in the thoracic or lumbar region leading to spinal nerve compression. Extra, fused or missing ribs and Sprengel anomaly are frequently seen.

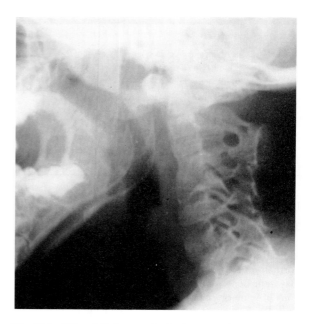

Fig. 59.2 Klippel-Feil anomaly. Radiograph of cervical spine. Note fusion of posterior elements of C1 to occiput and fusion and partial rotation of C2–C5.

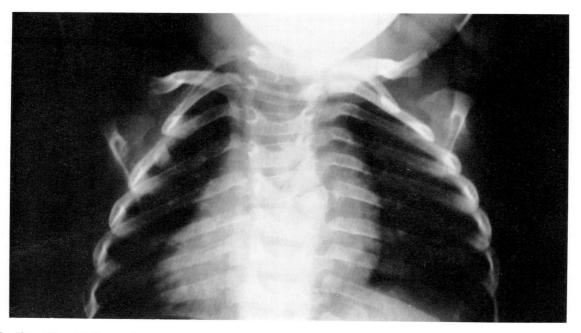

Fig. 59.1 Klippel-Feil anomaly. Radiograph of thoracic spine. Note right sixth thoracic, hemivertebrae and associated changes in T5.

Multiple system congenital anomalies are seen frequently with multiple vertebral fusion defects. Congenital heart disease may be present. Cleft palate or submucous cleft may be present in as many as 20% of the cases. Hearing loss (30%), with structural anomalies of the ossicles (Stark & Borton 1973), renal dysgenesis ranging from hypoplasia to bilateral agenesis, internal genital anomalies including vaginal atresia, and bicornuate uterus, limb anomalies, partial facial paralysis and ptosis are among the anomalies frequently reported (Gunderson et al 1967, Helmi & Pruzansky 1980, Nagib et al 1985).

Maroteaux (1979) has separated vertebral segmentation defects into anomalies of the cervical occipital region including vertebral blocks, malformations of the baso-occipital bone, abnormalities of the dens and abnormalities of the lumbosacral region. This distinction is useful, both in identifying which areas are involved and in considering the potential neurological complications.

In 1967, Gunderson distinguished three types of cervical vertebral fusion defect. These help to sort out familial types of vertebral fusion and the presence or absence of other system involvement. These are: type I – vertebral fusions containing massive fusion of many cervical and upper thoracic vertebrae (Figs 59.1 and 59.2); type II – those containing fusions of only one or two interspaces, usually C2–C3 or C5–C6; but there can be intrafamilial variability, and hemivertebrae and occipito-cervical fusion may be present; type III – patients in whom both cervical fusion and lower thoracic or lumbar fusion occur.

In type I (massive fusion of many cervical and upper thoracic vertebrae) most cases are sporadic and many have multiple anomalies of other organ systems. There are case reports of a second affected sib or a sib with multiple congenital anomalies, raising the possibility of a rare recessive gene being responsible for the anomalies. Family members may also have a small increased risk of neural tube defects or multiple vertebral anomalies (Wynne-Davies 1975).

In type II (fusion of only one or two interspaces, most commonly C2–C3 or C5–C6) there are usually no other anomalies. When the fusion is in the cervical area, genetic forms are relatively frequent. An autosomal dominant disorder is known in which there is C2–C3 fusion. Occipitocervical fusion may also be seen in some affected members of these families. Fusion of C5–C6 with narrowing of C5–C6 has been reported to occur in an autosomal recessive pattern in several families. Variable cervical fusion with kyphoscoliosis has been seen in other families in an apparent dominant pattern.

Type III (multiple vertebral segmentation anomaly including both cervical fusion and lower thoracic or lumber fusion) is often associated with multiple organ anomalies and neurological compromise. Usually, it is a sporadic occurrence. However, Wynne-Davies (1975) has recognized families with an apparent autosomal dominant inheritance with marked variability within the family as to which, and how many, vertebrae are affected. It is not clear whether this type is distinguishable or distinct from various spondylocostal dysplasias.

Differential diagnosis of Klippel-Feil anomaly includes Turner syndrome, Noonan syndrome, fetal alcohol syndrome, spondyloepiphyseal dysplasia congenita, spondylothoracic dysostosis, spondylocostal dysostosis and Goldenhar syndrome.

A subdivision of vertebral segmentation anomalies has been designated the Wildervanck or cervical-oculo-acoustic syndrome, which may well be an X–linked dominant lethal in males, since it appears to affect females exclusively (Kirkham 1969). It is characterized by congenital perceptive deafness, abducens paralysis with retraction of the bulb of one or both eyes (Duane syndrome), facial hypoplasia and asymmetry, fusion of cervical vertebrae and occasionally elbow hypoplasia.

The MURCS association is the observation that MUllerian duct aplasia, Renal hypoplasia, dysgensis or ectopia, and Cervical-thoracic Somite dysplasia occur together more frequently than would be expected by chance (Duncan et al 1979). Obviously some cases of Klippel-Feil will have this association, consequently all patients with Klippel-Feil should be screened for other associated anomalies.

The VATER association is the observation that Vertebral anomalies, Anal anomalies, Tracheal, Esophageal, and Radial ray defects occur together more often than expected by chance (Smith 1982). Since the original observation, renal, cardiac, limb anomalies and single umbilical artery were also noted to be seen with this group, giving rise to the acronym VACTERLS.

Spondylocostal and spondylothoracic dysostoses

There are a number of spondylocostal and spondylothoracic dysostoses in which abnormal spinal segmentation and malformations of the ribs occur. Clinically, these patients have a short neck and/or trunk. Other visceral malformations are not generally seen. This group of dysostoses falls into two major types: (1) mild varieties, which may be inherited as a dominant condition; and (2) more severe varieties, which may be inherited as autosomal recessive traits (Ayme & Preus 1986).

Dominantly inherited multiple segmentation anomalies of vertebrae have been reported. There may be hemivertebrae, fused vertebrae, butterfly vertebrae and various rib anomalies (Rimoin et al 1968). A family with mild ptosis has also been described by Faulk et al (1970). Because of marked variability within these families,

X-ray studies are needed to establish the possibility of hemivertebrae or fusion. The families with dominantly inherited Klippel-Feil anomaly (Gunderson et al 1967) may represent the same condition as the families with dominantly inherited spondylocostal dysostosis. The report of Wynne-Davies (1975) suggests that these families may be at a slightly increased risk for having children with neural tube defects.

The individuals with the recessively inherited types of multiple segmentation anomalies of vertebrae have all had marked shortening of the trunks. The diagnosis is readily apparent because the disproportion of the short trunk is dramatic when compared to the relatively long limbs; however, there appear to be several forms. In the Jarcho-Levin spondylothoracic dysostosis, (occipito-facial-cervico-thoracic-abdomino-digital dysplasia) the severe disproportion of the trunk and limbs gives a crab-like appearance on X-ray because of the marked platy-spondyly of the fused vertebrae (Perez Comas & Garcia Castro 1974). Many children with the Jarcho-Levin spondylothoracic dysostosis syndrome die during infancy, probably from respiratory complications. Jarcho-Levin syndrome has an excess of affected females and is primarily seen in Puerto Ricans (Poor et al 1983). Cantu et al (1971) have reported a family with less severe vertebral fusion, inherited as an autosomal recessive trait, in which survival is better, probably because the chest is larger. This may be the same condition as that reported by Norum and McKusick (1969). There are a number of other families consistent with autosomal recessive inheritance with moderately affected individuals (Bartsocas et al 1974, Franceschini et al 1974, Trindade & Nobrega 1977, Beighton & Horan 1981). A Mennonite family with spondylocostal dyplasia was also reported to have renal anomalies (Casamassima et al 1981). David and Glass (1983) reported affected sibs, one of whom developed a malignant cerebral tumour.

Prenatal diagnosis is probably possible in cases with severe vertebral involvement and short trunks (Tolmie et al 1987).

Differential diagnoses of the spondylocostal dysostoses include the Klippel-Feil syndrome, spondylo dysplasias, Poland syndrome, spondyloepiphysial dysplasia congenita and the short rib polydactyly syndromes.

Sprengel deformity (Sprengel sequence)

Sprengel deformity is characterized by a high, medially rotated scapula. It occurs as an isolated event unilaterally or bilaterally or in association with a variety of abnormalities. Sprengel deformity presumably results from a failure of the normal embryological descent of the scapula from the neck to the normal thoracic position during the second month of gestation. The scapula is usually hypoplastic, having the fetal shape of an equilateral triangle. Because it lies higher and closer to the midline, it may produce a lump in the upper back and lead to restricted movement of the shoulder. In 20–50% of cases, there is accumulation of connective tissue or even bony fusion between the scapula and ribs or vertebrae (Engel 1943). Even though 90% of cases are unilateral, associated anomalies occur in more than half of the cases. Scoliosis, hemivertebrae, fused vertebrae, spina bifida occulta, cervical ribs, missing ribs, fused ribs, clavicular anomalies and hypoplasia of the muscles of the shoulder girdle are seen. Association with situs inversus has been described, as have chest deformities and limb anomalies (Otter 1970). Many cases of Sprengel deformity seem to be only one manifestation of a more generalized disturbance of shoulder girdle and upper thorax (Warkany 1971).

Surgery may be needed, both to improve function of the shoulder and back, and to improve cosmetic appearance. Surgery usually involves removal of the scapulovertebral communication. Without surgery, exercise and stretching seem to be of little value. Most cases of Sprengel deformity are sporadic; however, a few families have been described with autosomal dominant transmission (Wilson et al 1971, Hodgson & Chiu 1981). Marked variability occurred in those families.

Osteo-onychodysostosis (nail-patella syndrome)

Osteo-onychodysostosis is a dominantly inherited condition with four major clinical features: dysplasia of the nails, absence or hypoplasia of the patella (Fig. 59.3), abnormalities of the elbow, and the presence of iliac horns (pyramidal spurs just outside the sacroiliac line) (Fig. 59.4). Nail-patella is linked to the ABO blood group locus on chromosome 9 (9q34) with about a 10% recombinant fraction. It is also very closely linked to adenylate kinase-1. The tendency to develop nephritis can be a serious complication and seems to have a familial aggregation (Maroteaux 1979).

The disorder is recognized at different ages, depending on the degree of involvement (Beals & Eckhardt 1969). Some patients have difficulty walking because of instability of the knee. Occasionally infants present with contractures of hips, knees, elbows, feet or fingers and may even have pterygium across the joints. Other individuals are basically asymptomatic and only recognized as a part of family studies. Height is usually within normal limits, but mildly short for the family.

The nails are hypo- and dysplastic. They may be small and concave, longitudinally grooved, abnormally split, pitted, softened, discoloured, brittle with triangular shaped lunula or even hypoplasia of the central part. The toes are rarely involved, while the thumb and index fingers are most often involved.

The patellae are small, laterally dislocated and may be bipartite or absent (Fig. 59.3). They may sublux or dislocate. Prominence of the medial femoral condyle, hypoplasia of the lateral femoral condyle and proximal tibial distortion are all seen. Hypoplasia of knee tendons

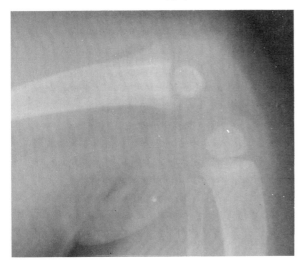

Fig. 59.3 Nail-patella syndrome (osteo-onychodysostosis) Radiograph of knee. Note absence of the patella, and proximal tibial distortion.

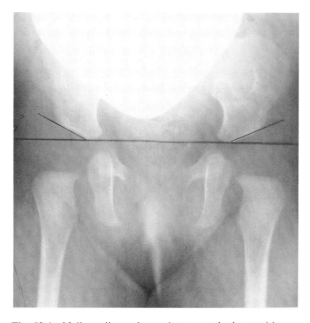

Fig. 59.4 Nail-patella syndrome (osteo-onychodysostosis) Radiograph of pelvis. Note flaring of iliac wings with definitive iliac horns.

and hypoplasia of the quadriceps and vastus medialis may contribute to instability of the knee.

At the elbow, hypoplasia of the capitellum, and relative hypertrophy of the medial condyle with hypoplasia of the radial head are present. Lateral or posterior subluxation of the radial head results in decreased pronation/supination and lack of full extension. Webbing at the elbow may be seen and the carrying angle is increased. Deltoid, triceps and brachio-radialis hypoplasia occur (Goldberg 1987). Hypoplasia of the lateral humeral condyle and head of the fibula may also be seem. These elbow and knee changes are usually bilateral (Valdueza 1973).

Iliac horns arising from the central area of the outer surface of the iliac wing are usually pyramidal in shape and are diagnostic (Fig. 59.4). The iliac horns may be asymmetrical but always occur bilaterally. They are palpable in 70% of patients but are usually of no medical significance. Flaring of the iliac crest and a small iliac angle are often seen, as well as concavity or even a notch in the anterior border of the iliac wing (Taybi & Lachman 1990).

Other skeletal anomalies include foot changes (equinovarus, calcaneo valgus or, most frequently, pes planum), dislocated hips, coxa valgus and contractures of other major joints (Lucas et al 1966).

The renal lesion in the nail-patella syndrome resembles chronic glomerulonephritis without infection (Beighton et al 1973). Clinically, the renal involvement presents with proteinuria. Uraemia develops in 30% of patients. Accumulation of abnormal collagen fibres and thickening of the basement membrane can be found in the glomeruli on autopsy. These changes may represent a basic structural defect present as part of the disease rather than a phenomenon which is secondary to glomerular sclerosis (Morita et al 1973). All patients should be screened for renal problems, especially those in families with a history of renal involvement (Bennet et al 1973).

Heterochromia of the iris, with a dark inner margin of the iris is frequently seen. Its significance is unclear. Hypoplasia and narrowing of the scapulae, clinodactyly and prominence of the outer portion of the clavicle can also be seen. Osteochondritis with loose bodies is often present in adolescence. A septum may be present in the synovia of the knee (Goldberg 1987).

Quadricepsplasty can be quite helpful in treating subluxation and dislocation of the patella. Radial head resection may relieve discomfort and prominence at the elbow but does not increase the range of movement (Yakish & Fu 1983).

Differential diagnosis includes distal arthrogryposis, Turner syndrome, trisomy 8 mosaicism and several other syndromes with arthrogryposis in which no patellae are present. Incontinentia pigmenti and ectodermal dysplasias have similar nail abnormalities but have skin changes which are seen in the nail-patella syndrome. Thus, an important distinguishing feature of the nail-patella syndrome is ectodermal involvement (nails) without changes in skin and hair.

Cerebro-costo-mandibular syndrome (Rib-Gap)

Rib gaps (consisting of uncalcified fibrous or cartilaginous tissues in the posterior part of the rib causing 'flail chest'), Pierre-Robin anomaly (micrognathia, cleft palate, glossoptosis) and vertebral dysplasia are the hallmarks of this syndrome (Langer & Herrmann 1974). Abnormalities of the heart and brain, extra skin at the neck, collapsing trachea, deafness, mental retardation, hydrocephaly, spina bifida, and polycystic kidneys have also been reported (McNicholl et al 1970, Silverman et al 1980, Hennekam et al 1985, Merlob et al 1987).

In infancy, X-rays shows gaps in the dorsal portions of the ribs with fragmented ossification and absence of normal costo-vertebral articulations. Lesions are bilateral but not necessarily symmetrical. Subluxation of the elbows is also occasionally seen. Most affected infants die in the newborn period of respiratory insufficiency due to a 'flail chest'. Mental retardation and microcephaly may be secondary to anoxia because of respiratory compromise (Langer & Herrman 1974). Most affected individuals fail to thrive and many have feeding problems because of the small jaw. They may require feeding gastrostomy.

Families consistent with both autosomal dominant (Leroy et al 1981) and autosomal recessive inheritance have been reported – and there is marked variability within families, such that one child may be mentally retarded while another is not. Prenatal diagnosis is probably possible and has been reported in one dominant family. Polyhydramnios has been seen, probably due to difficulty swallowing in utero because of the micrognathia.

Rib gaps may be seen in a number of conditions and are thus not pathognomonic for the diagnosis of cerebro-costo-mandibular syndrome. Differential diagnoses should include Goldenhar syndrome and oculovertebral syndrome. Cases with the Pierre-Robin anomaly and vertebral anomalies should have X-ray studies to look for rib gaps (Weyers & Thier 1978).

PREDOMINANTLY LIMB INVOLVEMENT

Acheiropodia

Acheiropodia is an autosomal recessively inherited condition with absence anomalies of both upper and lower limbs, usually with symmetrical involvement. Acheiropodia (absence of the hands and feet) has only been seen in inbred Brazilian kindreds of Portuguese origin (Freire-Maia 1981). The limb malformation involves a terminal transverse hemimelia (below the elbow) in the upper limbs, and a terminal transverse hemimelia of the distal third of the lower limbs. Some affected individuals have an elongated small bone at the tip of the stump, parallel to the humerus; others do not (Freire-Maia et al 1975). This inherited condition can be differentiated from other terminal transverse hemimelia conditions in that the latter usually have unilateral involvement of the upper limbs, and the lower limbs are rarely involved, whereas the defects in acheiropodia are usually uniform and bilateral, and involve both upper and lower limbs (Freire-Maia et al 1978). In addition there are no other associated abnormalities in acheiropodia. Prenatal diagnosis would be possible using ultrasound.

Differential diagnoses include the thalidomide syndrome, amniotic bands and Hanhart syndrome.

Tetraphocomelia – Cleft Palate syndrome (Robert syndrome, pseudothalidomide syndrome, SC syndrome)

This is a striking syndrome with autosomal recessive inheritance. Four limb reduction anomalies with shortening, fusion or absence of the long bones (tetraphocomelia), often with reduction in the number of fingers and occasionally toes (missing or fused metacarpals or phalanges) are seen, together with cleft lip and palate (usually bilateral, but occasionally only cleft palate or high palate). Midline facial haemangioma, mental retardation, intrauterine growth retardation, ocular hypertelorism, hypoplastic alar nasae, cloudy cornea and fine thin silvery-blond hair are often present. Occasionally relatively large clitoris or penis, cystic renal changes, or CNS structural changes (encephalocele, hydrocephaly) are seen (Herrmann & Opitz 1977, Romke et al 1987).

Chromosome studies show 'puffing' and localized separation of the centromeres in the heterochromatic, C banded regions of most chromosomes but particularly chromosomes 1, 9, 16 and Y (Tomkin & Sisken 1984). Prenatal diagnosis using ultrasound for structural anomalies or CVS for chromosome changes is possible.

Oro-Acral syndrome (Hanhart syndrome, aglossia adactylia, ankyloglossia superior)

Limb reduction (usually all four limbs with transverse amputations) and intraoral anomalies (usually a small or vestigial tongue, sometimes with adhesions of the tongue to the hard palate) comprise a distinctive combination which appears to be completely sporadic (Bersu et al 1976). Aetiology is unknown. Cleft palate may be present. Occasionally bony adhesions of the jaw occur.

The mandible is usually small and may be severely micrognathic (Garner & Bixler 1969). The mouth opening may be small and lead to feeding difficulties. Although the tongue may be rudimentary, speech is usually possible. The lower incisors may be absent.

The type of amputation varies from just absent digits to complete transverse below elbow and below knee loss (Nevin et al 1975). The humerus and femur are always preserved and lower limbs are usually spared when compared to the upper limbs (Goldberg 1987). Intelligence is usually normal. Occasionally Moebius syndrome is seen in association with oro-acral syndrome (Weidemann et al 1985). There is never complete lack of either tongue or limbs.

Radioulnar and humeroradial synostoses

Radioulnar and humeroradial synostosis (bony fusion at the elbow joint) can occur as an isolated anomaly or in association with several specific syndromes. Early in life there may appear to be a joint space on X-ray, but cartilaginous synostosis may already have occurred.

In isolated *radioulnar synostosis*, a proximal bony fusion of the radius and ulna is seen on X-ray and there is impaired pronation/supination of the arm. Consequent limitation of function is usually minimal. A number of families have been reported with dominant inheritance (Spritz 1978).

Radioulnar synostosis is seen in a number of chromosomal syndromes, particularly involving abnormal numbers of X and Y chromosomes. In addition, radioulnar synostosis can be seen in the Poland syndrome, SC or pseudothalidomide syndrome, the Pfeiffer syndrome, Nievergelt-Perlman syndrome or in association with the Kleeblatschadel deformity of the skull.

Clinically, patients with *humeroradial synostosis* have an immobile elbow joint, with decreased muscle in the upper arm, and bony fusion is seen on X-ray examination. Surgical manipulation may be necessary to improve function. Isolated humeroradial synostosis can be inherited as an autosomal recessive trait (Keutel et al 1970) as a dominant (Lenz & Rehmann 1976) or can be a sporadic occurrence.

Humeroradial synostosis is often a component of multiple synostosis syndromes, such as the brachymesosymphalangism syndrome, an autosomal dominantly inherited condition with coalition of the carpal and tarsal bones, brachydactyly and occasional vertebral anomalies. Hunter et al (1976) have reported an apparent case of the SC phocomelia syndrome or pseudothalidomide syndrome in which there was dwarfism with humeroradial synostosis. It is also reported in Pfeiffer syndrome,

femoral hypoplasia with unusual facies, Antley Bixler syndrome and femur fibula ulna complex.

Brachydactyly

Brachydactyly, or shortening of the digits due to abnormal development of either the phalanges or metacarpals, is seen as either an isolated malformation (in a variety of different forms) or in conjunction with anomalies of one or more other systems (Fitch 1979). Bell (1951) classified the isolated brachydactylies into nine definitive groups (A1–5, B, C, D, E) on the basis of her review of 124 pedigrees with 1336 individuals affected with brachydactyly. Familial reports of each type of isolated brachydactyly have shown an autosomal dominant pattern of inheritance. Poznanski (1974) and Baraitser and Burn (1983) have reported apparently autosomal recessive inheritance in type C as well.

Brachydactyly A is also called brachymesophalangia because there is a shortening of the middle phalanges. In brachydactyly type A1 (Farabee type), all middle phalanges are short or hypoplastic, and the proximal phalanges of the thumbs and halluces may be shortened. In the most severe cases, fingers are approximately one half their normal length. The third digit is usually least affected. Severe cases may have both cosmetic and functional problems. In brachydactyly type A2, middle phalanges are shortened but the shortening is predominantly seen in the second digits. The middle phalanx has a characteristic triangular shape as a result of a continuous epiphysis from proximal to distal ends on the shortened side. Consequently, growth of the phalanx is outward and results in angulation. Affected individuals may appear clinically normal. Type A3 is characterized by shortening of the middle phalanx of the fifth finger. Epiphyses may be cone-shaped and there is usually radial curving of the little finger resulting in clinodactyly. It is seen with increased frequency in orientals. In type A4 digits 2 and 5 are affected, with shortening of the middle phalanges. If digit 4 is affected, there is radial deviation. Club foot can be seen in these families. Finally, type A5 has shortening of all middle phalanges but is also associated with nail dysplasia and bifid distal phalanges of the thumb and hallux. Brachydactyly A5 can be confused with brachydactyly B; however, the latter is distinguished by hypoplasia of the distal phalanges (Temtamy & McKusick 1978). Osebold et al (1985) reported a sixth form of brachymesophalangia (A6) with mesomelic shortening of limbs and radial deviation of the index finger.

Differential diagnosis of brachydactyly type A includes a number of syndromes. Specifically, brachydactyly A2 is seen in Rubinstein-Taybi syndrome, Pfeiffer syndrome and Apert syndrome. Brachydactyly A3 is seen in Down syndrome, several conditions with X chromosomal abberrations, Russell-Silver syndrome, Coffin-Siris syndrome, oral-facial-digital (OFD) syndrome types I and II, oro-palato-digital syndrome (OPD), focal dermal hypoplasia, oculo-dental-digital syndrome (ODD), Holt-Oram syndrome, thrombocytopenia-absent radius syndrome (TAR), Noonan syndrome, Bloom syndrome, Seckel syndrome and Fanconi anaemia.

In *brachydactyly type B*, in addition to shortening of middle phalanges, there is shortening or complete absence of the terminal phalanges. Digits on the radial side of the hand are usually less severely affected than digits on the ulnar side of the hand (Temtamy & McKusick 1978). Abnormalities are consistently symmetrical and the feet are less severely affected. Soft tissue syndactyly, symphalangism, carpal and tarsal fusions, and shortening of metacarpals and metatarsals may be additional features. The additional abnormalities can be severely debilitating. Some authors have called brachydactyly B, symbrachydactyly, or apical atrophy because of the syndactyly, fusion of phalanges, and lack of terminal phalanges.

Differential diagnosis of brachydactyly B should include brachydactyly A4, the Sorsby syndrome, which is distinguished by macular coloboma, and occasional renal anomalies, and some families with symphalangism.

Brachydactyly type C has marked variability. However, characterisically, the middle and proximal phalanges of digits two and three, and the middle phalanges of digit five are shortened. It is striking that the fourth digit is basically normal and extends beyond the other digits. There may be marked ulnar deviation of the proximal phalanx of the index finger. Short metacarpals and symphalangism are occasionally seen, and there may be bifid phalanges and/or radial projections. There is only minimal involvement of the feet. Short stature may be an associated feature. X–ray studies show delayed maturation of ossification centres and hypoplasia, aplasia, or early fusion of the epiphyses (Temtamy & McKusick 1978). Baraitser and Burn (1983) reported sibs with consanguineous unaffected parents.

Brachydactyly type D is characterized by a shortened broad terminal phalanx of the thumbs and great toes. The abnormality is attributed to an early closure of the epiphysis at the base of the distal phalanx of the thumb (Temtamy & McKusick 1978). Reynolds et al (1983) reported the familial association of brachydactyly D and Hirschsprung disease. Gray and Hurt (1984) found incomplete penetrance in males but complete in females. 75% of affected individuals express the trait bilaterally.

Differential diagnoses of brachydactyly D should include heart-hand syndrome II (Tabatznik), Rubinstein-Taybi syndrome, Robinow syndrome and fibrodysplasia ossificans progressiva.

Finally, *brachydactyly type E* is characterized by shortening of one or all of the metacarpals or metatarsals. Terminal phalanges are often short, and hyperextensibility of the hands is common. The fourth digit is most frequently affected. There may be mild short stature (Riccardi & Holmes 1974) or mild generalized spondyloepiphyseal changes (Sybert et al 1979) associated with brachydactyly E.

Families with brachydactyly E associated with one of the following features have been reported: microcornea, keratoconus and hypertension. Differential diagnosis of brachydactyly E includes Turner syndrome, Albright syndrome, naevoid basal cell carcinoma syndrome, cryptodontic brachymetacarpalia, Ruvalcaba syndrome, Biemond syndrome type I, 5p-syndrome, and Tuomaala syndrome and acrodysostosis (Poznanski et al 1977).

Symphalangism

Symphalangism, or fusion of the phalanges, can be seen as an isolated finding (often post-traumatically) or inherited as an autosomal dominant trait. Both proximal (Strasburger et al 1965) and distal (Steinberg & Reynolds 1948) forms have been described. Families with distal symphalangism are rare, whereas proximal symphalangism is a much more common phenomenon. In addition, distal symphalangism tends to be an isolated anomaly and proximal symphalangism tends to occur with other associated abnormalities. Synostosis of the metacarpophalangeal joint has also been described, but only in one family (McKusick 1988).

In dominantly inherited proximal symphalangism usually more than one joint or finger is involved (Figs 59.5 and 59.6), but variability in the age of onset and severity is seen within families. Involvement of other bones can be seen, such as coalition or fusion of the tarsal and carpal bones, scoliosis, craniosynotosis and deafness in affected family members. Therefore careful evaluation of all joints, spine and skull should be done in family members of a patient affected with symphalangism. By contrast to other types of contractures and dysostotic processes, individuals with symphalangism may actually be made worse (i.e. have more rapid fusion) by vigorous physical therapy.

A difficult and as yet unanswered question is whether proximal dominantly inherited symphalangism is a different entity from dominantly inherited multiple synostosis, or simply represents variability of expression of a dominant gene. A number of kindreds with autosomal dominantly inherited proximal symphalangism and multiple synostosis syndrome have shown a

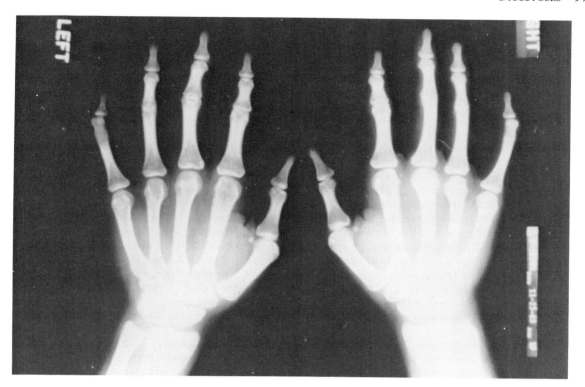

Fig. 59.5 Proximal symphalangism. Radiograph of dorsal view of hands. Note fusion of proximal phalanges on digits 4 and 5 and partial fusion of the proximal phalanges on digits 2 and 3.

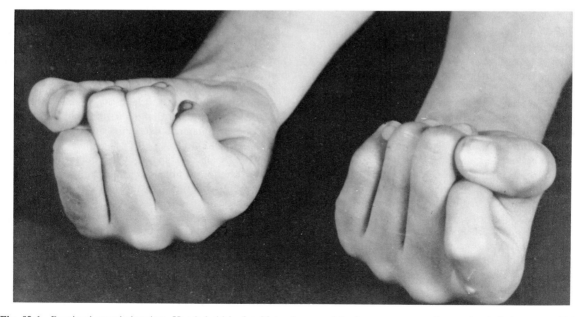

Fig. 59.6 Proximal symphalangism. Hands held in fist. Note absence of flexion creases over the proximal phalanges on digits 3, 4 and 5, and partial function of the proximal joint of digit 1 bilaterally.

conductive deafness with onset usually at the age of 2 or 3 years with progression throughout childhood (or at adolescence in multiple synostosis syndrome). A bony fusion of the stapes and petrous part of the temporal bone has been demonstrated at surgery in a number of patients. Excision of this fused area has frequently been successful in partial or complete restoration of hearing loss (Strasburger et al 1965). In these families affected individuals tend to have long narrow faces, and a prominent nose with a broad bridge and hypoplastic alae nasi. Fingers can be short and may even be missing the distal phalanx and nail.

Several theories have been proposed for the mechanism causing symphalangism. Most probably, symphalangism is caused by a developmental defect at the interzone of the phalanges prior to the time of joint cavity formation (Duken 1921). This absence of differentiation at the interzone allows cartilages to rest upon one another and ultimately to fuse to form a single cartilage rather than a joint space. Symphalangism may be present at birth; however, X-ray examination at birth may not show complete bony fusion but simply a narrowing of the interzone.

Differential diagnoses include Nievergelt Perlman syndrome, Fuhrman syndrome, diastrophic dysplasia, fibrodysplasia ossificans, Pillay syndrome, Apert syndrome, Pfeiffer syndrome and brachydactyly type A, B and C with or without short stature.

Polydactyly

Patients with polydactyly, or the presence of a supernumerary digit or a portion of an extra digit, can be classified into two major groups: those with preaxial addition or those with a postaxial addition (Flatt 1977, Goldberg 1987).

Isolated postaxial polydactyly has long been recognized as a specific entity and is very common in black individuals. Autosomal dominant inheritance with reduced penetrance or multifactorial inheritance among black families has been suggested because of the skipping of the trait in one or more generations. In the same family with apparent dominant inheritance, variability of expression is so marked that the gene is clinically manifested as fully developed extra digits (type A) in some black family members and simply as rudimentary supernumerary digits or postminimi (type B) in others (Temtamy & McKusick 1978).

Postminimi can be removed at birth by occluding the skin tag with a tight thread or string; the tag subsequently drops off. Adults so treated may often be unaware that they even had polydactyly and a careful family history should therefore be taken from parents. By contrast, extra digits involving bone or cartilage must be excised surgically to avoid osteomyelitis.

Preaxial polydactyly, on the other hand, is much less common than postaxial polydactyly and has been subdivided into four different categories by Temtamy and McKusick (1978): type 1 – preaxial thumb polydactyly; type 2 – polydactyly of a triphalangeal thumb; type 3 – polydactyly of an index finger; and type 4 – preaxial polydactyly and syndactyly. All types are inherited as autosomal dominant traits, but variability and reduced penetrance have been reported (Poznanski 1974).

Polydactyly is associated with a number of specific syndromes, the most notable of which are the chondrodyplasias, such as Ellis-van Creveld (chondroectodermal dysplasia), Jeune syndrome (asphyxiating thoracic dysplasia), the short rib/polydactyly syndromes, the acrocephalosyndactylies, hypothalamic hamartoblastoma syndrome (Hall et al 1980), Meckel syndrome, trisomy 13 and 18, Laurence-Moon-Biedl syndrome, Biemond syndrome type II, oral-facial-digital syndrome II and III, polydactyly with dental and vertebral anomalies (Rogers et al 1977, Czeizel & Brooser 1986) syndrome of polydactyly with myopia, polydactyly with imperforate anus and vertebral anomalies (Say & Gerald 1968), scalp defects and polydactyly (Fryns & Van den Berghe 1979), Kaufman syndrome, and several chromosomal anomalies. For the specific dysostotic changes found in other bones in these syndromes consult Taybi and Lachman (1990).

Syndactyly

Syndactyly or webbing of fingers can be complete or partial; it can be simple, with only skin binding the fingers together, or complicated, when there are fused bones, extra bones or shared structures such as nerves, vessels or nails (Goldberg 1987).

Isolated syndactyly has at least five forms. All five are inherited as autosomal dominant traits and are usually symmetrically bilateral. Variability of expression is seen (McKusick 1988).

Syndactyly type 1 (zygodactyly) is a cutaneous fusion of the third and fourth fingers and/or second and third toes. The webbing is usually to the nail base. Occasionally other digits can be affected.

Syndactyly type 2 (synpolydactyly, central polydactyly) is also complete cutaneous webbing of the third and fourth fingers with a partially duplicated digit hidden in the web. In the feet there is syndactyly of the fourth and fifth toes with a sixth toe in the web.

Syndactyly type 3 (ring finger) is complete cutaneous webbing between the fourth and fifth fingers. The middle phalanx of the fifth fingers may be hypoplasitc. The feet are usually normal.

Syndactyly type 4 (Hass) involves syndactyly of all fingers and the thumb, with finger flexion creating a cup-like hand. The feet may have lateral polydactyly.

Syndactyly type 5 (MC/MT synostosis) involves cutaneous syndactyly of the third and fourth fingers with synostosis of the metacarpals of digits 4 and 5. In the foot there is syndactyly of toes 2 and 3 and metatarsals 4 and 5.

Syndactyly can also be X–linked. It can be seen in the X–linked syndrome syndactyly with mental retardation, in a dominantly inherited condition with a horizontal earlobe groove, or in sporadic conditions such as amniotic bands and Poland anomaly. Syndactyly occurs in Smith Lemli Opitz, Apert, Pfeiffer, Carpenter, Saethre Chotzen, oral-facial-digital, Goltz and multiple pterygium syndromes.

Camptodactyly

Camptodactyly is clinically manifested by soft tissue flexion contractures of the fingers at one or several joints. Contractures may be present at birth or develop in childhood or even adulthood; they may be stationary or progressive, or may improve with physical therapy. Camptodactyly may be seen as an isolated anomaly, inherited as an autosomal dominant trait (Welch & Temtamy 1966, Flatt 1977), or occur as a feature in many syndromes. There can be extreme variability within families. Camptodactyly does not usually interfere with function unless it is very severe at birth or vigorous physical therapy is not begun early enough.

There are probably a number of different aetiologies of camptodactyly, one of which is misplaced, hypoplastic or absent tendons (Zadek 1934, Stevenson et al 1975). The types of contractures seen in camptodactyly often benefit from surgical repair by reattaching tendons or soft tissue release; and physical therapy with stretching exercises (Engber & Flatt 1977). Both fingers and toes can be affected. Some forms may represent early ageing, inflammatory response or deterioration of connective tissue which would lead to fibrosis and contracture of tendons as seen in diabetes.

Recently, several syndromes which include finger contractures along with many other features have been given a primary designation of camptodactyly, which is confusing. These include Tel Hashomer camptodactyly syndrome (camptodactyly, distinctive facial features, dermatoglyphic changes and musculoskeletal anomalies inherited in inbred Arab and Brazilian families as an autosomal recessive) (Pagnan et al 1988), Guadalajara camptodactyly I (camptodactyly, intrauterine growth retardation, mental retardation, unusual facies, musculoskeletal anomalies inherited as an autosomal recessive) (Cantu et al 1980) and Guadalajara camptodactyly II (camptodactyly, intrauterine growth retardation, mental retardation, short second toe and musculoskeletal changes inherited as an autosomal recessive) (Cantu et al 1985). In addition, camptodactyly has been reported as a recessive with ichthyosis (Baraitser et al 1983) and as a dominant with scoliosis (Baraitser 1982), with symphalangism (Ohdo et al 1981), and with brachydactyly (Edwards & Gale 1972).

Camptodactyly is seen as a feature of many other conditions. Differential diagnosis of isolated camptodactyly includes Dupuytren (late onset) and distal arthrogryposes (congenital). Conditions with autosomal dominant patterns of inheritance and distal contractures include Freeman-Sheldon or 'whistling face' syndrome, trismus pseudocamptodactyly, Hanley syndrome of camptodactyly, dwarfism, hypogonadism, pectus carinatum and Emery-Nelson syndrome, congenital contractural arachnodactyly and the distal arthrogryposes (Hall et al 1982). Recessively inherited conditions with camptodactyly include the multiple pterygium syndrome, Pena-Shokeir, Neu-Laxova, Zellweger syndrome, Kuskokwim syndrome, adducted thumb syndrome (Christian syndrome) and others. Camptodactyly is frequently associated with chromosomal anomalies.

Ectrodactyly

The term ectrodactyly ('ektromo' denoting abortion and 'daktylos' finger) should theoretically be reserved for a specific hand anomaly characterized by transverse terminal aphalangia or partial to total absence of distal segments of fingers. However, the term has been used for the split hand or lobster claw anomaly and in the EEC syndrome (ectrodactyly, meaning split hand, ectodermal dysplasia, clefting), and so has come to be misleadingly associated with split hand.

The 'true' ectrodactyly anomaly may involve one or more phalanges (aphalangia), one or more digits (adactylia) or the full hand (acheiria) and even part of the upper arm. More severe manifestations are hemimelia or amelia. All of these abnormalities are considered to represent various degrees of severity of the same anomaly and may be due to an intrauterine vascular occlusion or insufficiency. True ectrodactyly is usually sporadic and unilateral. Reports of familial ectrodactyly probably represent brachydactyly B. In a study by Birch-Jensen (1949), 19 individuals affected with true ectrodactyly had 51 normal children. However, a higher incidence of associated malformations in patients and their families has been reported (Grebe 1964). Certainly 'true' ectrodactyly can be seen with a wide variety of additional anomalies.

Several families have been reported with more than

one individual affected with terminal transverse amputations of digits or the whole limb, however no typical pattern of inheritance has emerged (Graham et al 1986, Soltan & Holmes 1986). It has been suggested that there may be a familial predisposition to in utero limb vascular accidents.

Differential diagnosis includes anmniotic band syndrome (Jones et al 1974).

The autosomal dominantly inherited form of isolated ectrodactyly (split hand, lobster claw or cleft hand) can be quite variable within a family and even involve absence of the long bones. Typically there is a medial cleft of the hand, the hand being divided into two portions. Often there is syndactyly of the remaining fingers and there can be absence of all but one digit. In the foot there can be medial clefting and absence analogous to the hand. Occasionally polydactyly or triphalangeal thumbs are seen. The limbs can be asymmetrically involved (Hoyme et al 1987). This form of ectrodactyly/split hand is remarkable for skipping generations. Typical pedigrees usually involve many spared individuals. Prenatal diagnosis is possible. Typical isolated familial ectrodactyly has also been reported as autosomal recessive and X-linked recessive (Verma et al 1976, Ahmad et al 1987). Associated nystagmus has been reported (Pilarski et al 1985).

The combination of ectodermal dysplasia (involving teeth, hair and nails), ectrodactyly (split hand), cleft lip/palate (EEC) is very striking (Pries et al 1974, Rosenmann et al 1976). There is probably also a variable dominant (Penchaszadeh & Negrotti 1976). The features can be quite different between affected members of the same family. The degree of keratosis and urinary tract involvement is also quite variable (Rollnick & Hoo 1988).

Adams Oliver syndrome or limb absence anomalies ('true' ectrodactyly) with scalp defects and with autosomal dominant inheritance has been reported in a number of families with variable expression (Fryns 1987). Scalp defects (cutis aplasia congenita) may be small or large and may occasionally overlie skull defects. The distal limb defects are terminal, transverse and may involve only the distal portion of the digits or may involve more of the limb with absence of hands or feet. Occasionally polydactyly is seen (Fryns & Van den Berghe 1979). Some cases have remarkable cutis marmorata telangiectasia (Toriello et al 1988) or cutis aplasia on other parts of the body. Brain structural and functional anomalies and renal anomalies (Buttiens & Fryns 1987) may be seen. The manifestations are so variable that it is easy to miss an affected relative unless there is careful examination; however an autosomal recessive form may exist (Koiffmann et al 1988). The assumption is that these anomalies are due to abnormal intrauterine vascular supply.

PREDOMINANT LIMB INVOLVEMENT WITH OTHER ASSOCIATED ABNORMALITIES

Catel Manzke syndrome

The combination of Pierre-Robin sequence (cleft palate, glossoptosis and micrognathia) together with bilaterally short second metacarpal and accessory proximal phalanx of the index finger giving radial clinodactyly of the index finger has come to be known as the Catel Manzke syndrome (Sundaram et al 1982). Affected individuals may also have dislocatable knees and congenital heart defects. There is an excess of affected males, and inheritance may well be X-linked recessive (Thompson et al 1986).

The Poland anomaly

The two major components of the Poland anomaly are unilateral symbrachydactyly and ipsilateral aplasia of the sternal head of the pectoralis major muscle. Clinically, there is unilateral absence of the normal anterior axillary fold and shortening or reduction of the digits associated with tissue webbing or syndactyly. There can be marked variability in the degree of reduction of the limb (David 1972). Most reports of the Poland anomaly indicate that cases have apparently been sporadic. Aetiology is unknown but early in utero vascular compromise has been proposed (Goldberg & Mazzei 1977, Bouwes Bavinck & Weaver 1986). Fuhrman described a family with apparent autosomal dominant inheritance (Temtamy & McKusick 1978) and David (1982) has reported second cousins affected.

The isolated malformations of either symbrachydactyly or unilateral aplasia of the sternal head of the pectoralis major muscle are also sporadic. David and Winter (1985) recently reported familial absence of pectoralis major and other chest muscles. Poland anomaly has been found to be more common in males (3:1). The right side is more commonly involved than the left (2:1) (Goldberg & Mazzei 1977). Analogous malformations have been seen in the lower limb. Several reported cases have been associated with the use of vascular constricting agents by the mother in early pregnancy (David 1972). The question of an increased risk for leukaemia in Poland anomaly has been raised (Sackey et al 1984).

The Poland anomaly has also been seen in association with other upper limb and trunk anomalies, such as radioulnar synostosis, Sprengel deformity, coalition of the carpal bones, camptodactyly, polydactyly, skin dimples, deficiencies of the rib cage, scoliosis and kyphosis. Other skeletal anomalies include cervical ribs, club foot, metatarsus adductus and syndactyly of the toes. Visceral anomalies reported include dextrocardia, herniation of the lungs, inguinal and umbilical hernias, cryptorchidism, ipsilateral hypoplasia of the kidney, coloboma of the optic disc, encephalocele, and microcephaly (Goldberg & Mazzei 1977).

Radiographs show syndactyly, polydactyly, hypoplasia of the long bones of the arm and hand, absence of the metacarpals and phalanges and relative hyperlucency of the ipsilateral hemithorax. Rib anomalies and lung herniation can also be seen (Taybi & Lachman 1990).

Because some patients have features similar to the Moebius syndrome, an overlap between these conditions is possible. If both conditions are secondary to intrauterine vascular compromise, it is not surprising that there would be overlap with regard to the amount and degree of involvement. Symbrachydactyly conditions and the acrocephalosyndactylies should be considered in the differential diagnosis.

Rubinstein-Taybi syndrome

Individuals affected with the Rubinstein-Taybi syndrome typically have broad toes and thumbs and a very specific facies with beaked nose (Rubinstein 1969). The facies is unusual even in infancy, and in addition to the prominent (beaked or pinched) nose, the columella is long and protrudes below the alae nasi. There is an antimongoloid slant to the eyes with arched eyebrows and a highly arched palate. The ears may be malrotated and usually have thickened helices (Berry 1987). The broad thumbs and toes are very characteristic and appear spatulate, short, stubby, flattened and wide. The broad-toed appearance is the result of both soft tissue and bony tissue changes which can be seen on X-ray of the terminal phalanx. Duplication of the proximal or distal phalanx of the thumb has been reported (Der Kaloustian 1972). All reported patients have been mentally retarded (with IQ estimates below 50); microcephaly is seen in over half the cases. EEG abnormalities have been reported, as has absence of the corpus callosum. Short stature is a common feature. In a study of 105 patients, approximately 80% were below the third percentile for height (Rubinstein 1969). In infancy the anterior fontanel may be large. In general, head size is below the 25th percentile. Other features that have been noted are cardiac malformations, joint laxity, increased deep tendon reflexes, stiff awkward gait, severe keloid formation, cryptorchidism, duplicated kidneys or ureters, absence of the kidney and hydronephrosis or hydroureter (Smith 1982).

X-ray changes include short and wide terminal phalanges of the thumbs and great toes, short, wide and tufted terminal phalanges in most fingers, flaring of the ilia and retardation of skeletal maturation (Taybi & Lachman 1990).

Aetiology of the Rubinstein-Taybi syndrome is unknown. Most cases are sporadic; however there are a few reports of familial cases (Berry 1987). Temtamy and McKusick (1978) favour a small chromosomal aberration. Familial recurrence, on the whole, is very rare. Thus, autosomal recessive inheritance seems unlikely. A new dominant mutation has been suggested, but paternal ages have not been significantly advanced. There may be aetiological heterogeneity.

Differential diagnoses include brachydactyly D, Robinow syndrome and chromosomal aberrations.

Coffin Siris syndrome

Sparse scalp hair, generalized hirsutism, intrauterine and postnatal growth retardation, mental retardation, coarse facial features, full lips and hypoplasitc distal phalanges and nails, particularly the fifth finger and lateral toes, characterize the Coffin Siris syndrome (Carey & Hall 1978). Affected individuals have recurrent respiratory problems and feeding difficulties (Lucaya et al 1981). Structural brain anomalies, partial gastric outlet obstruction, and cardiac anomalies have been reported (Bodurtha et al 1986). The aetiology is not known, but several sets of siblings have been reported (Haspeslagh et al 1984).

Fanconi anaemia (pancytopenia dysmelia)

Fanconi anaemia is characterized clinically by pancytopenia, hyperpigmentation, short stature and radial and renal defects. In some cases, not all of these clinical features are present and severity of the features present can be extremely variable (Glanz & Fraser 1982).

The pancytopenia is usually progressive. Average age of onset has been estimated as 8 years and all marrow elements are involved. However, anaemia may precede decrease in white blood cells or platelets or vice versa. Reports of the onset of haematological symptoms have varied from 17 months to 22 years. Fetal haemoglobin has been recorded as elevated, and in some cases there have been reduced numbers of erythrocytes and leucocytes, and decreased levels of platelet hexokinase (Schroeder et al 1976).

Hyperpigmentation of the skin is probably the most consistent clinical feature and appears as fine generalized hypermelanosis often presenting prior to haematological manifestations and increasing with age. Café-au-lait spots are also seen. Pre- and postnatal growth deficiency is present, frequently with microcephaly. About 20% of affected individuals are mentally retarded.

The most common bony defects are radial abnormalities with a hypoplastic, absent, digitalized or supernumerary thumb, hypoplasia of the first metacarpal, hypoplasia or absence of the radius and greater multiangular and navicular bones. Bifid thumbs, retarded skeletal maturation, osteoporosis, microcephaly with thick calvarium, syndactyly and hip dislocation have been reported (Esparza & Thompson 1966, Dosik et al 1970).

Patients should be evaluated for renal abnormalities, and those with external ear anomalies should also be evaluated for associated deafness. Other abnormalities that should be looked for on examination are spina bifida, Klippel-Feil anomalies, scoliosis, rib abnormalities, Sprengel deformity and flat or clubbed feet.

Complications usually result from pancytopenia with bleeding, pallor and recurrent infections. Therapy with testosterone and hydrocortisone has been helpful for the pancytopenia, although life expectancy is reduced. Affected individuals have a predisposition to leukaemia and other tumours. Cancer deaths may even be increased for heterozygotes (Swift & Hirschhorn 1971). Bone marrow transplantation may offer an alternative therapy for both pancytopenia and malignancy, although graft versus host reactions do occur.

Fanconi anaemia is inherited as an autosomal recessive trait; however genetic heterogeneity has been postulated, as well as the possibility that Fanconi syndrome is allelic to Blackfan Diamond syndrome. A high incidence of consanguinity and occurrence in sibs and cousins has been noted (Schroeder et al 1976). Intrafamilial variability of clinical features and age of onset does occur. There is an apparent excess of affected males. Chromosomal aberrations are seen, and include an increased number of chromatid breaks, gaps, exchange figures and endoreduplication. A defect in excessive UV induced disease has been demonstrated. Prenatal diagnosis has been reported as successful, through the susceptibility to chemically-induced chromatid breaks (Auerbach et al 1981).

Differential diagnosis should include TAR, Aase syndrome and the Holt-Oram syndrome.

Aase syndrome (Blackfan Diamond with thumb anomalies)

Triphalangeal thumbs with hypoplastic anaemia has been reported in several sets of sibs (Aase & Smith 1969). Growth deficiency is seen. Hypoplastic (normochromic normocyte) anaemia is present from infancy. Leucocytes and thrombocytes are normal, although fetal haemoglobin may be increased (Higginbottom et al 1978). No chromosome breakage is seen. Cardiac anomalies, cleft lip and mild mental retardation do occur. Steroid therapy may be effective (Pfeiffer & Ambs 1983).

Thrombocytopenia—absent radius syndrome (TAR) (thrombocytopenia radial aplasia syndrome)

Thrombocytopenia – absent radius – is considered to be an autosomal recessive trait, although consanguinity has not been reported and several families with affected relatives have been reported (Ward et al 1986, Schnur et al 1987). The cardinal clinical features are thrombocytopenia (usually with symptoms in the newborn period) and bilateral absence of the radius with the presence of both thumbs (i.e. each hand has five digits) (Hall 1987).

The thrombocytopenia is congenital and on a hypo-megakaryocytic basis. It is usually present at birth (90% are symptomatic during the first 4 months). Thrombocytopenia gradually improves over the first 2 years, and platelets may even be in a normal range in adulthood. Viral illnesses, particularly gastrointestinal viral illness, will often aggravate the thrombocytopenia. Leukaemoid reactions are seen in 60–70% of patients during the first year. Eosinophilia has been reported in 50% of the patients. Anaemia is thought to be the result of blood loss, but may be due to hypoplasia of red blood cells during the first year (Hall 1987).

The radius is absent bilaterally in all cases (Figs 59.7 and 59.8). The ulna is absent bilaterally in about 20% of the cases and is usually hypoplastic in other cases. Occasionally, the ulna is also absent. The humerus may be short and dysplastic. The thumbs are always present.

Anomalies of legs and hips are occasionally seen, e.g. dislocated hips, tibial torsion, abnormal tibiofibular joints, stiff knees, dislocation of the patella and camptodactyly of the toes with occasional club foot (Hall et al 1969). Congenital cardiac abnormalities are seen in one third of the cases, the most frequent being tetralogy of Fallot and septal defects. Mildly short stature is the rule.

Complications are related to thrombocytopenia and symptomatic bleeding. Death before one year of age occurred in 35–40% of patients in the past, mostly because of intracranial bleeding. This should be preventable by proper platelet transfusion (preferably from one donor). There may be delayed motor function because of hand anomalies; however, eventual good function can be expected. Other complications of skeletal anomalies include nerve compression of the wrist and arthritis. TAR patients seem to have an increased incidence of allergy to cow's milk which precipitates episodes of diarrhoea and low platelets.

Differential diagnosis should include Holt-Oram syndrome, pseudothalidomide syndrome and Fanconi anaemia. Prenatal diagnosis by demonstration of the absence of the radius using ultrasound has been successful (Luthy et al 1979).

Oral-facial-digital syndromes

The oral-facial-digital (OFD) syndrome has been subdivided into four types. They are somewhat similar clinically but have different patterns of inheritance and different associated anomalies (Majewski et al 1972, Baraitser 1986). In all types the clinical manifestations of

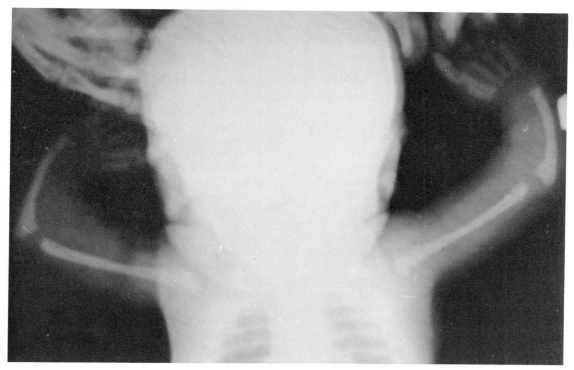

Fig. 59.7   Thrombocytopenia – absent radius syndrome (TAR). Radiograph of chest and upper limbs. Note absence of radius bilaterally, presence of thumb and shortening of ulna.

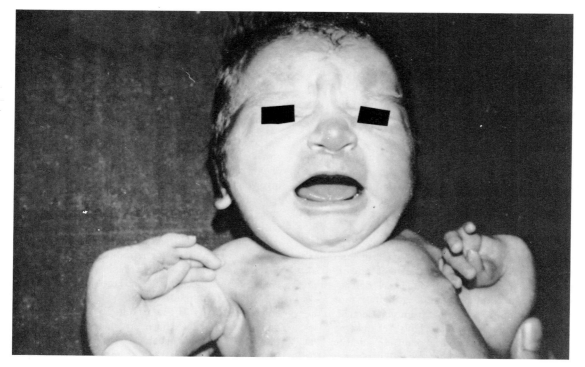

Fig. 59.8   Infant with TAR. Note curved short forearm, ulnar deviation of hand and presence of thumb bilaterally.

the face are striking, with hypertelorism, epicanthal folds, micrognathia, epidermoid cysts, hypotrichosis and hypertrophic frenula with clefts of the alveolar margin, lips and tongue. There is dystrophia canthorum, a broad nasal root and hypoplasia of the alar cartilage and malar bone (Maroteaux 1979).

OFD type I (Papillon-Leage) is clinically distinguished by cleft palate, frenular hypertrophy, thick alveolar bands, aplasia of nasal alae, ventral clefts and hamartomas of the tongue, dental anomalies, alopecia and evanescent milia in infancy. Mental retardation is seen in approximately 50% of the cases and is apparently associated with CNS malformations, such as agenesis of the corpus callosum. Polycystic renal anomalies have been seen in the kidneys of a number of autopsied cases.

OFD type II (Mohr) is clinically distinguished by normal intelligence, normal hair, normal teeth, no lateral oral frenula, conductive hearing loss, and short stature.

On X-ray, OFD type I is characterized by brachydactyly (due to short metacarpals, metatarsals and phalanges and usually showing an irregular distribution), clinodactyly, syndactyly, camptodactyly, cone-shaped epiphyses and an increased nasion-sella basion angle. Preaxial polydactyly has been seen in a few cases. In OFD type II, or Mohr syndrome, there is polysyndactyly of the toes, usually symmetrical with partial reduplication of the hallux, and postaxial polydactyly, primarily of the hand. Clinodactyly, brachydactyly, metaphyseal irregularity and flaring, and supernumerary sutures of the skull are also seen (Taybi & Lachman 1990).

OFD III is very similar to type I, but in addition has alternately see–saw winking of the eyelids.

OFD IV is a very similar to type II but in addition has short ribs, postaxial polydactyly, talipes, and severe tibial dysplasia. Both pre- and post-axial polydactyly are present.

OFD type I is inherited as an X–linked dominant trait with lethality in the male. All cases have been females with the exception of a phenotypic male who turned out to have an XXY karyotype. The other three forms of OFD appear to be inherited as autosomal recessive traits.

Differential diagnoses include Ellis-van Creveld syndrome, holoprosencephaly and frontonasal dysplasia.

Holt-Oram syndrome

The Holt-Oram syndrome is characterized by autosomal dominant inheritance (with penetrance of at least 90%), congenital heart disease and radial ray defects. The characteristic hand malformation is digitalization of a triphalangeal thumb so that the thumb is attached in the same plane as the other fingers. However in some cases the thumb is absent or rudimentary. In addition, the more severe cases show absence or hypoplasia of the radius, or even the ulna and humerus. Wrist radiographs are particularly important. Abnormal scaphoid bone and an abnormal first metacarpal to first distal phalanges ratio may identify otherwise apparently normal gene carriers (Gladstone & Sybert 1982). The most common cardiac defect is an atrial septal defect of the ostium secundum type. Cardiovascular abnormalities are also extremely variable. Other defects that have been described are patent ductus arteriosis, pulmonary hypertension, ventricular septal defect and transposition of the great vessels with a prolonged PR interval. Marked variability of limb and heart malformations may occur within the same family.

Complications are usually related to heart disease, and severe cases die within the first year of life (Kaufman et al 1974).

The bony changes which may be seen on X–ray are triphalangeal, hypoplastic, proximally placed or absent thumb, an abnormally shaped scaphoid bone, additional carpal bones or lack of ossification of the carpals, particularly the os centrale, a long ulnar styloid, carpal fusions, an apparent increase in length of the first metacarpal and shortening of the fifth middle phalanx with clinodactyly, a prominent or posterior projection of the medial epicondyle, clavicular hypoplasia, deformed humeral head and small rotated scapulae (Poznanski et al 1970a).

The Holt-Oram syndrome is distinct from other radial ray defect syndromes in that there are no abnormalities of the kidneys or gastrointestinal tract, no deafness, no ear malformations, no mental retardation and no specific haematological disorder. Differential diagnoses include Poland syndrome, heart-hand syndrome II (Tabatznik), Fanconi anaemia, TAR, the VACTERLS association and the thalidomide syndrome.

Focal femoral hypoplasia (proximal femoral focal deficiency, PFFD).

Variable deficiency of the proximal segment of the femur either unilaterally or bilaterally occurs with preservation of the distal part of the limb. There is a continuum of involvement starting most proximally, involving just the femoral head to involving the lower limb with complete absence of the femur. Severely involved cases may even fall into the femoral-fibula-ulna (FFU) complex. Some cases have unusual facies (see below). Typically, cases are sporadic with no known environmental insult.

When the pattern of long bone loss in the lower limb is analyzed, two specific patterns emerge: Femoral-Fibula-Ulna (FFU) complex and Femur-Tibia-Radius (FTR) complex. Among PFFD patients 50% also have a fibular deficiency and 25% have an ulna deficiency. Among these FFU patients usually all four limbs are involved, but there may be marked asymmetry to the point of appearing to be unilateral. Variations include coxa vara to complete femur absence, shortened ulna to humero-radial synostosis and small fibula to complete absence. Usually no spine or visceral anomalies are present. Hand and foot are relatively spared, but may also have a variety of anomalies (Goldberg 1987).

In the Femur-Tibia-Radius (FTR) pattern the deficiency at the distal end of the femur is most important. Loss of the tibia may be most striking, but any combination of loss may occur. This complex tends to involve specific genetic forms of lower limb deficiency as compared to PFFD and FFU which tend to be sporadic (Lewin & Opitz 1986). The FTR pattern was also seen in thalidomide embryopathy (Goldberg 1987).

Lewin and Opitz (1986) recently reviewed conditions with fibular aplasia or hypoplasia.

Femoral hypoplasia – unusual facies syndrome

A distinct pattern of malformation was characterized by Daentl et al in 1975 and was designated femoral hypoplasia – unusual facies syndrome (Fig. 59.9). Clinical features include femoral hypoplasia, usually on the severe end of the spectrum, and the unusual facial features of upslanting palpebral fissures, short nose with broad nasal tip, long philtrum, thin upper lip, micrognathia and cleft palate. In addition, renal anomalies, lower vertebral anomalies and deformed pelvis have been reported. With multiple surgery and the use of prosthetic devices, most patients are ambulatory and quite functional socially. Intelligence is completely normal. Occasionally with severe micrognathia, feeding and respiratory problems occur.

Some infants have been born to diabetic mothers, and the clinical similarities with the caudal regression syndrome might suggest a common aetiology (Assemany et al 1972). Shortening of the humerus, restricted motion at the elbows and Sprengel deformities found in some infants would suggest that this syndrome is not confined to the lower limbs and that a similar mechanism could be acting upon both upper and lower limbs. All reports so far have been of sporadic cases, but prenatal diagnosis could be offered for reassurance, using realtime ultrasound in an attempt to demonstrate presence of the femur.

Differential diagnosis includes proximal focal femoral hypoplasia without unusual facies, which is a relatively frequent sporadic orthopaedic anomaly.

Syndrome of multiple synostoses

The syndrome of multiple synostoses has been described as a highly variable dominant condition in which there can be synostosis of all the limb joints. Various combinations of synostoses can be seen within the family, with

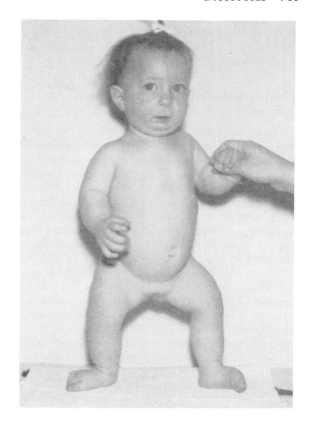

Fig. 59.9 Focal femoral hypoplasia with unusual facies syndrome. Note the short upper leg, short nose with broad nasal tip, long philtrum, thin upper lip, micrognathia and left equinovarus deformity of foot.

some affected individuals having nothing more than symphalangism while others may have fusion of elbows, wrists, fingers, metacarpals, metatarsals and coalition of the ankle bones (Herrmann 1974). Deafness may also be a feature, but characteristically fusions in the middle ear do not occur until adolescence. Growth is normally not affected. A typical facies has been described with a narrow nose, high nasal bridge, and hypoplasia of the alae nasi (Maroteaux 1979). As stated earlier, it is not yet clear whether this condition is distinct from autosomal dominant proximal symphalangism; however, the severity of involvement of distal phalanges (i.e. absence and hypoplasia of middle phalanges as well as consistency of carpal and tarsal coalitions) suggests it may be a distinct entity.

X-ray findings may show bony fusion of the joint, or early joint changes may be present simply as a narrowing of the joint space. The aetiological mechanism behind multiple synostoses is probably the same as for symphalangism. What determines which joints are affected is unknown. Differential diagnosis includes diastrophic dysplasia, fibrodysplasia ossificans, Pillay syndrome, Apert syndrome, Pfeiffer syndrome, brachydactylies A, B and C, and Emery-Nelson syndrome.

Hand-foot-genital syndrome (hand-foot-uterus syndrome)

The hand-foot-uterus syndrome is an autosomal dominantly inherited condition with variable expressivity (Poznanski et al 1970b). Clinical features include small feet with unusually short halluces and short abnormal thumbs. Females with the disorder have duplication anomalies of the genital tract and decreased fertility. Males have been reported with cryptorchidism and hypospadias; however, these seem to be distinct embryologically from the female genital duplication anomalies (Girdion & Prader 1976).

Radiographic findings include short first metacarpals and metatarsals, short fifth fingers with clinodactyly, trapezium-scaphoid fusion in the wrist, cuneiform-navicular fusion in the foot, an os centrale and a long ulnar styloid (Poznanski et al 1970b).

Genital tract anomalies are variable but are felt to represent different degrees of expression of the same underlying developmental problem. Duplication of the uterus varies in severity from a full double uterus to a uterus duplex unicornis. In addition, some patients have duplication of the cervix with septate vagina. These structural anomalies result in fertility complications; however normal pregnancies are possible.

Abnormalities are present at birth and can be detected by hysterosalpingogram, ultrasound or laparotomy. Congenital heart disease has been reported in some patients, therefore a careful cardiovascular examination is warranted.

Differential diagnosis includes Holt-Oram syndrome, trisomy 18, Ellis-van Creveld syndrome, and Cornelia de Lange syndrome.

Focal dermal hypoplasia (Goltz syndrome)

Focal dermal hypoplasia has been observed almost exclusively in females. It appears to be an X-linked dominant condition with lethality in males. Clinical features include cutaneous changes, skeletal defects, digital malformations, ocular anomalies and oral/dental anomalies (Ruiz et al 1974).

The most striking clinical features in all the cases of this syndrome are the widespread foci of dermal hypoplasia with herniation of fat (appearing as yellow-brown nodules), red streaking of the skin, and papillomas of the lips, gums, vulva and anus. The areas of dermal hypoplasia appear as atrophy or absence of skin, but the epidermis is intact. Telangiectasia and hypo- and hyperpigmentation are seen. Surgery is indicated for removal of lesions (e.g. angiofibromas) which are in areas prone to trauma. The hair is sparse, sometimes blonde or almost white in colour with patchy areas of alopecia. Nails may be absent, hypoplastic, dystrophic, spoon-shaped or grooved. Teeth are congenitally absent or malformed (Hall & Terezhal 1983).

Digital anomalies include syndactyly, polydactyly, camptodactyly and absence deformities. Most individuals are short in stature and have vertebral anomalies, kyphosis and scoliosis. The skull is described as rounded, and there is asymmetry of the face, trunk and limbs. A number of different ocular changes have been described. They include microphthalmia, colobomas, strabismus and nystagmus. The ears may be large and prominent. There is occasional mental retardation.

The degree of clinical severity varies widely. Some patients may have only skin changes or simply syndactyly, whereas others may show full manifestations of the syndrome with microphthalmus, bilateral coloboma of the iris, ectopia lentis, hypoplasia of the teeth and severe cutaneous, skeletal and digital malformations (Goltz et al 1970). Happle (Happle & Lenz 1977) has suggested the patchiness represents mosaicism with cell death of the cells which have the affected X activated. The rare cases of manifesting males would represent somatic mosaicism. The possibility of using fetoscopy for prenatal diagnosis exists, but has not been reported.

Differential diagnoses should include incontinentia pigmenti, congenital poikiloderma (Thomsen type), and naevus lipomatosus cutaneous superficialis.

Ulnar-mammary syndrome

The combination of ulnar ray defects, hypoplasia or aplasia of mammary glands, hypoplasia of nipples, hypoplasia of apocrine glands with reduction in body odour and genital anomalies in males, is reported to be inherited as a variably expressed autosomal dominant trait (Schinzel et al 1987).

The ulnar ray defect may be so mild as to involve only stiffness of the distal interphalangeal fifth finger joint or hypoplasia of the fifth fingernail, or may present with complete absence of one to three ulnar rays of fingers (Schinzel 1987). Carpals and tarsals may be involved, postaxial polydactyly may be seen and feet may show fibular hypoplasia of toes. Axillary and body hair is sparse, but pubic hair is normal. Nipple hypoplasia may lead to the inability to breast-feed. Affected males may have cryptorchidism, small penis and small testes with decreased sperm counts into adulthood. Male fertility is decreased.

Other visceral anomalies include subglottic stenosis, pyloric stenosis, anal stenosis, imperforate hymen, kidney malformations, hypodontia and pectoralis muscle hypoplasia.

REFERENCES

Aase J M, Smith D W 1969 Congenital anaemia and triphalangial thumbs: a new syndrome. Journal of Pediatrics 74: 471–474

Ahmad M, Abbas H, Haque S, Flatz G 1987 X–chromosomally inherited split hand/split foot anomaly in a Pakistani kindred. Human Genetics 75: 169–173

Assemany S, Muzzo S, Gardner L 1972 Syndrome of phocomelic diabetic embryopathy. American Journal of Diseases of Childhood 123: 489–491

Auerbach A, Adler B, Chaganti R S K 1981 Fanconi's anaemia: Prenatal diagnosis of 30 fetuses at risk. Pediatrics 76: 794–800

Ayme S,, Preus M 1986 Spondylocostal/spondylothoracic dysostosis: the clinical basis for prognosticating and genetic counselling. American Journal of Medical Genetics 24: 599–606

Baraitser M 1982 A new camptodactyly syndrome. Journal of Medical Genetics 19: 40–43

Baraitser M 1986 The orofaciodigital (OFD) syndromes. Journal of Medical Genetics 23: 116–119

Baraitser M, Burn J 1983 Recessively inherited brachydactyly type C. Journal of Medical Genetics 20: 128–129

Baraitser M, Burn J, Fixsen J 1983 A recessively inherited windmill-vane camptodactyly/ichthyosis syndrome. Journal of Medical Genetics 20: 125–127

Bartsocas C S, Kiossoglou K A, Papas C V, Xanthou-Tsingoglou M, Anagnostakis D E, Daskalopoulou H D 1974 Costovertebral dysplasia. Birth Defects X(9): 221–226

Beals R K, Eckhardt A L 1969 Hereditary Onycho-Osteodysplasia (Nail-Patella Syndrome). Journal of Bone and Joint Surgery 51–A: 505–515

Beighton P 1978 Inherited disorders of the skeleton. In: Emery A E H (ed) Genetics in medicine and surgery. Churchill Livingstone, New York

Beighton P, Horan F T 1981 Spondylocostal dysostosis in South African sisters. Clinical Genetics 19: 23–25

Beighton W M, Musgrave J E, Campbell R A et al 1973 The nephropathy of the nail-patella syndrome, clinicopathologic analysis of 11 kindred. The American Journal of Medicine 54: 304–320

Bell J 1951 On brachydactyly and symphalangism. In: Penrose L S (ed) Treasury of human inheritance. Cambridge University Press, London, 5: 1–31

Bennett W M, Musgrave J E, Campbell R A et al 1973 The nephropathy of nail-patella syndrome. American Journal of Medicine 54: 304–319

Bergsma D 1979 Birth defects compendium, 2nd edn. National Foundation March of Dimes. Alan Liss, New York

Berry A C 1987 Rubinstein-Taybi syndrome. Journal of Medical Genetic 24: 562–566

Bersu E T, Petterson J C, Charbonneau W J, Opitz J M 1976 Studies of malformation syndromes in man XXXXIA: Anatomical studies of the Hanhart syndrome – a pathologic hypothesis. European Journal of Pediatrics 122: 1–17

Birch-Jensen A 1949 Congenital deformities of the upper extremities. Ejnar Munsgaard, Copenhagen

Bodurtha J, Kessel A, Berman W, Hartenberg M 1986 Distinctive gastrointestinal anomaly associated with Coffin-Siris syndrome. Journal of Pediatrics 109: 1015–1017

Bouwes Bavinck J N, Weaver D D 1986 Subclavian artery supply disruption sequence: hypothesis of a vascular etiology for Poland, Klippel-Feil, and Mobius anomalies. American Journal of Medical Genetics 23: 903–918

Buttiens M, Fryns J P 1987 Apparently new autosomal recessive syndrome of mental retardation, distal limb deficiencies, oral involvement, and possible renal defect. American Journal of Medical Genetics 27: 651–660

Cantu J M, Urrusti J, Rosales G, Rojas A 1971 Evidence for autosomal recessive inheritance of costovertebral dysplasia. Clinical Genetics 2: 149–154

Cantu J M, Rivera H, Nazara Z, Rojas Q, Hernandez A, Garcia-Cruz D 1980 Guadalajara camptodactyly syndrome: A distinct probably autosomal recessive disorder. Clinical Genetics 18: 153–159

Cantu J M, Garcia-Cruz D, Gil-Viera J, Nazara Z, Ramirez M L, Sole-Pujol M T, Sanchez-Corona J 1985 Guadalajara camptodactyly syndrome type II. Clinical Genetics 28: 54–60

Carey J C, Hall B D 1978 The Coffin-Siris Syndrome: Five new cases including two siblings. American Journal of Diseases of Children. 132: 667–671

Casamassima A C, Morton C C, Nana W E, Kodroff M, Caldwell R, Kelley T, Wolf B 1981 Spondylocostal dysostosis associated with anal and urogenital anomalies in a mennonite sibship. American Journal of Medical Genetics 8: 117–127

Czeizel A, Brooser G 1986 A postaxial polydactyly and progressive myopia syndrome of autosomal dominant origin. Clinical Genetics 30: 406–408

Daentl D L, Smith D W, Scott C I, Hall B D, Gooding C A 1975 Femoral hypoplasia – unusual facies syndrome. Journal of Pediatrics 87: 107–111

David T J 1972 Nature and etiology of the Poland anomaly. New England Journal of Medicine 287: 487–489

David T J 1982 Familial Poland anomaly. Journal of Medical Genetics 19: 293–296

David T J, Glass A 1983 Hereditary costovertebral dysplasia with malignant cerebral tumour. Journal of Medical Genetics 20: 441–444

David T J, Winter R M 1985 Familial absence of the pectoralis major, serratus anterior, and latissimus dorsi muscles. Journal of Medical Genetics 22: 390–392

Der Kaloustian V M 1972 The Rubinstein-Taybi syndrome – clinical and muscle electron microscopy study. American Journal of Diseases of Children 123: 897

Dosik H et al 1970 Leukemia in Fanconi anaemia: cytogenetic and tumour virus susceptibility studies. Blood 3: 341–352

Duken J 1921 Ueber die Bezeihunger zwischen Assimilation Shypophalangie und Aplasie der Interphalangealgelenke. Virchows Archiv fur Pathologische Anatomie 233: 204

Duncan P A, Shapiro L R, Stangel J J, Klein R M, Addonizio J G 1979 The MURCS associate mullerian duct aplasia, renal aplasia and cervico/thoracic somite dyplasia. Journal of Pediatrics 95: 399–402

Edwards J A, Gale R P 1972 Camptobrachydactyl: A new autosomal dominant trait with two probable homozygotes. American Journal of Human Genetics 24: 464–474

Engber W D, Flatt A E 1977 Camptodactyly: An analysis of sixty six patients and twenty four operators. Journal of Hand Surgery 2: 216–224

Engel D 1943 The etiology of the undescended scapula and related syndromes. Journal of Bone and Joint Surgery 25: 613–625

Esparza A, Thompson W R 1966 Familial hypoplastic anaemia with multiple congenital anomalies (Fanconi syndrome) – report of three cases. Rhode Island Medical Journal 49: 103–110

Faulk W P, Epstein C J, Jones K L 1970 Familial posterior lumbosacral vertebral fusion and eyelid ptosis. American Journal of Diseases of Children 119: 510–512

Fitch N 1979 Classification and identification of inherited brachydactylies. Journal of Medical Genetics 16: 36–44

Flatt A 1977 Care of congenital hand anomalies. Mosby, New York

Franceschini P, Grassi E, Fabris C, Botetti G, Randaccio G 1974 The autosomal recessive form of spondylocostal dysostosis. Radiology 12: 673–675

Freire-Maia A 1981 Historical note: the extraordinary handless and footless families of Brazil – 50 years of acheiropodia. American Journal of Medical Genetics 9: 31–41

Freire-Maia A, Freire-Maia N, Morton N E, Azevedo E S, Quelce-Salgado A 1975 Genetics of archeiropodia (the handless and footless families of Brazil). VI. Formal genetic analysis. American Journal of Human Genetics 27: 521–527

Freire-Maia A, Laredo-Filho J, Freire-Maia N 1978 Genetics of acheiropodia (the handless and footless families of Brazil) X: Radiologic study. American Journal of Medical Genetics 2: 330–341

Fryns J P 1987 Congenital scalp defects with distal limb reduction anomalies. Journal of Medical Genetics 24: 493–496

Fryns J P, Van den Berghe H 1979 Congenital scalp defects associated with postaxial polydactyly. Human Genetics 49: 217–219

Garner L D, Bixler D 1969 Micrognathia, an associated defect of Hanhart syndrome, types II and III. Oral Surgery 27: 601–606

Girdion A, Prader A 1976 Hand-foot-uterus (HFU) syndrome with hypospadius: The hand-foot genital (HFG) syndrome. Pediatric Radiology 4: 96–102

Gladstone I, Sybert V P 1982 Holt-Oram Syndrome: penetrance of the gene and lack of maternal effect. Clinical Genetics 21: 98–103

Glanz A, Fraser F C 1982 Spectrum of anomalies in Fanconi anaemia. Journal of Medical Genetics 19: 412–416

Goldberg M J 1987 The Dysmorphic Child: an orthopedic perspective. Raven Press, New York

Goldberg M J, Mazzei R J 1977 Poland syndrome: a concept of pathogenesis based on limb bud embryology. Birth Defects 13 (3D): 102–115

Goltz R W, Henderson R R, Hitch J M, Ott J E 1970 Focal dermal hypoplasia syndrome. A review of the literature and report of two cases. Archives of Dermatology 101: 1–11

Gorlin R J, Pindborg J J, Cohen M M 1976 Syndromes of the head and neck, 2nd edn. McGraw-Hill, New York

Graham J M, Brown F E, Struckmeyer C L, Hallowell C 1986 Dominantly inherited unilateral terminal transverse defects of the hand (adactylia) in twin sisters and one daughter. Pediatrics 78: 103–106

Gray E, Hurt V K 1984 Inheritance of brachydactyly D. Journal of Heredity 75: 297–299

Grebe H 1964 Missbildungen der Gliedmassen. In: Becker P E (ed) Humangenetik II. Georg Thieme, Stuttgart.

Gunderson C H, Greenspan R H, Glaser G H, Lubs H A 1967 The Klippel-Feil syndrome: genetic and clinical reevaluation of cervical fusion. Medicine 46(6): 491–511

Hall E H, Terezhal G T 1983 Focal dermal hypoplasia. Journal of the American Academy of Dermatology 9: 443–451

Hall J G 1987 Thrombocytopenia and absent radius (TAR) syndrome. Journal of Medical Genetics 24: 79–83

Hall J G, Levin J, Kuhn J P Ottenheimer E J, van Berkun K A P, McKusick V A 1969 Thrombocytopenia with absent radius. Medicine 48–411

Hall J G, Pallister P D, Claaren S K et al 1980 Congenital hypothalmic hamartoblastoma, hypopituitarism, imperforate anus, and postaxial polydactyly – a new syndrome Part I: clinical, causal and pathogenetic considerations. American Journal of Medical Genetics 11: 185–239

Hall J G, Reed S D, Greene G 1982 Distal arthrogryposis: a newly recognized condition with distal congenital contractures and its variants. American Journal of Medical Genetics 11: 185–239

Happle R, Lenz W 1977 Striation of bones in focal dermal hypoplasia: manifestation of functional mosaicism. British Journal of Dermatology 96: 133–137

Haspeslagh M, Fryns J P, Van den Berghe H 1984 The Coffin-Siris Syndrome: Report of a family and further delineation. Clinical Genetics 26: 374–378

Helmi C, Pruzansky S 1980 Cranio-facial and extra cranial malformations in the Klippel-Feil syndrome. Cleft Palate Journal 17: 65–69

Hennekam R C M, Beemer F A, Huijbers W A R, Hustinx P A, Van Sprang F J 1985 The cerebro-costo-mandibular syndrome: third report of familial occurrence. Clinical Genetics 28: 118–121

Herrmann J 1974 Symphalangism and brachydactyly syndrome. Report of WL symphalangism-brachydactyly syndrome: Review of literature and classification. Birth Defects 10(5): 23–53

Herrmann J, Opitz J M 1977 The SC phocomelia and the Roberts syndrome: Nogologic aspects. European Journal of Pediatrics 125: 117–134

Higginbottom M C, Jones K L, Kung F H, Koch T K, Boyer J L 1978 The Aase syndrome in a female infant. Journal of Medical Genetics 15: 484–486

Hodgson S V, Chiu D C 1981 Dominant transmission of Sprengel's shoulder and cleft palate. Journal of Medical Genetics 18: 263–265

Hoyme H, Lyons Jones K, Nyhan W L, Pauli R M, Robinow M 1987 Autosomal dominant ectrodactyly and absence of long bones of upper or lower limbs: Further clinical delineation. Journal of Pediatrics 111: 538–543

Hunter A G, Cox D, Rudd N 1976 The genetics of and associated clinical findings in humero-radial synostosis. Clinical Genetics 9: 470–478

Jones K L, Hall B D, Hall J G, Ebbins A J, Massaud H, Smith D W 1974 A pattern of cranio-facial and limb defects secondary to aberrant tissue bands. Journal of Pediatrics 84: 90–95

Kaufman R, Rimoin D, McAlister W, Hartman A 1974 Variable expression of the Holt-Oram syndrome. American Journal of Diseases of Children 127: 21–25

Keutel J, Kinderman I, Mockel H 1970 Eine wahrscheinlich autosomal recessiv vertebti Skeletmissbildung mit Humeroradial synostose. Humangenetik 9: 43–53

Kirkham T H 1969 Cervico-oculo-acusticus syndrome with pseudopapilloedema. Archives of Disease in Childhood 44: 504–508

Koiffmann C P, Wajntal A, Huyke B J, Castro R M 1988 Congenital scalp skull defects with distal limb anomalies

(Adams-Oliver syndrome – McKusick 10030): Further suggestion of autosomal recessive inheritance. American Journal of Medical Genetics 29: 263–268

Langer L O, Herrmann J 1974 The cerebrocostomandibular syndrome. Birth Defects 10(4): 167–170

Lenz W, Rehmann I 1976 Distale Symphalangien mit Humeroradialsynostose Karpalsynostosen und Brachyphalangie des Daumens: ein dominantes Syndrome Zeitschrift Orthopedic 114: 202–211

Leroy J G, Devos E A, Vanden-Bulcke L J, Robbe N S 1981 Cerebro-costo-mandibular syndrome with autosomal dominant inheritance. Journal of Pediatrics 99: 441–443

Lewin S O, Opitz J M 1986 Fibular A/hypoplasia: Review and documentation of the fibular developmental field. American Journal of Medical Genetics Supplement 2: 215–238

Lucas G L, Opitz J M, Wiffler C 1966 Nail-Patella Syndrome Journal of Pediatrics 68: 273–287

Lucaya J, Garcia-Conesar J A, Bosch-Banyeras J M, Pono-Peradejordi G 1981 The Coffin Siris Syndrome: A report of four cases and review of the literature. Pediatric Radiology 11: 35–38

Luthy D, Hall J G, Graham B 1979 The use of fetal radiography in the prenatal diagnosis of thrombocytopenia with absent radius. Clinical Genetics 15: 495–499

McKusick V A 1988 Mendelian inheritance in man. Johns Hopkins University Press, Baltimore

McNicholl B, Egan-Mitchell B, Murray J P, Doyle J F, Kennedy J D, Crone L 1970 Cerebro-costo-mandibular syndrome. Archives of Disease in Childhood 45: 421–424

Majewski F, Lenz W, Pfeiffer R A, Tunte W 1972 Das oro-facio-digitale Syndrome. Zeitschrift Fur Kinderheilkunde 112: 89–112

Maroteaux P 1979 Bone diseases of children. J P Lippincott, Philadelphia

Maroteaux P 1983 Nomenclature des maladies osseuses constitutionnelles. Annales de Radiologie 26: 456–462

Merlob P, Schonfeld A, Grunebaum M, Mor N, Reisner S 1987 Autosomal dominant cerebro-costo mandibular syndrome: ultrasonographic and clinical findings. American Journal of Medical Genetics 26: 195–202

Morita T, Laughlin L, Kawrano K, Kimmelstiel P, Suzuki Y, Churg J 1973 Nail Patella syndrome. Archives of Internal Medicine 131: 271–277

Nagib M G, Maxwell R E, Chou S N 1985 Klippel-Feil syndrome in children: Clinical features and management. Child's Nervous System 1: 255–263

Nevin N C, Burrows D, Allen G, Kernokan D C 1975 Aglossia-adactylia syndrome. Journal of Medical Genetics 12: 89–93

Norum R A, McKusick V A 1969 Costovertebral anomalies with apparent recessive inheritance. Birth Defects 5: 326–329

Ohdo S, Yamauchi Y, Hayakawa K 1981 Distal symphalangism associated with camptodactyly. Journal of Medical Genetics 18: 456–458

Osebold W R, Remondini D J, Lester E L, Spranger J W, Opitz J M 1985 An autosomal dominant syndrome of short stature with mesomelic shortness of limbs, abnormal carpal and tarsal bones, hypoplastic middle phalanges, and bipartite calcanei. American Journal of Medical Genetics 22: 791–809

Otter G D 1970 Bilateral Sprengel's syndrome with situs inversus totalis. Acta Orthopaedica Scandinavica 41: 402–410

Pagnan N A B, Gollop R T, Lederman H 1988 The Tel Hashomer Camptodactyly Syndrome: Report of a New Case

and Review of Literature. American Journal of Medical Genetics 29: 411–417

Penchaszadeh V B, De Negrotti T C 1976 Ectrodactyly-ectodermal dysplasia-clefting (EEC) syndrome: dominant inheritance and variable expression. Journal of Medical Genetics 13: 281–284

Perez-Comas A, Garcia-Castro J M 1974 Occipito-facial-cervico-thoracic-abdomino-digital dysplasia: Jarcho-Levin syndrome of vertebral anomalies. Journal of Pediatrics 85: 388–391

Pfeiffer R A, Ambs E 1983 Das Aase-Syndrom: autosomal-rezessiv vererbte, konnatal insuffiziente Erythropoese und Triphalangie der Daumen. Monatsschrift fur Kinderheilkunde 131: 235–237

Pilarski R T, Pauli R M, Bresnick G H, Lebovitz R M 1985 Karsch-Neugebauer syndrome: split foot/split hand and congenital nystagmus. Clinical Genetics 27: 97–101

Poor M A, Alberti O, Gricom N T, Driscoss S G, Holmes L B 1983 Nonskeletal malformations in one of three siblings with Jarcho-Levin syndrome of vertebral anomalies. Journal of Pediatrics 103: 270–272

P.O.S.S.U.M. version 1.0 1987 The Murdoch Institute for Research into Birth Defects, Computer Power Pty Ltd., Melbourne

Poznanski A 1974 The hand in radiologic diagnosis. W G Saunders, Philadelphia

Poznanski A, Gall J, Stern A 1970a Skeletal manifestations of the Holt-Oram syndrome. Radiology 94: 45–53

Poznanski A K, Stern A M, Gall J C 1970b Radiographic findings in the hand-foot-uterus syndrome (HFUS). Radiology 95: 129–134

Poznanski A K, Werder E A, Giedion A, Martin A, Shaw H 1977 The pattern of shortening of the bones of the hand in PHP and PPHP – A comparison with brachydactyly E, Turner syndrome, and acrodysostosis. Pediatric Radiology 123: 707–717

Pries C, Mittelman D, Miller M, Solomon L M, Pashayan H M, Pruzansky S 1974 The EEC Syndrome. American Journal of Diseases of Children 127: 840–844

Reynolds J F, Barber J C, Alford B A, Chandler J G, Kelly T E 1983 Familial Hirschsprung's disease and type D brachydactyly: A report of four affected males in two generations. Pediatrics 71: 246–249

Riccardi V M, Holmes L B 1974 Brachydactyly Type E: Hereditary shortening of digits, metacarpals, metatarsals and long bones. Journal of Pediatrics 84: 251–254

Rimoin D L, Fletcher B D, McKusick V A 1968 Spondylocostal dysplasia. American Journal of Medicine 45: 948–953

Rogers J G, Levin L S, Dorst J P, Temtamy S M 1977 A postaxial polydactyly-dental-vertebral syndrome. Journal of Pediatrics 90: 230–235.

Rollnick B R, Hoo J J 1988 Genitourinary anomalies are a component manifestation in the ectodermal dysplasia, ectrodactyly, cleft lip/palate (EEC) syndrome. American Journal of Medical Genetics 29: 131–136

Romke C, Froster-Iskenius U, Heyne K et al 1987 Roberts syndrome and SC phocomelia. A single genetic entity. Clinical Genetics 321: 170–177

Rosenmann A, Shapiro T, Cohen M M 1976 Ectrodactyly, ectodermal dysplasia and cleft palate (EEC): Report of a family and review of the literature. Clinical Genetics 9: 347–353

Rubinstein J H 1969 The broad thumbs syndrome – progress report 1968. Birth Defects 5 (2): 25

Ruiz M R, Carnevale A, Tamayo L, de Montiel E M 1974

Focal dermal hypoplasia. Clinical Genetics 6: 36–45

Sackey K, Odone V, George S L, Murphy S B 1984 Poland's syndrome associated with childhood non-Hodgkin's lymphoma. American Journal of Diseases of Children 138: 600–601

Say B, Gerald P S 1968 A New Polydactyly/Imperforate-Anus/Vertebral-Anomalies Syndrome? Lancet September 21: 688

Schinzel A 1987 Ulnar-mammary syndrome. Journal of Medical Genetics 24: 778–781

Schinzel A, Illig R, Prader A 1987 The ulnar-mammary syndrome: an autosomal dominant pleiotropic gene. Clinical Genetics 32: 160–168

Schnur R E, Eunpu D L, Zackal E H 1987. Thrombocytopenia with absent radius in a boy and his uncle. American Journal of Medical Genetics 28: 117–123

Schroeder T M, Tilgen D, Jruger J, Vogel F 1976 Formal genetics of Fanconi anaemia. Human Genetics 32: 257–288

Silverman F N, Strefling A M, Stevenson D K, Lazarus J 1980 Cerebro-Costo-Mandibular syndrome. Journal of Pediatrics 97: 406–416

Smith D W 1982 Recognizable patterns of human malformation, 3rd edn. Saunders, Philadelphia

Soltan H C, Holmes L B 1986 Familial occurrence of malformations possibly attributable to vascular abnormalities. Journal of Pediatrics 108: 112–113

Spranger J, Benirschke K, Hall J G et al 1982 Errors of morphogenesis: Concepts and terms. Journal of Pediatrics 100: 160–165

Spritz R A 1978 Familial radioulnar synostosis. Journal of Medical Genetics 15: 160–162

Stark E W, Borton T E 1973 Klippel-Feil syndrome and associated hearing loss. Archives of Orolaryngology 97: 415–419

Steinberg A G, Reynolds E L 1948 Further data on symphalangism. Journal of Heredity 39: 23–27

Stevenson R E, Scott C I, Epstein M 1975 Dominantly inherited ulnar drift. Birth Defects 11(5): 75

Strasburger A K, Hawkins M R, Eldridge R, Hargrave R L, McKusick V A 1965 Symphalangism: genetic and clinical aspects. Bulletin of Johns Hopkins 117: 108–127

Sundaram V, Taysi K, Hartmann A F, Schaekilford G D, Risting J P 1982 Hyperphalangy and clinodactyly of index finger with Pierre Robin anomaly: Catel Manzke syndrome: a case report and review of the literature. Clinical Genetics 21: 407–410

Swift M R, Hirschhorn K 1971 Fanconi anaemia. Annals of Internal Medicine 65: 496–503

Sybert V P, Byers P H, Hall J G 1979 Variable expression in a dominantly inherited skeletal dysplasia with similarities to brachydactyly E and spondyloepiphyseal-spondyloperipheral dysplasia. Clinical Genetics 15: 160–166

Taybi H, Lachman R 1990 Radiology of syndromes, metabolic disorders and skeletal dysplasias, 3rd edn. Year Book Medical Publishers, Chicago

Temtamy S A, McKusick V A 1978 The genetics of hand malformations. Birth Defects XIV (3)

Thompson E M, Winter R M, Williams M J H 1986 A male infant with the Catel-Manzke syndrome and dislocatable knees. Journal of Medical Genetics 23: 271–275

Tolmie J L, Whittle M J, McNay M B, Gibson A A M, Connor J M 1987 Second trimester prenatal diagnosis of the Jarcho-Levin syndrome. Prenatal Diagnosis 7: 129–134

Tomkin D J, Sisken J E 1984 Abnormalities in the cell-division cycle in Roberts syndrome fibroblasts. American Journal of Human Genetics 36: 1332–1340

Toriello H V, Graff R G, Florentine M F, Lacina S, Moore W D 1988 Scalp and limb defects with cutis marmorata telangiectatica congentita: Adams Oliver syndrome? Journal of Medical Genetics 29: 269–276

Trindade C E P, de Nobrega F J 1977 Spondylothoracic dysplasia in two siblings. Clinical Pediatrics 16: 1097–1099

Valdueza A F 1973 The nail-patella syndrome. A report of three families. Journal of Bone and Joint Surgery 55b: 145–162

Verma I C, Joseph R, Bhargava S, Mehta S 1976 Split-hand and split-foot deformity inherited as an autosomal recessive trait. Clinical Genetics 9: 8–14

Ward R E, Bixler D, Provisor A J, Bader P 1986 Parent to child transmission of the thrombocytopenia absent radius (TAR) syndrome. American Journal of Medical Genetics Supplement 2: 207–214

Warkany J 1971 Congenital Malformations Yearbook, Chicago

Welch J P, Temtamy S A 1966 Hereditary contractures of the fingers (camptodactyly). Journal of Medical Genetics 3: 104–112

Weyers H, Thier C V 1978 Malformations mandibulofaciales et delimitation d'un syndrome oculo-vertébral. Journal de Genetique Humaine 7: 143–173

Wiedemann H R, Grossi K R, Dibbern H 1985 An Atlas of Characteristic Syndromes. Wolfe, London

Wilson M G, Mikity V G, Shinno N W 1971 Dominant inheritance of Sprengel's deformity. Journal of Pediatrics 79: 818–821

Winter R, Baraitser M, Somerville L 1985 Syndrome Program, Version 1.3 U.K. Medical Research Council & Institute of Child Health

Wynne-Davies R 1975 Congenital vertebral anomalies: aetiology and relationship to spina bifida cystica. Journal of Medical Genetics 12: 280–288

Yakish S D, Fu F H 1983 Long-term follow-up of the treatment of a family with nail-patella syndrome. Journal of Pediatric Orthopedics 3: 360–363

Zadek 1934 Congenital absence of the extensor pollicus longus of both thumbs. Operation and cure. Journal of Bone and Joint Surgery 16: 432–434

60. Arthrogryposes (multiple congenital contractures)

J. G. Hall

INTRODUCTION

Arthrogryposis multiplex congenita (AMC) is a term which has been used for almost a century to describe conditions with non-progressive multiple congenital joint contractures. The conditions which have been called arthrogryposis range from well-known syndromes to non-specific combinations of joint contractures. The term has become descriptive rather than diagnostic, and is now used in connection with a very heterogenous group of patients and disorders, all of which have in common multiple congenital joint contractures.

Although arthrogryposis is said to be a rare condition with an incidence of 1 in 5–10 000 liveborn, many kinds of congenital contractures, such as club feet and dislocated hips, are relatively common. One in 100–200 infants is born with some type of congenital contracture. The term arthrogryposis implies a more generalised involvement, with multiple joints having congenital contractures, and is most often reserved for non-progressive conditions which involve more than one part of the body.

The medical literature on arthrogryposis (multiple congenital joint contractures) is very confusing. Over the last 50 years, more than 300 articles have been published describing what is said to be arthrogryposis, but the term has been used very loosely, first as a diagnostic term, but more recently as a clinical sign or as a general category of disorders. In addition to the imprecise use of the term, the medical literature on arthrogryposis is confusing because many authors fail to describe clinical features of their cases. They have often lumped together a number of patients with congenital contractures who in actuality represent many different specific entities, and have then made generalisations about recurrence, management, prognosis and treatment. This chapter will attempt to sort out some of the major known clinical entities with congenital contractures, to describe a clinical approach to distinguishing heterogeneity, to discuss the investigation of the individual with congenital contractures, and to make some comments about genetics, recurrence risk, prenatal diagnosis and therapy.

It has become increasingly apparent, both from animal studies (Drachman & Coulombre 1962, DeMyer & Baird 1969, Moessinger 1983) and from human work (Smith 1982, Swinyard & Bleck 1985, Goldberg 1987) that anything which leads to decreased movement in utero may also lead to congenital contractures or fixation of joints which will then be present at birth.

The studies of Drachman and Coulombre (1962) demonstrated that temporary paralysis by curarisation of chick embryos at various times in development resulted in multiple congenital contractures. The immobilised chick developed fixation of various joints, depending on the time in morphogenesis that immobilisation occurred. DeMyer and Baird (1969) have shown that removal of amniotic fluid during gestation in rats could lead to limitation of movement of joints and subsequent contractures at birth. Moessinger (1983) noted that rat fetuses which had been paralysed in utero by curare developed a set of anomalies he designated the 'fetal akinesia deformation sequence.' He noted that these findings were similar to anomalies seen in the human Pena-Shokeir syndrome (Type 1) including multiple joint contractures, pulmonary hypoplasia, micrognathia, intrauterine growth retardation, short umbilical cord and polyhydramnios. These clinical features are seen in a number of specific conditions (Hall 1986). When any one of them is present the others should be looked for.

It appears that any process which limits movement during development of fetus or embryo may lead to congenital contractures. The in utero process may well be similar to the postnatal process of wearing a cast for a broken bone. When the cast is taken off, there is usually residual limitation of movement in joints which were immobilised. Swinyard (1982) has called this a 'collagenic response' with thickening of the joint capsule and fibre deposition in muscle tissue. The growing embryo or fetus which has superimposed limitation of movement

989

may develop even more marked contractures because the process of growth appears to accentuate the contractures. In this regard, most congenital contractures may be considered deformations rather than primary malformations (Spranger et al 1982). The timing during development probably plays a critical role in the severity of contractures, in the position of joints, and in the secondary changes which may occur in other organ systems (Hall 1986).

The potential causes of limitation of movement in utero fall into four categories: (1) *myopathic* processes including myopathies and abnormal muscle structure or function, such as absence of muscles and congenital myopathies; (2) *neuropathic* processes including abnormalities in nerve structure or function, either central or peripheral, such as meningomyelocele, failure of nerves to form, migrate or myelinate, and congenital neuropathies; (3) abnormal *connective tissue* including joint and tendon abnormalities, such as diastrophic dysplasia or abnormal tendon attachments; and (4) *limitation* of space or restriction of movement within the uterus, such as in the case of twins (Schinzel et al 1979), structural anomalies of the uterus, amniotic bands or chronic leakage of amniotic fluid.

APPROACH

An approach to sorting out various types of congenital contractures (Table 60.1) includes taking a careful history of the pregnancy and delivery, full family history, a detailed physical examination with definition and documentation of what parts of the body are involved in the process, a natural history of complications and response to therapy, laboratory data such as muscle biopsies, autopsy including CNS histopathology and chromosome studies, and photographs at various ages.

Table 60.1   Approach to congenital contractures

A. Clinical evaluation

I History

1. Pregnancy (anything decreasing in utero movement leads to congenital contractures)
   a. Illness in mother, chronic or acute (diabetes, myasthenia gravis, myotonic dystrophy, etc)
   b. Infections (rubella, rubeola, coxsackie, enterovirus, Akabane)
   c. Fever (above 39°C, determine timing in gestation)
   d. Nausea (viral encephalitis)
   e. Drugs (curare, robaxin, alcohol, dilantin, addictive drugs)
   f. Fetal movement (polyhydramnios, fetal kicking in one place, 'rolling' decreased)
   g. Oligohydramnios, chronic leakage
   h. Trauma during pregnancy (blow to the abdomen, attempted termination)
   i. Other complications during pregnancy such as bleeding, abnormal lie, threatened abortion.

2. Delivery history
   a. Presentation (breech, transverse)
   b. Length of gestation
   c. Initiation of labour
   d. Length of labour
   e. Traumatic delivery (limb, CNS)
   f. Intrauterine mass (twin, fibroid)
   g. Abnormal uterine structure or shape
   h. Abnormal placenta or membranes
   i. Time of year, geographical location.

3. Family history
   a. Marked variability within family
   b. Change with time – degenerate vs. improve
   c. Increased incidence of congenital contractures in second- and third-degree relatives

   d. Hyperextensibility or hypotonia present in family member
   e. R/O myotonic dystrophy, myasthenia gravis in parents (particularly mother)
   f. Consanguinity
   g. Advanced paternal age
   h. Increased stillbirths or miscarriages.

II Newborn evaluation

1. Description of contractures
   a. Which limbs and joints
   b. Proximal vs. distal
   c. Flexion vs. extension
   d. Amount of limitation (fixed vs. passive vs. active movement)
   e. Characteristic position at rest
      PHOTOGRAPHS!!
   f. Severity (firm vs. some give)
   g. Complete fusion or ankylosis vs soft tissue contracture.

2. Other anomalies (contractures are most obvious, look carefully for other anomalies)
   a. Deformities
      (i)   Genitalia (cryptorchid, lack of labia, microphallus)
      (ii) Limbs (pterygium, shortening, webs, cord wrapping, absent patella, dislocated radial heads, dimples)
      (iii) Jaw (micrognathia, trismus)
      (iv) Facies (asymmetry, flat bridge of nose, haemangioma)
      (v)   Scoliosis
      (vi) Dermatoglyphics (absent, distorted, crease abnormalities)

Table 60.1 Approach to congenital contractures (*contd.*)

(vii) Hernias, inguinal and umbilical
(viii) Other features of fetal akinesia sequence:
    (aa) intrauterine growth retardation
    (bb) pulmonary hypoplasia
    (cc) craniofacial anomalies (hypertelorism, cleft palate, depressed tip of nose, high bridge of nose)
    (dd) functional short gut with feeding problem.

b. Malformations
  (i) Eyes (small, corneal opacities, malformed, ptosis, strabismus)
  (ii) CNS (structural malformation, seizures, MR)
  (iii) Palate (high, cleft, submucous)
  (iv) Limb (deletion anomalies, radioulnar synostosis)
  (v) GU (structural anomalies of kidneys, ureters and bladder)
  (vi) Skull (craniosynostosis, asymmetry, microcephaly)
  (vii) Heart (congenital anomalies vs. cardiomyopathy)
  (viii) Lungs (hypoplasia vs. weak muscles or hypoplastic diaphragm)
  (ix) Tracheal and laryngeal clefts and stenosis
  (x) Changes in vasculature, haemangiomas, cutis marmorata, blue cold distal limbs
  (xi) Other visceral anomalies.

3. Other features
  a. Neurological examination (detailed)
    (i) Vigorous vs. lethargic
    (ii) Deep tendon reflexes (present vs. absent, slow vs. fast)
    (iii) Sensory intact or not.
  b. Muscle
    (i) Mass (normal vs. decreased)
    (ii) Texture (soft vs. firm)
    (iii) Fibrous bands
    (iv) Normal tendon attachments or not
    (v) Change with time.
  c. Connective tissue
    (i) Skin (soft, doughy, thick, extensible)
    (ii) Subcutaneous (decreased fat, increased fat)
    (iii) Hernias (inguinal, umbilical, diaphragmatic)
    (iv) Joints (thickness, symphalangism)
    (v) Tendon attachment and length.

III Course

1. Changes with time
  a. Developmental landmarks (motor vs. social and language)
  b. Growth of affected limbs
  c. Progression of contractures
  d. Lethal vs. CNS damage vs. stable vs. improvement
  e. Asymmetry (decreases or progresses)
  f. Trunk vs. limb changes
  g. Intellectual abilities
  h. Socialization.

2. Response to therapy
  a. Spontaneous improvement
  b. Response to physical therapy
  c. Response to casting
  d. Which surgery at which time
  e. Development of motor strength proportionate to limb size.

B. Laboratory evaluation

1. Tests
  a. Documentation of range of motion and position with photographs
  b. X-rays if:
    (i) bony anomalies (gracile, fusions, extra or missing carpals and tarsals)
    (ii) disproportionate
    (iii) scoliosis
    (iv) ankylosis
  c. CAT scan to evaluate CNS or muscle mass
  d. Ultrasonic evaluation of CNS or other viscera for anomalies or to establish potential muscle tissue
  e. MRI for presence of muscle mass obscured by contractures
  f. Chromosomes if:
    (i) multiple system involvement
    (ii) CNS abnormality (eye, microcephaly, MR, lethargic, degenerative)
    (iii) consider fibroblasts if lymphocytes were normal and patient has MR with no diagnosis
  g. Viral cultures $+/-$ specific antibodies in newborn or IgM levels
  h. Muscle biopsy in normal *and* affected areas at time of surgery in order to distinguish myopathic from neuropathic (do special histopathology and electron micrographic studies) – if CPK or unusual muscle response, do muscle biopsy earlier
  i. EMG in normal and affected area
  j. Nerve conduction in normal and affected area
  k. CPK if:
    (i) generalized weakness
    (ii) doughy or decreased muscle mass
    (iii) progressively worse
  l. Eye examination (opacities, retinal degeneration).

2. Autopsy
  a. Visceral anomalies
  b. CNS - brain neuropathology
  c. Spinal cord (number and size of anterior horn cells, presence or absence of tracts at various levels)
  d. Ganglion, peripheral nerve
  e. Eye (neuropathology)
  f. Muscle tissue from different muscle groups (EM & special stains)
  h. Fibrous bands replacing muscle
  i. Tendon attachments
  j. Other malformations, deformations or disruptions.

This kind of evaluation has proven to be important and necessary in distinguishing different types of arthrogryposis. Thus, in the course of the investigation of a patient with congenital contractures, definition of all these areas will be helpful in arriving at a specific diagnosis.

Histories

Pregnancy history, delivery history and family history are all extremely important, and several particular points should be kept in mind in their analysis.

Pregnancy history

The pregnancies of infants with multiple congenital contractures do have an increased frequency of complications (Fahy & Hall 1989). The question of intrauterine infections should always be considered in the evaluation of infants with congenital contractures, particularly with neurological impairment. Not infrequently, the mother has had an infection which could have led to secondary CNS damage and she is not even aware of it. It is appropriate to do IgM studies in the newborn with congenital contractures looking for increased levels which would indicate intrauterine infection and, in addition, specific titres can be measured (coxsackie, enterovirus, Akabane virus, etc.). Seasonal and geographical variables may be indicators of the particular viral infection which should be investigated. Maternal fever above 39°C for an extended period may lead to CNS damage. Secondary contractures may occur in the fetus because of abnormal nerve growth or migration associated with maternal hyperthermia (Smith et al 1978). Chronic maternal illness such as diabetes mellitus, myotonic dystrophy or myasthenia gravis are important because they have been associated with arthrogryposis in the newborn. A history of nausea in the mother is of importance as a high frequency of pregnancies which result in congenital contractures have been noted to be associated with excessive nausea at various times in pregnancy (Fahy & Hall 1989). It is not known whether the nausea is due to a maternal viral infection or to discomfort or irritation because of an abnormal positioning of the fetus. Both need to be considered. Use of drugs by the mother during the pregnancy which might lead to decreased movement of the fetus such as muscle relaxants, or drugs which may lead to potential CNS damage and secondarily affect fetal movement such as alcohol or vasoconstrictors, should be asked about specifically when taking a pregnancy history (Hall & Reed 1982, Swinyard 1982).

A careful pregnancy history frequently indicates abnormal fetal movement (decreased movement, movement in only one area, or a 'swimming motion').

Polyhydramnios during the pregnancy may indicate fetal compromise, e.g. that the fetus is not swallowing normally. Together with hydrops it is a poor prognostic sign. Oligohydramnios or chronic leakage of fluid may cause fetal constraint and secondary deformational contractures. An abnormal fetal lie may be a clue to intrauterine joint contractures. Prenatal diagnosis is possible using realtime ultrasonic evaluation of the fetus looking for movement. Since management of the pregnancy may be altered if arthrogryposis is diagnosed prenatally, the diagnosis should be considered in the face of an abnormal lie or polyhydramnios.

Delivery history

Delivery history is usually abnormal either because of an abnormal presentation or difficulty in delivery due to the fixed joints. It is not unusual for a fracture to occur during delivery (probably 5–10% of the time, Goldberg 1987). The presence of fractures in the newborn with arthrogryposis certainly does not specifically imply fragile bones, although some affected individuals do have thin gracile bones, particularly those with long-standing disuse. Babies with congenital contractures have been erroneously diagnosed as osteogenesis imperfecta by inexperienced individuals simply on the basis of fractures. The length of gestation is usually normal, although certain conditions with congenital contractures such as trisomy 18 may go post-delivery date, and other factors such as congenital infections and rupture of membranes may lead to early delivery. The length of labour is often prolonged because of difficulty in actually delivering due to the unusual position of the joints. Breech and transverse positioning are relatively common. Both CNS and limb trauma occur not infrequently during delivery. Many pregnancies end up needing caesarian sections.

Careful examination of the uterus for structural uterine anomalies or a uterine mass such as a fibroid is important if caesarian section is performed. The placenta, membranes, and cord insertion need to be examined looking for amniotic bands or signs of vascular compromise. The umbilical cord may be shortened or wrapped around a limb and may actually lead to compression of that limb.

Family history

A careful family history is important. There is marked variability within families as to severity of contractures; congenital contractures may actually have worked themselves out by the time parents of an affected child reach adulthood. Frequently family members have other kinds of tissue abnormalities such as hyperextensibility, dislocated joints, club feet and dislocated hips (Hall 1985). A surprising number of children with arthrogryposis have their multiple congenital contractures secondary to specific complications of a known genetic disorder. For instance, congenital contractures are occasionally seen in association with tuberous sclerosis and neurofibromatosis. Infants with multiple congenital contractures are born more often than by chance to mothers affected with myotonic dystrophy, myasthenia gravis and multiple sclerosis. Thus, careful family histories with special attention to relevant disorders should be taken. Consanguinity, multiple stillbirths or miscarriages and advanced paternal age should be asked about.

Physical examination

Careful newborn examination and documentation is important. Photographs at birth and regularly thereafter are extremely helpful. Position of contractures with active and passive range of motion should be carefully measured and described. It is important to document a description of whether the contractures are proximal or distal, in flexion or extension and the amount of limitation and characteristic position at rest. The presence of dimples overlying contractures is frequent and skin webs across joints with limitation of movement are common and may reflect something about the time of onset of the limitation of movement of that joint. It is important to describe tendon attachments, since 'misplaced' tendons and abnormal sesamoid bones in the tendons are frequently seen. Limitation of opening of the jaw (trismus) should be defined since it has significance for feeding and intubation.

A variety of secondary anomalies, including deformations and malformations, have been seen in children with congenital contractures. These anomalies may well give some clue to the underlying basic process, and to differential diagnosis. Careful documentation of the neurological status and muscle tissue presence and texture are important. Other connective tissue findings should be documented.

Course

The natural history and response to therapy is different with different forms of arthrogryposis. These differences are helpful in distinguishing specific entities, but may also indicate different types of therapy. For instance, physical therapy stretching contractures is usually indicated, but in diastrophic dysplasia this may actually lead to ankylosis of joints. Many forms of arthrogryposis respond well to simple physical therapy (e.g. the hands, in distal arthrogryposis) while others usually require surgical procedures in addition to physical therapy (e.g. most cases of amyoplasia). Prognosis for children with normal intelligence may be very good for living independent productive lives, in spite of severe handicaps. A rare form of arthrogryposis is prone to malignant hyperthermia, so anaesthesia should be undertaken with care in all children with congenital contractures (Froster-Iskenius et al 1988).

Therapy

Treatment of arthrogrypotic joints is a controversial topic, probably because there is no one completely successful approach (Thompson 1985, Goldberg 1987, Staheli et al 1987). It has become clear that vigorous physical therapy early is very important to avoid muscle atrophy. Splinting, combined with physical therapy, seems preferable to continuous casting. Night splints after surgical procedures to maintain increased range of movement are important. If surgery is undertaken, muscle biopsy should be performed. Malignant hyperthermia occurs rarely, so care should be taken to monitor temperature during surgery.

Laboratory tests

On the whole, laboratory tests have not been extremely useful in making a diagnosis in cases of congenital contractures. EMG, muscle biopsies, nerve conduction studies, and muscle enzyme studies are quite often interpreted as showing nonspecific changes, however if they indicate a myopathy (Banker 1986) they are very helpful in making a diagnosis. Muscle biopsies often show fatty and connective tissue replacement of muscle fibres, variation in fibre size, or decreased fibre diameter, all nonspecific signs of muscle atrophy. Radiographs are useful in ruling out specific bone dysplasias and in documenting scoliosis.

Autopsy

If a child with multiple congenital contractures dies, it is very important to do a complete autopsy. Very little information is available on the changes seen in arthrogryposis on autopsy (Clarren & Hall 1983, Herva et al 1985, Lindhout et al 1985, Banker 1986) and the pathogenetic associations of particular patterns is not yet clear. Spinal cord sections at multiple levels and muscle pathology from several sites need to be evaluated. The finding of specific changes has a great deal of significance for recurrence to the family. 'Misplaced' tendons are frequently seen. Whether these are primary or secondary changes is not yet clear. Thickening of joint capsules and fibrous fatty replacement of muscle are frequent.

GENETICS

There are some generalisations which can be made about the genetic aspects of arthrogryposis. In the past, when a child with arthrogryposis or congenital contractures was born to normal parents with an unremarkable family history, the parents were given an empiric 'polygenic/multifactorial' 5% recurrence risk that they might have another affected child. However, with careful documentation a specific diagnosis can be reached in probably half of the patients seen with arthrogryposis (Hall 1985). For instance, amyoplasia appears to have no recurrence risk at all. Distal forms of arthrogryposis may have as much as a 50% recurrence risk. At least three forms of X-linked recessive arthrogryposis exist (Hall et al 1982b). In the category of individuals with CNS involvement, consideration of a chromosomal anomaly must be excluded, this sometimes involves fibroblast chromosome studies (Reed et al 1985). Among children with arthrogryposis and CNS involvement, the recurrence risk may be as high as 25%, with an average risk of 10–15%. (This implies, of course, that there is a high incidence of autosomal recessive disorders within this category.) For those families where a specific diagnosis cannot be made, the empiric recurrence risk to unaffected parents of an affected child or to the affected individual with arthrogryposis is in the 3–5% range.

Prenatal diagnosis is possible in many conditions with congenital contractures, using realtime serial ultrasound studies to evaluate fetal movement (Miskin et al 1979, Hogge et al 1985, Bendon et al 1987, Baty et al 1988, Ohlsson et al 1988). Studies at 16, 20, 24 and 32 weeks are recommended. There is at least one reported case of failure to make the diagnosis in an infant with multiple joint contractures utilising realtime ultrasound during the second trimester (Benzie et al 1976). However, techniques have improved since that report. Care must be taken to look at each major joint for full range of motion. However, the timing of onset of in utero limitation of movement is probably different for different conditions. Norms for in utero movement have now been established. If arthrogryposis is diagnosed prenatally consideration of therapy to increase fetal movement (caffeine, increased maternal activity, etc.) in order to possibly increase lung volume and lessen severity of contractures at birth must be weighed against expected outcome. If a family is at risk for recurrence, prenatal diagnosis should be offered in subsequent pregnancies.

DIFFERENTIAL DIAGNOSIS

The differential diagnosis of congenital contractures is extensive. Tables 60.2, 60.3 and 60.4 outline most of the more common conditions which must be considered. Overall 5–10% of cases of arthrogryposis have been considered to be myopathic and 90–95% to be neuropathic (Banker 1986). With true malformations of the CNS and with in utero disuse, muscle biopsies appear neuropathic. Many specific conditions can be recognised by particular clinical features and/or by laboratory tests. The clinical approach we have found most useful has been to first distinguish three categories of congenital contractures on a clinical basis: (1) primarily musculoskeletal involvement; (2) musculoskeletal involvement plus other system malformations or anomalies; (3) musculoskeletal involvement plus central nervous system dysfunction and/or mental retardation. Tables 60.2, 60.3 and 60.4 are organized on the basis of this clinical approach. There is obvious overlap because some individuals with a condition may only have involvement of the limbs, and others in the same family or with the same condition may have more widespread involvement. Similarly, in some conditions with congenital joint contractures, a characteristic feature is mental retardation, but there may be affected individuals who do not have mental retardation. Nevertheless, we have found this approach to be the most useful for the clinician.

It is impossible to describe in detail all the conditions with congenital contractures, but it seems appropriate to emphasise several of the frequently observed conditions under the three categories.

FREQUENTLY OBSERVED CONDITIONS

Primarily limb involvement (see Table 60.2)

Amyoplasia

Amyoplasia is probably the most common condition with severe multiple congenital contractures and is referred to as 'classical arthrogryposis' by most orthopaedic specialists. One third of all patients in our large study of congenital contractures had amyoplasia (Hall et al 1983a, 1983b, Reid et al 1986, Goldberg 1987). Many forms of arthrogryposis have decreased muscle, hypoplastic muscle or loss of muscle, however when the term 'amyoplasia' is used, it is meant to refer only to this specific condition.

Amyoplasia is characterised by very specific positioning and symmetrical limb involvement, and usually involves all four limbs; however, occasionally only the arms or only the legs are involved. Affected individuals have fibrous bands and fatty tissue where muscles would normally be, suggesting that the muscle or muscle anlage was formed embryologically but failed to develop in a normal way. These patients usually have firmly fixed

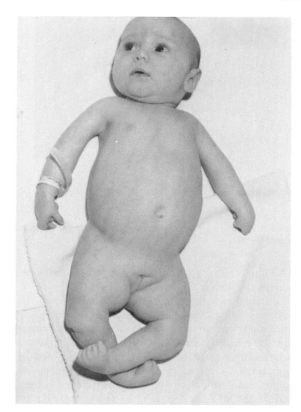

Fig. 60.1 Amyoplasia in a newborn. Note characteristic internally rotated shoulders with decreased muscle mass, extended elbows, hand contractures, equino varus deformities of the feet, dimples and flexion contractures at the knees. The face is round, the nose short and upturned; there is a midline facial haemangioma.

joints (Fig. 60.1) with a fusiform or cylindrical shape to the limbs in the newborn period. No flexion creases are present. The feet are almost always in equinovarus position, the wrists are almost always flexed, the shoulders are internally rotated, the elbows are extended and fixed at 180° at birth but may develop some flexion with growth. There may be slight webbing of skin across the hips which may be flexed or extended in abduction or adduction but are usually dislocated. The knees may be fixed in extension or flexion. Sensation is intact.

Early physical therapy is extremely important to loosen contractures that are present at birth and thereby give whatever muscle is present a chance to strengthen rather than atrophy. Surgery is important to align the limbs in positions of function (Goldberg 1987, Staheli et al 1987).

90% of individuals affected with amyoplasia have no other system involvement; however, there is a variety of other anomalies which can be seen in amyoplasia. 10% of patients with amyoplasia have abdominal wall defects (gastroschisis, or lateral wall hernias) or bowel atresia (Reid et al 1986). There is a very high frequency of haemangioma type birthmarks over the mid-face. The face is usually somewhat round and flat with mild micrognathia. About 5% of the cases have had amniotic bands or digit reduction anomalies on one or more limbs. A small number of children have a decrease in size of the distal digit; many have mild syndactyly or webbing of the digits. Often at birth, but definitely with time, there is undergrowth of an affected limb, much like the disuse atrophy seen in polio. Intelligence is within normal limits, unless there was trauma and/or anoxia at birth.

There appears to be an increased incidence of amyoplasia in identical twins with one normal twin and one affected twin; often the affected twin has only arms or only legs involved (Hall et al 1983b).

All cases of amyoplasia have been sporadic, and many affected individuals have reproduced, having unaffected children. Prenatal diagnosis in subsequent pregnancies can be offered for reassurance using serial realtime ultrasound to detect normal limb movement. Most probably, the condition is secondary to a type of vascular compromise during the mid trimester. Recurrence has not been observed.

Distal arthrogryposis

Distal arthrogryposis is characterised by a very specific positioning of hands in the newborn period, and primarily distal contractures of the limbs (McCormack et al 1980, Hall et al 1982a) (Fig. 60.2). There are other conditions which have distal contractures but this particular type has autosomal dominant inheritance and is characterized by being quite responsive to physical therapy. The hand positioning in the newborn is similar to that seen in trisomy 18, with a clenched fist and overlapping fingers (Fig. 60.3). With physical therapy the hand usually opens up, but there is often some residual ulnar drift of the fingers. Foot positioning is variable. Both equino varus and calcaneovalgus feet have been seen within the same family, as well as in a single individual. Both the hand and foot abnormalities appear to be due to misplaced tendons. There are a number of cases in which this has been documented at surgery. Occasionally, affected family members have contractures of the hips, knees and elbows. There can be marked variability in the involvement within a family.

Some individuals with primarily distal involvement of limbs have been reported as familial camptodactyly, contractural arachnodactyly, or Freeman–Sheldon syndrome because of the similarity of distal limb involvement and positioning. A number of sporadic cases have

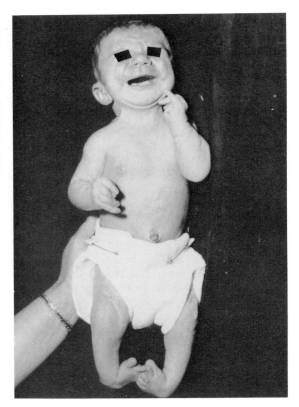

Fig. 60.2 Distal arthogryposis in a newborn. Note predominant distal contractures, with overlapping finger contractures, ulnar deviation and clubfeet.

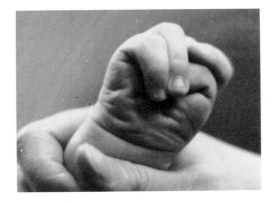

Fig. 60.3 Distal arthogryposis newborn hand. Note clenched fist and overlapping fingers similar to hand position in trisomy 18.

Another category with distal contractures has severe scoliosis (Pagnan & Gollop 1987) (Distal IID).

Still another subcategory of distal arthrogryposis has limitation of jaw movement, +/− micrognathia in association with more generalised congenital contractures. The hand contractures are in an unusual position with flexion of the wrist, hyperextension of the metacarpophalangeal joint, and flexion of the other finger joints. Approximately one third of these cases have mild mental retardation. All cases appear to be sporadic. There is a higher-than-expected incidence of other joint anomalies within the family, and it is not entirely clear whether or not the condition is sporadic or an extremely variable dominant disorder. It has been designated distal arthrogryposis with trismus (or Distal IIE) for want of a better term (Hall et al 1982a).

All forms of distal arthrogryposis seem relatively responsive to physical therapy and surgical procedures. Some individuals and families are so mildly affected that one is not able to recognize any residual deformity, and only by talking to the grandparents is it found that there were mild contractures at birth.

had advanced paternal age, suggesting new dominant mutations. Family studies are very helpful because observing the variability within a family allows proper classification.

Most affected individuals have no non-orthopaedic anomalies; however, there are several subcategories of distal arthrogryposis which may have additional physical abnormalities. It is not clear whether these are totally distinct categories or whether all types can be seen within the same family (Reiss & Sheffield 1986). One of these subtypes is often referred to as the Gordon syndrome, (Robinow & Johnson 1981) (designated Distal IIA in Hall et al 1982a) and has the additional features of cleft palate and short stature in some affected family members (approximately 30–50%). The degree of short stature and severity of clefting in an affected individual seems to be proportionate to the severity of involvement of the joints.

A second category of distal arthrogryposis (Distal IIC) that has additional anomalies comprises families which have cleft lip (Hall et al 1982a, Reiss & Sheffield 1986).

Bony fusion leading to apparent congenital contractures

Bony fusions may appear initially to be congenital contractures, and so are confused with arthrogryposis, particularly because the connection between the two bones may be cartilaginous and not ossified in the infant. Bony fusions are separated into fusions of phalanges (symphalangism), fusion of carpal or tarsal bones (coalitions) and fusions of long bones (synostoses). Usually radiographs will distinguish these conditions. However, symphalangism may be associated with more generalised contractures and is therefore considered separately.

Table 60.2 Primarily musculoskeletal involvement

Entity	Primary features	Contractures		Progression	Lab tests, X-rays, Autopsy findings	Inheritance	Incidence	References
		Body area	Position					
Absence of dermal ridges	1. absent dermal ridges 2. bilateral flexion contractures 3. bilateral webbing of toes 4. congenital milia	fingers toes	flexed	milia-transient (disappear at 6 months)	chromosomes normal; skin biopsy normal	AD	2 families with contractures, 10 families reported	Baird (1964) Reed & Schreiner (1983)
Absence of DIP creases	1. absent DIP creases 2. camptodactyly 3. palmar contracture	hands	flexed	progressive	X-rays; no bone fusion; chromosomes normal	AD	5 families	Fried & Mundel (1976) Lambert et al (1977) Ohdo et al (1981)
Amniotic bands (Streeter)	1. ring-like constrictions 2. amputations 3. +/- other visceral or craniofacial anomalies	limbs	variable	no	secondary to construction of bands	sporadic	frequent	Smith (1982)
Amyoplasia	1. loss of muscle tissue and replacement with fat and fibrous tissue 2. symmetrical contractures, always equinovarus feet, extended elbows 3. round face, midline haemangioma 4. normal intelligence 5. abdominal wall defects and bowel atresia (10%) 6. increased in monozygous twins	wrists elbows shoulders hips knees feet	flexion extension IR flexion, CDH +/- extension or flexion equinovarus	improves with therapy; usually needs surgery; normal IQ	spinal cord ↓ # anterior horn cells in some cases; muscle: variation in fibre diameter, small fibres, replacement muscle tissue with fat and CT	apparently sporadic	1/10 000 births; over 400 cases	Hall et al (1983a and 1983b) Reid et al (1986) Goldberg (1987)
Antecubital webbing	1. elbow dysplasia 2. antecubital web 3. +/- carpal wrist abnormalities	elbow +/- wrist	flexion carpal fusion	non-progressive	X-rays; +/- fusion humerus & ulna, +/- dysplasia condyle, +/- trochlear dysplasia	AD	4 families reported	Shun-Shin (1954) Mead & Martin (1963)
Campto-dactyly	1. camptodactyly 2. not always present at birth	fingers only +/- toes	fixed flexion	may be progressive	shortness of deep flexor tendons	AD	5 families	Welch & Temtamy (1966) Flatt (1977)
Campto-dactyly with arthropathy	1. camptodactyly 2. joint effusions +/- arthritis	fingers toes	stiff curved	slowly progressive	arthritis changes	AR	several families	Athreya & Schumacher (1978) Malleson et al (1981) Ochi et al (1983)

Table 60.2 Primarily musculoskeletal involvement (*contd.*)

Entity	Primary features	Contractures Body area	Position	Progression	Lab tests, X-rays, Autopsy findings	Inheritance	Incidence	References
Clasped thumbs, congenital (see also adducted thumb)	1. extensor muscles and tendons of thumb weak or absent	thumb (bilateral) occasionally 1st finger	flexed at MP and DIP joints, radial deviation (adducted)	surgical treatment, tendon transplant	hypoplastic tendon peripheral neuropathy	AD	100 families	White & Jenson (1952) Weckesser et al (1968)
Coalition	1. calcaneus-navicular 2. scaphoid-astragalus 3. talus-navicular 4. calcaneus-scaphoid	ankles toes	fusion +/- contractures		X-rays; synostosis; differential diagnosis: peroneal spastic foot	AD	relatively common	Bersani & Samilson (1957) Wray & Herndon (1963) Challis (1974) Gregersen & Petersen (1977) Tuncbilek et al (1985)
Contractures, continuous muscle discharge & titubation	1. contractures 2. myokymia 3. ataxia and titubation	hand feet all extremities	fixed flexion stiffened		abnormal muscle fibres (small)	AD	1 family	Hanson et al (1977)
Distal arthrogryposis	1. clenched hand with overlapping fingers at birth – opens to ulnar deviation (90%) 2. usually calcaneovalgus but all combinations (80%) of club feet 3. other major joint contractures	fingers hands elbows hips knees feet toes	clenched, overlap, then open and ulnar deviate +/- flexion or extension calcaneovalgus or equinovarus overlap, camptodactyly	good therapy response, improves with time, ulnar deviation of hands	X-ray; hip dislocation, mild scoliosis misplaced or hypoplastic tendons	AD (variable)	relatively common, more than 50 families	Sack (1978) Hall et al (1982a) McCormack et al (1980)
Distal arthrogryposis with scoliosis (Distal Type IID)	1. distal contracture 2. severe scoliosis +/- vertebral anomalies	fingers feet back	clenched variable stiff & scoliosis	scoliosis progressive	occasional hemi-vertebrae	AD	3 families	Hall et al (1982a) Baraitser (1982) Pagnan & Gollop (1987)

Syndrome	Features	Site	Clinical / functional	Progression	X-ray findings	Inheritance	Frequency / cases	References
Humero-radial synostosis (HRS)	Familial 1. AD 100% are bilateral AR 91% are bilateral Sporadic 2. 62% have hypoplasia of hand and 77% have involvement of ulna	hand wrist elbow shoulder hips knees feet	46% of sporadic humeroradial synostosis 38% of sporadic 25% of AR 50% of AD	surgery may improve function	X-rays; humeroradial synostosis	sporadic, AR and AD	sporadic) AD) AR	Keutel et al (1970) Straňák & Oberender (1971) Say et al (1973) Hunter et al (1976) Lenz & Rehmann (1976) Richieri Costa (1986)
Impaired pronation/supination of forearm (familial)	1. no synostoses	forearm	reduction of supination-pronation		X-rays: flattenting of radial head, but no displacement, no abnormal curvature of radial shaft or synostosis	AD	1 family	Thompson et al (1968)
Liebenberg syndrome	1. prominence of radial head 2. unusual slope of olecranon process 3. brachydactyly 4. streblomicrodactyly intercarpal fusion	elbows fingers wrists	limited ROM flexion, clinodactyly 5 flexion	non-progressive	X-ray: fusion triquetrum & pisiform	AD	10 affected/ 5 generations	Liebenberg (1973)
Poland anomaly	1. absent pectoral major (costal head) 2. ipsilateral limb deficiency	fingers or distal upper limb	radioulnar synostosis (occasional)	non-progressive	X-ray: hypoplasia of missing or absent phalanges, rib deficiencies	sporadic	over 200 reports	Goldberg & Mazzei (1977) McGillivray & Lowry (1977) David (1982)
Radioulnar synostosis	1. radioulnar synostosis short forearm	hand elbow (⅓ of cases)	pronation fixed 10–30° extension limitation, reduced pronation	non-progressive	X-rays: synostosis of proximal radius and ulna seen in chromosomal anomalies involving X and Y	sporadic and AD	over 250 cases reported	Hansen & Andersen (1970) Spritz (1978)
Symphalangism 'Cushing' (see also multiple synostosis)	1. proximal interphalangeal symphalangism – hands, feet 2. deafness variable 3. variable carpal and tarsal ankle bone fusion	fingers	clinodactyly ankylosis of 1st and 2nd phalanges, absent PIP creases inability to invert and evert ankle	fusions become worse with time	X-ray: PIP fusion +/− DIP fusion, +/− talus and naviculus fusion	AD	351 affected/10 generations	Strasburger et al (1965)

Table 60.2 Primarily musculoskeletal involvement (*contd.*)

Entity	Primary features	Contractures		Progression	Lab tests, X-rays, Autopsy findings	Inheritance	Incidence	References
		Body area	Position					
Symphalangism distal	1. symphalangism distal IP joint 2. synostosis metacarpals and metatarsals	fingers toes wrist ankles	limited movement distally	non-progressive	fusions of phalanges	AD		Matthews et al (1987)
Symphalangism/brachydactyly (see also multiple synostosis)	1. brachydactyly 2. symphalangism (proximal and distal) 3. +/− club feet 4. +/− craniosynostosis 5. +/− scoliosis just before menarche 6. missing distal fingers or nails	hands hips feet	flexed 'clubbed'	non-progressive	lab data normal; X-rays; carpal fusion; +/− flat vertebrae; +/− craniosynostosis	AR AD	2 patients 5 affected/3 generations 5 affected/2 generations	Walbaum et al (1970) Ventruto et al (1976) Sillence (1978) Schott (1978)
Symphalangism/brachydactyly Nievergelt-Pearlman type	1. radioulnar synostosis 2. coalitions of tarsals & carpals 3. symbrachyphalangism of fingers	hand elbows	clinocamptodactyly radioulnar synostoses talipes, tarsal synostoses	non-progressive	X-ray: radioulnar synostoses, carpal and tarsal synostoses	AD	more than 5 families	Fuhrmann et al (1966) Dubois (1970) Spranger et al (1974) Lenz & Rehmann (1976) Richieri Costa (1986)
Trismus pseudocamptodactyly	1. inability to open mouth fully 2. camptodactyly with wrist dorsiflexed but straightening with wrist flexion 3. mild S/S 4. about ¼ with feet or hips involved	fingers toes +/− feet jaw	flexed when hand is dorsiflexed pes cavus, equinovarus trismus		pathology: short finger, leg & foot flexor tendons, short muscles of mastication with secondary TM joint deficiency, thumb sparse	AD	7 families	Ter Haar & Van Hoof (1974) Mabry et al (1974)
X-linked resolving arthrogryposis	1. flexion contracture 2. camptodactyly 3. anterior rotation of shoulders	knee	flexion	resolving		X-linked	4 families	Hall et al (1982b)

Symphalangism

Symphalangism may occur secondary to trauma or as part of a bony dysplasia such as diastrophic dysplasia. There is also a well-known autosomal dominant condition with symphalangism. Some affected individuals and families with dominantly inherited symphalangism are born with congenital contractures as well as developing fusion of various bones (Goldberg 1987). Affected individuals may have dislocated hips, short stature and conductive deafness due to fusion of the stapes and the petrous bone (Strasburger et al 1965). There is a great deal of intrafamilial variability, but the diagnosis is made by the recognition of characteristic fusion of phalanges which may not be present or obvious in early childhood. Individuals in affected families should be carefully examined for subtle signs of physical involvement that might ordinarily be overlooked. Surgery may need to be different from that in other types of congenital contractures because of the expected fusion of bones. Physical therapy may exacerbate and hasten early fusion. A severe form of symphalangism has been described as multiple synostosis (Maroteaux et al 1972, Herrmann 1974) but may be part of the spectrum seen in dominantly inherited symphalangism. Deafness, a long nose and a prominent bridge, and missing distal phalanges are seen in these families.

Limb involvement with other system abnormalities
(see Table 60.3)

The second major category of conditions with congenital contractures is that in which there are congenital contractures of the limbs in association with anomalies or malformations of other parts of the body.

Freeman–Sheldon syndrome

Perhaps the most common of these is Freeman–Sheldon, or Whistling Face, syndrome (also known as craniocarpotarsal dystrophy) in which there are congenital contractures, primarily of the hands and feet with overlapping fingers and ulnar deviation, in association with limitation in mouth and facial movement secondary to fibrosis of facial muscles (Fig. 60.4). There may be a characteristic 'H' shaped connective tissue band on the chin. Affected individuals tend to have long faces with markedly decreased facial movement. Individuals with Freeman–Sheldon syndrome may also have scoliosis, mid-face hypoplasia, lateral coloboma of the alae nasae, ptosis and an antimongoloid slant of the eyes. Freeman–Sheldon syndrome appears to be more resistant to therapy than other forms of distal arthrogryposis. Vanek et al (1986) have suggested that Freeman–Sheldon syndrome may be

due to a congenital myopathy, although the changes they describe are also compatible with disuse.

It is clear that there is interfamilial and intrafamilial variability but that autosomal dominant inheritance is the most common mode of inheritance. On the other hand, there appears to be a recessive form which tends to be more severe (Alves & Azevedo 1977, Sanchez & Kaminker 1986, Wang & Lin 1987) and is even lethal in some affected individuals (Fitzsimmons et al 1984).

Contractural arachnodactyly

Contractural arachnodactyly is a well-defined condition with autosomal dominant inheritance characterized by congenital contractures, long, thin extremities, crumpling of the top of the helix of the ear and kyphoscoliosis (Ramos Arroyo et al 1985). Various chest deformities are

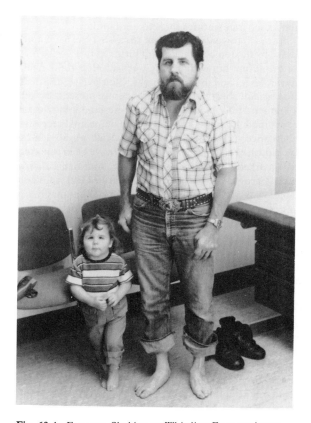

Fig. 60.4 Freeman-Sheldon or Whistling Face syndrome in father and daughter. Note hand and foot contractures, more severe in father who has a very small left foot. The eyes are deeply set with an antimongoloid slant, the mouth is small and there is a mild groove in the chin. Both have short stature and short necks.

seen as well, with pectus excavatum or carinatum. Marked inter- and intrafamilial variability is seen. Less than 10% of cases appear to be severely involved with progressive scoliosis. The other 90% of cases seem to improve with age. Recently there has been a suggestion of overlap with the Marfan syndrome, in that some individuals with contractural arachnodactyly may have structural abnormalities of the heart with mitral valve prolapse and/or aortic aneurysms (Bass et al 1981, Anderson et al 1984). Severely affected sporadic newborns have been reported with advanced bone age (Ho & Khoo 1979) and additional GI or vertebral anomalies (Currarino & Friedman 1986).

Multiple pterygium syndromes

Many newborns and children with arthrogryposis have webs (or pterygia) across the joints which have limited movement. However, there are several specific conditions with marked webbing (Hall et al 1982c) which are seen as separate entities in different families.

Multiple pterygium syndrome (Escobar type) is characterised by flexion contractures at birth. At birth webs may not be present but with ageing webs develop at the neck, elbows, knees and intracural areas. Cleft palate, deafness, scoliosis and short stature are frequently present, as well as segmentation anomalies of the vertebrae. Many cases are sporadic but most appear to have autosomal recessive inheritance (Escobar et al 1978, Hall et al 1982c, Thompson et al 1987). A few families have been reported with marked variability and possible dominant inheritance (Carnevale et al 1973, Frias et al 1973, Haspeslagh et al 1985, McKeown & Harris 1988). This may be a progressive condition as about 20% of individuals seem to get worse as they enter puberty, with decreasing pulmonary capacity and increasing thoracic lordosis (Hall et al 1982c, Thompson et al 1987). Recently, myopathic changes have been reported in a fairly typical case (Papadia et al 1987).

Lethal multiple pterygium syndrome (Gillin-Pryse-Davis type) is characterised by intrauterine growth retardation, severe flexion contractures, webs in utero, frequently with cystic hygromas and hydrops. Lungs are severely hypoplastic, so that survival does not occur. Polyhydramnios, ocular hypertelorism, cryptorchidism, cardiac hypoplasia and ambiguous genitalia in males are frequently seen. Subtypes related to bony fusions and the time during gestation when severity becomes obvious may exist (Hall 1984). Apparently most cases are autosomal recessive and can be diagnosed prenatally (Van Regemorter et al 1984, Herva et al 1985, Martin et al 1986). However there may be an X-linked recessive form (Tolmie et al 1987a).

Popliteal pterygium syndrome (Gorlin type) is characterised by dense webs in the popliteal area (often with the nerve and blood vessel in the web), cleft lip and palate, syndactyly, nail anomalies, reduction deformities of digits and other contractures. It is an autosomal dominant condition with marked variability in expression (Gorlin et al 1968, Escobar & Weaver 1978).

Bartsocas–Papas syndrome (lethal popliteal web syndrome) is characterised by severe popliteal webs, cleft lip and palate with facial clefts, hypoplasia of the nasal tip and genital area, syndactyly with missing distal digits, sparse hair and hypoplastic teeth. It is almost always lethal but, if the newborn period is survived, intelligence appears normal. Autosomal recessive inheritance seems likely and consanguinity, particularly with Mediterranean ancestry, has been observed (Bartsocas & Papas 1972, Distefano & Romeo 1974, Papadia et al 1984).

Multiple pterygium with malignant hyperthermia has been observed in several families. Scoliosis, torticollis, myopathic facies and cleft palate have been present (Kousseff & Nichols 1985, Robinson et al 1987, Froster-Iskenius et al 1988). CPKs are not necessarily elevated and muscle biopsy is compatible with disuse atrophy rather than a myopathy. The relationship to Kings syndrome is not clear since Kings syndrome has Noonan phenotype and malignant hyperthermia with elevated CPKs, but congenital contractures can be seen (McPherson & Taylor 1981).

Chondrodysplasias

A variety of chondrodysplasias (including camptomelic dysplasia, diastrophic dysplasia, Dyggve–Melchior–Clausen dysplasia, dyssegmental dysplasia, Kneist dysplasia, Larsen syndrome, metatropic dysplasia, osteogenesis imperfecta) also fall into this second category of congenital contractures associated with other system anomalies.

Congenital contractures with CNS anomalies or dysfunction (see Table 60.4)

The third category of conditions with congenital contractures is that in which there are congenital contractures of the limbs associated with CNS malformations or dysfunction (Fig. 60.5). Many relatively rare autosomal recessive lethal conditions fall into this category.

Pena-Shokeir phenotype

Pena and Shokeir described the combination of short fixed limbs and pulmonary hypoplasia. Subsequently many other families have been reported (Hall 1986) with the additional features of intrauterine growth retardation,

Table 60.3 Musculoskeletal involvement plus other system anomalies

Entity	Primary features	Contractures Body area	Position	Progression	Lab tests, X-rays, Autopsy findings	Inheritance	Incidence	References
Aase–Smith	1. camptodactyly 2. Dandy-Walker 3. hydrocephalus 4. cleft palate 5. scoliosis	hands elbows knees hips feet	flexion flexion flexion flexion equinovarus	non-progressive	autopsy neuroblastoma ventriculo-septal defect	AD	2 families	Aase & Smith (1968) Patton et al (1985)
Campto-dactyly-Guadalajara	1. camptodactyly 2. short stature 3. microcornea microphthalmia 4. microcephaly – mentally retarded 5. pectus excavatum	hands feet hips	flex equinovarus or planus dislocated	non-progressive	X-rays dislocated hips, scoliosis	AR	1 family	Cantu et al (1985)
Campto-dactyly London	1. camptodactyly 2. facial immobility 3. ichthyosis 4. short stature 5. scoliosis	fingers feet	flexed ulnar deviation vertical talus	non-progressive		AR	1 family	Baraitser (1982)
Campto-dactyly Tel Hashomer	1. camptodactyly 2. long thin nose & high broad bridge 3. short stature 4. prominent forehead 5. scoliosis 6. malformed toes	fingers	spindle shaped flexed	non-progressive	muscle hypoplasia type 2b fibres	AR	5 families	Goodman et al (1976) Pagnan et al (1988)
Congenital Fibre type disproportion with congenital contractures	1. generalised contractures 2. disuse			non-progressive	apparently related to disuse		sporadic frequent	Banker (1986)
Conradi-Hunermann (chondrodysplasia punctata)	1. hypertelorism, prominent forehead 2. cataracts (17%) 3. limb contractures (27%) 4. atrophoderma follicularis/alopecia	large joints +/− feet	flexion clubbed		X-ray: punctate calcifications, tubular bones – mildly short, scoliosis-abnormal vertebrae; pathology: epiphyses abnormal	AD X-linked dominant, lethal in males	65 patients reviewed by Spranger, 27% had contractures	Smith (1982) Spranger et al (1974) Happle (1981)

Table 60.3 Musculoskeletal involvement plus other system anomalies (*contd.*)

Entity	Primary features	Contractures Body area	Position	Progression	Lab tests, X-rays, Autopsy findings	Inheritance	Incidence	References
Contractural arachnodactyly	1. contractural arachnodactyly 2. kyphoscoliosis 3. crumpled ear helix 4. club foot +/− 5. +/− CHD 6. chest deformities	fingers elbows knees ankles	flexion PIP limitation supination & pronation flexed calcaneus with dorsiflexion adduction of forepart	improves with age (knees the worst) about 10% get worse with age	X-ray: bones gracile, kyphoscoliosis, advanced bone age	AD AR	at least 30 kindreds	Reeve et al (1960) Beals & Hecht (1971) Temtamy & McKusick (1978) Ho & Khoo (1979) Bass et al (1981) Ramos Arroyo et al (1985) Anderson et al (1984) Currarino & Friedman (1986)
Deafness and camptodactyly	1. neurosensory deafness 2. camptodactyly without fusion 3. proximally placed thumbs	fingers wrist elbow toes	flexed, camptodactyly limited pronation flexed lateral deviation	non-progressive	muscle mass decrease distally	AD	2 families	Stewart & Bertstron (1971) Akbarnia et al (1979)
Diastrophic dysplasia	1. dwarfism 2. joint contractures/ 'hitchhiker' thumb 3. scoliosis/vertebral instability 4. abnormal ears 5. cleft lip, +/− abnormal tracheal ring	thumb fingers hip +/− feet	adducted ankylosis PIP joint dislocated equinovarus	progressive (probably due to joint trauma)	X-ray: precocious calcification of cartilage, pathology: abnormal epiphyses, hypertrophic auricular cartilage and calcifications, specific histology	AR	over 100 cases	Lamy & Maroteaux (1960) Temtamy & McKusick (1978) Horton et al (1978) Lachman et al (1981)
Distal Arthrogryposis II with cleft lip & palate, Type IIC	1. distal contractures 2. cleft lip +/− palate	hands feet hips	clenched various positions dislocated	responds to therapy		AD	3 families	Hall et al (1982a) Reiss & Sheffield (1986)
Distal Arthrogryposis II with trismus (Distal IIE)	1. distal contractures 2. trismus 3. mild mental retardation in 1/3	hands feet	wrist flexed MCP extended, fingers flexed variable	responds to therapy		sporadic	50 cases	Hall et al (1982a)

Syndrome	Features	Site	Description	Progression	Other	Inheritance	Number	References
Freeman–Sheldon (Craniocarpotarsal dystrophy) (Whistling face syndrome)	1. pursed lips, small mouth 2. immobile face, ptosis 3. contractures with ulnar drift 4. 'H' on chin 5. notched alae nasi 6. scoliosis	hands feet hips	flexion opening with ulnar deviate calcaneal valgus dislocated	non-progressive	displaced tendons, fibrotic facial muscles	AD AR	60 families	Cox & Pearce (1974) Gorlin et al (1976) Alves & Azevedo (1977) Sanchez & Kaminker (1986) Wang & Lim (1987)
Freeman–Sheldon-like dysplasia	1. pursed lips 2. dislocated limbs 3. rhizomelic shortening with bowing 4. cervical kyphosis 5. short stature	elbows knees	flexed flexed	slowly progressive	X-ray: wide dumbbell shaped metaphysis platyspondyly	AR		Burton et al (1986)
Focal femoral dysplasia	1. cleft palate, long philtrum, short nose with hypoplastic alae nasae, micrognathia 2. shortened limbs – lower > upper 3. joint contractures 4. +/– unusual facies	elbow hips feet toes	fixed in flexion dislocated equinovarus clinodactyly	non-progressive	vertebral anomalies	sporadic (associated with maternal diabetes)	over 100 cases	Smith (1982) Gleiser et al 1978
Gordon syndrome (Distal Type IIa)	1. distal contractures 2. cleft palate (40%) 3. short stature	hands feet	clenched, overlapping fingers calcaneal valgus or equinovarus	respond well to therapy		AD	10 families	Hall et al (1982a) Robinow & Johnson (1981)
Hand foot uterus	1. contractures hands and feet 2. small thumbs and great toes 3. structural anomalies of uterus particularly duplication	hand feet	camptodactyly club	non-progressive	GU anomalies	AD	30 families	Stern et al (1970) Poznanski et al (1975)
Hanhart (aglossia adactyly, hypoglossia hypodactyly)	1. limb deficiency with transverse loss 2. small or absent tongue 3. +/– Moebius 4. fusion of knee or elbow joint	hands feet knee elbow	fused fused fused fused	non-progressive		sporadic	50 cases	Herrmann & Opitz (1974) Goldberg (1987) Bersu et al (1976)
Holt–Oram	1. abnormalities of shoulders, hands and wrists 2. cardiac defects (structural) 3. abnormal joint structure (rare)	hands wrists shoulders knee foot	usually hypoplasia, +/– synostosis hypoplasia genu valgum talocalcaneal synostosis (rare)		pathology: CHD	AD	200 cases	Poznanski et al (1970a) Brans & Lintermans (1972) Kaufman et al (1974) Gladstone & Sybert (1982)

Table 60.3 Musculoskeletal involvement plus other system anomalies (*contd.*)

Entity	Primary features	Contractures		Progression	Lab tests, X-rays, Autopsy findings	Inheritance	Incidence	References
		Body area	Position					
Kneist dysplasia	1. short trunk dwarfism, S/S 2. kyphoscoliosis 3. joint enlargement with limitation 4. myopia, deafness, cleft palate 5. +/− mucopolysacchariduria	hands fingers. hips ankles	flexed	progressive weakness	lab: some with high keratan sulphate excretion: X-ray: irregular ossification of epiphyses	AD heterogeneous	50 cases	Spranger et al (1974) Kim et al (1975)
King-Denborough Noonanlike multiple pterygium with malignant hyperthermia	1. contractures 2. torticollis 3. kyphosis scoliosis 4. cleft palate 5. pterygium with progressive weakness 6. malignant hyperthermia	hands knees hips	camptodactyly flexed dislocated	does respond to therapy, beware of anaesthesia	muscle biopsy does not always show myopathy CPK, high, low or normal	AR	rare	Goldberg (1987) Robinson et al (1987) Froster-Iskenius et al (1988)
Kuskokwim	1. multiple joint contractures 2. +/− pigmented nevi and ↓ corneal reflexes	elbows knees ankles feet	flexed +/− web		pathology: muscle atrophy; X-ray: +/− patella migration, normal, muscle and nerve function	AR	17 cases (7 Eskimo families)	Petajan et al (1969) Wright & Aase (1967)
Larsen syndrome	1. prominent forehead, hypertelorism, depressed nasal bridge, flat round face 2. multiple joint dislocations, particularly anterior knees 3. hand anomalies – long cylindrical fingers, broad at end 4. scoliosis +/−, vertebral anomalies, short stature +/−, cleft palate +/−, mid-cervical kyphosis/subluxation 5. cardiac septal defects 6. laryngeal & tracheal collapse	hands fingers elbow hips knees feet	hypermobile joints anterior dislocations of knee	diminished cartilage rigidity at birth, improved with time, continue to sublux	X-ray: dislocated patella, poor ossification of phalanges, CDH, juxtacalcaneal accessory bone, hypoplasia of humerus distally ↑ carpal ossification, cervical vertebral subluxation	AR & AD	50 cases	Spranger et al (1974) Goldberg (1987) Kiel et al (1983)

Condition	Features	Joint/site	Deformity	Course	Pathology / X-ray	Inheritance	Number	References
Metaphyseal dysplasia (Jansen)	1. small thorax 2. characteristic facies 3. flexion joint deformities 4. wide irregular metaphyses	knee hip	flexion	progressive	X-ray: hypercalcaemia, hyperostosis of calvarium, lack of metaphyseal ossification gives gross irregular cyst like areas	AD	very rare	Sutcliffe (1966) Spranger et al (1974)
Metatropic dysplasia	1. short stature/kyphoscoliosis 2. prominent joints with restricted mobility, but ↑ finger extensibility 3. pelvic hypoplasia	knee hip	flexed	progressive	X-ray: platyspondyly/kyphoscoliosis, pelvic hypoplasia, short limbs-metaphyseal flaring, epiphyseal irregularity, hyperplastic trochanters	AD & AR?	25 cases	Rimoin et al (1976) Smith (1982) Beck et al (1983) Belik et al (1985)
Moebius	1. facial diplegia (VI and VII nerves) 2. joint contractures, reduction anomalies 3. difficulty swallowing 4. chest & trunk absent muscles (e.g. pectoralis muscle)	hand knees foot	camptodactyly flexed, genu valgum clubbed	non-progressive	EMG: frontalis, orbicularis oculi, facial and external rectus no response; pathology: muscle hypoplasia	most sporadic, AD	100 cases	Sprofkin & Hillman (1956) Smith (1982) Sudarshan & Goldie (1985) Bavinck & Weaver (1986)
Multiple pterygium syndrome (Escobar Type)	1. multiple webs develop with time 2. joint contractures, camptodactyly 3. vertebral anomalies +/-, scoliosis 4. +/- cleft palate, deafness 5. antimongoloid slant, ptosis 6. progressive thoracic lordosis 7. restrictive lung disease 8. short stature	fingers hands elbows hips knees ankles feet	camptodactyly flexion deformities	2 forms: 1 non-progressive 1 progressive	pathology: skin, spinal cord & brain normal, muscle hypoplasia, fatty replacement, progressive respiratory dysfunction	AR most AD (rare)	60 families 4 families	Srivastava (1968) Escobar et al (1978) Hall et al (1982c) Thompson & Baraitser (1987) Frias et al (1973) Carnevale et al (1973) McKeown & Harris (1988)
Multiple synostosis (severe symphalangism WL syndrome) (also see symphalangism brachydactyly)	1. symphalangism 2. deafness from ossicular fusion 3. long nose with broad bridge 4. synostosis of elbows 5. coalition of tarsals and carpals 6. distal digit defects	finger ankle wrist elbow hips	fusion fusion fusion fusion dislocated	increasing fusions, progressive deafness	fusion of bones hemivertebra, fixed ossicles	AD	30 families	Maroteaux et al (1972) Herrmann (1974) Pedersen et al (1980) Higashi & Inoue (1983) Hurvitz et al (1985)
Myasthenia – with contractures	1. maternal myasthenia 2. pulmonary hypoplasia 3. kyphoscoliosis 4. hypotonia 5. small chin	multiple hand feet	flexion camptodactyly equinovarus	may markedly improve with anticholinesterase therapy		maternal transmission may affect more than 1 sib	many families	Holmes et al (1980) Moutard-Codou et al (1987)

Table 60.3 Musculoskeletal involvement plus other system anomalies (*contd.*)

Entity	Primary features	Contractures		Progression	Lab tests, X-rays, Autopsy findings	Inheritance	Incidence	References
		Body area	Position					
Nail Patella (Hereditary Onycho-osteodysplasia)	1. nail dysplasia 2. absent or hypoplastic patella 3. joint contractures 4. +/− kidney disease 5. Occasional elbow and knee webbing	fingers elbow knee foot	ulnar deviation (5th finger clino-campto-dactyly) flexed pes planus, talipes, equinovarus	non-progressive	X-ray: pathognomonic iliac horns, absent patella, subluxation of radial heads, linked to ABO blood group, renal failure (nephritis)	AD		Lucas (1967) Spranger et al (1974) Myers et al (1980) Hogh & MacNicol (1985)
Nemaline myopathy	1. hypotonic, respiratory problems 2. congenital heart disease 3. short 1st metacarpal, clinodactyly 4. bilateral talipes varus	fingers feet	clinodactyly talipes varus	lethal	autopsy: papillary muscle anomaly, myocardial scarring, hepatic fibrosis, pathology muscle: rods in muscle fibres	AD AR	at least 20 cases with contractures	McComb et al (1979) Bucher et al (1985) Papadia et al (1987)
Neurofibromatosis	1. neurofibromas 2. café-au-lait spots (multiple) 3. contractures +/− congenital	hands elbows hips knees feet	flexion	can be progressive	histopathology: neurofibromas	AD	1/3000 have NFD but contractures are rare	Relkin (1965) Kibbe et al (1965)
Oculo-dental-digital syndrome	1. small sunken eyes, thin nose 2. severe hypoplasia of enamel, microdontia 3. phalangeal hypoplasia, camptodactyly of 4th and 5th digits	fingers hallux	campto-todactyly abduction		chromosomes: normal; X-rays: absence of middle phalanges of toes, widening long and short tubular bones and ribs and clavicles	AD	30 cases	Gorlin et al (1976) Spranger et al (1974)
Ophthalmo-mandibulo-melic dysplasia	1. fusion of tem-poromandibular joint 2. eyes - blindness from corneal opacities 3. joint contractures, mild limb shortening	fingers hands elbows	campto-dactyly ulnar deviation radio-humero dislocation, limited extension		chromosomes: normal; X-rays: fusion temporomandibular joint, elbows fused	AD	father & 2 children	Pillay (1964)

Syndrome	Features	Site	Contractures	Course	X-ray / Pathology	Inheritance	Cases	References
Oral-cranial-digital syndrome (Juberg-Hayward)	1. cleft lip and palate 2. hypoplastic inflexible distally placed thumbs 3. bilateral elbow deformities 4. microcephalus, mild mental retardation 5. pituitary dysfunction	thumb elbow toes	IP inflexibility limited extension camptodactyly		X-rays: 1st metacarpals- small, radius dislocated; chromosomes: normal, low growth hormone	AR	3 families	Juberg (1969) Nevin et al (1981) Kingston et al (1982)
Oto-onchyo-peroneal	1. generalised contractures 2. unfolded ears 3. aplasia/dysplasia of nails 4. fibula aplasia/hypoplasia	hands hip knee ankle	camptodactyly dislocation dislocation fixed	non-progressive	X-rays: anterior bowing of tibia	AR vs X-recessive	2 boys in 1 family	Pfeiffer (1982)
Para-stremmatic	1. multiple contractures 2. twisted legs 3. bowed long bones 4. kyphoscoliosis	knees elbows hips	dislocated flexed flexed	slowly progressive	X-ray: coarse trabeculations, dense 'flocky woolly' areas, lacey border to pelvis	AD	6 families	Langer et al (1970) Spranger et al (1974) Horan & Beighton (1976)
Pfeiffer	1. craniosynostoses, brachycephaly 2. syndactyly 3. +/- contractures 4. +/- humeroradial synostosis	elbow +/- feet +/-	radioulnar synostosis mild calcaneovarus		X-ray: broad distal phalanges	AD	rare	Spranger et al (1974) Smith (1982)
Popliteal pterygium (fascia-genital popliteal Gorlin type)	1. popliteal web with cord at edge 2. cleft palate, cleft lip, lip pits, frenulae, intraoral web 3. syndactyly 4. nail anomalies, absence deformities of digits 5. equinovarus 6. +/- ankyloblepharon filiforme adnatum 7. short stature 8. genitalia with web and scrotal anomaly	knee +/- foot	flexion with web equinovarus	may require surgery to release – watch for nerve & vessel in web	pathology: free edge of web is cord-like & the web contains sciatic nerve and blood vessel	AD	at least 60 cases, 26 familial	Gorlin et al (1968) Escobar & Weaver (1978a, 1978b) Hall et al (1982b)
Pseudo-diastrophic	1. short stature 2. rhizomelic shortening 3. scoliosis and platyspondyly 4. elbow dislocation 5. finger dislocation 6. generalised contractures	fingers elbows hips knees feet	flexed flexed dislocated flexed equinovarus	non-progressive	X-rays: mild changes, thin bony histology: different from diastrophic	AR	10 cases	Eteson et al (1986)
Puretic-Murray syndrome	1. joint contractures 2. face/skull deformities 3. multiple fibromatosis 4. skin lesions 5. infections: skin, eyes, nose, ears	5th finger arms legs	camptodactyly fixed flexion contractures	progressive contractures from early infancy	histopathology: skin ↓ collagen, ↑ soluble protein, ↓ fat content, altered connective tissue	AR	30 families	Fayad et al (1987)

Table 60.3 Musculoskeletal involvement plus other system anomalies (*contd.*)

Entity	Primary features	Contractures Body area	Position	Progression	Lab tests, X-rays, Autopsy findings	Inheritance	Incidence	References
Sacral agenesis	1. lower limb aplasia with contractures 2. +/– others	shoulders hips feet	Sprengel flexion equinovarus		X-rays: absence sacrum	maternal diabetes	bony abnorm- alities in 1% of diabetic mothers	Blumel et al (1959) Assemany et al (1972) Smith (1982)
SED congenita	1. short trunk 2. myopia 3. lag in epiphyseal mineralization	elbows knees hips	joint limitation, flexion	progressive	X-rays: flat epiphyses, ↓ mineralisation of pubis, talus, calcaneus, knee centres	AD AR?	>50 cases	Spranger et al (1974) Smith (1982) Harrod et al (1984)
Stiff man/ stiff baby syndrome	1. alert tense facial expression 2. hiatus, diaphragmatic & umbilical hernias 3. feeding problems 4. intermittent generalised contractures	all joints	flexed	improves	EMG: exaggerated response	AD	several families	Lingham et al (1981)
Sturge- Weber	1. flat facial haemangioma 2. meningeal haemangioma with calcifications 3. MR +/– seizures 4. buphthalmos, glaucoma	large joints	paresis in 30% of cases, flexion		pathology: cerebral cortical atrophy, sclerosis, double contour convolutional calcifications seen on X-ray	sporadic		Smith (1982) Wiedemann et al (1985)
Trismus pseudo- campto- dactyly syndrome	1. trismus 2. limited movement of fingers when wrist dorsiflexed 3. dislocated hips 4. generalised contractures 5. short stature	fingers feet hips	limitation varus dislocated	non- progressive	pathology: shortened flexor tendons	AD	10 families	Mabry et al (1974) Ter Haar & Van Hoof (1974) O'Brien et al (1984) Tsukahara et al (1985)
Tuberous sclerosis	1. glioma-angioma lesions, phacomata, seizures 2. adenoma sebaceum, shagreen patch ↓ pigment patches 3. +/– joint contractures	fingers 1–3 feet toes	flexed equinovarus flexed	can be progressive	autopsy: brain-tuberous sclerosis lesions; X-rays: no bone changes	AD variable, most without contractures	10 cases	Sandbank & Cohen (1964)
VATER association	1. vertebral/vascular defects 2. anal atresia 3. tracheo-oesophageal fistula 4. oesophageal atresia 5. radial/renal defects	hand & arm	'clubbed'		chromosomes: normal; pathology: CHD, anal atresia, TE fistula, renal anomaly	sporadic		Temtamy & McKusick (1978) Smith (1982)

Syndrome	Clinical features	upper limb	flexion contractures	non-progressive	neurocrest anomaly	inheritance	families	references
Waardenberg (Klein/Waardenberg syndrome)	1. white patch or early greying hair 2. deafness 3. displaced inner canthus 4. heterochromia of iris 5. syndactyly & finger contractures 6. carpal fusions		flexion contractures	non-progressive	neurocrest anomaly		most families are AD	Goodman et al (1982) Preus et al (1983)
Weill–Marchesani syndrome	1. short stature 2. stiff joints 3. camptodactyly 4. carpal tunnel 5. small/dislocated lenses	fingers hips	flexion flexion	slowly progressive	carpal & tarsal tunnel from excessive connective tissue	AR	30 families	Gorlin et al (1974)
Winchester syndrome	1. craniofacial asymmetry & coarsening 2. brachydactyly & contractures 3. faint corneal opacities 4. malar flush, thick facial skin	fingers elbows knees toes	flexed	progressive	lab: not MPS; pathology: swelling and degeneration of mitochondria, dilation of endoplasmic reticulum, replacement bone with fibres, fibroblastic function disorder, osteolysis of tarsals & osteoporosis	AR	4 families	Hollister et al (1974) Goodman & Gorlin (1977)
X-linked moderately severe	1. generalised contractures 2. dimples over shins 3. small mouth 4. may have mild MR	fingers elbows knees hips	flexion flexion flexion flexion	slowly improves	short hypoplastic tendons	X-linked recessive		Hall et al (1982b) Gareis & Mason (1984)

Table 60.4 Musculoskeletal involvement plus central nervous system dysfunction and/or MR

Entity	Primary features	Contractures		Progression	Lab tests, X-rays, Autopsy findings	Inheritance	Incidence	References
		Body area	Position					
Adducted thumbs (also see Clasp thumb and X-linked hyrdocephaly)	1. thumbs flexed 2. micrognathia, cleft palate 3. craniosynostosis 4. microcephaly, dysmyelination 5. pectus excavatum	thumbs elbows wrists, knees feet	flexed, adducted limited extension clubbed, varus		chromosomes: normal; EMG; abnormal, cine-oesophagoscopy: abnormal; lab: proteinuria; pathology: displaced tendons, dysmyelination, long	AR	4 families	Christian et al (1971)
Antley–Bixler (X-Trapezoidocephaly)	1. unusual facies with frontal bossing 2. craniosynostosis 3. contractures – camptodactyly 4. radiohumeral synostosis 5. congenital contractures of femur 6. scoliosis	fingers wrist elbows ankles toes	flexed flexion at 190°, carpal synostosis radiohumeral synostosis tarsal synostosis flexed		ECG, EMG, lab: WNL; X-ray: radiohumeral synostoses, tarsal synostoses, choanal atresia	AR	10 families	Antley & Bixler (1975) Robinson et al (1982) Antley & Bixler (1983) Schinzel et al (1983) Herva & Seppanen (1983)
Bartsocas–Papas syndrome (Lethal popliteal pterygium)	1. contractures with marked webs 2. syndactyly leading to mitten hand and foot 3. cleft lip, nose and palate 4. abnormal skin around mouth and anal area 5. microcephalic 6. IUGR	all joints (particularly knee to foot)	flexion, web	usually lethal	perioral and perianal and distal limb skin dysplasia	AR	6 families	Bartsocas & Papas (1972) Distefano & Romeo (1974) Papadia et al (1987)
Bixler-microcephaly	1. IUGR 2. microcephaly 3. generalised flexion, contractures 4. seizures 5. large nose & eyes 6. cleft palate, small mandible 7. ↑ A P diameter 8. cup ears			lethal		AR	1 family 2 daughters	Bixler & Antley (1974)
Bowen-Conradi syndrome	1. IUGR 2. microcephaly 3. micrognathia 4. prominent nose 5. cloudy corneae 6. large ears 7. clinodactyly and rockerbottom feet	hand feet hips	ulnar valgus dislocated	lethal	absent vermis hypoplastic cerebellum	AR	10 families	Bowen & Conradi (1976) Hunter et al (1979)

Syndrome	Features	Joints/limbs	Foot deformity	Prognosis	Investigations / pathology	Inheritance	No. of cases	References
Campto-melic dysplasia	1. curvature & shortening of long bones, particularly femur & tibia 2. pretibial dimpling over curves 3. cleft palate 4. hypoplasia of facial bones, scapulae and fibula 5. +/− ambiguous genitalia 6. +/− craniosynostosis	hips elbows feet	CDH synostosis calcaneo-valgus or equinovarus	lethal, perinatal or death in infancy observed	X-rays, bowing of long bones, pathology; abnormal enchondral ossification; chromosomes: normal; ambiguous genitalia, fractures, platyspondyly	AR	100 cases	Thurmon et al (1973) Khajavi et al (1976) Houston et al (1983) Cooke et al (1985)
Cerebro-oculo-facio-skeletal (COFS) (Pena-Shokier II)	1. microcephaly, IUGR 2. cataracts, microphthalmia 3. micrognathia, abnormal ears 4. overlapping flexed fingers 5. calcaneovalgus 6. hypotonia	fingers elbows hips knees feet	flexed, medially deviated flexion; calcaneovalgus	lethal progressive degenerates	dysmyelinisation; chromosomes: normal, radiographs: platyspondyly, membranous cranial bones decreased ossification, osteoporosis; renal anomalies, osteopetrosis can be seen	AR	at least 40 cases	Preus et al (1977) Pena et al (1978) Scott-Emuakpor et al (1977) Siber (1984) Lerman Sagie et al (1987)
Clasp thumb and mental retardation	1. adducted thumb 2. +/− camptodactyly 3. +/− club foot 4. moderate to severe mental retardation 5. microcephaly to hydrocephaly +/− aqueductal stenosis	wide range of contractures		lethal to long life	malformation of neurons, hypoplastic thumb	X-linked recessive	very variable	Edwards (1961) Gareis & Mason (1984) Yeatman (1984)
Dyggve-Melchior-Clausen syndrome	1. camptodactyly 2. short trunk 3. mental retardation 4. short long bones 5. short neck	fingers stiff	claw-like	progressive	platyspondyly, irregular lacy iliac crest, vertebral notch	AR X-linked	50 cases	Bonafede & Beighton (1978) Yunis et al (1980)
Dysse-gmental dysplasia (Rolland Desbuquos)	1. short trunk 2. thick broad long bones 3. cleft palate 4. stiff joints		segmental dysplasia	lethal	segmental spinal defects	AR 2 subtypes	30 cases	Aleck et al (1987)
Faciocar-diomelic	1. IUGR 2. microstomia, epicanthal folds, abnormal ears, microglossia, glossoptosis 3. short/webbed neck 4. short limbs 5. CHD, complex 6. talipes varus	hands feet	radial deviation talipes or varus	lethal	lab, chromosomes: normal; pathology: complex CHD; X-ray: delayed bone age, shortened limbs, thumb hypoplasia, short metacarpals	AR with consan-guinity vs. X-linked	3 male sibs	Cantu et al (1975)

Table 60.4 Musculoskeletal involvement plus central nervous system dysfunction and/or MR (*contd.*)

Entity	Primary features	Contractures Body area	Position	Progression	Lab tests, X-rays, Autopsy findings	Inheritance	Incidence	References
Fetal alcohol syndrome	1. microcephaly/IUGR 2. characteristic facial features 3. joint contractures, palmar creases (73%) 4. +/− CHD (50%) 5. mental retardation	fingers elbow hips	limitation dislocation flexion	non-progressive	pathology: CNS abnormal; CHD	teratogen	over 200 cases	Jones & Smith (1973) Hanson et al (1976) Mulvihill & Yeager (1976) Clarren et al (1987)
FG syndrome	1. MR, large head 2. broad tall forehead with cowlick 3. hypotonia +/− joint contractures 4. imperforate anus and other GI abnormalities, including constipation 5. +/− CHD 6. seizures; CNS anomalies 7. +/− contractures 8. hyperactive	fingers wrists knees ankles feet	ulnar deviation radial deviation limited extension lateral displacement	non-progressive	chromosomes: normal; pathology: CNS abnormal; +/− agenesis of the corpus callosum	X-linked recessive	50 cases	Opitz & Kareggia (1974) Riccardi (1977) Neri et al (1984) Thompson (1985) Richieri-Costa (1986) Thompson & Baraitser (1987)
Fryns syndrome	1. coarse face, cloudy corneae 2. cleft palate, micrognathia 3. hypoplasia/aplasia lung 4. digitalisation thumbs 5. distal limb deformities & hypoplasia 6. GU anomalies 7. +/− absent diaphragm 8. omphalocele	fingers thumbs	flexion PIP digital- ization	lethal	chromosomes: normal; X-rays: hands and feet − rudimentary digit development; pathology: hypoplasia lungs and diaphragm, broad clavicles	AR	10 families	Fryns et al (1979) Meinecke & Fryns (1985)
Geleo-physic dysplasia	1. short stature & short bones 2. campto and brachydactyly 3. congenital heart anomalies, aortic stenosis 4. dislocated dysplastic hip 5. club feet 6. happy facial appearance 7. mental retardation	fingers hips feet	campto-dactyly dislocated clubbed	progressive	X-rays: dyostosis multiplex, inclusions in WBC and liver	AR		Koiffman et al (1984) Spranger et al (1984)
German syndrome	1. generalised contractures 2. oedema 3. fetal akinesis sequence 4. hypotonia 5. hypotonic facies 6. cleft or high palate 7. large ears 8. mental retardation	generalized	flexion	non-progressive, oedema improves	muscle microscopic glycogen, brain apparently normal	AR		Lewin & Hughes (1987)

Syndrome	Features	Contractures	Course	Pathology / CNS	Inheritance	Frequency	References
Hyper-thermia maternal	1. history of maternal fever >39°C for several hours 2. microcephaly 3. +/− microphthalmia 4. +/− cleft palate 5. mental retardation 6. +/− seizures 7. generalised contractures	flexion	non-progressive but may have cerebral palsy	CNS structural anomalies	teratogen		Clarren et al (1979) Fisher & Smith (1980) Smith (1982) Edwards (1986)
Ives micro-cephaly micromelia	1. IUGR 2. microcephaly 3. fused elbows 4. short forearm +/− 1 bone 5. hypoplastic hand missing whole digits	generalized flexion	lethal	pathology: renal dysplasia, decreased myelin	AR	several Cree families	Ives & Houston (1980)
Lenz-Majewski (hyper-ostotic dysplasia)	1. progressive osteosclerosis or osteopetrosis 2. synostosis and symphalangism 3. enamel abnormalities 4. broad ribs and clavicles 5. pinched nose +/− choanal atresia 6. large ears, prominent eyes 7. mental retardation 8. thin skin with prominent veins 9. delayed closure of fontanel	generalized flexion	progressive	choanol atresia	AD	4 sporadic cases	Lenz & Majewski (1969) Robinow et al (1977) Gorlin & Whitely (1983)
Leprech-aunism	1. IUGR 2. specific elfin facies 3. hirsutism 4. loose skin, dry 5. contractures	hands feet	flexion talipes varus	lethal	autopsy: renal hyperplasia, focal changes in liver, calcified deposits in kidneys, aberration of endocrine system, brain-normal, insulin receptor defect	AR	very rare	Donohue (1954) Der Kaloustian et al (1971) Elsas et al (1985)
Marden-Walker	1. blepharophimosis arachnodactyly 2. joint contractures, kyphosis, pectus 3. +/− hypotonia congenital 4. characteristic facies: immobile depressed nasal bridge, pursed lips 5. mental retardation s/s	wrists elbows hips knees ankles	flexion equinovarus	lethal	pathology: atrophic muscles, CHD, microcysts in kidneys, ↓ muscle fibre size; haematology and urine: normal	sporadic	10 cases	Fitch et al (1971) Jaatoul et al (1982) Jancar & Miele (1985) Gossage et al (1987)

Table 60.4 Musculoskeletal involvement plus central nervous system dysfunction and/or MR (*contd.*)

Entity	Primary features	Contractures Body area	Position	Progression	Lab tests, X-rays, Autopsy findings	Inheritance	Incidence	References
Martsolf syndrome	1. short stature 2. mental retardation 3. hypogonadism (small penis) 4. malocclusion 5. cataracts 6. hypermobile tapering fingers 7. adducted thumb 8. Arnold Chiari malformation 9. clubbed feet			non-progressive		AR or XR	2 families	Martsolf et al (1978) Sanchez et al (1985)
MASA	1. adducted thumbs 2. aphasia 3. shuffling gait 4. short stature 5. mental retardation			non-progressive		AR	2 families	Bianchine & Lewis (1974)
Megalo-cornea and skeletal anomalies	1. Megalocornea 2. unusual shaped hand 3. prominent forehead 4. saddle nose, large ears 5. micrognathia 6. gibbus/kyphoscoliosis 7. contractures distally 8. mental retardation 9. IUGR	flexion	campto-dactyly club foot		chromosome: normal; X-ray: kyphoscoliosis, thin cortical bone of skull	AR	4 families	Frank et al (1973) Neuhauser et al (1975)
Meningo-myelocele	1. spinal lesion 2. paralysis → joint contractures 3. others +/−	usually lower limbs depending on lesion position	flexed	can be lethal			multi-factorial	Smith (1982)
Mietens	1. corneal opacity, strabismus, nystagmus 2. flexion elbows 3. growth failure 4. mental retardation	elbows knees	flexed limited extension		X-rays: metacarpal bone age ↑, head of radius dislocated bilaterally, epiphyses absent, shortened ulna and radius, clinodactyly; chromosomes: normal	AR	4 families	Mietens & Weber (1966) Smith (1982)

Condition	Clinical features	Site	Deformity	Prognosis	Investigations/pathology	Inheritance	Cases	References
Miller-Dieker (lissencephaly)	1. lissencephaly – brain with smooth surface and large ventricles 2. seizures 3. IUGR 4. CHD 5. hypotonia 6. camptodactyly 7. microcephaly	hands	campto-dactyly generalized flexion contractures	lethal	chromosome 17 deleted; autopsy: lissencephaly, PDA, renal agenesis, duodenal atresion		several families	Stratton et al (1984) Dobyns et al (1985) Dobyns (1987)
Multiple pterygium lethal (Gillin Pryce Davis type)	1. multiple pterygium in utero 2. IUGR, polyhydramnios 3. contractures +/− bony fusion 4. facies with ocular hypertelorism 5. lung hypoplasia 6. cystic hygroma	hands elbows hips knees feet	flexion calcaneo-valgus	lethal may die in utero prenatally diagnosed	pathology: lung hypoplasia, cerebellar hypoplasia; chromosomes: normal	AR	15 families	Gillin & Pryse-Davis (1976) Hall (1984) Van Regemorter et al (1984) Herva & Seppanen (1985) Martin et al (1986) Tolmie et al (1987a)
Multiple sclerosis in mother	1. Maternal MS 2. multiple congenital contractures 3. flexion contractures	feet hips	equinovarus dislocated	non-progressive		possible teratogen		Livingstone & Sack (1984)
Myhre contractures with muscular hypertrophy	1. distal contractures 2. muscle hypertrophy 3. hearing loss 4. short stature 5. mental retardation	legs			X-ray: thickened calvarium, broad prominent mandible, broad ribs, flattened vertebra	AD	4 cases (?)	Myhre et al (1981) Soljak et al (1983)
Myotonic Dystrophy – Severe Congenital (SCMD)	1. mother with myotonic dystrophy 2. poor suck, difficulty swallowing 3. generalized hypotonia 4. facial diplegia 5. talipes equinovarus 6. cataracts, ptosis, MR	knees phalanges feet	frog position hyperex-tension talipes equinovarus	progressive; changes from normal muscle histology and EMG, life expectancy limited	biopsy: muscular dystrophy, pathology: abnormal CNS; mitral valve prolapse; prenatal diagnosis possible	AD (maternal effect)	over 75 cases	Harper (1975) Zellweger et al (1967) Zellweger (1973) Bell & Smith (1972) Swift & Finegold (1969)
Neu Laxova	1. lissencephaly, microcephaly, absence of corpus callosum 2. flexion deformities 3. short neck, hypertelorism, micrognathia, exophthalmos 4. syndactyly, oedema 5. IUGR, open eyes 6. ichthyotic skin changes	fingers wrists elbows hips knees ankles feet	overlapping flexed rocker bottom	lethal prenatally diagnosable	chromosomes: normal; pathology: lissencephaly, absent corpus callosum, cerebellar hypoplasia, lung hypoplasia, small placenta, short umbilical cord, skin with ichthyotic changes	AR	30 cases	Neu (1971) Laxova et al (1972) Lazjuk et al (1979) Curry (1982) Tolmie et al (1987b) Muller et al (1987)

Table 60.4 Musculoskeletal involvement plus central nervous system dysfunction and/or MR (*contd.*)

Entity	Primary features	Contractures Body area	Position	Progression	Lab tests, X-rays, Autopsy findings	Inheritance	Incidence	References
Neuro-muscular disease of larynx	1. IUGR 2. abnormal CNS 3. Pierre Robin facies 4. respiratory distress, absent arytenoid cartilage 5. no visceral malformations	hands feet 3rd finger	clubbed flexion	lethal	autopsy: absent L arytenoid cartilage, brain abnormal, neuro-myopathic changes in limb and laryngeal intrinsic muscles, normal chromosomes	sporadic		Schmitt (1978)
Nezelof syndrome (renal-hepatic)	1. joint contractures 2. liver disease (pigment overload and biliary stasis) 3. renal dysfunction	hand foot	'clubbed' calcaneus and talipes equinus	lethal	autopsy: rarefaction of anterior horn cells	AR	1 family	Nezelof et al (1979)
Oculo-dental-digital syndrome	1. small sunken eyes, thin nose 2. severe hypoplasia of enamel, microdontia 3. phalangeal hypoplasia, camptodactyly of 4th and 5th digits	fingers hallux	campto-dactyly abduction		chromosomes: normal; X-rays: absence of middle phalanges of toes, widening long and short tubular bones and ribs and clavicles	AD	30 cases	Gorlin et al (1963) Spranger et al (1974) Judisch et al (1979) Patton et al (1985)
Osteo-genesis imperfecta, congenital lethal 'crumpled bone type' (Type II)	1. short limbs 2. fractures – poor mineralisation, wormian bones 3. blue sclerae, shallow orbits, small nose 4. +/− contractures, hydrocephalus	wrists elbows knees feet	flexed flexed webbing	lethal, often stillborn	X-ray: wormian bones, fractures, cystic changes – long bones, flattened vertebrae, poor mineralization, crumpled bones. Type 1 collagen defect	AD	relatively common, 6% recurrence risk	Guha et al (1969) Sharma & Anand (1975) Sillence (1978) Byers et al (1988)
Oto-palato-digital Type II	1. deafness – conductive 2. dwarfism/bone dysplasia 3. adontia, soft cleft palate 4. characteristic facies: hypertelorism, frontal bossing 5. mild mental retardation 6. broad distal phalanges	fingers wrists elbows toes	broad distal phalanges limited supination limited extension clino-dactyly, broad distal phalanges		X-ray: facial bones hypoplastic; 2° ossification centre at base of metacarpals and tarsals, short metacarpals, broad distal phalanges, pectus excavatum	X-linked recessive	rare	Taybi (1962) Gorlin (1970) Brewster et al (1985) Vigneron et al (1987)
Palant syndrome	1. camptodactyly 2. cleft palate 3. mental retardation 4. broad nasal bridge 5. short stature 6. scoliosis	fingers wrist	campto-dactyly flexion				2 sibs	Palant et al (1971)

Syndrome	Clinical features	Site	Deformity	Lethality	Pathology / notes	Inheritance	Frequency	References
Pena-Shokeir phenotype (ankylosis, facial anomalies and pulmonary hypoplasia)	1. IUGR 2. CNS abnormalities 3. ankylosis of joints 4. pulmonary hypoplasia 5. polyhydramnios, small placenta, short umbilical cord 6. hypertelorism, micrognathia 7. fetal akinesia sequence	hands; elbow; hip; knee; feet	camptodactyly; flexed; ankylosis; clubbed	lethal in almost all cases, prenatally diagnosable	pathology: lung hypoplasia; chromosomes: normal; at least 6 different familial forms on basis of CNS changes	some sporadic, most AR	at least 70 cases	Punnett et al (1974) Pena & Shokeir (1970) Hunter et al (1979) Hall (1986) Moessinger (1983) Davis & Kalousek (1988)
Potter syndrome	1. renal agenesis 2. flattened face, large floppy ears, micrognathia, skin crease under eyes, wrinkled skin 3. joint contractures 4. oligohydramnios, lung hypoplasia, broad hands, club feet	hands; wrists; elbows; hips; knees; ankles; feet	'spade-like'; fixed; flexion; clubbed	lethal	chromosomes: normal; autopsy: +/− absent uterus and vagina, pulmonary hypoplasia, kidneys and ureters absent or rudimentary, fetal akinesia sequence	sporadic occasional AR/AD	not rare 1/3000–9000 births	Passarge & Sutherland (1965) Smith (1982) McPherson et al (1987)
Prader-Willi habitus, osteoporosis, hand contractures	1. MR 2. short stature 3. obesity 4. genital abnormalities 5. hand and feet contractures	hands; feet	flexed		X-ray: wormian bones, osteoporosis; chromosomes: normal; thyroid: normal	AR?	2 brothers	Urban et al (1979)
Restrictive dermopathy	1. flexion contractures 2. tight thin skin 3. open eyes and mouth			lethal: prenatally diagnosable	miniature constrained skin with inclusion	AR	5 families	Lowry et al (1985) Witt et al (1986) Holbrook et al (1987) Gillerot & Koulischer (1987)
Roberts syndrome (pseudo-thalidomide syndrome, SC syndrome)	1. microbrachycephalia, +/− craniosynostosis 2. limb reduction +/− humeroradial synostosis 3. +/− cleft lip and palate 4. characteristic facies 5. moderate to severe MR 6. +/− IUGR	elbows; knees; feet	radio-humeral synostosis; femorotibial fusion; talipes, calcaneovalgus	can be lethal	chromosomes: can have 'puffing' phenomena; pathology: CHD, renal anomalies	AR	over 30	Herrman et al (1969) Freeman et al (1974) Grosse et al (1975) Ladda et al (1978) Tomkins & Sisken (1984) Romke et al (1987)
Rudiger	1. camptodactyly 2. coarse facies 3. hydronephrosis and ureteral stenosis 4. cleft palate 5. short limbs 6. diaphragmatic hernia	finger; joints	camptodactyly; stiff				2 sibs	Rudiger et al (1971) Fitch et al (1978)

Table 60.4 Musculoskeletal involvement plus central nervous system dysfunction and/or MR (*contd.*)

Entity	Primary features	Contractures		Progression	Lab tests, X-rays, Autopsy findings	Inheritance	Incidence	References
		Body area	*Position*					
Rutledge	1. short limbs 2. club feet 3. camptodactyly 4. dislocated elbows and knees 5. micrognathia 6. ambiguous genitalia	fingers elbow knee feet	flexed dislocated dislocated clubbed	lethal	pathology: renal hypoplasia, hydrocephaly, unilobar lung	AR	3 cases	Rutledge et al (1984)
Schinzel Giedion	1. hypertrichosis 2. congenital heart defect 3. high prominent forehead 4. hydronephrosis 5. mental retardation 6. camptodactyly 7. club foot 8. choanal atresia 9. abundant skin	fingers feet	campto-dactyly clubbed flexion contractures	usually lethal		AR	3 families	Schinzel & Giedion (1978) Kelley et al (1982)
Smith-Lemli-Opitz (Type II-Severe)	1. camptodactyly and syndactyly +/- polydactyly 2. CNS structural anomalies 3. renal agenesis/cysts/dysplasia 4. pulmonary segmentation			lethal	multiple internal anomalies of all systems	AR	20 families	Curry et al (1987)
Schwartz-Jampel	1. small stature 2. myotonia 3. fixed facial expression, pinched 4. contractures; pectus carinatum 5. blepharophimosis; myopia 6. normal intelligence	fingers wrists hips toes +/- feet	limitation equinovarus	progressive: very mild at birth, gets worse during childhood	EMG: characteristic myotonic pattern not abolished by curare; X-ray: fragmentation and flattening of epiphyses and vertebrae, pectus, reduced muscle mass, hip movement, carpal turned, dislocated radial head, malignant hyperthermia	AR	at least 7 cases reported	Aberfeld et al (1965) Smith (1982) Goldberg (1987) Farrell et al (1987a)
Tricho-Rhino-Phalangeal syndrome Type II (Langer-Giedion)	1. bulbous nose 2. sparse hair 3. multiple exostoses 4. long philtrum 5. mental retardation 6. multiple contractures	fingers hip ankle	campto-dactyly bony limitation contractures limitation	progressive as exostoses grow	chromosomes: 8 deletion, exostosis on X-ray and pathology cone epiphysis on X-ray	acts like AD		Murachi et al (1981)

Syndrome	Clinical features	Location	Deformity	Prognosis	Investigations	Inheritance	Number	References
Trigonocephaly (C syndrome)	1. trigonocephaly (triangular shape) 2. metopic suture fusion 3. nose with broad root 4. anteverted nares 5. hypotelorism 6. club feet 7. contractures 8. dislocated hips 9. mental retardation	fingers knees elbows hips feet	campto- and clinodactyly flexed flexed dislocated clubbed	often lethal	chromosomes: normal	AR	8 families	Opitz et al (1969a) Say & Meyer (1981) Sargent et al (1985)
VSR syndrome	1. short stature 2. trigonocephaly 3. cleft palate 4. scoliosis 5. rhizomelic shortening		generalised flexion contractures	non-progressive		AD	1 family	Herrmann & Opitz (1974)
Van Benthem	1. cryptorchidism 2. chest deformity, pulmonary anomalies 3. hypoplasia of muscle and absence of subcutaneous fat 4. MR severe, dolichocephaly 5. flexed knees, arachnodactyly 6. IUGR and mental retardation	knees	flexed	lethal	chromosomes, lab: normal; pathology: subcutaneous fat, atrophic musculature	AR or X-linked	3 families	Van Benthem et al (1970), Van Benthem (1975)
Van Biervielt chest dysplasia	1. IUGR/psychomotor delay 2. craniofacial dysostosis 3. joint contractures 4. progeroid appearance 5. chest dysplasia	toes fingers elbows hips knees feet	campto-dactyly flexed limited extension clubbed	lethal	EEG abnormal; EMG normal; lab: CMV in saliva of 1 sib, chromosomes: normal	AR	2 sibs	Van Biervielt et al (1977)
Warburg syndrome (HARD +/−E, Cerebro-oculo-muscular syndrome)	1. hydrocephaly/large ventricles +/− 2. abnormal nerve migration with dysmyelination 3. retinal aplasia/dysplasia 4. microphthalmia/cataract 5. hypotonia 6. +/− encephalocele 7. muscle dystrophy 8. joint contractures 9. adducted thumbs		generalised contractures	lethal progression	lissencephaly, ocular hypoplasia, adductal cong. stenosis, muscular dystrophy changes	AR	40 families	Takada et al (1984) Williams et al (1984) Donnai & Farndon (1986) Farrell et al (1987b)
Weaver syndrome	1. macrosomia 2. accelerated skeletal maturation 3. camptodactyly 4. unusual facies	fingers +/− feet	campto-dactyly talipes equinovarus		X-ray: broad distal femurs and ulnae	sporadic	2 cases (1974)	Weaver et al (1974) Smith (1982)

Table 60.4 Musculoskeletal involvement plus central nervous system dysfunction and/or MR (contd.)

Entity	Primary features	Contractures		Progression	Lab tests, X-rays, Autopsy findings	Inheritance	Incidence	References
		Body area	Position					
Wieacker muscular atrophy and contractures	1. club feet 2. progressive distal atrophy 3. dyspraxia of eye and tongue muscles 4. mild mental retardation	feet	clubbed	progressive		X-linked recessive	1 family	Wieacker et al (1985) Wieacker et al (1987)
Zellweger syndrome (cerebrohepatorenal)	1. CNS impairment, IUGR 2. hypotonia +/− joint contractures 3. myopathic facies 4. hepatomegaly 5. high forehead with delayed closure of sutures	hands fingers knees feet	ulnar deviation flexed flexion clubbed	lethal	chromosomes: normal; X-ray: calcification density over ischium and hip joints, stippling of patella and hands; pathology: agenesis corpus callosum, lissencephaly, renal cysts; ECG, EEG: abnormal, abnormal liver function with iron deposits, peroxisomal disorder	AR	over 100 reports	Bowen et al (1964) Poznanski et al 1970b Moser et al (1984) Hajra et al (1985) Wilson et al (1986) Weese–Mayer et al (1987)
47XXY/ 48XXXY	1. bilateral aniridia/ exophthalmos/glaucoma 2. severe mental retardation 3. webbing 4. cryptorchidism 5. pes equinovarus	elbows knees	flexion, cubital webbing flexion, popliteal webbing	progressive		chromosome abnormality	1 case	Pashayan et al (1973)
48XXXX and 49XXXXY	1. mental retardation 2. scoliosis 3. hypertelorism 4. contractures, clinodactyly of fifth finger	hands elbows knees +/− feet	clinodactyly radioulnar synostosis flexed equinovarus, pes planus		X-ray: thick sternum, scoliosis, radioulnar synostosis	chromosome abnormality	4 cases	Smith (1982)
trisomy 4p	1. MR, IUGR 2. small spherical nose, nasal aplasia 3. scoliosis 4. S/S	fingers hand feet hallux	flexion clubbed varus, calcaneovalgus	1/3 die in childhood	X-ray: scoliosis; abnormal vertebrae, hips, iliac alae, sacrum, costal hypoplasia, decreased ossification	chromosome abnormality	23 cases	de Grouchy & Turleau (1977)

Syndrome	Clinical features	Site	Anomaly	Prognosis	Pathology	Diagnosis	Cases	References
trisomy 8 / trisomy 8 mosaicism	1. moderate MR 2. high prominent forehead, long face, thick everted lower lip, large ears 3. skeletal malformations 4. +/− cryptorchidism, testicular hypoplasia 5. deep palmar-plantar creases	hands elbows hips knees feet	campto-dactyly ankylosed arti-culations absent patellae clubbed, hallux valgus	normal lifespan	pathology: +/− cardiopathy, +/− renal anomaly	chromo-some abnormality	most mosaic at least 30 cases	de Grouchy & Turleau (1977) Yunis (1977)
trisomy 9	1. MR, brachycephaly 2. CHD 3. bulbous nose 4. abnormal genitalia	fingers hands feet	overlapping clubbed	lethal	pathology: PDA, VSD +/− cerebral abnormalities; X-ray: dislocation knees, elbows, hips	chromo-some abnormality	at least 10 cases	de Grouchy & Turleau (1977) Yunis (1977)
trisomy 9q	1. MR 2. small face, beaked nose, micrognathia 3. amyotrophy	fingers hips knees hallux	long, tapering index overlaps at right angle flexion hammertoe	retarded	pathology: amyotrophy	chromo-some abnormality	3 cases	de Grouchy & Turleau (1977)
trisomy 10q	1. MR/microcephaly 2. hypotonia 3. CHD	fingers lg. joint toes	taper dislocations hammer	1/2 die in first year	pathology: cardiac, renal malformations; X-ray: scoliosis	chromo-some abnormality	9 cases	de Grouchy & Turleau (1977)
trisomy 10p	1. IUGR, dolichocephaly 2. skeletal anomalies 3. lips inverted 4. hypotonia	finger hands elbows	campto-dactyly flexion	usually lethal	pathology: cardiac- 1/3, renal, ocular abnormalities; X-ray diaphyses, metaphyses are slender and narrow	chromo-some abnormality	9 cases	de Grouchy & Turleau (1977)
trisomy 11q	1. MR 2. +/− renal anomalies, cardiopathy 3. +/− agenesis corpus callosum 4. contractures	elbows hips +/− feet	synostosis, fixed flexion ABD clubbed	1/2 die within 1 year	X-ray: acetabulum dysplasia, radioulnar synostosis; pathology: visceral malformations +/−	chromo-some abnormality	14 cases	Yunis (1977) de Grouchy & Turleau (1977)

Table 60.4 Musculoskeletal involvement plus central nervous system dysfunction and/or MR (*contd.*)

Entity	Primary features	Contractures Body area	Position	Progression	Lab tests, X-rays, Autopsy findings	Inheritance	Incidence	References
trisomy 13	1. MR, microcephaly, holoprosencephaly 2. multiple visceral anomalies 3. bilateral cleft lip 4. microphthalmia 5. hexadactyly	fingers feet	overlapping calcaneo-valgus	mean life expectancy: 130 days	pathology: oculocerebral malformations, cardiac, renal abnormalities	chromo-some abnormality	1/4000-1/10 000 L.B.	Yunis (1977) de Grouchy & Turleau (1977)
partial trisomy 14 (proximal)	1. severe MR 2. prominent nose, MR, cupid bow mouth	fingers hips feet	flexion CDH	staturo-ponderal retardation	pathology: cardiopathy	chromo-some abnormality	at least 8 cases	Yunis (1977) de Grouchy & Turleau (1977)
trisomy 15 (proximal)	1. MR – IQ=20 2. seizures, hypotonia	fingers toes +/− feet	mal-positioned clubbed				15 cases	de Grouchy & Turleau (1977)
trisomy 18	1. corneal opacities/cataracts 2. abnormal ears 3. short neck, webbed 4. cryptorchidism 5. limb anomalies 6. visceral anomalies	fingers hands elbows hips knees feet	overlapping flexion calcaneo-valgus	lethal	pathology: cerebral, ocular, cardiac renal malformations; X-ray: +/− vertebral anomalies, CDH	chromo-some abnormality	1/8000 births	Yunis (1977) de Grouchy & Turleau (1977)

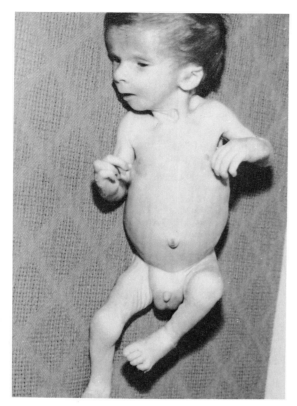

Fig. 60.5 Congenital contractures associated with central nervous system dysfunction. Note all limbs have flexion contractures, there is microcephaly with an abnormally shaped head and an unusual facies. The infant has micro-ophthalmia, abnormally shaped ears, a thin upper lip, long philtrum, and micrognathia and a large inguinal hernia.

polyhydramnios, short umbilical cord and unusual craniofacies being noted. This combination of features seems to be due to fetal akinesia (Moessinger 1983) suggesting the fetus must move in utero to have normal development. At least six familial subtypes can be distinguished on CNS pathology, suggesting that the external features represent a phenotype rather than a specific diagnosis. Prenatal diagnosis is possible in these families (Davis & Kalousek 1988).

Cerebro-oculo-facial-skeletal syndrome

Pena and Shokeir also described cerebro-oculo-facial-skeletal syndrome (COFS). This has led to a great deal of confusion since it seems to be one of the more common lethal conditions with contractures, characterised by structural abnormalities of the brain, dysmyelinisation,

and eye anomalies including microphthalmia and cataracts. The natural history of this degenerative condition is variable even within a family (Winter et al 1981). In some families, some affected individuals are born with contractures and others are spared at birth but develop contractures later in life (Scott–Emuakpor et al 1977). Renal anomalies, other visceral anomalies, and osteoporosis can be seen (Lerman-Sagie et al 1987). An X-linked recessive form may exist (Siber 1984).

Neu-Laxova syndrome

Neu-Laxova is a striking phenotype with dramatic contractures, intrauterine growth retardation, microcephaly, open eyes, tight ichthyotic skin and severe CNS anomalies (Curry 1982, Tolmie et al 1987b). Kyphosis, syndactyly, and hydrops are often seen. It is a lethal autosomal recessive and can be diagnosed prenatally (Muller et al 1987).

Restrictive dermopathy

Several recent reports describe a syndrome with contractures in which it appears that fetal skin fails to grow normally and thereby restricts movement, leading to secondary contractures. All families are compatible with autosomal recessive inheritance (Lowry et al 1985, Witt et al 1986, Holbrook et al 1987).

Chromosomal anomalies

Many chromosomal anomalies can have congenital contractures (Reed et al 1985). When no other diagnosis can be reached in a child with mental retardation and multiple congenital contractures, chromosome studies should be done. If the lymphocyte karyotype is normal, fibroblast chromosomal studies should be considered. Two chromosomal anomalies are particularly striking for the frequency of multiple congenital contractures.

Trisomy 18 Probably the most frequent condition in this category is trisomy 18, which is characterised by intrauterine growth retardation, visceral anomalies with extremely high incidence of heart disease, radial limb anomalies, short sternum, small pelvis, facial paralysis and a typical positioning of fingers with overlapping fingers, clenched fists and rocker bottom feet.

Trisomy 8 mosaicism Trisomy 8 mosaicism also frequently presents with congenital contractures and is often characterised by absence of patella and deep furrows in the palms or soles. Individuals with trisomy 8 mosaicism may only be identified with fibroblast karyotype.

In addition to chromosomal anomalies and specific syndromes (see Table 60.4) within this third category of arthrogryposis with CNS disorders, there is a very high incidence of lethality and death within the first two years of life. Autopsies are helpful in making a diagnosis.

SUMMARY

Multiple congenital contractures are relatively frequent and often part of recognizable syndromes. Marked heterogeneity does exist as seen in Tables 60.2, 60.3 and 60.4. Careful investigation should lead to a specific diagnosis in over half the cases, allowing more specific prognostication, counselling and therapy.

REFERENCES

Aase J M, Smith D W 1968 Dysmorphogenesis of joints, brain and palate: A new dominantly inherited syndrome. Journal of Pediatrics 73: 606–611

Aberfeld D C, Hinterbuchner L P, Schneider M 1965 Myotonia, dwarfism diffuse bone disease and unusual ocular and facial abnormalities (a new syndrome). Brain 88: 313

Akbarnia B A, Bowen J R, Dougherty J 1979 Familial arthrogrypotic-like hand abnormality and sensorineural deafness. American Journal of Diseases of Children 133: 403–405

Aleck K A, Grix A, Clericuzio C et al 1987 Dyssegmental dysplasias: Clinical, radiographic and morphologic evidence of heterogeneity. American Journal of Medical Genetics 27: 295–312

Alves A F, Azevedo E S 1977 Recessive form of Freeman-Sheldon's syndrome or 'whistling face'. Journal of Medical Genetics 14: 139–141

Anderson R A, Koch S, Camerini-Otero R D 1984 Cardiovascular findings in congenital contractural arachnodactyly: report of an affected kindred. American Journal of Medical Genetics 18: 265–271

Antley R, Bixler D 1975 X-trapezoidocephaly, midfacial hypoplasia and cartilage abnormalities with multiple synostoses and skeletal fractures. Birth Defects Original Article Series 11: 397–401

Antley R M, Bixler D 1983 Invited editorial comment: Developments in the trapezoidcephaly-multiple synostosis syndrome. American Journal of Medical Genetics 14: 149–150

Ardinger H H, Hanson J W, Harrod M J E et al 1985 Further delineation of Weaver syndrome. Journal of Pediatrics 108: 228–235

Assemany S, Muzzo S, Gardner L 1972 Syndrome of phocomelic diabetic embryopathy. American Journal of Diseases of Children 123: 489–491

Athreya B H, Schumacher R 1978 Pathological features of a familial arthropathy associated with congenital flexion contractures of fingers. Arthritis and Rheumatism 21: 429–437

Baird H W III 1964 Kindred showing congenital absence of dermal ridges and associated anomalies. Journal of Pediatrics 64:621–631

Baird H W III 1968 Absence of fingerprints in four generations. Lancet II:1250

Banker B Q 1986 Arthrogryposis mulitiplex congenita: Spectrum of pathologic changes. Human Pathology 17:656–671

Baraitser M 1982 A new camptodactyly syndrome. Journal of Medical Genetics 19:40–43

Baraitser M, Winter R M, Taylor D S I 1982 Lenz Microphthalmia-A case report. Clinical Genetics 22:99–101

Baraitser M, Burn J, Fixsen J 1983 A recessively inherited windmill-vane camptodactyly/ichthyosis syndrome. Journal of Medical Genetics 20: 125–127

Bartsocas C S, Papas C V 1972 Popliteal pterygium syndrome: Evidence for a severe autosomal recessive form. Journal of Medical Genetics 9: 222–226

Bass H N, March S M, Sparkes R S, Crandall B F 1981 Congenital contractural arachnodactyly Keratoconus and probably Marfan syndrome in the same pedigree. Journal of Pediatrics 98: 591–595

Baty B J, Cubberley D, Morris C, Carey J 1988 Prenatal diagnosis of distal arthrogyposis. American Journal of Medical Genetics 29: 501–510

Bavinck J N B, Weaver D D 1986 Subclavian artery supply disruption sequence: Hypothesis of a vascular etiology for Poland, Klippel-Feil, and Moebius anomalies. American Journal of Medical Genetics 23: 903–918

Beals R K, Hecht F 1971 Congenital contractural arachnodactyly. Journal of Bone & Joint Surgery 53a: 987–993

Beck M, Roubicek M, Rogers J G 1983 Heterogeneity of metatropic dysplasia. European Journal of Pediatrics 140: 231–237

Belik J, Anday E K, Kaplan F, Zackai E 1985 Respiratory complications of metatropic dwarfism. Clinical Pediatrics 24: 504–511

Bell D G, Smith D W 1972 Myotonic dystrophy in the neonate. Journal of Pediatrics 81: 83–86

Bendon R, Dignan P, Siddiqi T 1987 Prenatal diagnosis of arthrogryposis multiplex congenita. Journal of Pediatrics 111: 942–946

Benzie R J, Malone R, Miskin M, Runn N, Schofield P 1976 Prenatal diagnosis by fetoscopy with subsequent normal delivery: report of a case. Journal of Pediatrics 126: 287–288

Bersani F A, Samilson R L 1957 Massive familial tarsal synostosis. Journal of Bone & Joint Surgery 39a: 1187–1189

Bersu E T, Pettersen J C, Charbonneau W J, Opitz J M 1976 Studies of malformation syndromes of man XXXXIA: Anatomical studies in the Hanhart syndrome – A pathogenetic hypothesis. European Journal of Pediatrics 122: 1–17

Bianchine J W, Lewis R C 1974 The MASA syndrome: A new heritable mental retardation syndrome. Clinical Genetics 5: 298–306

Bixler D, Antley R M 1974 Microcephalic dwarfism in sisters. Birth Defects Original Article Series 10: 161–165

Blumel J, Evans B C, Eggers G 1959 Partial and complete agenesis or malformation of the sacrum with associated anomalies. Journal of Bone & Joint Surgery 41a: 497–518

Bonafede R P, Beighton P 1978 The Dyggve-Melchior-Clausen syndrome in adult siblings. Clinical Genetics 14: 24–30

Bowen P, Conradi G J 1976 Syndrome of skeletal and genitourinary anomalies with unusual facies and failure to thrive in Hutterite sibs. Birth Defects Original Article Series XII: 101–108

Bowen P, Lee C S N, Zellweger H, Lindenberg R 1964 A familial syndrome of multiple congenital defects. Bulletin of the Johns Hopkins Hospital 114: 402–414

Braham R L 1969 Multiple congenital anomalies with diaphyseal dysplasia (Camurati-Englemann's syndrome). Oral Surgery 27: 20–26

Brans Y W, Lintermans J P 1972 The upper limb cardiovascular syndrome. American Journal of Diseases of Children 124: 779–783

Brewster T G, Lachman R S, Kushner D C et al 1985 Otopalatal-digital syndrome, type II – An X-linked skeletal dysplasia. American Journal of Medical Genetics 20: 249–254

Bucher H U, Boltshauser E, Briner J 1985 Neonatal nemaline myopathy presenting with multiple joint contractures. European Journal of Pediatrics 144: 288–290

Burton B K, Sumner T, Langer L O et al 1986 A new skeletal dysplasia: Clinical, radiologic and pathologic findings. Journal of Pediatrics 109: 642–648

Byers P H, Tsipouras P, Bonadio J F, Starman B J, Schwarz R C 1988 Perinatal lethal osteogenesis (OI Type II). American Journal of Human Genetics 42: 237–248

Cantu J M, Hernandez A, Ramirez J, Bernal M, Rubio G, Urrusti J, Franco-Vazquez S 1975 Lethal faciocardiomelic dysplasia – a new autosomal recessive disorder. Birth Defects Original Article Series XI: 91–98

Cantu J M, Garcia-Cruz D, Gil-Viera J et al 1985 Guaralajara camptodactyly syndrome type II. Clinical Genetics 28: 54–60

Carnevale A, Hernandez A L, de los Cobos L 1973 Sindrome de pterigium familiar con probable transmission dominate ligada al cromosoma X. Revista de Investigacion Clinica 25: 237–244

Challis J 1974 Hereditary transmission of talonavicular coalition in association with anomaly of the little finger. Journal of Bone and Joint Surgery (a) 56: 1273–1276

Christian J C, Andrews P A, Conneally P M, Muller J 1971 The adducted thumbs syndrome (an autosomal recessive disease with arthrogryposis, dysmyelineation, craniostenosis and cleft palate). Clinical Genetics 2: 95–103

Clarren S K, Hall J G 1983 Neuropathologic findings in the spinal cords of 10 infants with arthrogryposis. Journal of Neurological Sciences 58: 89–102

Clarren S, Ellsworth C, Sumi M, Streissguth A, Smith D W 1978 Brain malformations related to prenatal exposure to ethanol. Journal of Pediatrics 92: 64–67

Clarren S K, Smith D W, Harvey M A S, Ward R H 1979 Hyperthermia– a progressive evaluation of a possible teratogenic agent in May. Journal of Pediatrics 95: 81

Clarren S K, Sampson P D, Larsen J et al 1987 Facial effects of fetal alcohol exposure: Assessment by photographs and morphometric analysis. American Journal of Medical Genetics 26: 651–666

Cooke C T, Mulcahy M T, Cullity G J et al 1985 Campomelic dysplasia with sex reversal: Morphological and cytogenic studies of a case. Pathology 17: 526–529

Cos D J, Simmons F B 1974 Midline vocal cord fixation in the newborn. Archives of Otolaryngology 100: 219

Cox D, Pearce W G 1974 Variable expressivity in craniocarpotarsal dysplasia. Birth Defects Original Article Series X: 243–248

Currarino G, Friedman J M 1986 A severe form of congenital contractural arachnodactyly in two newborn infants. American Journal of Medical Genetics 25: 763–773

Curry C J R 1982 Further comments on the Neu-Laxova syndrome. American Journal of Medical Genetics 15: 515–517

Curry C J R, Carey J C, Holland J S et al 1987 Smith-Lemli-Opitz syndrome – type II: Multiple congenital anomalies with male pseudohermaphroditism and frequent early lethality. American Journal of Medical Genetics 26: 45–57

David T J 1982 Familial Poland Anomaly. Journal of Medical Genetics 19: 293–296

Davis J E, Kalousek D K 1988 Fetal akinesia deformation sequence in previable fetuses. American Journal of Medical Genetics 29: 77–87

de Grouchy J, Turleau C 1977 Clinical atlas of human chromosomes. Wiley, New York

DeMyer W, Baird I 1969 Mortality and skeletal malformations from amniocentesis and oligohydramnios in rats: cleft palate, clubfoot, microstomia and adactyly. Teratology 2: 33–38

Der Kaloustian V, Kronfol N, Takla R, Habash A, Khazin A, Najjar S 1971 Leprechaunism. American Journal of Diseases of Children 122: 442–445

Distefano G, Romeo M G 1974 La sindrome dello pterigio popliteo (contributo casistico). Rivista Pediatrica Siciliana XXIX: 54–75

Dobyns W B 1987 Developmental aspects of Lissencephaly and the Lissencephaly syndromes. Birth Defects Original Article Series 23: 225–241

Dobyns W B, Gilbert E F, Opitz J M 1985 Letter to the Editor: Further comments on the Lissencephaly syndromes. American Journal of Medical Genetics 22: 197–211

Donnai D, Farndon P A 1986 Walker-Warburg syndrome (Warburg syndrome, HARD +/− E syndrome). Journal of Medical Genetics 23: 200–203

Donner M, Rapola J, Somer H 1975 Congenital muscular dystrophy: a clinico-pathological and follow-up study of 15 patients. Neuropaediatrie 6, 239–258

Donohue W L 1954 Dysendocrinism. Journal of Pediatrics 45: 739–748

Drachman D 1961 Arthrogryposis multiplex congenita. Archives of Neurology 5: 89–93

Drachman D G, Coulombre A J 1962 Experimental clubfoot and arthrogryposis multiplex congenita. Lancet II: 523–526

Dubois H J 1970 Nievergelt-Pearlman syndrome: Synostosis in feet and hands with dysplasia of elbows: Report of a case. Journal of Bone and Joint Surgery 52(b): 325–329

Edwards J H 1961 The syndrome of sex-linked hydrocephalus. Archives of Disease in Childhood 36: 486–493

Edwards M J 1986 Hyperthermia as a teratogen: a review of experimental studies and their clinical significance. Teratogenesis Carcinogenesis and Mutagenesis 6: 563–582

Elsas L J, Endo F, Strumlauf E, Elders J, Priest J H 1985 Leprechaunism: an inherited defect in a high-affinity insulin receptor. American Journal of Human Genetics 37: 73–88

Escobar V, Weaver D 1978a Popliteal pterygium syndrome: A

phenotypic and genetic analysis. Journal of Medical Genetics 15: 35–42

Escobar V, Weaver D D 1978b Facio-genito-popliteal syndrome. Birth Defects Original Article Series XIV: 185–192

Escobar V, Bixler D, Gleiser S, Weaver D D, Gibbs T 1978 Multiple Pterygium syndrome. American Journal of Diseases of Children 132: 609–611

Eteson D J, Beluffi G, Burgio G R, Belloni C, Lachman R S, Rimoin D L 1986 Pseudodiastrophic dysplasia: A distinct newborn skeletal dysplasia. Journal of Pediatrics 109: 635–641

Fahy M, Hall J G 1989 Obstetrical complications in arthrogryposis. (in preparation)

Farrell S A, Davidson R G, Thorp P 1987a Neonatal manifestations of Schwartz-Jampel syndrome. American Journal of Medical Genetics 27: 799–805

Farrell S A, Toi A, Leadman M L, Davidson R G, Caco C 1987b Prenatal diagnosis of retinal detachment in Walker-Warburg syndrome. American Journal of Medical Genetics 28: 619–624

Fayad M N, Yacoub A, Salman S et al 1987 Juvenile Hyaline fibromatosis: Two new patients and review of the literature. American Journal of Medical Genetics 26: 123–131

Fisher N L, Smith D W 1980 Hyperthermia as a possible cause for occipital encephalocele. Clinical Research 38: 116A

Fisk J 1974 Congenital ulnar deviation of the fingers with clubfoot deformities. Clinical Orthopedics and Related Research 104: 200–205

Fitch N, Levy E P 1975 Adducted thumb syndromes. Clinical Genetics 8: 190–198

Fitch N, Karpati G, Pinsky L 1971 Congenital blepharophimosis, joint contractures and muscular hypotonia. Neurology 21: 1214–1220

Fitch N, Srolovitz H, Robitaille Y et al 1978 Absent left hemidiaphragm, arhinencephaly and cardiac malformations. Journal of Medical Genetics 15: 399–401

Fitzsimmons J S, Zaldua V, Chrispin R 1984 Genetic heterogeneity in the Freeman-Sheldon syndrome: two adults with probable autosomal recessive inheritance. Journal of Medical Genetics 21: 364–368

Flatt A 1977 The care of congenital hand anomalies. C V Mosby, St. Louis

Frank Y, Ziprkowski M, Romano A et al 1973 Megalocornea associated with multiple skeletal anomalies: A new genetic syndrome? Journale de Genetique Humaine 21: 67–72

Freeman M V R, Williams D W, Schimke R N, Temtamy S A 1974 The Roberts syndrome. Clinical Genetics 5: 1–16

Frias J L, Holahan J R, Rosenbloom A L, Felman A H 1973 An autosomal dominant syndrome of multiple pterygium, ptosis and skeletal abnormalities. In: Fourth International Conference on Birth Defects, Vienna. Excerpta Medica, Amsterdam 19:41

Fried K, Mundel G 1976 Absence of distal interphalangeal creases of fingers with flexion limitation. Journal of Medical Genetics 13: 127–130

Froster-Iskenius U G, Waterson J R, Hall J G 1988 A recessive form of congenital contractures and torticollis associated with malignant hyperthermia. Journal of Medical Genetics 25: 104–112

Fryns J P, Moerman F, Goddeeris P, Boxxuyt C, Van den Berghe H 1979 A new lethal syndrome with cloudy corneae, diaphragmatic defects and distal limb deformities. Human Genetics 50: 65–70

Fuhrmann W, Steffens C, Rompe G 1966 Dominant erbliche doppelseitige dysplasie und synostose de Ellenbogengelenks. Humangenetik 3: 64–77

Gareis F, Mason J D 1984 X-linked mental retardation associated with bilateral clasp thumb anomaly. American Journal of Medical Genetics 17: 333–338

Gilbert E F, Optiz J M, Spranger J W, Langer L O, Wolfson J J, Viseskul C 1976 Chondrodysplasia Punctata – rhizomelic form: Pathologic and radiologic studies of three infants. European Journal of Pediatrics 123: 89–109

Gillerot Y, Koulischer L 1987 Letter to the editor: Restrictive dermopathy. American Journal of Medical Genetics 27: 239–240

Gillin M E, Pryse-Davis J 1976 Case report - pterygium syndrome. Journal of Medical Genetics 13: 249–251

Gladstone I, Sybert V P 1982 Holt-Oram Syndrome: penetrance of the gene and lack of maternal effect. Clinical Genetics 21: 98–103

Gleiser S, Weaver D D, Escobar V, Nicholas G, Escobedo M 1978 Femoral hypoplasia – unusual facies syndrome from another viewpoint. European Journal of Pediatrics 128: 1–5

Goldberg J H, Mazzei R J 1977 Poland syndrome: A concept of pathogenesis based on limb bud embryology. Birth Defects Original Article Series 13: 103–115

Goldberg M 1987 Arthrogryposis multiplex congenita and arthrogryposis syndromes. In: The Dysmorphic Child: an Orthopedic Perspective. Raven, New York

Goodman R M, Gorlin R J 1977 Atlas of the face in genetic disorders, 2nd edn. Mosby, Saint Louis

Goodman R M, Katznelson M B-M, Hertz M, Katznelson A 1976 Camptodactyly, with muscular hypoplasia, skeletal dysplasia, and abnormal palmer creases: Tel Hashomer camptodactyly syndrome. Journal of Medical Genetics 13: 136–141

Goodman R M, Lewithal I, Solomon A, Klein D 1982 Upper limb involvement in the Klein-Waardenburg syndrome. American Journal of Medical Genetics 11: 425–433

Gorlin R J 1970 Inheritance of the oto-palato-digital syndrome. American Journal of Diseases of Children 119: 377

Gorlin R J, Whitely C B 1983 Lenz-Majewski syndrome. Radiology 149: 129–131

Gorlin R J, Sedano H O, Cervenka J 1968 Popliteal pterygium syndrome: A syndrome comprising cleft lip-palate, popliteal and intercrural pterygia, digital and genital anomalies. Pediatrics 41: 503–509

Gorlin R J, L'Heureux P R, Shapiro I 1974 Weill-Marchesani syndrome in two generations: Genetic heterogeneity or pseudodominance? Journal of Pediatric Ophthalmology 11: 139–144

Gorlin R J, Pindborg J J, Cohen M M 1976 Syndromes of the head and neck, 2nd edn. McGraw Hill, New York

Gossage D, Perrin J M, Butler M G 1987 Brief clinical report and review: a 26-month old child with Marden-Walker syndrome and pyloric stenosis. American Journal of Medical Genetics 26: 915–919

Goutieres F, Aicardi J, Farkas E 1977 Anterior horn cell disease associated with pontocerebellar hypoplasia in infants. Journal of Neurology, Neurosurgery & Psychiatry 40: 370–378

Gregersen H N, Petersen G B 1977 Congenital malformation of the feet with low body height: A new syndrome, caused by an autosomal dominant gene. Clinical Genetics 12: 255–262

Grosse F R, Pandel C, Wiedemann H 1975 The

tetraphocomelia-cleft palate syndrome. Humangenetik 28: 353–356

Guha D K, Rashmi A, Khanduja P C, Kochhar M 1969 Intrauterine osteogenesis imperfecta with arthrogryposis multiplex and regional achondroplasia. Indian Pediatrics 6: 804–807

Hageman G, Smit L M E, Hoogland R A, Jennekens F G I, Willemse J 1986 Muscle weakness and congenital contractures in a case of congenital myasthenia. Journal of Pediatric Orthopedics 6: 227–231

Hajra A K, Datta N S, Jackson L G et al 1985 Prenatal diagnosis of Zellweger cerebrohepatorenal syndrome. New England Journal of Medicine 312: 445–446

Hall J G 1984 Editorial comment: the lethal multiple pterygium syndromes. American Journal of Medical Genetics 17: 803–807

Hall J G 1985 Genetic aspects of arthrogryposis. Clinical Orthopaedics 184: 44–53

Hall J G 1986 Invited editorial comment: Analysis of Pena Shokeir phenotype. American Journal of Medical Genetics 25: 99–117

Hall J G, Reed S D 1982 Teratogens associated with congenital contractures in humans and in animals. Teratology 25: 173–191

Hall J G, Reed S D, Greene G 1982a The distal arthrogryposis. American Journal of Medical Genetics 11: 185–239

Hall J G, Reed S D, Scott C I, Rogers J G, Jones K L, Camarano A 1982b Three distinct types of X-linked arthrogryposis seen in 6 families. Clinical Genetics 21: 81–97

Hall J G, Reed S D, Rosenbaun K, Guershanik J, Chan H, Wilson K 1982c Limb pterygium syndrome. A review and report of eleven patients. American Journal of Medical Genetics 12: 377–409

Hall J G, Reed S D, Driscoll E P 1983a Amyoplasia: A common sporadic condition with congenital contractures. American Journal of Medical Genetics 15: 571–590

Hall J G, Hermann J, McGillivray B, Partington M, Schinzel A, Shapiro J, Reed S D 1983b Part II. Amyoplasia: Twinning in amyoplasia – a specific type of arthrogryposis with an apparent excess of discordant identical twins. American Journal of Medical Genetics 15: 591–599

Hamanishi C, Ueba Y, Tsuji T et al 1986 Congenital aplasia of the extensor muscles of the fingers and thumb associated with generalised polyneuropathy: An autosomal recessive trait. American Journal of Medical Genetics 24: 247–254

Hansen O H, Andersen O 1970 Congenital radio-ulnar synostosis. Acta Orthopaedica Scandinavica 41: 225–230

Hanson J, Jones K L, Smith D W 1976 Fetal alcohol syndrome: Experience with 41 patients. Journal of the American Medical Association 235: 1458–1460

Hanson P A, Martinez L B, Cassidy R 1977 Contractures, continuous muscle discharges and titubation. Annals of Neurology 1: 120–124

Happle R 1981 Cataracts as a marker of genetic heterogeneity in chondrodysplasia punctata. Clinical Genetics 19: 64–66

Harper P 1975 Congenital myotonic dystrophy in Britain. Archives of Disease in Childhood 50: 514

Harrod M J E, Friedman J M, Currarino G, Pauli R M, Langu L O Jr. 1984 Genetic heterogeneity in spondyloepiphyseal dysplasia congenita. American Journal of Medical Genetics 18: 311–320

Haspeslagh M, Fryns J P, de Muelenaere A, Schauthet L, van den Bergh H 1985 Mental retardation with pterygia,

shortness and distinct facial appearance. Clinical Genetics 28: 550–555

Hecht F 1969 Inability to open mouth fully: An autosomal dominant phentotype with facultative camptodactyly and short stature. Birth Defects Original Article Series V: 96–102

Herrmann J 1974 Symphalangism and brachydactyly syndrome: Report of the WL symphalangism-brachydactyly syndrome: Review of the literature and classification. Birth Defects Original Article Series X: 23–53

Herrmann J, Opitz J M 1974 The VSR syndrome (Studies of malformation syndromes of man XXXII). Birth Defects Original Article Series 10: 227–239

Herrmann J, Feingold M, Tuffli G A, Opitz J M 1969 A familial dysmorphogenetic syndrome of limb deformities, characteristic facial appearance and associated anomalies: the "pseudothalidomide" or "SC-syndrome". Birth Defects Original Article Series V (3): 81–89

Herva R, Seppanen U 1985 Multisynostotic osteodysgenesis. Pediatric Radiology 15: 63–64

Herva R, Leisti J, Kirkinen P, Seppanen U 1985 A lethal autosomal recessive syndrome of multiple congenital contractures. American Journal of Medical Genetics 20: 431–439

Heselson N G, Cremin B J, Beighton P 1978 Lethal chondrodysplasia punctata. Clinical Radiology 29: 679–684

Heymans H S A, Oorthuys J W E, Nelck G, Wanders R J A, Schutgens R B H 1985 Rhizomelic chondrodysplasia punctata: Another peroxisomal disorder. New England Journal of Medicine 313: 187–188

Higashi K, Inoue S 1983 Conductive deafness, sympalangism, and facial abnormalities: The WL syndrome in a Japanese family. American Journal of Medical Genetics 16: 105–109

Ho N, Khoo T 1979 Congenital contractural arachnodactyly: report of a neonate with advanced bone age. American Journal of Diseases of Children 133: 639–640

Hogge W A, Golabi M, Filly R A, Douglas R, Golbus M S 1985 Letter to the editor: The lethal multiple pterygium syndromes: Is prenatal detection possible? American Journal of Medical Genetics 20: 441–442

Hogh J, MacNicol M F 1985 Foot deformities associated with onycho-osteodysplasia: A familial study and a review of associated features. International Orthopedics 9: 135–138

Holbrook K A, Dale B A, Witt D R, Hayden M R, Toriello H V 1987 Arrested epidermal morphogenesis in three newborn infants with a fatal genetic disorder (Restrictive dermopathy). Journal of Investigative Dermatology 88: 330–339

Hollister D W, Rimoin D L, Lachman R, Cohen A, Reed W, Westin G 1974 The Winchester syndrome: A nonlysosomal connective tissue disease. Journal of Pediatrics 84: 701–709

Holmes L B, Driscoll S G, Bradley W G 1980 Contractures in a newborn infant of a mother with myasthenia gravis. Journal of Pediatrics 96: 1067–1069

Horan F, Beighton P 1976 Parastremmatic dwarfism. Journal of Bone and Joint Surgery 58: 343–346

Horton W A, Rimoin D L, Lachman R S et al 1978 The phenotypic variability of diastrophic dysplasia. Journal of Pediatrics 93: 609–613

Houston C S, Opitz J M, Spranger J W et al 1983 The campomelic syndrome: Review, report of 17 cases, and follow-up on the currently 17-year-old boy first reported by Maroteaux et al in 1971. American Journal of Medical Genetics 15: 3–28

Hunter A G, Cox D W, Rudd N L 1976 The genetics of and

associated clinical findings in humeroradial synostosis. Clinical Genetics 9: 470–478

Hunter A G W, Woerner S J, Montalvo-Hicks L D C et al 1979 The Bowen-Conradi syndrome – A highly lethal autosomal recessive syndrome of microcephaly, micrognathia, low birth weight, and joint deformities. American Journal of Medical Genetics 3: 269–279

Hurvitz S A, Goodman R M, Hertz M, Katznelson M B-M, Sack Y 1985 The facio-audio-symphalangism syndrome: report of a case and review of the literature. Clinical Genetics 28: 61–68

Ives E J, Houston C S 1980 Autosomal recessive microcephaly and micromelia in Cree Indians. American Journal of Medical Genetics 7: 351–360

Jaatoul N Y, Haddad N E, Khoury L A 1982 Brief clinical report and review: The Marden-Walker syndrome. American Journal of Medical Genetics 11: 259–271

Jancar J, Mlele T J J 1985 The Marden-Walker syndrome: A case report and review of the literature. Journal of Mental Deficiency Research 29: 63–70

Jones K L, Smith D W 1973 Recognition of the fetal alcohol syndrome in early infancy. Lancet II: 999–1001

Juberg R C 1969 A new familial syndrome of oral, cranial and digital anomalies. Journal of Pediatrics 74: 755–762

Judisch G F, Martin-Casalo A, Hanson J W, Olin W H 1979 Oculodentodigital dysplasia: four new reports and a literature review. Archives of Ophthalmology 97: 878–884

Kaufman R L, Rimoin D L, McAlister W H, Hartman A F 1974 Variable expression of Holt-Oram syndrome. American Journal of Diseases of Children 127: 21–25

Kelley R I, Zackai E H, Charney E G 1982 Congenital hydronephrosis, skeletal dysplasia and severe developmental retardation: The Schinzel-Gidieon syndrome. Journal of Pediatrics 100: 943–946

Keutel J, Kindermann I, Mockell H 1970 Eine wahrscheinlich autosomal recessiv verebte Skeletmissbildung mit Humeroradialsynostose. Humangenetik 9: 43–53

Khajavi A, Lachman R S, Rimoin D L et al 1976 Heterogeneity in the campomelic syndromes: Long and short bone varieties. Birth Defects Original Article Series 12: 93–100

Kibbe M H, Kaufman B, Funk R L 1965 Arthrogryposis multiplex congenita associated with Von Recklinghausen's disease. Virginia Medical Monthly 95: 344–350

Kiel E A, Frias J L, Victoria B E 1983 Cardiovascular manifestations in the Larsen syndrome. Pediatrics 71: 942–946

Kim H J, Beratis N G, Brill P, Raab E, Hirschorn K, Matalon R 1975 Kniest syndrome with dominant inheritance and mucopolysacchariduria. American Journal of Human Genetics 27: 755–764

Kingston H M, Hughes I A, Harper P S 1982 Orocraniodigital (Juberg-Hayward) syndrome with growth hormone deficiency. Archives of Disease in Childhood 57: 790–792

Koiffmann C P, Wajntal A, Ursich M J M, Pupo A A 1984 Brief Clinical Report: Familial recurrence of geleophysic dysplasia. American Journal of Medical Genetics 19: 483–486

Koussaff B G, Nichols P 1985 A new autosomal recessive syndrome with Noonan-like phenotype, myopathy, with congenital contractures and malignant hyperthermia. Birth Defects Original Article Series 21: 111–117

Kunze J, Park W, Hansen K H, Hanefeld F 1983 Adducted

thumb syndrome, report of a new case and a diagnostic approach. European Journal of Pediatrics 141: 122–126

Lachman R, Sillence D, Rimoin D et al 1981 Diastrophic dysplasia: The death of a variant. Pediatric Radiology 140: 79–86

Ladda R L, Stoltzfus E, Gordon S, Graham W 1978 Craniosynostosis associated with limb reduction malformations and cleft lip/palate: A distinct syndrome. Pediatrics 61: 12–15

Lambert D, Nivelon-Chevallier A, Chapuis J L 1977 Absence of DIP fold causing difficulty in extending fingers. Journal of Medical Genetics 14: 466–467

Lamy M, Maroteaux P 1960 Le nanisme diastrophique. Presse Medicale 68: 1977–1980

Langer L O, Petersen D, Spranger J W 1970 An unusual bone dysplasia: Parastremmatic dwarfism. American Journal of Roentgenology 110: 550–560

Latta R J, Graham C B, Aase J, Scham S M, Smith D W 1971 Larsen's syndrome: A skeletal dysplasia with multiple joint dislocations and unusual facies. Journal of Pediatrics 78: 291–298

Laxova R, Ohara P T, Timothy A D 1972 A further example of a lethal autosomal recessive condition in sibs. Journal of Mental Deficiency Research 16: 139–143

Lazjuk G I, Cherstvoy E D, Lurie I W, Nedzved M K 1978 Pulmonary hypoplasia, multiple ankyloses and camptodactyly: One syndrome or some related forms. Helvetica Paediatrica Acta 33: 73–79

Lazjuk G I, Lurie I W, Ostrowskaja T I, Cherstvoy E D, Kirillova I A, Nedzved M K, Usoev S S 1979 Brief clinical observation: The Neu-Laxova syndrome– a distinct entity. American Journal of Medical Genetics 3: 261–267

Lenz W D, Majewski F 1974 A generalised disorder of the connective tissue with progeria, choanal atresia, symphalangism, hypoplasia of dentine and craniodiaphyseal hyperostosis. Birth Defects Original Article Series X (12): 133–136.

Lenz W, Rehmann I 1976 Distal symphalangien mit humeroradialsynostose, karpalsynostosen und brachyphalangie des daumens: ein dominantes syndrom. Zeitschrift fur Orthopadie und ihre Grenzgebiete 114: 202–211

Lerman-Sagie T, Levi Y, Kidron D, Grunebaum M, Nitzan M 1987 Brief clinical report: syndrome of osteopetrosis and muscular degeneration associated with cerebro-oculo-facio-skeletal changes. American Journal of Medical Genetics 28: 137–142

Lewin S O, Hughes H E 1987 Brief clinical report: German syndrome in sibs. American Journal of Medical Genetics 26: 385–390

Liebenberg F 1973 A pedigree with unusual anomalies of the elbows, wrist and hands in five generations. South African Medical Journal 47: 745–748

Lindhout D, Hageman G, Beemer F A, Ippel P F, Breslau-Siderius L, Willemse J 1985 The Pena-Shokeir Syndrome: Report of nine Dutch cases. American Journal of Medical Genetics 21: 655–668

Lingham S, Wilson J, Hart E 1981 Hereditary Stiff-baby syndrome. American Journal of Diseases of Children 135: 909–911

Livingstone I R, Sack G J 1984 Arthrogryposis multiplex congenita occurring with maternal multiple sclerosis. Archives of Neurology 41: 1216–1217

Lowry R B, MacLean R, MacLean D M, Tischler B 1971 Cataracts, microcephaly, kyphosis and limited joint movement in two siblings: a new syndrome. Journal of Pediatrics 79: 282–284

Lowry R B, Machin G A, Morgan D et al 1985 Congenital contractures, edema, hyperkeratosis and intrauterine growth retardation: A fatal syndrome in Hutterite and Mennonite kindreds. American Journal of Medical Genetics 22: 531–543

Lucas G L 1967 Hereditary onycho osteodysplasia (nail-patella syndrome) masquerading as arthrogryposis. Southern Medical Journal 60: 751–755

Lurie I W, Cherstvoy E D, Lazjuk G I, Nedzved M K, Usoev S S 1976 Further evidence for AR inheritance of COFS syndrome. Clinical Genetics 10: 343–346

Mabry C C, Barnett I S, Hutcheson M W, Sorenson H W 1974 Trismus pseudocamptodactyly syndrome: Dutch-Kentucky syndrome. Journal of Pediatrics 85: 503–508

McComb R D, Markesbery W R, O'Connor W N 1979 Fatal neonatal nemaline myopathy with multiple anomalies. Journal of Pediatrics 94: 47–51

McCormack M K, Coppola-McCormack P J, Lee M 1980 Autosomal-dominant inheritance of distal arthrogryposis. American Journal of Medical Genetics 6: 163–169

McGillivray B C, Lowry R B 1977 Poland syndrome in British Columbia: Incidence and reproductive experience of affected persons. American Journal of Medical Genetics 1: 65–74

McKeown C M E, Harris R 1988 An autosomal dominant multiple pterygium syndrome. Journal of Medical Genetics 25: 96–103

MacLeod P, Patriquin H 1974 The whistling face syndrome – cranio-carpo-tarsal dysplasia. Clinical Pediatrics 13: 184–189

McPherson E, Carey J, Kramer A, Hall J G, Pauli R M, Schimke R N, Tasin M H 1987 Dominantly inherited renal adysplasia. American Journal of Medical Genetics 26: 863–872

McPherson E W, Taylor C A Jr. 1981 The King syndrome: malignant hyperthermia, myopathy and multiple anomalies. American Journal of Medical Genetics 8: 159–165

Malleson P, Schaller J G, Dega F et al 1981 Familial arthritis and camptodactyly. Arthritis and Rheumatism 24: 1199–1204

Maroteaux P, Bourvet J P, Briard M L 1972 La maladie des synostoses multiples. La Nouvelle Presse Medicale 45: 3041–3047

Martin N J, Hill J B, Cooper D H, O'Brien G D, Masel J P 1986 Lethal multiple pterygium syndrome: three consecutive cases in one family. American Journal of Medical Genetics 24: 295–304

Martsolf J T, Hunter A G W, Haworth J C 1978 Severe mental retardation, cataracts, short stature, and primary hypogonadism in two brothers. American Journal of Medical Genetics 1: 291–299

Matthews S, Farnish S, Young I D 1987 Distal symphalangism with involvement of the thumbs and great toes. Clinical Genetics 32: 375–378

Mead C, Martin M 1963 Aplasia of the trochlea – an original mutation. Journal of Bone & Joint Surgery 45A: 379–382

Meinecke P, Fryns J P 1985 The Fryns syndrome: diaphragmatic defects, craniofacial dysmorphism, and distal digit hypoplasia: further evidence for autosomal recessive inheritance. Clinical Genetics 28: 516–520

Mietens C, Weber H 1966 A syndrome characterized by corneal opacity, nystagmus, flexion of elbows, growth failure and mental retardation. Journal of Pediatrics 69: 624–629

Miskin M, Rothberg R, Rudd N, Benzie R J, Shine J 1979 Arthrogryposis multiplex congenita: prenatal assessment with diagnostic ultrasound and fetoscopy. Journal of Pediatrics 95: 463–464

Moessinger A C 1983 Fetal akinesia deformation sequence: an animal model. Pediatrics 72: 857–863

Moser A E, Singh I, Brown F R et al 1984 The cerebrohepatorenal (Zellweger) syndrome: Increased levels and impaired degradation of very-long-chain fatty acids and their use in prenatal diagnosis. New England Journal of Medicine 310: 1141–1146

Moutard-Codou M L, Delleur M M, Dulac O et al 1987 Severe neonatal myasthenia with arthrogryposis. Presse Medicale 16: 615–618

Muller L M, de Jong G, Mouton S C E, Greef M J, Kirby P, Hewlett R, Jordaan H F 1987 A case of the Neu-Laxova syndrome: prenatal ultrasonographic monitoring in the third trimester and the histopathological findings. American Journal of Medical Genetics 26: 421–429

Mulvihill J J, Yeager A M 1976 Fetal alcohol syndrome. Teratology 13: 345–348

Murachi S, Nogami H, Oki T, Ogino T 1981 Familial tricho-rhino-phalangeal syndrome Type II. Clinical Genetics 19: 149–155

Myers H S, Gregory M, Beighton P 1980 Renal failure in a 44-year-old female. Urologic Radiology 1: 251–253

Myhre S A, Ruvalcaba H A, Graham C B 1981 A new growth deficiency syndrome. Clinic Genetics 20: 1–5

Neri G, Blumberg B, Miles P V, Opitz J M 1984 Sensorineural deafness in the FG syndrome: Report on four new cases. American Journal of Medical Genetics 19: 369–377

Neu R 1971 A lethal syndrome of microcephaly with multiple congenital anomalies in three siblings. Pediatrics 47: 610–612

Neuhauser G, Kaveggia E G, France T D, Opitz J M 1975 Syndrome of mental retardation, seizures, hypotonic cerebral palsy and megalocorneae, recessively inherited. Zeitschrift für Kinderheilkunde 120: 1–18

Neustein H S 1973 Nemaline myopathy. Archives of Pathology 96: 192–195

Nevin N C, Henry P, Thomas P T S 1981 A case of the orocraniodigital (Juberg-Hayward) syndrome. Journal of Medical Genetics 18: 478–480

Nezelof C, Dupart M, Jaubert F, Eliacha E 1979 A lethal familial syndrome associating arthrogryposis multiplex congenita, renal dysfunction and a cholestatis and pigmentary liver disease. Journal of Pediatrics 94: 258–260

Norman R M 1961 Cerebellar hypoplasia in Werdnig-Hoffman disease. Archives of Disease in Childhood 36: 96–101

Norman R M, Kay J M 1965 Cerebello-thalamo-spinal degeneration in infancy: An unusual variant of Werdnig-Hoffman disease. Archives of Disease in Childhood 40: 302–308

O'Brien P J, Gropper P T, Tredwell S J, Hall J G 1984 Orthopaedic aspects of the Trismus pseudocamptodactyly syndrome. Journal of Pediatric Orthopedics 4: 469–471

Ochi T, Iwase R, Okabe N, Fink C W, Ono K 1983 The pathology of the involved tendons in patients with familial arthropathy and congenital camptodactyly. Arthritis and Rheumatism 26: 896–900

Ohdo S, Yamauchi Y, Hayakawa K 1981 Distal

symphalangism associated with camptodactyly. Journal of Medical Genetics 18: 456–458

Ohlsson A, Fong K W, Rose T H, Moore D C 1988 Prenatal sonographic diagnosis of Pena-Shokeir syndrome type I, or fetal akinesia deformation sequence. American Journal of Medical Genetics 29: 59–65

Opitz J M, Kareggia E G 1974 Studies of malformation syndromes of man XXXIII: The FG syndrome. Zeitschrift für Kinderheilkunde 117: 1–18

Optiz J M, Johnson R C, McCreadie S R, Smith D W 1969a The C syndrome of multiple congenital anomalies. Birth Defects Original Article Series 5: 161–166

Opitz J M, Zurhein G, Vitale L et al 1969b The Zellweger syndrome. Birth Defects Original Article Series V: 144–160

Pagnan N A B, Gollop T R 1987 Brief clinical report: Distal arthrogryposis Type II D in three generations of a Brazilian family. American Journal of Medical Genetics 26: 613–619

Pagnan N A B, Gollop T R, Lederman H 1988 The Tel Hashomer camptodactyly syndrome: Report of a new case and review of the literature. American Journal of Medical Genetics 29: 411–417

Palant D I, Feingold M, Berkman M D 1971 Unusual facies, cleft palate, mental retardation, and limb abnormalities in siblings – a new syndrome. Journal of Pediatrics 78: 686–688

Papadia F, Zimbalatti F, Gentile L A, Rosca C 1984 The Bartsocas-Papas syndrome: Autosomal recessive form of popliteal pterygium syndrome in a male infant. American Journal of Medical Genetics 25: 575–579

Papadia F, Longo N, Serlenga L, Porzio G 1987 Progressive form of multiple pterygium syndrome in association with Nemalin-Myopathy: report of a female followed for twelve years. American Journal of Medical Genetics 26: 73–83

Parker N 1963 Dystrophia myotonica presenting as congenital facial diplegia. Medical Journal of Australia 2: 939–944

Pashayan H, Dallaire L, McLeod P 1973 Bilateral aniridia, multiple webs and severe mental retardation in a 47,XXY/48,XXXY mosaic. Clinical Genetics 4: 125–129

Passarge E 1965 Congenital malformations and maternal diabetes. Lancet I: 324–325

Passarge E, Sutherland J M 1965 Potter's syndrome. American Journal of Diseases of Children 109: 80–84

Patton M A, Sharma K, Winter R M 1985 The Aase-Smith syndrome. Clinical Genetics 28: 521–525

Pedersen J C, Fryns J P, Carpentier G, Heremans G, Van den Berghe H 1980 Multiple Synostosis Syndrome. European Journal of Pediatrics 134: 273–275

Pena S D, Shokeir M 1970 Syndrome of camptodactyly, multiple ankyloses, facial anomalies and pulmonary hypoplasia – further delineation and evidence for autosomal recessive inheritance. Birth Defects Original Article Series XXI: 201–208

Pena S D J, Shokeir M H K 1974 Autosomal recessive cerebro-oculo-facio-skeletal syndrome. Clinical Genetics 5: 285–293

Pena S D, Evans J, Hunter A G 1978 COFS syndrome revisited. Birth Defects Original Article Series XIV: 205–213

Petajan J H, Momberger G, Aase J 1969 Arthrogryposis syndrome. Kuskokwim disease in the Eskimo. Journal of the American Medical Association 209 (10): 1481

Pfeiffer R A 1982 The Oto-onycho-peroneal syndrome: A probably new genetic entity. European Journal of Pediatrics 138: 317–320

Pfeiffer R A, Ammerman M 1972 Das syndrom von Freeman and Sheldon. Zeitschrift für Kinderheilkunde 121: 43–53

Pillay V K 1964 Ophthalmo-mandibulo-melic dysplasia – a hereditary syndrome. Journal of Bone & Joint Surgery 46A: 858–862

Povysilova V, Macek M, Salichova J, Seemanova E 1976 Letalni syndrom mnohocetnyck malformaci u tri sourozencu. Ceskoslovenska Pediatrie 31: 190–194

Poznanski A K, Gall J C, Stern A M 1970a Skeletal manifestations of the Holt-Oram syndrome. Radiology 94: 45–53

Poznanski A K, Nosanchuk J S, Baublis J, Holt J F 1970b The cerebro-hepato-renal syndrome (CHRS) American Journal of Roentgenology, Radiotherapy & Nuclear Medicine 109(2): 313–322

Poznanski A K, Kuhns L R, Lapides J, Stern A M 1975 A new family with the hand-foot-genital syndrome – A wider spectrum of the hand-foot-uterus syndrome. Birth Defects Original Article Series II: 127–136

Preus M, Kaplan P, Kirkham T H 1977 Renal anomalies and oligohydramnios in the cerebro-oculo-facio-skeletal syndrome. American Journal of Diseases of Children 131: 62–64

Preus M, Linstrom C, Polomeno R C, Milot J 1983 Waardenburg syndrome – Penetrance of major signs. American Journal of Medical Genetics 15: 383–388

Punnett H, Kistenmacher M L, Valdes-Dapena M, Ellison R T 1974 Syndrome of ankylosis, facial anomalies and pulmonary hypoplasia. Journal of Pediatrics 85: 375–377

Ramos Arroyo M A, Weaver D D, Beals R K 1985 Congenital contractural arachnodactyly: report of four additional families and review of literature. Clinical Genetics 27: 570–581

Reed S D, Hall J G, Riccardi V M, Aylsworth A, Timmons C 1985 Chromosomal abnormalities associated with congenital contractures (arthrogryposis). Clinical Genetics 27: 353–372

Reed T, Schreiner R L 1983 Absence of dermal ridge patterns: Genetic heterogeneity. American Journal of Medical Genetics 16: 81–88

Reeve R, Silver H, Ferrier P 1960 Marfan's syndrome (arachnodactyly) with arthrogryposis (amyoplasia congenita). American Journal of Diseases of Children 99: 101–106

Reid C O M V, Hall J G, Anderson C et al 1986 Association of amyoplasia with gastroschisis, bowel atresia and defects of the muscular layer of the trunk. American Journal of Medical Genetics 24: 701–710

Reiss J A, Sheffield L J 1986 Distal arthrogryposis type II: a family with varying congenital abnormalities. American Journal of Medical Genetics 24: 255–267

Relkin R 1965 Arthrogryposis multiplex congenita. Report of 2 cases, review of literature. American Journal of Medicine 39: 871–876

Riccardi V M 1977 The FG syndrome: Further characterization, report of a third family, and of a sporadic case. American Journal of Medical Genetics 1: 47–58

Richieri-Costa A 1986 Brief clinical report: FG syndrome in a Brazilian child with additional previously unreported signs. American Journal of Medical Genetics supplement 2: 247–254

Richieri-Costa A, Pagnan N A G et al 1986 Humeroradial/Multiple synostosis syndrome in a Brazilian child with consanguineous parents: a new multiple synostosis syndrome? Revista Brasileira de Genetica 9: 115–122

Rimoin D, Siggers D, Lachman R, Silberberg R 1976 Metatropic dwarfism, the Kneist syndrome and the pseudoachondroplastic dysplasias. Clinical Orthopedics 114: 70–82

Robinow M, Johnson G F 1981 The Gordon syndrome: autosomal dominant cleft palate, camptodactyly, and club feet. American Journal of Medical Genetics 9: 139–146

Robinow M, Johanson A J, Smith T H 1977 The Lenz-Majewski hyperostotic dwarfism: A syndrome of multiple congenital anomalies, mental retardation, and progressive skeletal sclerosis. Journal of Pediatrics 91: 417–421

Robinson L K, Powers N G, Dunklee P, Sherman S, Jones K L 1982 The Antley-Bixler syndrome. Journal of Pediatrics 101: 201–205

Robinson L K, O'Brien N C, Puckett M C, Cox M A 1987 Multiple pterygium syndrome: a case complicated by malignant hyperthermia. Clinical Genetics 32: 5–9

Romke C, Froster-Iskenius U, Heyne K et al 1987 Roberts syndrome and SC phocomelia: A single genetic entity. Clinical Genetics 31: 170–177

Rudiger R A, Schmidt W, Loose D A, Passarge E 1971 Severe developmental failure with coarse facial features, distal limb hypoplasia, thickened palmar creases, bifid uvula, and ureteral stenosis: A previously unidentified familial disorder with lethal outcome. Journal of Pediatrics 79: 977–981

Rutledge J C, Friedman J M, Harrod M J E et al 1984 A new lethal multiple congenital anomaly syndrome: Joint contractures, cerebellar hypoplasia, renal hypoplasia, urogenital anomalies, tongue cysts, shortness of limbs, eye abnormalities, defects of the heart, gallbladder agenesis, and ear malformations. American Journal of Medical Genetics 19: 255–264

Sack G 1978 A dominantly inherited form of arthrogryposis multiplex congenita with unusual dermatoglyphics. Clinical Genetics 14: 317–323

Sanchez J M, Kaminker C P 1986 New evidence for genetic heterogeneity of the Freeman-Sheldon syndrome. American Journal of Medical Genetics 25: 507–511

Sanchez J M, Barreiro C, Freilij H 1985 Two brothers with Martsolf's syndrome. Journal of Medical Genetics 22: 308–310

Sandbank U, Cohen L 1964 Arthrogryposis multiplex congenita associated with tuberous sclerosis. Journal of Pediatrics 64: 571–574

Sargent C, Burn J, Baraitser M, Pembrey M E 1985 Trigonocephaly and the Opitz C syndrome. Journal of Medical Genetics 22: 39–45

Saulk J J, Delaney J R, Reaume C, Brandjord R, Witkop C F 1974 Electromyography of oral-facial musculature in craniocarpaltarsal dysplasia (Freeman-Sheldon syndrome). Clinical Genetics 6: 132–137

Say B, Meyer J 1981 Familial trigonocephaly associated with short stature and developmental delay. American Journal of Diseases of Children 135: 711–712

Say B, Balci S, Atasu M 1973 Humeroradial synostosis. Humangenetik 19: 341–343

Schinzel A, Giedion A 1978 A syndrome of severe midface retraction, multiple skull anomalies, clubfeet, and cardiac and renal malformations in sibs. American Journal of Medical Genetics 1: 361–375

Schinzel A, Smith D W, Miller J R 1979 Monozygotic twinning and structural defects. Journal of Pediatrics 95: 921–930

Schinzel A, Savoldelli G, Briner J et al 1983 Antley-Bixler

syndrome in sisters: A term newborn and a prenatally diagnosed fetus. American Journal of Medical Genetics 14: 139–147

Schmalbruch J, Kamieniecka Z, Arre M 1987 Early fatal nemaline myopathy: Case report and review. Developmental Medicine and Child Neurology 29: 800–804

Schmitt H P 1978 Involvement of the larynx in a congenital 'myopathy' unilateral aplasia of the arytenoid, micrognathia and malformation of the brain – A new syndrome. Virchows Archiv fur pathologische Anatomie und Physiologie und fur Klinische Medizin 381: 85–96

Schott G D 1978 Hereditary brachydactyly with nail dysplasia. Journal of Medical Genetics 15: 119–122

Scott C I, Louro J M, Laurence K M, Tolarova M, Hall J G, Reed S D, Curry J R 1981 Comments on the Neu Laxova syndrome and CAD Complex. American Journal of Medical Genetics 9: 165–175

Scott-Emuakpor, Heffelfinger J, Higgins J V 1977 A syndrome of microcephaly and cataracts in 4 siblings. American Journal of Diseases of Children 131: 167–170

Sharma N L, Anand J S 1975 Osteogenesis imperfecta with arthrogryposis multiplex congenita. Journal of the Indian Medical Association 43: 124–126

Shun-Shin M 1954 Congenital web formation. Journal of Bone & Joint Surgery 366(2): 268–271

Siber M 1984 X-linked recessive microencephaly, microphthalmia with corneal opacities, spastic quadriplegia, hypospadias and cryptorchidism. Clinical Genetics 26: 453–456

Sillence D 1978 Brachydactyly, distal symphalangism, scoliosis, tall stature and club feet: A new syndrome. Journal of Medical Genetics 15: 208–211

Smith D W 1974 The VATER association. American Journal of Diseases of Children 128: 767

Smith D W 1982 Recognizable patterns of human malformations. Saunders, Philadelphia

Smith D W, Clarren S K, Harvey M A 1978 Hyperthermia as a possible teratogenic agent. Journal of Pediatrics 92: 876–883

Smith R, Kaplan E 1968 Camptodactyly and similar atraumatic flexion deformities of the proximal interphalangeal joints of the fingers. Journal of Bone & Joint Surgery 50A: 1187–1203

Soljak M A, Aftimos S, Gluckman P D 1983 A new syndrome of short stature, joint limitation and muscle hypertrophy. Clinical Genetics 23: 441–446

Spranger J W, Langer L O, Wiedemann H K 1974 The atlas of bone dysplasias. Saunders, Philadelphia

Spranger J W, Schinzel A, Myers T, Ryan J, Giedion A, Opitz J 1980 Cerebro-arthro-digital syndrome. American Journal of Medical Genetics 5: 13–24

Spranger J, Bernischke K, Hall J G et al 1982 Errors of morphogenesis: concepts and terms. Journal of Pediatrics 100: 160–165

Spranger J, Gilbert E F, Arya S, Hoganson G M I, Opitz J 1984 Geleophysic Dysplasia. American Journal of Medical Genetics 19: 487–499

Spritz R A 1978 Familial radioulnar synostosis. Journal of Medical Genetics 15: 160–162

Sprofkin B E, Hillman J W 1956 Moebius syndrome: Congenital oculo-facial paralysis. Neurology 6: 50–54

Srivastava R 1968 Arthrogryposis multiplex congenita – a case report of two siblings. Clinical Pediatrics 7(11): 691–694

Staheli L T, Chew D E, Elliott J S, Mosca V S 1987

Management of hip dislocations in children with arthrogryposis. Journal of Pediatric Orthopaedics 7: 681–683

Stern A M, Gall J C, Perry B L et al 1970 The hand-foot-uterus syndrome. Journal of Pediatrics 77: 109–116

Stewart J M, Bertstron L 1971 Familial hand abnormality and sensori-neural deafness: A new syndrome. Journal of Pediatrics 78: 102–110

Straňák V, Oberender H 1971 Uber einen fall von ageborener synostosis humero-radialis bilateralis. Beitrage zur Orthopadie und Traumatologie 18(8): 460–464

Strasburger A K, Hawkins M R, Eldridge R, Hardgrave R L, McKusick V A 1965 Symphalangism: Genetic and clinical aspects. Bulletin of the Johns Hopkins Hospital 117: 108–127

Stratton R F, Dobyns W B, Airhart S D et al 1984 New chromosomal syndrome: Miller-Dieker syndrome and monosomy. Human Genetics 67: 193–200

Sudarshan A, Goldie W D 1985 The spectrum of congenital facial diplegia (Moebius syndrome). Pediatric Neurology 1: 180–184

Sugarman G I 1973 Syndrome of microcephaly, cataracts, kyphosis and joint contractures versus Cockayne's syndrome. Journal of Pediatrics 82: 351–352

Sutcliffe J 1966 Metaphyseal dysostosis. Annals of Radiology 9: 215–223

Swift M R, Feingold M J 1969 Myotonic muscular dystrophy: abnormalities in fibroblast culture. Science 165: 294–296

Swinyard C A, 1982 Concepts of multiple congenital contractures (arthrogryposis) in man and animals. Teratology 25: 247–259

Swinyard C A, Black E E 1985 The etiology of arthrogryposis (multiple congenital contractures). Clinical Orthopaedics & Related Research 194: 15–29

Takada K, Nakamura H, Tanaka J 1984 Cortical dysplasia in congenital muscular dystrophy with central nervous system involvement (Fukuyama type). Journal of Neuropathology & Experimental Neurology 43: 395–407

Taybi H 1962 Generalized skeletal dysplasia with multiple anomalies. American Journal of Roentgenology 88: 450–457

Taybi H 1975 Radiology of syndromes. Year Book Medical Publishers, Chicago

Temtamy S A, McKusick V A 1978 The genetics of hand malformations. Birth Defects Original Article Series XIV (3)

Ter Haar B G A, Van Hoof R F 1974 The Trismus-pseudocamptodactyly syndrome. Journal of Medical Genetics 11: 41–49

Thompson E, Baraitser M 1987 FG syndrome. Journal of Medical Genetics 24: 139–143

Thompson E M, Baraitser M, Lindenbaum R H, Zaidi Z H, Kroll J S 1985 The FG syndrome: 7 new cases. Clinical Genetics 27: 582–594

Thompson E M, Donnai D, Baraitser M, Hall C M, Pembrey M E, Fixsen J 1987 Multiple pterygium syndrome: evolution of the phenotype. Journal of Medical Genetics 24: 733–749

Thompson G H (ed) 1985 Symposium: arthrogryposis multiplex congenita. Clinical Orthopaedics and Related Research 194: 1–124

Thompson J S, McLaughlin P R, Heslin D J 1968 Impaired pronation supination of the forearm: An inherited condition. Journal of Medical Genetics 5: 48–75

Thurmon T, DeFraites E B, Anderson E E 1973 Camptomelic Dwarfism. Journal of Pediatrics 83: 841–843

Tolmie J L, Patrick A, Yates J R W 1987a A lethal multiple pterygium syndrome with apparent X-linked recessive inheritance. American Journal of Medical Genetics 27: 913–919

Tolmie J L, Mortimer G, Doyle D, McKenzie R, McLaurin J, Neilson J P 1987b The Neu-Laxova syndrome in female sibs: clinical and pathological features with prenatal diagnosis in the second sib. American Journal of Medical Genetics 27: 175–182

Tomkins D J, Sisken J E 1984 Abnormalities in the cell-division cycle in Roberts syndrome fibroblasts: A cellular basis for the phenotypic characteristics? American Journal of Medical Genetics 36: 1332–1340

Tsukahara M, Shinozaki F, Kajii T 1985 Trismus-pseudocamptodactyly syndrome in a Japanese family. Clinical Genetics 28: 247–250

Tuncbilek E, Besim A, Bakkaloglu A et al 1985 Carpal-Tarsal Osteolysis. Pediatric Radiology 15: 255–258

Urban M D, Rogers J G, Meyer W J 1979 Familial syndrome of mental retardation, short stature, contractures of the hands, and genital anomalies. Journal of Pediatrics 94(1): 52–55

Van Benthem L H 1975 Editorial Comment. Syndrome Indentification 3: 25–28

Van Benthem L H, Driessen O, Haneveld G, Rietema H 1970 Cryptorchidism, chest deformities and other congenital anomalies in three brothers. Archives of Disease in Childhood 45: 590–592

Van Biervelt J P, Hendricks G, Van Ertbruggen I 1977 Intrauterine growth retardation with craniofacial and brain anomalies and arthrogryposis. Acta Paediatrica Belgica 30: 97–103

Vanek J, Janda J, Amblerova V, Losan F 1986 Freeman-Sheldon syndrome: a disorder of congenital myopathic origin? Journal of Medical Genetics 23: 231–236

VanRegemorter N, Wilkin P, Englert Y, El Khazen N, Alexandre S, Rodesch F, Milaire J 1984 Lethal multiple pterygium syndrome. American Journal of Medical Genetics 17: 827–834

Ventruto V, Girolano R, Festa A, Romano A, Sebastio G, Sebastio L 1976 Family study of inherited syndrome with multiple congenital deformities: Symphalangism, carpal and tarsal fusion, brachydactyly, cranio-synostosis, strabismus, hip osteochondritis. Journal of Medical Genetics 13: 394–398

Vigneron J, Didier F, Vert P 1987 Le syndrome oto-palato-digital de Type II: Diagnostic prenatal par echoraphie. Journale de Genetique Humaine 35: 69–70

Walbaum R, Fontaine G, Lienhardt J, Piquet J J 1970 Surdite familiale avec osteo-onycho-dyplasia. Journal de Genetique Humaine 18: 101–108

Walbaum R, LeJeune M, Poupard B, Lacheretz M, Fontain G 1973 Le syndrome de Freeman-Sheldon (syndrome du Siffleur). Annals of Pediatrics 20: 357–364

Wang T, Lin S 1987 Further evidence for genetic heterogeneity of Whistling Face or Freeman-Sheldon syndrome in a Chinese family. American Journal of Medical Genetics 28: 471–475

Weaver D D, Graham C B, Thomas I T, Smith D W 1974 A new overgrowth syndrome with accelerated skeletal maturation, unusual facies and camptodactyly. Journal of Pediatrics 84: 547–552

Weckesser E, Reed J, Heiple K 1968 Congenital clasped thumb (congenital flexion adduction deformity of the thumb). Journal of Bone & Joint Surgery 50a(7): 1417–1428

Weese-Mayer D E, Smith K M, Reddy J K, Salafsky I, Poznanski A K 1987 Computerized tomography and ultrasound in the diagnosis of cerebro-hepato-renal syndrome of Zellweger. Pediatric Radiology 17: 170–172

Weinberg A G, Kirkpatrick J B 1975 Cerebellar hypoplasia in Werdnig-Hoffman disease. Developmental Medicine & Child Neurology 17: 511–516

Welch J P, Temtamy S A 1966 Hereditary contractures of the fingers (camptodactyly). Journal of Medical Genetics 3: 104–112

White J W, Jenson W E 1952 The infant's persistent thumb – clutched hand. Journal of Bone & Joint Surgery 34a(3): 680–688

Wieacker P, Wolff G, Wienker T F et al 1985 A new X-linked syndrome with muscle atrophy, congenital contractures and oculomotor apraxia. American Journal of Medical Genetics 20: 597–606

Wieacker P, Wolff G, Wienker T F 1987 Close linkage of the Wieacker-Wolff syndrome to the DNA segment DXYSI in proximal Xq. American Journal of Medical Genetics 28: 245–253

Wiedemann H R, Grossi K R, Dibbern H 1985 An Atlas of Characteristic Syndromes. Wolfe, London

Williams R S, Holmes L B 1980 The syndrome of multiple ankyloses and facial anomalies. Acta Neuropathologica 50: 175–179

Williams R S, Swisher C N, Jennings M, Ambler M, Caviness V S 1984 Cerebro-ocular dysgenesis (Walker-Warburg syndrome): Neuropathologic and etiologic analysis. Neurology 34: 1531–1541

Wilson G N, Holmes R G, Custer J et al 1986 Zellweger syndrome: Diagnostic assays, syndrome delineation, and potential therapy. American Journal of Medical Genetics 24: 69–82

Winchester P, Grossman H, Lim W, Dounes B S 1969 A new acidmucopolysaccaridosis with skeletal deformities simulating rheumatoid arthritis. American Journal of Roentgenology 106: 121–128

Winter R M, Donnai D, Crawford M D 1981 Syndromes of microcephaly, microphthalmia, cataracts and joint contractures. Journal of Medical Genetics 18: 129–133

Witt D R, Hayden M R, Holbrook K A, Dale B A, Baldwin V J, Taylor G P 1986 Restrictive dermatopathy: A newly recognized autosomal recessive skin dysplasia. American Journal of Medical Genetics 24: 631–648

Wray J B, Herndon C N 1963 Hereditary transmission of congenital coalition of the calcaneus to the navicular. Journal of Bone & Joint Surgery 45A: 365–372

Wright D G, Aase J 1967 The Kuskokwim syndrome. Birth Defects V: 91–95

Yeatman G W 1984 Mental retardation – clasped thumb syndrome. American Journal of Medical Genetics 17: 339–344

Young R S K, Gang D L, Zalneraitis E L, Krishnamoorty K S 1981 Dysmaturation in infants of mothers with myotonic dystrophy. Archives of Neurology 38: 716–719

Yunis E, Fontalvo J, Quintero L 1980 X-linked Dyggve-Melchior-Clausen syndrome. Clinical Genetics 18: 284–290

Yunis J J (ed) 1977 New chromosomal syndromes. Academic Press, New York

Zellweger H 1973 Early onset of myotonic dystrophy in infants. American Journal of Diseases of Children 125: 601–604

Zellweger H, Afifi A, McCormick W F, Mergner W 1967 Severe congenital muscular dystrophy. American Journal of Diseases of Children 114: 591–602

Zergollern L, Hitrec V 1976 Three siblings with Robert's syndrome. Clinical Genetics 9: 433–436

61. Common skeletal deformities

William A. Horton

INTRODUCTION

Familial aggregation of common skeletal deformities is well known. Often this is because the deformity is a component of a simply inherited syndrome, such as the scoliosis that usually occurs in diastrophic dysplasia, or the club foot that often accompanies spondyloepiphyseal dysplasia congenita. However, even after these syndromes are excluded and only the idiopathic variety of the deformities is considered, familial aggregation still exists. Much interest has been generated in attempting to define the role of genetic and non-genetic factors in these instances. Twin studies, family surveys, and analysis of individual pedigrees have been employed, and numerous potential environmental causes have been investigated. These various approaches have indicated that genetic factors play an important role in the aetiology of certain of the deformities and, in several instances, specific modes of inheritance have been identified. Genetic heterogeneity has frequently been uncovered. In certain cases, environmental factors have been incriminated and often their relationship to genetic predisposition defined. For some of them, however, the contribution of genetic factors remains undefined and in virtually all cases the precise mechanism by which these factors predispose to the deformities are poorly understood. The goal of this chapter is to examine the current knowledge concerning the inheritance of these common skeletal deformities.

IDIOPATHIC SCOLIOSIS

Scoliosis, curvature of the spine, results from a multitude of causes. Examples of specific causes include polio-myelitis with trunk paralysis, myelomeningocele, neuro-fibromatosis, and radiation therapy to one side of the trunk (Harrington 1977). Scoliosis is also frequently associated with congenital anomalies, such as hemivertebrae or abnormally segmented vertebral bodies and with certain of the skeletal dysplasias in which the spine is involved, such as the spondyloepiphyseal dysplasias and spondylometaphyseal dysplasias (Winter et al 1968, Rimoin 1975). In the vast majority of cases, however, the aetiology is obscure, and the term idiopathic scoliosis is used.

The incidence of idiopathic scoliosis in the population varies considerably, ranging from 0.2–2–8% (Riseborough & Wynne-Davies 1973, Harrington 1977). It usually appears and shows the greatest progression during periods of rapid growth, infancy and adolescence. The process may begin during the juvenile period as well, but worsens during adolescence. In so-called infantile scoliosis, the curve usually appears during the first year of life, is typically to the left side, often resolves without treatment, and occurs most frequently in boys. It is common in Great Britain, accounting for almost half of all cases of idiopathic scoliosis, but is uncommon in North America. Idiopathic scoliosis of the adolescent variety usually appears during the pubertal growth spurt, is to the right side and occurs predominantly in girls. Curves developing after the age of six years show the characteristics of adolescent scoliosis (Wynne-Davies 1968).

Familial aggregation of idiopathic scoliosis has long been recognized. Many forms of inheritance have been postulated including autosomal dominant, X–linked dominant and multifactorial inheritance (Wynne-Davies 1968, Filho & Thompson 1971, Cowel et al 1972, Riseborough & Wynne-Davies 1973, Bonaiti et al 1976, Czeizel et al 1978). Environmental factors have also been proposed to explain this phenomenon (DeGeorge & Fisher 1967).

There have been many reports of twins with at least one member of the pair having scoliosis. Fisher and DeGeorge (1967) questioned the validity of those reported prior to 1967 because of insufficient radiographic studies. Those described after that time are listed in Table 61.1. Seventeen of the pairs exhibited adolescent scoliosis, while in one case (#18) it was the infantile variety. Seven of the pairs were monozygotic; all were concordant and all were female. Of the ten pairs of

Table 61.1 Twin studies in scoliosis*

Authors	Zygosity	Twin 1	Twin 2
1. Fisher & DeGeorge (1967)	MZ	F-A	F-A
2. Fisher & DeGeorge (1967)	MZ	F-A	F-A
3. Fisher & DeGeorge (1967)	MZ	F-A	F-A
4. Fisher & DeGeorge (1967)	MZ	F-A	F-A
5. Fisher & DeGeorge (1967)	MZ	F-A	FA
6. Fisher & DeGeorge (1967)	MZ	F-A	F-A
7. Wynne-Davies (1968)	MZ	F-A	F-A
8. Fisher & DeGeorge (1967)	DZ	F-A	F-A
9. Fisher & DeGeorge (1967)	DZ	F-A	F-A
10. Fisher & DeGeorge (1967)	DZ	F-A	F-A
11. Fisher & DeGeorge (1967)	DZ	M-A	M-A
12. Wynne-Davies (1968)	DZ	M-A	M-U
13. Fisher & DeGeorge (1967)	DZ	F-A	M-A
14. Fisher & DeGeorge (1967)	DZ	F-A	M-U+
15. Fisher & DeGeorge (1967)	DZ	F-A	M-U
16. Fisher & DeGeorge (1967)	DZ	M-A	M-U
17. Wynne-Davies (1968)	DZ	F-A	M-U
18. Wynne-Davies (1968)	DZ	M-A	F-U

* All cases were adolescent scoliosis except for # 18 in which the affected boy had infantile scoliosis
+ Curve of less than 10°

Abbreviations: MZ = monozygotic; DZ = dizygotic;
F = Female; M = Male; A = Affected;
U = Unaffected

dizygotic twins with adolescent scoliosis, five were concordant and five were discordant. In the latter group four were of unlike sex, and in three cases it was the female who was affected. Thus, the concordance rate of 100% for monozygotic twins and 50% for dizygotic twins with adolescent scoliosis illustrates the importance of genetic factors in the aetiology of the deformity. However, the marked preference for females indicates that sex is a strong determinant as well. Similarly, the usual sex predilection for boys was observed in the one pair of infants with scoliosis.

A number of surveys have examined the incidence of scoliosis in family members (Table 61.2). They are difficult to compare because different methods and criteria for diagnosis were employed. For example, the diagnosis was made by a questionnaire in the survey of DeGeorge and Fisher (1967), while X-rays were used by Cowell et al (1972) and photofluorography by Czeizel et al (1978). Moreover, although most of the surveys focused on adolescent scoliosis, some included substantial numbers of or only children with infantile scoliosis (Wynne-Davies 1968, Connor et al 1987). Despite these differences, the surveys showed similar trends. For adolescent scoliosis the parents and sibs of patients with scoliosis were affected much more frequently than the general population, the incidence ranging from 3–35%

for parents and from 5–36% for sibs. The percentage of affected relatives was much lower in infantile scoliosis: no affected sibs in the study of Connor et al (1987) and 2.6% of first-degree relatives of infantile scoliosis patients, versus 12% in adolescent scoliosis in the survey of Wynne-Davies (1968). When the incidence of scoliosis among second and third degree relatives was examined, all the surveys showed a dramatic drop-off. Furthermore, females were consistently affected more often than males in all categories of relatives, and the frequency of affected relatives was the same for male and female probands (Riseborough & Wynne-Davies 1973, Czeizel et al 1978).

Several other observations were made in these surveys. For instance, plagiocephaly (moulding of the head) was common in patients with infantile scoliosis, particularly those with resolving scoliosis (Connor et al 1987). It was on the same side as the curve and was transient in almost all cases (Wynne-Davies 1968). Mental retardation was found in one third of patients with progressive infantile scoliosis, where additional malformations were observed in infants with congenital scoliosis (Wynne-Davies 1968, Riseborough & Wynne-Davies 1973, Connor et al 1987). However, except for the high incidence of scoliosis already mentioned, the frequency of the additional anomalies in relatives was the same as in the general population. A substantial elevation of maternal age was found for adolescent scoliosis in three of the surveys (DeGeorge & Fisher 1967, Wynne-Davies 1968, Riseborough & Wynne-Davies 1973), but it was noted to be normal by Filho and Thompson (1971). Finally, Wynne-Davies (1968) observed several instances in which typical infantile and adolescent scoliosis occurred in the same family.

These surveys confirm that genetic factors are important in the aetiology of idiopathic scoliosis, primarily of the adolescent variety (onset beyond 6 years). Moreover, the incidence figures in first-degree relatives and rapid drop-off in second and third-degree relatives indicate multifactorial inheritance. According to this model, the highest frequency of scoliosis should be found in the relatives of males, the least affected sex (Carter 1965). However, the incidence of affected relatives was found to be approximately the same for affected males and females. The model also predicts that the frequency of affected relatives is related to the severity of the condition in the proband. This was not assessed in most of the surveys because of the numerous variables that influence the degree of scoliosis, such as age and treatment, although Czeizel et al (1978) showed a trend in this direction. In a small number of patients they also observed that the scoliotic curve was slightly greater in offspring of affected fathers than those of affected mothers, and greater yet when both parents were affected.

Table 61.2 Scoliosis surveys in families

Author	DeGeorge & Fisher	Wynne-Davies	Filho & Thompson	Cowell et al	Riseborough & Wynne Davies	Bonaiti et al	Czeizel et al	Connor et al
Year	1967	1968	1971	1972	1973	1976	1978	1987
Location	New York	Edinburgh	Toronto	Wilmington	Boston	Paris	Budapest	Glasgow
No. probands	446	114	201	110	208	241	116	36
Method	Questionnaire	Exam	X-ray	X-ray	X-ray	Interview	Photo fluorography,	Exam
Criteria		'Rib hump'		10° curve	20° curve		10° curve	
Predominant type surveyed	Adolescent	Adolescent & infantile	Adolescent	Adolescent	Adolescent	Adolescent	Adolescent	Infantile
Incidence (%)								
Parents	19	3	6	35	11	7	3.4	
(male/female)	(6/13)			(29/42)	(3/18)	(5/9)	(3/4)	
Sibs	9	5	7	36	12	8	8	0
(male/female)					(4/17)	(5/12)	(7/10)	
All relatives								
first-degree			6.9	6.8	11.1	7.4	5.8	
second-degree			3.7	1.6	2.4	1.9	1.4	
third-degree			1.6	1.0	1.4	0.9	0.8	

There have also been many families reported in which members in several generations exhibited adolescent scoliosis (Garland 1934, Gilly et al 1963, Cowell et al 1972, Robin & Cohen 1975). Because no instance of male to male transmission was seen in seventeen families studied in depth, Cowell et al (1972) proposed X–linked dominant inheritance. Riseborough and Wynne-Davies (1973) however challenged this interpretation because father to son transmission had been observed in the families described by the other authors, and it had also been noted in one of their cases. Thus, families exhibiting autosomal dominant inheritance of scoliosis do exist.

In summary, genetic factors appear to play a definite role in the causation of idiopathic scoliosis. The observation that infantile and adolescent scoliosis appear within the same families suggests that common genetic factors are involved in both, although they seem to be much more important in the latter. Genetic heterogeneity exists with regard to adolescent scoliosis. In some families it appears to be transmitted as an autosomal dominant trait. In the majority, however, it seems to be inherited in a multifactorial manner. The female sex is a strong determinant in converting the genetic predisposition into clinical disease.

The mechanism through which genetic factors operate is unknown. An association between HLA-A19 and scoliosis was reported by Bradford et al (1977a). Several investigators have observed abnormalities in collagen and proteoglycan (Ponseti et al 1976, Bradford et al 1977b, Francis et al 1977, Bushell et al 1978, 1979, Uden et al

1980). In most of the studies the biochemical alterations were most marked at the region of greatest spinal curvature, making it difficult to determine if they were primary or secondary in nature. In one study, however, increased susceptibility of collagen to pepsin digestion was noted throughout the spine in patients with scoliosis compared to non-scoliotic individuals (Bushell et al 1978, 1979). The authors proposed that the observation reflected a subtle collagen defect which predisposes to scoliosis. Such a defect might be inherited.

SPONDYLOLISTHESIS

The slippage of a vertebral body forward over the one below it is called spondylolisthesis. It most commonly involves the fifth lumbar vertebra, although the fourth lumbar and occasionally other vertebrae may be affected. Patients are usually asymptomatic but may exhibit low back pain, stiffness or even neurological symptoms (Haukipuro et al 1978). In most instances the displacement is associated with, and thought to be due to, a defect in the pars interarticularis (posterior inferior process) of the vertebral arch (Wiltse 1962). This defect is designated spondylolysis, and five types have been defined: dysplastic (congenital), isthmic, degenerative, traumatic, and pathological, the most common being the isthmic type (Wiltse et al 1976). Spina bifida occulta often accompanies the dysplastic type (Blackburne & Velikas 1977). Spondylolysis occurs in 4–8% of the general population over six years of age; whereas spondylolisthesis is found approximately half as often (Haukipuro et al 1978, Wynne-Davies & Scott 1979). Familial aggregation of spondylolysis with and without displacement has been observed on several occasions. The dysplastic and isthmic forms of spondylolysis are found in these families. In reviewing spondylolysis Wynne-Davies and Scott (1979) noted that in most radiographic surveys of family members, about 27% of near relatives were affected. In their study, which was restricted to spondylolisthesis of the fifth lumbar vertebra, 19% of relatives had spondylolysis. However, when subdivided according to the type of spondylolysis in the proband, 33% and 15% of relatives of patients with the dysplastic and isthmic forms respectively were affected. They also noted that the relatives sometimes had the opposite type of spondylolysis to that found in the index case.

Several individual families have been reported containing multiple affected members (Wiltse 1962, Amuso & Mankin 1967, Haukipuro et al 1978, Shahriaree et al 1979). Wiltse (1962) postulated autosomal recessive inheritance with incomplete penetrance, but most authors have concluded that autosomal dominant inheritance is more likely. In one study the penetrance was 75% for spondylolysis and approximately 30% of those patients showed some degree of slippage (Haukipuro et al 1978).

The inherited abnormality appears to be a defect in the pars interarticularis of the vertebral arch. It can be either the dysplastic or isthmic type, although the latter is more common (Wynne-Davies & Scott 1979). Similarly, different vertebral bodies can be affected as evidenced by monozygotic twins who exhibited defects at different levels (Wiltse 1962). Radiographically, the defects become evident between the ages of five and seven years (Wiltse 1962). The process of fatigue fracture due to repeated stress and trauma, rather than an acute traumatic event, is thought to be responsible (Wiltse et al 1975). The slippage, if it occurs, usually appears during adolescence concomitantly with the pubertal growth spurt. The displacement is greater if spina bifida occulta or other vertebral anomalies are present (Blackburne & Velikas 1977). The occurrence of spina bifida seems to be aetiologically independent, however, since the incidence of spina bifida and other neural tube defects is no greater in the patients' relatives than in the general population (Wynne-Davies & Scott 1979).

CONGENITAL DISLOCATION OF THE HIP

Congenital dislocation of the hip (CDH) is characterized by the displacement of the femoral head outside the acetabulum prior to or slightly after birth. When lesser degrees of displacement occur so that the femoral head articulates with the outer margin of the acetabulum, the

Table 61.3 Incidence of CDH

Location	Incidence (per 1000)
Birmingham, England	0.6
Oslo, Norway	1.0
Salford, England	1.6
New York City, USA	1.6
Malmo, Sweden	1.7
Salt Lake City, USA	9.1
Jerusalem, Israel	9.8
Budapest, Hungary	27.5
Arizona, USA (Navajo Indian)	38.0

term congenital subluxation is used. Acetabular dysplasia refers to the development of an abnormally shallow acetabulum without actual displacement (Wedge & Wasylenko 1978). CDH is a common birth defect but the incidence varies considerably throughout the world (Table 61.3), ranging from 0.6 per 1000 Caucasians living in Birmingham, England, to 38 per 1000 North American Indians living in Arizona (Woolf et al 1968). Although much of the discrepancy is due to different methods of ascertainment, criteria for diagnosis, etc, environmental and genetic factors are thought to be important as well. For example, CDH is more common in infants born in the winter months (Wynne-Davies 1970, Bjerkreim & van der Hagen 1974). Presumably, the wrapping of the child for warmth keeps the hips in the extended position in which dislocation is more likely. The practice of swaddling an infant to a cradle board with hips extended and adducted for the first few months of life is thought to account for the high incidence of CDH in certain American Indian groups (Carter & Wilkinson 1964a). Intrauterine posture is very important as well; both breech presentation and being the first infant born to a mother predispose to CDH (Wynne-Davies 1970, Bjerkreim & van der Hagen 1974). The female sex is perhaps the major determining factor. CDH occurs approximately six times as often in females as in males. It is thought that the production of oestrone by the fetal ovary and possibly relaxin by the fetal uterus, both of which increase ligamentous laxity, account for this sex predilection (Carter & Wilkinson 1964a, Woolf et al 1968).

Familial aggregation of CDH has long been recognized. Twin studies have consistently shown a higher concordance rate for monozygotic than for dizygotic twins (Table 61.4). There have been several large surveys in which the incidence of CDH in relatives of probands with CDH has been determined (Table 61.5). In two of the recent studies the patients were divided into two groups: those having neonatal and those having late onset, depending upon whether the diagnosis was made

Table 61.4   Twin studies in CDH

Author(s)	Year	Concordance MZ	DZ
Idelberger	1951	10/29	3/109
Kambara & Saskawa	1954	15/21*	3/6+
Wynne-Davies	1970	1/2	1/3
Czeizel et al	1975a	3/6	0/11

* Twins classified as monochorionic
+ Twins classified as biovular

MZ = monozygotic; DZ = dizygotic

before or after the age of four weeks. This was because prior to 1960 it was not appreciated that CDH could be diagnosed in the neonatal period; most cases were detected when the child began to walk. Thus the prior studies had dealt primarily with the late-onset type and it was not known if the patients diagnosed in the neonatal period represented the same or perhaps an aetiologically different group.

The incidence of CDH was found to be much higher in relatives of patients with CDH than in the general population in all the surveys. For example, the incidence in sibs ranged from 2.2–14%, the highest being in Hungary, where the population incidence is high. In the two studies in which neonatal and late-onset CDH were separated, there were several instances in which both types were observed within the same family (Wynne-Davies 1970, Bjerkreim & van der Hagen 1974). Moreover, in one pair of dizygotic twins, both types of CDH were found.

The sex preference for females was observed in affected sibs. For instance, the 5% of affected sibs reported by Record and Edwards (1958) comprised 1%

Table 61.5   Family surveys of CDH

Author(s)	Year	Type	Incidence (%) Parents	Sibs	Children
Muller & Seddon	1953	NS*	1.3	2.2	3.4
Record & Edwards	1958	NS		5.0	
Carter & Wilkinson	1964a	NS		5.7	
Woolf et al	1968	NS	1.6	4.3	
Wynne-Davies	1970	Neonatal	0.8	13.5	
		Late onset	0.8	5.0	12.1
Bjerkreim & van der Hagen	1974	Neonatal	1.8	6.0	
		Late onset	2.7	8.5	
Czeizel et al+	1975a	NS	2.1	14.0	
		NS	2.3	14.0	

* NS = not specified
+ Surveys at two locations reported

brothers and 10% sisters. Similarly, the series of Carter and Wilkinson (1964a) consisted of 4% brothers and 7% affected sisters. In general the incidence of affected sibs was slightly greater when the proband was male (Woolf et al 1968, Bjerkreim & van der Hagen 1974, Cziezel et al 1975a) as would be expected in polygenic inheritance. However, in the two surveys in which the data were subjected to statistical analysis, no significant difference was found (Wynne-Davies 1970, Bjerkeim & van der Hagen 1974). A dramatic drop-off in the incidence of CDH in second- and third- degree relatives compared to first-degree relatives was observed by Wynne-Davies (1970), Bjerkreim and van der Hagen (1974), and Czeizel et al (1975a).

The genetic contribution to CDH appears to have two separate components. Based on the observation that the configuration of the acetabulum is determined by a multiple gene system (Record & Edwards, 1958), Carter and Wilkinson (1964a) postulated that acetabular dysplasia inherited in this fashion interacted with ligamentous laxity, possibly transmitted as an autosomal dominant trait, to predispose an infant to CDH. Subsequent studies by Wynne-Davies (1970) and Czeizel et al (1975b) confirmed that 'normal' parents of children with CDH have acetabula that measure radiographically as being more shallow than normal. In the first study the association was noted only for the late-onset type of CDH, however it was observed in both types in the latter investigation.

Several studies have demonstrated the occurrence of generalized joint laxity in infants with CDH (Carter & Wilkinson 1964a,b, Wynne-Davies 1970, Czeizel et al 1975b). This was observed especially for boys and, particularly, in the neonatal form. Furthermore, these studies showed that it was more common in family members than in the general population; but the mode of inheritance was difficult to determine, i.e. joint laxity is difficult to assess and quantify and tends to decrease with age. Carter and Wilkinson (1964a,b) postulated that this common form of joint laxity was an autosomal dominant trait. The basis for this speculation appears to have been a few families exhibiting autosomal dominant transmission of generalized joint laxity frequently associated with CDH (Carter & Sweetnam 1958, 1960). Horton et al (1980), however, recently demonstrated that these particular families probably had a separate autosomal dominant trait which they termed familial joint instability syndrome. This syndrome can be distinguished from simple joint laxity as seen in CDH by its tendency to present at birth and its association with dislocation of several major joints in addition to the hip. Moreover, the incidence of CDH is approximately equal in males and females with this syndrome. Thus it is not clear if the joint laxity in typical CDH is truly an autosomal dominant trait as postulated or may be simply the extreme of normal joint mobility, possibly inherited in a polygenic fashion. In either case, simple familial joint laxity is very common. It occurs in 5% of the normal population and conveys a small but definite risk for CDH (Carter & Wilkinson 1964b, Wynne-Davies 1970, Jessee et al 1980).

Thus, CDH appears to be inherited as a multifactorial trait. Acetabular dysplasia transmitted in a polygenic manner and ligamentous laxity inherited in a polygenic or autosomal dominant fashion interact with a number of factors to bring about CDH. The other factors include female sex (which probably indicates it has a hormonal basis) and others, as yet undefined, that influence the position of the hip before birth and during infancy. Although increased joint laxity may be associated with an early diagnosis and a shallow acetabulum with a later one, the two seem to act additively.

CLUB FOOT

Club foot is a relatively common congenital anomaly occurring at a rate of approximately one to three per 1000 live births (Cowell & Wein 1980). It occurs as a component of a number of syndromes, especially those involving the nervous and connective tissue systems, but also as an isolated developmental anomaly, idiopathic congenital club foot. The idiopathic variety shows familial aggregation, but its inheritance is confusing. Many types of transmission including autosomal recessive, X–linked recessive, autosomal dominant and multifactorial have been proposed (Ching et al 1969). Part of the confusion is due to the inclusion of patients with unrecognized syndromes in surveys of idiopathic congenital club foot. In addition, many investigators have considered club foot as a single entity, when in fact it is comprised of three distinct anomalies: talipes equinovarus, talipes calcaneovalgus, and metatarsus varus. The limited number of genetic studies in which this heterogeneity has been appreciated have indicated that the three forms are separate entities (Palmer 1964, Wynne-Davies 1964, Ching et al 1969, Palmer et al 1974).

Talipes equinovarus

Talipes equinovarus is characterized by adduction of the forefoot, inversion of the heel and plantar flexion of the forefoot and ankle. It is seen in males approximately twice as often as in females and about 18% of patients exhibit additional minor abnormalities of connective tissues such as joint laxity, hernias, etc. (Wynne-Davies 1964). In a study of 174 twin pairs Idelberger (1939) reported the concordance to be 3% in monozygotic twins

and 3% in dizygotic twins. In a survey of 110 families Palmer (1964) described 43 families in which at least two members had the deformity. Noting instances in which multiple members and three generations of a family were affected, together with the occurrence of male to male transmission and an equal ratio of affected males to females, he suggested that autosomal dominant transmission with reduced penetrance was responsible for the deformity at least in certain families. A segregation analysis of data from many of these families and others ten years later (Palmer et al 1974) suggested that multifactorial inheritance was more likely. However the incidence in second and third-degree relatives was higher than expected. This mode of transmission was supported by studies done by Carter (1965) in which he found that the incidence of talipes equinovarus was 2.1%, 0.61% and 0.20% in first-, second- and third-degree relatives, respectively. In addition, a survey of relatives of 340 patients revealed that 2.9% of relatives had talipes equinovarus, while talipes calcaneovalgus and metatarsus varus were very infrequent (Wynne-Davies 1964). Male relatives of affected females showed the highest rate. Thus, it appears that in most cases talipes equinovarus is inherited in the multifactorial manner. The risk of recurrence to sibs is approximately 3% (Wynne-Davies 1964, Palmer et al 1974). Autosomal dominant inheritance cannot be excluded in some families.

Talipes calcaneovalgus

In this anomaly there is dorsal flexion of the forefoot and the plantar surface of the foot faces laterally. It is mild, often correcting spontaneously, and it occurs more often in girls (male: female ratio 0.61:1). It is frequently seen in first-born children suggesting that uterine constraint might be an aetiological factor. Like talipes equinovarus other minor connective tissue abnormalities occur in approximately 18% of patients, especially congenital dislocation of the hip, which was present in nearly 5% of patients. The incidence of affected sibs is 4.5%, suggesting multifactorial inheritance (Wynne-Davies 1964).

Metatarsus varus

Inversion and adduction of the forefoot are found alone in this anomaly. It resembles talipes calcaneovalgus in many respects. Often mild, it may go unnoticed. Girls are affected slightly more frequently than boys, and it is observed in approximately 4.5% of sibs. Again multifactorial inheritance is suggested. It differs, however, in that patients do not exhibit additional minor connective tissue abnormalities, nor does there appear to be any excess of first-born infants (Wynne-Davies 1964).

Table 61.6 Juvenile osteochondroses

Region affected	Eponym	Inheritance
Capital femoral epiphysis	Legg-Perthes disease	–
Tibial tubercle	Osgood-Schlatter disease	–
Os calcis	Sever disease	–
Tarsal of navicular bone	Kohler disease	–
Head of second metatarsal	Freiberg disease	–
Vertebral bodies	Scheuermann disease	–
Medial aspect of proximal tibial epiphysis	Blount disease, tibia vara	AD
Subchondral areas of diarthroidal joints (particularly knee, hip, elbow and ankle)	Osteochondritis dissecans	AD
Capitellum of humerus	Panner disease	–
Patella	Larsen-Johansson disease	–

AD = Autosomal dominant

JUVENILE OSTEOCHONDROSES

The juvenile osteochondroses are a group of disorders in which localized noninflammatory arthropathies result from regional disturbances of skeletal growth (Table 61.6). There is ischaemic necrosis of either primary or secondary endochondral ossification centres (Pappas 1967). Most of the abnormalities occur sporadically, but familial forms have been described. Legg-Perthes disease, osteonecrosis of the capital femoral epiphysis, has received the greatest attention. It has been reported as an autosomal dominant trait (Wamoscher & Farhi 1963), a sex-influenced dominant trait with reduced penetrance (Wansbrough et al 1959) and as a multifactorial trait (Gray et al 1972). However, these studies were done, or in the case of Gray et al, data recorded, prior to the delineation of a number of simply inherited skeletal dysplasias which exhibit abnormal development of the capital femoral epiphyses. It seems likely that patients

with these conditions may have been included in the studies, especially patients with the mild form of multiple epiphyseal dysplasia (Ribbing), an autosomal dominant trait in which involvement may be restricted to the capital femoral epiphyses (Rimoin 1975). In the recent surveys in which attempts were made to exclude such patients (Fisher 1972, Harper et al 1976, Wynne-Davies & Gormley 1978) the frequency in relatives was found to be very low; approximately 1% of first-degree relatives were affected and the incidence in second- and third-degree relatives approached that of the general population. Moreover, in the three pairs of unselected monozygotic twins reported, all were discordant for Legg-Perthes disease (Wynnes-Davies 1980). Thus in the vast majority of cases, this condition is not inherited.

Blount disease, a growth disturbance of the medial aspect of the proximal tibial growth plate, occurs in both infancy and adolescence. Pedigrees consistent with autosomal dominant transmission have been reported in the infantile form (Sibert & Bray 1977). However Bathfield and Beighton (1978), in a survey of 231 sibs of 110 patients with the infantile form, found that only 10 were affected. They concluded that common environmental factors were largely responsible for the familial aggregation.

Osteochondritis dissecans involving multiple sites, especially the knees, hips, elbows and ankles, has been reported as an autosomal dominant trait in several families (Stougaard 1961, Hanley et al 1967, Mubarak & Carroll 1979). The condition is characterized by the separation of a small piece of articular cartilage and underlying bone to form a loose body within the joint. Overlap with other of the osteochondroses has been observed. For example, osteochondritis dissecans has been seen in patients with involvement of the tibial tubercle (Osgood-Schlatter disease), spine (Scheuermann disease), the medial aspect of the proximal tibial epiphyses (adolescent Blount disease), patella (Larsen-Johansson syndrome), and the capital femoral epiphyses (Legg-Perthes disease) (Tobin 1957, Hanley et al 1967). Thus it appears to be a generalized disorder affecting growing epiphyses and may be inherited in some families.

REFERENCES

Amuso S J, Mankin H J 1967 Hereditary spondylolisthesis and spina bifida, report of a family in which the lesion is transmitted as an autosomal dominant through three generations. Journal of Bone and Joint Surgery 49A: 507–513

Bathfield C A, Beighton P H 1978 Blount disease, a review of etiological factors in 110 patients. Clinical Orthopedics and Related Research 135: 29–33

Bjerkreim I, van der Hagen C B 1974 Congenital dislocation of the hip joint in Norway. V. Evaluation of genetic and environmental factors. Clinical Genetics 5: 433–448

Blackburne J S, Velikas E P 1977 Spondylolisthesis in children and adolescents. Journal of Bone and Joint Surgery 59B: 490–494

Bonaiti C, Feingold J, Briard M L, Lapeyre F, Rigault P, Guivarch J 1976 Genetique de la scoliose idiopathique. Helvetica Paediatrica Acta 31: 229–240

Bradford D S, Noreen H, Hallgren H M, Yunis E J 1977a

Histocompatibility determinants in idiopathic scoliosis. Clinical Orthopaedics and Related Research 123: 261–265

Bradford D S, Oegema T R, Brown D M 1977b Studies on skin fibroblasts of patients with idiopathic scoliosis. Clinical Orthopaedics and Related Research 126: 111–118

Bushell G R, Ghosh P, Taylor T K F 1978 Collagen defect in idiopathic scoliosis. Lancet 2: 94–95

Bushell G R, Ghosh P, Taylor T K F, Sutherland J M 1979 The collagen of the intervertebral disc in adolescent idiopathic scoliosis. Journal of Bone and Joint Surgery 61B: 501–508

Carter C O 1965 The inheritance of common congenital malformations. Progress in Medical Genetics 4: 59–84

Carter C, Sweetnam R 1958 Familial joint laxity and recurrent dislocation of the patella. Journal of Bone and Joint Surgery 40B: 664–667

Cater C, Sweetnam R 1960 Recurrent dislocation of the patella and of the shoulder, their association with familial joint laxity. Journal of Bone and Joint Surgery 42B: 721–727

Carter C O, Wilkinson J A 1964a Genetic and environmental factors in the etiology of congenital dislocation of the hip. Clinical Orthopedics and Related Research 33: 119–128

Carter C, Wilkinson J 1964b Persistent joint laxity and congenital dislocation of the hip. Journal of Bone and Joint Surgery 46B: 40–45

Ching G H S, Chung C S, Nemechek R W 1969 Genetic and epidemiological studies of clubfoot in Hawaii, ascertainment and incidence. American Journal of Human Genetics 21: 566–580

Connor J M, Conner A N, Connor R A, Tolmie J L, Yeung B, Goudie D 1987 Genetic aspects of early childhood scoliosis. American Journal of Medical Genetics 27: 419–424

Cowell H R, Wein B K 1980 Genetic aspects of club foot. Journal of Bone and Joint Surgery 62A: 1381–1384

Cowell H R, Hall J N, MacEwen G D 1972 Genetic aspects of idiopathic scoliosis. Clinical Orthopedics and Related Research 86: 123–131

Czeizel A, Szentpetery J, Tusnady G, Vizkelety T 1975a Two family studies on congenital dislocation of the hip after early orthopaedic screening in Hungary. Journal of Medical Genetics 12: 125–130

Czeizel A, Tusnady G, Vaczo G, Vizkelety T 1975b The mechanism of genetic predisposition in congenital dislocation of the hip. Journal of Medical Genetics 12: 121–124

Czeizel A, Bellyei A, Barta O, Magda T, Molnar L 1978 Genetics of adolescent idiopathic scoliosis. Journal of Medical Genetics 15: 424–427

DeGeorge F V, Fisher R L 1967 Idiopathic scoliosis, genetic and environmental aspects. Journal of Medical Genetics 4: 251–257

Filho N A, Thompson M W 1971 Genetic studies in scoliosis. Journal of Bone and Joint Surgery 53A: 199

Fisher R L 1972 An epidemiologic study of Legg-Perthes disease. Journal of Bone and Joint Surgery 54A: 769–778

Fisher R L, DeGeorge F V 1967 A twin study of idiopathic scoliosis. Clinical Orthopedics and Related Research 55: 117–126

Francis M J O, Smith R, Sanderson M C 1977 Collagen abnormalities in idiopathic adolescent scoliosis. Calcified Tissue Research 22: 381–384

Garland H G 1934 Hereditary scoliosis. British Medical Journal 1: 328

Gilly R, Stagnara P, Fredrich A, Dalloz C, Robert J M, Goldblatt B 1963 Les aspects medicaux de la scoliose structurale essentielle chez l'enfant. Lyon Med 95: 79–95

Gray I M, Lowrey R B, Renwick D H G 1972 Incidence and genetics of Legg-Perthes disease (osteochondritis deformans) in British Columbia, evidence of polygenic determination. Journal of Medical Genetics 9: 197–202

Hanley W B, McKusick V A, Barranco F T 1967 Osteochondritis dissecans with associated malformations in two brothers. Journal of Bone and Joint Surgery 49A: 925–937

Harper P S, Brotherton B J, Cochlin D 1976 Genetic risks in Perthes disease. Clinical Genetics 10: 178–182

Harrington P R 1977 The etiology of idiopathic scoliosis. Clinical Orthopedics and Related Research 126: 17–25

Haukipuro K, Keranen N, Koivisto E, Lindholm R, Norio R, Punto L 1978 Familial occurrence of lumbar spondylysis and spondylolisthesis. Clinical Genetics 13: 471–476

Horton W A, Collins D L, De Smet A A, Kennedy J A, Schimke R N 1980 Familial joint instability syndrome. American Journal of Medical Genetics 6: 221–228

Idelberger K 1939 Die Ergebnisse der zwillingeforschung beim angeborenen klumpfuss. Verhandlungen der Deutschen Orthopaedischen Gesellschaft 33: 272–276

Idelberger K 1951 Die erbpathologic der sogenannten angeborenen Hüftverrenkung, München und Berlin. Urban & Schwarzenberg

Jessee E F, Owen D S, Sagar K B 1980 The benign hypermobile joint syndrome. Arthritis and Rheumatism 23: 1053–1056

Kambara H, Sasakawa Y 1954 On twins with congenital dislocation of the hip. Journal of Bone and Joint Surgery 36A: 186–187

Mubarak S J, Carroll N C 1979 Familial osteochondritis dissecans of the knee. Clinics in Orthopedics and Related Research 140: 131–136

Muller G M, Seddon H J 1953 Late results of treatment of congenital dislocation of the hip. Journal of Bone and Joint Surgery 35B: 342–362

Palmer R M 1964 Hereditary club foot. Clinical Orthopedics 33: 138–146

Palmer R N, Conneally P M, Yu P L 1974 Studies of the inheritance of idiopathic talipes equinovarus. Orthopedic Clinics of North America 5: 99–108

Pappas A M 1967 The osteochondroses. Pediatric Clinics of North America 14: 549–570

Ponseti I V, Pedrini V, Wynne-Davies R, Duval-Beaupere G 1976 Pathogenesis of scoliosis. Clinical Orthopedics and Related Research 120: 268–280

Record R G, Edwards J H 1958 Environmental influences related to the aetiology of congenital dislocation of the hip. British Journal of Preventive and Social Medicine 12: 8–22

Rimoin D L 1975 The chondrodystrophies. Advances in Human Genetics 5: 1–118

Riseborough E J, Wynne-Davies R 1973 A genetic survey of idiopathic scoliosis in Boston, Massachusetts. Journal of Bone and Joint Surgery 55A: 974–982

Robin G C, Cohen T 1975 Familial scoliosis, a clinical report. Journal of Bone and Joint Surgery 57B: 146–147

Shahriaree H, Sajadi K, Rooholamini S A 1979 A family with spondylolisthesis. Journal of Bone and Joint Surgery 61A: 1256–1258

Sibert J R, Bray P T 1977 Probable dominant inheritance in Blount's disease. Clinical Genetics 11: 394–396

Stougaard J 1961 The hereditary factor in osteochondritis

dissecans. Journal of Bone and Joint Surgery 43B: 256–258

Tobin W J 1975 Familial osteochondritis dissecans with associated tibia vara. Journal of Bone and Joint Surgery 39A: 1091–1105

Uden A, Nilsson I M, Willner S 1980 Collagen changes in congenital and idiopathic scoliosis. Acta Orthopedica Scandinavica 51: 271–274

Wamoscher Z, Farhi A 1963 Hereditary Legg-Calve-Perthes disease. American Journal of Diseases of Children 106: 131–134

Wansbrough R M, Carrie A W, Walker F N, Ruckerbauer G 1959 Coxa plana, its genetic aspects and results of treatment with the long Taylor walking caliper. Journal of Bone and Joint Surgery 41A: 135–146

Wedge J H, Wasylenko M J 1978 The natural history of congenital dislocation of the hip. Clinical Orthopedics and Related Research 137: 154–162

Wiltse L L 1962 The etiology of spondylolisthesis. Journal of Bone and Joint Surgery 44A: 539–560

Wiltse L L, Widell E H, Jackson D W 1975 Fatigue fracture, the basic lesion in isthmic spondylolisthesis. Journal of Bone and Joint Surgery 57A: 17–22

Wiltse L L, Newman P H, Machab I 1976 Classification of spondylolisis and spondylolisthesis. Clinical Orthopedics and Related Research 117: 23–29

Winter R B, Moe J H, Eilers V E 1968 Congenital scoliosis, a study of 234 patients treated and untreated. Journal of Bone and Joint Surgery 50A: 1–47

Woolf C M, Koehn J H, Coleman S S 1968 Congenital hip disease in Utah, the influence of genetic and nongenetic factors. American Journal of Human Genetics 20: 430–439

Wynne-Davies R 1964 Family studies and the cause of congential club foot, talipes equinovarus, calcanovalgus and metatarsus varus. Journal of Bone and Joint Surgery 46B: 445–463

Wynne-Davies R 1968 Familial (idiopathic) scoliosis, a family survey. Journal of Bone and Joint Surgery 50B: 24–30

Wynne-Davies R 1970 A family study of neonatal and late diagnosis congenital dislocation of the hip. Journal of Medical Genetics 7: 315–333

Wynne-Davies R 1980 Some etiologic factors in Perthes' disease. Clinical Orthopedics and Related Research 150: 12–15

Wynne-Davies R, Gormley J 1978 The aetiology of Perthes' disease, genetic, epidemiological and growth factors in 310 Edinburgh and Glasgow patients. Journal of Bone and Joint Surgery 60B: 6–14

Wynne-Davies R, Scott J H S 1979 Inheritance and spondylolisthesis, a radiographic family survey. Journal of Bone and Joint Surgery 61B: 301–305

62. Marfan syndrome

R. E. Pyeritz

HISTORICAL PERSPECTIVE

In 1896 the French paediatrician A B-J Marfan described a nearly 6-year-old girl with long, thin fingers and limbs, which he termed dolichostenomelia (Marfan 1896); this girl also had multiple joint contractures and developed scoliosis. Several years later Achard (1902) described a patient who had loose-jointedness of the hands, hypognathism and dolichostenomelia and called the condition arachnodactyly. In retrospect, neither of these patients may have been affected by what now is called the Marfan syndrome. Over the next 40 years, other features of the syndrome were coupled with the skeletal. In 1914, subluxation of the ocular lenses was associated with the dolichostenomelic habitus (Boerger 1914), though two tall, loose-jointed sibs with ectopia lentis had been described many years before (Williams 1876). The heritable nature of the condition and primary involvement of tissue derived from embryonic mesoderm were first noted by Weve (1931), who also associated Marfan's name with the phenotype for the first time, calling the syndrome dystrophia mesodermalis congenita, typus Marfanis. The aortic complications of dissection and dilatation were clearly associated with the skeletal findings by Baer et al (1943) and by Etter and Glover (1943), though reports of congenital heart disease and arachnodactyly had appeared previously (Salle 1912, Piper & Irvine-Jones 1926). McKusick (1955) drew wider attention to the spectrum of the cardiovascular problems encountered in living patients and postmortem specimens; of more fundamental importance was his labelling of the Marfan syndrome as a heritable disorder of connective tissue, one of the first of a long line of conditions to be so designated (McKusick 1972). Beals and Hecht (1971) described the contractural arachnodactyly syndrome and suggested it as the condition that affected Marfan's original patient.

The aetiology, phenotype, clinical history and management of the Marfan syndrome have been studied extensively in the past decade (Pyeritz & McKusick 1979, 1981, Maumenee 1981, Sisk et al 1983, Pyeritz 1981, 1983, 1986a, 1989a, Gott et al 1986, Chan et al 1987).

Debate continues over whether Abraham Lincoln, who was tall, dolichostenomelic and loose-jointed, was affected by the Marfan syndrome (Gordon 1962, Schwartz 1964, Lattimer 1981). Other people of historical importance who had some outward features typical of the Marfan syndrome include the violinist Paganini (Schoenfeld 1978) and the pianist Rachmaninov (Young 1986). In recent years, several young athletes have died from aortic complications of Marfan syndrome diagnosed, unfortunately, only in retrospect. The death in 1986 of US Olympic Volleyball star Flo Hyman (Demak 1986) increased awareness of the condition among the general public, athletic coaches and trainers, and physicians throughout the world (Weiner & Pyeritz 1987).

THE MARFAN PHENOTYPE

The Marfan syndrome is defined solely by clinical features and mode of inheritance at the present time. The cardinal features defining the phenotype appear in three systems: the skeletal; the ocular; and the cardiovascular. A summary of the most prevalent manifestations observed in 50 consecutive patients is shown in Table 62.1.

Skeletal manifestations

Mean height in the Marfan syndrome is greater than that of either unaffected sibs or the population average for similar sex, age, race and cultural background (Fig. 62.1, Pyeritz et al 1985). The limbs are disproportionately long compared with the trunk (dolichostenomelia). The increased length of the limbs may be estimated if the lower segment length (top of the pubic ramus to floor) is divided into the upper segment length (height minus lower segment). This US/LS ratio varies with age during normal growth but, in the person affected by the Marfan syndrome, is usually at least two standard deviations below the mean for age, race and sex (Fig. 62.2). The US/LS ratio may be exaggerated by scoliosis or abnormal

Table 62.1   Features of the Marfan syndrome in 50 consecutive clinic patients. From Pyeritz and McKusick (1979)

Clinical feature	No. demonstrating feature
Ocular	35/50
ectopia lentis	30/50
myopia	17/50
Cardiovascular	49/50
mid-systolic click only	15/50
mid-systolic click and late systolic murmur	9/50
aortic regurgitant murmur	5/50
mitral regurgitant murmur only	3/50
prosthetic aortic valve	5/50
abnormal echocardiogram	48/50
aortic enlargement	42/50
mitral valve prolapse	29/50
prosthetic aortic valve	5/50
Musculoskeletal	50/50
arachnodactyly	44/50
US/LS 2SD below mean for age	36/47
pectus deformity	34/50
high, narrow palate	30/50
height>95 percentile for age	29/50
hyperextensible joints	28/50
vertebral column deformity	22/50
pes planus	22/50
Family history	40/47
additional documented cases of syndrome	40/47
sporadic cases (presumed new mutations)	7/47
unclear or unknown pedigree	3/50

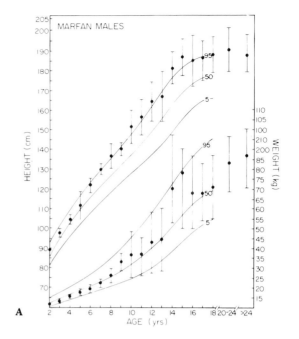

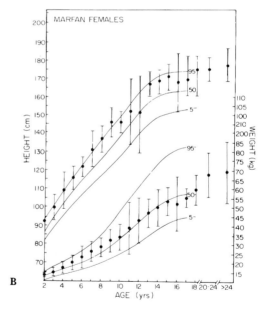

kyphosis. Arachnodactyly appears in numerous other syndromes and remains in large part a subjective feature. Attempts to provide a radiographic criterion by means of the length-to-width ratio of hand bones (metacarpal index) have not demonstrated enough improvement in diagnostic power to justify the time, cost and radiation exposure (Eldridge 1964, Emanuel et al 1977). Simple manoeuvres such as the thumb sign (Steinberg 1966) (positive if the thumb, when maximally opposed within the clenched hand, projects beyond the ulnar border, Fig. 62.3A) and the wrist sign (Walker & Murdoch 1970) (positive if the distal phalanges of the first and fifth digits of one hand overlap when wrapped around the opposite wrist, Fig. 62.3B), are helpful when positive but are subject to observer interpretation and may reflect the longitudinal laxity of the hand rather than arachnodactyly.

Longitudinal overgrowth of the ribs produces anterior chest deformity, either depression (pectus excavatum or funnel chest, Fig. 62.4A) or protrusion (pectus carinatum or pigeon breast, Fig. 62.4B) of the sternum. Both defects may be present in the same patient. The chest is often asymmetrical, with one set of costochondral junctions protruding more than the contralateral set. The deform-

Fig. 62.1   Growth in the Marfan syndrome. Plots of height and weight vs age of males (**A**) and females (**B**) who were not treated with hormones. Both cross-sectional and longitudinal data of about 200 caucasian patients were used in constructing these preliminary curves. The points show the means for persons grouped in one-year intervals and the bars show +/− one standard deviation. The curved lines show the 5, 50 and 95 percentiles of the unaffected population (Pyeritz et al 1985).

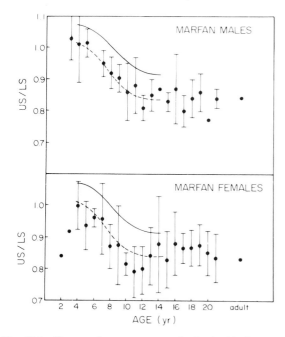

Fig. 62.2 Upper-to-lower segment ratios in the Marfan syndrome. The US/LS falls with increasing age through early puberty. The points show the means for caucasian patients grouped in one-year intervals and the bars show +/− one standard deviation. The solid curve is the mean and the dashed curve two standard deviations below the mean for unaffected caucasians (adapted from McKusick 1972).

ity is subject to considerable alteration during the time of rib growth.

Joint laxity is frequently present but has little diagnostic specificity. The fingers, wrists, elbows and knees (genu recurvatum) are commonly hyperextensible. Laxity of the carpal ligaments produces flat feet (pes planus with or without calcaneoplano valgus, Fig. 62.5). Some patients have limited extension or unequivocal congenital contractures, usually of fingers or elbows, which may coexist with laxity of other joints.

Scoliosis may occur at one or multiple sites along the vertebral column and generally worsens during periods of rapid growth, such as early adolescence (Robins et al 1975, Birch & Herring 1987). Mild degrees of curvature can best be appreciated clinically by observation of erect patients from behind as they bend forward at the hips with arms at full length and palms in contact; either the curve of the vertebral column will be more evident, or one shoulder will be higher than the other. Thoracic scoliosis is usually obvious on the routine chest radiograph. Kyphosis of the thoracic or thoraco-lumbar region often accompanies scoliosis, but in many patients, even in

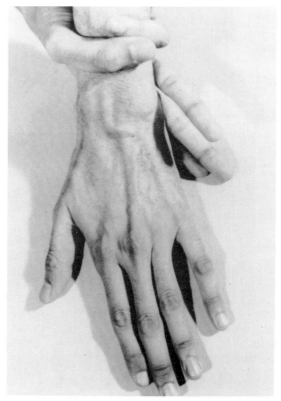

A   **B**

Fig. 62.3 Positive thumb (**A**) and wrist (**B**) signs in a 30-year-old man affected by the Marfan syndrome. Arachnodactyly is evident in B.

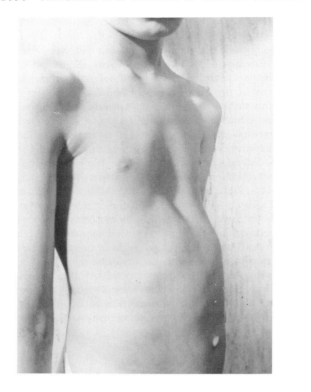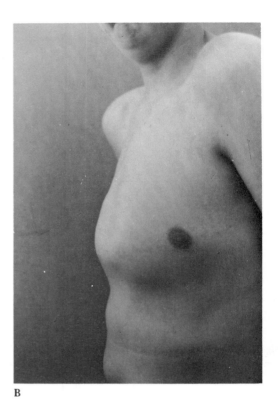

Fig. 62.4   Pectus excavatum (**A**) and carinatum (**B**) in two young adolescent boys affected by the Marfan syndrome.

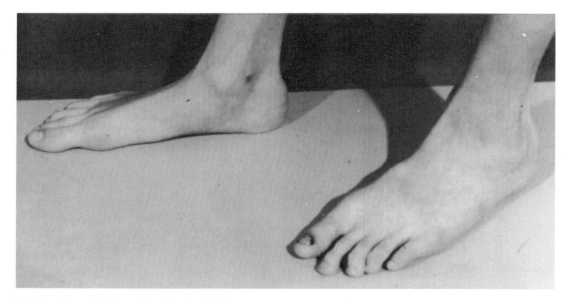

Fig. 62.5   Pes planus in a boy affected by the Marfan syndrome. Note the arachnodactyly and the long narrow foot.

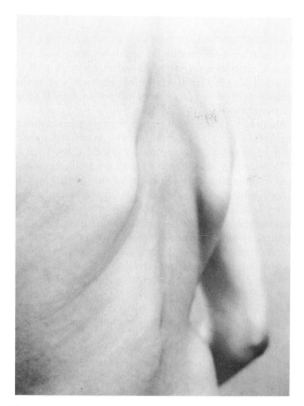

Fig. 62.6 Thoracic lordosis in the Marfan syndrome. The adolescent boy has a reversal of the usual thoracic kyphotic curve, resulting in a reduction of the anteroposterior diameter of the thorax. This type of deformity is present in the 'straight back syndrome'.

the absence of scoliosis, a straightening of the usually mild thoracic kyphosis (straight-back syndrome) or even a thoracic lordosis occurs, resulting in a reduced antero-posterior diameter of the chest (Fig. 62.6).

An abnormally deep socket of the hip joint (protrusio acetabuli) occurs in about 50% of Marfan patients (Kuhlman et al 1987), and occasionally causes disability. As patients survive longer through preventive cardio-vascular surgery, degenerative arthritis of the hip may become a more common problem.

The hard palate is often narrow and highly-arched, (described as 'gothic') and causes tooth crowding. Retro-gnathia is common and contributes to dental mal-occlusion.

Ocular manifestations

Subluxation of the lens (ectopia lentis) occurs in a proportion of cases variously estimated between 50–80%, is usually bilateral, and rarely progresses (McKusick 1972, Cross & Jensen 1975, Pyeritz & McKusick 1979, Maumenee 1981). The lens is most commonly displaced upward; the zonules remain intact and accommodation is possible (Fig. 62.7). Subluxation is usually present at the time of the first detailed ophthalmological examination (Cross & Jensen 1975) suggesting that the displacement freqently occurs in utero. Occasionally, the lens in the Marfan syndrome will dislocate into the anterior chamber (commonly as a result of trauma) and produce acute glaucoma. Most cases of glaucoma follow surgical

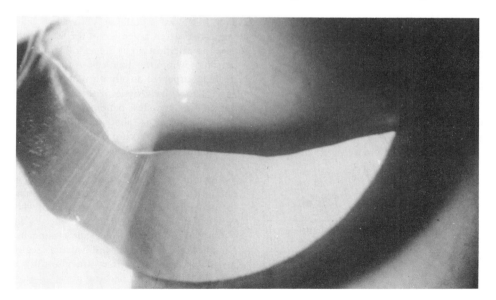

Fig. 62.7 Ectopia lentis in the Marfan syndrome. A photograph taken through a slit lamp of the lens of a young girl. The lens is dislocated supratemporally. Note the zonules which are stretched but intact.

Table 62.2 Axial length of the ocular globe in the Marfan syndrome (adapted from Maumenee 1981)

Age (yrs)	No. eyes measured	Mean length (mm ± S.D)	
1-8	20	23.5 ± 0.8	
9-14	23	24.5	
15+	43	25.3 ± 2.50	
All ages			
Without lens subluxation		23.4	
With lens subluxation		26.0	(p<0.01)

Normal eyes have a mean axial length of 23 mm at age 3 yrs and between 23.5-24.7 mm at ages over 15 yrs.

extirpation of the lens (Cross & Jensen 1975). A subluxed ocular lens is often not visible with the direct ophthalmoscope, but fluttering of the iris as the lens accommodates (iridodonesis) usually provides a clue to lens displacement. Any patient suspected of the Marfan syndrome must undergo a slit lamp examination with the pupils fully dilated.

The axial length of the globe is increased, which contributes to myopia, an increased risk of retinal detachment, and lens subluxation (Table 62.2). As with glaucoma, the prevalence of retinal detachment increases following lens extraction (Maumenee 1981). Studies of corneal shape (keratometry) show that nearly all patients with the Marfan syndrome have relatively flat corneas (Table 62.3). Myopia is frequent and may appear early and be severe. While abnormalities of the globe, retina, lens and cornea all may impair vision, a flat cornea tends to correct myopia.

Cardiovascular manifestations

The two most common cardiovascular features of the Marfan syndrome are mitral valve prolapse and dilatation of the ascending aorta. The former may result in mitral regurgitation, while the latter may result in aortic

Table 62.3 Corneal shape in the Marfan syndrome (adapted from Maumenee 1981)

Age (yrs)	No. eyes measured	Mean keratometer reading (diopter ± S.D)
1-8	37	40.9 ± 2.4
9-14	28	40.8 ± 2.3
15+	72	41.9 ± 1.7

Normal adult eyes have mean keratometer readings of 43.7 ± 0.2

regurgitation and predispose to aortic dissection and rupture. The mean age at death is reduced by 30–40% in persons with the Marfan syndrome, and nearly all of the precocious deaths result from a cardiovascular complication (Murdoch et al 1972a).

About 60% of patients have auscultatory signs of mitral or aortic valve pathology, but the rest may have normal cardiovascular physical findings (Table 62.1, Brown et al 1975, Pyeritz & McKusick 1979). Echocardiography has greatly enhanced the detection of the cardiovascular abnormalities, with a concomitant improvement in the ability to diagnose the Marfan syndrome. For example, whereas about one-third of the patients have single or multiple systolic clicks or systolic murmurs of presumed mitral origin, echocardiography shows that over 80% of all Marfan patients, irrespective of age or sex, have prolapse of at least the posterior mitral leaflet (Brown et al 1975, Pyeritz & McKusick 1979, Pyeritz & Wappel 1983). The prolapse is often pansystolic, with exaggerated leaflet excursion suggesting redundancy of valvular tissue.

M-mode echocardiography of the Marfan aorta (Fig. 62.8) in both children and adults readily shows that the diameter of the aortic root, measured at the level of the aortic valve cusps and relative to bodysurface area, is usually, but not always, greater than the upper limit of the normal range (Sisk et al 1983). Cross-sectional echocardiography often displays the ascending aorta for a distance of 4–6 cm above the aortic valve and may be the first clue that a clinically silent dissection has occurred. The mitral valve leaflets are often thickened and redundant. Mitral valve prolapse is often associated with mitral regurgitation, enlargement of the left atrium, and dilatation and calcification of the mitral annulus. Rarely will a person in whom the diagnosis of the Marfan syndrome is strongly suspected on other grounds (skeletal, ocular, and auscultatory) have none of these echocardiographic abnormalities. In a few patients, a technically satisfactory echocardiogram is unobtainable because of a severe pectus deformity or emphysema.

The chest radiograph is an insensitive technique for detecting early aortic root enlargement or dissection. Dilatation of the proximal ascending aorta is visible on the frontal radiograph only when substantial; mild to moderate enlargement is frequently hidden by the vertebral column and cardiac silhouette (Fig. 62.9).

No typical electrocardiographic abnormalities occur. Changes result from chronic valvular regurgitation, but usually after these lesions are clinically recognizable. Axis deviations occur because of rotation of the heart by severe pectus excavatum or thoracic lordosis.

On aortography, the dilated Marfan aorta is characteristic (Fig. 62.10). The enlargement is symmetrical and

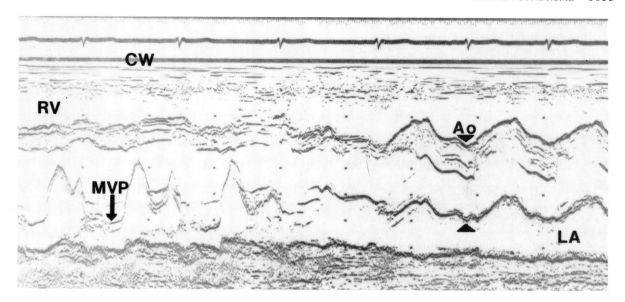

Fig. 62.8 Echocardiogram showing mitral valve prolapse and aortic dilatation. This 8-year-old boy had a normal clinical examination – no clicks or murmurs. Both leaflets of the mitral valve prolapse in mid-systole (MVP). The aortic root (Ao) has a diameter of 2.8 cm, greater than the upper limit of normal for either age or body surface. The right ventricle (RV), left atrium (LA) and chest wall (CW) are indicated.

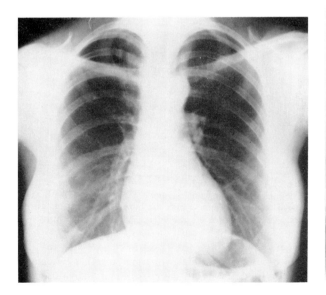

Fig. 62.9 Normal chest radiograph in the presence of aortic root dilatation. The proximal aorta of this 28-year-old woman affected by the Marfan syndrome measured 4.8 cm, nearly 50% greater than normal. This enlargement is hidden by the cardiac silhouette.

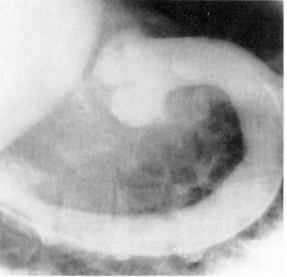

Fig. 62.10 Aortic root dilatation in the Marfan syndrome. The sinuses of Valsalva are symmetrically dilated to a moderate degree in this 37-year-old woman. While no aortic regurgitation is present, severe mitral regurgitation necessitated valve replacement in this patient.

begins in the sinuses of Valsalva. Rarely does the dilatation extend as far as the innominate artery, and the ascending aorta has a gourd-like appearance when contrast material is injected.

Other clinical manifestations

The predominant abnormality of the skin is the stria atrophica, most commonly found over the shoulders and buttocks (Fig. 62.11). Striae gravidarum can be marked in women with the Marfan syndrome. The skin is otherwise not unusually fragile or susceptible to bruising or poor healing, but may be hyperextensible. Frequently hernias occur, especially in the inguinal region. They may appear in early childhood, and a history of multiple repairs is not uncommon.

Spontaneous pneumothorax occurs in about 5% of Marfan patients (Hall et al 1984). Some patients have markedly reduced total lung capacity and residual volume ascribable to deforming kyphoscoliosis or pectus excavatum. Even in patients without thoracic distortion, forced vital capacity is consistently less than predicted based on height; however, the use of a more accurate predictor of thoracic size, such as the sitting height, shows that static lung volumes in the absence of severe scoliosis and pectus excavatum are not markedly abnormal (Streeten et al 1987).

Ectasia of the caudal dural sac is a common finding, evident on radiographs of the lumbosacral spine as bony erosions, especially of the neural foramina, and on axial CT or MRI scans as a widened neural canal (Pyeritz et al 1988). An extreme manifestation is an intrapelvic meningocele, which may present as a pelvic mass and be confused with an ovarian cyst or tumour. Dural ectasia is usually asymptomatic, but should be in the differential diagnosis of a Marfan patient with low back pain, lower radicular pain, or leg weakness.

It has been assumed that people with Marfan syndrome have no impairment of cortical function. We recently studied 30 unselected school-aged clinic patients and confirmed average intellectual and gross motor development. However, half of the young patients had one or more neuropsychological deficits, including learning disability, attention deficit disorder with or without hyperactivity, neuromaturational immaturity, and verbal-performance discrepancy (Hofman et al 1988). Joint laxity of the hand and wrist contributed to the latter deficit, but the pathogenesis of the rest of the problems is obscure.

DIAGNOSIS

Each of the clinical features of the Marfan syndrome occurs with variable frequency in the general population,

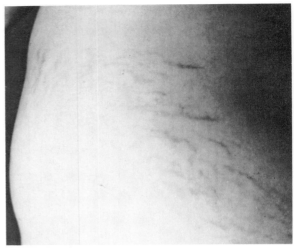

A

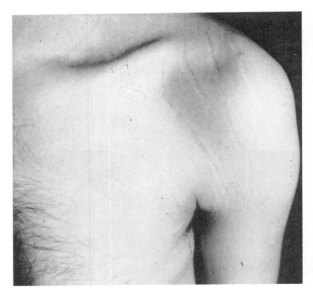

B

Fig. 62.11 Striae atrophicae in the Marfan syndrome. These characteristic skin lesions appear and expand with age. Striae usually first appear over the hip (**A**, an 8-year-old girl) and often occur over the shoulders (**B**, a 30-year-old man).

and occasionally several will occur together by chance alone. In determining which of such individuals are affected by a systemic connective tissue disorder, more diagnostic reliance is placed on the presence of hard manifestations (subluxed lenses, aortic dilatation, severe kyphoscoliosis and asymmetrical deformity of the anterior chest) than on soft features (myopia, mitral prolapse, tall stature, joint laxity and arachnodactyly). Exceptional cases, such as an individual with ectopia lentis and an aneurysm of the ascending aorta with a normal habitus and a negative family history may rate the diagnosis of the Marfan syndrome, even though only two criteria are present (Beighton et al 1988). On the other hand, the familial occurrence of scoliosis, pectus excavatum, and mitral valve prolapse merits consideration of the Marfan syndrome because three of the criteria are present, but may well represent the mitral valve prolapse syndrome (Bon Tempo et al 1975, Pyeritz et al 1979, Glesby & Pyeritz 1989).

Two laboratory tests are required of any person in whom the Marfan diagnosis is suspected: slit lamp examination of the eyes and echocardiography. The former is to establish whether ectopia lentis is present. Echocardiography is needed to determine if mitral valve prolapse and aortic root dilatation are present.

No single laboratory test can establish the diagnosis of the Marfan syndrome. No biochemical tests have proved to be either highly sensitive or specific for the Marfan syndrome.

Conditions which must be excluded routinely when considering the diagnosis of the Marfan syndrome include: homocystinuria; contractural arachnodactyly; a number of the Ehlers-Danlos variants; and familial mitral valve prolapse. A variety of other conditions include one or more of the clinical features of the Marfan syndrome, but would rarely be confused; these are listed in Table 62.4.

Homocystinuria must be excluded in any patient thought to have the Marfan syndrome because the pleiotropic manifestations of the two conditions include the same organ systems. Homocystinuria is ruled-out in most cases by a negative cyanide-nitroprusside test of the urine, an easy screening test for disulphide accumulation; positive reactions necessitate further evaluation by quantitative amino acid analysis of urine and plasma (Mudd et al 1989). Patients with the pyridoxine-responsive form of homocystinuria may have a mild phenotype and escape detection until adolescence or adulthood, especially if they unwittingly take regular multivitamin supplements that contain folate and B_6 (Mudd et al 1985). Such cystathionine beta-synthase-deficient patients may have a negative qualitative urine screen for disulphides.

Contractural arachnodactyly is a rare, autosomal dominant condition (Beals & Hecht 1971). Some patients who clearly have the Marfan syndrome also have congenital contractures and abnormal ears (Pyeritz 1986b). Any patient diagnosed as contractural arachnodactyly should have echocardiography and detailed ophthalmological examination.

Patients with Ehlers-Danlos Types I, II, or III may be

Table 62.4 Other conditions which have clinical features in common with the Marfan syndrome (adapted from Pyeritz et al 1979)

Skeletal
homocystinuria
congenital contractural arachnodactyly
osteogenesis imperfecta
mitral valve prolapse syndrome
pseudoxanthoma elasticum
eunuchoidism or delayed puberty
Klinefelter syndrome (47,XXY)
trisomy 8 (47,XX or XY, +8)
Goodman camptodactyly syndrome B
Stickler syndrome
syndrome of nerve deafness, eye anomalies, and marfanoid habitus
nemaline myopathy
syndrome of pigmentary degeneration, cataract, microcephaly and arachnodactyly
myotonic dystrophy
multiple endocrine adenomatosis, type III
fragilitas oculi
Achard syndrome
Ocular
homocystinuria
familial ectopia lentis
Weill-Marchesani syndrome
Ehlers-Danlos syndrome, type VI
Stickler syndrome
Cardiovascular
syphilitic aortitis
Ehlers-Danlos syndromes, types I-II and other variants
familial bicuspid aortic valve
mitral valve prolapse syndrome
osteogenesis imperfecta
Erdheim cystic medial necrosis
relapsing polychondritis
ankylosing spondylitis
Reiter syndrome

asthenic and have skeletal deformity (McKusick 1972, Leier et al 1980). Mitral valve prolapse occurs frequently, and occasionally the aortic root may dilate. Generally, the body proportions are not disturbed as in the Marfan syndrome. Severe joint laxity and skin elasticity argue against the Marfan syndrome.

Persons with the mitral valve prolapse syndrome lack ocular or severe aortic involvement but often have scoliosis, thoracic lordosis, asthenia, and pectus excavatum; these features are heritable as an autosomal dominant trait (Glesby & Pyeritz 1989).

Genetic heterogeneity undoubtedly exists in the Marfan syndrome (McKusick 1972, Pyeritz et al 1979). Discovery of a biochemical abnormality in one patient will enable definitive diagnosis in relatives; the same abnormality may not occur in another affected family and thus be of limited diagnostic utility. At the present time no biochemical or DNA marker has been unequivocally linked to the Marfan syndrome, and diagnosis remains based on phenotype.

NATURAL HISTORY AND PROGNOSIS

Skeletal

At birth affected children tend to be longer than normal, a discrepancy which persists, though the growth rate is no greater than their unaffected peers. The reduced upper to lower segment ratio compared with the normal population persists with increasing age (Fig. 62.3). The anterior chest deformity can change markedly during the course of growth of the ribs. A mild pectus excavatum in an infant can worsen in a matter of a few years, become asymmetrical, or convert to a carinatum defect.

Joint laxity can lead to recurrent dislocation, most commonly of the first metacarpal-phalangeal joint and the patella. Laxity of the ankle and foot produces instability and various foot deformities, in addition to pes planus. If they are ignored at an early age, severe life-long gait disturbances can result. Pes cavus may occasionally develop. Joint laxity of the fingers, elbows and knees often lessens with age. In later life degenerative arthritic changes are commonplace in joints that were once particularly lax. Protrusio acetabuli may predispose to functional problems of the hips.

Scoliosis develops gradually, but progresses most rapidly during the adolescent growth spurt (Robins et al 1975, Birch & Herring 1987).

Ocular

Subluxation of the lens usually does not progress. Because the zonules remain intact, there is little tendency for the lens to migrate into either the anterior or posterior humours (Cross & Jensen 1975). When the lens is present, retinal detachments rarely occur; however, once the lens is extirpated, retinal detachment becomes much more common (Maumenee 1981). The degree of myopia may change substantially during the time of growth as various ocular structures change shape.

Cardiovascular

Mitral valve prolapse may not be clinically or echocardiographically present during infancy but may be noted several years later. The degree of prolapse may worsen with age, and mitral regurgitation may appear and progress haemodynamically in some patients who initially had only prolapse (Pyeritz & Wappel 1983). Even in children the mitral regurgitation can become severe enough to warrant valve replacement (Phornphutkul et al 1973, Sisk et al 1983).

The size of the aortic root relative to body surface area is generally larger than normal even in infancy and increases with age at a rate greater than normal (Sisk et al 1983). Moreover, aortic root dilatation does not cease at skeletal maturity. The aortic root enlarges symmetrically in the sinus of Valsalva region and eventually above the sinotubular ridge. The so-called annulus of the aortic valve may also dilate; however, it is the dilatation in the region of the sinotubular ridge that results in eventual failure of the cusps of the aortic valve to appose (Pyeritz et al 1980). As the aorta continues to dilate, the regurgitant flow increases. The left ventricular response to aortic regurgitation in the Marfan syndrome is qualitatively similar to that with other causes of chronic aortic regurgitation, but the following sequence of events may evolve more rapidly in the Marfan syndrome. The left ventricle dilates to compensate for the increased stroke volume required. Eventually the myocardium begins to fail and irreversible myopathic changes follow. The end stage, if dissection or rupture of the aorta does not supervene, is death from congestive heart failure (McKusick 1955).

The dilated ascending aorta is more susceptible than the undilated aorta to traumatic dissection or rupture (McDonald et al 1981). Numerous cases of dissection or rupture, often associated with sudden death, have occurred in persons with the Marfan syndrome while they were playing contact sports such as basketball (Maron et al 1980, Demak 1986) or when they were involved in relatively minor deceleration injuries in automobile accidents.

Several dozen case reports describe the rupture or dissection of the aorta and other large arteries in pregnant women affected by the Marfan syndrome. Because of the increase in cardiac output which occurs during the midtrimester, the dilated ascending aorta is under more strain than in the nonpregnant condition. The largest retrospective survey examined 105 pregnancies in 26 Marfan women (Pyeritz 1981). Only one death occurred, that due to endocarditis in a woman with severe mitral valve disease which predated the pregnancy (McKusick 1972). Recently we have followed 18 Marfan women, all but one of whom had aortic root diameters less than 42 mm, through 24 pregnancies. None with minimal aortic dilatation had any vascular complication and echocardiography every six weeks showed no further aortic dilatation (Pyeritz unpublished). One woman with aortic regurgitation and moderate aortic dilatation suffered an acute dissection of the descending aorta.

The records of 257 Marfan patients at the Johns

Hopkins Hospital were examined for life expectancy and causes of death (Murdoch et al 1972a). The study was performed at a time when medical and surgical therapy had virtually no beneficial impact on patient survival. Survival had fallen to 50% for men at age 40 years and for women at age 48 years, a reduction in expected life span of about 30–40% for both sexes.

The mean age of death of the 72 deceased patients was 32 years. The immediate cause of death in over 90% was a cardiovascular complication. Dissection or rupture of the aorta and chronic aortic regurgitation with congestive heart failure accounted for the vast majority of the deaths.

AETIOLOGY AND PATHOGENESIS

Over 50 years ago the Marfan syndrome was hypothesized to be a generalized disorder of mesenchyme (Weve 1931), and was one of the original group of conditions classified as a heritable disorder of connective tissue (McKusick 1955). In the past decade, notable progress has been achieved in discovering the fundamental defects of connective tissue in an ever-expanding group of hereditary conditions (Prockop & Kivirikko 1984, Hollister 1987, Pyeritz 1987, Beighton et al 1988). Nonetheless, the cause of the Marfan syndrome has not been defined beyond the obvious heterozygosity for a mutant allele of a gene that in some way participates in metabolism of the extracellular matrix.

At various times, attention has been directed at collagen (Boucek et al 1981, Byers et al 1981, Halbritter et al 1981), glycosaminoglycan (Lamberg 1978, Appel et al 1979, Nakashima 1986), elastin (Gunja-Smith & Boucek 1981, Halme et al 1982), elastase (Derouette et al 1981) and smooth muscle (Simpson et al, 1980). Numerous histological, ultrastructural and biochemical alterations have been described, but none has come to be regarded as more than either a consequence of a more fundamental defect, or a defect restricted to the single patient from whom a specimen was obtained (Pyeritz & McKusick 1981). Advantage has been taken of autosomal dominant inheritance and complete penetrance of the disorder, and availability of cloned DNA probes to search for the cause of the Marfan syndrome by a candidate-gene linkage strategy (Francomano & Kazazian 1986, Gusella 1987). Thus far, the loci for the alpha1 (I), alpha2 (I), alpha1 (II), and alpha1 (III) procollagens have been excluded as the site of the mutation in several informative pedigrees, effectively excluding primary structural defects of the major fibrillar collagens (types I, II and III) as common causes of the Marfan syndrome (Dalgleish et al 1987, Ogilvie et al 1987, Tsipouras et al 1986, Francomano et al 1988).

In the past several years, attention has refocused on abnormalities of elastic fibres in the Marfan syndrome (Perejda et al 1985, Tsuji 1986). Elastic fibres are composed of an amorphous core of highly cross-linked elastin monomers and a surrounding array of microfibrils (Ross & Bornstein 1969). The biochemical composition of microfibrils is incompletely characterized, but one of the constituents is fibrillin, a high-molecular weight glycoprotein (Sakai et al 1986). Both immunohistopathological and biochemical investigations point to an abnormality of the microfibril fibre array as central to the pathogenesis, and perhaps the aetiology, of the Marfan syndrome (Hollister et al 1987).

Several animal models may have pertinence to the pathogenesis of the Marfan syndrome in humans. Feeding rats the lathyritic agent beta-aminoproprionitrile (BAPN) produces a phenotype resembling the Marfan syndrome with kyphoscoliosis, hernias, and aneurysms of the aorta. Dissection of the aorta in turkeys can be produced by adding BAPN to the feed (Barnett et al 1957).

Copper deficiency in swine or fowl leads to aortic rupture (O'Dell et al 1961). The histopathology and ultrastructure of the aortic wall in the Marfan syndrome, copper-deficient chicks, and BAPN-treated turkeys are similar (Simpson et al 1980).

GENETICS

A great many families in which multiple individuals affected by the Marfan syndrome occur have been studied; in some the phenotype can be traced through six generations (McKusick 1972). Male-to-male transmission occurs. All of these characteristics are consistent with autosomal dominant inheritance.

Reports of multiple affected sibs with ostensibly normal parents are rare and in no cases have both the parents been examined with sufficient detail to exclude their being mildly affected. Consanguinity has not been reported in these families.

No formal studies of the frequency of sporadic cases or of the evolutionary (or genetic) fitness of the Marfan syndrome have been published. McKusick (1972) estimated that 15% of patients had unaffected parents and most likely developed the Marfan syndrome from de novo mutation in a parental germ cell. Recently in our medical genetics clinic, of 138 consecutive Marfan patients, 41 had neither parent affected. While various biases influence which patients attend a clinic, these data suggest that sporadic cases account for 15–30% of all patients. The average age of the fathers of sporadic cases exceeds by some seven years that of fathers in the general population (Murdoch et al 1972b); the average age of the mothers of sporadic cases is not as advanced. This paternal age effect has been described in other autosomal dominant disorders such as achondroplasia. The progenitor cells of spermatozoa in the testes of older fathers have a longer time during which to mutate, through either exposure to mutagens, or DNA replication errors, and for mutations to accumulate, since each mitosis of a mutated spermatogonia returns a replicated cell to the progenitor pool.

The marked degree of variability of expression of the Marfan gene undoubtedly explains the claims of 'nonpenetrance' which appear in the older literature. When presumed cases of 'nonpenetrance' or 'formes frustes' in families in which other, well-documented cases of the Marfan syndrome occur are examined by sensitive methods (such as echocardiography), usually the assignment of the Marfan gene can be made with confidence.

The chromosomal location of a genetic locus determining the Marfan phenotype is unkown. The only attempts to determine a map position have been by means of linkage analysis. Several studies examined linkage between the Marfan phenotype and a variety of blood group antigens and serum protein markers. Two studies found no suspicions of linkage (Lynas & Merritt 1958, Schleutermann et al 1976), while one found a suggestion of linkage between the Marfan phenotype and Rh, with a lod score of $+1.17$ at a recombination fraction of 0.30 (Mace 1979).

Restriction fragment length polymorphisms of either candidate genes or anonymous chromosome probes may provide evidence for the chromosomal location of genes capable of producing the Marfan phenotype before the biochemical defects are discovered.

PREVALENCE

Based on what was thought to be complete ascertainment of the phenotype in Northern Ireland, the mutation rate of the 'Marfan locus' was calculated (Lynas & Merritt 1958). From this figure a minimal prevalance of 1–2 cases per 100 000 population was derived. However, the syndrome was clearly underdiagnosed three decades ago. Based on crude calculations of the size of the catchment area and the number of Marfan patients in the files of the Johns Hopkins Hospital, the prevalence was estimated as 4–6/100 000 (Pyeritz & McKusick 1979). Since the manifestations of the Marfan syndrome may extend from the limits of normal to the floridly 'classic' in which the diagnosis is unquestionable, the actual prevalence of the Marfan syndrome may exceed this estimate.

The Marfan syndrome occurs in all races and in all major ethnic groups that reside in the United States. Relative prevalences in ethnic groups elsewhere are unknown. Nothing is known about the geographical distribution of the Marfan syndrome, but no predilection is obvious in the United States.

PATHOLOGY

Gross pathology

Numerous reports of autopsies of patients affected by the Marfan syndrome appear in the literature (see McKusick 1972 for review). The aorta dilates in its most proximal region, the sinuses of Valsalva. The dilatation is symmetrical and may extend above the sinotubular junction. The diameter of the ascending aorta usually returns to normal before the innominate artery, unless a dissection is present. Dilatation of the sinotubular junction, at the upper aortic valve attachments, results in failure of the cusps to coapt.

When dissection of the aorta occurs, the entry tear in the intima is frequently several centimetres above the aortic annulus, in the area of greatest dilation. The dissection can either progress antegrade no further than the arch, progress through the arch into the descending aorta, or extend retrograde. In the latter case, attachments of the valve cusps may be torn, coronary ostia may be occluded, or rupture into the pericardial sac producing tamponade may occur. Any dissection can undergo rapid or gradual evolution. Intimal tears in the absence of dissection are common in the dilated proximal ascending aorta.

The valve cusps are usually diaphanous and redundant, and the mitral valve and annulus are prone to calcification. Fenestrations occur in a minority of aortic and mitral valve cusps. The aortic and mitral valves are prone to the development of bacterial endocarditis.

The proximal pulmonary artery is usually mildly dilated, but pulmonic regurgitation is uncommon.

Aneurysmal dilatation of coronary arteries has been reported but is uncommon. The coronary ostia may be abnormally high in the aortic root because of root dilatation.

No specific changes occur in the atria, ventricles or myocardium that are not attributable to the effects of chronic valvular regurgitation. Several patients have had clinical congestive heart failure out of proportion to their valvular disease and the existence of a cardiopathy associated with the Marfan syndrome has been suggested. Histopathological studies of such patients are lacking.

Reports of gross ocular pathology are few, and little can be said other than that the lenses tend to dislocate superiorly, the globes tend to be elongated in the anteroposterior direction, and the corneas are flatter than normal.

Published reports of gross pathology of bone, ligaments and tendons show no particular abnormalities.

Histology and ultrastructure

The aortic wall characteristically shows changes in the medial layer. The elastic fibres become progressively swollen, fragmented and reduced in number as the aortic diameter increases (Fig. 62.12). Lacunae appear in the media which are filled with basophilic proteoglycan. The term 'cystic medial necrosis' has been applied to these histological changes, but is a misnomer and its use should be discouraged. Neither necrosis nor cysts are present. These histopathological features are also seen in aortas from non-Marfan patients who had hypertension or aortic valve disease, and to a lesser degree may be a concomitant of ageing. The most reasonable explanation is that the histopathology indicates injury and repair regardless of the cause of the injury (Schlatmann & Becker 1977). Electron microscopic examination confirms focal elastin fibre degeneration and abnormalities of collagen fibres. The medial smooth muscle fibres

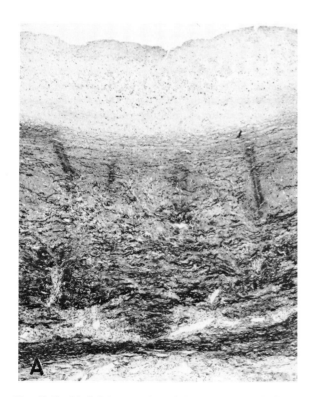

Fig. 62.12 Medial degeneration of the aorta in the Marfan syndrome.

appear shrunken and their basement membrane is greatly thickened.

Arteries elswhere in the body may show evidence of medial disorganization, but less than that present in the ascending aorta. The aortic and mitral valve usually show myxomatous degenerative changes.

Cartilage biopsies from the iliac crest in three adolescent patients were examined by transmission electron microscopy. The chondrocytes had dilated endoplasmic reticulum, cytoplasmic vacuoles and increased glycogen stores (Nogami et al 1979). Few reports of histological changes in other tissues exist.

MANAGEMENT

No specific therapy exists for the underlying defect in the Marfan syndrome. Therapeutic efforts are directed at first establishing an accurate diagnosis, determining which problems are present at the time of diagnosis, anticipating the problems which will likely arise in the future, and pursuing certain prophylactic measures for specific problems. The patients should have one physician, knowledgeable about the syndrome, who serves as the primary physician and refers to subspecialists as the need arises. The multidisciplinary approach is often best conducted in the setting of the academic medical institution (Pyeritz 1986a).

Skeletal

All children with any evidence of abnormal spinal curvature and all adults with a progressive deformity should be evaluated by an orthopaedic specialist semi-annually. Scoliosis greater than 20 degrees in children should be pursued aggressively with mechanical bracing and physical therapy. Spinal surgery is necessary when bracing fails to halt progression and in curves of greater than 45 degrees (Birch & Herring 1987).

Scoliosis tends to progress most during rapid growth, especially in early adolescence. If this adolescent growth spurt can be shortened the scoliosis may not progress so far. A second benefit of decreasing the length of time that the bones have to elongate is a reduction in adult body height. Girls can be treated before menarche with oestrogen on a daily basis to induce puberty and epiphyseal closure. Progestogen is added five days each cycle to prevent dysfunctional bleeding. No conclusive data are yet available to show whether scoliosis is abated by this approach. Adult height has clearly been reduced in women who begin therapy before the menarche (Fig. 62.13).

Other orthopaedic problems associated with joint instability should be managed by an orthopaedic surgeon

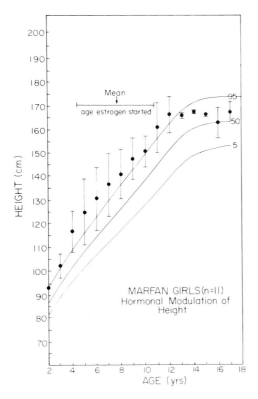

Fig. 62.13 Hormonal modulation of height in girls affected by the Marfan syndrome. In all cases treatment with ethinyl estradiol (0.05 mg/10 kg daily) and conjugated estrogen (Premarin[R], 10 mg on days 25-28 each menstrual cycle) was begun before menarche. Therapy was continued until the time menarche was likely to have occurred naturally or until bone maturation was well-advanced, whichever occurred first. Comparison with Figure 62.1B shows early cessation of growth and reduction in height of the treated girls.

familiar with connective tissue disorders. The major indication for repair of anterior chest deformity is cardiopulmonary compromise and should be deferred until late adolescence if possible (Arn et al 1989). Repair early in life provides many years for rib growth to depress the sternum and re-establish the deformity.

Ocular

The patient should be evaluated annually by an ophthalmologist experienced in connective tissue disorders. Emphasis should fall on the correction of amblyopia, the direction and degree of lens subluxation, anterior chamber abnormalities, and detection of retinal detachment. The earliest symptoms of retinal detachment and the necessity of seeking consultation immediately should be explained to patients and their families. The subluxed lens rarely requires extirpation, except when adequate correction of visual acuity is impossible, or in the rare instance of displacement into the anterior chamber (Maumenee 1981).

Cardiovascular

The frequency of cardiological evaluation depends on the severity of the manifestation. If the patient has only mitral valve prolapse and a mildly dilated aorta without any valvular regurgitation, then an annual examination including an echocardiogram and an EKG is sufficient. As the aorta dilates and as valvular regurgitation appears and progresses, more frequent examinations are indicated.

The dilated aorta is susceptible to rupture or dissection, either spontaneously or following modest trauma. The shearing forces of ventricular ejection may be the driving forces behind dissection and dilatation. For these reasons, some restriction of patient activity seems warranted. Patients should not engage in contact sports, activities requiring maximal exertion, or isometric exercise. Most prepubertal children do not require stringent restrictions. However, their interests and activities should be channelled away from competitive athletics.

The use of propranolol to delay or prevent severe aortic complications rests on several premises (Halpern et al 1971, Pyeritz 1986a). The first premise is that the risk of an aortic complication is proportionate to the diameter of the aorta. Since rupture and dissection depend on the tension or stress on the aortic wall, the Laplace relationship (wall tension is directly proportional to blood pressure and aortic radius and inversely proportional to wall thickness) applies. The second premise is that the ascending aortic dilatation is due to the repeated impulse of left ventricular ejection buffeting the intrinsically weak aortic wall. The final premise is that aortic enlargement can be prevented by reducing the static and dynamic forces acting on the proximal aorta. These premises led to the proposition that reducing stress on the proximal aorta over a long period of time would reduce the morbidity and mortality of the Marfan syndrome (Halpern et al 1971). Propranolol and related drugs reduce the rate of systolic aortic pressure rise through blockage of the beta-1 adrenergic receptors. Aortic dissection in turkeys, either spontaneous or induced by lathyritic agents, is preventable by oral administration of propranolol, independent of any effect on heart rate or blood pressure (Simpson et al 1968). Early results of propranolol therapy in a small group of Marfan patients, most of whom had aortic regurgitation, were not encouraging (Ose & McKusick 1977). Most of the subjects went on to die suddenly or require surgery. In retrospect the tension on the aortic wall, because of pre-existing dilatation, was already great, and propranolol probably had little effect. A prospective randomized trial of propranolol in patients with mild-to-moderate aortic dilatation showed two beneficial effects of chronic beta-blockade; the rate of aortic root enlargement was lessened and fewer patients developed aortic regurgitation or dissection during the course of the study (Pyeritz 1989b).

Surgical correction of the aorta and aortic valve is required: in an acute emergency due to rupture, dissection, or severe left ventricular decompensation; when early signs of left ventricular strain appear in the presence of severe regurgitation; and for substantial enlargement of the aorta even if the aortic regurgitation is mild. Some patients require mitral valve replacement alone, or in addition to aortic surgery. Use of a composite graft of prosthetic aortic valve sutured into one end of a Dacron conduit has resulted in a dramatic decrease in perioperative mortality of aortic surgery in the Marfan syndrome (Crawford 1983, Gott et al 1986).

All patients are at risk of endocarditis regardless of whether demonstrable valvular abnormalities exist. They should be instructed in routine antibiotic prophylaxis with dental and genitourinary procedures.

Counselling

The major issue in genetic counselling is straightforward, each affected person having a 50% probablity of passing the gene to any offspring. When the Marfan syndrome is diagnosed in a young child and the family history is negative, the parents must be counselled about the risk of having subsequent affected children. Both parents must be carefully examined to ensure that neither has signs of the Marfan gene before assurances are given that the risk that future offspring will be affected is slight.

Women affected by the Marfan syndrome must deal with two concerns. The first is the 50% risk that any offspring will inherit the syndrome. The second concerns the risk of cardiovascular problems during pregnancy. As described above, women with minimal aortic dilatation do well during pregnancy (Pyeritz 1981). However, as the diameter increases beyond 40 mm, or in the presence of aortic regurgitation, the risks become progressively larger. Women who decide to become pregnant are treated as high-risk pregnancies, and management of labour and delivery should minimize maternal haemodynamic stresses.

Parents should be counselled about the range of intra-familial variability possible in the Marfan syndrome. Affected offspring may be more or less severely involved than their parents.

Prevention

The only method of preventing the Marfan syndrome is through reproductive abstinence by affected parents. Even then, many new cases will appear through spontaneous mutation.

Prenatal diagnosis

No method now exists for prenatal diagnosis of the Marfan syndrome. The potential exists for prenatal diagnosis based either on a biochemical defect expressed in amniocytes or chorionic villi or linkage with restriction fragment length polymorphisms.

REFERENCES

Achard C 1902 Arachnodactylie. Bulletins et Memoires de la Societe Medicales Hôpital (Paris) 19: 834–840

Appel A, Horowitz A L, Dorfman A 1979 Cell-free synthesis of hyaluronic acid in Marfan syndrome. Journal of Biological Chemistry 254: 12199–12203

Arn P H, Scherer L R, Haller J A Jr., Pyeritz R E 1989 Clinical outcome of pectus excavatum in the Marfan syndrome and in the general population. Journal of Pediatrics 115: 954–958

Baer R W, Taussig H B, Oppenheimer E H 1943 Congenital aneurysmal dilatation of the aorta associated with arachnodactyly. Bulletin of the Johns Hopkins Hospital 72: 309–331

Barnett B D, Bird R H, Lalich J J 1957 Toxicity of beta-aminoproprinoitrile for turkey poults. Proceedings of the Society for Experimental Biology and Medicine 94: 67–70

Beals R K, Hecht F 1971 Congenital contractural arachnodactyly: a heritable disorder of connective tissue. Journal of Bone and Joint Surgery 53A: 987–993

Beighton P, de Paepe A, Danks D et al 1988 International nosology of heritable disorders of connective tissue.

American Journal of Medical Genetics 29: 581–599

Birch J G, Herring J A 1987 Spinal deformity in Marfan syndrome. Journal of Pediatric Orthopaedics 7: 546–552

Boerger F 1914 Uber zwei von Arachnodaktyllie. Zeitschrift fur Kinderheilkunde 12: 161–184

Bon Tempo C P, Ronan J A Jr, deLeon A C Jr et al 1975 Radiographic appearance of the thorax in systolic click-late systolic murmur syndrome. American Journal of Cardiology 36: 27–31

Boucek R J, Noble N L, Gunja-Smith Z et al 1981 A possible role for dehydrodihydroxylysinorleucine in collagen fibre and bundle formation. Biochemistry Journal 177: 853–860

Brown O R, DeMots H, Kloster F E, Roberts A, Menashe V D, Beals R K 1975 Aortic root dilatation and mitral valve prolapse in Marfan's syndrome: an echocardiographic study. Circulation 47: 587–596

Byers P H, Siegel R C, Peterson K E et al 1981 Marfan syndrome: abnormal alpha-2 chain in type I collagen. Proceedings of National Academy of Sciences USA 78: 7745–7749

Chan K-L, Callahan J A, Seward J B et al 1987 Marfan syndrome diagnosed in patients 32 years of age or older. Mayo Clinic Proceedings 62: 589–594

Crawford E S 1983 Marfan's syndrome: broadspectral surgical treatment of cardiovascular manifestations. Annals of Surgery 198: 487–505

Cross H E, Jensen A D 1975 Ocular manifestations in the Marfan syndrome and homocystinuria. American Journal of Ophthalmology 75: 405–420

Dalgleish R, Hawkins J R, Keston M 1987 Exclusion of the alpha2 (I) and alpha1 (III) collagen genes as the mutant loci in a Marfan syndrome family. Journal of Medical Genetics 24: 148–151

Demak R 1986 Marfan syndrome: a silent killer. Sports Illustrated 17 February p 30–35

Derouette S, Hornbeck W, Loisance D et al 1981 Studies on elastic tissue of aorta in aortic dissections and Marfan syndrome. Pathological Biology 29: 539–547

Eldridge R 1964 The metacarpal index: a useful aid in the diagnosis of the Marfan syndrome. Archives of Internal Medicine 113: 248–254

Emanuel R, Ng R A L, Marcomichekalis J et al 1977 Formes frustes of Marfan's syndrome presenting with severe aortic regurgitation: clinicogenetic study of 18 families. British Heart Journal 39: 190–197

Etter L E, Glover L P 1943 Arachnodactyly complicated by dislocated lens and death from rupture of dissecting aneurysm of the aorta. Journal of the American Medical Association 123: 88–89

Francomano C A, Kazazian H H Jr. 1986 DNA analysis in genetic disorders. Annual Review of Medicine 37: 377–395

Francomano C A, Streeten E A, Meyers D A et al 1988 Exclusion of fibrillar procollagens as causes of the Marfan syndrome. American Journal of Medical Genetics 29: 457–462

Glesby M J, Pyeritz R E 1989 Association of mitral valve prolapse and systemic abnormalities of connective tissue: a phenotypic continuum. Journal of the American Medical Association 262: 523–528

Gordon A M 1962 Abraham Lincoln – a medical appraisal. Journal of the Kentucky Medical Association 60: 249–253

Gott V L, Pyeritz R E, Magovern G J Jr. et al 1986 Surgical treatment of aneurysm of the ascending aorta in the Marfan syndrome: results of composite-graft repair in 50 patients. New England Journal of Medicine 314: 1070–1074

Gunja-Smith Z, Boucek R J 1981 Desmosines in human urine: amounts in early development and in Marfan's syndrome. Biochemical Journal 193: 915–918

Gusella J F 1987 Recombinant DNA techniques in the diagnosis of inherited disorders. Journal of Clinical Investigation 77: 1723–1726

Halbritter R, Aumailley M, Rackwitz R et al 1981 Case report and study of collagen metabolism in Marfan's syndrome. Klinische Wochenschrift 59: 83–90

Hall J, Pyeritz R E, Dudgeon D L et al 1984 Pneumothorax in the Marfan syndrome: Prevalence and therapy. Annals of Thoracic Surgery 37: 500–504

Halme T, Vihersaari T, Savunen T et al 1982 Desmosines in aneurysms of the ascending aorta (annulo-aortic ectasia). Biochimica et Biophysica Acta 717: 121–138

Halpern B L, Char F, Murdoch J L et al 1971 A prospectus on the prevention of aortic rupture in the Marfan syndrome with data on survivorship without treatment. Johns Hopkins Medical Journal 129: 123–129

Hofman K J, Bernhardt B A, Pyeritz R E 1988 Marfan syndrome: Neuro-psychologic aspects. American Journal of Medical Genetics 31: 331–338

Hollister D W 1987 Molecular basis of osteogenesis imperfecta. Current Problems in Dermatology 17: 76–94

Hollister D W, Sakai L Y, Pyeritz R E 1987 Abnormalities of the micro-fibrillar fiber system in Marfan syndrome. American Journal of Human Genetics 39: A7

Kuhlman J E, Scott W W Jr, Fishman E K et al 1987 Protrusio acetabuli in Marfan syndrome. Radiology 164: 415–417

Kuhlman J E, Scott W W Jr., Fishman E K, Pyeritz R E, Siegelman S S 1987 Protrusio acetabuli in Marfan syndrome. Radiology 164: 415–417

Lamberg S I 1978 Stimulatory effect of exogenous hyaluronic acid distinguishes cultured fibroblasts of Marfan's disease from controls. Journal of Investigative Dermatology 71: 391–395

Lattimer J K 1981 Lincoln did not have the Marfan syndrome: documented evidence. New York State Journal of Medicine 81: 1805–1813

Leier C V, Call T D, Fulkerson P K, Wooley C F 1980 The spectrum of cardiac defects in the Ehlers-Danlos syndrome. Annals of Internal Medicine 92: 171–178

Lynas N A, Merritt A D 1958 Marfan's syndrome in Northern Ireland. Annals of Human Genetics 22: 310–314

Mace M 1979 A suggestion of linkage between the Marfan syndrome and the rhesus blood group. Clinical Genetics 16: 96–102

McDonald G, Schaff H V, Pyeritz R E et al 1981 Surgical management of patients with the Marfan syndrome and dilatation of the ascending aorta. Journal of Thoracic and Cardiovascular Surgery 81: 180–186

McKusick V A 1955 The cardiovascular aspects of Marfan's syndrome: a heritable disorder of connective tissue. Circulation 11: 321–341

McKusick V A 1972 The Marfan syndrome. In: Heritable Disorders of Connective Tissue, 4th edn. Mosby, St. Louis p 61–223

Marfan A B 1896 Un cas de deformation congenital des quatre membres plus pronouncee aux extremities characterisée par l'allongement des os avec un certain degre d'amonassement. Bullitens et Memoires de la Societe Medicales Hopital (Paris) 13: 220–226

Maron B J, Roberts W C, McAllister H A et al 1980 Sudden death in young athletes. Circulation 62: 218–229

Maumenee I H 1981 The eye in the Marfan syndrome. Transactions of the American Ophthalmologic Society 79: 684–733

Mudd S H, Skovby F, Levy H L et al 1985 The natural history of homocystinuria due to cystathionine beta-synthase deficiency. American Journal of Human Genetics 36: 1–31

Mudd S H, Levy H L, Skovby F 1989 Disorders of transsulfuration. In: Scriver C R et al (eds) Metabolic Basis of Inherited Disease. McGraw-Hill, New York, p 693–734

Murdoch J L, Walker B A, Halpern B L et al 1972a Life expectancy and causes of death in the Marfan syndrome. New England Journal of Medicine 286: 804–808

Murdoch J L, Walker B A, Mckusick V A 1972b Parental age effects on the occurrence of new mutations for the Marfan syndrome. Annals of Human Genetics 35: 331–336

Nakashima Y 1986 Reduced activity of serum beta-glucuronidase in Marfan syndrome. Angiology 37: 576–580

Nogami H, Oohira A, Ozeki K, Oko T, Ogino T, Murachi S 1979 Ultrastructure of cartilage in heritable disorders of connective tissue. Clinical Orthopaedics 143: 251–259

O'Dell B L, Harfwick B L, Reynolds G et al 1961 Connective tissue defect in the chick resulting from copper deficiency. Proceedings for the Society of Experimental Biology and

Medicine 108: 402–405

Ogilvie D J, Wordsworth B P, Priestly I M et al 1987 Segregation of all four major fibrillar collagen genes in the Marfan syndrome. American Journal of Human Genetics 41: 1071–1082

Ose L, McKusick V A 1977 Prophylactic use of propranolol in the Marfan syndrome to prevent aortic dissection. Birth Defects 13(3C): 163–169

Perejda A J, Abraham P A, Carnes W H et al 1985 Marfan's syndrome: structural, biochemical and mechanical studies of the aortic media. Journal of Laboratory and Clinical Medicine 106: 376–383

Phornphutkul C, Rosenthal A, Nadas A C 1973 Cardiac manifestations of Marfan syndrome in infancy and childhood. Circulation 47: 587–596

Piper R K, Irvine-Jones E 1926 Arachnodactylia and its association with congenital heart disease. American Journal of Diseases of Children 31: 832–839

Prockop D J, Kivirikko K I 1984 Heritable diseases of collagen. New England Journal of Medicine 311: 376–386

Pyeritz R E 1981 Maternal and fetal complications of pregnancy in the Marfan syndrome. American Journal of Medicine 71: 784–790

Pyeritz R E 1983 Cardiovascular manifestations of heritable disorders of connective tissue. Progress in Medical Genetics 5: 191–302

Pyeritz R E 1986a The diagnosis and management of the Marfan syndrome. American Family Physician 34(6): 83–94

Pyeritz R E 1986b Arthrogryposis in the Marfan syndrome: an explanation for congenital contractural arachnodactyly. American Journal of Medical Genetics 25: 725–726

Pyeritz R E 1987 Heritable defects in connective tissue. Hospital Practice 22(2): 153–168

Pyeritz R E 1989a Conference report: First International Symposium on the Marfan Syndrome. American Journal of Medical Genetics 32: 233–238

Pyeritz R E 1989b Effectiveness of beta-adrenergic blockade in the Marfan syndrome: experience over 10 years. American Journal of Medical Genetics 32: 245

Pyeritz R E, McKusick V A 1979 The Marfan syndrome: Diagnosis and management. New England Journal of Medicine 300: 772–777

Pyeritz R E, McKusick V A 1981 Basic defects in the Marfan syndrome. New England Journal of Medicine 305: 1011–1012

Pyeritz R E, Wappel M A 1983 Mitral valve dysfunction in the Marfan syndrome. American Journal of Medicine 74: 797–807

Pyeritz R E, Murphy E A, McKusick V A 1979 Clinical variability in the Marfan syndrome. Birth Defects 15(5B): 155–178

Pyeritz R E, Brinker J A, Fortuin N J et al 1980 Annular dilatation does not cause aortic regurgitation in the Marfan syndrome. Clinical Research 78: 203A

Pyeritz R E, Murphy E A, Lin S J et al 1985 Growth and anthropometrics in the Marfan syndrome. In: Papadatos C J, Bartsocas C S (eds) Endocrine Genetics and Genetics of Growth. Alan Liss, New York, p 355–366

Pyeritz R E, Fishman, E K, Bernhardt B A et al 1988 Dural ectasiais: a common pleiotropic feature of the Marfan syndrome. American Journal of Human Genetics 43: 726–732

Robins P R, Moe J H, Winter R B 1975 Scoliosis in Marfan's syndrome: its characteristics and results of treatment in thirty-five patients. Journal of Bone and Joint Surgery 57A: 358–368

Ross R, Bornstein P 1969 The elastic fiber. Journal of Cell Biology 40: 366–381

Sakai L Y, Keene D R, Engvall E 1986 Fibrillin, a new 350-kD glycoprotein, is a component of extracellular microfibrils. Journal of Cell Biology 103: 2499–2509

Salle V 1912 Uber einen Fall von angeborener abnormer Grosse der Extremitaten mit einem an Akromegalie erinnernden Symptomenkomplex. Jahrbuch Kinderheilkunde 75: 540–550

Schlatmann T J M, Becker A E 1977 Pathogenesis of dissecting aneurysm of the aorta: Comparative histopathologic study of significance of medial changes. American Journal of Cardiology 29: 21–26

Schleutermann D A, Murdoch J L, Walker B A et al 1976 A linkage study of the Marfan syndrome. Clinical Genetics 10: 51–53

Schoenfeld M R 1978 Nicolo Paganini – musical magician and Marfan mutant. Journal of the American Medical Association 239: 40–42

Schwartz H 1964 Abraham Lincoln and the Marfan syndrome. Journal of the American Association 187: 473–479

Simpson C F, Kling J M, Palmer R F 1968 The use of propranolol for the protection of turkeys from the development of beta-aminoproprionitrile-induced aortic ruptures. Angiology 19: 414–418

Simpson C F, Boucek R J, Nobel N L 1980 Similarity of aortic pathology in Marfan's syndrome, copper deficiency in chicks and beta-aminoproprionitrile toxicity. Experimental and Molecular Pathology 32: 31–90

Sisk H E, Zahka K G, Pyeritz R E 1983 The Marfan syndrome in early childhood: analysis of 15 patients diagnosed at less than four years of age. American Journal of Cardiology 52: 353–358

Soulen R L, Fishman E, Pyeritz R E et al 1987 Evaluation of the Marfan syndrome: MR imaging versus CT. Radiology 165: 697–701

Steinberg I 1966 A simple screening test for the Marfan syndrome. American Journal of Roentgenology, Radium Therapy and Nuclear Medicine 97: 118–124

Streeten E A, Murphy E A, Pyeritz R E 1987 Pulmonary function in the Marfan syndrome. Chest 91: 408–412

Tsipouras P, Borressen A-L, Bamforth S et al 1986 Marfan syndrome: exclusion of genetic linkage to the COLIA2 gene. Clinical Genetics 30: 428–432

Tsuji T 1986 Marfan syndrome: demonstration of abnormal elastic fibres in skin. Journal of Cutaneous Pathology 13: 144–153

Walker B A, Murdoch J L 1970 The wrist sign: a useful physical finding in the Marfan syndrome. Archives of Internal Medicine 126: 276–277

Weiner J, Pyeritz R E 1987 Publicity about the Marfan syndrome was associated with increased referrals to genetics centers. American Journal of Human Genetics 39: A90

Weve H 1931 Uber arachnodakylie. Archiv Augenheilkunde 104: 1–46

Williams E 1873–1879 Rare cases, with practical remarks. Transactions of the American Ophthalmologic Society 2: 291

Young D A 1986 Rachmaninov and Marfan's syndrome. British Medical Journal 293: 20–27

63. Ehlers-Danlos syndrome

P. H. Byers   K. A. Holbrook

INTRODUCTION

The Ehlers-Danlos syndrome (EDS) is a group of disorders characterized by abnormalities of skin, joints and other connective tissues (Beighton 1970, McKusick 1972, Hollister 1978). In early descriptions of these disorders joint laxity and skin hyperextensibility were emphasized (Ehlers 1901, Danlos 1908), but as more patients were identified, skin fragility, easy bruising and the occasional complications of bowel and arterial rupture were recognized (Sack 1936, Gottron 1942, Barabas 1967). During the last ten years the clinical and genetic heterogeneity has been explained, in part, by biochemical and ultrastructural studies which distinguish at least ten distinct varieties of the syndrome (Table 63.1) (Hollister 1978, Bornstein & Byers 1980, Pinnell 1983, Byers 1989).

This chapter provides a detailed clinical, genetic and biochemical summary of the ten recognized Ehlers-Danlos types and the information about collagen structure, biosynthesis, heterogeneity and tissue distribution which serves as the basis for understanding the pathophysiology of some of these disorders.

COLLAGEN TYPES

The collagens are a family of evolutionary related, structurally similar proteins (Bornstein & Sage 1980, Mayne & Burgeson 1987, Byers 1989) which have distinguishing gene structure, amino acid sequence, tissue distribution and cells of origin (Table 63.2).

Each collagen molecule contains three α chains arranged in a triple-helical conformation that extends the length of the molecule which for fibrillar collagens (those known to be affected in several forms of the Ehlers-Danlos syndrome) are just over 1000 amino acid residues long. In the fibrillar collagens one third of all amino acids is glycine, which occurs in every third position such that the triple-helical domains can be described as $(Gly-X-Y)_{338}$, in which X and Y can be any amino acid except cysteine and tryptophan, but are often proline (X) and hydroxyproline (Y).

On the basis of protein and gene structure, collagens can be divided into four classes (Table 63.2): fibrillar collagens (types I, II, III, V and XI); basement membrane or long chain collagen with an interrupted triple-helix (type IV); short chain collagens with interrupted triple helix (types VI, VIII, IX, X); and extended chain collagens with interrupted triple-helix (type VII). Each collagen has a characteristic tissue distribution. The collagens which are the most abundant in skin and other soft tissues, and thus the primary candidates for mutations that may lead to the Ehlers-Danlos syndrome phenotypes, are types I, III, V and VI. Most type I collagen molecules are heteropolymers which consist of two $\alpha 1(I)$ chains and one very similar $\alpha 2(I)$ chain to form the molecules $[\alpha 1(I)]_2\alpha 2(I)$. Type I collagen is the primary constituent of the large fibrils seen in most connective tissues, provides the tensile strength of skin and tendon, and forms the organic matrix of bone, the transparent matrix of the cornea and the opaque tissue of the sclera, and in most of those tissues constitutes 75% or more of the collagen. Type III collagen is a homotrimer of the $\alpha 1(III)$ chain, $[\alpha 1(III)]_3$, and parallels type I collagen distribution in tissues, except that it is absent from bone matrix, it is a major constituent of the walls of hollow organs of the gastrointestinal tract, of blood vessels and of the uterus and in most tissues it makes up 15–20% of the collagen. Although the content of type III collagen in mature skin may be 15%, it may be a more abundant component of dermal collagen in the fetus and thus may have a role in the initial structuring of the tissue. Type V collagen is present in tissues as a mixed polymer and is ubiquitously distributed in parallel to type I collagen. Type VI collagen is a heteropolymer of its three constituent α chains and occurs as fine fibrils with a periodic structure. Its function is not well-defined. Type VII collagen forms anchoring fibril structures and type VIII collagen is probably important for endothelial integrity. Collagen types IX, X and XI are found only in cartilage.

Table 63.1 Ehlers-Danlos syndromes

Type	Clinical features	Inheritance	Biochemical disorder	Ultrastructural findings
I Gravis	Soft, velvety skin; marked skin hyperextensibility, fragility and easy bruisability; 'cigarette paper' scars; large-and small-joint hypermobility; frequent venous varicosities; hernia. Prematurity due to ruptured fetal membranes is common.	AD	Not known	Large collagen fibrils, many irregular in shape.
II Mitis	Soft skin, moderate skin hyperextensibility and easy bruisability; moderate joint hypermobility; varicose veins and hernia do occur but are less common than in type I. Prematurity is rare.	AD	Not known	Large collagen fibrils, many irregular in shape.
III Benign familial hypermobility	Skin is soft but otherwise minimally affected; joint mobility is markedly increased and affects large and small joints; dislocation is common.	AD	Not known	Large collagen fibrils, many irregular in shape.
IV Ecchymotic or arterial	Skin is thin or translucent or both; veins are readily visible over the trunk, arms, legs, and abdomen. Repeated ecchymosis with minimal trauma. Skin is not hyperextensible, and joints (except the small joints in the hands) are usually of normal mobility. Bowel rupture (usually affecting the colon) and arterial rupture are frequent and often lead to death.	AD(AR)	Decreased or absent synthesis of type III collagen, altered secretion of type III collagen due to rearrangements or point mutations in COL3A1 gene.	Thin dermis, small fibres, often engorged cells in dermis, fibrils of variable size.
V X-linked	Similar to EDS II; muscle haemorrhage may be more extensive.	XR	Not known	Not known
VI Ocular	Soft, velvety, hyperextensible skin; hypermobile joints; scoliosis, scarring less severe than in EDS I; some patients have ocular fragility and keratoconus.	AR	Lysyl hydroxylase deficiency	Small collagen bundles fibrils normal or similar to those in EDS I.
VII Arthrochalasis multiplex congenita	Soft skin; scars near normal. Marked joint hyperextensibility, congenital hip dislocation.	AD(AR)	Deletion of amino-terminal N-protease cleavage site in proα(I) or proα2(I)	Normal in proα2(I) mutations. Irregular fibrils in proα(I) mutations.
VIII Periodontal form	Marked skin fragility with abnormal, atrophic pigmented scars, minimal skin extensibility and moderate joint laxity. Aesthenic habitus, generalized periodontitis.	AD	Not known	Not known
IX Bladder diverticula, occipital horns	Skin hyperextensibility, joint hypermobility, bladder diverticula, broad clavicles, occipital horns, radio-ulnar synotosis, chronic diarrhoea.	XR	Defective copper utilization	Variable-sized collagen fibrils
X Fibronectin defect	Skin hyperextensibility, joint hypermobility, bruising.	AR	Fibronectin defect	Large collagen fibrils, many irregular in shape.

AD: Autosomal dominant
AR: Autosomal recessive
XR: X-linked recessive

Table 63.2 Collagen types, tissue distribution, molecular structure and gene location

Collagen type	Chains	Genes	Chromosomal location	Molecules	Tissue distribution
Fibrillar collagens					
I	$\alpha1(I)$	COLIA1	17q21-22	$[\alpha1(I)]_2\alpha2(I)$	Skin, tendon, bone, arteries
	$\alpha2(I)$	COLIA2	7q21-22		
				$[\alpha1(I)]_3$	Above, tumours, amniotic fluid
II	$\alpha1(II)$	COL2A1	12q131-132	$[\alpha1(II)]_3$	Cartilage, vitreous
III	$\alpha1(III)$	COL3A1	2q31-32	$[\alpha1(III)]_3$	Skin, arteries, uterus
V	$\alpha1(V)$	COL5A1		$[\alpha1(V)]_3$	Skin, placenta, vessels,
	$\alpha2(V)$	COL5A2	2q24- 31	$[\alpha2(V)]_3$	chorion, uterus
	$\alpha3(V)$	COL5A3		$[\alpha1(V)]_2\alpha2(V)$	
				$\alpha1(V)\alpha2(V)\alpha3(V)$	
XI	$\alpha1(XI)$	COL11A1	1p21	$\alpha1(XI)\alpha2(XI)\alpha1(II)$	Cartilage
	$\alpha2(XI)$	COL11A2			
Long chain/interrupted					
IV	$\alpha1(IV)$	COL4A1	13q34	$[\alpha1(IV)]_2\alpha2(IV)$	Basal laminae
	$\alpha2(IV)$	COL4A2	13q34	$[\alpha1(IV)]_3$	
				$[\alpha2(IV)]_3$	
Short chain/interrupted					
VI	$\alpha1(VI)$	COL6A1	21	Uncertain	Ubiquitous
	$\alpha2(VI)$	COL6A2	21		
	$\alpha3(VI)$	COL6A3	6		
VIII	$\alpha1(VIII)$	COL8A1			
IX	$\alpha1(IX)$	COL9A1		$\alpha1(IX)\alpha2(IX)\alpha3(IX)$	Cartilage
	$\alpha2(IX)$	COL9A2			
	$\alpha3(IX)$	COL9A3			
X	$\alpha1(X)$	COL10A1		$[\alpha1(X)]_3$	Cartilage
Extended chain/interrupted					
VII	$\alpha1(VII)$	COL7A1		$[\alpha1(VII)]_3$	Epithelial-mesenchymal junctions

BIOSYNTHESIS OF COLLAGENS

The biosynthesis of collagens is complex and involves many steps beyond gene transcription (see Table 63.3) (Prockop & Kivirikko 1984, Byers 1989). The genes that encode the fibrillar collagens have a complex structure and are 4–8 times the size of the functional mRNAs (Ramirez 1989). The 50 or more exons of the fibrillar collagen genes are arrayed over 18–38 kilobase pairs; the genes are transcribed and spliced in the nucleus and the mature mRNAs of 4800–7200 bp are transported to the cytoplasm where they are translated on membrane-bound polysomes. The precursor chains of the fibrillar collagens are 1350–1450 amino acids in length. Each chain is initiated by a signal sequence which facilitates transfer into the lumen of the rough endoplasmic reticulum and is cleaved during the vectoral insertion of the chain during synthesis.

As co- and post-translational events, certain lysyl residues in the Y-position and virtually all Y-position prolyl residues are hydroxylated by the enzymes lysyl and prolyl hydroxylase, respectively. These enzymes are dis-

tinct proteins which share cofactors (ferrous iron, ascorbate or other reducing compounds, and α-ketoglutarate). Prolyl hydroxylase is located within the lumen of the rough endoplasmic reticulum and the catalytic subunit is identical to disulphide isomerase which catalyzes disulphide interchain bond formation during protein folding and association; lysyl hydroxylase is probably located in the membrane of the rough endoplasmic reticulum. The degree of both prolyl and lysyl hydroxylation varies markedly in different collagen types and may vary from tissue to tissue for the same collagen. Following hydroxylation, some hydroxylysyl residues are glycosylated (the extent of glycosylation varies with collagen type) to form glucosyl-galactosylhydroxylysyl or galactosylhydroxylysyl residues, and oligosaccharide is added to single residues in the carboxyl-terminal propeptide of each chain of fibrillar collagen.

When the synthesis of the proα chain is completed the procollagen molecule is then assembled. The three constituent chains of each collagen first interact at sites within the carboxyl-terminal propeptide domain, the association is stabilized by interchain disulphide bonds,

Table 63.3   Nature and location of events during collagen biosynthesis

Event	Enzyme	Location*
Transcription	Many	Nucleus
Splicing	'Splicesome-complex'	Nucleus
Transport	Unknown	Nucleus-cytoplasm
Translation	Many	Cytoplasm/RER
Signal cleavage	Signal peptidase	RER membrane
Prolyl hydroxylation	Proline 4-hydroxylase Proline 3-hydroxylase	RER lumen RER lumen
Lysyl hydroxylation	Lysyl hydroxylase	RER lumen
Hydroxylysyl glycosylation	Collagen glucosyl transferase Collagen galactosyl transferase	RER lumen RER lumen
Heterosaccharide addition and modification	Many	RER lumen
Intrachain disulphide bond formation	Disulphide isomerase	RER lumen
Chain assembly	Not known	RER lumen
Interchain disulphide bond formation	Disulphide isomerase	RER lumen
Triple-helix propagation	Prolyl cis-trans isomerase	RER lumen
Transport to Golgi	Many (unknown)	RER/Golgi
Modification of heterosaccharide	Many	Golgi
Sulphation	Sulphotransferase	Golgi
Exocytosis	Many	Cell surface
Amino-terminal processing	Procollagen amino-protease	ECM
Carboxyl-terminal processing	Procollagen carboxyl-protease	ECM
Firbil formation	Non-enzymatic	ECM
Cross-linked formation	Lysyl oxidase	ECM

*RER = rough endoplasmic reticulum; ECM = extracellular matrix

and the triple-helix is propagated towards the amino-terminal end of the molecule. Post-translational hydroxylation and glycosylation of residues in the triple-helical core domain cease when a stable triple-helix is achieved. In turn, the stability of the triple-helix is dependent on complete hydroxylation of the available Y-position prolyl residues; in the absence of hydroxylation the melting temperature of the triple-helix is 27°C but with full hydroxylation it is about 42°C. Upon formation of stable triple-helix the procollagen molecule is transported to the Golgi where the heterosaccharide moiety of the carboxyl-terminal propeptide is modified. The procollagen molecule is transported to the cell surface in secretory vesicles which fuse with the cell membranes and release their contents. Once secreted, fibrillar procol-

lagens are processed by proteolytic cleavage to collagen by specific proteases which remove the amino-terminal and carboxyl-terminal propeptides. The extent of cleavage varies with collagen type and on location within a tissue. Type I procollagen is for the most part processed completely, although molecules in the papillary dermis are more likely to retain their amino-terminal extensions. Type III procollagen may be only partly processed and type IV procollagen is virtually unprocessed.

The extracellular molecules assemble into fibrils or other higher order structures where they become covalently cross-linked to form highly stable structures. The cross-link precursors are lysyl or hydroxylysyl residues which are oxidatively deaminated by lysyl oxidase (Siegel 1978). The resultant aldehydes then condense with adjacent lysyl or hydroxylysyl residues, or their respective aldehydes, to form covalent bifunctional cross-links; subsequently, polyfunctional cross-links involving additional lysyl or histidinyl residues can form (Eyre 1980). The extent of fibril formation and of cross-link formation differs with collagen type, location, and age. The structure of the collagen fibril, its aggregation into bundles, and the mechanical properties of tissues depend not only on cross-linking but also on interactions with several other macromolecules, most notably proteoglycans and glycoproteins (Lindahl & Höök 1978, Bornstein & Sage 1980).

The complexity of collagen biosynthesis, involving substantial post-transcriptional mRNA processing and cotranslational and post-translational protein processing provides many oppotunities for error. In the Ehlers-Danlos syndrome abnormalities in collagen gene expression and gene structure, and in intracellular and extracellular protein processing, have been implicated in pathogenesis of some of the types. These are described in some detail in the following sections.

EHLERS-DANLOS, TYPE I (GRAVIS)

The gravis variety, or type I EDS, is the classic, severe disorder characterized by marked skin hyperextensibility and joint hypermobility (Fig. 63.1). Typically, the skin is soft, velvety in texture, and can be extended several centimetres away from attachment sites. The skin has increased compliance but returns to its original shape promptly and is not lax. It is fragile and there is easy bruising. Trauma results in gaping wounds which may bleed less than expected, but which heal with characteristic atrophic 'cigarette paper' scars. Areas of repeated trauma, such as elbows, knees and shins, often have marked pigment deposition in addition to the characteristic scarring. 'Molluscoid pseudotumours', small (0.5–1.5 cm) accumulations of connective tissue may form in the skin and some individuals develop palpable subcutaneous calcified nodules.

As many as 50% of infants with EDS I are born 4–8 weeks premature. The cause of prematurity is uncertain, but may be related to early rupture of the fetal membranes, as a result of mechanical alterations secondary to the primary connective tissue defect. The diagnosis of EDS I can be made in the perinatal period and family members are often proficient in distinguishing affected from unaffected newborns. The affected infants have softer skin than normal, increased skin extensibility and small joint hypermobility. Bruising in the newborn period is unusual, but begins as children start to crawl and stand. At this time, skin fragility is also evident and characteristic scars may appear on the forehead, under

the chin, and on knees and elbows. Motor development may be somewhat slower than usual because the joint hypermobility often limits stability until muscle development is sufficient to overcome the ligamentous laxity. Intellectual development is normal.

Individuals with EDS I may have a variety of complications as a result of connective tissue involvement. Many people with the disorder have cardiovascular anomalies, the most common of which is the 'floppy' mitral valve. This common disorder may affect more than half of patients with EDS I. Other cardiac structural abnormalities are also seen and should be considered in all patients with the syndrome (Leier et al 1980). Vascular rupture is a rare event among patients with EDS I in contrast to those with EDS IV (see below), but is encountered occasionally. Pes planus is common and mild to moderate scoliosis, especially in the lumbar region, is seen in some patients. It is our impression that the ligamentous laxity is associated with earlier than usual degenerative arthritis. Pregnancy may be complicated by premature rupture of membranes of affected infants and by early labour for unknown reasons among some affected women carrying normal or affected children. Surgery in individuals with EDS VI is generally uncomplicated, although tissues are more friable than usual and care must be taken to assure complete haemostasis. Sutures should be left in place two or three times longer than usual.

EDS I is inherited in an autosomal dominant manner with relatively little variation in expression. Although there are no distinctive biochemical tests, the diagnosis is generally not ambiguous in families. In the sporadic case the diagnosis of EDS V (in males) or EDS VI must be considered.

The biochemical basis of EDS I is unknown. Histologically, the dermal structure is altered so that the usual orthogonal weave of collagen bundles is defective. The collagen bundles are small, but the constituent fibrils are 10–40% larger than normal (110–140 nm compared to 90–100 nm for controls) (Vogel et al 1979). Many fibrils are irregular in outline and some appear as poorly integrated structures (Fig. 63.2). The mechanism by which the formation of collagen fibrils and of higher order structures is changed is not clear, although alterations in regions of the collagen molecule which direct intermolecular interaction, or abnormalities in other macromolecules of the connective tissue matrix (e.g. proteoglycans or glycoproteins) might both produce disturbances of collagen fibril morphogenesis.

Shinkai et al (1976) studied one patient with EDS I and found abnormalities in the biosynthesis of proteoglycans. Sasaki and colleagues (1987) recently studied collagens synthesized by dermal fibroblasts grown from a woman

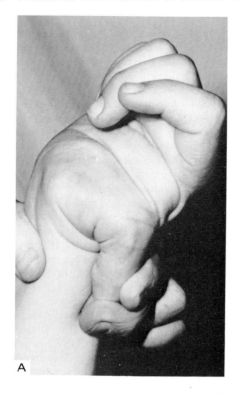

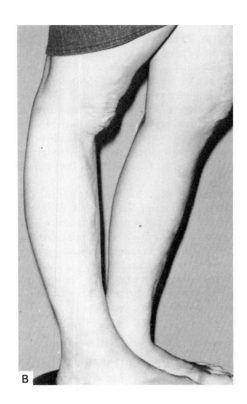

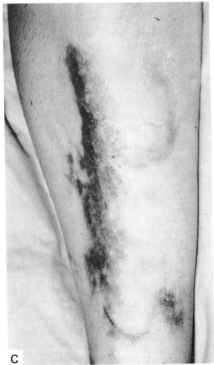

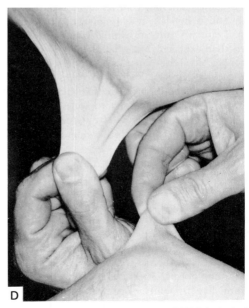

Fig. 63.1 The clinical features of type I EDS include **A** joint hypermobility; **B** and **C** abnormal 'cigarette paper' scars, and **D** skin hyperextensibility.

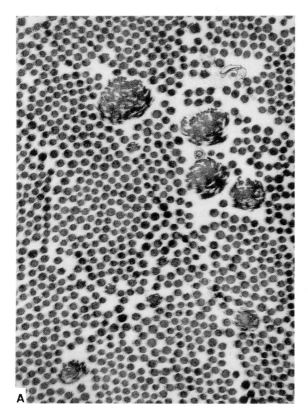

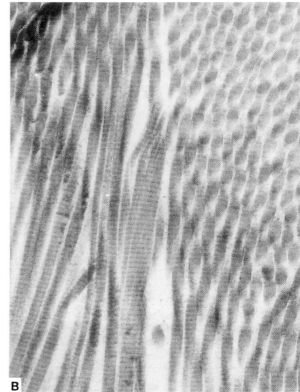

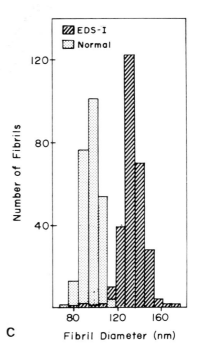

Fig. 63.2 Normal and abnormal appearing collagen fibrils are characteristics of the reticular dermis of individuals with dominant forms of the Ehlers-Danlos syndrome. The irregular, lobulated fibrils seen in cross section **A** correspond with the loosely aggregated conglomerate fibrils observed in longitudinal section **B**. **C** Histogram of collagen fibril diameters of normal individuals and of patients with type I Ehlers-Danlos syndrome.

they described as having Ehlers-Danlos syndrome, probably type I or II, and found that no proα2(I) chains were synthesized. As this woman had significant aortic root dilatation and aortic insufficiency it is not clear how her connective tissue disorder should be classified. It is clear, however, that such patients are rare among those with the usual forms of EDS and may constitute a small subset. The lack of synthesis of proα2(I) chains is most suggestive of homozygosity for a null allele or compound heterozygosity for two different COLIA2 alleles that decrease production (and thus autosomal recessive inheritance). In cells cultured from some patients with EDS type I, the efficiency with which the carboxyl-terminal propeptide is removed from type I procollagen seems to be markedly reduced. Fibrils made from collagen that retains the carboxyl-terminal propeptide may have a 'composite' character similar to those seen in skin from individuals with EDS type I, lending support to the hypothesis that some patients may have defects in the proteolytic conversion at the carboxyl-terminal end of the molecule. Again, such patients are likely to be rare. Linkage studies suggest that there are few families in which structural mutations in either the COLIA1 or the COLIA2 gene could be involved in the pathogenesis of EDS type I. It is likely then, that EDS I is a biochemically heterogeneous disorder, the phenotypic manifestation of a number of molecular abnormalities which alter fibril formation and stability (Holbrook & Byers 1986, 1989).

In the absence of definitive biochemical diagnostic tests, genetic counselling in the sporadic case can be difficult. Although there are no data available on the frequency of new dominant mutations in this disorder, if the clinical features are consistent with EDS I, and if EDS VI can be excluded, then it is likely that the patient has a disorder that is inherited in an autosomal dominant fashion.

EHLERS-DANLOS, TYPE II (MITIS)

The clinical features of EDS II, the mitis form, are similar to those of EDS I, but are milder. Skin is soft and velvety, but scarring and bruising are less than in EDS I, and joint hypermobility is less marked. Prematurity is rare and motor development is not as delayed as in EDS I. Like EDS I, EDS II is inherited in an autosomal dominant fashion and there is only modest variability in expression. The clinical course and natural history of the disorder are generally uncomplicated although many patients have the 'floppy' mitral valve syndrome and some develop early onset of degenerative arthritis. The ultrastructural features of the disease are similar to those of EDS I and the biochemical aetiology remains

unknown. Evaluation and counselling should parallel those in EDS I.

EHLERS-DANLOS, TYPE III (BENIGN FAMILIAL HYPERMOBILITY)

EDS III, benign familial hypermobility is an autosomal dominant disorder with variable expression in which the major clinical features are large and small joint hypermobility. This disorder has considerable variability both within and among families. Joint hypermobility is generally accompanied by soft skin, but skin hyperextensibility is absent and scars are normal. The joint hypermobility may be dramatic in some individuals (see Beighton 1970 for illustrations). The major problems associated with the disorder are recurrent joint dislocations. While surgical repair is generally satisfactory, recurrence is more common than in unaffected individuals.

The ultrastructural findings are similar to those in EDS I and EDS II (Sevenich et al 1980), but there are no distinctive biochemical findings. Counselling may present problems in sporadic cases. Because there is a wide range of normal in joint mobility (which can be augmented by training), establishing the diagnosis of EDS III may be difficult without a family history. Without a clear family history of EDS III, an individual with only modest joint laxity may represent normal variation.

EHLERS-DANLOS, TYPE IV (VASCULAR, ECCHYMOTIC, SACK-BARABAS)

EDS IV, the vascular or ecchymotic variety, was recognized as a distinct entity by Barabas in 1967, although Sack in 1936, and Gottron in 1942, probably described the same diseases. It is in this group of disorders, all due to abnormalities in metabolism of type III collagen, that some of the most extensive biochemical investigations have been done and in which heterogeneity is best recognized (Pope et al 1975, 1977, 1980, Byers et al 1979, 1981, Holbrook and Byers 1981, Clark et al 1980, Pyeritz et al 1984, Stolle et al 1985, Tsipouras et al 1986, Nicholls et al 1988, Superti-Furga & Steinmann 1988, Superti-Furga et al 1988, Temple et al 1988). Individuals with EDS IV have fragile, thin or translucent skin, through which the venous pattern is readily visible (Fig. 63.3), marked bruising, and a characteristic facies (Pope et al 1980). Some patients have soft skin which is mildly hyperextensible, but the majority have skin with normal texture and normal extensibility. Joint mobility is generally normal or hypermobility is limited to the small joints of the hands. In some patients with the 'acrogeric' form of the disorder, the skin over the distal extremities has an aged, atrophic appearance, and in others the skin on the

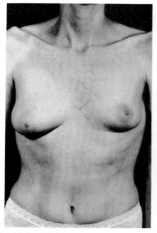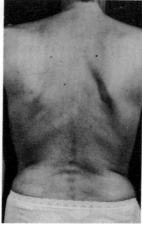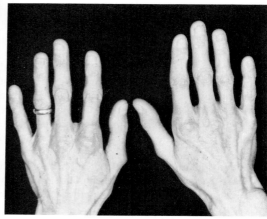

Fig. 63.3 This 26-year-old woman has type IV EDS. Her skin is extremely thin and the venous vasculature can be seen over the chest, abdomen and back. She has elastosis perforans serpiginosa over both antecubital regions, and skin over her hands appears markedly aged. (From Byers et al 1979).

hands has a fine, parchment quality. Venous varicosities are common and may be severe.

The major clinical complications are bowel, arterial and uterine rupture. Because of these dramatic complications, life expectancy is shortened to a mean of less than 40 years in both men and women (Byers & Superti-Furga, unpublished). Both autosomal dominant and autosomal recessive inheritance has been suggested, but autosomal recessive forms of EDS type IV appear to be rare and may result from mutations in genes other than COL3A1 (Pope et al 1977). The most frequent complication is bowel rupture which usually occurs distal to the splenic flexure along the antimesenteric border. The small intestine is rarely involved. Treatment is the same as for any acute bowel rupture, but because tissues of affected individuals are exceeding friable, surgical repair of any lesion is often difficult. Since the colon appears to be most susceptible to spontaneous rupture, consideration should be given to removal if rupture recurs.

Major vessel rupture is another life-threatening complication. The clinical presentation depends on the location of the ruptured artery so that haemorrhagic stroke, haemothorax, haemoperitoneum and compartmental syndromes may all result. Uterine rupture near term in pregnancy is an occasional complication (Rudd et al 1983).

The clinical features of the disorder are variable. In some patients the diagnosis can be made early in infancy because of marked bruising and thin skin. In other patients with a family history of the disorder the diagnosis may be suspected in infancy because of other complications such as cerebral haemorrhage. However in many

patients the diagnosis is not suspected unless there is a positive family history, and even then the signs of the disease may be limited to mild bruising during childhood. Vessel and bowel rupture may be seen in children, although they occur most commonly in the third to fifth decades.

A summary of our experience with 23 affected individuals from nine families helps to evaluate the natural history of the disorder. Nineteen of these people are found in five families in which EDS IV is inherited in an autosomal dominant manner; the remaining four are the only affected member in their respective families in which there is no history of consanguinity. Of the 23 affected individuals, seven are now dead, three as a result of arterial rupture (ages 46, 23 and 12 years), two as a consequence of ruptured bowel (both at 39 years), and two from uterine rupture at term in pregnancy (ages 32 and 22). Nine of the sixteen survivors are well and have had no major complications of their disease, the oldest of whom is in her mid-40s. Of the remaining seven, one has had a spontaneous pneumothorax, one has severe periodontal disease, one had a spontaneous bowel rupture at 33, one patient has had a bowel rupture at 6, epiphyseal bleed at 12, stroke at 23 and a compartmental bleed at 26; two patients had intracranial haemorrhage in the neonatal period but have done well since, and one patient had a pneumothorax at 20, a femoral artery compartmental bleed at 21, and three episodes of bowel rupture in his early 20s. It should be recognized that EDS IV is an underdiagnosed disorder and those patients having difficulties are most likely to be referred for diagnostic evaluation. As a result, determination of natural history from such families may bias presentations toward major complications.

The clinical diagnosis of EDS IV can be confirmed biochemically by the demonstration of decreased or absent type III collagen in affected tissues. Pathologically, dermis is thin and may be only 25% of normal thickness. There appears to be an increased amount of elastic fibres, but this is probably a relative increase since the total skin thickness is decreased. Collagen bundles are smaller than normal and, at the ultrastructural level, collagen fibrils are small in some patients and varied in size with a major component of small fibrils in others. Many patients have marked dilatation of the rough endoplasmic reticulum of dermal fibroblasts in situ, evidence of decreased secretion of synthesized proteins (Fig. 63.4).

Studies of dermal fibroblasts in culture from patients with EDS IV have demonstrated several alterations in type III collagen metabolism (Superti-Furga et al 1989). The first studies of such cells were consistent with absent synthesis since no type III procollagen was secreted by

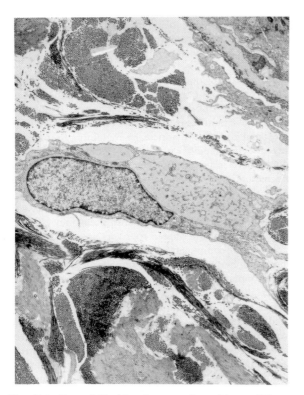

Fig. 63.4 Dermal fibroblast from a patient with type IV Ehlers-Danlos syndrome. Engorged cirsternae of the rough endoplasmic reticulum (RER) occupies a major portion of the cell.

the cells in culture and the cultured cells did not stain with antibodies to type III procollagen (Pope et al 1975, Gay et al 1976). Subsequent studies of cells from other patients have demonstrated a variety of mechanisms by which the synthesis, structure, secretion, stability or processing of type III procollagen is altered. In a small number of families the synthesis of type III procollagen is reduced, perhaps to about half the normal level and there is no evidence of intracellular storage. In these families, the phenotype may result from a 'non-functional' COL3A1 allele but no definitive studies have been performed. Frequently, there is evidence of marked alteration in the efficiency of secretion and accompanying overmodification of chains in the abnormal type III procollagen molecules (Byers et al 1981, Superti-Furga & Steinmann 1988, Superti-Furga et al 1988). In one such family a large deletion from within the domain of one COL3A1 allele that encodes the triple-helical portion of the chain has been identified (Superti-Furga et al 1988). Several classes of molecule can be synthesized, those which contain only normal chains and those which contain one, two or three abnormal chains. If the deletion results in an uninterrupted triple-helix then the molecules that contain the three abnormal chains may be secreted normally but may still have aberrant function. A third class of mutations, many of which may be point mutations that result in substitution for glycyl residues in the triple-helical domain of the proα1(III) chain, result in marked intracellular retention (often in the rough endoplasmic reticulum) of the abnormal molecules that are recognized because the triple-helical domain is markedly overmodified. Finally, there appears to be a fourth class of mutations which markedly destabilize the completed molecules and result in rapid intracellular breakdown of molecules that contain the mutant chains. In some instances it appears that these molecules can be rescued by incubation of cells at temperatures below 37°C (Superti-Furga & Steinmann 1988). At present there is no clear correlation between the nature of the mutation in COL3A1 and the clinical features of EDS type IV.

Although only about half of individuals with EDS type IV have a recognized family history, comparison of the types of molecular mutation identified among cells from sporadically affected individuals and those from families in which EDS type IV is inherited in an autosomal dominant fashion indicates that they are similar. Thus the vast majority of sporadically affected individuals appear to have new dominant mutations in one COL3A1 allele. Genetic counselling for the sporadically affected individual may depend on the ability to confirm the diagnosis at the biochemical and molecular genetic level. Prenatal diagnosis, by linkage analysis using polymorphic sites in the COL3A1 gene or by analysis of the structure, secretion and processing of type III procollagen synthesized by cells grown from chorionic villus biopsy samples, is feasible (see Tsipouras et al 1986 and Byers et al 1987 for discussions of prenatal diagnosis of inherited collagen disorders).

No medical treatment for EDS type IV has been shown to be effective.

EHLERS-DANLOS, TYPE V (X–LINKED VARIETY)

Type V EDS is an X–linked variety of the disorder, first described by Beighton (1970). Skin hyperextensibility is similar to that in EDS II, but joint mobility and bruising are less marked. The other typical features of EDS II, scars and pseudotumours, may be present and, in addition, intramuscular haemorrhage may occur. There has been considerable uncertainty and confusion as to the biochemical aetiology of this disorder. DiFerrante et al (1975a,b) described a family with an X-linked connective tissue disorder with some features of the Ehlers-Danlos syndrome, but clinically different from Beighton's patients. They measured lysyl oxidase activity in the medium of cultured dermal fibroblasts from these patients and found it to be decreased, although the methods used for enzyme determination may not have been reliable (Siegel et al 1979). Siegel et al (1979) examined Beighton's original X–linked families and could find no evidence of abnormalities in lysyl oxidase function or in cross-link generation. Thus, the biochemical basis of the X–linked form of EDS remains unknown.

Genetic counselling for the sporadic, moderately affected male with EDS may be difficult. Such individuals should be studied carefully for lysyl hydroxylase deficiency (EDS VI, an autosomal recessive disorder) by assay of skin collagen for hydroxylysine and of dermal fibroblasts for the enzyme. If these studies are negative, then, given a compatible clinical picture, the most likely diagnosis is EDS II, since it appears to be far more frequent than EDS V.

EHLERS-DANLOS, TYPE VI (OCULAR)

Type VI EDS was the first of the true molecular disorders of collagen metabolism to be recognized when Pinnell et al (1972) described two sisters with lysyl hydroxylase deficiency that resulted in hydroxylysine deficient collagen. The two sisters described in the initial report had smooth, hyperextensible, velvety skin, moderate scarring and bruising, large and small joint laxity, a Marfanoid habitus with moderately severe thoracic kyphoscoliosis, and keratoconus with ocular globe fragility (Fig. 63.5).

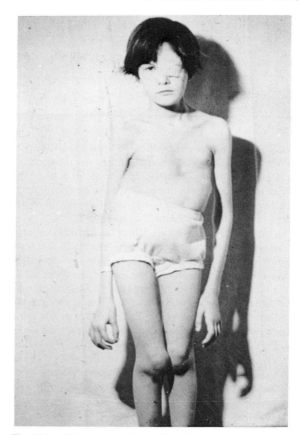

Fig. 63.5 This young girl has EDS VI, an autosomal recessive disorder characterized by reduced lysyl hydroxylation. She has a Marfanoid habitus, scoliosis, and lost her eye as a result of minor trauma. (Photograph courtesy of Dr Sheldon Pinnell, Duke University.)

Since the initial description, several other patients have been identified and there is clinical heterogeneity (Sussman et al 1974, Steinmann et al 1975, Elsas et al 1978, Krieg et al 1979, Dembure et al 1984, Ihme et al 1983, 1984). With only a small number of these patients identified, the natural history of the disorder is not known. One of the early patients described died suddenly, possibly as a result of an aortic rupture in her early 50s; an affected brother had died earlier from a gastrointestinal haemorrhage (Sussman et al 1974, McKusick 1988). Both had had intraocular haemorrhages previous to their fatal systemic haemorrhages. The other known patients are all less than 30 years old at this time. One patient died in his early 20s because of kyposcoliotic heart disease (Ihme et al 1984).

The histopathology in this disorder is not well

Table 63.4 Lysyl hydroxylase activity in cultured cells from a patient with EDS VI. Data from Sussman et al (1974)

	Lysyl hydroxylase ^{3}H cpm released	% control	Prolyl hydroxylase ^{3}H cpm released	% control
Control	850		11 100	
EDS VI	100	12	9800	88

described. In two patients collagen fibril morphology is said to be normal, although in one fibre organization may be disrupted (Pinnell et al 1972, Steinmann et al 1975). We examined skin from one patient with the disorder; she has normal fibril diameters but small fibres; there are many bizarre fibrils, such as seen in EDS I.

In most affected patients, there is virtually no hydroxylysine found in skin collagen: normally there are approximately 5 residues of hydroxylysine per 1000 amino acids but in most affected individuals there is less than 0.5 residue (Tables 63.4 and 63.5). Steinmann et al (1975) described a sib pair in whom hydroxylysine in skin was only modestly decreased, but who had virtually no measurable lysyl hydroxylase in cultured cells. All patients in whom it has been measured have very low lysyl hydroxylase levels in cultured cells (Tables 63.4 and 63.5). Parents of affected individuals generally have about half normal levels of the enzyme, consistent with autosomal recessive inheritance.

The major pathophysiological effect of decreased lysyl hydroxylation in collagen is a decrease in the production of stable intermolecular cross-links which alters the physical properties of tissues. It is not certain whether the enzymatic deficiency affects all tissue, since collagen in skin (types I and III) is markedly deficient, collagen in ligament (type I) is underhydroxylated, but cartilage (type II) has normal levels of hydroxylysine. Lysyl hydroxylase requires ascorbic acid, ferrous iron and α-ketoglutarate as cofactors. Studies by Quinn and Krane (1976) indicated that the interaction of the abnormal enzyme with ascorbate was altered. Subsequently, Elsas et al (1978) suggested that treatment of patients with ascorbate could increase urinary excretion of hydroxylysyl glycosides and produce subjective decrease in bruising, although no change in skin hydroxylysine content was demonstrable.

As is the case for most enzymatic defects, EDS VI is an autosomal recessive disorder. Thus, the risk of recurrence in a family with one affected child is 25% for each pregnancy. The risk for each affected person to have affected children is negligible unless he or she mates with a relative or other carrier. As indicated above, counselling concerning the natural history of the disorder remains uncertain because of the paucity of information. The clinical disorder may be additionally heterogeneous since two children with a similar presentation, including ocular globe fragility, have been described, who appear to have normal lysyl hydroxylation (Judisch et al 1976). Prenatal diagnosis of lysyl hydroxylase deficiency is feasible using amniotic fluid cells in culture to assay for the enzyme (Dembure et al 1984).

EHLERS-DANLOS, TYPE VII (ARTHROCHALASIS MULTIPLEX CONGENITA)

EDS type VII, arthrochalasis multiplex congenita, is characterized by extreme joint laxity, soft but non-fragile skin, minimal bruising and mild skin hyperextensibility (Lichtenstein et al 1973, 1974). Several of the affected individuals had bilateral congenital hip dislocation, which was difficult to stabilize, and at older ages had multiple dislocations of other joints.

When first described, all patients were thought to have abnormalities in the conversion of procollagen to collagen as a result of a defective amino-terminal procollagen peptidase (Lichtenstein et al 1973). It is now clear that most patients have mutations in either the COL1A1 or COL1A2 gene that interfere with proteolytic processing at the amino-terminal end of type I procollagen (Steinmann et al 1980, Eyre et al 1985, Cole et al 1986, 1987, Wirtz et al 1987, Weil et al 1988, 1989). Indeed, attempts to demonstrate defective enzyme have failed (Halila et al 1986).

In four individuals in which the mutation that results in EDS type VII has been characterized, three lack the sequences encoded by exon 6 in COL1A2 in about half the proα2(I) chains synthesized and the fourth lacks the

Table 63.5 Partial amino acid composition of skin from control and EDS VI. Data from Sussman et al (1974)

	Control	EDS VI
4-OHpro	81	76
Pro	118	114
Gly	316	300
Ala	122	134
Hylys	4.2	0.24
Lys	28	31

same sequence from the COL1A1 gene. Exon 6 from both genes contains the cleavage site for the amino-terminal procollagen peptidase. The defect in all four individuals results from an alteration in mRNA splicing such that an exon is deleted from the mature mRNA. When missing from a chain, the cleavage of the other chains in a molecule may be delayed. Furthermore, the remaining amino-terminal propeptide extension may interfere with normal fibrillogenesis (Cole et al 1987). Although ultrastructural studies of skin from some patients with EDS type VII have been surprisingly normal, fibrils in skin from a patient with a defect in proα1(I) chains have an abnormal structure (Cole et al 1987). It is possible that mutations that affect the structure of proα2(I) chains have less influence on fibrillogenesis than those in proα1(I) chains.

All the patients in whom mutations have been described are sporadic in their families. We are aware of one patient with a similar mutation in a dominant pedigree and, because of the nature of the mutation, this defect would be expected to be inherited in an autosomal dominant fashion. Other mutations which similarly affect the conversion of proα chains to α chains should occur, but technical reasons have facilitated discovery of the single exon deletions.

EHLERS-DANLOS, TYPE VIII (PERIODONTAL FORM)

Stewart and his colleagues (1977) described two families in which periodontal disease was accompanied by marked bruising, joint hypermobility and skin hyperextensibility and all were inherited in an autosomal dominant manner. Remarkably, affected individuals had lost most of their teeth to periodontal disease by their early twenties. There have been no published biochemical or ultrastructural studies of these patients. Interestingly, periodontal disease may be a feature of EDS VI. Thus careful biochemical studies will be needed to distinguish these two disorders.

EHLERS-DANLOS SYNDROME TYPE IX

EDS type IX is a rare X-linked recessive disorder characterized by lax and soft skin at birth, development of bladder diverticula during childhood, and the appearance of bony occipital horns during adolescence (Lazoff et al 1975, Byers et al 1980, Sartoris et al 1984). Although the affected males are of normal height, skeletal deformities which include short humeral bones, partial radio-ulnar synostosis which limits pronation and supination, and short broad clavicles are apparent on clinical and radiological examination. Most affected individuals have

mild chronic diarrhoea which appears to result from a defect in bowel motility, and some have symptomatic orthostatic hypotension. Intellect is generally measured as normal but some affected males have required special education and at least one affected male has moderate mental retardation (Blackston et al 1987). Carrier females are asymptomatic.

The basic defect in EDS type IX has not been identified. Serum copper and ceruloplasmin levels are low, often in a range similar to those seen in males with the Menkes syndrome. Cultured fibroblasts from individuals with EDS type IX have a normal rate of copper uptake but have very high intracellular copper levels apparently because they do not have normal rates of efflux (Kuivaniemi et al 1982, 1985, Peltonen et al 1983). Copper is a co-factor for many enzymes, including lysyl oxidase, tyrosine oxidase and dopamine β-hydroxylase. Lysyl oxidase levels in tissue and in the medium of fibroblasts cultured from individuals with EDS type IX are extremely low (Byers et al 1980, Kuivaniemi et al 1982) which probably accounts for the connective tissue abnormalities. Alterations in activity of other copper-dependent enzymes may explain the other features.

It is likely that EDS type IX and the Menkes syndrome represent allelic mutations.

EHLERS-DANLOS SYNDROME TYPE X

EDS type X is inherited in an autosomal recessive fashion and is characterized by mild joint hypermobility, slight increase in skin extensibility, and increased bruising (Arneson et al 1980). The disorder apparently results from an alteration in the structure of fibronectin that interferes both with normal platelet function (Arneson et al 1980) and with collagen fibril formation (Holbrook & Byers 1986). A single family has been described, so the frequency of the disorder is not known.

DIFFERENTIAL DIAGNOSIS AND PRENATAL DIAGNOSIS

The Ehlers-Danlos syndrome is a heterogeneous group of disorders of connective tissue manifest primarily as abnormalities of skin, joints, vessels and hollow organs. Disorders in type I and type III collagen have been identified, and the clinical disorders due to alterations in these two different molecules can be readily distinguished. Some of the clinical manifestations of the EDS are seen in certain other inherited connective tissue disorders so that careful medical history and physical examination are necessary to confirm the diagnosis. In the Marfan syndrome, for example, joint hypermobility is common but the associated features of arachnodactyly, lens subluxation and skeletal abnormalities help to distinguish the two syndromes (Pyeritiz & McKusick 1979). The Marfanoid hypermobility syndrome, because of the marked joint hypermobility, may be difficult to distinguish from EDS III unless the clinician is aware of both syndromes (Walker et al 1969). Some of the cutaneous manifestations of osteogenesis imperfecta (Sillence et al 1979), thin skin and easy bruising, are similar to those in some of the Ehlers-Danlos syndromes but the presence of marked bone fragility helps to distinguish the disorders. The differentiation between the true cutis laxa disorders and some varieties of the Ehlers-Danlos syndrome is occasionally confusing (see the discussion of EDS V, above). In cutis laxa, the elastic components of the skin are generally altered and the skin is lax and, in contrast to skin in the EDS, does not return to its original position rapidly.

Increased joint laxity and slow motor development are often seen in neuromuscular disorders and children with EDS I or EDS II are sometimes thought to have those conditions. Conversely, in the evaluation of joint laxity and slow motor development in children, the connective tissue disorders should be considered. Occasionally, individuals with EDS I, EDS II and EDS IV are thought to have bleeding disorders. In most instances careful haematological evaluations have yielded no identifiable abnormalities in haemostasis (but see discussion of EDS I above). Nonetheless, some individuals with EDS are considered to have unidentified disorders of haemostasis and it is not until the connective tissue problems are recognized that the correct diagnosis is made.

Prenatal diagnosis of those forms of the Ehlers-Danlos syndrome in which specific biochemical abnormalities are known is feasible by analysis of the structure of collagens synthesized by chorionic villus cells or by analysis of enzymes synthesized by cultured amniocytes (Dembure et al 1984, Byers et al 1987). It must be emphasized, however, that such attempts must be preceded by the accurate diagnosis of the defect in each family and, because different amniotic fluid cells synthesize and secrete different collagens (Crouch & Bornstein 1978), must be accompanied by careful studies of the appropriate type of normal amniotic fluid cells. Other potential problems in the prenatal diagnosis of disorders of collagen metabolism include the uncertainty about whether the collagen types synthesized and secreted by the developing fetal cells are the products of the same genes as expressed by adult cells, and similar questions about the relation of the developmentally active enzyme modifying systems to those of the adult.

The clinical descriptions and classification system for the Ehlers-Danlos syndrome that we have presented here do not include all the families that have been described with the disorder. It is sometimes difficult to classify new families with respect to this system, underlining the yet undescribed heterogeneity that still exists. We anticipate that, as more families are studied by biochemical techniques, many different disorders in metabolism of collagen (and other macromolecules) will be identified that will provide specific diagnostic criteria and more rational genetic counselling, and facilitate prenatal diagnosis of some of the very severe disorders.

Already, the study of these unusual connective tissue disorders has provided considerable insight into a number of facets of collagen metabolism: the importance of certain collagen cross-links, the regulation of collagen synthesis, and the manner in which development of some tissues is modulated. The application of many of the techniques of molecular biology promises insight into the structure of some of these abnormal genes and may provide even more detailed understanding of the disease mechanisms that will be useful in the clinical sphere.

REFERENCES

Arneson M A, Hammerschmidt D E, Furcht L T, King R A 1980 A new form of Ehlers-Danlos Syndrome: fibronectin corrects defective platelet function. Journal of the American Medical Association 244: 144–147

Barabas A P 1966 Ehlers-Danlos syndrome associated with prematurity and premature rupture of foetal membranes; possible increase in incidence. British Medical Journal 2: 682–684

Barabas A P 1967 Heterogeneity of the Ehlers-Danlos syndrome: description of three clinical types and a hypothesis to explain the basic defect. British Medical Journal 2: 612–614

Beighten P 1970 The Ehlers-Danlos syndrome. William Heinemann, London

Blackston R D, Hirschhorn K, Elsas L J 1987 Ehlers-Danlos syndrome (EDS), type IX: biochemical evidence for X-linkage. American Journal of Human Genetics 41: A49

Bornstein P, Byers P H 1980 Disorders of collagen metabolism. In: Bondy P K, Rosenberg L E (eds) Metabolic Control and Disease, 8th edn. W B Saunders Co, Philadelphia, p 1089–1153

Bornstein P, Sage H 1980 Structurally distinct collagen types. Annual Review of Biochemistry 49: 957–1004

Byers P H 1989 Disorders of collagen biosynthesis and structure. In: Scriver C R, Beaudet A L, Sly W S, Valle D (eds) The Metabolic Basis of Inherited Disease, 6th edn. McGraw-Hill, New York, p 2802–2845

Byers P H, Holbrook K A 1985 Molecular basis of clinical heterogeneity in the Ehlers-Danlos syndrome. Annals of the New York Academy of Sciences 460: 298–310

Byers P H, Narayanan A S, Bornstein P, Hall J G 1976. An X-linked form of cutis laxa due to deficiency of lysyl oxidase. Birth Defects: Original Article Series 12(5): 293–298

Byers P H, Holbrook K A, McGillivray B, MacLeod P M, Lowry R B 1979 Clinical and ultrastructural heterogeneity of type IV Ehlers-Danlos syndrome. Human Genetics 47: 141–150

Byers P H, Siegel R C, Holbrook K A, Narayanan A S, Bornstein P, Hall J G 1980 X–linked cutis laxa: defective collagen crosslink formation due to decreased lysyl oxidase activity. New England Journal of Medicine 303: 61–65

Byers P H, Holbrook K A, Barsh G S, Smith L T, Bornstein P 1981 Altered secretion of type III procollagen in a form of type IV Ehlers-Danlos syndrome: biochemical studies in cultured fibroblasts. Laboratory Investigation 44: 336–341

Byers P H, Wenstrup R J, Bonadio J F, Starman B, Cohn D H 1987 Molecular basis of inherited disorders of collagen biosynthesis: implication for prenatal diagnosis. Current Problems in Dermatology 16: 158–174.

Clark J G, Kuhn C, Uitto J 1980 Lung collagen in type IV Ehlers-Danlos syndrome: ultrastructural and biochemical studies. American Review of Respiratory Disease 122: 971–978

Cole W G, Chan D, Chambers G W, Walker I D, Bateman J F 1986 Deletion of 24 amino acids from the proα1(I) chain of type I procollagen in a patient with the Ehlers-Danlos syndrome type VII. Journal of Biological Chemistry 261: 5496–5503

Cole W G, Evans R, Sillence D O 1987 The clinical features of Ehlers-Danlos syndrome type VII due to a deletion of 24 amino acids from the proα1(I) chains of type I procollagen. Journal of Medical Genetics 24: 698–704

Crouch E, Bornstein P 1978 Collagen synthesis by human amniotic fluid cells in culture: characterization of a procollagen with three identical α1(I) chains. Biochemistry 17: 5499–5509

Danlos M 1908 Un cas de cutis laxa avec tumeurs par contusion chronique des coudes et des Mace de Lepinay. Bulletin of the Societe Francais Dermatologie 19: 70

Dembure P P, Priest J H, Snoddy S C, Elsas L J 1984 Genotyping and prenatal assessment of collagen lysyl hydroxylase deficiency in a family with Ehlers-Danlos syndrome, type VI. American Journal of Human Genetics 36: 783–790

DiFerrante N, Leachmann R D, Angelini D, Donnelly P W, Francis G, Almazan A 1975a Lysyl oxidase deficiency in Ehlers-Danlos syndrome type V. Connective Tissue Research 3: 48–53

DiFerrante N, Leachmann R D, Angelini P et al 1975b Ehlers-Danlos type V (X-linked form) lysyl oxidase deficiency. Birth Defects Original Article Series II (6) 31–37

Ehlers E 1901 Cutis laxa, Neigung zu hemorrhagien in der Haut, Loekerung mehrerer artikulationen. Dermatalogische Zeitschrift 8: 173

Elsas L J, Miller R L, Pinnell S R 1978 Inherited human collagen lysyl hydroxylase deficiency: ascorbic acid response. Journal of Pediatrics 92: 378–384

Epstein E H Jr 1974 α1(III)$_3$ human skin collagen: release by pepsin digestion and preponderance in fetal life. Journal of Biological Chemistry 249: 3325–3231

Eyre D R 1980 Collagen: molecular diversity in the body's protein scaffold. Science 207: 1315–1322

Eyre D R, Glimcher M J 1972 Reducible cross-links in hydroxylysine-deficient collagens of a heritable disorder of connective tissue. Proceedings of the National Academy of Sciences USA 69: 2594–2595

Eyre D R, Shapiro F D, Aldridge J F 1985 Heterozygous collagen defect in a variant of the Ehlers-Danlos syndrome type VII: evidence for a deleted amino telopeptide domain in the proα2(I) chain. Journal of Biological Chemistry 260: 11322–11329

Fessler J H, Fessler L I 1978 Biosynthesis of procollagen. Annual Review of Biochemistry 47: 129–162

Frischauf A M, Lerach H, Rosner C, Boedtker H 1978 Procollagen complementary DNA, a probe for messenger RNA purification and the number of type I collagen genes. Biochemistry 17: 3243–3249

Gay S, Martin G R, Müller P K, Timpl R, Kühn K 1976 Simultaneous synthesis of types I and III collagen by fibrolasts in culture. Proceedings of the National Academy of Sciences USA 73: 4037–4040

Gottron H 1942 Familiare acrogeria. Archives of Dermatology, Berlin, 181: 571–576

Halila R, Steinmann B, Peltonen L 1986 Processing of types I and III procollagen in Ehlers-Danlos syndrome type VII. American Journal of Human Genetics 39: 222–231

Holbrook K A, Byers P H 1981 Ultrastructural characteristics of the skin in a form of Ehlers-Danlos syndrome type IV: storage in the rough endoplasmic reticulum. Laboratory Investigation 44: 342–350

Holbrook K A, Byers P H 1986 Disease of the extracellular matrix: Structural alterations of collagen fibrils in skin. In: Uitto J, Perejda A (eds) Connective Tissue Disease: The Molecular Pathology of the Extracellular Matrix. Marcel Dekker, New York, p 101–140

Holbrook K A, Byers P H 1989 Skin is a window on heritable disorders of connective tissue. American Journal of Medical Genetics (in press)

Holbrook K A, Byers P H, Counts D F, Hegreberg G A 1980 Dermatosparaxis in a himalayan cat: ultrastructural studies of dermis. Journal of Investigative Dermatology 74: 100–104

Hollister D W 1978 Heritable disorders of connective tissue: Ehlers-Danlos syndrome. Pediatric Clinics of North America 25: 575–591

Ihme A, Krieg T, Nerlich A et al 1984 Ehlers-Danlos syndrome type VI: collagen type specificity of defective lysyl hydroxylation in various tissues. Journal of Investigative Dermatology 83: 161–165

Ihme A, Risteli L, Krieg T, Risteli J, Feldmann U, Kuuse K, Müller P K 1983 Biochemical characterization of variants of the Ehlers-Danlos syndrome type VI. European Journal of Clinical Investigation 13: 357–362

Judisch G F, Waziri M, Krachmer J H 1976 Ocular Ehlers-Danlos syndrome with normal lysyl hydroxylase activity. Archives of Ophthalmology 94: 1489–1491

Krieg T, Feldmann U, Kessler W, Müller P K 1979 Biochemical characteristics of Ehlers-Danlos syndrome type VI in a family with one affected infant. Human Genetics 46: 41–49

Kuivaniemi H, Peltonen L, Palotie A, Kaitila I, Kivirikko K I 1982 Abnormal copper metabolism and deficient lysyl oxidase activity in a heritable connective tissue disorder. Journal of Clinical Investigation 69: 730–733

Kuivaniemi H, Peltonen L, Kivirikko K I 1985 Type IX Ehlers-Danlos syndrome and Menkes syndrome: the decrease in lysyl oxidase activity is associated with a corresponding deficiency in the enzyme protein. American Journal of Human Genetics 37: 798–808

Lazoff S G, Rybak J J, Parker B R, Luzzatti L 1975 Skeletal dysplasia, occipital horns, diarrhoea and obstructive uropathy - a new hereditary syndrome. Birth Defects Original Article Series 11(2): 71–74

Leier C V, Call T D, Fulkerson P K, Wooley C F 1980 The spectrum of cardiac defects in the Ehlers-Danlos syndrome, types I and III. Annals of Internal Medicine 92: 171–178

Lichtenstein J R, Martin G R, Kohn L, Byers P H, McKusick V A 1973 Defects in conversion of procollagen to collagen in a form of Ehlers-Danlos syndrome. Science 182: 298–300

Lichtenstein J R, Kohn L D, Martin G R, Byers P H, McKusick V A 1974 Procollagen peptidase deficiency in a form of the Ehlers-Danlos syndrome. Transactions of the American Association of Physicians 86: 333–339

Lindahl V, Höök M 1978 Glycosaminoglycans and their binding to biological macro-molecules. Annual Review of Biochemistry 47: 385–412

McKusick V A 1972 Heritable disorders of connective tissue C V Mosby, St Louis

McKusick V A 1988 Mendelian inheritance in man. Catalogs of autosomal dominant, autosomal recessive, and X–linked phenotypes, 8th edn. Johns Hopkins University Press, Baltimore

Mayne R, Burgeson R E (eds) 1987 Structure and function of collagen types. Academic Press, Orlando.

Nicholls A C, De Paepe A, Narcisi P, Dalgleish R, DeKeyser F, Matton M, Pope F M 1988 Linkage of a polymorphic marker for the type III collagen gene (COL3A1) to atypical autosomal dominant Ehlers-Danlos syndrome type IV in a large Belgian pedigree. Human Genetics 78: 276–281

Peltonen L, Kuivaniemi H, Palotie A, Horn N, Kaitila I, Kivirikko K I 1983 Alterations in copper and collagen metabolism in the Menkes syndrome and a new subtype of the Ehlers-Danlos syndrome. Biochemistry 22: 6156–6163

Pinnell S R 1983 Disorders of collagen. In: Stanbury J B, Wyngaarden J B, Frederickson D S (eds). The Metabolic Basis of Inherited Disease. McGraw Hill, New York, p 1425–1449

Pinnell S R, Krane S M, Kenzora J E, Glimcher M J 1972 A heritable disorder of connective tissue: Hydroxylysine-deficient collagen disease. New England Journal of Medicine 866: 1013–1020

Pope F M, Martin G R, Lichtenstein J R, Penttinen R P, Gerson G, Rowe D W, McKusick V A 1975 Patients with Ehlers-Danlos type IV syndrome. Journal of Medical Proceedings of the National Academy of Sciences USA 72: 1314–1316

Pope F M, Martin G R, McKusick V A 1977 Inheritance of Ehlers- Danlos type IV syndrome. Journal of Medical Genetics 14: 200–204

Pope F M, Nicholls A C, Jones P M, Wells R S, Lawrence D 1980 EDS IV (acrogeria): new autosomal dominant and recessive types. Journal of the Royal Society of Medicine 73: 180–186

Prockop D J, Kivirikko K I 1984 Heritable diseases of collagen. New England Journal of medicine 311: 376–386

Pyeritz R E, McKusick V A 1979 The Marfan syndrome: diagnosis and management. New England Journal of Medicine 300: 772–775

Pyeritz R E, Stolle C A, Parfrey N A, Myers J C 1984 Ehlers-Danlos syndrome IV due to a novel defect in type III procollagen. American Journal of Medical Genetics 19: 607–622

Quinn R S, Krane S M 1976 Abnormal properties of collagen lysyl hydroxylase from skin fibroblasts of siblings with hydroxylysine-deficient collagen. Journal of Clinical Investigation 57: 83–93

Ramirez F 1989 Organization and evolution of the fibrillar collagen genes. In: Olsen B R, Nimni M E (eds) Collagen Vol. IV, Molecular Biology. CRC Press, Boca Raton

Rudd N L, Holbrook K A Nimrod C, Byers P H 1983 Pregnancy complications in type IV Ehlers-Danlos syndrome. Lancet 1: 50–53

Sack G 1936 Status dysvascularis; ein Fall von besonderer Zerreisslichkeit der Blutgefasse. Deutsches Archiv für Klinische Medizin 178: 663–669

Sartoris D J, Luzzatti L, Weaver D D, MacFarlane J D, Hollister D W, Parker B R 1984 Type IX Ehlers-Danlos syndrome: a new variant with pathognomonic radiographic features. Radiology 152: 665

Sasaki T, Arai K, Ono M, Yamaguchi T, Furuta S, Nagai Y 1987 Ehlers-Danlos syndrome. A variant characterized by the deficiency of proα2 chain of type I procollagen. Archives of Dermatology 123: 76–78

Sevenich M, Schultz-Ehrenburg U, Orfanos C G 1980 Ehlers-Danlos syndrome: a disease of fibroblasts and collagen fibrils. Archives of Dermatology and Research 267: 237–251

Shinkai H, Hirabayashi O, Tameki A, Matsubayashi S, Seno S 1976 Connective tissue metabolism in cultured fibroblasts of a patient with Ehlers-Danlos syndrome type I. Archives of Dermatology and Research 257: 113–122

Siegel R C 1978 Lysyl oxidase. International Review of Connective Tissue Research 8: 73–118

Siegel R C, Black C M, Bailey A J 1979 Cross-linking of collagen in the X–linked Ehlers-Danlos type V. Biochemical and Biophysical Research Communications 88: 281–287

Sillence D O, Senn A, Danks D M 1979 Genetic heterogeneity in osteogenesis imperfecta. Journal of Medical Genetics 16: 101–116

Steinmann B, Gitzelmann R, Vogel A, Grant M E, Harwood R, Sear C H J 1975 Ehlers-Danlos syndrome in two siblings with deficient lysyl hydroxylase activity in cultured skin fibroblasts but only mild hydroxylysine deficit in skin. Helvetica Pediatrica Acta 30: 255–274

Steinmann B, Tuderman L, Peltonen L, Martin G R, McKusick V A, Prockop D J 1980 Evidence for a structural mutation of procollagen type I in a patient with the Ehlers-Danlos syndrome type VII. Journal of Biological Chemistry 255: 8887–8893

Stewart R E, Hollister D W, Rimoin D L 1977 A new variant of the Ehlers-Danlos syndrome: an autosomal dominant disorder of fragile skin, abnormal scarring and generalized periodontitis. Birth Defects 13(3B): 85–93

Stolle C A, Pyeritz R E, Myers J C, Prockop D J 1985 Synthesis of an altered type III procollagen in a patient with type IV Ehlers-Danlos syndrome. Journal of Biological Chemistry 260: 1937–1944

Superti-Furga A, Steinmann B 1988 Impaired secretion of type III procollagen in Ehlers-Danlos syndrome type IV fibroblasts: correction of the defect by incubation at reduced temperature and demonstration of subtle alterations in the triple-helical region of the molecule. Biochemical and Biophysical Research Communications 150: 140–147

Superti-Furga A, Gugler E, Gitzelmann R, Steinmann B 1988 Ehlers-Danlos syndrome type IV: a multi-exon deletion in one of the two COL3A1 alleles affecting structure, stability, and processing of type III procollagen. Journal of Biological Chemistry 263: 6226–6232

Superti-Furga A, Steinmann B, Ramirez F, Byers P H 1989 Molecular defects of type III procollagen in Ehlers-Danlos syndrome type IV. Human Genetics 82: 102–108

Sussman M, Lichtenstein J R, Nigra T P, Martin G R, McKusick V A 1974 Hydroxylysine-deficient collagen in a patient with a form of the Ehlers-Danlos syndrome. Journal of Bone and Joint Surgery 56A: 1228–1234

Temple A S, Hinton P, Narcisi P, Pope F M 1988 Detection of type III collagen in skin fibroblasts from patients with Ehlers-Danlos syndrome type IV by immunofluorescence. British Journal of Dermatology 118: 17–26

Tsipouras P, Byers P H, Schwartz R C et al 1986 Ehlers-Danlos syndrome type IV: cosegregation of the phenotype to a COL3A1 allele of type III procollagen. Human Genetics 74: 41–46

Vogel A, Holbrook K A, Steinmann B, Gitzelmann R, Byers P H 1979 Abnormal collagen fibril structure in the gravis form (type I) of the Ehlers-Danlos syndrome. Laboratory Investigation 40: 201–206

Walker B A, Beighton P, Murdoch J L 1969 The Marfanoid hypermobility syndrome. Annals of Internal Medicine 71: 349–352

Weil D, Bernard M, Combata N, Wirtz M K, Hollister D W, Steinmann B, Ramirez F 1988 Identification of a mutation that causes exon-skipping during collagen pre-mRNA splicing in an Ehlers-Danlos syndrome variant. Journal of Biological Chemistry 263: 8561–8564

Wirtz M K, Glanville R W, Steinmann B, Rao V H, Hollister D W 1987 Ehlers-Danlos syndrome type VIIB. Journal of Biological Chemistry 262: 16376

64. Pseudoxanthoma elasticum and related disorders

R. M. Goodman

PSEUDOXANTHOMA ELASTICUM

Introduction

Pseudoxanthoma elasticum (PXE) is a genetically deter-mined heterogeneous disorder with clinical manifesta-tions that may involve many organ systems. Although this condition has been referred to by many names (Table 64.1), it was first described as an atypical xanthoma by Rigal (1881) and the first autopsy report was given by Balzer (1884). Subsequent clinicians have recognized that the skin involvement is the least serious of its clinical features. In addition to the xanthoma-like appearance of part of the skin, the most frequently encountered mani-festations include angioid streaks and other chorioretinal changes which frequently impair vision, and degener-ative vascular charges which account for upper gastro-intestinal haemorrhage, cardiovascular symptoms and a variety of neurological complications.

Attempts to relate the diverse clinical findings to a single pathological change led to the belief that PXE represents a genetic defect involving elastic or collagen fibres (McKusick 1972). Although the elastic fibre hypothesis is the oldest and currently the most widely held, much remains to be learned concerning the basic defect in this disorder (Goodman et al 1963).

Clinical features

Skin and mucosa

It has been commonly thought that recognizable skin changes do not appear before the second decade of life or later, however Goodman and co-workers (1963) noted that on careful questioning the majority of their patients were aware of skin changes between the ages of 3 and 12 years. One patient was told that lesions were present about the neck from birth. All areas of normal body folds are prone to involvement, especially the neck. The yellowish-appearing skin becomes thickened, pebbled and grooved, resembling coarse-grained Moroccan leather. With progression of the disease the skin develops

Table 64.1 Terms used for pseudoxanthoma elasticum

Date	Author	Term
1881	Rigal	Diffuse xanthelasma
1884	Balzer	Atypical xanthoma
1896	Darier	Pseudoxanthoma elasticum (PXE)
1929	Grönblad and Strandberg	Grönblad-Strandberg syndrome = angioid streaks plus skin lesions of PXE
1933	Lewis and Clayton	Elastosis atrophicans
1938	Böck	Elastosis dystrophica
1940	Témine	Elastorrhexie systématisée
1952	Tunbridge et al	Pseudo-xanthoma pseudo-elasticum

lax, redundant and inelastic features. About the face, exaggeration of the nasolabial folds and chin creases is often striking, producing a distinct, sagging facial appear-ance (Fig. 64.1). Extreme laxity of the skin in the neck, axillary folds (Fig. 64.2) and abdominal wall has caused some patients to seek surgical intervention.

In some individuals the skin changes are exceedingly mild despite pronounced pathological changes in the eye and cardiovascular system. In addition to the character-istic skin changes described, some patients may have a different skin lesion which consists of ring-shaped plaques of closely grouped hyperkeratotic papules, 1–2 mm in size. Frequently a hyperkeratotic cap becomes dis-lodged to leave a small haemorrhagic depression which has been termed reactive perforating elastoma or Miescher elastoma (Smith et al 1962).

Calcinosis cutis has been observed in some patients, and calcification in the middle and deeper layers of the dermis may be noted readily by radiographic techniques.

Mucosal lesions similar to the characteristic skin findings have been observed on the inner aspects of the lower lip, buccal mucosa and in the rectum and vagina. Endoscopic examinations have also shown like lesions in the stomach and bladder.

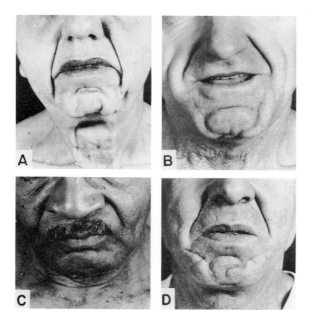

Fig. 64.1 Patients with PXE from three different families showing the prominent nasolabial folds as the skin about the face becomes lax. Altered skin changes about the neck can also be noted.

Eye

The best described and most characteristic ocular lesion of PXE consists of peripapillary or radial 'angioid streaks'. Although angioid streaks are not pathognomonic of PXE, they are recognized in approximately 85% of cases, and a comparably large portion of all individuals with these streaks have PXE.

Depending upon the depth of retinal pigmentation these streaks appear grey, red or maroon. Lack of pigmentation of the streaks may be demonstrated by applying sufficient pressure upon the eye to occlude the retinal artery. Pallor of the vascular retina produced by this manoeuvre decreases visual contrasts and may lead to a virtual disappearance of the streaks (Goodman et al 1963). In later stages, the streaks are bordered by proliferating scar tissue and retinal pigmentary epithelium. That angioid streaks are true cracks in Bruch's membrane beneath the retina is clinically substantiated by the observation of their tapering and their complimentary zigzag borders. They always underlie the retinal vessels.

Although probably not present at birth, these streaks usually develop in the second decade or later. They may persist for many years as the only ocular sign of PXE; however, chorioretinal changes usually appear. The development of haemorrhage or the appearance of chorioretinal scarring is an ominous sign.

Complete blindness does not usually occur but macular involvement frequently results in a diminution of visual acuity to 20/200, 20/400 or the ability only to see fingers at a few feet. When chorioretinal scarring and accompanying retinal pigment proliferation are exten-

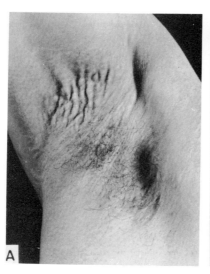

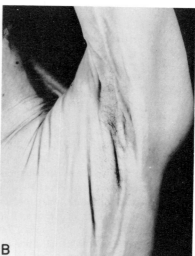

Fig. 64.2 Moderate (A) and marked (B) skin changes in the axilla.

sive, angioid streaks may be obscured, although indistinct remnants of streaks usually persist at the periphery of such scars.

Some patients show only pigmentary mottling of the fundus and this is thought to be the earliest finding of an alteration in Bruch's membrane.

Berlyne and co-workers (1961) reported that persons presumed to be heterozygous for the PXE gene had an abnormally prominent choroidal vascular pattern but other studies (Goodman et al 1963) have not been able to confirm this finding.

Gastrointestinal

The frequency of gastrointestinal haemorrhage in PXE is difficult to ascertain, but bleeding appears to be common and may be fatal. It may result from a peptic ulcer or hiatus hernia, but in most instances the source is not evident. Superficial ulceration and a friable oozing mucosal surface with diffusely scattered erosions have been seen by gastroscopy. Gastroscopy done in the absence of bleeding may show a yellowish papular gastric mucosa with lesions similar to those found in the oral and rectal mucosa. Redundancy of mucosal tissue of the lesser curvature of the stomach has been seen (Goodman et al 1963).

Upper gastrointestinal tract bleeding in PXE has been known to occur in children as early as age 3 years but in most instances onset is in adulthood. Massive gastrointestinal haemorrhage has been observed during pregnancy, suggesting that this state may be an influencing factor. In patients with upper gastrointestinal haemorrhage of unknown cause one should always look for the skin lesions noted in PXE.

The nature of the complex vascular anatomy of the stomach and its regulatory mechanism are fundamental to the understanding of the mucosal abnormalities and to the occurrence of gastrointestinal bleeding in PXE. As described by Bentley and Barlow (1952) the submucosal arterial plexus gives off spiralling branches which anastomose to form the mucosal plexus. These then arborize into a rich capillary bed. Arteriovenous shunts are present which can dilate to 140 μm in calibre and can, when open, direct blood away from the mucosa and lead to pallor of the surface. Although the mechanism for the control of flow in this system is not well understood, it seems reasonable that alteration in the elastic tissue of the vessels might impair the normal regulation of gastric blood flow. This alteration could account for poor constriction of vessels and inadequate shunting of blood away from the mucosa with persistence of vascular dilation and resultant diffuse oozing from the mucosal surface. This hypothesis (Goodman et al 1963) suggests

that upper gastrointestinal haemorrhage in PXE occurs as the result of an alteration in vascular elastic tissue and impairment of the normal mechanism for the regulation of gastric blood flow.

Another possible mechanism for haemorrhage is entirely speculative: proliferation and calcification of nodular lesions in the stomach may be followed by perforation and ulceration, such as occurs in the skin in lesions of elastoma perforans of PXE.

Abdominal angina has been reported in several patients with PXE due to stenosis of the coeliac artery. The symptoms are usually of pain coming on 40–50 minutes after a meal.

Cardiovascular

It has been known that the peripheral arteries are involved in the pathological process underlying PXE. Intermittent claudication has been described as early as the age of nine and in other cases before the age of 36 years.

Radial and/or ulnar pulses are frequently absent in this disorder, but ischaemic symptoms are rather unusual in the upper extremities despite the severe angiographic changes that can be observed (Fig. 64.3). The lack of upper extremity symptoms may be due to the fact that collateral circulation from the interosseous artery provides adequate filling of the arterial system in the hand.

Calcification of peripheral arteries is frequently observed in PXE. The most common site is the femoral artery. Although calcification of vessels tends to increase with age, as does that of the skin, it has been reported to occur as early as the age of nine years. The media is the predominant site of calcium deposition within the artery.

PXE patients are prone to premature atherosclerosis, and coronary arterial involvement can be demonstrated by the presence of angina pectoris, ECG changes demonstrating myocardial infarction and radiographic evidence of occlusive coronary artery disease. McKusick (1972) mentions an 11-year-old girl with angina pectoris who at the age of 18 years showed disease in three vessels and the following year had a triple graft replacement.

Lebwohl et al (1982) called attention to the fact that some PXE patients may develop mitral-valve prolapse. Pyeritz et al (1982) suggested that patients with PXE of the autosomal dominant type II may be more prone to mitral-valve prolapse because of their joint hypermobility and Marfanoid features.

The disease process in PXE may also involve the endocardium, heart valves and cardiac conduction system. Clinical manifestations may include cardiac enlargement, heart failure, arrhythmias and murmurs with

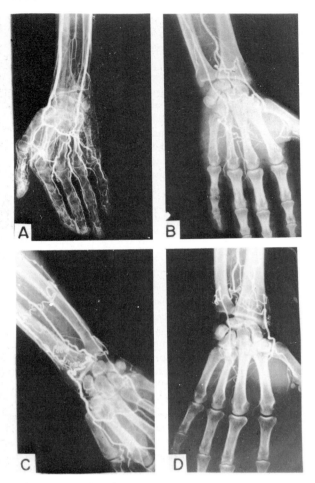

Fig. 64.3   A normal upper extremity arteriogram, **B–D** arteriograms in patients with PXE showing varying degrees of occlusive changes involving the radial, ulnar and digital arteries.

valve deformity which result from the endocardial thickening (McKusick 1972).

Hypertension is not uncommon in such patients and this has been shown to be due to renal vascular disease of the PXE type (McKusick 1972). The presence of hypertension can be an influencing factor in the tendency to haemorrhage. Excessive uterine bleeding and intra-articular haemorrhage with formation of haemarthroses have been reported in a few patients (Altman et al 1974).

Neurological

Various neurological signs and symptoms can be manifested in patients with PXE depending upon the location

and severity of the vascular lesion (Iqbal et al 1978). Patients may complain of paraesthesia and numbness. Aneurysms often involve the cerebral arteries with secondary complications. Subarachnoid haemorrhage has been a cause of death in some patients.

Frequent associations of prominent mental or psychiatric disturbances, such as forgetfulness or impaired memory, dull mentality, depression, psychoneurosis and mental deterioration, have been noted in association with PXE. The incidence of seizures is increased in this disorder but no specific EEG abnormality has been observed.

Pregnancy

Gastrointestinal bleeding is one of the most common complications during pregnancy in women with PXE (Lao et al 1984). Usually the bleeding originates from generalized mucosal oozing without an identifiable focus. The bleeding is usually severe enough to require blood transfusions. Other complications during pregnancy include congestive heart failure, epistaxis, preeclampsia, cerebral haemorrhage and premature delivery of a stillbirth or a fetus with intrauterine growth retardation (Elejalde 1984). From the above, one must conclude that pregnancy in women with one of the more severe forms of PXE deserves careful monitoring of both the patient and her developing fetus.

Diagnosis

At present the diagnosis of PXE is based on distinct clinical and histological changes as no precise biochemical alteration has been found. The combination of the characteristic skin changes with the presence of angioid streaks (Grönblad-Strandberg syndrome) is pathognomonic for the disorder. The involved skin shows characteristic histological changes involving masses of abnormal elastic-staining material within the mid-dermis and, less frequently, within the upper or lower dermis (Goodman et al 1963). For the most part, this material is granular but in places rodlike structures are observed (Fig. 64.4). Tuberculoid areas with giant cells are found in the area of degeneration. Calcification of the degenerated material occurs, and it has now been documented that calcium deposition in elastic fibres is the earliest demonstrable histopathological change in PXE (Goodman et al 1963). Elastic fibres surrounding the sweat glands (Fig. 64.4) are thought to be among the first to show this early change (Goodman et al 1963.)

Recently Lebwohl et al (1987) took skin biopsies from 10 patients with angioid streaks (35–73 years) and no skin changes of PXE. Six of these patients showed histological

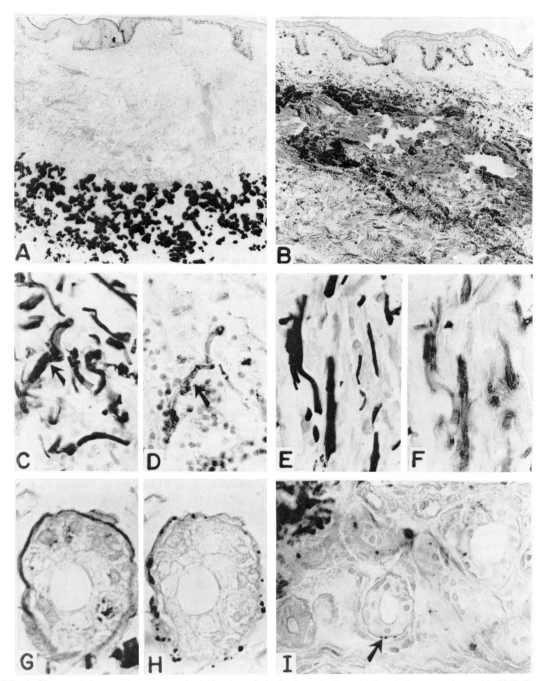

Fig. 64.4 **A** Characteristic granular pattern of calcification of elastic tissue in the mid-dermis from a patient with PXE. **B** Massive and nonspecific calcification in the skin of a patient with secondary hypercalcaemia due to leukaemia. **C** Elastic stain showing normal appearing elastic fibres in the skin of a patient with PXE. **D** Same fibres restained for calcium illustrating that some fibres are calcified despite the fact that they appear normal with the elastic stain. **E** and **F** The same as **C** and **D** in a patient with secondary hypercalcaemia due to leukaemia. **G** Elastic fibres surrounding a sweat gland from a patient with PXE. **H** Same sweat gland showing small foci of calcification in the elastic tissue. **I** Arrow points to small foci of calcification of elastic tissue about the sweat gland in a patient with transient idiopathic hypercalcaemia.

evidence of PXE. Thus, the mere absence of skin lesions should not be used to exclude the diagnosis of PXE.

Further clinical documentation of PXE may be obtained by visual examination of the mucosal surface of the oral cavity, stomach, rectum and vagina, or by noting the characteristic occlusive changes in the upper extremities using the technique of brachial artery angiography.

Differential diagnosis

Actinic or senile elastosis may outwardly resemble the skin lesions of PXE but such changes are limited to the exposed surfaces of the body and histologically are distinguishable from PXE.

Light et al (1986) have shown that patients undergoing long-term, high dose D-penicillamine therapy for various disorders may develop PXE-like skin changes.

Angioid streaks occur in 8–15% of patients with Paget disease of bone. This disease shares with PXE a predisposition to calcification of the media of arteries, and the angioid streaks in the two disorders are clinically and histologically indistinguishable (Schmorl 1931). However, the streaks in Paget disease are observed late in life when the bone changes are far advanced. A few cases with both Paget disease and PXE have been reported in detail as well as several less well documented cases (Woodcock 1952, Shaffer et al 1957).

It is estimated that 5% of all individuals homozygous for sickle-cell disease have angioid streaks (Goodman et al 1963). The pathology has not been defined, but description of abnormal elastic tissue in Bruch's membrane and the internal elastic lamella of ocular vessels may suggest involvement of the elastic tissue in this disorder – probably of the secondary type. Patients with both sickle-cell disease and PXE have been reported (Geereats & Guerry 1960, Goodman et al 1963).

Angioid streaks have been observed in one person with familial hyperphosphataemia and metastatic calcification (McPhaul & Engel 1961), in a patient with idiopathic thrombocytopenic purpura and in several instances of lead poisoning (De Simone & De Concilliis 1958). The mechanism of streak production in these disorders is not known.

Genetic

Incidence and prevalence

Although this genetically determined disorder should be thought of as being rare several hundred cases of PXE have been reported in the literature since the first case was described in 1881 by Rigal.

The frequency of PXE is not known. Berlyne and his group (1961) in England suggested that one case may occur among every 160 000 to 1 million persons. It is the impression of many (Goodman et al 1963, McKusick 1972) that it occurs more frequently than 1 in 160 000. (See section under Inheritance).

Sex ratio

Various observers have concluded, by tabulation of cases in the literature, that there is a preponderance of affected females (McKusick 1972). A review of 106 cases of PXE from the Mayo Clinic (Connor et al 1961) showed a 1:1.2 ratio of affected males to females. But within this group there were 32 cases with angioid streaks alone, the ratio then being 2.2:1 males to females. A major problem in ascertaining the sex distribution in PXE from reports in the literature is that females are more likely to seek medical advice when there is a cosmetic problem.

Inheritance

Extensive studies in the United Kingdom by Pope (1974a,b, 1975) have firmly established that there is genetic heterogeneity in PXE. At present there appear to be two autosomal dominant and two recessive forms (Table 64.2).

Recessive type I is the most common (the classic type) and resembles dominant type I, although the vascular and retinal degenerative changes are milder. Upper gastrointestinal haemorrhage tends to be more common in affected females.

Recessive type II is an extremely rare variant which exhibits generalized cutaneous laxity and infiltration without systemic complications. Pope (1975) found only three affected families out of some 140 examined in Britain and none were found in the previous literature.

Dominant type I is the most severe form exhibiting the characteristic skin changes with cardiovascular complications and degenerative retinopathy leading to a marked loss in vision.

Dominant type II is about four times more common than dominant type I. This form is characterized by a canary-yellow macular skin lesion, minimal vascular symptoms and mild retinal changes with prominent choroidal vessels. Increased extensibility of the skin, blue sclerae, high-arched palate and myopia are also observed in this type.

Consanguinity has been found in at least 20% of cases with the classic recessive type I. Altman and co-workers (1974) estimated the prevalence of all forms of PXE in the Seattle area to be greater than 1 in 70 000.

In a recent survey of PXE within South Africa and Zimbabwe, Viljoen and co-workers (1987) noted that out

Table 64.2 Clinical findings in autosomal dominant and recessive types of PXE (based on data presented by Pope 1974a,b).

Characteristics	Genetic types			
	Autosomal dominant		Autosomal recessive	
	Dominant I (%)	Dominant II (%)	Recessive I (%)	Recessive II (%)
Cutaneous changes				
Classic peau d'orange and flexural rash	100	25	75	
Macular rash		70	15	
General increase of extensibility	10	65	10	
General cutaneous PXE				100
Vascular disease				
Angina	55			
Claudication	55			
Hypertension	75	10	20	
Haematemesis	10	5	15	
Ophthalmic abnormalities				
Severe choroiditis	75	10	35	
Angioid streaks	35	50	50	
Washed-out pattern		15	2	
Prominent choroidal-vessels		20		
Myopia	25	50	5	
Blue sclerae	10	40	10	
Other findings				
High arched palate		55	15	
Joint hypermobility		35	5	

of 64 identifiable patients with PXE, 39 such patients of Afrikaner descent had manifestations that did not fit the classification of Pope (1975). They concluded that there is an 'Afrikaner' form characterized by autosomal recessive inheritance and mild skin changes with early and consistent retinal deterioration and eventual blindness. The eye features were age-related and severe visual impairment was usually apparent by the fourth decade of life. 40% of these patients also had severe hypertension and occasionally angina or intermittent claudication.

It is important to know that although the human elastin gene is located on the short arm of chromosome 2 (Emanuel et al 1985) few restriction fragment length polymorphism markers are yet available for linkage studies. Thus, it is not yet possible to prove heterogeneity in PXE and our only current methods of suggesting it are the clinical findings and mode of inheritance.

Genetic counselling and prenatal diagnosis

Every effort must be made to establish the precise type of PXE afflicting the patient before proper genetic coun-

selling is undertaken. Recurrence risks can then be given depending upon whether one is dealing with an autosomal dominant or recessive form or perhaps a new mutation.

Despite the fact that some investigators (Berlyne et al 1961, Altman et al 1974) have claimed that it is possible in some families to detect clinically those heterozygous for the type I recessive form of PXE, most do not believe that this is possible at present.

Prenatal diagonsis has not been done in this disorder but theoretically in the more severe forms it might be possible to use a skin biopsy from a commonly involved site to demonstrate early predisposition to calcification of the elastic tissue.

Basic defect

The basic defect in PXE is not known, although it is thought that the elastic fibre is primarily involved. It has been shown quite clearly that calcification of elastic fibres is not only frequent in PXE, but that it is always present in the various lesions which can be detected by light microscopy. Furthermore, it has been demonstrated that calcification is the earliest recognizable change, occurring in elastic fibres which appear normal under light microscopy (Goodman et al 1963, Reeve et al 1979). Such observations suggest that calcification represents a far more basic aspect of PXE than has been previously suspected (Akhtar & Brody 1975).

More recently the work of Gordon et al (1983) suggested that the abnormal presence of the zinc-dependent cysteine protease in PXE fibroblasts may be associated with the biochemical lesion in this disease. Electron microscopy of elastic fibres from patients with PXE has shown that the principal alterations are in the elastin moiety (Ross et al 1978). In contrast, the micro-fibrillar component of the elastic fibre appears to be normal.

It has been shown by in situ hybridization experiments (Emanuel et al 1985) that the elastin gene is located on the long arm of chromosome 2. With this information it might prove informative to perform in situ hybridization studies in patients with PXE to determine if there are submicroscopic alterations in the region of the elastin gene. It would also be instructive to note if patients with deletions or other abnormalities in this region have any of the clinical features of PXE.

Prognosis and treatment

In considering the prognosis in patients with PXE it is important to know the genetic type. In general, the earlier the onset in PXE, the more severe are the manifestations and thus the worse the prognosis. For the more severe forms of the disease life span is shortened by various vascular complications involving the cardiovascular, gastrointestinal and central nervous systems.

Unfortunately no curative form of therapy is known. There have been a few isolated reports claiming that X-ray therapy (Carlborg 1944) and tocopherol have produced improvement in the skin lesions (Stout 1951). Ocular lesions have been treated with vitamin C in conjunction with calcium, and iodine and bismuth treatment has occasionally been used for resolving haemorrhages in the fundi (Carlborg 1944). Although none of these treatments has been successful, there are certain supportive measures that are worth bearing in mind. Since the most disabling feature of this disease is progressive loss of vision, the use of visual aids is important. Redundant and unsightly skin folds about the neck can be improved by plastic surgery. Gastrointestinal haemorrhage should usually be treated conservatively, though surgical intervention may be life saving.

More recently Renie et al (1984) reported on a positive correlation between the overall severity of PXE and calcium intake during adolescence. Because of these observations there is a need for a properly controlled prospective trial of the effect of different levels of dietary calcium on the clinical expression of PXE, particularly in young patients. Until such a trial is conducted some think it is prudent to counsel patients with PXE, particularly children and adolescents, to avoid indulging in food and liquids with a high calcium content.

CUTIS LAXA

Introduction

The genetic form of cutis laxa is a very rare disorder of connective tissue often confused with the Ehlers-Danlos syndrome and the severe type of PXE. Kopp (1888) described the disorder in a father and son and Weber (1923) was the first to discuss the clinical differences between this disorder and the Ehlers-Danlos syndrome. Many designations have been used to describe cutis laxa and they include such terms terms as: chalazoderma, cutis pendula, dermatomegaly, dermatochalasia and systemic elastolysis when there are internal manifestations. Beighton (1972) recognized the presence of genetic heterogeneity in cutis laxa and commented on the clinical differences between the dominant and recessive forms.

Clinical features

Skin

Characteristically the skin has the appearance of being too large for the rest of the body and thus tends to sag extensively in those areas where it is normally loose, e.g. around the face and eyes (Goodman & Gorlin 1977). Frequently the skin is wrinkled and appears prematurely aged so that an affected pubertal child will look older than his or her unaffected parents (Fig. 64.5). At birth, the skin may be soft and loose and nurses may comment on noticing a different 'feel' to the skin when compared to other infants. Even from birth the pendulous skin over the abdomen may cover the genitalia.

Unlike the skin in the Ehlers-Danlos syndrome, the skin in cutis laxa shows no fragility, bruisability or hyperextensibility. Some observers have noted that as affected individuals grow they tend to fill out their loose skin.

Facial

A number of facial features are common to this disorder and they include the following: an unusually long upper

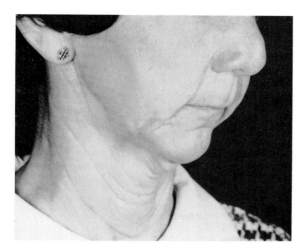

Fig. 64.5 Facial wrinkling in a 16-year-old girl with cutis laxa. (Courtesy of Professor P. Beighton.)

lip, hooking of the nose with shortening of the columella and unusually long ear lobes (Beighton 1970). Frequently the voice from birth may be deep and resonant in tone due to the laxity of the vocal cords. Micrognathia, delayed or bizarre tooth eruption and thickening of the oral and pharyngeal mucosa have also been observed. A variety of eye findings have been noted and these include ectropion of the lids, ocular hypertelorism, iris hypoplasia, blue sclerae and microcornea.

Internal manifestations

A variety of internal organ findings have been reported, but lung involvement with emphysematous changes is one of the more common and severe manifestations of the recessive form of the disorder (McKusick 1972). This may cause right ventricular enlargement, cor pulmonale and death at any early age. Pulmonary artery stenosis and extremely tortuous blood vessels along with dilation of the aorta have also been observed in the recessive form.

Inguinal, diaphragmatic, and umbilical hernias have been described as well as diverticulae of the oesophagus, stomach, intestine and bladder. Prolapse of the rectum and uterus has been reported.

Musculoskeletal changes include such findings as delayed somatic growth, hypotonia, late closure of the anterior fontanelle, hip dislocation and joint hyperextensibility.

Diagnosis

The clinical features are usually present at birth or in infancy with the skin changes giving a prematurely aged

appearance to the affected individual. A skin biopsy shows a reduced number of elastic fibres which are fragmented and granular (Goltz et al 1965).

X-ray studies may show various types of herniations, prolapses and diverticula, while arteriographic studies may reveal pulmonary artery stenosis, dilation of the aorta and kinking of peripheral vessels (Meine et al 1974).

Differential diagnosis

Cutis laxa may develop as a secondary manifestation in the later stages of certain infectious diseases affecting the dermis, or secondary to an allergic phenomenon such as a contact dermatitis or penicillin allergy (Rock et al 1979). In the acquired forms of cutis laxa the skin changes are like those of the congenital or genetic form but they begin in adulthood.

More recently Linares et al (1979) reported an infant with generalized cutis laxa born to a cystinuric mother who took penicillamine throughout pregnancy. By the age of nine months the infant had normal skin. They postulated that the D-penicillamine treatment may have produced low blood copper levels accounting for the connective tissue changes present at birth. Walshe (1979) challenged the interpretation of the copper studies done by Linares et al (1979) and felt the skin changes could not be attributed to copper depletion.

Cutis laxa confined to the anterior abdominal wall and thorax and present from birth may occur in association with dysplasia of the abdominal musculature, deformity of the thorax and mediastinal hernia.

Loose skin folds may develop in certain areas of the body in patients with the Ehlers-Danlos syndrome, PXE, neurofibromatosis, blepharochalasis and leprechaunism, but these disorders can usually be differentiated from cutis laxa by their other clinical manifestations and/or skin histopathological findings.

Two other genetic syndromes which have skin findings that should be considered in the differential diagnosis of cutis laxa are the wrinkly skin syndrome and geroderma osteodysplastica. These will be discussed subsequently.

Genetics

Incidence and prevalence

The genetic forms of cutis laxa are extremely rare and as of 1987 not more than 70 well documented cases have been reported in the medical literature. Almost all patients have been Caucasian.

Sex ratio

No unusual sex ratio has been noted.

Inheritance

Autosomal dominant and recessive forms of cutis laxa are well recognized. The most common and severe type is transmitted as an autosomal recessive and the parents are frequently consanguineous. In this form, congenital cutis laxa is associated with a generalized disorder of elastic tissue leading to various kinds of hernias, diverticula and infantile emphysema. Death usually occurs during the first year of life. There is obvious heterogeneity within the autosomal recessive group as evidenced by reports of cutis laxa occurring in other distinct syndromes. For example, De Barsy and co-workers (1968) described an infant girl who had cutis laxa, hypotonia, bilateral congenital athetosis, cloudy corneas and psychomotor retardation. Since this report both isolated and familial cases with these findings have been reported (Kunze et al 1985). The De Barsy syndrome is thought to be an autosomal recessive disorder. Anderson et al (1984) reported on a consanguineous family in which three of four sibs had severe congenital haemolytic anaemia of unknown cause and early onset of pulmonary emphysema. Two of the three affected sibs died of septic shock after splenectomy at ages 7 and 3½ years. The third sib, 20 years old at the time of their report, had severe pulmonary emphysema and cutis laxa. We have also seen a case of cutis laxa with a variety of findings suggesting a new syndrome transmitted as an autosomal recessive trait. Further reporting and documentation of all such cases is necessary before an adequate classification can be formulated.

A less commonly observed form is the relatively benign autosomal dominant type (Beighton 1972). The reported mild sporadic cases are probably of this type. An X-linked disorder associated with decreased lysyl oxidase activity, initially termed X-linked recessive cutis laxa (Byers et al 1976), is now designated Ehlers-Danlos type IX. Acquired forms of cutis laxa differ from genetic varieties in their mode of presentation, course and progression (see *Differential diagnosis* above).

Genetic counselling and prenatal diagnosis

As with any heritable disorder in which there is genetic heterogeneity, it is essential to know which form of the condition the patient is afflicted with before embarking on genetic counselling. Once this is established, recurrence risks can be given according to the mode of transmission be it autosomal dominant or recessive.

If a skin biopsy could be obtained using fetoscopy then a fetus at risk for the more severe autosomal recessive form of the disorder could possibly be diagnosed based on the histopathological features of cutis laxa.

Basic defect

The basic defect in all forms of cutis laxa is not known. Nevertheless, histopathological studies using both light (Goltz et al 1965) and electron miscroscopy (Hashimoto & Kanzaki 1975) have shown that it is primarily the elastic fibre that undergoes change. Some investigators have postulated that there is increased susceptibility of elastin to the action of elastase, due to a deficiency of elastase inhibitor resulting from a disturbance of copper metabolism (Goltz & Hult 1965). However, there is no evidence at present to support this hypothesis (Harris et al 1978).

Prognosis and treatment

The autosomal recessive form often leads to death early in childhood, due to cardiorespiratory complications. The dominant form is not a life-threatening condition in the early years of life but various complications, reflecting tissue weakness of internal organs, should be looked for as these patients age.

Plastic surgery should be considered to reduce the cosmetic disfigurement and to improve the psychosocial attitude of the patient. Periodic respiratory function studies should be done to ensure early diagnosis of associated emphysema. In children with heart failure, upper airway obstruction should be evaluated and tracheostomy considered.

WRINKLY SKIN SYNDROME

Clinical features

This genetic disorder of connective tissue was first described by Gazit and co-workers (1973) in three sibs of consanguineous parents.

At birth it was noted that all three affected sibs were hypotonic and small for dates although all were full-term. The most striking physical finding pertained to the skin. Over most of the body, except the face, the skin appeared dry and easily wrinkled, as noted about the abdomen in the sitting position (Fig. 64.6). Numerous skin wrinkles were noted on the dorsal and ventral surfaces of the hands (Fig. 64.7) and feet. This wrinkled appearance of the skin about the hands and feet was present from birth. A reduction in the elasticity of skin about the hands was noted but there appeared to be no altered skin elasticity in other parts of the body. A prominent venous pattern was observed on the anterior surface of the chest and the dorsal surface of the hands and feet. The skin did not sag, there was no evidence of abnormal scar tissue formation and no history of easy bruisability. The joints were not

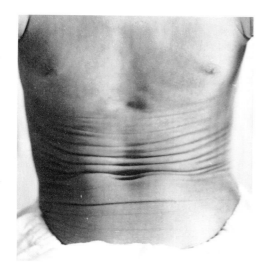

Fig. 64.6   Multiple abdominal skin wrinkles in a 9-year-old girl with the wrinkly skin syndrome.

hyperextensible. The two affected sibs had kyphosis, 'winging' of the scapulae and poor muscle development. In addition one of them had microcephaly with moderate mental retardation along with myopic changes with old chorioretinitis and partial optic atrophy.

Now that more cases of this disorder have been reported (Goodman et al 1982, Karrar et al 1983, Casamassima et al 1987) the characteristic clinical features have been delineated as wrinkling of the skin of the dorsum of the hands and feet, decreased elastic recoil of the skin in affected areas, an increased number of palmar and plantar creases, multiple musculoskeletal abnormalities, microcephaly and mental retardation. One patient had an atrial septal aneurysm (Casamassima et al 1987).

Diagnosis

At present the diagnosis of this syndrome is based primarily on the clinical features described above. Initially no distinct histopathological changes were observed from biopsied skin tissue studied under light microscopy (Gazit et al 1973). However, recently Casamassima et al (1987) reported atrophy of the epidermis and fragmentation of the elastic fibres in a skin biopsy taken from the wrinkled skin of the dorsum of the hand. Electron microscopy did not show any abnormalities.

Duksin et al (1983) reported on an Israeli child (9-year-old girl) with the wrinkly skin syndrome and demonstrated that her cultured skin fibroblasts had altered protein glycosylation, and procollagen to collagen conversion was impaired with procollagen chains accumulating in the growth medium. This biochemical finding, along with the recently described histopathological changes needs confirmation.

Differential diagnosis

The wrinkly skin syndrome can be distinguished from cutis laxa by clinical findings and skin biopsy. In cutis laxa the facial skin characteristically hangs loose giving a prematurely aged appearance to the patient. On skin biopsy in cutis laxa there are a diminished number of elastic fibres that are thin and fragmented. Clumping of fibres and ectopic aggregation of dense granules are also seen. Hyperextensible skin and joints in the various forms of the Ehlers-Danlos syndrome, along with ease in bruisability and poor scar tissue formation, differentiate this disorder from the wrinkly skin syndrome.

Genetics

This condition is transmitted as an autosomal recessive disorder. As of 1988 five affected unrelated families are

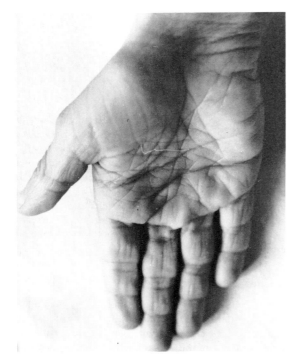

Fig. 64.7   Accentuated and multiple palmar creases in a 9-year-old girl with the wrinkly skin syndrome.

known to the author, three from Israel (Gazit et al 1973, Goodman et al 1982, one unpublished), one from Saudi Arabia (Karrar et al 1983) and one from a Moslem family from Malaysia (Casamassima et al 1987). In all instances the parents have been normal and consanguineous. The three families from Israel are of non-Ashkenazi Jewish ancestry. The above observations suggest that the gene for this disorder may be more common in populations of Middle Eastern origin.

The recurrence risk for this disorder is that of any other autosomal recessive disease. Prenatal diagnosis is not currently available.

Basic defect

The basic defect in this heritable disorder of connective tissue is not known.

Prognosis and treatment

Not enough is known about this syndrome to assess all its possible prognostic features. For example, there is no certainty that the microcephaly with mental retardation observed in one affected sib is part of the disorder. No special treatment other than symptomatic care is indicated.

GERODERMA OSTEODYSPLASTICA

Clinical features

This heritable disorder of connective tissue was first described by Bamatter and co-workers (1949) and is characterized by distinct facial and musculoskeletal findings.

The skin about the face gives the appearance of premature ageing due to excessive wrinkling and atrophic changes (Fig. 64.8). Eye abnormalities may include microcornea, myopia and keratoconus. Frequently these patients have micrognathia and various dental anomalies. Premature wrinkling of the skin is also common about the abdomen and dorsal surface of the hands and feet.

Musculoskeletal findings include the following: short stature, excessive length of the upper extremities, stooped posture due to kyphoscoliosis, 'winging' of the scapulae, pes planus, hyperextensible joints with ease in dislocation, muscular hypotonia with a protuberant abdomen and hernias.

Diagnosis

The diagnosis of this syndrome is a clinical one and many of the above clinical features are present from early childhood. X-ray studies show generalized osteoporosis, platyspondyly and multiple incremental lines within bones like growth rings of a tree (Brocher 1968). A skin

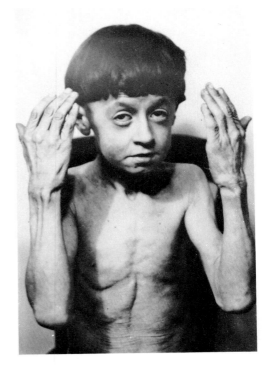

Fig. 64.8 A 10-year-old boy with geroderma osteodysplastica showing premature wrinkling of the skin. (Courtesy of Professor D. Klein.)

biopsy showed atrophy of the epidermis and fragmentation of the elastic fibres (Lisker et al 1979).

Differential diagnosis

This syndrome must be differentiated from cutis laxa and the wrinkly skin syndrome. The laxity of the skin in geroderma osteodysplastica is not generally as severe as that observed in cutis laxa, and the extensive skeletal changes known to be present in the former are not found in either cutis laxa or the wrinkly skin syndrome. A skin biopsy from a patient with the wrinkly skin syndrome does not show specific changes, whereas characteristic findings have been observed in both cutis laxa and geroderma osteodysplastica.

Genetics

In the original Swiss family reported by Bamatter et al (1949), Boreux (1969) postulated that the disorder might be inherited as an X-linked recessive trait with mild manifestations in the female. Hunter and co-workers (1978) reported two families with six affected children. Consanguinity and two fully affected females among the six children strongly support autosomal recessive transmission. Genetic heterogeneity in this rare syndrome is a possibility but actual verification must await reports of other families.

Genetic counselling must be based on the most likely mode of transmission for the family in question. Prenatal diagnosis has not been done in this disorder.

Basis defect

The basic defect in this syndrome is not known.

Prognosis and treatment

At present there is no evidence to suggest that affected individuals have a shortened life span. Because of their osteoporosis these patients are prone to fractures, espe-

cially of the vertebrae. Treatment for the osteoporosis is required. Possible orthopaedic intervention for correction of the kyphoscoliosis and plastic surgery for the facial skin involvement should be considered.

ACKNOWLEDGEMENTS

Supported by grants to R. M. Goodman from the National Foundation for Jewish Genetic Diseases and LA-CO Industries Inc. of the United States.

NOTE ADDED IN PROOF

Professor Goodman completely revised his chapter at proof stage but died in 1989 prior to the book's publication.

REFERENCES

Pseudoxanthoma elasticum

Akhtar M, Brody H 1975 Elastic tissue in pseudoxanthoma elasticum: ultrastructural study of endocardial lesions. Archives of Pathology 99: 667–671

Altman L K, Fialkow P J, Parker F, Sagebiel R W 1974 Pseudoxanthoma elasticum. Archives of Internal Medicine 134: 1048–1054

Balzer F 1884 Recherches sur les characters anatomiques du xanthelasma. Archives of Physiology 4: 65–80

Bentley F H, Barlow T E 1952 The vascular anatomy of the stomach. Modern Trends in Gastroenterology. Butterworth, London p 309

Berlyne G M, Bulmer H G, Platt R 1961 The genetics of pseudoxanthoma elasticum. Quarterly Journal of Medicine 30: 201–212

Böck J 1938 Zur Klinik und Anatomie der Gefässählichen Streifen im Augenhintergrund. Zeitschrift für Augenheilkunde 95: 1

Carlborg U 1944 Study of circulatory disturbances, pulse wave velocity and pressure pulses in large arteries in cases of pseudoxanthoma elasticum, and angioid streaks. A contribution to the knowledge of the function of the elastic tissue and the smooth muscles in larger arteries. Acta Medica Scandinavica 151: 1

Connor P J, Juergens J L, Perry H O, Hollenhorst R W, Edwards J E 1961 Pseudoxanthoma elasticum and angioid streaks, a review of 106 cases. American Journal of Medicine 30: 537–543

Darier J 1896 Pseudoxanthoma elasticum. Monatsh Prakt Dermatol 23: 609–617

De Simone S, De Concilliis U 1958 Strie angioidi della retina (considerazioni cliniche e patogenetiche). Archives of Otolaryngology 62: 161

Elejalde B R 1984 Manifestations of pseudoxanthoma elasticum during pregnancy: A case report and review of the literature. American Journal of Medical Genetics 18: 755–762

Emanuel B S, Cannizzaro L, Ornstein-Goldstein N et al 1985 Chromosomal localization of the human elastin gene. American Journal of Human Genetics 37: 873–882

Geereats W J, Guerry J 1960 Angioid streaks and sickle cell disease. American Journal of Ophthalmology 49: 450–470

Goodman R M, Smith E W, Paton D et al 1963

Pseudoxanthoma elasticum: A clinical and histopathological study. Medicine (Baltimore) 42: 297–334

Gordon S G, Hinkle L L, Shaw E 1983 Cysteine protease characteristics of proteoglycanase activity from normal and pseudoxanthoma elasticum (PXE) fibroblasts. Journal of Laboratory and Clinical Medicine 102: 400–410

Gronblad E 1929 Angioid streak — pseudoxanthoma elasticum: Vorläufige Mitteilung. Acta Ophthalmologica (Kbh) 7: 329

Iqbal A, Alter M, Lee S H 1978 Pseudoxanthoma elasticum: A review of neurological complications. Annals of Neurology 4: 18–20

Lao T T, Walters B N J, De Swiet M 1984 Pseudoxanthoma elasticum and pregnancy. Two case reports. British Journal of Obstetrics and Gynaecology 91: 1049–1050

Lebwohl M, Distefano D, Priokau P G, Uram M, Yannuzzi L A, Fleischmajer R 1982 Pseudoxanthoma elasticum and mitral-valve prolapse. New England Journal of Medicine 307: 228–231

Lebwohl M, Phelps R G, Yannuzzi L, Chang S, Schwartz I, Fuchs W 1987 Diagnosis of pseudoxanthoma elasticum by scar biopsy in patients without characteristic skin lesions. New England Journal of Medicine 317: 347–350

Lewis G M, Clayton M D 1933 Pseudoxanthoma elasticum and angioid streaks. Archives of Dermatology and Syphilology 28: 546–556

Light N, Meyrick R H, Stephens A, Kirby J D T, Fryer P R, Avery N C 1986 Collagen and elastin changes in D-penicillamine-induced pseudoxanthoma elasticum-like skin. British Journal of Dermatology 114: 381–388

McKusick V A 1972 Heritable disorders of connective tissue, 4th edn. C V Mosby, St Louis p 475–529

McPhaul J J Jr, Engel F L 1961 Heterotopic calcification, hyperphosphatemia and angioid streaks of the retina. American Journal of Medicine 31: 488–492

Pope F M 1974a Autosomal dominant pseudoxanthoma elasticum. Journal of Medical Genetics 11: 152–157

Pope F M 1974b Two types of autosomal recessive pseudoxanthoma elasticum. Archives of Dermatology 110: 209–212

Pope F M 1975 Historical evidence for the genetic heterogeneity of pseudoxanthoma elasticum. British Journal of Dermatology 92: 493–510

Pyeritz R E, Weiss J L, Renie W A, Fine S L 1982 Pseudoxanthoma elasticum and mitral-valve prolapse

(Letter). New England Journal of Medicine 307: 1451–1452

Reeve E B et al 1979 Development and calcification of skin lesions in thirty-nine patients with pseudoxanthoma elasticum. Clinics in Experimental Dermatology 3: 291–301

Renie W A, Pyeritz R E, Combs J, Fine S L 1984 Pseudoxanthoma elasticum: High calcium intake in early life correlates with severity. American Journal of Medical Genetics 19: 235–244

Rigal D 1881 Observation pour servir á l'histoire de la chéloide diffuse xanthelasmique. Annals of Dermatology and Syphilology 2: 491–501

Ross R, Fialkow P J, Altman L K 1978 Fine structure alterations of elastic fibers in pseudoxanthoma elasticum. Clinical Genetics 13: 213–223

Schmorl G 1931 Anatomische Befunde bei einem Fall von Osteopoikilic. Fortschritte auf dem Gebiete der Roentgenstrahlen und der Nuklearmedizin 44: 1–8

Shaffer B, Copelan H W, Beerman H 1957 Pseudoxanthoma elasticum. A case of Paget's disease and a case of calcinosis with arteriosclerosis as manifestations of the syndrome. Archives of Dermatology 76: 622–633

Smith E W, Malak J, Goodman R M, McKusick V A 1962 Reactive perforating elastoma: A feature of certain genetic disorders. Bulletin of the Johns Hopkins Hospital 11: 235–251

Stout O M 1951 Pseudoxanthoma elasticum with retinal angioid streaking, decidedly improved on tocopherol therapy. Archives of Dermatology and Syphilology 63: 510–511

Strandberg J 1929 Pseudoxanthoma elasticum. Zeitschrift für Haut – und Geschlechtskrankheiten 31: 689

Témine P 1940 Contribution à l'étude de l'elastorrhexie systématisée. Paris thesis et cie, Paris

Tunbridge R E, Tattersall R N, Hall D A, Astbury W T, Reed R 1952 The fibrous structure of normal and abnormal human skin. Clinical Science 11: 315

Viljoen D, Pope F M, Beighton P 1987 Heterogeneity of pseudoxanthoma elasticum: delineation of a new form? Clinical Genetics 32: 100–105

Woodcock C W 1952 Pseudoxanthoma elasticum, angioid streaks of retina and osteitis deformans. Archives of Dermatology and Syphilology 65:623

Cutis laxa

Anderson C E, Finkelstein J, Nyssbaum E et al 1984 Association of hemolytic anemia and early-onset pulmonary emphysema in three siblings. Journal of Pediatrics 105: 247–251

Beighton P 1972 The dominant and recessive forms of cutis laxa. Journal of Medical Genetics 9: 216–221

Beighton P, Bull J C, Edgerton M T 1970 Plastic surgery in cutis laxa. British Journal of Plastic Surgery 23: 285–290

Byers P H, Narayanan A S, Bornstein P 1976 An X-linked form of cutis laxa due to deficiency of lysyl oxidase; the collagen and elastin crosslinking enzyme. Birth Defects 36: 293–298

De Barsy A M, Moens E, Dierckx L 1968 Dwarfism, oligophrenia and degeneration of the elastic tissue in the skin and cornea. A new syndrome? Helvetica Paediatrica Acta 23: 305–313

Goltz R W, Hult A M 1965 Generalized elastolysis (cutis laxa) and Ehlers-Danlos syndrome (cutis hyperelastica); a comparative clinical and laboratory study. Southern Medical Journal 58: 848–854

Goltz R W, Hull A M, Goldfarb M, Gorlin R J 1965 Cutis laxa, a manifestation of generalized elastolysis. Archives of Dermatology 92: 373–387

Goodman R M, Gorlin R J 1977 Atlas of the face in genetic disorders. C V Mosby, St Louis p 106–107

Harris R B, Heaphy M R, Perry H O 1978 Generalized elastolysis (cutis laxa). American Journal of Medicine 65: 815–822

Hashimoto K, Kanzaki T 1975 Cutis laxa ultrastructural and biochemical studies. Archives of Dermatology 111: 861–873

Kopp W 1888 Demonstration zweier Falle von 'Cutis laxa'. Munchener Medizinische Wochenschrift 35: 259–260

Kunze J, Majewski F, Montgomery P, Hockey A, Karkut I, Riebel P 1985 DeBarsy syndrome – an autosomal recessive, progeroid syndrome. European Journal of Pediatrics 144: 348–354

Linares A, Farrant J J, Rodrigez-Alancon J, Diaz-Perez J L 1979 Reversible cutis laxa due to maternal D-penicillamine treatment. Lancet 2: 43

McKusick V A 1972 Heritable disorders of connective tissue, 4th edn. C V Mosby, St Louis p 372–389

Meine F, Grossman H, Forman W, Jackson D 1974 The radiographic findings in congenital cutis laxa. Radiology 113: 687–690

Rook A et al 1979 Textbook of dermatology, 3rd edn. Blackwell, London p 1626–1627

Walshe J M 1979 Congenital cutis laxa and maternal D-penicillamine. Lancet 2: 144–145

Weber F P 1923 Chalasodermia or "loose skin" and its relationship to subcutaneous fibroids or calcareous nodules. Urologic and Cutaneous Reviews 27: 407

Wrinkly skin syndrome

Casamassima A C, Wesson S K, Conlon C J, Weiss F H 1987 Wrinkly skin sydrome: Phenotype and additional manifestations. American Journal of Medical Genetics 27: 885–893

Duksin D, Gal A, Goodman R M 1983 Altered protein glycosylation and procollagen to collagen conversion in human fibroblasts. Laboratory Investigation 49: 346–352

Gazit E, Goodman R M, Katznelson M B, Rotem Y 1973 Wrinkly skin syndrome: A new heritable disorder of connective tissue. Clinical Genetics 4: 186–192

Goodman R M, Duskin D, Legum C et al 1982 The wrinkly skin syndrome and cartilage-hair hypoplasia (a new variant?) in sibs of the same family. In: Papadatos C J, Bartsocas C S (eds) Skeletal Dysplasias. Alan R Liss, New York 104: 205–214

Karrar Z A, Elidrissy A T H, Al Arabi K, Adam K A 1983 The wrinkly skin syndrome: A report of two siblings from Saudi Arabia. Clinical Genetics 23: 308–310

Geroderma osteodysplastica

Bamatter F 1949 Gérodermie ostéodysplastique héréditaire. Un nouveau biotype de la "progeria". Confinia Neurologica 9: 397

Boreux G 1969 A gérodermie ostéodysplastique à hérédité liée au sexes, nouvelle entité clinique et génétique. Journal de Génétique Humaine 17: 137–178

Brocher J E W 1968 Roentgenologische Befunde bei Geroderma osteodysplastica hereditaria. Fortschritte anf dem Gebiete der Roentgenstrahlen und der Nuklearmedizin 109: 185–198

Hunter A G 1978 Geroderma osteodysplastica: a report of two affected families. Human Genetics 40: 311–325

Lisker R, Hernandez A, Martinez-Lavin H et al 1979 Gerodermia osteodysplastica hereditaria: Report of three affected brothers and literature review. American Journal of Medical Genetics 3: 389–395

65. Peptic ulcer

J. I. Rotter   T. Shohat

INTRODUCTION

The familial aggregation of peptic ulcer disease and its association with such clear-cut genetic factors as blood group O and non-secretor status is well established. However, the genetics of this disorder or group of disorders was, until the last decade, poorly delineated . At one time polygenic inheritance was the prevailing hypothesis proposed for peptic ulcer, based primarily on the finding of blood group associations and the exclusion of a simple mode of inheritance for all ulcer disease. Genetic heterogeneity was proposed as an alternative hypothesis that could explain both the familial aggregation of peptic ulcer disease and the lack of a simple Mendelian pattern of inheritance (Rotter & Rimoin 1977). This concept states that peptic ulcer is not one disease, but a group of disorders with different genetic and environmental causes. Initially based on indirect evidence, genetic heterogeneity has now received direct support from genetic studies using subclinical markers such as serum pepsinogen I (Rotter 1980a,b). The unravelling of the genetic heterogeneity of peptic ulcer has important clinical and aetiological implications, for if what is termed a 'disease' is in reality a number of disorders that are grouped together because of some common clinical feature, these distinct disorders may differ markedly in genetics, pathophysiology, interaction with environmental agents, natural history and response to therapeutic and preventive measures.

This chapter will discuss the current state of knowledge regarding the genetic basis of peptic ulcer. The concept of polygenic inheritance will be contrasted with that of genetic heterogeneity, and the methods for delineating genetic heterogeneity in a common disease such as ulcer will be described.

DISEASE DEFINITION AND DIFFICULTIES FOR GENETIC STUDIES

A peptic ulcer is a circumscribed loss of tissue occurring in those parts of the gastrointestinal tract exposed to acid and pepsin – in the main, the lower oesophagus, stomach and upper intestine (duodenum) (Grossman et al 1981, Grossman 1981). Its typical symptom is epigastric abdominal pain, worse at night and relieved by meals. Such classical symptoms occur only in a portion of all ulcer patients, and many present with less classical abdominal pain or with an ulcer complication. Complications include bleeding into the gastrointestinal tract (which can range from chronic blood loss to a severe life threatening haemorrhage), perforation (extension of the ulcer through the full thickness of the wall of the gastrointestinal tract), and obstruction of gastric emptying (from scarring and/or oedema and spasm). The diagnosis of a peptic ulcer is usually made by upper gastrointestinal radiography using a contrast material such as barium sulphate, or by direct visualization by endoscopy.

An ulcer is generally thought to occur when there is an imbalance between the 'aggressive' forces of acid and pepsin and the less defined 'defensive' forces of mucosal resistance and regeneration. The goal of ulcer therapy, both medical and surgical, is to correct this imbalance in order to promote ulcer healing, relieve symptoms, and prevent complications and recurrences. This is usually done by agents or methods that either buffer the acid produced (e.g. antacids) or reduce acid secretion (e.g. cimetidine, vagotomy), though protective agents such as prostaglandins and sulphated disaccharides are also being developed. A complete discussion of ulcer diagnosis and therapy is beyond the scope of this chapter and the reader is referred to more complete references of this area (Grossman et al 1981, Taylor 1988, Soll & Isenberg 1989). Peptic ulcer tends to be an episodic, chronic disorder, characterized by symptomatic periods and pain-free intervals. The natural history of ulcer is still being defined, and this may well vary as the different diseases leading to an ulcer are delineated by clinical, physiological and genetic studies.

Peptic ulcer is among the most common of chronic diseases, occurring in 5–10% of the population in their lifetime (depending on such factors as geography, population, level of health care) (Langman 1979, Grossman 1980, 1981, Kurata & Haile 1984). This leads to a number of problems for genetic studies. Is a relative affected because he has the same genotype, shares the same environment, or has the chance occurrence of a common disorder? Even if peptic ulcer is a group of disorders, these disorders are sufficiently common for different forms to occur in the same family by chance alone. The age of onset of peptic ulcer varies markedly. Therefore, it is impossible to say whether an individual who is clinically unaffected at any given time will become affected later in life. Like many common diseases, genetic studies of peptic ulcer have suffered from confusion engendered by the varying definitions of 'affected' used by different investigators. 'Affected' has ranged from a person who has abdominal pain to one with an endoscopically demonstrated crater. Probably the greatest obstacle limiting genetic studies has been ignorance of the basic defects in various kinds of peptic ulcer and the corresponding lack of genetic markers that would disclose clinically unaffected individuals with the hereditary predisposition.

Despite these difficulties, we have known for many years that genetic factors play a role in the aetiology of peptic ulcer, based on three lines of evidence: family studies; twin studies; and blood group studies.

EARLY GENETIC EVIDENCE

Family studies

The first approach in looking for genetic factors in a common disease is to determine whether familial aggregation is present. One compares the incidence of the disease in relatives of patients with the incidence in the general population. If increased, this is often the first indication that genetic factors are important in a disease. Family aggregation was noted in the late 1800s, but as with many diseases, the majority of initial reports presented one or a few pedigrees with no control data. Subsequently, individuals with peptic ulcer were shown to have an 'increased family history' of the disease (McConnell 1966, 1980). Most reports indicated a positive family history in 20–50% of individuals with peptic ulcer, compared to 5–15% in controls. While this information has been used to support the importance of genetic factors, it is of little value in testing genetic hypotheses, since the prevalence of a positive family history will vary greatly; with the type of interview, family size, number of relatives included, and with the criteria used for defining an affected individual. A more accurate assessment of familial aggregation is obtained by comparing the prevalence of the disorder among specific relatives of an affected individual to that found among similar

relatives of a control group. This was done in several excellent studies (see Table 65.1). The consistent observation was that the frequency of peptic ulcer was 2–3 times greater in the first-degree relatives of peptic ulcer patients than in similar relatives of controls or the general population. Because these differences persisted across generations and social classes, genetic factors were presumed to explain these findings.

Twin studies

Familial aggregation can conceivably be due to common environmental as well as common genetic factors. Twin studies represent an approach to resolving the question of the relative influence of genetics and environment. The frequency of concordance (both members of the twin pair affected) of monozygotic (identical) twins is compared with that of dizygotic (fraternal) twins. Monozygotic twins share all genes, and should be concordant for disorders with pure genetic aetiology. Dizygotic twins share on average only half their genes and are no more alike genetically than any pair of sibs. If the characteristic being studied is genetically determined with no environmental influence, then one expects 100% concordance in monozygotic twins, and less in dizygotic twins. If the disorder is entirely environmental, one should see equal concordance between monozygotic and dizygotic twins. If an interaction between a genetic predisposition and an environmental agent is necessary for clinical expression, one would expect to find a higher concordance among monozygotic than dizygotic twins, but not 100%. For peptic ulcer the concordance in monozygotic twins is less than 100% but consistently exceeds that in dizygotic twins (Table 65.2). This difference persists when dizygotic twins are restricted to those pairs of like sex. From the twin studies we can conclude that a large part of the familial aggregation is due to genetic factors.

Blood group studies

The third line of evidence for genetic factors in ulcer came from studies of blood group associations. The goal of such disease association studies is to determine the prevalence of a disorder among individuals with well defined genetic traits, such as blood groups or serum enzyme polymorphisms (also known as qualitative gene markers). If there is a positive association between a given disease and a particular allele of a well defined genetic locus, then the genetically determined trait is usually considered to be of importance in the pathogenesis of the disorder under study. Soon after the original association between blood group A and gastric cancer was described,

Table 65.1 Peptic ulcer in families

Author	Proband's diagnosis	Relatives studied	Criteria	Relatives of ulcer proband	Relatives of controls or population controls
Doll & Buch 1950	Peptic ulcer	Brothers	Hospital	11.5%	4.6%
		Sisters	records (60%)	2.8%	0.9%
		Fathers	Patient's	16.4%	4.5%
		Mothers	account (40%)	4.3%	–
Wretmark 1953	Peptic ulcer	Brothers	History	15.0%	6.6–8.1%
		Fathers	from	14.8%	3.6%
		Mothers	proband	7.4%	1.2%
Kuenssberg 1962	Duodenal ulcer	Sons	History	7.9%	2.4%
		Daughters	from proband	5.1%	0.7%
Monson 1970a	Peptic ulcer	Fathers	History	24.5%	14.4%
		Mothers	from	9.5%	4.5%
		Brothers	proband	14.3%	6.5%
		Sisters		3.7%	1.6%
Jirasek 1971	Duodenal ulcer	Parents	History	14.7%	
		Sibs	from	9.9%	
	Duodenal Gastric	Parents	proband	10.0%	
	ulcer	Sibs		8.0%	1.5–4.8%
	Pyloric ulcer	Parents		8.0%	
		Sibs		7.1%	
	Gastric ulcer	Parents		12.1%	
		Sibs		6.8%	
Kubickova &	Duodenal ulcer	First-degree	History	9.5%	1.7%
Vesely 1972		Second-degree	from	2.9%	0.5%
		Third-degree	proband	1.4%	0.22%

the same group of investigators demonstrated that peptic ulcer was associated with blood group O (Aird et al 1954). Individuals with blood group O have a 30–40% greater incidence of peptic ulcer than those of the remaining blood groups (McConnell 1966, 1980, Mourant el al 1978). The blood group O association is particularly evident with duodenal ulcer and ulcers of the antrum and prepylorus, but not with ulcers of the body of the stomach (Vesely et al 1968). One might question whether this relatively small increased risk is real. Yet this observation has been repeated by many investigators in many countries, and in different racial and ethnic groups throughout the world. The physiological basis for the blood group O association remains unknown. Attempts have been made to relate it to the acid secretory capacity of the stomach, as defined by serum pepsinogen

Table 65.2 Peptic ulcer in twins

Author	Criteria	No. of pairs	Concordance MZ	DZ
Camerer (1936)	Often clinical	14	14%	14%
Huhn (1939)	Questionnaire, then X-ray	13	80%	0%
Doig (1957)	X-ray	10	50%	12.5%
Harvald & Hauge (1958)	Hospitalized	112	18%	7.2%
Marshall et al (1962)[*]	X-ray	58	14.3%	6.3%
Eberhard (1968)	X-ray	112	50.0%	14.1%
Pollin et al (1969)[†]	Medical records	837	11.3%	5.8%
Gotlieb–Jensen (1972)[‡].	X-ray of all twins	181	52.6%	35.7%

[*] Very young population.
[†] Duodenal ulcer only. Based on follow-up of US World War II veterans, whose care is still under the Veterans Administration.
[‡] An excellent detailed study using the Danish twin registry. Should be compared with Harvald and Hauge (1958), same twin source, to show what detailed investigation and an extra 10 years of follow-up reveals.

or maximal acid output, but no consistent relationship has been delineated (McConnell 1966, Langman 1973, Lam & Sircus 1975, Prescott et al 1976). A small yet statistically significant relationship has been reported between blood group O and ulcer complications, especially bleeding (Evans et al 1968, Lam & Sircus 1975, Lam & Ong 1976, Mourant et al 1978). Studies in Hong Kong, Scotland and Argentina further characterized this association, suggesting that the blood group O association seemed predominantly confined to the older onset group of duodenal ulcer patients (Gutierrez-Cabano 1983, Lam et al 1983b). The next polymorphic genetic marker found to be associated with peptic ulcer was nonsecretor status (Clarke et al 1956). Nonsecretors are 40–50% more likely to have a duodenal ulcer than secretors (McConnell 1966, Mourant et al 1978). The effect of the two genes, O and nonsecretor, on the risk for ulcer seem to be multiplicative (Doll et al 1961, Langman 1973). The relative risk for duodenal ulcer in a blood group O individual is 1.3 (30% increase over a non-O individual), and the relative risk for duodenal ulcer in a nonsecretor is 1.5 (increased 50% over a secretor). Individuals who are both O and nonsecretor have a relative risk for duodenal ulcer of approximately 2.5 (hence the term multiplicative).

Many other gene marker associations have been reported with peptic ulcer (Table 65.3) (reviewed in Rotter 1980b). As can be seen, some eight different genetic systems have been implicated at one time or another as predisposing to peptic ulcer, making peptic ulcer the most 'associated' disorder in man. Some of these associations, notably blood group O and blood group nonsecretor, are so well established that they are undeniably real. Others, such as Rh positivity, are of such small effect, relative risk 1.1 for duodenal ulcer, that they must remain of questionable importance. In the case of HLA antigens an increased incidence of the class I antigens B5, B12 and B35 has been observed (Ellis & Woodrow 1979, Gough et al 1982). It is possible that these associations might be more easily distinguished when subgroups of patients are examined. Indeed, when the HLA association was examined in a duodenal ulcer sample that was divided by age of onset, HLA B35 was found in 25% of patients with onset over age 30 and in none of the patients with onset of ulcer under 30 years (Goedhard et al 1983). The remaining associations listed in Table 65.3 have only been examined in a few or even single studies, and so must be considered tentative. What can we conclude about the genetics of ulcer from this wealth of association data? There are two major possibilities. One is that each of these genes has a small effect in predisposing to peptic ulcer, a true polygenic system. The other is that each predisposes to a specific subgroup of peptic ulcer. If the latter hypothesis is true then, as subgroups are delineated, one would expect stronger associations in certain subgroups, and no association in others. In contrast, if these predispositions are truly polygenic in nature, then these associations should occur across ulcer groups. Our understanding of the nature of these various associations in relation to peptic ulcer would be greatly enhanced if we were able to delineate the physiological basis of each of them. In the case of blood group O and nonsecretor status, the pathophysiological relationships to ulcer remain unknown after more than 20 years of study. This is probably because the degree of the association is so small. It has been

Table 65.3   Gene marker associations with peptic ulcer*

Polymorphic allele with increased risk for ulcer	Genetic marker system	Number of reports	Relative risk	Comments
0	ABO	>200	1.3	well established
nonsecretor	ABH secretor	~ 40	1.5	well established
RH⁺	Rh	~ 30	1.1	very small relative risk
taster	PTC tasting	2	1.4–2.7	
decreased α-1-antitrypsin activity	α-1-antitrypsin	5	1.4–3.0	? a partial explanation of ulcer pulmonary disease association
Pg^A	urinary pepsinogen phenotyping	2	2.4	? related to quantitative pepsinogen I
B5, B12, B35[†]	HLA	5 (1 negative)	2.1–2.9	? an immunologic form of ulcer
G6PD deficiency	glucose-6-phosphate dehydrogenase	1	2.2	

For references see Rotter 1980b
* Most associations are with duodenal ulcer; nonsecretor and alpha-1-antitrypsin are associated with duodenal and gastric ulcer.
[†] See Also Ellis & Woodrow 1979, Gough et al 1982, Goedhard et al 1983.

calculated that both O and nonsecretor combined contribute only 2.5–3% of the genetic variance to ulcer (Edwards 1965, Roberts 1965). In the case of α-1-antitrypsin deficiency, HLA antigens and urinary pepsinogen phenotype, there are clinical or theoretical clues for the association. Thus, even though the latter associations are still statistically tentative, the possibility of a pathophysiological relationship makes them of interest.

GENETIC INTERPRETATIONS – POLYGENIC VS GENETIC HETEROGENEITY

It has thus been clear for a number of years that genetic factors predispose to peptic ulcer, but the mode of inheritance of this genetic predisposition had not been resolved. For over a decade, the hypothesis of polygenic or multifactorial inheritance was used to explain the genetics of peptic ulcer (Roberts 1965, McConnell 1966, Cowan 1973). Peptic ulcer was placed in the polygenic category for two principal reasons. First, the inheritance of all ulcer disease could not be explained by any simple, single genetic defect – that is, the genetics of ulcer was not compatible with simple autosomal dominant, autosomal recessive or X–linked modes of inheritance. Second, the demonstration of the gene marker associations, blood group O and blood group nonsecretor status, provided some direct support for the polygenic hypothesis, since more than one gene seemed to contribute a small but measurable tendency towards peptic ulcer and the presence of both genes had a multiplicative effect. However, while there may be a polygenic contribution to peptic ulcer, the alternative mechanism of genetic heterogeneity is probably much more important.

Genetic heterogeneity was proposed as an alternative hypothesis that could explain both the familial aggregation of peptic ulcer disease and the lack of a simple Mendelian pattern of inheritance (Rotter et al 1976, Rotter & Rimoin 1977). Furthermore, genetic heterogeneity would better account for the varying physiological disturbances and diverse clinical manifestations that have been described in peptic ulcer patients. The concept of genetic heterogeneity states that a particular clinical disorder is, in reality, a group of distinct diseases with different aetiologies, both genetic and nongenetic which, by a variety of pathogenetic mechanisms, result in a similar clinical picture. In the absence of subclinical markers to help separate the different diseases, a number of distinct disorders may be lumped together in a common genetic analysis, masking the existence of subsets of a variety of simply inherited disorders, in such a way that the familial aggregation observed would appear to conform with the polygenic model. There has been an increasing realisation that peptic ulcer is not a single disorder, but a whole host of disorders with a common clinical manifestation, a hole in the lining of the gastrointestinal tract in those areas exposed to acid and pepsin (Grossman 1978, Rotter et al 1978, 1979d, 1980, Lam 1979).

Heterogeneity of a common disease can be demonstrated by the several methods listed in Table 65.4, and advances in all these areas have contributed to our knowledge of ulcer heterogeneity. These methods are being increasingly utilized to define the heterogeneity of many common gastrointestinal diseases (see Rotter et al 1980). The evidence for heterogeneity within peptic ulcer has accumulated rapidly over recent years, and this concept has gained increasingly widespread acceptance (Grossman 1978, Rotter et al 1979d, 1980, Lam 1979). It should be noted that many of the lines of evidence for ulcer heterogeneity are genetic. As will become apparent in our discussion, genetic methods are powerful tools for dissecting distinct disorders from a broad phenotype. Because of limitations of space, we can discuss each of these only briefly, and the interested reader is referred to more extensive reviews (Rotter et al 1980, Rotter 1980b, Rotter et al 1990).

GENETIC SYNDROMES WITH PEPTIC ULCER

The existence of well defined genetic and rare clinical syndromes that feature peptic ulceration is an important demonstration of genetic and aetiological heterogeneity. It also suggests that such heterogeneity may exist in common peptic ulcer. The existence of over 50 genetic syndromes with glucose intolerance, and in some cases frank diabetes, was an important early indicator of genetic heterogeneity within that group of disorders (Rimoin 1967, Rimoin & Schimke 1971, Rotter & Rimoin 1981). Besides the demonstration of heterogeneity, the study of such disorders serves an even more important function – such rare disorders may elucidate different pathogenetic mechanisms that can lead to the ulcer diathesis, and in the process teach us much about normal physiology and common pathophysiology. This is precisely what has occurred in at least one such syndrome – the Zollinger-Ellison (ZE) syndrome.

Multiple endocrine neoplasia syndrome, type I (MEN I)

MEN I is an autosomal dominant disorder characterized by pituitary, parathyroid and pancreatic adenomas (Ballard et al 1964, Rimoin & Schimke 1971, Schimke 1976). Its familial nature was first described by Wermer (1954). Soon after, Zollinger and Ellison (1955) reported a triad

Table 65.4 Methods of demonstrating heterogeneity in a common disease, peptic ulcer

Method	Example
1. Rare genetic syndromes with peptic ulcer	MEN I and ZE, systemic mastocytosis, ulcer-tremor-nystagmus (see also Table 65.5)
2. Ethnic variability	*Ulcer incidence and site* DU more frequent in Europe, GU more frequent in Japan *Complications* Stenosis common in African and Indian DU, haemorrhage most common in Europe
3. Clinical genetic studies	*Ulcer site* Increased familial risk is site specific, i.e. GU or DU runs in families or twin pairs
4. Clinical evidence	*Age of onset* Childhood DU vs adult DU Younger DU different complications than older DU
5. Heterogeneity of association with genetic polymorphisms	Blood group O associated with DU and not with GU of the body of the stomach
6. Physiological differences[†]	*GU vs DU* Acid secretion and serum pepsinogen I greater in DU than GU *Within DU* Acid hypersecretors and normosecretors Hyper PG I and normo PG I Increased and normal gastrin response Increased and normal rate of gastric emptying *Combined GU – DU* Positive gastrin-gastric acid correlation
7. Genetic studies utilizing physiological abnormalities as subclinical markers	Hyperpepsinogenaemic I DU vs Normopepsinogenaemic I DU Rapid emptying DU Antral G cell hyperfunction Abnormal PG I/PG II ratio

DU – duodenal ulcer; GU – gastric ulcer.
[†] – Includes biochemical, histological, immunological etc. See text and Rotter et al 1980, Rotter 1980a,b, 1981, Grossman et al 1981.

of: (1) fulminant peptic ulcer disease, with ulcers that could occur as far down the intestine as the jejunum and that would recur despite repeated operations; (2) gastric acid hypersecretion, with an elevated basal to maximal output ratio (greater than 0.6); and (3) non-beta islet cell tumours of the pancreas. This clinical syndrome was later shown to be due to secretion by the pancreatic tumours of the hormone gastrin, a major stimulant of acid secretion (Gregory et al 1960, 1967). All the features of the syndrome, which include gastric hyper-rugosity, hyperplasia, and hypersecretion, can be explained as consequences of the gastrin excess (Isenberg et al 1973). Thus, this syndrome aided in the elucidation of normal and abnormal gastric physiology. Until the association of ulcer disease with the endocrine tumours was recognized, the pattern of inheritance for multiple endocrine neoplasia elucidated, and the biochemical marker of increased plasma gastrin levels characterized, this specific entity was lost among the mass of peptic ulcer patients. The estimated prevalence of MEN I is 0.02–0.2 in 1000 (Lips et al 1984). The penetrance is probably complete: however, years may pass between the discovery of one neoplasm and the appearance of the next. Gastrinoma of the pancreas and associated ulcer disease may also occur as a sporadic somatic mutation without familial aggregation and without endocrine tumours in other organs. The sporadic and familial forms seem equally common (Rimoin & Schimke 1971, Lamers et al 1978, 1980). The diagnostic criterion of an elevated basal to maximal output ratio has essentially been replaced by the radioimmunoassay of gastrin in serum and the response of serum gastrin to a variety of stimuli, which include a protein meal, calcium and secretin (Lamers & van Tongeren 1977, Deveney et al 1977). With the distinctive marker of increased plasma gastrin as a tool, more and more patients are being diagnosed at a stage when they are clinically indistinguishable from 'common' peptic ulcer (Regan & Malagelada 1978). The gene for MEN I has recently been localized by linkage studies to chromosome 11 (Larsson et al 1988). This will enable prenatal diagnosis, as well as early diagnosis of first-degree relatives before any signs or symptoms have arisen. Until recently, the recommended therapy for this severe form of ulcer disease was total gastrectomy, but many patients are being treated successfully with H2 blockers such as cimetidine, often in combination with other agents (Grossman 1981, van Heerden et al 1986). In cases where treatment with H2-receptor antagonists fails, (as often happens with long-term treatment) Omeprazole®, which directly inhibits the hydrogen potassium ATPase, and thus reduces acid secretion by 77–100%, has been found to be very effective (Lamers et al 1984).

Systemic mastocytosis

Another multisystem syndrome that includes peptic ulcer as one of its manifestations is systemic mastocytosis, a disorder characterized by flushing, maculopapular rash, pruritus, abdominal pain and diarrhoea. Genetic factors would appear to be of major importance in this disorder, since six of eight reported monozygotic twin pairs have been concordant for the disorder (Selmanowitz et al 1970). A number of familial cases of systemic mastocytosis have been reported and both dominant and recessive modes of inheritance have been suggested (Shaw 1968, Selmanowitz et al 1970). However, a careful review of the pedigrees reported by Shaw (1968) clearly demonstrates examples of incomplete penetrance, and thus dominant susceptibility could reasonably be invoked to explain most pedigrees. This syndrome illuminates the role of another stimulant of acid secretion, histamine. These histamine excess syndromes can lead to gastric hypertrophy and gastric hypersecretion with high basal acid outputs, mimicking the Zollinger-Ellison syndrome, and to frank duodenal ulceration (Rotter 1980b). Erosive gastroduodenitis and elevated acid secretion can occur without elevated blood levels of histamine, but with elevated gastric tissue stores of the secretagogue. This observation by Ammann et al (1976) led them to conclude that it is the tissue, and not the serum, level of histamine that leads to gastrointestinal complications. This uncommon disorder demonstrates the important role of histamine in acid secretion, a role that has been confirmed by the discovery of the H-2 receptor (histamine receptor-2) blockers such as cimetidine, as potent inhibitors of gastric acid secretion (Grossman 1981, Grossman et al 1981). Therapy now includes the use of H-1 and H-2 blockers (Frieri et al 1985), though even together these are not always fully successful (Hirschowitz & Groarke 1979, Achord & Langford 1980).

Tremor-nystagmus-ulcer syndrome

Another distinct autosomal dominant syndrome associated with peptic ulcer consists of essential tremor, congenital nystagmus, duodenal ulcer, and a narcolepsy-like sleep disturbance. This was described in a family of Swedish-Finnish ancestry by Neuhauser et al (1976). Of 17 affected family members, 12 had essential tremor, 12 had nystagmus, and 8 had duodenal ulcer; the latter occurred almost exclusively in individuals with the neurological syndrome and sometimes preceding the onset of neurological symptoms. Basal and maximal gastric acid outputs were unremarkable (range 1.9–4.0 meq/hr and 23.4–58.4 meq/hr, respectively). Both essential tremor and narcolepsy appear most often to be dominant disorders (Pratt 1967, Baraitser & Parkes 1978), and it might be useful to ascertain such a disorder through neurology clinics. However, this clinical entity was not identified in a series of 50 narcolepsy cases (Parkes 1979). A strong association has been reported between HLA antigen DR2 and narcolepsy in all populations studied, with 98% of affected individuals carrying the DR2-DW2/DQW1 haplotype (Langdon et al 1984). It might be that involvement of either autoimmune immunological mechanisms or susceptibility to specific neurotropic viral agents (similar to the mechanism suggested for multiple sclerosis which is also strongly associated with DR2) leads to this syndrome.

Amyloidosis (Van Allen type)

Another dominant disorder accompanied by peptic ulcer is a distinct form of amyloidosis reported by Van Allen et al (1969). The term amyloidosis encompasses a variety of disorders which have in common the presence of infiltrates in various tissues of amyloid, a heterogeneous complex of insoluble proteins and/or protein polysaccharides. Amyloidosis can be secondary to chronic inflammation due to infections or autoimmune diseases, to deposition of immunoglobulin light chains in plasma cell dyscrasias, and in other cases can have a clear genetic basis. In fact, over a dozen hereditary disorders with amyloidosis as one of their cardinal features are recognized (Glenner et al 1978, McKusick 1988). In a large family of English-Scottish-Irish origin, Van Allen et al (1969) were able to identify 12 affected members in two generations, 8 of whom had confirmation of their amyloidosis by pathological studies. Male to male transmission supported dominant inheritance. Duodenal ulcer occured in 9 of the 12 affected individuals, with death due to perforation in one. The mechanism of the ulcer predisposition remains obscure, but it appears not to be due to local amyloid infiltration. Other prominent features were chronic progressive sensorimotor neuropathy, involving the lower extremities most prominently and usually the means of presentation, and amyloid nephropathy leading to renal failure as the usual cause of death. Onset was on the average in the mid 30s and death in the late 40s. Other features included deafness and cataracts. Nichols et al (1987) identified a protein homologous to apolipoprotein A-I as a major component of the amyloid in this kindred. Gimeno et al (1974) appeared to have identified a similarly affected individual, with a prominent family history of ulcer, deafness and renal disease.

Other syndromes

The relationship of peptic ulcer to the above mentioned syndromes appears clear. There are several additional genetic disorders in which an increased incidence of peptic ulcer has been suggested. These include hyperparathyroidism (this association may be solely through MEN I), cystic fibrosis, α-1-antitrypsin deficiency, carcinoid syndrome, 'stiff skin and multisystem disease', pachydermoperiostosis leuconychia-gallstone syndrome, gastrocutaneous syndrome and phenylketonuria (see Table 65.5) (Rotter 1980b, Lam et al 1981). Though less well established, each of these suggest the possibility of a different pathogenetic mechanism leading to peptic ulceration. In the case of hyperparathyroidism this may occur via increased acid secretion (Barreras 1973). Grossman (1972) has argued that the increased incidence of duodenal ulcer and gastric hypersecretion in hyperparathyroid patients, if it occurs, could well be due to the coexistent occurrence of parathyroid with gastrin tumours as part of MEN I. A systematic study of gastrin levels and their response to provocative agents in hyperparathyroid patients and their families is needed to answer this question. The association of duodenal ulcer and cystic fibrosis could occur through inadequate acid neutralization by deficient pancreatic secretions. The possible association of ulcer and α-1-antitrypsin deficiency is of interest because the association may be with both gastric and duodenal ulcer, and because it may serve as a model of deficient mucosal protection that could explain the more common association of chronic pulmonary disease with both gastric and duodenal ulcer (Rotter 1980b, Rotter et al 1982a). The carcinoid ulcer association may be a manifestation of MEN I, but there appears to be a specific risk for gastric ulcer, especially with bronchial carcinoids (Sandler et al 1961).

The multisystem 'stiff skin syndrome' is of interest because of the coincident manifestation of calcium renal stones and peptic ulcer (Stevenson et al 1979), which may have a common underlying mechanism in certain families (Rotter 1980b). Lam et al (1981) have identified a Chinese family with four male members in two generations affected with pachydermoperiostosis and peptic ulcer. Duodenal ulcer was documented in the two male sibs, and the father and paternal uncle had typical ulcer pain. Acid and meal stimulated gastrin studies were normal, and the only physiological abnormality identified was hyperpepsinogenaemia I. Ingegno and Yatto (1982) documented a syndrome combining leuconychia totalis (i.e. white nails), duodenal ulcer and/or gallstones. The association with gallstones in this syndrome rasies the pathophysiological possibility that abnormal biliary secretions are injurious to the duodenal mucosa. Another syndrome including peptic ulcer, hiatal hernia, and multiple lentigines (café-au-lait spots) was described in a French-Canadian kindred (Halal et al 1982). An increased incidence of peptic ulcer disease was suggested in patients with phenylketonuria; it was proposed that excess phenylalanine levels caused increased gastric acid secretion, leading to excess ulcer formation (Greeves et al 1988).

The recognition of these disorders is important not just for the implications for genetic heterogeneity, but because they illustrate that different pathogenetic mechanisms, e.g., excess gastrin or excess histamine, can result in peptic ulcer. Patients with these disorders should have specific genetic counselling and therapy. MEN I is an excellent example of how the alert physician, by making an accurate diagnosis, can then screen asymptomatic family members both by molecular linkage techniques and endocrine analysis to identify those who most probably carry the gene for the disease. The use of linkage requires certain affected family members to be available for study. In addition, highly accurate information can be obtained regarding the genetic status of family members who have no evidence for direct or subclinical disease. These individuals should be followed carefully for developing subclinical disease. By detecting the endocrine tumours early, it is possible to prevent or ameliorate many of their manifestations. The existence of these rare disorders also suggests that what we recognize as 'common' peptic ulcer may, in fact, comprise several disorders.

EPIDEMIOLOGICAL HETEROGENEITY – ETHNIC VARIABILITY

The marked ethnic variability in the prevalence, and especially in the clinical features, of peptic ulcer constitutes epidemiological evidence for heterogeneity (Susser 1967, Tovey & Tunstall 1975, Tovey 1979, Rotter 1980b, Moshal 1980). While duodenal ulcer is usually more common than gastric ulcer, this ratio varies widely over the globe; in a few countries, such as Japan, gastric ulcer is more frequent. The absolute incidence also varies

Table 65.5 Genetic syndromes with peptic ulcer

Syndromes	Location of ulcer	Pathogenetic mechanism	Associated clinical findings	Pattern of inheritance
Relationship established				
Multiple endocrine neoplasia type I	DU	Excess gastrin	Pituitary-acromegaly (GH), infertility (prolactin). Parathyroid-renal stones, hypercalcaemia (PTH). Pancreas-hypoglycaemia (insulin), diabetes (glucagon)	Autosomal dominant
Sporadic gastrinoma	DU	Excess gastrin		Somatic mutation
Systemic mastocytosis	DU	Excess histamine	Skin lesions, urticaria	? (both dominant and recessive pedigrees reported)
Ulcer-tremor-nystagmus	DU	Unknown	Essential tremor, nystagmus, narcolepsy	Autosomal dominant
Amyloidosis, type IV	DU, ?GU	Unknown	Sensorimotor neuropathy, nephropathy, hearing loss, cataracts	Autosomal dominant
Pachydermoperiostosis	DU	Unknown	Clubbing, thickened skin, increased periosteum of distal extremities	Autosomal dominant
Leuconychia-gallstones	DU	Damage by biliary secretions	White nails, cholelithiasis	Autosomal dominant
Relationship suggested but not established				
Hyperparathyroidism	DU	?Calcium increasing gastric secretion	Hypercalcaemia, renal stones	Familial form-autosomal dominant
Cystic fibrosis	DU	?Deficient pancreatic secretion	Pulmonary disease, malabsorption	Autosomal recessive
α-1-antitrypsin deficiency	DU, GU	?Deficient mucosal protection	Pulmonary disease, cirrhosis	Autosomal recessive
Carcinoid syndrome	?GU	?Excess-5-hydroxy-tryptophan	Flushing, cyanosis, diarrhoea, bronchoconstriction	? Autosomal dominant
Stiff skin syndrome	DU	Unknown	Stiff skin, joint enlargement, renal stones, diabetes	Autosomal dominant
Gastrocutaneous syndrome	DU	Unknown	Hiatal hernia, lentigines, café-au-lait spots, hyper-telorism, myopia	? Autosomal dominant
Phenylketonuria	DU, GU	?Excess phenyl-alanine causes increased gastric acid secretion	Mental retardation	Autosomal recessive

widely; e.g. the frequency of duodenal ulcer in Southwest American Indians is one fortieth that of United States whites. Male/female ratios also vary widely, from over 30 to 1 in rural Africal and India to about 2–3 to 1 in the United States. Most significantly, there is extensive ethnic and geographical variation in clinical characteristics, such as age of onset or complications. The incidence of young patients with duodenal ulcer is greatly increased in Hong Kong, compared to Scotland (Lam & Sircus 1975, Lam & Ong 1976). A younger mean age of duodenal ulcer is also found in the high ulcer incidence areas of Africa and India compared to the mean age of the United Kingdom (Tovey & Tunstall 1975, Tovey 1979). The complications of pyloric stenosis as an indication for surgery are much more frequent in the high prevalence areas of south India and the Nile Congo watershed, whereas haemorrhage and perforation are more frequent complications in Europe. There are other unique features of rural African and Indian ulcer, including the occurrence of a fibrous tumour-like inflammatory mass around the duodenal bulb, and an increased frequency of postbulbar ulceration and chole-dochoduodenal fistula. While there is certainly extensive phenotypic heterogeneity on an ethnic basis, much of it could be due to environmental differences, such as diet as well as to genetic differences between the populations.

CLINICAL SUGGESTIONS OF HETEROGENEITY – GASTRIC ULCER VS DUODENAL ULCER

The demonstration of clinical, physiological, or genetic differences within a disorder that can be consistently related to other clinical features such as ulcer location or age of onset can also suggest genetic heterogeneity. In the case of gastric ulcer and duodenal ulcer, much of the evidence to indicate that these are separate and distinct disorders has been gathered in this fashion, using the ulcer location as the dividing criterion and then comparing other features – age of onset, complications, male/female ratio, acid secretion, etc. (see Table 65.6) This separation was confirmed by the classic clinical genetic study of Doll and Kellock (1951). Starting with index cases with a radiographically defined ulcer site, Doll and Kellock painstakingly tracked down the actual radiographs of relatives who were reportedly also affected with peptic ulcer. They observed that the relatives of gastric ulcer probands had a three-fold increased prevalence of gastric ulcer compared to the general population. However, duodenal ulcer occurred no more frequently among these relatives than in the general

population. Likewise, the relatives of duodenal ulcer patients had three times as many duodenal ulcers compared to the control population, but no increased risk of gastric ulcer. Monson (1970a) confirmed these findings, observing twice as many duodenal ulcers as expected in the relatives of physicians with duodenal ulcer, yet no increase in gastric ulcer over that expected. This familial separation is termed independent segregation and is extremely strong evidence that gastric and duodenal ulcer are separate disorders.

Further genetic evidence validates this separation of gastric and duodenal ulcer. In the vast majority of like-sex twins concordant for peptic ulcer, the ulcer site has been observed to be identical (Gotlieb-Jensen 1972). Blood group association studies also support this division, since heterogeneity of genetic polymorphism association is observed. In numerous studies, blood group O is consistently found to be associated with duodenal ulcer (with or without associated gastric ulcer) but not with primary gastric ulcer (McConnell 1966, 1980, Langman 1973, Mourant et al 1978). Since blood groups are genetic polymorphisms that are inherited in a simple Mendelian fashion, these consistent differences in association are ascribed to genetic and hence aetiological differences between the disorders. Physiological data also support this separation, as maximum gastric acid output and serum pepsinogen I are usually normal or even subnormal in gastric ulcer patients, while on average both are increased in duodenal ulcer patients (Wormsley & Grossman 1965, Samloff et al 1975).

It might be appropriate here to deal with a common question. If gastric and duodenal ulcer are truly independent disorders, why do we observe the two together in the same patient more often than the product of the two prevalences in the population at large (Bonnevie 1975). The answer is probably further heterogeneity; that is, combined ulcer (gastric and duodenal) may well be a distinct form of ulcer disease separate from either

Table 65.6 Separation of gastric and duodenal ulcer

Method	Evidence
Clinical	Differences in age of onset, complications, male-female ratio
Clinical genetic	Independent segregation of gastric and duodenal ulcer
Heterogeneity of blood group associations	Blood group O associated with DU, pyloric and combined ulcer, but not with solitary gastric ulcer
Physiological	GU – Acid normosecretors, or subnormal (on the average)
	DU – Acid hypersecretors (on the average)
Ethnic variability	GU – more frequent in Japan
	DU – more frequent in Europe
Clinical genetic	Concordant twins – ulcer site concordant
Physiological	GU – normopepsinogenaemic I
	DU – hyperpepsinogenaemic I

primary gastric or primary duodenal ulcer. Support for this concept comes from the same study by Doll and Kellock (1951) which suggested independent segregation of combined ulcer, i.e. the prevalence of combined ulcer was greater in the relatives with combined disease than in the relatives of probands who had either a solitary gastric or solitary duodenal ulcer. Physiological studies by Lam and Lai (1978) also support this separation. They found a positive correlation between gastric acid output and gastrin response to a protein meal in such patients, and a negative correlation in gastric ulcer patients and controls.

Heterogeneity within duodenal ulcer has also been claimed on clinical grounds, most actively by Lam and co-workers (Lam 1979). Age of onset has been proposed as one dividing criterion. Childhood duodenal ulcer may well be distinct genetically from adult duodenal ulcer, analogous to the separation of juvenile from maturity onset diabetes (Rotter & Rimoin 1981). Investigators have been impressed by the frequency of a 'positive' family history (Cowan 1973), and one study has reported that the first- and second-degree relatives of childhood duodenal ulcer patients are affected with a frequency twice that of relatives of adult probands (Sedlackova & Seemanova 1973). In Hong Kong, Lam and Ong (1976) divided their duodenal ulcer patients on the basis of age of onset and found that their early-onset group (onset below age 20 years) had a significantly stronger family history, a frequency of blood group O similar to that of controls, more frequently presented with gastrointestinal bleeding as the first manifestation of the disease, and rarely had complications such as perforation, obstruction, intractable pain or secondary gastric ulcer, while, in contrast, their late-onset group (onset after age 30 years) had an infrequent family history of ulcer disease, an increased frequency of blood group O, presented less frequently with gastrointestinal bleeding, and had an increased frequency of complications such as perforation, pyloroduodenal stenosis, severe pain, virulent ulcer and secondary gastric ulcer. Similarly, Gutierrez-Cabano (1983) in Argentina showed that among patients whose symptoms began under age 40, there were significantly more subjects with blood A, B and AB, and a significantly stronger family history of dyspepsia, compared to those with later onset of symptoms, in whom blood group O was more frequent.

Another means of looking for heterogeneity clinically is to examine the association of ulcer with other diseases within families. Based on preliminary observations in certain families, we have proposed that the association of ulcer with certain chronic diseases may occur because of the inheritance of a common defect that predisposes to both diseases (Rotter et al 1979d). This may account for

observations of the family aggregation of ulcer disease and renal stones (without hyperparathyroidism), ulcer and coronary artery disease, and ulcer and chronic obstructive pulmonary diseases. In the latter case, it has often been assumed that the ulcer is secondary to the pulmonary disease, yet the association is both with chronic pulmonary disease and lung cancer (Bonnevie 1977), which have been shown to have a common familial component (Cohen et al 1977). Although cigarette smoking is associated with both lung disease and ulcer, it does not fully account for the association of lung lesions and ulcer (Monson 1970b). Furthermore, Kellow et al (1986) showed decreased pulmonary function in both smoking and nonsmoking patients with gastric or duodenal ulcer. In addition, we have observed that in many, if not most cases, the ulcer disease precedes the pulmonary disease (Rotter et al 1982a). a-1-antitrypsin deficiency may be a specific cause of this more general association (Rotter 1980b).

PHYSIOLOGICAL HETEROGENEITY

There is extensive evidence for physiological heterogeneity in peptic ulcer. For example, in gastric ulcer patients mean levels of acid secretion and of serum pepsinogen I are decreased, while in duodenal ulcer patients they are increased (Wormsley & Grossman 1965, Samloff et al 1975). It has been suggested that combined ulcer (gastric and duodenal ulcer) patients have a different pathophysiology, exhibiting a positive correlation of gastric acid output and gastrin response (Lam & Lai 1978). Physiological evidence for heterogeneity within duodenal ulcer includes: (1) the occurrence of duodenal ulcer in both acid hyperpepsinogenaemic and normosecretors; (2) the identification of hyperpepsinogenaemic I and normopepsinogenaemic I duodenal ulcer patients; (3) marked variability in the gastrin response to a protein meal; (4) the observation that the rate of gastric emptying differs among duodenal ulcer patients (Rotter & Rimoin 1977, Grossman 1978, Lam 1980, Rotter 1980b); (5) the demonstration of decreased mucosal defence in some patients, including decreased prostaglandin synthesis (Rachmilewitz et al 1986) and low mucosal bicarbonate secretions (Isemberg et al 1987); (6) the suggestion of an association of certain HLA antigens with duodenal ulcer (Rotter et al 1977a, Ellis & Woodrow 1979, Gough et al 1982, Goedhard et al 1983); (7) the report of antibodies to secretory IgA in certain duodenal ulcer patients (Kwitko & Shearman 1978, Kwitko et al 1988); and (8) the observation of acid stimulating antibodies (Dobi et al 1980, DeLazzari et al 1988). These latter observations hint that there may be immunological forms of peptic ulcer (Rotter 1980b, Rotter & Heiner 1981). Yet each of these abnormalities is found in some, but not all, ulcer patients. Thus, rather than looking for a single defect in all ulcer patients, we should be emphasizing the differences between patients as clues to delineate different disorders.

GENETIC STUDIES UTILIZING SUBCLINICAL MARKERS

Possibly the most powerful method to demonstrate genetic heterogeneity is to utilize family studies to test whether the reported physiological abnormalities have a genetic basis and, if so, whether they serve as subclinical markers (Rotter 1980a,b). Subclinical markers (predictors) are abnormalities proposed to have a role in the pathogenesis of the disease under study. They thus detect individuals with the abnormal genotype, in addition to those with overt disease. They are important in genetic studies, because in many disorders not all individuals with the mutant genotype manifest the disorder (reduced penetrance), the variability of the phenotype may be so great that the clinical features are too mild to be readily apparent (variable expressivity), or there may be delayed onset of the disease, such that the younger genetically predisposed individuals are clinically normal. Thus subclinical markers maximize the number of affected individuals that can be detected. Until we identified subclinical markers in peptic ulcer we could not detect individuals genetically predisposed to ulcer until its clinical manifestations were full blown.

Subclinical markers can also be used to detect heterogeneity within a clinical syndrome. Even if a given potential marker does not occur in all individuals with a clinically similar disorder, this does not mean that it is unimportant in a subgroup of these individuals who may have a distinct, but previously unrecognized disease. For example, sickling of the red cells is an excellent subclinical marker in some patients with anaemia, whereas G6PD levels are a subclinical marker in another group of individuals. If anaemia was considered a single disease, then both sickling and G6PD levels would be rejected as good subclinical markers since they do not occur in all affected individuals. Similarly, in peptic ulcer numerous biochemical and physiological abnormalities have been described in some, but not all ulcer patients (Rotter 1980a,b, Lam 1984). The proposition that distinct ulcer syndromes can be defined by the stratification of patients into groups according to different markers is being borne out by appropriate genetic-

physiological studies. This has been done for several physiological traits including serum pepsinogen I, gastric emptying, and gastrin response to a protein meal.

The most extensive studies have utilized the radioimmunoassay of serum pepsinogen I (PG I) developed by Samloff (1977, 1980, Samloff et al 1986). Human serum pepsinogens, the precursors of pepsin, have been separated into two immunochemically distinct groups, one of fast electrophoretic mobility which is confined to the acid secreting part of the stomach (pepsinogen I, PG I), and the other of slower mobility which is found throughout the stomach and in the first part of the duodenum (pepsinogen II, PG II).

Studies of some 120 duodenal ulcer sibships, in collaboration with Drs McConnell and Ellis of Liverpool, have shown that about half duodenal ulcer patients have hyperpepsinogenaemia I (hyper PG I) and the other half have normopepsinogenaemia I (normo PG I), both on a familial basis (Rotter et al 1979a). That is, the hyper PG I duodenal ulcer and normo PG I duodenal ulcer, for the most part, segregate independently. Both forms of duodenal ulcer exhibit an increased risk for sibs for ulcer (some 20–25% of the sibs affected) compared to the population risk. Thus both forms demonstrate familial aggregation whose basis is presumably genetic. Other risk factors did not distinguish between the two groups, such as blood groups, or the male/female ratio which was 3 to 1 in both groups. A small series of twins also supported this separation of hyper and normo PG I duodenal ulcer (Rotter et al 1977b), as did a study of PG I levels in the clinically normal sibs of the duodenal ulcer probands. The mean serum PG I of the normal sibs of the hyper PG I probands was significantly greater than that of the clinically normal sibs of the normo PG I probands. In fact, the mean PG I level in the clinically normal sibs of the hyper PG I probands was intermediate between that in probands and in healthy controls.

These sib studies and studies of extended families have also suggested that the familial aggregation of an elevated PG I is consistent with autosomal dominant inheritance (Rotter et al 1979a,b). In the sibships studied, 36 of 83 clinically normal sibs of hyper PG I probands had an elevated PG I (Rotter et al 1979a). Segregation analysis of the trait of an elevated PG I yielded segregation ratios bracketing the value of 0.5, supporting autosomal dominant inheritance of this trait. In the extended families studied, the vertical transmission of an elevated PG I was also characteristic of autosomal dominant inheritance. In each generation, approximately 50% of the offspring of members with an elevated PG I had an elevated PG I, all offspring of normo PG I members had a normal PG I, and there was male to male transmission of hyperpepsinogenaemia (Rotter et al

1979b). Further support has come from a family study done by Habibullah et al (1984) in the Indian sub-continent. They observed that first-degree relatives of hyper-pepsinogenaemic ulcer patients (assayed proteolytically) had serum pepsinogen values intermediate between that of patients and controls, and the transmission of hyperpepsinogenaemia was consistent with autosomal dominant inheritance. The results from a Japanese study (Sumii et al 1986) further support these findings. In this study it was shown again that hyperpepsinogenaemia I was inherited as an autosomal dominant trait in families with duodenal ulcer. In this latter study, as well as in Britain and the USA, there were a number of duodenal ulcer families in which normopepsinogenaemia I also segregated. Thus, these studies have delineated a major genetic factor, elevated serum pepsinogen I, that can identify individuals at risk and that may account for the major genetic predisposition of many, possibly even half, of duodenal ulcer patients. This does not mean that an elevated serum pepsinogen I itself predisposes to ulcer. More likly, it identifies those individuals with an increased mass of chief and parietal cells who are genetically predisposed on the basis of producing excess pepsin and acid. In family and sibling studies of hyperpepsinogenaemic I patients, some 40–75% of the relatives with an elevated pepsinogen I have clinical duodenal ulcer. Thus other factors, environmental and/or genetic, must also play a role in disease expression.

These accumulated studies suggest that there are at least two genetic subtypes of duodenal ulcer. In the hyper PG I type, the genetic predispostion to duodenal ulcer in apparently normal sibs can be identified by an elevated serum PG I level. The second type is characterized by normopepsinogenaemia I in both the ulcer proband and his or her sibs. This latter type of ulcer also appears to have a genetic basis, as demonstrated by its familial aggregation, but other markers must be sought to identify the individuals at risk. One should not conclude from these studies that there are only two forms of duodenal ulcer. One might predict that the use of other subclinical markers might further subdivide these broad groups. Additional studies utilizing other physiological characteristics are just starting to further subdivide the hyperpepsinogenaemic I and normopepsinogenaemic I duodenal ulcer groups. Thus, there appears to be a subgroup of the normopepsinogenaemic I class in which rapid gastric emptying seems to be the inherited physiological abnormality predisposing to ulcer (Rotter et al 1979c). Familial hyperpepsinogenaemic I duodenal ulcer also seems to be separable into different groups. A group of patients with a markedly exaggerated gastrin response to a protein meal from an antral souce (antral G cell hyperfunction) have also been shown to have hyperpepsinogenaemia I (Calam

et al 1979, Taylor et al 1981). In addition, it was shown that G-cell hyperfunction-hyperpepsinogenaemia I can be a component of familial G-cell hyperfunction hyperpepsinogenaemia I syndrome, or of familial peptic ulcer disease with normal or increased serum pepsinogen I levels without G-cell hyperfunction, thus demonstrating further heterogeneity of peptic ulcer disease (Lamers et al 1985). Both rapid emptying and postprandial hypergastrinaemia appeared to follow autosomal dominant inheritance patterns (Rotter et al 1982b). Combining physiological studies and family history in a cross sectional study, Lam and Ong (1980) have presented evidence that there may be more than one form of early onset ulcer. In the early-onset (symptoms before age 30) group, the postprandial gastrin response was significantly greater in those with a positive family history than in those with a negative family history and in the normosecretors versus the hypersecretors. Furthermore, among the early-onset patients, family-history-positive normosecretors had a significantly positive correlation between maximal acid output and postprandial gastrin reponse, while family-history-positive hypersecretors had a significantly negative correlation between these variables.

Thus pepsinogen I, gastric emptying, and gastrin response, have been demonstrated to be useful markers in genetic studies. There are a variety of additional potential subclinical markers for genetic studies of peptic ulcer (Rotter 1980a,b, Rotter et al 1985). Another marker examined in a family study has been maximum acid secretion. Fodor et al (1968) measured maximum acid output in 160 duodenal ulcer patients, 113 nonulcerated first-degree relatives, and 155 healthy controls without a family history of ulcer. Acid secretion in the family members was found to be intermediate between the ulcer patients and controls, regardless of blood group or secretor status. Since only the mean values were reported, we have no knowledge whether there was any segregation of elevated acid secretion, but the considerable overlap between normals and ulcer patients would complicate such analaysis. It would be worthwhile, however, to re-examine Fodor's data with modern genetic analytical techniques. Kekki et al (1985) have shown that peak acid output exhibits familial aggregation, with sibs (though not offspring) having higher levels than expected. Furthermore, familial aggregation of duodenal ulcer was found only among the hypersecretor families, supporting the role of acid in ulcer formation. A subclinical marker that should be examined is the pepsinogen I to pepsinogen II ratio. This is a sensitive measure of gastritis. Familial aggregation of an abnormal PG I/PG II ratio has been found in a few duodenal ulcer and gastric ulcer families (Rotter et al 1985). Another potential duodenal ulcer subclinical marker is duodenitis. The frequency of macroscopic duodenitis was found to be significantly higher in relatives of duodenal ulcer patients than in controls, suggesting a link between duodenitis and duodenal ulcer (Tarpila et al 1982).

It should be noted that the genetic-family method of studying potential markers is useful not only for demonstrating heterogeneity. Equally important, by showing cosegregation of the disease and the physiological marker in certain families, it can help demonstrate that a particular abnormality does in fact have a clear pathophysiological relationship to at least one type of peptic ulcer. Such studies can thus resolve any doubt about whether a given abnormality is a 'real' observation in peptic ulcer patients.

A GENETIC CLASSIFICATION

Thus, the accumulating evidence suggests that the genetic predisposition to peptic ulcer is not due principally to the cumulative effect of multiple, additive predisposing genes each with a small effect (the polygenic hypothesis), but rather that there are multiple forms of peptic ulcer, each with a different genetic basis. A classification of our evolving knowledge of peptic ulcer genetic and aetiological heterogeneity is shown in Table 65.7. It should be noted that polygenic inheritance and genetic heterogeneity are not necessarily mutually exclusive. There may well be a polygenic background upon which major predisposing genes act. While the

Table 65.7 Classification of peptic ulcer heterogeneity

I. Peptic ulcer associated with rare genetic syndromes
  A. Relationship established
    1. Multiple endocrine adenomatosis, Type I (gastrinoma)
    2. Systemic mastocytosis
    3. Tremor-nystagmus-ulcer syndrome
    4. Amyloidosis, type IV
    5. Pachydermoperiostosis
    6. Leuconychia-gallstones
  B. Relationship suggested
    1. Hyperparathyroidism
    2. Cystic fibrosis
    3. α-1-antitrypsin deficiency
    4. Carcinoid syndrome
    5. Stiff skin syndrome
    6. Gastrocutaneous syndrome
    7. Phenylketonuria
II. Oesophageal ulcer
III. Gastric ulcer
  A. Accompanied by chronic gastritis
  B. Secondary to use of non-steroidal anti-inflammatory agents
IV. Combined gastric and duodenal ulcer
V. Hyperpepsinogenaemic–I duodenal ulcer[†]
  A. Without postprandial hypergastrinaemia
  B. With postprandial hypergastrinaemia
  C. Secondary to retained antrum
VI. Normopepsinogenaemic–I duodenal ulcer
  A. Without rapid gastric emptying
  B. With rapid gastric emptying
VII. Childhood duodenal ulcer
  A. Normal acid secretion[*]
  B. Elevated acid secretion[*]
VIII. Immunological forms of duodenal ulcer[*]
  A. Antibody to secretory IgA
  B. Immunoglobulin stimulated acid secretion
IX. Peptic ulcer associated with other chronic diseases[*]
  A. Peptic ulcer and chronic lung disease
  B. Duodenal ulcer and renal stones (without hyperparathyroidism)
  C. Duodenal ulcer and coronary artery disease
  D. Duodenal ulcer and cirrhosis
X. Meckel's diverticulum

[†] Also usually acid hypersecretors.
[*] Tentative subdivision.
For further details, see Rotter 1980a,b, 1981, Rotter et al 1990 and the text.

studies mentioned above appear to be identifying major genes, such as hyperpepsinogenaemia I, which predispose to one form of peptic ulcer, this does not rule out the effect of genes such as blood group O, nonsecretor, and even male sex, as having an additional effect on the genetic predispositon. Such 'minor genes' may form the genetic background upon which the major disease-predisposing genes exert their effects. In addition, some of the various heterogeneous forms may be polygenic in origin, as has been suggested for childhood duodenal ulcer. Cowan (1973) proposed that childhood duodenal ulcer may be an example of polygenic inheritance in that these children have 'more genes' (stronger family history) and therefore their disease is 'more severe' (younger age of onset). An alternative explanation is that 'adult' and 'childhood' duodenal ulcer are different disorders, with different average ages of onset, as is the case for adult and juvenile diabetes. The genetic physiological approaches enumerated here should be able to resolve this question.

Genetic counselling

At the present time, how do we counsel our ulcer patients and their families? We tell our ulcer patients that about 20% of their first-degree relatives (parents, sibs, offspring) will also experience peptic ulcer disease in their lifetime.

Are the subclinical markers useful in genetic counselling? About 50% of patients with duodenal ulcer appear to have hyperpepsinogenaemia I, and some half of their sibs and half of their offspring also have this trait and therefore have an increased risk (40–60%) of developing duodenal ulcer. Should efforts be made to identify these individuals so they will know they have this susceptibility? Should such individuals be told to avoid risk factors such as smoking cigarettes, and to seek medical care promptly if symptoms suggestive of ulcer occur? Studies need to be done to determine whether such an effort is worthwhile. If we should discover specific environmental factors which act in concert with a given genetic trait, such as hyperpepsinogenaemia I, to convert genetic predisposition into clinical disease, then it would obviously be desirable to identify those with the genetic trait so they could be warned to avoid the environmental factor.

In the case of the rare genetic syndromes that feature peptic ulceration, especially multiple endocrine adenomatosis type I, a thorough search of all family members should be made for occult cases so the disease can be treated in its earliest stages before complications arise.

Future implications

The polygenic hypothesis suggests that all ulcer is a spectrum of one disease, and that pathophysiology and optimal therapy would be similar for all ulcer patients. In direct contrast, the implication of genetic heterogeneity is that the pathophysiology, and therefore optimal therapy, may well differ between different types of ulcer patients. Our goal as physicians and scientists is to recognize the full heterogeneity of this group of disorders, to develop specific methods for identifying individuals predisposed to each of the component disorders, and to define the specific environmental differences that lead to clinical expression in each kind of genetically predisposed individual. This may eventually lead to specific modes of therapy, prevention, and genetic counselling for each of the disorders that lead to the ulcer syndrome.

ENVIRONMENTAL FACTORS

We have shown throughout this chapter that genetic factors play a major role in the predisposition to peptic ulcer. However, there are certain environmental factors that can also predispose to peptic ulcer disease (Table 65.8). It is quite likely that individuals with the appropriate genetic constitution, when exposed to these environmental factors, develop ulcers. Cigarette smoking is associated with a two-fold increased incidence of gastric and duodenal ulcer (Harrison et al 1979), impairment of ulcer healing and predisposition to ulcer relapse (Korman et al 1983). Chronic usage of aspirin is an established cause for gastric ulcer (Piper et al 1982). In the last few years many studies have examined the role of non-steroidal anti-inflammatory drugs in the development of peptic ulcer. There is good evidence that such agents can cause duodenitis, exacerbate and cause ulcer and induce ulcer complications (Roth 1988). Interestingly Semble et al (1987) demonstrated that among

Table 65.8 Environmental factors in the aetiology of peptic ulcer

Positive evidence for an association with ulcer disease
    Cigarette smoking
    Regular use of aspirin
    Non-steroidal anti-inflammatory drugs
    High total doses or extensive use of steroids

Equivocal evidence
    Infectious agents – Herpes virus
                Campylobacter pyloridis
    Stress
    Coffee

Contradicting evidence
    Alcohol (except for alcoholic hepatic cirrhosis)
    Food and diets (except for possible protective effect of high fibre diets)

Modified from Grossman 1981, and Rotter et al 1990.

rheumatoid arthritis patients treated with non-steroidal anti-inflammatory agents, those most likely to develop ulcers had blood group O. This demonstrates a genetic-environmental interaction that requires further investigation. Stress has long been suggested as a factor in the development of peptic ulcers (Feldman et al 1986). Although many studies could not prove such association, Walker et al (1988) showed a significant relationship between serum pepsinogen I and negative personality traits and impaired coping ability, suggesting that chronic emotional stress can contribute to peptic ulcer, presumably through increased peptic cell mass and the neuronal stimulus of pepsinogen I. Infectious agents have also been implicated as aetiological agents for peptic ulcer, especially *Campylobacter pyloridis*. While there is convincing evidence that it causes gastritis (Bartlett 1988), its significance in the aetiology of gastric and duodenal ulcer disease is still not resolved.

REFERENCES

Archord J L, Langford H 1980 The effect of cimetidine and propantheline on the symptoms of a patient with systemic mastocytosis. American Journal of Medicine 69: 610–614

Aird I, Bentall H H, Mehigaro J A, Roberts J A F 1954 The blood groups in relation to peptic ulceration and carcinoma of the colon, rectum, breast and bronchus. British Medical Journal ii: 315–321

Ammann R W, Vetter D, Deyhle P, Tschen H, Sulser H, Schmid M 1976 Gastrointestinal involvement in systemic mastocytosis. Gut 17: 107–112

Ballard H S, Frame B, Hartsock R J 1964 Familial multiple endocrine adenoma-peptic ulcer complex. Medicine 43: 481–516

Baraitser M, Parkes J D 1978 Genetic study of the narcoleptic syndrome. Journal of Medical Genetics 15: 254–259

Barreras R F 1973 Calcium and gastric secretion. Gastroenterology 64: 1168–1184

Bartlett J G 1988 Campylobacter pylori: Fact or fancy? Gastroenterology 94: 229–238

Bonnevie O 1975 The incidence in Copenhagen County of gastric and duodenal ulcers in the same patient. Scandinavian Journal of Gastroenterology 10: 529–536

Bonnevie O 1977 Causes of death in duodenal and gastric ulcer. Gastroenterology 73: 1000–1004

Calam J, Taylor I L, Dockray G J, Simkin E, Cooke A, Rotter J I, Samloff I M 1979 Subgroup of duodenal ulcer patients with familial G-cell hyperfunction and hyperpepsinogenemia I. Gut 20: A934

Camerer J W 1936 Z. Menschl. Vererb-U. Konstit. Lehre 19: 416, quoted in Gotlieb-Jensen, 1972

Clarke C A, Edwards J W, Haddock D R W, Howel Evans A W, McConnell R B, Sheppard P M 1956 ABO blood group and secretor character in duodenal ulcer. British Medical Journal 725–731

Cohen B H, Diamond E L, Graves C G et al 1977 A common familial component in lung cancer and chronic obstructive pulmonary disease. Lancet ii: 523–526

Cowan W K 1973 Genetics of duodenal and gastric ulcer. Clinics in Gastroenterology 2: 539–546

DeLazzari F, Mirakian R, Hammond L, Venturi C, Naccarato R, Bottazzo G F 1988 Gastric cell c-AMP stimulating autoantibodies in duodenal ulcer disease. Gut 29: 94–100

Deveney C W, Deveney K S, Jaffe B M, Jones R S, Way L W 1977 Use of calcium and secretin in the diagnosis of gastrinoma (Zollinger-Ellison syndrome). Annals of Internal Medicine 87: 680–686

Dobi S, Gasztonyi F, Lenkey B 1980 Immunoglobulin stimulated superacidity in duodenal ulcer. Acta Medica Academiae Scientarium Hungaricae 37: 51–59

Doig R K 1957 Illness in twins: duodenal ulcer. Medical Journal of Australia 2: 617–619

Doll R, Buch J 1950 Hereditary factors in peptic ulcer. Annals of Eugenics 15: 135–146

Doll R, Kellock T D 1951 The separate inheritance of gastric and duodenal ulcer. Annals of Eugenics 16: 231–240

Doll R, Drane H, Newell A C 1961 Secretion of blood group substances in duodenal, gastric and stomach ulcer, gastric carcinoma and diabetes mellitus. Gut 2: 352–359

Eberhard G 1968 Peptic ulcer in twins. A study in personality, heredity and environment. Acta Psychiatrica Scandinavica. Supplement 205

Edwards J H 1965 The meaning of the associations between blood groups and disease. Annals of Human Genetics 29: 77–83

Ellis A, Woodrow J C 1979 HLA and duodenal ulcer. Gut 20: 760–762

Evans D A P, Horwich L, McConnel R B, Bullen M F 1968. Influence of the ABO blood groups and secretor status on bleeding and on perforation of duodenal ulcer. Gut 9: 311–322

Feldman M, Walker P, Green J, Weingarden K 1986 Life events, stress and psychological factors in men with peptic ulcer disease I. Gastroenterology 9: 1370–1379

Fodor O, Vestea S, Urcan S Popeicu S, Suhca L, Ienicca R, Cola A, Flea V 1968 Hydrochloric acid secretion capacity of the stomach as an inherited factor in the pathogenesis of duodenal ulcer. American Journal of Digestive Diseases 13: 260–265

Frieri M, Alling D W, Metcalfe D D 1985 Comparison of the therapeutic efficacy of cromolyn sodium with that of combined chlorpheniramine and cimetidine in systemic mastocytosis. Results of a double-blind clinical trial. American Journal of Medicine 78: 9–14

Gimeno A, Garcia-Alix D, Segovia de Arana J M, Mateos F, Sotelo M T 1974 Amyloidotic polyneuritis of type III (Iowa-Van Allen). European Neurology 11: 46–57

Glenner G G, Ignaczak T F, Page D L 1978 The inherited system amyloidoses and localized amyloid deposits. In: Stanbury J B, Wyngaarden J B, Frederickson D S (eds) The Metabolic Basis of Inherited Disease, McGraw-Hill, New York, p 1308–1339

Goedhard J G, Biemond I, Pena S A, Kreuning J, Schreuder G M T, Van Rood J J 1983 HLA and duodenal ulcer in the Netherlands. Tissue Antigens 22: 213–218

Gotlieb-Jensen K 1972 Peptic ulcer: Genetic and epidemiological aspects based on twin studies. Munksgaard, Copenhagen

Gough M J, Rajah S M, Giles G R 1982 HLA antigens in

relationships to duodenal ulceration, gastric acid secretion and clinical results following vagotomy. British Journal of Surgery 69: 105–107

Greeves L G, Carson D J, Dodge J A 1988 Peptic ulceration and phenylketonuria, a possible link? Gut 29: 691–692

Gregory R A, Tracy H J, French J M, Sircus W 1960 Extraction of a gastrin-like substance from a pancreatic tumour in a case of Zollinger-Ellison syndrome. Lancet i: 1045–1048

Gregory R A, Grossman M I, Tracy H J, Bentley P H 1967 Nature of the gastric secretagogue in Zollinger-Ellison tumours. Lancet ii: 543–544

Grossman M I 1972 Gastrointestinal hormones: some thoughts about clinical applications. Scandinavian Journal of Gastroenterology 7: 97–104

Grossman M I 1978 Abnormalities of acid secretion in patients with duodenal ulcer. Gastroenterology 75: 524–526

Grossman M I 1980 Peptic ulcer, definition and epidemiology. In: Rotter J I, Samloff I M, Rimoin D L (eds) The Genetics and Heterogeneity of Common Gastrointestinal Disorders. Academic Press, New York, p 21–29

Grossman M I (ed) 1981 Peptic Ulcer, A Guide for the Practising Physician. Year Book, Chicago

Grossman M I, Kurata J H, Rotter J I et al 1981 Peptic ulcer – new therapies, new diseases. Annals of Internal Medicine 95: 609–627

Gutierrez-Cabano C A 1983 ABO blood groups, onset age of ulcer symptoms, family history of dyspepsia and complications in duodenal ulcer. Acta Gastroenterologica Latino America 13: 171–178

Habibullah O M, Ali M M, Ishaq M 1984 Study of duodenal ulcer disease in 100 families using total serum pepsinogen as a genetic marker. Gut 25: 907–908

Halal F, Gervais M H, Baillargeon J, Lesage R 1982 Gastro-cutaneous syndrome: peptic ulcer/hiatal hernia, multiple lentigines/cafe-au-lait spots, hypertelorism, and myopia. American Journal of Medical Genetics 11: 161–176

Harrison A R, Elashoff J D, Grossman M I 1979 Smoking and health. A report to the Surgeon General. DHEW Publication no. 79-50066. Washington 1–21

Harvald B, Hauge M 1958 A catamnestic investigation of Danish twins. Acta Genetica 8: 287–294

Hirschowitz B I, Groarke J F 1979 Effect of cimetidine on gastric hypersecretion and diarrhea in systemic mastocytosis. Annals of Internal Medicine 90: 769–771

Huhn G 1939 Magenerkrankagen bei Zwillingen. Hamburg. Quoted in Gotlieb-Jensen 1972

Ingegno A P, Yatto R P 1982 Hereditary white nails (leukonychia totalis) duodenal ulcer and gallstones. New York State Journal of Medicine 82: 1797–1800

Isenberg J I, Walsh J H, Grossman M I 1973 Zollinger-Ellison syndrome. Gastroenterology 65: 140–165

Isenberg J I, Selling J A, Hogan L D, Koss M A 1987 Impaired proximal duodenal mucosal bicarbonate secretion in patients with duodenal ulcer. New England Journal of Medicine 316: 374–379

Jirasek V 1971 Hereditary factors in the etiology of peptic ulcer. Acta Universitatis Carolinae Medicae 17: 383–456

Kang J Y, Doran T, Crampton R, McClenehar W, Piper D W 1983 HLA antigens and peptic ulcer disease. Digestion 26: 99–104

Kekki M, Sipponen P, Siurala M 1985 Hypersecretion of gastric acid in a representative Finnish family sample. Scandinavian Journal of Gastroenterology 20: 478–484

Kellow J E, Tao Z, Piper D W 1986 Ventilatory function in chronic peptic ulcer. Gastroenterology 91: 590–595

Korman M G, Hansky J, Evans E R, Schmidt G T 1983 Influence of cigarette smoking on healing and relapse in duodenal ulcer disease. Gastroenterology 85: 871–874

Kubickova Z, Vesely K T 1972 The value of investigation of the incidence of peptic ulcer in families of patients with duodenal ulcer. Journal of Medical Genetics 9: 38–42

Kuenssberg E V 1962 Are duodenal ulcer and chronic bronchitis family diseases? Proceedings of the Royal Society of Medicine 55: 299–302

Kurata J H, Haile B M 1984 Epidemiology of peptic ulcer disease. Clinical Gastroenterology 13: 289–307

Kwitko A, Shearman D J C 1978 Antibodies to secretory IgA (SIgA) in duodenal ulcer disease. Gut 19: A437

Kwitko A O, Hetzel D J, LaBrooy J I, Shearman D J C 1980 Antibodies to secretory IgA in duodenal ulcer disease. Gastroenterology 78: 1202

Lam S K 1979 Duodenal-ulcer inheritance. Lancet i: 977–978

Lam S K 1980 Physiologic abnormalities and heterogeneity in peptic ulcer. In: Rotter J I, Samloff I M, Rimoin D L (eds) Genetics and Heterogeneity of Common Gastrointestinal Disorders. Academic Press, New York, p 67–80

Lam S K 1984 Pathogenesis and pathophysiology of duodenal ulcer. Clinics in Gastroenterology 13: 447–472

Lam S K, Lai C L 1978 Gastric ulcers with and without associated duodenal ulcer have different pathophysiology. Clinical Science and Molecular Medicine 55: 97–102

Lam S K, Ong G B 1976 Duodenal ulcers, early and late onset. Gut 17: 169–179

Lam S K, Ong G B 1980 Identification of two subgroups of familial early onset duodenal ulcer. Annals of Internal Medicine 93: 540–544

Lam S K, Sircus W 1975 Studies in duodenal ulcer, the clinical evidence for the existence of two populations. Quarterly Journal of Medicine 44: 369–387

Lam S K, Hui K K, Rotter J I, Samloff I M 1981 Pachydermoperiostosis and peptic ulcer. Gastroenterology 80: 1202

Lam S K, Hui W K, Ho J, Wong K P, Rotter J I, Samloff I M 1983a Pachydermoperiostosis, hypertrophic gastropathy, and peptic ulcer. Gastroenterology 84: 834–839

Lam S K, Koo J, Sircus W 1983b Early and late onset duodenal ulcer in Chinese and Scots. Scandinavian Journal of Gastroenterology 18: 651–658

Lamers C B H, Van Tongeren J H M 1977 Comparative study of the value of the calcium, secretin, and meal stimulated increase in serum gastrin in the diagnosis of the Zollinger-Ellison syndrome. Gut 18: 128–134

Lamers C B, Stadil F, Van Tongeren J H 1978 Prevalence of endocrine abnormalities in patients with the Zollinger-Ellison syndrome in their families. American Journal of Medicine 64: 607–612

Lamers C, Diemel C, Froeling P, Jansen J 1980 Heredity of hypergastrinemic hyperchlorlydria syndromes. In: Rotter J I, Samloff I M, Rimoin D L (eds) The Genetics and Heterogeneity of Common Gastrointestinal Disorders. Academic Press, New York, p 81–89

Lamers C B, Lind T, Moberg S, Jansen J B, Olbe L 1984 Omeprazole in Zollinger-Ellison syndrome. Effects of a single dose and of long-term treatment in patients resistant to histamine H_2-receptor antagonists. New England Journal of Medicine 310: 758–761

Lamers C B H W, Jansen J B M J, Rotter J I, Samloff I M 1985 Serum pepsinogen I in hereditary hypergastrinemic peptic ulcer syndromes. In: Kreuning J, Samloff I M, Rotter

J I, Eriksson A W (eds) Pepsinogens in Man: Clinical and Genetic Advances Liss, New York, p 273–281

Langdon N, Welsh K I, Van Dam M, Vaughan R W, Parkes W 1984 Genetic markers in narcolepsy. Lancet 2: 1178–1180

Langman M J S 1973 Blood groups and alimentary disorders. Clinics in Gastroenterology 2: 497–506

Langman M J S 1979 The Epidemiology of Chronic Digestive Disease. Edward Arnold, London

Larsson C, Skogseid B, Oberg K, Nakamura Y, Nordtgold M 1988 Multiple endocrine neoplasia type I maps to chromosome 11 and is lost in insulinoma. Nature 332: 85–87

Lips C J M, Vasen H F, Lamers C B 1984 Multiple endocrine neoplasia syndrome. CRC Critical Review of Oncology and Hematology 2: 117–184

McConnell R B 1966 The Genetics of Gastrointestinal Disorders. Oxford University Press, London

McConnell R B 1980 Peptic ulcer, early genetic evidence – families, twins, and markers. In: Rotter J I, Samloff I M, Rimoin D L (eds) The Genetics and Heterogeneity of Common Gastrointestinal Disorders. Academic Press, New York, p 31–41

McKusick V A 1988 Mendelian Inheritance in Man, Catalogue of Autosomal Dominant, Autosomal Recessive, and X-linked Phenotypes. Johns Hopkins University Press, Baltimore

Marshall A G, Hutchinson E O, Honisett J 1962 Heredity in common diseases, a retrospective survey of twins in a hospital population. British Medical Journal i: 1–6

Monson R R 1970a Familial factors in peptic ulcer, the occurrence of ulcer in relatives. American Journal of Epidemiology 91: 453–466

Monson R R 1970b Duodenal ulcer as a second disease. Gastroenterology 59: 712–716

Moshal M G 1980 Ethnic differences in duodenal ulceration. In: Rotter J I, Samloff I M, Rimoin D L (eds) The Genetics and Heterogeneity of Common Gastrointestinal Disorders. Academic Press, New York, p 91–110

Mourant A E, Kopec A C, Domaniewska-Sobczak K 1978 Blood Groups and Diseases: A Study of Associations of Diseases with Blood Groups and Other Polymorphisms. Oxford University Press, Oxford

Neuhauser G, Daly R F, Magnelli N C, Barreras R F, Donaldson R M, Opitz J M 1976 Essential tremor, nystagmus and duodenal ulceration. Clinical Genetics 9: 81–91

Nichols W C, Dwulet F E, Benson M D 1987 Apolipoprotein AI in Iowa type hereditary amyloidosis (FAP type IV). Clinical Research 35: 595A

Parkes J D 1979 Personal communication

Piper D W, McIntosh J H, Greig M, Shy C M 1982 Environmental factors and chronic gastric ulcer: a case control study of the association of smoking, alcohol, and heavy/analgesic ingestion with the exacerbation of chronic gastric ulcer. Scandinavian Journal of Gastroenterology 17: 721–729

Pollin W, Allen M G, Hoffer A, Stabenau J R, Hrubec Z 1969 Psychopathology in 15 909 pairs of veteran twins: evidence for a genetic factor in the pathogenesis of schizophrenia and its relative absence in psychoneurosis. American Journal of Psychiatry 126: 597–610

Pratt R T C 1967 The Genetics of Neurological Disorders. Oxford University Press, London

Prescott R J, Sircus W, Lai C L, Lam S K 1976 Failure to confirm evidence for existence of two populations with duodenal ulcer. British Medical Journal ii: 677

Rachmilewitz D, Ligumsky M, Fich A, Goldin E, Eliakim A, Karmeli F 1986 Role of endogenous gastric prostanoids in the pathogenesis and therapy of duodenal ulcer. Gastroenterology 90: 963–969

Regan P T, Malagelada J R 1978 A reappraisal of clinical, roentgenographic and endoscopic features of the Zollinger-Ellison syndrome. Mayo Clinic Proceedings 53: 19–23

Rimoin D L 1967 Genetics of diabetes mellitus. Diabetes 16: 346–351

Rimoin D L, Schimke R N 1971 Endocrine pancreas. In: Genetic Disorders of the Endocrine Glands. Mosby, St. Louis, p 150–216

Roberts J A F 1965 ABO blood groups, secretor status, and susceptibility to chronic diseases: An example of genetic basis for family predispositions. In: Neel J V, Shaw M W, Schull W J (eds) Genetics and the Epidemiology of Chronic Diseases. U.S. Government Printing Office, Public Health Service Publication No. 1163, p 77–86

Roth S H 1988 Nonsteroidal anti-inflammatory drugs: Gastropathy, deaths, and medical practice. Annals of Internal Medicine 109: 353–354

Rotter J I 1980a Genetic approaches to ulcer heterogeneity. In: Rotter J I, Samloff I M, Rimoin D L (eds) The Genetics and Heterogeneity of Common Gastrointestinal Disorders. Academic Press, New York, p 111–128

Rotter J I 1980b Peptic ulcer disease – more than one gene, more than one disease. In: Steinberg A G, Bearn A G, Motulsky A G, Childs B (eds) Progress in Medical Genetics, Volume 4 (new series). Saunders, Philadelphia, p 1–58

Rotter J I 1981 Gastric and duodenal ulcer are each many different diseases. Digestive Diseases and Sciences 26: 154–160

Rotter J I, Heiner D C 1981 Are there immmunological forms of duodenal ulcer? Journal of Clinical and Laboratory Immunology 7: 1–6

Rotter J I, Rimoin D L 1977 Peptic ulcer disease – a heterogeneous group of disorders? Gastroenterology 73: 604–607

Rotter J I, Rimoin D L 1981 Etiology of diabetes – genetics. In: Brownlee M (ed) Handbook of Diabetes Mellitus. Garland STPM Press, New York, p 3–93

Rotter J I, Gursky J M, Samloff I M, Rimoin D L 1976 Peptic ulcer disease – further evidence for gentic heterogeneity. Excerpta Medica International Congress Series, No. 397: 96

Rotter J I, Rimoin D L, Gursky J M, Teraski P I, Sturdevant R A L 1977a HLA-B5 associated with duodenal ulcer. Gastroenterology 73: 435–437

Rotter J I, Rimoin D L, Samloff I M, McConnell R B, Gotlieb-Jensen K, Gadeburg O, Hauge M 1977b The genetics of peptic ulcer disease – elevated serum group I pepsinogen concentrations in siblings and twins of ulcer probands. Gastroenterology 72: 1165

Rotter J I, Rimoin D L, Samloff I M 1978 Genetic heterogeneity in diabetes mellitus and peptic ulcer. In: Morton N E, Chung C S (eds) Genetic Epidemiology. Academic Press, New York, p 381–414

Rotter J I, Petersen G M, Samloff I M, McConnell R B, Ellis A, Spence M A, Rimoin D L 1979a Genetic heterogeneity of familial hyperpepsinogenemic I and normopepsinogenemic I duodenal ulcer disease. Annals of Internal Medicine 91: 372–377

Rotter J I, Sones J Q, Samloff I M, Richardson C T, Gursky J

T, Walsh J H, Rimoin D L 1979b Duodenal ulcer disease associated with elevated serum pepsinogen I, an inherited autosomal dominant disorder. New England Journal of Medicine 300: 63–66

Rotter J I, Rubin R, Meyer J H, Samloff I M, Rimoin D L 1979c Rapid gastric emptying – an inherited pathophysiologic defect in duodenal ulcer? Gastroenterology 76: 1229

Rotter J I, Rimoin D L, Samloff I M 1979d Genetic heterogeneity in peptic ulcer. Lancet i: 1088–1089

Rotter J I, Samloff I M, Rimoin D L (eds) 1980 The genetics and Heterogeneity of Common Gastrointestinal Disorders. Academic Press, New York.

Rotter J I, Monson R R, Grossman M I 1982a Duodenal ulcer and pulmonary disease, which comes first? (unpublished observations)

Rotter J I, Meyer J H, Rubin R, Samloff I M, Taylor I L 1982b Inherited rapid gastric emptying and duodenal ulcer disease. Clinical Research 30: 293A

Rotter J I, Petersen G M, Samloff I M 1985 Pepsinogens and other physiologic markers in genetic studies of peptic ulcer and related disorders. In: Kreuning J, Samloff I M, Rotter J I, Eriksson A W (eds) Pepsinogens in Man, Clinical and Genetic Advances. Liss, New York, p 227–244

Rotter J I, Petersen G M, Shohat T 1990 Peptic ulcer disease. In: King R A, Rotter J I, Motulsky A G (eds) The genetic basis of common diseases. Oxford University Press, New York, (in press)

Samloff I M 1979 Serum pepsinogens I and II. In: Berk J E (ed) Developments in Digestive Diseases. Lea and Febiger, Philadelphia, p 1–12

Samloff I M 1980 Pepsinogens and their relationship to peptic ulcer. In: Rotter J I, Samloff I M, Rimoin D L (eds) The Genetics and Heterogeneity of Common Gastrointestinal Disorders. Academic Press, New York, p 43–49

Samloff I M, Liebman W M, Panitch N M 1975 Serum group I pepsinogens by radioimmunoassay in control subjects and patients with peptic ulcer. Gastroenterology 69: 83–90

Samloff I M, Stemmermann G N, Heilbrun I K, Nomura A 1986 Elevated serum pepsinogen I and II levels differ as risk factors for duodenal ulcer and gastric ulcer. Gastroenterology 90: 570–576

Sandler M, Scheuler P J, Watt P J 1961 5-Hydroxytrytophan secreting bronchial carcinoid tumour. Lancet ii: 1067–1069

Schimke R N 1976 Multiple endocrine adenomatosis syndromes. In: Stollerman G E (ed) Advances in Internal Medicine, vol 21. Year Book, Chicago, p 249–265

Sedlackova M, Seemanova E 1973 Genealogical investigation in a group of children with duodenal ulcer. Review of Czechoslovak Medicine 19: 81–88

Selmanowitz V J, Orentreich N, Tiango C C, Demis D J 1970 Uniovular twins discordant for cutaneous mastocytosis. Archives of Dermatology 102: 34–41

Semble E L, Turner R A, Wu W C 1987 Clinical and genetic characteristics of upper gastrointestinal disease in rheumatoid arthritis. Journal of Rheumatology 14: 692–699

Shaw J M 1968 Genetic aspects of urticaria pigmentosa. Archives of Dermatology 97: 137–138

Soll A H, Isenberg J I 1989 Duodenal ulcer diseases. In: Sleisinger M H, Fordtran J S (eds) Gastrointestinal disease, pathophysiology, diagnosis and management. Saunders, Philadelphia, p 814–878.

Stevenson R E, Lucas T, Martin J R 1979 Stiff skin and multiple system disease in four generations. American Journal of Human Genetics 31: 84A

Sumii K, Uemura N, Inbe A et al 1986 Familial aggregation of duodenal ulcer and an autosomal dominant inheritance of hyperpepsinogenemia I. Hiroshima Journal of Medical Sciences 35(2): 171–175

Susser M 1967 Causes of peptic ulcer: A selective epidemiological review. Journal of Chronic Disease 20: 435–456

Tarpila S, Samloff I M, Pillarainen P, Vouristo M, Ihamaki T 1982 Endoscopic and clinical findings in first-degree relatives of duodenal ulcer patients and control subjects. Scandinavian Journal of Gastroenterology 17: 503–506

Taylor I L 1988 Duodenal ulcer disease. In: Gitnick G, Hollander D, Kaplowitz N, Samloff I M, Schoenfield L J (eds) Principles and Practice of Gastroenterology and Hepatology. Elsevier, New York, p 175–190

Taylor I L, Calam J, Rotter J I et al 1981 Family studies of hypergastrinemic, hyperpepsinogenemic I duodenal ulcer. Annals of Internal Medicine 95: 421–425

Tovey F I 1979 Progress report, peptic ulcer in India and Bangladesh. Gut 29: 329–347

Tovey F I, Tunstall M 1975 Progress report, duodenal ulcer in black populations in Africa south of the Sahara. Gut 16: 564–576

Van Allen M W, Frohlich J A, Davis J R 1969 Inherited predisposition to generalized amyloidosis, clinical and pathological study of a family with neuropathy, nephropathy, and peptic ulcer. Neurology 19: 10–25

van Heerden J A, Smith S L, Miller L J 1986 Management of the Zollinger-Ellison syndrome in patients with multiple endocrine neoplasia type I. Surgery 100: 971–977

Vesely K T, Kubickova Z, Duorakova M, Zvolankova K 1968 Clinical data and characteristics differentiating types of peptic ulcer. Gut 9: 57–68

Walker P, Luther J, Samloff I M, Feldman M 1988 Life events, stress and psychological factors in men with peptic ulcer disease. Gastroenterology 94: 323–330

Wermer P 1954 Genetic aspects of adenomatosis of endocrine glands. American Journal of Medicine 16: 363–371

Wormsley K G, Grossman M I 1965 Maximal histalog test in control subjects and patients with peptic ulcer. Gut 6: 427–435

Wretmark G 1953 The peptic ulcer individual, a study in heredity, physique and personality. Acta Psychiatrica Scandinavica and Neurologica (Supplement 84)

Zollinger R M, Ellison E H 1955 Primary peptic ulcerations of the jejunum associated with islet cell tumors of the pancreas. Annals of Surgery 143: 709–728

66. Developmental defects of the gastrointestinal tract

E. Passarge

INTRODUCTION

This chapter reviews the genetic aspects of developmental defects of the gastrointestinal tract. Since these usually occur as part of chromosomal or monogenic disorders, which are dealt with in other chapters, emphasis here is on isolated defects and the assessment of their risk of recurrence.

Congenital pyloric stenosis, previously described by the late Cedric O. Carter in the first edition of this book (Carter 1983) is now included. In order to facilitate the use of McKusick's catalogue of Mendelian phenotypes in man (McKusick 1988) I have included his numbers (McK —) with respect to the defects considered in this chapter.

DEFECTS OF THE GROSS INTESTINAL ANATOMICAL STRUCTURE

Developmental defects of the gastrointestinal tract may occur alone, limited to one or several sites of the tract, or they may be part of an overall developmental disorder. Clinically they usually lead to signs of obstruction, resulting from stenosis, atresia or impaired intestinal mobility, or to bleeding due to ulceration. Although familial occurrence has been observed in gastrointestinal malformations (see below), it may be noteworthy that Mendelian inheritance is unlikely in most instances. In syndromes with gastrointestinal involvement, the overall disorder determines the aetiology of the gastrointestinal maldevelopment. Hence, it is important to recognize the presence of associated non-gastrointestinal defects, which may provide a clue to the recognition of genetic factors.

Intestinal atresia

About one third of congenital atresias involve the oesophagus, with or without concomitant tracheal fistula. However, familial occurrence is rare. The duodenum is the site of atresia in about 10%. In some series, up to one third of patients with duodenal atresia have been found to have an additional chromosome 21 (trisomy 21) (Warkany 1971). Duodenal atresia (McK 22340) has been reported in three sibs (Mishalany et al 1970, 1971).

Four reports of the familial occurrence of jejunal atresia (McK 24360) could be consistent with a rare autosomal recessive gene. However, preferential reporting of rare familial coincidences seems just as likely. Multiple intestinal atresias (Familial intestinal polyatresia syndrome, FIPA, McK 24315), reported in an inbred kindred (Dallaire & Perreault 1974) and in a few other cases, could be the result of an autosomal recessive mutation. On the other hand, the so-called 'apple peel' syndrome (Martin et al 1976) could be explained on the basis of intrauterine mesenteric artery accidents which, in turn, could lead to multiple atresias. Farag and Teebi (1989) reported three sibs with apple peel jejunal atresia.

Malrotation

This is a common developmental failure, but little evidence for genetic factors is available. However, it is often part of a chromosomal or Mendelian disorder.

Duplication

Duplicated parts of the intestines are relatively common developmental defects, but genetic factors do not seem to be involved.

Gastroschisis and omphalocele

Gastroschisis (McK 23075) has been reported in sibs (Salinas et al 1979, Lowry & Baird 1982), but genetic factors seem very unlikely, at least in most cases. Baird and MacDonald (1981) assumed multifactorial inheritance to be possible.

Gastroschisis is an important feature of the abdominal wall disruption sequence ('Prune belly' complex, McK

10010). Although this has been reported in sibs (Gaboardi et al 1982), there is no evidence of genetic factors being involved in its aetiology (Pagon et al 1979).

In contrast, a few older observations suggest the possibility that omphalocele may occur in a pattern resembling autosomal dominant inheritance (McK 16475). Havalad et al (1979) have reported omphalocele in four males; two maternal half-brothers, and two grandsons of one of them (McK 31098). Nevertheless, in an isolated patient it would seem that the risk of recurrence is low.

Omphalocele is a feature in the syndromes of Beckwith-Wiedemann (McK 13065) and Shprintzen-Goldberg (omphalocele with hypoplasia of the pharynx and larynx, dysmorphic face and learning disability; Shprintzen & Goldberg 1979, McK 18221).

Diaphragmatic defects

Since the earlier reports of the familial occurrence of unilateral diaphragmatic agenesis (McK 22240, Passarge et al 1968) I have come to the conclusion that autosomal recessive inheritance is probably unlikely in most cases. This view is supported by recent studies of Norio et al (1984) and Czeizel and Kovacs (1985). Empirically a slightly increased risk of recurrence over the fairly high population incidence of about 1:1200 may be assumed. Prenatal recognition by ultrasonography and early surgical intervention may be useful to anticipate recurrence and improve the prognosis.

Anterior diaphragmatic hernia (McK 30695) has been reported in a family with two affected brothers and their maternal uncle (Lilly et al 1974). A few families with hiatus hernia (McK 14240) or congenital short oesophagus have been reported (Goodman et al 1969). Altogether there is little evidence for genetic factors in most cases.

Developmental defects of the pancreas

Annular pancreas (McK 16775) is a characteristic malformation in patients with Down syndrome. In spite of two reports of familial occurrence in a mother and three of her four children (Jackson & Apostolides 1978) and a mother and one child, genetic factors need not be considered in counselling.

In contrast, acute or subacute pancreatitis may occur as an autosomal dominant trait (McK 16780). However, this is a relatively rare cause of pancreatitis. A common ampulla of the biliary pancreatic ductus together with hypertrophy of the sphincter of Oddi may be an anatomical basis but has not been found in other studies (Layer et al 1985). Sibert (1978) studied 72 patients in seven families in England and Wales. The disorder showed a penetrance of 80% and occurred in two peaks of age of onset, one at 5, and one at 17 years, with a mean of 13–14. The second peak was considered to be due to genetic susceptibility to environmental factors such as alcohol. Only four of the 72 patients developed life-threatening disease. Early pancreatic calcification may be another feature of this form of pancreatitis.

Winter et al (1986) described two brothers with early-onset insulin-dependent diabetes and pancreatic insufficiency assumed to be due to congenital pancreatic hypoplasia.

Anorectal malformations

Congenital malformations of the anus and rectum include anal stenosis, atresia or ectopy. They occur at a frequency of about 1 per 5000 births. About half of the patients also show other associated developmental defects. Pinsky (1978) has listed at least 26 different patterns of malformations involving anorectal anomalies. These include Mendelian, chromosomal, and non-genetic conditions.

One of the most frequent associations is the VATER/VACTERL complex (McK 19235), an acronym for vertebral, anal, tracheo-esophageal, renal and radial limb anomalies, including cardiovascular and nonradial limb anomalies which may also be present. Pinsky (1978) emphasized the aetiological heterogeneity of these defects and warned of wrong estimates of the genetic recurrence risk unless the underlying phenotype is recognized.

A few reports of imperforate anus in multiple affected sibs (McK 20750) and possible X–linked inheritance (McK 30180) have been recorded. Usually, however, the risk of recurrence may be assumed not to be increased.

Imperforate anus is part of the Townes-Brock syndrome (McK 10748) of hand, foot, and ear anomalies associated with sensorineural deafness.

FUNCTIONAL INTESTINAL DEFECTS

A number of anatomical defects manifest themselves clinically primarily as malfunction. Achalasia, congenital pyloric stenosis, congenital intestinal aganglionosis (Hirschsprung disease) and intestinal pseudo-obstruction fall into this category. Empirical risk figures are available, derived from the increased familial recurrence.

Familial oesophageal achalasia

Six reports of familial occurrence are listed by McKusick (McK 20040) in addition to achalasia associated with microcephaly and mental deficiency in three sisters and a brother (Dumars et al 1980). However, it is doubtful that genetic factors are generally involved.

Intussusception

This is a frequent complication in Peutz-Jeghers syndrome and sometimes in cystic fibrosis. As an idiopathic event there is little to support possible genetic factors in the aetiology. Jolly et al (1982) reported five members in three generations (McK 14771). So-called segmental aganglionosis may cause intussusception (Lawrence & van Wormer 1961).

Congenital pyloric stenosis

For a detailed description of the clinical features, pathology, differential diagnosis, therapy, epidemiology and genetics the reader is referred to chapter 61, pages 879–885 of the first edition of this book (Carter 1983). The following section will summarize the genetic risk figures used in genetic counselling, based mainly on the work of Cedric O. Carter and his associates and a review by Dodge (1980).

Congenital pyloric stenosis is inherited as a multifactorial trait. Environmental factors have been suspected, because of seasonal variation in birth incidence, but have not yet been defined. A recent study from Atlanta, Georgia, did not show evidence for an increasing trend in population incidence or of a higher rate of pyloric stenosis in first-born infants (Lammer & Edmonds 1987).

The population incidence in Caucasians is about 1.5–3 per thousand live births, with a range of 0.5–4.5 reported in different studies in different geographical regions and ethnic groups (Carter 1983). Pyloric stenosis is rare in Asians (less than 1:10 000) and less common in populations of African origin (0.5 per 1000) compared to Caucasians. The sex ratio in Europeans is usually 4–5 males to 1 female, thus giving a birth frequency of about 1:200 in males and 1:1000 in females.

The familial aggregation of congenital pyloric stenosis can be seen from its occurrence among first-degree, second-degree, and third-degree relatives (Carter 1983) as summarized in Table 66.1.

Congenital intestinal aganglionosis (Hirschsprung disease)

Hirschsprung disease is an early childhood disease observed in about 1 per 5000 newborns with a sex ratio of 3.75 males to 1 female. The disease is characterized by chronic constipation leading to severe abdominal disten-

Table 66.1 Pyloric stenosis: Proportion (mean percent) of affected relatives

Affected relatives	Index patient Male	Female
Brothers	6.6	10.8
Sisters	2.8	3.8
Sons	5.5	18.9
Daughters	2.4	7
Male second-degree relatives	2.2	0.5
Female second-degree relatives	4.3	1.7
Male third-degree relatives	0.9	0.2
Female third-degree relatives	0.7	0.3
Population incidence	0.5	0.1

Data based on Carter (1983) with some alterations.

sion, megacolon, and possible secondary electrolyte disturbances. It may present in the neonatal period with ileus or sigmoid perforation. Although the first clinical description by Hirschsprung in 1887 was followed by good pathological studies in 1901 (Tittel 1901) and 1924 (Dalla Valle 1924), which demonstrated absence of intramural intestinal ganglion cells, it was not until 1948 that this was firmly established as the cause of the disease (Zuelzer & Wilson 1948, Swenson & Bill 1948). Since then, numerous studies have been devoted to the diagnosis, management, surgical procedures, and the genetic aspects (Ehrenpreis 1970, Weinberg 1974, Bolande 1975). Genetic factors are implicated by familial occurrence in 4% of cases. Genetic heterogeneity is suggested because congenital intestinal aganglionosis may occur as part of a variety of disorders, most notably trisomy 21, Waardenburg syndrome, cartilage hair dysplasia, phaeochromocytoma, and others.

Anatomical and embryological considerations

Intestinal mobility is controlled via three distinct enteric plexuses: the myenteric plexus of Auerbach, between the circular and longitudinal muscle layers of the muscularis propia, and two plexuses in the submucosal region. These are the superficial submucosal plexus of Meissner, just beneath the muscularis mucosa, and the deep submucosal plexus of Henle. The latter appears to be analogous to Auerbach's plexus (Baumgarten et al 1973, Weinberg 1974).

Ganglion cells of the normal myenteric plexuses are concentrated along the neural strands and the nodal points of a network of non-myelinated extrinsic nerve fibres. Nerve trunks are of vagal origin and largely acetylcholinesterase-positive. However, considerable morphological and histochemical heterogeneity appears to exist, and the complexities of the anatomical and physiological properties of enteric plexuses are not yet fully understood. As pointed out by Weinberg (1974), the enteric ganglion cells do not simply represent peripheral parasympathetic effector cells, but should be viewed as part of a complex neuroregulatory system (Baumgarten et al 1973).

Apparently intramural intestinal ganglion cells reach the alimentary tract by migrating from the cephalic neural crest between the 6th and 12th week of embryogenesis (Hüther 1954, Okamoto & Ueda 1967, Andrew 1971). This migration occurs in a defined time sequence with a cranial-caudal gradient. At 5 weeks' gestation, paired vagal fibres extend to the upper oesophagus, and there are a few fine fibres from the periaortic and pelvic plexuses, but ganglion cells are still absent. At 6 weeks, neuroblasts are present in the oesophagus outside the circular layer and the stomach. At 8 weeks (18 mm embryo) ganglion cells are present in the small intestine and the rectum, but not the colon. At 12 weeks (70 mm) the entire plexus is innervated, presumably by further caudal ganglion cell migration. The most critical period seems to be between weeks 8 and 12, when most of the distal plexus develops.

The neuroblasts first reaching the alimentary tract form the myenteric plexus. The submucosal plexus is formed by neuroblasts migrating from the myenteric plexus across the circular muscle layer into the submucosa (Okamoto & Ueda 1967). The submucosal plexus is also formed in the caudal direction, but later, during the third and fourth months of gestation. The outer longitudinal muscle layer develops from embryonic mesenchymal tissue after the myenteric plexus has been formed in the 12th week (Okamoto & Ueda 1967). In contrast to the apparently direct role of vagal nerve fibres, sympathetic and pelvic parasympathetic nerves are not involved in the development of the intramural plexus.

It should be noted that the intrinsic innervation of the anal canal differs from that of the intestines by a zone normally lacking ganglion cells (Weinberg 1974). This zone may extend up to about 14–18 mm above the pectinate line, followed by another 4–5 mm with a reduced number of ganglion cells. This normal hypoganglionic zone may thus extend for up to 23 mm until the normal plexus is reached.

Thus, a diagnostic rectal biopsy must be taken 20–30 mm above the pectinate line. The orientation of the specimen must be clearly marked and it should be pinned to a flat surface prior to fixation to allow sectioning perpendicular to the plane of the plexus (Weinberg 1974). A full-thickness biopsy of about 5 × 10 mm must be obtained to ensure that both layers of the muscle are present. Fragmented specimens pose considerable difficulties in interpretation. Different methods of biopsy including suction biopsy have been reviewed by Weinberg (1974).

Absence of intestinal ganglion cells

In classic Hirschsprung disease, ganglion cells of the mucosal and submucosal plexus are absent (*total aganglionosis*). The aganglionic segment extends from the supra-anal region (see above) up to the sigmoid colon in 80–90% of patients. In others, the aganglionic segment may reach up to the splenic flexure, and in some cases may involve the entire colon and small intestine. A reduced number of ganglion cells in the enteric plexus may be found in the distal colon, a condition called *hypoganglionosis* (Weinberg 1974). It is not clear whether this constitutes a disease entity in terms of a defined aetiology. Usually, however, a hypoganglionic segment represents the transition between the aganglionic segment and the normal bowel. Another condition is *segmental aganglionosis*. Pathological findings and embryological considerations make it unlikely that this is a developmental defect. It is more likely to be the result of a localized vascular accident (Yntema & Hammond 1954).

Genetics

Several systematic genetic studies (McK 24920) indicate an overall risk of recurrence of about 1–18% depending on the sex of the index patient, the sex of the sib at risk, and the length of the aganglionic segment (Bodian & Carter 1963, Madsen 1964, Emanuel et al 1965, Gordon et al 1966, Passarge 1967a,b, 1973, Garver et al 1985).

Passarge (1967a,b, 1972) suggested that multifactorial inheritance (McK 24920) could explain the familial occurrence. In particular, the high proportion of affected sibs of female index patients, i.e., the sex less often affected in the general population, would represent the so-called 'Carter effect' seen in congenital pyloric stenosis. However, individual observations have been made which suggest that in some families the risk of recurrence may rather correspond to a monogenic disorder, either autosomal recessive (Passarge 1967a,b, Talwalker 1976, MacKinnon & Cohen 1977) or autosomal dominant (Carter et al 1981, Carmi et al 1982, Cohen & Gadd 1982, Badner 1987, Lipson & Harvey 1987). Thus, caution should be exercised when applying empirically derived risk figures. Unfortunately no reliable signs exist in order to distinguish these possible high risk situations from the risks usually assumed to prevail.

Table 66.2 Congenital intestinal aganglionosis frequency of affected sibs*

Index patients	Affected sibs Brothers	Sisters
319 males	16/300 (5.3%)	7/305 (2.3%)
85 females	9/79 (11.4%)	11/81 (13.6%)

* Source of data: Bodian & Carter (1963), Madsen (1964), Passarge (1967a,b). Cases with aganglionosis as part of systemic disorders not included.

The familial incidence is generally higher when the aganglionic segment is long. However, in a few families both short and long segment involvement has been observed in affected relatives (Carmi et al 1982, Garver et al 1985, Lipson & Harvey 1987). Tables 66.2 and 66.3 summarize the recurrence risk to sibs.

Badner et al (1990) reported a study of 487 probands with aganglionosis and a complex segregation analysis of their families. For patients with aganglionosis beyond the sigmoid colon, the mode of inheritance was compatible with a dominant gene with incomplete penetrance, whereas for short colon involvement the inheritance was equally likely multifactorial or autosomal recessive with very low penetrance.

Aganglionosis of the entire bowel has been reported in about 10 families including affected sibs (MacKinnon & Cohen 1977, Talwalker 1976). At present it is not clear whether this is a separate entity, possibly with autosomal recessive inheritance, or the result of over-reporting of a rare coincidence. In some cases nerve fibres were also absent, in contrast to the usual form where ganglion cells are lacking but nerve trunks are present. Other observations are consistent with autosomal dominant inheritance (Carmi et al 1982, Cohen & Gadd 1982, Lipson & Harvey 1987, and others). Experience with surviving affected parents will eventually indicate if monogenic inheritance is responsible in a proportion of cases.

Table 66.3 Congenital intestinal aganglionosis frequency of affected sibs according to length of aganglionic segment*

Index patients	Affected Sibs Brothers	Sisters
Type I : 182 males	4/73 (5.5%)	1/172 (0.6%)
35 females	3/37 (8.1%)	1/35 (2.85%)
Type II: 28 males	10/148 (6.75%)	3/27 (11.1%)
15 females	2/11 (18.2%)	1/11 (9.1%)

* Source of data in Table 66.2. Length of aganglionic segment defined as type I for absence of intestinal ganglion cells caudal to the splenic flexure, and as type II for absence anywhere further rostral to this point.

Hirschsprung disease was not observed in 34 children of affected parents studied by Puri and Nixon (1977), but was in two and possibly four of 103 children reported by Carter et al (1981). Of these, three were born to parents with long segment disease. The authors considered there to be a genetic risk of about 2% for a parent with short segment disease and a high risk for a parent with long segment disease, bearing in mind that the length of the segment affected may differ in parent and child.

At least one attempt at prenatal diagnosis utilizing amniotic fluid disaccharidase analysis, ultrasound, and amniography has been unsuccessful (Jarmas et al 1983).

Evidence for genetic heterogeneity

Congenital intestinal aganglionosis may occur in a number of other disorders (Table 66.4). Several studies have shown that 2.5% of patients with Hirschsprung disease have trisomy 21 (Down syndrome). The reason for this rather frequent association, however, is not yet clear.

A number of associated malformations may occur in patients with Hirschsprung disease, in particular of the urinary tract (hydronephrosis, megalocystis, hydroureter), the gastrointestinal tract (anal stenosis or imperforate anus, colon and small bowel atresia), and cardiovascular system (septal defects) as well as cleft palate, polydactyly, and other malformations (de Bruyn et al 1982, Spouge & Baird 1985).

Table 66.4 Congenital intestinal aganglionosis, frequently observed in association with other disorders

Chromosomal disorders
Trisomy 21
Other chromosomal aberrations
Mendelian disorders
Deafness, different forms
Waardenburg syndrome
Cartilage hair dysplasia
Smith-Lemli-Opitz syndrome (Curry et al 1987)
Type D brachydactyly (Reynolds et al 1983)
Syndrome of congenital heart defect, broad halluces, and ulnar polydactyly in sibs (Laurence et al 1975)
Aarskog syndrome (Hassinger et al 1980)
Syndrome of microcephaly, hypertelorism, short stature and submucous cleft palate (Goldberg & Shprintzen 1981)
Other disorders
Neuroblastoma
Phaeochromocytoma
Rubella embryopathy
Colon atresia
Other congenital defects

Recent observations indicate that the association of microcephaly/mental retardation/cleft palate in some patients, and Hirschsprung disease (Goldberg & Shprintzen 1981) may be an autosomal recessive condition (Hurst et al 1988, Bankier 1989). Other reports include various clinical associations with Hirschsprung disease (Santos et al 1988, Hamilton & Bodurtha 1989). Two different interstitial deletions, 2p22 and 13q22–q32, have also been reported in congenital intestinal aganglionosis (Webb et al 1988, Lamont et al 1989).

In view of the neural crest origin of intramural intestinal ganglion cells, melanocytes, and the sensory components of the spinal and cranial nerves, several observations reporting the association of intestinal aganglionosis and Waardenburg syndrome (Omenn & McKusick 1979, Branski et al 1979, Shah et al 1981, Meire et al 1987) are of particular interest. With an estimated incidence of Waardenburg syndrome with deafness of 2 per 100 000 and of Hirschsprung disease of 2 per 10 000, the chance association would be only 4 per one billion. Omenn and McKusick (1979) have rightly pointed out that this association must be significant (McK 27758).

A similar association of pigmentary anomalies and intestinal aganglionosis has been observed in several mouse mutants. These are the recessive alleles *piebald*, *piebald-lethal* and *lethal-spotting* (Lane 1966). Homozygotes for *piebald-lethal* and *lethal-spotting* show a 100% incidence of aganglionosis. *Piebald* homozygotes and *piebald/piebald-lethal* compound heterozygotes have a 10% incidence for aganglionosis (Omenn & McKusick 1979). These murine disorders represent genetically determined disturbances in cells derived from the neural crest, although the direct effects of the mutant alleles on the neural crest are not yet clear.

Minutillo et al (1989) reported a patient with failure of automatic control of ventilation leading to lethal apnoea (Ondine's curse) associated with intestinal aganglionosis extending into the distal ileum. In view of similar observations in ten other patients cited by Minutillo and one other (Zerres 1990), this is likely to be an aetiologically relevant association. However no familial occurrence has yet been observed.

The occurrence of intestinal aganglionosis in such diverse disorders as trisomy 21 (chromosomal), Waardenburg syndrome and other forms of deafness (Mendelian), phaeochromocytoma (presumptive neural crest disorder), in addition to classic Hirschsprung disease (presumptive multifactorial) supports the contention that failure of the intramural intestinal ganglion cells to develop properly is aetiologically heterogeneous. It remains to be seen whether defects in migration from the neural crest account for all the observations. The complex development of the intramural intestinal neuroregulatory system leaves ample room for different genetic mechanisms leading to maldevelopment.

Intestinal pseudo-obstruction

Idiopathic intestinal pseudo-obstruction with megaduodenum and/or megacystis/microcolon has been reported in a few families as an autosomal dominant trait (McK 15531). Intestinal pseudo-obstruction may occur as part of a generalized disorder affecting smooth muscles (McK 27732), including ptosis palpebrae and ophthalmoplegia as reported in three sibs by Ionasescu et al (1983, 1984). McKusick (1988) lists a report of three infants showing argyrophil myenteric plexus deficiency with short small intestines, malrotation, and pyloric stenosis (McK 24318).

REFERENCES

Andrew A 1971 The origin of intramural ganglia. Journal of Anatomy 108: 169

Badner J A 1987 Evidence for dominant gene(s) in Hirschsprung Disease. American Journal of Human Genetics 41: A44

Badner J A, Sieber W K, Garver K L, Chakravati A 1990 A genetic study of Hirschsprung disease. American Journal of Human Genetics 46: 568–580

Baird P A, MacDonald E C 1981 An epidemiologic study of congenital malformations of the anterior abdominal wall in more than half a million consecutive live births. American Journal of Human Genetics 33: 470

Bankier A 1989 Hirschsprung's disease, distinctive facies, and microcephaly. Journal of Medical Genetics 26: 287

Baumgarten H G, Holstein A F, Stelzner F 1973 Nervous elements in the human colon of Hirschsprung's disease. Archives of Pathology and Anatomy 358: 113

Bodian M, Carter C O 1963 Family study of Hirschsprung's disease. Annals of Human Genetics 29: 261

Bodurtha J, Hamilton J, Nance W E 1987 Congenital central alveolar hypoventilation syndrome (CCHS) and Hirschsprung Disease (HD) in half siblings. American Journal of Medical Genetics 41: A50

Bolande R P 1975 Hirschsprung's disease, aganglionic or hypoganglionic megacolon. American Journal of Pathology 79: 189

Branski D, Neale J M, Brooks L J 1979 Hirschsprung's disease and Waardenburg's syndrome. Pediatrics 63: 803

Carmi R, Hawley P, Wood J W, Gerald P S 1982 Hirschsprung Disease in progeny of affected individuals: A case report and review of the literature. Birth Defects: Original Article Series Vol. 18, No 3B: 187

Carter C O 1983 Congenital Pyloric Stenosis In: Emery A E H, Rimoin D L (eds) Principles and Practice of Medical Genetics Ist edn. Churchill Livingstone, Edingburg, p 879–885

Carter C O, Evans K, Hickman V 1981 Children of those treated surgically for Hirschsprung's disease. Journal of Medical Genetics 18: 87

Ciment G, Weston J A 1983 Enteric neurogenesis by neural

crest-derived branchial arch mesenchymal cells. Nature 305: 424

Cohen I T, Gadd M A 1982 Hirschsprung's Disease in a Kindred: A Possible Clue to the Genetics of the Disease. Journal of Pediatric Surgery 17: 632

Curry C J R, Carey J C, Holland J S et al 1987 Smith-Lemli-Opitz syndrome-type II: multiple congenital anomalies with male pseudohermaphroditism and frequent lethality. American Journal of Medical Genetics 26: 45

Czeizel A, Kovacs M 1985 A family study of congenital diaphragmatic defects. American Journal of Medical Genetics 21: 105

Dallaire L, Perreault G 1974 Hereditary multiple intestinal atresia. Birth Defects. Original Article Series Vol. X, No. 4: 259

Dalla Valle A 1924 Contributo alle conoscenza della forma famigliare del megacolon congenito. Pediatria 32: 569

de Bruyn R, Hall CM, Spitz M 1982 Hirschsprung's disease and malrotation of the mid-gut. An uncommon association. British Journal of Radiology 55:554

Dodge J A 1980 Infantile hypertrophic pyloric stenosis. Definition, physiology and genetics. In Rotter J I, Samloff I M, Rimoin D L (eds) The Genetics and Heterogeneity of Common Gastrointestinal Disorders, Academic Press, New York p 419

Dumars K W, Williams J J, Steele-Sandin C 1980 Achalasia and microcephaly. American Journal of Medical Genetics 6: 309

Ehrenpreis T 1970 Hirschsprung's disease. Year Book Medical Publishers Inc, Chicago

Emanuel B, Padorr M P, Swenson O 1965 Familial absence of myenteric plexus (congenital megacolon) Journal of Pediatrics. 67: 381–386

Farag T I, Teebi A S 1989 Apple peel syndrome in sibs. Journal of Medical Genetics 26: 67

Gaboardi F, Sterpa A, Thiebat E, Cornali R, Manfredi M, Bianchi C, Giacomoni M A, Bertagnoli L 1982 Prune-belly syndrome: report of three siblings. Acta Paediatrica Helvetica 37: 283

Garver K L, Law J C, Garver B 1985 Hirschsprung disease: a genetic study. Clinical Genetics 28: 503

Goldberg R B, Shprintzen R J 1981 Hirschsprung megacolon and cleft palate in two sibs. Journal of Craniofacial Genetics and Developmental Biology 1: 185

Goodman R M, Wooley C F, Ruppert R D, Freimanis A K 1969 A possible genetic role in esophageal hiatus hernia. Journal of Heredity 60: 71–74

Gordon H, Torrington M, Louw J H, Cywes S 1966 Genetical study of Hirschsprung's disease. South African Medical Journal 40: 720–721

Hamilton J, Bodurtha J N 1989 Congenital central hypoventilation syndrome and Hirschsprung's disease in half sibs. Journal of Medical Genetics 26: 272

Hassinger D D, Mulvihill J J, Chandler J B 1980 Aarskog's syndrome with Hirschsprung's disease, midgut malrotation, and dental anomalies. Journal of Medical Genetics 17: 235

Havalad S, Noblett H, Speidel B D 1979 Familial occurrence of omphalocele suggesting sex–linked inheritance. Archives of Disease in Childhood 54: 142

Hirschsprung H 1887 Stuhlträgheit Neugeborener infolge von Dilatation und Hypertrophie des Colons. Jahrbuch Kinderheilkunde 27: 1

Hurst J A, Markiewicz M, Kumar D, Brett E M 1988 Unknown syndrome. Hirschsprung's disease, microcephaly, and iris coloboma: a new syndrome of defective neuronal migration. Journal of Medical Genetics 25: 494

Hüther W 1954 Die Hirschsprung'sche Krankheit als Folge einer Entwicklungsstörung der intramuralen Ganglien. Beiträge zur pathologischen Anatomie und zur allgemeinen Pathologie 114: 161

Ionasescu V, Thompson S H, Ionasescu R, Searby C, Anuras S, Christensen J, Mitros F, Hart M, Bosch P 1983 Inherited ophthalmoplegia with intestinal pseudo-obstruction. Journal of Neurological Sciences 59: 215

Ionasescu V V, Thompson H S, Aschenbrenner C, Anuras S, Risk W S 1984 Late-onset oculogastrointestinal muscular dystrophy. American Journal of Medical Genetics 18: 781

Jackson L G, Apostolides P 1978 Autosomal dominant inheritance of annular pancreas. American Journal of Medical Genetics 1: 319

Jarmas A L, Weaver D D, Padilla L M, Stecker E, Bender H A 1983 Hirschsprung Disease: Etiologic implications of unsuccessful prenatal diagnosis. American Journal of Medical Genetics 16: 163

Jolly D T, McKim J C, Corrin M H 1982 A family with intussusception and malignant hyperthermia. Canadian Medical Association Journal 127: 737

Lammer E J, Edmonds L D 1987 Trends in pyloric stenosis incidence, Atlanta, 1968 to 1982. Journal of Medical Genetics 24: 482

Lamont M A, Fitchett M, Dennis N R 1989 Interstitial deletion of distal 13q associated with Hirschsprung's disease. Journal of Medical Genetics 26: 100

Lane P W 1966 Association of megacolon with two recessive spotting genes in mouse. Journal of Heredity 57: 29

Laurence K M, Prosser R, Rocker I, Pearson J F, Richards C 1975 Hirschsprung's disease associated with congenital heart malformation, broad big toes, and ulnar polydactyly in sibs: a case for fetoscopy. Journal of Medical Genetics 12: 334

Lawrence A G, van Wormer D E 1961 Intussusception due to segmental aganglionosis. Journal of the American Medical Association 175: 909

Layer P, Balzer K, Goebell H 1985 Hereditary Pancreatitis. Presentation of an additional family. Hepato-gastroenterology 32: 31

Lilly J R, Paul M, Rosser S B 1974 Anterior diaphragmatic hernia: familial presentation. Birth Defects: Original Article Series Vol. X, 4: 257

Lipson A H, Harvey J 1987 Three-generation transmission of Hirschsprung's disease. Clinical Genetics 32: 175

Lowry R B, Baird P A 1982 Familial gastroschisis and omphalocele. American Journal of Human Genetics 34: 517

MacFayden U M, Young I D 1987 Annular pancreas in mother and son. American Journal of Medical Genetics 27: 987

Mackinnon A E, Cohen S J 1977 Total intestinal aganglionosis. An autosomal recessive condition? Archives of Disease in Childhood 52: 898

McKusick V A 1988 Mendelian Inheritance in man, 8th edn. The Johns Hopkins University Press, Baltimore and London

Madsen C M 1964 Hirschsprung's disease. Munksgaard, Copenhagen

Martin C E, Leonidas F C, Amoury R A 1976 Multiple gastrointestinal atresias, with intraluminal calcifications and cystic dilatation of bile ducts: A newly recognized entity resembling 'a string of pearls'. Pediatrics 57: 268

Meire F, Standaert L, De Laey J J, Zeng L H 1987

Waardenburg Syndrome, Hirschsprung megacolon, and Marcus Gunn ptosis. American Journal of Medical Genetics 27: 683

Minutillo C, Pemberton P J, Goldblatt J 1989 Hirschsprung's disease and Ondine's curse: further evidence for a distinct syndrome. Clinical Genetics 36: 200–203

Mishalany H G, Der Kaloustian V M, Ghandour M H 1970 Familial congenital duodenal atresia. Pediatrics 46: 629

Mishalany H G, Kaloustian V M, Ghandour M H 1971 Familial congenital duodenal atresia. Pediatrics 47: 633

Norio R, Kaariainen H, Rapola J, Herva R, Kekomaki M 1984 Familial congenital diaphragmatic defects: aspects of etiology, prenatal diagnosis, and treament. American Journal of Medical Genetics 17: 471

Okamoto E, Ueda T 1967 Embryogenesis of intramural ganglion of the gut and its relation to Hirschsprung's disease. Journal of Pediatric Sugery 2: 437

Omenn G S, McKusick V A 1979 The association of Waardenburg syndrome and Hirschsprung megacolon. American Journal of Medical Genetics 3: 217

Orr J D, Scobie W G 1983 Presentation and incidence of Hirschsprung's disease. British Medical Journal 287: 1671

Pagon R A, Smith D W, Shepard T H 1979 Urethral obstruction malformation complex: a cause of abdominal deficiency and the 'prune-belly'. Journal of Pediatrics 94: 900

Passarge E 1967a The genetics of Hirschsprung's disease. Evidence for heterogeneous etiology and a study of sixty-three families. New England Journal of Medicine 276: 138

Passarge E 1967b Quelques considerations etiologiques et génétiques sur la maladie de Hirschsprung. Médecine et Hygiène 25: 240

Passarge E 1972 Genetic heterogeneity and recurrence risk of congenital intestinal aganglionosis. Birth Defects, Original Article Series (G.I Tract.) Vol. VIII, 2: 63

Passarge E 1973 Genetics of Hirschsprung disease. Clinics in Gastroenterology 2: 507

Passarge E, Halsey H, German J 1968 Unilateral agenesis of the diaphragm. Humangenetik 5: 226

Pinsky L 1978 The syndromology of anorectal malformation (atresia, stenosis, ectopia). American Journal of Medical Genetics 1: 461

Puri P, Nixon H H 1977 Long-term results of Swenson's operation for Hirschsprung's disease. Progress in Pediatric Surgery 10: 87

Reynolds J F, Barber J C, Alford B A, Chandler J G, Kelly T E 1983 Familial Hirschsprung's Disease and Type D Brachydactyly: A report of four affected males in two generations. Pediatrics 71: 246

Salinas C F, Bartoshesky L, Othersen H B, Leape L, Feingold M, Jorgensen R J 1979 Familial occurrence of gastroschisis. American Journal of Diseases of Children 133: 514

Santos H, Mateus J, Leal M 1988 Hirschsprung disease associated with polydactyly, unilateral renalagenesis, hypertelorism and congenital deafness: a new autosomal recessive syndrome. Journal of Medical Genetics 25: 204

Shah K N, Dalal S J, Desai M P, Sheth P N, Joshi N C, Ambani L M 1981 White forelock, pigmentary disorder of irides, and long segment Hirschsprung disease: Possible variant of Waardenburg syndrome. Journal of Pediatrics 99: 432–435

Shprintzen R J, Goldberg R B 1979 Dysmorphic facies, omphalocele, laryngeal and pharyngeal hypoplasia, spinal anomalies, and learning disabilities in a new dominant malformation syndrome. Birth Defects Original Article Series XV(5B): 347–353

Shprintzen R J, Goldberg R B 1982 A recurrent pattern syndrome of craniosynostosis associated with arachnodactyly and abdominal hernias. Journal of Craniofacial Genetics and Developmental Biology 2: 65–74

Sibert J R 1978 Hereditary pancreatitis in England and Wales. Journal of Medical Genetics 15: 189

Spouge D, Baird P A 1985 Hirschsprung Disease in a large birth cohort. Teratology 32: 171

Swenson O, Bill A H 1948 Resection of rectum and rectosigmoid with preservation of the sphincter for benign spastic lesions producing megacolon. Surgery 24: 212

Talwalker V C 1976 Aganglionosis of the entire bowel. Journal of Pediatric Surgery 2: 213

Tittel K 1901 Über eine angeborene Mißbildung des Dickdarms. Wiener Klinische Wochenschrift 14: 903

Warkany J 1971 Congenital malformations. Notes and comments. Year Book Medical Publishers, Chicago

Webb G C, Keith C G, Campbell N T 1988 Concurrent de novo interstitial deletion of band 2p22 and reciprocal translocation (3;7) (p21;q22). Journal of Medical Genetics 25: 125

Weinberg A G 1974 Hirschsprung's disease – A pathologist's view. In "Perspectives in pediatric pathology" II. Year Book Medical Publishers, Chicago, p 207

Winter W E, Maclaren N K, Riley W J, Toskes P P, Andres J, Rosenbloom A L 1986 Congenital pancreatic hypoplasia: A syndrome of exocrine and endocrine pancreatic insufficiency. Journal of Pediatrics 109: 465

Yntema C C, Hammond W S 1954 Origin of intrinsic ganglia of trunk viscera from vagal neural crest in chick embryo. Journal of Comparative Neurology 101: 515

Zuelzer W W, Wilson J L 1948 Functional intestinal obstruction of congenital neurogenic basis in infancy. American Journal of Diseases of Children 75: 40

67. The polyposes

A. M. O. Veale

(Professor Veale died at the time the text was being prepared and his chapter has been updated by one of the editors — AEHE.)

Polypoid conditions of the gastrointestinal tract, particularly the colon and rectum, form an interesting group of diseases with familial polyposis coli, Peutz-Jeghers syndrome and Gardner syndrome showing simple Mendelian dominant inheritance. Other conditions appear to show familial aggregation of affected cases with the formal genetics remaining obscure. Of particular interest is the fact that adenomas of the colon and rectum in polyposis coli and Gardner syndrome are indistinguishable from isolated adenomas arising in the general population, and from those seen in association with cancer of the large bowel.

Just as the detailed study of inborn errors of metabolism yields a greater understanding of normal metabolic pathways, it may be that the polyposes contain clues concerning the pathogenesis of colorectal cancer. Collectively, the polyposes are not a common group of disorders when seen from the perspective of a general physician. To a geneticist though they are far from infrequent and their study, apart from the intrinsic interest and importance to the family members, may yield a greater understanding of carcinogenesis, notwithstanding the considerable evidence implicating environmental factors in the causative chain. Genetic and environmental causes are not mutually exclusive, and individual differences in cancer susceptibility are now being increasingly recognised (Harris et al 1980).

In this chapter we describe non-premalignant polyps, premalignant polyps and finally evidence that genetic factors play a role in the appearance of colorectal cancer.

A medical dictionary defines a polyp as: 'A morbid excrescence or protruding growth from a mucous membrane'. In considering polypoid conditions of the gastrointestinal tract it is helpful to bear this definition in mind, as it does not carry any implications with respect to the malignant potential that any given polyp may or may not have. This serves to remind us that in the investigation of a polyp the histology of the lesion is an essential piece of information required to arrive at a correct diagnosis.

Geneticists naturally tend to classify a group of diseases sharing some common feature (in this case, polyps) into those recognisable syndromes which are apparently not inherited, and those which are. There usually remains an indistinct group in which the inherited nature of its members is debatable. An alternative classification of polypoid lesions of the colon and rectum could be based on the malignant potential of the polyp, based on histological criteria, followed by consideration of a further genetic subdivision.

Non-malignant or non-premalignant conditions would thus include:

1. Isolated hamartomas of childhood
2. Hyperplastic polyps
3. Juvenile polyposis
4. Peutz-Jeghers syndrome
5. Other benign forms of polyposis

Premalignant polypoid conditions are as follows:

1. Isolated adenomas of the rectum and/or colon
2. Multiple adenomas of the colon and rectum with or without associated lesions elsewhere
3. Other forms of multiple polyps which are not adenomas.

In this classification the term 'adenoma' is used in a generic sense as a grouped term to include neoplastic polyps in general, such as an adenoma itself or tubular adenoma, the tubular-villous or papillary adenoma and the villous adenoma or villous papilloma.

NON-PREMALIGNANT POLYPS

Isolated hamartomas of childhood

These lesions are also known as juvenile, cystic or retention polyps, and are prone to torsion of their long pedicle and subsequent auto-amputation. The histological appearances are typical, with large amounts of loose connective tissue and cystic spaces containing mucus. Occasionally, a polyp of this kind may be found in association with multiple adenomas, but this is rare.

Hyperplastic polyps

These lesions are frequently seen on sigmoidoscopy and colonoscopy, but are not regarded as having any malignant potential. They present as small raised areas a few millimetres across which macroscopically are indistinguishable from the early appearance of an adenoma with which they are often found in association. The microscopic appearances, however, are quite different with lengthening of the tubules which are dilated with mucus leading to flattening of the epithelial cells. There is also a diminution in the number of goblet cells. The potential of these lesions, also known as metaplastic polyps, is not known, but they are at present regarded as benign even though they may be found in association with adenomas or carcinoma.

Juvenile polyposis

This condition, described by McColl et al (1964) and later by Veale et al (1966), is characterised by lesions more closely resembling the isolated hamartomas of childhood than those of an adenoma. The histological appearances show less connective tissue than is commonly seen in the isolated lesions, with more irregularity of branching of the glands.

Sachatello (1972) divided the condition into three subgroups, the first corresponding with the isolated lesions described above, the second with multiple lesions confined to the large bowel, and a third with polypoid lesions throughout the gastrointestinal tract. Bussey et al (1978), however, emphasise the rarity of multiple juvenile polyposis, and attempt no subdivision of cases, apart from those with and those without a history of other affected relatives. It is note worthy that in their series of just over 50 cases in 36 families, three quarters of the families were of 'isolated' cases, and one quarter had from 2–5 affected family members. Other congenital anomalies such as congenital heart defects, malrotation of the gut, Meckel's diverticulum and hydrocephalus were found in nearly 20% of cases. At first it was thought that these abnormalities were confined to cases with no family history (Bussey 1970), but this is no longer the case and the apparent distinction is blurred.

Even though the histological appearances in juvenile polyposis coli are not suggestive of any malignant potential, and the disease is in the meantime grouped with other non-malignant and non-premalignant conditions, there does seem to be some relationship with familial polyposis coli. In the first instance, although the majority of the lesions in juvenile polyposis coli show the typical histological appearances of the isolated cystic or retention polyp seen in childhood, a proportion show areas of epithelial atypia similar to that seen in adenomas. Secondly, in some families with juvenile polyposis coli there are relatives affected with multiple adenomatous polyposis and/or colonic or rectal carcinoma (Veale et al 1966, Smilow et al 1966, Bussey et al 1978). In a family where a parent had adenomatous polyposis and two offspring had juvenile polyposis it was suggested by Veale et al (1966) that this variation between parent and offspring could be due to an allelic gene received from the unaffected parent and interacting with the gene for adenomatous polyposis received from the affected parent. This was purely speculative and families described since have given little support to the notion. The exact relationship between adenomatous and juvenile polyposis probably requires much more extensive data covering several generations in order to elucidate the problem. In the meantime, it seems logical to continue to include juvenile polyposis in the 'non-malignant' category. One should also remember that the term 'juvenile' does not necessarily mean that the condition is found only in children. The term refers more to the primitive nature of the connective tissue in the polyp rather than to the age of the patient.

Peutz-Jeghers syndrome

First described by Peutz (1921) and then by Jeghers et al (1949) the genetics of this condition is clear cut. Inherited as a Mendelian dominant, the characteristic findings are polyps of the gastrointestinal tract, and spots of skin pigmentation. The polyps may be present throughout the entire gastrointestinal tract, but in over 90% of cases the small bowel is involved, and in about one third of cases the colon and rectum as well (Louw 1972). The skin pigmentation is shown as patches of melanin a few millimetres in diameter on the lips, oral mucosa and the hands and feet.

At first, it was thought that the polyps had considerable malignant potential, but Bartholomew and Dahlin (1958) and Bartholomew et al (1957) suggested that they were in fact local tissue malformations (hamartomas), and had little or no potential for undergoing malignant change. Bailey (1957) collected 67 cases from the literature and tabulated the distribution of the tumours together with details of their histology. In 13 cases there was an adenocarcinoma of the small intestine, and in three cases a carcinoma of the large bowel. This emphasises an important difference between Peutz-Jeghers syndrome and familial polyposis coli (adenomatosis) where the risk of malignancy is high. The probability of malignant degeneration in Peutz-Jeghers syndrome has continued to be argued and it may be that the cases where malignancy does occur are the result of the concomitant occurrence of adenomas. Bussey (1975) reports knowledge of 18 cases of definite cancer in patients with Peutz-Jeghers polyposis. Most of these cases occurred in the stomach and duodenum. Morson (1962) believes the risk of malignancy in Peutz-Jeghers polyps is low. The histological appearances of a Peutz-Jeghers polyp are in marked contrast to those seen in an adenoma. A tree-like proliferation of the muscularis mucosae is primarily involved in the formation of a Peutz-Jeghers polyp with the epithelium only secondarily involved. Furthermore, the epithelium is substantially normal with the same proportion of individual cells of different types in the same relationship to each other as in uninvolved epithelium. There is no increase in epithelial mitotic activity, or alteration in mucus secreting activity. For all these reasons the Peutz-Jeghers syndrome should be regarded as essentially a non-premalignant condition, especially as some of the few cases of malignancy reported were found to have associated adenomas (Dodds et al 1972). The principal symptoms of Peutz-Jeghers polyposis are those arising from intussusception and/or intestinal obstruction.

Lipomatosis

Swain et al (1969) reported a condition resembling a generalised colorectal polyposis where there were deposits of fat in the submucosa. So far this condition has only been observed in children. Ordinary lipomas may also occur in the gastrointestinal tract, and are usually not multiple. Ling et al (1959) reported a case with multiple lipomas throughout the alimentary tract.

Cystic pneumatosis

Macroscopically this condition can be confused with adenomatosis because multiple gas filled cysts project into the lumen of the large bowel. The cause is unknown.

Inflammatory polyps

Any condition of the large bowel leading to patchy destruction of the mucosa may result in the formation of irregular tags of tissue projecting into the lumen, e.g. bacillary and amoebic dysentery, hyperplastic tuberculosis, bilharzia infection and ulcerative colitis. The latter carries a small risk of malignancy (1–2%), but it is probably the underlying cause of the ulcerative colitis rather than the mucosal tags themselves which leads to this.

Benign lymphoid polyposis

This condition arises as a result of non-neoplastic hypertrophy of lymphoid tissue normally present in the gastrointestinal tract. It must be distinguished from the conditions described by Cornes (1960, 1961) where the polyposis is secondary to some other pathological process. Benign lymphoid polyps are more frequently seen in children or young adults. Louw (1968) has described the condition appearing in three sibs.

PREMALIGNANT POLYPS

Isolated adenomas of the colon and rectum

The occurrence of single adenomas in the colon and rectum in adult patients over the age of 40 is commonplace, and not infrequently the number may be more than one. Andren and Frieberg (1959) surveyed 3609 patients and found the incidence of adenomas increased steadily with age from 5% at 20 to nearly 15% at 70. Rider et al (1959) studied 9669 patients and found polyps in 537 (5.6%), a lower incidence than in other surveys. A most significant finding, however, was the re-examination of 372 of these patients with adenomas during a four to nine year follow up period. It was found that 41% of these patients had developed additional polyps. The authors concluded that new polyps were being formed faster in this group of patients than in the general population, and that they represented a group that were 'polyp prone'.

Woolf et al (1955) described a large family in which isolated adenomas (1–4) occurred in nearly 50% of the adult members. They felt that there was good evidence in this family to suggest that the appearance of isolated adenomas may have been due to the segregation of a single gene predisposing to adenoma formation. Lynch et al (1979) described two families in which there occurred the simultaneous appearance of patients with familial polyposis coli and others showing only isolated adenomas.

Bussey (1975) described the frequency of adenomas in a series of 1788 patients thought not to have familial intestinal polyposis. The vast majority had only a single lesion and only 15 patients had more than six. Very rarely patients with 60 or 70 adenomas have been reported, but have not been thought to have familial polyposis coli, although any patient with more than 100 adenomas almost certainly has this condition. A possible genetic explanation for the occurrence of isolated adenomas will be discussed later. (See: 'A genetic model'.)

Familial polyposis coli (Familial adenomatous polyposis)

This condition was probably first described in the eighteenth century and several times in the nineteenth. Lockhart-Mummery (1925) first drew attention to the relationship between polyposis and cancer, and other reviews have been provided by Dukes (1952), Reed and Neel (1955), Veale (1965), Pierce (1968) and Bussey (1975). Multiple adenomas (>100) of the colon and rectum occurring in childhood or in young adults is pathognomonic, although it must be remembered that the appearance of polyps may be delayed until middle or later life.

The average age at which patients with symptoms are first diagnosed is 35 years, and approximately 10% of such cases are not diagnosed until older than 50. Naturally, once an index case has been identified the investigation of relatives will yield positive cases who may be quite young. Polyposis affects both sexes equally and is inherited as an autosomal dominant trait. The risk of one or more of the adenomas undergoing malignant degeneration is virtually 100%. The condition should be treated surgically by total colectomy or sub-total colectomy with an ileorectal anastomosis and subsequent examination of the rectal stump at frequent intervals.

Until comparatively recently it was thought that the adenomatous lesions were confined to the colon and rectum, and that the occasional cases of polyposis of the entire gastrointestinal tract perhaps represented a distinct genetic entity (Yanemoto et al 1969). Hoffman and Goligher (1971) reviewed the matter, and Ross and Mara (1974) reported two additional cases, one with adenocarcinoma of the jejunum with an associated adenoma 0.8 cms in diameter, and the other with adenocarcinoma of the ileum with a 25 cm length of the resected ileum showing multiple adenomatous polyps. It seems that the gastrointestinal lesions in familial polyposis coli are *not* confined to the colon and rectum, and that one should be alert to the possibility of adenomas in the small bowel as well. Even though this may not be a frequent complication, it should be borne in mind particularly in those patients who have had a successful surgical treatment of the large bowel for a number of years.

The Gardner syndrome (see below) characteristically shows a number of associated lesions, but quite apart from this, patients with familial polyposis coli sometimes show other manifestations of neoplastic activity. In his series of polyposis families Veale (1965) reported 11 unrelated cases of polyposis, all with affected relatives, all from different kindreds, none of which was thought to be affected with Gardner syndrome. The associated lesions found were fibroma of uterus, carcinoma of the uterus, sebaceous cyst and frontal bone osteomas, abdominal wall desmoid and frontal osteomas, mesenteric lymphangioma, thyroid adenoma and two abdominal desmoids, multiple lipomas, hepatoma, medulloblastoma, keloid in abdominal scar, and an abdominal desmoid. In addition to these cases, there were five isolated cases of polyposis (no affected relatives) showing similar lesions, and another isolated case with chronic lymphocytic leukaemia. There seems to be little doubt that patients with polyposis have some kind of predisposition to other forms of neoplastic activity, particularly the formation of desmoid tumours in the abdominal wall following surgery (McAdam & Goligher 1970).

Gardner syndrome

The characteristic tetrad of gastrointestinal adenomas, fibromas, osteomas and epidermal cysts described by Gardner and Richards (1953) is much less frequent than the classical form of familial polyposis coli. In all respects, apart from the extra-colonic lesions, the two diseases are similar. In view of the fact that some patients with classical polyposis occasionally show some of the features of Gardner syndrome, and that in some kindreds assumed to have Gardner syndrome not all affected members show all the characteristic extra-colonic features, or when shown they are not necessarily affected to the same degree, it is not surprising to find that there is some debate with respect to whether the two genes are distinct (Smith 1968). Evidence in favour of Gardner syndrome being a separate disorder from familial polyposis coli is afforded by several large pedigrees with all affected members showing the characteristic lesions.

Utsunomiya and Nakamura (1975), however, were able to demonstrate occult osteomatous changes in the mandible not only in cases of Gardner syndrome, but also in the majority (19 out of 21 cases) of patients with polyposis coli. They now regard routine panoramic X-rays of the jaws as an essential part of their work-up of any polyposis family, and have been able to predict correctly the presence of colonic adenomatosis following such X-ray examination. As a result they have concluded that Gardner syndrome and classical familial polyposis coli should not be regarded as different aetiological categories, and that their findings are a further indication that familial polyposis coli can manifest other forms of neoplastic activity apart from that in the colon and rectum. Recent molecular studies indicate that the two disorders are infact allelic (Solomon 1990).

Cronkite-Canada syndrome

This is another form of polyposis of the colon and rectum with associated lesions. Originally described by Cronkite and Canada (1955) the characteristic lesions associated with general gastrointestinal polyposis were diffuse areas of skin pigmentation, alopecia and onychotrophia. All the cases described so far have been sporadic so it is difficult to know how to fit this syndrome in with the others. The condition is accompanied by intestinal malabsorption with disturbances of the plasma proteins and electrolytes. The prognosis is poor and a genetic causation remains to be proved.

Turcot syndrome

Turcot et al (1959) reported polyposis coli in association with malignant tumours of the central nervous system. Two sibs died at the ages of 17 and 21 from medulloblastoma and glioblastoma respectively. Previous polyposis had been diagnosed and treated surgically when the patients were aged 15 and 16. Two reports of isolated cases are cited by Bussey (1975) who also mentions another member of a polyposis family from the St Mark's Hospital series who died from a medulloblastoma. This patient was 'at risk' for developing polyposis, but at the time of death was not known to have been affected. This case from St Mark's is in addition to the one mentioned earlier (under 'Familial polyposis coli') where the patient was known to have had polyposis. It has been suggested that Turcot syndrome may be an autosomal recessive trait if it does indeed represent a condition distinct from polyposis coli.

Other rare syndromes

Cornes (1960, 1961) described cases with primary malignant lymphomas and carcinomas of the intestinal tract. These patients were found to have adenomas of the colon as well as malignant lymphomas, again demonstrating another facet in the relationship between adenoma formation and other neoplastic activity.

Von Recklinghausen disease (multiple neurofibromatosis) may occasionally produce multiple neurofibromas of the colon and rectum (Ghrist 1963) and one case of polyposis coli has been found subsequently to have had neurofibromatosis (Bussey 1975). A mixture of colonic neurofibromas and juvenile polyps has also been reported (Donnelly et al 1969).

BOWEL CANCER IN THE POPULATION

The importance of adenomas as a predisposing factor to colorectal cancer in polyposis coli and Gardner syndrome is undisputed. Similarly, the occurrence of small adenomas (1–4) in the colon or rectum of a person not a member of a polyposis family is regarded as not without significance with respect to the development of a sub-sequent carcinoma. Adenomas are correctly regarded as premalignant lesions, even though the risk may be small. It should also be noted that so far there is nothing histologically which serves to distinguish an adenoma in a polyposis patient from an isolated adenoma arising spontaneously, independent of polyposis. Naturally, there has been speculation about whether or not there is a tendency towards familial aggregation in cases of colorectal cancer. We have already seen that Woolf et al (1955) suggested that in at least one family there was a tendency for isolated adenomas to appear as if determined by a single gene similar to the polyposis gene, but with a less powerful action.

Similarly, Lynch et al (1966, 1967, 1973) have presented reports of families in which many members were affected with colorectal cancer, sometimes occurring in conjuction with cancer of the breast and endometrium. This has given rise to the notion of families which are 'cancer prone'. More generally, Macklin (1960) and Lovett (1976) have looked at the incidence of cancer in the relatives of unselected index cases with colorectal cancer and found that the incidence of colorectal cancer, particularly in first-degree relatives, is much increased. Apart from the obvious 'cancer prone' families, polyposis coli and Gardner syndrome, the increased incidence of colorectal cancer in the relatives of index cases has hitherto been ascribed as probably due to environmental factors for which there is quite impressive evidence.

Numerous studies have reported that the incidence of colon cancer shows a striking positive correlation with dietary factors such as meat and fat intake, and a negative correlation with dietary fibre intake. Vitamin A and alcohol intake also seem to be involved. There are striking international differences in colorectal cancer indicating that it is probably a disease of 'life style', the incidence being highest in Western European-like countries. Native born Japanese have a very low incidence of large bowel cancer, but on migration to Hawaii or the USA the incidence soon approaches that of the host population, although there is some protection afforded if the immigrants seek to retain their national dietary habits. Similarly McMichael (1980) has shown that European migrants from Italy, Yugoslavia and Greece have an increasing incidence of colorectal cancer depending on their length of stay in Australia. Seventh Day Adventists, who observe a strict dietary code, have also been much studied in the USA where it is found that their incidence of colorectal cancer is much lower than that of their non Seventh Day Adventist compatriots.

Considerable attention has been focused on the role of intestinal bacteria in the causation of bowel cancer, particularly the ratio of anaerobes to aerobes in the faecal flora of individuals from groups with marked differences in colorectal cancer incidence. Similarly, concentrations of acid and neutral steroids in the faeces have also differed in patients on high and low protein diets. In this connection Watne and Core (1975) have reported differences in the faecal steroids found in polyposis patients from those in the general population. More importantly, Wilkins and Hackman (1974) have reported that normal patients are divisible into two distinct classes based upon the analysis of neutral sterols in faeces, which may be a reflection of an underlying genetic heterogeneity. Much animal experimental work has been done on the induction of colorectal cancer, and Hill (1975) has suggested that in humans the role of cocarcinogen and carcinogen is fulfilled by unsaturated and saturated bile acids interacting with colonic anaerobic bacteria. There is considerable evidence to invoke environmental factors in the causation of bowel cancer, but there are still areas of controversy such as disputes over the role (if any) of dietary cholesterol. Furthermore, the Mormons of Utah represent a group with a very high protein and meat intake, and yet have a low incidence of colorectal cancer (Enstrom 1975). Dietary factors seem to have an 'immediate' effect in that immigrants assume the host population's incidence at a rate proportional to their exposure time but, surprisingly, there is no correlation in the host population between the incidence of colorectal cancer in spouses (Jensen et al 1980).

A colorectal cancer hypothesis

Quite apart from the study of colorectal cancer itself, the epidemiology of adenoma formation in populations is informative. Hill (1978) reported the size of adenomas in different populations (high and low incidences of colorectal cancer), together with the frequency with which malignancy was found in adenomas of different sizes. Small adenomas (<1 cm) were relatively much more frequent in Japan than in England, but the percentage of large adenomas showing malignant changes was the same (approximately 50%) in each group. The distribution of small adenomas is fairly uniform throughout the large bowel, but the distribution of large adenomas is similar to that of carcinoma, showing an increased frequency as the site considered passes more distally. Hill et al (1978) interpreted these findings as indicating that the factors predisposing to small adenoma formation are different from those which conspire to induce small adenomas to become large. They propose that adenomas will only arise in persons of an appropriate genotype, and that an environmental factor (A) will induce the formation of small adenomas uniformly throughout the large bowel. Environmental factor (B) will cause small adenomas to become large, but with an effect showing an increasing gradient as we pass from proximal to distal. Finally, agent (C) induces malignancy in a high proportion of large adenomas, a small proportion of small adenomas and, rarely, in normal mucosa.

Hill et al then comment on the nature of the three factors postulated. They suggest that (A) must be ingested preformed and be of uniform concentration throughout the large bowel.

Factor (B) is probably a bacterial metabolite of the bile acids (already implicated in the causation of colorectal cancer) or something else related to dietary intake of fat or meat.

Factor (C) remains unknown.

A genetic model

Of particular interest is the genetic component of the model proposed by Hill et al (1978). The predisposing genotype is designated pp where p is an allele of the polyposis coli gene P first postulated by Veale (1965). The hypothesis was proposed to explain the absence of parent/child correlations in polyposis families in connection with various age related parameters, such as appearance of polyps, onset of malignancy, and age at death from cancer. Sib/sib correlations were statistically consistent with a value of $+0.5$, whereas parent/child values approached zero. There was also a suggestion of bimodality in the age distributions so that two polyposis genotypes were postulated: Pp with earlier onset and $P+$ with later onset, each distribution showing considerable overlap with the other. This theory is sufficient to explain the zero parent/child correlations and the values of $+0.5$ for sibs. It was further suggested that non-polyposis patients of genotype pp of frequency 9% in the general population represented those persons predisposed to adenoma formation.

Formal consequences of this are:

1. There should be an increased incidence of colorectal cancer among index cases with the condition. This is now well documented (Lovett 1976).

2. There would be 'polyp prone' individuals of the population (Woolf et al 1955, Rider et al 1959, Brahme et al 1974).

3. We would expect that families would occur from time to time in which there was a predominance of pp individuals. Such families would show a high incidence of colorectal cancer, and have been reported (Warthin 1925, Macklin 1960, Lynch & Krush 1967, Lynch et al 1973).

4. If there were a large bowel 'cancer proneness' bestowed upon an individual by virtue of his genotype it might be that this could manifest itself in other organs.

Such an association in colon cancer families has been reported by Lynch et al (1966) and Lynch and Krush (1973) with respect to an increased frequency of endometrial cancer, breast cancer and multiple primary malignancies.

5. If 'cancer proneness' had a genetic basis there might be some manifestation of this in a tissue culture system.

Estimation of genetic parameters

If we assume the gene frequency of the p gene is u and $v = 1 - u$, then the frequency of the pp genotype will be u^2. Given that the probability of developing cancer when of genotype pp is x, the frequency of cancer patients = $u^2 x$ which, for colorectal cancer, is approximately 0.03 in England and Wales. Among the parents of index cases with colorectal cancer the frequency of persons with genotype pp and cancer will be ux. An estimate of this quantity can be obtained from data based on that of Lovett (1976), but with two families now known to have polyposis coli omitted. The series now consists of 207 sets of parents nearly all of whom are dead, and for which there is reliable hospital and/or death certificate information concerning their bowel cancer status. A total of 36 out of 414 parents are known to have had colorectal cancer giving a value of $ux = 0.087$. Solving these two equations gives values for u and x of 0.34 and 0.25 respectively.

It is also possible to use sib data to obtain other equations involving u and x, but here the matter is complicated because of the nonexistence of a suitable body of data. Lovett's (1976) amended series of index cases included 672 sibs of whom only 166 were dead. Among 104 of those who died in the period 1930–1970 there were 18 who died of colorectal cancer (17.31%) which is over five times the number of deaths expected. In view of the large number of sibs still alive, no formal segregation analysis was possible. Such an analysis is further complicated by the fact that the risk to sibs will vary between families due to the fact that the probabilities for parental genotypes will also vary with the incidence of cancer found among relatives. For example, the risk to a sib given no other family history of bowel cancer other than the index case is $(u + \frac{1}{2}v)^2 x$, whereas if one parent is known to have had cancer the risk is $(u + \frac{1}{2}v)x$. More complicated expressions arise when there are other affected relatives such as uncles and aunts or additional affected sibs.

Additional complications in segregation analysis are introduced by the inherent biases in ascertaining families (truncate selection). In the meantime it would appear that in order to investigate familial aggregation of cancer, the families of index cases should be followed with the same persistence as that bestowed on undoubted genetic conditions such as polyposis coli. Notwithstanding the importance of environmental influences as demonstrated by the studies on immigrants, the lack of correlation in incidence between spouses seems to indicate that such factors might require the appropriate genetic predisposition to be effective.

Polyps, cancer and ABO blood groups

The possibility that familial aggregations of large bowel cancer might be the result of a combination of environmental factors and of relatives tending to share some common genetic factor such as a blood group, has been suggested. McConnell (1966) cites 11 investigations into an association between the ABO blood groups and colorectal cancer, and concludes that the overall impression is that the ABO blood groups do not seem to be involved. Fleming et al (1967) investigated the association with polyps of the colon or rectum (373 patients) and found a significant excess of blood group O (p <0.001) in patients with papillary adenomas. These represented 21 patients, of whom 16 were group O. The distribution of blood groups in patients with tubular adenomas did not differ from controls. Vogel and Krüger (1968) concluded, from their survey of the literature, that blood group A was over-represented in colorectal cancer patients, but that this was weaker than the well known association with stomach cancer. Later studies by Bjelke (1973) reporting no consistent differences, are cited by Correa and Haenszel (1978).

Tissue culture systems

There has been considerable work done on the changes found in metabolic pathways within the cells which constitute the normal colonic and rectal mucosa. During differentiation of the cell types, various nucleic acid activities appear to be induced and others are repressed. Additional chemical changes are observed in tissue culture from cells derived from tubular and villous adenomas, but so far nothing has served to differentiate an adenoma from a polyposis coli or Gardner syndrome patient, and an isolated adenoma found in a non-polyposis patient. Danes (1975, 1976, 1979) has detected a major cytogenetic change in cultures of epithelial cells taken by skin biopsy in patients with Gardner syndrome. Such cultures have shown a greatly increased incidence of tetraploidy (30–40%) over the 2–3% found in normals. Similar findings were found in cell lines derived from colonic and rectal mucosa.

At first, the finding was thought to be confined to Gardner syndrome only and not polyposis coli. It appears, however, that some polyposis coli patients do show increased tetraploidy although Delhanty et al (1980) found the frequency similar in both polyposis coli and controls. Danes (1980) presented data showing results in controls, polyposis coli and Gardner syndrome. There does not seem to be any doubt that tetraploidy is much increased in Gardner syndrome, and only marginally so in polyposis coli. Of particular interest is the result in the controls where 7 out of 97 (7.2%) gave positive results.

Molecular genetics

Bodmer and colleagues (Bodmer et al 1987) have found close linkage between a DNA marker on chromosome 5 (5q21-22) and polyposis coli. The use of closely linked markers will now make possible presymptomatic detection as well as prenatal diagnosis. This same group (Solomon et al 1987) have found that in at least 20% of sporadic colorectal adenocarcinomas there is loss of one

of the alleles on chromosome 5q present in normal tissue and is thus comparable to retinoblastoma and Wilms tumour (Solomon 1990). However, the situation is not entirely clear because loss of material from 17p (Fearon et al 1987) and 18q (Muleris et al 1985) may also be involved in the progression from the benign to the malignant state in colorectal tumours. Furthermore, in colon carcinomas in familial polyposis coli, studies have revealed frequent allele loss on chromosomes 5, 6, 12 and 15 (Okamoto et al 1988). Loss of 5q tends to be an early event whereas deletions of 17p (and 18q etc.) come later (Anon 1989). It therefore seems clear that more than one chromosomal locus is involved in the development of familial and sporadic colon carcinomas. Nonetheless presymptomatic and prenatal diagnosis of familial adenomatous polyposis is now possible with a high degree of reliability using bridging DNA markers on chromosome 5 (Tops et al 1989, Solomon 1990).

REFERENCES

Andren L, Frieberg S 1959 Frequency of polyps of rectum and colon, according to age, and relation to cancer. Gastroenterology 36: 631

Anon 1989 Colon cancer: molecular analysis marches on. Lancet 1: 1236–1238

Bailey D 1957 Polyposis of the gastrointestinal tract: the Peutz Syndrome. British Medical Journal 2: 433

Bartholomew L G, Dahlin D C 1958 Intestinal polyposis and mucocutaneous pigmentation (Peutz-Jeghers syndrome). Minnesota Medicine 4: 848

Bartholomew L G, Dahlin D C, Waugh J M 1957 Intestinal pigmentation associated with mucocutaneous melanin pigmentation (Peutz-Jeghers syndrome). Gastroenterology 32: 434

Bjelke E 1973 Epidemiological studies of cancer of the stomach, colon, and rectum: With special emphasis on the role of diet. 1–5, University Microfilms, Ann Arbor, Michigan. Cited by Correa P, Haenszel W. In: Klein G, Weinhouse S (eds) 1978 Advances in cancer research 26, Academic Press, New York, San Francisco, London

Bodmer W F, Bailey C J, Bodmer J et al 1987 Localization of the gene for familial adenomatous polyposis on chromosome 5. Nature 328: 614–616

Brahme F, Ekelund G R, Norden J G, Wenckert A 1974 Metachronous colorectal polyps: Comparison of development of colorectal polyps and carcinomas in persons with and without histories of polyps. Diseases of the Colon and Rectum 17: 166–171

Bussey H J R 1970 Gastrointestinal polyposis. Gut 11: 970–978

Bussey H J R 1975 Familial polyposis coli. The Johns Hopkins University Press, Baltimore, London

Bussey H J R, Veale A M O, Morson B C 1978 Genetics of gastrointestinal polyposis. Gastroenterology 74: 1325–1330

Cornes J S 1960 Multiple primary cancers: Primary malignant lymphomas and carcinomas of the intestinal tract in the same patient. Journal of Clinical Pathology 13: 483

Cornes J S 1961 Multiple lymphomatous polyposis of the gastrointestinal tract. Cancer 14: 249

Correa P, Haenszel W 1978 The epidemiology of large bowel cancer. In: Klein G, Weinhouse S (eds) Advances in cancer research, Vol. 26, Academic Press, New York, San Francisco, London

Cronkite L W Jr, Canada W J 1955 Generalized intestinal polyposis: An unusual syndrome of polyposis, pigmentation, alopecia and onychotrophia. New England Journal of Medicine 252: 1011–1015

Danes B S 1975 The Gardner Syndrome: A study in cell culture. Cancer 36: 2337 (Supplement)

Danes B S 1976 Increased tetraploidy in cultured skin fibroblasts. Journal of Medical Genetics 13: 52

Danes B S 1979 In vitro evidence for adenoma-carcinoma sequence in large bowel. Lancet 2: 44–45

Danes B S 1980 In vitro tetraploidy in familial polyposis coli. Lancet 2: 200–201

Delhanty J D A, Pritchard M B, Bussey H J R, Morson B C 1980 Tetraploid fibroblasts and familial polyposis coli. Lancet 1: 1365

Dodds W J, Schulte W J, Hensley G T, Hogan W J 1972 Peutz-Jeghers syndrome and gastrointestinal malignancy. American Journal of Roentgenology 115: 374–377

Donnelly W H, Sieber W K, Yunis E J 1969 Polypoid ganglio-neurofibromatosis of the large bowel. Archives of Pathology 87: 537–541

Dukes C E 1952 Familial intestinal polyposis. Annals of Eugenics 17: 1

Enstrom J E 1975 Cancer mortality among Mormons. Cancer 36: 825–841

Fearon E R, Hamilton S R, Vogelstein B 1987 Clonal analysis of human colorectal tumors. Science 238: 193–196

Fleming T C, Caplan H W, Hyman G A, Kitchin F D 1967 ABO blood groups and polyps of the colon. British Medical Journal 2: 526–527

Gardner E J, Richards R C 1953 Multiple cutaneous and subcutaneous lesions occurring simultaneously with hereditary polyposis and osteomatosis. American Journal of Human Genetics 5: 139

Ghrist T D 1963 Gastrointestinal involvement in neurofibromatosis. Archives of Internal Medicine 112: 357–362

Harris C C, Mulvihill J J, Thorgierrson S S, Minna J D 1980 Individual differences in cancer susceptibility. Annals of Internal Medicine 92: 809–825

Hill M J 1975 The role of colon anaerobes in the metabolism of bile acids and steroids, and its relation to colon cancer. Cancer 36: 2387–2400

Hill M J 1978 Etiology of the adenoma-carcinoma sequence. In: Bennington J L (ed) The pathogenesis of colorectal cancer, W B Sanders Company, Philadelphia, London, Toronto. Ch 12, p 153–162

Hill M J, Morson B C, Bussey H J R 1978 Aetiology of adenoma-carcinoma sequence in large bowel. Lancet 1: 245–247

Hoffman D C, Goligher J C 1971 Polyposis of stomach and small intestine in association with familial polyposis coli. British Journal of Surgery 58: 126–128

Jeghers H, McKusick V A, Katz K H 1949 Generalised intestinal polyposis and melanin spots of the oral mucosa, lips and digits. New England Journal of Medicine 241: 993–1005, 1031–1036

Jensen O M, Bolander A M, Sigtryggsson P, Vercelli M, Nguyen-Dinh X, MacLennan R 1980 Large bowel cancer in married couples in Sweden. Lancet 1: 1161–1163

Ling C S, Leagus C, Stahlgren L H 1959 Intestinal lipomatosis. Surgery 46: 1054–1059

Lockhart-Mummery J P 1925 Cancer and heredity. Lancet 1: 427

Louw J H 1968 Polypoid lesions of the large bowel in children with particular reference to benign lymphoid polyposis. Pediatric Surgery 3: 195–209

Louw J H 1972 Polypoid lesions of the large bowel in children. South African Medical Journal 46: 1347–1352

Lovett E 1976 Family studies in cancer of the colon and rectum. British Journal of Surgery 63: 13–18

Lynch H T, Krush A J 1967 Heredity and adenocarcinoma of the colon. Gastroenterology 53: 517–527

Lynch H T, Krush A J 1973 Differential diagnosis of the cancer family syndrome. Surgery 136: 221

Lynch H T, Shaw M M, Magnuson C W, Larsen A L, Krush A J 1966 Hereditary factors in cancer: Study of two large mid Western kindreds. Archives of Internal Medicine 117: 206–212

Lynch H T, Guirgis H, Swartz M, Lynch J, Krush A J, Kaplan A R 1973 Genetics and colon cancer. Archives of Surgery 106: 669–675

Lynch H T, Lynch Patricia M, Follett Karen, Harris R E 1979 Familial polyposis coli: Heterogeneous polyp expression in two kindreds. Journal of Medical Genetics 16: 1–7

McAdam W A F, Goligher J C 1970 The occurrence of desmoids in patients with familial polyposis coli. British Journal of Surgery 57: 618–631

McColl I, Bussey H J R, Veale A M O, Morson B C 1964 Juvenile polyposis coli. Proceedings of the Royal Society of Medicine 57: 896–897

McConnell R B 1966 The genetics of gastro-intestinal disorders. Oxford Monographs on Medical Genetics, Oxford University Press, London

Macklin M T 1960 Inheritance of cancer of the stomach and large intestine in man. Journal of the National Cancer Institute 24: 551–571

McMichael A 1980 Personal communication

Morson B C 1962 Precancerous lesions of upper gastrointestinal tract. Journal of the American Medical Association 179: 311

Muleris M, Salmon R J, Zafrani B et al 1985 Consistent deficiencies of chromosome 18 and of the short arm of chromosome 17 in eleven cases of human large bowel cancer. Annals of Genetics 28: 206–213

Okamoto M, Sasaki M, Sugio K et al 1988 Loss of constitutional heterozygosity in colon carcinoma from patients with familial polyposis coli Nature 331: 273–277

Peutz J L A 1921 Over een zeer merkwaardige, gecombineerde familiaire polyposis van de slijmoliezen van den tractus intestinalis met die van de neuskeelholte en gepaard met eigenaardge pigmentaties van huid-en slijmoliezen. Maandschrift Geneesk. 10: 134–146

Pierce E R 1968 Some genetic aspects of familial multiple polyposis of the colon in a kindred of 1422 members. Diseases of the Colon and Rectum 11: 321–329

Reed T E, Neel J V 1955 A genetic study of multiple polyposis of the colon (with an appendix deriving a method of estimating relative fitness). American Journal of Human Genetics 7: 236

Rider J A, Kirsner J B, Moeller H C, Palmer W L 1959 Polyps of colon and rectum: Four year to nine year follow-up study of 537 patients. Journal of the American Medical Association 170: 633

Ross Janice E, Mara J E 1974 Small bowel polyps and carcinoma in multiple intestinal polyposis. Archives of Surgery 108: 736–738

Sachatello C R 1972 Polypoid disease of the gastrointestinal tract. Journal of the Kentucky Medical Association 70: 540–544

Smilow P C, Pryor C A Jr, Swinton N W 1966 Juvenile polyposis coli: A report of three patients in three generations of one family. Diseases of the Colon and Rectum 9: 248–254

Smith W G 1968 Familial multiple polyposis: Research tool for investigating the etiology of carcinoma of the colon? Diseases of the Colon and Rectum 11: 17–31

Solomon S 1990 Colorectal cancer genes. Nature 343: 412–414

Solomon S, Voss R, Hall V et al 1987 Chromosome 5 allele: Loss in human colorectal carcinomas. Nature 328: 616–619

Swain V A J, Young W F, Pringle E M 1969 Hypertrophy of the appendices epiploicae and lipomatous polyposis of the colon. Gut 10: 587–589

Tops C M, Wijnen J Th, Griffioen G et al 1989 Presymptomatic diagnosis of familial adenomatous polyposis by bridging DNA markers. Lancet ii: 1361–1363

Turcot J, Despres J P, St Pierre F 1959 Malignant tumours of the central nervous system associated with familial polyposis of the colon. Diseases of the Colon and Rectum 2: 465–468

Utsunomiya J, Nakamura T 1975 The occult osteomatous changes in the mandible of patients with familial polyposis coli. British Journal of Surgery 62: 45–51

Veale A M O 1965 Intestinal polyposis. Eugenics Laboratory, Memoir Series (40): London

Veale A M O, McColl I, Bussey H J R, Morson B C 1966 Juvenile polyposis coli. Journal of Medical Genetics 3: 5–16

Vogel F, Krüger J 1968 Statistische Beziehungen zwischen den ABO-Blutgruppen und Krankheiten mit Ausnahme der Infektionskrankheiten. Blut 16: 351–376

Warthin A S 1925 The further study of a cancer family. Journal of Cancer Research 9: 279–286

Watne A L, Core S S 1975 Fecal steroids in polyposis coli and ileorectostomy patients. Journal of Surgical Research 19: 157–161

Wilkins T, Hackman A 1974 Two patterns of neutral steroid conversion in the feces of normal North Americans. Cancer Research 34: 2250–2254

Woolf C M, Richards R C, Gardner E J 1955 Occasional discrete polyps of the colon and rectum showing an inherited tendency. Cancer 8: 403

Yanemoto R M, Slayback J B, Byron R L Jr, Rosen R B 1969 Familial polyposis of the entire gastrointestinal tract. Archives of Surgery 99: 427–434

68. Inherited disorders of bilirubin metabolism

Jayanta Roy Chowdhury   Pulak Lahiri   Namita Roy Chowdhury

Degradation of haem, a process essential for mammalian life, results in the formation of bilirubin. Bilirubin is a potentially toxic waste product, and elaborate metabolic processes for its detoxification and elimination have evolved in vertebrates. Appreciation of the chemical structure, mechanisms of transport, metabolism and excretion of bilirubin will facilitate the understanding of inherited disorders of bilirubin metabolism and the mechanism of bilirubin toxicity. It may also provide insight into the hepatic transport of many other organic anions that share the metabolic pathway with bilirubin.

FORMATION OF BILIRUBIN

Haem is the exclusive source of biliverdin and bilirubin. Formation of these two pigments is the predominant pathway of haem degradation in mammals. About 80% of bilirubin is derived from the haemoglobin of senescent erythrocytes (Berk et al 1969), the remainder mainly derived from other haemoproteins, such as myoglobin, tissue cytochromes, catalase, peroxidase and tryptophan pyrrolase. Following injection of radiolabelled glycine, a precursor of porphyrins, there are two peak periods of radiolabelled bilirubin in serum and bile. The first or 'early labelled peak' is seen within 72 hours; the second or 'late peak' coincides with the lifespan of erythrocytes (approximately 120 days in man and 50-60 days in rats). The initial component of the early labelled peak, contains about two thirds of the early labelled bilirubin, and is derived mainly fom hepatic haemoproteins, such as cytochrome P-450s and a pool of free haem in hepatocytes. The terminal component of the early-labelled peak, comprising of 3% of daily normal bilirubin production, is derived from breakdown of haem that is synthesized in the bone marrow, but not incorporated into erythrocytes ('ineffective erythropoiesis'); this component is greatly enhanced in patients with haemoglobinopathies, lead poisoning, megaloblastic anaemias and other conditions associated with increased ineffective erythropoiesis (Robinson et al 1966).

Haem oxygenase-mediated conversion of haem to biliverdin

The initial step in the formation of biliverdin involves the cleavage of the porphyrin ring of haem specifically at the α-methene bridge (Fig. 68.1). This reaction is catalyzed by the microsomal enzyme haem oxygenase and requires Fe^{2+} and a reducing agent, such as NADPH. Haem oxygenase activity is predominantly present in the spleen, where sequestration of senescent erythrocytes occurs (Tenhunen et al 1970), lower but detectable activity is observed in the liver and kidney. Haem oxygenase is thought to be rate-limiting in haem oxidation and in formation of bilirubin (Sassa et al 1979). However, evidence supporting a contrasting view has been recently presented (Cowan et al 1983, Posselt et al 1985). The initial reaction of O_2 with the α-bridge carbon of the porphyrin ring results in the formation of α-oxyhaem followed by ring cleavage and release of the α-bridge carbon as CO. This step is linked to the addition of two additional oxygen atoms that appear as the lactam oxygens of biliverdin and bilirubin.

Biliverdin reductase-catalyzed conversion of biliverdin to bilirubin

Most mammals convert biliverdin to bilirubin prior to excretion. Conversion of biliverdin to bilirubin is catalyzed by a cytosolic enzyme, biliverdin reductase, which requires NADH or NADPH for activity (Colleran & O'Carra 1977). These chemical reactions result in formation of bilirubin $IX\alpha$, which is the most abundant naturally occurring isomer (Blanckaert et al 1976).

SOLUBILITY OF BILIRUBIN AND ITS RELATION TO STRUCTURAL CONFORMATION

The bilirubin molecule has four acidic groups. The two carboxyl groups have pKs of 4.4, and the two lactam groups have pKs of 13.0. Despite these acidic groups,

1135

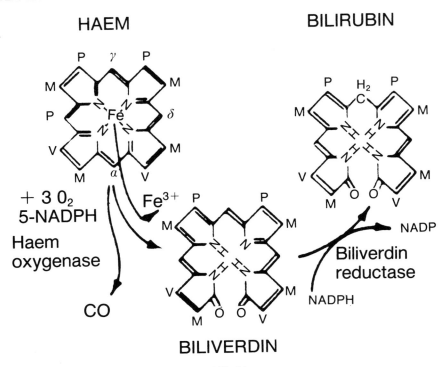

Fig. 68.1 Conversion of haem to biliverdin and biliverdin to bilirubin.

bilirubin is poorly soluble in water. X-ray diffraction studies show that the bilirubin IXα molecule has internal hydrogen bonding between each propionic acid side chain and the pyrrolic and lactam sites in the opposite half of the molecule. As both carboxylic groups, all NH groups, and the two lactam oxygens are engaged by hydrogen bonding, the molecule is insoluble in water (Bonnet et al 1976). Bilirubin is readily soluble in polar solvents, provided that the intramolecular hydrogen bonds can be interrupted. Thus, highly polar solvents, such as formamide and dimethylsulphoxide, are the best solvents for bilirubin. Internal hydrogen bonding may be disrupted by esterification of the propionic acid side chains; the resulting molecule (conjugated bilirubin) is water-soluble and is readily excreted in bile. Internal hydrogen bonding of the bilirubin requires that the carbon bridges within the two dipyrroic halves of the molecule are in Z configuration (bilirubin IXα-ZZ). Exposure of bilirubin in the circulation to light results in the conversion of bilirubin IXα-ZZ to geometric configurational isomers in which one or both carbon bridges within the two dipyrrolic halves of bilirubin are in E or 'cis-' configuration (ZE, EZ or EE isomers). Since the E configuration interferes with hydrogen bonding, the geometric isomers lack one or more internal hydrogen

bonds, are more polar than than bilirubin IXα-ZZ and can be excreted in bile without conjugation (McDonagh 1975, Lightner et al 1979). When injected into rats, the geometric isomers are readily excreted in bile where they revert to bilirubin IXα-ZZ (Lightner et al; 1979). Under some circumstances, the geometric isomers may undergo cyclization forming more stable structural isomers, e.g. E-cyclobilirubin (McDonagh et al 1982, Itoh & Onishi 1985). Formation of the geometric and structural isomers is imporant in phototherapy for unconjugated hyperbilirubinaemia.

TOXICITY OF BILIRUBIN

Clinical aspects

With rare exceptions, bilirubin-induced brain damage is limited to neonates or infants. Clinical manifestations range from fully developed kernicterus to subtle intellectual abnormalities which occur in later life. Kernicterus is usually diagnosed between the third and sixth day of life. The normal Moro reflex is lost. The cry is high-pitched and reflex opisthotonus occurs in response to a startling stimulus. Hypotonia and athetoid movements appear. This may progress to lethargy, atonia and death.

Survivors may develop chronic hearing loss, athetosis, paralysis of upward gaze and mental retardation, in various combinations. Infants with moderately high serum unconjugated bilirubin levels may not manifest overt kernicterus in infancy, but may have a higher incidence of impaired neurological or intellectual performance in later life (Naeye 1978).

Histopathological features

Bilirubin staining of the hippocampus, basal ganglia, and nuclei of the cerebellum and brain stem is found in infants who have died in acute kernicterus (Zuelzer & Mudgett 1950). In children dying in the chronic stage of the disorder such staining is not observed. Cytoplasmic degeneration, loss of Niss substance and fine vacuolation, and swelling of nuclear chromatin are found within 72 hours of the beginning of clinical manifestations (Vaughan et al 1950). Later, focal necrosis of neurons and glia appear. Gliosis of the affected areas is seen in chronic cases (Vaughan et al 1950). Since the structural changes are not present from the onset of kernicterus, these may not be the primary pathophysiological events in bilirubin encephalopathy. Kernicterus cannot always be differentiated from other causes of encephalopathy in neonates, such as cerebral haemorrhage, without pathological documentation (Lucey 1982). Conversely, bilirubin staining of the brain also occurs in other forms of brain injury, and does not establish the diagnosis of kernicterus in the absence of neuronal degenerative changes (Turkel et al 1982).

Determinants of the bilirubin content of the brain

The exchange of water-soluble substances and proteins between blood and brain is restricted by anatomical and functional mechanisms, collectively termed the blood-brain barrier (Rappaport 1976). Immaturity of the blood-brain barrier in neonates has been implicated in kernicterus. However, at present there is little evidence to support the concept of an immature blood-brain barrier in the neonate (Purpura & Carmichael 1960, Cornford et al 1982). Experimentally, the blood-brain barrier can be unilaterally and reversibly opened without causing brain damage by infusion of hypertonic urea (Laas & Helmke 1981) or arabinose (Rappaport 1976). In newborn rats, this results in the rapid entrance of intravenously-administered albumin-bound bilirubin into the brain. Following the reversal of the opening of the blood-brain barrier, bilirubin is rapidly cleared from the brain (Levine et al 1985). However, damaged and oedematous brains may bind bilirubin (Lee & Gartner 1983). This may slow down bilirubin clearance making the brain more vulnerable to bilirubin toxicity.

Biochemical mechanism of bilirubin toxicity

Bilirubin is known to inhibit a large number of biochemical mechanisms. These include inhibition of DNA (Schiff et al 1983), RNA and protein synthesis in neural tissues (Nandi Majumdar 1974) and protein synthesis in the liver (Nandi Majumdar & Greenfield 1974). Bilirubin also inhibits carbohydrate metabolism in the brain (Katoh et al 1975), uncouples oxidative phosphorylation and inhibits ATPase activity of brain mitochondria (Mustafa et al 1969). Bilirubin inhibits hydrolytic enzymes (Strumia 1959), dehydrogenases (Flitman & Worth 1966) and enzymes involved in electron transport (Noir et al 1972). It is not clear which, if any, of these mechanisms are primarily responsible for bilirubin-induced encephalopathy. Bilirubin has been shown to inhibit cAMP-dependent protein kinase activity in vitro (Constantopoulos & Matsaniotis 1976) and non-cAMP-dependent protein kinase activity in vivo (Morphis et al 1982). In a cell-free system, bilirubin irreversibly inhibits $Ca+$-activated, phospholipid-dependent protein kinase (protein kinase C) activity and cAMP-dependent protein kinase activity (Sano et al 1985). Inhibition of protein kinase C by bilirubin may interrupt protein phosphorylation in the brain and thus play a role in the pathogenesis of kernicterus.

BILIRUBIN TRANSPORT IN THE PLASMA

Bilirubin circulates bound to albumin (Odell 1959), which protects cells against the potential toxicity of bilirubin (Bowen et al 1959, Mustafa et al 1969). Under physiological conditions, bilirubin is present almost exclusively bound as the dianion to a primary binding site on albumin, with smaller amounts on one or two secondary sites (Berde et al 1979, Brodersen 1979, Cowan et al 1983). Binding of other ligands to albumin may influence its binding capacity for bilirubin. Sulphonamides, anti-inflammatory drugs, and cholangiographic contrast media displace bilirubin competitively from albumin and increase the risk of kernicterus in jaundiced newborn babies (Odell 1973, Brodersen 1978a). Because of the influence of many metabolites and drugs on albumin binding of bilirubin and its transfer from plasma to the central nervous system, measurement of unbound plasma bilirubin concentration, rather than the total bilirubin level, may more accurately estimate the risk of brain damage from unconjugated bilirubin (Odell 1959). Methods for quantitation of unbound bilirubin in serum include gel chromatography (Kapitulnik et al 1974a), peroxidase treatment (Brodersen et al 1979), electrophoresis on cellulose acetate (Athanassiadis et al 1974), and fluorimetry of serum with or without detergent treatment (Lamolla et al 1979). Alternatively, the amount of unoccupied bilirubin binding sites on albumin, termed the reserve bilirubin binding capacity, can be determined by titration of serum with bilirubin or competitive binding by albumin-binding dyes (Brodersen 1978b, Hsia et al 1978). Front-face fluorimetry for determination of bound albumin and reserve bilirubin binding capacity (Lamolla et al 1979) in whole blood appears to be simple and promising. Despite inaccuracies, several empirical tests for determination of reserve bilirubin binding capacity of serum albumin clinically correlate with brain damage (Porter & Waters 1966) and may be useful in clinically assessing the risk of bilirubin toxicity.

METABOLISM AND EXCRETION OF BILIRUBIN BY THE LIVER

Hepatic uptake and storage of bilirubin

Although the high-affinity binding to albumin inhibits the entry of bilirubin into most tissues, bilirubin is rapidly transferred from plasma into the liver. Albumin does not accompany bilirubin into the hepatocyte. Bilirubin uptake appears to be a specific hepatic function requiring the recognition of bilirubin by a plasma membrane receptor (Goresky 1975, Scharschmidt et al 1975). Competition for hepatic uptake in vivo occurs among bilirubin, indocyanine green (ICG) (Scharschmidt et al 1975), sulphobromophthalein (BSP) (Scharschmidt et al 1975), and conjugated bilirubin but not with bile acids (Scharschmidt et al 1975, Paumgartner & Reichenn 1976). A 55 000 dalton organic anion-binding glycoprotein (OABP) isolated from liver plasma membrane preparations is considered to be a putative surface receptor for bilirubin (Reichen & Berk 1979, Wolkoff & Chung 1980, Stremmel et al 1983, Stremmel & Berk 1986). The relation between this protein and another bromosulphophthalein-binding 170 000 dalton protein (bilitranslocase) isolated by another group of investigators (Lunazzi et al 1982), is not known.

Whether free or albumin-bound bilirubin interacts with the hepatocyte prior to hepatic uptake is controversial (Van der Sluijs et al 1987). Based on kinetic studies, it has been proposed that the albumin-bilirubin complex interacts with an albumin receptor on the hepatocyte (Forker & Luxon 1981, Weisiger et al 1981, 1982). However, studies with isolated perfused liver (Barnhart & Clarenburg 1973, Stollman et al 1983) and in intact analbuminaemic rats (Inoue et al 1985) indicate that albumin binding does not facilitate hepatic bilirubin

uptake and the search for a hepatic albumin receptor provided no evidence for a specific liver cell binding protein for albumin (Stremmel et al 1983).

Transport of bilirubin across the sinusoidal membrane of the hepatocyte is bidirectional. Glutathione-S transferases, collectively termed ligandins, are abundant proteins in the hepatocyte cytosol which bind bilirubin with high affinity (Ketterer et al 1967, Levi et al 1969a, Morey & Litwack 1969, Litwack et al 1971, Fleischner et al 1972, 1977, Habig et al 1974, Kamisaka et al 1975a,b, Kirsch et al 1975, Goldstein & Arias 1976, Lichter et al 1976, Benson et al 1977, Prohaska & Ganther 1977, Bhargava et al 1980). Following uptake into the liver, and until its excretion into the bile, bilirubin is stored in the hepatocyte bound to ligandins. Hepatic ligandin concentration does not affect the influx rate of bilirubin, but increases net bilirubin uptake by decreasing the efflux from hepatocyte to blood (Wolkoff et al 1979a, Wolkoff 1980).

Conjugation of bilirubin

Before excretion in bile, the propionic acid carboxyl groups of bilirubin are esterified with sugar groups, usually with glucuronic acid (Fevery et al 1972), forming mono- and diconjugates (Fig. 68.2) (Jansen & Billing 1971). Bilirubin diglucuronide is the major pigment in human bile (Fevery et al 1972). In addition to glucuronides, glucosides, glucoside-glucuronide mixed conjugates and xylosides have been described in human bile (Onishi et al 1980). Glucuronidation of bilirubin is catalyzed by the microsomal enzyme uridinediphosphoglucuronoside glucuronosyltransferase (UDP-glucuronosyltransferase, EC 2.4.1.17), which catalyzes the transfer of the glucuronosyl moiety of UDP-glucuronic acid to a variety of hormones, endogenous metabolites and xenobiotics, forming O-, N-, S- and C-glucuronides (Dutton 1966). UDP-glucuronosyltransferase consists of a family of related isoforms that are integral proteins of the endoplasmic reticulum of liver cells (Roy Chowdhury et al 1985). In addition, lower levels of enzyme activity are present in the kidney, small intestine and adrenal glands (Roy Chowdhury et al 1985). The transferases require membrane lipids for their activity (Jansen & Arias 1975).

Individual isoforms of UDP-glucuronosyltransferase differ in perinatal development, effect of enzyme inducers and inherited functional defect in mutant animals. The transferase activity towards 4-nitrophenol and other simple phenolic substrates develops in late fetal life in rats, whereas activity towards bilirubin and steroid substrates develops after birth (Wishart 1978). In rats, 3-methylcholanthrene treatment induces the transferase activity towards the 'late-fetal' group of substrates (Bock

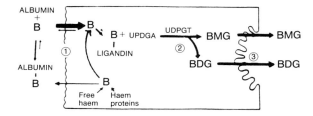

Fig. 68.2 Summary of hepatic transport and metabolism of bilirubin. In the plasma, bilirubin is avidly bound to albumin. At the sinusoidal surface, bilirubin dissociates from albumin and is transported into the liver cell by facilitated diffusion (1). An additional fraction of bilirubin is produced in the hepatocyte from haemoproteins and free haem. Transport of bilirubin across the sinusoidal membrane is bidirectional; binding to ligandins inhibits the efflux of bilirubin from the hepatocyte. Conjugation of bilirubin with glucuronic acid, catalyzed by a specific isoform of the endoplasmic reticulum enzyme UDP-glucuronosyltransferase (2), results in the formation of bilirubin diglucuronide and monoglucuronide. Conjugated bilirubin is transported across the bile canaliculus (3) by an energy-consuming process that may be shared by other organic anions, except bile salts; this step is thought to be rate-limiting in bilirubin throughput.

et al 1973), whereas the transferase activity towards bilirubin is specifically induced by clofibrate (Lillienblum et al 1982). Treatment of rats with triiodothyronine results in a 3-fold increase in the transferase activity towards 4-nitrophenol, whereas activity towards bilirubin is decreased by 80% (Roy Chowdhury et al 1983). Mutant rats with inherited deficiency of bilirubin-UDP-glucuronosyltransferase activity (Gunn strain) cannot form bilirubin glucuronides but form acyl- and N-glucuronides and glucuronides of several phenolic substrates, such as thyroxine and tetrahydrocortisol (Drucker 1968); glucuronidation of simple phenols occurs at a rate lower than normal (Mowat & Arias 1970). Several forms of UDP-glucuronosyltransferase have been chromatographically separated (Burchell 1977, 1981, Gorski & Kasper 1977, Bock et al 1978, 1979, Falany & Tephly 1983, Falany et al 1983). Structural and functional studies of purified rat liver UDP-glucuronosyltransferase isoforms (Roy Chowdhury et al 1986a) and cloning of their corresponding cDNAs (Iyanagi et al 1986, Jackson & Burchell 1986, Mackenzie 1986) indicate the presence of 7–11 isoforms of rat liver UDP-glucuronosyltransferases. These isoforms differ in their range of subtrates; one of these forms appears to be specific for bilirubin (Burchell & Blanckaert 1984, Roy Chowdhury et al 1984, 1986a,b).

Biliary excretion of bilirubin

Excretion of conjugated bilirubin across the bile canalicular membrane occurs against a concentration gradient, by an energy-dependent process. Patients with the Dubin-Johnson syndrome and mutant Corriedale sheep (Alpert et al 1969), and rats (Jansen et al 1985) with analogous functional defects have reduced transport maxima for various organic anions including bilirubin, but not for infused taurocholate (Alpert et al 1969), suggesting the presence of at least two pathways for organic anion excretion by the liver: one for bile salts, another for other organic anions. Kinetic studies of taurocholate and BSP excretion suggest that there may be interaction of bile salt receptors and receptors for other organic anions at the level of canalicular excretion (Forker 1977). Self-aggregation and incorporation of bilirubin in mixed micelles (Scharschmidt & Schmid 1978) may occur in bile and decrease the bilirubin concentration in the aqueous phase.

Degradation of bilirubin in the intestine

Conjugated bilirubin is not substantially absorbed in the intestine (Lester & Schmid 1963). In some circumstances, there may be enhanced excretion of unconjugated bilirubin into the intestine or conjugated bilirubin may undergo β-glucuronidase-catalyzed or nonenzymic hydrolysis. Absorption of unconjugated bilirubin from the intestine may contribute to neonatal hyperbilirubinaemia (Brodersen & Hermann 1963). Degradation of bilirubin by intestinal bacteria results in the formation of urobilinogen and related products (Stoll et al 1977). Most of the urobilinogen is absorbed in the intestine and undergoes enterohepatic circulation; the remainder appears in the stool or is excreted by the kidney. Urobilinogen is colourless; its oxidation product, urobilin, contributes to the colour of normal urine and stool.

In total biliary obstruction, urinary excretion becomes the major pathway of bilirubin excretion (Fulop et al 1965). Renal excretion of conjugated bilirubin depends on glomerular filtration of a small, nonprotein-bound fraction of conjugated bilirubin (Fulop et al 1965). There is evidence for tubular reabsorption but not tubular secretion of bilirubin (Gollan et al 1978).

QUANTIFICATION OF SERUM UNCONJUGATED AND CONJUGATED BILIRUBIN

Serum bilirubins can be quantified as intact tetrapyrroles or after conversion to azoderivatives. Reaction of bilirubin with diazo reagents converts the tetrapyrrole to diazotized azopyrroles and formaldehyde (Hutchinson et al 1972). Van den Bergh and Muller (1916) discovered that on the basis of the rate of reaction with diazotized sulphanilic acid, serum bilirubins can be classified into two species. One reacts within minutes ('direct' van den Bergh reaction) and the other reacts rapidly only when accelerator substances, such as methanol or caffeine, are present ('indirect' reaction) (Van den Bergh & Muller 1916). The direct-reacting fraction represents largely conjugated bilirubin, while unconjugated bilirubin gives the indirect reaction (Talafant 1956). Despite some limitations, modifications of the van den Bergh reaction are commonly used for clinical determination of bilirubin conjugates (Heirwegh et al 1974, Trotman et al 1982). The direct diazo reaction overestimates the levels of conjugated bilirubin; solutions of crystalline bilirubin may show as much as 10-15% of total pigment as direct reacting. Thus, in most clinical laboratories a direct-reacting bilirubin concentration of less than 15% of total is considered within normal limits, although in normal serum bilirubin is almost entirely unconjugated. In addition, the diazo reaction does not differentiate between noncovalently albumin-bound conjugated bilirubin and the fraction of bilirubin that becomes irreversibly bound to serum proteins, particularly albumin, during conjugated hyperbilirubinaemia (Lauff et al 1983, Poon & Hinberg 1985) because both fractions give direct diazo reaction.

More accurate quantification of bilirubin and its conjugates can be performed by high pressure liquid chromatography of underivatized bile pigments (Jansen et al 1977, Roy Chowdhury et al 1978, 1979, 1981, Onishi et al 1980, Roy Chowdhury & Roy Chowdhury 1982, Spivak & Carey 1985, Roy Chowdhury & Arias 1986) or products of their alkaline methanolysis (Blanckaert et al 1980). By reverse-phase chromatography of partially deproteinated serum, covalently protein-bound bilirubin and the various forms of non-covalently bound bilirubin can be simultaneously quantitated (Lauff et al 1983).

Recently, a slide test (Ektachem) for determination of conjugated, unconjugated and irreversibly protein-bound bilirubin has been introduced (Dappen et al 1983, Kubasick et al 1985).

Results obtained by these methods have been validated in patients by comparison with results obtained by high pressure liquid chromatography .

Front-face fluorimetric analysis offers another convenient method for determination of total and albumin-bound bilirubin, and reserve bilirubin-binding capacity from as little as 0.1 ml of whole blood (Brown et al 1980).

Abnormalities of uptake of bilirubin from the circula-

tion, intracellular binding or storage, conjugation or biliary excretion may result in hyperbilirubinaemia. Complex clinical disorders, such as hepatitis or cirrhosis, may affect multiple processes. In several genetic disorders the transfer of bilirubin from blood to bile is disrupted at a specific step, resulting in varied degrees of hyperbilirubinaemia of the unconjugated or conjugated type.

DISORDERS CHARACTERIZED BY PREDOMINANTLY UNCONJUGATED HYPERBILIRUBINAEMIA

Neonatal hyperbilirubinaemia

Serum bilirubin concentration in neonates is normally higher than that in adults. Half of all neonates become clinically jaundiced during the first five days of life. Serum bilirubin is predominantly unconjugated. Exaggeration of this 'physiological jaundice' can result in marked jaundice, with an attendant risk of kernicterus. In 4000 consecutive infants, 16% had maximal serum bilirubin concentrations of 10 mg/dl or above, and in 5% bilirubin concentrations exceeded 15 mg/dl (Hardy & Peebles 1971). In normal, full-term babies, a peak serum bilirubin concentration of 5-6 mg/dl is reached in approximately 72 hours with subsequent decrease until normal levels are attained in 7–10 days (Gartner et al 1977). Physiological hyperbilirubinaemia of the newborn may result from a combination of increased bilirubin production and delayed maturation of hepatic mechanisms for disposal of bilirubin.

Increased endogenous carbon monoxide production (Maisels et al 1971), early-labelled peak from erythroid and nonerythroid sources (Hardy & Peebles 1971) and decreased erythrocyte half-life (Vest et al 1965) indicate increased bilirubin production in the neonate. The increased bilirubin load may be exaggerated in haemolytic diseases of the fetus. Rh incompatibility between mother and fetus used to be a common cause of kernicterus ('erythroblastosis fetalis'), until prevention of this disease by administration of anti-Rh immunoglobulins to the mother (Freda et al 1964, Clarke et al 1971). Major blood group (ABO) incompatibility remains a common cause of exaggerated neonatal hyperbilirubinaemia, which often requires treatment (Hsia & Gellis 1954, Haberman et al 1960).

Hepatic bilirubin uptake occurs at a lower rate than in the adult during the first two days of life; the lower uptake may extend beyond it. Increase of bilirubin uptake to adult levels coincides with the development of adult levels of hepatic ligandin (Levi et al 1969b, 1970, Grodsky et al 1970) which influences the net hepatic bilirubin uptake. Hepatic bilirubin uptake may result from delayed closure of the ductus venosus, which allows the bilirubin-enriched portal blood to bypass the liver (Odell 1967).

UDP-glucuronosyltransferase activity towards bilirubin is deficient in the fetal liver and rapidly develops to adult levels during the first few days of life (Brown & Zuelzer 1958). Deficiency of UDP-glucuronyltransferase activity may be prolonged and exaggerated in some genetic disorders due to inhibitory factor(s) in maternal milk or serum (see below).

During the late newborn period, as in adults, canalicular excretion appears to be rate-limiting in the hepatic disposition of bilirubin. Therefore, an increase in the bilirubin load results in the accumulation of conjugated bilirubin (Hsia et al 1952).

Maternal milk jaundice

Plasma bilirubin concentrations in breast-fed infants are generally higher than those in formula-fed babies (Arthur et al 1966). Bilirubin levels in breast-fed infants occasionally rise to maximum concentrations of 15–24 mg/dl within 10–19 days of life. Discontinuation of breast-feeding promptly ameliorates jaundice, which otherwise disappears within one month. This syndrome is benign; none of these infants develop kernicterus (Arias et al 1964a).

Neonatal unconjugated hyperbilirubinaemia related to breast-feeding is associated with an inhibitor of UDP-glucuronyltransferase activity in maternal milk but not maternal serum (Holton & Lathe 1963, Arias et al 1964a, Hargreaves & Piper 1964). Degree of inhibition of hepatic UDP-glucuronosyltransferase activity (Arias & Gartner 1964) by human milk correlates with the free fatty acid concentration of the milk. The inhibitory activity of free fatty acids, in vitro, is proportional to the number of double bonds in unsaturated fatty acids and inversely proportional to the chain length of saturated fatty acids (C_{10} to C_{18}) (Foliot et al 1976). A lipolytic enzyme, which is present in some maternal milk samples, may be responsible for the increased concentration of free fatty acids in the milk (Foliot et al 1976). Free fatty acid concentration and the inhibitory effect of maternal milk on UDP-glucuronosyltransferase activity increase on storage and are destroyed by heating at 56°C (Foliot et al 1976).

A progestational steroid, $3\alpha,20\beta$-pregnanediol, isolated from the milk of mothers of infants with the maternal milk jaundice syndrome, inhibited o-aminophenol glucuronidation by guinea pig liver microsomes (Arias et al 1964a) and bilirubin glucuronidation by rat and rabbit liver (Arias et al 1964a, Hargreaves & Piper 1964), but not

by human liver (Holton & Lathe 1963). Women whose infants have prolonged jaundice associated with breast-feeding have increased amounts of 3,2-pregnanediol in their urine (Johnson 1975). However, experimental feeding of the steroid to healthy infants yielded contradictory results (Arias & Gartner 1964, Ramos et al 1966).

Transient familial neonatal hyperbilirubinaemia

In this syndrome, jaundice occurs within the first four days of life (Lucey & Driscol 1961, Arias et al 1965a). Peak serum bilirubin concentrations of 8.9–65 mg/dl are usually reached within seven days. An unidentified inhibitor of UDP-glucuronosyltransferase activity was found in the serum of mothers of these infants with this syndrome (Arias et al 1965a). One infant died at 36 hours. This condition is clinically distinguished from jaundice associated with maternal milk by earlier onset, greater severity of hyperbilirubinaemia and occasional incidence of kernicterus.

Treatment of neonatal unconjugated hyperbilirubinaemia

Bilirubin encephalopathy usually occurs with plasma bilirubin concentrations of 20 mg/dl or above; however kernicterus can occur at lower bilirubin levels. The goal of treatment is to decrease serum bilirubin concentrations to an acceptable level until the capacity of the liver to dispose of bilirubin matures. Exchange transfusion and phototherapy are commonly used modes of management (see 'Treatment of Crigler-Najjar Syndrome, Type I'). Prevention of intestine reabsorption of bilirubin by ingestion of agar (Poland & Odell 1971) or activated charcoal also decreases serum bilirubin concentrations; however, efficacy of this treatment is not established (Brodersen & Hermann 1963).

Inherited disorders associated with increased bilirubin production

Increased bilirubin load can cause hyperbilirubinaemia in the presence of normal liver function, however the serum bilirubin level rarely exceeds 3–4 mg/dl. Higher levels may be observed when there is coexistent hepatobiliary dysfunction (Berk et al 1975a, 1980). Common inherited disorders associated with haemolysis and consequent bilirubin over-production include sickle-cell anaemia, hereditary spherocytosis, and toxic or idiosyncratic drug reactions in susceptible individuals. Serum bilirubin is nearly all unconjugated.

However, in massive haemolysis, bilirubin production may transiently exceed the maximum excretory capacity of the liver for conjugated bilirubin, resulting in the accumulation of conjugated bilirubin in serum (Schalm & Weber 1964, Snyder et al 1967). Ineffective erythropoiesis associated with thalassaemia and other haematological disorders may lead to hyperbilirubinaemia (Robinson et al 1962). Congenital dyserythropoietic anaemias are a group of rare hereditary disorders characterized by normoblastic hyperplasia of the bone marrow, secondary haemochromatosis and ineffective erythropoiesis with unconjugated hyperbilirubinaemia (Israels & Zipursky 1959, Verwilghen et al 1969, 1973, Berendsohn et al 1974).

Crigler-Najjar syndrome, type I

Crigler-Najjar syndrome (Crigler & Najjar 1952), type I, is a rare disorder characterized by severe unconjugated hyperbilirubinaemia resulting from a virtual absence of UDP-glucuronosyltransferase activity towards bilirubin (Table 68.1). The syndrome occurs in all races, is transmitted as an autosomal recessive trait (Childs et al 1959, Szabo & Ebrey 1963, Arias et al 1969), and is often associated with consanguinity. Crigler-Najjar syndrome

was originally described in six infants in three related families (Crigler & Najjar 1952). Each infant manifested severe nonhaemolytic unconjugated hyperbilirubinaemia within the first few days of life. Five of the six infants died of kernicterus by the age of 15 months. The single surviving infant did not exhibit signs of neurological damage until 15 years of age, when he suddenly developed kernicterus and died within 6 months (Childs & Najjar 1956, Childs et al 1959). A female cousin of this infant also had this syndrome and developed neurological symptoms at age 18. She died at the age of 24 (Blaschke et al 1974a, Berk et al 1975b, 1980). This family has a high level of consanguinity and several members of the family have other recessively inherited traits, such as Morquio syndrome, homocystinuria, metachromatic leukodystrophy and bird-headed dwarfism (Sleisenger et al 1967).

Approximately 100 other patients with Crigler-Najjar syndrome, type I have been described, the majority of whom died with kernicterus during the neonatal period (Schmid 1972, Wolkoff et al 1979b, Berk et al 1980). Several individuals survived infancy, but succumbed to kernicterus at puberty or early adulthood (Crigler &

Table 68.1   Principal characteristics of inherited disorders associated with unconjugated hyperbilirubinaemia

Characteristic	Crigler-Najjar syndrome, type I	Crigler-Najjar syndrome, type II	Gilbert syndrome
Serum bilirubin level	20-50 mg/dl	8-20 mg/dl	1-5 mg/dl
Serum aminotransferase γ-glutamyltranspeptidase and alkaline phosphatase activities	Normal	Normal	Normal
Serum bile acid levels	Normal	Normal	Normal
Plasma BSP retention (at 45 min)	Normal	Normal	Usually normal, elevated in some
Oral cholecystogram	Normal	Normal	Normal
Bile	Pale; may contain variable amounts of unconjugated bilirubin	Increased proportion of bilirubin monoglucuronide	Increased proportion of bilirubin monoglucuronide
Liver histology	Normal	Normal	Normal
Hepatic bilirubin-UDP-glucuronosyl transferase activity	Absent	Markedly reduced or undetectable	Reduced by 40-70%
Effect of phenobarbital on serum bilirubin level	Slight or no reduction	Marked reduction	Marked reduction
Prevalence	Rare	Uncommon	5% or more of the population
Inheritance	Autosomal recessive	Autosomal recessive (?)	Autosomal dominant (?)
Prognosis	Kernicterus	Usually benign	Benign
Animal model	Gunn rat	-	Bolivian squirrel monkey; mutant Southdown sheep (?)

Najjar 1952, Childs & Najjar 1956, Sleisenger et al 1967, Verwilghen et al 1969, Schmid 1972, Berk et al 1975b). With modern treatment of neonatal hyperbilirubinaemia, larger numbers of these patients survive into childhood. The patients have normal physical examinations, apart from jaundice and neurological impairment, and lack hepatosplenomegaly.

Biochemical abnormalities

The serum bilirubin level is usually 20–25 mg/dl, but may be as high as 50 mg/dl (Crigler & Najjar 1952, Childs & Najjar 1956, Childs et al 1959, Arias 1962, Szabo & Ebrey 1963, Arias et al 1969, Schmid 1972, Blaschke et al 1974a, Berk et al 1975b, Wolkoff et al 1979b). Serum bilirubin is all unconjugated. Bilirubin is not excreted in urine, but the urine may be yellow due to the presence of pigment (Kapitulnik et al 1974b). Serum bilirubin concentrations fluctuate; lower levels occur in summer and on exposure to sun, and higher levels are observed during intercurrent illness (Schmid & Hammaker 1963, Bloomer et al 1971a, Blaschke et al 1974a, Wolkoff et al 1979b). The bile may be pale (Arias et al 1969); however, the colour may be deeper due to the excretion of increased amounts of unconjugated bilirubin following phototherapy (see below). Bilirubin excreted in bile is virtually all unconjugated, and only traces of conjugated bilirubin may be found by sensitive tests. Stool colour is normal, although faecal urobilinogen excretion is reduced (Crigler & Najjar 1952, Billing et al 1964a, Arias et al 1969). Bilirubin production (Schmid & Hammaker 1963, Billing et al 1964, Blaschke et al 1974a), haematocrit, bone marrow morphology and red cell survival (Arias et al 1969, Bloomer et al 1971a, Blaschke et al 1974a) are normal. Routine liver function tests yield normal results. Plasma disappearance of BSP (Crigler & Najjar 1952, Blaschke et al 1974a) and ICG (Blaschke et al 1974a) are normal. Despite the high serum bilirubin concentrations, there is normal radiological visualization of the biliary tree by cholecystographic agents.

Liver histology

Architecture and cellular morphology of the liver are normal. 'Pigment plugs' in bile canaliculi and bile ducts (Crigler & Najjar 1952, Blaschke et al 1974a, Wolkoff et al 1979b) may result from biliary excretion of unconjugated bilirubin as an effect of phototherapy, with subsequent precipitation in the bile canaliculi. Electron microscopy of the liver reveals no ultrastructural abnormality (Novikoff & Essner 1960, De Brito et al 1966,

Miniopaluello et al 1968, Huang et al 1970, Rothmaler & Lowe 1970).

Animal model of Crigler-Najjar syndrome, type I

A mutant strain of Wistar rats with nonhaemolytic unconjugated hyperbilirubinaemia was originally described by Gunn (1938). Later, this mutant strain was found to have a deficiency of UDP-glucuronosyltransferase activity towards bilirubin, resulting in the lack of excretion of conjugated bilirubin in the bile (Schmid et al 1958, Schmid & Hammaker 1963, Blanckaert et al 1977a). The availability of Gunn rats has resulted in major advances in understanding bilirubin metabolism transport, and encephalopathy. Jaundice in these animals is inherited as an autosomal recessive trait (Gunn 1938). Heterozygotes are anicteric. Serum bilirubin concentration in homozygous Gunn rats ranges from 3–20 mg/dl in colonies maintained at various institutions. As in Crigler-Najjar syndrome, serum bilirubin is all unconjugated (Schmid et al 1958), there is no bilirubinuria, and bile is pale and only traces of nonglucuronide and glucuronide conjugates of bilirubin have been detected in bile (Blanckaert et al 1977a). Liver histology is normal by light microscopy (Schmid et al 1958) and shows minor nonspecific structural modifications of the endoplasmic reticulum on electron microscopy (De Brito et al 1966).

Although Gunn rats excrete only minor amounts of exogenously administered bilirubin in bile (Cornelius 1969, Blanckaert et al 1977b, Roy Chowdhury & Arias 1981), they normally excrete exogenously administered conjugated bilirubin (Gutstein et al 1968, Shupeck et al 1978) and organic anions, such as sulphobromophthalein (Blanckaert et al 1977a) and phenol red (Howan & Guarino 1974), that do not require glucuronidation. Although Gunn rats lack UDP-glucuronosyltransferase activity towards bilirubin, transferase activity for aniline (Arias 1961a), steroid substrates (Drucker 1968) and thyroid hormone (Flock et al 1965) are normal. The transferase activity towards 4-nitrophenol is present at a lower level, but is restored to normal upon addition of diethylnitrosamine in vitro (Mowat & Arias 1970). Five UDP-glucuronosyltransferase isoforms were purified from Gunn rat liver by chromatofocusing, affinity chromatography and hydrophobic interaction chromatography (Roy Chowdhury et al 1987). An immunoreactive protein similar in molecular weight and charge to the bilirubin-specific isoform was isolated from Gunn rats; however, this form is enzymatically inactive. Another isoform, that normally catalyzes glucuronidation of 4-nitrophenol and methylumbelliferone has a greatly reduced level of activity; this activity was restored to normal by addition of diethylnitrosamine in vitro. Three other isoforms, which are normally active towards steroid substrates, have normal transferase activity in Gunn rats.

The Gunn rat is the only experimental animal in which endogenously produced bilirubin results in neuropathological lesions and neurological deficits (Schmid et al 1958, Blanc & Johnson 1959, Wolkoff et al 1979b). Cytoplasmic neuronal changes develop on the third day of life. By two weeks, degeneration of Purkinje cells and other neurons is evidenced by enlargement of mitochondria and formation of membranous cytoplasmic bodies. By eight days of age many mitochondria contain glycogen (Schutta & Johnson 1967, Rose & Johnson 1972). Despite the presence of these degenerative lesions in all Gunn rats, only half exhibit gross disturbances of gait (Wolkoff et al 1979b). Clinically healthy Gunn rats do not have yellow staining of the brain. Administration of sulphadimethoxine, a drug that competes with bilirubin for binding to albumin, to 14-day-old animals results in yellow staining in the brain and neurological deterioration (Schutta & Johnson 1969).

Gunn rats have a renal concentration defect and are sensitive to water deprivation (Odell et al 1967, Cowger 1973). The renal medullary bilirubin concentration is high and interferes with sodium and water transport (Odell et al 1967, Cowger 1973, Call & Tisher 1975). Occasionally, renal papillary necrosis occurs (Call & Tisher 1975). The concentration defect may be partially reversed upon lowering serum bilirubin by treatment of Gunn rats with cholestyramine, agar, or phototherapy (Odell et al 1967, Axelsen 1973). Similar concentrating problems have not been described in patients with Crigler-Najjar syndrome, type I, although bilirubin is deposited in the kidney (Gardner & Konigsmark 1969, Axelsen 1973). Hereditary hydronephrosis and renal cysts occur in some Gunn rats as concomitant genetic abnormalities (Lozzio et al 1967), and are unrelated to the disorder in bilirubin metabolism.

Treatment of Crigler-Najjar syndrome, type I

Treatment is designed to reduce serum bilirubin levels. Unlike results in patients with Crigler-Najjar syndrome, type II, and Gilbert syndrome (see below), the serum bilirubin level and hepatic bilirubin glucuronidation activity do not respond to phenobarbital administration (Arias et al 1969, Gorodischer et al 1970, Karon et al 1970, Bloomer et al 1971a, Blaschke et al 1974a). Since bilirubin is tightly bound to serum albumin, it can be efficiently removed from the body by plasmapheresis (Blaschke et al 1974a, Berk et al 1975b, Wolkoff et al 1979b). Plasmapheresis results in an immediate but

transient decrease in serum bilirubin levels. Phototherapy leads to geometric and structural isomerization of bilirubin, resulting in its increased excretion into bile (see 'Solubility of bilirubin and its relation to structural conformation'). Phototherapy has received widespread acceptance as the major therapeutic modality for icteric newborns whose serum bilirubin concentrations place them at risk for kernicterus (Callahan et al 1970, Gorodischer et al 1970, Karon et al 1970, Behrman et al 1974, Lund & Jacobsen 1974, Berk et al 1975b, Blaschke et al 1974a, Wolkoff et al 1979b). Experience with phototherapy in older children and adults is limited to patients with Crigler-Najjar syndrome, type I. After children reach 3 or 4 years of age, phototherapy becomes relatively less effective due to thickening of the skin, increased pigmentation, and decreased surface area in relation to body mass (Wolkoff et al 1979b).

Experimental treatment methods

Chronic phlebotomy in Crigler-Najjar syndrome, type I, was used in one patient to reduce the average age of circulating erythrocytes and hence reduce bilirubin production (Berk et al 1976). Although this procedure resulted in a decrease in bilirubin production, the effect was offset by an unexpected reduction in plasma bilirubin clearance. The plasma bilirubin level remained unaffected.

Affinity chromatography of bilirubin-containing blood on albumin-conjugated agarose gel has been suggested for removal of plasma bilirubin (Plotz et al 1974, Scharschmidt et al 1974, Berk et al 1975b). Although effective in reducing hyperbilirubinaemia in Gunn rats, difficulties due to removal of formed elements are encountered with simian or human blood (Scharschmidt et al 1977a,b).

Crigler-Najjar syndrome, type I, is a single enzyme deficiency disease, and UDP-glucuronosyltransferase replacement is a possible future treatment. Transplantation of a normal Wistar rat kidney, which contains bilirubin UDP-glucuronosyltransferase activity, into homozygous Gunn rats resulted in excretion of bilirubin glucuronides in bile and rapid decrease in serum bilirubin concentration (Roy Chowdhury et al 1978). However, since enzyme activity is undetectable in human kidney, renal transplantation cannot be recommended for the treatment of Crigler-Najjar syndrome, type I.

Subcutaneous transplantation of rat hepatoma cells (Rugstad et al 1970) and portal venous infusion of hepatocytes (Sebrow et al 1980) isolated from heterozygous Gunn rats resulted in transient biliary excretion of bilirubin glucuronides in homozygous Gunn rats and reduction of plasma bilirubin concentration. Transplantation of small pieces of normal rat liver into homozygous Gunn rats was also reported to reduce serum bilirubin concentration (Mukherjee & Krasner 1973); however, attempts at confirmation of these results were unsuccessful (Van Houwelingen & Arias 1976).

Intraperitoneal injection of isolated normal liver cells bound to collagen-coated dextran microcarriers has been successfully used to provide bilirubin-UDP-glucuronosyltransferase activity to Gunn rats (Demetriou et al 1986a,b,c). The injected microcarriers with attached hepatocytes rapidly form conglomerates on the anterior surface of the pancreas and develop their own blood supply (Demetriou et al 1986b). When normal rat hepatocytes were transplanted into congeneic recipients, conjugated bilirubin was present in bile for at least six weeks and serum bilirubin progressively decreased to near normal levels over the course of four weeks (Demetriou et al 1986a,b,c).

Because, at present, there is no other effective long-term treatment for patients with this condition, liver transplantation has been proposed as definite therapy (Liver Transplantation Consensus Conference 1983). Although this procedure is not without risk there has been a report of successful orthotopic liver transplantation in a 3-year-old girl with Crigler-Najjar syndrome, type I (Kaufman et al 1986). Serum bilirubin rapidly declined to normal levels after transplantation

Crigler-Najjar syndrome, type II (Arias syndrome)

This condition is phenotypically similar to Crigler-Najjar syndrome, type I, except that the serum bilirubin concentration is usually below 20 mg/dl (Table 68.1) (Arias 1962, Berk et al 1975a) and the clinical course is usually benign. In the original series described by Arias (Arias 1962), of the eight patients with chronic unconjugated hyperbilirubinaemia between 14 and 52 years of age, four had clinical jaundice before the age of one year and in one patient jaundice was noted only at the age of 30 years. In these patients, serum bilirubin concentration ranged from 8–18 mg/dl. Hepatic glucuronosyltransferase activities towards bilirubin, o-aminophenol and 4-methylumbelliferone were low or absent in all cases. Erythrocyte life span was normal. One 43-year-old patient had a neurological syndrome resembling kernicterus and died at the age of 44; autopsy revealed a histologically normal liver. The brain was small, lacked bilirubin staining, but demonstrated the typical histology of kernicterus. All other patients were clinically normal, despite continuous icterus.

Neurological abnormality in Crigler-Najjar syndrome, type II has been described in several other cases. Of three brothers who had this syndrome for over 50 years, two were neurologically normal, while the third had a slight bilateral intention tremor and nonspecific abnormalities on electroencephalogram (Gollan et al 1975a). These nonspecific neurological changes had not been noted previously. Another patient, a 15-year-old male, was icteric from the second day of life (Gordon et al 1976). Total serum bilirubin was 24 mg/dl at 10 months and averaged approximately 15 mg/dl thereafter. Although the physical development was normal, psychological testing revealed a perceptual deficit and slightly subnormal intelligence. At age 13, following surgery for acute appendicitis, the serum bilirubin rose to 40 mg/dl, and the patient developed diplopia, generalized seizures, confusion and an abnormal electroencephalogram. After treatment for hyperbilirubinaemia and recovery from surgery, serum bilirubin level returned to 15 mg/dl. His neurological status returned to baseline and has remained that way.

Biochemical abnormalities

As in Crigler-Najjar syndrome, type I, the only biochemical abnormality in the serum is elevated serum bilirubin. Serum bilirubin is unconjugated and is usually less than 20 mg/dl but may be as high as 40 mg/dl during fasting (Gollan et al 1975a) or intercurrent illness (Gordon et al 1976). There is no bilirubinuria. The bile is pigmented, although less than 50% of estimated daily bilirubin production is excreted into bile (Arias et al 1969, Gordon et al 1976). Although over 90% of conjugated bilirubin in normal bile is bilirubin diglucuronide, the major pigment in this syndrome is bilirubin monoglucuronide (Arias 1962, Liver Transplantation Consensus Conference 1983). The change in the proportion of bilirubin conjugates in bile may be related to greatly reduced hepatic bilirubin-UDP-glucuronosyltransferase activity, which may be too low to detect by in vitro assays (Gordon et al 1976, Fevery et al 1977).

Effect of induction of bilirubin-UDP-glucuronosyltransferase activity

Hyperbilirubinaemia is reduced following treatment with phenobarbital (Arias et al 1969) or other liver microsomal enzyme inducers (Thompson et al 1969, Hunter et al 1971, Black et al 1974, Blaschke et al 1974b, Orme 1974). The response to phenobarbital treatment in this syndrome contrasts with the lack of effect of the drug in Crigler-Najjar syndrome, type I (Arias et al 1969). Assay of bilirubin-UDP-glucuronosyltransferase activity is relatively insensitive, and increased enzyme activity has only rarely been demonstrated (Black et al 1974, Gollan et al 1975a). In some patients, clinical differentiation of these two types of Crigler-Najjar syndrome is difficult (Blaschke et al 1974b).

Inheritance

Crigler-Najjar syndrome, type II commonly occurs in families (Arias 1962, Arias et al 1969). However, there is no evidence of consanguinity, and the pattern of inheritance is not certain. Both autosomal dominant transmission with incomplete penetrance (Arias 1962, Arias et al 1969) and autosomal recessive transmission (Hunter et al 1973, Blaschke et al 1974b) have been suggested. In one study of three families, parents and sibs of affected individuals had mild unconjugated hyperbilirubinaemia consistent with Gilbert syndrome (see below) (Hunter et al 1973, Blaschke et al 1974b), suggesting that Crigler-Najjar syndrome, type II, may be a homozygous form of Gilbert syndrome (Smith et al 1967). However, the precise relationship of this syndrome with Gilbert syndrome is conjectural. Detailed analysis of bilirubin conjugates in the bile of patients and their families may clarify the inheritance of this disorder (Gordon et al 1976, Fevery et al 1977).

Gilbert syndrome

This syndrome, also termed constitutional hepatic dysfunction or familial nonhaemolytic jaundice, is a common disorder characterized by mild, chronic and unconjugated hyperbilirubinaemia (Table 68.1) (Gilbert & Lereboullet 1901, Gilbert et al 1907). Familial occurrence is common (Thompson 1981). Autosomal dominant inheritance is likely (Powell et al 1967), although most patients present as sporadic cases. Gilbert syndrome is usually diagnosed in young adults who present with mild, unconjugated hyperbilirubinaemia (serum bilirubin concentration usually less than 3 mg/dl (Foulk et al 1959). Serum bilirubin level fluctuates with time, and increases during intercurrent illness. The physical examination is otherwise normal. Some patients complain of vague constitutional symptoms, including fatigue and abdominal discomfort (Foulk et al 1959), these symptoms may be manifestations of anxiety. Apart from serum bilirubin level, other liver function tests including serum alkaline phosphatase or aminotransferase activities and oral cholecystography, yield normal results. Liver histology, at light microscopic and ultrastructural levels is normal; however, liver biopsy is usually not needed for diagnosis. Often a nonspecific accumulation of lipofuscin

pigment is seen in the centrilobular zones (Novikoff & Essner 1960, Sagild et al 1962).

Transport defect in Gilbert syndrome

The precise mechanism of unconjugated hyperbilirubinaemia in Gilbert syndrome is not known. Reduced plasma bilirubin clearance has been demonstrated in Gilbert syndrome (Billing et al 1964b, Black et al 1974, Scharschmidt 1978). Multicompartmental analysis suggests that reduced plasma clearance results from reduction in hepatic bilirubin uptake as well as bilirubin conjugation (Billing et al 1964b, Berk et al 1970, Cobelli 1975, Okolicsanyi et al 1978). Thus, two seemingly unrelated biochemical abnormalities appear to coexist in this syndrome. Although reduced hepatic bilirubin-UDP-glucuronosyltransferase activity has been observed consistently in Gilbert syndrome (Arias 1962, Arias et al 1969, Black & Billing 1969, Hunter et al 1971, Felsher et al 1973, Bellet & Raynana 1974, Auclair et al 1976), the enzyme activity in the liver of patients with this syndrome appears to be in excess of that needed to conjugate normal bilirubin production. Thus, the relationship of UDP-glucuronosyltransferase deficiency to hyperbilirubinaemia is not clear. However, the in vitro determination of the enzyme activity may not truly reflect its physiological availablility. Studies on hepatic bilirubin uptake have yielded contradictory results (Billing et al 1964b, Goresky et al 1978, Scharschmidt 1978). It is likely that Gilbert syndrome represents an heterogeneous group of disorders, some of which have an anion uptake defect. Plasma disappearance of organic anions other than bilirubin is usually normal. However, two subsets of the syndrome with abnormal plasma clearance of BSP (Berk et al 1972, Cartel et al 1975, Cobelli et al 1981) and ICG (Martin et al 1976) have been reported. In one group, reduced BSP and ICG plasma disappearance suggests reduced hepatic uptake. In the second group, compartmental analysis revealed a defect in BSP transport at a later stage in the transport process. BSP is conjugated in the liver with glutathione, whereas ICG is excreted into bile intact; none of these compounds depends on hepatic UDP-glucuronosyltransferase activity for excretion.

Intercurrent illness, physical exertion and stress result in increased serum bilirubin levels in Gilbert syndrome. A relationship to the menstrual cycle has been reported in two women (Yamaguchi et al 1975).

Caloric deprivation exaggerates the hyperbilirubinaemia (Felsher et al 1970, Barrett 1971a, Bloomer et al 1971b, Bensinger et al 1973, Owens & Sherlock 1973 , Felsher & Carpio 1975, Felsher 1976, Gollan et al 1976,

Okolicsanyi et al 1981). Serum bilirubin levels in normal individuals (Felsher et al 1970, Barrett 1971a, Bensinger et al 1973, Owens & Sherlock 1973, Felsher & Carpio 1975, Felsher 1976, Gollan et al 1976, Okolicsanyi et al 1981) and in individuals with other hepatobiliary disorders also rise with fasting (Owens & Sherlock 1973, Felsher & Carpio 1975). Although serum bilirubin response following a 48-hour fast has been used as a diagnostic test for Gilbert syndrome, a significant percentage of false positive and negative results make this test of limited value. Fasting-induced hyperbilirubinaemia appears to result from reduced hepatic clearance of bilirubin from plasma rather than increased production of bilirubin (Bloomer et al 1971b, Black et al 1974, Kirshenbaum et al 1976). Fasting does not reduce hepatic bilirubin-UDP-glucuronosyltransferase activity in vitro in normal rats (Barrett 1971b), however the availability of UDP-glucuronic acid in vivo may be decreased because of a reduction of UDP-glucose dehydrogenase activity (Felsher et al 1979). Fasting exacerbates hyperbilirubin-aemia in homozygous Gunn rats (Barrett 1971b, Bloomer et al 1971b, Gollan et al 1975b, 1979), suggesting that it must also affect hepatic disposition of bilirubin at a step other than conjugation. Fasting hyperbilirubinaemia may result from a combination of several factors, and roles for increased serum nonesterified fatty acids (Cowan et al 1977) and reduced hepatic content of the cytosolic ligandin and Z protein (Stein at el 1976) have been suggested.

Although intravenous nicotinic acid administration has been proposed as a provocative diagnostic test for Gilbert syndrome (Fromke & Miller 1972, Davidson et al 1975), like fasting, it does not clearly separate patients with Gilbert syndrome from normal subjects or those with hepatobiliary disease (Fromke & Miller 1972, Davidson et al 1975). Nicotinic acid administration does not increase serum bilirubin level after splenectomy (Fromke & Miller 1972), suggesting that nicotinic acid-induced unconjugated hyperbilirubinaemia is probably due to enhanced bilirubin formation in the spleen, resulting from increased erythrocyte fragility and enhanced splenic haem oxygenase activity (Ohkubo et al 1979).

Gilbert syndrome is conventionally diagnosed in individuals with mild unconjugated hyperbilirubinaemia without evidence of haemolysis or structural liver disease. Although haemolysis is not a part of the syndrome, a significant proportion of patients exhibit evidence for concomitant haemolysis. Combination of both factors results in higher, more clinically apparent bilirubin levels than in individuals with either abnormality alone. In a study of 14 patients with chronic haemolysis due to

hereditary spherocytosis (Berk et al 1981), seven had reduced plasma clearance of radio-labelled bilirubin. The diagnosis of Gilbert syndrome in these patients was supported by family studies and low hepatic bilirubin-UDP-glucuronosyltransferase activity. Following elective splenectomy, which corrected the haemolytic state, the low preoperative bilirubin clearance values improved in all seven patients, and became normal in five. These patients may represent a latent form of Gilbert syndrome which is unmasked by increased bilirubin production during haemolysis.

Similar to findings in patients with Crigler-Najjar syndrome, type II, and heterozygous Gunn rats, bile from patients with Gilbert syndrome has an increased proportion of bilirubin monoglucuronide (Table 68.1) (Rugstad et al 1970, Goresky et al 1978, Van Steenbergen et al 1979, Sebrow et al 1980). The abnormal pattern of biliary bilirubin conjugates may be related to reduced hepatic bilirubin-UDP-glucuronosyltransferase activity. The findings suggest that Crigler-Najjar syndrome, type II and Gilbert syndrome may represent different degrees of phenotypic expression of a common biochemical defect. Increased proportion of bilirubin monoglucuronide in bile in these syndromes may serve as a useful marker for diagnosis and studies of inheritance.

Incidence and inheritance of Gilbert syndrome

Serum bilirubin levels in the general population follow a skewed (Vaughan & Haslewood 1938, Alwall et al 1946, O'Hagen et al 1957, Bailey et al 1977) or bimodal distribution (Powell et al 1967, Owens & Evans 1975), rather than a Gaussian distribution. This makes it difficult to set a precise upper limit of normal serum bilirubin concentration, and thereby define Gilbert syndrome in an uniform fashion. Thus the exact incidence of this common disorder is not known. Serum bilirubin levels in males are significantly higher than in females (Werner et al 1970, Wilding et al 1972, Owens & Evans 1975), which may account, in part, for the reported higher incidence of Gilbert syndrome in males (Foulk et al 1959, Powell et al 1967). A clinically inapparent latent form of the disorder has been described (Berk et al 1981). Unconjugated hyperbilirubinaemia to levels of 5–8 mg/dl may occur in both Gilbert syndrome and Crigler-Najjar syndrome, type II. Differentiation of these disorders based upon serum bilirubin levels, hepatic bilirubin UDP-glucuronyltransferase activity and bilirubin mono-glucuronide content of bile may be arbitrary.

It is clear that Gilbert syndrome is a genetic disorder (Gilbert et al 1907, Damashek & Singer 1941, Alwall 1946, Meulengracht 1947, Baroody & Shugart 1956,

O'Hagen et al 1957, Powell et al 1967, Thompson 1981). Although autosomal dominant inheritance has been suggested for Gilbert syndrome (Damashek & Singer 1941, O'Hagen et al 1957, Powell et al 1967), the difficulties inherent in diagnosing the disorder make this conclusion somewhat tenuous. Additional family studies using markers such as bilirubin monoglucuronide content of bile may provide more conclusive information as to inheritance.

Animal models for Gilbert syndrome

Mutant Southdown sheep: This mutant strain exhibits photosensitivity, which is inherited as an autosomal recessive trait (Cunningham et al 1942, Hancock 1950). These animals have unconjugated hyperbilirubinaemia and photodermatitis resulting from retention of phylloerythrin, the end product of chlorophyll metabolism that is normally excreted by the liver into bile (Clare 1945, Cornelius & Gronwall 1968). Plasma clearance of intravenously administered bilirubin, BSP, cholate, ICG and ^{131}I-labelled rose bengal (Meulengracht 1947) is reduced. BSP transport maximum and storage capacity are also low (Cornelius & Gronwall 1968, Gronwall 1970). The mutant sheep may have increased bilirubin production from nonerythroid sources, including hepatic haem (Mia et al 1970a). As in patients with Gilbert syndrome, plasma disappearance studies with intravenously administered [14C]bilirubin in these sheep suggest reduced hepatic influx of bilirubin (Mia et al 1970b). However, in contrast to patients with Gilbert syndrome, mutant sheep had significantly increased efflux from liver to plasma and normal hepatic sequestration rates. Moreover, bilirubin-UDP-glucuronosyltransferase activity is normal in mutant sheep (Meulengracht 1947). The mechanism of unconjugated hyperbilirubinaemia in these animals most likely differs from that in patients with Gilbert syndrome.

Bolivian squirrel monkey: Bolivian squirrel monkeys have higher post-cibal serum unconjugated bilirubin concentration and a greater degree of fasting hyperbilirubinaemia than does a closely related Brazilian population (Portman et al 1984a). Compared to the Brazilian population, Bolivian monkeys have slower plasma clearance of intravenously administered bilirubin, a lower level of hepatic bilirubin-UDP-glucuronosyltransferase activity and a higher bilirubin monoglucuronide to diglucuronide ratio in bile (Portman et al 1984a). The two populations of squirrel monkeys have comparable erythrocyte life span and hepatic glutathione-S-transferase activity (Portman et al 1984a). In these respects, the Bolivian squirrel monkeys are a model of human Gilbert syndrome. Fasting hyperbilirubinaemia is rapidly reversed by oral or intravenous administration of carbo-

hydrates, but not by lipid administration (Portman et al 1984b).

Treatment of Gilbert syndrome

Gilbert syndrome is a benign, cosmetic disorder. Once the diagnosis is made, only reassurance is necessary. Under some special circumstances, clinical jaundice may be ameliorated by a course of phenobarbital therapy.

DISORDERS OF BILIRUBIN METABOLISM THAT CAUSE PREDOMINANTLY CONJUGATED HYPERBILIRUBINAEMIA

Dubin-Johnson syndrome

This syndrome, described by Dubin and Johnson (1954), and Sprinz and Nelson (1954), is characterized by mild, predominantly conjugated hyperbilirubinaemia (Table 68.2) and a black liver. For the most part, these patients are asymptomatic, although occasionally mild constitutional complaints such as vague abnominal pains and weakness occur (Dubin 1958, Shani et al 1970a). Pruritus is absent in Dubin-Johnson syndrome, and serum bile acid levels are normal (Cohen et al 1972, Javitt et al 1978). The degree of icterus is increased by intercurrent illness, oral contraceptives, and pregnancy (Cohen et al 1972). Except for jaundice, physical examination is normal. An occasional patient may have hepatosplenomegaly. The Dubin-Johnson syndrome is rarely detected before puberty, although cases have been reported in neonates (Ivicic & Sosovec 1975, Kondo et al 1975, Nakata et al 1979). The disorder may be noted for the first time during pregnancy or use of oral contraceptives, which increase the mild hyperbilirubinaemia to a level at which jaundice becomes apparent (Cohen et al 1972).

Biochemical abnormalities

Serum bilirubin is usually between 2–5 mg/dl but can be as high as 20–25 mg/dl. Bilirubinuria is frequent and 50% or more of total serum bilirubin is conjugated. In most other hepatobiliary disorders bilirubin monoglucuronide is the predominant conjugated bilirubin in serum. In contrast, in Dubin-Johnson syndrome, bilirubin diglucuronide is the major conjugated bile pigment in serum. The serum bilirubin level fluctuates, and frequently individual determinations may be normal. As is the case in all hepatobiliary disorders in which conjugated bilirubin is chronically retained in the plasma, a portion of the retained bile pigments become irreversibly bound to plasma albumin. The irreversibly protein-bound pigments give a direct van den Bergh reaction and can be quantitated by high pressure liquid chromatography of the serum. As in normal human bile, bilirubin diglucuronide is the predominant form of bilirubin excreted in the bile of patients with this disorder. Complete blood count and routine laboratory tests including serum albumin and cholesterol levels, prothrombin time, serum transaminase and alkaline phosphatase activities are normal (Dubin 1958, Wolf et al 1960, Butt et al 1966, Shani et al 1970a, Cohen et al 1972, Kondo et al 1974). Serum bile salt levels are normal. Oral cholecystography, even using a 'double dose' of contrast material, may not visualize the gallbladder, although visualization may occur 4–6 hours after intravenous injection of iodipamide (Mandema et al 1960, Dittrich & Seifert 1962, Morita & Kihava 1971).

Histological appearance of the liver

On direct inspection, the liver is black. Light microscopy reveals normal histology except for accumulation of a pigment which, on electron microscopy, appears as electron-dense granules contained within lysosomes (Essner & Novikoff 1960, Oppermann et al 1971). Composition of these granules is not known. It has been suggested that they are composed of poorly defined lipofuscins (Callard et al 1971, Oppermann et al 1971, Kermarec et al 1972) or melanin-like pigments (Ehrlick et al 1960, Wegmann et al 1960, De Saram et al 1969, Sosnnet et al 1969). In the mutant Corriedale sheep, an animal model of Dubin-Johnson syndrome (see below), the hepatic pigment histochemically resembles melanin (Arias et al 1964b). Following infusion of [³H] epinephrine into the mutant Corriedale sheep, there is reduced biliary excretion of radioactivity and incorporation of the isotope into the hepatic pigment (Arias et al 1965b,c Arias 1968), suggesting that the pigment is related to melanin. However, electron spin resonance (ESR) spectroscopy suggests that this pigment differs from authentic melanin (Swartz et al 1979a) and may be composed of polymers of epinephrine metabolites (Arias & Blumberg 1979, Swartz et al 1979b). Computerized tomography of the liver showed higher attenuation values in patients with Dubin-Johnson syndrome as compared to normal controls, although there was considerable overlap between the two groups (Rubinstein et al 1985). The possible relationship of the liver cell pigment to this finding is not known. The degree of hepatic pigmentation may vary in individuals with the Dubin-Johnson syndrome (Wolf et al 1960, Arias 1961b). During attacks of coincidental diseases, such as acute viral hepatitis, the pigment is cleared from the liver, and reaccumulates slowly after recovery (Hunter et al 1964, Masuda 1965, Varma et al 1970, Ware et al 1972, 1974).

Defect of organic anion transport

Uptake of organic anions, as measured by initial plasma disappearance of bilirubin (Gilbert & Lereboullet 1901, Billing et al 1964b), BSP (Schoenfield et al 1963, Shani et al 1970a, Cohen et al 1972, Erlinger et al 1973, Kondo et al 1974, Abe & Okuda 1975), dibromsulphalein (DBSP) (Erlinger et al 1973), ICG (Erlinger et al 1973, Schoenfield et al 1963), and ¹²⁵I-labelled rose bengal (Erlinger et al 1973), following intravenous administration, are usually normal in Dubin-Johnson syndrome. Plasma BSP concentration 45 minutes after intravenous administration, may be normal or may show mild retention (Schoenfield et al 1963, Shani et al 1970a, Cohen et al 1972, Kondo et al 1974); however in approximately 90% of patients, there is a secondary increase in the plasma BSP concentration at 90 minutes after intravenous administration (Charbonnier & Brisbois 1960, Mandema et al 1960, Shani et al 1970a, Cohen et al 1972, Kondo et al 1974). A similar secondary rise has been described following intravenous administration of unconjugated bilirubin (Schoenfield et al 1963, Swartz et al 1979a). The secondary rise is due to reflux of conjugated BSP or bilirubin from the liver cell into the circulation (Charbonnier & Brisbois 1960, Sosnnet et al 1969). This rise does not occur for organic anions such as DBSP, ¹²⁵I-labelled rose bengal, and ICG, that are not conjugated prior to excretion by the hepatocyte (Schoenfield et al 1963, Erlinger et al 1973). Although the secondary rise of plasma BSP is highly characteristic of Dubin-Johnson syndrome, it may be found in other hepatobiliary disorders and is, therefore, not diagnostic (Rodes et al 1972).

Maximum BSP transport during constant intravenous infusion is reduced to only 10% of normal in Dubin-Johnson syndrome; however, the hepatic storage capacity is normal (Wheeler et al 1960, Shani et al 1970b, Cohen et al 1972). In a patient with Dubin-Johnson syndrome who had a biliary fistula (Gutstein et al 1968), dehydrocholate choleresis did not augment biliary BSP excretion. BSP transport is normal in phenotypically normal parents and children (i.e., carriers) (Shani et al 1970b, Cohen et al 1972).

Abnormalities of urinary porphyrin excretion

Of the two isomeric forms of coproporphyrin, isomers I and III, coproporphyrin III is the precursor of haem, whereas isomer I porphyrins are metabolic byproducts without known function and are excreted into urine and bile (Kaplowitz et al 1972). In urine, coproporphyrin isomer I normally comprises approximately 75% of total urinary coproporphyrins. In Dubin-Johnson syndrome, total urinary coproporphyrin excretion is normal, but over 80% is coproporphyrin I (Ben-Ezzer et al 1971, Wolkoff et al 1973, Kondo et al 1976). This pattern is diagnostic of Dubin-Johnson syndrome. Urinary coproporphyrin excretion proved useful in diagnosing Dubin-Johnson syndrome in two neonates (Kondo et al 1975, Nakata et al 1979). Although neonates normally have elevated urinary content of coproporphyrin I as compared to adults, levels are not as high as seen in Dubin-Johnson syndrome (Wolkoff & Arias 1974). In unaffected parents and children of patients with Dubin-Johnson syndrome (obligate heterozygotes), there is a 50% reduction of urinary coproporphyrin III excretion, resulting in a 40% reduction of total urinary coproporphyrin excretion (Ben-Ezzer et al 1973, Wolkoff et al 1973, Kondo et al 1976). The proportion of coproporphyrin I in urine was intermediate between results in controls and in patients with Dubin-Johnson syndrome.

Normally, daily biliary coproporphyrin excretion is approximately three times that of daily urinary excretion. In normal bile, porphyrin isomer I constitutes approximately two thirds of the total (Kaplowitz et al 1972). In most hepatobiliary disorders, including cholestasis, urinary coproporphin excretion is increased (Aziz et al 1964, Ben-Ezzer et al 1971) the proportion of isomer I in urine is usually less than 65%. Dubin-Johnson syndrome is unique in that total urinary coproporyphyrin is normal, but the proportion of isomer I is over 80%. The mechanism of this unique excretory pattern is not known, and an alteration in hepatic porphyrin biosynthesis has been postulated (Wolkoff et al 1973, Wolkoff & Arias 1974). Hepatic uroporphyrin III cosynthetase activity, required for the formation of coproporphyrin III (Wolkoff et al 1973), is normal in blood cells and liver from patients with Dubin-Johnson syndrome (Shimzu et al 1977). Intravenous administration of aminolevulinic acid (ALA), results in very little change in the coproporphyrin III content of urine and bile in patients with Dubin-Johnson syndrome, as compared with results in normal control subjects (Shimzu et al 1978, Kondo et al 1979). The mechanism of abnormal coproporphyrin excretion and the relationship of the porphyrin abnormality to the conjugated hyperbilirubinaemia which characterizes the syndrome, is not clear at present.

Incidence and inheritance

Dubin-Johnson syndrome has been described in both sexes in virtually all races (Beker & Read 1958, Dubin 1958, Berkowitz et al 1960, Wolf et al 1960, Arias 1961b, Hislop 1964, Burnscox 1965, Banerjee 1970, Shani et al 1970a, Vaughan et al 1970, Cohen et al 1972, Schmid 1972, Kondo et al 1974). It is frequent (1:1300) in Persian Jews (Shani et al 1970a) in whom it is associated with

clotting factor VII deficiency (Seligsohn et al 1969, 1970, Levanon et al 1972). The disorder is clearly familial, but the data in the initial descriptions did not fit an autosomal dominant pattern, and carriers could not be detected even with constant infusion studies of BSP transport (Shani et al 1970b, Cohen et al 1972). However, using urinary coproporphyrin excretion, Dubin-Johnson syndrome is clearly inherited as an autosomal recessive trait. A study of BSP and bilirubin metabolism in 173 sibs of 44 patients with Dubin-Johnson syndrome indicated a similar mode of inheritance (Edwards 1975). The overlap of results in carriers with those in controls (Ben-Ezzer et al 1973, Wolkoff et al 1973, Kondo et al 1976) makes determination of urinary coproporphyrin excretion less useful in deciding whether an individual carries the gene for the syndrome.

Animal models of Dubin-Johnson syndrome

Mutant Corriedale sheep: A mutant strain of Corriedale sheep exhibits mild conjugated hyperbilirubinaemia, hepatic pigmentation, and reduced biliary excretion of organic anions, such as conjugated bilirubin, BSP, ICG, phylloerythrin, iodopanoic acid and ^{125}I-labelled rose bengal (Arias et al 1964b, 1965b,c, Cornelius et al 1965, 1968, Arias 1968, Mia et al 1970c, Gronwall 1970). Retention of phylloerythrin results in photosensitivity (Cornelius et al 1968, Cornelius 1969). Biliary excretion of bile salts is normal. In contrast to the findings in normal sheep, taurocholate infusion does not stimulate biliary excretion of BSP (Arias 1968, Alpert et al 1969). Biliary excretion of the organic cation procainamide ethobromide is normal in mutant sheep, as is renal excretion of PAH (Alpert et al 1969). Studies suggesting that the hepatic pigment granules are related to melanin have been discussed above. The disorder is transmitted as an autosomal recessive trait.

Hereditary chronic conjugated hyperbilirubinaemia in mutant rats

A mutant rat strain with conjugated hyperbilirubinaemia, inherited as an autosomal recessive characteristic, has recently been described (Jansen et al 1985). Serum bilirubin levels are elevated to 5-10 mg% with over 90% bilirubin glucuronides. As in Dubin-Johnson syndrome, serum γ-glutamyltransferase, alkaline phosphatase, aminotransaminase activities, cholesterol and phospholipid levels are normal. Plasma clearance of dibromosulphthalein and ouabain are reduced to 7% and 37% of normal respectively, due to severely impaired hepatic excretion. Initial uptake of these compounds is normal. In isolated perfused normal liver 75% of infused tracer dose of dibromosulphthalein is excreted in bile within 60 minutes. In contrast, only 1.5% of the dose is recovered in the bile in the mutant strain; the remainder is retained in the liver and in the perfusate. Biliary excretion of cholate, bile salts and organic cations is normal.

Liver histology is normal in the mutant rats with chronic conjugated hyperbilirubinaemia. In contrast to the findings in Dubin-Johnson syndrome, no pigmentation is found in the liver; this may reflect the fact that this mutation occurred in an albino strain. Other features that differentiate this disorder from the Dubin-Johnson syndrome include an absence of a secondary plasma rise of BSP during plasma clearance studies and a five-fold increase in serum bile acid levels. Urinary coproporphyrin I, although elevated, represents only 20% of the total. Normal rats have only 5% of urinary coproporphyrin as isomer I, so that the elevation seen in mutant rats may be comparable to that seen in patients with the Dubin-Johnson syndrome.

Rotor syndrome

This syndrome is also characterized by chronic, mild, predominantly conjugated hyperbilirubinaemia (Rotor et al 1948). Physical examination is normal, except for jaundice. Apart from the hyperbilirubinaemia, liver function tests including serum alkaline phosphatase and transaminase activities, and cholesterol levels are normal. In contrast to the findings in Dubin-Johnson syndrome, the liver is not hyperpigmented.

Organic anion excretion defect

Compared to Dubin-Johnson syndrome, there is a greater (over 25%) and more consistent plasma retention of BSP 45 minutes after intravenous injection of 5 mg/kg body weight of the dye in Rotor syndrome (Porush et al 1962, Pereira-Lima et al 1966, Peck et al 1969, Wolpert et al 1977, Kawasaki et al 1979, Shimzu et al 1981). There is no secondary rise of plasma BSP level in Rotor syndrome 90 minutes after the injection, and conjugated BSP is not found in plasma (Abe & Okuda 1975, Wolpert et al 1977, Kawasaki et al 1979). Although the gallbladder is not usually visualized during oral cholecystography in Dubin-Johnson syndrome, it is usually visualized in Rotor syndrome (Porush et al 1962, Pereira-Lima et al 1966). There is also marked plasma retention of unconjugated bilirubin (Schiff et al 1959, Kawasaki et al 1979), and ICG (Kawasaki et al 1979) when these substances are injected intravenously. Phenotypically normal obligate heterozygotes for Rotor syndrome have mildly abnormal BSP retention at 45 minutes (Wolpert et al 1977).

Transport maximum and relative hepatic storage capacity for BSP have been determined in patients with Rotor and Dubin-Johnson syndrome, using a constant infusion technique (Wolpert et al 1977, Kawasaki et al 1979). In Dubin-Johnson syndrome the storage capacity is normal while the transport is nearly absent. In contrast, in Rotor syndrome, hepatic storage capacity is reduced to 10–25% of normal and the transport maximum is reduced by half (Wolpert et al 1977, Kawasaki et al 1979). In phenotypically normal obligate heterozygotes the transport maximum and hepatic storage capacity are intermediate between those in patients with Rotor syndrome and controls (Wolpert et al 1977). In a variant of the Rotor syndrome, termed 'hepatic storage disease', there is a modest reduction in the transport maximum and a greater reduction in hepatic storage capacity (Hadchouel et al 1971, Dhumeaux & Berthelot 1975).

Urinary coproporphyrin excretion

In contrast to the findings in Dubin-Johnson syndrome, total urinary coproporphyrin is increased by 250–500% in Rotor syndrome compared to normal subjects, and the proportion of coproporphyrin I in urine is approximately 65% of total (Wolkoff et al 1976, Shimizu et al 1981). In some families, over 80% of urinary coproporphyrins may exist as an isomer I (Rapacini et al 1986). Similar results are seen in many other hepatobiliary disorders (Localio et al 1941, Aziz et al 1964, Koskelo et al 1966, 1967, Koskelo & Toivonen 1968, Ben-Ezzer et al 1971). Phenotypically normal obligate heterozygotes have a coproporphyrin excretory pattern which is intermediate between that of normal subjects and patients with Rotor syndrome. The urinary coproporphyrin abnormality in Rotor syndrome is most likely caused by a reduced biliary excretion of coproporphyrins, with increased renal excretion of the porphyrins retained in plasma. The nature of the organic anion transport defect in Rotor syndrome is unknown.

Incidence and inheritance

Although it has been described in several nationalities and races, Rotor syndrome is rare. The finding of abnormal BSP transport in obligate heterozygotes suggested an autosomal recessive pattern of inheritance (Wolpert et al 1977). A more complete genetic analysis was performed following determination of urinary coproporphyrin excretion in patients with Rotor syndrome and phenotypically normal relatives (Wolkoff et al 1976, Shimizu et al 1981). With respect to urinary coproporphyrin excretion, Rotor syndrome is inherited as an autosomal recessive characteristic and is distinct from

Table 68.2 Principal characteristics of inherited disorders associated with conjugated hyperbilirubinaemia

Characteristic	Dubin-Johnson syndrome	Rotor syndrome
Serum bilirubin level	Usually 2-5 mg/dl, occasionally up to 20 mg/dl; predominantly direct	Usually 2-5 mg/dl, occasionally up to 20 mg/dl; predominantly direct
Serum aminotransferase, γ-glutamyltranspeptidase and alkaline phosphatase activities	Normal	Normal
Serum bile acid levels	Normal	Normal
Plasma BSP retention	Normal or elevated at 45 min; secondary rise at 90 min.	Elevated at 45 min; no secondary rise
Oral cholecystogram	Usually no visualization	Usually normal
Urinary coproporphyrins	Total excretion is normal; over 80% is isoform I	Total excretion increased; proportion of isoform I increased, but less than 80% of total
Liver histology	Grossly black; centrilobular pigmentation, otherwise normal	Normal; no pigmentation
Prevalence	Uncommon (1:1300 in Persian Jews)	Rare
Inheritance	Autosomal recessive	Autosomal recessive
Prognosis	Benign	Benign
Animal model	Mutant Corriedale sheep; mutant rats with inherited defect or organic anion excretion	-

Dubin-Johnson syndrome (Table 68.2) (Wolkoff et al 1976, Shimizu et al 1981).

Benign recurrent intrahepatic cholestasis

This rare disorder is characterized by recurrent attacks of cholestasis (Summerskill & Walshe 1959). For 2–4 weeks prior to the onset of jaundice, patients experience malaise, anorexia, and pruritus (Williams et al 1964, Spiegel et al 1965, Ruymann et al 1970, De Pagter et al 1976). Subsequently, patients become icteric and may have an enlarged tender liver. There is no splenomegaly and patients are afebrile (Summerskill & Walshe 1959, Tygstrup 1960, Kuhn 1963, Shapiro & Isselbacher 1963, Williams et al 1964, Schubert et al 1965, Spiegel et al 1965, Summerskill 1965, Tygstrup & Jensen 1969, Ruymann et al 1970, De Pagter et al 1976). The onset of symptoms is usually in adolescence or early adulthood (De Pagter et al 1976), although this disorder has been described as presenting in infancy (Tygstrup 1960, Tygstrup & Jensen 1969, Ruymann et al 1970, De Pagter et al 1976) as well as in middle age (Summerskill 1965). The clinical presentation may suggest biliary obstruction, and in the past many of these patients underwent one or more exploratory laparotomies. Typically, episodes of cholestasis last from a few weeks to several months (De Pagter et al 1976), and intervals between attacks may range from several months to years. In a given patient, recurrent attacks resemble each other as to symptoms and duration. Prolonged cholestasis may lead to steatorrhoea and weight loss, requiring parenteral administration of fat-soluble vitamins. Between episodes of cholestasis, patients are clinically normal. No negative influence on longevity has been noted. The disorder runs in families, but the mode of inheritance is not known (De Pagter et al 1976).

Biochemical abnormalities

During a cholestatic episode, serum bile acids, alkaline phosphatase activity and conjugated bilirubin concentration increase to abnormal levels (Schubert et al 1965, Spiegel et al 1965, Biempica et al 1967, Van Berge Henegouwen et al 1974, Endo et al 1979). Serum transaminases may be mildly elevated, and the prothrombin time may be elevated because of malabsorption of vitamin K. Plasma disappearance of unconjugated bilirubin is normal, but conjugated bilirubin level increases as it refluxes from the liver (Williams et al 1964, Brodersen & Tygstrup 1967, Bloomer et al 1974, Summerfield et al 1980).

During the attacks, liver biopsy shows characteristic features of intrahepatic cholestasis (Summerskill & Walshe 1959, Tygstrup 1960, Kuhn 1963, Shapiro &

Isselbacher 1963, Williams et al 1964, Dickson et al 1965, Schubert et al 1965, Spiegel et al 1965, Summerskill 1965, Biempica et al 1967, Tygstrup & Jensen 1969, Ruymann et al 1970, Beudoin et al 1973, Lesser 1973, De Pagter et al 1976, Summerfield et al 1980). Electron-microscopic examination reveals marked distortion and reduction in the number of bile canalicular microvilli, almost complete disappearance of nucleoside phosphatase activity, and reduction in the number of acid phosphatase-rich lysosomes are normal (Biempica et al 1967, Ruymann et al 1970, Beudoin et al 1973). These changes are not specific for this disorder and may be seen in other forms of cholestasis. Between attacks, biochemical studies and liver histology are normal (Biempica et al 1967, Ruymann et al 1970, Beudoin et al 1973). The pathogenesis of this disorder is unknown. No effective measures for preventing or shortening the cholestatic episodes are known.

ACKNOWLEDGEMENT

This work was supported by National Institutes Health grants DK 34357 to JRC and DK 39137 to NRC.

REFERENCES

Abe H, Okuda K 1975 Biliary excretion of conjugated sulfobromophtalein (BSP) in constitutional conjugated hyperbilirubinemias. Digestion 13: 373

Alpert S , Mosher M, Shanske A, Arias I M 1969 Multiplicity of hepatic excretory mechanisms for organic anions. Journal of General Physiology 53: 238

Alwall N 1946 On hereditary non-hemolytic bilirubinemia. Acta Medica Scandinavica 123: 560

Alwall N, Laurell C B, Nilsby I 1946 Studies on heredity in cases of "Non-hemolytic hyperbilirubinemia without direct van den Bergh reaction" (hereditary, non-hemolytic bilirubinemia). Acta Medica Scandinavica 124: 114

Arias I M 1961a Ethereal and N-linked glucuronide formation by normal and Gunn rats in vitro and in vivo. Biochemical and Biophysical Research Communications 6: 81

Arias I M 1961b Studies of chronic familial non-hemolytic jaundice with conjugated bilirubin in the serum with and without an unidentified pigment in the liver cells. American Journal of Medicine 31: 519

Arias I M 1962 Chronic unconjugated hyperbilirubinemia without overt signs of hemolysis in adolescents and adults. Journal of Clinical Investigation 41: 2233

Arias I M 1968 Chronic idiopathic jaundice. In: Bock K (ed) Ikterus. FK Schattauer Verlag, Stuttgart, p 65

Arias I M, Blumberg W 1979 The pigment in Dubin-Johnson syndrome. Gastroenterology 77: 820

Arias I M, Gartner L M 1964 Production of unconjugated hyperbilirubinemia in full-term newborn infants following administration of pregnane-3(alpha), 20(beta)-diol. Nature 203: 1292

Arias I M, Gartner L M, Seifter S, Furman M 1964a Prolonged neonatal unconjugated hyperbilirubinemia associated with breast feeding and a steroid, pregnana-3(alpha), 20(beta)-diol,m in maternal milk that inhibits glucuronide formation in vitro. Journal of Clinical Investigation 43: 2037

Arias I M, Bernstein L, Toffler R, Cornelius C, Novikoff A B, Essner E 1964b Black liver disease in Corriedale sheep: A new mutation affecting hepatic excretory function. Journal of Clinical Investigation 43: 1249

Arias I M, Wolfson S, Lucey J F, Mckay R J Jr 1965a Transient familial neonatal hyperbilirubinemia. Journal of Clinical Investigation 44: 1442

Arias I M, Bernstein L, Roffler R, Ben-Ezzer J 1965b Biliary and urinary excretion of metabolites of

7-H^5-epinephrine in mutant Corriedale sheep with hepatic pigmentation. Gastroenterology 48: 495

Arias I M, Bernstein L, Roffler R, Ben-Ezzer J 1965c Black liver diseases in Corriedale sheep: Metabolism of tritiated epinephrine and incorporation of isotope into the hepatic pigment in vivo. Journal of Clinical Investigation 44: 1026

Arias I M, Gartner L M, Cohen M, Ben-Ezzer J, Levi A J 1969 Chronic nonhemolytic unconjugated hyperbilirubinemia with glucuronyl transferase deficiency: Clinical, biochemical, pharmacologic, and genetic evidence for heterogeneity. American Journal of Medicine 47: 395

Arthur L J H, Bevan B R, Holton J B 1966 Neonatal hyperbilirubinemia and breast feeding. Developmental Medicine and Child Neurology 8: 279

Athanassiadis S, Chopra D R, Fisher M, Mckenna J 1974 An electrophoretic method for detection of unbound bilirubin and reserve bilirubin binding capacity in serum of newborns. Journal of Laboratory and Clinical Medicine 83: 968

Auclair C, Hakim J, Boivin P, Troube H, Boucherrot J 1976 Bilirubin and paranitrophenol glucuronyl transferase activity of the liver in patients with Gilbert's syndrome. Enzyme 21: 97

Axelsen R A 1973 Spontaneous renal papillary necrosis in the Gunn rat. Pathology 5: 43

Aziz M A, Schwartz S, Watson C J 1964 Studies of coproporphyrin. VIII. Reinvestigation of the isomer distribution in jaundice and liver diseases. Journal of Laboratory and Clinical Medicine 63: 596

Bailey A, Robinson D, Dawson A M 1977 Does Gilbert's disease exist? Lancet 1: 931

Banerjee A K 1970 Dubin-Johnson syndrome: a family study. Medical Journal of Malaysia 25: 21

Barnhart J L, Clarenburg R 1973 Factors determining clearance of bilirubin in perfused rat liver. American Journal of Physiology 225: 497

Baroody W G, Shugart R T 1956 Familial nonhemolytic icterus. American Journal of Medicine 20: 314

Barrett P V D 1971a The effect of diet and fasting on the serum bilirubin concentration in the rat. Gastroenterology 4: 572

Barrett P V D 1971b Hyperbilirubinemia of fasting. Journal of the American Medical Association 217: 1349

Behrman R E, Brown A K, Currie M R et al 1974 Committee on phototherapy in the newborn. Final report of the committee. Division of Medical Sciences, Assembly of Life Sciences, National Research Council, National Academy of

Sciences, Washington, D.C.

Beker S, Read A E 1958 Familial Dubin-Johnson syndrome. Gastroenterology 35: 387

Bellet H, Raynana A 1974 An assay of bilirubin UDP glucuronyl transferase on needle biopsies applied to Gilbert's syndrome. Clinica Chimica Acta 53: 51

Ben-Ezzer J, Rimington C, Shani M, Seligsohn U, Sheba C, Szeinberg A 1971 Abnormal excretion of the isomers of urinary coproporphyrin by patients with Dubin-Johnson syndrome in Israel. Clinical Science 40: 17

Ben-Ezzer J, Blonder J, Shani M, Seligsohn U, Post C A, Adam A, Szeinberg A 1973 Dubin-Johnson syndrome. Abnormal excretion of the isomers or urinary coproporphyrin by clinically unaffected family members. Israel Journal of Medical Sciences 9: 1431

Bensinger T A, Maisels M J, Marlson D E, Conrad M E 1973 Effects of low caloric diet on endogenous carbon monoxide production: Normal adults and Gilbert's syndrome. Proceedings of the Society for Experimental Biology and Medicine 144: 417

Benson A M, Talalay P, Jakoby W B 1977 Relationship between the soluble glutathione-dependent ^{5}-3-kestosteroid isomerase and the glutathione S-transferases of the liver. Proceedings of the National Academy of Sciences USA 74: 158

Berde C B, Hudson B S, Simoni R D, Sklar L A 1979 Human serum albumin: spectroscopic studies of binding and proximity relationships for fatty acid and bilirubin. Journal of Biological Chemistry 254: 391

Berendsohn S, Lowman J, Sundberg D, Watson C J 1974 Idiopathic dyserythropoietic jaundice. Blood 24: 1

Berk P D, Howe R B, Bloomer J R, Berlin N I 1969 Studies of bilirubin kinetics in normal adults. Journal of Clinical Investigation 48: 2176

Berk P D, Bloomer J R, Howe R B, Berlin N I 1970 Constitutional hepatic dysfunction (Gilbert's syndrome): A new definition based on kinetic studies with unconjugated radiobilirubin. American Journal of Medicine 49: 296

Berk P D, Blaschke T F, Waggoner J G 1972 Defective BSP clearance in patients with constitutional hepatic dysfunction (Gilbert's syndrome). Gastroenterlogy 63: 472

Berk P D, Wolkoff A W, Berlin N I 1975a Inborn errors of bilirubin metabolism. Medical Clinics of North America 59: 803

Berk P D, Martin J F, Blaschke T F, Scharschmidt B F, Plotz P H 1975b Unconjugated hyperbilirubinemia: Physiological evaluation and experimental approaches to therapy. Annals of Internal Medicine 82: 552

Berk P D, Scharschmidt B F, Waggoner J G, White S C 1976 The effect of repeated phlebotomy on bilirubin turnover, bilirubin clearance and unconjugated hyperbilirubinaemia in the Crigler-Najjar syndrome and the jaundiced Gunn rat: Application of computers to experimental design. Clinical Science and Molecular Medicine 50: 333

Berk P D, Jones E A, Howe R B, Berlin N I 1980 Disorders of bilirubin metabolism. In: Bondy P K, Rosenberg L E (eds) Metabolic Control and Disease, 8th edn. Saunders, Philadelphia, p 1009

Berk P D, Berman M D, Blitzer B L et al 1981 Effect of splenectomy on hepatic bilirubin clearance in patients with hereditary spherocytosis: Implications for the diagnosis of Gilbert's syndrome. Journal of Laboratory and Clinical Medicine 98: 37

Berkowitz D, Entine J, Chunn L 1960 Dubin-Johnson

syndrome: Report of a case occurring in a Negro male. New England Journal of Medicine 262: 1028

Bendoin M, Feldmann G, Erlinger S, Benhamou J-P 1973 Benign recurrent cholestasis. Digestion 9: 49

Bhargava M, Ohmi N, Listowsky I, Arias I M 1980 Structural catalytic, binding, and immunological properties associated with each of the two subunits of rat liver ligandin. Journal of Biological Chemistry 255: 718

Biempica L, Gutstein S, Arias I M 1967 Morphological and biochemical studies of benign recurrent cholestasis. Gastroenterology 52: 521

Billing G H, Gray C H, Kulcycka A, Manfield P, Nicholson D C 1964a The metabolism of ^{14}C-bilirubin in congenital nonhaemolytic hyperbilirubinaemia. Clinical Science 27: 163

Billing B H, Williams R, Richards T G 1964b Defects in hepatic transport of bilirubin in congenital hyperbilirubinaemia. An analysis of plasma bilirubin disappearance curves. Clinical Science 27: 245

Black M, Billing B H 1969 Hepatic bilirubin UDP glucuronyltransferase activity in liver disease and Gilbert's syndrome. New England Journal of Medicine 280: 1266

Black M, Fevery J, Parker D, Jacobsen J, Billing B H, Carson E R 1974 Effect of phenobarbitone on plasma (^{14}C) bilirubin clearance in patients with unconjugated hyperbilirubinaemia. Clinical Science and Molecular Medicine 46: 1

Blanc W A, Johnson L 1959 Studies on kernicterus. Journal of Neuropathology and Experimental Neurology 18: 165

Blanckaert N, Fevery J, Compernolle F 1976 Synthesis and separation by thin-layer chromatography of bilirubin-IX isomers. Their identification as tetrapyrroles and dipyrrol anthranilate azo derivates. Biochemical Journal 155: 405

Blanckaert N, Fevery J, Heirwegh K P N, Compernolle F 1977a Characterization of the major diazopositive pigments in bile of homozygous Gunn rats. Biochemical Journal 164: 237

Blanckaert N, Heirwegh K P M, Zaman Z 1977b Comparison of the biliary excretion of the four isomers of bilirubin-IX in Wistar and homozygous Gunn rats. Biochemical Journal 164: 229

Blanckaert N, Kabra P M, Farina F A, Stafford B E, Marton L M, Schmidt R 1980 Measurement of bilirubin and its mono- and diconjugates in human serum by alkaline methanolysis and high performance liquid chromatography. Journal of Laboratory and Clinical Medicine 96: 198

Blaschke T F, Berk P D, Scharschmidt B F, Guyther J R, Vergalla J, Waggoner J G 1974a Crigler-Najjar syndrome: An unusual course with development of neurologic damage at age eighteen. Pediatric Research 8: 573

Blaschke T F, Berk P D, Rodkey F L, Scharschmidt B F, Collison H A, Waggoner J G 1974b Effects of glutethimide and phenobarbital on hepatic bilirubin clearance, plasma bilirubin turnover, and carbon monoxide production in man. Biochemical Pharmacology 23: 2795

Bloomer J R, Berk P D, Howe R B, Berlin N I 1971a Bilirubin metabolism in congenital nonhemolytic jaundice. Pediatric Research 5: 256

Bloomer J R, Barrett P V, Rodkey F L, Berlin N I 1971b Studies on the mechanisms of fasting hyperbilirubinemia. Gastroenterology 61: 479

Bloomer J R, Berk P D, Howe R B 1974 Hepatic clearance of unconjugated bilirubin in colestatic liver diseases. American Journal of Digestive Diseases 19: 9

Bock K, Frohling W, Remmer H, Rexer B 1973 Effects of phenobarbital and 3-methyl cholanthrene on substrate specificity of rat liver microsomal UDP glucuronyl transferase. Biochimica et Biophysica Acta 327: 46

Bock K W, Kittel J, Josting G 1978 Purification of rat liver UDP glucuronyl transferase: Separation of two enzyme forms with different substrate specificity and differential inducibility. In: Aitio A (ed) Conjugation Reactions in Drug Biotransformation. Elsevier, Amsterdam, p 357

Bock K W, Josling D, Lilenblum W M, Pfeil H 1979 Purification of rat liver glucuronyl transferase-separation of two enzyme forms inducible by 3-methyl-cholanthrene or phenobarbital. European Journal of Biochemistry 98: 19

Bonnet R J, Davis E, Hursthouse M B 1976 Structure of bilirubin. Nature 262: 326

Bowen W R, Porter E, Waters W F 1959 The protective action of albumin in bilirubin toxicity in newborn puppies. American Journal of Diseases of Children 98: 568

Brodersen R 1978a Binding of bilirubin and other ligands to human serum albumin. In: Peters T, Sjoholm I (eds) Albumin: Structure, Biosynthesis, Function, Pergamon, Oxford, p 61

Brodersen R 1978b Determination of the vacant amount of high affinity bilirubin binding site on serum albumin. Acta Pharmacologica et Toxicologica 42: 153

Brodersen R 1979 Bilirubin solubility and interaction with albumin and phospholipid. Journal of Biological Chemistry 254: 2364

Brodersen R, Hermann L S 1963 Intestinal reabsorption of unconjugated bilirubin: a possible contributing factor in neonatal jaundice. Lancet 1: 1242

Brodersen R, Tygstrup N 1967 Serum bilirubin studies in patients with intermittent intrahepatic cholestasis. Gut 8: 46

Brodersen R, Cashore W, Wennberg R P, Ahlfors C E, Rasmussen L F, Shusterman D 1979 Kinetics of bilirubin oxidation with peroxidase, as applied to studies of bilirubin-albumin binding. Scandinavian Journal of Clinical and Laboratory Investigation 39: 143

Brown A K, Zuelzer W W 1958 Studies on the neonatal development of the glucuronide conjugating system. Journal of Clinical Investigation 37: 332

Brown A K, Einsinger J, Blumberg W E, Flores J, Boyle G Lamola A A 1980 A rapid fluorometric method for determining bilirubin levels and binding in the blood of neonates: comparison with other methods. Pediatrics 65: 767

Burchell B 1977 Purification of UDP glucuronyl transferase from untreated rat liver. FEBS Letters 78: 101

Burchell B 1981 Identification and purification of multiple forms of UDP-glucuronosyltransferase. Reviews in Biochemical Toxicology 3: 1

Burchell B, Blanckaert N, 1984 Bilirubin mono- and diglucuronide formation by purified rat liver microsomal bilirubin-UDP-glucuronyl transferase. Biochemical Journal 223: 461

Burnscox C J 1965 The Dubin-Johnson syndrome in a Timorese. Medical Journal of Malaysia 19: 311

Butt H R, Anderson V E, Foulk W T, Baggenstoss A H, Schoenfield L J, Dickson E R 1966 Studies of chronic idiopathic jaundice (Dubin-Johnson syndrome). II. Evaluation of a large family with the trait. Gastroenterology 51: 619

Call N B, Tisher C C 1975 The urinary concentrating defect in the Gunn strain of rat. Role of bilirubin. Journal of

Clinical Investigation 55: 319

Callahan E W, Thaler M, Karon M, Bauer K, Schmid R 1970 Phototherapy of severe unconjugated hyperbilirubinemia: formation and removal of labelled bilirubin derivatives. Pediatrics 46: 841

Callard P, Ganter P, Kalifat S R, Dupuy-Coin A M, Delarve J 1971 Etude cytochimique et ultrastructurale de pigment d'un cas de maladie de Dubin-Johnson. Virchows Archiv Abteilung B Zellpathologie 7: 63

Cartel G V M, Chisesi T, Cazzavillian M, Barbui T, Battista R, Dini E 1975 Bromsulphthalein-Ausscheidung und Hyperbilirubinaemia beim Gilbert Syndrome. Deutsche Zeitschrift fur Verdauungs- und Stoffwechselkrankheiten 35: 169

Charbonnier A, Brisbois P 1960 Etude chromatographique de la BSP au cours de l'epreuve clinique d'epuration plasmatique de ce colorant. Revue Internationale Hepatologie 10: 1163

Childs B, Najjar V A 1956 Familial nonhemolytic jaundice with kernicterus: A report of two cases without neurological damage. Pediatrics 18: 369

Childs B, Sidbury J B, Migeon C J 1959 Glucuronic acid conjugation by patients with familial non-hemolytic jaundice and their relatives. Pediatrics 23: 903

Clare N T 1945 Photosensitivity diseases in New Zealand. IV. Photosensitizing agent in Southdown photosensitivity. New Zealand Journal of Science and Technology 27A: 23

Clarke C A, Donohoe W T A, Finn R et al 1971 Combined study: Prevention of Rh hemolytic disease: Final results of the "high risk" clinical trial. A combined study from centers in England and Baltimore. British Medical Journal 2: 607

Cobelli C 1975 Modelling, identification and parameter estimation of bilirubin kinetics in normal, hemolytic and Gilbert's states. Computers and Biomedical Research 8: 522

Cobelli C, Ruggeri A, Toffolo G, Okolicsanyi L, Venuti M, Orlando R 1981 BSP vs bilirubin kinetics in Gilbert's syndrome. In: Okolicsanyi L (ed) Familial Hyperbilirubinemia. Wiley, New York, p 121

Cohen L, Lewis C, Arias I M 1972 Pregnancy, oral contraceptives, and chronic familial jaundice with predominantly conjugated hyperbilirubinemia (Dubin-Johnson syndrome). Gastroenterology 62: 1182

Colleran E, O'Carra P 1977 Enzymology and comparative physiology of biliverdin reduction. In: Berk P D, Berlin N I (eds) The Chemistry and Physiology of Bile Pigments. U.S. Government Printing Office, Washington, D.C. p 69

Constantopoulos A, Matsaniotis N 1976 Bilirubin inhibition of protein kinase: its prevention by cyclic AMP. Cytobios 17: 17

Cornelius C E 1969 Organic anion transport in mutant sheep with congenital hyperbilirubinemia. Archives of Environmental Health 19: 852

Cornelius C E, Gronwall R R 1968 Congenital photosensitivity and hyperbililrubinemia in Southdown sheep in the United States. American Journal of Veterinary Research 29: 291

Cornelius C E, Arias I M, Osburn B I 1965 Hepatic pigmentation with photosensitivity: A syndrome in Corriedale sheep resembling Dubin-Johnson syndrome in man. Journal of the American Veterinary Medical Association 146: 709

Cornelius C E, Osburn B I, Gronwall R R, Cardinet G H 1968 Dubin-Johnson syndrome in immature sheep.

American Journal of Digestive Diseases 13: 1072

Cornford E M, Braun L D, Oldendrop W H, Hill M A 1982 Comparison of lipid-mediated blood-brain barrier penetrability in neonates and adults. American Journal of Physiology 243–C161

Cowan B E, Kwong L K, Vreman H J, Stevenson D K 1983 The effect of tin-protoporphyrin on the bilirubin production rate in newborn rats. Pediatric Pharmacology 3: 95

Cowan R E, Thompson R P H, Kaye J P, Clark G M 1977 The association between fasting hyperbilirubinaemia and serum non-esterified acids in man. Clinical Science and Molecular Medicine 53: 155

Cowger M L 1973 Bilirubin encephalopathy. In: Gaull G (ed) Biology of brain dysfunction. Plenum, New York, vol 2, p 265

Crigler J F, Najjar V A 1952 Congenital familial non-hemolytic jaundice with kernicterus. Pediatrics 10: 169

Cunningham I J, Hopkirk C S M, Filmer J F 1942 Photosensitivity diseases in New Zealand. I Facial eczema: Its clinical, pathological and biochemical characteristics. New Zealand Journal of Science and Technology 24A: 185

Damashek W, Singer K 1941 Familial nonhemolytic jaundice. Constitutional hepatic dysfunction with indirect van den Bergh reaction. AMA Archives of Internal Medicine 67: 259

Dappen G M, Sundberg M W, Wu T W, Babb B E, Schaeffer J R 1983 A diazo-based dry film for determination of total bilirubin in serum. Clinical Chemistry 29: 37

Davidson A R, Rojas-Bueno A, Thompson R P H, Williams R 1975 Reduced caloric intake and nicotinic acid provocation tests in diagnosis of Gilbert's syndrome. British Medical Journal 2: 480

De Brito T, Borges M A, Dasilva L C 1966 Electron microscopy of the liver in nonhemolytic acholuric jaundice with kernicterus (Crigler-Najjar) and in idiopathic conjugated hyperbilirubinemia (Rotor). Gastroenterlogia 106: 325

Demetriou A A, Levenson S M, Whiting J et al 1986a Replacement of hepatic functions in rats by transplantation of microcarrier-attached hepatocytes. Science 233: 1190

Demetriou A A, Levenson S M, Whiting J et al 1986b Organization, morphology and function of microcarrier-attached transplanted hepatocytes in rats. Proceedings of the National Academy of Sciences USA 83: 7475

Demetriou A A, Whiting J, Levenson S M et al 1986c New method of hepatocyte transplantation and extracorporeal liver support. Annals of Surgery 204: 259

De Pagter A G F, Van Berge Henegouwen G P, Bokkel-Huinnuk J A, Brandt K-H 1976 Familial benign recurrent intrahepatic cholestasis. Gastroenterlogy 71: 202

De Saram W G, Gallagher C H, Goodrich B S 1969 Melanosis of sheep liver. I. Chemistry of the pigment. Australian Veterinary Journal 45: 105

Dhumeaux D, Berthelot P 1975 Chronic hyperbilirubinemia associated with hepatic uptake and storage impairment: A new syndrome resembling that of the mutant Southdown sheep. Gastroenterology 69: 988

Dickson E R, Fleischer J, Summerskill W H J 1965 Ultrastructural changes of the liver in benign recurrent cholestasis. Mayo Clinic Proceedings 40: 288

Dittrich H, Seifert E 1962 Uber das verhalten des pigmentes sowie der biligrafin auscheidung bei einem patienten mit Dubin-Johnson syndrome. Acta Hepatosplenologica 9: 45

Drucker W D 1968 Glucuronic acid conjugation of tetrahydrocortisone p-nitrophenol in the homozygous Gunn rats. Proceedings of the Society for Experimental Biology and Medicine 129: 308

Dubin I N 1958 Chronic idiopathic jaundice: A review of fifty cases. American Journal of Medicine 23: 268

Dubin I N, Johnson F B 1954 Chronic idiopathic jaundice with unidentified pigment in liver cells: A new clinocopathologic entity with a report of 12 cases. Medicine (Baltimore) 33: 155

Dutton G J 1966 The biosynthesis of glucuronide. In: Dutton G J (ed) Glucuronic Acid Free and Combined. Academic Press, New York, p 185

Edwards R H 1975 Inheritance of the Dubin-Johnson-Sprinz syndrome. Gastroenterology 68: 734

Ehrlick J C, Novikoff A B, Platt R, Essner E 1960 Hepatocellular lipofuscin and the pigment of chronic idiopathic jaundice. Bulletin of the New York Academy of Medicine 36: 488

Endo T, Uchida K, Amuro Y, Higashino K, Yamamura Y 1979 Bile acid metabolism in benign recurrent intrahepatic cholestasis. Comparative studies on the icteric and anicteric phases of a single case. Gastroenterology 76: 1002

Erlinger S, Dhumeaux D, Desjeux J F, Benhamou J P 1973 Hepatic handling of unconjugated dyes in the Dubin-Johnson syndrome. Gastroenterology 64: 106

Essner E, Novikoff A B 1960 Human hepatocellular pigments and lysosomes. Journal of Ultrastructure Research 3: 3764

Falany C N, Tephly T R 1983 Separation, purification and characterization of three isozymes of UDP-glucuronyl transferase from rat liver microsomes. Archives of Biochemistry and Biophysics 227: 248

Falany C N, Roy Chowdhury J, Roy Chowdhury N, Tephly T R 1983 Steroid 3- and 17-OH-UDPglucuronosyltransferase activities in rat and rabbit liver microsomes. Drug Metabolism and Disposition 11: 426

Felscher B F 1976 Effect of changes in dietary components on the serum bilirubin in Gilbert's syndrome. American Journal of Clinical Nutrition 7: 705

Felscher B F, Carpio N M 1975 Caloric intake and unconjugated hyperbilirubinemia. Gastroenterology 69: 42

Felscher B F, Rickard D, Redeker A G 1970 The reciprocal relation between caloric intake and the degree of hyperbilirubinemia in Gilbert's syndrome. New England Journal of Medicine 283: 170

Felscher B F, Craig J R, Carpio N 1973 Hepatic bilirubin glucuronidation in Gilbert's syndrome. Journal of Laboratory and Clinical Medicine 81: 829

Felscher B F, Carpio N M, Van Couvering K 1979 Effect of fasting and phenobarbital on hepatic UDP-glucuronic acid formation in the rat. Journal of Laboratory and Clinical Medicine 93: 414

Fevery J, Van Damme B, Michiels R, De Groote J, Heirwegh K P M 1972 Bilirubin conjugates in bile of man and rat in the normal state and in liver disease. Journal of Clinical Investigation 51: 2482

Fevery J, Blanckaert N, Heirwegh K P M, Preaux A-M, Berthelot P 1977 Unconjugated bilirubin and an increased proportion of bilirubin monoconjugates in the bile of patients with Gilbert's syndrome and Crigler-Najjar syndrome. Journal of Clinical Investigation 60: 970

Fevery J, Verwilghen R, Tan T G, Degroote J 1980 Glucuronidation of bilirubin and the occurrence of pigment gallstones in patients with chronic haemolytic diseases.

European Journal of Clinical Investigation 10: 219

Fleischner G, Robbins J, Arias I M 1972 Immunological studies of Y protein: a major cytoplasmic organic anion binding protein. Journal of Clinical Investigation 51: 677

Fleischner G M, Robbins J B, Arias I M 1977 Cellular localization of ligandin in rat, hamster and man. Biochemical and Biophysical Research Communications 74: 992

Flitman R, Worth N H 1966 Inhibition of hepatic alcohol dehydrogenase by bilirubin. Journal of Biological Chemistry 251: 669

Flock E V, Bollman J L, Owen C A, Zollman P E 1965 Conjugation of thyroid hormones and analogues by the Gunn rat. Endocrinology 77: 303

Foliot A, Ploussard J P, Housett E, Christoforov B, Luzean R, Odievre M 1976 Breast milk jaundice: In vitro inhibition of rat liver bilirubin-uridine diphosphate glucuronyl transferase activity and Z protein-bromosulfophthalein binding by human breast milk. Pediatric Research 10: 594

Forker E L 1977 Canalicular anion transport. Effect of bile acid-independent choleretics. In: Berk P D, Berlin N I (eds) Bile Pigments, Chemistry and Physiology. U.S. Department of Health, Education and Welfare, Bethesda, Maryland, p 383

Forker E L, Luxon B A 1981 Albumin helps mediate removal of taurocholate by rat liver. Journal of Clinical Investigation 67: 1517

Foulk W T, Butt H R, Owen C A, Whitcomb F F 1959 Constitutional hepatic dysfunction (Gilbert's disease): Its natural history and related syndrome. Medicine 38: 25

Freda V J, Gorman J G, Pollack W 1964 Successful prevention of experimental Rh sensitization in man with an anti Rh gamma 2 globulin antibody preparation. Transfusion 4: 26

Fromke V L, Miller D 1972 Constitutional hepatic dysfunction (CHD: Gilbert's disease): a review with special reference to a characteristic increase and prolongation of the hyperbilirubinemic response to nicotinic acid. Medicine (Baltimore) 51: 451

Fulop M, Sandson J, Brazeau P 1965 Dialyzability, protein binding, and renal excretion of plasma conjugated bilirubin. Journal of Clinical Investigation 44: 666

Gardner W A, Konigsmark B 1969 Familial nonhemolytic jaundice: bilirubinosis and encephalopathy. Pediatrics 43: 365

Gartner L M, Lee K, Vaisman S, Lane D, Zaraful I 1977 Development of bilirubin transport and metabolism in the newborn Rhesus monkey. Journal of Pediatrics 90: 513

Gilbert A, Lereboullet P 1901 La cholamae simple familiale. Semaine Médicale 21: 241

Gilbert A, Lereboullet P, Herscher M 1907 Les trois cholemies congenitals. Bulletins et Memoires de la Societe Medicale des Hopiteaux de Paris 24: 1203

Goldstein E J, Arias I M 1976 Interaction of ligandin with radiographic contrast media. Investigative Radiology 11: 594

Gollan J L, Huang S M, Billing B, Sherlock S 1975a Prolonged survival in three brothers with severe type II Crigler-Najjar syndrome. Ultrastructural and metabolic studies. Gastroenterology 68: 1543

Gollan J L, Hatt K J, Billing B H 1975b The influence of diet on unconjugated hyperbilirubinemia in the Gunn rat. Clinical Science and Molecular Medicine 49: 229

Gollan J L, Bateman C, Billing B H 1976 Effect of dietary composition on the unconjugated hyperbilirubinemia of Gilbert's syndrome. Gut 5: 335

Gollan J L, Dallinger K J C, Billing B H 1978 Excretion of conjugated bilirubin in the isolated perfused rat kidney. Clinical Science and Molecular Medicine 54: 381

Gollan J L, Hole D R, Billing B H 1979 The role of dietary lipid in the regulation of unconjugated hyperbilirubinemia in Gunn rats. Clinical Science 57: 327

Gordon E R, Shaffer E A, Sass-Kortsak A 1976 Bilirubin secretion and conjugation in the Crigler-Najjar syndrome type II. Gastroenterology 70: 761

Goresky C A 1975 The hepatic uptake process: its implication for bilirubin transport. In: Goresky CA, Fisher M M (eds) Jaundice. Plenum, New York p 159.

Goresky C A, Gordon E R, Shaffer E A, Parie P, Carassavas D, Aronoff A 1978 Definition of a conjugation dysfunction in Gilbert's syndrome: Studies of the handling of bilirubin loads and of the pattern of bilirubin conjugates secreted in bile. Clinical Science and Molecular Medicine 1: 63

Gorodischer R, Levy G, Krasner J, Yaffe S J 1970 Congenital nonobstructive, nonhemolytic jaundice: effect of phototherapy. New England Journal of Medicine 282: 375

Gorski J P, Kasper C B 1977 Purification and properties of microsomal UDP glucuronyl transferase from rat liver. Journal of Biological Chemistry 252: 1336

Grodsky G M, Kolb H J, Fanska R E, Nemechek C 1970 Effect of age of rat on development of hepatic carriers for bilirubin: A possible explanation for physiologic jaundice and hyperbilirubinemia in the newborn. Metabolism 3: 246

Gronwall R 1970 Sulfobromophthalein sodium excretion and hepatic storage in Corriedale and Southdown sheep with inherited hepatic dysfunction. American Journal of Vetinary Research 31: 2131

Gunn C H 1938 Hereditary acholuric jaundice in a new mutant strain of rats. Journal of Heredity 29: 137

Gutstein S, Alpert S, Arias I M 1968 Studies of hepatic excretory function. IV. Biliary excretion of sulfobromophthalein in a patient with Dubin-Johnson syndrome and a biliary fistula. Israel Journal of Medical Sciences 4: 46

Haberman S, Kraft E J, Leucke P E, Peach R O 1960 ABO isoimmunization: The use of the specific Coombs and best elution tests in the detection of hemolytic disease. Journal of Pediatrics 56: 471

Habig W H, Pabst M J, Fleischner G, Gatmaitan Z, Arias I M, Jakoby W B 1974 The identity of glutathione S-transferase B with ligandin, a major binding protein of liver. Proceedings of the National Academy of Sciences 10: 3879

Hadchouel P, Charbonnier A, Lageron A, Leominier F, Rautureau M, Scotto J, Carol J 1971 A Propos d'une Nouvelle forme d'ictere chronique idiopathique. Hypothese physio-pathologique. Revue Medico-Chirurgicale des Maladies du Foie 46: 61

Hancock J 1950 Congenital photosensitivity in Southdown sheep. A new sublethal factor in sheep. New Zealand Journal of Science and Technology 32A: 16

Hardy J B, Peeples M O 1971 Serum bilirubin levels in new born infants. Distributions and associations with neurological abnormalities during the first year of life. Johns Hopkins Medical Journal 128: 265

Hargreaves T, Piper R F 1964 Breast milk jaundice: Effect of inhibitory breast milk and 3(alpha), 20(beta)-diol, in maternal milk that inhibits glucuronide formation in vitro. Journal of Clinical Investigation 43: 2037

Heirwegh K P M, Fevery J B, Meuwissen J A T P, De Groote J, Compernolle F, Desmet V, Van Roy F P 1974 Recent advances in the separation and analysis of diazo-positive bile pigments. Methods of Biochemical Analysis 22: 205

Hislop D M C 1964 A case of Dubin-Johnson syndrome in a North American Cree Indian with suggestive evidence of familial occurrence. Medical Services Journal (Canada) 10: 61

Holton J B, Lathe G H 1963 Inhibitors of bilirubin conjugation in newborn infant serum and male urine. Clinical Science 25: 499

Howan E R, Guarino A M 1974 Biliary excretion of phenol red by Wistar and Gunn rats. Proceedings of the Society for Experimental Biology and Medicine 146: 46

Hsia D Y-Y, Gellis S S 1954 Studies on erythroblastosis fetalis due to ABO incompatibility. Pediatrics 13: 503

Hsia D Y-Y, Patterson P, Allen F H, Diamond L K, Gellis S S 1952 Prolonged obstructive jaundice in infancy: General Survey of 156 cases. Pediatrics 10: 243

Hsia J C, Kwan N H, Er S S, Wood D J, Chance G W 1978 Development of a spin assay for reserve bilirubin loading capacity of human serum. Proceedings of the National Academy of Sciences USA 75: 1542

Huang P W H, Rozdilsky B, Gerrard J W, Goluboff N, Holmannch 1970 Crigler-Najjar syndrome in four of five siblings with post-mortem findings in one. Archives of Pathology 90: 536

Hunter F M, Sparks R D, Flinner R L 1964 Hepatitis with resulting mobilization of hepatic pigment in a patient with Dubin-Johnson syndrome. Gastroenterology 47: 631

Hunter J, Thompson R P H, Rake M O, Williams R 1971 Controlled trial of phetharbital, a non-hypnotic barbiturate, in unconjugated hyperbilirubinaemia. British Medical Journal 2: 497

Hunter J O, Thompson R P H, Dunn P M, Williams R 1973 Inheritance of type II Crigler-Najjar hyperbilirubinemia. Gut 14: 46

Hutchinson D W, Johnson B, Knell A J 1972 The reaction between bilirubin and aromatic diazo compounds. Biochemical Journal 127: 907

Inoue M, Hirata E, Morino Y, Roy Chowdhury J, Roy Chowdhury N, Arias I M 1985 The role of albumin in the hepatic transport of bilirubin: Studies in mutant analbuminemic rats. Journal of Biochemistry 97: 737

Israels L G, Zipursky A 1959 Primary shunt hyperbilirubinemia due to an alternate path of bilirubin production. American Journal of Medicine 27: 693

Itoh S, Onishi S 1985 Kinetic study of the photochemical changes of (ZZ)-bilirubin IX bound to human serum albumin. Demonstration of (EZ)-bilirubin IX as an intermediate in photochemical changes from (ZZ)-bilirubin IX to (EZ)-cyclobilirubin IX. Biochemical Journal 226: 251

Ivicic L, Sosovec V 1975 Vrodena benigni konjugovena hyperbilirubinemia S pigmentom peceni (Dubin-Johnson syndrom) u novorodenca. Ceskoslovenska Pediatrie (Praha) 30: 287

Iyanagi T, Hanium M, Sogawa K, Fuji-Kuriyama Y, Watanabe S, Shively J, Anan K 1986 cloning and characterization of cDNA encoding 3-methylcholanthrene-inducible rat mRNA for UDP-glucuronosyltransferase. Journal of Biological Chemistry 261: 15607

Jackson M R, Burchell B 1986 The full length coding sequence of rat liver androsterone UDP-glucuronyltransferase cDNA and comparison with other members of the gene family. Nucleic Acids Research 14: 779

Jansen F H, Billing B H 1971 Identification of monoconjugates of bilirubin in bile as amide derivatives. Biochemical Journal 125: 917

Jansen P L M, Arias I M 1975 Delipidation and reactivation of UDP glucuronosyl transferase from rat liver. Biochimica et Biophysica Acta 391: 28

Jansen P L M, Roy Chowdhury J, Fischberg E B, Arias I M 1977 Enzymatic conversion of bilirubin monoglucuronide to diglucuronide by rat liver plasma membranes. Journal of Biological Chemistry 252: 2710

Jansen P L M, Peters W H, Lamers W H 1985 Hereditary chronic conjugated hyperbilirubinemia in mutant rats caused by defective hepatic anion transport. Hepatology 5: 573

Javitt N B, Kondo T, Kuchiba K 1978 Bile acid excretion in Dubin-Johnson syndrome. Gastroenterology 75: 931

Johnson J D 1975 Neonatal nonhemolytic jaundice. New England Journal of Medicine 292: 194

Kamisaka K, Listowsky I, Gatmaitan Z, Arias I M 1975a Interactions of bilirubin and other ligands with ligandin. Biochemistry 14: 2175

Kamisaka K, Habig W H, Ketley J N, Arias M, Jakoby W B 1975b Multiple forms of human glutathione S-transferase and their affinity for bilirubin. European Journal of Biochemistry 60: 153

Kapitulinik J, Valaes T, Kaufmann N A, Blondheim S H 1974a Clinical evaluation of Sephadex gel filtration in estimation of bilirubin binding in serum in neonatal jaundice. Archives of Disease in Childhood 49: 886

Kapitulnik J, Kaufmann N A, Goitein K, Cividalli G, Blondheim S H 1974b A pigment found in the Crigler-Najjar syndrome and its similarity to an ultrafilterable photo-derivative of bilirubin. Clinica Chimica Acta 57: 231

Kaplowitz N, Javitt N, Kappas A 1972 Coproporphyrin I and III excretion in bile and urine. Journal of Clinical Investigation 51: 2895

Karon M, Imach D, Schwartz A 1970 Effective phototherapy in congenital nonobstructive, nonhemolytic jaundice. New England Journal of Medicine 282: 377

Katoh R, Kashiwamata S, Niwa F 1975 Studies on cellular toxicity of bilirubin. Effect on the carbohydrate metabolism in the young rat brain. Brain Research 83: 81

Kaufman S S, Wood R P, Shaw B W, Markin R S, Rosenthal P, Gridelli B, Vanderhood J A 1986 Orthotopic liver transplantation for type I Crigler-Najjar syndrome. Hepatology 6: 1259

Kawasaki H, Kinwa N, Irisa T, Hirayama C 1979 Dye clearance studies in Rotor's syndrome. American Journal of Gastroenterology 71: 380

Kermarec J, Duplay H, Daniel R 1972 Etude histochimique et ultrastructurale comparative des pigments de la melanose colique et du syndrome de Dubin-Johnson. Annales de Biologie Clinique 30: 567

Ketterer B, Ross-Mansell P, Whitehead J K 1967 The isolation of carcinogen-binding protein from livers of rats given 4-dimethyl aminoazobenzene. Biochemical Journal 103: 316

Kirsch R, Kamisaka K, Fleishner G, Arias I M 1975 Structural and functional studies of ligandin, a major renal organic anion binding protein. Journal of Clinical Investigation 55: 1009

Kirshenbaum G, Shames D M, Schmid R 1976 An expanded model of bilirubin kinetics: effect of feeding, fasting and phenobarbital in Gilbert's syndrome. Journal of Pharmacokinetics and Biopharmaceutics 2: 115

Kondo T, Kuchiba K, Ohtsuka Y, Yanagisawa W, Shiomura T, Taminato T 1974 Clinical and genetic studies on Dubin-Johnson syndrome in a cluster area in Japan. Japanese Journal of Human Genetics 18: 378–392

Kondo T, Yagi R, Kuchiba K 1975 Dubin-Johnson syndrome in a neonate. New England Journal of Medicine 292: 1028

Kondo T, Kuchiba K, Shimizu Y 1976 Coproporphyrin isomers in Dubin-Johnson syndrome. Gastroenterology 70: 1117

Kondo T, Kuchiba K, Shimizu Y 1979 Metabolic fate of exogenous delta-aminolevulinic acid in Dubin-Johnson syndrome. Journal of Laboratory and Clinical Medicine 94: 421

Koskelo P, Toivonen I 1968 Urinary excretion of coproporphyrin isomers I and III and aminolaevulinic acid in normal pregnancy and obstetric hepatosis. Acta Obstetricia et Gynecologica Scandinavica 47: 292

Koskelo P, Eisala A, Toivonen I 1966 Urinary excretion of porphyrin precursors and coproporphyrin in healthy females on oral contraceptives. British Medical Journal 1: 652

Koskelo P, Toivonen I, Adlercreutz H 1967 Urinary coproporphyrin isomer distribution in Dubin-Johnson syndrome. Clinical Chemistry 13: 1006

Kubasik N P, Mayer T K, Baskar A G, Sine H E, D'Souza J P 1985 The measurement of fractionated bilirubin by Ektachem Film Slides. Method validation and comparison of conjugated bilirubin measurements with direct bilirubin in obstructive and hepatocellular jaundice. American Journal of Clinical Pathology 84: 518

Kuhn H A 1963 Intrahepatic cholestasis in two brothers. German Medical Monthly 8: 185

Laas R, Helmke K 1981 Regional cerebral blood flow following unilateral blood-brain barrier alteration induced by hyperosmolar perfusion in the albino rat. In: Cervos-Navarro J, Fritschka E (eds) Cerebral Circulation and Metabolism. Raven Press, New York, p 317

Lamolla A A, Eisinger J, Blumberg W E, Palet S C, Flores J 1979 Fluorometric study of the partition of bilirubin among blood components: Basis for rapid microassays of bilirubin and bilirubin binding capacity in whole blood. Analytical Biochemistry 15: 25

Lauff J J, Kasper M E, Ambros R T 1983 Quantitative liquid chromatographic estimation of bilirubin species in pathological serum. Clinical Chemistry 29: 800

Lee K-S, Gartner L M 1983 Management of unconjugated hyperbilirubinemia in the newborn. Seminars in Liver Disease 3: 52

Lesser P B 1973 Benign familial recurrent intrahepatic cholestasis. American Journal of Digestive Diseases 18: 259

Lester R, Schmid R 1963 Intestinal absorption of bile pigments. II. bilirubin absorption in man. New England Journal of Medicine 269: 178

Levanon M, Rimon S, Shani M, Ramot B, Goldberg E 1972 Active and inactive factor-VII in Dubin-Johnson syndrome with factor-VII deficiency, hereditary factor-VII deficiency and on coumadin administration. British Journal of Haematology 23: 669

Levi A J, Gatmaitan Z, Arias I M 1969a Two hepatic cytoplasmic protein fractions, Y and Z, and their possible role in the hepatic uptake of bilirubin, sulfobromophthalein and other anions. Journal of Clinical Investigation 48: 2156

Levi A J, Gatmaitan Z, Arias I M 1969b Deficiency of hepatic organic anion-binding protein as a possible cause of nonhaemolytic unconjugated hyperbilirubinemia in the new born. Lancet 2: 139

Levi A J, Gatmaitan Z, Arias I M 1970 Deficiency of hepatic organic anion-binding protein, impaired organic anion uptake by liver and "physiologic" jaundice in newborn monkeys. New England Journal of Medicine 283: 1136

Levine R L, Fredericks W R, Rappaport S I 1985 Clearance of bilirubin from rat brain after reversible osmotic opening of the blood-brain barrier. Pediatric Research 19: 1040

Lichter M, Fleischner G, Kirsch R, Levi A J, Kamisaka K, Arias I M 1976 Ligandin and Z protein in binding of thyroid hormones by the liver. American Journal of Physiology 230: 1113

Lightner D A, Wooldrige T A, McDonagh A F 1979 Photobilirubin. An early bilirubin photoproduct detected by absorbance difference spectroscopy. Proceedings of the National Academy of Sciences 76: 29

Lillienblum W, Walli A K, Bock K W 1982 Differential induction of rat liver microsomal UDP-glucuronosyl-transferase activities by various inducing agents. Biochemical Pharmacology 31: 907

Litwack G, Ketterer B, Arias I M 1971 An abundant liver protein which binds steroids, bilirubin, carcinogens and a number of exogenous anions. Nature 234: 466

Liver Transplantation-Consensus Conference 1983 Journal of the American Medical Association 250: 2961

Localio S A, Schwartz M S, Gannon C F 1941 The urinary/fecal coproporphyrin ratio in liver disease. Journal of Clinical Investigation 20: 7

Lozzio B B, Chernoff A L, Machedo E R, Lozzio S H 1967 Hereditary renal disease in a mutant strain of rats. Science 156: 1742

Lucey J F 1982 Bilirubin and brain damage - a real mess. Pediatrics 69: 381

Lucey J F, Driscol J J 1961 Physiological jaundice re-examined. In: Sass-Kostsak A (ed) Kernicterus. Toronto, University of Toronto Press p 29

Lunazzi G, Tiribelli C, Gazzin B, Sottocasa G 1982 Further studies on bilitranslocase, a plasma membrane protein involved in hepatic organic anion uptake. Biochemica et Biophysica Acta 685: 177

Lund H T, Jacobsen J 1974 Influence of phototherapy on the biliary bilirubin excretion patterns in newborn infants with hyperbilirubinemia. Journal of Pediatrics 85: 262

McDonagh A F 1975 Thermal and photochemical reactions of bilirubin IX. Annals of the New York Academy of Sciences 244: 553

McDonagh F, Palma L A, Lighner D A 1982 Phototherapy for neonatal jaundice. Stereospecific and regiospecific photoisomerization of bilirubin bound to human serum albumin and NMR characterization of intramolecularly cyclized photoproducts. Journal of the American Chemical Society 104: 6867

Mackenzie P I 1986 Rat liver UDP-glucuronosyl-transferase: Sequence and expression of a cDNA encoding a phenobarbital-inducible form. Journal of Biological

Chemistry 261: 6119

Maisels M J, Pathak A, Nelsen N M, Nathan D G, Smith C A 1971 Endogenous production of carbon monoxide in normal and erythroblastic newborn infants. Journal of Clinical Investigation 50: 1

Mandema E, De Fraiture W H, Nieweg H O, Arends A 1960 Familial chronic idiopathic jaundice (Dubin-Sprinz disease), with a note on bromsulphalein metabolism in this disease. American Journal of Medicine 28: 42

Martin J F, Vierling J M, Wolkoff A W, Scharschmidt B F, Vergalla J, Waggoner J G 1976 Abnormal hepatic transport of indocyanine green in Gilbert's syndrome. Gastroenterlogy 70: 385

Masuda M 1965 On the relation between Dubin-Johnson syndrome and Rotor type; a case of Dubin-Johnson syndrome complicated with serum hepatitis. Revue Internationale Hepatologie 15: 1227

Meulengracht E 1947 A review of chronic intermittent juvenile jaundice. Quarterly Journal of Medicine 16: 83

Mia A S, Cornelius C E, Gronwall P R 1970a Increased bilirubin production from sources other than circulating erythrocytes in mutant Southdown sheep. Proceedings of the Society for Experimental Biology and Medicine 136: 227

Mia A S, Gronwall R R, Cornelius C E 1970b Bilirubin ^{14}C turnover in normal and mutant Southdown sheep with congenital hyperbilirubinemia. Proceedings of the Society for Experimental Biology and Medicine 133: 955

Mia A S, Gronwall R R, Cornelius C E 1970c Unconjugated bilirubin transport in normal and mutant Corriedale sheep with Dubin-Johnson syndrome. Proceedings of the Society for Experimental Biology and Medicine 135: 33

Miniopaluello F, Gautier A, Magnenat P 1968 L'ultrastructure due foie human dans un cas de Crigler-Najjar. Acta Hepatosplenologica 15: 65

Morey K S, Litwack G 1969 Isolation and properties of cortisol metabolite binding proteins of rat liver cytosol. Biochemistry 8: 4813

Morita M, Kihara T 1971 Intravenous cholecystography and metabolism of meglumine iodipamide (biligrafin) in Dubin-Johnson syndrome. Radiology 99: 57

Morphis I, Constantopoulos A, Matsaniotis N, Papaphilis A 1982 Bilirubin-induced modulation of cerebral protein phosphorylation in neonate rabbits in vivo. Science 218: 156

Mowat A P, Arias I M 1970 Observations of the effect of diethyl nitrosamine on glucuronide formation. Biochimica et Biophysica Acta 212: 175

Mukherjee A B, Krasner J 1973 Induction of an enzyme in genetically deficient rats after grafting of normal liver. Science 183: 68

Mustafa M G, Cowger M L, Kind T E 1969 Effects of bilirubin on mitochondrial reactions. Journal of Biological Chemistry 244: 6403

Naeye R L 1978 Amniotic fluid infections, neonatal hyperbilirubinemia and psychomotor impairment. Pediatrics 62: 497

Nakata F, Oyanagi K, Fujiwara M et al 1979 Dubin-Johnson syndrome in a neonate. European Journal of Pediatrics 132: 299

Nandi Majumdar A P 1974 Bilirubin encephalopathy. Effect on RNA polymerase activity and chromatin template activity in the brain of the Gunn rat. Neurobiology 4: 425

Nandi Majumdar A P, Greenfield S 1974 Evidence of defective protein synthesis in liver in rats with congenital hyperbilirubinemia. Biochimica et Biophysica Acta 335: 250

Noir B A, Boveris A, Garazo Pereira A M, Stoppani A O M 1972 Bilirubin: A multi-site inhibitor of mitochondrial respiration. FEBS Letters 27: 270

Novikoff A B, Essner E 1960 The liver cell. American Journal of Medicine 19: 102

Odell G B 1959 The dissociation of bilirubin from albumin and its clinical implications. Journal of Pediatrics 55: 268

Odell G B 1967 "Physiologic" hyperbilirubinemia in the neonatal period. New England Journal of Medicine 277: 193

Odell G B 1973 Influence of binding on the toxicity of bilirubin. Annals of the New York Academy of Sciences 226: 225

Odell G B, Natzschka J C, Storey G 1967 Bilirubin nephropathy in the Gunn strain of rat. American Journal of Physiology 212: 931

O'Hagen J E, Hamilton T, De Breton E G, Shaw A E 1957 Human serum bilirubin. Clinical Chemistry 3: 609

Ohkubo H, Musha H, Okuda K 1979 Studies on nicotinic acid interaction with bilirubin metabolism. Digestive Diseases and Sciences 24: 700

Okolicsanyi L, Ghidini O, Orlando R, Cortellazzo S, Benedetti G, Naccarato R, Manitto P 1978 An evaluation of bilirubin kinetics with respect to the diagnosis of Gilbert's syndrome. Clinical Science and Molecular Medicine 54: 535

Okolicsanyi L, Orlando R, Venuti M, Dalbrun G, Cobelli C, Ruggeri A, Salvat A 1981 A modeling study of the effect of fasting on bilirubin in Gilbert's syndrome. American Journal of Physiology 240: 266

Onishi S, Itho S, Kawade N, Isobe K, Sugiyama S 1980 An accurate and sensitive analysis by high pressure liquid chromatography of conjugated and unconjugated bilirubin IX and in various biological fluids. Biochemical Journal 185: 281

Oppermann A, Carbillet J-P, Gisselbrecht H, Pageant G, Clement D 1971 Syndrome de Dubin-Johnson: donnees ulstructurales. Semaine des Hopitaux de Paris 47: 2721

Orme M L E 1974 Increased glucuronidation of bilirubin in men and rat by administration of antipyrine (phenazone). Clinical Science and Molecular Medicine 46: 511

Owens D, Evans J 1975 Population studies on Gilbert's syndrome. Journal of Medical Genetics 12: 152

Owens D, Sherlock S 1973 Diagnosis of Gilbert's syndrome: Role of reduced caloric intake test. British Medical Journal 3: 559

Paumgartner G, Reichenn J 1976 Kinetics of hepatic uptake of unconjugated bilirubin. Clinical Science and Molecular Medicine 51: 169

Peck O C, Rey D F, Snell A M 1969 Familial jaundice with free and conjugated bilirubin in the serum and without liver pigmentation. Gastroenterology 39: 625

Pereira-Lima J E, Utz E, Rosenberg I 1966 Hereditary nonhemolytic conjugated hyperbilirubinemia without abnormal liver cell pigmentation. A family study. American Journal of Medicine 40: 628

Plotz P H, Berk P D, Scharschmidt B F, Gordon J K, Vergalla J 1974 Removing substances from blood by affinity chromatography. I. Removing bilirubin and other albumin-bound substances from plasma and blood with albumin-conjugated agarose beads. Journal of Clinical

Investigation 53: 778

Poland R L, Odell G B 1971 Physiologic jaundice: The enterohepatic circulation of bilirubin. New England Journal of Medicine 284: 1

Poon R, Hinberg I H 1985 Indican interference with six commercial procedures for measuring total bilirubin. Clinical Chemistry 31: 92

Porter E G, Waters W J 1966 A rapid micromethod for measuring the reserve albumin binding capacity in serum for newborn infants with hyperbilirubinemia. Journal of Laboratory and Clinical Medicine 67: 660

Portman O W, Roy Chowdhury J, Roy Chowdhury N, Alexander M, Cornelius C E, Arias I M 1984a A non-human primate model for Gilbert's syndrome Hepatology 4: 175

Portman O W, Alexander M, Roy Chowdhury J, Roy Chowdhury N, Cornelius C E, Arias I M 1984b Effects of nutrition on hyperbilirubinemia in Bolivian squirrel monkeys. Hepatology 4: 454

Porush J G, Delman A J, Feuer M M 1962 Chronic idiopathic jaundice with normal liver histology. Archives of Internal Medicine 109: 102

Posselt A M, Cowan B E, Kwong L K, Vreman H J, Stevenson D K 1985 Effect of tin protoporphyrin on the excretion rate of carbon monoxide in newborn rats after hematoma formation. Journal of Pediatric Gastroenterology 4: 650

Powell L W, Hemingway E, Billing B H, Sherlock S 1967 Idiopathic unconjugated hyperbilirubinemia (Gilbert's syndrome): A study of 42 families. New England Journal of Medicine 277 : 1108

Prohaska J R, Ganther H E 1977 Glutathione peroxidase activity of glutathione S-transferases purified from rat liver. Biochemical and Biophysical Research Communications 76: 437

Purpura D P, Carmichael M W 1960 Characteristics of blood-brain barrier to gamma-aminobutyric acid in neonatal cat. Science 131: 410

Ramos A, Silberberg M, Stern I 1966 Pregnanediols and neonatal hyperbilirubinemia. American Journal of Diseases of Children 111: 353

Rapacini G L, Topi G C, Anti M et al 1986 Porphyrins in Rotor syndrome: A study on an Italian family. Hepato-Gastroenterology 33: 11

Rappaport S I 1976 Blood-Brain Barrier in Physiology and Medicine. Raven Press, New York

Reichen J, Berk P D 1979 Isolation of an organic anion binding protein from rat liver plasma membrane fractions by affinity chromatography. Biochemical and Biophysical Research Communications 91: 484

Robinson S, Vanier T, Desforges J F, Schmid R 1962 Jaundice in thalassemia minor: A consequence of "ineffective erythropoiesis". New England Journal of Medicine 267: 512

Robinson S H, Tsong M, Brown B W, Schmidt R 1966 The sources of bile pigment in the rat: studies of the 'early-labelled' fraction. Journal of Clinical Investigation 45: 1569

Rodes J, Zubizarreta A, Bruguera M 1972 Metabolism of the bromsulphalein in Dubin-Johnson syndrome. Diagnostic value of the paradoxical in plasma levels of BSP. Digestive Diseases 17: 545

Rose A L, Johnson A 1972 Bilirubin encephalopathy: Neuropathological and histochemical studies in the Gunn rat model. Neurology 22: 420

Rothmaler G, Lowe H 1970 Elektronenoptische untersuchungen der lever bei einem fall von knogenitalem nichtamolytischen ikterus (morbus Crigler-Najjar). Pediatric Radiology 7: 135

Rotor A B, Manahan L, Florentin A 1948 Familial nonhemolytic jaundice with direct van den Bergh reaction. Acta Medica Philippina 5: 37

Roy Chowdhury J, Arias I M 1981 Dismutation of bilirubin. Methods in Enzymology 77: 192

Roy Chowdhury J, Arias I M 1986 Disorders of bilirubin conjugation. In: Ostrow J D (ed) Bile Pigments and Jaundice. Marcel Dekker, New York, p 317

Roy Chowdhury J, Roy Chowdhury N 1982 Quantitation of bilirubin and its conjugates by high pressure liquid chromatography. Falk Hepatology 11: 1649

Roy Chowdhury J, Fischberg E B, Daniller A, Jansen P L M, Arias I M 1978 Hepatic conversion of bilirubin monoglucuronide to bilirubin diglucuronide in uridine diphosphate glucuronyl transferase deficient man and rat by bilirubin glucuronoside glucuronosyl transferase. Journal of Clinical Investigation 21: 191

Roy Chowdhury J, Roy Chowdhury N, Bhargava M, Arias I M 1979 Purification and partial characterization of rat liver bilirubin glucuronoside glucuronosyl transferase. Journal of Biological Chemistry 254: 8336

Roy Chowdhury J, Roy Chowdhury N, Wu G, Shouval R, Arias I M 1981 Bilirubin monoglucuronide and diglucuronide formation by human liver in vitro: Assay by high pressure liquid chromatography. Hepatology 1: 622

Roy Chowdhury J, Roy Chowdhury N, Moscioni A D, Tukey R, Tephly T R, Arias I M 1983 Differential regulation by triiodothyronine of substrate-specific uridinediphosphoglucuronate glucuronyl transferases in rat liver. Biochimica et Biophysica Acta 761: 58

Roy Chowdhury J, Roy Chowdhury N, Arias I M 1984 UDP-glucuronyltransferase deficiency in man and animals. Biochemical Society Transactions 12: 81–83

Roy Chowdhury J, Novikoff P M, Roy Chowdhury N, Novikoff A B 1985 Distribution of UDP-glucuronosyl transferase in rat tissue. Proceedings of the National Academy of Sciences, USA 82: 2990

Roy Chowdhury J, Roy Chowdhury N, Falany C N, Tephly T W, Arias I M 1986a Isolation and characterization of multiple forms of rat liver UDP-glucuronoate glucuronosyltransferase. Biochemical Journal 233: 827

Roy Chowdhury N, Arias I M, Lederstein M, Roy Chowdhury J 1986b Substrates and products of purified rat liver bilirubin-UDP-glucuronosyl-transferase. Hepatology 6: 123-128

Roy Chowdhury N, Gross F, Moscioni A D, Kram M, Arias I M, Roy Chowdhury J 1987 Isolation and purification of multiple normal and functionally defective forms of UDP-glucuronosyltransferase from livers of inbred Gunn rats. Journal of Clinical Investigation 79: 327

Rubinstein Z J, Seligsohn U, Modan M, Shani M 1985 Hepatic computerized tomography in the Dubin-Johnson syndrome: increased liver density as a diagnostic aid. Computerized Radiology 9: 315

Rugstad H E, Robinson S M, Yannoni C, Tasjia A H 1970 Transfer of bilirubin uridine diphosphate glucuronyl transferase to enzyme deficient rats. Science, 170: 553

Ruymann F B, Takeuchi A, Boyce H W 1970 Idiopathic, recurrent cholestasis. Pediatrics 45: 812

Sagild U, Dalgard O Z, Tygstrup N 1962 Constitutional hyperbilirubinemia with unconjugated bilirubin in the serum and lipochrome-like pigment granules in the liver. Annals of Internal Medicine 56: 308

Sano K, Nakamura H, Tamotsu M 1985 Mode of inhibitory action of bilirubin on protein kinase C. Pediatric Research 19: 587

Sassa S, Kappas A, Bernstein S E, Alvares A P 1979 Heme biosynthesis and drug metabolism in mice with hereditary hemolytic anemia. Journal of Biological Chemistry 254: 729

Schalm L, Weber A P 1964 Jaundice with conjugated bilirubin in hyperhaemolysis. Acta Medica Scandinavica 176: 549

Schapiro R H, Isselbacher K J 1963 Benign recurrent intrahepatic cholestasis. New England Journal of Medicine 268: 708

Scharschmidt B F 1978 Bilirubin kinetics in Gilbert's syndrome: Clinical applications and pathophysiological implications. In: Okolicsanyi L (ed) Familial Hyperbilirubinemia. Wiley, New York, p 99

Scharschmidt B F, Schmid R 1978 The "micellar sink". A quantitative assessment of the association of organic anions with mixed micelles and other macromolecular aggregates in rat bile. Journal of Clinical Investigation 62: 1122

Scharschmidt B F, Plotz P H, Berk P D, Waggoner J G, Vergalla J 1974 Removing substances from blood by affinity chromatography. II. Removing bilirubin from the blood of jaundiced rats by hemoperfusion over albumin-conjugated agarose beads. Journal of Clinical Investigation 53: 786

Scharschmidt B F, Waggoner J G, Berk P D 1975 Hepatic organic anion uptake in the rat. Journal of Clinical Investigation 56: 1280

Scharschmidt B F, Martin J F, Shapiro L J, Plotz P H, Berk P D 1977a Hemoperfusion through albumin-conjugated agarose gel for the treatment of neonatal jaundice in Rhesus monkeys. Journal of Laboratory and Clinical Medicine 89: 101

Scharschmidt B F, Martin J F, Shapiro L J, Plotz P H, Berk P D 1977b The use of calcium chelating agents and prostaglandin El to eliminate platelet and white blood cell losses resulting from hemoperfusion through uncoated charcoal, albumin-agarose gel, and neutral and cation exchange resin. Journal of Laboratory and Clinical Medicine 90: 110

Schiff L, Billing B H, Oikawa Y 1959 Familial nonhemolytic jaundice with conjugated bilirubin in the serum. New England Journal of Medicine 260: 1315

Schiff D, Chan G, Poznasky M J 1983 Bilirubin toxicity in neural cell lines N115 and NBR10A. Pediatric Research 19: 908

Schmid R 1972 Hyperbilirubinemia. In: Stanbury J B, Wyngaarden J B, Fredrickson D S (eds) The Metabolic Basis of Inherited Disease, 3rd edn. McGraw-Hill, New York, p 1141

Schmid R, Hammaker L 1963 Metabolism and disposition of C^{14}-bilirubin in congenital nonhemolytic jaundice. Journal of Clinical Investigation 42: 1720

Schmid R, Axelrod J, Hammaker L, Swarn R L 1958 Congenital jaundice in rats due to a defective glucuronide formation. Journal of Clinical Investigation 37: 1123

Schoenfield L J, McGill D B, Hunton D B, Foulk M J, Butt H R 1963 Studies of chronic idiopathic jaundice (Dubin-Johnson syndrome). I. Demonstration of hepatic excretory defect. Gastroenterology 44: 101

Schubert W K, Garancis J, Perrin E 1965 Idiopathic benign recurrent cholestasis: Biochemical and histologic changes induced by cholestyramine therapy (abstract). Clinical Research 13: 409

Schutta H S, Johnson L 1967 Bilirubin encephalopathy in the Gunn rat: a fine structure study of the cerebellar cortex. Journal of Neuropathology and Experimental Neurology 26: 377

Schutta H S, Johnson L 1969 Clinical signs and morphologic abnormalities in Gunn rats treated with sulfadiethoxine. Journal of Pediatrics 75: 1070

Sebrow O, Gatmaitan Z, Orlandi F, Roy Chowdhury J, Arias I M 1980 Replacement of hepatic UDP glucuronyltransferase activity in homozygous Gunn rats. Gastroenterology 78: 1332

Seligsohn U, Shani M, Ramot B, Adam A, Sheba C 1969 Hereditary deficiency of blood clotting factor VII and Dubin-Johnson syndrome in an Israeli family. Israel Journal of Medical Sciences 5: 1060

Seligsohn U, Shani M, Ramot B, Adam A, Sheba C 1970 Dubin-Johnson Syndrome in Israel. II. Association with factor-VII deficiency. Quarterly Journal of Medicine 39: 569

Shani M, Seligsohn U, Gilon E, Sheba C, Adam A 1970a Dubin-Johnson syndrome in Israel. I. Clinical laboratory, and genetic aspects of 101 cases. Western Journal of Medicine 39: 549

Shani M, Gilon E, Ben-Ezzer J, Sheba C 1970b Sulfobromophthalein tolerance test in patients with the Dubin-Johnson syndrome and their relatives. Gastroenterology 59: 842

Shimizu Y, Kondo T, Kuchiba K, Urata G 1977 Uroporphyrin III cosynthetase in liver and blood in the Dubin-Johnson syndrome. Journal of Laboratory and Clinical Medicine 89: 517

Shimizu Y, Ida S, Naruto H, Urata G 1978 Excretion of porphyrins in urine and bile after the administration of delta-aminolevulinic acid. Journal of Laboratory and Clinical Medicine 92: 795

Shimizu Y, Naruto H, Ida S, Kohakura M 1981 Urinary coproporphyrin isomers in Rotor's syndrome. A study in eight families. Hepatology 1: 173

Shupeck M, Wolkoff A W, Scharschmidt B F, Waggoner J G, Berk P D 1978 Studies of the kinetics of purified conjugated bilirubin-3H in the rat. American Journal of Gastroenterology 70: 259

Sleisenger M H, Kahn I, Barniville H, Rubin W, Ben Ezzer J, Arias I M 1967 Nonhemolytic unconjugated hyperbilirubinemia with hepatic glucuronyl transferase deficiency: a genetic study in four generations. Transactions of the Association of American Physicians 80: 259

Smith P M, Middleton J E, Williams R 1967 Studies on the familial incidence and clinical history of patients with chronic unconjugated hyperbilirubinemia. Gut 8: 449

Snyder A L, Satterlee W, Robinson S H, Schmid R 1967 Conjugated plasma bilirubin in jaundice caused by pigment overload. Nature 213: 93

Sosnnet J, Steichen-De Falque M, Brisbois P 1969 Isolement et proprietes d'une melanine obtenue a partir de melanogenes urinaires dans un cas de maladie de Dubin-Johnson. Clinica Chimica Acta 24: 325

Spiegel E L, Schubert W, Perrin E, Schiff L 1965 Benign recurrent intrahepatic cholestasis with response to cholestyramine. American Journal of Medicine 39: 682

Spivak W, Carey M C 1985 Reverse-phase h.p.l.c. separation, quantification and preparation of bilirubin and its conjugates from native bile. Biochemical Journal 225: 787

Sprinz H, Nelson R S 1954 Persistent nonhemolytic hyperbilirubinemia associated with lipochrome-like pigment in liver cells: Report of four cases. Annals of Internal Medicine 41: 952

Stein L B, Mishkin S, Fleischner G, Gatmaitan Z, Arias I M 1976 Effect of fasting on hepatic ligandin, Z protein, and organic anion transfer from plasma in rats. American Journal of Physiology 231: 1371

Stoll M S, Lim C D, Gray C H 1977 Chemical variants of the uroblins. In: Berk P D, Berlin N I (eds) Bile Pigments, Chemistry and Physiology. U.S. Government Printing Office, Washington, D.C. p 483

Stollman Y R, Gartner U, Theilman L, Ohmi N, Wolkoff A W 1983 Hepatic bilirubin uptake in the isolated perfused liver is not facilitated by albumin binding. Journal of Clinical Investigation 72: 718

Stremmel W, Berk P D 1986 Hepatocellular uptake of sulfobromophthalein and bilirubin is selectively inhibited by an antibody to the liver plasma membrane sulfobromophthalein/bilirubin binding protein. Journal of Clinical Investigation 78: 822

Stremmel W, Gerber M A, Glezerov V, Thung S N, Kochwa S, Berk P D 1983 Physicochemical and immunohistological studies of a sulfobromophthalein and bilirubin-binding protein from rat liver plasma membrane. Journal of Clinical Investigation 71: 1796

Strumia E 1959 Effect of bilirubin on some hydrolases. Bollettino-Societe Italiana Biologia Sperimentale 35: 2160

Summerfield J A, Scott J, Berman M, Ghent C, Bloomer J R, Berk P D, Sherlock S 1980 Benign recurrent intrahepatic cholestasis: studies of bilirubin kinetics, bile acids, and cholangiography. Gut 21: 154

Summerskill W H J 1965 The syndrome of benign recurrent cholestasis. American Journal of Medicine 38: 298

Summerskill W H J, Walshe J M 1959 Benign recurrent intrahepatic obstructive jaundice. Lancet 2: 686

Swartz H M, Sarna T, Varma R R 1979a On the nature and excretion of the hepatic pigment in the Dubin-Johnson syndrome. Gastroenterology 76: 958

Swartz H M, Sarnat T, Varma R R 1979b The pigment in Dubin-Johnson syndrome. Gastroenterology 77: 821

Szabo L, Ebrey P 1963 Studies on the inheritance of Crigler-Najjar syndrome by the menthol test. Acta Paediatrica Hungarica 4: 153

Talafant E 1956 Properties and composition of bile pigment giving direct diazo rection. Nature 178: 312

Tenhunen R, Marver H S, Schmid R 1970 The enzymatic catabolism of hemoglobin: Stimulation of microsomal heme oxygenase by hemin. Journal of Laboratory and Clinical Medicine 75: 410

Thompson R P H 1981 Genetic transmission of Gilbert's syndrome. In: Okolicsanyi L (ed) Familial Hyperbilirubinemia. Wiley, New York, p 91

Thompson R P H, Pilcher C W T, Robinson J, Strathers G M, McLean A E M, Williams R 1969 Treatment of unconjugated jaundice with dicophane. Lancet 2: 4

Trotman B W, Roy Chowdhury J, Wirt G D, Bernstein S E 1982 Azodi-pyrrole analysis of unconjugated and conjugated bilirubin using diazotized ethylanthranilate in dimethylsulfoxide. Analytical Biochemistry 121: 175

Turkel S B, Miller C A, Guttenberg M E, Moynes D R,

Hodgman J E 1982 A clinical pathologic reappraisal of kernicterus. Pediatrics 69: 267

Tygstrup N 1960 Intermittent possibly familial intrahepatic cholestatic jaundice. Lancet 1: 1171

Tygstrup N, Jensen B 1969 Intermittent intrahepatic cholestasis of unknown etiology in five young males from the Faroe Islands. Acta Medica Scandinavica 185: 523

Van Berge Henegouwen G P, Bonndt K-H, De Pagter A G F 1974 Is an acute disturbance in hepatic transport of bile acids the primary cause of cholestasis in benign recurrent intrahepatic cholestasis? Lancet 1: 1249

Van den Bergh, A A H, Muller P 1916 Ueber eine direkte und eine indirekte Diazoreaktion auf Bilirubin. Biochemische Zeitschrift 77: 90

Van der Sluijs P, Postema B, Meijer D K F 1987 Lactosylation of albumin reduces uptake of dibromosulphthalein in perfused rat liver and dissociation rate from albumin in vitro. Hepatology 7: 688

Van Houwelingen C A J, Arias I M 1976 Attempts to induce hepatic uridine diphosphate glucuronyl transferase in genetically deficient Gunn rats by grafting of normal liver tissue. Pediatric Research 10: 830

Van Steenbergen W, Kutz K, Fevery J 1979 Effects of conjugation, bile flow and bile acid load on the apparent maximal excretion of bilirubin ("Tm"). In: Preisig R, Paumgartner G (eds) The Liver. Proceedings of the 3rd Gstaad Symposium, p 208

Varma R R, Grainger J M, Scheuer P J 1970 A case of the Dubin-Johnson syndrome complicated by acute hepatitis. Gut 11: 817

Vaughan J M, Haslewood G A D 1938 The normal level of plasma bilirubin. Lancet 1: 133

Vaughan J P, Marubbio A T, Maddocks I, Cooke R A 1970 Chronic idiopathic jaundice in Papua and New Guinea: A report of nine patients with Dubin-Johnson's syndrome or Rotor's syndrome. Transactions of the Royal Society of Tropical Medicine and Hygiene 64: 287

Vaughan V C, Allen F C, Diamond L K 1950 Erythroblastosis fetalis. IV. Further observation on kernicterus. Pediatrics 6: 706

Verwilghen R, Verhaegen H, Waumanns P, Beert J 1969 Ineffective erythropoiesis with morphological abnormal erythroblasts and unconjugated hyperbilirubinemia. British Journal of Haematology 17: 27

Verwilghen R, Lewis S, Dacie J, Crookston J, Crookston M 1973 Hempas: congenital dyserythropoietic anaemia (type II). Quarterly Journal of Medicine 42: 257

Vest M, Strebel L, Hauensiein D 1965 The extent of "shunt" bilirubin and erythrocyte survival in the newborn infant measured by the administration of (^{15}N) glycine. Biochemical Journal 95: 11c

Ware A J, Eigenbrodt E H, Shoey J, Combes B 1972 Viral hepatitis complicating the Dubin-Johnson syndrome. Gastroenterology 63: 331

Ware A, Eigenbrodt E, Naftalis J, Combes B 1974 Dublin-Johnson syndrome and viral hepatitis. Gastroenterology 67: 560

Wegmann R, Rangier M, Eteve J, Charbonnier A, Caroli J 1960 Melanose hepatosplenique avec ictere chronique a bilirubine directe: maladie de Dubin-Johnson? Etude clinique et biologique de la maladie. Etudie histochimique, chimique et spectographique du pigment anormal. Semaine des Hopitaux de Paris 26: 1761

Weisiger R, Gollan J, Ockner R 1981 Receptor for albumin

on the liver cell surface may mediate uptake of fatty acids and other albumin-bound substances. Science 211: 1048.

Weisiger R A, Gollan J L, Ockner R K 1982 The role of albumin in hepatic uptake processes. In: Popper H, Schaffner F (eds) Progress in Liver Disease. Grune & Stratton, New York, p 71

Werner M, Tolls R E, Hultin J V, Mellecker J 1970 Influence of sex and age on the normal range of eleven serum constituents. Zeitschrift fur Klinische Chemie und Klinische Biochemie 8: 105

Wheeler H O, Meltzer J I, Bradley S E 1960 Biliary transport and hepatic storage of sulfobromophthalein sodium in the unanesthetized dog, in normal man, and in patients with hepatic disease. Journal of Clinical Investigation 39: 1131

Wilding P, Rollasen J G, Robinson D 1972 Patterns of change for various biochemical constituents detected in well population screening. Clinica Chimica Acta 41: 375

Williams R, Cartter M A, Sherlock S, Sgheuer P J, Hill K R 1964 Idiopathic recurrent cholestasis: A study of the functional and pathological lesions in four cases. Quarterly Journal of Medicine 33: 387

Wishart G J 1978 Functional heterogeneity of UDP glucuronosyltransferase as indicated by its differential development and inducibility by glucocorticoids. Biochemical Journal 174: 485

Wolf R L, Pizette M, Richman A, Dreiling D A, Jacobs W, Fernandez O, Popper H 1960 Chronic idiopathic jaundice: A study of two afflicted families. American Journal of Medicine 28: 32

Wolkoff A W 1980 The glutathione S-transferases: their role in the transport of organic anions from blood to bile. In:

Javitt N B (ed) Liver and Biliary Tract Physiology I. University Park Press, Baltimore, p 151

Wolkoff A W, Arias I M 1974 Coproporphyrin excretion in amniotic fluid and urine from premature infants: A possible maturation defect. Pediatric Research 8: 591

Wolkoff A W, Chung C T 1980 Identification, purification and partial characterization of an organic anion binding protein from rat liver cell plasma membrane. Journal of Clinical Investigation 65: 1152

Wolkoff A W, Cohen L E, Arias I M 1973 Inheritance of the Dubin-Johnson syndrome. New England Journal of Medicine 288: 113

Wolkoff A W, Wolpert E, Pascasio F N, Arias I M 1976 Rotor's syndrome: A distinct inheritable pathophysiologic entity. American Journal of Medicine 60: 173

Wolkoff A W, Goresky C A, Sellin J, Gatmaitan Z, Arias I M 1979a Role of ligandin in transfer of bilirubin from plasma into liver. American Journal of Physiology 236: E638

Wolkoff A W, Chowdhury J R, Gartner L A et al 1979b Crigler-Najjar syndrome (Type I) in an adult male. Gastroenterology 76: 3380

Wolpert E, Pascasio F M, Wolkoff A W, Arias I M 1977 Abnormal sulfobromophthalein metabolism in Rotor's syndrome and obligate heterozygotes. New England Journal of Medicine 296: 1099

Yamaguchi K, Okuda Y, Yanemitsu H, Tsukada Y, Shigata H 1975 Cyclic premenstrual unconjugated hyperbilirubinemia. Report of two cases. Annals of Internal Medicine 83: 514

Zuelzer W W, Mudgett R T 1950 Kernicterus. Etiologic study based on an analysis of 55 cases. Pediatrics 6: 452

69. Cystic fibrosis

W. M. McCrae   R. Williamson

INTRODUCTION

Cystic fibrosis (CF) is the most common inherited disease in Caucasian populations and one of the commonest causes of death in childhood. Although described in 1938 (Andersen) and now a very familiar problem to all paediatricians, the molecular defect has only recently been identified (Riordan et al 1989). There is abundant evidence that cystic fibrosis is inherited as an autosomal recessive trait. The expected occurrence of 1 in 4 among sibs has been demonstrated in a number of studies (e.g. Danks et al 1965). It seems likely therefore that all the features of the disease should be attributable to a defect of a single protein. It is possible, however, that more than one mutant allele may be responsible for the disorder recognised as cystic fibrosis. This concept has some attraction for the clinician who is aware of the wide variation in the way in which the disease may present and the differences in the manner and speed with which the condition progresses to the fully developed phenotype. The observation of genetic differences between cystic fibrosis with and without meconium (Mornet et al 1988) gives weight to the suggestion that differences in the clinical presentation of cystic fibrosis may be the result of multiallelism (i.e. different mutations occurring at the same locus). Recent molecular evidence indicates that different mutations at the same locus may well determine the severity of pulmonary disease in cystic fibrosis (Santis et al 1990).

INCIDENCE

For many years standard textbooks have given the incidence of cystic fibrosis for Caucasian populations as approximately 1 in 2500, with an equal sex distribution. This implies a carrier rate of 1 in 20–25 and thus approximately 1 in 400–600 marriages would be at risk of producing an affected child.

These estimates were based in part on autopsy records. Between 2–4% of autopsies in children's hospitals are performed on patients with cystic fibrosis. For the most part, however, the estimates were computed from the number of cases which made themselves clinically manifest and were satisfactorily diagnosed.

It is now clear that these estimates are too low. In studies in which populations of newborns are universally screened for cystic fibrosis the incidence has been found to be at least 1 in 1800 (Stephan et al 1975). It has been claimed in other Caucasian populations that the incidence may be even higher (Sweet 1977). The difference from previous estimates is probably due to the inclusion of cases of cystic fibrosis where the expression of the disease is so mild that it would not have been recognised under normal circumstances.

Cystic fibrosis is principally a disease of Caucasian children, although it has also been diagnosed in Blacks, Indians, American Indians and Japanese. The incidence in these races, although probably very low, is not known precisely. It is of interest that although previously unknown in Arabs, 17 cases were discovered in Baghdad by a single clinical team in a few months (Al-Hassani 1976).

BASIC DEFECT

The clinical features of cystic fibrosis are the result of: (a) an abnormality of all exocrine glands; and (b) a susceptibility to respiratory infection, the site of the infection being the lower respiratory airways.

The genetics of the condition suggests that these abnormalities should all result from a defect of a single abnormal protein.

Cystic fibrosis is an epithelial disease. The organs of the epithelium develop in response to an interaction with mesenchymal cells, so that cystic fibrosis could perhaps be caused by a mesenchymal defect. The epithelial glands, however, are initially normal in structure, disruption of a gland occurring in the course of the disease as a result of a defect in secretion. Epithelial glands are acinar-ductal structures. As the disease progresses alterations in the secretions which increase their viscosity lead to obstruction of the ducts and subsequent structural damage. The vas deferens and associated structures, however, represent a special case in that ductal blockage, injury and reabsorption occur during embryonic development resulting in sterility in males. In cystic fibrosis the embryonic development of all other organs is normal.

The cause of the abnormality in secretion is unknown but is being investigated at the various levels of: (a) control of secretion; (b) intracellular events associated with secretion and (c) the biochemistry of exocrine gland products. Most evidence now implicates a basic defect in epithelial ion transport though its precise nature is still not clear (Cuthbert 1989).

Spock et al (1967) reported that serum from cystic fibrosis patients disorganised the beat of cilia in explants of respiratory mucosa from rabbit trachea. This observation has since been confirmed using other animal tissues including oyster gills (Bowman et al 1969) and fresh water mussels (Besley et al 1969). Investigation suggests that the factor inhibiting ciliary movement is a heat labile protein with a molecular weight of between 2500 and 10 000 daltons usually bound to IgG (Wilson & Fundenberg 1978). Unfortunately the assay methods for this factor have given inconsistent results and the significance of the factor in relation to the pathology of the disease has not been established. However this factor has attracted great research interest. It has been shown that a similar substance can be isolated from culture medium of long-term lymphoid lines and peripheral blood leucocytes from those harbouring the CF gene (Wilson & Fundenberg 1978).

The main cause of death in cystic fibrosis is the severe chronic lower respiratory tract infection. This susceptibility to infection cannot be explained by any defect in immune function. Both B-cell and T-cell systems are normal. There is, however, some conjecture about the role of the alveolar macrophage. A defect in its function could explain both the occurrence and the site of infection since it has a major role in maintaining the sterility of the lower respiratory tract.

PATHOLOGY

Pancreas

In 15–20% of cases there is no defect of pancreatic function at the time of diagnosis; in the others the degree of impairment varies widely. The initial defect is a failure of production of water and bicarbonate. The pancreatic enzymes continue to be produced but the resulting secretion becomes increasingly viscous until ductules become blocked. The related acini undergo dilatation and rupture, with escape of enzymes into the supporting structures where a fibrous reaction is provoked.

The absence of pancreatic secretions from the lumen of the upper intestine produces a form of malabsorption which has certain characteristics. Only those ingestants which require digestion before absorption are affected. Iron absorption is not impaired and indeed, because of the abnormally low pH in the upper jejunum, iron absorption is enhanced. Anaemia is not a feature of the disease. Absence of pancreatic lipase results in particularly severe steatorrhoea. Fat globules can often be seen on examination of the stool. This is not the case in any of the other common causes of malabsorption in childhood.

Liver and bile ducts

The initial abnormality in the liver is the accumulation of excess mucus in the bile ducts which dilate and proliferate (Oppenheimer & Esterly 1975). Increased fibrosis is provoked in the portal areas and these areas expand and become linked together. The cirrhosis then progresses until it becomes clinically significant by causing portal hypertension. Hepatocellular injury is not a prominent feature. Enzyme measurements and other liver function tests are not helpful in following the progress of the disease. Of those reaching adult life some 20% will have evidence of portal hypertension. Jaundice is unusual and presents only very late in the disease.

Intestine

Meconium ileus

Approximately 10% of cases of cystic fibrosis present in the neonatal period with meconium ileus. The intestinal obstruction is caused by inspissation of the meconium in the distal ileum. The plug of putty-like material produced has a high protein content as the result of absence of proteolytic enzymes, secretion of abnormally viscid mucus and reduced water secretion by the pancreas and biliary system. The obstruction may be complicated by volvulus or perforation. The presence of the plug during late stages of embryonic development may also result in a degree of atresia of the lower gut.

Mucus production

Throughout the gut, goblet cells are distended and the crypts are often filled by eosinophilic material. These abnormalities can be demonstrated by rectal biopsy.

The distension of Brunner glands can be demonstrated radiologically following a barium meal.

Rectal prolapse

Rectal prolapse is a common complication of untreated cystic fibrosis in the first two or three years of life. This is due to a number of factors, the chief of which are the near vertical course of the rectum at this age, diarrhoea, cough and diminution of ischiorectal fat resulting from poor nutrition. Cystic fibrosis should be suspected whenever rectal prolapse occurs in this age group (Schwachman 1975).

Sweat glands

As is the case in other serous glands, the sweat gland in cystic fibrosis is structurally normal. The sweating rate is also normal but variable. At very low sweating rates the sodium and chloride concentrations approach normal values. At high sweating rates produced by heat, exercise or stimulation by pilocarpine, the sodium and chloride concentrations become abnormally high (i.e. above 70 mmol/l) due to defective absorption of these ions from the fluid secreted at the base of the gland as it passes outwards through the duct (di Sant'Agnese et al 1953).

In hot climates this defect may be a troublesome predisposing factor to heat exhaustion.

As this abnormality of sweating is characteristic of cystic fibrosis its chief importance is as diagnostic evidence of the disease.

Reproductive system

Approximately 97% of male cystic fibrosis patients are sterile. The anatomical basis is bilateral absence or atrophy of the epididymis, vas deferens and seminal vesicles (see above). Aspermia is accompanied by a reduced semen volume. The patients are not impotent (Landing et al 1969).

In females delayed menarche is common. Fertility is reduced to about one-fifth of normal, probably due to abnormal viscosity of the cervical mucus. Maternal mortality is also increased (Cohen et al 1980).

Pulmonary disease

In cystic fibrosis the lungs are peculiarly susceptible to infection both by common pathogenic bacteria and also by organisms which do not behave as pathogens in normal subjects. Along with the progress of the infection there is a concomitant alteration in the secretion of mucus which is both promoted by the presence of infection and at the same time increases the susceptibility to further infections by interference with lung drainage. It is the state of the lung pathology which determines the quality of the patient's life, and respiratory infection is the usual cause of death.

At birth the lungs are structurally normal. For reasons unknown but conceivably due to a defect of alveolar macrophage function, the peripheral airways become infected. At first the common pathogens are *Haemophilus influenzae* and *Staphylococcus aureus*. Later in the course of the illness, especially after there has been extensive use of antibiotics, the most troublesome organism is pseudomonas. In most cases the pseudomonas is present in its usual 'rough' form but in time the dominant organism becomes the mutant mucoid pseudomonas which is almost never found as a pathogen except in the cystic fibrosis lung.

In response to the presence of infection there is hypertrophy in the mucus-secreting tissues in the airway. Submucous glands hypertrophy. The proportion of goblet cells in the respiratory mucosa increases and the goblet cells are found more peripherally in the small airways than in the normal lung. The presence of excess mucus prediposes to further infection. The pathology which begins as bronchiolitis progresses to chronic bronchitis and bronchiectasis.

The respiratory dysfunction is the result of airway obstruction. Vital capacity is reduced, while residual volume and functional residual capacity are increased (Wood et al 1976).

Cardiovascular disease

With longer survival of the patients cardiovascular complications are being encountered more frequently. These complications can be expected when the vital capacity has fallen below 60% of normal. The combination of low pO_2 and pulmonary hypertension leads to right ventricular hypertrophy and failure. It has been noted that the low pO_2 affects the contractility of both ventricles so that left ventricular function also deteriorates in the late stage of the disease (Goldring et al 1964).

Diabetes mellitus

The incidence of diabetes mellitus increases with age, and results from increasing encroachment on the islet cells as the pancreatic lesion progresses. Its prevalance in the total population of cystic fibrosis patients is approximately 1 in 100.

This diabetes is mild and easily controlled. It is not accompanied by ketosis, retinopathy, neuropathy or other complications. It does not adversely affect the prognosis of the cystic fibrosis patient (Kellman & Larsson 1975).

DIAGNOSIS

Sweat test

The significance and relationship of elevated sweat sodium and chloride to the disease were first described in 1953 (di Sant'Agnese et al 1953). Elevated sweat electrolyte concentrations occur in a few other conditions — severe malnutrition, diabetes insipidus, adrenal insufficiency and glucose-6-phosphatase deficiency — but these are conditions which could not be confused clinically with cystic fibrosis. More troublesome is the elevation of sweat electrolytes which occurs with ageing. Normal adults (i.e. over 17 years) at high sweating rates may occasionally have values for sweat sodium and chloride which lie within the range usually associated with cystic fibrosis. In childhood, however, the sweat test is a good diagnostic tool provided it is done with meticulous care and by a laboratory with frequent experience of the test and good quality control (Howell 1976, Schwachman & Mohmoodian 1979).

The method of testing now preferred is that of pilocarpine iontophoresis (Gibson & Cooke 1959). Both sodium and chloride should be measured as a check. A difference of more than 30 mmol/l between the concentration of either of the two ions in repeat tests indicates technical error.

Most clinicians would accept that a concentration of sodium over 70 mmol/l and chloride over 60 mmol/l (measured in a minimum collection of 100 mg of sweat) are significantly abnormal, and consistent with the diagnosis of cystic fibrosis. If the test has been performed correctly very similar results should be obtained if the test is repeated under similar conditions. Schwarz (1974) noted that in cystic fibrosis sodium loss resulting from diarrhoea, and the malnutrition due to malabsorption, may cause increased aldosterone production which may lower the sodium concentration in sweat and raise the potassium concentration. Thus, when the disease is treated, the sodium level may rise and the potassium fall. These changes are of interest but not sufficient to cause confusion in clinical practice.

Pancreatic function tests

Pancreatic function tests are not usually required for the diagnosis of cystic fibrosis. The tests are unpleasant for the child. Pancreatic achylia may occur in other conditions such as familial chronic pancreatitis and Schwachman syndrome. Conversely, pancreatic function may be normal in as many as 15–20% of cases at presentation.

Early in the course of the disease blood immunoreactive trypsin (IRT) levels are markedly elevated. This test is highly sensitive, detecting >98% of patients, including those with normal pancreatic function assessed by the older stool trypsin or meconium albumin methods. CF infants presenting with meconium ileus may fail to show increased IRT levels.

With advancing pancreatic disease, blood IRT concentrations fall into and below the range found in normal children at a rate which is highly variable between patients. IRT testing is therefore not a useful diagnostic tool beyond the neonatal period. It is currently under evaluation at several centres as a neonatal screening test. Abnormal IRT results must always be followed up by a sweat test, which remains the only reliable diagnostic test, apart from molecular studies (see later).

TREATMENT

There is no specific therapy. Treatment is supportive only, but can significantly improve both the quality and duration of life (Dodge 1989). The main burden of the disease results from the respiratory component. Infection has not been effectively prevented by the use of prophylactic antibiotics or by vaccine. It is not possible to maintain a sterile lower respiratory tract for any length of time. In the long term the best that can be achieved is to maintain a balance between the patient and the invading pathogens so that the infection remains contained and the patient is able to grow and develop normally and lead a normal life.

Exercise promotes chest drainage and the patients should be encouraged to take an active part in some form of sport (e.g. swimming, trampolining, squash). Lung function is improved by regular postural drainage and physiotherapy. It is also possible that physiotherapy, by helping to clear the airways of excess secretions, also lessens the frequency of infection. To be effective physiotherapy must be carried out twice or three times daily. At first, in the young child, this is done by the parents, but it is helpful if friends or relatives are willing to learn the necessary techniques and give occasional relief to the parents in their prolonged burden of care. As the patient gets older the physiotherapy techniques can be altered so that the patient becomes progressively less dependent on the help of others. The teenager can carry out his treatment quite independently, except during exacerbation of infection. Continuing guidance to the family by an experienced physiotherapist is an essential part of management, and it is important for the morale of both patient and family that independence, in relation to physiotherapy, should be achieved as soon as possible.

Exacerbation of infection should be treated as early as possible with appropriate antibiotics. To this end it is best if the patient is seen frequently by a paediatrician (e.g. every four weeks) and that the paediatrician should have the support of a bacteriologist with knowledge of the special problems of cystic fibrosis. When early in the disease the infecting organism is staphylococcus, haemophilus or pneumococcus, a wide range of antibiotics is available. In the later stages of the disease when the principal pathogen is a mucoid pseudomonas, antibiotic treatment is less satisfactory. At present the best prospects seem to be offered by a combination of one of the newer aminoglycosides such as Tobramycin and one of the new penicillins, Ticarcillin or Azlocillin. Even with these drugs complete eradication of the organism is unusual, but with energetic use of intravenous antibiotics and physiotherapy, good clinical improvement can be achieved.

The cardiovascular complications of cystic fibrosis are now seen more frequently than before because of longer survival. They are difficult to prevent and the effectiveness of treatment has so far not been adequately studied.

The progress of liver disease likewise cannot be prevented. When portal hypertension results, however, shunt operations can be carried out very successfully without the complication of encephalopathy which is met with in other forms of liver disease such as alcoholic cirrhosis.

The nutritional problems of cystic fibrosis are usually easily managed. Almost all patients can be maintained on a normal diet. It is helpful if the diet is rich in protein. Occasionally when the pancreatic deficiency is very severe it may be necessary to restrict the dietary fat. Pancreatic extracts are given in sufficient dosages to secure adequate digestion and absorption. The effectiveness of treatment may be judged by the patient's growth and weight gain, as well as the character of the stools. When steatorrhoea is not adequately controlled the stools are foul smelling and persistence of this smell may cause social embarrassment to the patient. The dosage of pancreatic enzymes should be increased until this problem is removed. The effectiveness of enzyme treatment can be improved if an alkali is also given orally to secure a more normal pH in the upper jejunum.

PROGNOSIS

The prognosis in cystic fibrosis is very variable and difficult to forecast for the individual patient. Where two or more sibs are affected experience with an older child gives no guidance as to the course of illness and subsequent outcome in later children.

The course of the illness is influenced by social conditions, the aggressiveness of management and the standard of comprehensive care. However the best guide to prognosis is the extent of irreversible pulmonary involvement at the time of diagnosis. Those who present with established pulmonary disease in the first month of life do badly; those who present later, but yet before pulmonary disease is obvious, do relatively well. In one large series (Stern et al 1976) the mean follow-up time from diagnosis was over 14 years.

FAMILY EFFECTS OF CYSTIC FIBROSIS

When cystic fibrosis is diagnosed the whole family becomes involved. If the genetics of the disease is adequately explained to and fully understood by the parents, then there should be no recrimination between them and in this sense the disease should have no disruptive effects on the family.

The divorce rate in affected families is in fact no greater than in the general population.

Many parents have feelings of guilt which may remain troublesome even after the fullest discussion over several years.

Parents are anxious and often depressed. In the author's experience 70% of mothers of cystic fibrosis children are receiving antidepressant drugs at any one time. Some anxieties can be alleviated. Many mothers go in constant fear of further pregnancy. Advice from an expert in contraception can be helpful. Many parents have not been fully informed about the course of the disease and the manner in which death is likely to occur. They are often in constant fear of the child's sudden death. Reluctance of paediatricians to discuss the subject of the child's death before the event is unhelpful.

Financially the disease may be a burden to the family even where medical services are provided free of cost. Travel, even to free clinics, may be expensive, but more important is the impulse in parents to indulge their affected child in ways which lead to insupportable expense.

The child too suffers emotionally. In early childhood behaviour disorders are extremely common as a result of the parents' reluctance to discipline the affected child, about whom they have disturbing feelings of guilt. At school performance tends to be poor, not because of breaks in attendance caused by the illness, but through low standards of expectation by parents and teachers because of the child's disability. The emotional pressures become cumulative as the patient matures. There is the increasing realisation of the threat of physical disorder, as well as impending difficulties in employment resulting from a combination of poor physique and poor educational attainments. This distressing period is often made worse by increasing isolation. Retardation of growth and development, as well as increase in symptoms, may make it impossible to hide the condition and 'differences' from peers. At this stage of the illness rejection of treatment and support is common, as a result of a feeling of hopelessness.

THE MOLECULAR GENETICS OF CYSTIC FIBROSIS

The first linkage with CF was found by Eiberg et al (1985), to the polymorphic serum enzyme paroxonase, but the gene coding for this enzyme was not localised chromosomally. The location was determined by the use of restriction fragment length polymorphisms (RFLPs) with DNA probes, published simultaneously by different groups (Knowlton et al 1985, Scambler et al 1985, Tsui et al 1985, Wainwright et al 1985, White et al 1985). These studies demonstrated that the CF locus is situated near to the middle of the long arm of chromosome 7.

A collaborative study demonstrated that two of the linked probes, the DNA coding for the oncogene *MET* and the random probe J3.11, are fortuitously within one centiMorgan of the CF locus, and flank the mutant allele (Beaudet et al 1986). Cell lines containing *MET* and J3.11 were constructed, containing a portion of human chromosome 7q in a mouse background, by chromosome mediated gene transport, followed by selection for transformation (Scambler et al 1986). These lines would therefore be expected to contain the mutant CF allele as well. A DNA sequence which codes for a protein was isolated from the human transgenome in one of these cell lines (Estivill et al 1987). RFLPs recognised by this sequence are in marked linkage disequilibrium with CF, and it is estimated that they are within a few tens of thousands of base pairs of the CF locus, but the gene is not CF itself (Estivill et al 1987, Beaudet et al 1988, Farrall et al 1988, Wainwright et al 1988).

However, because the markers are in linkage disequilibrium with CF, they are very useful for prenatal diagnosis and carrier testing in families, and can be used to provide a more accurate risk of being a carrier for members of the general population (Farrall et al 1986, 1987). They will also be useful when using polymerase chain reaction techniques with small amounts of human material (Kogan et al 1987).

The linkage disequilibrium also demonstrates that the great majority, at least 85%, of CF chromosomes contain the same set of DNA polymorphisms as surround the mutation which causes the disease (Estivill et al 1987). This is explained most easily as the result of inheritance of a single mutation which occurred originally in one person, and then spread (whether by founder effect or selection) in Caucasian populations. There is some evidence supporting a second mutation at the same locus, which occurs less frequently and only in Southern Mediterranean populations (Estivill et al 1988). There are also data which suggest that a second and interacting mutation at the same locus, in the presence of the pre-existing CF mutation, may cause cases which present with meconium ileus (Mornet et al 1988).

ISOLATION OF THE CF GENE

Recently the gene which carries the mutation-causing CF has itself been identified (Kerem et al 1989, Riordan et al 1989, Rommens et al 1989). The protein product has been named the CF transmembrane regulator (CFTR), an ATP-dependent transport system protein, which may be involved in regulating chloride flux. The findings indicate that about 70% of mutant CF chromosomes in Canada have a specific deletion of 3 base pairs in the coding sequence, causing the loss of a phenylalanine residue at amino acid position 508 of the putative product. The other CF chromosomes, whose proportions vary in different countries, have at least three other mutations (as determined from the allele haplotypes).

The detection of the specific mutation causing CF will allow direct diagnosis at the DNA level. This will be important not only in prenatal diagnosis but possibly in population screening for heterozygous carriers. The characterisation of the gene, and determining the function of the corresponding gene product, will clearly lead to a better understanding of the pathogenesis of this disease, and hopefully to the design of more effective treatments (Lancet 1990).

REFERENCES

Al-Hassani 1976 Personal communication

Andersen D H 1938 Cystic fibrosis of the pancreas and its relation to coeliac disease: A clinical and pathological study. American Journal of Diseases of Children 56: 344–399

Beaudet A, Bowcock A, Buchwald M et al 1986 Linkage of cystic fibrosis to two tightly linked DNA markers: joint report from a collaborative study. American Journal of Human Genetics 39: 681–693

Beaudet A, Spence J, Montes M et al 1988 Experience with new DNA markers for the diagnosis of cystic fibrosis. New England Journal of Medicine 318: 50–51

Besley G T N, Patrick A D, Norman A P 1969 Inhibition of motility of gill cilia of *Dreissena* by plasma of cystic fibrosis patients and parents. Journal of Medical Genetics 6: 278–280

Bowman B H, Lockart L H, McCombe M L 1969 Oyster ciliary inhibition by cystic fibrosis factor. Science 164: 325–326

Cohen L F, di Sant'Agnese P A, Freidlander J 1980 Cystic fibrosis and pregnancy. Lancet 2: 842–844

Cuthbert A W 1989 Defects in epithelial ion transport in cystic fibrosis. In: Goodfellow P (ed) Cystic fibrosis. Oxford University Press, Oxford, p 24–40

Danks D M, Allan J, Anderson C M 1965 Genetic study of fibrocystic disease of the pancreas. Annals of Human Genetics 28: 323–356

di Sant'Agnese P A, Darling R C, Perera G A, Shea E 1953 Abnormal electrolyte composition of sweat in cystic fibrosis of the pancreas. Clinical significance and relationship to disease. Pediatrics 12: 549–563

Dodge J A 1989 Management of cystic fibrosis. In: Goodfellow P (ed) Cystic fibrosis. Oxford University Press, Oxford, p 12–23

Eiberg H, Mohr J, Schmiegelow K 1985 Linkage relationships of paraxonase (PON) with other markers: indication of PON cystic fibrosis synteny. Clinical Genetics 28: 265–271

Estivill X, Farrall M, Scambler P J et al 1987 A candidate for the cystic fibrosis locus isolated by selection for methylation-free islands. Nature 326: 840–845

Estivill X, Scambler P J, Wainwright B J et al 1987 Patterns of polymorphism and linkage disequilibrium for cystic fibrosis. Genomics 1: 257–263

Farrall M, Law H-Y, Rodeck C H et al 1986 Experience with first trimester prenatal diagnosis of cystic fibrosis using linked DNA probes. Lancet i : 1402–1405

Farrall M, Estivill X, Williamson R 1987 Indirect cystic fibrosis carrier detection. Lancet ii: 156–157

Farrall M, Wainwright B J, Feldman G L et al 1988 Recombination between IRP and cystic fibrosis. American Journal of Human Genetics 43: 471–475

Gibson L E, Cooke R E 1959 A test for the concentration of electrolytes in sweat in cystic fibrosis of the pancreas utilising pilocarpine by iontophoresis. Pediatrics 23: 545–549

Goldring R M, Fishman A P, Turino G M, Cohen H I, Denning C R, Anderson D H 1964 Portal hypertension and cor pulmonale in cystic fibrosis of the pancreas. Journal of Pediatrics 65: 501–524

Heeley A F, Heeley M E, Richmond S W J 1983 The value of blood trypsin measurement by RIA in the early diagnosis of cystic fibrosis. In: Albertine A, Crosigni P G (eds). Progress in perinatal medicine. Elsevier/Excerpta Medica, Amsterdam

Howell D A (Chairman) 1976 Committee for a study for evaluation of testing for cystic fibrosis. Journal of Pediatrics 88: 711–750

Kellman N I, Larsson Y 1975 Insulin release in cystic fibrosis. Archives of Disease in Childhood 50: 205–209

Kerem B, Rommens J M, Buchanan J A et al 1989 Identification of the cystic fibrosis gene: genetic analysis. Science 245: 1073–1080

Knowlton R G, Cohen-Haguenauer O, Van Cong N et al 1985 A polymorphic DNA marker linked to cystic fibrosis is located on chromosome 7. Nature 318: 380–382

Kogan S C, Doherty M, Gitschier J 1987 An improved method for prenatal diagnosis of genetic diseases by analysis of amplified DNA sequences. Application to Hemophilia A. New England Journal of Medicine 317: 985–990

Lancet Editorial 1990 Cystic fibrosis: prospects for screening and therapy. Lancet 1: 79–80

Landing B H, Wells T R, Wang G 1969 Abnormality of the epididymis and vas deferens in cystic fibrosis. Archives of Pathology 88: 569–580

Mornet E, Serre J L, Farrall M, Simon-Bouy B, Estivill X, Williamson R, Boue A 1988 Genetic differences between cystic fibrosis with and without meconium ileus. Lancet i: 376–378

Nadler H L, Wodnicki J M, O'Flynn N E 1969 Cultivated amniotic fluid cells and fibroblasts from families with cystic fibrosis. Lancet 2: 84–85

Oppenheimer E H, Esterly J R 1975 Hepatic changes. Young

infants with cystic fibrosis. Journal of Pediatrics 86: 683–684

Poustka A, Pohl T M, Barlow D P et al 1987 Construction and use of human chromosome jumping libraries from NotI-digested DNA. Nature 325: 353–355

Riordan J R, Rommens J M, Kerem B et al 1989 Identification of the cystic fibrosis gene: cloning and characterization of complementary DNA. Science 245: 1066–1073

Rommens J M, Iannuzzi M C, Kerem B et al 1989 Identification of the cystic fibrosis gene: chromosome walking and jumping. Science 245: 1059–1065

Santis G, Osborne L, Knight R et al 1990 Genetic influences on pulmonary severity in cystic fibrosis. Lancet 1: 294

Scambler P J, Farrall M, Stanier P et al 1985 Linkage of COL1A2 collagen gene to cystic fibrosis and its clinical implications. Lancet ii: 1241–1242

Scambler P J, Law H-Y, Williamson R et al 1986 Chromosomal mediated gene transfer of six DNA markers linked to the CF locus on human chromsome seven. Nucleic Acids Research 14: 7159–7174

Schwarz V 1974 The development of the sweat glands and their function. In: Daves J, Dobbing J (eds) Scientific foundation of paediatrics. Heinemann, London, p 544–546

Schwachman H 1975 Gastro-intestinal manifestation of cystic fibrosis. Pediatric Clinics of North America 224: 787–805

Schwachman H, Mohmoodian A 1979 Quality of sweat test performance in the diagnosis of cystic fibrosis. Clinical Chemistry 25(1): 158–161

Solomon E, Bodmer W 1979 Evolution of sickle variant gene. Lancet i: 923

Spock A, Heick H M C, Cress H et al 1967 Abnormal serum factor in patients with cystic fibrosis of the pancreas. Pediatric Research 1: 173–177

Stephan V, Busch E W, Kollberg H, Hellsing K 1975 Cystic fibrosis detection by means of a test-strip. Pediatrics 55: 35–38

Stern R C, Boar T F, Doershuk C F, Tucker A S, Primiano F F, Matthews L W 1976 Course of cystic fibrosis in 95 cases. Journal of Pediatrics 89: 406–411

Sweet E M 1977 Cause of delayed respiratory distress in childhood. Proceedings of the Royal Society of Medicine 70: 863–866

Tsui L C, Buckwald M, Braman J C 1985 Cystic fibrosis locus defined by a genetically linked polymorphic DNA marker. Science 230: 1054–1057

Wainwright B J, Scambler P J, Schmidtke J 1985 Localisation of cystic fibrosis locus to human chromosome 7 cen-q22. Nature 318: 384–385

Wainwright B J, Scambler P J, Stanier P et al 1988 Isolation of a human gene with protein sequence similarity to human and murine int-1 and the *Drosophilia* segment polarity mutant *wingless*. EMBO Journal 7: 1743–1748

White R, Woodwards S, Leppert M et al 1985 A closely linked genetic marker for cystic fibrosis. Nature 318: 382–384

Wilson G B, Fundenberg H H 1978 Separation of ciliary dyskinesis substances found in serum and secreted by cystic fibrosis leucocytes and lymph cell lines, using protein. A-Sepharose C L-4B. Journal of Laboratory and Clinical Medicine 93: 463–482

Wood R E, Boat T F, Doeshuk C F 1976 Cystic fibrosis. State of the art. American Review of Respiratory Disease 113: 833–875

70. Asthma and other allergic conditions

J. A. Raeburn

INTRODUCTION

Allergy of the respiratory tract is a very common condition and causes considerable morbidity and mortality. As many as 10% of the population may be affected in childhood (Williams & McNicol 1975, Soothill 1976) but, as the child grows, there is a reduction in the disproportionate narrowing of the airways; therefore asthma symptoms may moderate. There are many different causes of asthma, but a useful clinical classification is into an extrinsic type, provoked by a wide range of external allergens, and intrinsic asthma which develops later in life without allergic sensitivity and in the absence of a family history. In contrast, patients with extrinsic asthma frequently have a positive family history of allergic disorders. The clinical distinction between these two main types of asthma is often disputable and many genetic studies suffer from the consequent difficulty in classification. However, the high prevalence of asthma and the strong familial tendency suggest that a genetic approach might lead to useful methods of prevention.

Extrinsic asthma and other forms of atopy are very difficult to study from a genetic viewpoint because the patient's clinical state, and the levels of various markers (such as IgE), are the end result of the lifelong interaction between immunological constitution (under considerable genetic control) and previous environment (see Blumenthal et al 1986). Therefore before making attempts to identify specific loci which are involved in the genetic control of, for example, IgE, it is essential to make allowance for differences in the environmental factors which confront the individual, such as exposure to specific sensitising agents (Gerrard et al 1978). Our own studies of factors influencing phagocytic cells showed that venous blood from men who were occupationally exposed to coal dust for many years had higher leucocyte counts, higher serum levels of lysozyme and a higher half-time for phagocytosis than did blood from the age-matched controls (Table 70.1).

Allergic disorders of the respiratory tract and of other

Table 70.1 Influence of environment on phagocytic cells and their products. Ranges in parenthesis are 95% confidence limits.

	Dust-exposed men (miners)	Normal controls
Mean age (SE)	53.2 (1.5)	51.9 (4.2)
Mean time underground	37 years	Nil
Mean total leucocytes ($\times$ 10^9/l)	7.60 (6.98-8.22)	6.48 (5.96-7.00)
Mean serum lysozome level (μg/ml)	9.5 (7.97-11.01)	8.1 7.47-8.81)
Half-time for phagocytosis (min)	88.4 (64.9-111.9)	26.1 19.1-32.2)

regions, particularly the skin, often coexist either in an individual patient or in one family (Reeves 1977). This phenomenon suggests that the inherited feature is the immunological response to certain external allergens. However, there are many enigmatic aspects; for example, in patients with both asthma and atopic eczema why do exacerbations of asthma often coincide with improvement in the eczema and vice versa? Another unsolved question is that the abnormal reactivity can be localised to one site in one affected family member and to another site in his affected relatives. In this chapter we will concentrate on respiratory allergy, principally allergic rhinitis and asthma, and on atopic dermatitis. All three conditions are very common and they are frequently associated.

INVESTIGATIONS IN ATOPIC DISEASES

Atopic disorders suffer from the lack of reliable markers of disease, whether clinical, immunological or biochemical. Therefore there are no accurate figures for the population incidence, estimates varying between 2–20%

Table 70.2 Plan of investigation of the atopic family

A Clinical information
  i) Allergic history of the proband
  ii) Allergic history of the first and second-degree relatives
  iii) Distribution of affected family members
  iv) Other conditions, e.g. susceptibility to infection in family members and index patient
B Side room tests
  i) Skin prick tests
  ii) Eosinophil counts in blood (and sputum)
C Specialist investigations
  i) Total serum IgE level
  ii) Antigen-specific IgE levels (based on radioallergosorbent tests)
  iii) Provocation tests

(Seah & Wilkinson 1974). Table 70.2 lists the main information required in the investigation of an atopic patient; the extent to which such investigations are completed will depend on the severity of the condition in the index patient or his family. The various investigations need not be described in detail here (see Reeves 1977), but it is worth stressing that unless a personal and family history that is accurate and detailed has been obtained, the specialist investigations will provide little useful information.

Skin prick tests can be performed simultaneously on many members of the family and can give semi-quantitative information about the degree of atopy (Pepys 1975). The solutions used in prick testing can be chosen on the basis of known precipitants of atopic attacks, but usually a wide range of allergens, as well as a control solution, will be tested in each patient, thus giving a profile of the skin reactivity. However reactivity in the asthmatic's skin may differ from the bronchial reactivity. A further limitation is that children below three years of age have a reduced skin reactivity to histamine and allergens (Aas 1975). Loeffler and colleagues (1973) showed that there is good correlation between serum IgE levels and the skin test reactions; for example, only 11% of subjects with negative skin tests had elevated serum levels of IgE (over 800

units/ml) whereas 83% of skin test positive subjects had elevated levels.

Immunoglobulin E and atopy

The great majority of patients who have elevated IgE levels suffer from the common atopic disorders, but there is considerable overlap between atopic and non-atopic populations (see Table 70.3 based on Adkinson 1976 and Barnetson et al 1980). Of the atopic patients, the highest serum IgE levels occur in atopic eczema; in patients with allergic asthma, or hay fever, levels are much lower (Barnetson et al 1980). Barnetson and his colleagues also noted that the very high IgE concentrations occurred in atopic eczema patients who had food allergies and positive allergen-specific responses to foods. This observation, coupled with the considerable variation of IgE levels in each group, suggests that in atopy there are many disease subgroups within which IgE variation could be much smaller. It is likely that such subgroups could be the result of genetic heterogeneity. Additional markers of atopy are therefore required in order to subclassify the range of allergy.

GENETIC STUDIES IN ALLERGY

There are three major approaches to such studies. Firstly, there are population studies to establish prevalence and incidence figures and any disease or genetic marker associations. Secondly, twin studies can evaluate the relative importance of genetic and environmental factors. Finally, family studies can establish the genetic basis and mode of inheritance. When coupled with studies of DNA-based polymorphic markers it is likely that future family studies will identify the chromosomal location of specific allergic response genes, and this will provide a means of tracking such genes in asymptomatic members of the family.

Reports of a familial basis for asthma date back to the last century and the various authors have suggested either autosomal dominant or autosomal recessive inheritance, as well as multifactorial transmission (Bias 1973,

Table 70.3 Total serum IgE levels in different adult populations

Population	No. studied	Range of IgE levels (international units per ml)	Geometric mean
Non-atopic adults	102	1–3824	26.7
Unselected adults (allergy not excluded)	73	2.5–7896	43.8
Asthma /hay fever adults	28	10–1900	160
Atopic eczema adults	32	40–45 000	2800

Schwartz 1952, Adkinson 1920). There has been a similar dispute for all atopic disorders and for many years the prevalent view ranged from autosomal dominant (Spain & Cooke 1924) to autosomal recessive inheritance (Tips 1954). Recently the heterogeneity of atopy has been better appreciated and Kaufman and Frick (1976) suggested the multifactorial mode of inheritance, following a prospective study which attempted to classify different types of allergy as well as the varying environmental influences, particularly diet. Despite these contradictions about the mode of inheritance, all studies show firstly that allergy is very common, and secondly that the recurrence risk is high if a parent or sib is affected.

The genetic heterogeneity of atopic disorders is almost certainly very marked and is reminiscent of the heterogeneity recognised in diabetes ten years ago. Some families undoubtedly show inheritance fully compatible with a single gene, autosomal dominant disorder. In all atopic diseases, however, susceptible individuals may fail to express the condition if they do not encounter the appropriate antigen(s) at a specific phase of their immunological development. Figure 70.1 shows the pedigree of a family suffering from severe asthma which in most individuals is triggered by mild respiratory infections. At the age of 21 the monozygotic twins in the second generation (II) were thought to be discordant for asthma. The onset of that disease in one twin was at age 14 and in the other was at 24. In this family autosomal dominant inheritance is the likely cause of the susceptibility to asthma but the disease does not develop spontaneously, it requires an appropriate environmental trigger.

Sibbald and Turner-Warwick (1979) have emphasized the importance of distinguishing the two main clinical subtypes of asthma in any genetic studies of the disease. Their study of 416 probands showed that asthma occurred in 13.3% of first-degree relatives of extrinsic (atopic) asthmatics and in 7.6% of first-degree relatives of intrinsic (non-atopic) asthmatics, a highly significant reduction in the latter group (p < 0.001). However it is frequently difficult to classify asthma as either extrinsic or intrinsic and the above authors recognised at least two intermediate groups. They were unable to determine the mode of inheritance, but in a separate study, Sibbald (1980) showed that there is probably no genetic basis for differences between males and females as regards the prevalence of asthma.

Lubs (1972) carried out a postal survey of those twins recorded at the Swedish twin registry to ascertain the prevalence of allergic disorders and to determine the heritability. There were responses from both twins in 74.5% of the register population, providing data on almost 7000 twin pairs. Table 70.4 summarises the data

Table 70.4 Allergic disorders in twins (based on Lubs 1972)

Disease group	Prevalence (%)	Concordance (%)*	
		Monozygotic	*Dizygotic*
Asthma	3.8	19.0	4.8
Hay fever	14.8	21.4	13.6
Eczema	2.5	15.4	4.0
Asthma or hay fever or eczema	18.2	24.4	16.2

* The concordance for monozygotic twins in each disease group significantly exceeded that for dizygotic twins (p < 0.01 in all four comparisons).

for asthma, hay fever and eczema. The concordance rate for monozygotic twins in this study was lower (15.4–24.4%) than in previous, but much smaller, twin samples. Nevertheless the differences between these values and the concordance rates for dizygotic twins (4–16.2%) strongly suggest a hereditary component. These data can only apply to the populations from which the twins were derived and similar large studies of prevalence are needed for any population in which genetic approaches to prevention are anticipated. An interesting observation in Lubs' (1972) study is that migraine, classified as an allergic disorder, had a prevalence of 8% and also showed increased concordance in monozygotic twins. Oakshot (personal communication 1980) has found that the incidence of migraine is increased in families affected by the common atopic diseases.

GENETIC COUNSELLING IN ALLERGIC DISORDERS

In view of the genetic and clinical heterogeneity of all allergic disorders the estimation of recurrence risks is problematical. The author's approach is to take a careful family history, noting the ocurrence of any type of allergy in the first- and second-degree relatives of the proband. In preparing pedigrees note is also taken of diseases which may be associated with atopy such as immune deficiency syndromes or autoimmune disorders. Where there are affected family members it is useful to enquire about the age of onset and any known precipitating factors, because this information gives an indication of possible methods of prevention.

Having examined the pedigree and all clinical data a Mendelian form of inheritance may be suggested which forms the basis of a risk estimate. For example, the offspring of the asthmatic son of the identical twin in Figure 70.1 would have a 50% risk of inheriting the susceptibility. X-linked recessive atopic diseases have not

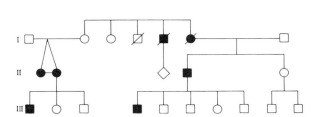

Fig. 70.1 The affected members of this family had asthma which was usually precipitated by an upper respiratory infection of viral type. Unless the consequent bronchoconstrictive symptoms were energetically treated, usually with short-term high doses of steroids, the subsequent exacerbations of asthma could persist for many months. Autosomal dominant inheritance of a susceptibility gene is the simplest model to explain this family.

yet been described, but in the differential diagnosis of severe eczema in the young male, the X-linked Wiskott-Aldrich syndrome should be considered.

Autosomal recessive inheritance is a possibility if the atopic disorders occur only in one sibship, and two possible syndromes are 'asthma associated with aspirin intolerance' (occasionally with nasal polyposis) (McKusick 1988, No. 20855) or 'asthma with short stature and elevation of serum levels of IgA', (McKusick 1988, No. 20860). Cystic fibrosis (CF) families show an increase of atopy in both homozygotes and obligate heterozygotes for the causative gene. This phenomenon has not yet been adequately explained but the genetic counsellor should perhaps consider the possibility of cystic fibrosis in the offspring of a couple, both of whom are atopic. In the near future it is likely that the CF gene will have been sequenced and there will therefore be probes which can detect this gene in heterozygotes. Thus the clinical suspicion of the carrier state in an atopic subject will be directly open to investigation.

There is still a great need for accurate clinical descriptions of families with rare syndromes in which allergic disease coexists with other genetic handicaps. As the human gene map is increasingly explored, such families may provide valuable evidence for the location of immune response genes. For example, the syndrome of oculo-palato-cerebal dwarfism, probably autosomal recessive, has severe asthma as one of the main manifestations (Frydman et al 1985).

Having excluded those atopic families which show a Mendelian form of inheritance, empiric risk figures can be used to estimate the chances of further individuals being affected. Table 70.5, based on data from van Arsdel and Motulsky (1959), Leigh and Marley (1967), Lubs (1972) and Gerrard et al (1976), gives the risk of atopies in a child some of whose first-degree relatives are affected.

In assessing the risk of asthma two other aspects need consideration. Firstly, if a proband has asthma *plus* either allergic rhinitis or eczema, then the risk to first-degree relatives is doubled (Lubs 1972). Secondly, in the adult age groups the risk of asthma increases by a factor of two from age 45 to 65 years (Leigh & Marley 1967). The empiric figures from Table 70.5 will give an approximate risk of atopic diseases in certain situations, which will help parents to make decisions about their future family. In addition, the figures will help clinicians to identify high risk subjects *before* atopic diseases have developed, so that preventive management can be instituted. Genetic counselling in the field of allergy will therefore involve an accurate diagnosis, careful pedigree analysis, calculation of appropriate Mendelian or empiric risk figures, discussion with the consultand(s) and an active approach to prevention.

THE PREVENTION OF ALLERGIC DISEASES

For most allergic diseases the susceptible individual is clinically and immunologically normal at birth and prenatally. However Taylor et al (1973) showed that about half of the infants at high risk of atopy on genetic grounds had low IgA levels at the age of three months and an 'overshoot' at one year. The infants with this 'transient IgA deficiency' were much more likely to develop infantile atopy than other 'high risk' babies who had normal IgA levels throughout. Since the transient IgA deficiency precedes the development of reaginic allergy (Soothill 1976), IgA studies may identify the atopic subjects at a stage at which intervention may be considered. For example, Matthew et al (1977) have shown that a simple allergen avoidance regimen, based

Table 70.5 Empiric risk of atopic disease in children with affected first-degree relatives

Disease	Affected sib, normal parents (%)	One parent affected (%)	Both parents affected (%)
Asthma[†]	10	26	34
Hay fever[*]	6	12	insufficient data
Atopic dermatits[†]	14	34	57
Any atopic disease	20	35	50

† The risk given is the risk of the same atopic disease.
* The risk given is the risk of asthma in the child whose first-degree relatives have hay fever — the risk of hay fever is much higher but the clinical consequences are less severe.

on breast feeding, could significantly reduce the incidence of atopic dermatitis at six months and also at one year of age. Whether this initial allergen avoidance can permanently reduce the individual's risk of atopy remains to be seen. There have, however, been disappointing initial results in a controlled study which excluded cow's milk and eggs from the diet of pregnant women whose fetuses were at high risk of allergy. The trial group of women avoided these foods from 28 weeks of gestation until delivery of the baby. When the offspring were aged 18 months there was no significant decrease in allergies in the offspring of diet-treated mothers compared with the normal diet group (Falth-Magnusson & Kjellman 1987). As well as dietary measures, avoidance of inhaled antigens from animal or plant dusts can also be instigated, in addition to therapy, such as disodium cromoglycate, which may prevent histamine release into lung tissue following antigen exposure. Transient IgA deficiency is unlikely to detect all individuals with susceptibility to atopic diseases.

An additional approach is based on a search for either linkage to the HLA loci or association with specific HLA haplotypes. Ragweed pollinosis is always associated with intense skin reactivity to antigen E, the major antigen of ragweed pollen. Affected subjects all have severe hay fever following contact with ragweed pollen, and often concomitant asthma. Analyses of several studies of HLA types in this disease have shown associations with HLA B7, Dw2 and DR2 (Braun 1978, Marsh et al 1982). However, although some families showed linkage with HLA, others definitely did not (Blumental et al 1986). Thus HLA testing (now utilising polymorphic DNA-based probes) will detect 'at risk' subjects in *some* ragweed-sensitive families. Prospective studies in susceptible families will provide a further model for the prevention of allergic diseases.

HLA studies in asthma families have shown no association with a particular HLA antigen. Early studies suggested a small increase in the AI-B8 haplotype, but the results were no longer statistically significant when correction was made for the number of antigens studied (Braun 1978). Turton et al (1979) confirmed the lack of association with known antigens of the A, B and C loci in 40 extrinsic asthma patients, as well as in 41 patients with intrinsic asthma and 41 with allergic bronchopulmonary aspergillosis. In addition, the haplotype segregation in the sibs of probands with or without asthma did not differ from that predicted. These negative results are disappointing but they indicate the need for study of other immunological and genetic markers in asthma.

For many subjects at risk of respiratory allergy the best prospects for disease prevention lie in measures taken in early infancy or childhood. Some, however, will be free from any form of allergy until adult life, when contact with new agents provokes specific sensitisation. An appropriate area for application of preventive management would be in the field of industrial health, where a wider knowledge of atopic disorders will indicate which individuals should avoid specific situations (e.g. some asthma subjects should not work in factories producing biological detergents). If genetic studies or immunological markers could be used prospectively to identify high risk individuals the possibilities for prevention would be very great in industries which range from coal mining to synthetic chemical manufacture. Although some allergic diseases may be mild, a careful study of allergy may suggest ways of preventing life-threatening asthma states or chronic handicapping atopic dermatitis.

ACKNOWLEDGEMENTS

It is a pleasure to acknowledge the help of several colleagues in the preparation of this chapter, particularly Dr I P Gormley and Professor A E H Emery.

REFERENCES

Aas K 1975 Diagnosis of immediate type respiratory allergy. Pediatric Clinics of North America 22: 1: 33–42

Adkinson J 1920 The behaviour of bronchial asthma as an inherited character. Genetics 5: 363–418

Adkinson N F 1976 Measurement of total serum immunoglobin E and allergen-specific IgE antibody. In: Rose N R, Friedman H (eds) Manual of Clinical Immunology, Ch 79, p 590–602

Barnetson R StC, Merrett T G, Ferguson A 1980 Hyperimmunoglobulinaemia E in atopy (Abstract) In: Preud'homme J L, Hawken V A L (eds) 4th International Congress of Immunology. French Society of Immunology, Paris, Ch 13.1.02

Bias W B 1973 The genetic basis of asthma. In: Austen K F, Lichtenstein L M (eds) Asthma: Physiology,

Immunopharmacology and Treatment, Academic Press, New York p 39–44

Blumenthal M N, Yunis E, Mendell N, Elston R C 1986 Preventive allergy: Genetics of IgE-mediated diseases. Journal of Allergy and Clinical Immunology 78: 962–968

Braun W E 1978 Current status of HLA and disease associations. In: HLA and Disease, A comprehensive review. CRC Press Inc., Boca Raton, Ch 7, p 29–33

Falth-Magnusson K, Kjellman N-I M 1987 Development of atopic diseases in babies whose mothers were receiving exclusion diets during pregnancy – A randomised study. Journal of Allergy and Clinical Immunology 80: 868–875

Frydman M, Kaushansky A, Leshem I, Savir H 1985 Oculo-palato-cerebral dwarfism – a new syndrome. Clinical Genetics 27: 414–419

Gerrard J W, Vickers P, Gerrard C D 1976. The familial incidence of allergic disease. Annals of Allergy 36: 10–15

Gerrard J W, Rao D C, Morton N E 1978 A genetic study of Immunoglobulin E. American Journal of Human Genetics 30: 46–58

Kaufman H S, Frick O L 1976 The development of allergy in infants of allergic parents: a prospective study concerning the role of heredity. Annals of Allergy 37: 410–415

Leigh D, Marley E 1967 Bronchial Asthma. Pergamon Press, Oxford

Loeffler J A, Cawley L P, Moeder M 1973 Serum IgE levels correlation with skin test reactivity. Annals of Allergy 31: 331–336

Lubs E M L 1972 Empiric risks for genetic counselling in families with allergy. Journal of Pediatrics 80: 26–31

McKusick V A 1988 Mendelian inheritance in man – Catalog of autosomal dominant, autosomal recessive and X-linked phenotypes, 8th edn. The Johns Hopkins University Press, Baltimore.

Marsh D, Hsu S H, Roebler M et al 1982 HLA DW2 – a genetic marker for human immune response to short ragweed allergen RAS: I. Response resulting primarily from natural antigenic exposure. Journal of Experimental Medicine 155: 1439–1451

Matthew D J, Taylor B, Norman A P, Turner M W, Soothill J F 1977 Prevention of eczema. Lancet 1: 321–324

Pepys J 1975 Skin testing. British Journal of Hospital Medicine 14: 412–417

Reeves W G 1977 Atopic disorders. In: Holborow E J, Reeves W G (eds) Immunolgy in Medicine. Academic Press, London, Ch 22, p 749–779

Schwartz M 1952 Heredity in Bronchial Asthma. Munksgaard, Copenhagen

Seah P P, Wilkinson D S 1974 Eczema. In: Fry L, Seah P P (eds) Immunological aspects of skin diseases. MTP, Lancaster, England, Ch 6, p 234–284

Sibbald B 1980 Genetic basis of sex diferences in the prevalence of asthma. British Journal of Diseases of the Chest 74: 93–94

Sibbald B, Turner-Warwick M 1979 Factors influencing the prevalence of asthma among first degree relatives of extrinsic and intrinsic asthmatics. Thorax 34: 332–337

Soothill J F 1976 Some intrinsic and extrinsic factors predisposing to allergy. Proceedings of the Royal Society of Medicine 69: 439–442

Spain W C, Cooke R A 1924 Studies in specific hypersensitiveness. Journal of Immunology 9: 521–569

Taylor B, Normal A P, Orgel H A, Stokes C R, Turner M W, Soothill J F 1973 Transient IgA deficiency and pathogenesis of infantile atopy. Lancet 2: 111–113

Tips R L 1954 A study of the inheritance of atopic hypersensitivity in man. American Journal of Human Genetics 6: 328–343

Turton C W G, Morris L, Buckingham J A, Lawler S D, Turner-Warwick M 1979 Histocompatibility antigens in asthma: population and family studies. Thorax 34: 670–676

van Arsdel P P, Motulsky A G 1959 Frequency and heritability of asthma and allergic rhinitis in college students. Acta Genetica 9: 101–114

Williams H E, McNicol K N 1975 The spectrum of asthma in children. Pediatric Clinics of North America 22: 43–52

71. Alpha$_1$-antitrypsin deficiency and related disorders

Jack Lieberman

ALPHA$_1$-ANTITRYPSIN (AAT)

An inherited deficiency of alpha$_1$-antitrypsin (AAT) is currently the best understood of the genetic abnormalities affecting the lungs. The molecular defect of the AAT molecule is known (Jeppson 1976, Owen & Carrell 1976, Yoshida et al 1976, Owen & Carrell 1977, Yoshida et al 1977, Owen et al 1978, Yoshida et al 1979a,b); the major disease syndromes resulting from the defect have been described (Eriksson 1965, Lieberman 1969); the specific chromosome and DNA sequence of the responsible gene have been identified (Colau et al 1984, Long et al 1984, Schroeder et al 1985, Rabin et al 1986); the gene has been cloned (Schroeder et al 1985, Rabin et al 1986); genetically engineered AAT has been synthesized (Courtney et al 1984, Rosenberg et al 1984, George et al 1984, Janoff et al 1986, Ledley & Woo 1986); treatment regimens with synthetic or pooled AAT have been initiated (Glaser et al 1983, Coan et al 1985, Cohen 1986a,b, Boswell & Carrell 1986); and plans are being made for replacing the defective gene through viral mediated gene transfer therapy (Ledley & Woo 1986).

The discovery of AAT deficiency, by Laurell and Eriksson in 1963 in addition to leading to the genetic research stated above, has had tremendous impact on the field of pulmonology in general: it has emphasized the role of cellular proteases in the pathogenesis of disease; it has clarified the role of AAT as one of the body's defence mechanisms; it has led to a clear understanding of the pathogenesis of pulmonary emphysema; and has provided a tool for geneticists to study inheritance patterns and gene mapping.

At the time that Laurell and Eriksson (1963) discovered five patients who lacked an alpha$_1$-globulin peak on serum protein electrophoresis, it was known that the alpha$_1$-globulin peak was composed primarily of the AAT glycoprotein. Measurement of AAT activity via the serum-trypsin-inhibitory-capacity (STIC) revealed a marked deficiency in the five patients. Three of these five had emphysema, as did 9 of 14 additional cases with pronounced AAT deficiency reported later by Eriksson (1964). Measurement of STIC in relatives of the patients clearly demonstrated that the defect was inherited through two codominant autosomal genes, with heterozygotes having intermediate STIC levels (approximately 60% of normal) and deficient homozygotes having approximately 15% of normal activity levels. These observations were quickly confirmed worldwide by many investigators.

The typical clinical picture of a patient with severe AAT deficiency is that of a man or woman between 20 and 60 years of age with insidious progression of shortness of breath leading to a picture of panacinar emphysema. Such emphysema typically involves the basilar portions of the lungs most seriously, as reflected on chest radiography and by perfusion and ventilation lung scans. Pulmonary function measurements typically show obstructive changes with increased residual volumes, increased compliance, reduced airflow from the lungs (FEV$_1$), and reduced diffusing capacity. Some patients may present with symptoms of bronchial asthma (Makino et al 1970), chronic bronchitis (Falk & Smith 1971), or bronchiectasis (Longstreth et al 1975). A family history of obstructive lung disease is frequently obtained from subjects with AAT deficiency.

Lung disease in association with AAT deficiency did not initially appear to be an important clinical entity, since early studies had suggested that only 1% of emphysema patients had severe AAT deficiency. More recently, however, these studies have led to a concept of protease/antiprotease imbalance leading to lung damage, so that the mechanism described for the development of lung disease with the genetic deficiency probably plays a role in the pathogenesis of emphysema in general. Thus, the importance of the genetic defect goes far beyond the number of subjects inheriting the abnormality. In addition, the concept that the carrier (heterozygous) state may also predipose to the development of lung disease increases the numbers of potentially affected individuals with the inherited deficiency state from 0.04% of the population (deficient homozygotes) to approximately 5% of the population (Lieberman 1969). This disclosure in 1969 raised a burst of clinical interest in AAT deficiency with arguments still raging regarding the susceptibility of the heterozygote to the detrimental effects of cigarette smoking in causing lung disease.

Role of AAT as a protective protein

Alpha$_1$-antitrypsin is a broad spectrum inhibitor of proteolytic enzymes (Table 71.1), and constitutes essentially the entire α_1-globulin peak on serum protein electrophoresis. The circulating protein is primarily synthesized by the liver; its relatively low molecular weight of 50 000 daltons enables its passage into most tissue spaces of the body. AAT binds and inhibits proteases released from cells (leucocytes and macrophages) participating in infectious or inflammatory processes. In the lung leucocytes release proteolytic enzymes, either through cellular death or during the act of phagocytosis. When levels of AAT are inadequate, either because of a genetic defect or deactivation by oxidants or by an overwhelming release of proteases, the uninhibited proteolytic enzymes digest the alveolar septi and produce the pathological picture which we recognize as pulmonary emphysema. Experimental support of this concept was provided by demonstrating that leucocyte proteases are capable of digesting lung tissue, and that AAT strongly inhibits this activity (Lieberman & Gawad 1971, Janoff et al 1972).

Other protective actions of AAT have been suspected over the years; for example, Arora et al (1978) demonstrated an immunosuppressive action for AAT, so that an AAT deficiency would enhance an immunological response to an antigen with increased numbers of leucocytes and increased release of proteases. Another effect was demonstrated by Mirsky and Foley (1945) who showed that trypsin inhibitors have an antibiotic action and, conversely, that certain antibiotics such as penicillin had a weak but definite antiproteolytic action. Thus, a rise of antiprotease levels in blood during certain pathological states could play an important role in resistance to infection.

It is of great interest that the lung appears to be the organ most dependent upon the protective action of AAT. It has been shown that the lung preferentially incorporates AAT (Ishibashi et al 1978, Moser et al 1978) and tends to retain active AAT for longer periods of time than other mammalian tissues, perhaps indicating the need in lungs for this type of protection. Lungs are most frequently exposed to infectious and inflammatory responses because of direct contact with the environment and the imposed exposure to irritants like cigarette smoke. In addition, leucocytes are known to sequester within the pulmonary capillaries at the lung bases as a natural phenomenon (Bierman et al 1955), and do so more strikingly during acute trauma to the lungs, sometimes causing complete occlusion of pulmonary capillaries as in 'shock lung' (Ratliff et al 1971, Wittels et al 1974). Such storage of leucocytes in the lung's basilar capillaries could be the reason for enhanced emphysematous damage to the bases of the lungs in AAT deficient individuals. Alveolar macrophages also contain proteases, the level of which may be increased in those who smoke cigarettes (Kuhn & Senior 1978)

Table 71.1 Enzymes inhibited or not inhibited by AAT

Enzyme	Reference
Enzymes inhibited	
Trypsin	Eriksson (1965)
Chymotrypsin	Bloom & Hunter (1978)
Elastase	Turino et al (1969)
Granulocyte proteases (elastase, chymotrypsin-like enzyme, and collagenase)	Lieberman & Kaneshiro (1972)
Plasmin (in vitro)	Laurell (1975)
Human factor XI(PTA)	Heck & Kaplan (1974)
Renin	Scharpe et al (1976)
Urokinase	Clemmensen & Christensen (1976)
Bacterial subtilisin	Wicher & Dolovich (1971)
Acrosomal proteinase	Schumacher (1971)
Thrombin	Machovich et al (1977)
Enzymes not inhibited	
Kallikrein	Heck & Kaplan (1974)
Plasminogen activator	Heck & Kaplan (1974)
Papain ⎫	
Ficin ⎬ Plant proteases	Sasaki et al (1974)
Bromelain ⎭	
Plasmin (in vitro)	Laurell (1975)
Hyaluronidase	
Pepsin	Lieberman (1971)
Anhydrotrypsin	Moroi et al (1975)

Polymorphism of alpha$_1$-antitrypsin

AAT is a polymorphic protein for which approximately 60 variants have been described to date. The method for distinguishing these variants usually involves a form of isoelectric focusing on polycrylamide, starch or agarose gels (Fig. 71.1). Not all 60 variants are of clinical significance other than to investigators studying inheritance patterns of populations. Only a few need be remembered as being associated with disease.

The terminology used to distinguish the AAT variants was originated by Fagerhol (1968); the Protease Inhibitor

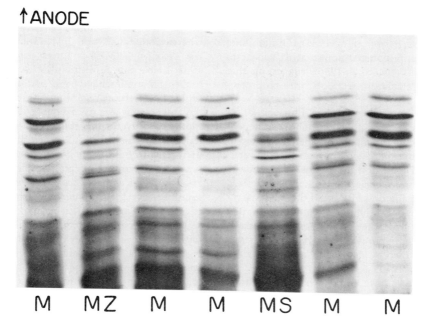

↑ANODE

M   MZ   M   M   MS   M   M

Fig. 71.1 Pi type patterns as seen on isoelectric focusing gels (pH 3.0–5.0).

system is abbreviated as the 'Pi' system. Each variant is assigned a letter in the alphabet according to its mobility at acid pH of isoelectric focusing. The normal, most common, form in Pi^M, having medium mobility. Variants moving faster in the electric field are assigned letters lower in the alphabet; those moving more slowly are assigned letters later in the alphabet. The most common variants associated with disease include the Pi^Z, Pi^S, and null gene (PiQO). Heterozygotes for the various types are designated as PiMZ, PiMS, PiSZ, etc. Homozygous states may be designated simply as PiM, or PiZ, etc. The Z variant is the most common cause of AAT deficiency (Table 71.2). A homozygous ZZ phenotype causes a severe deficiency of AAT (15% of normal); the heterozygous MZ phenotype causes an intermediate deficiency (approximately 60% of normal); the rare homozygous null gene (PiQOQO) causes total absence of AAT. The SZ phenotype is also of clinical significance, resulting in less than 40% of normal plasma AAT levels, it also predisposes to lung disease.

Effect of smoking on protease/antiprotease balance

The concept of protease/antiprotease imbalance suggests that a relative acquired AAT deficiency may contribute to the development of emphysema whether a genetic deficiency of AAT exists or not. Smokers in general have been found to have significantly higher mean serum

levels of AAT than non-smokers (Rees et al 1975, Lellouch et al 1979, 1985, Ashley et al 1980, Bridges et al 1985), suggesting that cigarette smoke is capable of initiating increased synthesis and release of AAT from the liver in the role of AAT as an acute-phase-reactant-protein. On the other hand, evidence has accumulated to indicate that cigarette smoke can suppress AAT activity directly in vitro, and can induce a functional deficiency of antiprotease in the lower respiratory tract (Janoff & Carp 1977, Carp & Janoff 1978, Gadek et al 1979, Janoff et al 1979a, Pryor et al 1985, 1986). This has been shown to result from an oxidant in cigarette smoke affecting the methionine-based active centre, so that a reducing agent

Table 71.2 Characteristics of the Pi^Z variant of AAT

PiZZ phenotype – causes severe deficiency of AAT
PiMZ phenotype – causes intermediate deficiency of AAT
Hepatic globules – PiZZ and PiMZ associated with hepatocytic globules – PAS positive, diastase resistant, immunologically related to AAT, in RER under the electron microscope
Acid gradient electrophoresis
  Slow mobility; low concentration
Increased heat lability
Reduced content of sialic acid
  None in PiZ from liver
  Half normal in PiZ from serum
Serum levels do not rise in response to oestrogens or other 'acute-phase-reactant' stimuli

is capable of restoring the elastase-inhibitory-capacity (Janoff et al 1979a) or preventing the loss of inhibitor in vitro to begin with (Pryor et al 1986). Glutathione, ascorbic acid and unprotonated amino acids appear to have this function (Pryor et al 1986), suggesting that ingestion of ascorbic acid, for example, may be protective.

On the protease side of the imbalance, Blue and Janoff (1978) showed that human polymorphonuclear leucocytes released their content of elastase when incubated in vitro in the presence of cigarette smoke condensate. Hinman et al (1980) and Kuhn and Senior (1978) showed that macrophages from cigarette smokers synthesized and secreted greater amounts of elastase than did macrophages from non-smokers. Thus, it would appear that cigarette smoking increases the production and release of cellular protease, and simultaneously reduces elastase-inhibitory activity, thereby producing a functional or relative deficiency of AAT.

Not all investigators have confirmed these findings: Abboud et al (1983) found that chronic smoking did not affect neutrophil elastase release in vitro, and Stone et al (1983) did not find a reduction in AAT activity in the lower respiratory tract of cigarette smokers. Janoff and Chan (1984) suggest that Stone's negative results may be time-related, since the loss of AAT activity occurs a short time after exposure to cigarette smoke; Abboud et al (1984, 1985) suggest that the effect may depend upon the total amount of cigarette consumption. Abboud also found inhibition of AAT only within one hour of exposure to cigarette smoking. Cox and Billingsley (1984) found no significant difference between non-smokers' and smokers' serum or plasma AAT, but this conclusion was no different from those reports actually showing an increase in serum AAT in smokers. The effect of oxidants, according to most studies, is localized to the lungs, and is best studied through measurements of AAT in broncho-alveolar-lavage fluid (BAL) (Abboud et al 1985).

Role of intermediate AAT deficiency in predisposing to pulmonary disease

The increased susceptibility of individuals with a severe (homozygous) deficiency of AAT to develop pulmonary emphysema is universally accepted. However, the role of an intermediate deficiency (PiMZ) as a risk factor is not universally accepted. In this regard it seems to me that the argument is rather academic, if we believe that an acquired or relative deficiency of AAT contributes to the pathogenesis of emphysema. Wouldn't a baseline intermediate-deficiency-level of AAT be more likely to result in an imbalanced protease/antiprotease system than would a normal level of AAT? The normal type of AAT

is also capable of responding to 'stress' such as infection by achieving even higher AAT levels in the blood, whereas individuals with the Z variant of AAT are either less responsive (MZ) or unresponsive (ZZ) (Kueppers 1968, Lieberman & Mittman 1973).

Clinical studies have been performed in attempts to settle the question regarding the role of intermediate AAT deficiency as a risk factor. The type of study that is most supportive of this role is that in which the prevalence of intermediate AAT deficiency was determined in patients with pulmonary emphysema. This was the first type of study to incriminate the intermediate deficiency as a risk factor with 4–25% of patients in various studies found to have the intermediate deficiency, as compared to 2.6–5% in controls (Lieberman 1969, Matzen et al 1977, Lochon et al 1978, Lebeau & Rochemaure 1978). Our most recent survey included 965 patients with various forms of Chronic-Obstructive-Pulmonary-Disease (COPD) in whom 8% had the MZ phenotype (Lieberman et al 1986) in contrast to 2.9% of control subjects (P < 0.0005). This is a smaller prevalence than the 18% with the intermediate deficiency that we found before (Lieberman 1969), but the earlier study was limited specifically to patients with diagnosed pulmonary emphysema.

Klasen et al (1986) also found a significantly higher number of PiZZ and PiMZ individuals in a flaccid lung (emphysema) population (1.5% and 5.3% respectively vs 0.1% and 2.5% in controls). They concluded that the excess risk due to the heterozygous deficiency alone is negligible compared to MM individuals, but is highly influenced by environmental and possibly other genetic factors.

The other type of study that has been most successful in demonstrating the potential risk of AAT heterozygotes for developing emphysema is the longitudinal study in which pulmonary function is measured over long periods of time in patients subdivided by AAT phenotype and by their smoking history. Ostrow and Cherniack (1972) have shown that changes in lung elasticity due to aging may be accelerated in the heterozygous state. Kanner et al (1979) found that COPD patients with higher levels of AAT had less deterioration in FVC and FEV_1 over a 2–6 year period. More recently, Eriksson et al (1985) found a significantly higher mean annual decrease in FEV_1 in smoking heterozygotes than in non-smoking heterozygotes. However, during the six years covered by the study, they did not detect an increased prevalence of clinical obstructive lung disease. The non-smoking heterozygotes did not differ from either smoking or non-smoking PiM controls.

A third type of survey has been less successful in demonstrating the AAT heterozygous state as a risk factor for the development of lung disease. These studies involve measurements of pulmonary function among random, usually healthy, individuals with an MZ, intermediate deficiency state as compared to those with normal AAT levels (Larsson et al 1977, Chan-Yeung et al 1978, Kozarevic et al 1978, Buist et al 1979, Kanner et al 1979, McDonagh et al 1979, Horton et al 1980, Pride et al 1980, Eriksson et al 1985). An exception was the study of Larsson et al (1977) who found that smoking heterozygotes showed a significant loss of elastic recoil, enlarged residual volumes and increased closing capacity, but no signs of obstructive ventilatory impairment. These subjects were 50-year-old Swedish men, and most of the smoking MZ individuals reported mild exertional dyspnoea.

In the USA, a collaborative study involved 143 PiMZ heterozygous subjects from random populations, plus matched PiM controls from the same population (Bruce et al 1984). These subjects completed questionnaires regarding respiratory symptoms. The authors concluded that the MZ phenotype alone carries no greater risk of developing lung disease than does the normal M phenotype, irrespective of age, smoking, or sex. This study was criticized by Kauffmann (1985) who stated that PiMZ subjects seem to remove themselves from risk factors like tobacco, occupational exposure to dust, or air pollution, thereby resulting in selection bias.

Stjernberg et al (1984) studied 518 workers at a sulphite pulp factory in Northern Sweden, looking for symptoms of chronic bronchitis. They found a significant increase of the MZ phenotype in individuals with chronic bronchitis as compared to the area's population in general (8.5% vs 2.1%) but no significant difference between the frequency of MZ in employees with bronchitis and those without respiratory symptoms (8.5% vs 3.4%). This study is suggestive, but statistically inconclusive, of some predisposition to bronchitis in MZ individuals. In a similar study, Horne et al (1986) had employees from the Saskatchewan country grain elevators answer questionnaires and undergo pulmonary studies. 28 men with the PiMZ phenotype were case matched with others of type PiM. The MZ group had three times as many individuals with abnormal chest radiographs and poorer pulmonary function tests than the control group, suggesting that the PiMZ individuals may be at higher risk of COPD than PiM individuals, but only in the presence of other risk factors such as grain dust exposure. It has been my contention for many years that individuals with an MZ phenotype were only prone to develop lung disease if they were smokers or worked in industry where they were exposed to unusual amounts of dusts or respiratory irritants.

The final method utilized for evaluating the possible risk of intermediate AAT deficiency in the pathogenesis of pulmonary emphysema involves the detection of hepatocytic globules (AAT retention particles) at autopsy. Eriksson et al (1975) found macroscopic emphysema in 50% of 26 subjects having positive liver inclusions, as compared to a prevalence of 18% with macroscopic emphysema among 100 lacking such liver globules. In this type of study, one assumes that the majority of individuals with AAT hepatocytic globules at autopsy are heterozygous for the Z gene; the validity of this assumption has been questioned inasmuch as others have found similar globules in elderly, ill males with an MM phenotype (see below).

It would appear from all that has been written regarding the role of intermediate antitrypsin deficiency in the pathogenesis of pulmonary emphysema that nothing definite can be decided by surveys of healthy populations. An increased prevalence of intermediate AAT deficiency among patients with pulmonary emphysema, plus logic, must dictate what our attitude should be in consulting with patients who have this degree of deficiency. Certainly the heterozygote is better protected than the deficient homozygote, and the severely deficient person may be somewhat better protected than the individual with absolutely no antitrypsin in his body (homozygous for the null gene) (Cox & Levison 1988). I consider those with intermediate AAT deficiency to have an increased predisposition to lung damage as compared to those with a normal AAT phenotype, and I warn them that they must not smoke cigarettes nor expose themselves to unusual lung pollutants or irritations. Other genetic or environmental factors may also contribute to the development of lung disease in some individuals with intermediate AAT deficiency (Kueppers et al 1977).

AAT deficiency and the liver

Site of synthesis

It is obvious that the liver is the major site of synthesis of AAT (Kueppers 1971), although other sites of localization and synthesis have been detected, including the pancreatic islet cells (Ray et al 1977, Ray & Desmet 1978a,b, McElrath et al 1979, Ray & Zumwalt 1986a,b), mast cells (Ray & Desmet 1978a,b), polymorphonuclear leucocytes (Bribiesca & Horta 1978), platelets (Bagdasarian & Colman 1978), the surface of mitogen-stimulated human lymphocytes (Lipsky et al 1979) and monocytes and macrophages (Van Furth et al 1983, Lamontagne et al 1985, Takemura et al 1986). The presence of intra-hepatocytic globules composed essentially of pure AAT of the Z variant was first described by Sharp (1971) in children with juvenile cirrhosis. These globules, which stained with PAS, were immunoreactive for AAT and were diastase resistant. Similar globules were later detected in the livers of adults carrying the Z variant of AAT, both with and without liver disease (Gordon et al 1972, Lieberman et al 1972, Hultcrantz & Mengarelli 1984), suggesting that the liver globules were specific for the Z variant, although the M-Duarte variant was found to have similar globules (Lieberman et al 1976a). The globules have been shown to contain either active (Glaser et al 1977, Bathurst et al 1984) or inactive AAT (Matsubara et al 1974) within rough endoplasmic reticulum (RER) as seen under the electron microscope (EM). The retention of PiZ AAT by the liver appears to result from an amino acid substitution that prevents completion of the carbohydrate side chains, or cleavage of the propeptide in the Golgi vesicles to give the mature protein (Carrell & Owen 1976, Nemeth et al 1983).

Similar globules may be seen in diseased liver from individuals with normal AAT, but these can usually be distinguished from the PiZ liver globules by their loose or compact granular composition within lysosomal structures rather than within dilated RER (Reintoft 1979). However, there have been a total of six patients with PiM phenotype reported to have AAT globules in their livers (Fisher et al 1976, Bradfield & Blenkinsopp 1977, Carlson et al 1981). These have been elderly patients with elevated levels of AAT and severe underlying disease. This may be due to the accumulation of AAT in the liver of older ill patients with a normal AAT phenotype exceeding the liver's capacity to secrete AAT (Berninger et al 1985).

Juvenile hepatitis and cirrhosis

The association of AAT deficiency and idiopathic juvenile cirrhosis was first reported by Sharp et al (1969) who found seven children with juvenile cirrhosis to be homozygous deficient for AAT. An intensive screening of 200 000 infants by Sveger (1976) in Norway revealed 120 with severe AAT deficiency, of whom 14 had prolonged obstructive jaundice, 9 had severe clinical and laboratory evidence of liver disease, and 5 laboratory evidence of liver disease only. The others with severe AAT deficiency did not have clinical liver disease, but approximately half had some abnormal liver function tests.

The variability of the liver disease in infants with severe AAT deficiency suggests that additional provocative factors maybe involved. Such factors may induce hepatic inflammation that would ordinarily be limited by normal levels of AAT. It has been suggested that the hepatitis antigen (HAA) may be a factor in these individuals (Lieberman et al 1972). Porter et al (1972) found that three of five infants with neonatal hepatitis and severe AAT deficiency had Australia antigen in their serum and that Australia antigen or antibody was present in one or both parents of these children and in the parents

of even those children whose serum was negative. Bradfield and Wells (1978) postulated that Kupffer cells and their intracellular proteolytic enzymes may be the link between AAT deficiency and liver damage. Release of proteolytic enzymes from the Kupffer cells into the liver parenchyma during phagocytosis could cause damage when AAT is deficient.

Another recent observation was that breast feeding may offer some protection against disease with AAT deficiency (Udall et al 1985). In this study, only one of 12 breast-fed infants (8%) with AAT deficiency developed severe liver disease, whereas eight of 20 bottle-fed infants (40%) developed severe liver disease. These authors postulate that human milk contains protease inhibitors, including antitrypsin. The antiproteases in ingested milk are protected from destruction by the more alkaline pH of the stomach of human infants, thereby reaching the small intestine where they can neutralize intestinal proteases and provide passive protection of extra-intestinal organs such as the liver from the absorbed enzymes. Enzyme absorption from the intestine has been found to occur in the neonate (Udall et al 1982).

Portasystemic shunts in AAT deficient infants also seem to protect against severe liver disease (Sotos et al 1981, Starzl et al 1983, Alagille 1984). Starzl et al (1983) have noted reversal of hepatic AAT deposition after portacaval shunts. Postoperative liver biopsy material from two of three children showed an apparent reduction in the quantity of AAT particles in the hepatocytes. The authors believe that a general reduction in RER and depression of many biosynthetic processes, including a reduction in the synthesis of AAT and reduced numbers of retained AAT globules, occurs after portacaval shunt, without causing any change in the serum level of AAT.

Adult cirrhosis and hepatoma

Most reports describing liver disease in adults with AAT deficiency have been individual case reports, so that the risks of developing cirrhosis and liver cancer in AAT-deficient adults could not be estimated. More recently, Cox and Smyth (1983) studied 115 adults with AAT deficiency (mostly PiZ). In this series of adults, five had biopsy- or autopsy-proven cirrhosis, and one had definite biochemical evidence of liver disease with a scan compatible with cirrhosis. The risk of developing liver disease was 6.2% for men between 41 and 50 years, but 15.4% for those between 51 and 60 years of age. For women, the risk of developing liver disease appeared to be low. In such patients the presence of liver disease was usually overshadowed by the patients' chest symptoms, and in fact many patients with AAT deficiency have died from lung disease by 50 years of age.

Eriksson et al (1986) conducted a population-based autopsy study to establish whether patients with homozygous AAT deficiency were at increased risk for cirrhosis and primary liver cancer; they found a relationship with both which was statistically significant only for male patients.

Other diseases and AAT

In addition to emphysema, infantile hepatitis and hepatocellular carcinoma, the list of diseases reported in association with AAT deficiency has been growing over the years (see Table 71.3). In some instances only a single case was reported, whereas with others multiple conflicting reports have appeared. Glomerulonephritis and angiitis or vasculitis may be associated with AAT deficiency, but confirmatory reports are needed. A number of reports claim that rheumatoid arthritis is associated with AAT deficiency, but the number of negative reports in this regard is quite large. Fibrosing alveolitis, panniculitis, periodontal disease, anterior uveitis and psoriasis have all been reported in association with AAT deficiency, but confirmation is required. In most instances, the rationale behind an association between AAT deficiency and a specific tissue damage is thought to be the lack of protection against proteolysis during an inflammatory process.

Genetics of alpha₁-antitrypsin

Prevalence of specific Pi variants

AAT is inherited via two codominant autosomal genes. The Pi^M allele is the major type detected in all populations studied (gene frequency varies between 0.859 and 1.000). The AAT genetic variants, however, may differ in their occurrence among various populations (Table 71.4). The Pi^S, Pi^Z, Pi^F, Pi^X and Pi^M subtype distributions especially have been noted to vary in this manner:

1. The Pi^S allele has its highest prevalence in Spain and Portugal, with the next highest rates seen in Frenchmen from the middle South of France and in French Canadians. This association tends to suggest that the French Canadians originate predominantly from the middle South of France, whose people in turn may have an ethnic relationship to the people of Spain and Portugal. Similarly, the Pi^S allele is more predominant in the southern part of the Netherlands (below the Rhine) than the northern part (Dijkman et al 1980). Since prehistoric times, the Rhine has formed the ethnic border between Saxons and Franks and this may be the reason for differences in Pi types between populations on the two banks of the river. Dijkman et al also observed

Table 71.3 Diseases reported in association with AAT

Disease	Reference
Multiple cases studied (cumulative)	
Angiitis and glomerulonephritis	Brandrup & Ostergaard (1978)
	Miller & Kuschner (1969)
	Lubec et al (1976)
	Moroz et al (1976a, 1976b)
Rheumatoid arthritis	*For an association:*
	Cox & Huber (1976, 1980)
	Buisseret et al (1977)
	Arnaud et al (1977c, 1979a, 1979b)
	Against an association:
	Geddes et al (1977)
	Sjoblom & Wollheim (1977)
	Karsh et al (1979)
	Brackertz & Kueppers (1977)
	Walsh & McConkey (1977)
Fibrosing alveolitis	Geddes et al (1977)
Panniculitis	Rubinstein et al (1977)
Anterior uveitis	Brewerton et al (1978)
	Brown et al (1979) – negative report
Peptic ulcer	Andre et al (1974)
	Blenkinsopp (1978) – negative report
	Lieberman (1969) – negative report
Psoriasis	Beckman et al (1980a)
Thrombocytopenia and/or platelet function defects	Miale et al (1977)
Reduced C4	Le Prévost (1975)
Pre-albumin deficiency	Premachandra & Yu (1979)
IgA deficiency	Casterline et al (1978)
	Robert et al (1979)
Paraproteinaemias	Ananthakrishnan et al (1979)
Autism	Walker-Smith & Andrews (1972)
Coeliac disease	Walker-Smith & Andrews (1972)
Glucose intolerance	Santiago et al (1974)
Chronic pancreatitis	Novis et al (1975)
	Lankisch et al (1978) – negative report
Periodontal disease	Peterson & Marsh (1979)
Hepatocellular carcinoma	Lieberman (1974)
	Palmer & Wolfe (1976)
Single case reports or a family study	
Multisystem fibrosis	Palmer et al (1978)
Extrahepatic bile duct hypoplasia	Christen et al (1975)
Pemphigus vulgaris	Benitez-Bribiesca et al (1972)
Severe combined immuno-deficiency	Gelfand et al (1979)
Hypercholesterolaemia	Victorino et al (1978)
Multiple sclerosis	Samad & O'Connell (1972)
Growth hormone deficiency	Schydlower et al (1979)
Multiple endocrine adenomatosis	Eberle et al (1979a)
Cystathioninuria and renal iminoglycinuria	Halal et al (1979)
Pancreatic fibrosis	Freeman et al (1976)
Mannosidosis	Perelman et al (1975)
Intestinal mucosal atrophy	Greenwald et al (1975)
Cardiomyopathy	Torp (1975)

Table 71.4 Gene frequencies for Pi^M, Pi^S, Pi^Z and Pi^F for various populations

Population	No.	Pi^M	Pi^S	Pi^Z	Pi^F	Reference
Spain	378	0.866	0.112	0.012	0.003	Fagerhol & Tenfjord (1968)
	576	0.881	0.114	0.005	0	Goedde et al (1970)
Portugal	36	0.859	0.141	0	0	Fagerhol & Tenfjord (1968)
	189	0.920	0.059	0.023	0	Geada et al (1976)
	330	0.865	0.115	0.018	0	Martin et al (1976)
Greece	504	0.960	0.028	0.002*	0.006	Fertakis et al (1974)
	400	0.959	0.003	0.016	0.013	Kellermann & Walter (1970)
Germany	262	0.967	0.023	0.019	0.010	Goedde et al (1970)
	517	0.879	0.021	0.009	0.090	Kellermann & Walter (1970)
	200	0.980	0.020	0.003	0.003	Kueppers (1971)
	229	0.961	0.024	0.011	0.004	Kuhn & Spielmann (1979)
Italy (North)	202	0.951	0.030	0.010	0.007	Klasen et al (1978)
Poland	3560	0.982	0.016	0.001	0.001	Szczeklik et al (1974)
France						
Normandy	394	0.901	0.066	0.022	0.009	Morin et al (1975)
Lyon	1653	0.902	0.071	0.014	0.004	Arnaud et al (1977a)
Brittany	280	0.896	0.075	0.023	0.004	Sesboue et al (1978)
Other	1520	0.910	0.079	0.006*	0.001	Robinet-Levy & Rieunier (1972)
	934	0.983	0.019	0.001*	0.006	Vandeville et al (1972)
French-Canadians	390	0.892	0.092	0.006	0	Joly et al (1980)
United Kingdom	5237	0.930	0.050	0.014*	0	Cook (1975)
Southern England	926	0.924	0.048	0.022	0.002	Arnaud et al (1979a)
Northern Ireland	1000	0.936	0.039	0.020	0.002	Blundell et al (1975)
Netherlands	708	0.956	0.030	0.005	0.006	Klasen et al (1977)
	1474	0.828	0.016	0.012	0.002	Hoffman & van den Broek (1976) Dijkman et al (1980)
Finland	548	0.966	0.017	0.014	0.002	Arnaud et al (1977b)
	223	0.9955	0	0.005	0	Fagerhol et al (1969)
	300	0.972	0.015	0.013	0	Beckman et al (1980b)
Norway	2830	0.946	0.023	0.016	0.013	Fagerhol (1967)
Sweden	1869	0.981	0.010	0.008	0.0003	Beckman et al (1980b)
Lapps						
Finnish	468	0.996	0.003	0.001	0	Fagerhol et al (1969)
Norwegian	302	0.992	0	0.008	0	Fagerhol et al (1969)
Swedish	217	0.995	0.005	0	0	Beckman et al (1980b)
Canada	426	0.928	0.048	0.016	0	Moroz et al (1976)
	360	0.960	0.036	0.004	0	Ostrow et al (1978)
USA (Whites)	1381	0.937	0.043	0.014	0.001	Lieberman et al (1976b)
	1933	0.948	0.036	0.012	0	Pierce et al (1975)
Japan	100	1.000	0	0	0	Roberts et al (1977)
	1271	1.000	0	0	0	Miyake et al (1979)
Malaysia						
Malaysians†	908	0.979	0.015	0	0	Lie-Injo et al (1978)
Chinese	371	0.981	0.019	0	0	Lie-Injo et al (1978)
Indians	231	0.976	0.024	0	0	Lie-Injo et al (1978)
Blacks						
Mozambique	274	0.982	0.002	0	0.164	Kellerman & Walter (1970)
American	186	0.989	0.008	0	0	Lieberman et al (1976b)
American	204	0.980	0.010	0.005	0	Pierce et al (1975)
Bantu	132	1.000	0	0	0	Vandeville et al (1974)
The Gambia (West Africa)	701	1.000	0	0	0	Welch et al (1980)
New Zealand Maori	487	0.959	0.005	0.035	0.001	Janus et al (1975)
American Indians	230	0.939	0.039	0.004*	0.010	Vandeville et al (1972)
Thailand	852	0.963	0.018	0.011	0.006	Pongpaew & Schelp (1980)

*Pi^Z may be underestimated due to technical limitations
† Pi^X = 0.007

clustering of AAT deficiency in small rural communities in which the populations move relatively little and consanguinity may have played a role. As one travels further north in Europe, the prevalence of Pi^S decreases considerably. The Pi^S gene is absent among Orientals and African Blacks.

2. The Pi^Z allele, in contrast to the Pi^S, has a reduced prevalence in the south of Europe, and also in Lapps from Finland, Norway or Sweden, and among the Dutch from northeast Holland. The Pi^Z is essentially absent in African Blacks, Orientals and Indians. On the other hand, it has an unusually high frequency among the Maoris of New Zealand. Janus et al (1975) discussed the possible association of the high Pi^Z frequency in Maoris with the high incidence of chronic respiratory disease and liver disease in these people. The incidence of cirrhosis and hepatomas in male Maoris ranks third highest in the world, after Polynesian Hawaiian and Hawaii Chinese. Janus and Carrell (1975) performed clinical studies of the diseases found in Maoris with severe AAT deficiency, but studies in heterozygotes have not been reported.

Of all the variants discovered to date, approximately 60 in number (Kamboh 1985), the Pi^Z variant is most commonly associated with deficient serum AAT levels. Studies of diseases associated with specific AAT variants must take into account the prevalence of that variant in the country or area in which the population is being studied, requiring that an appropriate control study be performed.

3. The Pi^F variant has an overall lower frequency than Pi^S or Pi^Z wherever it has been studied, but seems to be essentially missing from Spain and Portugal. Apparent Pi^F AAT bands sometimes appear with old sera, so that the frequency of Pi^F may be overestimated in some studies (Martin et al 1976).

4. The Pi^X allele is quite rare in most populations, but has increased frequency in Malaysians (frequency = 0.007), although it is not present among the Chinese or Indians of the same country (Lie-Injo et al 1978).

5. Subtypes of the normal Pi^M allele have been described, broadening the utilization of AAT as a genetic tool for studying and comparing populations. Five such subtypes are recognized (M1–M5); the currently acceptable terminology labels the fastest moving (toward the anode on isoelectric focusing) as M1, and the slowest moving as M2, with the two intermediate-moving subtypes as M3 and M4. Evidence of a fifth subtype of Pi^M was most recently reported, with the M5 band located between M1 and M3 (Cox et al 1980, Weidinger et al 1985). In spite of an attempt by the International Nomenclature Committee to standardize the Pi^M subtype nomenclature inconsistencies have appeared in the literature, leading to some confusion (Kueppers 1981). Distribution of the various Pi^M subtypes among various populations has been reported worldwide, and has been tabulated in excellent fashion by Kamboh (1985). The only significant regional variations were reported from China, where the frequency of the M2 allele was found to increase from North to South China (Kamboh 1985); in Australia where the M2 allele was found to be high in the Aboriginal population and low in white Australian blood donors and in Vietnamese immigrants (Clark 1982); in the Amerindians of Brazil, where complete absence of the M2 allele and relatively high frequency of the M3 allele was found (Frants & Eriksson 1978); and in the American Black population, where a low frequency of the M2 allele was found (Kueppers 1978).

Molecular structure and function of AAT variants

AAT is an inhibitor of serine proteases in general, but in man its critical targets are the proteases released from polymorphonuclear leucocytes, especially leucocyte elastase and cathepsin G (Travis & Salvesen 1983). The reactive structure of AAT is formed by a methionine amino acid at position 358 located on an exposed loop of the molecule where it attracts and binds the target enzymes (Fig. 71.2) (Owen et al 1983). The enzyme-inhibitor complex remains locked together until it is removed and catabolized within the circulatory system. AAT is therefore a suicidal protein with a normal circulatory life of six days, but whose synthesis can increase dramatically in the acute-phase state.

A single amino acid at the reactive site of the inhibitor determines its specificity. The normal presence of a methionine allows it to fit into the active centre of elastase; the presence of an arginine rather than a methionine converts the inhibitor into an antithrombin (Owen et al 1983) and kallikrein inhibitor (Schapira et al 1985). Replacement of the methionine by valine or leucine also produces a highly effective inhibitor of elastase. However, this replacement causes the inhibitor to be resistant to oxidation and to neutrophil inactivation. These latter types of mutants can be produced through genetic engineering, and are being investigated for their potential prophylactic use, and for treating acute shock syndromes (Welter et al 1986). The shock syndromes are regarded as a fulminant form of neutrophil-induced tissue damage.

The naturally occurring variants of AAT that are associated with AAT deficiency states are also the result of a single amino acid replacement, but not at the reactive site of the inhibitor (Table 71.5). The Z variant has a glutamic acid replaced by a lysine at the S342 site, whereas the S variant has a glutamic acid replaced by a

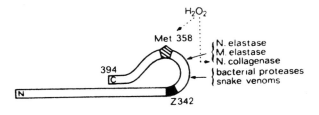

Fig. 71.2 Schematic structure of alpha$_1$-antitrypsin to show the exposed loop containing the reactive centre and hinged near the Z-mutation position 342. The exposed loop is susceptible to proteolytic cleavage, and this provides a physiological and pathological switch enabling the irreversible inactivation of the protein. AAT has a second reversible switch, inasmuch as its reactive-site methionine (Met) can be readily oxidized to give loss of elastase inhibitory activity. The stimulated neutrophil utilizes both switches to nullify inhibitory activity within its immediate environment. Abbreviations: N = neutrophil; M = macrophage. (Printed with permission of Robin W. Carrell and the publishers Journal of Clinical Investigation 78: 1427–1431 (1986).)

valine at the S264 site. The glutamic acids act to stabilize the molecule. Reduced stability of the Pi^S variant contributes to its somewhat low level due to its proteolysis. The blood levels of the Pi^Z variant are more severely reduced because 85% of the newly synthesized inhibitor appears to be blocked in its production within the rough endoplasmic reticulum at a stage just prior to the final processing of its carbohydrate side chains and its entry into the Golgi secretion apparatus. Blockage of Pi^Z appears to be accompanied by its increased proteolytic degradation (Bathurst et al 1984). The retained Pi^Z within the liver gives rise to the hepatocytic globules seen in such livers. Carrell believes that the liver damage is a direct consequence of the intracellular accumulation of the Z variant. He believes that the build-up of Z antitrypsin within the cell represents overloading of the

proteolytic system, with necrosis and cell death occurring in those periportal hepatocytes with the greatest accumulation of material (Hultcrantz & Mengarelli 1984).

The block in the processing of the carbohydrate site chains of the Z variant was detected prior to the discovery of the amino acid replacement (Hercz et al 1978) with sialic acid being reduced from seven residues per molecule in Pi^M to three residues per molecule in Pi^Z from serum, and totally lacking in Pi^Z from liver. Yoshida and Wessels (1978) also found that the sialic acid content varied within the multiple components of the human AAT seen in acid-starch electrophoresis, with the three major components containing eight, seven and six sialic acid residues per molecule respectively.

The Z variant of AAT in the liver has been noted to have a tendency to aggregate (Eriksson & Larsson 1975). Cox et al (1986) showed that the Z protein in plasma also had a tendency to aggregate, possibly contributing to the typical liver inclusions and plasma deficiency of Pi^Z.

Genetic benefits of AAT deficiency

AAT deficiency has been suspected of enhancing reproductive capacity, since penetration of cervical mucus and fertilization of the ovum by spermatozoa involve the enzymatic action of both acrosomal hyaluronidase and proteases. Increased proteolytic activity by sperm or reduced inhibition could increase penetrability of the ovum and thereby increase fertility. The content of proteolytic enzyme inhibitors in cervical mucus also varies with the menstrual cycle, so that the protease inhibitor level is lowest during the female's most fertile interval (Schumacher & Pearl 1965). Thus, an inborn reduction in protease inhibitory activity could enhance the opportunity for sperm penetration and fertilization.

Fagerhol and Gedde-Dahl (1969) found a deficiency of the normal MM × MM genotype combinations in families selected for large family size, suggesting that individuals with AAT variants may have a high fertility. They found that heterozygosity for AAT occurred more frequently among mothers than fathers.

An increased number of individuals with reduced AAT activity were also detected among twins and parents of twins (Lieberman et al 1979); both monozygotic and dizygotic twins had the same prevalence of AAT deficiency. It is possible that both increased fertility and twinning may be heterozygote advantages in AAT deficiency states.

It is of interest that smoking by women is associated with decreased fertility (Ashley 1987). Ashley postulates that the increases in AAT induced by smoking could be responsible for this phenomenon, through the higher levels of AAT in the genital secretions which would

Table 71.5 Amino acid substitutions in variants of AAT

AAT variant	Reference	Pi^M	Amino acid variant
Z	Yoshida et al (1976) Jeppson (1976)	Glutamic acid	Lysine
S	Yoshida et al (1977) Owen & Carrell (1976)	Glutamic acid	Valine
B Alhambra	Yoshida et al (1979a)	Glutamic acid Lysine Pi^{M1}	Aspartic acid Aspartic acid
M2	Yoshida et al (1979b)	Glutamic acid	Aspartic acid

impede fertility. This effect of smoking on fertility would be reversible.

Chromosome localization and structure

The gene controlling AAT synthesis has been localized to chromosome 14 (Cox et al 1982, Darlington et al 1982, Lai et al 1983, Colau et al 1984, Long et al 1984, Schroeder et al 1985, Rabin et al 1986). The specific region on chromosome 14 to which the gene is localized lies between q24.3 and q32.1 (Cox et al 1982). The human chromosomal AAT gene has been cloned (Leicht et al 1982) and used as a hybridization probe; the probe has indicated that the authentic AAT gene resides within the 9.6-kb fragment (Lai et al 1983).

Prenatal detection of AAT deficiency

Before 1984 prenatal diagnosis of AAT deficiency could only be accomplished by Pi typing of fetal blood obtained by fetoscopy during the second trimester of pregnancy (Feppsson et al 1981), since the fetal AAT phenotype is fully expressed in fetal plasma in midpregnancy. The procedure involved passage of the fetoscope through the abdominal wall lateral to the placental margin with puncture, or preferably cannulation, of a large vessel near the insertion of the umbilical cord into the placenta. The technique is potentially hazardous, with a significant risk of fetal loss. Sampling and testing of amniotic fluid only is inappropriate as the amniotic fluid proteins are mainly of maternal origin (Feppsson et al 1981).

With the development of recombinant DNA technology, it became possible to develop synthetic oligonucleotide probes specific to the M and Z alleles (Kidd et al 1983, 1984). The probes hybridise to the area of mutational sequence causing the deficiency; hybridisation is impaired by a single base-pair mismatch between the probe and the AAT allele. Successful use of these probes requires parental samples for comparison, because any clinically silent mutation in the DNA sequence under study would result in a mismatch and an erroneous result. Large quantities of DNA, in the order of $10\,\mu g$, are needed for study, and specific conditions for probe hybridisation are required (Kidd et al 1984).

Another molecular approach which avoids some of the difficulties in the use of oligonucleotide probes involves the use of restriction fragment length polymorphisms (RFLPs) (Hejtmancik et al 1986). A most useful linkage disequilibrium exists between the Z allele and a unique haplotype identified by means of AvaII digests and a 6.5 kilobase AAT probe; a unique Southern blot band pattern, designated 371, is seen exclusively with DNA from PiZZ individuals (Cox & Mansfield 1985, Cox et al

1985, Cox & Billingsley 1986, Cox & Mansfield 1987). Cox and Mansfield (1987) found this unique 371 haplotype in all 32 PiZZ patients studied, but in none of 32 controls. It now appears possible to make a direct prenatal diagnosis of PiZZ AAT deficiency by analysis of fetal DNA, without requiring DNA from parents or sibs. However they recommend that parents and sibs always be studied, as a precaution, since the 371 haplotype might occur with non-Z alleles or the Z allele may produce another haplotype. Other DNA polymorphisms have also been identified; the one with the MaeIII enzyme appears promising especially with chorionic villus sampling (Cox & Billingsley 1986).

But we should consider when, and in whom, neonatal diagnosis of AAT deficiency should be performed. The procedure is usually performed with the concept in mind that a therapeutic abortion would take place should the homozygous defect be detected. With AAT deficiency, however, only a small proportion of deficient individuals encounters major problems in early life, and the later development of lung disease can be modified by avoidance of cigarette smoking and, more recently, through use of synthetic or blood-derived AAT injections (Editorial 1985). However, the development of liver disease in PiZZ children shows a strong positive intrafamilial correlation. If one PiZZ sib has severe liver disease, the risk to a subsequent PiZZ sib may be as high as 40–78% (Psacharopoulos et al 1983, Cox & Mansfield 1987) whereas only 3% of PiZZ infants develop clinical liver disease in general (Sveger 1978). Prenatal diagnosis, therefore, would seem appropriate in families with a history of infant liver disease. Of course there are AAT alleles other than M and Z which could complicate interpretation of DNA polymorphism, suggesting that accurate Pi-typing of parental samples is essential before prenatal diagnosis is ever considered.

Neonatal screening for AAT deficiency

Like prenatal testing for AAT deficiency, the need for neonatal screening has also been debated at some length. Screening programmes have usually employed heel-prick blood collected on filter paper, then assayed for AAT concentration by electroimmunoassay and Pi-typing by isoelectric focusing (Laurell & Sveger 1975, Sveger 1978, O'Brien et al 1978, Dijkman et al 1980). O'Brien et al (1978) screened 107 038 infants by measuring the serum-trypsin-inhibitory-capacity (STIC), finding an incidence of 1 in 5000 with a PiZZ phenotype. It is of interest that 9 of the 21 PiZ infants detected were missed on an initial sample obtained upon the day of discharge from the hospital, but were identified by a sample drawn 4–6 weeks later. Most of these tests could not identify infants with an intermediate AAT deficiency.

The psychological factors involved in such neonatal screening programmes were studied intensively in Sweden (McNeil et al 1985, Thelin et al 1985a,b). Nationwide screening for AAT deficiency had been conducted upon 200 000 newborn in Sweden from November 1972 to September 1974. During this time 171 infants with AAT deficiency were identified, and the genetic type was confirmed at about three months of age. Neonatal screening for AAT deficiency was subsequently discontinued due to negative psychological effects on the parents and the parent-child relationship (McNeil et al 1985). A retrospective investigation of early events and reactions, and a concurrent investigation of long-term effects on the parents, child and family were then conducted. The investigators found that most parents felt that they had received unclear or inadequate information, and that AAT deficiency represented an imminent, serious danger to the child's health (Thelin et al 1985a). Most of the parents reported having immediate negative emotional reactions of worry, anxiety and fear, which were often long-lasting and strong, especially in the mothers. After the initial appointment, however, many of the parents were somewhat relieved about the problem and felt positive about the fact that their child's AAT deficiency had been identified at this age. However they continued to be upset about the repeated blood tests of the child's liver function (Thelin et al 1985b). The parents felt that they should have been informed in advance that analysis for AAT deficiency was to be performed on the same blood sample taken for PKU testing, so that they would have been prepared emotionally for the eventuality of the abnormality being detected.

A screening programme to detect AAT deficiency in older children was undertaken by Lieberman et al in Long Beach, California (1976b). The 13-year-old students and their parents were most receptive of the programme; of the 1841 students, 3.04% of the Caucasians had a PiMZ phenotype. These students and their families were warned against cigarette smoking and exposure to extremes of air pollution (i.e. in employment); no long-term follow-up study was undertaken.

Treatment of AAT deficiency

Replacement therapy

Recent developments have elevated replacement therapy of AAT deficiency to an immediately available, practical level for use in patient care (Boswell & Carrell 1986, Cohen 1986a,b). Two products have been submitted for clinical use; one is isolated from human plasma, and the other is synthesized from an AAT gene introduced into a micro-organism utilizing recombinant DNA methods. The question of to whom these treatments should be made available, and what would constitute proof of efficacy, were addressed at a meeting between the FDA and the Lung Division of the NHLBI and The National Institute of Health. Since proof of efficacy would be exceedingly costly and difficult to procure, it was decided that efficacy would be established if the product raised AAT plasma concentrations to at least those levels found in patients with the MZ phenotype, and if active AAT inhibitor were found in lung-wash fluids of treated patients. It was decided that only patients with the severe ZZ form of AAT deficiency should be treated, but only if smoking were discontinued, and only in those with already demonstrable lung disease.

Blood derived AAT

Coan et al (1985) from The Miles Laboratories in Berkeley, California, described their method for preparing purified AAT from Cohn fraction IV-1. The methods used in the purification were gentle and the resulting product behaved almost identically to AAT from plasma. The protein was heat treated at 60°C for 10 hours to lower the risk of transmission of plasma-borne diseases. Half life studies in animals showed that the protein behaved normally with a half life of 68 hours.

Wewers et al (1987a) evaluated the feasibility, safety, and biochemical efficacy of intermittent infusions of human AAT in the treatment of patients with AAT deficiency. 21 patients were given 60 mg of AAT per kilogram of body weight once a week for up to six months. After a steady state was reached, the trough serum levels for the group was 126 ± 1 mg per decilitre as compared to 30 ± 1 mg per decilitre before treatment, and the levels of anti-elastase activity were equivalent. The AAT level in the epithelial-lining fluid of the lungs rose from $0.46 \pm 0.16 \, \mu M$ before treatment to $1.89 \pm 0.17 \, \mu M$ at six days after infusion ($P < 0.0001$). The only adverse reactions to the 507 infusions were four episodes of self-limited fever. No changes in lung function were observed over the six month treatment period; none were expected. This study demonstrated that infusions of AAT derived from plasma were safe and could reverse the biochemical abnormalities in serum and lung fluid that characterize this disorder. The authors concluded that, together with lifetime avoidance of cigarette smoking, replacement therapy with AAT may be a logical approach to long-term medical treatment.

Wewers et al (1987b) performed a similar study in a patient with the Null-Null phenotype for AAT deficiency with similar results. Their findings demonstrated that AAT provides more than 85% of the antineutrophil elastase protection for the lower respiratory tract, and that this protection can be modulated by the blood levels of AAT.

Recombinant DNA-derived AAT

A genetically engineered version of the AAT protein has been granted orphan drug status by the Food and Drug Administration. The potential value of the gene-cloned products is that the methionine at the reactive centre of AAT can be replaced by valine, protecting it from inactivation by neutrophil oxidants. This type of AAT product would be useful, not only in emphysema patients, but in treatment of the shock lung syndromes associated with massive neutrophil activation (George et al 1984, Rosenberg et al 1984, Janoff et al 1986). The mutant AAT only has a short half life because, by being expressed in yeast, it has no carbohydrate side chains (George et al 1984). Human AAT has also been produced in biologically active forms in *Escherichia coli* (Courtney et al 1984, Tessier et al 1986).

Synthetic elastase inhibitors

Another form of replacement therapy involves the use of potent low-molecular weight elastase-inhibitors. These may have a number of potential advantages in the treatment of pulmonary emphysema, in that a lower concentration of inhibitors in the lung may be required, which could be of importance if direct drug delivery to the lung by inhalation were to become the chosen dosage route (Roberts & Surgenor 1986). These synthetic inhibitors would also have advantages in terms of specificity, ability to inhibit the alpha₂-macroglobulin elastase complex, and stability to cigarette smoke. Alpha₂-macroglobulin does not completely suppress the enzymatic activity of a protease bound to it and may slowly release the free enzyme, acting as a persistent source of elastolytic activity. Inhibition of such bound elastase by the synthetic inhibitors would be another protective avenue not available with the other forms of human AAT replacement. Previous approaches to the treatment of AAT deficiency utilizing synthetic elastase inhibitors were limited by the potential toxicity of the compound when administered over prolonged intervals (Powers et al 1977).

Stimulation of AAT production by the liver

Since AAT is an acute-phase-reactive protein synthesized by the liver, a number of attempts have been made to raise deficient levels of the inhibitor through pharmacological stimulation of protein synthesis by the liver.

Lieberman and Mittman (1973) and Kueppers (1968) studied the ability of diethylstilbesterol and typhoid vaccine respectively to stimulate AAT levels in AAT deficient individuals. Subjects with the MZ phenotype showed half the normal response to these stimuli, but those with the ZZ severe deficiency did not respond at all.

Gadek et al (1980) used the synthetic androgen Danazol (Danol®) and found that it induced the hepatocyte to increase production of various proteins, with AAT levels rising from a mean of 30 mg/dl to 45 mg/dl in individuals with the homozygous Z or MduarteZ phenotypes. The AAT level in one SZ subject rose from 83 mg/dl to 160 mg/dl, indicating that the S variant is more capable of responding to Danazol than is the Z variant; similar observations were made by Lieberman and Mittman with diethylstilbesterol (1973). It was thought that Danazol might prove effective in treating AAT deficiency and further trials were undertaken (Wewers et al 1986). Of 43 Z patients treated with Danazol for one month, 23 (53%) responded with an average increase of AAT concentration of 52% over the pretreatment concentration, without major side-effects. Stanazol, another synthetic androgen, caused minimal increases in serum AAT concentration in seven homozygous patients. Thus, the absolute increase in serum AAT levels resulting from synthetic androgen therapy is minimal, inconsistent among patients, and probably ineffective in protecting lungs from further damage.

Another hormonal agent, Tamoxifen, which binds to intracytoplasmic oestrogen receptors, was also evaluated as a possible means of increasing AAT synthesis and/or secretion (Wewers et al 1987c). Treatment of 30 Z homozygotes with 10 mg twice daily for 30 days produced only minor increases in serum AAT levels far below the level of 80 mg/dl considered 'protective'.

Liver transplantation

Sharp et al (1969) were the first to show that AAT deficiency can be corrected completely by liver transplantation. Unfortunately, few of these patients survived for any length of time, although survival has increased significantly in recent years (Martorana et al 1982b). With liver transplantation, the phenotype of the recipient becomes that of the donor. For individuals with severe liver disease in association with AAT deficiency, a liver transplant may be lifesaving, but the AAT phenotype of the donor should be considered prior to the transplant.

Laboratory methods for detecting AAT deficiency

A laboratory manual has been prepared by Talamo et al (1978) that contains methodology and references for most of the still current procedures used for testing AAT.

Serum protein electrophoresis

Serum protein electrophoresis is a readily available procedure capable of giving a rough estimate of AAT concentration (Lieberman et al 1969). The severe deficiency can be diagnosed directly on the electrophoretic scan. A missing or plateau configuration of the α_1-globulin peak on cellulose-acetate-electrophoresis is usually diagnostic of severe AAT deficiency. An intermediate deficiency state can also be suspected by careful quantitation of the α_1-globulin peak, although this is difficult and inaccurate (Lieberman et al 1969).

Immunological assays

Radial immunodiffusion is most commonly used in clinical laboratories for quantitating serum AAT. The method requires a specific antibody against human AAT, plus accurate standards for quantitation. Electroimmunodiffusion is a more rapid method using similar concepts of antigen-antibody interaction (Laurell 1966).

Enzyme assays

Specific enzyme assays that evaluate AAT activity are more rapid than radial immunodiffusion, but not easier to perform, and do not require standards with each run. Inhibitory capacity for either trypsin or elastase can be measured (Lieberman 1969). To date, no inactive antitrypsin variant has been found, so that the enzyme assays and immunological assays can be used interchangeably. Should an inactive variant of AAT be discovered, then both types of quantitative procedure will be required for its detection.

Problems arise with the quantitative measurements when intermediate (heterozygous) deficiencies are being sought, because the acute-phase-reactive properties of AAT cause its blood levels to fluctuate in response to acute illnesses. The AAT levels in individuals with a severe deficiency do not respond to these stresses, but the levels with an intermediate deficiency can rise into the low normal range.

AAT phenotyping

AAT phenotyping was developed by Fagerhol of Norway (1968). He determined that AAT was a polymorphic protein with molecular variants that had different mobilities on acid-starch gel electrophoresis. With this procedure the AAT protein breaks up into at least five peaks in the acid gradient; these include three major peaks and two minor peaks. The pattern of these peaks is similar for most variants of AAT, but the variants usually differ in their mobility towards the anode. The difference in mobility of these peaks may be due to differences in sialic acid content (Yoshida & Wessels 1978), but each peak retains AAT activity (Langley & Talamo 1975). The major AAT variants have been described above. The location of the major bands for each of the variants are depicted in Figure 71.3 (Cox et al 1980).

Other means have been developed for identifying Pi^z gene carriers utilizing monoclonal antibody specific for this Pi type (Wallmark et al 1984). Antibodies are used in an ELISA procedure permitting easy and accurate identification of such individuals.

Animal models for AAT deficiency

The largest body of literature pertaining to experimental production of emphysema in animals relates to the use of aerosolized proteases. Karlinsky and Snider (1978) reviewed the status of this work in 1978. The two enzymes most effective for producing emphysema in animals are papain and elastase. The emphysema-inducing effect of papain was shown to result from the elastolytic content of the enzyme rather than its esterolytic activity. Papain products lacking the elastolytic activity were not effective for producing experimental emphysema. It appears that the destruction of lung elastin underlies the production of pulmonary emphysema, both in experimental animals and man.

In the hamster, Schuyler et al (1978) employed intravenous pancreatic elastase, producing significant loss of elastic recoil at low volumes, but with normal histology and mean linear intercept of the lungs. These observations suggested that submicroscopic lesions may antedate the earliest morphological evidence of emphysema, resembling ageing in the lung. Larger doses of intravenous elastase caused immediate fatal, haemorrhagic pulmonary oedema.

Martorana et al (1982a) utilized aerosolized papain in dogs in a six month study. The mean linear intercept and internal surface area of the lungs were significantly different in these animals from controls given saline aerosols, but no progression of the changes occurred between three and six months. A significant correlation was found at six months between the anatomical measurements and pulmonary arteriolar pressure and resistance, suggesting that the structural changes of the lung were responsible for pulmonary haemodynamic alterations.

Two other groups of investigators showed that young, growing hamsters are less susceptible to elastase injury than adult hamsters (Lucey & Clark 1982, Martorana et al 1982b). Martorana et al (1982b) believed that alveolar multiplication in the young animals may be responsible for less progression of the emphysematous process.

Another approach to experimental AAT deficiency

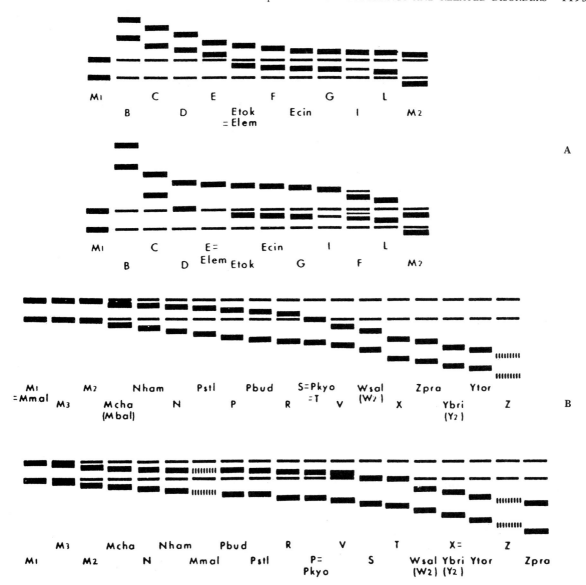

Fig. 71.3 Pi variants showing the two major bands of each variant. Top: acid starch gel electrophoresis. Bottom: isoelectric focusing in acrylamide. Narrow bands indicate position of M1. Dashed bands indicate deficiency alleles; **A** variants anodal to M; **B** variants cathodal to M. (From Cox et al (1980) with permission of the author and publisher.)

was undertaken by Blackwood et al (1979) who administered D-galactosamine to rats intraperitoneally. The rats developed a transient reduction in serum elastase inhibitory capacity, thereby enhancing the development of emphysema from intravenous injections of pancreatic elastase. The severity of the emphysema correlated with the trypsin and elastase-inhibitory capacities at the time of the elastase injection. Bolmer and Kleinerman (1987) found that rats treated with galactosamine had AAT containing 2–3 fewer moles of sialic acid, three fewer moles of neutral sugar, and two fewer moles of amino sugar per mole of anti-protease than AAT from controls. These alterations were similar to those seen in humans with genetically determined AAT deficiency.

GENETIC VARIATION IN PROTEASE CONTENT OF LEUCOCYTES

Studies with AAT indicate that an imbalance of the protease-inhibitor levels can result in damage to lung tissue and the development of pulmonary emphysema. A logical extension of the AAT investigations, therefore, would be a study of leucocytic protease relationships to the pathogenesis of pulmonary emphysema. Galdston et al (1973) measured the leucocyte lysosomal elastase-like esterase in family members of two AAT deficient probands and in 12 control subjects with normal AAT and free of lung disease. Two levels of elastase activity were found among the family members; one level like that in the control group and the other, one-half this level. The investigators interpreted this to mean that the lower level of leucocytic elastase activity reflected a genetic variation that was protective for some members with reduced AAT. In other words, normal elastase-like esterase was associated with an unfavourable clinical course in the presence of intermediate or low AAT (Galdston et al 1973, 1977). In a subsequent study Galdston et al (1977) reported that individuals with chronic obstructive pulmonary disease, of either MM, MZ or ZZ phenotypes, differed from healthy controls of the same Pi types by having greater mean leucocyte-lysosomal elastase-like activity than controls of the same Pi types without lung disease. The individuals with lung disease also had a greater number of polymorphonuclear leucocytes and a history of having smoked a greater number of cigarettes within their lifetimes. However, in these individuals the elastase-like activity was unrelated to the number of leucocytes, suggesting that the enzyme level was an associated variable of COPD and not necessarily a result of the disease.

Later Galdstone et al (1979) suggested that more elastase becomes bound to alpha$_2$-macroglobulin (α_2M) when antitrypsin is deficient, and that elastase bound to α_2M retains some of its elastolytic activity. Thus, in the presence of normal M serum, only about 6% of the neutrophil elastase activity is retained towards elastin, whereas approximately 12% of the activity is retained in the presence of Z serum. The authors postulated that increased binding of elastase to α_2M when AAT is deficient may increase the turnover of soluble elastin and contribute to lung damage.

Lam et al (1979) also found greater neutrophil-elastase content in patients with abnormal lung function and a PiMZ phenotype than in those with normal lung function and the same Pi type. They concluded that the neutrophil elastase content was a significant risk factor in MZ deficient subjects, and that neutrophil elastase and smoking interact to produce abnormal lung function in PiMZ subjects.

A slightly different concept was suggested by Martin and Taylor (1979) who had examined 71 patients with COPD and 46 healthy controls. They found that leucocytic elastase activity from patients with lung disease interacted abnormally with AAT so that increased residual activity was present despite adequate amounts of AAT for total inhibition. This was seen in 33 of 71 patients with COPD, as compared to 6 of 46 normal control subjects. This observation is somewhat similar to Galdston's findings of an increased reaction with α_2M and increased residual elastase activity when AAT is deficient.

Kramps et al (1980) found higher leucocyte elastase-like activity in 16 PiMM patients with emphysema than in healthy control subjects. These authors concluded that increased levels of leucocyte elastase may be a contributing factor in persons without AAT deficiency, but not in persons with AAT deficiency. In contrast, Abboud et al (1979) did not find significant differences in mean lysosomal elastase or protease activity between COPD patients and controls with normal AAT, although a few of their COPD patients did have higher concentrations of neutrophil-elastase. In patients with AAT deficiency however, both the elastase and protease content per 10^8 neutrophils was significantly higher in homozygous and heterozygous Pi^Z COPD patients as compared to normal subjects and PiM COPD patients. Abboud et al concluded that the concentration of neutrophil elastase and protease may be an important risk factor in patients with Z or MZ phenotypes and in a few patients with M phenotype.

Despite this number of supportive, though somewhat contradictory reports, a number of negative reports were also published. Klayton et al (1975) measured a series of leucocyte enzymes and found none of them to be associated with the development of COPD or with smoking history in heterozygotes, but they did find that cigarette smoking was a significant determinant of the development of COPD in heterozygotes. Similarly, Taylor and Kueppers (1977) found no differences in concentration of leucocytic elastase between patients with COPD and controls, but they found an almost fourfold increase in the prevalence of a slow electrophoretic type of elastase in the COPD patients. They concluded that there may be a qualitative rather than a quantitative difference in elastase which could play a role in the pathogenesis of COPD in patients with normal AAT phenotypes.

One can conclude from these studies that there is some significance to variation in leucocyte elastase activity that may play a role in the pathogenesis of pulmonary disease. Additional work in this area is indicated.

LEUCOCYTE CHEMOTACTIC FACTOR INACTIVATOR

Normal human serum contains an inactivator of chemotactic factors for neutrophil leucocytes (Berenberg & Ward 1973). Ward and Talamo (1973) found that human serum deficient in AAT was also deficient in this naturally occurring chemotatic-factor-inactivator. The serum-donors with this combined deficiency all had severe pulmonary emphysema. The deficiency of chemotactic-factor-inactivator was not observed in patients with clinically similar pulmonary disease who had normal AAT.

Ward and Talamo (1973) did not believe that AAT and chemotactic-factor-inactivator are identical, since AAT works by binding to the enzymes in stoichiometric fashion whereas the chemotactic-factor-inactivator appears to destroy the chemotactic factor in an enzymatic manner. Thus, according to Ward and Talamo, our concepts of how AAT deficiency works in predisposing to pulmonary emphysema should be modified to take into account a deficiency of the chemotactic-factor-inactivator.

Grady et al (1979) suggest that proteases themselves may have chemotactic activity. They found that a variety of inhibitors of serine-proteases and also protease substrates inhibit chemotaxis of human polymorphonuclear leucocytes in addition to inhibiting the esterase activity of these cells. They claim that serine-protease-activity may function during induction of chemotaxis, so that inhibition of enzyme activity also inhibits chemotaxis. This information could shed more light on the association of AAT with a deficiency of chemotactic-factor-inactivator, but implicates AAT as playing the role of a chemotactic-factor-inactivator contrary to the beliefs of Ward and Talamo.

Lam et al (1980) also measured the serum chemotactic-factor-inactivator in 22 subjects with chronic airflow obstruction and in 19 healthy subjects with PiM and PiMZ phenotypes. They observed that subjects with chronic airflow obstruction had significantly lower chemotactic-factor-inactivator activity than normal subjects, irrespective of the AAT phenotype. However, the lowest levels were found in those with chronic airflow obstruction and a PiZZ phenotype. Lam et al (1980) believe that the deficiency of serum chemotactic-factor-inactivator may be important in the pathogenesis of chronic airflow obstruction, particularly in those with severe AAT deficiency.

REFERENCES

Aagenaes O, Matlary A, Elgjo K, Munthe E, Fagerhol M 1972 Neonatal cholestasis in alpha₁-antitrypsin deficient children. Acta Paediatrica Scandinavica 61: 632–642

Aarskog D, Fagerhol M L 1970 Protease inhibitor (Pi) phenotypes in chromosome abberrations. Journal of Medical Genetics 7: 367–370

Aarskog D, Aarseth P, Fagerhol M K 1978 Alpha₁-antitrypsin (Pi) types in recurrent miscarriages. Clinical Genetics 13: 81–84

Abboud R T, Rushton J M, Grzybowski S 1979 Interrelationships between neutrophil elastase, serum alpha₁-antitrypsin, lung function and chest radiography in patients with chronic airflow obstruction. American Review of Respiratory Disease 120: 31–40

Abboud R T, Johnson A J, Richter A M, Elwood R K 1983 Comparison of in vitro neutrophil elastase release in nonsmokers and smokers. American Review of Respiratory Disease 128: 507–510

Abboud R T, Richter A N, Fera T, Johal S 1984 Is α₁-protease inhibitor inactivated by smoking? Science 224: 755–756

Abboud R T, Fera T, Richter A, Tabona M Z, Johal S 1985 Acute effect of smoking on the functional activity of alpha₁-protease inhibitor in bronchoalveolar lavage fluid. American Review of Respiratory Disease 131: 79–85

Abramowsky C R, Cebelin M, Choudury A, Izant R J 1980 Undifferentiated (embryonal) sarcoma of the liver with alpha₁-antitrypsin deposits: Immunohistochemical and ultrastructural studies. Cancer 45: 3108–3113

Alagille D 1984 Alpha₁-antitrypsin deficiency. Hepatology 4: 11S–14S

Ananthakrishnan R, Biegler B, Dennis P M 1979 Alpha₁-antitrypsin phenotypes in paraproteinaemias. Lancet 1: 561–562

Andre F, Andre C, Lambert R, Descos F 1974 Prevalence of alpha₁-antitrypsin deficiency in patients with gastric or duodenal ulcer. Biomedicine 21: 222–224

Arnaud P, Cellier C C, Vittoz P, Creyssel R 1977a Alpha₁-antitrypsin (Pi) phenotypes in a Finnish population. Scandinavian Journal of Clinical and Laboratory Investigation 37: 339–343

Arnaud P Koistinen J, Wilson G B, Fudenberg H H 1977b Alpha₁-antitrypsin (Pi) phenotypes in a Finnish population Scandinavian Journal of Clinical and Laboratory Investigation 37: 339–343

Arnaud P, Galbraith R M, Faulk W P, Ansell B M 1977c Increased frequency of the MZ phenotype of alpha₁-protease inhibitor in juvenile chronic polyarthritis. Journal of Clinical Investigation 69: 1442–1444

Arnaud P, Galbraith R M, Faulk W P, Black C 1979a Pi phenotypes of alpha₁-antitrypsin in Southern England: Identification of M subtypes and implications for genetic studies. Clinical Genetics 15: 406–410

Arnaud P, Galbraith R M, Faulk W P, Black C, Hughes G V 1979b Alpha$_1$-antitrypsin in adult rheumatoid arthritis. Lancet I: 1236–1237

Arora P K, Miller H C, Aronson L D 1978 α-antitrypsin is an effector of immunological stasis. Nature 274: 589–590

Ashley M J 1987 Smoking, Alpha-1-antitrypsin and decreased fertility in women. Medical Hypotheses 22: 277–285

Ashley M J, Corey P, Chan-Yeung M 1980 Smoking, dust exposure, and serum alpha$_1$-antitrypsin. American Review of Respiratory Disease 121: 783–788

Bagdasarian A, Colman R W 1978 Subcellular localization and purification of platelet α_1-antitrypsin. Blood 51: 139–156

Bathurst I C, Travis J, George P M, Carrell P M, Carrell R W 1984 Structural and functional characterization of the abnormal Z alpha 1-antitrypsin isolated from human liver. FEBS Letters 177: 179–183

Baumstark J S, Lee C T, Luby R J 1977 Rapid inactivation of α_1-protease (α_1-antitrypsin) by elastase. Biochimica et Biophysica Acta 482: 400–411

Beckman G, Beckman L, Liden S 1980a Association between psoriasis and the α_1-antitrypsin deficiency gene Z. Acta Dermatovenereologica 60: 163–164

Beckman G, Backman L, Nordenson I 1980b, Alpha$_1$-antitrypsin phenotypes in Northern Sweden. Human Heredity 30: 129–135

Benitez-Bribiesca L B, Horta R F 1978 Immunofluorescent localization of alpha$_1$-antitrypsin in human polymorphonuclear leucocytes. Life Science 21: 99–104

Benitez-Bribiesca L B, Attias J L, de la Vega G 1972 Pemphigus vulgaris associated with alpha$_1$-antitrypsin deficiency. Sobretiro de Patologia X: 41–48

Berenberg J L, Ward P A 1973 Chemotactic factor inactivator in normal human serum. Journal of Clinical Investigation 52: 1200–1206

Berninger R W, DeLellis R A, Kaplan M M 1985 Liver disease and the Pi Elemberg M phenotype of alpha$_1$-antitrypsin. American Journal of Clinical Pathology 83: 503–506

Bierman H R, Kelly K H, Cordes F L 1955 The sequestration and visceral circulation of leucocytes in man. Annals of the New York Academy of Sciences 59: 850–862

Blackwood R A, Cerreta J M, Mandl I, Turino G M 1979 Alpha$_1$-antitrypsin deficiency and increased susceptibility to elastase-induced experimental emphysema in a rat model. American Review of Respiratory Disease 120: 1375–1379

Blenkinsopp W K 1978 Alpha$_1$-antitrypsin bodies Pi^Z phenotype, and peptic ulcer. Gut 19: 157–158

Bloom J W, Hunter M J 1978 Interactions of α_1-antitrypsin with trypsin and chymotrypsin. Journal of Biological Chemistry 253: 547–559

Blue M L, Janoff A 1978 Possible mechanisms of emphysema in cigarette smokers. Release of elastase from human polymorphonuclear leucocytes by cigarette smoke condensate in vitro. American Review of Respiratory Disease 117: 317–325

Blundell G, Frazer A, Cole R B, Nevin N C 1975 Alpha$_1$-antitrypsin phenotypes in Northern Ireland. Annals of Human Genetics 38: 289–294

Bolmer S D, Kleinerman J 1987 Galactosamine-induced α_1-antitrypsin deficiency in rats. Alterations in plasma glycoproteins and α_1-antitrypsin carbohydrate compositions. American Journal of Pathology 126: 209–219

Boswell D R, Carrell R 1986 α_1-antitrypsin: Molecules and medicine. A meeting report. TIBS 11: 102–103

Brackertz D, Kueppers F 1977 Alpha-1-antitrypsin phenotypes in rheumatoid arthritis. Lancet 2: 934–935

Bradfied J W B, Blenkinsopp W K 1977 Alpha-2-antitrypsin globules in the liver and PiM phenotype. Journal of Clinical Pathology 30: 464–466

Bradfield J W B, Wells M 1978 Liver disease caused by lysosomal enzymes released from Kupffer cells. Lancet 1: 836

Brandrup F, Ostergaard P A 1978 α_1-antitrypsin deficiency associated with persistent cutaneous vasculitis. Archives of Dermatology 114: 921–924

Brewerton D A, Webley M, Murphy A H, Ward A M 1978 The α_1-antitrypsin phenotype MZ in acute anterior uveitis. Lancet 1: 1103

Bridges R B, Kimmerl D A, Wyatt R J, Rehm S R 1985 Serum antiproteases in smokers and nonsmokers. Relationships to smoking status and pulmonary function. American Review of Respiratory Disease 132: 1162–1169

Brown J H, Pollock S H 1970 Inhibition of elastase and collagenase by anti-inflammatory drugs. Proceedings of the Society for Experimental Biology and Medicine 135: 792–795

Brown W T, Mamelok A E, Bearn A G 1979 Anterior uveitis and alpha$_1$-antitrypsin. Lancet 2: 644

Bruce R M, Cohen B H, Diamond E L et al 1984 MS collaborative study to assess risk of lung disease in PiMZ phenotype subjects. American Review of Respiratory Disease 130: 386–390

Buisseret P D, Penbrey M E, Lessof M H 1977 α_1-antitrypsin phenotypes in rheumatoid arthritis and ankylosing spondylitis. Lancet 2: 1358–1359

Buist A S, Sexton G J, Azzam A M H, Adams B-E 1979 Pulmonary function in heterozygotes for alpha$_1$-antitrypsin deficiency: A case control study. American Review of Respiratory Disease 120: 759–766

Campra J L, Craig J R, Peters R L, Reynold T B 1973 Cirrhosis associated with partial deficiency of alpha$_1$-antitrypsin in an adult. Annals of Internal Medicine 78: 233–238

Carlson J, Eriksson S, Hagerstrand I 1981 Intra- and extracellular alpha$_1$-antitrypsin in liver disease with special reference to Pi phenotypes. Journal of Clinical Pathology 34: 1020–1025

Carp H, Janoff A 1978 Possible mechanisms of emphysema in smokers. In vitro suppression of serum elastase-inhibitory capacity by fresh cigarette smoke and its prevention by antioxidants. American Review of Respiratory Disease 118: 617–621

Carrell R W 1986 α_1-antitrypsin. Molecular pathology, leukocytes, and tissue damage. Journal of Clinical Investigation 78: 1427–1431

Carrell R W, Owen M C 1976 α_1-antitrypsin: Structure, variation and disease. Essays in Medical Biochemistry 4: 83–119

Carrico R J, Lieberman J, Yeager F 1976 The source of a minor alpha$_1$-antitrypsin in variant serum. American Review of Respiratory Disease 114: 53–57

Casterline C L, Evans R, Battista V C, Talamo R C 1978 Selective IgA deficiency and Pi ZZ-antitrypsin deficiency. Chest 73: 885–886

Chan C H, Steer C J, Vergalla J, Jones E A 1978 Alpha$_1$-antitrypsin deficiency with cirrhosis associated with the protease inhibitor phenotype SZ. American Journal of Medicine 65: 978–986

Chan-Yeung M, Ashley M J, Corey P, Maledy H 1978 Pi

phenotypes and the prevalence of chest symptoms and lung function abnormalities in workers employed in dusty industries. American Review of Respiratory Disease 117: 239–245

Chapuis-Cellier C, Arnaud P 1979 Preferential transmission of the Z deficient allele of α_1-antitrypsin. Science 205: 407–408

Christen H, Bau J, Halsband H 1975 Hereditary alpha$_1$-antitrypsin deficiency associated with congenital extrahepatic bile duct hypoplasia. Klinische Wochenschrift 53: 90–91

Clark P 1982 Alpha-1-protease inhibitor phenotypes in Australia. Human Heredity 32: 225–227

Clemmensen I, Christensen F 1976 Inhibition of urokinase by complex formation with human α_1-antitrypsin. Biochimica et Biophysica Acta 429: 591–599

Coan M H, Brockway W J, Equizabal H, Krieg T, Fournel M 1985 Preparation and properties of alpha$_1$-proteinase inhibitor concentrate from human plasma. Vox Sang 48: 333–342

Cohen A B 1979 Opportunities for the development of specific therapeutic agents to treat emphysema. American Review of Respiratory Disease 120: 723–727

Cohen A B 1986a Editorial The clinical usefulness of different forms of alpha-1-protease inhibitor. American Review of Respiratory Disease 133: 349–350

Cohen A B 1986b Unraveling the mysteries of alpha$_1$-antitrypsin. New England Journal of Medicine 314: 778–779

Colau B, Chuchana P, Bollen A 1984 Revised sequence of full-length complementary DNA coding for human α_1-antitrypsin. DNA 3: 327–330

Cook P J L 1975 The genetics of α_1-antitrypsin: a family study in England and Scotland. Annals of Human Genetics 38: 275–287

Courtney M, Buchwalder A, Tessier L-H et al 1984 High-level production of biologically active human α_1-antitrypsin in Escherichia coli. Proceedings of the National Academy of Sciences 81: 669–673

Cox D W 1975 Deficiency allele of α_1-antitrypsin PiMmalton (abstract). American Journal of Human Genetics 27: 29A

Cox D W 1980 Transmission of Z allele from heterozygotes for α_1-antitrypsin deficiency. American Journal of Human Genetics 32: 455–457

Cox D W, Billingsley G D 1984 Oxidation of plasma alpha$_1$-antitrypsin in smokers and nonsmokers and by an oxidizing agent. American Review of Respiratory Disease 130: 594–599

Cox D W, Billingsley G D 1986 Restriction enzyme MaeIII for prenatal diagnosis of α_1-antitrypsin deficiency. Lancet 2: 741–742

Cox D W, Huber O 1976 Rheumatoid arthritis and α_1-antitrypsin. Lancet 1: 1216–1217

Cox D W, Huber O 1980 Association of severe rheumatoid arthritis with heterozygosity for alpha$_1$-antitrypsin deficiency. Clinical Genetics 17: 153–160

Cox D, Levison H 1988 Emphysema of early onset associated with a complete deficiency of α_1-antitrypsin (null homozygotes). American Review of Respiratory Disease 137: 371–375

Cox D W, Mansfield T 1985 Prenatal diagnosis for alpha$_1$-antitrypsin deficiency. Lancet 1: 230

Cox D W, Mansfield T 1987 Prenatal diagnosis of α_1-antitrypsin deficiency and estimates of fetal risk for disease. Journal of Medical Genetics 24: 52–59

Cox D W, Smyth S 1983 Risk for liver disease in adults with alpha$_1$-antitrypsin deficiency. American Journal of Medicine 74: 221–227

Cox D W, Johnson A M, Fagerhol M K 1980 Report of nomenclature meeting for α_1-antitrypsin. Human Genetics 53: 429–433

Cox D W, Markovic V D, Teshima I E 1982 Genes for immunoglobulin heavy chains and for α_1-antitrypsin are localized to specific regions of chromosome 14q. Nature 297: 428–430

Cox D W, Woo S L C, Mansfield T 1985 DNA restriction fragments associated with α_1-antitrypsin indicate a single origin for deficiency allele piZ. Nature 316: 79–81

Cox D W, Billingsley G D, Callahan J W 1986 Aggregation of plasma Z type α_1-antitrypsin suggests basic defect for the deficiency. FEBS Letters 205: 255–260

Darlington G J, Astrin K H, Muirhead S P, Desnick R J, Smith M 1982 Assignment of human α_1-antitrypsin to chromosome 14 by somatic cell hybrid analysis. Proceedings of the National Academy of Sciences 79: 870–873

Dickinson P, Zinneman H H, Swaim W R, Doe R P, Seal U S 1969 Effects of testosterone treatment on plasma proteins and amino acids in men. Journal of Clinical Endocrinology and Metabolism 29: 837–841

Dijkman J H, Penders T J, Kramps J A, Sonderkamp H J A, van den Broek W G M, ter Haar B G A 1980 Epidemiology of alpha$_1$-antitrypsin deficiency in the Netherlands. Human Genetics 53: 409–413

Doeglas H M G, Bleumink E 1975 Protease inhibitors in plasma of patients with chronic urticaria. Archives of Dermatology III: 979–985

Eberle V F, Assmus C, Martino G A 1979a Familie mit multipler endokriver Adenomatose (MEA, Type I) und einigen zustatzlichen Besonderheiten alpha-1-antitrypsinmangel. Klinische Wochenschrift 57: 499–509

Eberle V F, Adler G, Kern H F, Martini G A 1979b Polypoid gastric heterotopy of the small intestine in a patient with primary hyperparathyroidism and alpha$_1$-antitrypsin deficiency belonging to a MEA-family. Zeitschrift fur Gastroenterologie 1: 354–365

Editorial 1985 Treatment for α_1-antitrypsin deficiency. Lancet ii: 812–813

Eriksson S 1964 Pulmonary emphysema and alpha$_1$-antitrypsin deficiency. Acta Medica Scandinavica 175: 197–205

Eriksson S 1965 Studies in α_1-antitrypsin deficiency. Acta Medica Scandinavica 177: Supplementum 432, p 85

Eriksson S 1978 Proteases and protease inhibitors in chronic obstructive lung disease. Acta Medica Scandinavica 203: 449–455

Eriksson S, Larsson C 1975 Purification and partial characterization of PAS-positive inclusion bodies from the liver in alpha-1-antitrypsin deficiency. New England Journal of Medicine 292: 176–180

Eriksson S, Moestrup T, Hagerstrand I 1975 Liver, lung and malignant disease in heterozygous (PiMZ) α_1-antitrypsin deficiency. Acta Medica Scandinavica 198: 243–247

Eriksson S, Lindell S-E, Wiberg R 1985 Effects of smoking and intermediate α_1-antitrypsin deficiency (PiMZ) on lung function. European Journal of Respiratory Disease 67: 279–285

Eriksson S, Carlson J, Velez R 1986 Risk of cirrhosis and primary liver cancer in alpha$_1$-antitrypsin deficiency. New England Journal of Medicine 314: 736–739

Evans H E, Keller S, Mandl I 1972 Serum trypsin inhibitory capacity and the idiopathic respiratory distress syndrome.

Journal of Pediatrics 81: 588–592

Fagerhol M K 1967 Serum Pi types in Norwegians. Acta Pathologica et Microbiologica Scandinavica 70: 421–428

Fagerhol M K 1968 The Pi system. Genetic variants of serum. Series Haematologica 1: 153–161

Fagerhol M K 1976 The genetics of alpha₁-antitrypsin and its implications. Postgraduate Medical Journal 52, Supplement 2: 73–83

Fagerhol M K, Gedde-Dahl T 1969 Genetics of the Pi serum types. Human Heredity 19: 354–359

Fagerhol M K, Tenfjord O W 1968 Serum Pi types in some European, American, Asian and African populations. Acta Pathologica et Microbiologica Scandinavica 72: 601–608

Fagerhol M K, Eriksson A W, Monn E 1969 Serum Pi types in some Lappish and Finnish populations. Human Heredity 19: 360–364

Falk G A, Smith J P 1971 Chronic bronchitis: A seldom noted manifestation of homozygous alpha₁-antitrypsin deficiency. Chest 60: 166–169

Fallat R J, Powell M R, Kueppers F, Lilker E 1973 ¹³³Xe ventilatory studies in α_1-antitrypsin deficiency. Journal of Nuclear Medicine 14: 5–13

Feppsson J O, Cordesius E, Gustavii B, Lofberg L, Franzen B, Stromberg P, Sveger T 1981 Prenatal diagnosis of alpha₁-antitrypsin deficiency by analysis of fetal blood obtained at fetoscopy. Pediatric Research 15: 154–256

Fertakis A, Tsourapas A, Douratsos D, Angelopoulos B 1974 Pi phenotypes in Greeks. Human Heredity 24: 313–316

Fineman R M, Kidd K K, Johnson A M, Breg W R 1976 Increased frequency of heterozygotes for α_1-antitrypsin variants in individuals with either sex chromosome mosaicism of trisomy 21. Nature 260: 320–321

Fisher R L, Taylor L, Sherlock S 1976 α_1-antitrypsin deficiency in liver disease: The extent of the problem. Gastroenterology 71: 646–651

Frants R R, Eriksson A W 1978 Reliable classification of six PiM subtypes by separator isoelectric focusing. Human Heredity 28: 201–209

Frants R R, Eriksson A W 1980 Pi M subtypes of α_1-antitrypsin in isolate studies. In: Eriksson A W, Forsius H R, Nevanlinna H R, Workman P L, Norio R K (eds). Population Structure and Genetic Disorders. Academic Press, London, p 199–210

Freeman H J, Weinstein W M, Shnitka T K, Crockford P M, Herbert F A 1976 Alpha₁-antitrypsin deficiency and pancreatic fibrosis. Annals of Internal Medicine 85: 73–76

Gadek J E, Fells G A, Crystal R G 1979 Cigarette smoking induces functional antiprotease deficiency in the lower respiratory tract of humans. Science 206: 1315–1316

Gadek J E, Fulmer J D, Gelfand J A, Frant M M, Petty T L, Crystal R G 1980 Danazol-induced augmentation of serum α_1-antitrypsin levels in individuals with marked deficiency of this antiprotease. Journal of Clinical Investigation 66: 82–87

Galdston M, Janoff A, Davis A L 1973 Familial variation of leukocyte lysosomal protease and serum α_1-antitrypsin as determinants in chronic obstructive pulmonary disease. American Review of Respiratory Disease 107: 718–727

Galdston M, Melnick E L, Goldring R M, Levytska V, Curasi C A, Davis A L 1977 Interactions of neutrophil elastase, serum trypsin inhibitory activity, and smoking history as risk factors for chronic obstructive pulmonary disease in patients with MM, MZ and ZZ phenotypes for alpha₁-

antitrypsin. American Review of Respiratory Disease 116: 837–846

Galdston M, Levytska V, Leener I E, Twumasi D Y 1979 Degradation of tropelastin and elastin substrates by human neutrophil elastase, free and bound to alpha₂-macroglobulin in serum of the M and Z (Pi) phenotypes for alpha₁-antitrypsin. American Review of Respiratory Disease 119: 435–441

Geada H M, Albino J P, Manso C 1976 Polymorphism of α_1-antitrypsin in a Portuguese population. Human Genetics 32: 109–113

Gedde-Dahl T, Fagerhol M K, Cook P J L, Noades J 1972 Autosomal linkage between the Gm and Pi loci in man. Annals of Human Genetics 35: 393–399

Gedde-Dahl T, Cook P J, Fagerhol M K, Pierce J A 1975 Improved estimate of the Gm-Pi linkage. Annals of Human Genetics 39: 43–50

Geddes D M, Webley M, Brewerton D A 1977 α_1-antitrypsin phenotypes in fibrosing alveolitis and rheumatoid arthritis. Lancet 2: 1049–1051

Gelfand E W, Cox D W, Lin M T, Dosch H M 1979 Severe combined immune-deficiency disease in patients with α_1-antitrypsin deficiency. Lancet 2: 202

George P M, Travis J, Vissers M C M, Winterbourn C C, Carrell R W 1984 A genetically engineered mutant of α_1-antitrypsin protects connective tissue from neutrophil damage and may be useful in lung disease. Lancet 2: 1426–1428

Gitlin D, Perricelli A 1970 Synthesis of serum albumin, prealbumin, alpha feroprotein, alpha₁-antitrypsin and transferrin by the human yolk sac. Nature 228: 995–997

Glaser C B, Karic L, Fallat R J, Stockert R 1977 Alpha₁-antitrypsin. Plasma survival studies in the rat of the normal and homozygous deficient forms. Biochemica et Biophysica Acta 495: 87–92

Glaser C B, Busby T F, Ingham K C, Childs A 1983 Thermal denaturation of alpha₁-protease inhibitor. Stabilization by neutral salts and sugars. American Review of Respiratory Disease 128: 77–81

Glasgow A H, Cooperband S R, Schmid K, Parker J T, Occhino J C, Mannick J A 1971 Inhibition of secondary immune responses by immunoregulatory alphaglobulin. Transplantation Proceedings III: 835–837

Goedde H W, Benkmann H G, Christ I, Singh S, Hirth L 1970 Gene frequencies of red cell adenosine deaminase adenylate kinase, phosphoglucomutase, acid phosphatase and serum α_1-antitrypsin (Pi) in a German population. Humangenetik 10: 235–243

Goetz I E, Weinstein C, Roberts E 1972 Effects of protease inhibitors on growth of hamster tumour cells in culture. Cancer Research 32: 2469–2474

Gordon H W, Dixon J, Rogers J C, Mittman C, Lieberman J 1972 Alpha₁-antitrypsin accumulation in livers of emphysematous patients with α_1-AT deficiency. Human Pathology 3: 361–370

Grady P G, Davis A T, Shapira E 1979 The effect of some protease substrates and inhibitors on chemotaxis and protease activity of human polymorphonuclear leucocytes. Journal of Infectious Diseases 140: 999–1003

Greenwald A J, Johnson D S, Oskvig R M, Aschenbrener C A, Randa D C 1975 α_1-antitrypsin deficiency, emphysema, cirrhosis, and intestinal mucosal atrophy. Journal of the American Medical Association 231: 273–276

Halal F, Scriver C R, Cox D W, Jaber L, Varsano I 1979 Cystathionuria, renal iminoglycinuria and α_1-antitrypsin deficiency in the same family: relevance in medical practice. CMA Journal 121: 64–67

Heck L W, Kaplan A P 1974 Substrates of Hageman factor. I. Isolation and characterization of human factor XI (PTA) and inhibition of the activated enzyme of α_1-antitrypsin. Journal of Experimental Medicine 140: 1615–1630

Hejtmancik J F, Ward P A, Mansfield T, Sifers R N, Harris S, Cox D W 1986 Prenatal diagnosis of α_1-antitrypsin deficiency by restriction fragment length polymorphisms, and comparison with oligonucleotide probe analysis. Lancet 2: 767–769

Hercz A, Katona E, Cutz E, Wilson J R, Barton M 1978 α_1-antitrypsin: The presence of excess mannose in the Z variant isolated from liver. Science 201: 1229–1232

Hinman L M, Stevens C A, Matthay R A, Gee J B L 1980 Elastase and lysozyme activities in human alveolar macrophages. Effects of cigarette smoking. American Review of Respiratory Disease 121: 263–271

Hoffman J J M L, van den Broek W G M 1976 Distribution of alpha$_1$-antitrypsin phenotypes in two Dutch population groups. Human Genetics 32: 43–48

Hood J M, Koep L J, Peters R L, Schroter G P J, Weil R, Redeker A G, Starzl T E 1980 Liver transplantation for advanced liver disease with alpha$_1$-antitrypsin deficiency. New England Journal of Medicine 302: 272–275

Horne S L, Tennent R K, Cockcroft D W, Cotton D J, Dosman J A 1986 Pulmonary function in Pi M MZ grainworkers. Chest 89: 795–799

Horton F O, Mackenthun A V, Anderson P S, Patterson C D, Mannarsten J F 1980 Alpha$_1$-antitrypsin heterozygotes (Pi type MZ). A longitudinal study of the risk of development of chronic air flow limitation. Chest 77: 261–263

Hultcrantz R, Mengarelli S 1984 Ultrastructural liver pathology in patients with minimal liver disease and alpha-1-antitrypsin deficiency. A comparison between heterozygous and homozygous patients. Hepatology 4: 937–945

Iammarino R M, Wagener D K, Allen R C 1979 Segregation distortion of the α_1-antitrypsin Pi Z allele. American Journal of Human Genetics 31: 508–517

Ishibashi H, Shibata K, Okubo H, Tsuda-kawamura K, Yanase T 1978 Distribution of α_1-antitrypsin in normal granuloma, and tumor tissues in rats. Journal of Laboratory and Clinical Medicine 91: 575–583

Janoff A, Carp H 1977 Possible mechanisms of emphysema in smokers. Cigarette smoke condensate suppresses protease inhibition in vitro. American Review of Respiratory Disease 116: 65–72

Janoff A, Chan S-K 1984 Is α_1-protease inhibitor inactivated by smoking? Science 224: 775 (letter)

Janoff A, Dearing R 1980 Prevention of elastase-induced experimental emphysema by oral administration of a synthetic elastase inhibitor. American Review of Respiratory Disease 121: 1025–1029

Janoff A, Sandhaus R A, Hospelhorn V D, Rosenberg R 1972 Digestion of lung proteins by human leucocyte granules in vitro. Proceedings of the Society for Experimental Biology and Medicine 140: 516–519

Janoff A, Carp H, Lee D K, Drew R T 1979a Cigarette smoke inhalation decreases α_1-antitrypsin activity in rat lung. Science 206: 1313–1314

Janoff A, White R, Carp H, Harel S, Dearing R, Lee D 1979b Lung injury induced leucocytic proteases. American Journal of Pathology 97: 111–129

Janoff A, George-Nascimento C, Rosenberg S 1986 A genetically engineered mutant human alpha-1-proteinase inhibitor is more resistant than the normal inhibitor to oxidative inactivation by chemicals, enzymes, cells, and cigarette smoke. American Review of Respiratory Disease 133: 353–356

Janus E D, Carrell R W 1975 Alpha$_1$-antitrypsin deficiency in New Zealand. New Zealand Medical Journal 81: 461–467

Janus E D, Joyce P R, Sheat J M, Carrell R W 1975 Alpha$_1$-antitrypsin variants in New Zealand. New Zealand Medical Journal 12: 289–291

Jeppsson J O 1976 Amino acid substitution in α_1-antitrypsin PiZ. FEBS Letters 65: 195–197

Johnson D A 1980 Ozone inactivation of human α_1-proteinase inhibitor. American Review of Respiratory Disease 121: 1031–1038

Joly J, Richer G, Boisvert F, Laverdiere M 1980 Alpha$_1$-antitrypsin phenotypes in French Canadian newborns. Human Heredity 30: 1–2

Jones E A, Vergalla J, Steer C F, Bradley-Moore P R, Vierling J M 1978 Metabolism of intact and desialylated α_1-antitrypsin. Clinical Science and Molecular Medicine 55: 139–148

Kamboh M I 1985 Review Article. Biochemical and genetic aspects of human serum α_1-proteinase inhibitor protein. Disease Markers 3: 135–154

Kanner R E, Renzetti A D, Klauber M R, Smith C B, Golden C A 1979 Variables associated with changes in spirometry in patients with obstructive lung diseases. American Journal of Medicine 67: 44–50

Karlinsky J B, Snider G L 1978 Animal models of emphysema. American Review of Respiratory Disease 117: 1109–1133

Karsh J, Vergalla J, Jones E A 1979 Alpha$_1$-antitrypsin phenotypes in rheumatoid arthritis and systemic lupus erthematosus. Arthritis and Rheumatism 22: 111–113

Kaufmann F 1985 Selection bias of PiMZ subjects. American Review of Respiratory Disease 131: 800–801

Kellermann G, Walter H 1970 Investigations on the population genetics of the α_1-antitrypsin polymorphism. Humangenetik 10: 145–150

Kelly J K, Taylor T V, Milford-Ward A 1979 Alpha$_1$-antitrypsin Pi S phenotype and liver cell inclusion bodies in alcoholic hepatitis. Journal of Clinical Pathology 32: 706–709

Kern W H, Mikkelsen W P, Turrill F L 1969 Significance of hyaline necrosis in liver biopsies. Surgery, Gynecology and Obstetrics 129: 749–754

Kidd V J, Wallace R B, Itakura K, Woo S L C 1983 α_1-antitrypsin deficiency detection by direct analysis of the mutation in the gene. Nature 304: 230–234

Kidd V J, Golbus M S, Wallace R B, Itakura K, Woo S L C 1984 Prenatal diagnosis of α_1-antitrypsin deficiency by direct analysis of the mutation site in the gene. New England Journal of Medicine 310: 639–642

Klasen E C, Franken C, Voleers W S, Bernini L F 1977 Population genetics of α_1-antitrypsin in the Netherlands. Human Genetics 37: 303–313

Klasen E C, D'Andrea F, Bernini L F 1978 Phenotype and gene distribution of alpha$_1$-antitrypsin in a North Italian population. Human Heredity 28: 474–478

Klasen E C, Biemond I, Laros C D 1986 α_1-antitrypsin deficiency and the flaccid lung syndrome. The heterozygote controversy. Clinical Genetics 29: 211–215

Klayton R, Fallat R, Cohen A B 1975 Determinants of chronic obstructive pulmonary disease in patients with intermediate levels of alpha$_1$-antitrypsin. American Review of Respiratory Disease 112: 71–75

Kleinerman J, Ranga V, Rynbrandt D, Sorensen J, Powers J C 1980 The effect of the specific elastase inhibitor, alanyl prolyl alanine chloromethylketone, on elastase-induced emphysema. American Review of Respiratory Disease 121: 381–387

Kozarevic D, Laban M, Budimir M, Vojvodic N, Roberts A, Gordon T, McGee D L 1978 Intermediate alpha$_1$-antitrypsin deficiency and chronic obstructive pulmonary disease in Yugoslavia. American Review of Respiratory Disease 117: 1039–1043

Kramps J A Bakker W, Dijkman J H 1980 A matched-pair study of the leucocyte elastase-like activity in normal persons and in emphysematous patients with and without alpha$_1$-antitrypsin deficiency. American Review of Respiratory Disease 121: 253–261

Kueppers F 1968 Genetically determined differences in the response of alpha$_1$-antitrypsin levels in human serum to typhoid vaccine. Humangenetik 6: 207–214

Kueppers F 1971 Alpha$_1$-antitrypsin: Physiology, genetics and pathology. Humangenetik 11: 177–189

Kueppers F 1978 Inherited differences in alpha$_1$-antitrypsin. In: Litwin S D (ed) Lung biopsy in health and disease; genetic determinants of pulmonary disease. Marcel Dekker ch 2, p 23–74

Kueppers F 1981 PiM subtypes in COPD. Chest 80: 247 (letter)

Kueppers F, Black L F 1974 α_1-antitrypsin and its deficiency. American Review of Respiratory Disease 110: 176–194

Kueppers F, Fallat R J 1969 α_1-antitrypsin deficiency: A defect in protein synthesis. Clinica Chimica Acta 24: 401–403

Kueppers F, Fallat R, Larson R K 1969 Obstructive lung disease and alpha$_1$-antitrypsin deficiency gene heterozygosity. Science 165: 899–901

Kueppers F, O'Brien P, Passarge E, Rudiger H W 1975 Alpha$_1$-antitrypsin phenotypes in sex chromosome mosaicism. Journal of Medical Genetics 12: 263–264

Kueppers F, Dickson E R, Summerskill W H J 1976 Alpha$_1$-antitrypsin phenotypes in chronic active liver disease and primary biliary cirrhosis. Mayo Clinic Proceedings 51: 286–288

Kueppers F, Miller R D, Gordon H, Hepper N G, Offord K 1977 Familial prevalence of chronic obstructive pulmonary disease in a matched pair study. American Journal of Medicine 63: 336–342

Kuhn C, Senior R M 1978 The role of elastases in the development of emphysema. Lung 155: 185–197

Kuhn P, Spielmann W 1979 Investigations on the Pi polymorphism in a German population. Forensic Science International 14: 135

Lai E C, Kao F-T, Law M L, Woo S L C 1983 Assignment of the α_1-antitrypsin gene and a sequence-related gene to human chromosome 14 by molecular hybridization. American Journal of Human Genetics 35: 385–392

Lam S, Abboud R T, Chan-Yeung M, Rushton J M 1979 Neutrophil elastase and pulmonary function in subjects with intermediate alpha$_1$-antitrypsin deficiency, and chronic obstructive lung disease. American Review of Respiratory Disease 119: 941–951

Lam S, Chan-Yeung M, Abboud R, Kreutzer D 1980 Interrelationships between serum chemotatic factor inactivator, alpha$_1$-antitrypsin deficiency, and chronic obstructive lung disease. American Review of Respiratory Disease 121: 507–512

Lamontagne L R, Stadnyk A W, Gauldie J 1985 Synthesis of alpha$_1$-protease inhibitor by resident and activated mouse alveolar macrophages. American Review of Respiratory Disease 131: 321–325

Langley C E, Talamo R 1975 Antitryptic activity of alpha$_1$-antitrypsin Pi bands in starch gel. In: Peeters N (ed) Protides of the biological fluids. Pergamon Press, New York, p 497–500

Lankisch P G, Koop H, Winckler K, Kaboth U 1978 α_1-antitrypsin in pancreatic disease. Digestion 18: 138–140

Larsson C, Eriksson S, Dirksen H 1977 Smoking and intermediate alpha$_1$-antitrypsin deficiency and lung function in middle-aged men. British Medical Journal 2: 922–926

Laurell C-B 1966 Quantitative estimation of proteins by electrophoresis in agarose gel containing antibodies. Analytical Biochemistry 15: 45–52

Laurell C B 1975 Relation between structures and biologic function of the protease inhibitors in the extracellular fluid. In: Peeters N (ed) Protides of the biological fluids. Pergamon Press, New York, p 3–12

Laurell C B, Eriksson S 1963 The electrophoretic α_1-antitrypsin deficiency. Scandinavian Journal of Clinical and Laboratory Investigation 15: 132–140

Laurell C B, Eriksson S 1965 The serum α_1-antitrypsin in families with hypo-α_1-antitrypsinemia. Clinica Chimica Acta 11: 395–398

Laurell C B, Sveger T 1975 Mass screening of newborn Swedish infants for α_1-antitrypsin deficiency. American Journal of Human Genetics 27: 213–217

Laurell C B, Nossling B, Jeppsson J O 1977 Catabolic rate of α_1-antitrypsin of Pi type M and Z in man. Clinical Science and Molecular Medicine 52: 457–461

Lebeau A, Rochemaure J 1978 Variations du taux d'alpha$_1$-antitrypsine chez les sujets atteints de broncho-pneumopathies aigues. Roles du phenotype Pi et de la fonction hepatique. La Nouvelle Presse Medicale 7: 3521–3525

Ledley F D, Woo S L C 1986 Molecular basis of α_1-antitrypsin deficiency and its potential therapy by gene transfer. Journal of Inherited Metabolic Disease 9 (Suppl 1): 85–91

Leicht M, Long G L, Chandra T et al 1982 Sequence homology and structural comparison between the chromosomal human α_1-antitrypsin and chicken ovalbumin genes. Nature 297: 655–659

Lellouch J, Claude J R, Thevenin M 1979 α_1-antitrypsine et tabac, une etude de 1296 hommes sains. Clinica Chimica Acta 95: 337–345

Lellouch J, Claude J-R, Martin J-P, Orssaud G, Zaoui D, Bieth J G 1985 Smoking does not reduce the functional activity of serum alpha-1-proteinase inhibitor. American Review of Respiratory Disease 132: 818–820

Le Prévost C, Frommel D, Dupuy J M 1975 Complement studies in alpha$_1$-antitrypsin deficiency in children. Journal of Pediatrics 87: 571–573

Lieberman J 1969 Heterozygous and homozygous alpha$_1$-

antitrypsin deficiency in patients with pulmonary emphysema. New England Journal of Medicine 281: 279–284

Lieberman J 1971 Alpha₁-antitrypsin and pepsin inhibition. New England Journal of Medicine 285: 524

Lieberman J 1973 Alpha₁-antitrypsin deficiency. Medical Clinics of North America 57: 691–706

Lieberman J 1974 Emphysema, cirrhosis, and hepatoma with alpha₁-antitrypsin deficiency. Annals of Internal Medicine 81: 850–851

Lieberman J 1980a Alpha₁-antitrypsin. In: Schmidt R M (ed) Handbook series in clinical laboratory science section I: Hematology, volume III, p 195–204

Lieberman J 1980b Alpha₁-antitrypsin deficiency. In: Simmons D H (ed) Current pulmonology, volume 2. Houghton Mifflin, ch 2, p 41–68

Lieberman J, Gawad M A 1971 Inhibitors and activators of leucocytic protease in purulent sputum. Journal of Laboratory and Clinical Medicine 77: 713–727

Lieberman J, Kaneshiro W 1972 Inhibition of leucocytic elastase from purulent sputum by alpha₁-antitrypsin. Journal of Laboratory and Clinical Medicine 80: 88–101

Lieberman J, Mittman C 1973 Dynamic response of α_1-antitrypsin variants to diethylstilbestrol. American Journal of Human Genetics 25: 610–617

Lieberman J, Mittman C, Schneider A S 1969 Screening for homozygous and heterozygous α_1-antitrypsin deficiency. Protein electrophoresis on cellulose acetate membranes. Journal of the American Medical Association 210: 2055–2060

Lieberman J, Mittman C, Kent J R 1971 Screening for heterozygous α_1-antitrypsin deficiency. III. A provocative test with diethylstilbestrol and effect of oral contraceptives. Journal of the American Medical Association 217: 1198–1206

Lieberman J, Mittman C, Gordon H W 1972 Alpha₁-antitrypsin in the livers of patients with emphysema. Science 175: 63–65

Lieberman J, Silton R M, Agliozzo C M, McMahon J 1975a Hepatocellular carcinoma and intermediate α_1-antitrypsin deficiency (MZ phenotype). American Journal of Clinical Pathology 64: 304–310

Lieberman J, Kaneshiro W, Gaidulis L 1975b Interference with alpha₁-antitrypsin studies in stored serum by presumed bacterial proteases. Journal of Laboratory and Clinical Medicine 86: 7–16

Lieberman J, Gaidulis L, Klotz S D 1976a A new deficient variant of α_1-antitrypsin (Mduarte). Inability to detect the heterozygous state by antitrypsin in phenotyping. American Review of Respiratory Disease 113: 31–36

Lieberman J, Gaidulis L, Roberts L 1976b Racial distribution of α_1-antitrypsin variants among junior high school students. American Review of Respiratory Disease 114: 1194–1198

Lieberman J, Gaidulis L, Schleissner L A 1976c Intermediate alpha₁-antitrypsin deficiency resulting from a null gene (M-phenotype). Chest 70: 532–535

Lieberman J, Borhani N O, Feinleib M 1979 α_1-antitrypsin deficiency in twins and parents-of-twins. Clinical Genetics 15: 29–36

Lieberman J, Winter B, Sastre A 1986 Alpha₁-antitrypsin Pi-types in 965 COPD patients. Chest 89: 370–373

Lie-Injo L E, Ganesan J, Herrera A, Lopez C G 1978 α_1-antitrypsin variants in different racial groups in Malaysia.

Human Heredity 28: 37–40

Lipsky J J, Berninger R W, Hyman L R, Talamo R C 1979 Presence of alpha₁-antitrypsin on mitogen-stimulated human lymphocytes. Journal of Immunology 122: 24–26

Lochon B, Vercaigne D, Lochon C, Fournier M, Martin J P, Derenne J P, Pariente R 1978 Emphysema pan-lobulaire: relations avec le taux d'alpha₁-antitrypsin serique le phenotype Pi et le systeme H.L.A. La Nouvelle Presse Medicale 7: 1167–1170

Long G L, Chandra T, Woo S L C, Davie E W, Kurachi K 1984 Complete sequence of the cDNA for human α_1-antitrypsin and the gene for the S variant. Biochemistry 23: 4828–4837

Longstreth G F, Weitzman S A, Browning R J, Lieberman J 1975 Bronchiectasis and homozygous alpha₁-antitrypsin deficiency. Chest 67: 233–235

Lubec V G, Weissenbacher G, Balzar E, Bugajer-Gleitmann H 1976 Alpha₁-antitrypsin bei Kindern mit glommerularen Nierenkrankheiten. Wiener Klinische Wochenschrift 88: 271–274

Lucey E C, Clark B D 1982 Differing susceptibility of young and adult hamster lungs to injury with pancreatic elastase. American Review of Respiratory Disease 126: 877–881

McDonagh D J, Nathan S P, Knudson R J, Lebowitz M D 1979 Assessment of alpha₁-antitrypsin deficiency heterozygosity as a risk factor in the etiology of emphysema. Journal of Clinical Investigation 63: 299–309

Macdougall B R D, McMaster P, Calne R Y, Williams R 1980 Survival and rehabilitation after orthotopic liver transplantation. Lancet 1: 1326–1328

McElrath M J, Galbraith R M, Allen R C 1979 Demonstration of alpha₁-antitrypsin by immunofluorescence on paraffin-embedded hepatic and pancreatic tissue. Journal of Histochemistry and Cytochemistry 27: 794–796

Machovich R, Borsodi A, Blasko G, Orakzai S A 1977 Inactivation of α and β-thrombin by antithrombin-III, α_2-macroglobulin and α_1-proteinase inhibitor. Biochemical Journal 167: 393–398

McNeil T F, Thelin T, Aspegren-Jansson E, Sveger T, Harty B 1985 Psychological factors in cost-benefit analysis of somatic prevention. Acta Paediatrica Scandinavica 74: 427–432

Makino S, Reed C E 1970 Distribution and elimination of exogenous alpha₁-antitrypsin. Journal of Laboratory and Clinical Medicine 75: 742–746

Makino S, Chosy L, Valdivia E, Reed C E 1970 Emphysema with hereditary alpha₁-antitrypsin deficiency masquerading as asthma. Journal of Allergy 46: 40–48

Martin J P, Sesboue R, Charlionet R, Ropartz C, Pereira M T 1976 Genetic variants of serum α_1-antitrypsin (Pi types) in Portuguese. Human Heredity 26: 310–314

Martin W J, Taylor J C 1979 Abnormal interaction of α_1-antitrypsin and leucocyte elastolytic activity in patients with chronic obstructive pulmonary disease. American Review of Respiratory Disease 120: 411–419

Martorana P A, Wusten B, van Even P, Gobel H, Schaper J 1982a A six month study of the evolution of papain-induced emphysema in the dog. A morphometric and pulmonary hemodynamic investigation. American Review of Respiratory Disease 126: 898–903

Martorana P A, van Even P, Schaper J 1982b The effect of lung growth on the evolution of elastase-induced emphysema in the hamster. Lung 160: 19–27

Matsubara S, Yoshida A, Lieberman J 1974 Material isolated from normal and variant human liver that immunologically crossreacts with alpha$_1$-antitrypsin. Proceedings of the National Academy of Sciences 71: 3334–3337

Matzen R N, Bader P I, Block W D 1977 Alpha$_1$-antitrypsin deficiency in clinic patients. Annals of Clinical Research 9: 88–92

Miale T D, Lawson D L, Demian S, Teague P O, Wolfson S L 1977 Possible involvement of blood platelet/megakaryocyte system in alpha$_1$-antitrypsin deficiency. Lancet 2: 93–94

Mihas A A, Hirschowitz B I 1976 Alpha$_1$-antitrypsin and chronic pancreatitis. Lancet 2: 1032–1033

Miller F, Kuschner M 1969 Alpha$_1$-antitrypsin deficiency, emphysema, necrotizing angiitis and glomerulonephritis. American Journal of Medicine 46: 615–623

Mirsky I A, Foley G 1945 Antibiotic actions of trypsin inhibitors. Proceedings of the Society for Experimental Biology and Medicine 59: 34–35

Mittman C 1978 The PiMZ phenotype: Is it a significant risk factor for the development of chronic obstructive lung disease? American Review of Respiratory Disease 118: 649–652

Mittman C 1980 Additional supporting data. American Journal of Human Genetics 32: 457–458

Mittman C, Lieberman J 1973 Screening for α_1-antitrypsin deficiency. Israel Journal of Medical Sciences 9: 1311–1318

Mittman C, Lieberman J, Marasso F, Miranda A 1971 Smoking and chronic obstructive lung disease in alpha$_1$-antitrypsin deficiency. Chest 60: 214–221

Miyake K, Suzuki H, Oka H, Oda T, Harada S 1979 Distribution of α_1-antitrypsin phenotypes in Japanese. Description of Pi M subtypes by isoelectric focusing. Japanese Journal of Human Genetics 24: 55–62

Morihara K, Tsuzuki H, Oda K 1979 Protease and elastase of Pseudomonas aeruginosa: inactivation of human plasma α_1-proteinase inhibitor. Infection and Immunity 24: 188–193

Morin T, Feldmann G, Benhamou J P, Martin J P, Rueff B, Ropartz C 1975 Heterozygous alpha$_1$-antitrypsin deficiency and cirrhosis in adults, a fortuitous association. Lancet 1: 250–251

Moroi M, Yamasaki M, Aoki N 1975 Association of human α_1-antitrypsin with anhydrotrypsin. Journal of Biochemistry (Tokyo) 78: 925–928

Moroz S P, Cutz E, Cox D W, Sass-Kortsak A 1976a Liver disease associated with alpha$_1$-antitrypsin deficiency in childhood. Journal of Pediatrics 88: 19–25

Moroz S P, Cutz E, Balfe J W, Sass-Kortsak A 1976b Membranoproliferative glomerulonephritis in childhood cirrhosis associated with alpha$_1$-antitrypsin deficiency. Pediatrics 57: 232–238

Moser K M, Kidikoro Y, Marsh J, Sgroi V 1978 Biologic half-life and organ distribution of radiolabeled human PiM and PiZ alpha$_1$-antitrypsin in the dog. Journal of Laboratory and Clinical Medicine 91: 214–222

Moskowitz R W, Heinrich G 1971 Bacterial inactivation of human serum alpha$_1$-antitrypsin. Journal of Laboratory and Clinical Medicine 77: 777–785

Nemeth A, Strandvik B, Glaumann H 1983 Alpha-1-antitrypsin deficiency and juvenile liver disease. Ultrastructural observations compared with light microscopy and routine liver tests. Virchows Archiv B 44: 15–33

Noades J E, Cook P J L 1976 Family studies with the Gm:Pi linkage group. Cytogenetics and Cell Genetics 16: 341–344

Novis B H, Bank S, Young G O, Marks I N 1975 Chronic pancreatitis and alpha$_1$-antitrypsin. Lancet 2: 748

O'Brien M L, Buist N R M, Murphey W H 1978 Neonatal screening for alpha$_1$-antitrypsin deficiency. Journal of Pediatrics 92: 1006–1010

O'Neill F J 1974 Limitation of nuclear division by protease inhibitors in cytochalasin-B-treated tumor cells. Journal of the National Cancer Institute 52: 653–657

Ostrow D N, Cherniack R M 1972 The mechanical properties of the lungs in intermediate deficiency of α_1-antitrypsin. American Review of Respiratory Disease 106: 377–383

Ostrow D N, Manfreda J, Tse K S, Dorman T, Cherniack R M 1978 Alpha$_1$-antitrypsin phenotypes and lung function in a moderately polluted northern Ontario community. Canadian Medical Association Journal 118: 669–672

Owen M C, Carrell R W 1976 Alpha$_1$-antitrypsin: molecular abnormality of S variant. British Medical Journal 1: 130–131

Owen M C, Carrell R W 1977 Alpha-1-antitrypsin: Sequence of the Z variant tryptic peptide. FEBS Letters 79: 245–247

Owen M C, Iorier M, Carrell R W 1978 Alpha-1-antitrypsin: Structural relationships of the substitutions of the S and Z variants. FEBS Letters 88: 234–236

Owen M C, Brennan S O, Lewis J H, Carrell R W 1983 Mutation of antitrypsin to antithrombin. α_1-antitrypsin Pittsburg (358 Met-Arg). A fatal bleeding disorder. New England Journal of Medicine 309: 694–698

Palmer P E, Wolfe H J 1976 α_1-antitrypsin deposition in primary hepatic carcinoma. Archives of Pathology and Laboratory Medicine 100: 232–236

Palmer P E, Safaii H, Wolfe H J 1976 Alpha$_1$-antitrypsin and alpha-fetoprotein. Protein markers in endodermal sinus (yolk sac) tumors. American Journal of Clinical Pathology 65: 575–582

Palmer P E, Wolfe H J, Kostas C I 1978 Multisystem fibrosis in alpha$_1$-antitrypsin deficiency. Lancet 1: 221–222

Perelman R, Nathanson M, Lepastier G, Lesavre Ph, Plainfosse B, Chirazi S, Seringe Ph 1975 Mannosidose associée a l'absence d'alpha-1-antitrypsin. Annales de Pediaterie 22: 385–396

Peterson R J, Marsh C L 1979 The relationship of alpha$_1$-antitrypsin to inflammatory periodontal disease. Journal of Periodontology 50: 31–35

Pierce J A, Eradio B, Dew T A 1975 Antitrypsin phenotypes in St. Louis. Journal of the American Medical Association 231: 609–612

Pitt E, Lewis D A 1979 Stimulatory action of steroidal anti-inflammatory drugs on plasma alpha$_1$-antitrypsin levels in the rat. British Journal of Pharmacology 66: 454–455

Pongpaew P, Schelp F P 1980 Alpha$_1$-protease inhibitor phenotypes and serum concentrations in Thailand. Human Genetics 54: 119–124

Porter C A, Mowat A P, Cook P J L, Haynes D W G, Shilken R W 1972 α_1-antitrypsin deficiency and neonatal hepatitis. British Medical Journal 2: 435–439

Powers J C, Gupton B F, Harley A D, Nishino N, Whitley R J 1977 Specificity of porcine pancreatic elastase, human leucocyte elastase and cathepsin G. Inhibition with peptide chloromethyl ketones. Biochimica et Biophysica Acta 485: 156–166

Premachandra B N, Yu S Y 1979 Association of prealbumin deficiency with alpha$_1$-antitrypsin deficiency. Metabolism 28: 890–894

Pride N B, Tattersall S F, Pereira R P, Hunter D, Blundell G 1980 Lung distensibility and airway function in intermediate alpha$_1$-antitrypsin deficiency (PiMZ). Chest 77: 253–255

Pryor W A, Dooley M M, Church D F 1985 Human α-1-proteinase inhibitor is inactivated by exposure to sidestream cigarette smoke. Toxicology Letters 28: 65–70

Pryor W A, Dooley M M, Church D F 1986 The inactivation of α-1-proteinase inhibitor by gas-phase cigarette smoke: Protection by antioxidants and reducing species. Chemico Biological Interactions 57: 271–283

Psacharopoulos H T, Mowat A P, Cook P J L, Carlile P A, Portmann B, Rodeck C H 1983 Outcome of liver disease associated with α_1-antitrypsin deficiency (PiZ). Archives of Disease in Childhood 58: 882–887

Putnam C W, Porter K A, Peters R L, Ashcavai M, Redeker A-G, Starzl T-E 1977 Liver replacement for alpha$_1$-antitrypsin deficiency. Surgery 81: 258–261

Rabin M, Watson M, Kidd V, Woo S L C, Breg W R, Ruddle F H 1986 Regional location of α_1-antichymotrypsin and α_1-antitrypsin genes on human chromosome 14. Somatic Cell and Molecular Genetics 12: 209–214

Ratliff N B, Wilson J W, Mikat E, Hackel D B, Graham T C 1971 The lung in hemorrhagic shock. IV. The role of neutrophilic polymorphonuclear leukocytes. American Journal of Pathology 65: 325–332

Ray M B, Desmet V J 1978a Immunohistochemical immunoreactivity in islet cells of adult human pancreas. Cell and Tissue Research 185: 63–68

Ray M B, Desmet V J 1978b Immunohistochemical demonstration of alpha-1-antitrypsin in the islet cells of human pancreas. Cell and Tissue Research 187: 69–77

Ray M B, Zumwalt R 1986a Islet-cell hyperplasia in genetic deficiency of alpha-1-proteinase inhibitor. American Journal of Clinical Pathology 85: 681–687

Ray M B, Zumwalt R E 1986b Identification of alpha-1-proteinase inhibitor-containing cells in pancreatic islets. Cell and Tissue Research 243: 677–680

Ray M B, Desmet V J, Gepts W 1977 Alpha-1-antitrypsin immunoreactivity in islet cells of adult human pancreas. Cell and Tissue Research 185: 63–68

Rees E D, Hollingsworth J W, Hoffman T R, Black H, Hearn T L 1975 Smoking and disease. Effect on serum antitrypsin in hospitalized patients. Archives of Environmental Health 30: 402–408

Reintoft I 1977 Alpha-1-antitrypsin deficiency. Experience from an autopsy material. Acta Pathologica et Microbiologica Scandinavica 85: 649–655

Reintoft I 1979 Alpha-1-antitrypsin globules in livers from a medicolegal autopsy material. Acta Pathologica et Microbiologica Scandinavica 87: 447–450

Robert J, Souillet G, Chapuis-Cellier C, Ghipponi J, Bienvenu J, Frobert Y, Carron R 1979 Immunite non specifique et role aggravant d'un phenotype abnormal de l'alpha-1-antitrypsin chez les enfants atteints de deficit selectiv en IgA. La Nouvelle Presse Medicale 8: 2659–2662

Roberts A, Kagan A, Rhoads G C, Pierce J A, Bruce R M 1977 Antitrypsin and chronic obstructive pulmonary disease among Japanese-American men. Chest 72: 489–491

Roberts N A, Surgenor A E 1986 Comparison of peptide aldehydes with α_1-antitrypsin as elastase inhibitors for use in emphysema. Biochemical and Biophysical Research Communications 139: 896–902

Robinet-Levy M, Rieunier M 1972 Techniques d'identification des groupes Pi. Premieres statistiques languedociennes. Revue Francaise de Transfusion et Immuno-Hematologie 15: 61–72

Rodriquez J R, Seals J E, Radin A, Lin J S, Mandl I, Turino G M 1975 The role of leukocyte elastase in the pathogenesis of obstructive lung disease. American Review of Respiratory Disease 111: 929

Rosenberg S, Bar P J, Najarian R C, Hallewell R A 1984 Synthesis in yeast of a functional oxidation-resistant mutant of human α_1-antitrypsin. Nature 312: 77–80

Rubinstein H M, Jaffer A M, Kudrna J C, Lertratanakul Y, Chandrasekhar A J, Slater D, Schmid F R 1977 Alpha$_1$-antitrypsin deficiency with severe panniculitis. Report of two cases. Annals of Internal Medicine 86: 742–744

Samad I A, O'Connell C J 1972 Serum alpha$_1$-antitrypsin deficiency. Chest 61: 307–308

Sandhaus R A, Janoff A 1974 Degradation of human α_1-antitrypsin by hepatocyte acid cathepsin. American Review of Respiratory Disease 110: 263–272

Santiago J V, Dew T A, Haymond M, Williamson J R, Kilo C, Kipnis M, Pierce J A 1974 Glucose intolerance in α_1-antitrypsin deficiency. Journal of Clinical Investigation 53: 70A

Sasaki M, Yamamoto H, Iida S 1974 Interaction of human serum proteinase inhibitors with proteolytic enzyme of animal, plant and bacterial origin. Journal of Biochemistry (Tokyo) 75: 171–177

Schapira M, Ramus M-A, Jallat S, Carvallo D, Courtney M 1985 Recombinant α_1-antitrypsin Pittsburgh (Met^{358}-Arg) is a potent inhibitor of plasma kallikrein and activated Factor XII gragment. Journal of Clinical Investigation 76: 635–637

Scharpe S, Eid M, Cooreman W, Lauwers A 1978 α_1-antitrypsin an inhibitor of renin. Biochemical Journal 153: 505–507

Schmitt M G, Phillips R B, Matzen R N, Rodey G 1975 α_1-antitrypsin deficiency. A study of the relationship between the Pi system and genetic markers. American Journal of Human Genetics 27: 315–321

Schroeder W T, Miller M F, Woo S L C, Saunders G F 1985 Chromosomal localization of the human α_1-antitrypsin gene (Pi) to 14q31–32 American Journal of Human Genetics 37: 868–872

Schumacher G F B 1971 Inhibition of rabbit sperm acrosomal protease by human alpha$_1$-antitrypsin and other protease inhibitors. Contraception 4: 67–78

Schumacher G F B, Pearl M J 1965 Alpha$_1$-antitrypsin in cervical mucus. Fertility and Sterility 19: 91–99

Schuyler M R, Rynbrandt D J, Kleinerman J 1978 Physiologic and morphologic observations of the effects of intravenous elastase on the lung. American Review of Respiratory Disease 117: 97–102

Schydlower M, Waxman S H, Patterson P H 1979 Coexistence of deficiency in alpha$_1$-antitrypsin and in growth hormone. New England Journal of Medicine 300:366

Sesboue R, Charlionet R, Vercaigne D, Guimbretiere J, Martin J P 1978 Genetic variants of serum alpha$_1$-antitrypsin (Pi types) in Bretones. Human Heredity 28: 280–284

Sharp H L 1971 Alpha$_1$-antitrypsin deficiency. Hospital Practice, May: 83–96

Sharp H L, Bridges R A, Krivit W, Freier E F 1969 Cirrhosis associated with alpha$_1$-antitrypsin deficiency: A previously unrecognized inherited disorder. Journal of Laboratory and Clinical Medicine 73: 934–939

Shulman N R 1952 Studies on the inhibition of proteolytic enzymes by serum. Journal of Experimental Medicine 95: 605–618

Sjoblom K G, Wollheim F A 1977 Alpha$_1$-antitrypsin phenotypes and rheumatic diseases. Lancet 2: 41

Snider G L, Hayes J A, Franzblau C, Kagan H M, Stone P J, Korthy A 1974 Relationship between elastolytic activity and experimental emphysema inducing properties of papain preparations. American Review of Respiratory Disease 110: 254–262

Sotos J F, Cutler E A, Romshe C A et al 1981 Successful spleno-renal shunt and splenectomy in two patients with alpha-1-antitrypsin deficiency. Journal of Pediatric Surgery 16: 12–16

Starzl T E, Porter K A, Francavilla A, Iwatsuki S 1983 Reversal of hepatic alpha-1-antitrypsin deposition after postacaval shunt. Lancet 2: 424–426

Stjernberg N, Beckman G, Beckman G, Beckman L, Nystrom L, Rosenhall L 1984 Alpha-1-antitrypsin types and pulmonary disease among employees at a sulphite pulp factory in northern Sweden. Human Heredity 34: 337–342

Stone P J, Calore J K, McGowan S E, Bernardo J, Snider G L, Franzblau C 1983 Smokers do not have less functional alpha$_1$-protease inhibitor in their lower respiratory tracts than nonsmokers. Chest 83S: 65S–66S

Sveger T 1976 Liver disease in alpha$_1$-antitrypsin deficiency detected by screening of 200 000 infants. New England Journal of Medicine 294: 1316–1321

Sveger T 1978 α_1-antitrypsin deficiency in early childhood. Pediatrics 62: 22–25

Szczeklik A, Turowska B, Mysik G C, Opolska B, Nizankowska E 1974 Serum alpha$_1$-antitrypsin in bronchial asthma. American Review of Respiratory Disease 109: 487–490

Takemura S, Rossing T H, Perlmutter D H 1986 A lymphokine regulates expression of alpha-1-proteinase inhibitor in human monocytes and macrophages. Journal of Clinical Investigation 77: 1207–1213

Talamo R C 1975 Basic and clinical aspects of the alpha$_1$-antitrypsin. Pediatrics 56: 91–99

Talamo R C et al 1978 Alpha$_1$-antitrypsin laboratory manual. U.S. Department of Health, Education and Welfare. DHEW Publication No. (NIH) 78–1420

Talerman A, Haije W G, Baggerman L 1977 Alpha$_1$-antitrypsin (AAT) and alphafoetoprotein (AFP) in sera of patients with germ-cell neoplasms: Value as tumour markers in patients with endodermal sinus tumour (yolk sac tumour). International Journal of Cancer 19: 741–746

Taylor J C, Kueppers F 1977 Electrophoretic mobility of leucocyte elastase of normal subjects and patients with chronic obstructive pulmonary disease. American Review of Respiratory Disease 116: 531–536

Terblanche J, Koep L J, Starzl T E 1979 Liver transplantation. Medical Clinics of North America 63: 507–521

Tessier L-H, Jallat S, Sauvageot M, Crystal R G, Courtney M 1986 RNA structural elements for expression in Escherichia coli. α_1-antitrypsin synthesis using translation control elements based on the cII ribosome-binding site of phage lambda. FEBS Letters 208: 183–188

Thelin T, McNeil T F, Aspegren-Jansson E, Sveger T 1985a Psychological consequences of neonatal screening for α_1-antitrypsin deficiency. Parental reactions to the first news of their infants' deficiency. Acta Paediatrica Scandinavica 74: 787–793

Thelin T, McNeil T F, Aspegren-Jansson E, Sveger T 1985b Psychological consequences of neonatal screening for α_1-antitrypsin deficiency (AID). Acta Paediatrica Scandinavica 74: 841–847

Torp A 1975 Myocardial biopsy in a case of cardiomyopathy and partial α_1-antitrypsin deficiency with liver engagement. Acta Medica Scandinavica 197: 137–140

Touraine J L, Malik M C, Perrot H, Maire I, Revillard U P, Grosshans E, Traeger J 1979 Maladie de Fabry: deux malades amellores par la greffe de cellules de foie foetal. La Nouvelle Presse Medicale 8: 1499–1503

Travis J, Salvesen G S 1983 Human plasma proteinase inhibitors. Annual Review of Biochemistry 52: 655–709

Triger D R, Millward-Sadler G H, Czaykowski A A, Trowell J, Wright R 1976 Alpha$_1$-antitrypsin deficiency and liver disease in adults. Quarterly Journal of Medicine 45: 351–372

Turino G M, Senior R M, Garg B D, Keller S, Levi M M, Mandl I 1969 Serum elastase inhibitor deficiency and α_1-antitrypsin deficiency in patients with obstructive emphysema. Science 165: 709–711

Tuttle W C, Jones R K 1975 Fluorescent antibody studies of alpha$_1$-antitrypsin in adult human lung. American Journal of Clinical Pathology 64: 477–482

Udall H N, Bloch K J, Walker W A 1982 Transport of proteases across the neonatal intestine and development of liver disease in infants with alpha$_1$-antitrypsin deficiency. Lancet 1: 1441–1443

Udall J N, Dixon M, Newman A P, Wright J A, James B, Bloch K J 1985 Liver disease in α_1-antitrypsin deficiency. A retrospective analysis of the influence of early breast-vs bottle-feeding. Journal of the American Medical Association 253: 2679–2682

Vandeville D, Martin J P, Lebreton J P, Ropartz C 1972 Le systeme Pi dans les populations Normande et Amerindienne. Revue Francaise de Transfusion et Immuno-Hematologie 15: 213–218

Vandeville D, Martin J P, Ropartz C 1974 α_1-antitrypsin in polymorphism of a Bantu population: Description of a new allele PiL. Humangenetik 21: 33–38

Van Furth R, Kramps J A, Diesselhof-DenDulk M M C 1983 Synthesis of α_1-antitrypsin by human monocytes. Clinical and Experimental Immunology 51: 551–557

Victorino R, Silveira J C B, Geada H, Moura M C 1978 Familial hypercholesterolaemia with alpha$_1$-antitrypsin deficiency. British Medical Journal 1: 413–414

Walker-Smith J, Andrews J 1972 Alpha$_1$-antitrypsin, autism, and coeliac disease. Lancet 2: 883–884

Wallmark A, Alm R, Eriksson S 1984 Monoclonal antibody specific for the mutant PiZ α_1-antitrypsin and its application in an ELISA procedure for identification of PiZ gene carriers. Proceedings of the National Academy of Sciences 81: 5690–5693

Walsh L, McConkey B 1977 Alpha$_1$-antitrypsin and rheumatoid arthritis. Lancet 2: 564–565

Ward P A, Talamo R C 1973 Deficiency of the chemotactic factor inactivator in human sera with α_1-antitrypsin deficiency. Journal of Clinical Investigation 52: 516–519

Weidinger S, Jahn W, Cujnik F, Schwarzfischer F 1985 Alpha-1-antitrypsin: Evidence for a fifth PiM subtype and a new deficiency allele PiZ Augsburg. Human Genetics 71: 27–29

Weitkamp L R, Cox D W, Johnston E, Guttormsen S A, Schwartz R H, Bias W B, Hsu S H 1976 Data on the genetic linkage relationships between red cell acid phosphatase and alpha$_1$-antitrypsin variants Z, S, I, and F.

Cytogenetics and Cell Genetics 16: 359–363

Weitkamp L R, Cox D, Guttormsen S, Johnston E, Hempgling S 1978 Allelic specific heterogeneity in the Pi:Gm linkage group. Cytogenetics and Cell Genetics 22: 647–650

Welch M H, Richardson R H, Whitcomb W H, Hammarsten J F, Guenter C A 1969 The lung scan in α_1-antitrypsin deficiency. Journal of Nuclear Medicine 10: 687–690

Welch S G, McGregor I A, Williams K 1980 α_1-antitrypsin (Pi) phenotypes in a village population from the Gambia, West Africa. Human Genetics 53: 223–235

Welter H F, Siebeck M, Wiesinger H, Seemuller U, Jochum M, Fritz H 1986 Cloned eglin prevents development of shock lung in experimental septicemia. Journal of Cellular Biochemistry Suppl 10A: 273 (Abstract)

Wewers M D, Gadek J E, Keogh B A, Fells G A, Crystal R G 1986 Evaluation of danazol therapy for patients with PiZZ alpha-1-antitrypsin deficiency. American Review of Respiratory Disease 134: 476–480

Wewers M D, Casolaro M A, Sellers S E, Swayze S C, McPhaul K M, Wittes J T, Crystal R G 1987a Replacement therapy for alpha₁-antitrypsin deficiency associated with emphysema. New England Journal of Medicine 316: 1055–1062

Wewers M D, Casolaro M A, Crystal R G 1987b Comparison of alpha-1-antitrypsin levels and antineutrophil elastase capacity of blood and lung in a patient with alpha-1-antitrypsin phenotype null-null before and during alpha-1-antitrypsin augmentation therapy. American Review of Respiratory Disease 135: 539–543

Wewers M D, Brantly M L, Casolaro M A, Crystal R G 1987c Evaluation of tamoxifen as a therapy to augment alpha-1-antitrypsin concentrations in Z homozygous alpha-1-antitrypsin-deficient subjects. American Review of Respiratory Disease 135: 401–402

Wicher V, Dolovich J 1971 Interactions of Bacillus subtilis alkaline proteinases with α_2-macroglobin and α_1-antitrypsin. International Archives of Allergy and Applied Immunology 40: 779–788

Wittels E H, Coalson J J, Welch M H, Guenter C A 1974 Pulmonary intravascular leucocyte sequestration. A potential mechanism of lung injury. American Review of Respiratory Disease 109: 502–509

Ying Q L, Zhang M L, Liang C C et al 1985 Geographical variability of alpha-1-antitrypsin alleles in China: A study on six Chinese populations. Human Genetics 69: 184–187

Yoshida A, Wessels M 1978 Origin of the multiple components of human α_1-antitrypsin. Biochemical Genetics 16: 641–649

Yoshida A, Lieberman J, Gaidulis L, Ewing C 1976 Molecular abnormality of human alpha₁-antitrypsin variant (Pi-ZZ) associated with plasma activity deficiency. Proceedings of the National Academy of Sciences 73: 1324–1328

Yoshida A, Ewing C, Wessels M, Lieberman J, Gaidulis L 1977 Molecular abnormality of Pi S variant of human alpha₁-antitrypsin. American Journal of Human Genetics 29: 233–239

Yoshida A, Chillar R, Taylor J C 1979a An α_1-antitrypsin variant, Pi B Alhambra with rapid anodal electrophoretic mobility. American Journal of Human Genetics 31: 555–563

Yoshida A, Taylor J C, van den Broek W G M 1979b Structural difference between the normal PiM₁ and the common PiM₂ variant of human α_1-antitrypsin. American Journal of Human Genetics 31: 564–568

Yu S D, Gan J C 1978 Effects of progressive desialylation on the survival of human plasma α_1-antitrypsin in rat circulation. International Journal of Biochemistry 9: 107–115

72. Congenital heart defects

Virginia V. Michels   Vincent M. Riccardi

INTRODUCTION

Congenital heart defects include all structural malformations of the heart and intrathoracic great vessels resulting from errors in morphogenesis. The term congenital heart defect (CHD) does not generally include morbid processes (diseases) that occur after the embryological heart has formed, whether or not they are congenital and/or heritable. This chapter will include discussion of congenital structural malformations, but except for endocardial fibroelastosis and some conduction defects, will exclude diseases such as the Marfan syndrome in which abnormal supporting and connective tissue may result in secondary gross structural abnormalities.

Congenital heart defects are aetiologically heterogeneous. A CHD may occur as an isolated event in an otherwise normal infant as a result of a localized error of morphogenesis. Alternatively, CHDs may occur in conjunction with other abnormalities as part of a syndrome, a sequence or association. A 'syndrome' is defined as a recognized pattern of malformation that presumably has a single aetiology and is not the consequence of a *localized* error in morphogenesis. A 'sequence' refers to a malformation together with consequent structural changes in one or more additional tissues or organs. An 'association' is a recognized pattern of malformations that occur together more frequently than by chance alone, but the pattern is not considered to constitute a syndrome or sequence. The determination that a CHD is an isolated abnormality, or is part of a syndrome, sequence or association does not suggest the nature of the aetiology for the defect. The aetiology of a specific instance of a CHD may be a single gene defect, multifactorial, teratogenic, chromosomal or unknown. Multifactorial means that the defect is determined by multiple genetic and nongenetic factors, each making a relatively small contribution to the phenotype (Nora & Fraser 1981). The evaluation of an individual with a CHD must take into account these various aetiologies, in addition to whether the defect is isolated or associated with other abnormalities.

As with any medical problem, a thorough medical history, including details of maternal health, pregnancy, developmental milestones, and family history must be obtained. During the physical examination, in addition to the cardiac findings, specific attention should be directed to evidence for other major or minor congenital defects. Individual minor findings may be inconsequential to the overall health of the individual, but they may provide valuable clues about the diagnosis and/or aetiology. In some instances, examination of other family members may be necessary to establish a correct diagnosis. Laboratory tests and specialized procedures necessary for diagnosis of the specific cardiac lesion are obviously indicated. Depending on the results of the history and physical examination, the patient may require chromosome analysis, viral cultures, serum antibody titres, ophthalmological examination, skeletal radiographs, intravenous pyelography, computerized axial tomography of the brain, audiometric evaluation, or formal psychometric testing. Clearly, the evaluation and care of a patient with a CHD is not limited to concerns about the cardiac status, but must take into account all potential or actual associated abnormalities, and must be viewed in the context of aetiological heterogeneity.

The incidence of CHDs among all births (stillbirths and live births) is approximately 8.1 per 1000 (Mitchell et al 1971) and 30% of these patients have extracardiac malformations. For stillborns, the incidence is 27.5 per 1000 and many of these stillborn infants have multiple congenital anomalies with a chromosomal or other aetiology (Mitchell et al 1971). In a series of consecutive spontaneous abortions between 8 and 28 weeks' gestation, 24 per 1000 had a CHD. However, if only those stillborns with normal karyotypes were considered, 11 per 1000 had a CHD (Ursell et al 1985). Among live borns, the prevalence of CHDs ranges between 3.7–7.7 per 1000 (Ferencz et al 1985). Among infants surviving beyond one year of age, the prevalence of CHDs is 5.0 per 1000 (Mitchell et al 1971).

The incidence of CHDs is similar for all major ethnic groups (Mitchell et al 1971) and for males and females (Richards et al 1955), although there is a differential sex ratio for certain types of CHDs. The overall frequency of non-cardiac malformations among patients with a CHD varies considerably (9–42%), depending on the method of ascertainment. In one comprehensive study that included both live clinic patients and autopsied subjects, 25% had an additional major malformation; one-third of those with an additional malformation had a recognizable syndrome. Of those with a recognizable syndrome, 6% had chromosome abnormalities and 1.7% had rubella (Greenwood et al 1975). Since the time of that study, the incidence of CHDs due to rubella has decreased dramatically.

In spite of the variable rates of associated non-cardiac malformations in different studies, in most patients CHDs are isolated lesions. Conversely, associated non-cardiac defects are approximately ten times more frequent than in the general population, in which the incidence of major birth defects is approximately 3%. Therefore, one must have a high index of suspicion about other anomalies in infants who present with a CHD, and it is imperative that the physician consider the possibility that the heart defect is only the most obvious element of a multisystem disorder. In general, the most common malformations associated with a CHD involve the musculoskeletal system (8.8%). Central nervous system disorders are present in 8.5%, renal-urinary tract malformations in 5.3%, and gastrointestinal anomalies in 4.2% (Greenwood et al 1975). Approximately 1.8% of patients with a CHD have a cleft palate. Although this is a relatively low rate of association, it represents a ten-fold increase in the incidence of cleft palate over that in the general population. Conversely, patients with congenital defects of other organ systems may have a statistically increased risk for a cardiac defect. For example, there is an increased frequency of CHDs in patients with oesophageal malformations (Smith 1982).

When additional congenital malformations are found, it is important to determine the nature of the multisystem involvement. Abnormalities in two or more systems may result from two primary abnormalities, or they may constitute a field defect. A 'field defect' is defined as a constellation of two or more malformations that result from a developmental error in a single embryological field. The DiGeorge sequence is an example of a field defect in which a primary abnormality in the fourth branchial arch and third and fourth pharyngeal pouches results in hypoplasia of the thymus and parathyroid glands, in addition to aortic arch or conotruncal anom-

alies. Similarly, secondary consequences of a primary malformation must be considered. Secondary defects are generally deformations, which are alterations in the shape and/or structure of an originally normally formed part. For example, it has been postulated that premature closure of the foramen ovale may result in some cases of hypoplastic left heart because of decreased blood flow through the left ventricle.

Occasionally, one must consider coincidence when two types of disease or birth defect are present in the same individual. For example, neurofibromatosis is not usually associated with CHDs, but case reports of this association have appeared in the literature (Neiman et al 1974). The incidence of CHDs is 8 per 1000 and the incidence of neurofibromatosis is approximately 1 per 4000. Therefore, one could expect a chance association of these two conditions in approximately 1 per 500 000 live births. Furthermore, since 14% of all infants have a minor anomaly, it is not uncommon to find a minor defect coincidentally in persons with 'isolated' CHDs (Smith 1982).

Whether other defects associated with CHDs are due to an underlying chromosomal or single gene defect, coincidence, secondary consequences, or field defects may be readily apparent in some cases and unclear in others. Repeated evaluations may be required, especially in infants with apparently isolated CHDs, to ensure that the defect is not part of an unsuspected multisystem disorder. For example, patients with a CHD as part of the DiGeorge sequence may not manifest the biochemical abnormalities of parathyroid hypoplasia until late in childhood.

AETIOLOGY

Known causes of congenital heart defects, particularly those associated with non-cardiac malformations, include chromosome abnormalities, single gene defects and teratogens. Until recently, it generally was accepted that over 90% of *isolated* congenital heart defects (CHDs not associated with non-cardiac malformations) had a multifactorial aetiology. Recently, this concept has been questioned (multifactorial aetiology is discussed below under 'Isolated CHDs').

Chromosome abnormalities

Approximately 6% of all CHDs are due to chromosome abnormalities (Greenwood et al 1975). Conversely, the incidence of CHDs among persons with chromosome abnormalities is approximately 30% (Wladimiroff et al 1985). As expected, patients with autosomal chromosomal anomalies virtually always have multiple congenital anomaly/mental retardation syndromes. Those with X chromosome anomalies usually have additional somatic features. Many of the recognized chromosomal syndromes that include CHDs are listed in the Tables referred to under specific heart defects. Most chromosomal syndromes do not have a single type of associated CHD; rather, many types of CHD can be seen with a single chromosomal syndrome. This has led some investigators to regard the CHDs in chromosomal syndromes as nonspecific. However, the well known association of atrioventricular canal in Down syndrome and aortic coarctation in the Turner syndrome should alert us to the probable existence of specific genes on specific chromosomes that predispose to particular types of congenital heart defects. A better localization and understanding of such genes should provide important clues to the genetic control of the development of the heart. This is particularly true as chromosomal deletion and duplication syndromes become more precisely defined at the chromosomal and DNA levels. Therefore, in spite of the *relative* non-specificity of CHDs and our current inability to understand how the chromosomal genotype relates to phenotype, one must emphasize the importance of continuing efforts to record accurately and to understand our clinical observations in this regard. Chromosomal syndromes associated with CHDs are listed in Tables 72.1–72.12.

Single gene defects

Approximately 3% of CHDs are due to single gene defects (Nora & Nora 1978). These gene defects can cause isolated CHDs, or they can have pleiotropic effects that result in CHDs plus other malformations. Familial occurrence of an isolated CHD may be an important clue that the defect is due to a single gene defect, although this is not necessarily so. CHDs within a family could also have a multifactorial or teratogenic aetiology, or each could be a chance occurrence. Examples of familial occurrence are discussed under the individual CHDs in the following sections.

The prototype for an autosomal dominant defect that causes CHDs plus other malformations is the Holt-Oram syndrome. Atrial septal defect (ASD) is the most common cardiac lesion in this syndrome, and hypoplasia with proximal placement of the thumb are the most frequent skeletal defects. However, other cardiac defects, including ventricular septal defect, and more severe abnormalities of the upper extremity can occur, even within the same family. Because expression can be highly variable, careful examination of other family members should be performed to detect previously unsuspected cases. Variable expression should also be taken into account when

genetic counselling is given, since future family members may be more or less severely affected. There are many other autosomal dominant conditions that cause CHDs. Examples of these syndromes are listed in Tables 72.1–72.12.

Autosomal recessive genes can also be responsible for isolated CHDs or CHDs as part of multisystem disorders. The Ellis-van Creveld syndrome is an example of a disorder in which approximately 50% of patients have a cardiac defect, most commonly an ostium primum ASD. Some other autosomal recessive disorders that may be associated with CHDs are listed in Tables 72.1–72.12.

X-linked disorders that include CHDs are not common. There may be an X-linked recessive syndrome of midline defects characterized by stenosis of the aqueduct of Sylvius, hypospadias, and/or heart defects such as tetralogy of Fallot (ToF) (Toriello & Higgins 1985). Other syndromes are listed in Tables 72.1–72.12.

Teratogens

It has been estimated that only 1% of CHDs are due to recognized teratogens (Nora & Nora 1978). Most teratogens that cause CHDs also cause non-cardiac malformations, although exceptions exist. For example, rubella can cause isolated patent ductus arteriosus, and lithium appears sometimes to cause isolated Ebstein anomaly. The teratogenic aetiology of a CHD is usually identified by the specific malformation pattern, in conjunction with the history of intrauterine exposure. The timing and intensity of the exposure partially determine whether or not a cardiac malformation will occur, but maternal and embryonic genetic susceptibility factors also probably play a role.

The only well-documented infectious teratogen that can cause CHDs is the rubella virus. The types of defects include PDA, ventricular septal defect (VSD), ASD, ToF, and peripheral pulmonary branch stenosis (PBS). Heart defects occur in 50–65% of affected infants (Jackson 1968). Most affected infants have additional non-cardiac abnormalities such as deafness, cataract, chorioretinitis or haematological abnormalities. The diagnosis of congenital rubella syndrome should be supported by serum viral antibody titres or, preferably, positive cultures. The incidence of congenital rubella is decreasing in many countries because of widespread use of immunization. Cytomegalovirus (CMV) has also been cited as a cause of CHDs, such as ToF (Boon et al 1972), ASD, and pulmonary and mitral valve stenosis (Feingold & Pashayan 1983). However, CMV infection is very common and is often acquired during birth or in the immediate postnatal period, so that positive cultures do not necessarily indicate that birth defects were caused by the virus. There has been at least one case report of intrauterine infection with *Borrelia burgdorferi*, the agent of Lyme disease, which may have resulted in CHDs (Schlesinger et al 1985).

Several pharmacological agents can cause CHDs. Thalidomide is notorious for its induction of limb defects in exposed fetuses. 5–10% of exposed patients also had CHDs, especially ToF, VSD, ASD, and truncus arteriosus, but aortic coarctation, PDA, pulmonary stenosis (PS), transposition of the great arteries (TGA) and total anomalous pulmonary venous return (TAPVR) have also been reported (Jackson 1968). The failure of this agent to induce birth defects in many animals serves as a constant reminder that no drug should be considered totally safe in pregnancy on the basis of negative animal data, and that no drug should be given to a pregnant woman unless it is necessary for her own health or the health of the fetus. This mandate also applies to drugs that have been used in humans for many years without documented teratogenic effects. Variable susceptibility to a given agent is well documented among inbred strains of laboratory animals, and similar variations in susceptibility may also exist in humans. For some medications the overall incidence of induced defects may be so low that teratogenicity would be difficult to document in epidemiological studies. Furthermore, combinations of drugs could have a teratogenic effect that may not be present when either drug is tested alone.

On the other hand, some therapeutic agents cannot be withdrawn safely during pregnancy in spite of suspected or known teratogenicity. Some of the anticonvulsants are teratogenic. Trimethadione results in cardiac defects such as TGA, ToF and hypoplastic left heart (HPLH), along with other characteristic features in 15–30% of exposed infants (Nora & Nora 1978). This agent can often be replaced by a safer anticonvulsant, and this should be done in post-pubertal females prior to childbearing. This approach can prevent exposure of the fetus in an unplanned or unsuspected pregnancy.

Hydantoins pose a risk for CHDs that is two- to three-fold increased over the general population risk (Committee on Drugs: American Academy of Pediatrics 1979). Other features of the fetal hydantoin syndrome may be present in 10% or more of exposed infants. Frequently this drug is necessary for seizure control, and it is generally accepted that the ill-effects of seizures on mother and fetus are probably greater than the teratogenic risks of the drug. Women of childbearing age who are taking hydantoin should be counselled about its possible teratogenic effects before a pregnancy is undertaken. There is evidence that a woman who has had a child with fetal hydantoin syndrome is at even greater risk for a subsequently affected child than other women

taking hydantoins who have had healthy children. The anticonvulsant primidone has also been suggested to be teratogenic, resulting in facial dysmorphism and CHDs (Myhre & Williams 1981).

Exposure to coumarin derivatives during pregnancy results in abnormal live borns in approximately 17–29% of pregnancies (Iturbe-Alessio et al 1986). Although CHDs are relatively infrequent in affected infants, PDA and peripheral branch stenosis have occurred (Hall et al 1980). In one study, coumarin resulted in birth defects when used in the first seven weeks of pregnancy, but not when heparin was substituted for anticoagulation in weeks 6–12 (Iturbe-Alessio et al 1986). It should be noted that a mother with a CHD may be treated with an anticoagulant, and the offspring is not only at risk for CHDs on a teratogenic basis but also on a genetic basis (Hall et al 1980).

Alcohol may be the non-therapeutic drug that is most frequently ingested by pregnant women. Alcohol induces CHDs in some exposed fetuses; VSD is most common, but ASD, ToF, and other defects can also occur. The overall incidence of the fetal alcohol syndrome in the general population may be 0.1–3.3 per 1000 (Smith 1982), with CHD present in 29–70% of affected infants (Fang et al 1987). Heavy alcohol drinkers, defined as women consuming a daily average equivalent of 45 ml or more absolute alcohol, had offspring with a higher incidence of major anomalies compared to more moderate drinkers. A 'safe' level of alcohol intake during pregnancy has not been established.

Lithium, used in the treatment of depression, was first recognized as a teratogen because of the increased number of babies born with Ebstein anomaly, a relatively rare CHD. In one study of 143 infants exposed in utero, 13 (9%) had malformations, including 10 with CHDs. Of the ten with CHDs, four had Ebstein anomaly plus other cardiac malformations (Weinstein & Goldfield 1975). More recently, data from the Swedish registry revealed four exposed infants with CHDs when 0.2 were expected, but none had Ebstein anomaly (Kallen 1987).

Retinoic acid, a vitamin A derivative used in the treatment of acne and other dermatological disorders, is a relatively potent teratogen. In one prospective study of 36 infants with first trimester exposure, five had malformations including conotruncal and aortic cardiac malformations, microtia or anotia, cleft palate, thymic hypoplasia, retinal and optic nerve abnormalities, and/or CNS malformations (Lammer et al 1985).

Use of aspirin in pregnancy has been reported as being associated with various types of CHDs, but confounding factors such as maternal fever or viral illness make it difficult to determine if aspirin itself is a teratogen (Zierler & Rothman 1985). Several other agents including phenobarbitol, amphetamines, meprobamate and oral contraceptives have been suggested as causing birth defects, but proof of their teratogenicity in humans is lacking and various studies have given conflicting results (Milkovich & van den Berg 1974, Hartz et al 1975, Heinonen et al 1977, Zierler & Rothman 1985).

Non-pharmacological chemical teratogens exist in the environment. For example, prenatal exposure to methyl-mercury causes microcephaly and brain damage (Smith 1982). However, no specific environmental chemical has been specifically linked to CHDs to date. It is conceivable that chemical pollutants or exposure to chemicals in the workplace may some day be shown to cause some CHDs.

Several maternal diseases are associated with an increased risk for CHDs. The incidence of birth defects in infants of diabetic mothers is 6–9% (Miller et al 1981); of those infants with malformations, 25% have CHDs (Ballard et al 1984). The risk for malformations is disproportionately higher when the diabetes is poorly controlled (Miller et al 1981). Few studies have supported an association between gestational diabetes and an increased risk for birth defects (Gabbe 1986).

Maternal collagen vascular diseases such as systemic lupus erythematosus (SLE) that are associated with antibody to the soluble tissue ribonucleoprotein antigen, Ro(SS-A), can result in congenital heart block in the offspring. Partial or complete atrioventricular block can occur (Reed et al 1983). In one study, 10% of control mothers and 50% of mothers who had infants with congenital complete heart block had demonstrable serum antibody to Ro(SS-A), even though less than half of the seropositive mothers had evidence of clinical SLE (Taylor et al 1986). The antibody can also be demonstrated in the serum of some infants with heart block when they are tested at less than three months of age (Taylor et al 1986). Histological findings in babies who died with heart block have included immunofluorescent evidence of antibody in cardiac tissue (Taylor et al 1986), AV node discontinuity (Litsey et al 1985), and generalized or conduction system myocardial fibrosis (Reed et al 1983). Infants affected with heart block can also have structural heart defects such as pulmonary valve stenosis, PDA, or TGA (Litsey et al 1985). However, not all babies born to mothers with anti-Ro(SS-A) antibodies have heart disease, suggesting that this factor is not specific and that other factors may be necessary for fetal heart disease to occur (Taylor et al 1986).

Elevated maternal serum phenylalanine, as seen in women with phenylketonuria who are not being treated with a low-phenylalanine diet, can result in significant birth defects. Microcephaly and mental retardation are most frequently observed but 19% have CHDs (Lenke & Levy 1980). ToF is most frequent, followed by VSD,

aortic coarctation, PDA, single ventricle and ASD (Lenke & Levy 1980). National collaborative studies are now in progress to determine the effects on fetal development of dietary therapy instituted prior to conception in women with PKU. The small amount of data on pregnancy outcome in women treated prior to conception is encouraging (Bush & Dukes 1985, Murphy et al 1985).

Maternal hyperthermia has been implicated as causing CHDs in at least one retrospective study; however the teratogenicity of hyperthermia in humans remains unproven (Warkany 1986). Amniotic band rupture is an example of a physical force that can result in ectopia cardis and other secondary CHDs (Kaplan et al 1985).

Teratogens associated with CHDs are listed in Tables 72.1–72.12.

Unknown aetiology

There are many infants with cardiac defects as part of multiple malformation disorders of unknown aetiology. Some patterns of malformation of unknown cause are recognized as representing particular syndromes, for example, the Cornelia de Lange syndrome. Other patterns of malformation are simply observed together more commonly than expected by chance alone, as in the VATER or VACTERL association. Still other multiple malformation disorders may not be categorized into currently recognized patterns. When no specific teratogen, chromosome abnormality, or single gene defect is identified, most multiple congenital anomaly disorders occur on a sporadic basis with a recurrence risk of 3% or less in siblings.

RISKS FOR CHD IN RELATIVES

When the proband has a CHD that is due to a chromosomal, single gene or teratogenic aetiology, recurrence risks for relatives are in keeping with the standard principles of genetic counselling.

Recurrence risks in relatives of patients with isolated CHDs presumed to be of multifactorial aetiology are currently being re-evaluated. Previous risk figures based on several series of patients were generally found to be 2–4% for all first-degree relatives, with slightly lower risks of 1% for more rare defects (Nora & Nora 1978). However, in a recent prospective study of 233 women who had CHDs, the frequency of CHDs in their 372 live-born offspring was found to be 15%. If instances in which the child's VSD closed spontaneously are eliminated, the prevalence was 14.2%, and if families with more than two affected relatives are eliminated, the prevalence was 12%. When the data were analyzed according to the type of

CHD in the mother, those with left ventricular outflow lesions had the highest risk (26%) (Whittemore et al 1982). Another smaller prospective study of 41 women resulted in no affected offspring (Allan et al 1986).

In one recent retrospective study of 219 parents with CHDs, the overall prevalence of CHDs in their 385 live-born offspring was 10.4%. When defects such as mitral valve prolapse and Wolff-Parkinson-White were excluded, the risk was 8.8% (Rose et al 1985). However, another recent retrospective study of 166 parents with CHDs showed a prevalence of CHDs of 4.9% in their 246 children (Czeizel et al 1982). In a third retrospective study of affected fathers, none of 52 offspring had a CHD (Ferencz 1986), while in a prospective study of 151 fathers with 308 children, 12.3% had CHDs (Whittemore et al 1987). Most of these studies (except for the most recent study of Whittemore et al 1987) plus previously reported series in which parental sex could be identified have been reviewed and used to generate revised recurrence risk data (Nora & Nora 1987). In these studies, affected women generally had higher risks for their offspring than did men; however, the study published after this review article suggested no statistical difference in recurrence risk for mothers compared to fathers (Whittemore et al 1987). Two very large subsequently published studies (Zellers et al 1989, Driscoll et al 1989) revealed lower risks of 1–3% for children born to affected parents. These lower risks are similar to those originally established by Nora & Nora (1978). The specific recurrence risks from these studies are summarized under the individual CHDs discussed below.

Recent studies have continued to show an overall recurrence risk of approximately 2–4% in siblings (Allan et al 1986). There have not been any recent reports of large series of sibling recurrence risks for individual CHDs to contradict earlier studies.

Genetic counselling for recurrence risks in relatives must take into account the discrepancies in various studies, and the possibility that these risk figures may undergo continuing revision over the next several years. Unless future data show otherwise, the risk for a person with two affected first-degree relatives is approximately double the risk when one is affected.

ISOLATED CONGENITAL HEART DEFECTS

Isolated CHDs are defined here as those unassociated with other major non-cardiac malformations. Overall, 73% of live-born infants with CHDs do not have serious non-cardiac malformations (Ferencz et al 1987). Although approximately 20% of CHDs are multiple, for example, VSD plus PDA (Richards et al 1955), these are considered 'isolated' CHDs in the sense that non-cardiac malformations are not present. The exact aetiology of most isolated CHDs is unknown. There is no significant difference in incidence by race, season of birth, birth order, maternal age, or socioeconomic status (Newman 1985).

Isolated CHDs may have a single gene, teratogenic, or multifactorial aetiology. Traditionally, it has been accepted that the majority (>90%) of isolated CHDs are of multifactorial aetiology (Nora & Nora 1978). This concept has been challenged recently, however, partly because of reports of higher than expected recurrence risks for children born to affected parents. Unfortunately, some authors who have addressed this question confuse the concepts of polygenic and multifactorial aetiology, and fail to consider that the multifactorial model includes the interaction of the polygenic predisposition with environmental factors. Some of the controversial points of the multifactorial model, as they relate to data on isolated CHDs, are as follows.

First, it has been suggested that recurrence risks for first-degree relatives are sometimes higher than expected, and that this is incompatible with the prediction that the risk for first-degree relatives approximates the square root of the frequency in the general population (Boughman et al 1987). However, this criticism fails to take into account that the prediction risks in this model assumed 100% heritability, while the heritability of CHDs is only 30–35% (Newman 1985).

Second, the fact that some of the more severe forms of congenital heart defects have lower recurrence risks than milder forms has been viewed by some (Boughman et al 1987) to be incompatible with predictions based on the multifactorial model, which holds that the recurrence risk is greater when the defect is more severe. However, it is possible that this concept *does apply within a given category of defect*. For example, the risk for a relative of a patient with a more severe form of tetralogy of Fallot may be greater than for a patient with VSD and mild PS. To our knowledge, such detailed recurrence risk data are not available. The fact that approximately 40–75% of CHDs are concordant or similar among first-degree relatives (Rose et al 1985), suggests that different genes may predispose to different heart defects. Interpretation of these data on apparent concordance is hampered by our lack of understanding of how genes control the development of the heart. Thus some phenotypic endpoints, for example VSD, can presumably result from many different factors, whether genetic or non-genetic, and the heart may have a limited number of responses to different insults, each of which result in the same defect. Conversely, apparently different defects may obscure a common pathogenetic mechanism, perhaps because of altered timing of the insult or modifying effects of other genes or intrauterine factors such as maternal blood flow.

Third, it has been noted that the differential recurrence risks according to sex ratios do not always conform to the Carter effect. For example, in one study the recurrence risk for children born to mothers with ASD was 12.3% versus 3.5% for affected fathers, even though ASD is more common in females. However, for the other two lesions in this study (coarctation of the aorta and aortic stenosis), the recurrence risks conformed to those expected (Rose et al 1985). It is more difficult to reconcile the data on ASD with what is expected from the multifactorial model. One could speculate that this deviation from the expected is only seen in live borns and that, if all conceptuses could be studied, the prediction would be verified. It is important to remember that the fact that several specific defects (ASD, aortic coarctation and others) *do have* a differential sex ratio suggests a genetic effect related to the X and Y chromosomes on the development of CHDs. For example, it is possible that aortic coarctation is more common in females with Turner syndrome and in males because a gene(s) on the X chromosome is important in controlling normal development of the aorta.

Fourth, some observations that recurrence risks are significantly higher for offspring than for siblings is not compatible with the multifactorial model. The reason why the offspring risks are so much higher in some studies is not known. Bias of selection may have been a factor in the prospective studies, since women who already had one or more healthy children may have been less likely to enrol in the study (Whittemore et al 1982). Retrospective studies (Rose et al 1985) could be biased for ascertainment of familial cases, since families with affected children would be more likely to remain in contact with the medical centre and were more likely to be located for the follow-up study.

Finally, several studies from which recurrence risks were derived did not specifically separate groups of infants with or without additional non-cardiac malformations. It is known that some CHDs, such as endocardial cushion defects, PDA and ASD, are frequently associated with non-cardiac defects, while TGA and aortic atresia are relatively infrequently associated with non-cardiac defects. Future studies on recurrence risks should pay careful attention to this type of information, since it is mainly for isolated CHDs that one would expect the multifactorial model to apply.

Although data from twin studies are often biased, when data from multiple studies are combined, concordance for CHDs is 15% for monozygous and 5% for dizygous twins (Newman 1985). Clearly, genetic factors cannot be the only determinant of CHDs, but the twin data available do not negate the possibility of a genetic effect.

Conceptually, it is appealing to accept that a polygenic effect on development of CHDs exists. That there must be a multitude of genes that can influence the development of the heart is apparent by the number of different chromosome disorders and single gene defects that are associated with CHDs. Most CHDs are not specific for a particular chromosomal or single gene syndrome. However, the disproportionate frequency of some defects in some syndromes such as an AV canal with Down syndrome or ASD with the Holt-Oram syndrome, suggests that particular genes tend to predispose to particular defects. This observation and the less than 100% concordance rate for specific defects in relatives with isolated CHDs, suggest that a multitude of genes can produce a limited number of abnormal responses that we recognize as phenotypic endpoints. Perhaps after the genetic control of the embryology of the heart is understood, the apparent discrepancies with the multifactorial model will be resolved.

Additional observations that are compatible with a multifactorial aetiology of some isolated CHDs include those indicating that CHDs are more frequent in some inbred populations. For example, in one study of an inbred population, the risk for a CHD in offspring of first cousins was 3.2%, while the risk for offspring of non-consanguineous parents was 1.2%. Furthermore, the relative frequencies of CHDs observed, with VSD being most common, were similar to those in the general population (Gev et al 1986). Thus the authors believe that it is premature to abandon the multifactorial model, although continued study of the genetic and environmental determinants of CHDs is needed. In these studies, aetiological heterogeneity must be considered.

Single gene mutations are a relatively uncommon cause of isolated CHDs. A positive family history is usually, but not always, the clue that leads one to suspect Mendelian heritability. For example, families with atrial septal defects in multiple generations suggest autosomal dominant inheritance in some cases (McKusick 1988). In other instances, it is the nature of the heart defect itself that raises suspicion that the defect is heritable. For example, secundum type ASD with prolonged atrioventricular conduction should lead one to consider a single gene aetiology even if a positive family history is not obtained (McKusick 1988).

A positive family history for a given defect, however, does not in itself prove that the condition is inherited as a single gene defect. For example, a family with four siblings having primum type ASD has been reported (Yao et al 1968); the parents were normal. This family situation suggests, but does not prove, autosomal recessive inheritance; a multifactorial or teratogenic aetiology still are possible. Similarly, there are reports of many other types of heart defect affecting two or more family members. These reports include families with Ebstein anomaly (McKusick 1988), hypoplastic left heart (McKusick 1988); coarctation of the aorta (McKusick 1988); and patent ductus arteriosus (McKusick 1988), to name a few. Although a single gene defect may be responsible for the heart defect in some of these families, multiple occurrences could be due to multifactorial or common environmental factors.

Teratogens must also be considered as a cause of isolated CHDs. For example, rubella virus usually causes multiple defects; however, 21% of infants with congenital rubella had single defects, many of which were isolated PDA. Drugs are often implicated as teratogenic agents, but relatively few are well documented as having this effect. It is usually more difficult to prove that an isolated CHD in a human is due to a specific drug than when the heart defect is part of a characteristic syndrome. Lithium as a cause of the Ebstein anomaly is an exception.

Other factors to consider in the pathogenesis of CHDs include maternal health as discussed above under 'Teratogens'. Maternal cyanotic CHD with accompanying hypoxia does not appear to result in a higher incidence of offspring with CHD than in mothers with non-cyanotic disease, although the former group has a higher frequency of spontaneous abortions, low birth weight and premature infants (Whittemore et al 1982).

VENTRICULAR SEPTAL DEFECT

Ventricular septal defect (VSD) occurs in 0.86–2.2 per 1000 live births (Ferencz et al 1985) and accounts for approximately 25% of CHDs (Boughman et al 1987). It has been suggested that the incidence of VSD in live births has increased during the time period 1970 to 1980 (Layde et al 1980). However, concomitant with this apparent increase, the mean age of diagnosis decreased from 2.2 to 0.2 years; spontaneous closures increased from 0.1 to 1.4 per 1000, and patients tended to have smaller lesions. This suggests that earlier and more intensive study accounts for the apparent increase (Spooner et al 1986). VSD is more frequent in low birth weight and premature infants, and the sex ratio is one (Newman 1985).

There are at least four types of VSD. *Type I*, or subarterial VSD, may be a conotruncal defect related to failure of fusion of the proximal conal cushions. This type is often associated with aortic insufficiency due to aortic valve cusp prolapse. *Type II*, perimembraneous VSD, may represent abnormal fusion of the muscular inflow and outflow septa. *Type III* is the atrioventricular canal type septal defect that occurs behind the posterior

leaflet of the tricuspid valve in the inflow portion of the right ventricle where the anterior and posterior endocardial cushions normally fuse. *Type IV*, muscular defect, may be caused by excessive cell death (Clark 1986b).

Major noncardiac malformations are present in 20% of patients with VSD; included in these series were persons with single gene defects and chromosome abnormalities (Levy et al 1978, Ferencz et al 1987). However, the majority of VSDs are isolated defects, possibly of multifactorial aetiology.

The overall risk for a CHD in a sibling of a person with VSD, when no other family members have CHD, is approximately 3% (Nora & Nora 1978, Czeizel et al 1982), but detailed risk figures for large series of each of the four types of VSD are unavailable. In one study of 179 patients with Type II VSD, the frequency of CHDs in siblings was 5.8%, while in 24 Type IV VSD patients, there were no affected siblings. There were insufficient numbers of Type I and III VSDs to study (Boughman et al 1987). More detailed data of this type will be important if we are to reach a more complete understanding of the aetiology of VSDs and provide more accurate genetic counselling.

The concordance rate for VSD in monozygous twins is 10% and heritability has been estimated to be 30–50% (Newman 1985).

The risk for offspring of persons with VSD had been believed to be approximately 4% (Nora & Nora 1978). However, one prospective study of mothers with VSD showed a 22% risk for offspring versus a 10% risk for children born to affected fathers (Whittemore et al 1987). Some of the children's VSDs closed spontaneously. It is difficult to understand why previous studies had consistently shown much lower risk figures. One possible explanation may be the prolonged (three year) follow-up in the study cited above, in which the children had annual examinations by the cardiologist (Whittemore et al 1987). Based on four recent series, both prospective and retrospective, it has been tentatively concluded that the recurrence risk among the offspring of mothers with VSD is 9.5% and for fathers, 2.1% (Nora & Nora 1987). However, a recent large retrospective study of 151 fathers with VSD who had 318 children showed only 10 (3.1%) with a CHD; of 382 children born to 190 affected mothers, only 11 (2.9%) had a CHD (Driscoll et al 1989).

The concordance for the type of heart defect when the proband has a VSD is approximately 25–50% (Corone et al 1983, Boughman et al 1987). Detailed concordance data for each type of VSD are needed. When two first-degree relatives have a CHD, the risk for recurrence approximately doubles. There are no documented instances of isolated VSD due to a single gene defect, but there are many single gene and chromosomal syndromes

Table 72.1 Disorders sometimes associated with ventricular septal defects

Chromosomal

Partial trisomy 1p	Elejalde et al 1984
Partial monosomy 1q	Garver et al 1976
Partial trisomy 2q	de Grouchy & Turleau 1984
Partial trisomy 3p	de Grouchy & Turleau 1984
Partial monosomy 4p	de Grouchy & Turleau 1984
Partial trisomy 4p	Yunis 1977
Partial monosomy 4q	de Grouchy & Turleau 1984
Partial monosomy 5p	Lammer & Opitz 1986
Partial trisomy 5p	Kleczkowska et al 1987
Partial trisomy 5q	de Grouchy & Turleau 1984
Partial monosomy 7p	de Grouchy & Turleau 1984
Partial monosomy 7q	Pfeiffer 1984
Mosaic trisomy 8	Nora & Nora 1978
Partial trisomy 8q	Townes & White 1978
Partial monosomy 9p	Smith 1982
Tetrasomy 9p	Yunis 1977
Partial trisomy 9q	de Grouchy & Turleau 1984
Mosaic trisomy 9	de Grouchy & Turleau 1984
Trisomy 10p	Snyder et al 1984
Partial monosomy 10p	Prieto et al 1978
Partial monosomy 10q	Shapiro et al 1985
Partial trisomy 10q	Yunis 1977
Partial monosomy 11q	Frank & Riccardi 1977
Partial trisomy 11;22	Lin et al 1986a
Trisomy 13	de Grouchy & Turleau 1984
Partial monosomy 13q	Nora & Nora 1978
Partial trisomy 14q	Nikolis et al 1983
Ring 15	Otto et al 1984
Partial trisomy 15q	de Grouchy & Turleau 1984
Partial monosomy 16q	Elder et al 1984
Partial monosomy 17p	Stratton et al 1984
Trisomy 18	de Grouchy & Turleau 1984
Partial monosomy 18q	Nora & Nora 1978
Ring 20	Burnell et al 1985
Partial trisomy 20p	Smith 1982
Trisomy 21	Smith 1982
Ring 21	de Grouchy & Turleau 1984
Partial monosomy 22	Lammer & Opitz 1986
Partial tetrasomy 22p and 22q	de Grouchy & Turleau 1984
Triploidy	Smith 1982

Single gene

Autosomal dominant

Aase-Smith syndrome	McKusick 1988
Hay Wells ectodermal dysplasia	Smith 1982
Holt-Oram syndrome	Smith 1982
Shprintzen velo-cardio-facial syndrome	McKusick 1988
Waardenburg syndrome	Smith 1982

Autosomal recessive

Carpenter acrocephalopolysyndactyly	Smith 1982
Hydrometrocolpos-polysyndactyly	Goecke et al 1981
Smith-Lemli-Opitz syndrome	Curry et al 1987
Spondylo-epimetaphyseal dysplasia with joint laxity	Beighton et al 1984

X-linked recessive

FG syndrome	Opitz et al 1982

Teratogenic

Alcohol	Fang et al 1987
Lithium	Weinstein & Goldfield 1975
Maternal diabetes	Grix 1982
Maternal phenylketonuria	Newman 1985
Phenytoin	Nakane et al 1980

Table 72.1   Disorders sometimes associated with ventricular septal defects (*contd.*)

Retinoic acid	Lammer et al 1985
Rubella	Jackson 1968
Trimethadione	Feldman et al 1977
Valproic acid	Ardinger et al 1986
Heterogeneous or uncertain aetiology	
Aase syndrome	Smith 1982
Asplenia syndrome	McKusick 1988
Beckwith-Wiedemann syndrome	Greenwood et al 1975
Cardiomelic dysplasia with mesoaxial hexadactyly	Martinez et al 1981
CHARGE association	Smith 1982
Cornelia de Lange syndrome	Smith 1982
DiGeorge sequence	Smith 1982
Distichiasis-vascular anomaly association	Goldstein et al 1985
Goldenhar syndrome	Smith 1982
Gonadal dysgenesis-scalp defects syndrome	Brosnan et al 1980
Hirschsprung-Ulnar polydactyly syndrome	McKusick 1988
Kabuki make-up syndrome	Ohdo et al 1985
Larson syndrome	Kiel et al 1983
Linear sebaceous nevus syndrome	Smith 1982
Locking finger-short stature syndrome	McKusick 1988
Mental retardation-blepharophimosis syndrome	Ohdo et al 1986
Pierre Robin sequence	Greenwood et al 1975
Polysplenia syndrome	McKusick 1988
Polysyndactyly-cardiac syndrome	McKusick 1988
Postaxial acrofacial dyostosis (Miller) syndrome	Donnai et al 1987
Rubinstein-Taybi syndrome	Smith 1982
Simpson dysmorphia syndrome	McKusick 1988
Splenogonadal fusion-peromelia syndrome	Loomis et al 1982
VATER association	Feingold & Pashayan 1983
Williams syndrome	Smith 1982

that are associated with VSD. Some syndromal and teratogenic causes of VSD are listed in Table 72.1.

ATRIAL SEPTAL DEFECT

Atrial septal defects (ASDs) occur with an incidence of 0.24–0.49 per 1000 live births (Ferencz et al 1985). In live borns, ASD is associated with major non-cardiac malformations in 30% of cases (Ferencz et al 1987). ASDs account for approximately 10% of all CHDs at birth and 12–15% of CHDs in children and adults (Campbell 1970). ASD is the only cardiac defect in approximately 84% of cases (Sanchez Cascos 1972). Of the two common types of ASD, ostium secundum defects are more common. The male:female ratio is 1:1.6 (Arena & Smith 1978). Secundum defects seem to result from an abnormality in the degenerative process in the septum primum that normally forms the ostium secundum, such that the opening which forms is too large; alternatively, the defect may result from malposition of the ostium secundum in relation to the septum secundum that ordinarily covers it. A third possibility is that the septum secundum forms improperly, so that the ostium secundum is unguarded. The secundum type of defect is separated from the atrioventricular valves by septal tissue while the ostium primum defect has no septal tissue separating it from the atrioventricular valves; this latter results from failure of the septum primum to fuse with the atrioventricular canal cushion tissue. The primum defect is often accompanied by a cleft of the mitral and/or tricuspid valve(s). Ostium primum defects are closely related to atrioventricular canal defects in which there is a common channel between both atria and ventricles in addition to cleft mitral and tricuspid valves. Ostium primum ASD and AV canal defects result from abnormal development of the endocardial cushions (Jackson 1968) and are discussed more fully in the following section on 'Endocardial Cushion Defects'.

Most isolated ASDs are probably of multifactorial aetiology. The recurrence risk for siblings of persons with secundum ASD is 2.5–3.2% (Nora & Nora 1978, Czeizel et al 1982) when no other family members are affected. In keeping with predictions based on multifactorial inheritance, the risk for siblings of male patients is 5% and of female patients, 2.5% (Sanchez Cascos 1972). The risk for affected offspring was previously reported to be 1.5–2.5% (Nora & Nora 1978), but recent studies suggest significantly higher recurrence risks for

Table 72.2   Disorders sometimes associated with atrial septal defects

Chromosomal

Partial trisomy 1q	Hindi et al 1986
Partial trisomy 3p	de Grouchy & Turleau 1984
Partial monosomy 4p	Nora & Nora 1978
Partial monosomy 4q	de Grouchy & Turleau 1984
Partial trisomy 4q	de Grouchy & Turleau 1984
Partial monosomy 5p	Nora & Nora 1978
Partial trisomy 5q	de Grouchy & Turleau 1984
Partial monosomy 7p	Schomig-Spingler et al 1986
Partial monosomy 7q	Fryns et al 1985
Partial monosomy 8p	Yunis 1977
Mosaic trisomy 8	Nora & Nora 1978
Partial monosomy 10p	Shokeir et al 1975
Partial trisomy 10q	Yunis 1977
Partial trisomy 11p	Waziri et al 1983
Partial trisomy 11;22	Lin et al 1986a
Partial monosomy 13q	de Grouchy & Turleau 1984
Trisomy 13	de Grouchy & Turleau 1984
Partial trisomy 15q	de Grouchy & Turleau 1984
Partial trisomy 16p	de Grouchy & Turleau 1984
Partial trisomy 16q	de Grouchy & Turleau 1984
Partial monosomy 17p	Stratton et al 1984
Partial trisomy 17q	de Grouchy & Turleau 1984
Trisomy 18	de Grouchy & Turleau 1984
Trisomy 21	Nora & Nora 1978
Tetrasomy 22p—>q11	Wilson et al 1984
Monosomy X	Nora & Nora 1978
49,XXXXY	Nora & Nora 1978
Triploidy	Smith 1982

Single gene

Autosomal dominant

Alagille arteriohepatic dysplasia	Gellis et al 1979
Holt-Oram syndrome	Smith 1982
Robinow syndrome	Smith 1982

Autosomal recessive

Ellis-van Creveld syndrome	Smith 1982
McDonough syndrome	Garcia-Sagredo et al 1984
Robert phocomelia syndrome	Smith 1982
Smith-Lemli-Opitz syndrome	Curry et al 1987
Spondylo-epimetaphyseal dysplasia with joint laxity	Beighton et al 1984
Thrombocytopenia absent radius syndrome	Hall 1987

Teratogenic

Alcohol	Fang et al 1987
Maternal phenylketonuria	Lenke & Levy 1980
Phenytoin	Nakane et al 1980
Retinoic acid	Lammer et al 1985
Rubella	Jackson 1968

Heterogeneous or uncertain aetiology

Asplenia syndrome	McKusick 1988
Beckwith-Wiedemann syndrome	Greenwood et al 1975
CHARGE association	Smith 1982
Coffin-Siris syndrome	Carey & Hall 1978
Larsen syndrome	Kiel et al 1983
Macrocranium-mental retardation-skeletal abnormalities syndrome	Cantú et al 1982
Mental retardation-blepharophimosis syndrome	Ohdo et al 1986
Pierre Robin-clubfoot syndrome	McKusick 1988
Polysplenia syndrome	McKusick 1988
Polysyndactyly cardiac syndrome	McKusick 1988
Thanatophoric dysplasia	Smith 1982
VATER association	Khoury et al 1983
White forelock-malformation syndrome	McKusick 1988
Williams syndrome	Smith 1982

offspring. In one prospective study, the risk for offspring born to affected mothers was 10.9% (Whittemore et al 1982), while in two retrospective studies the risk was 12.3% (Rose et al 1985) to 15.6% (Czeizel et al 1982). For affected fathers the risk for children was 3.5–10% in retrospective studies (Czeizel et al 1982, Rose et al 1985). Considering both older and more recent studies, it has been suggested that the risk for affected mothers' offspring is 4–4.5% and for affected fathers' offspring, 1.5% (Nora & Nora 1987).

Since ASDs are more common in females, the multifactorial model predicts that recurrence risks should be higher for affected fathers' offspring, which is the opposite of what has been observed. Future studies should carefully record the rate of spontaneous abortion and the sex ratio of both affected and unaffected offspring; theoretically, affected fathers could have more severely affected conceptuses that might be more likely to abort spontaneously.

The concordance rate for type of heart defects when the proband has ASD is approximately 35% (Corone et al 1983).

Autosomal dominant transmission of isolated secundum ASD in some families is well documented (McKusick 1988). In addition, there is an autosomal dominant syndrome of secundum type ASD with atrioventricular conduction defects that range from first degree to complete atrioventricular block (McKusick 1988). In patients with non-familial secundum ASDs, the frequency of first degree atrioventricular block is in the range of 6–19% (Kahler et al 1966).

Secundum ASD occurs in 70% of patients with the Holt-Oram syndrome and can be accompanied by right bundle branch block, or first degree AV block and bradycardia (Goldstein & Brown 1980). The accompanying limb defects range from severe phocomelia to carpal bone abnormalities detectable only by X-ray. The severity of skeletal defects does not correlate with the severity of cardiac defects (Gladstone & Sybert 1982). ASD is part of many other syndromes and malformation complexes, as listed in Table 72.2. In one series, 15% of patients had extracardiac abnormalities (Sanchez Cascos 1972).

ENDOCARDIAL CUSHION DEFECTS

Endocardial cushion defects (ECDs) occur in 0.13–0.68 per 1000 live births (Ferencz et al 1985); and account for approximately 4–8.5% (Mitchell et al 1971, Boughman et al 1987) of CHDs. Associated non-cardiac malformations, mainly Down syndrome, occur in approximately 75% of live borns with an ECD (Ferencz et al 1987). The overall male to female ratio is one (Arena & Smith 1978),

but for primum ASD alone, 64% of cases are female (McKusick 1988). Families which have several members with ECDs are known (Yao et al 1968, Michels, personal observation, 1987); some family members have a complete AV canal while others have ostium primum ASD or only a cleft mitral valve. Except for these unusual families, the recurrence risk is low, with recurrence risks among siblings of 1.4–2% (Nora & Nora 1978, Emanuel et al 1983). Recent studies suggest a relatively high risk of 9.6% for offspring of an affected parent. When only affected mothers are considered, the risk is even higher (14.3%) (Emanuel et al 1983) but relatively few offspring of affected fathers have been studied (Nora & Nora 1987).

A list of conditions associated with ECDs is shown in Table 72.3.

CONOTRUNCAL DEFECTS

Abnormalities related to faulty conotruncal septation include tetralogy of Fallot (ToF), VSD with pulmonic stenosis, transposition of the great arteries (TGA), truncus arteriosus and double outlet right ventricle (DORV). The incidence of this group of defects is 0.58–0.89 per 1000 live births (Ferencz et al 1985). ToF accounts for 7.5% of all CHDs occurring in 0.26–0.36 per 1000 live births (Ferencz et al 1985). Approximately 30% of live borns with ToF also have major non-cardiac malformations (Ferencz et al 1987). VSD with pulmonic stenosis (PS) accounts for 7.3% of CHDs and occurs in 0.20 per 1000 live births (Mitchell et al 1971). TGA accounts for 4.6% of CHDs, occurring in 0.21–0.38 per 1000 live births (Ferencz et al 1985); only 8% of live borns with TGA have major non-cardiac malformations (Ferencz et al 1987). Other conotruncal defects account for 4% of CHDs (Boughman et al 1987); the incidence of truncus arteriosus is 0.03–0.07 per 1000 and of DORV is 0.03–0.07 per 1000 live births (Ferencz et al 1985). Approximately 30% of live-born infants with truncus arteriosus have additional non-cardiac malformations (Ferencz et al 1987).

Conotruncal septation refers to the division of the single primitive heart tube into two distinct outflow tracts that result from the fusion of two swellings that arise in the truncal region at 30 days' gestation. The swellings grow towards each other in a spiral fashion and fuse to form the septum that divides the truncus arteriosus into the pulmonary artery and aorta. At the same time, two additional swellings in the conus region grow towards each other and fuse to form the division between the outflow tracts, just below the aortic and pulmonary valves (Miller & Smith 1979). Evidence that conotruncal septa-

Table 72.3 Disorders sometimes associated with endocardial cushion defects

Chromosomal	
Partial monosomy 8p	Yunis 1977
Mosaic trisomy 9	Yunis 1977
Partial trisomy 10q	Yunis 1977
Partial trisomy (11;22)	Lin et al 1986a
Mosaic trisomy 14	Kaplan et al 1986
Mosaic ring 15	Gimelli et al 1983
Trisomy 21	Nora & Nora 1978
Monosomy 22	Lammer & Opitz 1986
Triploidy	Blackburn et al 1982
Single gene	
Autosomal dominant	
Alagille arteriohepatic dysplasia	Gellis et al 1979
Holt-Oram syndrome	Gladstone & Sybert 1982
Autosomal recessive	
Ellis-van Creveld syndrome	Feingold & Pashayan 1983
Hydrolethalus syndrome	McKusick 1988
Hydrometrocolpos-polysyndactyly syndrome	Goecke et al 1981
Smith-Lemli-Opitz syndrome	Curry et al 1987
Teratogenic	
Alcohol	Loser & Majewski 1977
Maternal diabetes mellitus	Grix 1982
Heterogeneous or uncertain aetiology	
Asplenia syndrome	Smith 1982
Cardiomelic-dysplasia with mesoaxial hexodactyly syndrome	Martinez et al 1981
CHARGE association	Smith 1982
Dandy-Walker-Facial dysmorphism syndrome	Ritscher et al 1987
Limb reduction-ichthyosis syndrome	Smith 1982
Pierre Robin sequence	Greenwood et al 1975
Pilotto syndrome	Pena 1982
Polysplenia syndrome	Smith 1982

tion is under genetic control arises from studies of the Keeshond dog model (Van Mierop et al 1977). These data and those from human pedigrees (Pitt 1962) are consistent with multifactorial inheritance of conotruncal septation defects. However, in some cases with strongly positive family histories, a single gene defect with incomplete penetrance may be responsible and the recurrence risk may be higher than the usually quoted risk figures derived from large series of patients (Miller & Smith 1979).

Transposition of the great arteries seems to be due to complete lack of rotation of the conotruncal septum. The conotruncal wall itself is presumed to be involved in this failure of rotation, since the coronary ostia remain associated with the aorta (Jackson 1968). The recurrence risk for siblings is 2% (Nora & Nora 1978). Insufficient data on risks to children of affected persons are available. Concordance for TGA among first-degree relatives ranges from 8–25% (Corone et al 1983). The male to female ratio of TGA is 2.6:1 (Arena & Smith 1978). TGA is particularly common in infants of diabetic mothers, and the empiric recurrence risk for a CHD in offspring of

diabetics is 5% (Nora & Nora 1978). As previously noted, TGA can occur in the offspring of mothers with collagen-vascular disease (Litsey et al 1985).

Tetralogy of Fallot is an abnormality of conotruncal septation that seems to result from unequal partitioning of the conus at the expense of the right ventricular outflow tract and pulmonary trunk (Van Mierop et al 1977). The recurrence risk for siblings is approximately 2.5% (Nora & Nora 1978). Based on several studies, it has been suggested that the risk for children born to affected mothers is 2.5% and to fathers, 1.5% (Nora & Nora 1978). The male to female ratio for ToF is 1.4:1, so that the slightly higher risks for children born to affected mothers is compatible with the multifactorial model. The concordance rate for ToF among first-degree relatives is 31–35%, but there are also positive correlations for ToF with VSD, PS and TGA (Corone et al 1983).

Pulmonary atresia has a prevalence of 0.04–0.08% per 1000 live births (Ferencz et al 1985) and it accounts for 1.5% of CHDs (Mitchell et al 1971). The recurrence risk among siblings is 1%, but data for significant numbers of offspring of an affected parent are unavailable.

Table 72.4 Disorders sometimes associated with conotruncal defects

Chromosomal

Partial monosomy 1q	de Grouchy & Turleau 1984
Partial trisomy 1q	de Grouchy & Turleau 1984
Partial trisomy 3p	Reiss et al 1986
Partial trisomy 3q	Wilson et al 1985
Partial monosomy 4p	Pober et al 1988
Partial monosomy 4q	de Grouchy & Turleau 1984
Partial trisomy 4q	de Grouchy & Turleau 1984
Partial monosomy 8p	de Grouchy & Turleau 1984
Partial trisomy 8q	de Grouchy & Turleau 1984
Partial monosomy 9p	Yunis 1977
Partial trisomy 9q	de Grouchy & Turleau 1984
Mosaic partial trisomy 9	Nora & Nora 1978
Partial monosomy 10p	Berger et al 1977
Partial monosomy 10q	Mulcahy et al 1982
Partial trisomy 10q	Yunis 1977
Partial monosomy 11q	McPherson & Meissner 1982
Ring 11	Cousineau et al 1983
Partial trisomy (11;22)	Lin et al 1986a
Partial tetrasomy 14q	Johnston et al 1986
Partial trisomy 16p	de Grouchy & Turleau 1984
Trisomy 13	Smith 1982
Trisomy 18	Smith 1982
Partial monosomy 20p	Garcia-Cruz et al 1985
Partial trisomy 20p	Smith 1982
Mosaic trisomy 20	Djalali et al 1985
Partial trisomy 20q	Sax et al 1986
Trisomy 21	Levy et al 1978
Partial monosomy 22p and 22q	Kelley et al 1982
Triploidy	Blackburn et al 1982

Single gene

Autosomal dominant

Alagille arteriohepatic dysplasia	Gellis et al 1979
Holt-Oram syndrome	Greenwood et al 1975
Preauricular pits, broad forehead, ToF syndrome	Jones & Waldman 1985
Sphrintzen velo-cardio-facial syndrome	Lammer & Opitz 1986

Autosomal recessive

Carpenter syndrome	Smith 1982
Cohen syndrome	Friedman & Sack 1982
McDonough syndrome	Garcia-Sagredo et al 1984
Thrombocytopenia absent radius syndrome	Feingold & Pashayan 1983

X-linked recessive

Midline defect syndrome	Toriello & Higgins 1985

Teratogenic

Alcohol	Levy et al 1978
Maternal connective tissue disease	Litsey et al 1985
Maternal diabetes mellitus	Ballard et al 1984
Maternal phenylketonuria	Lenke & Levy 1980
Phenytoin	Clark 1986a
Retinoic acid	Lammer et al 1985
Rubella	Jackson 1968
Thalidomide	Jackson 1968
Trimethadione	Smith 1982
Valproic acid	Ardinger et al 1986

Heterogeneous or uncertain aetiology

Asplenia syndrome	Smith 1982
Beckwith-Wiedemann syndrome	Greenwood et al 1977
Bremer lethal malformation syndrome	McKusick 1988
CHARGE association	Smith 1982
Cleft-limb-heart syndrome	McKusick 1988
Cloacal extrophy	Pober et al 1988
Coffin-Siris syndrome	Carey & Hall 1978

Table 72.4 Disorders sometimes associated with conotruncal defects (*contd.*)

Cornelia de Lange syndrome	Pober et al 1988
DiGeorge sequence	Lammer & Opitz 1986
Genito-palato-cardiac syndrome	Greenberg et al 1987
Goldenhar syndrome	Feingold & Pashayan 1983
Kabuki make-up syndrome	Ohdo et al 1985
Kouseff syndrome	McKusick 1988
Limb reduction-icthyosis syndrome	Smith 1982
Nager acrofacial dyostosis	Thompson et al 1985
Noonan syndrome	Feingold & Pashayan 1983
Pierre Robin sequence	Greenwood et al 1975
Polysplenia syndrome	Smith 1982
Rubinstein-Taybi syndrome	Levy et al 1978
VATER association	Khoury et al 1983

The male to female ratio for truncus arteriosus is 1.6:1, and the recurrence risk among siblings is 1% (Nora & Nora 1978) to 6% (Pierpont et al 1988). Recurrence risk data for large numbers of patients with less common conotruncal defects are not available.

Overall, conotruncal defects are relatively frequent effects of teratogens such as thalidomide, retinoic acid and phenytoin. They also occur as the most frequent CHDs in several conditions such as the DiGeorge and Goldenhar sequences and the CHARGE association. These and other disorders that are sometimes associated with conotruncal defects are listed in Table 72.4.

PATENT DUCTUS ARTERIOSUS

The prevalence of patent ductus arteriosus (PDA) is 0.14–0.77 per 1000 live births (Ferencz et al 1985). Excluding babies born at less than 38 weeks' gestation, PDA accounts for 2.6% of all CHDs (Boughman et al 1987).

The ductus develops from the sixth embryonic arch (Boon & Roberts 1976). Perinatal factors related to prematurity or to high altitude hypoxia may delay closure of an intrinsically normal ductus arteriosus. When these factors are not present, most instances of PDA may have a multifactorial aetiology. The recurrence risk among siblings is approximately 3% (Nora & Nora 1978). The risk for children born to affected mothers varies from 3.5–10.8% in different reported series (Whittemore et al 1982, Nora & Nora 1987). The risk for the offspring of affected fathers is believed to be lower, approximately 2.5% (Nora & Nora 1987). The male to female ratio of PDA is 1:1.9 (Arena & Smith 1978), so that the apparently higher risk for offspring of affected mothers is the opposite of that expected with multifactorial aetiology. The concordance for PDA among affected first-degree relatives is approximately 50% (Corone et al 1983).

PDA has been reported in several generations of some families, suggestive of an autosomal dominant pattern of inheritance in these unusual cases (Martin et al 1986). Several conditions sometimes associated with PDA are listed in Table 72.5.

COARCTATION OF THE AORTA

The prevalence of coarctation of the aorta is 0.24–0.51 per 1000 live births (Ferencz et al 1985). Approximately 20% of live borns with the defect have non-cardiac malformations (Ferencz et al 1987). Aortic coarctation accounts for 5–7% of CHDs (Boon & Roberts 1976, Boughman et al 1987). The coarctation usually occurs opposite the ductus arteriosus. There are two theories regarding the development of this defect. The more popular theory is that the aorta fails to grow at a localized point; the second possibility is that a localized segment of the aorta contains ductus-like tissue that undergoes constriction at birth on the same basis as the normal ductus (Jackson 1968).

Most cases of isolated aortic coarctation have been considered to have a multifactorial aetiology. The recurrence risk among siblings is approximately 2% (Nora & Nora 1978). The risk for children born to an affected parent was previously believed to be 2–3% (Nora & Nora 1978). Recent studies suggest a higher risk, especially for the offspring of affected mothers, of 6.5% in both prospective (Allan et al 1986) and retrospective (Rose et al 1985) studies. Considering all the data, the offspring risk figures suggested for genetic counselling for affected mothers is 4% and for affected fathers, 2% (Nora & Nora 1987). The male to female ratio is 2.3:1 (Arena & Smith 1978) so that a higher risk for affected mothers' offspring is compatible with multifactorial aetiology. The concordance rate for aortic coarctation is 35–50% (Corone et al 1983).

Table 72.5 Disorders sometimes associated with patent ductus arteriosus

Chromosomal

Partial trisomy 3q	de Grouchy & Turleau 1984
Partial trisomy 3p	de Grouchy & Turleau 1984
Partial monosomy 4p	Nora & Nora 1978
Partial monosomy 4q	de Grouchy & Turleau 1984
Partial monosomy 5p	Nora & Nora 1978
Partial trisomy 6p	de Grouchy & Turleau 1984
Partial monosomy 6q	Yamamoto et al 1986
Partial monosomy 7p	Schomig-Spingler et al 1986
Partial monosomy 8p	Brocker-Vriends et al 1986
Mosaic trisomy 8	Nora & Nora 1978
Partial monosomy 9p	Smith 1982
Mosaic trisomy 9	Bowen et al 1974
Partial monosomy 10q	Lewandowski et al 1978
Partial trisomy 10q	Yunis 1977
Partial trisomy 11q	Yunis 1977
Partial trisomy (11;22)	Lin et al 1986a
Trisomy 13	Nora & Nora 1978
Partial deletion 17p	Stratton et al 1984
Partial monosomy 18p	de Grouchy & Turleau 1984
Trisomy 18	de Grouchy & Turleau 1984
Trisomy 21	Nora & Nora 1978
Monosomy 22	Lammer & Opitz 1986
49,XXXXY and 49,XXXXX	de Grouchy & Turleau 1984
Triploidy	Blackburn et al 1982

Single gene
　Autosomal dominant

Alagille arteriohepatic dysplasia	Gellis et al 1979
Hay Wells ectodermal dysplasia	Smith 1982
Holt-Oram syndrome	Smith 1982
Sphrintzen syndrome	Meinecke et al 1986

　Autosomal recessive

Camptomelic dysplasia	Feingold & Pashayan 1983
Carpenter syndrome	Smith 1982
McDonough syndrome	Garcia-Sagredo et al 1984
Meckel-Gruber syndrome	Smith 1982
Smith-Lemli-Opitz syndrome	Curry et al 1987

Teratogenic

Alcohol	Streissguth et al 1985
Hydantoin	Smith 1982
Lithium	Weinstein & Goldfield 1975
Maternal collagen vascular disease	Litsey et al 1985
Maternal diabetes mellitus	Ballard et al 1984
Maternal phenylketonuria	Lenke & Levy 1980
Retinoic acid	Lammer et al 1985
Rubella	Jackson 1968
Thalidomide	Jackson 1968
Trimethadione	Zackai et al 1975
Valproic acid	Ardinger et al 1986

Heterogeneous or uncertain aetiology

Asplenia syndrome	Hurwitz & Caskey 1982
Beckwith-Wiedemann syndrome	Greenwood et al 1977
C syndrome	Opitz et al 1969
Cardiomelic dysplasia with mesoaxial hexadactyly syndrome	Martinez et al 1981
CHARGE association	Smith 1982
Coffin-Siris syndrome	Carey & Hall 1978
DiGeorge sequence	Lammer & Opitz 1986
Goldenhar syndrome	Smith 1982
Gorlin Chaudhry Moss syndrome	McKusick 1988
Kabuki make-up syndrome	Ohdo et al 1985
Larsen syndrome	Kiel et al 1983

Table 72.5 Disorders sometimes associated with patent ductus arteriosus (*contd.*)

Nager acrofacial dyostosis	Thompson et al 1985
Noonan syndrome	Yunis 1977
Pierre Robin sequence	Greenwood et al 1975
Pilotto syndrome	Pena 1982
Rubinstein-Taybi syndrome	Smith 1982
Thanatophoric dysplasia	Smith 1982
VATER association	Khoury et al 1983
Williams syndrome	Kelly & Barr 1975

There has been at least one four-generation family suggested as having autosomal dominant aortic coarctation (Beekman & Robinow 1985), but these data could also be explained by a multifactorial aetiology.

Coarctation occurs in approximately 15% of patients with the Turner syndrome, in which the frequency of this defect seems to correlate with the severity of neck webbing (Clark 1984). Patients with the Turner syndrome also seem to be at increased risk for aortic dilation and rupture (Lin et al 1986b). Additional disorders sometimes associated with aortic coarctation are listed in Table 72.6.

AORTIC VALVE DEFECTS

Aortic stenosis (AS) can be valvular, subvalvular or supravalvular. The prevalence of aortic stenosis in live births is 0.11–0.34 per 1000 (Ferencz et al 1985) and it accounts for approximately 3% of CHDs (Boughman et al 1987). 20% of live-born infants with AS have non-cardiac malformations (Ferencz et al 1987). Valvular AS is usually associated with abnormal development of the valve leaflets. In 85% of cases there is a bicuspid aortic valve, and in 14% there is no apparent separation into leaflets. Only rarely are there three normal leaflets with fusion at the commissures. Severe stenosis can result in secondary effects that include hypoplasia of the ascending aorta and left ventricular endocardial thickening (Hoffman 1977).

The recurrence risk for AS among siblings is 2% (Nora & Nora 1978). The risk for offspring was previously believed to be 4% (Nora & Nora 1978), but subsequent studies suggested higher risks; for affected women, the risk to offspring was as high as 13–18%, while the risk for affected fathers' offspring was 3% (Nora & Nora 1987). More recently, the risk for offspring of 123 affected males, was found to be 3/227 children (1.3%) and for offspring of 33 females is 0/66 children. (Driscoll et at 1989). The concordance for AS among first-degree relatives with CHDs is approximately 50% (Corone et al 1983). The male to female ratio is 4:1 (Arena & Smith

1978), so that a higher risk for affected women's offspring is expected.

Subvalvular stenosis may be due to a thin membranous diaphragm or a thick fibromuscular obstruction. The aortic valve may be secondarily thickened due to abnormal blood flow caused by the obstruction. In other cases, aortic subvalvular obstruction may be a secondary consequence of an abnormally placed papillary muscle and mitral valve. Subaortic stenosis may also be due to diffuse hypertrophy of the left ventricle (hypertrophic subaortic stenosis) as seen in hypertrophic cardiomyopathy (McKusick 1988). Reports of familial subvalvular aortic stenosis that are not related to cardiomyopathy are rare (McKusick 1988).

Supravalvular AS (SVAS) is a narrowing that occurs in the aorta just above the coronary arteries; it is infrequent as an isolated lesion and usually occurs as part of the infantile hypercalcaemia syndrome of Williams (Smith 1982) or as an isolated autosomal dominant condition. Although some investigations believe that isolated autosomal dominant SVAS is a mild expression of the Williams syndrome, this probably is not so. The Williams syndrome is usually sporadic, and instances of patients with the Williams syndrome reputedly occurring in families with isolated SVAS are not well documented, either with regard to the facial dysmorphism or with regard to the SVAS (Schmidt et al 1989).

Bicuspid aortic valve without congenital AS is common, occurring in approximately 1% of the population (McKusick 1988). These individuals are at increased risk for bacterial endocarditis and for calcific aortic stenosis. In a series of adult patients with pure aortic stenosis requiring surgical excision, a congenitally bicuspid valve was present in 46% of patients. The mean age at which surgery was performed was 59 years. A unicommissural valve was found in 6% with a mean age at surgery of 48 years. The male to female ratio of patients requiring surgery was 3.4:1 (Subramanian et al 1984).

Conditions sometimes associated with aortic valve defects are listed in Table 72.7.

Many patients with valvular or subvalvular AS have

Table 72.6 Disorders sometimes associated with coarctation of the aorta

Chromosomal	
Partial trisomy 4q	de Grouchy & Turleau 1984
Partial monosomy 7q	Fryns et al 1985
Partial monosomy 9p	Yunis 1977
Mosaic trisomy 9	Nora & Nora 1978
Partial monosomy 10p	de Grouchy & Turleau 1984
Partial trisomy (11;22)	Lin et al 1986a
Partial monosomy 16q	Rivera et al 1985
Trisomy 18	Smith 1982
Ring 21	de Grouchy & Turleau 1984
Monosomy X	Nora & Nora 1978
Single gene	
Autosomal dominant	
Alagille arteriohepatic dysplasia	Gellis et al 1979
Autosomal recessive	
Meckel-Gruber syndrome	Smith 1982
Smith-Lemli-Opitz sydrome	Curry et al 1987
Teratogenic	
Alcohol	Smith 1982
Hydantoin	Smith 1982
Isotretinoin	Rosa et al 1986
Lithium	Weinstein & Goldfield 1975
Maternal diabetes mellitus	Grix 1982
Maternal phenylketonuria	Smith 1982
Rubella	Greenwood et al 1975
Thalidomide	Jackson 1968
Heterogeneous or uncertain aetiology	
Beckwith-Wiedemann syndrome	Best & Hoekstra 1981
Cornelia de Lange syndrome	Greenwood et al 1975
Goldenhar syndrome	Smith 1982
Kabuki make-up syndrome	Ohdo et al 1985
Linear sebaceous nevus syndrome	Smith 1982
Pierre Robin sequence	Greenwood et al 1975
Robinow syndrome	Butler & Wadlington 1987
Rubinstein-Taybi syndrome	Greenwood et al 1975
VATER association	Mapstone et al 1986

some degree of aortic regurgitation. In a series of adult patients with a mean age of 56 years (age range 3rd–8th decade) with aortic stenosis and insufficiency requiring surgery, congenital bicuspid valve was present in 19% of patients. 6%, with a mean age of 41 years, had an unicommissural valve. The male to female ratio of patients with these complications was 3:1 (Subramanian et al 1985).

The familial occurrence of bicuspid aortic valve is 17–34%. There is some evidence that the trait is autosomal dominant with reduced penetrance (McKusick 1988). Biscuspid aortic valve is present in 20–40% of patients with the Turner syndrome (Natowicz & Kelley 1987). Other conditions sometimes associated with bicuspid aortic valves are listed in Table 75.8.

MITRAL VALVE DEFECTS

Isolated congenital mitral stenosis is very rare. It may be associated with abnormal mitral valve cusps or cusps that appear normal but are fused. Obstruction may also result from a parachute mitral valve in which the chordae tendinae are attached to a single papillary muscle. Mitral valve stenosis more commonly occurs in conjunction with other CHDs such as aortic coarctation or VSD. In a series of patients undergoing valve replacement for mitral stenosis (with or without mitral insufficiency), only 1% had congenital defects (Olson et al 1987). Mitral stenosis has been reported in syndromes such as the Williams syndrome (Driscoll et al 1974) and geleophysic dwarfism (McKusick 1988), and has also occurred with chromosome abnormalities such as partial trisomy 1q (Hindi et al 1986). Mitral atresia is usually associated with complex heart defects. It can result from intrauterine lithium exposure (Weinstein & Goldfield 1975) and with chromosome abnormalities such as trisomy 13 (Smith 1982).

Congenital mitral regurgitation is rare, occurring in 0.05 per 1000 live births and accounting for 0.6% of CHDs (Mitchell et al 1971). Mitral insufficiency may

Table 72.7 Disorders sometimes associated with aortic stenosis

VALVULAR	
Chromosomal	
Partial trisomy 1q	Hindi et al 1986
Partial trisomy 2p	de Grouchy & Turleau 1984
Partial trisomy 2q	de Grouchy & Turleau 1984
Partial monosomy 7p	de Grouchy & Turleau 1984
Partial trisomy (11;22)	Lin et al 1986a
Partial monosomy 18p	de Grouchy & Turleau 1984
Monosomy X	Nora & Nora 1978
Single gene	
Autosomal dominant	
LEOPARD syndrome	Goldstein & Brown 1980
Autosomal recessive	
Gelophysic dwarfism	McKusick 1988
Smith-Lemli-Opitz syndrome	Curry et al 1987
Teratogenic	
Hydantoin	Smith 1982
Rubella	McKusick 1988
Heterogeneous or uncertain aetiology	
Pfeiffer-Palm-Teller syndrome	McKusick 1988
Williams syndrome	McKusick 1988
SUBVALVULAR	
Chromosomal	
Partial trisomy 17q	de Grouchy & Turleau 1984
Single gene	
Autosomal recessive	
Weill-Marchesani syndrome	McKusick 1988
Uncertain aetiology	
Onat syndrome	McKusick 1988

occur on the basis of abnormal insertion of short chordae tendinae, accessory commissures, or underdevelopment of valve leaflets. A cleft of the mitral valve may occur as an isolated lesion, but more commonly it is associated with an endocardial cushion defect or other lesions. In the past, rheumatic fever was probably the most frequent aetiology of mitral regurgitation, but congenital lesions now account for a higher proportion. The murmur of congenital mitral regurgitation may appear later in life, leading to the erroneous assumption that the lesion is acquired. A possible autosomal dominant disorder of mitral regurgitation, conductive deafness due to stapes footplate fixation, and fused cervical vertebrae has been reported in four generations of a family (McKusick 1988). Mitral insufficiency can also occur with bone disorders such as autosomal recessive spondylo-epimeta-physeal dysplasia with joint laxity (Beighton et al 1984).

Mitral valve prolapse is the most common abnormality of the mitral valve, occurring in 5% of the population. The frequency is highest (17%) in young women, but decreases with increasing age. Persons with MV prolapse tend to have a tall and thin body habitus (Savage et al 1983). It is interesting that MV prolapse also seems to occur more frequently in patients with anorexia nervosa,

Table 72.8 Disorders sometimes associated with bicuspid aortic valve

Chromosomal	
Partial trisomy 1q	Hindi et al 1986
Trisomy 13	Smith 1982
Trisomy 18	de Grouchy & Turleau 1984
Monosomy X	Natowicz & Kelley 1987
Teratogenic	
Retinoic acid	Lammer et al 1985
Heterogeneous or uncertain aetiology	
CHARGE association	Hittner et al 1979
DiGeorge sequence	Weinberg & Wright 1978
Robinow syndrome	Butler & Wadlington 1987

possibly due to a size disproportion between the normal leaflets and the small left ventricle (Meyers et al 1986). The occurrence of MV prolapse in 30% of first-degree relatives of affected patients is compatible with autosomal dominant inheritance (McKusick 1988). MV prolapse is present with increased frequency in many connective tissue disorders such as the Marfan and Ehlers-Danlos syndromes, pseudoxanthoma elasticum, osteogenesis imperfecta and the Stickler syndrome (Liberfarb & Goldblatt 1986). It can also be associated with other structural CHDs such as ASD (McKusick 1988) and the Holt-Oram syndrome (Gladstone & Sybert 1982). A possible X-linked disorder of congenital mitral and aortic insufficiency has been reported (Monteleone & Fagan 1969) and one of the authors (VVM) has observed a similar family.

PULMONARY VALVE DEFECTS

The prevalence of pulmonary stenosis (PS) in live births is approximately 0.16-0.66 per 1000 live births (Ferencz et al 1985), and accounts for 10.5% of CHDs (Mitchell et al 1971). Approximately 15% of affected live borns have non-cardiac malformations (Ferencz et al 1987).

Pulmonary stenosis can be valvular, subvalvular, or supravalvular. In valvular stenosis, the valve usually is normally formed but the cusps are thickened and fused (Hoffman 1977). Secondary consequences of PS can include infundibular hypertrophy and hypoplasia of the pulmonary arterial system.

The recurrence risk for PS among siblings of an affected patient is 3.5% (Nora & Nora 1978). The risk for offspring is 4-6.5% for affected mothers and 2% for affected fathers (Nora & Nora 1987). In a recent large study, the risk to offspring of 92 affected males was 3 per 169 children (1.8%) and to offspring of 106 affected females was 8 per 204 children (3.9%) (Driscoll et al 1989). The male to female ratio is one (Arena & Smith 1978), so that the recurrence risk data for offspring are not supportive of multifactorial aetiology. The concordance of PS in first-degree relatives with CHDs is approximately 35% (Corone et al 1983)

A few families with multiple instances of PS, with or without other cardiac defects such as ASD, have been reported; however, it is not clear that these represent single gene defects (Ciuffo et al 1985). A family in which four of five sibs had both PS and congenital nephrotic syndrome has been reported (McKusick 1988).

Isolated subvalvular PS is rare, but it may occur because of a discrete subpulmonic fibromuscular ring or aberrant muscular bands that may be associated with a VSD. It most commonly occurs in association with the tetralogy of Fallot. Supravalvular PS is uncommon and may be caused by discrete diaphragms, diffuse constrictions or hypoplasia of the pulmonary arteries.

Conditions sometimes associated with pulmonary stenosis are listed in Table 72.9.

TRICUSPID VALVE DEFECTS

Isolated tricuspid stenosis is extremely rare. Usually it is associated with hypoplastic right ventricle and pulmonic atresia with intact ventricular septum.

Tricuspid atresia is more common and virtually always associated with some degree of hypoplasia of the right ventricle. Tricuspid atresia has a prevalence of 0.05-0.09 per 1000 live births (Ferencz et al 1985). 10% of affected live borns have non-cardiac malformations (Ferencz et al 1987). Tricuspid atresia accounts for 1.6% of CHDs (Boughman et al 1987). The recurrence risk among siblings is 1%, but offspring recurrence risk data are unavailable (Nora & Nora 1978). This defect can be seen in chromosomal disorders, such as partial trisomy (11;22) (Fraccaro et al 1980).

The Ebstein anomaly is a malformation characterized by downward displacement of the tricuspid valve with anomalous attachment of the posterior and septal leaflets to the right ventricular wall. The frequency of Ebstein anomaly is less than 0.4 per 1000 live births, and it accounts for 1.1-1.7% of CHDs (Boughman et al 1987, Ferencz et al 1987). Approximately 25% of live-born patients have associated non-cardiac malformations (Ferencz et al 1987). The recurrence risk among siblings is 1% (Nora & Nora 1978). Mild Ebstein's anomaly associated with persistent atrial standstill has been reported in a father and son (Piérard et al 1985). It can result from intrauterine lithium exposure (Weinstein & Goldfield 1975) and can occur with chromosome abnormalities such as trisomy 21 (Levy et al 1978) and partial deletion 17p (Stratton et al 1984).

The increased frequency of this uncommon form of CHD in infants born to mothers taking lithium led to the discovery that lithium is teratogenic. As discussed previously, lithium also can cause other forms of CHDs such as tricuspid atresia and ASD (Nora & Nora 1978).

HYPOPLASTIC HEART

Hypoplastic left heart (HPLH) is characterized by underdevelopment of the left ventricle and aortic and mitral valves. It occurs in 0.10-0.25 per 1000 live births (Ferencz et al 1985) and accounts for 7-9% of CHDs (Natowicz & Kelley 1987). The male to female ratio is 2:1 (Child & Dennis 1977). Although instances of affected siblings have led some to postulate an autosomal recessive

Table 72.9 Disorders sometimes associated with pulmonary stenosis

VALVULAR STENOSIS
Chromosomal

Partial monosomy 5p	Lammer & Opitz 1986
Partial monosomy 8p	de Grouchy & Turleau 1984
Mosiac trisomy 8	Yunis 1977
Partial monosomy 9p	Smith 1982
Tetrasomy 9p	Yunis 1977
Partial monosomy 10p	Shokeir et al 1975
Partial trisomy (11;22)	Lin et al 1986a
Trisomy 13	Smith 1982
Partial trisomy 15q	de Grouchy & Turleau 1984
Partial monosomy 17p	Dobyns et al 1983
Trisomy 18	Nora & Nora 1978
Monosomy 22	Lammer & Opitz 1986

Single gene
  Autosomal dominant

Alagille arteriohepatic dysplasia	Gellis et al 1979
Holt-Oram syndrome	Smith 1982
LEOPARD syndrome	Smith 1982

  Autosomal recessive

Carpenter syndrome	Smith 1982
McDonough syndrome	Garcia-Sagredo et al 1984
Meckel-Gruber syndrome	Smith 1982

Teratogenic

Alcohol	Loser & Majewski 1977
Hydantoin	Smith 1982
Maternal collagen vascular disease	Litsey et al 1985
Maternal diabetes mellitus	Grix 1982
Retinoic acid	Lammer et al 1985
Rubella	McKusick 1988
Thalidomide	Jackson 1968

Heterogeneous or uncertain aetiology

Acro-renal-ocular syndrome	Halal et al 1984
Asplenia syndrome	Smith 1982
Cardiomelic dysplasia with mesoaxial hexodactyly syndrome	Martinez et al 1981
DiGeorge sequence	Mallette et al 1982
Noonan syndrome	Smith 1982
Polysplenia syndrome	Smith 1982
Rhizomelic syndrome	McKusick 1988
Rubinstein-Taybi syndrome	McKusick 1988
Williams syndrome	Smith 1982

INFUNDIBULAR STENOSIS
Chromosomal

Partial trisomy 3p	Reiss et al 1986
Partial trisomy (11;22)	Lin et al 1986a
Monosomy 22	Lammer & Opitz 1986

Single gene
  Autosomal recessive

Kartagener syndrome	Schidlow et al 1982

Teratogenic

Maternal diabetes mellitus	Ballard et al 1984
Rubella	Jackson 1968

Heterogeneous or uncertain aetiology

Branchial arch syndrome	McKusick 1988
Noonan syndrome	Feingold & Pashayan 1983

Table 72.10   Disorders sometimes associated with hypoplastic left heart

Chromosomal	
Partial monosomy 1q	Wright et al 1986
Partial monosomy 4p	Natowicz & Kelley 1987
Partial monosomy 4q	Natowicz & Kelley 1987
Partial monosomy 11q	Natowicz & Kelley 1987
Partial trisomy 12p	Natowicz & Kelley 1987
Trisomy 13	Natowicz & Kelley 1987
Trisomy 18	Natowicz & Kelley 1987
Trisomy 21	Natowicz & Kelley 1987
Monosomy X	Natowicz & Kelley 1987
46,X,i(Xq)	Shah et al 1985
Single gene	
Autosomal dominant	
Apert syndrome	Natowicz & Kelley 1987
Holt-Oram syndrome	Natowicz & Kelley 1987
Autosomal recessive	
Ellis-van Creveld syndrome	Natowicz & Kelley 1987
Saldino Noonan chondrodysplasia	Natowicz & Kelley 1987
Smith-Lemli-Opitz syndrome	Natowicz & Kelley 1987
Teratogenic	
Maternal diabetes mellitus	Miller et al 1981
Maternal phenylketonuria	Fisch et al 1969
Retinoic acid	Lammer et al 1985
Trimethadione	Zackai et al 1975
Heterogeneous or uncertain aetiology	
Asplenia syndrome	Natowicz & Kelley 1987
Beckwith-Wiedemann syndrome	Greenwood et al 1975
DiGeorge sequence	Greenwood et al 1975
Faciocardiomelic syndrome	Cantu et al 1975
Polysplenia syndrome	Natowicz & Kelley 1987
VATER association	Natowicz & Kelley 1987

aetiology, most series of patients show a sibling recurrence risk of 1–2% (Brownell & Shokeir 1976, Natowicz & Kelley 1987). One recent study of recurrence rates in siblings found that 13.5% were affected (Boughman et al 1987). Between 10% and 37% of infants with HPLH have extracardiac anomalies (Ferencz et al 1987, Natowicz & Kelley 1987). A list of conditions sometimes associated with HPLH is shown in Table 72.10.

Hypoplastic right heart (HPRH) is usually associated with tricuspid atresia or with pulmonary atresia with intact ventricular septum. HPRH with hypoplasia of the tricuspid valve is rare, but is more frequently familial than when associated with tricuspid atresia (Davachi et al 1967).

DEXTROCARDIA

Dextrocardia can occur with normal placement of other organs or in conjunction with visceral situs inversus. Dextrocardia with normal visceral situs is almost always associated with other CHDs, but the heart is often structurally normal in other respects when associated with visceral situs inversus (Miller & Divertie 1972). The frequency of situs inversus is 0.10–0.14 per 1000 among children and adults (Soltan & Li 1974, Layton 1976) while the frequency of isolated dextrocardia is 0.03–0.06 per 1000. Approximately 15% of persons with situs inversus have the autosomal recessive Kartagener immotile cilia syndrome (Goldstein & Brown 1980). Although patients with Kartagener syndrome occasionally have heart defects such as TGA, the majority have normal hearts except for the abnormal situs. Rarely, patients with Kartagener syndrome have asplenia or polysplenia (Schidlow et al 1982). Other conditions sometimes associated with dextrocardia are listed in Table 72.11.

Congenital absence of the spleen has an incidence of 0.02 per 1000 (Rose et al 1975) and is associated with CHDs in 63–97% of cases (Kirby & Bockman 1984). The types of CHDs that have been associated with asplenia are shown in Tables 72.1–72.5 and 72.9–72.13. The association of CHDs and asplenia or hypoplastic spleen is sometimes referred to as the Ivemark syndrome. Some authors have suggested that at least some cases of Ivemark syndrome are autosomal recessive (Hurwitz & Caskey 1982), while in other series the recurrence risk is approximately 5% (Rose et al 1975).

Table 72.11   Disorders sometimes associated with dextrocardia

Chromosomal	
Partial trisomy 2p	de Grouchy & Turleau 1984
Partial trisomy 10p	de Grouchy & Turleau 1984
Partial trisomy 10q	Yunis 1977
Trisomy 13	Smith 1982
Trisomy 18	Smith 1982
Triploidy	Blackburn et al 1982
Single gene	
Autosomal dominant	
Holt-Oram syndrome	Zhang et al 1986
Autosomal recessive	
Kartagener syndrome	Nora & Nora 1978
Multiple ptergyium-malignant	
hyperthermia syndrome	Robinson et al 1987
Thrombocytopenia-absent radius	Hall 1987
Heterogeneous or uncertain aetiology	
Asplenia syndrome	Rose et al 1975
Poland-Mobius syndrome	Bosch-Banyeras et al 1984
Polysplenia syndrome	Rose et al 1975
VATER association	Khoury et al 1983

Although some investigators consider the Ivemark asplenia syndrome to be an entity distinct from polysplenia, there have been families where one sib has polysplenia and another has asplenia (Rose et al 1975). Approximately 40% of patients with polysplenia have malposition of the cardiac apex, but in general the CHDs tend to be less severe with polysplenia than with asplenia (Rose et al 1975). Some of the CHDs seen with polysplenia are listed in Tables 72.1–72.4 and 72.9–72.13.

It has been suggested that polysplenia is due to premature development of body curvature in the embryo, while asplenia is due to delayed curvature (Hutchins et al 1983). In mice, a single gene may control situs such that an autosomal recessive mutation results in random situs (Layton 1976). In humans, one unusual family with isolated dextrocardia showed a pattern compatible with X-linked inheritance (McKusick 1988).

SINGLE VENTRICLE

Single ventricle is a rare disorder that may be due to failure of development at the bulbar ventricular loop stage. It occurs in approximately 0.05 per 1000 live births and accounts for 0.9% of CHDs (Mitchell et al 1971). In one series of 223 patients with univentricular heart, including single or common ventricle, the risk for CHD in siblings was 11/388 (2.8%) (Weigel et al 1989). In one reported family, a child had single ventricle and the mother had truncus arteriosus (Shapiro et al 1981). Conditions that have been associated with single ventricle are shown in Table 72.12.

TOTAL ANOMALOUS PULMONARY VENOUS RETURN

Total anomalous pulmonary venous return (TAPVR) occurs in 0.06–0.08 per 1000 live births (Ferencz et al 1985) and accounts for 1.6% of CHDs (Boughman et al 1987). Approximately 10% of live-born infants with the disorder also have major non-cardiac malformations (Ferencz et al 1987). The male to female ratio is one (Arena & Smith 1978). Occasional family occurrences have been reported (McKusick 1988). TAPVR is frequently associated with additional complex CHDs and is almost always present in cases of the Ivemark asplenia syndrome (Hutchins et al 1983). Other conditions

Table 72.12 Disorders sometimes associated with single ventricle

Chromosomal	
Trisomy 18	Levy et al 1978
Trisomy 21	Weigel et al 1989
Monosomy X	Weigel et al 1989
Single gene	
Autosomal dominant	
Holt-Oram syndrome	Zhang et al 1986
Teratogenic	
Maternal diabetes mellitus	Miller et al 1981
Maternal phenylketonuria	Lenke & Levy 1980
Retinoic acid	Lammer et al 1985
Heterogeneous or uncertain aetiology	
Asplenia syndrome	Smith 1982
Polysplenia syndrome	Smith 1982

Table 72.13 Disorders sometimes associated with total anomalous pulmonary venous return

Chromosomal	
Partial monsomy 4p	Lazjuk et al 1980
Partial tetrasomy 22(p—>q11)	Wilson et al 1984
Monosomy X	Clark 1984
Single gene	
Autosomal dominant	
Holt-Oram syndrome	Gladstone & Sybert 1982
Autosomal recessive	
Smith-Lemli-Opitz syndrome	Curry et al 1987
Teratogenic	
Maternal diabetes mellitus	Miller et al 1981
Rubella	Greenwood et al 1975
Thalidomide	Jackson 1968
Heterogeneous or uncertain aetiology	
Asplenia syndrome	Smith 1982
CHARGE association	Hittner et al 1979
Polysplenia syndrome	Smith 1982

sometimes associated with TAPVR or partial anomalous venous return are shown in Table 72.13.

ENDOCARDIAL FIBROELASTOSIS

Endocardial fibroelastosis (EFE) is probably the end result of several different pathogenic mechanisms. It can occur as a primary defect as one form of dilated cardiomyopathy, or secondary to other CHDs that result in severe obstruction, such as AS. Idiopathic EFE usually occurs in young infants and may sometimes be congenital. The incidence of idiopathic EFE is 0.17–0.23 per 1000 (Mitchell et al 1971, Goldstein & Brown 1980). EFE represents a heterogeneous group of disorders, with some cases due to metabolic abnormalities such as carnitine deficiency or to maternal anti-Ro(SS-A) antibody (Litsey et al 1985). Viral aetiologies, including mumps, have previously been considered as causes of EFE, but there is no adequate documentation of this (Hoffman 1977). Several families with patterns suggestive of X-linked and autosomal recessive inheritance have been reported (McKusick 1988). However, some of these sibs may have had an unrecognized metabolic or teratogenic cause for their EFE. The empiric recurrence risk, when the disorder is idiopathic, is approximately 7% (Goldstein & Brown 1980). Rarely, EFE occurs as part of a multiple congenital anomaly syndrome, as in the facio-cardio-renal syndrome (Eastman & Bixler 1977).

CARDIAC CONDUCTION DEFECTS

Cardiac conduction defects may accompany structural CHDs; for example, first-degree atrioventricular (AV) block frequently occurs with ECD.

In adults, most cardiac conduction defects are due to acquired diseases such as atherosclerosis, although some are due to hereditary storage diseases such as Fabry disease or amyloidosis. However, conduction defects, whether of prenatal, congenital or adult onset, are sometimes due to intrinsic defects of the conducting system that are unassociated with other apparent structural or cardiac muscle diseases. Some of these defects are heritable, while others may be due to teratogens or maternal connective tissue disease.

The Jervell and Lange-Nielsen syndrome is an autosomal recessive condition characterized by severe congenital deafness, a prolonged QT interval and large T-wave, and a propensity to syncope and sudden death due to ventricular fibrillation. The frequency in the general population is 0.3 per 1000, but this disorder may be present in 1% of deaf children (Goldstein & Brown 1980). The Romano-Ward syndrome is similar, but is not associated with deafness and is transmitted as an autosomal dominant condition. The onset of symptoms usually occurs before the age of 3 years, but may occur as early as the first day of life (Horn et al 1986). Alternatively, symptoms may occur after age 30 years (Goldstein & Brown 1980). Penetrance is approximately 90%. Many patients present with seizures secondary to ventricular arrhythmias which can result in a significant delay in diagnosis. In two cases, postmortem examination revealed enlargement and degeneration of ventricular Purkinje cells (Hashiba 1978).

The LEOPARD syndrome is an autosomal dominant disorder characterized by growth retardation, lentigines, deafness and cardiac conduction defects characterized by a prolonged PR interval, left anterior hemiblock, widening of the QRS complex or complete heart block. Sudden death may occur. Hypertrophic cardiomyopathy or subpulmonic stenosis may also be present (Goldstein & Brown 1980).

There are several rare but well-documented autosomal

dominant gene defects with cardiac conduction defects as their major manifestation. These include: a disorder of bundle branch block with or without atrial arrhythmias, ventricular premature systoles, Wolff-Parkinson-White syndrome and risk for premature death (McKusick 1988); isolated complete right bundle branch block (McKusick 1988); progressive adult-onset AV block with loss of R waves and syncope (McKusick 1988); and brachydactyly type C with intraventricular conduction defects or sick sinus syndrome (McKusick 1988). Numerous additional familial conduction defects that may or may not represent simple gene defects have been reported, including: congenital AV block due to absent AV node in sibs, resulting in neonatal death (Goldstein & Brown 1980); congenital AV dissociation in three sibs due to 'lazy' sinoatrial pacemaker (McKusick 1988); and progressive bundle branch block in sibs (McKusick 1988).

The Wolff-Parkinson-White (WPW) syndrome with pre-excitation due to congenital accessory AV pathways has been noted as occurring in multiple members of families on several occasions. The accessory pathways are believed to be due to failure of irradiation of the remnants of AV pathways during development. The frequency of pre-excitation syndrome in the general population is 0.015 per 1000, but among first-degree relatives of affected patients the prevalence was 0.005 per 1000. Conversely, for probands with WPW, 3.4% had an affected relative (Vidaillet et al 1987). It was suggested that these data support autosomal dominant inheritance, in particular because of several large families with occurrence in two or more generations. WPW can be seen in other disorders such as tuberous sclerosis (Jayakar et al 1986) and familial dilated cardiomyopathy (Schmidt et al 1988).

PRENATAL DIAGNOSIS

Real-time two-dimensional ultrasonic scanners with high resolution imaging capabilities can be used to visualize the fetal heart as early as 12–16 weeks' gestation (Wladimiroff et al 1985). In some cases, the ultrasound (US) examination of the fetus will be performed specifically looking for CHDs because of increased risk based on a positive family history. In one such study (Allan et al 1986) 1021 pregnant women were studied; in over 90% the US examination was performed at 18 weeks' gestation. Twenty fetuses with CHDs were detected prenatally; four cases of CHD were detected only postnatally. In other instances, fetal CHD will be identified because of fetal hydrops or intrauterine growth retardation. In these situations it is important to establish, as well as possible, whether or not additional non-cardiac malformations are also present. Such investigations may

include amniocentesis for fetal karyotype; in one study of patients referred for level-four US for a variety of reasons, the frequency of chromosome abnormalities among those with structural CHDs was 38% (Wladimiroff et al 1985).

The types of CHD detected by US of the fetus are numerous and include hypoplastic left heart (DeVore et al 1982), hypoplastic right heart with pulmonary atresia (Kleinman et al 1980) aortic valve atresia (Silverman et al 1984), and idiopathic endocardial fibroelastosis (Bovicelli et al 1984) to name a few. However, an apparently normal US examination, particularly early in pregnancy, does not definitely exclude the possibility of a CHD in the fetus; for example, cases of VSD have been missed (Wladimiroff et al 1985).

When a fetus is diagnosed as having a CHD, the information can be used to ensure that the baby is delivered in a tertiary care centre that can provide appropriate care. In some cases of severe CHD the parents may opt for termination of the pregnancy. In many cases, a normal US examination of the fetal heart will provide a measure of reassurance to anxious parents at increased risk for having a child with a CHD.

Cardiac dysrhythmias may occur in a fetus with a CHD or with a structurally normal heart (Stewart et al 1983). US is a useful tool for monitoring the clinical status of fetuses with dysrhythmias. The first sign of fetal heart failure may be pericardial effusion, which can be detected by US (DeVore et al 1982). Eventually, fetal hydrops and intrauterine death can occur. Fetal arrhythmias can be effectively treated in some cases by administration of anti-arrhythmic medications to the mother; the clinical response in terms of resolution of the hydrops can be monitored by US (Wiggins et al 1986). Such diagnosis and treatment has been accomplished as early as 24 weeks' gestation (Wiggins et al 1986).

CONCLUSION

Since the first edition of this chapter was published, significant advances have been made in the area of prenatal diagnosis of CHDs, and many fetal dysrhythmias have been shown to be amenable to successful intrauterine treatment. However, other areas that previously had been thought to be understood, such as the presumed multifactorial aetiology of CHDs, have recently become unsettled. It is likely that our understanding of the pathogenesis of CHDs will continue to evolve as recurrence risks in relatives are redefined, and as single gene and chromosome abnormalities associated with CHDs become mapped and better understood at the DNA level. It is hoped that our evolving understanding of CHDs will eventually take us to our ultimate goal, the prevention of CHDs.

REFERENCES

Allan L D, Crawford D C, Chita S K, Anderson R H, Tynan M J 1986 Familial recurrence of congenital heart disease in a prospective series of mothers referred for fetal echocardiography. American Journal of Cardiology 58: 334–337

American Academy of Pediatrics, Committee on Drugs, Anticonvulsants and Pregnancy 1979. Pediatrics 63: 331–333

Ardinger H H, Clark E B, Hanson J W 1986 Cardiac malformations associated with fetal valproic acid exposure. Proceedings of the Greenwood Genetic Center 5: 162

Arena J F P, Smith D W 1978 Sex liability to single structural defects. American Journal of Diseases of Children 132: 970–972

Ballard J L, Holroyde J, Tsang R C, Chan G, Sutherland J M, Knowles H C 1984 High malformation rates and decreased mortality in infants of diabetic mothers managed after the first trimester of pregnancy (1956–1978). American Journal of Obstetrics & Gynecology 148: 1111–1118

Beekman R H, Robinow M 1985 Coarctation of the aorta inherited as an autosomal dominant trait. American Journal of Cardiology 56: 818–819

Beighton P, Gericke G, Kozlowski K, Grobler L 1984 The manifestations and natural history of spondylo-epi-metaphyseal dysplasia with joint laxity. Clinical Genetics 26: 308–317

Berger R, Larroche J C, Toubas P L 1977 Deletion of the short arm of chromosome No. 10. Acta Paediatrica Scandinavica 66: 659–662

Best L G, Hoekstra R E 1981 Wiedemann-Beckwith syndrome: autosomal-dominant inheritance in a family. American Journal of Medical Genetics 9: 291–299

Blackburn W R, Miller W P, Supreneau D W, Cooley N R, Zellweger H, Wertelecki W 1982 Comparative studies of infants with mosaic and complete triploidy: an analysis of 55 cases. Birth Defects: Original Article Series 18: 251–274

Boon A R, Roberts D F 1976 A family study of coarctation of the aorta. Journal of Medical Genetics 13: 420–433

Boon A R, Farmer M B, Roberts D F 1972 A family study of Fallot's tetralogy. Journal of Medical Genetics 9: 179–192

Bosch-Banyeras J M, Zuasnabar A, Puig A, Catala M, Cuatrecasas J M 1984 Poland-Mobius syndrome associated with dextrocardia. Journal of Medical Genetics 21: 70–71

Boughman J A, Berg K A, Astemborski J A et al 1987 Familial risks of congenital heart defect assessed in a population-based epidemiologic study. American Journal of Medical Genetics 26: 839–849

Bovicelli L, Picchio F M, Pilu G et al 1984 Prenatal diagnosis of endocardial fibroelastosis. Prenatal Diagnosis 4: 67–72

Bowen P, Ying K L, Chung G S H 1974 Trisomy 9 mosaicism in a newborn infant with multiple malformations. Journal of Pediatrics 85: 95–97

Bröcker-Vriends A H J T, Mooij P D, Van Bel F, Beverstock G C, Van De Kamp J J P 1986 Monosomy 8p: an easily overlooked syndrome. Journal of Medical Genetics 23: 153–154

Brosnan P G, Lewandowski R C, Toguri A G, Payer A F, Meyer W J 1980 A new familial syndrome of 46,XY gonadal dysgenesis with anomalies of ectodermal and mesodermal structures. Journal of Pediatrics 97: 586–590

Brownell L G, Shokeir M H K 1976 Inheritance of hypoplastic left heart syndrome (HLHS): further observations. Clinical Genetics 9: 245–249

Burnell R H, Stern L M, Sutherland G R 1985 A case of ring 20 chromosome with cardiac and renal anomalies. Australian Paediatric Journal 21: 285–286

Bush R T, Dukes P C 1985 Women with phenylketonuria: successful management of pregnancy and implications. New Zealand Medical Journal 78: 181–183

Butler M G, Wadlington W B 1987 Robinow syndrome: report of two patients and review of literature. Clinical Genetics 31: 77–85

Campbell M 1970 Natural history of atrial septal defect. British Heart Journal 32: 820–826

Cantú J M, Hernandez A, Ramirez J 1975 Lethal facio-cardiomelic dysplasia – a new autosomal recessive disorder. Birth Defects: Original Article Series 11: 91–98

Cantú J M, Sanchez-Corona J, Hernandes A, Nazara Z, Garcia-Cruz D 1982 Individualization of a syndrome with mental deficiency, macrocranium, peculiar facies and cardiac and skeletal anomalies. Clinical Genetics 22: 172–179

Carey J C, Hall B D 1978 The Coffin-Siris syndrome: five new cases including two siblings. American Journal of Diseases of Children 132: 667–671

Child A H, Dennis N R 1977 The genetics of congenital heart disease. Birth Defects: Original Article Series 13: 85–91

Ciuffo A A, Cunningham E, Traill T A 1985 Familial pulmonary valve stenosis, atrial septal defect, and unique electrocardiogram abnormalities. Journal of Medical Genetics 22: 311–313

Clark E B 1984 Neck web and congenital heart defects: a pathogenic association in 45 X-O Turner syndrome? Teratology 29: 355–361

Clark E B 1986a Cardiac embryology: its relevance to congenital heart disease. American Journal of Diseases of Children 140: 41–44

Clark E B 1986b Mechanisms in the pathogenesis of congenital cardiac malformations. In: Pierpont M E, Moller J H (eds) The genetics of cardiovascular disease. Martinus-Nijoff, Boston

Corone P, Bonaiti C, Feingold J, Fromont S, Berthet-Bondet D 1983 Familial congenital heart disease: how are the various types related? American Journal of Cardiology 51: 942–945

Cousineau A J, Higgins J V, Scott-Emuakpor A B, Mody G 1983 Ring-11 chromosome: phenotype-karyotype correlation with deletions of 11q. American Journal of Medical Genetics 14: 29–35

Curry C J R, Carey J C, Holland J S et al 1987 Smith-Lemli-Opitz syndrome-type II: multiple congenital anomalies with male pseudohermaphroditism and frequent lethality. American Journal of Medical Genetics 26: 45–57

Czeizel A, Pornoi A, Peterffy E, Tarcal E 1982 Study of children of parents operated on for congenital cardiovascular malformations. British Heart Journal 47: 290–293

Davachi F, McLean R H, Moller J H, Edwards J E 1967 Hypoplasia of the right ventricle and tricuspid valve in siblings. Journal of Pediatrics 71: 869–874

de Grouchy J, Turleau C 1984 Clinical atlas of human chromosomes, 2nd edn. John Wiley, New York

DeVore G R, Donnerstein R L, Kleinman C S, Platt L D, Hobbins J C 1982 Fetal echocardiography. II. The diagnosis and significance of a pericardial effusion in the fetus using real-time – directed M-mode ultrasound. American Journal of Obstetrics and Gynecology 144:

693-700

Djalali M, Steinbach P, Schwinger E, Schwanitz G, Tettenborn U, Wolf M 1985 On the significance of true trisomy 20 mosaicism in amniotic fluid culture. Human Genetics 69: 321-326

Dobyns W B, Stratton R F, Parke J T, Greenberg F, Nussbaum R L, Ledbetter D H 1983 Miller-Dieker syndrome: lissencephaly and monosomy 17p. Journal of Pediatrics 102: 552-558

Donnai D, Hughes H E, Winter R M 1987 Postaxial acrofacial dysostosis (Miller) syndrome. Journal of Medical Genetics 24: 422-425

Driscoll D J, Friedberg D Z, Gallen W J 1974 Idiopathic hypercalcemic syndrome with mitral stenosis. Wisconsin Medical Journal 73: S115-S116

Driscoll D J, Michels V V, Gersony W M et al 1989 Occurrence of congenital heart defects in offspring of patients with ventricular septal defect, aortic stenosis, or pulmonary stenosis: Results of the Second Natural History Study of Congenital Heart Defects. Journal of American College of Cardiology 13: 136A.

Eastman J R, Bixler D 1977 Facio-cardio-renal syndrome: a newly delineated recessive disorder. Clinical Genetics 11: 424-430

Elder F F B, Ferguson J W, Lockhart L H 1984 Identical twins with deletion 16q syndrome: evidence that 16q12.2-q13 is the critical band region. Human Genetics 67: 233-236

Elejalde B R, Opitz J M, Mercedes de Elejalde M et al 1984 Tandem Dup (1p) within the short arm of chromosome 1 in a child with ambiguous genitalia and multiple congenital anomalies. American Journal of Medical Genetics 17: 723-730

Emanuel R, Somerville J, Inns A, Withers R 1983 Evidence of congenital heart disease in the offspring of parents with atrioventricular defects. British Heart Journal 49: 144-147

Fang T-T, Bruyere H J Jr, Kargas S A, Nishikawa T, Takagi Y, Gilbert E F 1987 Ethyl alcohol-induced cardiovascular malformations in the chick embryo. Teratology 35: 95-103

Feingold M, Pashayan H 1983 Genetics and birth defects in clinical practice, 1st edn. Little Brown, Boston

Feldman G L, Weaver D D, Lovrien E W 1977 The fetal Trimethadione syndrome: report of an additional family and further delineation of this syndrome. American Journal of Diseases of Children 131: 1389-1392

Ferencz C 1986 Offspring of fathers with cardiovascular malformations. American Heart Journal 111: 1212-1213

Ferencz C, Rubin J D, McCarter R J et al 1985 Congenital heart disease: prevalence at live birth. The Baltimore-Washington infant study. American Journal of Epidemiology 121: 31-36

Ferencz C, Rubin J D, McCarter R J et al 1987 Cardiac and noncardiac malformations: observations in a population-based study. Teratology 35: 367-378

Fisch R O, Doeden D, Lansky LL, Anderson J A 1969 Maternal phenylketonuria: detrimental effects on embryogenesis and fetal development. American Journal of Diseases of Children 118: 847-858

Fraccaro M, Lindsten J, Ford C E, Iselius L 1980 The 11q;22q translocation: a European collaborative analysis of 43 cases. Human Genetics 56: 21-51

Frank J, Riccardi V M 1977 The 11q-syndrome. Human Genetics 35: 241-246

Friedman E, Sack J 1982 The Cohen syndrome: report of five new cases and review of the literature. Journal of

Craniofacial Genetic Development Biology 2: 193-200

Fryns J P, Kleczkowska A, Limbos C, Vandecasseye W, Van den Berghe H 1985 Centric fission of chromosome 7 with 47,XX,del(7)(pter-->cen::q21-->qter)+cen fr karyotype in a mother and proximal 7q deletion in two malformed newborns. Annales de Genetique 28: 248-250

Gabbe S G 1986 Gestational diabetes mellitus. New England Journal of Medicine 315: 1025-1026

Garcia-Cruz D, Rivera H, Barajas L O et al 1985 Monosomy 20p due to a de novo del(20)(p12.2): clinical and radiological delineation of the syndrome. Annales de Genetique 28: 231-234

Garcia-Sagredo J M, Lozano C, Ferrando P, San Roman C 1984 Mentally retarded siblings with congenital heart defect, peculiar facies and cryptorchidism in the male: possible McDonough syndrome with coincidental (X;20) translocation. Clinical Genetics 26: 117-124

Garver K L, Ciocco A M, Turack N A 1976 Partial monosomy or trisomy resulting from crossing over within a rearranged chromosome 1. Clinical Genetics 10: 319-324

Gellis S S, Feingold M, Dubner D W, Kreidberg M B, Allport R B 1979 Arteriohepatic dysplasia. American Journal of Diseases of Children 133: 206-207

Gev D, Roguin N, Freundlich E 1986 Consanguinity and congenital heart disease in the rural Arab population in northern Israel. Human Hereditary 36: 213-217

Gimelli G, Cuoco C, Porro E 1983 Prenatal diagnosis, fetal pathology and cytogenetic analysis of a 46,XX/47,XX,+15 mosaic. Prenatal Diagnosis 3: 75-79

Gladstone I Jr, Sybert V P 1982 Holt-Oram syndrome: penetrance of the gene and lack of maternal effect. Clinical Genetics 21: 98-103

Goecke T, Dopfer R, Huenges R, Conzelmann W, Feller A, Majewski F 1981 Hydrometrocolpos, postaxial polydactyly, congenital heart disease, and anomalies of the gastrointestinal and genitourinary tracts: a rare autosomal recessive syndrome. European Journal of Pediatrics 136: 297-305

Goldstein J L, Brown M S 1980 Genetics and cardiovascular disease. In: Braunwald E (ed) Heart disease: a textbook of cardiovascular medicine, Vol 2, W B Saunders, Philadelphia, p 1683-1722

Goldstein S, Qazi Q H, Fitzgerald J, Goldstein J, Friedman A P, Sawyer P 1985 Distichiasis, congenital heart defects and mixed peripheral vascular anomalies. American Journal of Medical Genetics 20: 283-294

Greenberg F, Gresik M V, Carpenter R J, Law S W, Hoffman L P, Ledbetter D H 1987 The Gardner-Silengo-Wachtel or genito-palato-cardiac syndrome: male pseudohermaphroditism with micrognathia, cleft palate, and conotruncal cardiac defect. American Journal of Medical Genetics 26: 59-64

Greenwood R D, Rosenthal A, Parisi L, Fyler D C, Nadas A S 1975 Extracardiac abnormalities in infants with congenital heart disease. Pediatrics 55: 485-492

Greenwood R D, Sommer A, Rosenthal A, Craenen J, Nadas A S 1977 Cardiovascular abnormalities in the Beckwith-Wiedemann syndrome. American Journal of Diseases of Children 131: 293-294

Grix A Jr 1982 Malformations in infants of diabetic mothers. American Journal of Medical Genetics 13: 131-137

Halal F, Homsy M, Perreault G 1984 Acro-Renal-Ocular syndrome: autosomal dominant thumb hypoplasia, renal ectopia, and eye defect. American Journal of Medical Genetics 17: 753-762

Hall J G 1987 Thrombocytopenia and absent radius (TAR) syndrome. Journal of Medical Genetics 24: 79–83

Hall J G, Pauli R M, Wilson K M 1980 Maternal and fetal sequelae of anticoagulation during pregnancy. American Journal of Medicine 68: 122–140

Hartz S C, Heinonen O P, Shapiro S, Siskind V, Slone D 1975 Antenatal exposure to meprobamate and chlordiazepoxide in relation to malformations, mental development, and childhood mortality. New England Journal of Medicine 292: 726–728

Hashiba K 1978 Hereditary QT prolongation syndrome in Japan: genetic analysis and pathological findings of the conducting system. Japanese Circulation Journal 42: 1133–1150

Heinonen O P, Sloan D, Monson R R, Hook E B, Shapiro S 1977 Cardiovascular birth defects and antenatal exposure to female sex hormones. New England Journal of Medicine 296: 67–70

Hindi A, Beneck D, Greco M A, Wolman S R 1986 18q+, the progeny of a balanced translocation t(1;18)mat: case report with necropsy findings. Journal of Medical Genetics 23: 263–266

Hittner H M, Hirsch N J, Kreh G M, Rudolph A J 1979 Colobomatous microphthalmia, heart disease, hearing loss, and mental retardation – a syndrome. Journal of Pediatric Ophthalmology and Strabismus 16: 122–128

Hoffman J I E 1977 Circulatory system. In: Rudolph A M (ed) Pediatrics, 16th edn. Appleton-Century-Crofts, New York, Chapter 27

Horn C A, Beekman R H, Dick M II, Lacina S J 1986 The congenital long QT syndrome: an unusual cause of childhood seizures. American Journal of Diseases of Children 140: 659–661

Hurwitz R C, Caskey C T 1982 Ivemark syndrome in siblings. Clinical Genetics 22: 7–11

Hutchins G M, Moore G W, Lipford E H, Haupt H M, Walker M C 1983 Asplenia and polysplenia malformation complexes explained by abnormal embryonic body curvature. Pathological Research Practice 177: 60–76

Iturbe-Alessio I, Carmen Fonseca M D, Mutchinik O, Angel Santos M, Zajarias A, Salazar E 1986 Risks of anticoagulant therapy in pregnant women with artifical heart valves. New England Journal of Medicine 315: 1390–1393

Jackson B T 1968 The pathogenesis of congenital cardiovascular anomalies. New England Journal of Medicine 279: 25–29, 80–89

Jayakar P B, Stanwick R S, Seshia S S 1986 Tuberous sclerosis and Wolff-Parkinson White syndrome. Journal of Pediatrics 108: 259

Johnston K, Golabi M, Schonberg S et al 1986 Bilateral ectrodactyly of feet and tibial aplasia associated with an unusual chromosome abnormality: tetrasomy 14q121 to 14pter. Proceedings of the Greenwood Genetic Center 5: 176

Jones M C, Waldman J D 1985 An autosomal dominant syndrome of characteristic facial appearance, preauricular pits, fifth finger clinodactyly, and tetralogy of Fallot. American Journal of Medical Genetics 22: 135–141

Kahler R L, Braunwald E, Plauth W H, Morrow A G 1966 Familial congenital heart disease. American Journal of Medicine 40: 384–399

Kallen B 1987 Search for teratogenic risks with the aid of malformation registries. Teratology 35: 47–52

Kaplan L, Matsuoka R, Gilbert E F, Opitz J M, Kurnit D M 1985 Ectopia cordis and cleft sternum: evidence for mechanical teratogenesis following rupture of the chorion or yolk-sac. American Journal of Medical Genetics 21: 187–189

Kaplan L C, Wayne A, Crowell S, Latt S A 1986 Trisomy 14 mosaicism in a liveborn male: clinical report and review of the literature. American Journal of Medical Genetics 23: 925–930

Kelley R I, Zackai E H, Emanuel B S, Kistenmacher M, Greenberg F, Punnett H H 1982 The association of the DiGeorge anomalad with partial monosomy of chromosome 22. Journal of Pediatrics 101: 197–200

Kelly J R, Barr E S 1975 The elfin facies syndrome. Oral Surgery 40: 205–218

Khoury M J, Cordero J F, Greenberg F, James L M, Erickson J D 1983 A population study of the VACTERL association: evidence for its etiologic heterogeneity. Pediatrics 71: 815–820

Kiel E A, Frias J L, Victorica B E 1983 Cardiovascular manifestations in the Larsen syndrome. Pediatrics 71: 942–946

Kirby M L, Bockman D E 1984 Neural crest and normal development: new perspective. Anatomical Record 209: 1–6

Kleczkowska A, Fryns J P, Moerman P H, Van den Berghe K, Van den Berghe H 1987 Trisomy of the short arm of chromosome 5: autopsy data in a malformed newborn with inv dup(5)(p13.1-->p15.3). Clinical Genetics 32: 49–56

Kleinman C S, Hobbins J C, Jaffe C C, Lynch D C, Talner N S 1980 Echocardiographic studies of the human fetus: prenatal diagnosis of congenital heart disease and cardiac dysrhythmias. Pediatrics 65: 1059–1067

Lammer E J, Opitz J M 1986 The DiGeorge anomaly as a developmental field defect. American Journal of Medical Genetics Supplement 2: 113–127

Lammer E J, Chen D T, Hoar R M et al 1985 Retinoic acid embryopathy. New England Journal of Medicine 313: 837–841

Layde P M, Dooley K, Erickson J D, Edmonds L D 1980 Is there an epidemic of ventricular septal defects in the U.S.A? Lancet I: 407–408

Layton W M Jr 1976 Random determination of a developmental process. Journal of Heredity 67: 336–338

Lazjuk G I, Lurie I W, Ostrowskaja T I et al 1980 The Wolf-Hirschhorn syndrome. Clinical Genetics 18: 6–12

Lenke R R, Levy H L 1980 Maternal phenylketonuria and hyperphenylalaninemia: an international survey of the outcome of untreated and treated pregnancies. New England Journal of Medicine 303: 1202–1208

Levy R J, Rosenthal A, Fyler D C, Nadas A S 1978 Birthweight of infants with congenital heart disease. American Journal of Diseases of Children 132: 249–254

Lewandowski R C Jr, Kukolich M K, Sears J W, Mankinen C B 1978 Partial deletion 10q. Human Genetics 42: 339–343

Liberfarb R M, Goldblatt A 1986 Prevalence of mitral-valve prolapse in the Stickler syndrome. American Journal of Medical Genetics 24: 387–392

Lin A E, Bernar J, Chin A J, Sparkes R S, Emanuel B S, Zackai E H 1986a Congenital heart disease in supernumerary der(22),t(11;22) syndrome. Clinical Genetics 29: 269–275

Lin A E, Lippe B M, Geffner M E et al 1986b Aortic dilation, dissection, and rupture in patients with Turner syndrome. Journal of Pediatrics 109: 820–826

Litsey S E, Noonan J A, O'Connor W N, Cottrill C M,

Mitchell B 1985 Maternal connective tissue disease and congenital heart block: demonstration of immunoglobulin in cardiac tissue. New England Journal of Medicine 312: 98–100

Loomis K F, Moore G W, Hutchins G M 1982 Unusual cardiac malformations in splenogonadal fusion-peromelia syndrome: relationship to normal development. Teratology 25: 1–9

Loser H, Majewski F 1977 Type and frequency of cardiac defects in embryofetal alcohol syndrome. Report of 16 cases. British Heart Journal 39: 1374–1379

McKusick V A 1988 Mendelian inheritance in man, 8th edn. Johns Hopkins University Press, Baltimore

McPherson E, Meissner L 1982 11q- syndrome: Review and report of two cases. Birth Defects: Original Article Series 18: 295–300

Mallette L E, Cooper J B, Kirkland J L 1982 Transient congenital hypoparathyroidism: possible association with anomalies of the pulmonary valve. Journal of Pediatrics 101: 928–931

Mapstone C L, Weaver D D, Yu P-L 1986 Analysis of growth in the VATER association. American Journal of Diseases of Children 140: 386–390

Martin R P, Banner N R, Radley-Smith R 1986 Familial persistent ductus arteriosus. Archives of Disease in Childhood 61: 906–907

Martinez y Martinez R, Corona-Rivera E, Jimenez-Martinez M, Ocampo-Campos R, Garcia-Maravilla S, Cantu J M 1981 A new probably autosomal recessive cardiomelic dysplasia with mesoaxial hexadactyly. Journal of Medical Genetics 18: 151–154

Meinecke P, Beemer F A, Schinzel A, Kushnick T 1986 The velo-cardio-facial (Shprintzen) syndrome: clinical variability in eight patients. European Journal of Pediatrics 145: 539–544

Meyers D G, Starke H, Pearson P H, Wilken M K, Ferrell Jr 1986 The cause of mitral valve prolapse in anorexia nervosa. Clinical Research 34: 898A

Milkovich L, van den Berg B J 1974 Effects of prenatal meprobamate and chlordiazepoxide hydrochloride on human embryonic and fetal development. New England Journal of Medicine 491: 1268–1270

Miller E, Hare J W, Cloherty J P et al 1981 Elevated maternal hemoglobin A$_{1c}$ in early pregnancy and major congenital anomalies in infants of diabetic mothers. New England Journal of Medicine 304: 1331–1334

Miller M E, Smith D W 1979 Conotruncal malformation complex: examples of possible monogenic inheritance. Pediatrics 63: 890–892

Miller R D, Divertie M B 1972 Kartagener's syndrome. Chest 62: 130–135

Mitchell S C, Korones S B, Berendes H W 1971 Congenital heart disease in 56,109 births: incidence and natural history. Circulation 43: 323–332

Monteleone P L, Fagan L F 1969 Possible X-linked congenital heart disease. Circulation 39: 611–614

Mulcahy M T, Pemberton P J, Thompson E, Watson M 1982 Is there a monosomy 10qter syndrome? Clinical Genetics 21: 33–35

Murphy D, Saul I, Kirby M 1985 Maternal phenylketonuria and phenylalanine restricted diet: studies of 7 pregnancies and of offsprings produced. Irish Journal of Medical Science 154: 66–70

Myhre S A, Williams R 1981 Teratogenic effects associated with maternal primidone therapy. Journal of Pediatrics 99: 160–162

Nakane Y, Okuma T, Takahashi R et al 1980 Multi-institutional study on the teratogenicity and fetal toxicity of antiepileptic drugs: a report of a collaborative study group in Japan. Epilepsia 21: 663–680

Natowicz M, Kelley R I 1987 Association of Turner syndrome with hypoplastic left-heart syndrome. American Journal of Diseases of Children 141: 218–220

Neiman H L, Mena E, Holt J F, Stern A M, Perry B L 1974 Neurofibromatosis and congenital heart disease. American Journal of Roentgenology, Radium Therapy and Nuclear Medicine 122: 146–149

Newman T B 1985 Etiology of ventricular septal defects: an epidemiologic approach. Pediatrics 76: 741–749

Nikolis J, Ivanovic K, Kosanovic M 1983 Tandem duplication of chromosome 14 (q24—>q32) in male newborn with congenital malformations. Clinical Genetics 23: 321–324

Nora J J, Fraser F C 1981 (eds) Medical Genetics: Principles and Practice, 2nd edn. Lea & Febiger, Philadelphia, p 501

Nora J J, Nora A H 1978 The evolution of specific genetic and environmental counseling in congenital heart diseases. Circulation 57: 205–213

Nora J J, Nora A H 1987 Maternal transmission of congenital heart diseases: new recurrence risk figures and the questions of cytoplasmic inheritance and vulnerability to teratogens. American Journal of Cardiology 59: 459–463

Ohdo S, Madokoro H, Sonoda T, Nishiguchi T, Kawaguchi K, Hayakawa K 1985 Kabuki make-up syndrome (Niikawa-Kuroki syndrome) associated with congenital heart disease. Journal of Medical Genetics 22: 126–127

Ohdo S, Madokoro H, Sonoda T, Hayakawa K 1986 Mental retardation associated with congenital heart disease, blepharophimosis, blepharoptosis, and hypoplastic teeth. Journal of Medical Genetics 23: 242–244

Olson L J, Subramanian R, Ackermann D M, Orzulak T A, Edwards W D 1987 Surgical pathology of the mitral valve: a study of 712 cases spanning 21 years. Mayo Clinic Proceedings 62: 22–34

Opitz J M, Johnson R C, McCreadie S R, Smith D W 1969 The C Syndrome of multiple congenital anomalies. Birth Defects: Original Article Series 5: 161–166

Opitz J M, Kaveggia E G, Adkins W N Jr et al 1982 Studies of malformation syndromes of humans XXXIIIC: The FG syndrome – further studies on three affected individuals from the FG family. American Journal of Medical Genetics 12: 147–154

Otto J, Back E, Furste H O, Abel M, Bohm N, Pringsheim W 1984 Dysplastic features, growth retardation, malrotation of the gut, and fatal ventricular septal defect in a 4-month-old girl with ring chromosome 15. European Journal of Pediatrics 142: 229–231

Pena S D J 1982 Cleft lip and palate, congenital heart disease, scoliosis, short stature, and mental retardation: the Pilotto syndrome. Birth Defects: Original Article Series 18: 183–186

Pfeiffer R A 1984 Interstitial deletion of a chromosome 7 (q11.2q22.1) in a child with a splithand/splitfoot malformation. Annales de Genetique 27: 45–48

Pierpont M E A, Gobel J W, Moller J H, Edwards J E 1988 Cardiac malformations in relatives of children with truncus arteriosus or interruption of the aortic arch. American Journal of Cardiology 61: 423–427

Piérard L A, Henrard L, Demoulin J-C 1985 Persistent atrial

standstill in familial Ebstein's anomaly. British Heart Journal 53: 594–597

Pitt D B 1962 A family study of Fallot's tetrad. Australian Annals of Medicine 11: 179–183

Pober B R, Nelson K, Holmes L B 1988 Tetralogy of Fallot: Heterogeneity in a newborn population. Proceedings of the Greenwood Genetic Center vol. 7, p 190–191

Prieto F, Badia L, Moreno J A, Barbero P, Asensi F 1978 10p- syndrome associated with multiple chromosomal abnormalities. Human Genetics 45: 229–235

Reed B R, Lee L A, Harmon C, Wolfe R, Wiggins J, Peebles C, Weston W L 1983 Autoantibodies to SS-A/Ro in infants with congenital heart block. Journal of Pediatrics 103: 889–891

Reiss J A, Sheffield L J, Sutherland G R 1986 Partial trisomy 3p syndrome. Clinical Genetics 30: 50–58

Richards M R, Merritt K K, Samuels M H, Langmann A G 1955 Congenital malformations of the cardiovascular system in a series of 6053 infants. Pediatrics 15: 12–32

Ritscher D, Schinzel A, Boltshauser E, Briner J, Arbenz U, Sigg P 1987 Dandy-Walker (like) malformation, atrio-ventricular septal defect and a similar pattern of minor anomalies in 2 sisters: a new syndrome? American Journal of Medical Genetics 26: 481–491

Rivera H, Vargas-Moyeda E, Moller M, Torres-Lamas A, Cantu J M 1985 Monosomy 16q: a distinct syndrome: apropos of a de novo del(16)(q2100q2300). Clinical Genetics 28: 84–86

Robinson L K, O'Brien N C, Puckett M C, Cox M A 1987 Multiple pterygium syndrome: a case complicated by malignant hyperthermia. Clinical Genetics 32: 5–9

Rosa F W, Wilk A L, Kelsey F O 1986 Teratogen update: vitamin A congeners. Teratology 33: 355–364

Rose V, Izukawa T, Moes C A F 1975 Syndromes of asplenia and polysplenia: a review of cardiac and non-cardiac malformations in 60 cases with special reference to diagnosis and prognosis. British Heart Journal 37: 840–852

Rose V, Gold R J M, Lindsay G, Allen M 1985 A possible increase in the incidence of congenital heart defects among the offspring of affected parents. Journal of the American College of Cardiology 6: 376–382

Sanchez Cascos A 1972 Genetics of atrial septal defect. Archives of Disease in Childhood 47: 581–588

Savage D D, Garrison R J, Devereux R B et al 1983 Mitral valve prolapse in the general population. 1. Epidemiologic features: The Framingham study. American Heart Journal 106: 571–576

Sax C M, Bodurtha J N, Brown J A 1986 Case report: partial trisomy 20q(20q13.13->qter). Clinical Genetics 30: 462–465

Schidlow D V, Katz S M, Turtz M G, Donner R M, Capasso S 1982 Polysplenia and Kartagener syndrome in a sibship: association with abnormal respiratory cilia. Journal of Pediatrics 100: 401–403

Schlesinger P A, Duray P H, Burke B A, Steere A C, Stillman M T 1985 Maternal-fetal transmission of the Lyme disease spirochete, Borrelia burgdorferi. Annals of Internal Medicine 103: 67–69

Schmidt M A, Michels V V, Edwards W D, Miller F A 1988 Familial dilated cardiomyopathy. American Journal of Medical Genetics 31: 135–143

Schmidt M A, Ensing G J, Michels V V, Carter G A, Hagler D J, Feldt R H 1989 Autosomal Dominant Supravalvular aortic stenosis: Large Three-Generation Family. American Journal of Medical Genetics 32: 384–389

Schomig-Spingler M, Schmid M, Brosi W, Grimm T 1986 Chromosome 7 short arm deletion, 7p21—>pter. Human Genetics 74: 323–325

Shah A, Fay J E, Ford S, Holden J J A 1985 46,X,i(Xq) karyotype in a patient with hypoplastic left heart. Clinical Genetics 28: 178–179

Shapiro S R, Ruckman R H, Kapur S et al 1981 Single ventricle with truncus arteriosus in siblings. American Heart Journal 102: 456–459

Shapiro S D, Hansen K L, Pasztor L M et al 1985 Deletions of the long arm of chromosome 10. American Journal of Medical Genetics 20: 181–196

Shokeir M H K, Ray M, Hamerton J L, Bauder F, O'Brien H 1975 Deletion of the short arm of chromosome No. 10. Journal of Medical Genetics 12: 99–113

Silverman N H, Enderlein M A, Golbus M S 1984 Ultrasonic recognition of aortic valve atresia in utero. American Journal of Cardiology 53: 391–392

Smith C 1971 Recurrence risks for multifactorial inheritance. American Journal of Human Genetics 23: 578–588

Smith D W 1982 Recognizable patterns of human malformation, 3rd edn. W B Saunders, Philadelphia

Snyder F F, Lin C C, Rudd N L, Shearer J E, Heikkila E M, Hoo J J 1984 A de novo case of trisomy 10: gene dosage studies of hexokinase, inorganic pyrophosphatase and adenosine kinase. Human Genetics 67: 187–189

Soltan H C, Li M D 1974 Hereditary dextrocardia associated with other congenital heart defects: report of a pedigree. Clinical Genetics 5: 51–58

Spooner E W, Farina M A, Hook E B 1986 Evaluation of a temporal increase in ventricular septal defects. Proceedings of the Greenwood Genetic Center 5: 129–130

Stevenson C, Franken E A, Ha-Upala S, Christian J C 1971 Familial occurrence of single ventricle. Archives of Diseases in Childhood 46: 730–731

Stewart P A, Tonge H M, Wladimiroff J W 1983 Arrhythmia and structural abnormalities of the fetal heart. British Heart Journal 50: 550–554

Stratton R F, Dobyns W B, Airhard S D, Ledbetter D H 1984 New chromosomal syndrome: Miller-Dieker syndrome and monosomy 17p13. Human Genetics 67: 193–200

Streissguth A P, Clarren S K, Jones K L 1985 Natural history of the fetal alcohol syndrome: a 10-year follow-up of eleven patients. Lancet II: 85–91

Subramanian R, Olson L J, Edwards W D 1984 Surgical pathology of pure aortic stenosis: a study of 374 cases. Mayo Clinic Proceedings 59: 683–690

Subramanian R, Olson L J, Edwards W D 1985 Surgical pathology of combined aortic stenosis and insufficiency: a study of 213 cases. Mayo Clinic Proceedings 60: 247–254

Taylor P V, Scott J S, Gerlis L M, Esscher E, Scott O 1986 Maternal antibodies against fetal cardiac antigens in congenital complete heart block. New England Journal of Medicine 315: 667–672

Thompson E, Cadbury R, Baraitser M 1985 The Nagar acrofacial dysostosis syndrome with the tetralogy of Fallot. Journal of Medical Genetics 22: 408–410

Toriello H V, Higgins J V 1985 X-linked midline defects. American Journal of Medical Genetics 21: 143–146

Townes P L, White M R 1978 Inherited partial trisomy 8q (22—>qter). American Journal of Diseases of Children 132: 498–501

Ursell P C, Byrne J M, Strobino B A 1985 Significance of cardiac defects in the developing fetus: a study of spontaneous abortuses. Circulation 72: 1232–1236

Van Mierop L H S, Patterson D F, Schnarr W R 1977 Hereditary conotruncal septal defects in Keeshond dogs: embryologic studies. American Journal of Cardiology 40: 936–950

Vidaillet H J Jr, Pressley J C, Henke E, Harrell F E Jr, German L D 1987 Familial occurrence of accessory atrioventricular pathways (preexcitation syndrome). New England Journal of Medicine 317: 65–70

Warkany J 1986 Teratogen update: hyperthermia. Teratology 33: 365–371

Waziri M, Patil S R, Hanson J W, Bartley J A 1983 Abnormality of chromosome 11 in patients with features of Beckwith-Wiedemann syndrome. Journal of Pediatrics 102: 873–876

Weigel T J, Driscoll D J, Michels V V 1989 Occurrence of congenital heart defects in siblings of patients with univentricular heart and tricuspid atresia. American Journal of Cardiology 64: 768–771

Weinberg A G, Wright C G 1978 Stapedial hypoplasia in partial DiGeorge's syndrome. American Journal of Diseases of Children 132: 815–816

Weinstein M R, Goldfield M D 1975 Cardiovascular malformations with lithium use during pregnancy. American Journal of Psychiatry 132: 529–531

Whittemore R, Hobbins J C, Engle M A 1982 Pregnancy and its outcome in women with and without surgical treatment of congenital heart disease. American Journal of Cardiology 50: 641–651

Whittemore R, Wells J A, Wright M R 1987 Recurrence of congenital heart defects in progeny of affected men vs. women. Pediatric Research 21: 197A

Wiggins J W Jr, Bowes W, Clewell W et al 1986 Echocardiographic diagnosis and intravenous digoxin management of fetal tachyarrhythmias and congestive heart failure. American Journal of Diseases of Children 140: 202–204

Wilson G N, Baker D L, Schau J, Parker J 1984 Cat eye syndrome owing to tetrasomy 22pter—>q11. Journal of Medical Genetics 21: 60–63

Wilson G N, Dasouki M, Barr M Jr 1985 Further delineation of the dup(3q) syndrome. American Journal of Medical Genetics 22: 117–123

Wladimiroff J W, Stewart P A, Sachs E S, Niermeijer M F 1985 Prenatal diagnosis and management of congenital heart defect: significance of associated fetal anomalies and prenatal chromosome studies. American Journal of Medical Genetics 21: 285–290

Wright L L, Schwartz M F, Schwartz S, Karesh J 1986 An unusual ocular finding associated with chromosome 1q deletion syndrome. Pediatrics 77: 786

Yamamoto Y, Okamoto N, Shiraishi H, Yanagisawa M, Kamoshita S 1986 Deletion of proximal 6q: A clinical report and review of the literature. American Journal of Medical Genetics 25: 467–471

Yao J, Thompson M W, Trusler G A, Trimble A S 1968 Familial atrial septal defect of the primum type: a report of four cases in one sibship. Canadian Medical Association Journal 98: 218–219

Yunis J J 1977 New chromosomal syndromes. Academic Press, New York

Zackai E H, Mellman W J, Neiderer B 1975 The fetal trimethadione syndrome. Journal of Pediatrics 87: 280–284

Zellers T M, Driscoll D J, Michels V V 1989 Prevalence of congenital heart disease in offspring of parents with Fallot's tetralogy. Journal of the American College of Cardiology 13: 240A

Zhang K-Z, Sun Q-B, Cheng T O 1986 Holt-Oram syndrome in China: a collective review of 18 cases. American Heart Journal 111: 572–577

Zierler S, Rothman K J 1985 Congenital heart disease in relation to maternal use of Bendectin and other drugs in early pregnancy. New England Journal of Medicine 313: 347–352

73. Coronary heart disease

Gerd Utermann

CLINICAL DESCRIPTION — COMPLICATIONS — NATURAL HISTORY — PATHOGENESIS

Cardiovascular diseases are the most important cause of morbidity and mortality in all highly industrialized countries. Roughly half of all cardiovascular deaths are due to coronary heart disease which accounts for 30–40% of the total mortality in men aged 45–75 years in the US and western Europe. Among the clinical expressions of coronary heart disease are congestive heart failure, conduction defect, arrhythmia, angina pectoris and myocardial infarction. Most cases of sudden unexpected death also result from coronary heart disease. Coronary heart disease is a consequence of atherosclerosis of coronary arteries.

According to a WHO definition, atherosclerosis is 'a variable combination of changes in the arterial wall consisting of the focal accumulation of lipids, complex carbohydrates, blood and blood products, fibrous tissue and calcium deposits associated with changes in the media' (Classification of Atherosclerosis Lesions, Report of Study Group on Definition of Terms 1958). The fundamental element of atherosclerosis is the athero-sclerotic plaque. Three classic types of lesion are recognized: the fatty streak, the fibrous plaque, and the so-called 'complicated lesion' (McGill 1984). Growing evidence suggests that fatty streaks are precursors of fibrous plaques. Fatty streaks occur in the aorta in childhood, and later also in coronary arteries. The yellow colour of these lesions is due to the presence of lipid deposits found primarily within macrophages and smooth muscle cells (Smith & Smith 1976).

Many factors are involved in atherogenesis and different hypotheses have been advanced to explain how an atherosclerotic plaque starts. One of these, the response-to-injury hypothesis, dates back to the pioneer-ring work of Virchow (1856). This hypothesis is still the conceptual framework for most recent hypotheses on atherogenesis and has been modified and extended by many investigators (McGill 1984, Ross 1986, Steinberg 1987). The principal cell types involved in atherogenesis are vascular endothelial cells, monocyte-macrophages, smooth muscle cells and platelets. The relationship between these four cell types in plaque formation is far from clear, although an overall picture is emerging. According to the injury hypothesis, the primary event in the pathogenesis of atherosclerosis is endothelial damage as a result of mechanical, chemical, immunological or toxic injury. Endothelial cells normally form a non-thrombogenic barrier. They determine the nature of plasma constituents, including lipoproteins, that reach the subendothelial space. Factors such as hyperlipidae-mia, the increased shear in hypertension, or toxic agents contained in cigarette smoke may injure the endothelium and alter the nature of the endothelial barrier to the passage of blood constituents into the arterial wall (Ross 1986). Monocyte/macrophages have been implicated in the early stages of atherogenesis. Their chemotactic, mutagenic, and endocytotic properties make them prime candidates for triggering early key atherogenic events. They are attracted by chemotactic substances that are released from endothelial cells and, in experimental hypercholesterolaemia, attach randomly to the arterial endothelium. Subendothelial migration and localisation of monocytes are the earliest recognizable events in fatty streak formation.

Macrophages in the subendothelial space may injure neighbouring cells by forming toxic substances including superoxide anion and lysosomal hydrolases. They can also oxidize lipids in membranes and lipoproteins and thereby could injure the overlying endothelium. Further, monocyte/macrophages interact intensively with lipoproteins and may develop the appearance of foam cells. In particular they take up modified lipoproteins by specific receptor-mediated endocytosis (Brown & Gold-stein 1983a). Such modified lipoproteins are believed to be generated in vivo during long-standing hyperlipidae-mia. Whether or not macrophages become overloaded with lipids and form foam cells depends on the balance between influx and efflux of lipids. In contrast to other cell types that regulate receptor-mediated uptake of cholesterol according to the cell's demand, macrophages cannot down-regulate their receptors even when massive amounts of lipid are stored in their cytoplasm, (Brown & Goldstein 1983a). On the contrary, there seems to be a positive autoregulation of the human monocyte receptor for modified low density lipoprotein (LDL) that could accelerate cellular cholesterylester accumulation and foam cell formation. Moreover macrophages are able to do both, oxidize LDL and take up oxidized LDL by receptor-mediated endocytosis. However monocyte/macrophages under appropriate conditions can also rapidly secrete the large amount of cholesterylesters that they have stored in the cytoplasm and deliver it to high density lipoprotein (HDL). The significance of apolipoprotein in E/phospholipid complexes secreted by lipid-laden macrophages (Basu et al 1983) for cholesterol removal is still unclear. Importantly, however, not only elevated LDL but also low HDL levels and other forms of dyslipoproteinaemia might result in lipid accumulation in macrophages. Finally, macrophages also secrete different growth factors specific for connective tissue cells such as smooth muscle cells.

Fatty streaks enlarge by continuous invasion of monocytes, which become foamy macrophages, and by gradual accumulation of smooth muscle cells that migrate from the media into the intima. In experimental animals the proliferative activity of arterial intimal smooth muscle cells begins within a few days of starting a cholesterol-rich diet (Ross 1986). By a complicated and only poorly understood series of events fatty streaks may be converted into fibrous plaques. Smooth muscle cells are the predominant cell type in these lesions. Their proliferation is a key event in atherogenesis. In addition to migrating and multiplying they are able to form massive amounts of connective-tissue matrix. Moreover, they can also accumulate cholesterylesters and become foam cells.

Lipoproteins can be taken up by smooth muscle cells by receptor-mediated endocytosis or may be trapped in the intracellular matrix by glycosaminoglycans produced by the cells. LDL and also very low density lipoprotein (VLDL) have been shown to bind to specific connective tissue elements of the arterial intima, such as glycosaminoglycans and elastic fibres. LDL provides the excessive amounts of cholesterylester which accumulate in the lesion. The lipid material which accumulates in the intima of lesions has the physicochemical and immunochemical properties of lipoproteins. In particular, there are rather remarkable quantities of intact LDL in the diseased artery wall (Smith 1975). This may reflect the importance of chronic hyperlipidaemia, especially elevated LDL, in the process of atherosclerosis.

Fibrous plaques, with central lipid-rich cores surrounded by smooth muscle cells and connective tissue layers consisting of basement membranes and glycosaminoglycans, appear in the third decade of life. These undergo vascularization, haemorrhage, ulceration and calcification. Eventually thrombi will cover the surface of the lesion, occlude the artery and cause ischaemic necrosis in affected organs (McGill 1984).

Even though a uniform hypothesis to explain the cause and pathogenesis of atherosclerosis does not at present exist, some factors have been identified. One of these is particularly interesting in the context of this section: plasma cholesterol or, more precisely, plasma lipoproteins (Steinberg 1987). The reason for this is that a number of mutations involving the lipoproteins of blood plasma are known in man and some of these have remarkably high frequency in the population (Goldstein et al 1973). These mutations include two unique monogenic dominant disorders of lipoprotein metabolism that are associated with a considerably elevated risk of premature coronary heart disease. Moreover, single polymorphic gene loci have recently been identified that participate in the control of plasma lipid and lipoprotein levels in man and that are involved in the aetiology of multifactorial hyperlipidaemia (Utermann 1987, 1988, Utermann et al 1987). For this reason, this chapter will mainly be concerned with the genetic control of plasma lipids and its disturbances – the genetic dyslipidaemias.

RISK FACTOR CONCEPT

A series of large epidemiological studies performed over the last decade throughout the world have established what is called the risk factor concept (Dawber 1980, Keys 1980). According to this concept, hypercholesterolaemia, high consumption of cigarettes, and hypertension are first-order independent risk factors for coronary heart disease. They are today attributed with a causal relation to atherosclerosis. A second less significant risk factor category includes diabetes mellitus, gout, adiposity, lack of exercise and stress. Epidemiological studies by themselves cannot establish causal relationships, but the role of risk factors in atherosclerosis has been validated through the combined approaches of epidemiology, experimental pathology and clinical investigation. In particular the study of human mutations involving the lipoproteins of blood plasma have shed light on the role of lipoproteins in atherosclerosis. There is general agreement on the positive linear or curvilinear relationship between cholesterol level and the incidence of coronary heart disease. The role of triglycerides is still a matter of controversy (Lippel et al 1981). Cholesterol in plasma is present in different kinds of lipoprotein particles (see lipoproteins) and these are not equivalent with respect to coronary risk; whereas cholesterol in LDL is positively correlated with premature coronary heart disease, a negative correlation of cholesterol in HDL with coronary atherosclerosis has been established in epidemiological studies, and a protective effect against coronary heart disease has been attributed to HDL (Miller 1978). Conventionally, plasma lipids and lipoproteins are analysed in fasting subjects. However humans, for most of their lives, are not fasting. Zilversmit (1979) has therefore postulated that degradation products of triglyceride-rich lipoproteins (=remnants) present in postprandial plasma may have a pronounced atherogenic effect. Indeed one human disorder of lipoprotein metabolism (type III hyperlipoproteinaemia), where remnant-like lipoproteins accumulate even in the fasting state, is associated with premature atherosclerosis.

GENETICS OF CORONARY HEART DISEASE — GENERAL ASPECTS

As early as 1897 Osler realized the familial aggregation of heart attacks. Present-day knowledge suggests that this aggregation is largely due to clustering of genetically-determined risk factors in certain families. The contribution of genetic factors to the development of coronary heart disease has been documented, since Osler's original observation, by several studies during the last decades (Slack & Evans 1966, Slack 1969, 1975, Robertson & Cumming 1979, Glueck et al 1985, Goldbourt & Neufeld 1986). From these studies it has emerged that coronary heart disease is a multifactorial disorder. No single gene locus for coronary heart disease exists. Rather, different environmental and genetic factors interact in a highly complex and still poorly understood fashion in the pathogenesis of coronary atherosclerosis. Moreover, the interaction patterns will be different in different individuals; whereas heavy smoking will be the major precipitating agent in one individual, genetically determined hypercholesterolaemia will be the major cause for premature coronary heart disease in others. Nora et al (1980) calculated that the heritability of ischaemic heart disease that produced myocardial infarction before 55 years of age was 0.63. In other words, the contribution of heredity appeared to exceed the contribution of the environment. In their series of patients the risk was greater with a family history of ischaemic heart disease than with a cholesterol level in the highest quintile. 15% of patients in their study had a monogenic hyperlipidaemia. However, even when families with monogenic hyperlipidaemias were eliminated, heritability was still 0.56, indicating that genetic control of factors that did not result in overt hyperlipidaemia or that did not operate through lipoprotein pathways were also important. The complexity of the issue becomes even more evident if we consider that the different risk factors again are under multifactorial control. In particular this has been shown for plasma cholesterol and lipoprotein levels (see genetic control of plasma cholesterol).

Some genetic factors affecting the susceptibility to coronary heart disease must operate through such risk factors as blood lipid concentrations and blood pressure. Others presumably will act at the cellular level. However, such genes have not yet been identified. Fibrinogen levels in plasma are also associated with premature coronary heart disease. In a recent study Hamsten et al (1987) have estimated genetic and cultural heritability of plasma fibrinogen levels by path analysis in 170 families. They calculated that 51% of the variance was accounted for by genetic heritability. This finding supports the view that plasma fibrinogen is a primary risk factor for coronary heart disease. The results of a search for genetic factors in hypertension are still limited. It has been demonstrated by family and twin studies that hereditary factors are involved in hypertension (Miller & Grim 1983) and most data favour the assumption of multifactorial inheritance of blood pressure. However no single genes responsible for high blood pressure that could be used to predict an individual's risk to develop hypertension have yet been identified, except in very rare cases. One example is in hypertension caused by the autosomal dominantly inherited phaeochromocytoma. By contrast, several genetic disorders of plasma lipid metabolism have been delineated (Table 73.1).

PLASMA LIPOPROTEINS

Only a brief general description of the major human lipoproteins and the metabolism of lipoproteins can be given here. Recent reviews covering the topic are available for more detailed information (Dolphin 1985, Schaefer & Levy 1985).

Three major lipoprotein classes, different in particle size, chemical composition and physicochemical properties, are present in the plasma of healthy fasting subjects and can be separated by ultracentrifugation. These are the very-low-density lipoproteins (VLDL, < 1.006 g/ml), the low-density lipoproteins (LDL, 1.019–1.063 g/ml) and the high-density lipoproteins (HDL, 1.063–1.21 g/ml). These fractions in general correspond to pre-beta-(VLDL), beta- (LDL) and alpha-1-lipoproteins (HDL) as separated by electrophoretic methods. In certain forms of dys- or hyperlipoproteinaemia other lipoproteins may occur in fasting plasma, including chylomicrons and intermediate density lipoproteins (IDL, 1.006–1.019 g/ml). The electrophoretic system has been used for the classification of hyperlipidaemias into phenotypes I (hyperchylomicronaemia), IIa (hyperbetalipoproteinaemia), IIb (hyperbeta-plus hyperprebetalipoprotein-

Table 73.1   The genetic dyslipoproteinaemias

I) *Autosomal recessive forms*	*Primary defects / remarks*
1) Familial hyperchylomicronaemia (HLP type I)	a) LPL-deficiency
	b) Apo C-II mutants and deficiencies
2) Hepatic lipase deficiency	HTGL-deficiency
3) Cholesterylester storage disease	Lysosomal acid cholesterylester hydrolase
4) Lecithin-cholesterol-acyltransferase deficiency	LCAT deficiency
5) Fish-eye disease	Unknown
6) Familial hyperalphalipoproteinaemia (Japanese type)	Cholesterylester-transfer protein deficiency
7) Tangier disease	Defective intracellular trafficking of HDL-receptor
8) HDL-deficiency with planar xanthomatosis	Mutation in A-I gene
9) Familial apo A-I/C-III-deficiency types I, II	Inversion in apo A-I/C-III/A-IV gene cluster (Type I)
10) Primary dysbetalipoproteinaemia	Apolipoprotein E2 (arg$_{158}$ → cys)
11) Abetalipoproteinaemia	Unknown, probably not in apo B gene
12) Normotriglyceridaemic abetalipoproteinaemia	Unknown, deficiency of apo B-100
13) Anderson disease (Chylomicron retention disease)	Unknown, deficiency of apo B-48
14) Sitosterolaemia with xanthomatosis	Unknown
15) Cerebrotendinous xanthomatosis	Defects in bile acid synthesis
II) *Autosomal dominant forms*	
1) Familial hypercholesterolaemia	Multiple defects in LDL-receptor gene
2) Familial combined hyperlipidaemia (hyperapobetalipoproteinaemia)	Unknown, overproduction of VLDL apo B, dominant?
3) Familial defective apolipoprotein B-100	Apo B-structure
4) Familial hypobetalipoproteinaemia	Apo B-structure (e.g. apo B-37)
5) Familial hypoalphalipoproteinaemia type Milano and other apo A-I-mutants	Apo A-I structure
6) Hyperlipoproteinaemia type III	Some rare Apo E structural abnormalities or Apo E deficiency
Homozygous for autosomal dominant forms	
1) Homozygous familial hypercholesterolaemia	
2) Homozygous hypobetalipoproteinaemia	
III) *Multifactorial forms / genetics unclear*	
1) Polygenic hypercholesterolaemia	Multiple, association with apo E-4
2) Familial hypertriglyceridaemia	Unknown
3) Hyperlipoproteinaemia type III	Apo E2 Arg$_{158}$ → cys homozygosity, plus other defects
4) Familial type V hyperlipidaemia	Unknown, association with apo E alleles
5) Familial hyper-Lp(a) lipoproteinaemia	Unknown, apo(a) structure?
6) Familial hypoalphalipoproteinaemia	Unknown
7) Familial hyperalphalipoproteinaemia	Unknown

Abbreviations: LCAT = lecithin-cholesterol-acyltransferase; LPL = lipoprotein lipase;
              HTGL = hepatic triglyceride-lipase; Apo = apolipoprotein

aemia), III (dysbetalipoproteinaemia), IV (hyperprebeta-lipoproteinaemia), and V (hyperprebeta-plus hyper-chylomicronaemia), each characterized by elevation of one or more distinct lipoprotein fractions (Fredrickson et al 1967, 1968). However this classification is a phenotypic and not a genetic one.

The major constituents of lipoproteins are cholesterol (free and esterified), triglyceride, phospholipid and protein. All lipoproteins contain the major lipid classes but in different characteristic concentrations. The various protein moieties or apolipoproteins however are preferentially present in certain lipoproteins and are

important programmers of lipoprotein metabolism (Dolphin 1985). Several apolipoproteins have been described and characterized. In recent years their genes have been cloned and sequenced and their gene structure and localization has been elucidated (Breslow 1985, Li et al 1988).

HDL contains apo A-I and apo A-II as major protein constituents. Minor proteins in HDL are apo C-I, apo C-II, apo C-III, apo D and apo E. Apo A-I, the most abundant apoprotein in HDL, acts as a cofactor for the plasma enzyme lecithin-cholesterol acyltransferase (LCAT). LDL contains almost exclusively apo B-100.

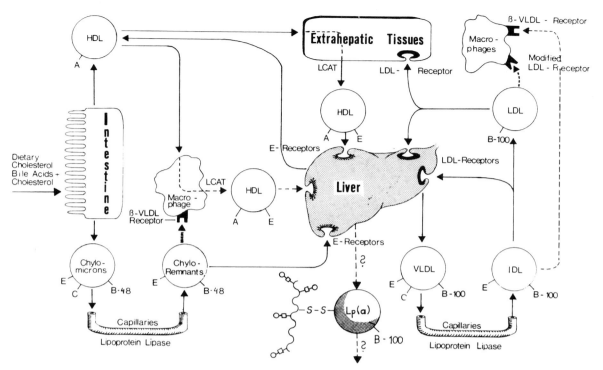

Fig. 73.1 Major pathways of cholesterol in human plasma.

Apo B-100 is also a major protein constituent of VLDL, together with apo C-I, C-II, C-III and apo E. Plasma chylomicrons have a protein composition similar to VLDL but human lymph chylomicrons have a remarkably different composition containing apo B-48, apo A-I and apo A-IV as major apoprotein. Apo E and apo B-100 are both recognized by a specific high affinity cell surface receptor (LDL-receptor) and are involved in the catabolism of lipoproteins by cells (Brown & Goldstein 1983b, 1986).

The plasma lipoproteins represent a highly dynamic system where the different lipoprotein particles are metabolically interrelated (Fig. 73.1). Lipoproteins are secreted as precursor molecules of circulating plasma lipoproteins, primarily by the liver (VLDL and nascent HDL; Havel 1985), and by the intestine (chylomicrons and nascent apo A-I rich HDL; Green et al 1978). In plasma, precursor lipoproteins are rapidly converted to mature lipoproteins by the combined action of enzymes (lipases, LCAT), by exchange of apolipoproteins and lipids and by interaction with cells. One of the most important metabolic pathways is the conversion of endogenous VLDL to LDL (Eisenberg et al 1978). Upon entry into the plasma compartment VLDL accepts apo C from HDL. One of the C apoproteins (apo C-II) is an

activator of lipoprotein lipase (LPL). In a first step the core triglycerides of VLDL are hydrolysed at the capillary endothelium by the action of apo C-II activated lipoprotein lipase and apo C is transferred back to HDL. The triglyceride and apo C poor particles generated have a density intermediate between VLDL and LDL and are designated IDL. These are either taken up by the liver via receptor-mediated endocytosis or they are further degraded to LDL. Most or all LDL in normal human plasma represents a catabolic product of VLDL. A similar pathway exists for chylomicrons that are the transport vehicles for exogenous fat and are assembled in the intestine and released into the lymph. Upon entry into the plasma compartment lymph chylomicrons lose apo A-I and apo A-IV. Apo A-I is transferred to HDL. Apo A-IV occurs in human plasma mainly as 'free apoprotein' but about 20% is present in HDL. In exchange, chylomicrons acquire apo C and apo E from plasma lipoproteins (Dolphin 1985). These plasma chylomicrons are then degraded into remnants by lipoprotein lipase. Finally, chylomicron remnants are taken up and degraded by liver cells through an apo E receptor-mediated mechanism (Havel 1985). The degradation of triglyceride-rich lipoproteins is tightly connected with the metabolism of HDL. There is not only the described transfer of surface components (apoproteins, phospholipids) to HDL during lipolysis and upon entry of chylomicrons into the plasma, but there also occurs a unidirectional transfer of cholesterylester from HDL to IDL/LDL that is facilitated by the cholesterylester transfer protein (CETP). Most of the core lipid cholesterylester is present in LDL in human plasma but is formed by the LCAT mediated esterification of HDL-cholesterol (Glomset & Norum 1973). Together the pathways involved in transporting cholesterol from peripheral cells to the liver are called reversed cholesterol transport. The metabolic interrelationship between the different classes of lipoproteins explains the multiple lipoprotein abnormalities that may emerge as a consequence of a single gene mutation in each of several lipoprotein disorders.

GENETIC CONTROL OF PLASMA CHOLESTEROL

Elevated plasma cholesterol concentrations, and particularly an elevation of cholesterol in LDL, is one major independent risk factor for coronary heart disease. There is considerable variation of cholesterol concentration within and between populations. One of the first to note and correlate this observation with the incidence of coronary heart disease was the Dutch physician De Lange (1933). Differences between ethnic groups are believed to be largely due to different environments, especially nutrition, rather than to genetic differences (Keys 1975), though this view has recently been challenged by findings from the apo E system (Utermann 1985, 1987). A significant genetic influence on serum lipid and lipoprotein levels including cholesterol, triglycerides, phospholipids, and the major lipoprotein classes from fasting plasma has been observed in twin studies. The genetic effect is particularly pronounced for cholesterol. Moreover, significant correlation of cholesterol was found in several family studies (Berg 1983, Namboodiri et al 1985). Sing and Orr (1978) have estimated that only approximately 20% of the observed correlation between sibs living in the same household is attributable to shared environments. This argues for a high quantitative contribution from genetic factors. Quantitative data on the contribution of genetic factors to plasma cholesterol or lipoprotein levels obtained by an 'unmeasured genotype' approach should be considered with great reservation. Several workers have tried by statistical methods to identify 'major genes' acting on either cholesterol or triglyceride levels (Ott 1979). The inherent difficulties of such an approach have been discussed by Hewitt et al (1979) and Boerwinkle et al (1986).

CANDIDATE GENES AFFECTING THE NORMAL VARIATION OF PLASMA LIPOPROTEIN LEVELS: POLYMORPHISMS OF APOLIPOPROTEIN E AND LP(a) GLYCOPROTEIN

As a consequence of the risk factor concept, any gene affecting the concentration or possibly even the relative distribution of plasma lipids and lipoproteins can be considered as contributing to susceptibility or resistance to coronary heart disease. Such genetic systems have recently been discovered, namely the polymorphisms of apolipoprotein E and of the Lp(a) glycoprotein (= apo(a)). Apo E is a major constituent of chylomicrons, VLDL, remnants, and of a subfraction of HDL. Apo E binds with high affinity to the LDL receptor and possibly also the the so-called remnant-receptor and is thereby involved in the receptor-mediated catabolism of lipoproteins (Brown & Goldstein 1983b, 1986). The protein exhibits genetic polymorphism that may be demonstrated by isoelectric focusing of delipidated sera, followed by immunoblotting (Utermann 1987). The apo E polymorphism is under the control of three common alleles, $\varepsilon 2$, $\varepsilon 3$ and $\varepsilon 4$ at one gene locus. These alleles determine the six phenotypes apo E-4/4, apo E-4/3, apo E-4/2, apo E-3/3, apo E-3/2 and apo E-2/2 (Fig. 73.2). The three gene products apo E 3, apo E 4 and (cys112 → arg) and apo E 2 (arg158 → cys) differ by single aminoacid substitutions and by their functional properties. Compared to apo E 3, which is the most frequent isoform in all populations studied so far, apo E 2 (arg158 → cys) has less than 2% of the binding activity to the LDL receptor and its plasma clearance is delayed. Apo E 4, on the contrary, exhibits enhanced in vivo catabolism. These functional differences explain the significant effects of the apo E polymorphism on lipid and lipoprotein levels (Utermann 1987, Boerwinkle & Utermann 1988). In all studied populations the average effect of the $\varepsilon 2$ allele is to lower plasma cholesterol by about 15 mg/dl. The average effect of the $\varepsilon 4$ allele is to increase plasma cholesterol by 5–10 mg/dl. The alleles at the apo E gene locus thus determine overlapping cholesterol distributions in the population. In westernized populations from 4% (Germany) to 20% (Iceland) of the total variance in plasma cholesterol levels is explained by variability at the apo E locus. Recent data have shown that subjects with different apo E types also have different responses to diet and drug therapy (Weintraub et al 1987, Davignon et al 1988). The apo E locus is also involved in the aetiology of some multifactorial disorders of plasma lipid metabolism such as type III hyperlipidaemia and polygenic hypercholesterolaemia (see below). The practical consequences of these, and

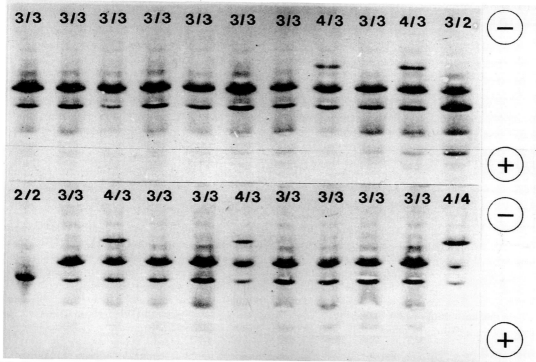

Fig. 73.2 Demonstration by immunoblotting of the common apo E phenotypes (from Menzel & Utermann 1986).

related findings, are that apo E typing is indicated in patients with severe forms of mixed hyperlipidaemia or excessive hypertriglyceridaemia to establish the diagnosis and to guide therapy.

The homozygous apo E-2/2 phenotype, that has a frequency of around 1% in most populations, is associated with a specific form of dyslipoproteinaemia. This has been termed primary dysbetalipoproteinaemia and is characterized by elevation of cholesterol-rich VLDL, presence of a so-called beta-VLDL fraction and low concentration of LDL. This phenotype is explained by the functional abnormality of the receptor-binding defective apo E 2 (arg158 → cys). Primary dysbetalipo-proteinaemia is the most frequent monogenic dyslipopro-teinaemia known in man and is transmitted as an autosomal recessive trait (Utermann et al 1977). With few exceptions (see type III hyperlipoproteinaemia) homozy-gous apo E-2/2 subjects with primary dysbetalipoprotein-aemia have subnormal total cholesterol concentrations (on the average 30–40 mg/dl below the population mean). The typical lipoprotein distribution seen in apo E-2/2 subjects corresponds to the lipoprotein pattern seen in subjects with hyperlipoproteinaemia type III. In fact, most patients with the classical type III disorder reported so far are of phenotype apo E-2/2 (Utermann 1987, 1988). This intriguing observation has raised the ques-tion of what factors determine, in a homozygous apo E-2/2 individual, whether there will be hypo-cholesterolaemia or type III hyperlipoproteinaemia. This question will be discussed later (see hyperlipoproteinae-mia type III). The significant effect of the apo E alleles on plasma lipids implies a major role of the apo E locus on the development of human atherosclerosis and coronary heart disease. Two studies have described an associ-ation of the apo E polymorphism with coronary heart disease (Cumming & Robertson 1984, Lenzen et al 1986).

A further genetic system that has implications for human atherosclerosis is the Lp(a)-system (for review see Utermann 1989). The Lp(a)-antigen was first described by Berg (1963) as part of the LDL fraction and was found in about 35% of persons in north-west Europe. The original population and family studies suggested that the polymorphism is under the control of a single autosomal gene locus with one dominant allele, Lp^a, and a silent allele, Lp^d. Later data suggested that Lp(a) is a quantitative genetic trait (Albers et al 1974, Sing et al 1974, Hasstedt & Williams 1986). Lp(a) lipoprotein concentrations in the population range from virtually undetectable to more than 200 mg/dl (hyper Lp(a) lipoproteinaemia) and their distribution is highly skewed.

The Lp(a) lipoprotein consists of an LDL-like particle containing apo B-100 and of the specific high molecular weight Lp(a)-glycoprotein (apo(a)) that are linked by a single disulphide bond. Apo(a) has an extremely high homology with plasminogen. It has been speculated that the Lp(a) lipoprotein provides a link between lipid metabolism and the clotting system (Brown & Goldstein 1987). The Lp(a) glycoprotein is genetically polymorphic. At least seven alleles at an autosomal locus control the size polymorphism of apo(a) (Utermann et al 1987). There exists an extremely strong association of apo(a) phenotypes with Lp(a) lipoprotein concentrations in plasma (Utermann et al 1987). A large fraction of Lp(a) level variance can be explained by variability at the apoprotein(a) locus. The Lp(a) locus also affects cholesterol levels significantly (Boerwinkle et al 1989).

There is now growing evidence that the Lp(a) lipoprotein is positively associated with coronary heart disease (Dahlen 1988). Subjects below 60 years with Lp(a) concentrations above 30 mg/dl have a two-fold elevated risk for premature myocardial infarction. The risk is especially high in subjects with concomitant elevation in LDL-cholesterol. Patients with LDL-cholesterol in the upper quintile of the population and Lp(a) levels above 30 mg/dl have a 5 to 6-fold increased risk of suffering from premature myocardial infarction (Armstrong et al 1986). Determination of Lp(a) lipoprotein concentration and probably Lp(a) phenotyping may soon become part of the risk assessment for coronary heart disease and stroke.

Several studies performed over recent years have described associations of RFLPs in candidate genes (mainly apolipoproteins) with lipid levels and coronary heart disease (Lusis 1988). However, most findings have to be confirmed by more extensive studies, and none have yet any practical consequences.

GENETIC DYSLIPIDAEMIAS

Autosomal recessive forms

There are several autosomal recessive inborn errors of plasma lipoprotein metabolism known to occur in humans. These are listed in Table 73.1. All of these, except primary dysbetalipoproteinaemia, are very rare and not all are associated with premature atherosclerosis.

Most of these disorders are characterized by both abnormal lipid levels (either subnormal or elevated), *and* by an abnormal distribution and composition of lipoproteins (= dyslipoproteinaemia). Defects may be in genes for lipolytic enzymes, apolipoproteins, lipid transfer proteins, or receptors. As a general rule disorders with HDL-deficiency are associated with a high risk for atherosclerois, whereas those with apo B-deficiency are not. Among those associated with premature atherosclerosis are Tangier disease, the combined deficiency of apo A-I and apo C-III, HDL-deficiency with planar xanthomatosis, and familial lecithin-cholesterol acyltransferase deficiency. The major clinical findings and lipoprotein abnormalities in these disorders are summarized in Table 73.2. These disorders have recently been reviewed by Schaefer (1984).

Clinical signs like corneal clouding and/or xanthomatosis in combination with low total- and HDL-cholesterol levels are highly indicative of a genetic HDL-deficiency syndrome. All severe atherogenic HDL-deficiency disorders have in common an almost complete (<2% of normal) or complete absence of apo A-I from plasma. In Tangier patients plasma cholesterol levels are usually below 120 mg/dl, whereas triglycerides tend to be elevated. HDL plasma levels are low and the concentration of apo A-I, the major apoprotein of normal HDL, tends to be less than 2% of controls, despite normal apo A-I synthesis and a virtually normal apo A-I protein- and gene-structure (Makrides et al 1988). Patients with Tangier disease have deposits of cholesterylesters in tonsils, bone marrow, liver, spleen, peripheral nerves and arterial wall (Ferrans & Frederickson 1975). The primary biochemical defect in Tangier disease is unknown. Overdegradation of normal HDL due to a defect in a retroendocytosis pathway has been postulated as the underlying abnormality (Schmitz et al 1985). The clinical hallmarks of Tangier disease are typical orange-yellow tonsils that allow distinction of this disease from other HDL-deficiency disorders. Heterozygous carriers of the Tangier gene, who have roughly half normal HDL levels, do not develop premature atherosclerosis.

Familial apo A-I/C-III deficiency (Norum et al 1982) has been described in only two families. One variant involves a DNA insertion in an intron of the apo A-I gene (Karathanasis et al 1983). Clinically and biochemically this disorder is clearly different from Tangier disease. It may however be identical with the apo A-I deficiency with planar xanthomatosis described by Gustafson et al (1979). Whether it is justified to distinguish two clinical variants of the disorder (Schaefer et al 1985) or whether there is variable expression of the same principal defect (absence of apolipoproteins A-I and C-III from plasma) is presently unclear. The only apo A-I mutant that is clearly

Table 73.2 Major clinical and laboratory findings in the recessive dyslipoproteinaemias

Form	Lipid and lipoprotein abnormalities	Characteristic clinical and laboratory findings	Premature coronary heart disease
Familial hyper-chylomicronaemia	Triglycerides grossly elevated; low total plasma cholesterol; severe hyperchylomicronaemia; low LDL- and HDL-levels	Eruptive xanthomas, pancreatitis	None
Hepatic lipase deficiency	Similar to HLP type III; presence of beta-VLDL; triglyceride-rich LDL and HDL	Eruptive skin xanthomas, linear yellow discolouration of the palmar creases, obesity	Unclear
Cholesterylester-storage disease	LDL elevated, type IIa or IIb	Hepatosplenomegaly	Moderate
Lecithin-cholesterol acyltransferase deficiency	Deficiency of cholesterylesters in plasma; abnormal chemical and physical properties of all major lipoproteins. HDL contains discoidal particles	Corneal opacities, anaemia, proteinuria, late nephropathy. Sea-blue histiocytes in spleen and bone marrow	Present in many patients
Fish eye disease	Reduced levels of HDL	Corneal opacities	Late atherosclerosis
Familial hyperalphalipoproteinaemia (Japanese type)	HDL$_2$ markedly elevated	None	None
Tangier disease	Low plasma total cholesterol; deficiency of HDL, apo A-I and apo A-II. Abnormal LDL; abnormal chylomicron remnants	Hypoplastic orange tonsils, splenomegaly, storage of cholesterylester in RES; relapsing neuropathy; corneal opacities	Unclear
HDL-deficiency with planar xanthomas	Severe HDL-deficiency; absent apo A-I	Planar xanthomas, diffuse corneal opacities	Severe
Familial apo A-I/C-III deficiency, type I, type II	Severe HDL-deficiency; absence of apo A-I and C-III	Planar xanthomas (type I), mild diffuse corneal opacities (I,II)	Severe
Primary dysbetalipoproteinaemia	Low or normal plasma total cholesterol; mild hypertriglyceridaemia; cholesterol-rich VLDL; presence of beta-VLDL; low LDL	Apo E-2/2 phenotype	None
Abetalipoproteinaemia and homozygous hypobetalipoproteinaemia	Extremely low plasma total cholesterol and triglyceride; chylomicrons, VLDL and LDL absent from plasma; deficiency of apo B-100 and apo B-48	Fat malabsorption, retinitis pigmentosa, acanthocytosis, ataxic neuropathy	None
Normotriglyceridaemic abetalipoproteinaemia	Low plasma cholesterol; absence of VLDL, LDL and B-100	Ataxic gait	None
Anderson disease (Chylomicron retention disease)	Absence of chylomicrons and B-48	Fat malabsorption, retinitis pigmentosa, ataxic neuropathy	None
Sitosterolaemia with xanthomatosis	Increased plant sterols (sitosterol, camposterol) in LDL and HDL. Facultative hypercholesterolaemia	Tendon and tuberous xanthomas, abnormal red blood cells	Severe

Table 73.2 Major clinical and laboratory findings in the recessive dyslipoproteinaemias (*contd.*)

Form	Lipid and lipoprotein abnormalities	Characteristic clinical and laboratory findings	Premature coronary heart disease
Cerebrotendinous xanthomatosis	Low HDL of abnormal composition; cholesterol increased in plasma lipoproteins	Progressive neurological dysfunction (dementia, spinal cord paresis, cerebellar ataxia); tendon xanthomas, cataracts	Severe
X-linked recessive form X-linked ichthyosis (Steroid-sulphatase deficiency)	LDL and VLDL with cholesterolsulphate and abnormal mobility in electrophoresis	Ichthyosis, corneal opacities	Unknown

associated with a clinical disorder is Apo A-I Iowa which results in hereditary amyloidasis (Nichols et al 1988).

A deficiency of cholesterylesters in plasma, subnormal HDL levels and an abnormal HDL composition characterize familial LCAT deficiency. Lecithin-cholesterol-acyltransferase is a plasma enzyme that catalyzes the transfer of a fatty acid residue preferentially from the β-position of phosphatidylcholine to the hydroxyl group of cholesterol (Glomset 1968). Patients with familial deficiency of the enzyme exhibit multiple lipoprotein abnormalities (Gjone et al 1978). HDL, the main site of acyltransferase-catalysed cholesterylester formation in human plasma, is anomalously heterogeneous and contains a population of cholesterylester-poor disc-shaped precursors of the spherical HDL in normal plasma (Utermann et al 1980). The lipoprotein abnormalities in familial LCAT-deficiency result in storage of cholesterol in several tissues. Clinically the disorder is characterized by anaemia, corneal opacity (Fig. 73.3) and proteinuria with late renal insufficiency. Some patients have to be treated by haemodialysis or undergo kidney transplantation. However transplantation does not seem to be very helpful since the transplanted organ may be filled with lipid shortly after transplantation. Many of the hitherto described patients had atherosclerosis (Gjone et al 1978).

Autosomal dominant forms

The dominant forms of familial hyperlipidaemia are among the most common genetic disorders in man and are clearly associated with the occurrence of premature coronary heart disease. The present genetic classification of dominant familial hyperlipidaemia is based primarily on the pioneering work of Goldstein and co-workers (1973). Three frequent familial disorders of lipoprotein metabolism were delineated by family studies in survivors

of myocardial infarction and 20% of survivors under age 60 years had one of these disorders. These are familial hypercholesterolaemia, familial hypertriglyceridaemia and familial combined hyperlipidaemia. Ascertainment of affected kindreds in the work of Goldstein et al (1973) has been criticised repeatedly (Hewitt et al 1979, Ott 1979, Williams & Lalouel 1982), since the selection and classification procedure used would tend to produce results suggestive of major gene effects even when no such genes operate. The appearance of monogenic segregation of cholesterol (LDL-cholesterol), with or without associated xanthomatosis, is however undisputed and the discovery of the LDL-receptor defects in familial hypercholesterolaemia has provided unequivocal evidence for the monogenic causation of this disease (Brown & Goldstein 1986). The data providing evidence for a monogenic mechanism in familial combined hyperlipidaemia are less convincing, especially since there is a lack of any specific biochemical marker for this disorder. Most

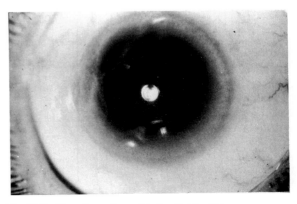

Fig. 73.3 Eye of a patient with familial lecithin-cholesterol-acyltransferase (LCAT)-deficiency and diffuse corneal clouding (courtesy of Dr W. Schoenborn).

investigators do not consider familial hypertriglyceridaemia a monogenic condition. The grouping of genetic
hyperlipidaemias will nonetheless follow the one originally proposed by Goldstein et al (1973), with slight
modifications.

Familial hypercholesterolaemia

Familial hypercholesterolaemia is the best example of a
monogenic disorder where the mutant gene produces
both hypercholesterolaemia and atherosclerosis. The
disease exists in two forms, the heterozygous form that
has a frequency of about 1-2/1000 in most populations
and the rare homozygous form that is present in about
1/1 000 000 of newborn children. Considerably higher
frequencies of heterozygous familial hypercholesterolaemia were observed in South Africans of Dutch origin
(1/200) (Gevers et al 1987).

Heterozygous familial hypercholesterolaemia The
triad of hypercholesterolaemia, xanthomatosis and
angina pectoris has been recognized as a dominantly
inherited syndrome since the work of Müller (1939).
Familial hypercholesterolaemia is characterized chemically by a 2-fold elevation of cholesterol in LDL. Mean
plasma cholesterol concentrations are about 350 mg/100
ml but range from 270 to 550 mg/100 ml. VLDL
cholesterol and triglycerides may also occasionally be
elevated. Electrophoresis of plasma followed by staining
for lipids results in a type IIa, or less frequently IIb,
phenotype. The elevation of LDL-cholesterol is seen
even in childhood and is the earliest detectable manifestation of the gene, usually being already present at birth
(Kwiterovich et al 1974). The Lp(a) lipoprotein levels are
increased about three-fold in patients with FH (Utermann et al 1989) and those with very high levels have the
highest risk for developing coronary heart disease.

Clinical symptoms of the disorder are tendinous
xanthomas (Fig. 73.4), preferentially of the Achilles
tendon, xanthelasma, arcus lipoides corneae and coronary atherosclerosis. These symptoms usually develop in
the 2nd, 3rd and 4th decades of life. By the 3rd decade
arcus cornea and tendon xanthomas are present in about
half of heterozygotes. Tuberous xanthomas may be
present but are rare. However, none of these symptoms is
obligatory even though as many as 80% of affected
subjects ultimately develop xanthomas. In contrast to
other forms of familial hyperlipidaemia, patients with
familial hypercholesterolaemia are not obese and do not
have glucose intolerance or hyperuricaemia. The fatal
complications of the progressive atherosclerosis are
myocardial infarction and cerebral stroke. Stone et al
(1974) have investigated over 1000 subjects from 116

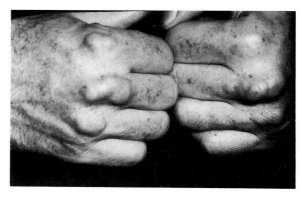

Fig. 73.4 Xanthomas at the extensor tendons of the hand
of a patient with familial hypercholesterolaemia.

kindreds with familial hypercholesterolaemia. In their
study the cumulative probability of coronary heart
disease by age 60 years was 52% in affected males and
33% in affected females, and the risk for coronary heart
disease was about 3–4 times higher in affected subjects
compared to intrafamilial controls. The mean age of
onset of symptomatic coronary heart disease is about 45
years in affected males and 53 years in affected females
(Harlan et al 1966). The high risk of premature
atherosclerosis in carriers of the gene for familial
hypercholesterolaemia is also evident from studies of
survivors of myocardial infarction. Independent studies
in Finland, Great Britain, and the US have shown that, in
unselected survivors, the frequency of familial hypercholesterolaemia is 3–6% compared to 0.1–0.2% in the
general population (Patterson & Slack 1972, Goldstein
et al 1973, Nikkila & Aro 1973).

The primary biochemical defect in familial hypercholesterolaemia has been elucidated by cell culture
studies using fibroblasts from homozygotes for the
disease and from normal controls. In normal humans
about 80% of LDL is degraded by receptor-mediated
endocytosis. The high affinity LDL-receptor is present in
hepatic and several extrahepatic tissues. This receptor is
deficient or functionally abnormal in homozygotes for
familial hypercholesterolaemia (Brown & Goldstein
1986). Heterozygotes for familial hypercholesterolaemia
have one normal allele specifying functionally normal
receptors and one abnormal allele at the LDL receptor
gene locus. Presence of only half the number of
functionally normal receptors results in impaired degradation of LDL and in accumulation of LDL in the
plasma compartment (Bilheimer et al 1979, Brown &
Goldstein 1986). Thus familial hypercholesterolaemia is
transmitted as an autosomal dominant trait. The domin-

ant gene is highly penetrant at all ages (90–100%) when either total cholesterol or LDL-cholesterol is used as a marker for the disease. In affected families a bimodal distribution of cholesterol and LDL-cholesterol is observed. There is however some overlap between normal and affected family members. Measurement of LDL-receptor activity on fibroblasts or lymphocytes also shows a bimodal distribution and may be used as an additional criterion to establish the diagnosis (Bilheimer et al 1978). The gene for the human LDL-receptor encompasses 45 kilobases of DNA on the short arm of chromosome 19 (Francke et al 1984). Recently Humphries et al (1985) have used RFLP-analysis with LDL-receptor cDNA to identify carriers in affected families by linkage.

Treatment of familial hypercholesterolaemia starts with a fat-modified diet. A diet low in cholesterol and low in fat with a ratio of polyunsaturated to saturated fatty acids close to 2 is recommended. However such a diet alone is usually not sufficient to lower effectively LDL-cholesterol levels and therefore drugs are commonly added to the dietary regime. The most effective drugs for lowering plasma cholesterol levels in familial hypercholesterolaemia are the bile acid sequestering agents cholestyramine and cholestipol that disrupt the enterohepatic cycle and that may reduce plasma cholesterol by 30% or more (Levy et al 1973) and the inhibitors of HMG CoA-reductase that block the endogenous synthesis of cholesterol (Brown & Goldstein 1986). Both groups of substances may be used to good effect in combination. The atherogenic effects of high LDL levels may be caused, at least in part, by modified LDL, e.g. oxidized LDL. Substances that lower cholesterol and that are antioxidants (e.g. probucol) have therefore been proposed for the treatment of familial hypercholesterolaemia. Further alternatives are neomicin or combinations of the bile acid sequestrants with niacin (Schaefer & Levy 1985). In patients with severe forms plasma exchange therapy has been used (Thompson et al 1980).

In the differential diagnosis of the disorder other forms of hypercholesterolaemia have to be considered. There are secondary hypercholesterolaemia, polygenic hypercholesterolaemia and the hypercholesterolaemia seen in one third of patients with familial combined hyperlipidaemia. Patients with these disorders rarely develop xanthomas, in particular no xanthomas of the Achilles tendon. Even in the absence of visible or palpable xanthomas, demonstration by X-ray or ultrasound of the thickening of the Achilles tendon has turned out to be a valuable clinical criterion for differential diagnosis of familial hypercholesterolaemia (Blankenhorn & Mayers 1969, Mabuchi et al 1977). Tendon xanthomas that are clinically indistinguishible from those in familial hypercholesterolaemia may develop in patients with autosomal recessive cerebrotendinous xanthomatosis. However, these individuals have normal LDL-cholesterol and may be distinguished by other clinical features such as cataracts and mental deterioration. Similarly xanthelasma and arcus corneae can also be observed in patients with normal cholesterol levels and may occur as a familial trait.

In an isolated patient with hypercholesterolaemia, but without characteristic clinical symptoms, it is frequently not possible to make the diagnosis. Due to the high degree of heterogeneity of the gene defect it will also not be feasible to diagnose the disease in a single patient by DNA analysis (see under homozygous familial hypercholesterolaemia). However, in some populations with a rather uniform genetic background, e.g. Africaans speaking South Africans, Finns, Franco-Canadians and Lebanese this may become possible (Gevers et al 1987, Hobbs et al 1987, Lehrman et al 1987, Aalto-Setälä et al 1988).

As a consequence of the autosomal dominant mode of transmission every first-degree relative of a proband with familial hypercholesterolaemia has a 50% risk of having inherited the mutant gene and of being at risk for premature atherosclerosis and coronary heart disease. Therefore once the diagnosis of familial hypercholesterolaemia has been established in a patient a family study is indicated to possibly identify affected relatives before manifestation of clinical complications. The potential of such an approach has been demonstrated by a large Norwegian population genetic study on xanthomatosis and hypercholesterolaemia. In this study 30% of patients ascertained through a propositus with xanthomatosis came from only seven large kindreds, each showing classical dominant inheritance of the trait (Heiberg 1976).

Homozygous familial hypercholesterolaemia. Rarely, two heterozygotes for familial hypercholesterolaemia marry and produce a homozygous child. This condition is much more devastating than the heterozygous form of the disease. Plasma LDL levels are elevated roughly 6-fold in these children compared to controls. Total plasma cholesterol levels range from 600–1200 mg/100 ml. There is massive deposition of cholesterol in tissues, and myocardial infarction generally occurs in the first two decades of life. Gross hypercholesterolaemia is present at birth and persists throughout life. Cutaneous xanthomas that have a unique yellow-orange colour may be present at birth and have been found by age 4 in virtually every patient. Tendon xanthomas and arcus corneae develop in childhood. A typical form of the xanthomatous infiltration of the aortic valve may result in aortic valvular stenosis. Occasionally mitral regurgitation and mitral stenosis have been observed due to xanthomatous plaquing and thickening of the endocardial surfaces of the mitral valve. Histological examination has revealed that the cholesterol in the xanthoma is present within histiocytic foam cells, mostly in the form of cytoplasmic droplets that are not bound to membranes. Upon autopsy typical atherosclerotic plaques are found in the arteries, but in addition there are intimal infiltrations of xanthomatous foam cells similar in histological appearance to those in the tuberous xanthomas. Severe atherosclerosis occurs not only in the coronary arteries but in the thoracic and abdominal aorta and in the major pulmonary arteries as well. Further clinical and laboratory findings are painful and inflamed joints, cardiac murmurs and persistently elevated sedimentation rate. Generalised atherosclerosis results in death from myocardial infarction usually before 30 years of age (Goldstein & Brown 1983). However in a large series of patients from Japan six exceeded the third decade (Mabuchi et al 1978).

The homozygotes held the key to solving the primary biochemical defect in familial hypercholesterolaemia and at the same time to elucidating the biochemical mechanism underlying a dominantly inherited disorder (heterozygous familial hypercholesterolaemia). By studying fibroblasts from homozygous children Goldstein and Brown (1974) were able to demonstrate a genetic defect in the LDL-receptor in familial hypercholesterolaemia. Moreover, elucidation of this defect has led to the detection of the LDL-receptor pathway and its relation to human atherosclerosis (Brown & Goldstein 1986).

By measuring the binding, uptake and degradation of LDL in fibroblast culture the receptor defects in familial hypercholesterolaemia were originally categorized into receptor negative (R^{b^o} allele), receptor defective (R^{b^-} allele) and internalization defective (R^{i^-}). In contrast to receptor negative subjects that have virtually no detectable receptors in binding studies, those of the receptor defective form still have receptor binding in the range of 2–10% of controls. Notably the clinical course of the disease is less severe in receptor defective patients and survival is significantly longer (Goldstein & Brown 1983). By extrapolation one may conclude that this relationship holds also in heterozygotes, explaining part of the variability in age of onset and severity of clinical symptoms. However, severity of atherosclerosis is also highly variable among homozygous subjects that share the same molecular defect. Among French Canadians with the same deletion in the LDL-receptor gene one patient died of myocardial infarction at the age of 3 years whereas another lived to the age of 33 years.

The LDL-receptor gene has recently been cloned and assigned to the short arm of chromosome 19 (Francke et al 1984). Almost 20 different defects causing familial hypercholesterolaemia have been described in the LDL-receptor gene (Brown & Goldstein 1986, Hobbs et al 1987, Lehrman et al 1987). Characterization of the many natural mutations and of some produced by in vitro mutagenesis has permitted dissection of the receptor protein into functional domains (Brown & Goldstein 1986, Russell et al 1986). The LDL-receptor at present is the best characterized receptor protein. It contains five functional domains, 1. the cytoplasmic domain that is responsible for the clustering of the receptor in coated pits, 2. the membrane spanning domain, 3. a domain rich in O-linked sugar, 4. a domain of high homology to the EGF-receptor, and 5. the cysteine-rich ligand-binding domain. Four major classes of mutants exist (Fig. 73.5). Class 1 mutants do not synthesize receptors. Class 2 mutants represent defects in the processing and transport of the receptors through the endoplasmic reticulum and through the Golgi compartments. Few or no receptors occur at the cell surface. Class 3 is characterized by binding defective receptors that occur at the cell surface. Class 4 mutations do bind LDL normally but receptors are unable to cluster in coated pits and to internalize LDL. Most patients with 'homozygous' familial hypercholesterolaemia are genetic compounds.

The parents of homozygous probands are obligate heterozygotes and have the dominant form of familial

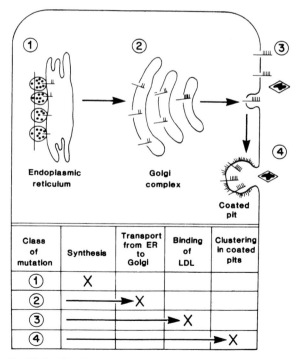

Class of mutation	Synthesis	Transport from ER to Golgi	Binding of LDL	Clustering in coated pits
①	X			
②	⟶	X		
③	⟶		X	
④	⟶			X

Fig. 73.5 Classification of mutations in the human LDL-receptor (from Brown & Goldstein 1986, with permission).

hypercholesterolaemia. The frequency of parental consanguinity was at least 33% in a study from Japan (Mabuchi et al 1978). Occasionally parents of homozygotes with normal lipid levels have been observed. They could be identified as heterozygotes by receptor studies. Therapy for homozygous familial hypercholesterolaemia is still far from being optimal. Drugs like cholestyramin may reduce plasma cholesterol levels by 20–30%. This is insufficient in view of the high starting levels and is not sufficient to prevent myocardial infarction. Moreover many of the children do not tolerate the drug regime. In this situation portacaval shunt and plasma exchange therapy have been used either alone or in combination as effective therapeutic intervention in homozygous familial hypercholesterolaemia (Bilheimer et al 1975, Thompson et al 1980, Starzl et al 1983). More recently extracorporal LDL-elimination has been introduced as a powerful alternative (Lupien et al 1976, Stoffel & Demant 1981). Liver transplantation has been performed in a homozygous child with severe atherosclerosis (Bilheimer et al 1984).

The LDL-receptor is expressed on amniotic cells in early pregnancy. This has made possible the successful prenatal diagnosis of homozygous familial hypercholesterolaemia in one case at risk (Brown et al 1978).

Familial combined hyperlipidaemia

Familial combined hyperlipidaemia (multiple type hyperlipidaemia) is probably the most frequent monogenic familial hyperlipidaemia but was not recognised as a distinct genetic entity until 1973 (Glueck et al 1973, Goldstein et al 1973, Nikkilä & Aro 1973, Rose et al 1973). The disorder is believed to be inherited as an autosomal dominant trait. The characteristic feature of familial combined hyperlipidaemia is its pleomorphic manifestation even among relatives in the same family. Roughly one third of affected individuals have hypercholesterolaemia (elevated LDL), one third have hypertriglyceridaemia (elevated VLDL) and another third have both hypercholesterolaemia and hypertriglyceridaemia (elevated LDL and VLDL). Accordingly patients may present with a type IIa, IIb, IV or rarely a type V phenotype. In a given individual the type of hyperlipoproteinaemia may change spontaneously. Mean plasma lipid levels are significantly increased but tend to show a lesser degree of elevation than in either familial hypercholesterolaemia or familial hypertriglyceridaemia. However, lipid levels may be normal at one time and abnormal at another. The lipid abnormality is rarely expressed before the age of 25 years.

Hyperapobetalipoproteinaemia, a condition characterized by an elevation of apo B in LDL and by the presence of small, dense LDL particles, may be identical with familial combined hyperlipidaemia (Grundy et al 1987). Familial combined hyperlipidaemia is associated with obesity, hyperinsulinaemia and glucose intolerance. Xanthomas do not occur. Patients with excessive hypertriglyceridaemia may develop pancreatitis. The most severe complication of combined hyperlipidaemia is coronary atherosclerosis. In independent studies from Finland and the US 11–20% of survivors of myocardial infarction under age 60 years had this disorder (Goldstein et al 1973, Nikkilä & Aro 1973). The prevalence in the general population has been estimated as high as 1–2% in one study but lack of a unique marker for the disorder makes this figure very uncertain. The occurrence of phenotypically different lipoprotein patterns in familial combined hyperlipidaemia is believed to be the expression of one single dominant gene. In a study of 47 families with combined hyperlipidaemia identified among survivors of myocardial infarction 50% of first-degree relatives above age 25 years had hyperlipidaemia, consistent with a dominant mechanism.

The primary biochemical lesion underlying the disorder is unknown. Subjects with hypercholesterolaemia from kindreds with combined hyperlipidaemia have a functionally normal LDL-receptor. Kinetic studies suggest that patients have an increased influx of apo B containing lipoproteins into the plasma compartment (Grundy et al 1987). Studies using RFLPs in the apo B gene have failed to detect linkage of familial combined hyperlipidaemia with apo B. Hence the defect is not in the apo B gene in those families studied so far. Heterozygotes for LPL-deficiency have lipoprotein abnormalities resembling familial combined hyperlipidaemia. Hence a subset of familial combined families may have heterozygous LPL-deficiency (Babirak et al 1989). To date no specific biochemical test exists for diagnosis of familial combined hyperlipidaemia. Due to this lack of any specific marker for the disorder the diagnosis is not possible in an individual patient. The only method available to differentiate combined hyperlipidaemia from other forms of primary hyperlipidaemia is by family studies. This approach for identification has also been used in the original delineation of the disorder and this has necessarily biased the subsequent genetic analysis. Hence the single-gene inheritance of familial combined hyperlipidaemia cannot be considered proven. Reanalysis of the original data from Seattle, using complex segregation analysis, supports multifactorial inheritance (Williams & Lalouel 1982). However four large pedigrees, each showing vertical transmission over three generations and the expected 1:1 segregation, have been reported in the literature. The data from these kindreds are most easily explained by single-gene inheritance. Results from a large Amish pedigree with hyperapobetalipoproteinaemia were also consistent with a dominant/

single locus model for this disorder (Beaty et al 1986). In any event suspicion of familial combined hyperlipidaemia or hyperapobetalipoprotein in a given patient should lead to determinations of plasma lipids in first-degree adult relatives since, independent from the mode of inheritance, the risk for first-degree relatives of a proband with this (these) disorder(s) of also having hyperlipidaemia is around 50%.

Treatment of combined hyperlipidaemia depends on the phenotypic expression of the disease. For individuals with pure hypercholesterolaemia (type IIa) or pure hypertriglyceridaemia (type IV) the same rules as described for familial hypercholesterolaemia or familial hypertriglyceridaemia respectively may be used as a guide. In obese probands with the IIb or IV phenotypes, treatment begins with the prudent diet, emphasizing weight reduction as well as fat modification. The most promising drug is nicotinic acid, since this agent lowers both cholesterol and triglycerides, probably by inhibiting the synthesis of hepatic apo B containing lipoproteins. Fibrates may also be appropriate. Sometimes a combination of resin and nicotinic acid or fibrate may be required to correct both the hypercholesterolaemia and the hypertriglyceridaemia. The combined use of gemfibrozil, and the HMG CoA-reductase inhibitor lovastatin has also been shown to be very effective in patients with combined hyperlipidaemia (Schaefer & Levy 1985, Grundy et al 1987).

Familial defective apo B-100

The counterpart of the LDL-receptor defect in familial hypercholesterolaemia is a defect in the ligand for the receptor, apo B-100. Recently patients with a binding-defective LDL have been identified (Innerarity et al 1987) that have a mutation in codon 3500 of the apo B gene. Hypercholesterolaemia seems to be moderate in these patients. The prevalence in the population of this dominantly inherited disorder is presently unknown, as is the spectrum of lipid and clinical abnormalities in this defect.

Polygenic hyperlipidaemia/multifactorial hyperlipidaemia

Familial type III hyperlipoproteinaemia

Familial type III hyperlipoproteinaemia (broad-beta-disease) is a disorder of lipoprotein metabolism associated with grossly elevated concentrations of both cholesterol and triglycerides in plasma. Lipid levels are extremely sensitive to caloric intake and consequently there is considerable variability of cholesterol and triglyceride levels in a given patient. Usually, however, cholesterol concentrations are over 300 mg/100 ml and triglyceride levels tend to exceed those of cholesterol. Chylomicrons that are rich in cholesterylesters may be present in fasting plasma. The characteristic lipoprotein abnormality of the type III disorder is the accumulation in plasma of lipoprotein particles that are intermediate in density, size, chemical composition and electrophoretic mobility between triglyceride-rich lipoproteins and LDL. Electrophoresis of type III plasma followed by staining for lipids therefore frequently reveals a broad unresolved band extending between beta- and pre-beta lipoproteins. Upon preparative ultracentrifugation the abnormal lipoproteins in part float with VLDL and are demonstrated by electrophoresis as a beta-migrating subfraction. The abnormal lipoprotein is therefore called 'floating-beta lipoprotein' or beta-VLDL. Beta-VLDL is enriched in apo E and depleted of apo C (Havel & Kane 1973). In over 95% of patients apo E exhibits a structural variant designated as the apo E-2/2 phenotype (Utermann 1985, Utermann et al 1987).

Hyperlipoproteinaemia type III is a disorder of the adult and is rarely seen before the age of 20 years. There are only few documented cases where type III hyperlipoproteinaemia already existed in childhood. Clinically the disorder is associated with xanthomatosis, coronary heart disease and peripheral vascular disease (Borrie 1969, Moser et al 1974, Mishkel et al 1975, Morganroth et al 1975). The most typical clinical features seen in about 60% of patients are planar yellowish lipid deposits in the creases of the palm (xanthoma striata palmaris). Tuberous xanthomas are present in a fraction of type III subjects (Fig. 73.6). Tendon xanthomas are rare in type III. Eruptive xanthomas, xanthelasma and arcus corneae may occur but are also comparatively rare. 33% of patients have coronary heart disease and 27% exhibit peripheral vascular disease. About 50% of patients have glucose intolerance. It must however be mentioned that all present data on the prevalence of clinical signs are biased by the selection of patients that are exclusively from clinical material. Thus 100% of patients ascertained by a dermatologist will present with xanthomas (Borrie 1969). There exist no data on patients randomly selected from the population. The increased risk for premature coronary heart disease is however evident from the frequency of type III hyperlipoproteinaemia among survivors of myocardial infarction. In this group the frequency is about 1/100 (Utermann 1985) compared to 1/5000 in the general population (Brown et al 1983). Men tend to present earlier with clinical symptoms than women. In a large series of patients from the NIH, ischaemic vascular disease was diagnosed at a mean age of 39 years in men, but 10 years later in women.

The familial occurrence of the type III disorder has been known since the early pioneering work of Fredrickson and co-workers (1967), but for many years there were

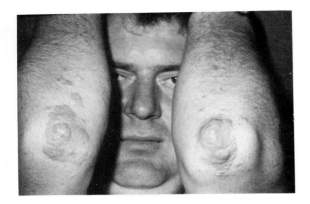

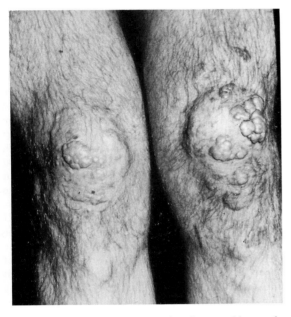

Fig. 73.6 Tuberous xanthomas at the elbows and knees of patients with familial type III hyperlipidaemia (courtesy of Dr H. Kaffarnik).

conflicting results on its genetic mode of transmission. The key to the clarification of the complicated genetics of type III hyperlipidaemia came from the discovery of a polymorphism of apolipoprotein E which is determined by three autosomal alleles ε4, ε3 and ε2 (see polymorphism of apo E). With few exceptions all patients with classical type III studied so far have been homozygous for the allele ε2 (phenotype apo E-2/2) suggesting an autosomal recessive mode of inheritance. However in most populations roughly 1% of subjects are homozygous apo E-2/2, whereas the frequency of classic type III is only about 1/5000. Moreover most individuals

of phenotype apo E-2/2 present with hypo- rather than hypercholesterolaemia, but all have in common the same type of dyslipoproteinaemia characterized by the presence of beta-VLDL and designated primary dysbetalipoproteinaemia (Utermann et al 1977, 1987). It had been estimated that no more than 2% of apo E-2/2 individuals ever develop clinical signs of the type III disorder and an additional mechanism resulting in the hyperlipidaemia in type III patients had to be anticipated. Therefore it was proposed that type III hyperlipoproteinaemia is caused by the simultaneous but independent inheritance of the ε2 allele and of other defects that produce hyperlipidaemia. Comparative studies of 19 kindreds ascertained through a proband of phenotype apo E-2/2 gave direct support for this two-factor-hypothesis. Probands with type III hyperlipoproteinaemia came from families where various phenotypic forms of hyperlipidaemia were present in about 50% of all adult first-degree relatives of probands (Utermann et al 1979). Hyperlipidaemia and apo E-phenotypes segregated independently in the families and some kindreds showed evidence for coexistence of monogenic familial combined hyperlipidaemia. On the other hand hyperlipidaemia was not observed in kindreds where the probands were normocholesterolaemic. From these observations it has been concluded that type III hyperlipoproteinaemia is caused by at least two non-allelic genes. Depending on the form of the co-inherited hyperlipidaemia the disorder will be dimeric in some, and polygenic in other patients. Vertical transmission of the dyslipoproteinaemia has been observed in many kindreds and had previously been taken as evidence for a monogenic dominant mechanism. However, this phenomenon represents pseudodominance that is due to the high frequency of the ε2 allele in most populations (Utermann et al 1977, Utermann 1987).

As mentioned earlier, lipid levels in type III patients are very sensitive to caloric intake. Most patients respond well to dietary or drug therapy. On a strict regime cholesterol concentration may be lowered to a normal level and xanthomas may disappear. Moreover hormonal factors such as hyperthyroidism and oestrogen treatment can completely eliminate the hyperlipidaemia, whereas hypothyroidism markedly exaggerates the lipoprotein abnormalities. Hypothyroidism as well as severe nephropathy are possible among exogeneous factors that may precipitate type III hyperlipoproteinaemia in a subject of apo E-2/2 phenotype, a phenomenon previously described as secondary type III hyperlipoproteinaemia. Since the degree of hyperlipidaemia and of clinical symptoms is under the control of different genes interacting with endogenous and environmental factors, type III hyperlipoproteinaemia ultimately has to be defined as a multifactorial disorder (Fig. 73.7).

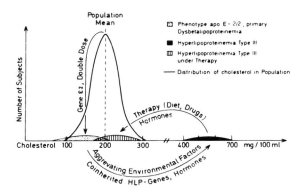

Hyperlipoproteinemia Type III : Model of a Multifactorial Disorder

Fig. 73.7 Model explaining the aetiological factors in type III hyperlipidaemia.

The genetic two-factor concept of type III hyperlipo-proteinaemia predicts that more than one defect operates in subjects with the classical type III disorder. One of these is shared by most type III subjects and also operates in subjects with simple uncomplicated dysbetalipoproteinaemia. This defect relates to the structural abnormality of apo E. The abnormal beta-VLDL and the cholesterol-rich chylomicrons present in type III plasma are considered degradation products (remnants) of triglyceride-rich lipoproteins that accumulate due to a defect in the catabolic conversion of remnants to LDL. Apo E normally plays a key role in the degradation of remnants. Apo E is a ligand for the LDL receptor and is possibly recognized by a hepatic apo E receptor (remnant-receptor, Mahley et al 1986). The accumulation of remnant lipoproteins in familial dysbetalipoproteinaemia and in type III hyperlipoproteinaemia is caused by a defect in apo E. The apo E-2 form of the protein represents a non-functional mutant that is not recognized by the LDL(B/E)-receptor (Schneider et al 1981). Several other mutants affecting receptor binding have been identified in the apo E gene of patients with type III hyperlipoproteinaemia (Mahley et al 1986). In one family, type III has resulted from apo E deficiency (Schaefer et al 1986). The metabolic block in remnant removal of E 2/2 homozygotes, however, does not usually result in hyperlipoproteinaemia type III, but a second independent defect is required for the development of hyperlipidaemia. Some rare mutants of apo E (e.g. E-3 Leiden, Havekes et al 1986), apparently result in dominant mutations of hyperlipoproteinaemia type III (Mann et al 1989, Rall et al 1989). Whereas apo E from type III subjects is probably not recognized by the hepatic receptors for apo E (LDL-receptor, remnant receptor) leading to the accumulation of remnants, it has been demonstrated that beta-VLDL is recognized by a specific receptor present on macrophages (Mahley et al 1980). These cells may bind and internalize the beta-VLDL and become overloaded with cholesterylester in type III hyperlipoproteinaemia and develop into foam cells. Foam cells that probably are derived from macrophages form the basis of xanthomas and have been found upon autopsy in coronary vessels, on the endocardial surface, in the spleen and in the bone marrow of patients with type III disorder.

Demonstration by electrophoresis of beta-VLDL was the original diagnostic test for the type III disorder. However this lipoprotein abnormality is not pathognomonic for hyperlipoproteinaemia type III and alternative clinical-chemical tests have been proposed, based on the abnormal lipid-chemical composition of VLDL in the type III disorder. Generally patients with type III hyperlipidaemia have a ratio of VLDL cholesterol to plasma triglyceride that is above 0.30, as compared with a ratio below 0.25 in normal subjects. The observation of the structural apo E abnormality in type III hyperlipoproteinaemia provides the basis for the specific diagnosis of the disorder. Demonstration of the apo E-2/2 phenotype or other structural and/or functional defects of apo E in a hyperlipidaemic individual proves unequivocally the diagnosis of the type III disorder (Utermann 1985, 1987) (Table 73.3).

An excellent response to therapy is the rule in most patients with type III hyperlipoproteinaemia. Treatment consists of caloric restriction, restriction of dietary cholesterol (300 mg/ 24 hours or less) and fat, and avoidance of alcohol. Upon weight reduction there is frequently a dramatic decrease in plasma lipid levels. In cases where plasma lipid levels remain elevated even after ideal weight is achieved, clofibrate, gemfibrocil or niacin are drugs of choice to reduce them to normal. Regression of xanthomas and of peripheral vascular disease has been reported as a consequence of hypolipidaemic therapy (Zelis et al 1970).

Genetic counselling in hyperlipoproteinaemia type III can help to early recognition of family members at risk. The risk for relatives of probands is two-fold. Given that the co-existing hyperlipidaemia is one of the monogenic dominant forms, the risk for a first-degree relative of having also inherited the 'hyperlipidaemic gene' is 1/2. The risk for the development of the type III disorder is different for sibs and for children of a proband. In the most frequent situation both parents of a proband will be heterozygous carriers of the apo $\varepsilon 2$ allele and the risk for any of their children to be homozygous apo E-2/2 will be 1/4. The combined risk to co-inherit both $\varepsilon 2$ alleles and the hyperlipidaemic gene will then be 1/8. The risk for children of a proband can be calculated from the known

Table 73.3 Apolipoprotein E mutants*

Designation	Structure	LDL-receptor binding	Association with HLP
E-0	abnormal mRNA's	—	Type III hyperlipidaemia
E-1	$Arg_{158} \rightarrow Cys; Gly_{127} \rightarrow Asp$	4 %	Type III hyperlipidaemia
E-1$_{Bethesda}$	—	—	Type III hyperlipidaemia
E-2	$Arg_{158} \rightarrow Cys$	< 2 %	Type III hyperlipidaemia
E-2	$Arg_{136} \rightarrow Ser$	n.d.	Type III hyperlipidaemia
E-2	$Arg_{145} \rightarrow Cys$	45 %	Type III hyperlipidaemia
E-2	$Lys_{146} \rightarrow Gln$	40 %	Type III hyperlipidaemia
E-3	'wild type'	100 %	No
E-3	$Cys_{112} \rightarrow Arg; Arg_{142} \rightarrow Cys$	< 20 %	Type III hyperlipidaemia
E-3	$Ala_{99} \rightarrow Thr; Ala_{152} \rightarrow Pro$	n.d.	Unknown
E-3$_{Leiden}$	no Cys	~ 50 %	Type III hyperlipidaemia
E-4	$Cys_{112} \rightarrow Arg$	100 %	Hypercholesterolaemia/type V-hyperlipidaemia
E-4$_{Innsbruck}$	no Cys; His +/−?	n.d.	Unknown
E-5	lower mol. wt.	n.d.	Hyperlipidaemia?
E-7(Suita)	—	n.d.	Hyperlipidaemia?

*Data from Yamamura et al 1984, Havekes et al 1986, Mahley et al 1986, Menzel and Utermann 1986, Wardell et al 1987

frequency of the ε2 allele in the population. In most Caucasian populations a proband with type III disorder has a chance of about 16% of having a spouse heterozygous for the ε2 allele and any child from this mating has a risk of 1/2 of being homozygous apo E-2/2 and independently of 1/2 of inheriting the 'hyperlipidaemic gene'. Hence the risk for children of a proband of developing hyperlipoproteinaemia type III in later life is about 4%. Actually the risk is rather higher, since there is a 1% chance that the spouse is also homozygous apo E-2/2 and furthermore the spouse may also contribute 'hyperlipidaemic genes' due to the high frequency of these genes in the population. In some families with rare apo E mutants (Table 73.3) the risk for first-degree relatives may be 50% due to the dominant character of the defect. Therefore apo E phenotyping is recommended in families of type III probands. This permits the early detection of relatives that are at risk of developing type III hyperlipoproteinaemia in later life. A follow-up of the at-risk individuals then permits early therapeutic intervention in those that start to develop the disorder.

Polygenic hypercholesterolaemia

Plasma cholesterol levels are under the control of many different genes and environmental factors that altogether result in a nearly Gaussian distribution of cholesterol level in the population. The presence in one individual of several genes, each tending to moderately elevate plasma cholesterol, theoretically should result in polygenic hypercholesterolaemia. Indeed Goldstein and co-workers (1973) in a study of survivors of myocardial infarction were able to identify a group of patients with elevated plasma cholesterol levels, but no evidence for bimodality

of plasma cholesterol concentrations was seen in the families of affected probands. Instead, the distribution of cholesterol in these families is unimodal, but shifted towards a higher mean level. This form was defined as polygenic hypercholesterolaemia.

In patients with primary hypercholesterolaemia (not familial) the ε4 allele of the apo E polymorphism is significantly increased. This allele is associated with elevated LDL-cholesterol in the general population. It may be one of several genes contributing to polygenic hypercholesterolaemia (Utermann 1987, 1988).

The disorder can be delineated only by family studies. The classical clinical features of familial hypercholesterolaemia, such as xanthomas and corneal arcus, do not occur in polygenic hypercholesterolaemia, but the disorder is likely to be associated with premature atherosclerosis. There are no studies on the prevalence of clinical symptoms in this group of patients. A frequency for familial hypercholesterolaemia cannot be given since it depends on the arbitrary definition of upper limits for normal cholesterol levels.

Familial hypertriglyceridaemia

Familial hypertriglyceridaemia is an adult disorder. Only 10–20% of individuals who carry the genes for familial hypertriglyceridaemia develop hyperlipidaemia before the age of 20 years, and expression of the disorder in children is extremely rare. A moderate elevation of triglycerides in VLDL is characteristic for the disorder (Goldstein et al 1973). Hyperchylomicronaemia is rare. Lipoprotein electrophoresis exhibits a type IV or rarely a type V pattern. Xanthomas usually do not develop. Familial hypertriglyceridaemia is associated with diabetes mellitus and obesity. Family studies on probands with familial hypertriglyceridaemia and diabetes mellitus have provided evidence that the hyperlipidaemia is transmitted independently from diabetes mellitus. However, patients that have both familial hyperlipidaemia and diabetes mellitus are more severely affected. A similar relationship may exist between hypertriglyceridaemia and pancreatitis (Brunzell & Schott 1973). Besides untreated diabetes several other factors, including alcohol abuse and oestrogen therapy, may lead to gross elevation of triglycerides, hyperchylomicronaemia and pancreatitis in patients with familial hypertriglyceridaemia (Fredrickson et al 1978). Acquired severe hypertriglyceridaemia will sometimes represent an exacerbation on the basis of a mild pre-existing familial hypertriglyceridaemia. However it will be impossible to differentiate in most individual cases since at present there exists no specific biochemical marker for familial hypertriglyceridaemia. The most severe clinical consequence of the familial hyperlipidaemia is atherosclerosis, leading to cerebral vascular disease and coronary heart disease. The role of triglyceride as an independent risk factor for atherosclerosis is still disputed. However, the fact that 5% of unselected survivors of myocardial infarction under the age of 60 years have familial hypertriglyceridaemia demonstrates that at least this form of hypertriglyceridaemia may be associated with a high risk for premature coronary artery disease (Brunzell et al 1976), although this view is not generally shared.

Family data on the inheritance of familial hypertriglyceridaemia have been considered compatible with an autosomal dominant mode of transmission (Goldstein et al 1973). About 40% of first-degree and 25% of second-degree adult blood relatives of probands also have hypertriglyceridaemia. However, subsequent studies suggested a multifactorial aetiology of familial hypertriglyceridaemia (Williams & Lalouel 1982). The frequency of the disorder has been estimated in the order of 2–3/1000 (Goldstein et al 1973). According to another study this figure underestimates the frequency of familial hypertriglyceridaemia (Motulsky & Bowman 1975). The primary biochemical defects in familial hypertriglyceridaemia are unknown. Overproduction of endogenous triglycerides as well as delayed catabolism of VLDL have both been observed. Mean LPL levels are lower than in controls but there is no deficiency of LPL (Krauss et al 1974). Most probably familial hypertriglyceridaemia represents a heterogenous group of biochemically distinct disorders that all have in common an elevation of VLDL. The discovery of a genetic variant of apo A-I that is associated with mild hypertriglyceridaemia and low HDL-cholesterol concentration (Franceschini et al 1980) may represent an example for such a specific biochemical entity.

Since most patients with familial hypertriglyceridaemia are obese, weight reduction is feasible for most of them and the first prescription should be dietary. This alone may result in a fall of triglyceride levels. The restriction of simple carbohydrates has been recommended and ethanol intake should be avoided. Failure of dietary intervention to lower plasma triglycerides is an indication for drug therapy. Clofibrate, fibrate derivatives and nicotinic acid are most effective (Carlson & Olsson 1979). In patients with a type V pattern, where chylomicrons are also elevated, fat restriction is the most important therapeutic intervention. Norethindrone acetate and nicotinic acid have been reported to be effective in otherwise untreated patients with a type V.

Isolated hypertriglyceridaemia is also seen in one third of patients with monogenic familial combined hyperlipidaemia (Goldstein et al 1973). At present there exist no specific criteria to recognize familial hypertriglyceridaemia in a single patient. Hence differentiation of the familial hypertriglyceridaemia from other genetic or non-genetic forms of hypertriglyceridaemia is not possible except by extended family studies. If a patient presents with a combination of hypertriglyceridaemia and premature vascular disease, a family study is indicated to identify family members who may be at risk.

Familial hyper*alphalipoproteinaemia and familial* hypo*alphalipoproteinaemia*

Genetic factors explain a large fraction of the variability in HDL-cholesterol levels in the population. The extremes of the spectrum are called hyper- and hypoalphalipoproteinaemia respectively. The familial aggregation of hyperalphalipoproteinaemia was first observed by Glueck et al (1975). These authors arbitrarily defined a concentration of cholesterol in HDL exceeding 70 mg/100 ml as hyperalphalipoproteinaemia and noticed that among blood relatives of probands about 50% had elevated HDL-cholesterol levels. Familial hyperalphalipoproteinaemia is not a disorder, but rather the opposite. In families affected with hyperalphalipoproteinaemia Glueck and colleagues observed a significantly lower degree of coronary atherosclerosis and the mean age at death of individuals with the trait was higher when compared with the population mean. From these data it was concluded that hyperalphalipoproteinaemia is a longevity syndrome (Glueck et al 1976). From the segregation of the trait in families an autosomal dominant mode of inheritance could be anticipated. However this assumption is not consistent with the correlation of HDL-cholesterol levels between family members (Glueck et al 1976). At present the genetics of familial hyperalphalipoproteinaemia is unclear but the trait is most probably under polygenic control. Moreover, there seem to exist different forms of hyperalphalipoproteinaemia. Whereas hyperalphalipoproteinaemia has occurred as a familial trait with evidence for a major gene effect in Caucasians, most cases among American Blacks have been sporadic (Siervogel et al 1980). A Japanese family with hyperalphalipoproteinaemia, a deficiency of cholesterylester transfer protein activity and evidence for autosomal recessive inheritance has been described (Koizumi et al 1985). Marked hyperalphalipoproteinaemia associated with premature corneal clouding was observed in an orphan Japanese patient (Matsuzawa et al 1984).

Primary hypoalphalipoproteinaemia has been defined as a condition where HDL-cholesterol levels are below the 10th percentile of the relevant age-, sex- and race-specific distribution and where no primary disease causing low HDL exists. The condition is clearly associated with end-points of atherosclerosis e.g. myocardial infarction. Hypoalphalipoproteinaemia has been described as a familial trait.

In pedigrees ascertained through probands with low HDL-cholesterol, dominant inheritance was suggested by segregation ratios of dichotomized levels (Third et al 1984), but complex segregation analysis supported recessive inheritance (Byard et al 1984). A major gene for primary hypoalphalipoproteinaemia has been suggested by Borecki et al (1986), and a dominant major locus resulting in low HDL-cholesterol was revealed in two out of 55 Utah pedigrees selected through probands with early coronary heart disease, stroke, or hypertension (Hasstedt et al 1986). Ordovas et al (1986) have claimed that a polymorphic Pst I site in the apo A-I gene region is associated with familial hypoalphalipoproteinaemia. If confirmed, this finding indicates that the apo A-I gene or a gene close by is the major gene for familial hypoalphalipoproteinaemia.

A unique monogenic form of hypoalphalipoproteinaemia is present in heterozygous carriers of the apo A-I (arg173 → cys) mutant (apo A-I Milano, Franceschini et al 1980).

REFERENCES

Aalto-Setälä K, Gylling H, Miettinen T, Kontula K 1988 Identification of a deletion in the LDL receptor gene. FEBS Letters 230: 31–34

Albers J J, Wahl P, Hazzard W R 1974 Quantitative genetic studies of the human plasma Lp(a) lipoprotein. Biochemical Genetics 11: 475–486

Armstrong V W, Cremer P, Eberle E, Manke A, Schulze F, Wieland H, Kreuzer H, Seidel D 1986 The association between serum Lp(a) concentrations and angiographically assessed coronary atherosclerosis. Atherosclerosis 62: 249–257

Babirak S P, Iverius P-H, Fujimoto W Y, Brunzell J D 1989 Detection and characterization of the heterozygote state for lipoprotein lipase deficiency. Arteriosclerosis 9: 326–334

Basu S K, Goldstein J L, Brown M S 1983 Independent pathways for secretion of cholesterol and apolipoprotein E by macrophages. Science 219: 871–873

Beaty T H, Kwiterovich M Jr, Khoury J, White S, Bachorik P S, Smith H H, Teng B, Sniderman A 1986 Genetic analysis of plasma sitosterol, apoprotein B and lipoproteins in a large Amish pedigree with sitosterolemia. American Journal of Human Genetics 38: 492–504

Berg K 1963 A new serum type system in man: The Lp system. Acta Pathologica and Micobiologica Scandinavia 59: 369–382

Berg K 1983 Genetics of coronary heart disease. In: Steinberg A G, Bearn A G, Motulsky A R, Childs B (eds) Progress in Medical Genetics, Saunders, Philadelphia p 35–90

Bilheimer D W, Goldstein J L, Grundy S M, Brown M S 1975 Reduction in cholesterol and low density lipoprotein synthesis after portocaval shunt surgery in a patient with homozygous familial hypercholesterolaemia. Journal of Clinical Investigation 56: 1420–1430

Bilheimer D W, Ho Y K, Brown M S, Anderson R G W,

Goldstein J L 1978 Genetics of the low density lipoprotein receptor. Journal of Clinical Investigation 61: 678–696

Bilheimer D W, Stone N J, Grundy S M 1979 Metabolic studies in familial hypercholesterolaemia. Evidence for a gene-dosage effect in vivo. Journal of Clinical Investigation 64: 524–533

Bilheimer D W, Goldstein J L, Grundy S M, Starzl T E, Brown M S 1984 Liver transplantation to provide low-density-lipoprotein receptors and lower plasma cholesterol in a child with homozygous familial hypercholesterolaemia. New England Journal of Medicine 311: 1658–1664

Blankenhorn D H, Mayers H J 1969 Radiographic determination of Achilles tendon xanthoma size. Metabolism 18: 882–886

Boerwinkle E, Utermann G 1988 Simultaneous effects of the apolipoprotein E polymorphism on apolipoprotein E, apolipoprotein B, and cholesterol metabolism. American Journal of Human Genetics 42: 104–112

Boerwinkle E, Chakraborty R, Sing C F 1986 The use of measured genotype information in the analysis of quantitative phenotypes in man. I. Models and analytical methods. Annals of Human Genetics 50: 181–194

Boerwinkle E, Menzel H J, Kraft H G, Utermann G 1989 Genetics of the quantitative Lp(a) lipoprotein trait III. Contribution of Lp(a) glycoprotein phenotypes to normal lipid variation. Human Genetics 82: 73–78

Borecki I B, Rao D C, Third J L H, Laskarzewski P M, Glueck C J 1986 A major gene for primary hypoalphalipoproteinaemia. American Journal of Human Genetics 38: 373–381

Borrie P 1969 Type III hyperlipoproteinaemia. British Medical Journal 2: 665–667

Breslow J L 1985 Human apolipoprotein molecular biology and genetic variation. Annual Review of Biochemistry 54: 699–727

Brown M S, Goldstein J L 1983a Lipoprotein metabolism in the macrophage: Implications for cholesterol deposition in atherosclerosis. Annual Review of Biochemistry 52: 223–261

Brown M S, Goldstein J L 1983b Lipoprotein receptors in the liver. Journal of Clinical Investigation 72: 743–747

Brown M S, Goldstein J L 1986 A receptor-mediated pathway for cholesterol homeostasis. Science 232: 34–47

Brown M S, Goldstein J L 1987 Plasma lipoproteins: Teaching old dogmas new tricks. Nature 330: 113–114

Brown M S, Goldstein J L, Vandenberghe K, Fryns J P, Kovanen P T, Eckels R E, van den Berghe H, Cassiman J J 1978 Prenatal diagnosis of homozygous familial hypercholesterolaemia: Expression of a genetic receptor disease in utero. Lancet I: 526–529

Brown M S, Goldstein J L, Fredrickson D S 1983 Familial type 3 hyperlipoproteinaemia (Dysbetalipoproteinaemia). In: Stanbury J B, Wyngaarden J B, Fredrickson D S, Goldstein J L, Brown M S (eds) The Metabolic Basis of Inherited Disease, 5th edn. McGraw Hill, New York, p 655–671

Brunzell J D, Schott H G 1973 The interaction of familial and secondary causes of hypertriglyceridemia: Role in pancreatitis. Transactions of the Association of American Physicians 86: 245–253

Brunzell J D, Schott H G, Motulsky A G, Bierman E L 1976 Myocardial infarction in the familial forms of hypertriglyceridemia. Metabolism 25: 313–320

Byard P J, Borecki I B, Glueck C J, Laskarzewski P M, Third J L H C, Rao D C 1984 A genetic study of hypoalphaproteinemia. Genetic Epidemiology 1: 43–51

Carlson L A, Olsson A G 1979 Effect of hypolipidemic drugs on serum lipoproteins. In: Eisenberg S, Karger S (eds) Progress in Biochemical Pharmacology Vol 15, Lipoprotein Metabolism. AG, Basel, p 238–257

Cumming A M, Robertson F W 1984 Polymorphism at the apoprotein-E locus in relation to risk of coronary disease. Clinical Genetics 25: 310–313

Dahlen G H 1988 Lipoprotein(a) in relation to atherosclerotic diseases. In: Recent Aspects of Diagnosis and Treatment of Lipoprotein Disorders: Impact on Prevention of Atherosclerotic Diseases. Liss, New York p 27–36

Davignon J, Gregg R E, Sing C F 1988 Apolipoprotein E polymorphism and atherosclerosis. Arteriosclerosis 8, (1): 1–21

Dawber T R 1980 The Framingham Study. Cambridge, Harvard University Press

De Lange C D 1933 Significance of geographic pathology in race problems in medicine. Geneeskundig tijdschrift voor Nederlandsch-Indie 73: 1026

Dolphin P J 1985 Lipoprotein metabolism and the role of apolipoproteins as metabolic programmers. Canadian Journal of Biochemistry and Cell Biology 63 (8): 850–869

Eisenberg S, Chajek T, Deckelbaum R 1978 Molecular aspects of lipoproteins interconversion. Pharmacological Research Communications 10: 729–738

Ferrans V J, Fredrickson D S 1975 The pathology of Tangier disease. A light and electron microscopic study. American Journal of Pathology 78: 101–158

Franceschini G, Sirtori C R, Capurso A, Weisgraber K H, Mahley R W 1980 A-I-Milano Apoprotein. Journal of Clinical Investigation 66: 892–900

Francke U, Brown M S, Goldstein J L 1984 Assignment of the human gene for the low density lipoprotein receptor to chromosome 19: synteny of a receptor, a ligand, and a genetic disease. Proceedings of the National Academy of Sciences USA 81: 2826–2830

Fredrickson D S, Levy R J, Lees R S 1967 Fat transport in

lipoproteins: an integrated approach to mechanism and disorders. New England Journal of Medicine 276: 34–44, 94–103, 148–156, 215–225, 273–281

Fredrickson D S, Levy R J, Lees R S 1968 A comparison of heritable abnormal lipoprotein patterns as defined by two different techniques. Journal of Clinical Investigation 47: 2446–2457

Fredrickson D S, Goldstein J L, Brown M S 1978 The familial hyperlipoproteinaemias. In: Stanbury J B, Wyngaarden J B, Fredrickson D S (eds) Metabolic Basis of Inherited Disease, 4th edn. McGraw Hill, New York, p 604–655

Gevers W, Casciola L A F, Fourie A M, Sanan D A, Coetzee G A, van der Westhuyzen D R 1987 Familial hypercholesterolaemia in South Africa. Biological Chemistry, Hoppe-Seyler, 368, p 1233–1243

Gjone E, Norum K R, Glomset J A 1978 Familial lecithin-cholesterol acyltransferase deficiency. In: Stanbury J B, Wyngaarden J B, Fredrickson D S (eds) The Metabolic Basis of Inherited Disease, 4th edn. McGraw Hill, New York, p 589–603

Glomset J A 1968 The plasma lecithin-cholesterol acyltransferase reaction. Journal of Lipid Research 9: 155–167

Glomset J A, Norum K R 1973 The metabolic role of lecithin-cholesterol acyltransferase: Perspectives from pathology. Advances in Lipid Research 11:1

Glueck C J, Fallat R, Buncher C R, Tsang R, Steiner P 1973 Familial combined hyperlipoproteinaemia. Studies in 91 adults and 95 children from 33 kindreds. Metabolism 22: 1403–1428

Glueck C J, Fallat R W, Millet F, Gartside P, Elston R C, Go R C P 1975 Familial hyperalphalipoproteinemia: Studies in eighteen kindreds. Metabolism 52: 1544–1568

Glueck C J, Gartside P, Fallat R W, Sielski J, Steiner P M 1976 Longevity syndromes: familial hypobeta and familial hyperalphalipoproteinemia. Journal of Laboratory and Clinical Medicine 88: 941–957

Glueck C J, Laskarzewski P, Rao D C, Morrison J A 1985 Familial aggregations of coronary risk factors. In: Connor W, Bristow D (eds) Complications of Coronary Artery Disease. Lippincott, Philadelphia p 173–193

Goldbourt U, Neufeld H M 1986 Genetic aspects of arteriosclerosis. Arteriosclerosis 6: 357–377

Goldstein J L, Brown M S 1974 Binding and degradation of low density lipoproteins by cultured human fibroblasts. Journal of Biological Chemistry 249: 5153–5162

Goldstein J L, Brown M S 1983 Familial hypercholesterolemia. In: Stanbury J B, Wyngaarden J B, Fredrickson D S, Goldstein J L, Brown M S (eds) Metabolic Basis of Inherited Disease, 5th edn. McGraw Hill, New York, p 672–712

Goldstein J L, Schrott H G, Hazzard W R, Bierman E L, Motulsky A G 1973 Hyperlipidemia in coronary heart disease. III. Genetic analysis of lipid levels in 176 families and delineation of a new inherited disorder, combined hyperlipidemia. Journal of Clinical Investigation 52: 1544–1568

Green P H R, Tall A R, Glickman R M 1978 Rat intestine secretes discoid high density lipoprotein. Journal of Clinical Investigation 61: 528–534

Grundy S M, Chait A, Brunzell J D 1987 Familial combined hyperlipidemia workshop. Arteriosclerosis 7: 203–207

Gustafson A, McConathy W J, Alaupovic P, Curry M D, Persson B 1979 Identification of lipoprotein families in a variant of human plasma apolipoprotein A deficiency. Scandinavian Journal of Clinical Laboratory Investigation 39: 377–387

Hamsten A, de Faire U, Iselius L, Blombäck M 1987 Genetic and cultural inheritance of plasma fibrinogen concentration. Lancet 2: 988–990

Harlan W R, Graham J B, Estes H 1966 Familial hypercholesterolemia: a genetic and metabolic study. Medicine 45: 77–110

Hasstedt S J, Williams R R 1986 Three alleles for quantitative Lp(a). Genetic Epidemiology 3: 53–55

Hasstedt S J, Ash O K, Williams R R 1986 A re-examination of major locus hypotheses for high density lipoprotein cholesterol level using 2,170 persons screened in 55 Utah pedigrees. American Journal of Medical Genetics 24: 57–67

Havekes L, de Wit E, Gevers Leuven J, Klasen E, Utermann G, Weber W, Beisiegel U 1986 Apolipoprotein E3-Leiden. A new variant of human apolipoprotein E associated with familial type III hyperlipoproteinemia. Human Genetics 73: 157–163

Havel R J 1985 Role of the liver in atherosclerosis. Arteriosclerosis 5: 569–580

Havel R J, Kane J P 1973 Primary dysbetalipoproteinemia: predominance of a specific apoprotein species in triglyceride-rich lipoproteins. Proceedings of the National Academy of Sciences, U.S.A. 70: 2015–2019

Heiberg A 1976 Inheritance of xanthomatosis and hyper-β-lipoproteinemia: A study of 7 large kindreds. Clinical Genetics 9: 92–111

Hewitt D, Jones G J L, Godin G J, Wraight D, Breckenridge W C, Little J A, Steiner G, Mishkel M A 1979 Nature of the familial influence on plasma lipid levels. Atherosclerosis 32: 381–396

Hobbs H H, Brown M S, Russell D W, Davignon J, Goldstein J L 1987 Deletion in the gene for the low-density-lipoprotein receptor in a majority of French Canadians with familial hypercholesterolemia. New England Journal of Medicine 317 (12): 734–737

Humphries S E, Kessling A M, Horstehmke B et al 1985 A common DNA polymorphism of the low density lipoprotein (LDL) receptor gene and its use in diagnosis. Lancet 1: 1003–1005

Innerarity T L, Weisgraber K H, Arnold K S, Mahley R W, Krauss R M, Vega G L, Grundy S M 1987 Familial defective apolipoprotein B-100: Low density lipoproteins with abnormal receptor binding. Proceedings of the National Academy of Sciences, U.S.A. 84: 6919–6923

Karathanasis S K, McPherson J, Zannis V I, Breslow J L 1983 An inherited polymorphism in the human apolipoprotein A-I gene locus related to the development of atherosclerosis. Nature 301: 718–720

Keys A 1975 Coronary heart disease. The global picture. Atherosclerosis 22: 149–192

Keys A 1980 Seven Countries: A multivariate analysis of death and coronary heart disease. Harvard University Press, Cambridge, p 1–381

Koizumi J, Mabuchi H, Yoshimura A et al 1985 Deficiency of serum cholesteryl-ester transfer activity in patients with familial hyperalphalipoproteinemia. Atherosclerosis 58: 75–186

Krauss R M, Levy R I, Fredrickson D S 1974 Selective measurement of two lipase activities in postheparin plasma from normal subjects and patients with hyperlipoproteinemia. Journal of Clinical Investigation 54: 1107–1124

Kwiterovich P O, Fredrickson D S, Levy R J 1974 Familial hypercholesterolemia (one form of familial type III hyperlipoproteinemia). A study of its biochemical, genetic and clinical presentation in childhood. Journal of Clinical Investigation 53: 1237–1249

Lehrman M A, Schneider W J, Brown M S, Davis C G, Elhammer A, Russell D W, Goldstein J L 1987 The Lebanese allele at the low density lipoprotein receptor locus. Journal of Biological Chemistry 262/1: 401–410

Lenzen H J, Assmann G, Buchwalsky R, Schulte H 1986 Association of apolipoprotein E polymorphism, low-density lipoprotein cholesterol, and coronary artery disease. Clinical Chemistry 32/5: 778–781

Levy R I, Fredrickson D S, Stone N J et al 1973 Cholestyramine in type II hyperlipoproteinemia. A double-blind trial of cholestrylamine in type II hyperlipoproteinemia. Annals of Internal Medicine 79: 51

Li W H, Tanimura M, Luo C C, Datta S, Chan L 1988 The apolipoprotein multigene family: biosynthesis, structure, structure-function relationships, and evolution. Journal of Lipid Research 29: 245–271

Lippel K, Tyroler H, Eder H, Gotto A Jr., Vahouny G 1981 Relationship of hypertriglyceridemia to atherosclerosis. Arteriosclerosis 1/6: 406–417

Lupien P J, Moorjami S, Awad J 1976 A new approach to the management of familial hypercholesterolemia: removal of plasma-cholesterol based on the principle of affinity chromatography. Lancet I: 1261–1265

Lusis J A 1988 Genetic factors affecting blood lipoproteins: the candidate gene approach. Journal of Lipid Research 29: 397–429

Mabuchi H, Ito S, Haba T et al 1977 Discrimination of familial hypercholesterolemia and secondary hypercholesterolemia by Achilles tendon thickness. Atherosclerosis 28: 61–68

Mabuchi H, Tatami R, Haba T et al 1978 Homozygous familial hypercholesterolemia in Japan. American Journal of Medicine 65: 290–297

McGill Jr H 1984 Persistent problems in the pathogenesis of atherosclerosis. Arteriosclerosis 4: 443–451

Mahley R W, Innerarity T L, Brown M S, Ho Y K, Goldstein J L 1980 Cholesterylester synthesis in macrophages: Stimulation by β-very low density lipoproteins from cholesterol-fed animals of several species. Journal of Lipid Research 21: 970–980

Mahley R W, Innerarity T L, Weisgraber K H et al 1986 Cellular and molecular biology of lipoprotein in metabolism: Characterization of lipoprotein receptor-ligand interactions. Cold Spring Harbor Symposia on Quantitative Biology, Volume LI: 821–828

Makrides S, Ruiz-Opazo N, Hayden M, Nussbaum A L, Breslow J L, Zannis V I 1988 Sequence and expression of Tangier apo A-I gene. European Journal of Biochemistry 173: 465–471

Mann W A, Gregg R E, Sprecher D L, Brewer H B Jr. 1989 Apolipoprotein E-1$_{Harrisburg}$: a new variant of apolipoprotein E dominantly associated with type III hyperlipoproteinemia. Biochimica et Biophysica Acta 1005: 239–244

Matsuzawa Y, Yamashita S, Kameda K, Kubo M, Tarui S, Hara I 1984 Marked hyper-HDL-cholesterolemia associated with premature corneal opacity. Atherosclerosis 53: 207–212

Menzel H J, Utermann G 1986 Apolipoprotein E phenotyping from serum by Western blotting. Electrophoresis 7: 492–495

Miller J Z, Grim C E 1983 Heritability of blood pressure. In:

Kotchen T A, Kotchen J M (eds) Clinical approaches to high blood pressure in the young. John Wright, PSG Inc, Littleton, p 79–80

Miller N E 1978 The evidence for the antiatherogeneity of high density lipoprotein in man. Lipids 13: 914–919

Mishkel M A, Nazir D I, Crowther S 1975 A longitudinal assessment of lipid ratios in the diagnosis of type III hyperlipoproteinemia. Clinica Chimica Acta 53: 121–136

Morganroth J R, Levy R I, Fredrickson D S 1975 The biochemical, clinical and genetic features of type III hyperlipoproteinemia. Annals of Internal Medicine 82: 158–174

Moser H, Slack J, Borrie P 1974 Type III hyperlipoproteinemia: A genetic study with an account of the risk of coronary death in first degree relatives. In: Schettler G, Weizel A (eds) Atherosclerosis III. Springer, Berlin, p 854

Motulsky A P, Bowman H 1975 Screening for the hyperlipidemias. In: Milunsky A (ed) The prevention of genetic disease and mental retardation. Saunders, Philadelphia, p 303–316

Müller C 1939 Angina pectoris in hereditary xanthomatosis. Archives of Internal Medicine 69: 675–700

Namboodiri K K, Kaplan E B, Heuch I et al 1985 The collaborative lipid research clinics family study. Biological and cultural determinants of familial resemblance for plasma lipids and lipoproteins. Genetic Epidemiology 2: 227–254

Nichols W C, Dwulet F E, Liepnieks J, Benson M D 1988 Variant apolipoprotein AI as a major constituent of a human hereditary amyloid. Biochemical and Biophysical Research Communications 156: 762–768

Nikkilä E A, Aro A 1973 Family study of serum lipids and lipoproteins in coronary heart disease. Lancet 1: 954–959

Nora J J, Lortscher R H, Spangler R D, Nora A H, Kimberling W J 1980 Genetic-epidemiologic study of early-onset ischemic heart disease. Circulation 61: 503–508

Norum R A, Lakier J B, Goldstein et al 1982 Familial deficiency of apolipoproteins A-I and C-III and precocious coronary-artery disease. New England Journal of Medicine 306: 1513–1519

Ordovas J M, Schaefer E J, Salem D et al 1986 Apolipoprotein A-I gene polymorphism associated with premature coronary artery disease and familial hypoalphalipoproteinemia. New England Journal of Medicine 314: 671–677

Osler W 1897 Lectures on Angina pectoris and allied states. Appleton-Century Crofts, New York

Ott J 1979 Detection of rare major genes in lipid levels. Human Genetics 51: 79–91

Patterson D, Slack J 1972 Lipid abnormalities in male and female survivors of myocardial infarction. Lancet 1: 393

Rall S C Jr., Newhouse Y M, Clarke H R G et al 1989 Type III hyperlipoproteinemia associated with apolipoprotein phenotype E-3/3: structure and genetics of a rare apolipoprotein E3 variant. Journal of Clinical Investigation 83: 1095–1101

Robertson F W, Cumming A M 1979 Genetic and environmental variation in serum lipoproteins in relation to coronary heart disease. Journal of Medical Genetics 16: 85–100

Rose H G, Krantz P, Weinstock M, Juliano J, Haft J I 1973 Inheritance of combined hyperlipoproteinemia: Evidence for a new lipoprotein phenotype. American Journal of Medicine 54: 148

Ross R 1986 The pathogenesis of atherosclerosis — an update. New England Journal of Medicine 314/8: 488–500

Russell D W, Lehrman M A, Südhof T C, Yamamoto T, Davis C G, Hobbs H H, Brown M S, Goldstein J L 1986 The LDL receptor in familial hypercholesterolemia: Use of human mutations to dissect a membrane protein. Cold Spring Harbour Symposia on Quantitative Biology, Volume LI, p 811–819

Schaefer E J 1984 Clinical, biochemical and genetic features of familial disorders of high density lipoproteins. Arteriosclerosis 4: 303–322

Schaefer E J, Levy R I 1985 Pathogenesis and management of lipoprotein disorders. New England Journal of Medicine 312/20: 1300–1310

Schaefer E J, Ordovas J M, Law S W et al 1985 Familial apolipoprotein A-I and C-III deficiency, variant II. Journal of Lipid Research 26: 1089–1101

Schaefer E J, Gregg R E, Ghiselli G, Forte T M, Ordovas J M, Zech L A, Brewer Jr H B 1986 Familial apolipoprotein E deficiency. Journal of Clinical Investigation 78: 1206–1219

Schmitz G, Assmann G, Robenek H, Brennhausen B 1985 Tangier disease: A disorder of intracellular membrane traffic. Proceedings of the National Academy of Sciences, U.S.A. 82: 6305–6309

Schneider W J, Kovanen P T, Brown M S et al 1981 Familial dysbetalipoproteinemia. Journal of Clinical Investigation 68: 1075–1085

Siervogel R M, Morrison J A, Kelly K, Mellies M, Gartside P, Glueck C J 1980 Familial hyper-alpha-lipoproteinemia in 26 kindreds. Clinical Genetics 17: 13–25

Sing C F, Orr J D 1978 Analysis of genetic and environmental sources of variation in serum cholesterol in Tecumseh, Michigan. IV. Separation of polygene from common environment effects. American Journal of Human Genetics 30: 491–504

Sing C F, Schultz J S, Shreffler D C 1974 The genetics of the Lp antigen. II. A family study and proposed models of genetic control. Annals of Human Genetics 38: 47–56

Slack J 1969 Risks of ischaemic heart disease in familial hyperlipoproteinemic states. Lancet II: 1380–1383

Slack J 1975 The genetic contribution to coronary heart disease through lipoprotein concentrations. Postgraduate Medical Journal 51/8: 27–32

Slack J, Evans K A 1966 The increased risk of death from ischaemic heart disease in first degree relatives of 121 men and 96 women with ischaemic heart disease. Journal of Medical Genetics 3: 239

Smith E 1975 Development of the atheromatous lesion. In: Wolf S, Wethessen N T (eds) The smooth muscle of the artery. Advances in Experimental Biology and Medicine 57. Plenum Press, New York, p 254

Smith E B, Slater R S 1972 Relationship between low density lipoprotein in aortic intima and serum lipid levels. Lancet 1: 463–469

Smith E B, Smith R H 1976 Early changes in aortic intima. In: Paoletti R, Gotto A M Jr (eds) Atherosclerosis Reviews, Vol 1. Raven Press, New York, p 119–136

Starzl T E, Chase H P, Ahrens E H Jr et al 1983 Portacaval shunt in patients with familial hypercholesterolemia. Annals of Surgery 198: 273–283

Steinberg D 1987 Lipoproteins and the pathogenesis of atherosclerosis. Circulation 76/3: 508–514

Stoffel W, Demant T 1981 Selective removal of apolipoprotein B containing serum lipoproteins from blood plasma. Proceedings of the National Academy of Sciences, U.S.A. 78: 611–615

Stone N J, Levy R I, Fredrickson D S, Verter J 1974 Coronary artery disease in 116 kindreds with familial type II hyperlipoproteinemia. Circulation 49: 476–488

Third J L H C, Montag J, Flynn M, Freidel J, Laskarzewski P, Glueck C J 1984 Primary and familial hypoalphalipoproteinemia. Metabolism 33: 136–146

Thompson G R, Myant N B, Kilpatrick D, Oakley C M, Raphael M J, Steiner R E 1980 Assessment of long-term plasma exchange for familial hypercholesterolemia. British Heart Journal 43: 680–688

Utermann G 1985 Genetic polymorphism of apolipoprotein E — Impact on plasma lipoprotein metabolism. In: Crepaldi G, Tiengo A, Baggio G (eds) Excerpta Medica: Diabetes, obesity and hyperlipidemias — III. International Congress Series, Amsterdam p 1–28

Utermann G 1987 Apolipoprotein E polymorphism in health and disease. American Heart Journal 113: 433–440

Utermann G 1988 Apolipoprotein polymorphism and multifactorial hyperlipidemia. Journal of Inherited Metabolic Disease 11: Suppl. 1: 74–86

Utermann G 1989 The mysteries of lipoprotein(a). Science 246: 904–910

Utermann G, Hees M, Steinmetz A 1977 Polymorphism of apolipoprotein E and occurrence of dysbetalipoproteinemia in man. Nature 269: 604–607

Utermann G, Pruin N, Steinmetz A 1979 Polymorphism of apolipoprotein E. III. Effect of a single polymorphic gene locus on plasma lipid levels in man. Clinical Genetics 15: 63–72

Utermann G, Menzel H J, Adler G, Dieker P, Weber W 1980 Substitution in vitro of lecithin-cholesterol-acyltransferase. Analysis of changes in plasma lipoproteins. European Journal of Biochemistry 107: 225–241

Utermann G, Menzel H J, Kraft H G, Duba H C, Kemmler H G, Seitz C 1987 Lp(a) Glycoprotein phenotypes. Journal of Clinical Investigation 80: 458–465

Utermann G, Hoppichler F, Dieplinger H, Seed M, Thompson G, Boerwinkle E 1989 Defects in the low density lipoprotein receptor gene affect lipoprotein (a) levels: Multiplicative interaction of two gene loci associated with premature atherosclerosis. Proceedings of the National Academy of Sciences, USA 86: 4171–4174

Virchow R 1856 Phlogose und Thrombose im Gefaβsystem. Gesammelte Abhandlungen zur wissenschaftlichen Medizin. Meidinger Sohn, Frankfurt am Main, p 458

Wardell M R, Brennan S O, Janus E D, Fraser R, Carrell R W 1987 Apolipoprotein E2-Christchurch (136 Arg — Ser). Journal of Clinical Investigation 80: 483–490

Weintraub M S, Eisenberg S, Breslow J L 1987 Dietary fat clearance in normal subjects is regulated by genetic variation in apolipoprotein E. Journal of Clinical Investigation 80: 1571–1577

Williams W R, Lalouel J M 1982 Complex segregation analysis of hyperlipidemia in a Seattle sample. Human Heredity 32: 24–36

Yamamura T, Yamamoto A, Sumiyoshi T, Hiramori K, Nishioeda Y, Nambu S 1984 New mutants of apolipoprotein E associated with atherosclerotic diseases but not to type III hyperlipoproteinemia. Journal of Clinical Investigation 74: 1229–1237

Zelis R, Mason D R, Braunwald E, Levy R I 1970 Effects of hyperlipoproteinaemias and their treatment on the peripheral circulation. Journal of Clinical Investigation 49: 1007

Zilversmit D B 1979 Atherogenesis: A postprandial phenomenon. Circulation 60: 473–485

74. The cardiomyopathies

R. Emanuel   R. Withers

INTRODUCTION

The genetically determined condition now generally known as hypertrophic cardiomyopathy first made its appearance on the clinical scene in 1947 when described by William Evans as Familial Cardiomegaly (Evans 1949). Little was then heard of this entity until Teare's description in 1958 of Asymmetrical Hypertrophy of the Heart in Young Adults (Teare 1958). Recognition did not become widespread until the early 1960s, a time when the study of haemodynamics was of primary interest in cardiology; hence the abnormal ventricular function and the mechanism of left ventricular outflow obstruction seen in a percentage of cases became a matter of controversy and received more attention than the fundamental problems of inheritance and pathogenesis (Criley et al 1965, Ross et al 1966, White et al 1967).

An early difficulty encountered with the cardiomyopathies was one of classification which, if based on aetiology as all sound classifications must be, became impossibly cumbersome and of little value (Hudson 1970, Emanuel 1970) for the vast majority of cases had to be labelled 'idiopathic'.

Goodwin and his co-workers were much aware of this problem and evolved both a definition and classification which with slight modification was accepted by the World Health Organization and International Society and Federation of Cardiology Task Force. They also suggested the term 'congestive' cardiomyopathy should be replaced by 'dilated' cardiomyopathy (Report of WHO/ISFC 1980). Thus, by definition, such conditions as acromegalic heart disease, thyrotoxic heart disease and the end stages of coronary artery disease associated with considerable cardiomegaly and failure are excluded. Goodwin originally divided the cardiomyopathies into two main types dependent on the pathophysiology of the left ventricle. In the first type, hypertrophic cardiomyopathy (with or without obstruction to left ventricular outflow), the main features were massive hypertrophy of the left ventricle, particularly the interventricular sep-

tum, associated with a small left ventricular cavity. The primary haemodynamic fault was in ventricular filling due to decreased compliance of the thickened, abnormal ventricular muscle. In the second type, dilated cardiomyopathy, there was a degree of left ventricular hypertrophy although the salient features were gross dilatation of the left ventricular cavity and normal coronary arteries. In this group the main haemodynamic fault was 'pump failure' with reduction in the ejection fraction. The classification recognized two other subgroups, both rare, and designated them 'constrictive' and 'restrictive' (Goodwin 1970).

By definition, the aetiology of the cardiomyopathies is unknown, but in hypertrophic cardiomyopathy genetic factors are recognised to be important. Familial cases are common (Braunwald et al 1964, Cohen et al 1964, Emanuel et al 1971) and autosomal dominant inheritance has been reported by many authors (Brigden 1957, Hollman et al 1960, Walther et al 1960, Paré et al 1961, Treger & Blount 1965, Emanuel 1971, Emanuel et al 1971). In dilated cardiomyopathy some evidence is forthcoming of a familial nature in about 2% of cases. Several authors (Michels et al 1985, Goldblatt et al 1987) have given evidence for familial aggregation, and the consanguinity reported in a large Portuguese pedigree suggests an autosomal recessive mode of inheritance. There is little evidence for a familial tendency in restrictive cardiomyopathy. Heart muscle disease may be associated with other conditions which have a genetic component. These have been reviewed briefly (Emanuel & Withers 1986). Further comments on the cardiomyopathies will be confined to hypertrophic cardiomyopathy which may occur with or without obstruction to left ventricular outflow.

CLINICAL FEATURES

Clinically, the disease is often asymptomatic and diagnosed at routine examination, which may have been prompted because some other member of the family had been found to be affected, or died unexpectedly. When symptoms are present they include angina and dyspnoea from left ventricular dysfunction, and arrhythmias, the frequency of which has only been appreciated recently with the advent of ambulatory monitoring (Savage et al 1979, McKenna et al 1980). In addition, syncope and sudden death are not uncommon, and evidence is accumulating that these events are generally due to a ventricular tachyarrhythmia, frequently ventricular fibrillation (Goodwin & Krikler 1976). One of the most difficult tasks which confront the physician in this disease is to identify those cases with an increased risk of unexpected death. There is no sure way of doing this, but sinister features include a short history of paroxysmal arrhythmias and an elevated end diastolic pressure in the left ventricle. It also appears that males with a positive family history are at increased risk. The presence of a gradient across the left ventricular outflow does not increase the hazard of sudden demise; in fact, there is some evidence suggesting that cases without obstruction have a worse prognosis (Frank & Braunwald 1968, Goodwin 1970, Maron et al 1978a, 1978c).

The clinical features of the disease include normal development in infancy and childhood and varying degrees of left ventricular hypertrophy, particularly of the interventricular septum. When there is obstruction to left ventricular outflow, there is an ejection murmur simulating that heard in aortic valve stenosis. The hypertrophic process also involves the papillary muscles to a greater or lesser degree, and mitral valve function may be abnormal, giving rise to mitral valve prolapse and regurgitation. Thus, late systolic or pansystolic murmurs at the apex are not uncommon. In some cases, mitral regurgitation is the dominant feature and may be misdiagnosed, particularly in children, as rheumatic mitral regurgitation. Similarly, if obstruction to left ventricular outflow dominates the clinical picture, the diagnosis of aortic valve disease may be entertained. The quality of the arterial pulse, however, is usually sufficient to lead to the correct diagnosis. In hypertrophic cardiomyopathy, obstruction to left ventricular outflow does not occur until mid or late systole, hence the upstroke of the arterial pulse is normal or sharp, whereas in fixed aortic valve stenosis, obstruction to left ventricular outflow is present throughout systole producing the classical slow rising or plateau pulse (Hardarson et al 1973, Goodwin 1974).

Echocardiography

When echocardiographic examination of the interventricular septum became possible (Assad-Morell et al 1974,

Sawaya et al 1974) it was soon evident that this was the single most important investigation in hypertrophic cardiomyopathy. It not only depicted the anatomy of the individual case but also gave considerable insight into the haemodynamics. In addition, it proved invaluable for population screening where asymptomatic septal hypertrophy may be the only abnormality (Maron et al 1984, Greaves et al 1987).

The classical echocardiographic findings in hypertrophic cardiomyopathy include a thickened and relatively immobile interventricular septum with an interventricular septum/posterior left ventricular wall thickness ratio in excess of 1.3, although this figure is by no means precise as the interventricular septum thickens with age (Marcomichelakis et al 1983). In addition, this degree of septal thickening in relation to the posterior left ventricular wall is not specific for hypertrophic cardiomyopathy. It is often seen in infants, occasionally in normal adults, as well as athletes. It also occurs in a number of pathological conditions (Emanuel & Withers 1983). Other classical echocardiographic features include a small left ventricular cavity, a high ejection fraction, systolic anterior movement of the mitral valve and midsystolic closure of the aortic valve.

Electrocardiography

The electrocardiogram may be misleading, for it can be normal in children and young adults with hypertrophic cardiomyopathy. Generally, however, it shows some degree of left ventricular hypertrophy and, not infrequently, left atrial hypertrophy. There may be Q waves with ST and T wave changes in both the anterior and anteroseptal leads, or left bundle branch block (Savage et al 1978). If, therefore, the patient is a middle-aged man with angina and only slight ventricular enlargement, it is all too easy to make the erroneous diagnosis of coronary artery disease, missing the underlying hypertrophic cardiomyopathy which would immediately become evident on the echocardiogram.

Chest X-ray

The chest X-ray is not particularly helpful. It is often normal or shows only a minor increase in heart size. Occasionally in the posteroanterior view an additional convexity may be seen on the left cardiac border, just above the ventricular arc. When present this represents unusual hypertrophy of the interventricular septum (Jefferson & Rees 1980). Late in the disease in a small percentage of cases the left ventricle dilates (see below), then there may be an appreciable increase in the cardiothoracic ratio.

All the above findings are infinitely better defined by echocardiography.

Other investigations

A number of other investigations are commonly used to study special aspects of the disease, the commonest of which is cardiac catheterization and left ventricular angiography (Meerschwam 1969). Myocardial biopsy is favoured at some centres, but has added little to our fundamental understanding of the pathophysiology (Olsen 1983). Computer tomography (Stone et al 1984) and magnetic resonance (Farmer et al 1985) are both attractive in showing the underlying anatomy but add little, if anything, to echocardiographic findings and are certainly more costly. Excluding echocardiography perhaps the most important investigation is ambulatory monitoring in view of the frequency and prognostic importance of ventricular arrhythmias (McKenna et al 1980, 1985).

Pathophysiology

The fundamental cause of myofibril hypertrophy and disarray, which are the hallmarks of hypertrophic cardiomyopathy, is unknown. There may well be complex genetically determined abnormalities involving catecholamines, calcium, thyroid and parathyroid metabolism (Davies 1984, Opie et al 1985, Symons et al 1985).

There has been much controversy about the mechanism of the obstruction to left ventricular outflow seen in some cases of hypertrophic cardiomyopathy. The degree of obstruction may vary from beat to beat and can often be provoked by inotropic agents in cases where there is little or no obstruction in the resting state. It is now generally agreed that a number of factors, which include abnormal ventricular contraction, the distorted ventricular cavity with abnormal alignment and contraction of the papillary muscles, systolic anterior movement of the mitral valve and the hypertrophied interventricular septum, all play a part depending on the degree to which each abnormality is present in any particular case (Falicov & Resnekov 1977, Wigle et al 1985). The most important determinant may yet prove to be the amount and distribution of the abnormal myocardial fibres within the heart (Maron et al 1974, Henry et al 1974).

Myocardial histology

Histological examination of the myocardium shows complete loss of the normal orderly pattern. In hypertrophic cardiomyopathy the muscle bundles are arranged in a totally disordered fashion and are interspersed with tracts of connective tissues. The myocardial fibres themselves are short in length and run in all directions, often forming small whorls. The fibres are considerably larger in diameter than normal, often measuring around $90-100 \mu m$ (normal $5-12 \mu m$). An additional histological feature consists of large, bizarre-shaped nuclei, each surrounded by a clear zone, the so-called 'perinuclear halo', which is rich in glycogen. The adjacent myocardial fibrils often have a motheaten appearence (Fig. 74.1). Although the main concentration of abnormal fibres is usually found in the interventricular septum, they are scattered throughout the myocardium involving the walls of all four cardiac chambers to a greater or lesser degree (Van Noorden et al 1971, Olsen 1973). More recently attention has been drawn to the presence of abnormal intramural coronary arteries in infants and adults with hypertrophic cardiomyopathy which has been found in cases with and without obstruction to left ventricular outflow. The significance of this arterial abnormality and its relation to myofibril hypertrophy and disarray is at present unknown (Maron et al 1986).

Course and prognosis

Complications occurring during the course of the disease include arrhythmias, which may be fatal; also emboli which can arise from either the left or right side of the heart and therefore present as systemic or pulmonary emboli. Infective endocarditis has been documented in a number of cases, but is rare (Vecht & Oakley 1968). An increased frequency of mitral ring calcification has been reported (Kronzon & Glassman 1978), but this observation has not been confirmed by others (Kessler & Rahim 1979). The frequency of mitral ring calcification in relation to age and to the presence or absence of mitral regurgitation has also been studied in hypertrophic cardiomyopathy (Motamed & Roberts 1987). In a minority of cases with long-standing disease, particularly those with midcavity obstruction, there may be some dilatation or regional hypokinesis of the ventricle, but this is never sufficient to obscure the underlying nature of the disease and should not lead to the misdiagnosis of dilated cardiomyopathy (Fighali et al 1987, Spirito et al 1987).

Hypertrophic cardiomyopathy may be associated with congenital heart disease, particularly bicuspid aortic valve and secundum atrial septal defects (Honey & Gold 1971, Shem-tov et al 1971, Block et al 1973, Somerville & Beçu 1977, Feizi et al 1978). There also appears to be an association, which is unexplained, between hypertrophic cardiomyopathy and the systemic myopathies (Meerschwam & Hootsmans 1971), Friedreich disease (Gach 1971, Van der Hauwaert & Dumoulin 1976), Turner syndrome (Nghiem et al 1972), Noonan syndrome (Phornphutkul

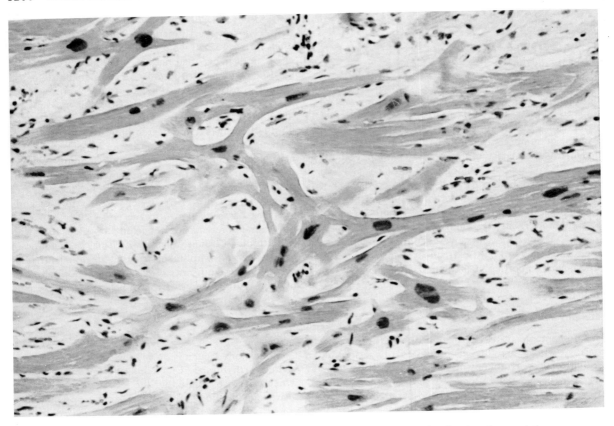

Fig. 74.1   Photomicrograph of the myocardium from a case of hypertrophic cardiomyopathy showing characteristic derangement of normal architecture with marked hypertrophy and branching of myocardial fibres. Many of the nuclei are large and bizarrely shaped. There is also considerable interstitial fibrosis. Haematoxylin and eosin × 124.

et al 1973, Hirsch et al 1975, Jackson et al 1979) and lentiginosis (Polani & Moynahan 1972, Somerville & Bonham-Carter 1972).

The natural history of the disease is extremely variable and the prognosis in any one case difficult to determine. Many affected individuals die unexpectedly in childhood, adolescence or middle life, and a few develop cardiac failure, while others remain asymptomatic for decades. Now that the disease is well recognized it is not uncommon to find patients with hypertrophic cardiomyopathy surviving into their 60s and 70s, many such cases having been previously considered to have coronary artery disease or rheumatic heart disease (Hardarson et al 1973, Goodwin 1974).

Therapy

The treatment of hypertrophic cardiomyopathy is unsatisfactory. The prime objectives must be improvement of ventricular function, particularly diastolic filling and the prevention of arrhythmias. Beta adrenergic beta-blocking agents, calcium channel blocking agents and disopyramide have all been greeted with varying degrees of enthusiasm, but have been found wanting, particularly in the prevention of ventricular arrhythmias and sudden death. They may, however, give symptomatic relief from angina. Amiodarone is the only antiarrhythmic which has been shown to reduce the frequency of potentially fatal arrhythmias and thus improve survival (McKenna et al 1985). The exact role of surgery has still to be defined, but good results have been reported following ventricomyotomy-myectomy, particularly for the relief of intractable angina and cardiac failure in those cases where there is important obstruction to left ventricular outflow. More recently cardiac transplantation has improved survival in cases which would previously have been considered beyond surgical help (Report of the Council of the British Cardiac Society 1984, Starnes et al 1987).

The subject of therapy, excluding the place of cardiac transplantation, has been well reviewed by Wigle et al (1985). Other therapeutic points include the need for antibiotic cover prior to dentistry etc. owing to the risk, albeit small, of infective endocarditis. The maintenance of sinus rhythm, particularly in the elderly, for the loss of atrial transport dramatically reduces the ejection fraction of the myopathic ventricle. In many patients, cardiac failure develops rapidly after the onset of atrial fibrillation. This, therefore, is one of the rare diseases in which repeated cardioversion may be required. In view of the embolic risk, prophylactic anticoagulants should be used prior to restoring sinus rhythm and, if the patient is having frequent paroxysmal arrhythmias, anticoagulants should form a permanent part of treatment.

GENETICS

As stated above, early studies (Davies 1952, Campbell & Turner-Warwick 1956, Brigden 1957, Bercu et al 1958, Teare 1958, Garrett et al 1959, Hollman et al 1960, Walther et al 1960, Brent et al 1960, Paré et al 1961, Schrader et al 1961, Stampbach et al 1961, Braunwald et al 1964, Bishop et al 1962, Wigle et al 1962, Wood et al 1964, Estes et al 1963, Björk & Orinius 1964, Cohen et al 1964, Treger & Blount 1965, Maurice et al 1966, Horlick et al 1966, Weber et al 1966, Meerschwam 1969) indicated that a familial tendency existed in hypertrophic cardiomyopathy. Many of the studies reported pedigrees in which the disease appeared to be transmitted as an autosomal dominant trait, for example that of Brigden (1975). In some families, however, dominant inheritance could only be entertained if variable expressivity and incomplete penetrance were also assumed. On the other hand, there were many instances where the condition appeared to be sporadic. A glance at the nomenclature used in these early studies reveals a plethora of synonyms due to variable expression of the disorder, many of which are still in current use (Maron & Epstein 1979b).

Recent family studies

In 1971, we attempted a genetic study (Emanuel et al 1971), based on clinical findings, of 671 first-degree relatives of 97 index patients. 558 of the relatives were clinically examined. Looking at the types of mating which produced the probands, we identified 76 families in which neither parent was affected, 12 families in which one parent was affected, and one family in which both parents were affected. The remaining 8 families were excluded because of doubtful diagnosis in the parents. Analysis of the 12 families with one affected

parent was consistent with dominant inheritance. For some of the 67 families in which neither parent was affected the proband could be considered to have received a new mutation, although for other families there was evidence of affected relatives. On the other hand, in those families with only one affected member, or with affected sibs, recessive inheritance might have been responsible for the condition. Our data seemed to confirm this latter possibility because the number of affected individuals did not differ significantly from that expected on the recessive hypothesis. It is interesting that Yamaguchi et al (1977) studied 67 probands and their families, and found one group of families having 64% consanguinity and giving a segregation ratio of 0.196 which they suggested involved a recessive gene. However, congestive rather than hypertrophic cardiomyopathy seemed to be characteristic of this group. Branzi et al (1985) have commented on the possible genetic heterogeneity of hypertrophic cardiomyopathy. Their evidence suggests the possibility of autosomal recessive inheritance to account for 67% of their probands who were isolated or sporadic cases.

Echocardiographic studies led to the concept of isolated asymmetric septal hypertrophy (IASH) being part of the clinical spectrum of hypertrophic cardiomyopathy (HC) (Emanuel et al 1983). Clark et al (1973) showed that ASH frequently associated with other evidence of HC was inherited as an autosomal dominant trait with high penetrance. This led to subsequent contributions to the genetics of hypertrophic cardiomyopathy (Bingle et al 1975, Maron et al 1979a, ten Cate et al 1979, van Dorp et al 1976) assuming that fully developed hypertrophic cardiomyopathy and isolated asymmetric septal hypertrophy had the same genetic cause.

However, ASH occurs in some normal adults (Bulkley et al 1977, Maron et al 1978c), it is present in congenital heart disease, especially in those cases where the right ventricle is involved (Maron et al 1975, Larter et al 1976, Maron et al 1979a), and is not uncommon in fixed aortic valve stenosis (Maron et al 1979c).

We attempted to investigate the association between ASH and hypertrophic cardiomyopathy. We examined two types of family (Emanuel et al 1983), in both of which the probands had confirmed hypertrophic cardiomyopathy. There were 12 families of the first type in which one of the parents showed clinical signs of the disease. In the second type of family, of which there were 7, both parents of each proband were clinically normal, but one had echocardiographic evidence of ASH. 114 out of the 119 first-degree relatives were examined or, if dead prior to the study, were investigated through necropsy or operation reports to establish the presence or absence of heart disease. In the first type of family, where both the proband and one parent had hypertrophic cardio-myopathy, the matings produced 34 offsprings, 19 of whom had hypertrophic cardiomyopathy with ASH and one of whom had ASH as the only anomaly. We have called this latter condition isolated asymmetric septal hypertrophy (IASH). In the second type of family, where one of the parents had IASH, 11 out of 24 offspring had hypertrophic cardiomyopathy, and 1 in 24 had IASH. In both types, the numbers of affected offspring do not differ significantly from those expected in dominant inheri-tance. We concluded that IASH and hypertrophic cardiomyopathy, when they occur in the same family, are different manifestations of the same condition trans-mitted as an autosomal dominant trait.

The simplest genetic concept would be of a single autosomal dominant gene which could be expressed in a mild form as IASH or in a more severe form as HC. It is improbable, however, that this hypothesis is correct, for isolated sporadic cases are too common and this would demand an unacceptably high mutation rate. In addition, families in which the disease involves more than half the first-degree relatives are not rare. These two factors virtually exclude uncomplicated autosomal dominant inheritance. Moreover, the variation of expression within a family would remain unexplained. This led us to suggest that there were modifying genes or environ-mental factors which could affect the expression of a single autosomal dominant gene. We proposed (Emanuel & Withers 1986) a polygenic threshold model, with a threshold for ASH which was different from the threshold for HC. This model required information about the incidence of both conditions and recently this has been forthcoming. Hada et al (1987) have suggested that the prevalence of ASH might be as high as 22/12 841 or 0.17%. From a study in the northern region of the United Kingdom Bennett et al (1987) have estimated the minimum prevalence of hypertrophic cardiomyopathy to be 3.33/100 000. These values give some indication of the threshold levels in the model. Incidentally, the genetic basis for ASH is further complicated by reports such as Moller's (Moller et al 1979) in which two cases of ASH occurred in a family where other members had a dominantly inherited dilated cardiomyopathy.

HLA studies

Several studies have investigated the relationship between the HLA system and cardiomyopathy. In a Japanese population Matsumori et al (1979) found an association between HLA-B7 and the disease within families although the frequency of HLA-B12 and HLA-B5 was less than found in controls (MacArthur &

McKenna 1980). A European study (Bloch et al 1980) compared 32 white patients with echocardiographically-diagnosed hypertrophic cardiomyopathy, with a group of control subjects. In 20 of 32 identified patients the diagnosis was confirmed by left heart catheterization. The frequency of HLA-B12 was again less in the disease group than in the controls, but the difference was not statistically significant. Meanwhile, Matsumori et al (1981) had examined the HLA-DR antigens and found, after correction, a significant ($P=0.028$) association between HLA-DRw4 and hypertrophic cardiomyopathy in patients with the obstructive form of the disease. Other authors (Gardin et al 1982, Mourant et al 1982, Haugland et al 1986) could find no evidence to suggest linkage disequilibrium between a particular HLA marker and a hypertrophic cardiomyopathy susceptibility gene. Strong associations did exist but became insignificant after correction for all the antigens studied. Indeed in a large Norwegian family (Haugland et al 1986) all members of generation 4 were found to be healthy and it was suggested that other factors, in addition to genetic predisposition, may be necessary for clinical hypertro-phic cardiomyopathy to develop.

This does not mean that linkage to the HLA complex is not present. Burn et al (1988), using recombinant DNA technology, have studied 10 informative families. They have shown that the short arm of chromosome 6 is a likely site for a possible hypertrophic cardiomyopathy gene, being 12 centiMorgans from the major histocom-patibility locus (lod score = 3.04). Further work using additional informative families offers the promise of gene location.

More recently, a Canadian family of 78 members has been studied using various DNA probes (Jarcho et al 1989). One probe, CRI-L436, has shown linkage to a gene for familial hypertrophic cardiomyopathy (lod score = +9.37 where $\theta=0$). Mapping studies with this and other probes suggest that the gene for familial hypertrophic cardiomyopathy is located on chromosome 14 band q1 and is closely linked to a locus for the α chain of the T-cell receptor. Three further families support this linkage model (combined lod score = +1.8). The authors point out that other genes believed to play a part in cardiac hypertrophy have also been mapped to chromosome 14. For example, genes for the heavy chains (α and β) of cardiac myosin have been mapped to chromosome 14q11.2-q13. However, the non-assignment of genes for abnormal adrenergic function or calcium antagonist receptors means that it is not yet possible to test aetio-logical hypotheses involving these functions. The use of probe CRI-L436 and other probes will eventually allow affected children to be distinguished before the disease becomes evident, thus offering early diagnosis.

Biochemical studies

What is lacking at the moment in hypertrophic cardio-myopathy is any knowledge of a fundamental biochemical abnormality associated with the mutant gene. A start on such an investigation has been made by Liew et al (1980). They examined myocardial tissue from the left ventricular septum of patients with hypertrophic cardiomyopathy who were undergoing ventriculomyotomy-myectomy. Six out of nine patients had a positive family history for hypertrophic cardiomyopathy with a dominant mode of inheritance. They compared the electrophoretic patterns of the histones in these patients with those from patients with normal hearts and from patients with acquired infundibular hypertrophy. The nuclear histones in the three groups were identical but the nuclear non-histone proteins showed distinct differences between the hypertrophic cardiomyopathic group and the other two groups. The altered non-histone proteins did not exhibit the patterns of the major contractile proteins. Furthermore, these nuclear proteins most probably did not come from non-muscle cells, i.e. connective tissue nuclei.

The function of these non-histone proteins is not known. One protein (pH 5.1, M_r 54 000) was markedly increased and another (pH 4.9 M_r 58 000) was greatly reduced in the hypertrophic cardiomyopathic hearts. Several other protein fractions were also decreased. These latter fractions were also reduced in the cardiomyopathy of Syrian hamsters. The authors concluded that the electrophoretic patterns in hypertrophic cardiomyopathy and the very early stage of hamster cardiomyopathy are strikingly similar. The fact that several proteins were affected suggests that they are regulated simultaneously, and thus the primary defect may be one of gene regulation. This may account for the variability in expression of the phenotype and the difficulties found in establishing any really clear diagnostic criteria for hypertrophic cardiomyopathy.

REFERENCES

Assad-Morell J L, Tajik A J, Giuliani E R 1974 Echocardiographic analysis of the ventricular septum. Progress in Cardiovascular Diseases 17: 219–237

Bennett C P, Burn J, Moore G 1987 Prevalence of hypertrophic cardiomyopathy in the Northern Region. Journal of Medical Genetics 24: 243

Bercu B A, Diettert G A, Danforth W H, Pund E E, Ahlvin R C, Belliveau R R 1958 Pseudoaortic stenosis produced by ventricular hypertrophy. American Journal of Medicine 25: 814–818

Bingle G J, Dillon J, Hurwitz R 1975 Asymmetric septal hypertrophy in a large Amish kindred. Clinical Genetics 7: 225–261

Bishop J M, Campbell M, Wyn Jones E 1962 Cardiomyopathy in four members of a family. British Heart Journal 24: 715–725

Björk G, Orinius E 1964 Familial cardiomyopathies. Acta Medica Scandinavica 176: 407–424

Bloch A, Crittin J, Barras C, Jeannet M 1980 Hypertrophic cardiomyopathy and HLA. New England Journal of Medicine 302: 1033

Block P C, Powell W J, Dinsmore R E, Goldblatt A 1973 Coexistent fixed congenital and idiopathic hypertrophic subaortic stenosis. American Journal of Cardiology 31: 523–526

Branzi A, Borneo G, Specchia S et al 1985 Genetic heterogeneity of hypertrophic cardiomyopathy. International Journal of Cardiology 7: 129–134

Braunwald E, Lambrew C T, Rockoff S D, Ross J, Morrow A G 1964 Idiopathic hypertrophic subaortic stenosis. I. A description of the disease based upon an analysis of 64 patients. Circulation 30: Supplement IV: 3–119

Brent L B, Aburano A, Fisher D L, Moran Th L, Myers J D, Taylor J W 1960 Familial muscular subaortic stenosis. Circulation 21: 267–280

Brigden W 1957 Uncommon myocardial diseases: the non-coronary cardiomyopathies. Lancet 2: 1179–1184

Bulkley B H, Weisfeldt M L, Hutchins G M 1977 Asymmetric septal hypertrophy and myocardial fiber disarray: features of normal developing and malformed hearts. Circulation 56: 292–298

Burn J, Bennett C P, Hunter S, McKenna W J 1988 Tentative localisation of the gene responsible for hypertrophic cardiomyopathy. British Heart Journal 59: 98–99

Campbell M, Turner-Warwick M 1956 Two more families with cardiomegaly. British Heart Journal 18: 393–402

Clark C E, Henry W L, Epstein S E 1973 Familial prevalence and genetic transmission of idiopathic hypertrophic subaortic stenosis. New England Journal of Medicine 289: 709–714

Cohen J, Effat H, Goodwin J F, Oakley C M, Steiner R E 1964 Hypertrophic obstructive cardiomyopathy. British Heart Journal 26: 16–32

Criley J M, Lewis K B, White J I Jr, Ross R S 1965 Pressure gradients without obstruction. A new concept of hypertrophic subaortic stenosis. Circulation 32: 881–887

Davies L G 1952 A familial heart disease. British Heart Journal 14: 206–212

Davies M J 1984 The current status of myocardial disarray in hypertrophic cardiomyopathy. British Heart Journal 51: 361–363

Emanuel R 1970 A classification for the cardiomyopathies. American Journal of Cardiology 26: 438–439

Emanuel R 1971 Hypertrophic obstructive cardiomyopathy. In: CIBA Study Group No. 37, J & A Churchill, London, p 54

Emanuel R, Withers R F J 1983 Genetics of the cardiomyopathies. In: Yu P N, Goodwin J G (eds) Progress in Cardiology. Lea & Fabiger, p 211–223

Emanuel R, Withers R 1986 Idiopathic cardiomyopathies. In: Pierpont M E, Moller J H (eds) Genetics of Cardiovascular Disease. Martinus Nijhoff Publishing, 143–159

Emanuel R, Withers R F J, O'Brien K 1971 Dominant and recessive modes of inheritance in idiopathic cardiomyopathy. Lancet ii: 1065–1067

Emanuel R, Marcomichelakis J, Withers R F J, O'Brien K 1983 The inheritance of asymmetric septal hypertrophy. British Heart Journal 49: 309–316

Estes H, Whalen R E, Roberts S R, McIntosh D D 1963 The electrocardiographic and vectorcardiographic findings in idiopathic hypertrophic subaortic stenosis. American Heart Journal 65: 155–161

Evans W 1949 Familial cardiomegaly. British Heart Journal 11: 68–82

Falicov R E, Resnekov L 1977 Mid ventricular obstruction in hypertrophic obstructive cardiomyopathy. New diagnostic and therapeutic challenge. British Heart Journal 39: 701–705

Farmer D, Higgins C B, Yee E, Lipton M J, Wah D, Ports T 1985 Tissue characterization by magnetic resonance imaging in hypertrophic cardiomyopathy. American Journal of Cardiology 55: 230–232

Feizi O, Farrer-Brown G, Emanuel R 1978 Familial study of hypertrophic cardiomyopathy and congenital aortic valve disease. American Journal of Cardiology 41: 956–964

Fighali S, Krajcer Z, Edelman S, Leachman R D 1987 Progression of hypertrophic cardiomyopathy into a hypokinetic left ventricle: higher incidence in patients with midventricular obstruction. Journal of the American College of Cardiology 9: 288–294

Frank S, Braunwald E 1968 Idiopathic hypertrophic subaortic stenosis. Clinical analysis of 126 patients with emphasis on the natural history. Circulation 37: 759–788

Gach J V 1971 Hypertrophic obstructive cardiomyopathy and Friedreich's ataxia. British Heart Journal 38: 1291–1298

Gardin J M, Gottdiener J S, Radvany R, Maron B J, Lesch M 1982 HLA linkage vs. association in hypertrophic cardiomyopathy. Evidence for the absence of an association in a heterogeneous Caucasian population. Chest 81: 466–472

Garrett G, Hay W J, Richards A G 1959 Familial cardiomegaly. Journal of Clinical Pathology 12: 355–361

Goldblatt J, Melmed J, Rose A G 1987 Autosomal recessive inheritance of idiopathic dilated cardiomyopathy in a Madeira Portuguese Kindred. Clinical Genetics 31: 249–254

Goodwin J F 1970 Congestive and hypertrophic cardiomyopathies. A decade of study. Lancet i: 731–739

Goodwin J F 1974 Prospects and predictions for the cardiomyopathies. Circulation 50: 210–219

Goodwin J F, Krikler D M 1976 Arrhythmia as a cause of sudden death in hypertrophic cardiomyopathy. Lancet ii: 937–940

Goodwin J F, Oakley C M 1972 The cardiomyopathies. British Heart Journal 34: 545–552

Greaves S C, Roche A H G, Neutze J M, Whitlock R M L, Veale A M O 1987 Inheritance of hypertrophic cardiomyopathy: A cross sectional and M Mode Echocardiographic Study of 50 families. British Heart Journal 58: 259–266

Hada Y, Sakamoto T, Amano K et al 1987 Prevalence of hypertrophic cardiomyopathy in a population of adult Japanese workers as detected by echocardiographic screening. American Journal of Cardiology 59: 183–184

Hardarson T, De la Calzada C S, Curiel R, Goodwin J F 1973 Prognosis and mortality of hypertrophic obstructive cardiomyopathy. Lancet ii: 1462–1467

Haugland H, Ohm O-J, Boman H, Thorsby E 1986 Hypertrophic cardiomyopathy in three generations of a large Norwegian family: A clinical, echocardiographic and genetic study. British Heart Journal 55: 168–175

Henry W L, Clark C E, Epstein S E 1973 Asymmetric septal hypertrophy: echocardiographic identification of the pathognomic anatomic abnormality of IHSS. Circulation 47: 225–233

Henry W L, Clark C E, Roberts W C, Morrow A G, Epstein S E 1974 Differences in distribution of myocardial abnormalities in patients with obstructive and non-obstructive asymmetric septal hypertrophy (ASH): Echocardiographic and gross anatomy findings. Circulation 50: 447–455

Hirsch H D, Gelband H, Garcia O, Gottlieb S, Tamer D M 1975 Rapidly progressive obstructive cardiomyopathy in infants with Noonan's syndrome. Report of two cases. Circulation 52: 1161–1165

Hollman A, Goodwin J F, Teare D, Renwick J W 1960 A family with obstructive cardiomyopathy (asymmetrical hypertrophy). British Heart Journal 22: 449–456

Honey M, Gold R G 1971 Congenital physiologically corrected transposition with hypertrophic cardiomyopathy. British Heart Journal 33: 214–219

Horlick L, Petkovich N J, Bolton C F 1966 Idiopathic hypertrophic subvalvular stenosis. American Journal of Cardiology 17: 419–425

Hudson R E B 1970 The cardiomyopathies: order from chaos. American Journal of Cardiology 25: 70–77

Jackson G, Anand I S, Oram S 1979 Asymmetric septal hypertrophy and propranolol treatment in a case of Ullrich-Noonan syndrome. British Heart Journal 42: 611–614

Jarcho J A, McKenna W, Pare P et al 1989 Mapping a gene for familial hypertrophic cardiomyopathy to chromosome 14ql. New England Journal of Medicine 321: 1372–1378

Jefferson K, Rees S 1980 Clinical cardiac radiology, 2nd edn. Butterworth, London p 263

Kessler K M, Rahim A 1979 Mitral anular calcification and idiopathic hypertrophic subaortic stenosis (letter). American Journal of Cardiology 44: 579

Kronzon I, Glassman E 1978 Mitral ring calcification in idiopathic hypertrophic subaortic stenosis. American Journal of Cardiology 42: 60–66

Larter W E, Allen H D, Sahn D J, Goldberg S J 1976 The asymmetrically hypertrophied septum: further differentiation of its causes. Circulation 53: 19–27

Liew C C, Sole M J, Silver M D, Wigle E D 1980 Electrophoretic profiles of nonhistone nuclear proteins of human hearts with muscular subaortic stenosis. Circulation Research 46: 513–519

MacArthur C, McKenna W 1980 HL-A and hypertrophic cardiomyopathy (letter). American Heart Journal 99: 542–543

McKenna W J, Chetty S, Oakley C M, Goodwin J F 1980 Arrhythmia in hypertrophic cardiomyopathy. Exercise and 48 hour ambulatory electrocardiographic assessment with and without beta-adrenergic blocking therapy. American Journal of Cardiology 45: 1–5

McKenna W J, Oakley C M, Krikler D M, Goodwin J F 1985 Improved survival with amiodarone in patients with hypertrophic cardiomyopathy and ventricular tachycardia. British Heart Journal 53: 412–416

Marcomichelakis J, O'Brien K, Emanuel R, Withers R 1983 Echocardiographic changes in the thickness of the interventricular septum and posterior left ventricular wall occurring with age in a normal male population. International Journal of Cardiology 4: 405–415

Maron B J, Ferrans V J, Henry W L, Clark C E, Redwood D R, Roberts W C, Morrow A C, Epstein S E 1974 Differences in distribution of myocardial abnormalities in patients with obstructive and nonobstructive asymmetric septal hypertrophy (ASH): light and electron microscopic findings. Circulation 50: 436–446

Maron B J, Edwards J E, Ferrans V J, Clark C E, Lebowitz E A, Henry W L, Epstein S E 1975 Congenital heart malformations associated with disproportionate ventricular septal thickening. Circulation 52: 926–932

Maron B J, Lipson L C, Roberts W C, Savage D D, Epstein S E 1978a "Malignant" hypertrophic cardiomyopathy: identification of a subgroup of families with unusually frequent premature death. American Journal of Cardiology 41: 1133–1140

Maron B J, Roberts W C, Edwards J E, McAllister H A Jr., Foley D D, Epstein S E 1978b Sudden death in patients with hypertrophic cardiomyopathy: characterization of 26 patients without functional limitation. American Journal of Cardiology 41: 803–810

Maron B J, Verter J, Kapur S 1978c Disproportionate ventricular septal thickening in the developing normal human heart. Circulation 57: 520–526

Maron B J, Edwards J E, Moller J H, Epstein S E 1979a Prevalence and characteristics of disproportionate ventricular septal thickening in infants with congenital heart disease. Circulation 59: 126–133

Maron B J, Epstein S E 1979b Hypertrophic cardiomyopathy. A discussion of nomenclature. American Journal of Cardiology 43: 1242–1244

Maron B J, Gottdiener J A, Roberts W C, Hammer W J, Epstein S E 1979c Nongenetically transmitted disproportionate ventricular septal thickening associated with left ventricular outflow obstruction. British Heart Journal 41: 345–349

Maron B J, Nichols P F, Pickle L W, Wesley Y E, Mulvihill J J 1984 Patterns of inheritance in hypertrophic cardiomyopathy: Assessment by M-Mode and 2-D echocardiography. American Journal of Cardiology 53: 1087–1094

Maron B J, Wolfson J K, Epstein S E, Roberts W C 1986 Intramural ("small vessel") coronary artery disease in hypertrophic cardiomyopathy. Journal of the American College of Cardiology 8: 545–557

Matsumori A, Hirose K, Wakabayashi A, Kawai C, Nabeya N, Sakurami T, Tsuji K 1979 HL-A and hypertrophic cardiomyopathy. American Heart Journal 97: 428–431

Matsumori A, Kawai C, Wakabayishi A et al 1981 HLA-DRW4 antigen linkage in patients with hypertrophic obstructive cardiomyopathy. American Heart Journal 101: 14–16

Maurice P, Ben-Ismail M, Penther Ph, Ferrane J, Lenègre J 1966 Les myocardiopathies obstructives. I. Etude clinique et radiologique. Archives des Maladies du Coeur et des Vaisseaux 59: 375–390

Meerschwam I S 1969 Hypertrophic obstructive cardiomyopathy. Excerpta Medica, Amsterdam, p 20

Meerschwam I S, Hootsmans W J M 1971 An electromyographic study in hypertrophic obstructive cardiomyopathy. In: Wolstenholme F E W, O'Connor M (eds) Hypertrophic obstructive cardiomyopathy, CIBA Foundation study group No. 37, J & A Churchill, London, p 55

Michels V V, Driscoll D J, Miller F A 1985 Familial aggregation of idiopathic dilated cardiomyopathy. American Journal of Cardiology 55: 1232–1233

Moller P, Lunde P, Hovig T, Nitter-Hauge S 1979 Familial cardiomyopathy. Autosomally dominantly inherited congestive cardiomyopathy with two cases of septal hypertrophy in one family. Clinical Genetics 16: 233–243

Motamed H E, Roberts W C 1987 Frequency and significance of mitral anular calcium in hypertrophic cardiomyopathy: Analysis of 200 necropsy patients. American Journal of Cardiology 60: 877–884

Mourant A J, Kafetz K M, Brigden W W et al 1982 HLA antigen associations in hypertrophic cardiomyopathy. Tissue Antigens 20: 389–393

Nghiem Q X, Toledo J R, Schreiber M H, Harris L C, Lockhart L L, Tyson K R T 1972 Congenital idiopathic hypertrophic subaortic stenosis associated with a phenotypic Turner's syndrome. American Journal of Cardiology 30: 683–689

Olsen E G J 1973 The pathology of the heart. Intercontinental Medical Book Corporation, New York, p 171–187

Olsen E G J 1983 Anatomic and light microscopic characterisation of hypertrophic obstructive and non-obstructive cardiomyopathy. European Heart Journal (Supp. F) 4: 1–8

Opie L H, Walpoth B, Barsacchi R 1985 Calcium and catecholamines: Relevance to cardiomyopathies and significance in therapeutic strategies. Journal of Molecular and Cellular Cardiology 17: 21–34

Paré J A P, Fraser R G, Pirozynski W J, Shanks J A, Stubington D 1961 Hereditary cardiovascular dysplasia. A form of familial cardiomyopathy. American Journal of Medicine 31: 37–62

Phornphutkul C, Rosenthal A, Nadas A S 1973 Cardiomyopathy in Noonan's syndrome: report of 3 cases. British Heart Journal 35: 99–102

Polani P E, Moynahan E J 1972 Progressive cardiomyopathic lentiginosis. Quarterly Journal of Medicine 41: 205–225

Report of the Council of the British Cardiac Society 1984 Cardiac transplantation in the United Kingdom. British Heart Journal 52: 679–682

Report of the WHO/ISFC Task Force 1980 The definition and classification of cardiomyopathies. British Heart Journal 44: 672–673

Roberts W C 1973 Operative treatment of hypertrophic obstructive cardiomyopathy. The case against mitral valve replacement. American Journal of Cardiology 32: 377–381

Ross J Jr, Braunwald E, Gault J H, Mason D T, Morrow A G 1966 The mechanism of the intraventricular pressure gradient in idiopathic hypertrophic stenosis. Circulation 34: 558–578

Savage D D, Seides S F, Clark C E, Henry W L, Maron B J, Robinson F C, Epstein S E 1978 Electrocardiographic findings in patients with obstructive and nonobstructive hypertrophic cardiomyopathy. Circulation 58: 402–408

Savage D D, Seides S F, Maron B J, Myers D J, Epstein S E 1979 Prevalence of arrhythmias during 24-hour electrocardiographic monitoring and exercise testing in patients with obstructive and nonobstructive hypertrophic cardiomyopathy. Circulation 59: 866–875

Sawaya J, Longo M R, Schlant R C 1974 Echocardiographic interventricular septal wall motion and thickness: a study in health and disease. American Heart Journal 87: 681–688

Schrader W H, Pankey G A, Davis R B, Theologides A 1961

Familial idiopathic cardiomegaly. Circulation 24: 599–606

Shem-tov A, Deutsch V, Hahini J H, Neufeld H N 1971 Cardiomyopathy associated with congenital heart disease. British Heart Journal 33: 782–793

Somerville J, Beçu L 1977 Congenital heart disease associated with hypertrophic cardiomyopathy. Johns Hopkins Medical Journal 140: 151–162

Somerville J, Bonham-Carter R E 1972 The heart in lentiginosis. British Heart Journal 34: 58–66

Spirito P, Maron B J, Borrow R O, Epstein S E 1987 Occurrence and significance of progressive left ventricular wall thinning and relative cavity dilatation in hypertrophic cardiomyopathy. American Journal of Cardiology 60: 123–129

Starnes V A, Stinson E B, Oyer P E, Valantine H, Baldwin J C, Hunt S A, Shumway N E 1987 Cardiac transplantation in children and adolescents. Circulation 76 (Supp. V) V43–V47

Stempbach O, Wyler F, Rentsch M, Schüpbach P 1961 Diagnostische und hämodynamische Probleme bei der Aortenstenose. Cardiologia, Basel, 38: 112–141

Stone D L, Petch M C, Verney G I, Dixon A K 1984 Computed tomography in patients with hypertrophic cardiomyopathy. British Heart Journal 52: 136–139

Symons C, Fortune F, Greenbaum R A, Dandona P 1985 Cardiac hypertrophy, hypertrophic cardiomyopathy and hyperparathyroidism — an association. British Heart Journal 54: 539–542

Teare R D 1958 Asymmetrical hypertrophy of the heart in young adults. British Heart Journal 20: 1–8

ten Cate F J, Hugenholtz P G, van Dorp W G, Roelandt J 1979 Prevalence of diagnostic abnormalities in patients with genetically transmitted asymmetric septal hypertrophy. American Journal of Cardiology 43: 731–737

Treger A, Blount S G 1965 Familial cardiomyopathy. American Heart Journal 70: 40–53

Van der Hauwaert L G, Dumoulin M 1976 Hypertrophic cardiomyopathy in Friedreich's ataxia. British Heart Journal 38: 1291–1298

van Dorp W G, ten Cate F J, Vletter W B, Dohmen H, Roelandt J 1976 Familial prevalence of asymmetric septal hypertrophy. European Journal of Cardiology 4: 349–357

Van Noorden S, Olsen E G J, Pearse A G E 1971 Hypertrophic obstructive cardiomyopathy. A histological, histochemical and ultrastructural study of biopsy material. Cardiovascular Research 5: 118–131

Vecht R J, Oakley C M 1968 Infective endocarditis in three patients with hypertrophic obstructive cardiomyopathy. British Medical Journal ii: 455–459

Walther R J, Madoff I M, Zinner K 1960 Cardiomegaly of unknown cause occurring in a family. New England Journal of Medicine 263: 1104–1110

Weber D J, Gould L, Schaffer A I 1966 A family with idiopathic myocardial hypertrophy. American Journal of Cardiology 17: 419–425

White R I, Criley J M, Lewis K B, Ross R S 1967 Experimental production of intracavity pressure differences. Possible significance in the interpretation of human hemodynamic studies. American Journal of Cardiology 19: 806–817

Wigle E D, Heimbecker R O, Gunton R W 1962 Idiopathic ventricular septal hypertrophy causing muscular subaortic stenosis. Circulation 26: 325–340

Wigle E D, Sasson Z, Henderson M A, Ruddy T D, Fulop J, Rakowski H, Williams G W 1985 Hypertrophic Cardiomyopathy. The importance of the site and the extent of hypertrophy. A review. Progress in Cardiovascular Disease 28: 1–83

Wood R S, Taylor W J, Wheat M W, Schiebler G L 1962 Muscular subaortic stenosis in childhood. Pediatrics 30: 749–758

Yamaguchi M, Toshima H, Yamase T, Ikeda Y, Koga Y, Yoshioka H, Ito M, Fujino T, Yasuda H 1977 A family study of idiopathic cardiomyopathy. Proceedings of the Japan Academy 53: Series B 209–214

75. Congenital and hereditary urinary tract disorders

J. Zonana   J. H. DiLiberti

Congenital and hereditary urinary tract disorders cover a wide spectrum, ranging from gross abnormalities of morphogenesis to more subtle derangements of renal function. The discussion of these disorders is organized as outlined in Table 75.1. Hereditary and congenital urinary tract disorders frequently present during infancy and childhood but some are discovered during adult life and occasionally an affected individual remains asymptomatic for an entire lifetime. The latter situation creates considerable difficulty for genetic analysis. Many renal disorders are clearly hereditary, following well-recognized Mendelian patterns of inheritance. Others, especially those with abnormal structural differentiation, have only recently been shown to have a genetic component. Heterogeneity has been recognized with increasing frequency in most of these disorders.

STRUCTURAL ABNORMALITIES OF THE URINARY TRACT

Renal agenesis

Bilateral and unilateral renal agenesis are discussed together, since it now appears that they may have common aetiologies. Bilateral renal agenesis has a reported (Potter 1965, Ratten et al 1973, Carter et al 1979) incidence of 0.12–0.3 per 1000 total births with a male to female ratio of approximately 2.7. Estimates of the incidence of unilateral agenesis range from 1:52 to 1:1286 (Museles et al 1971, Bernstein et al 1975). Bilateral renal agenesis frequently results in stillbirth, with a reported (Potter 1965) 38% prenatal loss in one series. Severe oligohydramnios is present, with rare exceptions. Live-born infants are frequently both premature and small for gestational age and most die within hours of birth as the result of respiratory insufficiency.

The central pathological finding is bilateral absence of the kidney, ureters and renal arteries, with a hypoplastic bladder lacking ureteral orifices (Potter 1965). Occasionally ureteric remnants may be present but these cases are still classified as bilateral renal agenesis (Carter et al 1979). Females have associated uterine and proximal vaginal agenesis with normal gonads, while in males the vas deferens and seminal vesicles are absent.

The frequent additional malformations, believed to be secondary to severe oligohydramnios, have been termed (Potter 1974, Thomas & Smith 1974) the 'oligohydramnios triad'. They are also found in association with severe oligohydramnios of non-renal origin and are absent in rare cases of bilateral renal agenesis without oligohydramnios (Bain & Scott 1960, Mauer et al 1974, Hjalmarson & Sabel 1978). Pulmonary hypoplasia, with arrest of alveolar development at the 12–16 week developmental stage, is directly related to the presence of oligohydramnios (Hislop et al 1979). The characteristic facial appearance of premature senility, broad epicanthal folds, blunt nose, micrognathia, and low set posteriorly rotated ears, as well as the clubfeet and bowed legs, are all believed to be deformations secondary to oligohydramnios and uterine constraint.

The majority of cases of bilateral renal agenesis involve only the primary renal and internal genital malformations, with secondary malformations due to oligohydramnios. Some infants, however, display a broader range of

Table 75.1 Congenital and hereditary urinary tract disorders

I. Structural abnormalities of the urinary tract
  A. Renal
    1. Agenesis
    2. Dysplasia
    3. Cystic
  B. Collecting system
  C. Malformation syndromes and associated urinary tract anomalies
II. Neoplasia
III. Functional abnormalities of the nephron
  A. Glomerular
    1. Nephrotic syndrome
    2. Nephritis
  B. Tubular

malformations with involvement of the anus, external genitalia, or even sirenomelia. These defects are not secondary to the renal agenesis but are considered (Buchta et al 1973, Carter et al 1979) an extension of an abnormal 'single developmental' field complex. Another small group of infants have multiple congenital anomalies of distant organ systems, including malformations of the heart or spine. The heterogeneity of associated malformations may help to distinguish distinct aetiologies.

Unilateral renal agenesis involves absence of a single kidney and the ipsilateral ureter and artery. The bladder has no ureteral orifice on the involved side, while the contralateral kidney may be completely normal, but is frequently ectopic (Bernstein et al 1975). Abnormalities of hydronephrosis, dysplasia or pyelonephritis have been reported in contralateral kidneys (Holmes 1972, Carter et al 1979), however, these series are biased by the inclusion of predominantly hospitalized patients. Many people with unilateral renal agenesis are totally asymptomatic and are only discovered accidentally or by family studies.

A high rate of complete or partial uterine duplication, up to 35%, is associated with unilateral agenesis. Approximately 43% of women with abnormalities of uterine duplication have unilateral renal agenesis (Semmens 1962, Fried et al 1978, Magee et al 1979). The spectrum of genital anomalies may extend to complete vaginal atresia, as seen in the Mayer-Rokitansky-Kuster anomaly (Biedel et al 1984, Opitz 1987). Absence of the vas deferens, seminal vesicle cysts or cryptorchidism may be found in males (Knudsen et al 1979, Ogreid & Hatteland 1979). Therefore, absence of the vas deferens in males or a duplicated uterus in females are indications for a renal ultrasound examination. Similarly, discovery of unilateral renal agenesis in a female should prompt the appropriate uterine examinations. Occasional patients with additonal non-renal malformations, including imperforate anus, vertebral and sacral defects, demonstrate heterogeneity and may represent distinct disorders (Holmes 1972, Emanuel et al 1974).

Discussion of the possible pathogenesis of renal agenesis centres on several key morphogenetic events. The kidney develops from two sources, the mesonephric duct, which gives rise to the ureteric bud, and the metanephric blastema (Potter 1972). The ureteral bud undergoes multiple divisions and forms the ureter, pelvis, calyces and collecting tubules. It also induces the metanephric blastema to proliferate and develop into nephrogenic cells and stroma. Severe disturbances in development or complete agenesis of the mesonephric duct, or of the subsequent ureteric bud, will result in renal agenesis. This theory has support from both clinical correlations and animal models. Embryological studies (Cramer &

Gill 1975, Marshall et al 1978) of the ACI rat, which has a high frequency of spontaneous renal agenesis, and of arsenate-induced renal agenesis (Burk & Beaudoin 1977) in other rat strains, confirm the postulated pathogenic mechanisms. Abnormalities of the vas deferens and seminal vesicle occur as a consequence of their derivation from the mesonephric duct. Since paramesonephric duct (Müllerian duct) formation is also dependent upon normal mesonephric duct development, associated uterine and vaginal abnormalities can be explained in a similar way (Marshall & Beisel 1978).

Renal agenesis has multiple aetiologies (Fitch 1977, Curry et al 1984). Until recent observations, both bilateral and unilateral renal agenesis were thought to be aetiologically unrelated, sporadic and nongenetic disorders. A number of families with multiple affected members have been reported (Madisson 1934, Schmidt et al 1952, Baron 1954, Arends 1957, Hilson 1957, Rosenfeld 1959, Gorvoy et al 1962, Rizza & Downing 1971, Whitehouse & Mountrose 1973, Kohn & Borns 1973, Buchta et al 1973, Cain et al 1974, Hack et al 1974, Zonana et al 1976, Carter et al 1979, Schimke & King 1980, Curry et al 1984, Biedel et al 1984, Roodhooft et al 1984, McPherson et al 1987). Individuals within the same family have had unilateral or bilateral renal agenesis or dysplasia. Concordant monozygotic twins have been described, (Mauer et al 1974, Carter et al 1979, Yates et al 1984, Wilson & Hayden 1985). Individuals with unilateral agenesis have had dysplasia, duplication or hydronephrosis of the contralateral kidney. Renal agenesis, both bilateral and unilateral, can be pathogenetically related, and are at the extreme end of a spectrum of ureteric bud malformations. In the familial cases, many of the pedigrees appear consistent with an autosomal dominant pattern of inheritance with variable expression, and this genetic trait has been termed 'hereditary renal adysplasia' (Buchta et al 1973, McPherson et al 1987).

Family studies utilizing ultrasound examination or IVP to detect subclinical renal anomalies have only recently been undertaken. Close relatives of most previously described 'sporadic' cases have not received adequate renal evaluation. In families purported (Buchta et al 1973, Bois et al 1975, Schinzel et al 1978) to display autosomal recessive or multifactorial inheritance, clinically normal parents have frequently not been adequately examined. A possible X-linked recessive form of bilateral renal agenesis has been postulated (Pashayan et al 1977) on the basis of one family study. An extensive population survey (Carter et al 1979), not utilizing radiological methods, found an empiric recurrence risk of 3.5% for bilateral renal agenesis. This rate was considered too high for multifactorial inheritance based on the reported incidence in the general population. This study did confirm the aetiological relationship of agenesis and dysplasia, both unilateral and bilateral. An ultrasound study of 111 first-degree relatives of probands with bilateral renal agenesis (BRA), bilateral renal dysplasia (BRD), and unilateral agenesis with contralateral dysplasia (URA/URD), revealed that 9% had some related urogenital anomaly, with a recurrence risk of 4.4% for renal malformations among sibs of the probands (Roodhooft et al 1984). One study estimated an empirical recurrence risk of 15–20% for BRA/BRD in the offspring of affected or obligate heterozygotes for hereditary renal adysplasia (McPherson et al 1987).

Most familial cases of bilateral and unilateral renal agenesis have malformations limited to the urinary tract, internal genitalia and those secondary to oligohydramnios, although this is not an invariable finding. Cases with multiple malformations should be examined for specific syndromes. Although chromosome defects are occasionally observed in patients with renal agenesis and multiple anomalies (Egli & Stadler 1973, Curry et al 1984, Schinzel 1984) (Table 75.2) chromosome studies in the majority of cases are normal. Multiple single gene disorders are also associated with renal agenesis (Table 75.3). One example, the branchio-oto-renal dysplasia syndrome, is an autosomal dominant disorder which may have either unilateral or bilateral renal agenesis or dysplasia (Fitch & Srolovitz 1976, Melnick et al 1976, 1978). Associated anomalies include preauricular pits, branchial cleft fistulas and hearing loss. A proband with renal agenesis, along with immediate family members, should be examined for these abnormalities. This syndrome may be responsible for many of the early observa-

Table 75.2 Urinary tract abnormalities associated with chromosomal disorders (Warkany et al 1966, Egli & Stadler 1973, Smith 1976, Bergsma 1979, Schinzel 1984)

Chromosomal abnormality	Renal abnormality	Estimated frequency of urinary tract malformation
4p-	Agenesis, hypoplasia	33%
5p-	Horseshoe kidney, agenesis	occasional*
8 trisomy mosaicism	Hydronephrosis, duplication	common
9 trisomy mosaicism	Hydronephrosis, cysts	common
13q-	Hydronephrosis, vesicoureteral junction obstruction	Uncommon*
13 trisomy	Cysts, hydronephrosis, horseshoe kidney, ureteral duplication	60-80%
18q-	Horseshoe kidney, unilateral agenesis, hydronephrosis	40%
18 trisomy	Horseshoe kidney, ectopia, ureteral duplication, cortical cysts, hydronephrosis	70%
18 ring	Hydronephrosis, tubular dilatation	20%
21q-	Unilateral agenesis	Uncertain*
21 trisomy	Agenesis, hypoplasia, horseshoe kidney	3-7%
22 trisomy (pter→q11) (Cat eye syndrome – coloboma anal atresia)	Agenesis, horseshoe kidney	Common
45,X (Plus other Turner karyotype abnormalities)	Horseshoe kidney, duplication of collecting system, abnormal rotation	60-80%
XXXXY	Hydronephrosis	10%
XXXXX	Hypoplasia, dysplasia	Uncertain*
Triploidy	Hydronephrosis, cysts	Uncertain*

* Reported renal abnormalities may be coincidental.

Table 75.3 Non-chromosomal syndromes and associated urinary tract malformations

Disorder	Urinary tract abnormality	Inheritance
Acral-renal association (Dieker & Opitz 1969)	Agenesis, duplication	
Apert syndrome (Smith 1982)	Hydronephrosis, polycystic kidney	AD
Brancho-oto-renal (Widdershoven 1983)	Unilateral agenesis	AD
Cerebrohepatorenal (Zellweger) (Danks 1975)	Cortical cysts, dysplasia	AR
Chondroectodermal dyplasia (Blackburn & Belliveau 1971)	Renal tubular dilation	AR
Congenital rubella syndrome (Menser et al 1967)	Polycystic, duplication, unilateral agenesis	
Cryptophthalmos (Varnek 1978)	Aplasia	AR
de Lange syndrome (France et al 1969)	Hypoplasia, dyplasia, cysts	
Ectrodactyly (EEC syndrome) (London et al 1985)	Aplasia, hydronephrosis hydroureter, cysts, dyplasia	AD
Ectromelia-ichthyosis (Cullen et al 1969)	Polycystic kidney, hydronephrosis	AR
Ehlers-Danlos (McKusick 1972)	Haematuria, hypoplasia, cortical cysts, uretero-pelvic obstruction	AD
Fanconi pancytopenia (McDonald & Goldschmidt 1959)	Hypoplasia, agenesis, ectopia, horseshoe kidney	AR
Fetal alcohol syndrome (Qazi et al 1979)	Horseshoe kidney, duplication, hypoplasia	
Fetal trimethadione syndrome (Zackai et al 1975)	Unilateral agenesis	
Hemihypertrophy (Gorlin et al 1976)	Ipsilateral renal enlargement, cysts, hydronephrosis, Wilms tumour	
Ivemark (Ivemark et al 1959)	Dysplasia	AR
Johanson-Blizzard (Johanson & Blizzard 1971)	Hydronephrosis	AR
Klippel-Feil (Duncan 1977)	Agenesis, ectopia	AD
Laurence-Moon-Biedl (Nadjini et al 1969)	Hydronephrosis, hypoplasia (also nephropathy)	AR
Lenz microphthalmia (Gorlin et al 1976)	uni- and bilateral agenesis, dyplasia, hydroureter	XLR
Lipodystrophy generalized congenital (Reed et al 1965)	Hydronephrosis, hydroureter, enlarged kidney	AR
Lissencephaly (Miller 1963)	Agenesis	AR
Marfan syndrome (Loughridge 1959)	Duplication, ectopia	AD
Meckel syndrome (Fried et al 1971)	Polycystic dyplastic kidney	AR
Multiple lentigines syndrome (Swanson et al 1971)	Unilateral agenesis, hydronephrosis	AD
MURCS Association (Duncan et al 1979)	Agenesis, ectopia	
Myelomeningocele (Cameron 1956)	Horseshoe kidney, cysts, hydronephrosis	
Neurofibromatosis (Feinman & Yakovac 1970)	Renal artery stenosis	AD
Ochoa (Elejalde 1979)	Hydronephrosis, hydroureter, bladder diverticula	AD
Oculoauriculovertebral dyplasia (Goldenhar) (Sugiura 1971)	Aplasia, duplication, ectopia	
Oculorenal associations (several types) (Senior et al 1961, Loken et al 1961, Fairley et al 1963)	Dysplasia, cysts, nephronophthisis	AR
Opitz BBB (Noe et al 1985)	Reflux	AD
Oral-facial-digital (type I) (Doege et al 1964)	Cortical cysts	XLR
Oro-cranial-digital (Juberg & Hayward 1969)	Horseshoe kidney	AR
Osteo-onycho-dyplasia (Cohen & Berant 1976)	Duplication	AD
Perlman (Greenberg et al 1986)	Dysplasia, hyperplasia, nephropathy, Wilms tumour	AR
Prune belly (Pagon et al 1979)	Hydronephrosis, hydroureter, posterior urethral valves	
Roberts (Freeman et al 1974)	Horse kidney, cysts	AR
Rokitansky (Caldamone & Rabinowitz 1981)	Agenesis, ectopia, horseshoe kidney, dysplasia, duplication	AR
Rubinstein-Taybi (Rubinstein 1979)	Agenesis, ureteral duplication, hydronephrosis	
Russell-Silver (Haslam et al 1973)	Ureteropelvic-junction obstruction, reflux	
Saethre-Chotzen (Bartsocas et al 1970)	Duplication	AD
Thalidomide embryopathy (Warkany 1971)	Unilateral agenesis, rotation anomalies, hydronephrosis, duplication, horseshoe kidney	
Thanatophoric dysplasia (Smith 1982)	Horseshoe kidney, hydronephrosis	AD
Tuberous sclerosis (Anderson & Tanner 1969)	Cysts, dysplasia	AD
VATER association (Barry & Auldist 1974)	Unilateral agenesis, hypoplasia, dysplasia	
Von Hippel-Lindau (Simon & Thompson 1955)	Cysts	AD
Wiedemann-Beckwith (Beckwith 1969)	Hyperplasia, medullary dysplasia	AD
Williams (Chantler et al 1966)	Renal artery stenosis	AR

tions (Hilson 1957) of associated ear and renal malformations.

Renal agenesis is also associated with multiple malformation syndromes of unknown aetiology. The VATER association of vertebral anomalies, anal atresia, tracheo-oesophageal fistula and renal abnormalities is one of the more common of these disorders (Quan & Smith 1973). It usually occurs sporadically, although some pedigrees appear to be consistent with an autosomal dominant pattern of inheritenace (Kurnit et al 1978). Patients with renal agenesis and their families should be examined for possible associated defects.

At the present time it would be reasonable to recommend renal ultrasound examination of all first-degree relatives of probands with renal agenesis and, on occasion, due to incomplete penetrance, even second-degree relatives. The only exception would be cases of known aetiology with a small risk of recurrence, such as those of chromosomal aetiology. If additional affected members are discovered, the pedigree should be analysed for a distinct pattern of inheritance and additional family members studied as necessary. Bilateral renal agenesis has a significant empiric recurrence risk of 3–5% and prenatal diagnosis should be offered in subsequent pregnancies. The risk of bilateral renal agenesis in the offspring of an individual with unilateral renal agenesis is unknown. The counselling is further complicated when there are no other affected family members.

Prenatal diagnosis

Prenatal diagnosis of congenital renal abnormalities is available through ultrasound examination, but at the same time one must be aware of its diagnostic limitations (Kaffe et al 1977b, Miskin 1979, Grannum et al 1980, Dubbins et al 1981, Schmidt et al 1982, Romero et al 1985, Morse et al 1987). Using this method, severe oligohydramnios can be identified as early as 16 weeks' gestation. Failure to visualize the fetal bladder over a defined period of time may indicate inadequate urine formation. Conversely, detection of a large distended bladder may indicate distal urethral obstruction. Actual identification of the kidneys and abnormal renal structures, such as renal cysts, may also be accomplished (Kaffe et al 1977a, Bartley et al 1977, Balfour & Lawrence 1980, Grannum et al 1980). The kidneys can be visualized as early as 18–20 weeks' gestation and sonographic measurements of the ratio of kidney to abdominal circumference have been published (Grannum et al 1980, Jeanty et al 1982). Reports of third trimester diagnosis of renal agenesis, dysplasia or polycystic disease are more numerous (Keirse & Meerman 1978, Mendoza et al 1979, Older et al 1979). Diagnosis

late in pregnancy may still aid in obstetrical management and early neonatal care.

Maternal serum and amniotic fluid alphafetoprotein measurements have been examined (Balfour & Lawrence 1980, Seller & Child 1980) as possible diagnostic aids but the levels may be elevated in the presence of oligo-hydramnios, whether or not there is a fetal renal abnormality. Maternal serum alphafetoprotein screening of the general population has allowed the diagnosis of some sporadic cases of BRA and BRD as well. Alphafetoprotein has also been elevated in cases of fetal obstructive uropathy (Vinson et al 1977, Nevin et al 1978, Dean & Bourdeau 1980). In contrast, the serum alphafetoprotein levels measured at birth in infants with bilateral renal agenesis were normal (Ainbender & Brown 1976).

The wide variability of expression of ureteral bud abnormalities in some families must be emphasised when prenatal diagnosis is considered. Less severe forms of renal dysplasia, not detected by present prenatal diagnostic methods, may still present significant renal functional problems to the infant. Fetal adrenal glands can be misdiagnosed as kidneys, leading to a false negative diagnosis. Prenatal diagnosis of these disorders must be approached cautiously, since diagnostic methods are still being explored.

Renal dysplasia

Renal dysplasia results from abnormal metanephric development, with altered structural organisation and ductal differentiation (Bernstein 1978). Dysplasia is essentially a histological diagnosis with distinct diagnostic criteria including abnormal ductal and mesenchymal elements, such as cartilaginous metaplasia, primitive glomeruli and ducts which may undergo cystic dilatation (Bernstein 1971, Risdon et al 1975, Pardo-Mindan et al 1978). The histology of dysplasia is thought to be distinct from that found in the polycystic disorders. In the past, there has been a good deal of confusion about the terminology and description of these two groups of disorders. Renal dysplasia is heterogeneous, both in functional and structural involvement. The affected kidney may be cystic or solid, hypoplastic or enlarged. Associated malformation of the ureters, bladder or urethra are found in 90% of cases (Bernstein 1978).

Dysplasia is frequently accompanied by renal hypoplasia, but two forms of hypoplasia not associated with dysplasia occur (Bernstein 1968). The Ask-Upmark kidney, with segmental hypoplasia, is congenital but no familial cases have been reported (Arant et al 1979). The other disorder, oligomeganephronie, characterized by extreme glomerular hypertrophy and severe hypoplasia, also does not appear to be inherited.

Renal dysplasia has been separated into three clinical types (Bernstein 1978). The first type, obstructive renal dysplasia, is frequently bilateral and most commonly associated with posterior urethral valves. Prune belly syndrome, or an ectopic ureterocele, can also be an associated malformation (Gribetz & Leiter 1978). The dysplasia is postulated to be secondary to obstruction with increased hydrostatic pressure interfering with normal metanephric differentiation. This type of dysplasia is usually sporadic.

The second category of dysplasia includes the multicystic and aplastic kidney. The multicystic kidney is enlarged and distorted with numerous cysts, while the aplastic kidney is small and solid (Pathak & Williams 1964, Newman et al 1972). Either may be unilateral or bilateral, with the contralateral kidney, in unilateral cases, having a high incidence of renal and ureteral ectopia. The multicystic kidney usually lacks renal function, with total ureteropelvic obstruction. Many small aplastic kidneys have a patent renal pelvis and ureter. Theories of pathogenesis are controversial and obstruction has again been postulated to be the primary defect with secondary renal dysplasia. However, abnormal ureteric bud formation could be responsible for both obstruction and abnormal metanephric induction, resulting in dysplasia. Bilateral involvement, if associated with severe oligohydramnios, results in an infant with a phenotype consistent with the 'oligohydramnios tetrad'. Unilateral involvement usually has a good clinical prognosis, although opinions on management differ (Hartman et al 1986).

The final clinical category involves the association of renal dysplasia with distinct syndromes (Curry et al 1984) which must be considered when dysplasia is associated with unusual non-renal malformations. A complete list of these disorders is beyond the scope of this review but many are listed in Table 75.3. The Meckel syndrome, an autosomal recessive disorder, is an illustrative example with variable features of encephalocele, polydactyly, cleft palate and cystic dysplasia of the kidneys (Fried et al 1971, Mecke & Passarge 1971). The kidneys may be enlarged or hypoplastic with cysts and fibrosis present secondarily to markedly abnormal metanephric differentiation (Bernstein et al 1974). Prenatal diagnosis of this disorder has been accomplished (Chemke et al 1977, Kaffe et al 1977b, Shapiro et al 1977, Friedrich et al 1979, Nevin et al 1979) using both alphafetoprotein levels, elevated in the presence of an encephalocele, and sonographic detection of oligohydramnios and cystic kidneys. Both techniques should be utilized because of the variable occurrence of encephalocele and detectable renal involvement.

Although most cases of multicystic and aplastic dysplasia appear to be sporadic only a few adequate family studies utilizing sonographic or radiograhic techniques have been performed. Families with affected siblings (Cole et al 1976, Krous & Wenzl 1980) and also pedigrees consistent with possible autosomal dominant inheritance with variable expression (Buchta et al 1973, Zonna et al 1976, Schimke & King 1980, Roodhooft et al 1984) have been reported. The gene expression within a family may range from renal duplication to severe dysplasia. Complete renal agenesis is now recognized as the most extreme expression of this abnormal gene influencing ureteric bud development, and the genetic trait has been termed 'hereditary renal adysplasia'. The familial cases of dysplasia are clinically and pathologically indistinguishable from sporadic cases.

Further work will be necessary to define the contribution of genetic factors and their heterogeneity in the different types of dysplasia. In the second category, multicystic and aplastic kidneys, an ultrasound investigation of first-degree relatives should be recommended. Estimates of the empiric recurrence risk for significant bilateral renal malformations in families who have had a previous child with bilateral dysplasia or a bilateral combination of agenesis and dysplasia has varied in three studies from 0–4.5% (Roodhooft et al 1984, Al Saadi et al 1984, Bankier et al 1985). Prenatal diagnosis of severe dysplasia has been accomplished by sonography during the second and third trimester (Bartley et al 1977, Mendoza et al 1979, Older et al 1979, Grannum et al 1980, Cass et al 1981, Grupe 1987, Rizzo et al 1987), but one must be aware that both false positive and negative diagnoses have been made. The kidney to abdominal circumference ratio may be elevated in cases with multicystic kidneys and reduced in those with aplastic or hypoplastic kidneys. Abnormal renal structures, including cysts, may be detectable during the later part of the second trimester.

Structural abnormalities of the ureter

Less severe ureteral malformations also have a hereditary basis. A duplication anomaly of the urinary tract involves a duplex kidney with separate calyceal systems. The two ureters may join, as a bifid ureter, or open independently into the bladder (Churchill et al 1987). The reported (Privett et al 1976) incidence of duplication anomalies varies from 1:50 to 1:300, with approximately 20% bilateral involvement. The overall clinical prognosis for patients with a duplication anomaly is good. It can be associated with hydronephrosis, ureterocele and pyelonephritis, but the great majority of individuals are asymptomatic. Abnormal division during ureteric bud formation can be postulated as the pathogenetic mechanism. Affected females outnumber males by two to one and several studies (Girsh & Karpinski 1956, Whitaker & Danks 1966, Atwell et al 1974) have reported an apparent autosomal dominant pattern of inheritance with variable expression. Duplications are a relatively minor ureteric bud abnormality and may be the result of a single gene abnormality. They can be associated with more severe disturbance of ureteric bud morphogenesis, which may be inherited as an apparent autosomal dominant trait and involve either a different gene locus or be allelic disorders (Perlman et al 1976).

An abnormal vesicoureteral junction may also result from abnormal ureteric bud morphogenesis and cause vesicoureteral reflux. The clinical significance of ureteral reflux has been widely debated (Woodard & Rushton 1987). Many pedigrees have been published (Mulcahy et al 1970, Miller & Caspari 1972, Mobley 1973, Fried et al 1975, Lewy & Belman 1975, Sengar et al 1979, Chapman et al 1985, Van den Abbeele et al 1987) and autosomal dominant inheritance with variable expression appears to be the mode of inheritance. A 45% incidence of reflux was recently reported in 60 asymptomatic sibs of 54 probands (mean age 4.2 years) (Van den Abbeele et al 1987). It has been recommended that all young asymptomatic first-degree relatives should be screened by radionuclide scanning to detect asymptomatic reflux. This should allow early monitoring and treatment of affected individuals.

MALFORMATION SYNDROMES AND ASSOCIATED URINARY TRACT ABNORMALITIES

Malformations of the urinary tract are observed in association with, or are an integral part of, a wide variety of syndromes. The available data for many syndromes contain bias of ascertainment, making the validity of some associations uncertain. The high frequency of urinary tract anomalies in the general population confounds this issue further, since the incidence of urinary tract malformations in some syndromes does not appear to be significantly higher (Kissane 1966, Egli & Stadler 1973, Royer et al 1974, Berry & Chantler 1986). Among the disorders discussed or tabulated below there may be chance associations which are not truly indicative of increased risk for urinary tract malformations. Well-documented syndromes with associated urinary tract malformations have been divided into chromosomal and non-chromosomal categories.

Urinary tract malformations occur with increased frequency in patients with many of the well-defined chromosomal syndromes (Table 75.2). As more patients are studied some of the less common syndromes will undoubtedly also be shown to have an increase in associated urinary tract malformations. Of the two most common syndromes, the Turner and Down syndromes, urinary tract anomalies are more numerous in the former, with an overall frequency of about 60% (Reveno & Palubinskas 1966, Hung & Lopresti 1968, Persky & Owens 1971, Egli & Stadler 1973, Litvak et al 1978). In contrast, the risk for patients with trisomy 21 is about 3–7%, only a modest increase over general population figures (Kissane 1966, Egli & Stadler 1973, Royer et al 1974). The identification of a chromosome anomaly in an individual with a urinary tract malformation would generally decrease the chances of recurrence for that malformation in other family members, unless a structural rearrangement is present and one of the parents is a balanced translocation carrier.

Urinary tract anomalies commonly observed in the Turner syndrome include horseshoe kidney, duplication of the collecting system, positional and rotational anomalies, multicystic kidney, and agenesis (Reveno & Palubinskas 1966, Hung & Lopresti 1968, Persky & Owen 1971, Egli & Stadler 1973, Litvak et al 1978). Horseshoe kidneys and duplication are the most common lesions and each is present in about 20% of patients. In patients with Turner syndrome there is no clear correlation between the nature of the X chromosome abnormality and the type or frequency of urinary tract lesions, except perhaps for a slightly lower reported frequency of malformations associated with mosaic 45,X karyotypes (Egli & Stadler 1973). The natural history of urinary tract anomalies in the Turner syndrome, as well as in the general population, is uncertain. Most patients apparently remain asymptomatic, but little information has been published about older individuals. The reported increase in urinary tract infections in chromosomally normal patients with similar urinary tract malformations suggests the need for careful long-term follow-up (Kunin et al 1960, Smellie et al 1964). Obstructive lesions of the urinary tract require prompt correction. All patients with the Turner syndrome should have intravenous pyelography and serum creatinine determinations in the initial evaluation. In prepubertal children an excellent estimate of glomerular filtration rate can be obtained by relating height to plasma creatinine level (Schwartz et al 1976), avoiding the need to do bothersome and frequently inaccurate 24-hour creatinine clearance studies. Periodic screening for asymptomatic urinary tract infections may be beneficial (Kunin 1971). Patients with the Turner syndrome and urinary tract abnormalities are also at risk for hypertension (Haddad & Wilkins 1959). Blood pressure should be measured regularly paying careful attention to technique and age-related standards.

Urinary tract malformations associated with non-chromosomal syndromes are summarized in Table 75.3. The large number of disorders precludes individual discussion in this chapter. Many of the urinary tract anomalies are similar to those discussed above and the same general diagnostic approach and follow-up methods are appropriate. The realization that a renal malformation is part of a single gene disorder may alter the recurrence risk dramatically for other family members.

NEOPLASTIC DISORDERS

Renal tumours generally occur sporadically but are found with increased frequency in association with some malformation syndromes and inherited diseases. Familial cases without obvious associated underlying diseases have also been reported. (Table 75.4).

The most common neoplastic condition affecting the kidney during childhood is Wilms tumour, a solid retroperitoneal neoplasm arising from embryonic renal tissue. The first conditions clearly proven to bear an increased risk of Wilms tumour were sporadic aniridia and hemihypertrophy (Miller et al 1964). A similar association was later demonstrated for the Wiedemann-Beckwith syndrome of omphalocele, visceromegaly, and macroglossia (Beckwith 1969). More recently, patients with the Drash syndrome of renal insufficiency, gonadal neoplasia and ambiguous genitalia (Manivel et al 1987), the Perlman syndrome of fetal gigantism, renal dysplasia and multiple congenital anomalies (Greenberg et al 1986), and possibly the Sotos syndrome (Maldonado et al 1984), have also been found to share this risk.

The increased risk for Wilms tumour, perhaps a 33% incidence (Turleau et al 1984), is almost exclusively associated with sporadic aniridia, often combined with ambiguous genitalia in males, external ear malformations, microcephaly, coarse (perhaps characteristic) facies and mental retardation. The discovery of small deletion on the short arm of chromosome 11 (at 11p13) in many of these cases has helped to clarify the Wilms-aniridia relationship considerably (Riccardi et al 1978, Yunis & Ramsay 1980, Turleau et al 1984). Rare families with autosomal dominant aniridia and Wilms tumour appear to carry the 11p deletion (Yunis & Ramsay 1980). More commonly, autosomal dominant anirida is caused by a gene which has been mapped to chromosome 2p (Ferrell et al 1980). For these patients the risk of developing Wilms tumour is apparently not increased.

Wilms tumour also occurs on a familial basis unassociated with other anomalies (Fitzgerald & Hardin 1955, Brown et al 1972, Knudson & Strong 1972, Cordero et al 1980). The reported frequency of familial Wilms tumour varies greatly with no obvious explanation for the observed differences (Knudson & Strong 1972, Cordero et al 1980). Familial Wilms tumour appears to be bilateral more often than expected (Knudson & Strong 1972, Bond 1975). The histological appearance of familial Wilms tumour includes subcapsular dysplasia, an abnormality not observed in sporadic or syndrome-associated Wilms tumours (Miller 1980).

Screening for early detection of Wilms tumour is prudent when a patient at increased risk has been identified. No agreement has been reached, however, on how screening should be done and whether it is efficacious. Intravenous pyelography at frequent intervals is unsatisfactory from the standpoint of radiation exposure, cost, risk, and discomfort to the patient. In addition, large tumours have been discovered shortly after a normal pyelogram. Abdominal ultrasound examination has few of these objections and coupled with frequent, careful abdominal examinations and evaluation for haematuria,

Table 75.4   Renal tumours associated with hereditary disorders or malformation syndromes

Tumour type	Syndrome	Inheritance of primary condition	Risk of developing tumour
Hamartoma	Tuberous sclerosis	AD	50–60 %
Renal cell carcinoma:			
	Von Hippel-Lindau	AD	?
	Familial	AD ? (see text)	?
	Translocation	Chromosomal	?
Wilms tumour:			
	Aniridia	Chromsomal ?	see text
	Drash	AD	?
	Familial Wilms	AD?	?
	Hemihypertrophy	Sporadic	?
	Perlman	AR	100% ?
	Sotos	AD	?
	Wiedemann-Beckwith	AD	?

should be an acceptable screening approach. A reasonable protocol consists of abdominal examination and urinalysis every one to two months, with ultrasound examinations at two to four month intervals during the period of highest risk, birth to 4 years of age, depending of course on the degree of risk.

Surgery, radiotherapy and chemotherapy have dramatically improved survival with reported cure rates of 50–95% depending on the stage of the tumour (D'Angio et al 1984). Female survivors of Wilms tumour who were treated with radiation appear to have higher than expected risks during pregnancy due to an increased incidence of prematurity and perinatal death (Li et al 1987).

Familial cases of renal cell carcinoma are occasionally reported (Rusche 1953, Guirguis 1973). Some of these families may also have von-Hippel-Lindau disease, known to be associated with this tumour (Kaplan et al 1961). Of interest in light of the 11p deletion-Wilms tumour association noted above, however, are two reports of renal cell carcinoma associated with apparently balanced translocations involving chromosome 3 (Cohen et al 1979, Pathak et al 1982).

Accumulating evidence suggests that both Wilms tumour and renal cell carcinoma frequently result from the loss of important tumour-suppressing DNA sequences (Friend et al 1988), thus supporting and expanding the scope of the 'two hit' hypothesis first postulated by Knudson and Strong (1972) as an explanation for the role of 'mutation' in the aetiology of Wilms tumour. In children with aniridia and Wilms tumour the first 'hit' is the 11p13 deletion. Subsequently a second, somatic, event removes the tumour-suppressing effect at an as-yet-undetermined locus in this region. This mechanism appears to explain not only Wilms tumours associated with sporadic aniridia but also tumours in the Wiedemann-Beckwith (Koufos et al 1985), Drash and Perlman syndromes (Dao et al 1987). In each disorder the 11p region has been implicated suggesting that closely related molecular mechanisms are responsible for all four disorders. The corollary that sporadic cases of Wilms tumour result from loss of heterozygosity as a consequence of somatic events (mutation, recombination, or rearrangement) has also been demonstrated (Dao et al 1987).

Evidence for loss of DNA sequences on the short arm of chromosome 3 in sporadic cases of renal cell carcinoma suggests that the same mechanism is operational for this tumour as well (Zbar et al 1987, Friend et al 1988). In all likelihood then, the families noted above with translocations involving chromosome 3 have an unbalanced rearrangement, undetectable by cytogenetic techniques, resulting in the loss of a tumour-suppressing locus.

NEPHROPATHY

Nephropathy (including nephritis) occurs as part of a heterogeneous group of disorders, some of which involve only the kidney, while others affect multiple organ systems. Profound impairment of renal function often results in the need for dialysis and/or transplantation. Glomerular lesions are always present but histological abnormalities in other parts of the kidney are also frequently evident. Hereditary disorders associated with nephritis or nephropathy are summarized in Table 75.5.

The prototypic hereditary nephropathy is the Alport syndrome, characterized by recurrent haematuria, progressive renal insufficiency and hearing loss (Alport 1927). Haematuria is usually the earliest manifestation and may follow respiratory infections as early as the first few months of life. Microscopic haematuria is usually evident between episodes of intermittent gross haematuria, which may be severe enough to cause renal colic. Proteinuria is usually mild early in the course of the disease. A variety of non-renal abnormalities have been reported in association with familial nephritis, most notably sensorineural hearing loss, cataracts and platelet anomalies. Although previously thought to represent variability within a single disorder, more recent evidence suggests the existence of as many as six different conditions (Hasstedt et al 1986, Atkin et al 1988). The association of familial nephritis with hyperprolinaemia does not appear to represent a distinct disorder (Kopelman et al 1964, Efron 1965).

The natural history of familial nephritis is variable, although affected males generally have a more severe and more rapidly progressive disease than females. Some of the reported variability may be a consequence of genetic heterogeneity. Following the onset of haematuria, glomerular filtration decreases and proteinuria, but rarely the nephrotic syndrome, develops. Uraemia may occur in a few years or as much as several decades later. Patients at risk for familial nephritis may be identified by the presence of microscopic haematuria, but in the absence of a family history the earliest manifestations in the child may be decreased appetite and activity, poor growth, and pallor. Occasionally hypertensive encephalopathy and seizures are the first signs of uraemia. Affected males usually have end-stage renal disease by the third or fourth decade and, untreated, die of uraemia (Gubler et al 1981). Females rarely progress to uraemia, usually experiencing intermittent episodes of haematuria along with some decrease in glomerular filtration rate. The occasional female with a severe clinical course emphasizes the need for regular medical observation of all cases. The complications observed in the Alport syndrome and other forms of familial nephropathy are generally those seen in end-stage renal disease and, unfortunately, no specific therapy exists. Dialysis and/or transplantation have been used successfully.

Differentiating familial nephropathy from sporadic forms is difficult in the absence of a positive family history. Numerous causes of recurrent haematuria including infections, calculi, tumours, nonfamilial benign recurrent haematuria, and other types of nephritis must be considered. In patients with strong evidence for nephropathy a renal biopsy is often helpful, but the findings may not be pathognomonic. The most characteristic renal biopsy findings in familial progressive nephritis are split, lamellated or irregularly thickened glomerular basement membranes (found on electron microscopy) and interstitial foam cells (Bernstein 1979, Gubler et al 1981). Other conditions associated with familial nephritis must be sought, in particular high frequency hearing loss, ocular abnormalities, and abnormalities of platelet size and function.

The pathogenesis of the Alport syndrome is unknown, but available data support the hypothesis of a primary basement membrane defect (Spear 1984). No primary immune-mediated abnormalities have been demonstrated, but some glomeruli have secondary deposition of immunoglobulins and complement (Spear et al 1970). Although Alport syndrome was previously thought to follow an autosomal dominant inheritance pattern, more recent mapping with DNA markers suggests X–linkage (Atkin et al 1988). Several loci may be involved in producing the Alport phenotype, however, and kindreds with autosomal dominant inheritance of progressive nephritis may exist.

Genetic counselling for progressive nephritis depends greatly upon careful evaluation of all potentially informative family members. Although some cases are presumed to result from new mutations many affected individuals will have one or more family members with some demonstrable evidence of the Alport syndrome. All examined individuals should have urinalysis, serum creatinine determinations, and audiological and ophthalmological examinations, except perhaps in kindreds known not to have associated ocular or hearing abnormalities. Recurrence risks for X–linked disorders should be used unless strong evidence for an alternative inheritance pattern is available for a particular family. Variability of expression must be emphasized, particularly the differences between affected males and females. Prenatal diagnosis is currently unavailable but some families might choose to identify fetal sex and carry only female fetuses to term. The small but definite risk of severe nephritis in affected females must be clearly understood in this situation. More refined mapping of the locus or loci which produce the Alport syndrome should soon make prenatal diagnosis feasible, at least for families who happen to have informative DNA markers.

Several other inherited varieties of familial nephropathy are known (Table 75.5). Hereditary immune nephritis is distinguished from the Alport syndrome by earlier development of proteinuria and sudden onset of oliguric renal failure with evidence of consumption coagulopathy and low levels of the third component of the complement system (Teisberg et al 1973). Patients with familial deficiency of the second component of complement (C2) develop mild mesangial nephritis without evidence of systemic disease (Sobel et al 1979). Progressive glomerulonephritis, leading to uraemia, occurs in association with two familial skeletal disorders, the nail-patella syndrome (osteo-onycho-dysplasia) and asphyxiating thoracic dysplasia. Of particular concern is the extremely rapid progression to end-stage disease seen occasionally in the nail-patella syndrome (Bennett et al 1973). Transplantation has been successful in patients with each disorder.

Table 75.5 Syndromes with nephritis or nephropathy

Syndrome	Inheritance
Alport syndrome (Atkin et al 1988)	
Type 1 Juvenile onset, deafness, cataracts	Dominant
Type 2 Juvenile onset, deafness, cataracts	XLR
Type 3 Adult onset, deafness	XLR
Type 4 Adult onset	XLR
Type 5 Deafness, thrombocytopathia	Autosomal
Type 6 Juvenile onset, cataracts	Autosomal
APRT deficiency (nephropathy, stones) (Kamatani et al 1987)	AD
Dento-renal-amelogenesis imperfecta (Lubinsky et al 1985)	AR
Drash syndrome (nephritis, pseudohermaphrodite, Wilms) (Manivel et al 1987)	AD
Fabry (Desnick & Bishop 1989)	XLR
Jeune (asphyxiating thoracic dystrophy) (Donaldson & Warner 1985)	AR
Laurence-Moon-Biedl (Linne et al 1986)	AR
Lemieux-Neemeh (deafness, neuropathy, nephritis) (Hanson et al 1970)	AD
Mainzer-Saldino (retinal dysplasia, nephropathy, skeletal anomalies) (Cantani et al 1985)	AR
Nezelof (arthrogryposis, nephropathy, hepatic disease) (Nezelof et al 1979)	AR
Osteolysis and chronic progressive glomerulopathy (Torg & Steel 1968, Hardegger et al 1985)	AD
Perlman (gigantism, renal dysplasia, Wilms tumour) (Greenberg et al 1986)	AR
Senior (retinitis pigmentosa, nephronophthisis) (Senior 1973)	AR
Spondylometaphyseal dysplasia (Carter et al 1985)	AR
Wiskott-Aldrich (Spitler et al 1980)	XLR

In addition to disorders with clearly defined Mendelian patterns of inheritance, a variety of acquired renal disorders appear to have either significant underlying genetic factors involved in the pathogenesis of the disorder, or else have genetic forms which mimic the usual acquired variety. Accumulating evidence suggests that a fairly common disease, IgA nephropathy (Berger disease), has a strong genetic component (Edigo et al 1987, O'Connell et al 1987). In the haemolytic-uraemic syndrome, the incidence of reported familial cases is higher than expected, as is the severity compared with non-familial cases (Rogers et al 1986, Kaplan & Proesmans 1987). A defect in prostacyclin metabolism may be involved in its pathogenesis (Turi et al 1986).

REFFERENCES

Ainbender E, Brown E 1976 Bilateral renal agenesis and serum α fetoprotein. The Lancet 1 (1 January): 99

Alport A C 1927 Hereditary familial congenital haemorrhagic nephritis. British Medical Journal 1: 504–506

Al Saadi A A, Yoshimoto M, Bree R et al 1984 A family study of renal dysplasia. American Journal of Medical Genetics 19: 669–677

Anderson D, Tanner R L 1969 Tuberous sclerosis and chronic renal failure. American Journal of Medicine 47 (July): 163–168

Arant B S Jr, Sotelo-Avila C, Bernstein J 1979 Segmental 'hypoplasia' of the kidney (Ask-Upmark). The Journal of Pediatrics 95 (6 December): 931–939

Arends N W 1975 Bilateral renal agenesis in siblings. Journal of the American Osteopathic Association 56: 681

Atkin C L, Hasstedt S J, Menlove L et al 1988 Mapping of Alport syndrome to the long arm of the X chromosome. American Journal of Human Genetics 42: 249–255

Atwell J D, Cook P L, Howell C J, Hyde I, Parker B C 1974 Familial incidence of bifid and double ureters. Archives of Diseases in Childhood 49: 390–393

Bader J L, Li F P, Gerald P S, Leikin S L, Randolph J G 1979 11p chromosome deletion in four patients with aniridia and Wilm's tumour (Abstract 850) Proceedings of the American Association of Cancer Research 20: 210

Bain A, Scott J 1960 Renal agenesis and severe urinary tract dysplasia. British Medical Journal 1: 841

Balfour R P, Laurence K M 1980 Raised serum AFP levels and fetal renal agenesis. The Lancet 1 (1 February): 317

Bankier A, De Campo M, Newell R, Rogers J G, Danks D M 1985 A pedigree study of perinatally lethal renal disease. Journal of Medical Genetics 22: 104–111

Baron C 1954 Bilateral agenesis of the kidneys in two consecutive infants. American Journal of Obstetrics and Gynecology 67: 667

Barry J E, Auldist A W 1974 The VATER association. American Journal of Diseases of Children 128: 769–771

Bartley J A, Golbus M S, Filly R A, Hall B D 1977 Prenatal diagnosis of dysplastic kidney disease. Clinical Genetics 11: 375–378

Bartsocas C S, Weber A L, Crawford J D 1970 Acrocephalosyndactyly type III Chotzen's syndrome. Journal of Pediatrics 77: 267–272

Beckwith J B 1969 Malformation syndromes. Birth Defects: Original Article Series V (2): 188–196

Bennett W M, Musgrave J E, Campbell R A et al 1973 The nephropathy of the nail-patella syndrome. American Journal of Medicine 54(3): 304–319

Bergsma D (ed) 1979 Birth defects compendium, 2nd edn. Alan Liss, New York

Bernstein J 1968 Developmental abnormalities of the renal parenchyma - renal hypoplasia and dysplasia. In: Sommers S C (ed) Pathology Annual. Appleton Century-Crofts, New York, ch 3, p 213–247

Bernstein J 1971 The morphogenesis of renal parenchymal maldevelopment (renal dysplasia). Pediatric Clinics of North America 18 (2 May): 395–407

Bernstein J 1978 Renal hypoplasia and dysplasia. In: Edelmann C M Jr (ed) Pediatric Kidney Disease. Little Brown and Company, Boston, vol II, ch 39, p 541

Bernstein J 1979 Hereditary renal disease. Monographs of Pathology, ch 13, 295–326

Bernstein J, Brough A J, McAdams A J 1974 The renal lesion in syndromes of multiple congenital malformations. Birth Defects: Original Article Series X(4): 35–43

Bernstein J, Fleischmann L E, Risdon R A Crocker J F S, Schimke R N 1975 Structural Maldevelopment of the kidney. In: Rubin M I (ed) Pediatric nephrology. The Williams and Wilkins Company, Baltimore, ch 13, p 337–373; 670; 721–728

Berry A C, Chantler C 1986 Urogenital malformations and disease.British Medical Bulletin 42: 181–186

Biedel C W, Pagon R A, Zapata J O 1984 Mullerian anomalies and renal agenesis: autosomal dominant urogenital adysplasia. Journal of Pediatrics 104: 861–863

Blackburn M G Belliveau R E 1971 Ellis–van Creveld syndrome. The American Journal Diseases of Children 122: 267–270

Bois E, Feingold J, Benmaiz H, Briard M L 1975 Congenital urinary tract malformations: epidemiologic and genetic aspects. Clinical Genetics 8: 37–47

Bond J V 1975 Bilateral Wilms's tumour: age at diagnosis, associated congenital anomalies and possible pattern of inheritance. The Lancet 2: 482–484

Braun W E, Strimlan C V, Negron A G et al 1975 The association of W17 with familial renal cell carcinoma. Tissue Antigens 6 (2 Aug): 101–104

Brown W T, Puranik S R, Altman D H et al 1972 Wilms tumour in three successive generations. Surgery 72: 756–761

Buchta R M, Viseskul C, Gilbert E F, Sarto G E, Opitz J M 1973 Familial bilateral renal agenesis and hereditary renal adysplasia. Zeitschrift fur Kinderheilkunde 115: 111–129

Burk D, Beaudoin A R 1977 Arsenate-induced renal agenesis in rats. Teratology 16: 247–260

Cain et al 1974 Familial renal agenesis and total dysplasia, American Journal of Diseases of Children 128: 377

Caldamone A A, Rabinowitz R 1981 Crossed fused renal ectopia, orthotopic multicystic dysplasia and vaginal agenesis. Journal of Urology 126: 105–107

Cameron A H 1956 The spinal cord lesion in spina bifida cystica. The Lancet 2 (July): 171–174

Cantani A, Bamonte G, Ceccoli D 1985 Familial juvenile nephrophthisis. A review and differential diagnosis. Clinical Pediatrics 25: 90–95

Carter C O, Evans K, Pescia G 1979 A family study of renal agenesis. Journal of Medical Genetics 16: 176–188

Carter P, Burke J R, Searle J 1985 Renal abnormalities and spondylometaphyseal dysplasia. Australian Paediatric Journal 21: 115–117

Cass A, Veeraraghavan K, Smith S, Tsai S, Godec C, Bendel R 1981 Prenatal diagnosis of fetal urinary tract abnormalities by ultrasound. Urology 18: 197–202

Chantler C, Davies D H, Joseph M C 1966 Cardiovascular and other associations of infantile hyperglycemia. Guy's Hospital Reports 115: 221–241

Chapman C J, Bailey R R, Janus E D, Abbott G D, Lynn K L 1985 Vesicoureteric reflux: segregation analysis. American Journal of Medical Genetics 20: 577–584.

Chemke J, Miskin A, Rav-Acha Z, Porath A, Sagiv M, Katz Z 1977 Prenatal diagnosis of Meckel syndrome: alpha-feto protein and beta-trace protein in amniotic fluid. Clinical Genetics 11: 285–289

Churchill B, Abara E O, McLorie G 1987 Ureteral duplication, ectopy and ureteroceles. Pediatric Clinics of North America 34: 1273–1289

Cohen A J, Li F P, Berg S et al 1979 Hereditary renal cell carcinoma associated with chromosomal translocation. New England Journal of Medicine 301: 592–595

Cohen N, Berant M 1976 Duplications of the renal collecting system in the hereditary osteo-onycho-dysplasia syndrome. The Journal of Pediatrics 89 (2 August): 261–263

Cole B R, Kaufman R L, McAlister W H, Kissane J M 1976 Bilateral renal dysplasia in three siblings: report of a survivor. Clinical Nephrology 5(2): 83–87

Cordero J F, Li F P, Holmes L B, Gerald P S 1980 Wilms tumour in five cousins. Pediatrics 66(5): 716–719

Cramer D V, Gill T J 1975 Genetics of urogenital abnormalities in ACI inbred rats. Teratology 12: 27–32

Cullen S I, Harris D E, Carter C H, Reed W B 1969 Congenital unilateral ichthyosiform erythroderma. Archives of Dermatology 99 (June): 724–729

Curry C J R, Jensen K, Holland J, Miller L, Hall B D 1984 The Potter sequence: a clinical analysis of 80 cases. American Journal of Medical Genetics 19: 679–702

D'Angio G J, Evans A E, Breslow N 1984 Results of the Third National Wilms' Tumor Study. Proceedings of the American Association for Cancer Research 25: 183

Danks D M 1975 Cerebrohepatorenal syndrome of Zellweger. Journal of Pediatrics 86 (3): 382–387

Dao D D, Schroeder W T, Chao L et al 1987 Genetic mechanisms of tumour-specific loss of 11p DNA sequences in Wilms tumor. American Journal of Human Genetics 41: 202–217

Dean W M, Bourdeau E J 1980 Amniotic fluid α fetoprotein in fetal obstructive uropathy. Pediatrics 66 (4 October): 537–539

Desnick R J, Bishop D F 1989 Fabry's disease. In: Scriver C R et al (eds) The Metabolic Basis of Inherited Disease. McGraw Hill, New York, p 1751–1796

Dieker H, Opitz J M 1969 Associated acral and renal malformations. Birth Defects: Original Article Series V (3): 68–77

Doege T C, Thuline H C, Priest J H, Norby D E, Bryant J S 1964 Studies of a family with the oral facial digital syndrome. New England Journal of Medicine 271: (November): 1073–1080

Donaldson M D C, Warner A A 1985 Familial juvenile nephronophthisis, Jeune's syndrome, and associated disorders. Archives of Disease in Childhood 60: 426–434

Dubbins P A, Kurtz A B, Wapner R J, Goldberg B B 1981 Renal agenesis: Spectrum of in-utero findings. Journal of Clinical Ultrasound 9: 189–193

Duncan P A 1977 Embryologic pathogenesis of renal agenesis associated with cervical vertebral anomalies (Klippel-Feil phenotype). Birth Defects: Original Article Series XIII (3D): 91–101

Duncan P A, Shapiro L R, Stangel J J, Klein R M, Addonizio J C 1979 The MURCS associations: Mullerian duct aplasia, renal aplasia, and cervicothoracic somite dysplasia. The Journal of Pediatrics 95 (3 September): 399–402

Edelmann C M Jr (ed) 1978 Pediatric kidney disease, vol II. Little Brown, Boston, p537–586

Edigo J, Julian B A, Wyatt R J 1987 Genetic factors in primary IgA nephropathy. Nephrology, Dialysis, Transplantation 134–142

Elfron M L 1965 Familial hyperprolinemia. New England Journal of Medicine 272 (June): 1243–1254

Egli F, Stadler G 1973 Malformations of kidney and urinary tract in common chromosomal aberrations. Humangenetik 18: 1–32

Elejalde B R 1979 Genetic and diagnostic considerations in three families with abnormalities of facial expression and congenital urinary obstruction. American Journal of Medical Genetics 3: 97–108

Emanuel B, Nachman R, Aronson N, Weiss H 1974 Congenital solitary kidney. American Journal of Diseases of Children 127 (January): 17–19

Fairley K F, Leighton P W, Kincaid-Smith P 1963 Familial visual defects associated with polycystic kidneys and medullary sponge kidney. British Medical Journal 1: 1060–1063

Feinman N L, Yakovac W C 1970 Neurofibromatosis in childhood. Journal of Pediatrics 76(3): 339–346

Ferrel R E, Chakravarti A, Hittner H M, Riccardi V M 1980 Autosomal dominant aniridia: probable linkages to acid phosphatase-1 on chromosome 2. Proceedings of the National Academy of Sciences 77: 1580–1582

Fitch N 1977 Heterogeneity of bilateral renal agenesis. Canadian Medical Association Journal 116 (February): 381–382.

Fitch N, Srolovitz H 1976 Severe renal dysgenesis produced by a dominant gene. American Journal of Diseases of Children 130 (December): 1356–1357

Fitzgerald W L, Hardin H C Jr 1955 Bilateral Wilms Tumor in Wilms Tumor family: case report. Journal of Urology 73: 468–474

France N E, Crome L, Abraham J M 1969 Pathological features in the deLange syndrome. Acta Paediatrica Scandinavica 58: 470–480

Francke U, Riccardi V, Hittner M, Barges W 1978 Interstitial del (11p) as a cause of the aniridia-Wilms tumor association: band localization and a heritable basis. American Journal of Human Genetics 30: 81a

Francke U, Holmer L B, Atkins L, Riccardi V M 1979

Aniridia-Wilms' tumor association: evidence for specific deletion of 11p13. Cytogenetics and Cell Genetics 24: 185–192

Freeman M V R, Williams D W, Schimke R N et al 1974 The Roberts syndrome. Clinical Genetics 5: 1–16

Fried A M, Oliff M, Wilson E A, Whisnant J 1978 Uterine anomalies associated with renal agenesis: role of gray scale ultrasonography. American Journal of Roentgenology 131 (December): 973–975

Fried K, Liban E, Lurie M, Friedman S, Reisner S H 1971 Polycystic kidneys associated with malformations of the brain, polydactyly and other birth defects in new born sibs. Journal of Medical Genetics 8 (September): 285–290

Fried K, Yuval E, Eidelman A, Beer S 1975 Familial primary vesicoureteral reflux. Clinical Genetics 7: 144–147

Friedrich U, Hansen K B Hauge M et al 1979 Prenatal diagnosis of polycystic kidneys and encephalocele (Meckel-syndrome). Clinical Genetics 15: 278–286

Friend S H, Dryja T P, Weinberg R A 1988 Oncogenes and tumor-suppressing genes. New England Journal of Medicine 318: 618–622

Girsh L S, Karpinski F E Jr 1956 Urinary tract malformations: their familial occurrence, with special reference to double ureter, double pelvis and double kidney. The New England Journal of Medicine 254 (18 May): 854–855

Gorlin R J, Pinborg J J, Cohen M M 1976 Syndromes of the head and neck, 2nd edn. McGraw-Hill, New York

Gorvoy J D, Smulewiez J et al 1962 Unilateral renal agenesis in two siblings. Pediatrics 29: 270

Grannum P, Bracken M, Silverman R, Hobbins J C 1980 Assessment of fetal kidney size in normal gestation by comparison of ratio of kidney circumference to abdominal circumference. American Journal of Obstetrics and Gynecology 136 (2 January): 249–254

Greenberg F, Stein F, Gresik M V, Finegold M J, Carpenter R J, Riccardi V M, Beaudet A L 1986 The Perlman familial nephroblastomatosis syndrome. American Journal of Medical Genetics 24: 101–110

Gribetz M E, Leiter E 1978 Ectopic ureterocele, hydroureter, and renal dysplasia. Urology XI (2 February): 131–133

Grupe W E 1987 The dilemma of intrauterine diagnosis of congenital renal disease. Pediatric Clinics of North America 34: 629–638

Gruskin A B, Baluarte H J, Cote M L, Elfenben I B 1974 The renal disease of thoracic asphyxiant dystrophy. Birth Defects: Original Article Series X (4): 44–50

Gubler M, Levy M, Broyer M, Naizot C, Gonzales G, Perrin D, Habib R 1981 Alport's syndome. A report of 58 cases and a review of the literature. American Journal of Medicine 70: 493–505

Guirguis A B 1973 Renal cell carcinoma: unusual occurrence in four members of one family. Urology 2: 283–285

Hack M Jaffe J, Blankstein J, Goodman R M, Brish M 1974 Familial aggregation in bilateral renal agenesis. Clinical Genetics 5: 173–177

Haddad H M, Wilkins L 1959 Congenital anomalies associated with gonadal aplasia: review of 55 cases. Pediatrics 23: 885–902

Hanson P, Farber R E, Armstrong R A 1970 Distal muscle wasting, nephritis, and deafness. Neurology 20: 426–434

Hardegger F, Simpson L A, Segmueller G 1985 The syndrome of idiopathic osteolysis: Classification, review and case report. Journal of Bone and Joint Surgery 67B: 89–93

Hartman G E, Smolik L M, Shochat S J 1986 The dilemma

of the multicystic dysplastic kidney. American Journal of Diseases of Children 140: 925–928

Haslam R H A, Berman W, Heller R M 1973 Renal abnormalities in the Russell–Silver syndrome. Pediatrics 51(2): 216–222

Hasstedt S J, Atkin C L, Alberto C S J, Jr 1986 Genetic heterogeneity among kindreds with Alport syndrome. American Journal of Human Genetics 38: 940–953

Hilson D 1957 Malformation of ears as sign of malformation of genito-urinary tract. British Medical Journal 2 (October): 785–789

Hislop A, Hey E, Reid L 1979 The lungs in congenital bilateral renal agenesis and dysplasia. Archives of Disease in Childhood 54: 32–38

Hjalmarson O, Sabel K G 1978 Bilateral renal aplasia without Potter's syndrome. Acta Paediatrica Scandinavica 67: 212–213

Holmes L B 1972 Unilateral renal agenesis: common, serious, hereditary. Pediatric Research 6(4): 419

Hung W, Lopresti J 1968 The high frequency of abnormal excretory urograms in young patients with gonadal dysgenesis. Journal of Urology 98: 697–700

Hurley R M, Dery P, Nogrady M B, Drummond K N 1975 The renal lesion in the Laurence-Moon-Biedl syndrome. Journal of Pediatrics 87: 206–209

Ivemark B I, Oldfelt V, Zetterstrom R 1959 Familial dysplasia of kidneys, liver and pancreas: a probably genetically determined syndrome. Acta Paediatrica Scandinavica 48: 1–11

Jeanty P, Dramaix-Wilmet M, Elkhazen N, Hubinont C, Van Regemorter N 1982 Measurement of fetal kidney growth on ultrasound. Radiology 144: 159–162

Jenkin R D T 1976 The treatment of Wilms' tumor. Pediatric Clinics of North America 23: 147–160

Johanson A, Blizzard R 1971 A syndrome of congenital aplasia of the alae nasi, deafness, hypothyroidism, dwarfism, absent permanent teeth and malabsorption. Journal of Pediatrics 79: 982–987

Juberg R C, Hayward J R 1969 A new familial syndrome of oral, cranial and digital anomalies. Journal of Pediatrics 74: (May): 755–762

Kaffe S, Godmilow L, Walker B A, Hirchhorn K 1977a Prenatal diagnosis of bilateral renal agenesis. Obstetrics and Gynecology 49 (4 April): 478–480

Kaffe S, Rose J S, Godmilow L, Walker B A, Kerenyi T, Beratis N, Reyes P, Hirschhorn K 1977b. Prenatal diagnosis of renal anomalies. American Journal of Medical Genetics I: 241

Kamatani N, Terai C, Kuroshima S 1987 Genetic and clinical studies on 19 families with adenine phosphoribosyl transferase deficiencies. Human Genetics 75: 163–168

Kaplan B S, Proesmans W 1987 The hemolytic uremic syndrome of childhood and its variants. Seminars in Hematology 24: 148–160

Kaplan C, Sayre G P, Greene L F 1961 Bilateral nephrogenic carcinomas in Lindau-von Hippel disease. Journal of Urology 86: 36–42

Kaufman D B, McIntosh R M, Smith F G Jr, Vernier R L 1970 Diffuse familial nephropathy: a clinicopathologic study. Journal of Pediatrics 77(1): 37–47

Keirse M J N C, Meerman R H 1978 Antenatal diagnosis of Potter syndrome. Obstetrics and Gynecology 52 (1 July): 64s–67s

Kissane J M 1966 Congenital malformations. In: Heptinstall R H (ed) Pathology of the kidney. Little Brown, Boston

Knudson A G Jr, Strong L C 1972 Mutation and cancer: a model for Wilms tumor of the kidney. Journal of the National Cancer Institute 48: 313

Knudsen J B, Brun B, Hans C E 1979 Familial renal agenesis and urogenital malformations. Scandinavian Journal of Urology and Nephrology 13: 109–112

Kohn G, Borns P F 1973 The association of bilateral and unilateral renal aplasia in the same family. The Journal of Pediatrics 83 (1 July): 95–97

Kopelman H, Asatoor A W, Milne M D 1964 Hyperprolinemia and hereditary nephritis. Lancet 2 (November): 1075–1079

Koufos A, Hansen M F, Copeland N G, Jenkins N A, Lampkin B C, Cavenee W K 1985 Loss of heterozygosity in three embryonal tumors suggests a common pathogenetic mechanism. Nature 316: 330–334

Krous H F, Wenzl J E 1980 Familial renal cystic dysplasia associated with maternal diabetes mellitus. Southern Medical Journal 73 (1 January): 85–86

Kunin C M 1971 Epidemiology and natural history of urinary tract infection in school age children. Pediatric Clinics of North America 18(2 May): 509–528

Kunin C, Southall I, Paquin A J 1960 Epidemiology of urinary tract infections. New England Journal of Medicine 263: 817–823

Kurnit D M, Steele M W, Pinsky L, Dibbins A 1978 Autosomal dominant transmission of a syndrome of anal, ear, renal, and radial congenital malformations. The Journal of Pediatrics 93 (2 August): 270–273

Lemieux G, Neemeh J A 1967 Charcot-Marie-Tooth disease and nephritis. Canadian Medical Association Journal 96 (November): 1193–1198

Lewy P R, Belman A B 1975 Familial occurrence of nonobstructive, noninfectious vesicoureteral reflux with renal scarring. The Journal of Pediatrics 86 (6 June): 851–856

Li F P, Gimbrere K, Gelber R D et al 1987. Outcome of pregnancy in survivors of Wilms' tumor. JAMA 257: 216–219

Linne T, Wikstad I, Zetterstrom R 1986 Renal involvement in the Laurence-Moon-Biedl syndrome. Functional and radiological studies. Acta Paediatrica Scandinavica 75: 240–244

Litvak A S, Rousseau T G, Wrede L D, Mabry C C, McRoberts J W 1978 The association of significant renal anomalies with Turner's syndrome. The Journal of Urology 120 (December): 671–672

Loken A C, Hansson O, Halvorsen S, Jolstor N J 1961 Hereditary renal dysplasia and blindness. Acta Paediatrica Scandinavica 50 (March): 177–184

London R, Heredia R M, Israel J 1985 Urinary tract involvement in the EEC syndrome. American Journal of Diseases of Children 139: 1191–1193

Loughridge L W 1959 Renal abnormalities in the Marfan syndrome. Quarterly Journal of Medicine 28: 531–547

Lubinsky M, Angle C, Marsh P W 1985 Syndrome of amelogenesis imperfecta, nephrocalcinosis, impaired renal concentration, and possible abnormality of calcium metabolism. American Journal of Medical Genetics 20: 233–243

McConville J M, West C D McAdams A J 1966 Familial and nonfamilial benign hematuria. Journal of Pediatrics 69 (August): 207–214

McDonald R, Goldschmidt B 1959 Pancytopenia with congenital defects (Fanconi's anaemia). Archives of Diseases of Children 34: 367–372

McKusick V A 1972 Heritable disorders of connective tissue, 4th edn. C V Mosby, St Louis

McKusick V A 1988 Mendelian inheritance in man. 8th edn. The Johns Hopkins University Press, Baltimore

McPherson E, Carey J, Kramer A, Hall J G, Pauli R M, Schimke R N, Tasin M H 1987 Dominantly inherited renal adysplasia. American Journal of Medical Genetics 26: 863–872

Madisson V H 1934 Ueber das fehler beider nieren. Zentralblatt fur Allgemeine Pathologie 60: 1

Magee M C, Lucey D T, Fried F A 1979 A new embryologic classification for uro-gynecologic malformations: the syndromes of mesonephric duct induced Mullerian deformities. The Journal of Urology 121 (March) 265–267

Maldonado V, Gaynon P S, Poznanski A K 1984 Cerebral gigantism associated with Wilms' tumor. American Journal of Diseases of Children 138: 486–488

Manivel J C, Sibley R K, Dehner L P 1987 Complete and incomplete Drash syndrome: A clinicopathologic study of five cases of a dysontogenetic-neoplastic complex. Human Pathology 18: 80–89

Margileth A M, Filipesen N 1974 Initial urinary tract bacterial infection: an overview of clinical features, management and outcome in 64 children. Clinical Proceedings of Children's Hospital National Medical Center 30: 175

Marshall F F, Beisel D S 1978 The association of uterine and renal anomalies. Obstetrics and Gynecology 51 (5 May): 559–562

Marshall F F, Garcia-Bunuel R, Beisel D S 1978 Hydronephrosis, renal agenesis, and associated genitourinary anomalies in ACI rats. Urology XI (1 January): 58–61

Mauer S M, Dobrin R S, Vernier R L 1974 Unilateral and bilateral renal agenesis in monoamniotic twins. The Journal of Pediatrics 84 (2 February): 236–238

Mecke S, Passarge E 1971 Encephalocele, polycystic kidneys, and polydactyly as an autosomal recessive trait simulating certain other disorders: the Meckel syndrome. Annales de Génétique 14 (2): 97–103

Melnick M, Bixler D, Nance W E, Silk K, Yune H 1976 Familial branchio-oto-renal dysplasia: a new addition to the branchial arch syndromes. Clinical Genetics 9: 25–34

Melnick M, Hodes M E, Nance W E, Yune H, Sweeney A 1978 Branchio-oto-renal dysplasia and brancho-oto-dysplasia: two distinct autosomal dominant disorders. Clinical Genetics 13: 425–442

Mendoza S A, Griswold W R, Leopold G R, Kaplan G W 1979 Intrauterine diagnosis of renal anomalies by ultrasonography. American Journal of Diseases of Children 133 (October): 1042–1043

Menser M, Robertson S E J, Dorman D C, Gillespie A M, Murphy A M 1967 Renal lesions in congenital rubella.. Pediatrics 40 (November): 901–904

Miller H C, Caspari E W 1972 Ureteral reflux as genetic trait. Journal of the American Medical Association 220 (6 May): 842–843

Miller J Q 1963 Lissencephaly in two siblings. Neurology 13 (October): 841–850

Miller R W 1980 Birth defects and cancer due to small chromosomal deletions. Journal of Pediatrics 96: 1031

Miller R W, Franmeni J F Jr, Manning M D 1964 Association

of Wilms tumor with aniridia hemihypertrophy and other congenital malformations. New England Journal of Medicine 270: 922–927

Miskin M 1979 Prenatal diagnosis of renal agenesis by ultrasonography and maternal pyelography. American Journal of Roentgenology 132 (June): 1025

Mobley D F 1973 Familial vesicoureteral reflux. Urology 2: 514–518

Morse R P, Rawnsley E, Crowe H C, Marin-Padilla M, Graham J M J 1987 Bilateral renal agenesis in three consecutive siblings. Prenatal Diagnosis 7: 573–579

Mulcahy J J, Kelalis P P, Stickler G B, Burke E C 1970 Familial vesicoureteral reflux. Journal of Urology 104: 762–764

Museles M, Gaudry C L Jr, Bason W M 1971 Renal anomalies in the newborn found by deep palpation. Pediatrics 47: 97–100

Nadjini B, Flanagan M J, Christian J R 1969 Laurence-Moon-Biedl syndrome. American Journal of Diseases of Children 117: 352–356

Nevin N C, Ritchie A, McKeown F, Roberts G 1978 Raised alpha-fetoprotein levels in amniotic fluid and maternal serum associated with distension of the fetal bladder caused by absence of the urethra. Journal of Medical Genetics 15: 61–78

Nevin N C, Thompson W, Davison G, Horner W T 1979 Prenatal diagnosis of the Meckel syndrome. Clinical Genetics 15: 1–4

Newman L, Simms K, Kissane J, McAlister W H 1972 Unilateral total renal dysplasia in children. American Journal of Roentgenology, Radiotherapy and Nuclear Medicine 116 (December): 778–784

Nezelof C, Dupart M C, Jaubert F 1979 A lethal familial syndrome associating arthrogryposis multiplex congenita, renal dysfunction, and a cholestatic and pigmentary liver disease. Journal of Pediatrics 94: 258–260

Noe H N, Peeden J N, Jerkins G R, Wilroy R S 1985 Hypertelorism — Hypospadias Syndrome. Journal of Urology 132: 951–952

O'Connell P J, Harris M, Ibels L S, Eckstein R P, Thomas M A 1987 Familial IgA nephropathy: A study of renal disease in an Australian aboriginal family. Australian and New Zealand Journal of Medicine. 17: 27–33

Ogreid P, Hatteland K 1979 Cyst of seminal vesicle associated with ipsilateral renal agenesis. Scandinavian Journal of Urology and Nephrology 13: 113–116

Older R A, Hinman C G, Crane L M, Cleeve D M, Morgan C L 1979 In utero diagnosis of multicystic kidney by gray scale ultrasonography. American Journal of Roentgenology 133 (July): 130–131

Opitz J M 1987 Editorial comment: Vaginal atresia (von Mayer-Rokitansky-Kuster or MRK anomaly) in hereditary renal adysplasia (HRA). American Journal of Medical Genetics 26: 873–876

Pagon R A, Smith D W, Shepard T H 1979 Urethral obstruction malformation complex: a cause of abdominal muscle deficiency and the 'prune belly'. Journal of Pediatrics 94: 900–906

Pardo-Mindan F J, Pablo C L, Vazquez J J 1978 Morphogenesis of glomerular cysts in renal dysplasia. Nephron 21: 155–160

Parsa K P, Lee D N, Zamboni L, Glassock R J 1976 Hereditary nephritis, deafness and abnormal thrombopoiesis: study of a new kindred. American Journal

of Medicine 60(5): 665–672

Pashayan H M, Dowd T, Nigro A V 1977 Bilateral absence of the kidneys and ureters. Journal of Medical Genetics 14: 205–209

Pathak I G, Williams D I 1964 Multicystic and cystic dysplastic kidneys. British Journal of Urology 36: 318–331

Pathak S, Strong L C, Ferrell RE, Trindade A 1982 Familial renal cell carcinoma with a 3;11 chromosome translocation limited to tumor cells. Science 217: 939–941

Perlman M, Williams J, Ornoy A 1976 Familial ureteric bud anomalies. Journal of Medical Genetics 13: 161–163

Persky L, Owens R 1971 Genitourinary tract abnormalities in Turner's syndrome. Journal of Urology 105: 309–313

Pilepich M V, Berkman E M, Goodchild N T 1978 HLA typing in familial renal carcinoma. Tissue Antigens 11: 487–488

Potter E L 1965 Bilateral absence of ureters and kidneys: a report of 50 cases. Obstetrics and Gynecology 25: (1 January) 3–12

Potter E L 1972 Normal and abnormal development of the kidney. Year Book Medical Publishers, Chicago, p 3–24

Potter E L 1974 Oligohydramnios: further comment. The Journal of Pediatrics 84 (6 June): 931–932

Privett J T J, Jeans W D, Roylance J 1976 The incidence and importance of renal duplication. Clinical Radiology 27: 521–530

Qazi Q, Masakawa A, Milman D, McGann B, Chua A, Haller J 1979 Renal anomalies in fetal alcohol syndrome. Pediatrics 63 (6 June): 886–889

Quan L, Smith D W 1973 The VATER association. Journal of Pediatrics 82: 104

Randolph M F, Morris K 1974 Instant screening for bacteriuria in children: analysis of dipstick. Journal of Pediatrics 84(2): 246–248

Ratten G J, Beischer N A, Fortune D W 1973 Obstetric complications when the fetus has Potter's syndrome. I clinical considerations. American Journal of Obstetrics and Gynecology 115 (7 April): 890–896

Reed W B, Dexter R, Corley C, Fish C 1965 Congenital lipodystrophic diabetes with acanthosis nigricans. Archives of Dermatology 91: 326–334

Reveno J, Palubinskas A J 1966 Congenital renal abnormalities in gonadal dysgenesis. Radiology 86: 49–51

Riccardi V M, Sujansky E, Smith A C, Francke U 1978 Chromosomal imbalance in the aniridia-Wilms' tumor association: 11p interstitial deletion. Pediatrics 61(4): 604–610

Risdon R A, Young L W, Chrispin A R 1975 Renal hypoplasia and dysplasia: a radiological and pathological correlation. Pediatric Radiology 3: 213–225

Rizza J M, Downing S E 1971 Bilateral renal agenesis in two female siblings. American Journal of Diseases of Children 121: 60

Rizzo N, Gabrielli S, Pilu G, Perolo A, Cacciari A, Domini R, Bovicelli L 1987 Prenatal diagnosis and obstetrical management of multicystic dysplastic kidney disease. Prenatal Diagnosis 7: 109–118

Rogers M F, Rutherford G W, Alexander S A, DiLiberti J H 1986 A population based study of hemolytic uremic syndrome in Oregon 1979–1982. American Journal of Epidemiology 123: 137–142

Romero R, Cullen M, Grannum P, Jeanty P, Reece E A, Venus I, Hobbins J C 1985 Antenatal diagnosis of renal anomalies with ultrasound. III. Bilateral renal agenesis.

American Journal of Obstetrics and Gynecology 151: 38–43

Roodhooft A M, Birnholz J C, Holmes L B 1984 Familial nature of congenital absence and severe dysgenesis of both kidneys. New England Journal of Medicine 310: 1341–1345

Rosenfeld L 1959 Renal agenesis. Journal of the American Medical Association 170: 1247

Royer P, Habib R, Mathieu H, Broyer M 1974 Pediatric nephrology. W B Saunders Company, Philadelphia

Rubinstein J H 1979 Broad thumb-hallux syndrome. In: Bergsma D (ed), Birth Defects Compendium, 2nd edn. Alan Liss, New York, p 157

Rusche C 1953 Silent adenocarcinoma of the kidneys with solitary metastases occurring in brothers. Journal of Urology 70 (August): 146–151

Schimke R N, King C R 1980 Hereditary urogenital adysplasia. Clinical Genetics 18: 417–420

Schinzel A 1984 Catalogue of unbalanced chromosome aberrations in man. Walter de Gruyter, Berlin

Schinzel A, Homberger C, Sigrist T 1978 Bilateral renal agenesis in 2 male sibs born to consanguineous parents. Journal of Medical Genetics 15: 314–316

Schmidt E C, Hartley A A, Bower R 1952 Renal aplasia in sisters. Archives of Pathology 54: 403

Schmidt W, Schroeder T M, Buchinger G, Kubli F 1982 Genetics, pathoanatomy and prenatal diagnosis of Potter I syndrome and other urogenital tract diseases. Clinical Genetics 22: 105–127

Schwartz G J, Haycock G B, Edelman C M Jr, Spitzer A 1976 A simple estimate of glomerular filtration rate in children derived from body length and plasma creatinine. Pediatrics 58(2): 259–263

Seller M J, Berry A C 1978 Amniotic fluid alpha-fetoprotein and fetal renal agenesis. The Lancet 1 (1 March): 660

Seller M J, Child A H 1980 Raised maternal serum alpha-fetoprotein, oligohydramnios and the fetus. The Lancet 1 (1 February): 317

Semmens J P 1962 Congenital anomalies of the female genital tract: functional classification based on review of 56 personal cases and 500 reported cases. Obstetrics and Gynecology 19: 328

Sengar D P S, Rashid A, Wolfish N M 1979 Familial urinary tract anomalies: association with the major histocompatibility complex in man. The Journal of Urology 121 (February): 194–197

Senior B 1973 Familial retinal-renal dystrophy. American Journal of Diseases of Children 125: 442–447

Senior B, Friedman A I, Brando J L 1961 Juvenile familial nephropathy with tapeto retinal degeneration. American Journal of Ophthalmology 52 (November): 625–633

Shapiro L J, Kaback M M, Toomey K E, Sarti D, Luther P, Cousins J 1977 Prenatal diagnosis of the Meckel syndrome. Birth Defects: Original Article Series XIII(3): 267–272

Shaw R F, Glover R A 1961 Abnormal segregation in hereditary renal disease with deafness. American Journal of Human Genetics 13 (March): 89–97

Simon H B, Thompson G J 1955 Congential renal polycystic disease: clinical and therapeutic study of 366 cases. Journal of the American Medical Association 159 (October): 657–662

Smellie J M, Hodson C J, Edwards D, Normand I C S 1964 Clinical and radiological features of urinary infection in children. British Medical Journal 2: 1222–1226

Smith D W 1976 Recognizable patterns of human malformation: genetic embryologic and clinical aspects, 2nd edn. W B Saunders, Philadelphia

Smith D W 1982 Recognizable patterns of human malformation: genetic, embryologic and clinical aspects, 3nd edn. W B Saunders, Philadelphia

Sobel A T, Moisy G, Hirbec G et al 1979 Hereditary C2 deficiency associated with non-systemic glomerulonephritis. Clinical Nephrology 12(3): 132–136

Spear G S 1973 Alport's syndrome: a consideration of pathogenesis. Clinical Nephrology I (November-December): 336–337

Spear G S 1984 Hereditary Nephritis (Alport's Syndrome) — 1983. Clinical Nephrology 21: 3–6

Spear G S, Whitworth J M, Konigsmark B W 1970 Hereditary nephritis with nerve deafness: immunofluorescent studies on the kidney with a consideration of discordant immunoglobulin-complement immunofluorescent reactions. American Journal of Medicine 49(1) 52–63

Spitler L E, Wray B B, Mogerman S, Miller J J, O'Reilly R J, Lagios M 1980 Nephropathy in the Wiskott-Aldrich syndrome. Pediatrics 66(3): 391–398

Sugiura 1971 Congenital absence of the radius with hemifacial microsomia, ventricular septal defect and crossed renal ectopia. Birth Defects: Original Articles Series VII (7): 109–116

Swanson S L, Santen R J, Smith D W 1971 Multiple lentigenes syndrome: new findings of hypogonadotrophism, hyposomia and unilateral renal agenesis. Journal of Pediatrics 78 (6 June): 1037–1039

Teisberg P, Grottom K A, Myhre E, Flatmark A 1973 In vivo activation of complement in hereditary nephropathy. Lancet 2: 356–358

Thomas I T, Smith D W 1974 Oligohydramnios, cause of the nonrenal features of Potter's syndrome, including pulmonary hypoplasia. The Journal of Pediatrics 84 (6 June): 811–814

Torg J S, Steel H H 1968 Essential osteolysis with nephropathy: A review of the literature and a case report of an unusual syndrome. Journal of Bone and Joint Surgery [A] 50: 1629–1638

Turi S, Beattie T J, Belch J J F, Murphy A V 1986 Disturbances of prostacyclin metabolism in children with hemolytic-uremic syndrome and in first degree relatives. Clinical Nephrology 25: 193–198

Turleau C, de Grouchy J, Tournade M F, Gagnadoux M F, Junien C 1984 Del 11p/aniridia complex. Report of three patients and review of 37 observations from the literature. Clinical Genetics 26: 356–362

Van den Abbeele A D, Treves S T, Lebowitz R L, Bauer S, Davis N M T, Retik A, Colodny A 1987 Vesicourerteral reflux in asymptomatic siblings of patients with known reflux: radionuclide cystography. Pediatrics 79: 147–153

Varnek L 1978 Crytophthalmos, dyscephaly, syndactyly and renal aplasia. Acta Ophthalmologica 56: 302–313

Vinson P C, Goldenberg R L, Davis R O, Finley S C 1977 Fetal bladder neck obstruction and elevated amniotic alpha-fetoprotein. New England Journal of Medicine 297: 1351

Warkany J 1971 Congenital malformations. Year Book Medical Publishers, Chicago, p 92

Warkany J, Passarge E, Smith L B 1966 Congenital malformations in autosomal trisomy syndromes. American

Journal of Diseases of Children 112 (December): 502–517

Whitaker J, Danks D M 1966 A study of the inheritance of duplication of the kidneys and ureters. The Journal of Urology 95 (February): 176–178

Whitehouse W, Mountrose U 1973 Renal agenesis in nontwin siblings. American Journal of Obstetrics and Gynecology 116: 880

Widdershoven J 1983 Renal disorders in the brancho-oto-renal syndrome. Helvetica Paediatrica Acta 38: 513–22

Wilson R D, Hayden M R 1985 Brief Clinical report: bilateral renal agenesis in twins. American Journal of Medical Genetics 21: 147–152

Woodard J R, Rushton H G 1987 Reflux uropathy. Pediatric Clinics of North America 34: 1349–1364

Yates J W, Mortimer G, Connor J M, Duke J E 1984 Concordant monozygotic twins with bilateral renal agenesis. Journal of Medical Genetics 21: 66–67

Yunis J J, Ramsay N K C 1980 Familial occurrence of the aniridia-Wilms tumor syndrome with deletion 11p13–14.1, Journal of Pediatrics 96(6): 1027–1030

Zackai E, Mellman W J, Neiderer B, Hanson J 1975 The fetal trimethadione syndrome. Journal of Pediatrics 87: 280–284

Zbar B, Brauch H, Talmadge C, Linehan M 1987 Loss of alleles of loci on the short arm of chromosome 3 in renal cell carcinoma. Nature 327: 721–724

Zonana J, Rimoin D, Lachman R, Sarti D, Kaback M 1976 Renal agenesis — a genetic disorder? Pediatric Research 10: 420

76. Renal cystic diseases

Stanley C. Jordan   *Hooshang Kangarloo*

INTRODUCTION

Cystic diseases of the kidney are a common cause of end stage renal disease (ESRD), accounting for more than 10% of all ESRD patients (Grantham 1983). Autosomal dominant (adult) polycystic kidney disease (ADPKD) is among the most common dominant diseases in man, with a frequency of 1 per 1000 live births (Reeders et al 1986a). The current annual cost of end stage care (dialysis and transplantation) for cystic renal diseases in the United States is appoximately $200 million. In addition to the risk of renal failure, patients with ADPKD are at increased risk for cerebral haemorrhage and cystic disease of the liver (Levey et al 1983). No specific therapy is currently available to prevent cyst development or the progression to ESRD. The morbidity and cost of caring for patients with cystic kidney disease has encouraged research into causes and potential therapies. To date, no common pathogenic mechanism has been identified and no single therapy has emerged that is universally effective in treating renal cysts. However, research has provided many new and exciting insights into our understanding of these disorders. The expression of renal cystic disease requires genetic, environmental and constitutional factors working together (Gardner 1988).

Approximately 20% of patients have asynchronous expression of ADPKD (Delaney et al 1985). This suggests that other factors (i.e. environmental or constitutional) may be equally important in the clinical expression of ADPKD. Certainly, if environmental or constitutional factors that regulate expression of the abnormal gene products contribute to ADPKD, their modification could serve as a useful adjunctive therapy for renal cystic disorders (Gardner 1988).

Both environmental and genetic factors play an important role in the ultimate pathogenesis of cystic kidney diseases. A discussion of experimental data from both human and animal model systems will outline these considerations. This will be followed by more specific discussion of the clinical, laboratory and radiographic features of specific cystic renal diseases.

Genetic considerations in renal cystic diseases

Reports from the early part of the twentieth century were the first to establish the hereditary nature of renal cystic diseases. Subsequent reports established the recessive (ARPKD or infantile polycystic kidney disease) and the dominant (adult polycystic kidney disease or ADPKD) (Cairns 1925, Lieberman et al 1971, Milutinovic et al 1984). Recent data have also established that the neph-ronophthisis – medullary cystic disease complex (N-MCD) exhibits clear hereditary patterns (Strauss 1962, Gardner 1971). In addition, heritable polycystic kidney disease has been described in a number of animal models (Solomon 1973, Iverson et al 1982, Werder et al 1984, Fry et al 1985, Takahashi et al 1986).

One of the most important developments in the past few years is the demonstration by Reeders et al (1985, 1986a,b) of two genetic markers on chromosome 16 which are closely linked to ADPKD. These investigators showed that the ADPKD gene is located on the short arm of chromosome 16 and is closely linked to two other genetic markers (alpha-globin cluster and phosphoglyco-late phosphatase loci) on the short arm of chromosome 16. To date, no information is available on the nature of the abnormal gene product that leads to the manifestation of ADPKD. Presumably, this product allows for abnormal compliance of the tubular basement membrane, allowing cystic dilation to occur. The importance of recognizing the location of the ADPKD gene lies in the ability to provide genetic counselling to individuals who carry this gene who wish to become pregnant, and to recognize affected fetuses in utero. Reeders et al (1986b) have recently reported the successful prenatal diagnosis of ADPKD in a 9-week-old fetus using the highly polymorphic DNA probe genetically linked to the ADPKD locus. This was accomplished by isolating DNA from fetal cells obtained by chorionic villus sampling.

Southern blotting with the DNA probe confirmed the fetus was affected and therapeutic abortion was performed. The fetus was examined at necropsy and the kidneys showed both glomerular and tubular cysts in the renal cortex. The authors concluded that effective prenatal diagnosis of ADPKD is now practical. However, Romeo at al (1988) have recently reported an Italian family in which a second genetic locus for ADPKD was described. In this family classic linkage of ADPKD with the alpha-globin gene on chromosome 16 could not be demonstrated. The authors stated that these data have important implications for the use of genetic markers in the diagnosis of ADPKD. Since no definable linkage pattern currently exists for newly described ADPKD patients, a linkage based test cannot be reliably used until linkage relationships have been independently established in the family under study. The authors concluded that when genetic marker data are used to aid in genetic counselling, one must always take into account the possibility that the patient may have the unlinked type, although the possibility is remote (Romeo et al 1988).

Environmental factors in renal cystic disease

Although a strong genetic influence is clearly important in the development of renal cystic disease, environmental conditions are of importance in other types of acquired and induced renal cystic diseases (Gardner 1988). The best example of acquired renal cystic disease (ARCD) is the cystic disease seen in patients on chronic dialysis (Leichter et al 1988). The aetiology of ARCD in dialysis patients is unknown (Gardner 1988).

Renal cystic disease may also result from chronic exposure to chemicals and drugs that are known to be 'cystogenic'. (Thomas et al 1957, Darmady et al 1970, Vargas et al 1970, Gardner et al 1976, Resnick et al 1976, Hestbech et al 1977, Evan & Gardner 1979, Dobyan et al 1981, Christensen et al 1982, Gardner & Evan 1983, Evan et al 1984, Kanwar & Carone 1984, Butkowski et al 1985, Gardner et al 1986, 1987, Gardner 1988). Known cystogens include the following: diphenylamine (and other antioxidants) (Thomas et al 1957, Darmady et al 1970, Gardner 1971, Solomon 1973, Gardner et al 1976, Resnick et al 1976, Evan & Gardner 1979, Iverson et al 1982, Gardner & Evan 1983, Kanwar & Carone 1984, Werder et al 1984, Butkowski et al 1985, Fry et al 1985, Reeders et al 1985, 1986b, Takahashi et al 1986, Leichter et al 1988); alloxan and streptozotocin (diabetogenic agents) (Evan et al 1984); lithium chloride (Hestbech et al 1977, Christensen et al 1982); and cis-platinum (Dobyan et al 1981). All of the above agents have the capability of producing cysts in otherwise normal kidneys (Gardner 1988). The cystogens produce uniform and bilateral

renal cysts. In contrast, ADPKD may present with unilateral or asymmetrical cysts which would tend to contradict the idea that an endogenous cystogenic substance is the abnormal gene product of the ADPKD genes and is responsible for the clinical manifestations of the disease (Gardner 1988).

Environmental influences in hereditary renal cystic disease

The asymmetrical expression of renal cysts in ADPKD has led to the speculation that environmental influences may play an important role in the phenotypic expression of this genetically determined disease. The susceptibility of genetically determined renal cystic disease to environmental influences was first shown in the CFW wd mouse model (Gardner & Evan 1984, Werder et al 1984). In a laboratory environment, approximately 70% of these animals develop renal cysts; however, when maintained in a germ-free environment, none develop renal cysts (Gardner & Evan 1984, Werder et al 1984, Gardner 1988). Keeping animals in a germ-free environment is also known to reduce the cystogenicity of specific antioxidant agents (Dobyan et al 1981, Gardner et al 1986). These investigators have also shown (Gardner et al 1987) that injecting the CFW wd mouse with endotoxin abrogates the protective effect of a germ-free environment on renal cyst development and is associated with renal interstitial inflammation and leucocytosis (Gardner et al 1987, Gardner 1988). The role of interstitial inflammation in the genesis of human polycystic kidney disease is unknown (Gardner 1988).

Endogenous conditions associated with renal cystic disease

Endogenous conditions such as obstruction to flow with subsequent transduction of abnormal glomerular tubular back pressure can result in the development of renal cystic disease. The best example of this is the development of a unilateral congenital multicystic-dysplastic kidney which is a non-heritable form of renal dysplasia (Hartman et al 1986, Gardner 1988). Other examples include the resolution of renal cysts in cystic kidneys of cpk/cpk mice when these kidneys are maintained in vitro (Avner et al 1986) and, finally, the demonstration of altered morphogenesis of cystic kidneys following dialysis or transplantation (Gardner 1988).

Aetiology of renal cyst development

Although there is no clear consensus regarding the pathophysiology of renal cyst development, there are three hypotheses that have evolved from clinical and laboratory observations. The first proposes increased tubular basement membrane compliance as the primary defect (Grantham 1983, Gardner 1988). This is suggested by the defective structure of the membrane (Gardner 1988) and the increased incidence of cysts (hepatic, pancreatic), vascular and cardiac abnormalities, cerebral aneurysms, prolapsed mitral valve, and colonic diverticulae (Darmady et al 1970, Scheff et al 1980, Gabow et al 1984, Kanwar & Carone 1984, Butkowski et al 1985, Hossack et al 1987) in patients with ADPKD; all suggest a common structural abnormality in the basement membrane. The second hypothesis regards the reversal of normal sodium and water transport out of renal tubular cells. This would result in an influx of sodium and water rather than efflux from the affected nephrons. Experimental evidence exists to support this contention since sodium/potassium ATPase mediates cyst formation in metanephric organ cultures (Avner et al 1985, Gardner 1988). The third hypothesis suggests that epithelial cell hyperplasia with micropolyp formation results in nephron obstruction. Dilation of the nephrons occurs secondary to increased intraluminal pressure (Gardner 1988).

There are significant limitations in each hypothesis. For example, if increased compliance of the tubular basement membrane was the sole cause of cystic kidneys, then one would expect that each nephron would behave in a similar fashion (i.e. each nephron should offer no resistance to dilation). This is not true since dilation pressure varies from nephron to nephron (Gardner 1988). In addition, deformability of tubular basement membrane is similar to that of normal nephrons (Grantham et al 1987). Experimental evidence is also lacking to support net inward movement of solute and water into renal cysts (Perrone 1985). The obstruction hypothesis with epithelial hyperplasia seems to be the most likely explanation (Gardner 1988), but has been criticized for not explaining how a non-compliant basement membrane becomes deformed.

CLINICAL, GENETIC AND RADIOLOGICAL FEATURES OF THE MAJOR CYSTIC KIDNEY DISEASES

Autosomal recessive (infantile) polycystic kidney disease (ARPKD)

ARPKD is the most common renal cystic disease seen in children and is not confined to infants. Initially clinicians considered the disorder fatal; however, more recent experience indicates that many patients may survive into adulthood, especially those with minimal renal involvement and more severe hepatic involvement (hepatic fibrosis and portal hypertension) (Resnick & Vernier 1986). The diagnosis of ARPKD should be confined to those individuals who present with bilateral renal cystic disease or renal tubular ectasia and congenital hepatic fibrosis of varying degrees. As with other types of renal cystic disease, the clinical features and degree of pathological involvement may vary from family to family depending on the age at presentation and the extent of organ involvement (Resnick & Vernier 1986).

ARPKD is characterized by lack of parental involvement (no kidney or liver abnormalities) and a 25% chance of sibling involvement. The importance of confirming the diagnosis for the purpose of genetic counselling cannot be overemphasized since there is a 25% risk for all future pregnancies. ARPKD can be reliably detected in utero by ultrasound.

Lieberman et al (1971) have demonstrated the variable expression of ARPKD and have described the presentation in infants and older children. They also showed that ARPKD shared similar features with congenital hepatic fibrosis, but that there were sufficient differences to separate these two entities. More recently (Alvanez et al 1981) a review of a large number of children with congenital hepatic fibrosis demonstrated renal cystic abnormalities in most patients. This study suggests that congenital hepatic fibrosis and ARPKD represent different clinical manifestations of the same autosomal recessive genetic disorder with varying severity of renal and hepatic involvement (Resnick & Vernier 1986). The locus for the gene responsible for ARPKD and congenital hepatic fibrosis has not yet been identified.

Clinical features

These children usually present at birth with large bilateral renal masses. The delivery is usually complicated by dystocia caused by the fetal abdominal mass, and oligohydramnios which is secondary to decreased fetal urine production. The initial clinical problems include development of bilateral pneumothorax, pulmonary hypoplasia and other classic manifestations of the fetal compression syndrome which may include the classic Potter facies. The major causes of morbidity and mortality in these infants are respiratory problems resulting from pulmonary hypoplasia and pneumothorax. Complications include hypoxia, severe acidosis and early death. Renal insufficiency is unusual initially but progresses with time (Resnick & Vernier 1986). The liver may be mildly enlarged, but hepatic fibrosis is always present. Despite the presence of hepatic fibrosis, liver function studies are normal. Oesophageal varices and clinically detectable liver dysfunction do not occur until later in life (Resnick & Vernier 1986).

Radiographic findings

Radiographs of the abdomen show enlarged kidneys bilaterally (Fig. 76.1). The kidney function depends on the degree of renal involvement by the polycystic disease. Very poor renal function appears in the newborn type and the collecting systems are usually not seen satisfactorily. The nephrographic phase is often prolonged, as long as a week, and shows a radiolucent mottled appearance, which is the result of numerous small cysts. The dilated tubules may appear as a 'brush border' perpendicular to the surface of the kidney. The diagnosis is obvious in this form of polycystic disease of the young.

In the childhood type, better renal function occurs. Medullary tubular ectasia leads to stasis of the excreted contrast material in the dilated ducts and gives the 'brush border' appearance (Fig. 76.2). The pelvicalyceal systems and ureters appear normal. Differentiation from the ADPKD presenting in childhood may be difficult by excretory urography. However, the demonstration of periportal fibrosis by ultrasonography or liver biopsy favours the diagnosis of ARPKD.

Ultrasonographic findings

Grey-scale ultrasonography identifies the nephromegaly and multiple small uniform cysts, which give the kidney an increased echogenicity (Fig. 76.3). The normal central echoes of the pelvicalyceal system are not seen. However, ultrasonography provides the best means of evaluation of the liver. The demonstration of liver cysts and/or periportal fibrosis assures the proper diagnosis. The liver cysts appear as simple cysts, but the periportal fibrosis imparts a highly echogenic character to the liver.

Magnetic resonance imaging (MRI)

Large kidneys as well as dilated tubules and cysts are well identified on T1-weighted SE sequences. This modality is useful to diagnose associated haemorrhage (Fig. 76.4).

Pathology

Renal biopsy is neither necessary nor desirable in confirming the diagnosis of typical ARPKD. However, it

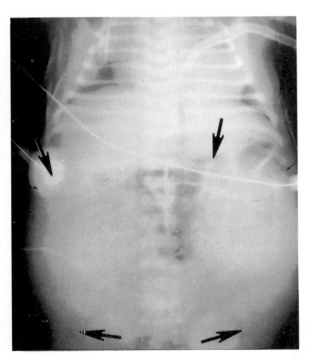

Fig. 76.1 An abdominal film in an infant with ARPKD 24 hours after intravenous injection of contrast material. The kidneys are large (arrows) and occupy almost the entire abdomen. When kidneys are severely affected, lungs are hypoplastic and infants suffer from pneumothorax. In this infant, chest tubes are placed to treat bilateral pneumothorax.

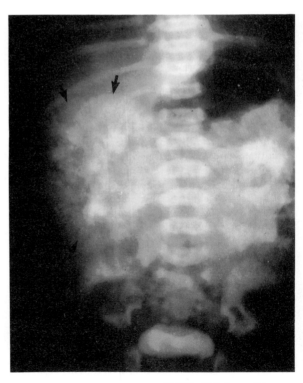

Fig. 76.2 An older child with ARPKD. This is a milder form than Figure 76.1. The film was taken after intravenous injection of contrast material. Notice dilated tubules (arrows)

may be useful, along with liver biopsy, to confirm the diagnosis in unusual cases.

Pathological features of ARPKD include medullary ductal dilation with scattered small cortical cysts with varying degrees of tubulointerstitial fibrosis. The kidneys are massively enlarged with numerous small cysts on the surface. Periductal fibrosis and proliferation or ectasia of biliary duct epithelium constitute the hepatic changes which are invariably present in this disorder.

It is theorized that initially the ureteric bud and metanephrogenic blastema develop normally and give rise to normal nephrons. But at some time during the last half of intrauterine life, the proximal collecting tubules develop large saccules and diverticula, and the more terminal tubules become enlarged, leading to Potter tubular gigantism.

Autosomal dominant (adult) polycystic kidney disease (ADPKD)

ADPKD is a highly penetrant, autosomal dominant form of renal cystic disease that commonly begins in the fourth or fifth decade of life, but is being diagnosed with increased frequency in infancy and childhood. Cole et al (1987) recently reported that 12.5% of infants presenting with polycystic kidney disease in the first year of life had ADPKD, while 35% had confirmed ARPKD (infantile variety). The remaining patients had insufficient data to categorize the type of polycystic kidney disease with certainty. The genetic transmission and location of the abnormal gene for this disorder have been previously discussed. Although autosomal dominant inheritance is well recognized, many patients may lack a positive family history. This may reflect spontaneous mutations, inadequate family history, or a prolonged latent period for expression of the disease (Resnick & Vernier 1986). The use of abdominal ultrasound and computerized axial tomography (CT-scan), both noninvasive radiological techniques, are the preferred methods of documenting ADPKD and screening family members for renal and hepatic cysts (Scheff et al 1980). In addition, prenatal ultrasound can identify affected infants in utero. More effective prenatal diagnosis is currently available using a highly polymorphic DNA probe closely linked to the ADPKD locus (Reeders et al 1986a,b). One must, of course, be aware of the genetic heterogeneity recently demonstrated in this condition (Romeo et al 1988).

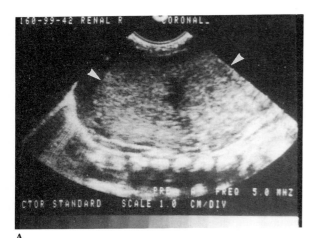

A

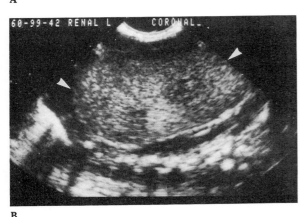

B

Fig. 76.3 Longitudinal sonograms of right **A** and left **B** kidneys show enlarged kidneys. Both kidneys show increased echogenicity which is a typical finding in the infantile form of polycystic disease. This increased echogenicity is a result of multiple interfaces created by dilated tubules.

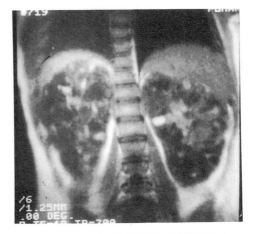

Fig. 76.4 Coronal MRI (SE 300/18) of ARPKD shows enlarged kidneys and some cysts. MRI is helpful to define complications such as haemorrhage but is not essential for diagnosis.

Clinical features

ADPKD usually presents in the third to fifth decade of life with haematuria, hypertension, abdominal pain, abdominal mass, and uraemia. These features are rarely seen in ADPKD children. Renal concentrating defects and microhaematuria are frequent findings.

Radiographic findings

Radiographs of the abdomen show bilateral renal enlargement. Occasionally, calculi, 'milk of calcium' or, rarely, arcuate or amorphous calcification may be seen in the kidneys, liver or spleen. Excretory urography with nephrotomography usually demonstrates multiple lucent masses with distortion of the pelvicalyceal system. Retrograde pyelography shows distortion and displacement of the pelvicalyceal system, stretching of the intrarenal arteries and multiple large and small cysts in the cortex and medulla in the nephrographic phase (Fig. 76.5). Visualization of these small cortical cysts, which give an inhomogeneous nephrographic appearance, in addition to the larger cysts, will differentiate this entity from multiple simple cysts, which show a homogeneous nephrogram with no evidence of multiple small cortical cysts.

Lack of visualization of these small cysts does not exclude the diagnosis of ADPKD. The demonstration of cysts in other organs, such as the liver, is strong evidence for the diagnosis of ADPKD.

Ultrasonographic findings

Ultrasonography shows nephromegaly and multiple discrete cysts, which are larger than the infantile type, distributed throughout the kidney. Adjacent cysts distort the normal central echogenic pelvicalyceal system. Other organs that may also be involved, such as the liver, spleen, ovaries, uterus, pancreas and bladder, are easily surveyed. MRI findings are similar to ultrasonographic findings (Fig. 76.6).

Pathology

ADPKD is characterized by asymmetrical renal enlargement with dilated cysts scattered over the kidney surface. Microscopic examination shows focal tubular dilation, tubular cysts of varying size, and cystic dilation of Bowman's capsule (Fig. 76.8 A & B). This is in contrast to the medullary tubular dilation seen in ARPKD. In addition, cysts may be found in other organs (liver, pancreas, ovary, lung), vascular abnormalities such as cerebral aneurysms and prolapsed mitral valve and diverticula of the colon have been described (Resnick & Vernier 1986). Hepatic fibrosis (a constant finding in ARPKD) is not seen in ADPKD. In difficult cases, a percutaneous liver biopsy may help differentiate ADPKD from ARPKD in an infant or small child.

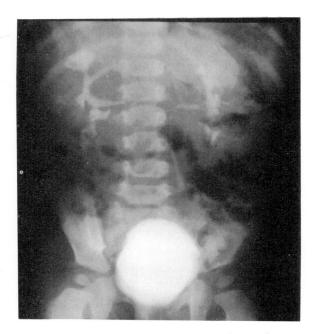

Fig. 76.5 ADPKD. An abdominal film 15 minutes after injection of contrast material shows enlarged kidneys. Collecting systems are deformed by presence of multiple cysts in the kidneys.

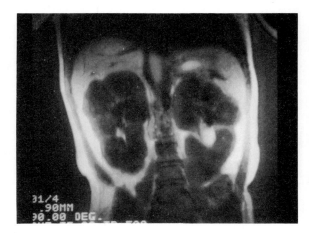

Fig. 76.6 MRI of a child with ADPKD shows enlarged kidneys containing large cysts.

Medullary cystic disease – familial juvenile nephronopthisis complex

Medullary cystic disease (MCD) is an important cause of ESRD in children, accounting for 15% of patients receiving paediatric kidney transplants in some studies (Garel et al 1984, Resnick & Vernier 1986). MCD is a chronic, progressive disorder characterized clinically by the slow onset of hyposthenuria (inability to concentrate the urine), anaemia, and growth retardation. Pathologically, this disease is characterized by small kidneys

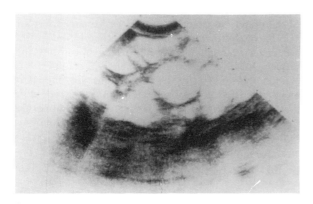

A

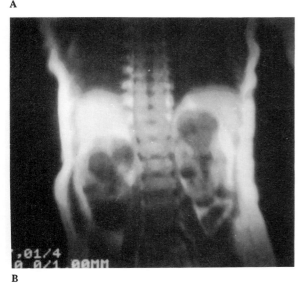

B

Fig. 76.7   Longitudinal sonogram **A** and a coronal (SE 28/500) MRI scan **B** of a child with tuberous sclerosis show multiple large cysts involving kidneys. This appearance is very similar to ADPKD. Tuberous sclerosis should be considered when the appearance of ADPKD is seen in any child.

with severe tubulointerstitial disease, with or without renal medullary cysts (Resnick & Vernier 1986). The terminology defining this syndrome is confusing, since it is called both medullary cystic disease and familial juvenile nephronopthisis (Smith & Graham 1945, Fanconi et al 1951, Strauss 1962). The differences in terminology depend on whether medullary cysts are present (MCD) or whether medullary tubulointerstitial fibrosis is present (familial juvenile nephronopthisis [FJN]) (Resnick & Vernier 1986).

MCD has two distinct genetic and age related forms. The first is an autosomal recessive disorder that occurs in children and is frequently associated with nonrenal manifestations. The associated abnormalities include the following: (1) ophthalmological (colobomas, nystagmus,

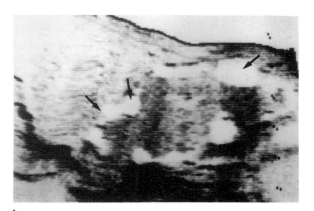

A

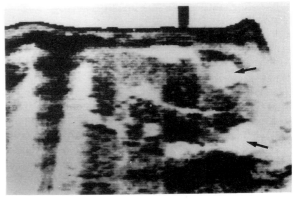

B

Fig. 76.8 A & B   Sonograms of glomerulocystic disease. Both kidneys are large and show increased echogenicity. Both kidneys contain multiple cysts (arrows). In glomerulocystic disease, cysts are the result of dilated Bowman's capsule.

retinitis pigmentosa, myopia strabismus, hyperopia, optic nerve atrophy, and tapetoretinal degeneration) (Loken et al 1961, Senior et al 1961, Rayfield & McDonald 1972, Waldherr et al 1982, Resnick & Vernier 1986); (2) mental retardation and cerebellar ataxia (Popovie-Rolovic et al 1976); (3) skeletal abnormalities (cone-shaped epiphyses) (Popovie-Rolovic et al 1976) and (4) hepatic fibrosis (Mainzer et al 1970). Consanguinity has been frequently reported in the childhood variety (Herdman et al 1967).

The other form of MCD is inherited as an autosomal dominant trait, has its onset in adulthood, and is not associated with other renal or nonrenal abnormalities (Resnick Vernier 1986). Sporadic cases of both autosomal dominant and autosomal recessive MCD are known to occur. Renal abnormalities in asymptomatic relatives of affected individuals have, on occassion, been demonstrated (Giselson et al 1970).

Clinical features

Patients presenting with FJN/MCD complex usually show an insidious onset of renal failure associated with polyuria, polydypsia, anaemia (out of proportion to the renal failure), and growth retardation (Resnick & Vernier 1986). Other associated symptoms include sodium and potassium wasting, associated with salt-craving or muscle weakness, secondary to profound hypokalaemia. Bone pain caused by renal osteodystrophy may be an initial presenting symptom. Enuresis is also a common presenting symptom secondary to polyuria. This symptom is often misdiagnosed as being caused by a sleep disorder or psychological disturbance and treated inappropriately. Oedema and hypertension are rare, primarily due to the salt wasting that occurs in this disease (Resnick & Vernier 1986).

Pathology

Small scattered medullary cysts with or without tubulo-interstitial disease are the characteristic findings in the FJN/MCD complex. However, the tubulointerstitial disease is nonspecific and cysts may be present or absent (Herdman et al 1967, Sherman et al 1971). The cysts are located in the collecting ducts and distal convoluted tubules, while the proximal tubules and loop of Henle are normal (Sherman et al 1971). The recent demonstration of Tamm-Horsfall protein (THP) surrounding many tubules is interesting. THP is a glycoprotein originating in the ascending limb of Henle's loop and the distal convoluted tubule (Resnick et al 1978, Resnick & Vernier 1986). The presence of THP indicates distal tubule damage. In addition, THP is phlogistic and has been associated with renal interstitial inflammation.

The pathogenesis of FJN/MCD is unknown, but the genetic predisposition is well established. The tubular defect coded for by as yet undiscovered genes could result in tubular death and dysfunction with extrusion of THP into the renal interstitium. The phlogistic nature of THP would then allow interstitial fibrosis to develop, thus completing the phenotypic expression of this disease.

OTHER CYSTIC RENAL DISEASES

Renal dysplasia

The kidneys require a normal progression and branching of the ureteric bud and ampulla (the expanded forward portion of the dividing tubule) to properly induce the metanephrogenic blastema to form nephrons. If this process is disturbed, maldevelopment will result.

The following terms and definitions are offered to avoid confusion. Plasia originates from the Greek word plassein, meaning to form. Dysplasia means abnormal formation. Severe dysplasia with apparent absence of the kidneys is called aplasia.

Multicystic kidney

The basic defect in the pathogenesis of a multicystic kidney is abnormal development of the advancing ureteric bud. This causes abnormal induction of the nephrogenic tissue, with subsequent formation of primitive, dysplastic tissues. This maldevelopment occurs very early in embryonic life, resulting in atresia of the ureter, pelvis or both. The two forms of multicystic

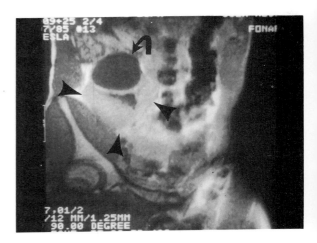

Fig. 76.9 Simple cysts. An MRI coronal scan (SE 28/500) of a child shows a pelvic kidney (arrowheads) containing a large simple cyst (arrow).

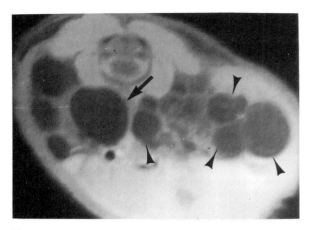

Fig. 76.10 Bilateral multicystic disease. Axial MRI scan of a stillborn infant shows bilateral cystic renal dysplasia. On one side, the kidney is replaced with varying size cysts (arrowheads), but on the other side an enlarged pelvis (arrow) is seen. This patient represents both classical (pelvi-infundibular atresia) and hydronephrotic types of multicystic disease.

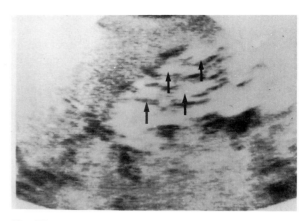

Fig. 76.11 Longitudinal sonogram in a patient with typical multicystic disease. Kidney is replaced by numerous cysts (arrows).

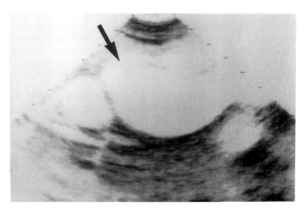

Fig. 76.12 Hydronephrotic multicystic disease. Enlarged pelvis (arrow) and smaller cysts are visible in this sonogram. It may be difficult to differentiate this form of multicystic disease from hydronephrosis.

kidney include pelvi-infundibular atresia and hydro-nephrosis (Fig. 76.10).

In the more common form, the atresia involves the infundibulopelvic region. As a result, the subsequent growth and branching of the ureteral bud is markedly altered. This severe renal disorganization is seen patho-logically as 'a cluster of grapes' with no resemblance to a normal kidney. Central cores of solid tissue with recog-nizable dysplastic elements are surrounded by many cysts, ranging from a few millimetres to several centi-metres in diameter. There is almost always an associated severe stenosis or atresia of the ureter. These cysts may or may not intercommunicate, depending on whether the proximal portion of the pelvis is present or obliterated.

In the hydronephrotic form of multicystic kidney, the atretic process involves only the ureter. The cysts in this form represent the dilated pelvicalyceal system, and they communicate through the dilated renal pelvis.

If one accepts the theory of an intrauterine obstruction as the major cause for development of a multicystic kidney, it is possible to explain focal and segmental forms of the disease, the focal form resulting in scattered areas of dysplasia secondary to collecting-duct obstruction, and the segmental form resulting in dysplasia of one moiety of a duplex collecting system.

Most multicystic kidneys manifest clinically as an abdominal mass in a healthy neonate, infant or child. In fact, a multicystic kidney is the most common cause of an abdominal mass in a neonate. Rarely, the mass is

undetected until adult life and is discovered incidentally during a urological examination for an unrelated condi-tion. In the adult, calcification may be seen in the walls of the cysts; this does not occur in children. No hereditary tendency has been described.

Up to one-third of patients with a multicystic kidney have some form of obstructive uropathy involving the contralateral kidney. Therefore, it is essential to evaluate the entire urinary system with ultrasonography and excretory urography.

Ultrasonography usually demonstrates a large mass with multiple cystic areas of varying size separated by echogenic septa (Figs 76.11 and 76.12). There is no identifiable renal parenchyma or pelvicalyceal system, i.e. a well-defined ellipsoid and relatively sonolucent band of homogenous echogenicity surrounding a linear, central, more echogenic band.

The flank mass may be identified on the scout film of the abdomen. During the total-body opacification phase of the excretory urogram, opacification of the cyst walls may be seen as a result of their vascular supply. Subsequently, during the early excretory phase, faint, thin, curvilinear densities ('calyceal crescents') appear as a result of stasis of the contrast material in compressed collecting tubules that lie adjacent to the cysts. On delayed films, irregular puddled opacification may be seen in the small or medium-sized cystic spaces, probably due to tubular reabsorption of water and therefore concentration of the contrast material. The renal artery is either very hypoplastic or absent. The bladder is normal. MRI shows hypointense cystic masses.

Multiple cysts associated with lower urinary tract obstruction

In children with congenital urinary outlet obstruction, the kidneys usually have small cortical cysts as well as renal dysplasia. These renal cysts are probably the result of increased pressure on the ampullae during fetal development of the kidney. The most common cause in males is a posterior urethral valve. Other less common causes are an ectopic ureterocele or, rarely, urethral atresia. Patients present with advanced renal failure, bilateral flank masses (the hydronephrotic kidneys), and a lower abdominal mass (dilated bladder).

Ultrasonography (Fig. 76.14) and excretory urography demonstrate bilateral hydroureteronephrosis and a dilated, trabeculated bladder. The pelvicalyceal system, although markedly dilated, normally develops and communicates with the ureters.

The cause of the outlet obstruction is usually identified by a voiding cystourethrogram. With a posterior urethral valve, the prostatic urethra is markedly dilated and the obstruction is at or just below the verumontanum. There is often associated vesicoureteral reflux. Cystic dysplasia may also be segmented, caused by obstruction in part of the collecting system (Fig. 76.13).

Cortical cysts

Cystic lesions occurring primarily in the cortex are classified as follows: cysts associated with trisomy syndromes or tuberous sclerosis, simple cysts, and multilocular cysts.

Cysts associated with the trisomy syndromes are very small cysts seen only histologically and with no clinical or radiographic importance.

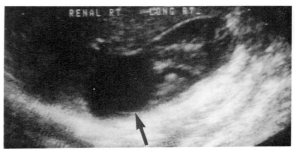

A

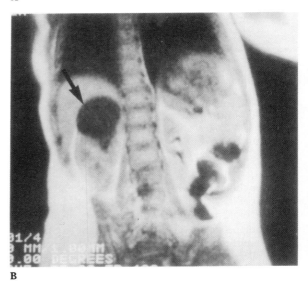

B

Fig. 76.13 Segmental multicystic disease. Cystic dysplasia may be segmental secondary to obstruction of part of the collecting system. Longitudinal sonogram **A** and a coronal MRI scan **B** show cystic dysplasia of right upper pole.

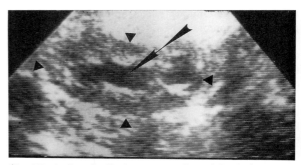

Fig. 76.14 Longitudinal sonogram of renal dysplasia secondary to distal obstruction. Both kidneys show a similar appearance with increased echogenicity and mild dilation of pelvis (arrow). This is difficult to differentiate from mild hydronephrosis. A more classic form is massive bilateral dilation as a result of distal obstruction.

Although renal masses in patients with tuberous sclerosis are usually hamartomas (angiomyolipomas), renal cysts can occur, and may enlarge to the extent of markedly impairing renal function. Accurate diagnosis is usually accomplished following excretory urography, angiography, ultrasonography and MRI (Fig. 76.7).

Simple (serous) renal cysts can be solitary or multiple and are very likely acquired lesions. Although simple cysts are primarily lesions of adults, they can occur in childhood and even in neonates. They contain serous fluid and do not inherently communicate with the collecting system, although they may rupture into it.

Excretory urography shows a round radiolucent mass usually bulging from a border of the kidney. Nephro-tomography will demonstrate a thin rim surrounding the cyst, and the 'beak sign,' which is a result of compression of normal renal parenchyma by the slow-growing lesion. Ultrasonography shows a round sonolucency without internal echoes, a sharply defined, smooth border and an increased through transmission. Simple cysts are also clearly seen on MRI (Fig. 76.9).

Since the possibility of a hypovascular cystic Wilms tumour always exists and true simple cysts are rare in children, a cyst puncture under sonographic or fluoroscopic guidance is necessary for laboratory analysis of the fluid. At the same time, contrast material can be injected into the cyst and the entire wall carefully evaluated by multiple cross-table radiographs with the patient in prone, supine, and both decubitus positions. Following these procedures, if the nature of the lesion is still suspicious, exploratory surgery is indicated to avoid misdiagnosing a cystic Wilms tumour as a simple cyst.

Multilocular cysts are the least common of all congenital cystic lesions of the kidney. The aetiology of the lesion is not known. This entity has been classified by some authors as a cystic hamartoma and by others as a benign multilocular cystic nephroma (benign form of Wilms tumour). Usually manifested in childhood as an asymptomatic abdominal mass discovered during a routine physical examination, it is a unilateral lesion involving only a portion of the kidney and sharply demarcated from the normal remaining renal parenchyma by a fibromuscular capsule. Pathologically, the lesion is composed of multiple loculi varying in size and separated from one another by septa composed of compact fibrous and smooth muscle tissue. There is no communication among the loculi or with the renal pelvis.

The excretory urogram identifies the lesion as a sharply demarcated lucent area displacing the pelvicalyceal system. Angiographically, the lesion is relatively avascular, but vessels within the cyst may opacify, simulating a neoplasm.

Medullary cysts

Cystic lesions occurring primarily in the medulla include medullary sponge kidney, medullary cystic disease, pyelogenic cysts and papillary necrosis (medullary type).

Medullary sponge kidney (renal tubular ectasia)

Medullary sponge kidney is a developmental abnormality of the kidney limited to the medulla. The disease has no significant familial incidence and is usually discovered in the third or fourth decade of life because of the associated complication of infection, haematuria, or calculus formation. There have been reports of association of medullary sponge kidney with hemihypertrophy, Ehlers-Danlos syndrome, congenital hypertrophic pyloric stenosis, and Caroli disease.

Pathologically, the collecting ducts in the renal pyramids are ectatic, and associated with small cysts, 1–3 mm in diameter, that communicate with the collecting ducts and may be considered as offshoots or segmentally dilated portions of the ducts.

Radiographic findings. Nephrocalcinosis (calcification in the renal pyramids) may be present on abdominal radiographs and is seen in up to 50% of patients with medullary sponge kidney. The excretory urogram shows typical streaks (and rounded collections) of opacified urine in the ectatic collecting ducts (and cysts) into the renal pyramids. These findings are present bilaterally in 60–80% of patients. In the remaining 20–40% of patients, the abnormalities are limited to one kidney or even to a single pyramid. However, the pathological changes are present throughout the kidneys bilaterally, but are too small to be detected radiographically. The tubular ectasia may lead to overall enlargement of the pyramids, with an appearance of papillary hypertrophy manifested by splaying and elongation of the calyces. The kidneys are usually normal in size, but may be slightly enlarged, and, in the absence of complications, function normally. On the other hand, with loss of renal parenchyma due to infection or obstruction by renal calculi, the kidneys may be small and have decreased function.

It is often difficult to differentiate minimal tubular ectasia from the normal pyramidal blush seen with high-dose urography. In those instances in which discrete collections or streaks of contrast material, although few, can be demonstrated, the diagnosis of medullary sponge kidney is more likely since the normal pyramidal blush tends to be indistinct.

Although ultrasonography may show scattered areas of dense echogenicity representing nephrocalcinosis, and possibly small cysts, accurate diagnosis is established by the excretory urogram.

Pyelogenic cysts (calyceal diverticulum)

A pyelogenic cyst is a small cavity in a renal column, frequently located medial to the corticomedullary junction. The cyst is connected to the adjacent calyx. The pathogenesis of this lesion is unknown.

The cysts are usually asymptomatic; however, complications such as infection and calculus formation can occur. Of all the cystic lesions of the kidney 'milk of calcium' is found most commonly in a calyceal diverticulum. At excretory urography, the cyst opacifies after visualization of the pelvicalyceal system. The connecting isthmus may or may not be visualized.

THERAPY OF CYSTIC RENAL DISEASES

Because the pathogenesis of all cystic renal diseases remains poorly understood, therapeutic considerations are based on existing theories of cyst formation. In a disease such as FJN/MCD, therapy would also include sodium, potassium and vitamin D replacement to substitute for renal tubular dysfunction as well as preparing patients for end-stage care. Patients with more common renal cystic disease such as ADPKD may benefit from cyst puncture (Rovsing procedure). Cyst decompression would not only relieve refractory pain, but may reduce hypertension and progressive renal dysfunction by alleviating pressure on adjacent normal nephrons (Bennett et al 1987). Families of patients diagnosed as having heritable renal cystic diseases are anxious to know the risk of the disorder in asymptomatic members. The benefit of early diagnosis of untreatable renal cystic diseases in unaffected children is debatable.

Other experimental forms of therapy (amiloride administration, cyst puncture, and deroofing) (Bennett et al 1987, Uchic et al 1987) have no proven effectiveness to date. If haematuria becomes life-threatening or the pain unbearable, focal embolization or nephrectomy may be considered. Cysts do not recur in the transplanted kidney.

REFERENCES

Alvanez F, Bernard O, Brunelle F et al 1981 Congenital hepatic fibrosis in children. Journal of Pediatrics 99: 370

Avner E D, Sweeney W E, Finegold D N, Piesco N P, Ellis D 1985 Sodium-potassium ATPase activity mediates cyst formation in metanephric organ culture. Kidney International 28: 447–455

Avner E D, Sweeney W E Jr., Piesco N P, Ellis D 1986 Regression of genetically determined polycystic kidney disease in murine organ culture. Experientia 42: 77–80

Bennett W, Elzinga L, Golper T, Barry J 1987. Reduction of cyst volume for symptomatic management of autosomal dominant polycystic kidney disease. Journal of Urology 137: 620–622

Butkowski R J, Carone F A, Grantham J J, Hudson B G 1985 Tubular basement membrane changes in 2-amino-4.5-diphenylthiazole-induced polycystic disease. Kidney International 28: 744–751

Cairns H W B 1925 Heredity in polycystic disease of the kidneys. Quarterly Journal of Medicine 18: 359–392

Christensen S, Ottosen P, Olsen S 1982 Severe functional and structural changes caused by lithium in the developing rat kidney. Acta Pathologica Microbiologica et Immunologica Scandinavica 80: 257–267

Cole B, Conley S, Stapleton F B 1987 Polycystic kidney disease in the first year of life. Journal of Pediatrics 111: 693–699

Darmady E M, Offer J, Woodhouse M A 1970 Toxic metabolic defect in polycystic disease of kidney. Lancet 1: 547–550

Delaney V B, Adler S, Burne F J, Licinia M, Segal D P, Fraley D S 1985 Autosomal dominant polycystic kidney disease: presentation, complications, and prognosis. American Journal of Kidney Disease 5: 104–111

Dobyan D C, Hill D, Lewis T, Bulger R E 1981 Cyst formation in rat kidney induced by cis-platinum administration. Laboratory Investigation 45: 260–268

Evan A P, Gardner K D 1979 Nephron obstruction in nordihydroguaiaretic acid-induced renal cystic disease. Kidney International 15: 7–19

Evan A P, Mong S A, Gattone V H, Connors B A, Aronoff G R, Luft F C 1984 The effect of streptozotocin and streptozotocin-induced diabetes on the kidney. Renal Physiology 7: 78–89

Fanconi G, Hanhant E, von Albertini A et al 1951 Die familiare juvenile nephronophthisis. Helvetica Paediatrica Acta 6: 1

Fry J L, Koch W E, Jennette J C, McFarland E, Fried F A, Mandell J 1985 A genetically determined murine model of infantile polycystic kidney disease. Journal of Urology 134: 828–833

Gabow P A, Inklerman D W, Holmes J H 1984 Polycystic kidney disease: Prospective analysis of nonazotemic patients and family members. Annals of Internal Medicine 101: 238–247

Gardner K D 1971 Evolution of clinical signs in adult-onset cystic disease of the renal medulla. Annals of Internal Medicine 74: 47–54

Gardner K D Jr. 1988 Cystic kidneys. Kidney International 33: 610–621

Gardner K D, Evan A P 1983 Renal cystic disease induced by diphenylthiazole. Kidney Inernational 24: 43–52

Gardner K D, Evan A P 1984 Cystic kidneys: An enigma evolves. American Journal of Kidney Disease 3: 403–413

Gardner K D, Solomon S, Fitzgerrel W W, Evan A P 1976 Function and structure in the diphenylamine-exposed kidney. Journal of Clinical Investigation 57: 796–806

Gardner K D, Evan A P, Reed W P 1986 Accelerated renal cyst development in deconditioned germfree rats. Kidney International 29: 1116–1123

Gardner K D, Reed W P, Evan A P, Zedalis J, Hylarides M D, Leon A A 1987 Endotoxin provocation of experimental renal cystic disease. Kidney International 32: 329–334

Garel I A, Habib R, Pariente D et al 1984 Juvenile Nephronophthisis: Sonographic appearance in children with severe uremia. Radiology 151: 93

Giselson N, Heinegaard D, Holmberg C–G et al 1970 Renal medullary cystic disease or familial juvenile nephronophthisis. A renal tubular disease. Biochemical findings in two siblings. American Journal of Medicine 48: 174

Grantham J J 1983 Polycystic kidney disease: A predominance of giant nephrons. American Journal of Physiology 244: F3–F10

Grantham J J, Donoso V S, Evan A P, Carone F A, Gardner K D 1987 Intrinsic viscoelastic properties of tubule basement membranes in experimental renal cystic disease. Kidney International 32: 187–197

Hartman G E, Smokik L, Shochat S 1986 The dilemma of the multicystic dysplastic kidney. American Journal of Diseases of Children 140: 925–928

Herdman R C, Good R A, Vernier R L 1967 Medullary cystic disease in two siblings. American Journal of Medicine 43: 335

Hestbech J, Hansen H E, Amdisen A, Olsen S 1977 Chronic renal lesions following long-term treatment with lithium. Kidney International 12: 205–213

Hossack K F, Leddy C L, Schrier R W, Gabow P A 1987 Incidence of cardiac abnormalities associated with autosomal dominant polycystic kidney disease (ADPKD) (Abstract). Kidney International 31: 203

Iverson W O, Fetterman G H, Jacobson E R, Olsen J H, Senior D F, Schobert E E 1982 Polycystic kidney and liver disease in spring-bok: 1. Morphology of the lesions. Kidney International 22: 146–155

Kanwar Y S, Carone F A 1984 Reversible changes of tubular cell and basement membrane in drug-induced renal cystic disease. Kidney International 26: 35–43

Leichter H E, Dietrich R, Salusky I B, Foley J, Cohen A, Kangarloo H, Fine R N 1988 Acquired cystic disease in children undergoing long-term dialysis. Pediatric Nephrology. 2: 8–11

Levey A S, Pauker S G, Kassirer J P 1983 Occult intracranial aneurysms in polycystic kidney disease. New England Journal of Medicine 308: 986–994

Lieberman E, Salinas-Madrigal L, Gwinn J L, Brennan L P, Fine R N, Landing B H 1971 Infantile polycystic disease of the kidneys and liver. Medicine 50: 277–318

Loken A C, Hanssen O, Halvorsen J et al 1961 Hereditary renal dysplasia and blindness. Acta Paediatrica. 50: 177

Mainzer F, Saldino R M, Ozonoff M D et al 1970 Familial nephropathy associated with retinitis pigmentosa, cerebellar ataxia, and skeletal abnormalities. American Journal of Medicine 49: 556

Milutinovic J, Fialkow P J, Agoda L Y, Phillips L A, Rudd T G, Bryant J L 1984 Autosomal dominant polycystic kidney disease: Symptoms and clinical findings. Quarterly Journal of Medicine 212: 511–522

Perrone R D 1985 In vitro function of cyst epithelium from human polycystic kidney. Journal of Clinical Investigation 76: 1688–1691

Popovie-Rolovic M, Calic-Penisic N, Bunjevacki G 1976 Juvenile nephronophthisis associated with retinal pigmentary dystrophy, cerebellar ataxia, and skeletal abnormalities. Archives of Disease in Childhood 51: 801

Rayfield E J, McDonald F D 1972 Red and blonde hair in renal medullary cystic disease. Archives of Internal Medicine 130: 72

Reeders S T, Breuning M H, Davies K E et al 1985 A highly polymorphic DNA marker linked to adult polycystic kidney disease on chromosome 16. Nature 317: 542–543

Reeders S T, Breuning M H, Corney G et al 1986a Two genetic markers closely linked to adult polycystic kidney disease on chromosome 16. British Medical Journal 292: 851–853

Reeders S T, Gal A, Propping P et al 1986b Prenatal diagnosis of autosomal dominant polycystic kidney disease with a DNA probe. Lancet 2: 6–8

Resnick J, Vernier R L 1986 Renal cystic disease and renal dysplasia. In: Holliday M A, Barratt T M, Vernier R L (eds) Pediatric Nephrology 2nd edn. Williams & Wilkins, Baltimore

Resnick J S, Brown D M, Vernier R L 1976 Normal development and experimental models of cystic renal disease. In: Gardner K D (ed) Cystic Disease of the Kidney, Wiley, New York, pp 221–241

Resnick J, Sisson S, Vernier R L 1978 Tamm-Horsfall protein. Abnormal localization in renal disease. Laboratory Investigation 38: 550

Romeo G, Costa G, Catizone L et al 1988 A second genetic locus for autosomal dominant polycystic kidney disease. Lancet ii: 8–10

Scheff R T, Zuckerman G, Hartner H, Delmez J, Koehler R 1980 Diverticular disease in patients with chronic renal failure due to polycystic kidney disease. Annals of Internal Medicine 92: 202–204

Senior B, Friedman A I, Brando J L 1961 Juvenile familial nephropathy with tapetoretinal degeneration. American Journal of Ophthalmology 52: 625

Sherman F E, Studnicki F M, Fetterman G H 1971 Renal lesions of familial juvenile nephronophthisis examined by microdissection. American Journal of Clinical Pathology 55: 391

Smith C H, Graham J B 1945 Congenital medullary cysts of kidneys with severe refractory anemia. American Journal of Diseases of Children 69: 369

Solomon S 1973 Inherited renal cysts in rats. Science 181: 451–452

Strauss M B 1962 Clinical and pathological aspects of cystic disease of the renal medulla. An analysis of eighteen cases. Annals of International Medicine 57: 373–381

Takahashi H, Ueyama Y, Hibino T, Kuwahara Y, Suzuki S, Hioki K, Tamaoki N 1986 A new mouse model of genetically transmitted polycystic kidney disease. Journal of Urology 135: 1280–1283

Thomas J O, Cox A J, DeEds F 1957 Kidney cysts induced by diphenylamine. Stadford Medical Bulletin 15: 90–93

Uchic M, Kornhaus J, Grantham J A, McAkeer J, Cragoe E J, Grantham J J 1987 Amiloride and amiloride analogues retard the enlargement of MDCK-cysts grown in hydrated collagen (abstract). Kidney International 31: 184

Vargas L, Friederici H H R, Maibenco H C 1970 Cortical sponge kidneys induced in rats by alloxan. Diabetes 19: 33–44

Waldherr R, Lennert T, Weber H-P et al 1982 The nephronophthisis complex: A clinicopathologic study in children. Virchows Archiv 394: 235

Werder A A, Amos M A, Nielsen A H, Wolfe G H 1984 Comparative effects of germ-free and ambient environments on the development of cystic kidney disease in CFW wd mice. Journal of Laboratory and Clinical Medicine 103: 399–407

77. The nephrotic syndromes

R. Norio

INTRODUCTION

The nephrotic syndrome (NS) is a *clinical* diagnosis. It is characterised by oedema, proteinuria, hypoalbuminaemia and hyperlipaemia, and sometimes by microscopic haematuria and arterial hypertension. Response to treatment with steroids or cytotoxic drugs and survival time in the nonresponders vary greatly. Several pathogenetic pathways may lead to NS. Their common denominator is the altered permeability of the glomerular filtration barrier; its details are poorly known.

The classification of NS is largely based on renal histology. This has produced a variety of *descriptive* diagnoses. Clinical genetics, however, endeavours to find an *aetiological* diagnosis. This is difficult for renal disease in general, and for the nephrotic syndromes in particular. An essential prerequisite is to take all the findings into account, not only one or two details, however important. Also the microscopic picture alone seldom provides a specific aetiological diagnosis. Very few histological renal findings are pathognomonic for a particular disease; they indicate the progression of the disease rather than give an accurate aetiological diagnosis. This is obvious if several specimens can be studied from the same patient at different ages. In fact, naming a renal disease only by aid of the microscope has led to a confusing diversity in the nomenclature, not only in the descriptions of individual patients but also in classifications.

The main interest of this chapter is directed towards the primary nephrotic syndromes, often without known cause. They mostly affect the paediatric age groups. NS may be called secondary if it occurs as a part of a renal or some other disease entity or is caused by a known exogenous factor. Most adult NS patients belong to this group. Thus, NS occurs associated with many systemic diseases such as anaphylactoid purpura, amyloidosis, diabetes, lupus erythematosus, and sickle-cell disease. Known or assumed causes for NS are infections such as maternal syphilis (Hill et al 1972, Kaschula et al 1974, Repetto et al 1982) and toxoplasmosis (Shahin et al 1974), cytomegalovirus (de Luca et al 1964) or E. coli (Flatz 1964). In Africa the epidemiology of NS differs greatly from that in non-tropical countries, being apparently caused by malaria and possibly also by other infections (Lancet Editorial 1980, Adu et al 1981). Cases of NS have been attributed to toxic agents like mercury (Worthen et al 1959), insect sting (Tareyeva et al 1982), or maternal steroid-chlorpheniramine treatment (Anand et al 1979). Nephrosis has been found to be a part of some less known syndromes (Shapiro et al 1976, Robain & Deonna 1983, Andermann et al 1986, Palm et al 1986). Among the renal diseases reported to be associated with or complicated by NS, several 'nephritic' disorders, at least in their advanced phases, are common, and nail-patella syndrome (Similä et al 1970) is rare. Renal vein thrombosis is nowadays regarded not as a cause but a complication of NS (Kaplan et al 1978, Lau et al 1980, Chugh et al 1981, Panicucci et al 1983). For further details of secondary NS as well as for other specific features of NS, the reader is referred to textbooks of nephrology.

It is difficult to find a practical grouping for primary NS for the purposes of clinical genetics. Only a few aetiological groups are known. Any attempt at too strict and systematic a classification would lead to confusion and unwarranted conclusions. A suitable balance between nosological splitting and lumping (McKusick 1969) must be found. A few clearly defined aetiological entities can be split off, whereas other nephrotic syndromes might be left lumped together as heterogeneous but clinically useful groups, until such time as additional knowledge allows for further splitting.

In this chapter the following grouping according to age at onset of NS is used:
Congenital nephrotic syndromes (CN)
— congenital nephrotic syndrome of Finnish type (CNF)
— other types (CNO)
Infantile nephrotic syndromes (IN)
— diffuse mesangial sclerosis (DMS) alone or as a part of the Drash syndrome
— other types (INO)

Nephrotic syndromes of later onset (LN)

This grouping, modified from the terms used by White (1973), is a relative one, with compromises and overlapping among the groups. It may, however, be useful as regards treatment, prognosis, genetic counselling and prenatal diagnosis. Before placing a patient in any of the groups, the possibility of a 'secondary' causative factor must be taken into account.

CONGENITAL NEPHROTIC SYNDROMES (CN)

Congenital nephrotic syndromes are present at birth, at least latently, and become manifest by the age of three months. In this group the congenital nephrotic syndrome of Finnish type is the only distinct aetiological entity known.

Congenital nephrotic syndrome of Finnish type (CNF)

Since the 1950s (Hallman et al 1956) this disease has raised active interest among Finnish paediatricians because it has proved to be exceptionally common in Finland. By 1973, 151 patients were known, and the number now exceeds 200. The incidence in Finland is about 1 in 8000 (Huttunen 1976). However, CNF has been reported from all over the world (Norio 1966, Hallman et al 1970), most cases among Caucasians, but also among Blacks (Eiben et al 1954, George et al 1976), American Indians (George et al 1976), Japanese (Kobayashi et al 1961, Yamamoto et al 1961), Indians (Rajamma et al 1974), Tunisians (Khrouf et al 1982) and Maoris (Kendall-Smith et al 1968). More than 150 CNF or CNF-like cases have been published outside Finland. Of the cases of NS manifesting in the first year of life, one half in North America (according to George et al 1976) and one third in France (judging by the series of Habib & Bois 1973) may have CNF.

The clinical picture of CNF varies only slightly (Hallman et al 1970, 1973, Huttunen 1976, Hallman & Rapola 1978, Mahan et al 1984, Rapola 1987). As proof of the congenital character of CNF, the placenta is always abnormally large, amounting to more than 25% of the birth weight (Fig. 77.1). The majority of patients are born prematurely — 90% of them before the 39th week of gestation — and are small for dates. Signs of perinatal asphyxia, such as meconium-stained amniotic fluid, low Apgar score and respiratory distress, are common; some patients die perinatally before the diagnosis of CNF has been made. Malformations are not a part of CNF; broad cranial sutures may be a sign of delayed ossification, and flexed ankles may indicate muscular weakness.

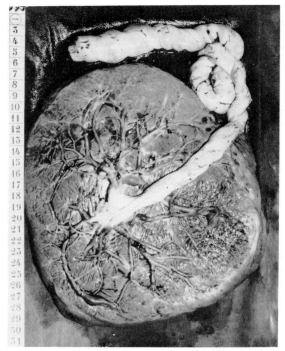

Fig. 77.1 Large placenta of newborn CNF infant; weight 1850 g, measurements 25 × 22 × 6 cm.

Proteinuria probably always begins in utero. Oedema is detectable from birth in one quarter of the cases, during the first week of life in half, and by the age of three months in all cases.

The clinical picture is totally different depending on whether the patient is treated conservatively and symptomatically according to general principles applied to nephrosis, or aggressively, with the aim of renal transplantation.

In the first alternative the outcome is always fatal, in half the cases by 6 months, in 75% by 12 months and always by 4 years of age. The patients fail to thrive; they never learn to walk or speak. Distension of the abdomen, due to meteorism and ascites, is a very characteristic sign; herniae are common. After the first few months the appearance is dystrophic rather than oedematous (Fig. 77.2). High susceptibility to infections and complete resistance to corticosteroids and antimetabolites are the rule.

The laboratory findings are similar to those of NS in general. Proteinuria is massive and in most patients selective (Huttunen et al 1980b). Microscopic haematuria occurs often; leucocytes, amino acids and glucose may also be found in the urine. The values of blood urea nitrogen are in general normal, sometimes slightly raised but seldom distinctly elevated.

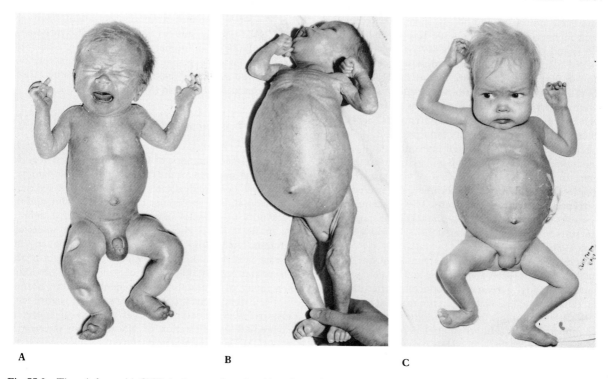

Fig. 77.2   Three infants with CNF: **A** a boy, age 2 weeks with oedema of the face and particularly of the lower limbs; **B** a severely affected girl, age 7 months, with a typical opisthotonic position, greatly distended abdomen, dystrophic but not oedematous appearance, and right inguinal hernia; **C** a girl, age 2 years 2 months, with milder course and longer survival than average.

The cause of death is often infections, never uraemia, but the precise cause of death remains unknown in nearly half the cases. Thromboembolic complications have been found at autopsy in a fifth of the recent cases.

The possibility of renal transplantation seems to have led the treatment of CNF into a new era. The first successful attempts were reported from Minneapolis in 1973 (Hoyer et al). In 1984 the same group (Mahan et al) published results from 17 transplantation patients with a two-year survival rate of 82% and a surprisingly good quality of life in most of the survivors. A necessary prerequisite for transplantation is a long and aggressive preoperative treatment including hyperalimentation, dialysis and often bilateral nephrectomy (Mahan et al 1984, Guillot et al 1980). The purpose of these procedures is to prevent and supplement the massive protein loss via urine and thus to make growth, psychomotor development and resistance to infections possible. Successful results have also been published from France (Floret et al 1976). In Finland nine transplantations were performed in the 1960s and 70s, all unsuccessful, probably because of the lack of sufficient preoperative treatment. The first successful renal transplantation on a Finnish CNF

patient was performed in 1987. Since then, five others have been performed, all successfully (Holmberg et al 1989).

The kidneys are large compared to the weight of the patient. The histological alterations are polymorphic and progressive; no single finding is pathognomonic or necessary for the diagnosis (Hallman et al 1973, Hallman & Rapola 1978, Huttunen et al 1980a). Dilatations of the proximal, but sometimes also distal, tubules are the most characteristic findings. Their amount varies greatly, from an occasional dilatation to a universal dispersion throughout the renal cortex. The tubular epithelium is tall in the beginning, but flat and atrophic in advanced cases. In the glomeruli, proliferation of mesangial cells and increase of PAS- and silver-positive matrix are characteristic: this mesangial sclerosis does not cause narrowing of the capillaries except in the very advanced cases. In a part of the glomeruli, periglomerular onion-like fibrosis gradually leads to obstruction and total hyalinization. Immature glomeruli with condensed tufts and wide Bowman's space are often seen in young patients, but they are also seen in normal infants of the same age (Huttunen et al 1980a). In the interstitium round cell infiltration and fibrosis increase with age. For electron microscopic findings see Rapola and Savilahti (1971) and Hallman and Rapola (1978).

CNF is an autosomal recessive disease. In a series of 57 Finnish families (Norio 1966) the sex ratio was 1.07 and the proportion of affected sibs very close to 0.25. Of the parental marriages 16 were shown to be consanguineous, even if remotely in most cases. 43 parents (38%) were related to parents of other CN families.

The ancestry was distributed unevenly in a large area which has been permanently populated for less than 500 years. In fact CNF was the first of the rare recessive disorders, now about 30 in number, discovered to be overrepresented among the Finns. This concentration of recessive disorders is due to the peculiar population structure of Finland (Norio et al 1973, Norio & Nevanlinna 1980, Norio 1981).

Heterozygous manifestations are not known. Kniker and Prindiville (1969) and Kniker and Sweeney (1972) reported slightly increased amounts of glomerular basement membrane like material in the urine of relatives of CNF patients, but this finding could not be substantiated in Finnish patients (Huttunen et al 1976).

CNF families can be helped by prenatal diagnosis since alphafetoprotein (AFP) concentration is very high (more than 10 SD) in the amniotic fluid and often also in maternal serum (Aula et al 1978), due to fetal proteinuria. Up to 1990 over 100 pregnancies of families with a previous CN baby have been monitored in Finland without a single false result (Aula 1990). In the AFP-screening of maternal serum of 54 299 Finnish pregnancies from central and eastern Finland, in addition to 19 fetuses with a neural tube defect, as many as 27 fetuses with confirmed CNF and three suspected cases have been found (Ryynänen et al 1983, Ryynänen 1988). CNF is one possibility to be taken into account in pregnancies with a 'false-positive' AFP-result; this diagnosis can be confirmed from ultrastructural and light microscopic findings of the fetal kidneys (Rapola et al 1984). Prenatal diagnosis may not be possible in most other forms of congenital or infantile nephrosis (Spritz et al 1978, Rapola & Hallman 1979).

The pathogenesis of CNF is not yet definitely solved. The reported immunological abnormalities of earlier studies (Kouvalainen 1963, Lange et al 1963) have not been confirmed (Hoyer et al 1967, Rapola & Savilahti 1971, Griswold & McIntosh 1972) and are thus apparently secondary. Glomeruli are present in nearly twice the normal number (Tryggvason & Kouvalainen 1975). The increased permeability of the glomerular basement membrane could be due to a genetically determined failure in its synthesis (Norio 1966, Mahieu et al 1976, Tryggvason 1977). Recently Vernier et al (1983) demonstrated a decrease of anionic sites in the renal basement membrane in CNF, possibly due to the failure of synthesis of glomerular heparan sulphate or proteoglycan. This could provide a logical explanation for the early fetal proteinuria as well as for the lack of recurrence of the disease after renal transplantation (Mahan et al 1984).

Other kinds of congenital nephrotic syndrome (CNO)

An undisputed diagnosis of CNF brings with it very decisive consequences for the infant and his or her family: a rapid and certain death or heroic treatment by renal transplantation, a recurrence risk of 25% for sibs, and the possibility of prenatal diagnosis. Therefore, a definite diagnosis of CNF should not be made on uncertain grounds. According to the Finnish experience, the disease is very unlikely to be CNF if the weight of the placenta is normal, if age at onset is more than 3 months, if primary psychomotor development is within normal limits, if the patient shows overt uraemia or is alive with 'original' kidneys at the age of 4 years or more. A 'congenital' manifestation of NS need not necessarily imply CNF but may also be due to either an exogenous or an unknown 'idiopathic' aetiology. Because of considerable overlap with related disorders these will be discussed together with 'Infantile nephrotic syndromes' (Norio & Rapola 1989).

INFANTILE NEPHROTIC SYNDROMES (IN)

Diffuse mesangial sclerosis (DMS)

In the group of NS manifesting at 3 to 12 months of age, the histopathological diagnosis of diffuse mesangial sclerosis (DMS) appears in at least two clinical forms, 'idiopathic' and as a component of the Drash syndrome. Their aetiological relationship is still uncertain. Habib and Bois (1973) introduced the concept when reporting six patients from France. More than 20 other patients with possible DMS have been described (Rossenbeck et al, Family 1, 1966, Hallman et al 1973, Kaplan et al 1974, Richard et al 1975, Seelig et al 1975, Gonzales et al 1977, Rumpelt & Bachmann 1980, Kikuta et al 1983, see further references in Urbach et al 1985).

Nothing exceptional is known about the pregnancy or perinatal features; the placenta, in particular, has not been reported to be abnormally large (a possible exception is patient 1 described by Rossenbeck et al 1966). Age of manifesting oedema or proteinuria has mostly been 1–13 months, though in one case it was at 2 weeks (Rumpelt & Bachmann 1980). The patients develop progressive renal insufficiency, which is often also the cause of death. The disease is resistant to steroids or cytotoxic drugs, and the outcome is always fatal, usually by the age of 4 years.

The histological picture is characteristic, perhaps pathognomonic, and differs distinctly from that seen in CNF. All glomeruli are affected. The capillary tufts are small and contracted and Bowman's space seems correspondingly wide. The number of glomerular cells is not increased. Instead, mesangial PAS- and silver-positive sclerosing fibrils are a constant finding, and the capillaries are severely occluded. Epithelial crescents may be present. Tubular atrophy and dilatations are common, as is interstitial fibrosis. Rumpelt and Bachmann (1980) have described a 'cloudy pattern' alteration of the glomerular basement membrane by electron microscopy.

In two families reported by Habib and Bois and in three other probable DMS families (Rossenbeck, Gonzales) two or three sibs have been affected. This suggests autosomal recessive inheritance. Attempts at prenatal diagnosis have not been reported; it may not be possible.

Habib and her group (1985, 1989) also drew attention to the Drash syndrome (Drash et al 1970, Eddy & Mauer 1985), a combination of male pseudohermaphroditism, Wilms tumour and DMS. Most of the patients reported by them had more or less ambiguous genitalia, XY karyotype, and testes. Many questions still require answers such as the relevance of patients with the XX karyotype, mode of inheritance, aetiological associations with 'idiopathic' DMS, and others. Rapola (1987) reported an exceptional Finnish Drash patient with large placenta and heavy proteinuria at birth, XY karyotype and female phenotype with slight clitorimegaly. He stressed the importance of chromosomal analysis and accurate inspection of the genitalia in patients with CN or IN.

Other kinds of infantile nephrotic syndrome (INO)

Nephrotic syndrome is a rare disease during the first year of life. At that age the cause may also be exceptional. If an individual patient does not fit into the narrow limits of CNF or DMS, or if an undisputed exogenous cause cannot be traced, very little can be said about the clinical course, response to treatment, prognosis, aetiology, and risk of recurrence in subsequent sibs. It seems that INO is often associated with overt histological glomerular changes and poor prognosis, and is often familial. The clinical features may appear in all possible combinations. A congenital manifestation — even with a large placenta — may, in contrast to CNF, be compatible with normal growth and development, considerably longer survival (Vernier et al 1957, Gantner 1965, Habib & Bois 1973) and even complete recovery (Anand et al 1979). More-over, the onset may be 'late' but the course rapidly fatal (Nagi & Nouri 1974). In familial cases, affected members of a sibship may show wide variation in age at onset, course, prognosis and survival (Mehls & Schärer 1970). One unanswered question is whether the CNF gene in a non-Finnish genetic background might, in a proportion of cases, cause a milder disorder with longer survival (and terminal renal failure) (Hoyer et al 1973, Moncrieff et al 1973, Family 2) than is the rule in Finland. However, different recessive genes are probably responsible for many cases of INO.

Many attempts at a histological classification may in the clinical sense be confusing rather than helpful. However, the classifications of Habib and Bois (1973) and Kaplan et al (1974) are also useful clinically. Many authors use the word 'microcystic' when speaking of the tubular dilatations typical of CNF. When Oliver (1960) introduced this term he did not give detailed clinical data on his patients, nor did he use it as a synonym for CNF. Unfortunately the term has come to have various meanings. As a histological term, 'microcystic' may lead to confusion with 'true' polycystic diseases of the kidney. Tubular dilatations are not seen in every renal biopsy specimen of CNF patients. Instead, they can be found in many other entities, e.g. DMS. Oliver himself reported patients who died 'in many instances of terminal renal failure'. The term microcystic renal disease should obviously be abandoned as a synonym for CNF (Hallman et al 1973).

It is reasonable to try conventional treatment of NS in cases of INO, although the results are uncertain. Genetic counselling in families with INO must be done cautiously, bearing in mind the possibility of autosomal recessive transmission.

NEPHROTIC SYNDROMES OF LATER ONSET (LN)

'Idiopathic' nephrotic syndrome usually manifests after the first year of life. The majority, about 80% or more of the cases, belong histologically to the group with 'minimal (glomerular) changes'; of these, over 90% respond, to varying degree, to treatment with steroids or cytotoxic agents. The rest show various histological glomerular changes and their prognosis is distinctly poorer.

It is usually assumed that 'idiopathic' nephrotic syndrome, here called nephrotic syndrome of later onset (LN), is a non-familial disease. However, surprisingly many familial cases have been reported. By 1968 I had found 79 familial cases in the literature (Norio 1969). In the series of their own patients Mehls and Schärer (1970) from Germany described 12 familial cases out of 135 (?) (9%), Bader et al (1974a,b) from Indiana, USA, 14 out of

70 (20%), and Gekle et al (1975) from Germany 4 out of 73 (5%). Moncrieff et al (1973) reported at least 20 familial cases from Great Britain, Gonzales et al (1977) 24 cases from France, and White (1973) 40 cases out of about 1850 (2%) through an inquiry in 24 European paediatric departments. The majority of the familial cases were pairs of sibs, including 13 pairs of twins, all apparently monozygous (those reported by 1968, see Norio 1969, Roy & Pitcock 1971, Bader et al 1974a,b). As yet, no familial LN cases are known in Finland.

The clinical data on familial LN found in the literature are fragmentary, difficult to combine and, in part, even contradictory. Without presenting a detailed analysis of them, some conclusions, even if uncertain, may be justified:

1. Marked histological glomerular alterations are observed in a far greater proportion of patients (about half of those reported by White 1973) than in the nonfamilial cases; prognosis is worse than average in these cases.
2. The prognosis for patients with minimal changes is similar to that in non-familial cases.
3. The histological grouping of an individual patient may change during the course of the disease.
4. The clinical features (age at onset, histological picture and prognosis) are often similar in affected sibs, but there are numerous exceptions to this rule, even in identical twins (Bader et al 1974a,b).
5. A male preponderance is evident also in familial LN.

Aetiologically, LN is certainly heterogeneous. As in most common disorders, the exact role of heredity has not been discovered. The familial cases of 'usual' LN have occurred mostly in pairs, i.e. only two affected sibs per family. Monozygous twins, all concordantly affected, have been overrepresented and no dizygous concordant twin pairs with LN have been reported. Some cases of LN in two consecutive generations or in near collateral relatives are also known (Norio 1969, White 1973, Gekle et al 1975). Based on these facts I suggested the possibility of a polygenic basis for at least a proportion of LN cases (Norio 1969). The analysis of Bader et al (1974a,b) gives support to this assumption.

Besides the 'usual' familial LN there are several reports of 'unusual' families with juvenile and infantile, or even congenital cases in the same sibship (Moncrieff et al 1973, Families V & VI). Also, the course of the disease may vary greatly between sibs, ranging from symptomless proteinuria to a rapidly fatal outcome, and from minimal glomerular changes to severe histological alterations. In these exceptional cases, sibships with more than two affected sibs have been reported, and sometimes also parental consanguinity (Devin 1960, Fanconi & Illig 1960, Fournier et al 1963). Probably different autosomal recessive genes are responsible in these cases.

The treatment of familial LN patients is similar to that of non-familial cases. Renal biopsy may give valuable clues to the course and prognosis. For genetic counselling Bader et al (1974a,b) have estimated a surprisingly high recurrence risk of 6% for the sibs of a patient. A convenient figure for general use is perhaps less than 5%, though many nephrologists might even be inclined towards a smaller risk figure, say less than 2%. However, overt glomerular alterations in a renal biopsy might indicate a greater risk of recurrence than in cases with minimal changes because patients with overt glomerular changes are particularly frequent among familial cases. Further, in many hereditary disorders the majority of patients are sporadic and only the minority are familial. Hence a proportion of non-familial LN patients with overt glomerular changes may in fact be genetic.

CONCLUSIONS

The nephrotic syndrome is aetiologically heterogeneous. To achieve an accurate diagnosis the patient should be evaluated on a broad basis rather than concentrating on one or two features only (e.g. renal histology). If a distinct exogenous aetiology is not demonstrable, age at onset may serve as a first criterion for further grouping.

In cases manifesting congenitally (or during the first 3 months of life) the congenital nephrotic syndrome of Finnish type, and in those manifesting during the first year of life diffuse mesangial sclerosis must be taken into consideration. The former diagnosis must be made on strict criteria only, because it means a hopeless prognosis with conservative treatment, a challenge for renal transplantation, a recurrence risk of 25% in sibs and the possibility of prenatal diagnosis. In other, rare and poorly understood nephrotic syndromes during the first year of life, course and prognosis may vary greatly, often being severe. Familial occurrence is not unusual and autosomal recessive inheritance is possible, if not probable.

The 'usual' or 'idiopathic' nephrotic syndrome usually manifests after the first year of life. In at least some of these patients heredity may play an important role in aetiology, probably in some polygenic manner. The recurrence risk in sibs is greater than is universally assumed: perhaps less than 5% in general, but greater in cases with overt histological glomerular alterations.

REFERENCES

Adu D, Anim-Addo Y, Foli A K, Blankson J M, Annobil S H, Reindorf C A, Christian E C 1981 The nephrotic syndrome in Ghana: Clinical and pathological aspects. Quarterly Journal of Medicine, New Series I: 297–306

Anand S K, Northway J D, Vernier R L 1979 Congenital nephrotic syndrome: report of a patient with cystic tubular changes who recovered. Journal of Pediatrics 95: 265

Andermann E, Andermann F, Carpenter S et al 1986 Action myoclonus-renal failure syndrome: a previously unrecognised neurological disorder unmasked by advances in nephrology. Advances in Neurology 43: 87–103

Aula P 1990 Personal communication

Aula P, Rapola J, Karjalainen O, Lindgren J, Hartikainen A L, Seppälä M 1978 Prenatal diagnosis of congenital nephrosis in 23 high-risk families. American Journal of Diseases of Children 132: 984

Bader P I, Grove J, Trygstad C W, Nance W E 1974a Familial nephrotic syndrome. American Journal of Medicine 56: 34

Bader P I, Grove J, Nance W E, Trygstad C W 1974b Inheritance of idiopathic nephrotic syndrome. Birth Defects: Original Article Series, vol X, No 4: 73

Chugh K S, Malik N, Uberoi H S et al 1981 Renal vein thrombosis in nephrotic syndrome — a prospective study and review. Postgraduate Medical Journal 57: 566–570

de Luca G, Delendi N, D'Andrea S 1964 Un raro caso di nefrosi congenita e malattia da inclusioni citomegaliche Nota I. Minerva Pediatrica 16: 1164

Devin P 1960 Syndromes néphrotiques familiaux et congénitaux. Thèse médicale Nancy No 27

Drash A, Sherman F, Hartmann W H, Blizzard R M 1970 A syndrome of pseudohermaphroditism, Wilms' tumor, hypertension, and degenerative renal disease. Journal of Pediatrics 76: 585–593

Eddy A A, Mauer S M 1985 Pseudohermaphroditism, glomerulopathy, and Wilms' tumor (Drash syndrome): frequency in end-stage renal failure. Journal of Pediatrics 106: 584–587

Eiben R M, Kleinerman J, Cline J C 1954 Nephrotic syndrome in a neonatal premature infant. Journal of Pediatrics 44: 195

Fanconi G, Illig R 1960 Das familiäre Vorkommen der Lipoid-nephrose und der Nephronophthise. Moderne Probleme der Pädiatrie 6: 298

Flatz G 1964 Nephrotisches Syndrom und Pyknocytose bei einem jungen Säugling. Monatsschrift für Kinderheilkunde 112: 102

Floret D et al 1976 Transplantation rénale à l'age de 2 ans 4 mois pour syndrome néphrotique congénital. La Nouvelle Presse Médicale 5: 2701

Fournier A, Paget M, Pauli A, Devin P 1963 Syndromes néphrotiques familiaux. Syndrome néphrotique associé à une cardiopathie congénitale chez quatre soeurs. Pédiatrie 18: 677

Gantner J 1965 Das idiopathische nephrotische Syndrom im Säuglingsalter an Hand von vier eigenen Beobachtungen. Helvetica Paediatrica Acta 20: 374

Gekle D, Buchinger G, Könitzer I 1975 Untersuchungen zur Familiarität des nephrotischen Syndroms. Monatsschrift für Kinderheilkunde 123: 106

George C R P, Hickman R O, Stricker G E 1976 Infantile nephrotic syndrome. Clinical Nephrology 5: 20

Gonzales G, Kleinknecht C, Gubler M C, Lenoir G 1977 Syndromes néphrotiques familiaux. La Revue de Pédiatrie 13: 427

Griswold W, McIntosh R M 1972 Immunological studies in congenital nephrosis. Journal of Medical Genetics 9: 245

Guillot M, Broyer M, Cathelineau L, Boulegue D, Dartois A M, Folio D, Guimbaud P 1980 Nutrition entérale à debit constant en néphrologie pédiatrique. Archives de Françaises de Pédiatrie 37: 497–505

Habib R, Bois E 1973 Hétérogénéité des syndromes néphrotiques a debut précoce du nourisson (syndrome néphrotique 'infantile'). Etude anatomoclinique et génétique de 37 observations. Helvetica Paediatrica Acta 28: 91

Habib R, Loirat C, Gubler M C, Niaudet P, Bensman A, Levy M, Broyer M 1985 The nephropathy associated with male pseudohermaphroditism and Wilms' tumor (Drash syndrome): a distinctive glomerular lesion - report of 10 cases. Clinical Nephrology 24: 269–278

Habib R, Gubler M C, Niaudet P, Gagnadoux M F 1989 Congenital/infantile nephrotic syndrome with diffuse mesangial sclerosis: relationship with Drash syndrome. In: Bartsocas C S (ed) Genetics of kidney disorders (Progress in clinical and biological research Vol 305). Alan R Liss, New York, p 193

Hallman N, Hjelt L, Ahvenainen E K 1956 Nephrotic syndrome in newborn and young infants. Annales Paediatriae Fenniae 2: 227

Hallman N, Norio R, Kouvalainen K, Vilska J, Kojo N 1970 Das kongenitale nephrotische Syndrom. Ergebnisse der Inneren Medizin und Kinderheilkunde 30: 3

Hallman N, Norio R, Rapola J 1973 Congenital nephrotic syndrome. Nephron 11: 101

Hallman N, Rapola J 1978 Congenital nephrotic syndrome. In: Edelman C M Jr (ed) Pediatric kidney disease. Little Brown, Boston, vol 2, ch 54, p 711

Hill L L, Singer D B, Falletta J, Stasney R 1972 The nephrotic syndrome in congenital syphilis. An immunopathy. Pediatrics 49: 260

Holmberg C, Jalanko H, Leijala M, Salmela K, Koskimies O 1989 Active treatment of 23 patients with congenital nephrotic syndrome of the Finnish type (abstract). Pediatric Nephrology 3: C227

Hoyer J R, Michael A F Jr, Good R A, Vernier R L 1967 The nephrotic syndrome of infancy: clinical, morphologic and immunologic studies of four infants. Pediatrics 40: 233

Hoyer J R et al 1973 Successful renal transplantation in 3 children with congenital nephrotic syndrome. Lancet 1: 1410

Huttunen N-P 1976 Congenital nephrotic syndrome of Finnish type: study of 75 patients. Archives of Disease in Childhood 51: 344

Huttunen N-P, Hallman N, Rapola J 1976 Glomerular basement membrane antigens in congenital and acquired nephrotic syndrome in childhood. Nephron 16: 401

Huttunen N-P, Rapola J, Vilska J, Hallman N 1980a Renal pathology in congenital nephrotic syndrome of Finnish type: a quantitative light microscopic study on 50 patients. International Journal of Pediatric Nephrology 1: 10

Huttunen N-P, Vehaskari M, Viikari M, Laipio M-L 1980b

Proteinuria in congenital nephrotic syndrome of the Finnish type. Clinical Nephrology 13: 12

Kaplan B S, Bureau M A, Drummond K N 1974 The nephrotic syndrome in the first year of life: is a pathologic classification possible? Journal of Pediatrics 85: 615

Kaplan B S, Chesney R W, Drummond K N 1978 The nephrotic syndrome and renal vein thrombosis. American Journal of Diseases of Children 132: 367

Kaschula R O C, Uys C J, Kuijten R H, Dale J R P, Wiggelinkhuizen J 1974 Nephrotic syndrome of congenital syphilis. Archives of Pathology 97: 289

Kendall-Smith I M, Pullon D H H, Tomlinson B E 1968 Congenital nephrotic syndrome in Maori siblings. New Zealand Medical Journal 68: 156

Khrouf N, Koraichi H, Brauner R, Ben Jilani S, Hamza M, Hamza B 1982 Les syndromes néphrotiques infantiles. A propos de six cas observés en Tunisie. Annales de Pédiatrie 29: 215–218

Kikuta Y, Yoshimura Y, Saito T, Ishihara T, Yokoyama S, Hayashi T 1983 Nephrotic syndrome with diffuse mesangial sclerosis in identical twins. Journal of Pediatrics 102: 586–589

Kniker W T, Prindiville T 1969 Increased urinary glomerular basement membrane products: a measure of renal inflammation or altered metabolism. Pediatric Research 3: 513

Kniker W T, Sweeney M 1972 Increased urinary basement membrane-like products (BMP) in infants with congenital nephrosis (CN) and their healthy relatives. Clinical Research 20: 115

Kobayashi N, Imahori K, Wakao H 1961 The congenital nephrotic syndrome, a case report and a review. Paediatria Universitatis Tokyo 6: 27

Kouvalainen K 1963 Immunological features in the congenital nephrotic syndrome. A clinical and experimental study. Annales Paediatriae Fenniae, suppl 22

Lancet editorial 1980. Nephrotic syndrome in the tropics. 2: 461

Lange K, Wachstein M, Wasserman E, Alptekin F, Slobody L B 1963 The congenital nephrotic syndrome, an immune reaction? American Journal of Diseases of Children 105: 338

Lau S O, Tkachuck J Y, Hasegawa D K, Edson J R 1980 Plasminogen and anti-thrombin III: Deficiencies in the childhood nephrotic syndrome associated with plasminogenuria and antithrombinuria. Journal of Pediatrics 96: 390

McKusick V A 1969 On lumpers and splitters, or the nosology of genetic disease. Birth Defects: Original Article Series vol 5, No 1: 23

Mahan J D, Mauer S M, Sibley R K, Vernier R L 1984 Congenital nephrotic syndrome: Evolution of medical management and results of renal transplantation. Journal of Pediatrics 105: 549–557

Mahieu P, Monnens L, van Haelst U 1976 Chemical properties of glomerular basement membrane in congenital nephrotic syndrome. Clinical Nephrology 5: 134

Mehls O, Schärer K 1970 Familiäres nephrotisches Syndrom. Monatsschrift für Kinderheilkunde 118: 328

Moncrieff M W, White R H R, Glasgow E F, Winterborn M H, Cameron J S, Ogg C S 1973 The familial nephrotic syndrome: II. A clinicopathological study. Clinical Nephrology 1: 220

Nagi N A, Nouri L 1974 Infantile nephrotic syndrome. Postgraduate Medical Journal 50: 237

Norio R 1966 Heredity in the congenital nephrotic syndrome. A genetic study of 57 Finnish families with a review of reported cases. Annales Paediatriae Fenniae 12: suppl 27

Norio R 1969 The nephrotic syndrome and heredity. Human Heredity 19: 113

Norio R 1981 Diseases of Finland and Scandinavia. In: Rothschild H (ed) Biocultural aspects of disease. Academic Press, New York, p 359

Norio R, Nevanlinna H R 1980 Rare hereditary diseases and markers in Finland. In: Eriksson A W, Forsius H R, Nevanlinna H R, Workman P L, Norio R (eds) Population structure and genetic disorders. Academic Press, London, p 567

Norio R, Rapola J 1989 Congenital and infantile nephrotic syndromes. In: Bartsocas C S (ed) Genetics of kidney disorders (Progress in Clinical and Biological Research vol 305). Alan R Liss, New York, p 179

Norio R, Nevanlinna H R, Perheentupa J 1973 Hereditary diseases in Finland; rare flora in rare soil. Annals of Clinical Research 5: 109

Oliver J 1960 Microcystic renal disease and its relation to 'infantile nephrosis'. American Journal of Diseases of Children 100: 312

Palm L, Hägerstrand I, Kristofferssen U, Blennow G, Brun A, Jörgensen C 1986 Nephrosis and disturbances of neuronal migration in male siblings – a new hereditary disorder? Archives of Disease in Childhood 61: 545–548

Panicucci F, Sagripanti A, Vispi M, Pinori E, Lecchini L, Barsotti G, Giovanetti S 1983 Comprehensive study of haemostasis in nephrotic syndrome. Nephron 33: 9

Rajamma K, Balasundaram D, Rao B N 1974 Congenital nephrotic syndrome: a case report. Indian Pediatrics 11: 149

Rapola J 1987 Congenital nephrotic syndrome. Pediatric Nephrology 1: 441–446

Rapola J, Hallman N 1979 AFP and congenital nephrosis Finnish type. Lancet 1: 274

Rapola J, Savilahti E 1971 Immunofluorescent and morphological studies in congenital nephrotic syndrome. Acta Paediatrica (Uppsala) 60: 253

Rapola J, Sariola H, Ekblom P 1984 Pathology of fetal congenital nephrosis: immunohistochemical and ultra-structural studies. Kidney International 25: 701–707

Repetto H A, Vazquez L A, Russ C, Costa J A 1982 Late appearance of nephrotic syndrome in congenital syphilis. Journal of Pediatrics 100: 591–592

Richard P, Déchelette E, Gilly J, Bouvier R, Larbre F 1975 Syndrome néphrotique infantile. A propos de 14 observations. Pédiatrie 30: 581

Robain O, Deonna T 1983 Pachygyria and congenital nephrosis disorder of migration and neuronal orientation. Acta Neuropathologica 60: 137–141

Rossenbeck H G, Margraf O, Hofmann D 1966 Uber das infantile nephrotische Syndrom bei kongenitaler Glomerulonephritis. Deutsche Medizinische Wochenschrift 91: 348

Roy S III, Pitcock J A 1971 Idiopathic nephrosis in identical twins. American Journal of Diseases of Children 121: 428

Rumpelt H J, Bachmann H J 1980 Infantile nephrotic syndrome with diffuse mesangial sclerosis: a disturbance of glomerular basement membrane development? Clinical Nephrology 13: 146

Ryynänen M 1988 Personal communication

Ryynänen M, Seppälä M, Kuusela P et al 1983 Antenatal

screening for congenital nephrosis in Finland by maternal serum alpha-fetoprotein. British Journal of Obstetrics and Gynaecology 90: 437

Seelig H P, Seelig R, Schärer K 1975 Immunhistologische Untersuchungen bei der diffusen mesangialen Sklerose mit nephrotischem Syndrom im Säuglingsalter. Zeitschrift für Kinderheilkunde 120: 111

Shahin B, Papadopoulou Z L, Jenis E H 1974 Congenital nephrotic syndrome associated with congenital toxoplasmosis. Journal of Pediatrics 85: 366

Shapiro L R, Duncan P A, Farnsworth P B, Lefkowitz M 1976 Congenital microcephaly, hiatus hernia and nephrotic syndrome: An autosomal recessive syndrome. Birth Defects: Original Article Series, vol XII, No 5: 275–278

Similä S, Vesa L, Wasz-Höckert O 1970 Hereditary onycho-osteodysplasia (the nail-patella syndrome) with nephrosis-like renal disease in a newborn boy. Pediatrics 46: 61.

Spritz R A, Soiffer S J, Siegel N J, Mahoney M J 1978 False-negative AFP screen for congenital nephrosis Finnish type. Lancet 2: 1251

Tareyeva I E, Nikolaev A J, Janushkevitch T N 1982 Nephrotic syndrome induced by insect sting. Lancet II: 825

Tryggvason K 1977 Composition of the glomerular basement membrane in the congenital nephrotic syndrome of the Finnish type. European Journal of Clinical

Investigation 7: 177

Tryggvason K, Kouvalainen K 1975 Number of nephrons in normal human kidneys and kidneys of patients with the congenital nephrotic syndrome. A study using a sieving method for counting of glomeruli. Nephron 15: 62

Urbach J, Drukker A, Rosenmann E 1985 Diffuse mesangial sclerosis – light, immunofluorescent and electronmicroscopy findings. International Journal of Pediatric Nephrology 6: 101–104

Vernier R L, Brunson J, Good R A 1957 Studies on familial nephrosis. American Journal of Diseases of Children 93: 469

Vernier R L, Klein D J, Sisson S P, Mahan J D, Oegema T R, Brown D M 1983 Heparan sulfate-rich anionic sites in the human glomerular basement membrane. Decreased concentration in congenital nephrotic syndrome. New England Journal of Medicine 309: 1001–1009

White R H R 1973 The familial nephrotic syndrome. I. A European survey. Clinical Nephrology 1: 216

Worthen H C, Vernier R L, Good R A 1959 Infantile nephrosis. American Journal of Diseases of Children 98: 731

Yamamoto Y, Kuroda T, Kanamura S, Sawada S 1961 A case of 'congenital nephrotic syndrome.' Annales Paediatrica Japonica 7: 391.

78. Haemoglobinopathies and thalassaemias

J. A. Phillips   H. H. Kazazian, Jr.

INTRODUCTION

The biosynthesis of haemoglobin in the erythrocyte is one of the most striking examples of cellular specialization known in nature. Inherited disorders of haemoglobin synthesis, such as the haemoglobinopathies and the thalassaemia syndromes, are common and significant clinical conditions. The purpose of this chapter is to summarize briefly current knowledge of the structure, function, and biosynthesis of normal haemoglobin, then to discuss clinical diseases which result from qualititative (haemoglobinopathies) or quantitative (thalassaemia syndromes) defects in globin synthesis.

NORMAL HUMAN HAEMOGLOBIN

Haemoglobin is a tetramer with a molecular weight of 64 500. It consists of two α and two non-α globin polypeptide chains, each of which has a single covalently bound haem group. Each of the four haem groups is made up of an iron atom bound within a protoporphyrin IX ring.

In man, the six known different globin polypeptide chains are designated α, β, γ, δ, ϵ, and ζ. Each chain consists of a specific sequence of amino acids linked by peptide bonds. The α-chains contain 141 amino acids, while the β, γ, δ, and ϵ-chains have 146 residues. The ϵ, γ, and δ-chains are more similar to β-chains than to α-chains, differing from β at 36, 39, and 10 positions respectively (Bunn et al 1977a, Baralle et al 1980). The two globins, ϵ and ζ, are found in embryonic erythrocytes. The ϵ gene encodes an embryonic β-like chain, and the ζ sequence encodes an embryonic α-like chain.

The haemoglobin composition of erythrocyte lysates can be quantified by zone electrophoresis. Different haemoglobin tetramers, their structure, percentage in normal adult lysate, and conditions in which levels are increased, are seen in Table 78.1 (Bunn et al 1977a). Haemoglobin A ($\alpha_2\beta_2$) is usually 92% of the total haemoglobin in normal adults. Haemoglobin A_2 ($\alpha_2\delta_2$) constitutes about 2.5%, and it is evenly distributed in normal red cells; it may be increased in β-thalassaemias and megaloblastic anaemia and decreased in iron deficiency and sideroblastic anaemias.

Hb A_{1c} differs from Hb A by the post-translational addition of a glucose at the NH_2-terminus of the β chain, hence the tetramer's structure is $\alpha_2(\beta$-N-glucose$)_2$. The percentage of Hb A_{1c} (5% in normals) is related to the intracellular concentration of glucose and the red cell lifespan. In diabetic patients, the concentration of Hb A_{1c} is increased about two-fold because of the elevated glucose concentration in their red cells (Bunn et al 1977a).

Table 78.1 Human haemoglobins

Hb name	Synonym	Structure	% in adults	Conditions in which increased
A	Adult Hb	$\alpha_2\beta_2$	92	
A_{1c}		$\alpha_2(\beta$-N-glucose$)_2$	5	Diabetes mellitus
A_2		$\alpha_2\delta_2$	2.5	β-thalassaemia
F	Fetal Hb	$\alpha_2\gamma_2$	< 1	Newborn, β-thalassaemia, and marrow stress
H		β_4	0	Some α-thalassaemias
Barts		γ_4	0	Some α-thalassaemias
Gower 1	Embryonic Hb	$\zeta_2\epsilon_2$	0	Early embryos (< 8 weeks)
Gower 2	Embryonic Hb	$\alpha_2\epsilon_2$	0	Early embryos (< 8 weeks)
Portland	Embryonic Hb	$\zeta_2\gamma_2$	0	Early embryos (< 8 weeks) and $\alpha°$-thalassaemia (hydrops fetalis)

Data from Bunn et al 1977b. Human Hemoglobins. Saunders, Philadelphia

While HbF ($\alpha_2 \gamma_2$) comprises the bulk of haemoglobin (50–85%) in human newborns, it declines rapidly after birth, reaching concentrations of 10–15% by 4 months of age. Subsequently the decline is slower and adult levels of <1% are reached by 3–4 years of age. Fetal haemoglobin may be increased in β- and δβ-thalassaemia, hereditary persistence of fetal haemoglobin, D_1 trisomy, some cases of thyrotoxicosis, megaloblastic and aplastic anaemia, leukaemia and various malignancies involving marrow, sickle-cell anaemia, and during pregnancy (Cooper & Hoagland 1972). Hb F is measured by resistance to alkali, electrophoresis, or column chromatography.

Hbs Gower I ($\zeta_2\varepsilon_2$), Gower II ($\alpha_2\varepsilon_2$), and Portland ($\zeta_2\gamma_2$) are embryonic haemoglobins found in fetuses before 7–10 weeks of gestation. At 4–5 weeks of gestation, a simultaneous decrease in ζ- and ε-chain production and an increase in α- and γ-chain production occur (Kazazian 1974). β-chain synthesis in reticulocytes accounts for 4% of non-α synthesis at 5 weeks of gestation and gradually increases thereafter (Kazazian & Woodhead 1973). While the time of the decrease in ε- and ζ-chains coincides with the switch from yolk sac to hepatic-derived erythrocytes, the restriction of embryonic chain synthesis to yolk sac cells and the converse restriction of γ- and β-chains to hepatic cells have not been proven.

Hbs H and Barts are tetramers of β- and γ-chains, respectively, and both function very poorly in transporting oxygen. These two haemoglobins may be increased in some types of α-thalassaemia.

Primary and secondary structures

The primary structure of each globin chain is its amino acid sequence; 141 amino acids in α- and ζ-chains and 146 amino acids in β-, γ-, δ-, and ε-chains. The primary structure of α- and β-chains is seen in Figure 78.1.

The relationship between adjacent amino acids along the chain enables interactions which can result in one of two basic configurations of secondary structure: the α-helix or β-pleated-sheet. The α-helix, stabilized by hydrogen bonding between carbonyl and amino groups, has 3.6 amino acid residues per turn. About 75% of haemoglobin in its native state is in the α-helix form, as shown in Figure 78.1. The β-pleated-sheet configuration predominates in other molecules, such as immunoglobulins and chymotrypsin.

At specific locations in the haemoglobin subunits, the rodlike α helix is interrupted by nonhelical segments which allow folding. On X–ray crystallography, the confirmations of α and β haemoglobin subunits are seen to be similar. The β-globin chain has eight helical segments, A through H, and the secondary structure of the α-globin corresponds to that of the β-globin except for the absence of residues forming the D helical region (Fig. 78.1). The histidine residue at position 8 of the F helical segment (F8) is linked covalently to the haem iron molecule. This histidine residue is located at position 87 in the α-chain and 92 in the β-chain, and mutations altering it have important pathological consequences. Amino acids with charged side groups, e.g. lysine, arginine, and glutamic acid, lie on the external surface, while uncharged residues tend to be oriented toward the interior of the molecule (Rieder 1974).

Tertiary and quaternary structures

Tertiary structure refers to the configuration of a protein subunit in three-dimensional space, while quaternary structure refers to the relationships of the four subunits of haemoglobin to each other. The haemoglobin tetramer has been shown by X-ray crystallography to be an oblate spheroid with a diameter of 5.5 nm and a single axis of symmetry. The globin chains are folded so that the four haem groups are in surface clefts equidistant from each other. The four subunits forming the tetramers are labeled α_1, α_2, β_1, and β_2. While there is no contact between the two β-chains, each α-chain touches both β-chains. Bonds across the $\alpha_1\beta_1$ interface are firmer than those at the $\alpha_1\beta_2$ interface and changes from oxy- to deoxyhaemoglobin involve more extensive movement at the $\alpha_1\beta_2$ interface. The quaternary structure changes markedly in going from oxy- to deoxyhaemoglobin, and this accounts for many of the observed changes in physical properties. Haemoglobin mutations resulting in amino acid substitutions at these points can markedly alter specific functional properties (Rieder 1974).

Functional properties

For haemoglobin to fulfill its physiological role, it must bind oxygen with a certain affinity. One measure of oxygen affinity is P_{50}, or the partial pressure of oxygen in mm Hg which is required for 50% saturation of haemoglobin: a haemoglobin with increased P_{50} has decreased oxygen affinity (Fig. 78.2). Oxygen affinity is also affected by a number of environmental factors including temperature, pH, organic phosphate concentration, and pCO_2 (see Fig. 78.2) (Bellingham 1976).

The sigmoid shape of the oxyhaemoglobin dissociation curve reflects haem-haem interaction; i.e., successive oxygenation of each haem group in the tetramer increases the oxygen affinity of the remaining unoxygenated haem groups. The basis of haem-haem interaction is the decrease in the atomic radius of the haem iron that occurs with oxygenation allowing the iron atom to fit into the plane of the porphyrin ring. This alteration is amplified by a series of conformational changes which affect the other haem groups (Bellingham

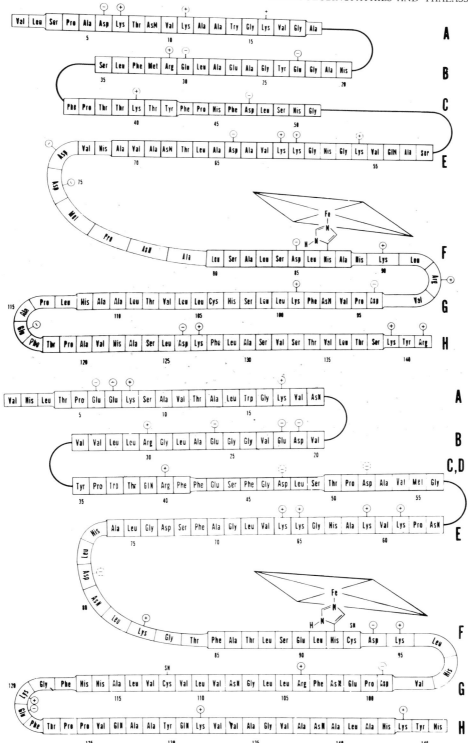

Fig. 78.1 The primary and secondary structures of globin chains Top: α-chain. Bottom: β-chain. Residues in squares are in α-helix configuration and nonhelical residues are in rectangles. (From Murayama M 1971 In: Nalbandian R M (ed) Molecular aspects of sickle cell hemoglobin. Charles Thomas, Springfield, Il. By permission of Charles C. Thomas, Publisher.)

1976). The resulting sigmoid oxyhaemoglobin dissociation curve has great physiological importance because it enables large amounts of oxygen to be bound or released with a small increase or decrease in oxygen tension. In contrast to Hb A, Hb H (β_4) and Hb Barts (γ_4) lack subunit interaction and have a hyperbolic rather than sigmoid oxyhaemoglobin dissociation curve which prevents oxygen release at physiological oxygen tensions.

The Bohr effect is a change in oxygen affinity of haemoglobin with a change in pH. This effect is beneficial at the tissue level where the lower pH de-

creases the oxygen affinity and promotes oxygen release (Fig. 78.2). Oxygen uptake in the lungs is enhanced by the opposite changes in pH and pCO_2.

Red cells have unusually high concentrations of 2,3-diphosphoglycerate (2,3-DPG). One molecule of 2,3-DPG sits in a pocket in deoxyhaemoglobin bound to specific β-chain residues (1,2,82, and 143 of both β-chains). The importance of the binding is that 2,3-DPG stabilizes the deoxy form of haemoglobin in preference to the oxy form, thereby lowering the oxygen affinity of the molecule. The γ chain of Hb F lacks the β^{143} histidine residue, and the resultant decrease in binding of 2,3-DPG to Hb F accounts for the increased oxygen affinity of fetal red cells compared to that of adult red cells (Bellingham 1976).

HAEMOGLOBIN BIOSYNTHESIS

Genetics

In man there are eight different genetic loci which code for the six globin genes (Lawn et al 1978, Orkin 1978, Bernards et al 1979, Proudfoot & Baralle 1979, Lauer et al 1980, Baralle et al 1980). In addition, there are at least three pseudogenes which have sequences similar to other globin genes but which differ in that they are not expressed into globin proteins (Fritsch et al 1980, Proudfoot & Maniatis 1980). Normally, globin tetramers are formed of two α or α-like chains and two non-α-chains; a schematic representation of the interaction of the products of these genes is shown in Figure 78.3. Since humans are diploid, i.e. have a pair of each non-sex chromosome or autosome, they have two genes for each autosomal locus. For example, there are two loci encoding the structure of the α-chain, thus there are four α-

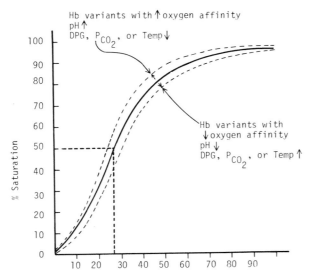

Fig. 78.2 The oxyhaemoglobin dissociation curve and effect of different factors on oxygen affinity.

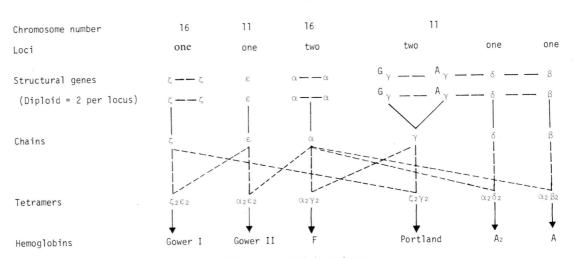

Fig. 78.3 Schematic representation of the various globin genes and their products.

chain genes. In contrast, there is only a single β-globin locus; therefore, two β genes (Fig. 78.3). The relative numbers of α and β loci are important in understanding the different inheritance patterns of α- and β-thalassaemias, as well as the different relative amounts of variant haemoglobins in individuals carrying a variant α- or β-globin gene. These quantitative differences correlate directly with the clinical severity of the various disorders.

The region of chromosome 11 (11p15.5) containing the β-like genes (ε, $^G\gamma$, $^A\gamma$, δ, β) has been thoroughly mapped by restriction endonuclease analysis (Fig. 78.4) and sequenced (Baralle et al 1980, Slightom et al 1980, Spritz et al 1980, Lawn et al 1980, Efstradiadis et al 1980). Each of the genes contains two intervening sequences (IVSs) which interrupt the coding sequence at the junctions of the codons for amino acids 30–31 and 104–105. The first IVS is 122–130 base pairs (bp), while the second is 850–904 bp in length. The entire β-gene cluster spans about 50 kilobases (kb) and contains one ε, two γ, one δ, and one β locus plus one pseudogene locus (Fritsch et al 1980). The pseudogene (Ψβ) has sequences which are similar to β-gene sequences, but differs in having altered sequences which prevent production of functional globin chains. Pseudogenes comprise a minority of the single gene sequences in both the α- and β-gene regions. Single gene sequences, in turn, comprise only about 7 kb of the 50 kb of DNA in the β-gene region, while the remaining 43 kb are flanking sequences, which presumably have some unknown regulatory role. In this regard, nucleotides within the 4 kb 5′ to the δ locus have been suggested to be important in γ-gene regulation, since their deletion in some forms of hereditary persistence of fetal haemoglobin is associated with increased γ-gene expression (Fritsch et al 1979).

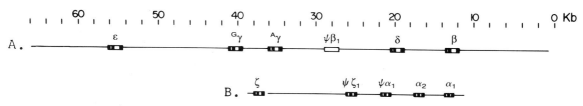

Fig. 78.4 Globin genes complexes. **A** β-gene complex on chromosome 11. **B** α-gene complex on 16. Distances along the chromosome are measured in kilobases (kb) at top.

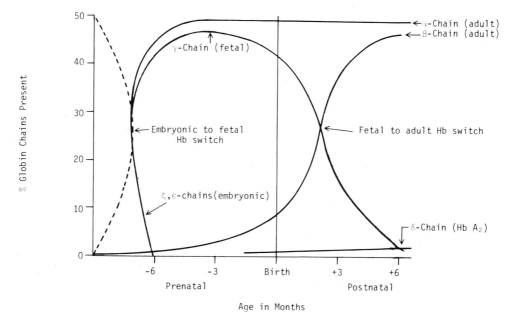

Fig. 78.5 Qualitative and quantitative changes in globin chains during human development. Note that the percentage of β-chains accumulated in early fetal development is much less than the percentage of β-chains synthesized during fetal development. (Modified from Bunn H F, Forget B G, Ranney H M 1977 In: Human haemoglobins. WB Saunders, Philadelphia, ch 1, p 4.)

More recently, sequences in the 20 kb upstream of the ε globin gene have been shown to be critical for position-independent expression of the β-globin gene in transgenic mice (Grosveld et al 1987).

The α-gene complex contains two α loci which have 3.6 kb between their centres, one ζ locus one pseudo-α locus ($\Psi\alpha_1$), and one pseudo-ζ locus. The pseudo-zeta locus results from a single nucleotide substitution which is polymorphic in some populations. Thus, some individuals have a $\Psi\zeta_1$ locus and others have a second functional ζ gene at that site. Figure 78.4B depicts this complex which is on chromosome 16 and it should be noted that in each case about 4 kbs separate the ζ_1, $\Psi\alpha_1$, α_2 and α_1 loci, suggesting the existence of discrete duplication units in the DNA (Proudfoot & Maniatis 1980). α-genes have smaller intervening sequences than are found in the β-like genes; IVS I contains 114 bp, while IVS II contains 132 bp.

Ontogeny

The globin genes are expressed at different times and in different relative amounts during human development (Fig. 78.5). The sequence of appearance of the various globin chains is helpful in understanding the timing of onset of clinical manifestations of the haemoglobinopathies and thalassaemias. For example, a deficiency of α- or γ-chain synthesis and α- or γ-variants with abnormal functions should be observed at birth, while a deficiency of β chains may not cause symptoms until several months of age. Finally, levels of β-chain variants, such as Hb S, progressively increase over the first months, so that the onset of clinical manifestations may be delayed until the latter half of the first year life.

Globin biosynthesis

The genetic information for every normal and abnormal

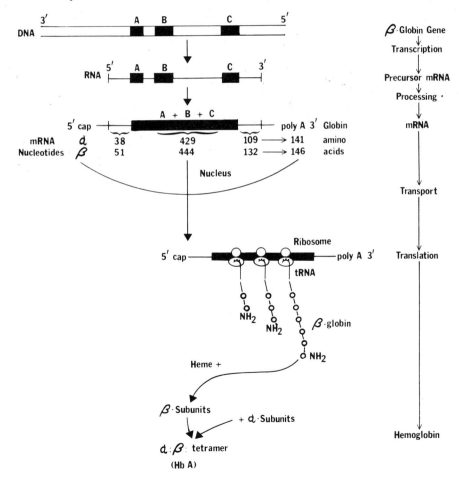

Fig. 78.6 Steps involved in haemoglobin biosynthesis. Understanding of the order and function of various steps is incomplete.

globin chain is encoded in the nucleotide sequence of the DNA. These sequences, or genes, are located at specific loci on chromosomes 16 and 11 (Deisseroth et al 1977, Scott et al 1979, Gusella et al 1979, Deisseroth et al 1978).

As mentioned above, IVSs reside between the portions of the globin genes that are translated into protein. These IVSs are present in the gene and in the RNA transcribed from the gene which is called messenger RNA precursor (pre-mRNA) (Fig. 78.6). Pre-mRNA undergoes excision of the intervening sequences and splicing of the translated portions (Tilghman et al 1978). Studies of the function of hybrid SV 40-β-globin genes in cultured monkey kidney cells suggest that IVS excision is crucial to mRNA transport from the nucleus to the cytoplasm (Hamer & Leder 1979).

Further processing occurs at each end of this RNA molecule (Kazazian et al 1977). At the 5'-end, guanosine is added in a special triphosphate linkage, and this guanosine and the next two nucleotides are then methylated. These 5'-end modifications are called capping and methylation and while their function is not completely known, they have been shown to be vital for initiation of translation of many mRNAs, including globin mRNAs. The 3'-end modification involves the addition of about 150 adenylic acid nucleotides [poly(A)]. Poly(A) addition may also be important for the transport of mRNA to the cytoplasm and its subsequent stability. With ageing of the mRNA, the poly(A) 'tail' shortens (Merkel et al 1976).

Once the processed mRNA has been transported to the cytoplasm, it binds to ribosomes. The first step in translation (initiation) requires the binding of mRNA to the two ribosome subunits, amino acyl-tRNA, guanosine triphosphate, and protein intiation factors. Initiation occurs at the 5', or capped, end of mRNA which corresponds to the NH_2-terminal end of the globin chain. Protein synthesis then proceeds toward the COOH-terminal end. Four to six chains of varying length (nascent chains) undergo translation on the same mRNA simultaneously. When these nascent chains have attained full length, a termination codon is reached. Since no tRNA is available for decoding this codon, polypeptide synthesis stops and, with the assistance of protein termination factors, the polypeptide chain is released from the ribosome and its mRNA. About one third of the mature mRNA sequence is not used for translation, but these untranslated nucleotides which are located at both ends of the molecule may have other regulatory functions (Kazazian et al 1977).

The protein chain assumes its secondary and tertiary structures due to interactions resulting from its amino acid sequence. Next, haem is bound and, in combination with other polypeptide subunits, the quaternary haemoglobin molecule is formed. These steps are shown in Figure 78.6.

HUMAN HAEMOGLOBIN VARIANTS

Molecular aetiology

Abnormal haemoglobins result from mutations which

Table 78.2 Molecular basis of haemoglobinopathies

Mutation	Example	Clinical manifestation
Nucleotide base substitutions to a codon for:		
another amino acid	Hb S ($\beta^{6Glu \rightarrow Val}$)	Sickling
	Hb C$_{Harlem}$ ($\beta^{6Glu \rightarrow Val} + \beta^{73 Asp \rightarrow Asn}$)	Sickling
termination	Hb McKees Rock ($\beta^{145 Tyr \rightarrow Termination}$)	Increased oxygen affinity and polycythemia
amino acid instead of termination	Hb Constant Spring ($\alpha^{Termination \rightarrow Gln}$)	Decreased synthesis (thalassaemia-like)
Nucleotide base deletions		
Single base deletion → frame shift	Hb Wayne ($\alpha^{139-141 [Lys-Tyr-Arg]} \rightarrow Asn-Thr-Val...$)	Normal
Triplet deletion → single amino acid	Hb Leiden ($\beta^{6 \text{ or } 7 Glu \rightarrow 0}$)	Unstable
Multiple codon	Hb Gun Hill ($\beta^{91-95 [Leu-His-Cys-Asp-Lys] \rightarrow 0}$)	Unstable
Crossover	Hb Lepore ($\delta\beta$-fusion with segments of δ and β lost)	Decreased synthesis (thalassaemia-like)
Whole gene	α-Thalassemia$_1$ and α-thalassemia$_2$ combination	Hb H disease
Nucleotide base additions		
Two bases added → frame shift	Hb Cranston ($\beta^{144[Tyr-His]} \rightarrow [Ser-Ile-Thr]$)	Unstable
Multiple codon	Hb Grady (9 bases → 3 additional amino acids)	Normal

change the sequence or number of nucleotides within the globin gene involved, or from mispairing during meiosis giving fusion of two different genes. Mutation can cause substitution, addition, or deletion of one or more amino acids in the polypeptide sequence of the affected globin (Table 78.2).

Single base changes can result in single amino acid substitutions e.g. Hb S (β^6Glu→Val), shortened chains due to premature termination of translation e.g. Hb McKees Rock [$\beta^{145 \, (Tyr \to Term)}$], or elongated chains. Elongated chains result when the terminator codon undergoes a mutation to a codon for an amino acid such as UAA→CAA in Hb Constant Spring. Two other elongated chains are Hb Icaria and Hb Koya Dora, both of which also have 31 additional residues and differ from Hb Constant Spring only at residue 142 (Bunn et al 1977b).

Single base deletions or additions can cause a frame shift in the normal reading process (Seid-Akhavan et al 1976). For example, in the α^{Wayne} variant a single base deletion (A) causes the following codons to be read out of phase:

Lys		Tyr		Arg		Term
(AAA	–	UAC	–	CGU)	–	UAA

	Asn		Thr		Val	
→	(AAU	–	ACC	–	GUU)	...

Deletions of three, or multiples of three, nucleotides in the DNA cause deletions of one or more amino acids. It is interesting that of 13 examples of this type, all are β-chain variants, including Hb Leiden ($\beta^{6 \, or \, 7 \, Glue}$→0) and Hb Gun Hill [$\beta^{91-95 \, (Leu-His-Cys-Asp-Lys)}$→0]. Deletions of segments of genes may be due to nonhomologous crossing-over after mispairing in meiosis. This mechanism accounts for the Lepore globins (δβ fusion chains), anti-Lepore globins (βδ fusion chains), and Kenya globin (γβ fusion chain) (Kazazian et al 1977).

Known variants

The numbers of known haemoglobin variants resulting from changes in the nucleotide base number or sequence in DNA are now as shown in Table 78.3 (Internat. Hgb. Info. Ctr. 1984). Most of these mutants were detected by zone electrophoresis which separates haemoglobins on the basis of charge differences resulting from the amino acid substitutions. Since many mutations which do not change the protein's charge are not detected by this method, many undetected haemoglobin variants must still exist in the population. The number of β variants (232) is approximately twice that of α variants (126), even though there are two α loci and a single β locus. Also, the percentage of β-chain variants which have abnormal physical properties (47%) is twice that of the α-chain variants (19%). The great majority of these mutants arise from a single base substitution which results in a single

Table 78.3 Known haemoglobin variants (International Haemoglobin Information Center 1984)*

Globin chain	Total variants	Clinically silent	Abnormal properties		Ferric Hb
			Unstable	Abnormal oxygen affinity	
α	126	102 (81%)	16 (12%)	6 (5%)	2 (2%)
β	232	122 (52%)	68 (30%)	39 (16%)	3 (1%)
γ	38	36 (95%)	1 (3%)	–	1 (3%)
δ	15	15 (100%)	–	–	–
Totals	411	275 (66%)	85 (22%)	45 (11%)	5 (1%)

*Fusion variants are not included. Compiled from information from Bunn & Forget (1986).
(Note: The percentages may be greater than 100 because some variants have more than one abnormal property.)

Table 78.4 Clinical manifestations of haemoglobin mutants

Type	Example	Clinical manifestation
Sickling	Hb S	Sickling due to decreased solubility
Unstable	Hb Bristol	Anaemia with Heinz body formation
Abnormal oxygen affinity		
Decreased	Hb Kansas	Mild anaemia possible
Increased	Hb Chesapeake	Polycythaemia due to decreased oxygen transport
M haemoglobin	Hb M$_{Boston}$	Cyanosis due to ferric haemoglobin
Decreased synthesis	Hb Lepore	Thalassaemia

Table 78.5   Inheritance risks for a haemoglobin variant

Parents	Homozygous normal (%)	*Offspring* Heterozygous (%)	Homozygous affected (%)
Both normal	100	0	0
Normal/Heterozygous	50	50	0
Normal/Homozygous	0	100	0
Both heterozygous	25	50	0
Heterozygous/Homozygous	0	50	25
Both homozygous	0	0	50
			100

amino acid substitution. Many of these substitutions, even some of those which produce abnormal physical properties in the variant haemoglobin, are clinically silent and were detected only by population screening. Other substitutions cause: (1) instability of the tetramer; (2) deformity of the 3-dimensional structure; (3) inhibition of ferric iron reduction; (4) alteration of the residues which interact with haem, with 2,3 DPG, or at the α-β subunit contact site; or (5) abnormality of other properties of the molecule resulting in a variety of clinical phenotypes (Table 78.4).

The location of the amino acid changed by the mutation can often be correlated with the resultant phenotype. Unstable haemoglobin variants are caused by several types of changes in the primary sequence which affect the secondary, tertiary, or quaternary structure. These substitutions tend to be at residues in the interior of the molecule, at contact points between chains, at residues which interact with the haem groups (Rieder 1974), or when a proline residue replaces another amino acid within an α helical region (Hb Genova [β^{28} (B10)$^{Leu \rightarrow Pro}$], Hb Abraham Lincoln [β^{32}(B14)$^{Leu \rightarrow Pro}$]), resulting in disruption of the helix. Hb Philly [β^{35}(C1)$^{Tyr \rightarrow Phe}$] is also unstable, secondary to a missing α hydrogen bond normally found between the α_1 and β_1 subunits. Many other unstable haemoglobins are the result of mutations affecting residues which bind haem or are in the hydrophobic haem cleft, e.g. Hb Gun Hill [$\beta^{91-95 \ (Leu-His-Cys-Asp-Lys) \rightarrow 0}$] and Hb Hammersmith ($\beta^{42}$ $^{Phe \rightarrow Ser}$).

Substitutions on the surface of the molecule usually do not affect tertiary structure or haem-haem interaction, but they may permit molecular interactions which decrease solubility under certain conditions [Hb S β^6 $^{Glu \rightarrow Val}$]. Substitution of tyrosine for either of the histidines which bind the iron molecule (E7 or F8) results in increased stability of the ferric (oxidized) iron state seen in M haemoglobins, M-Boston [α^{58}(E7)$^{His \rightarrow Tyr}$] and M-Iwate [β^{87}(F8)$^{His \rightarrow Tyr}$]. Substitution at an $\alpha_1\beta_1$ subunit contact point, such as β^{99}, can disturb haem-haem interactions causing increased oxygen affinity and poly-

cythaemia, as with Hb Kempsey [β^{99}(G1)$^{Asp \rightarrow Asn}$] (Reider 1974).

Inheritance of haemoglobinopathies

Variants of α, β, γ or δ globins result from mutations affecting their respective genes. All the variants for β chains, for example, are coded by alleles since they result from different genes found at the single β-chromosomal locus. Heterozygotes for a haemoglobin containing an abnormal β globin have an abnormal as well as a normal β gene at that locus, and their status is often described by the term 'trait'. Since most variants are rare, they usually occur in the heterozygous state and, if they cause clinical symptoms, are examples of autosomal dominant conditions. When both alleles code for the same common β variant, the individual is then homozygous and is said to have the 'disease' state. However, the term 'sickle-cell disease' is often used to describe a similar phenotype that is seen when any of several genotypes (SS, SC S/β-thal, SD$_{Punjab}$, or SO$_{Arab}$) are exposed to a certain environment (hypoxia). Furthermore, under conditions of severe hypoxia a person with the AS genotype or 'trait' can also manifest symptoms of the sickle-cell 'disease' phenotype. This distinction between the genotype (homozygous and heterozygous) and the phenotype (trait and disease) is an important one. Also, it should be noted that patterns of inheritance of haemoglobin variants are more precisely expressed in terms of genotypes than in terms of phenotypes.

Inheritance risks from matings of individuals who are normal, heterozygous, or homozygous for variant haemoglobins are shown in Table 78.5. Since there are multiple alleles for each locus, a person heterozygous for two alleles at the same locus (usually referred to as a genetic compound) may be seen, e.g. Hb SC individual. A mating between an AA and an SC individual can result in AS or AC, but not AA or SC, offspring. However, a mating of an AS and an AC individual can result in offspring who are AA, AS, AC, or SC. This pattern of Mendelian inheritance is called codominant inheritance.

SICKLE CELL ANAEMIA AND RELATED DISORDERS

Molecular basis

The sickle cell gene results from a point mutation which causes the amino acid substitution $\beta^{6 \text{ Glu}\rightarrow\text{Val}}$; therefore, Hb S is $\alpha_2^A\beta_2^{6 \text{ Glu}\rightarrow\text{Val}}$. The frequency of sickle trait (Hb AS) among United States Blacks at birth is about 8%, and the incidence of sickle-cell anaemia at birth should be around 0.16%, or 1 per 625 births (Motulsky 1973). This contrasts with the higher carrier frequencies seen in some areas of Africa (up to 30%) which are due to the protective advantage conferred by the carrier state against falciparum malaria. As expected, the prevalence of sickle-cell anaemia differs in these two populations. The prevalence of sickle-cell anaemia among all Blacks in the United States is about 1 per 1875, considerably lower than expected from the incidence at birth. It is still lower in some underdeveloped regions of Africa, despite the higher incidence of the trait, due to higher mortality in infancy (Motulsky 1973).

Pathophysiology of sickling

Substitution of valine for glutamic acid at the β^6 residue causes a change on the surface of the deoxygenated β^s chain which allows it to interact in a special way with other β chains. This interaction results in the formation by $\alpha_2^A\beta_2^s$ tetramers of a 14-stranded helical polymer with a diameter of 15–17nm. The parallel alignment of these rod-like polymers, in turn, causes the deformation seen in sickled erthrocytes. In sickle-cell anaemia the sickling process may begin when the oxygen saturation of Hb S is decreased to 85%, but it does not occur in heterozygotes (Hb AS) until the oxygen saturation of haemoglobin is decreased to 40% (Nathan & Pearson 1974). In addition to a decrease in oxygen tension, a reduction in pH or an increase in 2,3-DPG also promotes sickling. These factors probably interact in patients with sickle-cell anaemia since their blood normally has an increased 2,3-DPG concentration.

The viscosity of oxygenated sickle-cell blood is increased, primarily due to irreversibly sickled cells, but also due to increased gamma globin levels. When the blood becomes deoxygenated, viscosity increases further due to the cellular rigidity which occurs with sickling. This, in turn, increases the exposure time of erythrocytes to a hypoxic environment, and the lower tissue pH decreases the oxygen affinity which further promotes sickling. The end result is occlusion of capillaries and arterioles and infarction of surrounding tissues. Haemolysis probably occurs secondary to increased mechanical fragility of deformed cells and membrane damage.

Clinical aspects of sickle-cell disease

As can be seen from Figure 78.5, β-chain production usually does not reach sufficient levels to cause symptoms

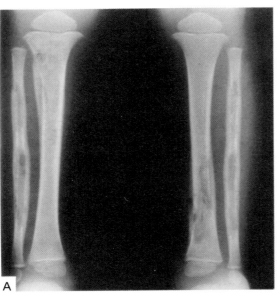 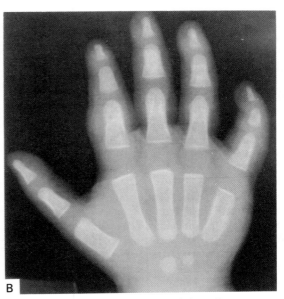

Fig. 78.7 Radiographic changes in sickle-cell anaemia. **A** Changes in the tibias and fibulas secondary to *Salmonella* osteomyelitis. **B** Hand-and-foot syndrome with soft tissue swelling and focal areas of cortical destruction and periosteal new bone formation. (Courtesy of Dr John Dorst.)

until the second half of the first year of life. As higher concentrations of Hb S are reached in erythocytes, the cells become susceptible to haemolysis and a progressive haemolytic anaemia with splenomegaly is seen. The increased rate of erythropoiesis leads to erythroid marrow expansion and increased folic acid requirements. However the two major problems for young children with SS disease are infections and vaso-occlusive crises.

Children with sickle-cell anaemia have increased susceptibility to potentially life-threatening bacterial infections including sepsis and meningitis caused by *Streptococcus pneumoniae* and *Haemophilus influenzae*. The relative risk of sickle-cell anaemia patients compared with that of normals for pneumococcal *H. influenzae* and all bacterial meningitis is 579:1, 116:1, and 309:1, respectively (Barrett-Connor 1971). These patients are also susceptible to bacterial pneumonia (often pneumococcus), osteomyelitis (*Salmonella* and *Staphylococcus*) (Fig. 78.7), and urinary tract infections (*Escherichia coli* and *Klebsiella*). Increased susceptibility is also seen for *Shigella* and *Mycoplasma pneumoniae*. Several factors that contribute to this susceptibility are functional hyposplenism, impaired antibody response, decreased opsonization, impaired complement activation in the properdin pathway, and abnormal chemotaxis.

Bacterial infection is the most common reason for hospitalisation of paediatric sickle-cell anaemia patients and often leads to the diagnosis (Barrett-Connor 1971). Serious bacterial infections are seen in approximately one third of children with sickle-cell anaemia before 4 years of age. Infection, not crisis, is the most common cause of death in these children, although infections often precipitate crises.

Vaso-occlusive crises begin in infancy with dactylitis, or hand-and-foot syndrome (Fig. 78.7). Later crises may involve the periosteum, bones, or joints, resulting in infarction which must be differentiated from osteomyelitis and septic arthritis. Vaso-occlusive crises and sepsis are difficult to differentiate and often coexist in younger children.

Pulmonary crises with pleural pain and fever may be due to either infection, in situ thrombosis, or embolism. Other clinical manifestations include splenic sequestration, abdominal and aplastic crises, cholelithiasis, hepatic infarcts, occlusion of cerebral vessels, ocular changes, haematuria, hyposthenuria, hyponatraemia, priapism, and skin ulcers (Cooper & Hoagland 1972, Nathan & Pearson 1974).

Diagnosis

The peripheral blood smear of sickle cell anaemia patients may have normal, irreversibly sickled, target, and nucleated red cells. Howell-Jolly bodies and red cell fragments are also present, especially after functional asplenia develops (Fig. 78.8A). The clinical history of crises or severe infections with anaemia, abnormal red cell morphology on peripheral smear with a normal or elevated mean corpuscular volume, positive sickling test, and Hb S (greater than 80%) and Hb F on haemoglobin electrophoresis, makes the diagnosis of sickle-cell anaemia probable. However, family studies indicating that both parents have sickle cell trait are helpful to exclude S/β-thalassaemia and S/hereditary persistence of fetal haemoglobin. In addition, sibs should also be tested to identify and treat previously undiagnosed cases.

Treatment

At present there is no safe drug to ameliorate the condition, but a number of antisickling agents are under trial (Dean & Schechter 1978). Recently hydroxyurea has been given experimentally to sickle-cell anaemia patients. This drug increases fetal haemoglobin production, presumably through its effect in speeding erythroid precursors through their maturation steps. The drug appears to reduce the number of painful crises and haemolysis in uncontrolled studies with a small number of patients (Charache et al 1987), but it is not yet in general use. Infections should be treated promptly with antibiotics, and some centres advocate prophylactic antibiotic treatment. A polyvalent pneumococcal polysaccharide has been shown to afford some protection against sytemic infections due to *Streptococcus pneumoniae* in sickle-cell disease and in splenectomized patients (Ammann et al 1977); however, multiple clinical failures as well as side-effects have been reported (Akhonkhai et al 1979, Giebiuk et al 1979).

The associated anaemia is usually tolerated well, but if folate deficiency occurs the anaemia becomes more severe and is associated with macrocytosis, hypersegmented granulocytes, and a decrease in percentage of reticulocytes. Folate deficiency is prevented easily by daily folic acid supplement. Transfusions are seldom indicated for uncomplicated anaemia, but exchange transfusions can be effective for life-threatening vaso-oclusive crises (cerebral) or in preparation for surgery. Crises should be managed with vigorous hydration because of the patient's inability to concentrate urine and the increased viscosity of his blood. Acidosis and hypoxia should be treated, and analgesics should be given for the accompanying severe pain.

Prevention

During genetic counselling, *AS* × *AS* couples are advised of their 25% risk for having children with sickle-cell disease; certain couples may request prenatal diagnosis. In the past several years methods for the prenatal detection of sickle-cell anaemia have been improved to the point where they are now applicable to all couples at risk.

Between 1975 and 1979, about 50 couples at risk for sickle-cell anaemia had prenatal diagnosis using fetal blood obtained by techniques of fetoscopy or placental aspiration (Hobbins & Mahoney 1974, Alter et al 1976).

Synthetic studies were used to detect the types of β-chains produced in fetal red cells. The significant risk of fetoscopy (6% fetal mortality), its limited availability, and the variable clinical course of the disease have combined to limit widespread use of these methods (Alter 1979).

In 1978, Kan discovered that restriction endonuclease studies of DNA from fetal amniocytes could also enable prenatal diagnosis of sickle-cell anaemia in a substantial proportion of cases (Kan & Dozy 1978). The applicability

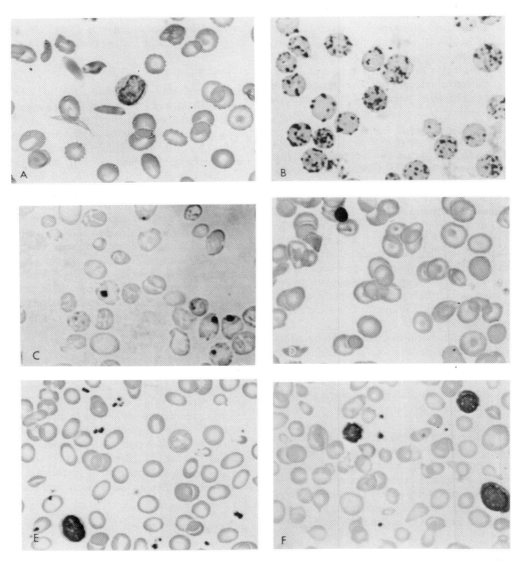

Fig. 78.8 Peripheral blood smears from patients with various disorders of globin synthesis. **A** Homozygous sickle-cell anaemia. **B** Unstable Hb Zurich with Heinz bodies. **C** Hb H disease. **D** Sickle/β-thalassaemia. **E** β-thalassaemia trait. **F** Homozygous β-thalassaemia. **B** and **C** were prepared as follows: whole blood with EDTA was incubated at 41°C for 3–6 hours, then a 1:1 mixture of blood and 0.5% rhodanile blue in 0.9% saline was made and immediately smeared. Haemoglobin precipitates formed secondary to heating are seen. (Courtesy of Dr William Zinkham).

of this test was expanded (Phillips et al 1980a) through the use of other polymorphic restriction endonuclease sites near the β locus. When family studies were carried out to assign DNA 'markers' to the respective $β^{A-}$ and $β^{S-}$ bearing chromosomes of both parents, prenatal diagnosis could be accomplished in 90% of pregnancies by amniocentesis alone (Phillips et al 1980a).

In 1982 it was found that the restriction enzyme Mst II (or Cvn I) cut the $β^A$-globin gene at codons 5–7 of the gene, but failed to cut the $β^S$-globin gene at this point (the mutation site). Prenatal diagnosis could then be accomplished in all couples at risk without family studies. Now gene amplification techniques, (polymerase chain reaction) developed at the Cetus Corporation (Saiki et al 1988), in conjunction with Mst II, allow prenatal diagnosis of sickle-cell anaemia in a few days without Southern blotting (Chehab et al 1987).

Interactions with sickle haemoglobin

Heterozygotes for Hb S (AS) are generally asymptomatic, however severe hypoxia (oxygen saturation less than 40%) can induce sickling. The loop of Henle provides an environment in which both the pH and oxygen tension are decreased sufficiently to cause sickling, resulting in microinfarctions, haematuria, and hyposthenuria. Exposure to hypoxia can also cause splenic and other organ infarcts in sickle trait individuals.

Hb C trait is found in about 3% of American Blacks at birth, Hb SC disease in 1 per 833, and Hb C disease in about 1 per 1250 (Motulsky 1973). Patients with SC disease tend to have a variable course with most of the complications occurring less frequently than in SS disease. Other haemoglobin variants which interact with S are D_{Punjab}, O_{Arab}, C_{Harlem} and β-thalassaemia. Clinical manifestations tend to be severe in patients with Hb SS, Hb SD_{Punjab} and Hb SO_{Arab}; moderate in those with Hb SC, Hb S/β-thal and Hb CC; and mild or absent in individuals with Hb AS and Hb AC trait.

UNSTABLE HAEMOGLOBIN VARIANTS

Molecular basis

At least 85 unstable haemoglobin variants are known (Table 78.3). Among these, β-variants are four times more frequent than α-variants (68:16), a discrepancy which may be due to the smaller percentage of unstable haemoglobin and hence milder clinical symptoms associated with the α-chain variants. An individual with a single variant α gene has three normal α genes, so that the percentage of unstable haemoglobin in the red cells is very small (5–20%). In contrast, an individual with a variant β gene has only a single normal β gene; so the unstable haemoglobin containing the variant β chain makes up a greater proportion of the total cellular haemoglobin synthesized (20–40%) (Bunn et al 1977c). Because the gene frequencies for these variants are extremely low, almost all affected individuals seen are heterozygotes.

The increased propensity of unstable haemoglobins to denature can result from several types of mutations. As mentioned previously, the α-helix of α- or β-globin can be disrupted by proline replacing another amino acid within the helix. There are at least ten examples of this type of disruption of primary and secondary structure, including Hb Bibba ($α^{136 \ Leu→Pro}$) and Hb Genova ($β^{28 \ Leu→Pro}$) (Rieder 1974). Deletions of amino acid residues alter primary and secondary structures as well as conformation of the haemoglobin molecules, and eight of the ten variants of this type are unstable, e.g. Hb Leiden ($β^{6 \ or \ 7 \ Glu→0}$) and Hb Gun Hill [$β^{91-95 \ (Leu-His-Cys-Asp-Lys)→0}$] (Bunn et al 1977c). Interference with interchain contacts permits the αβ dimers to dissociate into monomers, e.g. Hb Philly ($β^{35 \ Tyr→Phe}$) and Hb Tacoma ($β^{30 \ Arg→Ser}$) lack hydrogen bonds normally linking the α and β subunits. Substitutions which affect haem binding or disturb the hydrophobic haem pocket (certain non-polar residues in the CD, E, F, and FG regions) decrease the molecule's stability (Fig. 78.1). There are over 30 such mutations, and most result in unstable haemoglobins, such as Hb Bristol ($β^{67 \ Val→Asp}$) and Hb Köln ($β^{98 \ Val→Met}$) (Rieder 1974). Finally, globin chain elongation can result in instability due to hydrophobic properties of the extended chain, e.g. Hb Cranston ($β^{144-151}$) (Bunn et al 1977c).

These variant haemoglobins tend to denature spontaneously; and the globin subunits precipitate in the red cell, forming aggregates or Heinz bodies. The Heinz bodies adhere to the red cell membrane and result in decreased pliability of the cell. Inflexible erythrocytes are then selectively trapped by the reticuloendothelial system.

Clinical aspects of unstable haemoglobins

Patients often present in infancy or early childhood with a haemolytic anaemia, jaundice and splenomegaly, or later with cholelithiasis. Some variants also cause cyanosis due to their abnormal properties, i.e. propensity to form methaemoglobin or decreased oxygen affinity. Clinical severity varies with different unstable variants; for β-variants, symptoms appear after the γ to β transition in haemoglobin synthesis (Fig. 78.5).

Diagnosis

The peripheral smear may be normal or hypochromic. Staining with a supravital stain, such as 1% methyl violet, demonstrates preformed Heinz bodies (Fig. 78.8B). Heat instability of the variant haemoglobin is demonstrated by the formation of a haemoglobin precipitate when a haemolysate is incubated at 50°C or higher, or at 37°C in 17% isopropanol. Haemoglobin electrophoresis by usual methods may detect only about one half of unstable variants since the charge of these variants is often unaltered by the substitutions. Oxygen saturation curves of whole blood may indicate normal (20% of the unstable variants), decreased (30%), or increased (50%) oxygen affinity (Bunn et al 1977c).

Treatment

Treatment is generally supportive. If haemolysis is severe, prophylactic folate may be indicated. Oxidant drugs, such as sulphonamides, increase haemolysis in some patients and should be avoided. Transfusions are indicated only in the treatment of aplastic crises. While splenectomy may result in improvement of the anaemia, it also increases the risk of septicaemia, especially in young patients. Because of the mortality associated with septicaemia in splenectomized patients, the physician should reserve splenectomy for selected patients. Splenectomy should be postponed until the patient is at least six years of age, and the administration of pneumococcal vaccine and prophylactic antibiotics should be considered (Bunn et al 1977c).

HAEMOGLOBIN VARIANTS WITH ALTERED OXYGEN AFFINITY

Molecular basis

The oxygen dissociation curve shown in Figure 78.2 is sigmoid shaped due to haem-haem interactions. Mutations which affect haem-haem interaction, the Bohr effect, or deoxyhaemoglobin-2,3-DPG interaction can change the shape or position of the oxygen dissociation curve. Mutations affecting the $\alpha_1\beta_2$ subunit contact point can alter haem-haem interaction by causing the deoxyhaemoglobin conformation to be less stable. These mutations result in increased stability of the oxyhaemoglobin conformation and increased oxygen affinity [Hb Kempsey ($\beta^{99\ Asp\to Asn}$)]. Alternatively, the oxyghaemoglobin conformation can be destabilized by mutations affecting the $\alpha^{94}\beta^{102}$-contact point resulting in decreased oxygen affinity [Hb Kansas ($\beta^{102\ Asn\to Thr}$)]. Substitutions at the COOH-terminal ends of globin chains can lead to instability of the deoxyhaemoglobin conformations and increased oxygen affinity [Hb Bethesda ($\beta^{145\ Tyr\to His}$)] as well as a reduction in the Bohr effect. 2,3-DPG binds to residues $\beta^{1,\ 2,\ 82,\ and\ 143}$ in the

deoxygenated form. Substitutions altering these residues tend to have increased oxygen affinity [Hb F (γ globin has a serine for histidine substitution at position 143)] (Bellingham 1976).

The variants with increased oxygen affinity cause a shift to the left of the oxygen dissociation curve (Fig. 78.2), resulting in less oxygen delivery per gram of haemoglobin. To compensate, haemoglobin concentration and/or blood flow increases in order to partially restore oxygen delivery to the tissues (Bellingham 1976). Some variants with increased oxygen affinity do not cause polycythaemia due to the small fraction of the total haemoglobin they comprise, or to compensatory changes in the shape of the oxygen dissociation curve. Variants with decreased oxygen affinity have a shift to the right and increased oxygen delivery per gram of haemoglobin. As a result, the haemoglobin concentration is normal or decreased [Hb Beth Israel ($\beta^{102\ Asn\to Ser}$)] (Nagel et al 1976).

Clinical aspects and diagnosis

Because the gene frequencies for nearly all variant haemoglobins are very low, patients are nearly always heterozygotes. β-chain variants outnumber α-chain variants by 2:1 (Table 78.3). The great majority of patients are asymptomatic, and when oxygen affinity is increased the major finding is polycythaemia with erythrocytosis, normal white blood cell and platelet counts, and absence of splenomegaly. Since about half of these variants cannot be detected on routine electrophoresis, whole blood oxygen affinity studies are required for diagnosis. Some concern has been raised regarding the risk to fetuses of mothers who have variants with increased oxygen affinity. The little data available regarding the outcome of such pregnancies does not, in general, seem to indicate increased fetal mortality (Bellingham 1976).

Treatment

The condition is generally considered benign. It is important to avoid chemical treatment of the compensatory polycythaemia unless haematocrit levels are high enough to cause increased viscosity.

M HAEMOGLOBIN VARIANTS

Molecular basis

There are five known variants of M haemoglobin, four of which result from substitution of tyrosine for histidine at positions α^{58}, α^{87}, β^{63}, and β^{92}[M-Boston ($\alpha^{58\ His\to Tyr}$), M-Iwate ($\alpha^{87His\to Try}$), M-Saskatoon ($\beta^{63\ His\to Tyr}$) and M-Hyde

Table 78.6 Characteristics of certain thalassaemia states

Condition	Parents	Inheritance risk (%)	Haemoglobin electrophoresis	DNA sequences	mRNA
Heterozygotes					
Silent carrier (α-thalassaemia$_2$)	α-thal$_2$, normal	50	1–2% γ_4 (birth)	3α	Slight ↓ α
α-Thal trait (α-thalassaemia$_1$)	Both α-thal$_2$ or α-thal$_1$, normal	25 50	5% γ_4 (birth)	2α	↓↓ α
Hb H	α-thal$_1$, α-thal$_2$	25	4–30% β_4 (adults) 20–40% γ_4 (birth)	1α	↓↓↓ α
β^+-Thalassaemia	β^+/β, normal	50	Hb A$_2$ ↑, slight ↑ F, or 5–12% F	2β	↓ β
β°-Thalassaemia	β°/β, normal	50	Hb A$_2$ ↑, slight ↑ F	2β	0 or ↓ β
$\delta\beta^\circ$-Thalassaemia	$\delta\beta^\circ$/δβ, normal	50	5–20% Hb F	1β and 1δ	↓ δ and β
δβ-Lepore	Lepore/β, normal	50	Slight ↑ Hb F, normal or ↓ A$_2$, and 5–15% Lepore	1δ, 1β, and 1δβ-Lepore	↓ δβ-Lepore
Hb Constant Spring (CS)	Hb CS heterozygote, normal	50	1–2% γ_4 (birth), 0.5–1% Hb CS	3α α^{CS}	↓ CS
Homozygotes					
Hydrops fetalis (α°-thalassaemia$_1$)	Both α-thal$_1$	25	80% γ_4 (birth) 10% $\delta_2\gamma_2$, 10% β_4	0α	0α
β°-Thalassaemia	Both β°/β	25	↑ Hb F + A$_2$, OA	2β	0 or ↓ β
β^+-Thalassaemia	Both β^+/β, or one β^+/β and one β°/β	25	↑ Hb F + A$_2$, ↓ A	2β	↓ β
$\delta\beta^\circ$-Thalassaemia	Both $\delta\beta^\circ$/δβ	25	100% Hb F OA, and OA$_2$	0 β, 0 δ	0 δ and 0 β
δβ-Lepore	Both Lepore/β	25	75% Hb F, 25% Lepore	2δβ-Lepore	↓ δβ-Lepore
Hb Constant Spring (CS)	Both Hb CS heterozygotes	25	5–6% Hb CS	2α 2α^{CS}	↓ CS

Data from Orkin SH, Nathan DG 1976 Current topics in genetics: The thalassaemias. New England Journal of Medicine 295:710 and Weatherall DJ 1976 The molecular basis of thalassaemia. Johns Hopkins Medical Journal 139:205

Park ($\beta^{92\ His \rightarrow Tyr}$)]. The substituted tyrosine may form a stable bond with the ferric form of the haem iron. This bond prevents interaction of the ferric iron of the affected α- or β-chain with oxygen, but it does not render the globin-haem unit unstable. Both α-variants (M-Boston and M-Iwate) have decreased oxygen affinity, two of the β-variants (M-Hyde Park and M-Saskatoon) have normal affinity, and the final β-variant (M-Milwaukee-I) has decreased oxygen affinity (Bellingham 1976, Bunn 1974).

Clinical aspects

M haemoglobin variants, like other rare haemoglobin disorders, are inherited in an autosomal dominant pattern. The age of onset of cyanosis differs depending on whether the α- or β-chain is affected. With α-chain variants, cyanosis is seen at birth; while β-globin variants develop cyanosis when γ to β switching is nearly complete, at about 6 months of age (Fig. 78.5).

Diagnosis

The blood is chocolate brown and does not change colour on exposure to oxygen. Usually there is no anaemia, and routine electrophoresis may be normal. Spectral analysis allows differentiation of M haemoglobins from methaemoglobin secondary to diaphorase I deficiency. The latter is a red cell enzyme deficiency which is inherited as an autosomal recessive (Bunn 1974). Because the modes of inheritance for M haemoglobins and diaphorase deficiency differ, usually one parent of a patient with the former is affected, while both parents of a patient with the latter disorder are unaffected.

Treatment

No treatment is indicated; however, the diagnosis should be made so that extensive cardiac and pulmonary evaluations can be avoided.

THALASSAEMIAS: QUANTITATIVE DISORDERS OF GLOBIN SYNTHESIS

The thalassaemia syndromes are genetic disorders characterised by absent or deficient synthesis of one or more of the normal globin chains. Absent globin synthesis is designated with an 'o' superscript, e.g. β^o-thalassaemia, while the presence of some (but not enough) of the gene product is noted by a '+' superscript, e.g. β^+-thalassaemia. When there is partial synthesis of the affected globin chain, it is usually structurally normal; therefore, the defect is a quantitative one secondary to unbalanced globin synthesis. This contrasts with the haemoglobinopathies in which the variant haemoglobins are qualitatively or structurally abnormal. Thalassaemia is distributed primarily among people of Mediterranean, African, Middle Eastern, Asian Indian, and Chinese and Southeast Asian descent, but sporadic cases have been reported in many ethnic groups. (Orkin & Nathan 1976, Bunn & Forget 1986).

Molecular basis

As discussed previously, and shown in Figure 78.6, glo-

bin biosynthesis has many steps, each of which has the potential for regulating the amount of globin chains produced. The thalassaemia syndromes provide examples of defects at essentially all different steps. First, deletion of the DNA sequences coding for the structural gene occurs in most α-thalassaemias and in certain rare types of β-thalassaemia, one of which is common in Asian Indians (Bunn & Forget 1986) (Table 78.6). Evidence has accumulated that the chromosome in most Blacks, Filipinos, and some Chinese, which has one of the two α genes deleted, arose by a mispairing of the 5' α gene of one chromosome 16 with the 3' α gene of its homologue and subsequent unequal crossing-over (Fig. 78.9) (Orkin et al 1979, Phillips et al 1980b). The reciprocal chromosome, one containing three α genes, has been observed in Mediterraneans and Blacks (Goossens et al 1980). In Chinese, about one third of chromosome 16s containing a single functional α-globin gene originated from a simple deletion of the 5' α gene, while another third have a nondeletion defect (Embury et al 1980). Chromosomes lacking both α genes have been studied in Asian subjects, and they have large deletions which remove $\psi\zeta_1,\psi\alpha$, and both α genes while leaving the ζ gene intact (Pressley et al 1980). A large number of different deletions in the α-

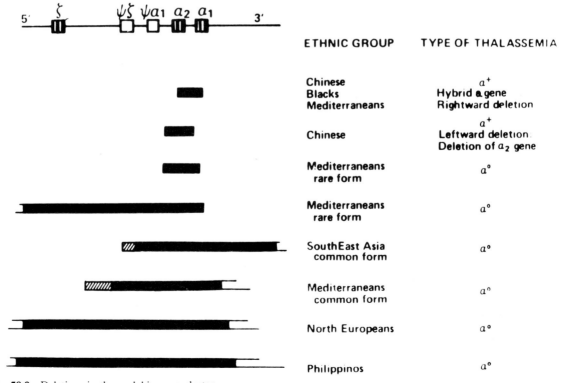

ETHNIC GROUP	TYPE OF THALASSEMIA
Chinese Blacks Mediterraneans	α^+ Hybrid α gene Rightward deletion
Chinese	α^+ Leftward deletion Deletion of α_2 gene
Mediterraneans rare form	α^o
Mediterraneans rare form	α^o
SouthEast Asia common form	α^o
Mediterraneans common form	α^o
North Europeans	α^o
Philippinos	α^o

Fig. 78.9   Deletions in the α-globin gene cluster.

globin gene complex have been observed (Bunn & Forget 1986) (Fig 78.9).

In 1988 we knew of 51 point mutations in the β-globin gene and three deletions affecting only the β-globin gene which produce 'simple' β-thalassaemia (Orkin & Kazazian 1984). The location of these abnormalities in the gene and their effect on gene expression are shown in Figure 78.10 and Table 78.7. The mutations produce defects in transcription, RNA splicing, RNA modification, translation via frameshifts and nonsense codons, or they may produce a highly unstable β-globin.

Transcription mutations are all relatively mild and are commonly observed in β-thalassaemia intermedia. They are single nucleotide substitutions in the TATA box at -30 from the transcription start site, in the ACACCC distal promoter region at -90, but none have yet been observed in the CCAAT box at -70. *RNA splicing mutations* occur at splice junctions, in consensus sequences around splice junctions, in introns to produce new donor and acceptor splice sites, and in cryptic splice

sites in exons. These latter mutations alter sequences which are similar to donor splice sites at the 5' ends of introns but which are not normally used for splicing. By making these sequences resemble more closely the consensus sequence for a donor splice site these mutations activate the cryptic site, and its use leads to production of abnormal RNA and slowed normal splicing. With regard to splice site mutations, it is worth noting the marked discrepancy between the number of different alleles in the consensus donor sequence of intron-1 (9) and the consensus donor sequence of intron-2 (1). *RNA modification defects* are found at both the 5' end or cap site and the 3' end in the RNA cleavage and polyadenylation signal. The cap site mutation which changes the first A residue to a C may work either by reducing transcription itself or slowing the 5' capping process which may reduce mRNA stability. The mutations in the AATAAA signal at the 3' end of the transcript markedly reduce RNA cleavage and lead to elongated mRNA molecules which are probably unstable. *Frame-*

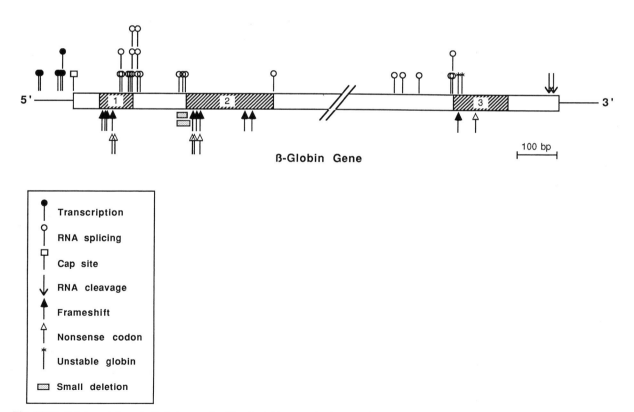

β-Globin Gene

Transcription
RNA splicing
Cap site
RNA cleavage
Frameshift
Nonsense codon
Unstable globin
Small deletion

Fig. 78.10 Point mutations in β-thalassaemia. The β-globin gene is shown with numbered hatched areas representing the coding regions or exons. Boxed open areas between the exons are introns and boxed open areas at the 5'- and 3'-ends of the gene are untranslated regions which appears in the messenger RNA. The various types of mutations are depicted by different symbols; For example, 22 of the 51 mutations affect RNA splicing and are shown as ♀.

Table 78.7   Point mutations in β-Thalassaemia (Total number = 51, April 1988)

Mutant class	Type (0 = β°, + = β⁺)	Origin
I. Nonfunctional mRNA		
a. Nonsense mutants:		
1) codon 17 (A-T)	0	Chinese
2) codon 39 (C-T)	0	Mediterranean, European
3) codon 15 (G-A)	0	Asian Indian
4) codon 121 (A-T)	0	Polish
5) codon 37 (G-A)	0	Saudi Arabian
6) codon 43 (G-T)	0	Chinese
b. Frameshift mutants:		
7) −2 codon 8	0	Turkish
8) −1 codon 16	0	Asian Indian
9) −1 codon 44	0	Kurdish
10) +1 codons 8/9	0	Asian Indian
11) −4 codons 41/42	0	Asian Indian, Chinese
12) −1 codon 6	0	Mediterranean
13) +1 codons 71/72	0	Chinese
14) +1 codons 106/107	0	American Black
15) −1 codon 76	0	Italian
16) −1 codon 37	0	Kurdish
II. RNA Processing mutants		
a. Splice junction changes:		
1) IVS-1 position 1 (G-A)	0	Mediterranean
2) IVS-1 position 1 (G-T)	0	Asian Indian, Chinese
3) IVS-2 position 1 (G-A)	0	Med., Tunisian, Am. Black
4) IVS-1 position 2 (T-G)	0	Tunisian
5) IVS-1 3′-end -17 bp	0	Kuwaiti
6) IVS-1 3′-end -25 bp	0	Asian Indian
7) IVS-2 3′-end (A-G)	0	American Black
8) IVS-2 3′-end (A-C)	0	American Black
b. Consensus changes		
9) IVS-1 position 5 (G-C)	+	Asian Indian
10) IVS-1 position 5 (G-T)	+	Mediterranean, European
11) IVS-1 position 5 (G-A)	+	Algerian
12) IVS-1 position 6 (T-C)	+	Mediterranean
13) IVS-1 position -1 (G-C) (codon 30)	?	Tunisian
14) IVS-1 position -3 (C-T) (codon 29)	?	Lebanese
15) IVS-2 3′-end CAG-AAG	+	Iranian, Egyptian
16) IVS-1 3′-end TAG-GAG	+	Saudi Arabian
c. Internal IVS changes		
17) IVS-1 position 110 (G-A)	+	Mediterranean
18) IVS-1 position 116 (T-G)	0	Mediterranean
19) IVS-2 position 705 (T-G)	+	Mediterranean
20) IVS-2 position 745 (C-G)	+	Mediterranean
21) IVS-2 position 654 (C-T)	0	Chinese
d. Coding regions substitutions		
affecting processing:		
22) codon 26 (G-A)	E	S.E. Asian, European
23) codon 24 (T-A)	+	American Black
24) codon 27 (G-T)	Knossos	Mediterranean
III. Transcriptional mutants		
1) −88 C-T	+	Am. Black, As. Indian
2) −87 C-G	+	Mediterranean
3) −31 A-G	+	Japanese
4) −29 A-G	+	American Black, Chinese
5) −28 A-C	+	Kurdish
6) −28 A-G	+	Chinese
IV. RNA cleavage + polyadenylation mutants		
1) AATAAA - AACAAA	+	American Black
2) AATAAA - AATAAG	+	Kurdish

Table 78.7 Point mutations in β-Thalassaemia (Total number = 51, April 1988) *(contd.)*

Mutant class	Type (0 = β°, + = β⁺)	Origin
V. Cap site mutants		
1) +1 A-C	+	Asian Indian
VI. Unstable globins		
1) β^Indianapolis (codon 112)	+	European
2) β^Showa-Yakushiji (codon 110)	+	Japanese

shift mutations are deletions or additions of 1, 2, or 4 nucleotides which change the ribosome reading frame and cause premature termination of translation. Likewise, nonsense codon mutations directly stop translation. *Missense mutations* may rarely produce β-thalassaemia when they lead to a highly unstable β-globin. This is the case with β^Indianapolis, and β^Showa-Yakushiji. *Most deletions* in the β-globin cluster affect more than the β-globin gene and produce δβ-thalassaemia, γδβ-thalassaemia, or HPFH syndromes. One 619 bp deletion affects the β-globin gene and is the most common β-thalassaemia allele in Asian Indians. Two other small deletions of the β-globin gene have been seen rarely. The Lepore deletions which produce fusion δβ globins due to unequal crossing-over between mispaired δ- and β-globin genes are also causes of a β-thalassaemia phenotype. A β-thalassaemia gene not associated with mutation in the β-globin gene and not associated with the β-globin gene cluster has been reported, but no further information or substantiation has appeared. The mutations themselves are population specific as summarized in Table 78.8.

Pathophysiology

In the thalassaemia syndromes there is reduced or absent synthesis of the affected globin chain; the unaffected chain continues to be synthesized at relatively normal levels. The result is an imbalance which causes aggregation and precipitation of excess unpaired chains. In β-thalassaemia, free α-chains aggregate; the aggregates are highly insoluble and form inclusions in nucleated erythroid precursors in the bone marrow. These inclusion bodies cause intramedullary haemolysis (ineffective

Table 78.8 β-Thalassaemia mutations are population specific

Mediterranean:	15 alleles (6 account for 93%)
Chinese/S.E. Asian:	9 alleles (4 account for 91%)
Indian:	10 alleles (5 account for 90%)
Black:	9 alleles
N African/Middle Eastern:	12 alleles plus Mediterranean alleles

erythropoiesis). In contrast, in α-thalassaemia the γ₄(Hb Barts) and β₄(Hb H) tetramers that form are more soluble. Thus, in severe α-thalassaemias, inclusions are seen in mature erythrocytes and the ineffective erythropoiesis of β-thalassaemia is absent. In any severe thalassaemia, removal of these inclusions from erythrocytes by the reticuloendothelial system damages the cells and produces 'teardrop' forms. Splenomegaly can be secondary to splenic congestion or hypersplenism. After the spleen is removed, cell destruction continues at a decreased rate in the liver, and the number of red cell inclusions may increase greatly. The large number of erythroid precursors expands the marrow cavities, and bone deformities, thinning, and occasional pathological fractures result (Fig. 78.11) (Nathan 1972).

Iron accumulation results from increased gastrointestinal absorption stimulated by the anaemia, blood transfusions, and decreased utilization for haemoglobin synthesis. The deposition of excess iron causes damage to the heart, pancreas, and other tissues.

Folic acid requirements are increased in thalassaemia. If deficiencies develop, they may worsen the anaemia.

Clinical features

α-thalassaemia

Patients are often of Mediterranean or Oriental descent, but the frequency of mild α-thalassaemia is also high in Blacks. When the mutation affects both α loci on the same chromosome 16, the genotype is called α-thal₁ (--). When a single locus on only one of the number 16 chromosomes is affected, the genotype is α-thal₂ (α-).

Four clinical types are seen, depending upon the number of α genes affected. The most severe form is α°thal (α-thal₁ homozygote) (--/--), or hydrops fetalis with Hb Barts. This condition is found usually in Oriental infants who are spontaneously aborted or die of severe hydrops shortly after birth. In the usual case, over 80% of the haemoglobin is Hb Barts (γ₄), which has a very high oxygen affinity, causing severe tissue hypoxia; the remainder is Hb Portland (ζ₂γ₂) and Hb H (β₄). Both parents carry the α-thal₁ trait (Forget & Kan 1974).

Fig. 78.11 Radiographic changes in homozygous β-thalassaemia. **A** Thickened parietal calvaria with outer table destruction and 'hair-on-end' appearance. Note absent pneumatization of maxillary sinuses and coincidental epidermoidoma. **B** Widened medullary cavities, cortical thinning and coarse trabeculation secondary to intramedullary hyperplasia. (Courtesy of Dr John Dorst.)

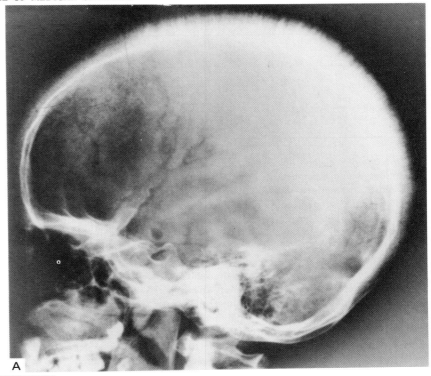

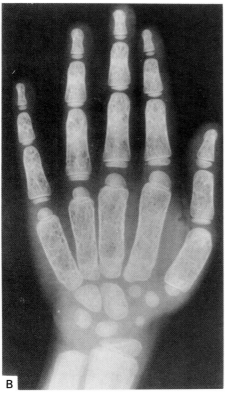

The frequency of Hb H disease ($--/\alpha-$) is high in Southeast Asians, Greeks and Italians. The anaemia varies with an average range of 8–10 gm of haemoglobin per 100 ml of blood, and reticulocytes make up 5–10% of red cells. Splenomegaly and, occasionally, hepatomegaly are found. The red cells are microcytic [decreased mean corpuscular volume (MCV)] and their haemoglobin content is decreased [decreased mean corpuscular haemoglobin (MCH)], but the concentration of haemoglobin per cell is normal [normal mean corpuscular haemoglobin concentration (MCHC)]. On the peripheral smear, poikilocytosis, polychromasia, and target cells are seen. The β_4 tetramer (Hb H) inclusions are seen easily following incubation with 1% brilliant cresyl blue, or after splenectomy they can be seen occasionally with methylene blue reticulocyte stain or Wright's stain (Fig. 78.8C) (Forget & Kan 1974). Studies of globin chain synthesis suggest an α/β ratio of 0.3 to 0.4, rather than 1, and most individuals have a genotype comprised of α-thal$_1$ and α-thal$_2$ ($--/\alpha-$) (Fig. 78.12). This imbalance causes 20% or higher levels of Hb Barts at birth and Hb H levels of 4–30% after the switch from γ- to β-chain synthesis is complete. Both tetramers precipitate causing an inclusion body haemolytic anaemia. Deficient α-chain synthesis causes a drop in Hb A$_2$ ($\alpha_2\delta_2$) levels to 1–1.5%.

Deficient α-chain synthesis is secondary to a deficiency of α-globin mRNA caused by deletion of three of the four α genes. Usually, one of the parents of such a patient has α-thal$_1$ (--) and the other has α-thal$_2$ (α-). The inheritance risk for Hb H disease in offspring from such matings is 25% with each pregnancy (Table 78.6) (Wasi et al 1974).

Heterozygous α-thal$_1$ individuals (Fig. 78.12) are usually of Oriental or Mediterranean descent. They are relatively asymptomatic, but have a mild microcytic anaemia (10–12 gm of haemoglobin per 100 ml of blood) and mild poikilocytosis and anisocytosis. The diagnosis of α-thal trait should be considered seriously when the MCV and MCH are low, the MCHC is relatively normal and the patient is not iron deficient, and the haemoglobin electrophoresis is normal. At birth, Hb Barts may reach 5% in cord blood. The α/β synthesis ratio is 0.6 to 0.75, and the genotype in Orientals is usually a single mutation which deletes both α genes on the same chromosome (Fig. 78.12). A second type of α-thal gene which is dysfunctional but not deleted has been found in Chinese and Cypriots (Kan et al 1977, Orkin et al 1979). Blacks have mild elevation of Hb Barts (>2%) in 2–5% of newborns (Wasi et al 1974), and such individuals have been shown to have an α-thal trait phenotype. Restriction endonuclease studies have shown that the α-thal trait phenotype in Blacks is usually due to deletion of a single α gene on both chromosome 16s (trans) (α-thal$_2$ homozygote) (α-/α-), in contrast to the usual oriental genotype [deletion of both α genes on one chromosome 16 (cis, or α-thal$_1$ heterozygote) ($\alpha\alpha/$--)] (Dozy et al 1979b).

Silent carriers have α-thal$_2$ genotypes with the deletion of a single α gene ($\alpha\alpha/\alpha$-) in affected Orientals, and in 28% of Blacks (Dozy et al 1979b). The haematological findings are normal because the reduction of α mRNA is insufficient to produce significant globin chain imbalance (α/β = 0.8 to 0.9) (Fig. 78.12). Among Southeast Asians there is also a second relatively common α-thal$_2$ allele, the $\alpha^{Constant\ Spring}$ gene. This gene encodes an abnormal α-chain which has 31 additional amino acids at the COOH-terminal end and which is synthesized at about 3% of the rate of normal α-chains (Bunn et al 1977b).

β-thalassaemia

In contrast to the α-thalassaemia states in which there are four levels of severity, the β-thalassaemias can be considered as having two degrees of severity: β-thalassaemia

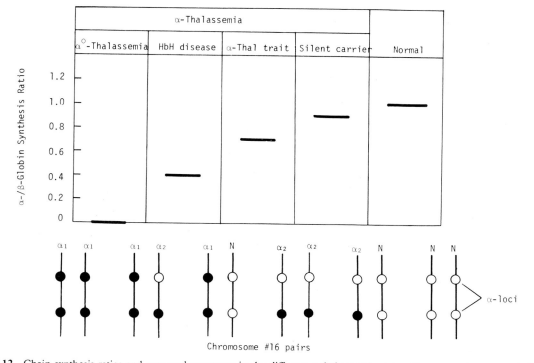

Fig. 78.12 Chain synthesis ratios and proposed genotypes in the different α-thalassaemia states. Genotypes: $\circ$ = normal, N = normal, $\bullet$ = abnormal, α_1 = α-thal$_1$, α_2 = α-thal$_2$, α_1N could also be $\alpha_2\alpha$s22. (Modified from Nathan D G 1972 Thalassaemia. New England Journal of Medicine 286: 586)

major (Cooley's anaemia) results from two β-thalassaemia genes at the β-globin locus; β-thal trait results from a single β-thal gene.

β-thalassaemia major is a severe disease. At birth, affected infants are relatively normal because the change from γ-chain synthesis to β-chain synthesis has not occurred (Fig. 78.5). However, by 6 months of age the infant develops a severely microcytic haemolytic anaemia with aniso- and poikilocytosis, polychromasia, and tear drop red cells (Fig. 78.8F) (Forget & Kan 1974). The failure in β-globin production due to absent or greatly decreased β mRNA leads to imbalance in α- and β-globin synthesis. Subsequent precipitation of free α-chains results in inclusion bodies which damage the erythrocyte membrane and lead to destruction of nucleated red cells in the marrow. The reticulocyte count is usually no greater than 5–10% because of massive destruction of erythroid precursors in the marrow. To maintain an adequate haemoglobin level, transfusions are usually required every four to eight weeks. Affected children develop hepatosplenomegaly secondary to extramedullary haematopoiesis, and a characteristic Oriental facial appearance due to excessive intramedullary haematopoiesis. The bones have expanded marrow cavities resulting in pathologic fractures and a 'hair-on-end' appearance on skull films (Fig. 78.11). Other complications include cholelithiasis, susceptibility to infections, secondary hypersplenism, and delayed growth and maturation (Nathan 1972, Forget & Kan 1974).

The major causes of mortality are haemochromatosis and overwhelming infections following splenectomy, the former due to excessive iron deposition as a result of blood transfusions and increased gastrointestinal absorption (Bannerman et al 1964). Excess iron deposited in the heart, pancreas, liver, and other organs damages tissue and leads to cardiac failure, arrhythmias, diabetes mellitus, and liver failure. Given antibiotic and transfusion therapy, many patients survive until their twenties (Forget & Kan 1974). Greek and Italian homozygotes generally follow this course.

Affected Blacks often have a milder disease (β-thalassaemia intermedia). Transfusions are not usually required in these patients even though α/β synthesis ratios are similar to those observed in Mediterranean homozygotes (Weatherall 1976). β-thalassaemia intermedia is also seen occasionally in other groups, particularly Portuguese, and is correlated with: (1) particular mutations in the β-globin gene which are mild; or (2) the concomitant presence of an α-thalassaemia state.

Individuals with β-thal trait (heterozygous β-thalassaemia) are usually asymptomatic. They have a mild anaemia (10–11 gm of haemoglobin per 100 ml of blood) with decreased MCV (55–70) and MCH (16–22 pg). Microcytosis, anisocytosis, poikilocytosis, and targeting and stippling of the red cells can be seen on the blood smear (Fig. 78.8E) (Forget & Kan 1974). On physical examination there is mild to moderate splenomegaly in about half of the cases.

Differential diagnosis

In the general practice of medicine many patients present with a mild microcytic anaemia. Nearly all of them have iron deficiency anaemia or a thalassaemia trait. In heterozygous thalassaemia, the peripheral smear may be more abnormal than that of iron deficiency, and the MCV and MCH are decreased; but the MCHC is normal in contrast to the decreased MCHC seen in advanced iron deficiency anaemia. Also, the MCV in thalassaemia traits tends to be lower in relation to the red cell count than the MCV in iron deficiency. This difference is the basis of the Mentzer index [MCV/red cell count (RBC)]. MCV/RBC values of less than 11.5 suggest thalassaemia trait, while values greater than 13.5 suggest iron deficiency anaemia (Mentzer 1973). A much more definitive approach is to measure Hb A_2 in patients with microcytosis (Fig. 78.13). Patients with microcytosis and normal Hb A_2 should have serum iron or ferritin determinations; a low value suggests iron deficiency anaemia, while a normal iron or ferritin value suggests α-thal trait (diagnosis is confirmed when documentation is obtained in first-degree relatives). When microcytosis and an increased Hb A_2 are found, β-thal trait is the tentative diagnosis (Pearson et al 1973). Confirmation of the diagnosis is obtained by family studies and chain synthesis ratios. A possible simple alternative for differentiating iron deficiency from thalassaemia trait in patients with low MCVs is to measure the degree of anisocytosis with an electronic red cell counter. Anisocytosis is significantly greater in patients with iron deficiency than those with thalassaemia trait (Bessman & Feinstein 1979).

As seen in Table 78.6, β-thal heterozygotes can have different haemoglobin patterns. The most common is that of β^0-thal or β^+-thal with an increased Hb A_2 (usually 4–6%) and a normal or slightly increased Hb F (2–5%). In the rare δβ-thal trait, the Hb A_2 is normal, but Hb F is usually increased. Finally, Hb Lepore trait has 5–15% Hb Lepore, which contains a δβ fusion chain, and a slight elevation of Hb F (Orkin & Nathan 1976, Forget & Kan 1974). Chain synthesis studies in most β-thal heterozygotes yield α/β ratios of 1.5 to 2.5.

The term β-thalassaemia intermedia is sometimes used to describe individuals who are mild homozygotes; Black β^+-thal homozygotes with a mild clinical course are an example. Family studies in many have confirmed that the

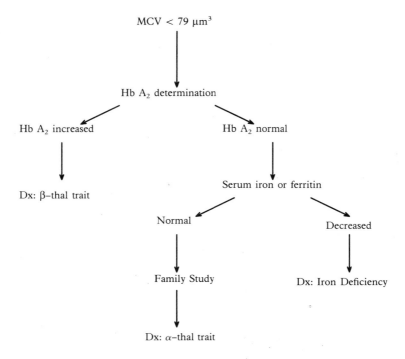

Fig. 78.13 Approach to screening for thalassaemia trait. Note that since this approach was designed as a guide for screening of adults, other causes of microcytosis, such as lead poisoning in children, are not considered. (Modified from Pearson H A, O'Brien R T, McIntosh S 1973 Screening for thalassaemia trait by electronic measurement of MCV. New England Journal of Medicine 288: 351)

presumed β^+-thal homozygotes had, in fact, inherited two different β-thal alleles and thus were actually genetic compounds. Homozygous $\delta\beta$-thalassaemia also tends to be clinically mild because, for unknown reasons, Hb F production is higher in this condition than in other β-thal states and compensates for the absent Hb A and Hb A_2. One can also find the combination of α-thal and β-thal traits in the same individual. This condition is mild because the resulting α/β synthesis ratio is more normal and there are fewer free α-chains to cause haemolysis.

δβ-thalassaemia, or F thalassaemia

Homozygous $\delta\beta$-thalassaemia usually occurs in Greeks and, as stated above, tends to be a mild disorder. The term F thalassaemia is used because homozygotes have 100% Hb F and lack Hb A and Hb A_2. The mild anaemia and haemolysis are due to increased γ-chain synthesis, which makes the imbalance between synthesis of α-chains and non-α-chains less than that seen in other β-thalassaemias. Patients with heterozygous $\delta\beta$-thalassaemias have mild microcystosis and 5–20% Hb F on electrophoresis (Table 78.6).

Hb Lepore thalassaemia

As previously mentioned, Hb Lepore is a variant haemoglobin containing a $\delta\beta$-fusion chain. Originally this chain probably resulted from nonhomologous crossing-over between the linked δ- and β-genes during meiosis. Three different Lepore variants are described which differ in the point at which the $\delta\beta$-fusion occurs. Hb Lepore has an electrophoretic mobility similar to that of Hb S, and it forms 5–15% of the total haemoglobin of heterozygotes (Table 78.6). Decreased Hb Lepore synthesis may be secondary to instability of the $\delta\beta$-mRNA. Heterozygotes are clinically similar to β°-thal heterozygotes and Hb Lepore homozygotes, or Lepore/β°-thal genetic compounds are similar to β°-thal homozygotes (Forget & Kan 1974).

γβ-thalassaemia

Two full-term newborns with haemolytic, hypochromic anaemia and microcytosis have been described. Hb H and Hb Barts were absent, and globin synthesis studies revealed a deficiency of γ- and β-synthesis in relation to α-synthesis. With time, the peripheral smears and morphology improved and resembled those of the fathers and other relatives with heterozygous β-thal. These cases are probably examples of heterozygous γβ-thalassaemia (Kan et al 1972, Van der Ploeg et al 1980). Restriction endonuclease mapping of DNA of one child has shown a large deletion which removes all the ε, ^{G}γ, ^{A}γ, and δ genes from one chromosome 11. Interestingly, the deletion ends 2 kb 5' to the β gene, yet that β gene, while present, is not expressed (Van der Ploeg et al 1980). In other cases a deletion has eliminated the entire β-globin gene cluster.

δ°-thalassaemia

Heterozygous and homozygous δ°-thalassaemia have, respectively, decreased and absent Hb A_2. However, anaemia and changes in peripheral smears are not seen due to the normal low level of δ-chain production (Fig. 78.5).

Hereditary persistence of fetal haemoglobin

Hereditary persistence of fetal haemoglobin (HPFH) can occur in many different forms due to different mutations. HPFH heterozygotes differ from thalassaemia heterozygotes in that they have no imbalance between the synthesis of α- and non-α-chains (i.e., γ- and β-chains). The HPFH syndromes are characterised by an asymptomatic heterozygous state without microcytosis. The elevated Hb F ranges from 10–15% in the Greek type to 3–30% in certain types in Blacks. The proportion of γ-chain type (^{G}γ versus ^{A}γ) varies among patients with different HPFHs and usually, but not always, the Hb F is homogeneously distributed within red cells, in contrast to δβ- and other thalassaemias (Kazazian 1974). In a few cases, HPFH heterozygotes have two populations of cells: one contains Hb F; the other lacks Hb F. These patients are said to have heterocellular HPFH, as opposed to the bulk of patients who have pancellular HPFH (Boyer et al 1977).

The β and δ genes adjacent to the HPFH gene are often inactive and, in fact, may be deleted in Blacks with two HPFH types, but both are present and active in other HPFH cases involving Blacks. In these latter cases, point mutations at −202 and −175 upstream of the ^{G}γ-globin gene have been found. In other ethnic groups point mutations in the same region 5' to the ^{A}γ-globin gene have produced non-deletion HPFH. The differences between HPFH and δβ-thalassaemia are subtle, but in δβ-thal the clinical picture and blood smears are somewhat more abnormal and the Hb F has a more heterogeneous cellular distribution. HPFH homozygotes have mild hypochromia, microcytosis, and morphologi-

cal changes in the red cells; 100% of the haemoglobin is F, and there is no anaemia. In some of these cases, α/γ chain synthesis ratios of 1.5 occur, similar to the α/β ratios seen in milder β-thal trait. It has been hypothesised that a suppression region for γ-chain synthesis is located between the ^{A}γ- and δ-loci and that HPFH, but not δβ-thalassaemia mutations, inhibit its function. However, suppression and activation regions in the β-globin gene cluster appear multiple in number, and a clear picture has not yet emerged.

Interaction of thalassaemia with haemoglobin variants

Thalassaemia and structural variant haemoglobin genes may or may not interact. An interacting thalassaemia gene is one which causes an increased level of the variant haemoglobin chain in the individual heterozygous for the variant gene and a thalassaemia gene at the same locus. When the presence of both the thalassaemia and variant genes does not increase the level of the haemoglobin variant, then the thalassaemia is noninteracting.

α-thalassaemia and α-variants

α-thalassaemia$_1$-Hb Q ($α^{47\ Asp→His}$). The genetic compound of α-thal$_1$ (--) and Hb Q is found mainly in Thailand. The clinical picture is similar to that of Hb H disease, but there is an absence of Hb A synthesis which is expained by the fact that the $α^Q$ allele occurs on a chromosome from which the second α gene is deleted ($α^{Q}$-) (Lie-Injo et al 1979).

α-thalassaemia – Hb G-Philadelphia ($β^{68Asn→Lys}$). Heterozygotes for Hb G-Philadelphia, the most common α-variant in Blacks, have been studied, and the amount of the variant seems to be trimodal (22%, 30%, and 41% of the total haemoglobin) (Baine et al 1976). Individuals with 30% Hb G have been shown to have chromosomal homologues containing: (1) a single $α^G$ gene and; (2) two normal $α^A$ genes ($αα/α^G$-); and those with 41% Hb G have one chromosome containing a single $α^G$ gene and another with a single $α^A$ gene ($α$-/$α^G$-) (Sancar et al 1980). Individuals with 22% Hb G have three normal $α^A$ genes in addition to an $α^G$ gene ($αα/α^Gα$).

β-thalassaemia and β-variants

In S/β-thalassaemia, the β-thal gene interacts with the $β^S$ gene in the heterozygote to increase the level of Hb S near homozygous SS levels. The S/β-thal heterozygote has a milder clinical course than the SS homozygote, and splenomegaly is a common physical finding. Anaemia is present in S/β-thal and is characterised by microcytic red and target cells with occasional sickled forms (Fig. 78.8). Haemoglobin electrophoresis reveals 60–90% Hb S, 0–30% Hb A, 1–20% Hb F, and increased Hb A_2 (Forget & Kan 1974). The percentages of Hb S and Hb A vary depending on whether the β-thal gene is β^+ or β°.

β-thalassaemia – Hb C is seen among Blacks. Splenomegaly and an increased Hb C level differentiate this genetic compound from that of Hb C heterozygote.

β-thalassaemia – Hb E is a common disease in Thailand. It results in a clinical picture similar to that of homozygous β-thalassaemia.

Management of thalassaemia

Prevention

Matings which can give rise to various types of α- and β-thalassaemias are outlined in Table 78.6. The parents of homozygous α- or β-thalassaemia offspring are themselves heterozygotes. As such, with each pregnancy there is a 25% risk of producing another homozygous offspring.

For maximum benefit of genetic counselling, heterozygotes should be identified before they bear affected children. Thalassaemia heterozygotes can be diagnosed tentatively by appropriate studies (MCV, haemoglobin electrophoresis, serum iron) (Fig. 78.13). Once the condition is diagnosed, the heterozygote should be informed of its presence, its inheritance, and the potential for affected children from certain matings, so that he or she has an accurate grasp of the risk. In some cases this would result in the testing of mates who would be identified as noncarriers, and hence these couples would be at no risk for homozygous offspring. The risk of having a homozygous offspring when both parents are heterozygotes is shown in Table 78.6; other parents might be at risk for genetic compounds in their offspring.

Prenatal diagnosis may be desired by certain heterozygous couples at risk. The procedure has become widely used; but while it leads to in utero diagnosis, it is not a treatment, but merely a preventive measure. From 1975–1980, prenatal diagnosis of various thalassaemias was done exclusively by analysis of fetal blood. The feasibility of this procedure was based on a number of factors. First, β-chains are synthesized by erythroid precursors as early as 5 weeks of fetal age (Fig. 78.5). Second, normal standards of β-chain synthesis at 18–20 weeks' gestation are known. Third, fetal cells can be obtained (with a 6% risk of fetal death at present) by either transabdominal placental puncture under ultrasonography or from fetal vessels visualized by fetoscopy (Alter 1979). Fourth, small numbers of fetal reticulocytes can be separated from maternal red cells by differential

agglutination or by preferential lysis of maternal cells. The fetal blood sample can be incubated with radioactive leucine, and the relative synthesis of α, β (or variant β-chains), and γ-chains can be determined using chromatographic separation (Alter 1979). By 1980 about 1000 pregnancies had been tested for β-thalassaemia in this way (Alter 1979). The procedure has usually resulted in adequate fetal blood samples (>90%) with few technical errors.

In 1978 prenatal diagnosis by restriction endonuclease mapping of DNA came into general use. Fetal amniocytes were obtained for study by amniocentesis, which carries a very low risk of fetal mortality (<0.5%). DNA analysis was first carried out on fetuses at risk for α-thalassaemia and δβ-thalassaemia in whom deletions could be detected (Orkin et al 1978, Dozy et al 1979a). In 1980 polymorphic restriction endonuclease sites in the β-globin gene complex were used for prenatal detection of various β-thalassaemias not due to deletions. Kan et al (1980) first showed that a Bam HI site 3' to the β gene was useful for prenatal diagnosis of a certain β°-thalassaemia allele in Sardinian couples at risk. Later, Little et al (1980) demonstrated that other polymorphic sites in the γ genes could be valuable in this undertaking in non-Sardinian couples. Using a combination of known DNA polymorphisms and linkage analysis, it became possible to carry out prenatal diagnosis for various β-thalassaemia states, by amniocentesis alone, in 75% of pregnancies at risk in which the couple had a previous child (Kazazian et al 1980).

As the various mutations producing β-thalassaemia were characterized (see Fig. 78.10) and oligonucleotide hybridization techniques were developed for detecting specific nucleotide changes in genomic DNA, prenatal diagnosis by direct mutation detection came into routine use in Sardinia (Rosatelli et al 1985). Recently, the development of the polymerase chain reaction technique has allowed amplification of β-globin gene sequences by a million fold. This technique can then be coupled with oligonucleotide hybridization in dot blots, restriction digestion of amplified product, or direct nucleotide sequencing of the amplified product (Wong et al 1987) to allow direct detection of mutations in general prenatal diagnosis of β-thalassaemia. At Johns Hopkins, in July 1989, the last 100 consecutive prenatal diagnoses of β-thalassaemia were carried out in various ethnic groups by direct detection of the mutations involved.

Therapy

Anaemia. Treatment for severe β-thalassaemia is primarily symptomatic. If anaemia is severe enough, transfusions are required to maintian adequate levels of haemoglobin. There are two approaches. First, transfusion may be given when the patient's haemoglobin drops below 8 gm per 100 ml to avoid symptoms secondary to anaemia. Second, hypertransfusion, or repeated transfusions, may be given as frequently as needed to maintain the haemoglobin at a minimum of 10 gm per 100 ml. The latter approach may require 2–3 units every 2–4 weeks in adults (Forget & Kan 1974). Evidence suggests that children maintained on hypertransfusion (haemoglobin greater than 9.5–10 gm per 100 ml) are more active, have fewer infections, and have less frequent complications of cardiac dysfunction, hypersplenism, and bone and dental changes. However, there is conflicting evidence as to whether this therapy can aid the child to attain normal growth (Forget & Kan 1974, Weiner et al 1978).

Iron accumulation. Both methods of transfusion increase the iron overload. Iron chelation therapy with deferoxamine has been used to attempt to prevent this side-effect of chronic transfusion. The route of administration is important, since 750 mg of deferoxamine IM (with oral ascorbic acid in patients over 5 years old) resulted in urinary clearance of iron ranging from 2.2–44.8 mg per 24 hours (prior to treatment, excretion was 0.1–2.5 mg per 24 hours). Subcutaneous infusions of 1.5 gm deferoxamine over 18 hours further increased iron excretion 2.4-fold, and large doses given intravenously increased clearance over that obtained by subcutaneous infusion (Propper et al 1977, Cohen & Schwartz 1978). The iron excretion attained following intravenous or slow subcutaneous infusion of deferoxamine is far better than excretion when deferoxamine is injected intramuscularly. Other data suggest that in children, while 20 mg of deferoxamine B per kg of body weight given daily by IM injection might reduce the daily iron accumulation somewhat, if the deferoxamine is given by overnight infusion, it allows iron balance to be reached even when the child has large transfusion requirements (Weiner et al 1978). The relative effectiveness of different doses in thalassaemia patients of different ages has been reported (Graziano et al 1978). These experimental data all suggest that chelation therapy is applicable to clinical practice.

Other side-effects of transfusions include hepatitis and cytomegalovirus infections. Also, isoimmunization to minor blood groups may occur, but careful selection of donors may decrease this risk. Sensitization to white cell or plasma antigens may be decreased by using blood with the white cells removed. Urticaria may be treated with antihistamines, as well as epinephrine, prior to and during transfusion. Febrile reactions may require antipyretics and occasionally, if severe, steroids (Nathan 1972).

Finally, the increased rate of erythropoiesis can lead to increased folic acid requirements. If a folate deficiency occurs, it may cause increased anaemia; however, a deficiency is easily avoided by daily oral administration of folic acid.

Infection. Splenectomy may be avoided by hypertransfusion therapy; however, splenectomy may be necessary to alleviate hypersplenism with worsening of the anaemia or pain due to progressive splenomegaly or infarction of the spleen. As discussed under sickle-cell disease, splectomized children, especially those under 6 years of age, are at risk for life-threatening infections. Pneumococcal vaccine, as well as prophylactic penicillin, should be used in such children, and suspected infections should be treated aggressively (Forget & Kan 1974, Ammann et al 1977).

Bone marrow transplantation. This has been used successfully not only in aplastic anaemia and leukaemia, but also for thalassaemia. A large number of affected children have received transplants, with many cures, although there are clearly risks involving graft rejection, morbidity, and death.

Future treatment

Theoretical approaches to thalassaemia treatment which may become possible include induction of expression of the deficient globin chain, stabilization of the appropriate mRNA, or activation of non-expressed γ genes to reduce the globin chain imbalance. Methods for insertion of DNA into eukaryotic cells are being developed, but technical as well as ethical problems remain. The chances of applying such techniques to the treatment of thalassaemia syndromes or the haemoglobinopathies still seem five years removed at this time.

REFERENCES

Alter B P 1979 Prenatal diagnosis of hemoglobinopathies and other hematologic disorders. Journal of Pediatrics 95: 501

Alter B P, Modell C B, Fairweather D, Hobbins J C, Mahoney M J, Frigoletto F D, Sherman A S, Nathan D G 1976 Prenatal diagnosis of hemoglobinopathies. New England Journal of Medicine 295: 1437

Akhonkhai V I, Landesman S H, Fikrig S M, Schmalzer E A, Brown A K, Cherubin C E, Schiffman G 1979 Failure of pneumococcal vaccine in children with sickle cell disease.

New England Journal of Medicine 301: 26

Ammann A J, Addiego J, Wara D W, Lubin B, Smith W B, Mentzer W C 1977 Polyvalent pneumococcal-polysaccharide immunization of patients with sickle-cell anemia and patients with splenectomy. New England Journal of Medicine 297: 897

Baine R M, Rucknagel D L, Dublin P A Jr, Adams J G III 1976 Trimodality in the proportion of hemoglobin G Philadelphia in heterozygotes. Evidence for heterogeneity in the number of human alpha chain loci. Proceedings of the National Academy of Sciences USA 73: 3636

Bannerman R M, Callender S T, Hardisty R M, Smith R S 1964 Iron absorption in thalassemia. British Journal of Haematology 10: 490

Baralle E F, Shoulders C C, Proudfoot N J 1980 The primary structure of the human ε-globin gene. Cell 21: 621

Barrett-Connor E 1971 Bacterial infection and sickle cell anemia. Medicine 50: 97

Bellingham A J 1976 Haemoglobins with altered oxygen affinity. British Medical Bulletin 32: 234

Bernards R, Little P F R, Annison G, Williamson R, Flavell R A 1979 Structure of human $^G\gamma$-$^A\gamma$-δ-β globin gene locus. Proceedings of the National Academy of Sciences USA 76: 4827

Bessman J D, Feinstein D I 1979 Quantitative anisocytosis as a discriminant between iron deficiency and thalassemia minor. Blood 53: 288

Boyer S H, Margolet L, Boyer M L, et al 1977 Inheritance of F cell frequency in heterocellular hereditary persistence of fetal hemoglobin: An example of allelic exclusion. American Journal of Human Genetics 26: 256

Bunn H F 1974 The structure and function of human hemoglobins. In: Nathan D G, Oski F A (eds) Hematology of infancy and childhood. W B Saunders, Philadelphia, ch 13, p 412

Bunn H F, Forget B G 1986 Hemoglobin: Molecular, genetic and clinical aspects. W B Saunders, Philadelphia

Bunn H F, Forget B G, Ranney H M 1977a Hemoglobin structure. In: Human hemoglobins. W B Saunders, Philadelphia, ch 1, p 4

Bunn H F, Forget B G, Ranney H M 1977b Human hemoglobin variants. In: Human hemoglobins. W B Saunders, Philadelphia, ch 6, p 193

Bunn H F, Forget B G, Ranney H M 1977c Unstable hemoglobin variants-congenital Heinz body hemolytic anemia. In: Human hemoglobins. W B Saunders, Philadelphia, ch 8, p 282

Charache S, Dover G J, Moyer M A, Moore J W 1987 Hydroxyurea-induced augmentation of fetal hemoglobin production in patients with sickle cell anemia. Blood 69: 109

Chehab F, Doherty M, Cai S, Kan Y W, Cooper S, Rubin E 1987 Detection of sickle cell anemia and thalassemias. Nature 329: 293

Cohen A, Schwartz E 1978 Iron chelation therapy with deferoxamine in Cooley anemia. Journal of Pediatrics 92: 643

Cooper H A, Hoagland H C 1972 Subject review. Fetal hemoglobin. Mayo Clinic Proceedings 47: 402

Dean J, Schechter A N 1978 Sickle cell anemia: Molecular and cellular bases of therapeutic approaches. New England Journal of Medicine 299: 863

Deisseroth A, Nienhuis A, Turner P et al 1977 Localization of the human α-globin structural gene to chromosome 16 in somatic cell hybrids by molecular hybridization assay. Cell 12: 205

Deisseroth A, Nienhuis A, Lawrence J, Giles R, Turner P, Ruddle F H 1978 Chromosomal localization of human β globin gene on human chromosome 11 in somatic cell hybrids. Proceedings of the National Academy of Sciences USA 75: 1456

Dozy A M, Forman E N, Abuelo D N, et al, 1979a Prenatal diagnosis of homozygous α-thalassemia. Journal of the American Medical Association 241: 1610

Dozy A M, Kan Y W, Embury S H et al 1979b α-globin gene organisation in blacks precludes the severe form of α-thalassemia. Nature 280: 605

Efstradiadis A, Posakony J W, Maniatis T et al 1980 The structure and evolution of the human β-globin gene family. Cell 21: 653

Embury S H, Miller J A, Dozy A M, Kan Y W, Chan V, Todd D 1980 Two different molecular organizations account for the single α-globin gene of the α-thalassemia-2 genotype. Journal of Clinical Investigation 66: 1319

Forget B F, Kan Y W 1974 Thalassemia and the genetics of hemoglobin. In: Nathan D G, Oski F A (eds) Hematology of infancy and childhood. W B Saunders, Philadelphia, ch 7, p450

Fritsch E F, Lawn R M, Maniatis T 1979 Characterisation of deletions which affect the expression of fetal globin genes in man. Nature 279: 598

Fritsch E F, Lawn R M, Maniatis T 1980 Molecular cloning and characterization of the human β-like globin gene cluster. Cell 19: 959

Giebiuk G S, Schiffman G, Krivit W, Quie P G 1979 Vaccine type pneumococcal pneumonia: occurrence after vaccination in an asplenic patient. Journal of the American Medical Association 241: 2736

Goossens M, Dozy A M, Embury S H et al, 1980 Triplicated α-globin loci in man. Proceedings of the National Academy of Sciences USA 77: 518

Graziano J H, Markenson A, Miller D R et al 1978 Chelation therapy in β-thalassemia major. I. Intravenous and subcutaneous deferoxamine. Journal of Pediatrics 92: 648

Grosveld F, van Assendelft G B, Greaves D R, Kollias G 1987 Position independent high level expression of the human β-globin gene in transgenic mice. Cell 51: 975

Gusella J, Varsanyi-Breiner A, Kao F-T et al 1979 Precise localization of the human β-globin gene complex on chromosome 11. Proceedings of the National Academy of Sciences USA 76: 5239

Hamer D, Leder P 1979 Splicing and the formation of stable RNA. Cell 18: 1299

Hobbins J C, Mahoney M J 1974 *In utero* diagnosis of hemoglobinopathies. New England Journal of Medicine 290: 1065

International Hemoglobin Information Center 1984 List of Hemoglobin Variants. Augusta, Georgia

Kan Y W, Dozy A M 1978 Antenatal diagnosis of sickle cell anemia by DNA analysis of amniotic fluid cells. Lancet ii: 910

Kan Y W, Forget B G, Nathan D G 1972 Gamma-beta thalassemia. A cause of hemolytic disease of the newborn. New England Journal of Medicine 286: 129

Kan Y W, Dozy A M, Trecartin R, Todd D 1977 Identification of a non-deletion defect in α thalassemia. New England Journal of Medicine 297: 1081

Kan Y W, Lee K Y, Furbetta M, Angius A, Cao A 1980 Polymorphism of DNA sequence in the β-globin gene region. New England Journal of Medicine 302: 185

Kazazian H H Jr. 1974 Regulation of human fetal hemoglobin production. Seminars in Hematology 11: 525

Kazazian H H Jr, Woodhead A P 1973 Hemoglobin A synthesis in the developing fetus. New England Journal of Medicine 289: 58

Kazazian H H Jr, Cho S, Phillips J A III 1977 The mutational basis of the thalassemia syndromes. Progress in Medical Genetics 2: 165

Kazazian H H Jr, Phillips J A III, Boehm C D, Vik T A, Mahoney M J, Ritchey A K 1980 Prenatal diagnosis of β-thalassemia by amniocentesis: Linkage analysis of multiple polymorphic restriction endonuclease sites. Blood 56: 926

Lauer J, Shon C–K J, Maniatis T 1980 The chromosomal

arrangement of human α-like globin genes: sequence homology and α-globin gene deletions. Cell 20: 119

Lawn R M, Fritsch E F, Parker R C, Blake G, Maniatis T 1978 The isolation and characterization of linked δ- and β-globin genes from a cloned library of human DNA. Cell 15: 1157

Lawn R M, Efstradiadis A, O'Connell G, Maniatis T 1980 The nucleotide sequence of the human β-globin gene. Cell 21: 647

Lie-Injo L E, Dozy A M, Kan Y W, Lopes M, Todd D 1979 The α-globin gene adjacent to the gene for Hb Q-$\alpha^{74\ Asp\rightarrow His}$ is deleted, but not that adjacent to the gene for Hb G $\alpha^{30\ Glu\rightarrow Gln}$; Three-fourths of the α-globin genes are deleted in Hb Q-α-thalassemia. Blood 54: 1407

Little P F R, Annison G, Darling S, Williamson R, Camba L, Modell B 1980 Model for antenatal diagnosis of β-thalassemia and other monogenic disorders by molecular analysis of linked DNA polymorphisms. Nature 285: 144

Mentzer W C 1973 Differentiation of iron deficiency from thalassemia trait. Lancet 1: 882

Merkel C G, Wood T G, Lingrel J B 1976 Shortening of the poly(A) region of mouse globin messenger RNA. Journal of Biological Chemistry 251: 5512

Motulsky A G 1973 Frequency of sickling disorders in US Blacks. New England Journal of Medicine 288: 31

Nagel R L, Lynfield J, Johnson J et al 1976 Hemoglobin Beth Israel. A mutant causing clinically apparent cyanosis. New England Journal of Medicine 295: 125

Nathan D G 1972 Thalassemia. New England Journal of Medicine 296: 586

Nathan D G, Pearson H A 1974 Sickle cell syndromes and hemoglobin C disease. In: Nathan D G, Oski F A (eds) Hematology of infancy and childhood. W B Saunders Philadelphia, ch 14, p 419

Orkin S H 1978 The duplicated human α globin genes lie close together in cellular DNA. Proceedings of the National Academy of Sciences USA 74: 560

Orkin S H, Kazazian H H Jr. 1984 The mutation and polymorphism of the human β-globin gene and its surrounding DNA. Annual Review of Genetics 18: 131

Orkin S H, Nathan D G 1976 Current concepts in genetics. The thalassemias. New England Journal of Medicine 295: 710

Orkin S H, Alter B P, Altay C et al 1978 Application of endonuclease mapping to the analysis and prenatal diagnosis of thalassemia caused by globin-gene deletion. New England Journal of Medicine 299: 166

Orkin S H, Old J M, Lazarus H, Altay C, Gurgey A, Weatherall D J, Nathan D G 1979 The molecular basis of α-thalassemias: Frequent occurrence of dysfunctional α loci among non-Asians with Hb H disease. Cell 17: 33

Pearson H A, O'Brien R T, McIntosh S 1973 Screening for thalassemia trait by electronic measurement of mean corpuscular volumes. New England Journal of Medicine 288: 351

Phillips J A III, Panny S R, Kazazian H H Jr et al 1980a Prenatal diagnosis of sickle cell anemia by restriction endonuclease analysis: Hind III polymorphisms in γ-globin genes extend test applicability. Proceedings of the National Academy of Sciences USA 77: 2856

Phillips J A III, Vik T A, Scott A F, et al 1980b Unequal crossing-over: A common basis of single α-globin genes in Asians and American Blacks with Hemoglobin H disease. Blood 55: 1066

Pressley L, Higgs D R, Clegg J B, Weatherall D J 1980 Gene deletions in α-thalassemia prove that the 5' ζ locus is functional. Proceedings of the National Academy of Sciences USA 77: 3586

Propper R D, Cooper B, Rufo R R et al 1977 Continuous subcutaneous administration of deferoxamine in patients with iron overload. New England Journal of Medicine 297: 418

Proudfoot N J, Baralle F 1979 Molecular cloning of the human ϵ-globin gene. Proceedings of the National Academy of Sciences USA 76: 5435

Proudfoot N J, Maniatis T 1980 The structure of a human α-globin pseudogene and its relationship to α-globin gene duplication. Cell 21: 537

Rieder R F 1974 Human hemoglobin stability and instability. Molecular mechanisms and some clinical correlations. Seminars in Hematology 11: 423

Rosatelli C, Tuveri T, DiTucci A, Falchi A M, Scalas M T, Monni G, Cao A 1985 Prenatal diagnosis of β-thalassemia with the synthetic-oligomer technique. Lancet i: 241

Saiki R K, Gelfand D H, Stoffel B et al 1988 Primer-directed enzymatic amplification of DNA with a thermostable DNA polymerase. Science 239: 487

Sancar G B, Tatsis B, Cedeno M M, Rieder R F 1980 Proportion of hemoglobin G Philadelphia ($\alpha_2^{68\ Asn\rightarrow Lys}\beta_2$) in heterozygotes determined by α-globin gene deletions. Proceedings of the National Academy of Sciences USA 77: 6874

Scott A F, Phillips J A III, Migeon B R 1979 DNA restriction endonuclease analysis for the localization of the human β and δ globin genes on chromosome 11. Proceedings of the National Academy of Sciences USA 76: 4563

Seid-Akhavan M, Winter W P, Abramson R K, Rucknagel D L 1976 Hemoglobin Wayne: A frameshift mutation detected in human hemoglobin alpha chains. Proceedings of the National Academy of Sciences USA 73: 882

Slightom J L, Blechl A E, Smithies O 1980 Human fetal $^G\gamma$ and $^A\gamma$ globin genes: Complete nucleotide sequences suggest that DNA can be exchanged between these duplicated genes. Cell 21: 627

Spritz R A, DeRiel J K, Forget B G, Weissman S M 1980 Complete nucleotide sequence of the human δ-globin gene. Cell 21: 639

Tilghman S M, Curtis P J, Tiemeier D C, Leder P, Weissmann C 1978 The intervening sequence of a mouse β-globin gene is transcribed within the 15S β-globin mRNA precursor. Proceedings of the National Academy of Sciences USA 75: 1309

Van der Ploeg L H T, Konings A, Oort M, Roos D, Bernini L, Flavel R A 1980 γ-β-thalassemia studies showing that deletion of the γ and δ genes influences β-globin gene expression in man. Nature 283: 637

Wasi D, Na-Nakorn S, Pootrakul S-N 1974 The α thalassemias. Clinical Hematology 3: 383

Weatherall D J 1976 The molecular basis of thalassemia. Johns Hopkins Medical Journal 139: 205

Weiner M, Karpatkin M, Hart D et al 1978 Cooley anemia: High transfusion regimen and chelation-therapy, results, and perspective. Journal of Pediatrics 92: 653

Wong C, Dowling C E, Saiki R K, Higuchi R G, Erlich H A, Kazazian H H Jr 1987 Characterization of β-thalassemia mutations using direct genomic sequencing of amplified single copy DNA. Nature 330: 384–386

79. Hereditary red blood cell disorders (Excluding haemoglobinopathies and thalassaemias)

Bertil E. Glader

INTRODUCTION

This chapter focuses on genetic diseases which are primarily expressed as disorders of the red blood cell (RBC). Some of these conditions cause haemolytic anaemia (enzyme and membrane disorders), some are associated with impaired RBC production (hypoplastic, megaloblastic, sideroblastic and dyserythropoietic anaemias) and some, although not associated with anaemia, cause clinical problems due to abnormal erythrocyte function (methaemoglobinaemia). This section also describes assorted genetic disorders which have no significant effect on RBC physiology and do not cause anaemia, although the diagnosis of these inherited conditions is suggested by erythrocyte enzyme or shape abnormalities. The important genetic disorders caused by haemoglobin abnormalities are discussed elsewhere in this text (Chapter 78).

HAEMOLYSIS CAUSED BY HEREDITARY RBC ENZYME DISORDERS

The majority of erythrocyte enzyme abnormalities associated with haemolysis are caused by deficiency of an enzyme critical for RBC function. The enzyme deficiency in these cases may be a consequence of decreased enzyme synthesis or progressive enzyme instability as cells age (the latter is important since mature anucleate erythrocytes are incapable of new protein synthesis). In rare cases, haemolysis is not caused by an enzyme deficiency, but is a consequence of increased enzyme activity which secondarily has deleterious effects on cell metabolism (e.g. adenosine deaminase excess). In addition to enzymopathies that cause haemolysis, some enzyme deficiencies have no adverse effects on RBC function (e.g. lactic dehydrogenase and 6-phosphogluconate dehydrogenase deficiency), or if they occur in patients with haemolytic anaemia, it is not clear that the enzyme deficiency and haemolysis are causally related (e.g. glutathione peroxidase, glutathione reductase and

adenylate kinase deficiencies) (Beutler 1979). The major causes of haemolysis due to hereditary RBC enzyme defects are abnormalities in the hexosemonophosphate (HMP) shunt and glutathione metabolism, glycolytic enzyme deficiencies, and abnormalities in purine and pyrimidine metabolic enzymes (Fig. 79.1).

Disorders of the hexosemonophosphate shunt pathway and glutathione metabolism

General considerations

The hexosemonophosphate (HMP) shunt pathway metabolizes 5–10% of glucose utilized by red blood cells, and this is critical for protecting RBCs against oxidant injury. The HMP pathway is the only source of reduced nicotinamide adenine dinucleotide phosphate (NADPH), a co-factor important in glutathione metabolism. Red blood cells contain relatively high concentrations of reduced glutathione (GSH), a sulphydryl containing tripeptide (glytamylcysteinylglycine) which functions as an intracellular reducing agent that protects cells against oxidant injury. Oxidants, such as superoxide anion (O_2^-) and hydrogen peroxide (H_2O_2), are produced by exogenous factors (i.e. drugs, infection) and are also formed within red cells as a consequence of reactions of haemoglobin with oxygen. However, when these oxidants accumulate within RBCs, cellular proteins are altered, thereby causing lethal cell injury. Under normal circumstances this does not occur since GSH, in conjunction with the enzyme glutathione peroxidase (GSH-Px), rapidly inactivates these compounds. During the oxidant detoxification process, however, GSH itself is converted to oxidized glutathione (GSSG), and GSH levels fall. In order to sustain protection against persistent oxidant injury, GSH levels must be maintained, and this is accomplished by glutathione reductase (GSSG-Rx) which catalyzes reduction of GSSG to GSH. This reaction requires the NADPH generated by glucose-6-phosphate dehydrogenase (G6PD), the first enzymatic

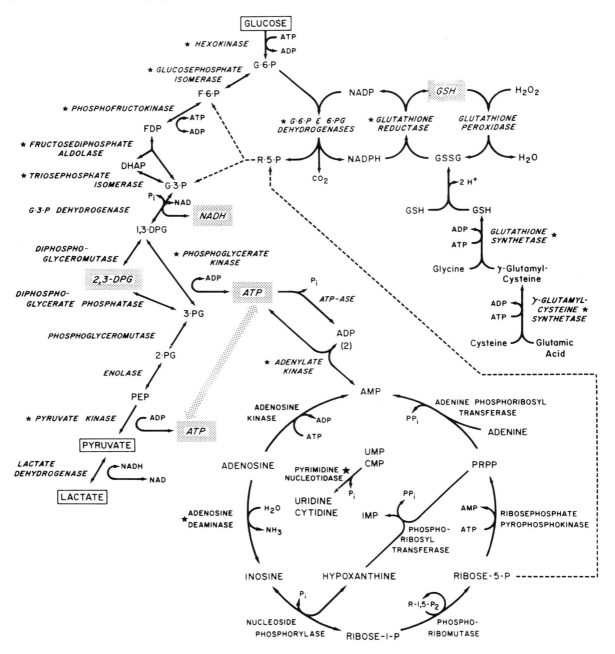

Fig. 79.1 Overall energy, oxidant and nucleotide metabolism of mature erythrocytes. Specific reactions and pathways are discussed in text. Enzymes associated with hereditary haemolytic anaemia are indicated by the asterisk (*). (From Valentine W N, Tanaka K R, Paglia D E 1983 In: Stanbury, Wyngaarden, Fredrickson, Goldstein, Brown (eds) The Metabolic Basis of Inherited Disease, 5th edn. McGraw Hill, New York; by permission of the author and publishers.)

reaction of the HMP shunt. Thus, it is this tight coupling of the HMP shunt and glutathione metabolism that is responsible for protecting intracellular proteins from oxidative assault. Haemolytic disorders associated with abnormalities of the HMP shunt and glutathione metabolism have been reported in four different settings: (1) G6PD deficiency; (2) decreased GSSG-Rx activity; (3) GSH-Px deficiency; and (4) deficiencies of GSH synthetic enzymes.

Glucose-6-phosphate dehydrogenase (G6PD) deficiency

This is the most common red blood cell enzyme abnormality associated with haemolysis (Beutler 1983). It has been estimated that this RBC enzyme disorder affects millions of people throughout the world, the highest frequency occurring in Mediterranean countries, Africa and China (Luzzatto 1975). Approximately 10–15% of all Blacks in the United States are deficient in erythrocyte G6PD activity (Boyer et al 1962), and this is not dissimilar from the 20% incidence reported in Nigeria. In contrast, the incidence of G6PD deficiency in Mediterranean individuals is much more variable, ranging from approximately 2% in Sicily to over 20% on the Greek Island of Rhodes. It is intriguing that the world-wide distribution of G6PD deficiency is similar to that for malaria, and it has been hypothesized that the gene for G6PD deficiency may be protective against malaria (Motulsky 1960). Partial indirect support for this is that G6PD deficiency in Sardinia is more common at sea level than at higher elevations, and this also parallels the endemicity of malaria. In adddition, it has been observed that female heterozygotes for G6PD deficiency (who therefore have normal *and* G6PD-deficient RBCs) have more malaria parasites in normal erythrocytes than in G6PD-deficient cells (Luzzatto et al 1969). A possible biochemical explanation for this phenomenon relates to the fact the G6PD-deficient RBCs have slightly elevated levels of oxidized glutathione, an extremely potent inhibitor of protein synthesis (Kosower & Kosower 1970).

Haemolysis occurs primarily in G6PD-deficient males and the magnitude of haemolysis is much more severe in Caucasians. In most individuals with G6PD deficiency, there is no anaemia in the steady state, reticulocyte counts are normal, but RBC survival may be slightly decreased. However, episodic exacerbations of haemolysis accompanied by anaemia occur in association with the administration of certain drugs, infections and the ingestion of fava beans.

Drugs: The discovery of G6PD deficiency as a cause of haemolysis originally followed the observation that Black soldiers developed haemolysis after receiving primaquine phosphate for malaria prophylaxis (Carson et al 1956). Subsequently, numerous other drugs have been implicated as causative agents and the common denominator of these drugs is that they interact with haemoglobin and oxygen, thus accelerating the intracellular formation of H_2O_2 and other oxidizing radicals.

Infections: Hepatitis, salmonellosis and pneumonia are established inciting causes of haemolysis in G6PD deficiency, but virtually any type of bacterial or viral infection can lead to accelerated destruction of G6PD-deficient red cells. As a possible explanation for this relationship between infection and haemolysis, it has been proposed that the oxidants generated by phagocytosing macrophages diffuse into the extracellular medium and thereby pose an oxidative threat to G6PD-deficient erythrocytes (Baehner et al 1971).

Favism: Haemolysis following exposure to fava beans occurs in G6PD-deficient Caucasians and Orientals, but is not seen in Blacks (Stamatoyannopoulos et al 1966). It occurs primarily in children, and it is the most common cause of haemolysis in G6PD-deficient Sicilian children. Haemolytic episodes occur primarily in the spring months when fresh fava beans are plentiful, and it is thought that unstable pyrimidine glycosides (isouramil and divicine) in fava beans are the active oxidants responsible for haemolysis (Chevion et al 1982). Favism does not occur in all susceptible G6PD individuals, and it is thought that an additional genetic factor is involved, presumably related to how fava bean oxidants are metabolized.

Neonatal haemolysis due to G6PD deficiency is well documented in Caucasians and Orientals, and this usually occurs in the absence of any obvious exogenous oxidant stress. In one study from Greece, approximately 30% of all exchange transfusions for hyperbilirubinaemia were done in G6PD-deficient infants (Valaes et al 1969). Moreover, severe intrauterine haemolytic anaemia leading to hydrops fetalis has been reported in a term male Chinese infant with severe G6PD deficiency (Mentzer & Collier 1975). Black infants with G6PD deficiency manifest no increased incidence or severity of hyperbilirubinaemia and/or haemolysis, although hyperbilirubinaemia may be more common in premature Black infants with G6PD deficiency (O'Flynn & Hsia 1963, Eshaghpour et al 1967).

In some cases of Caucasian G6PD deficiency, there is a concurrent decrease in the enzyme activity of leucocytes as well as erythrocytes. In general, this is of little clinical significance, although rarely the magnitude of leucocyte G6PD deficiency is sufficiently severe to be associated with impaired leucocyte function and increased infections (Gray et al 1973). The presumed biochemical basis for this is that G6PD deficiency leads to decreased amounts of NADPH generation and, thus, to impaired leucocyte oxidase activity and H_2O_2 production.

More than 150 different variants of G6PD have been described, each of which differs in its biochemical properties (e.g. kinetic activity, electrophoretic mobility, pH optima and/or affinity for substrate and/or co-factor) (Beutler 1983). Most known G6PD variants are enzymatically normal and do not cause clinical problems. The normal enzyme, G6PD^B, is found in almost all Caucasians and a majority of Blacks. It has normal catalytic activity and is not associated with haemolysis. The four most commonly encountered variants include the following. (1) G6PD^{A+} is found in 20% of American Blacks. It has normal catalytic properties and does not cause haemolysis. It differs from G6PD^B in that it has a much faster electrophoretic mobility. The structure of G6PD^{A+} differs from that of G6PD^B by the substitution of one amino acid, an asparagine for aspartate (Yoshida 1967). (2) G6PD^{A-} is the common variant associated with haemolysis, and is found in 10–15% of American Blacks. Its electrophoretic mobility is identical to that of G6PD^{A+}. This is an unstable enzyme and its catalytic activity is decreased in older RBCs (Yoshida et al 1967). Hence, this variant is designated G6PD^{A-} compared with G6PD^{A+}. (3) G6PD Mediterranean is the most common *abnormal* variant found in Caucasians, particularly those whose origins are in the Mediterranean area. The electrophoretic mobility of G6PD Mediterranean is identical to that of G6PD^B, but its catalytic activity is markedly reduced. (4) G6PD Canton is a variant seen in Orientals. Its biochemical properties are very similar to those of G6PD Mediterranean (Luzzatto 1975).

As normal red blood cells age, the intracellular activity of the G6PD^B decreases. Despite this loss of enzyme activity, however, normal old red blood cells contain sufficient G6PD activity to generate NADPH and thereby maintain GSH levels in the face of oxidant stress (Fig. 79.2). The defect in Blacks with G6PD deficiency is due to increased enzyme instability of G6PD^{A-} such that young red blood cells have relatively normal enzyme activity, whereas older red cells are severely G6PD deficient (Piomelli et al 1968). The clinical correlate of this is that haemolysis in patients with G6PD^{A-} is generally mild and is limited to the older deficient erythrocytes. In contrast, the enzymatic defect in G6PD Mediterranean is due to a much greater enzyme instability, and red blood cells of all ages are grossly deficient. Consequently, the entire red blood cell population of individuals with G6PD Mediterranean is susceptible to oxidant-induced injury, and this can lead to severe haemolysis.

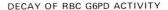

DECAY OF RBC G6PD ACTIVITY

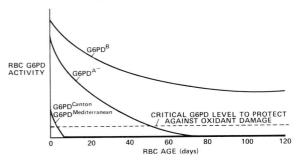

Fig. 79.2 Decay of erythrocyte G6PD activity in normal individuals (G6PD^B), and accelerated loss of activity associated with the common abnormal variants occurring in Blacks (G6PD^{A-}), Caucasians (G6PD^{Mediterranean}), and Orientals (G6PD^{Canton}).

The clinical observation that the severity of haemolysis caused by G6PD deficiency is worse in males than in females is consistent with the fact that the gene for G6PD is located on the X chromosome (Childs et al 1958). Males have only one type of G6PD, whereas females can have two different biochemical types of enzyme. According to the Lyon hypothesis, however, only one X chromosome is active in any given somatic cell (Lyon 1961). Thus, although females may have two different G6PD variants, any given red blood cell contains only one type of G6PD. Dependent upon the degree of lyonization, the mean red blood cell enzyme activity in females who carry a gene for G6PD deficiency may be normal, moderately reduced, or grossly deficient. A female with 50% normal G6PD activity has 50% normal red cells and 50% of G6PD-deficient red cells. The G6PD-deficient cells in females, however, are as vulnerable to haemolysis as are enzyme-deficient red blood cells in males.

G6PD-deficient erythrocytes exposed to oxidants (infection, drugs, fava beans) become depleted of GSH. This reaction is central to the cell injury in this disorder since once GSH is depleted there is further oxidation of other RBC sulphhydryl-containing proteins. Oxidation of haemoglobin leads to the formation of sulphhaemoglobin and Heinz bodies while oxidation of membrane sulphhydryl groups leads to the accumulation of membrane polypeptide aggregates, presumably due to disulphide bond formation between spectrin molecules and between spectrin and other membrane proteins (Johnson et al 1979). The end result of all these changes is the production of rigid, non-deformable erythrocytes that are susceptible to stagnation and destruction by reticuloendothelial macrophages. Moreover, some patients with unstable haemoglobinopathies may also manifest oxidant injury, since these abnormal haemoglobins are inordinately susceptible to mild oxidant stress. In most cases, however, oxidant injury is associated with G6PD deficiency.

The diagnosis of G6PD deficiency is suggested by the presence of episodic haemolytic anaemia in association with drugs or infection. Spherocytes, dense cells and cells that look as if a bite has been removed (due to splenic removal of Heinz bodies) are occasionally seen on routine Wright-stained peripheral blood smears (Fig. 79.3A). Brilliant cresyl blue supravital stains of the peripheral blood may reveal Heinz bodies during haemolytic episodes (Fig. 79.3B). The diagnosis of G6PD deficiency is made by a specific spectrophotometric assay or screening test which utilizes haemolysate as a source of enzyme. Regardless of the specific test used, however, false-negative reactions may occur if the most enzymatically deficient red blood cells have been removed by haemolysis. This is not generally critical in testing male Caucasians, but it certainly is a problem in diagnosing some Caucasian females and Blacks of both sexes,

especially during the reticulocytosis following acute haemolysis. In these cases, family members can be studied. An alternative approach to diagnosis is to wait until the haemolytic crisis is over and re-evaluate the patient at the time his red blood cell mass has been repopulated with cells of all ages (approximately two to three months).

In most cases, there is no specific treatment for haemolysis due to G6PD deficiency. Red blood cell transfusions are appropriate in those rare circumstances in which signs and symptoms of anaemia indicate severe cardiovascular compromise. In the usual case, however, therapeutic endeavours are directed towards minimizing potential sources of oxidant stress. The most common drugs implicated are some of the sulphonamide antibiotics and antimalarial drugs (Table 79.1). Aspirin was formerly thought to contribute to haemolysis in these patients, but current thought is that aspirin-induced red blood cell destruction is an extremely rare event, if it occurs at all (Glader 1976). Since aspirin is commonly taken for fever during infections, it seems more likely that the association between aspirin and haemolysis is due to infection rather than to the drug. Many other

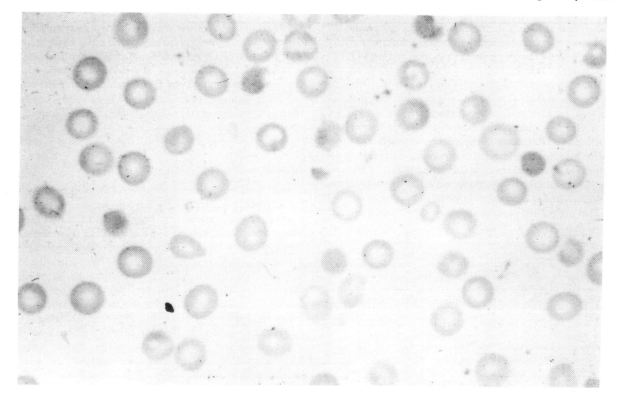

Fig. 79.3A Peripheral smear (Wright stain) from an individual with G6PD deficiency during a haemolytic episode. Note appearance of some RBCs which appear to have a 'bite' removed. Some spherocytes are also present.

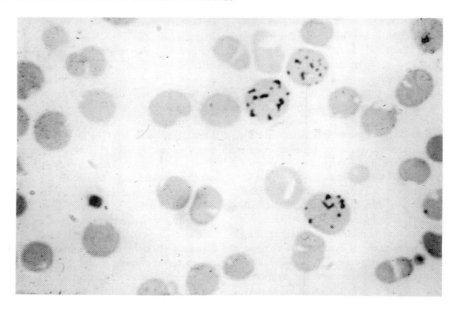

Fig. 79.3B Heinz bodies in G6PD deficient red cells seen following incubation of fresh blood with brilliant cresyl blue.

drugs have also been implicated as causes of haemolysis, but in most cases normal therapeutic concentrations of these drugs can be given safely to individuals with G6PD deficiency (Table 79.2).

While most individuals with G6PD deficiency have an almost normal RBC survival, and haemolytic anaemia only occurs with oxidant stress, there are rare individuals with G6PD variants who manifest chronic haemolysis (Yoshida 1973). Common clinical characteristics of these patients include mild anaemia, neonatal jaundice, gallstones and splenomegaly (Luzzatto 1975). Although these individuals always have evidence of haemolysis (reticulocytosis, hyperbilirubinaemia), the same factors which trigger haemolysis in other G6PD-deficient in-

dividuals also exacerbate the rate of cell destruction in these cases of chronic non-spherocytic haemolytic anaemia. In cases of G6PD variants associated with chronic non-spherocytic haemolysis, there is no specific biochemical abnormality which characterizes the enzyme defect. In some of these cases associated with chronic haemolysis, splenectomy often reduces the rate of red cell destruction.

Glutathione reductase (GSSG-Rx) deficiency

Partial deficiency of erythrocyte GSSG-Rx activity, although not associated with haemolysis, has been described in a variety of haematological disorders, malignancies, liver disease and malnutrition. However, it now appears that most GSSG-Rx deficiencies reported to date are a reflection of riboflavin deficiency, since flavin adenine-dinucleotide (FAD) is an essential co-factor for maximal GSSG activity (Beutler 1969). Only one clear case of haemolysis associated with GSSG-Rx deficiency has been described (Loos et al 1976). In this patient, a 22-year-old woman, erythrocyte GSSG-Rx levels were undetectable, and enzyme activity was not altered when FAD was added to the incubation medium. Her only haematological problem was an episode of haemolysis associated with the ingestion of fava beans. Interestingly, the patient's two haematologically normal siblings also had undetectable levels of erythrocyte GSSG-Rx, but

Table 79.1 Drugs and chemicals associated with significant haemolysis in subjects with erythrocyte G6PD deficiency

Acentanilid	Primaquine
Methylene blue	Sulphacetamide
Nalidixic acid (Neg-Gram)	Sulphamethoxazole (Gantanol)
Naphthalene	Sulphanilamide
Niridazole (Ambilhar)	Sulphapyridine
Nitrofurantoin (Furadantin)	Thiazolesulphone
Pamaquine	Toluidine blue
Pentaquine	Trinitrotoluene (TNT)
Phenylhydrazine	

Modified from Beutler (1983)

Table 79.2 Drugs which can be given safely in normal therapeutic concentrations to individuals with erythrocyte G6PD deficiency without chronic nonspherocytic haemolysis

Acetaminophen (Tylenol®)	Phenylbutazone
Acetophenetidine (phenacetin)	Phenytoin
Acetylsalicylic acid (aspirin)	Probencid (Benemid®)
Aminopyrine (Pyramidon®, amidopyrine)	Procainamide hydrochloride (Pronesty®)
Antazoline (Anistine®)	Pyrimethamine (Daraprim®)
Antipyrine	Quinidine
Ascorbic acid (Vitamin C)	Quinine
Benzhexol (Artane®)	Streptomycin
Chloramphenicol	Sulphadiazine
Chlorguanide (Proguanil®, Paludrine®)	Sulphaguanidine
Chloroquine	Sulphamerazine
Colchicine	Sulphamethoxypyridazine (Kynex®)
Diphenylhydramine (Benedryl®)	Sulphisoxazole (Gantrisin®)
Isoniazide	Trimethoprim
L-dopa	Tripelennamine (Pyribenzamine®)
Menadione sodium bisulphate (Hykinone®)	Vitamin K
p-aminobenzoic acid	

Modified from Beutler (1983)

they had no history of haemolysis. An additional interesting observation in this family with GSSG-Rx deficiency was that the proband and one of her siblings had cataracts, and it has been suggested that cataracts may be due to oxidant injury of lens protein in the presence of reduced GSSG-Rx levels. In this family, where three individuals had virtually complete GSSG-Rx deficiency, only one patient haemolyzed after ingesting fava beans, while the other two had no evidence of haemolysis. It would thus appear that only minimal amounts of GSSG-Rx are necessary to sustain adequate levels of reduced glutathione, and it has been questioned whether hereditary deficiency of GSSG-Rx is a cause of haemolytic anaemia (Beutler 1979). In cases where GSSG-Rx deficiency is due to suboptimal FAD levels, supplemental riboflavin administration will correct the systemic vitamin deficiency and increase GSSG-Rx activity, but there is usually no correction of any underlying haematological disorder (Beutler 1969).

Glutathione peroxidase (GSH-Px) deficiency

Several cases of haemolysis in association with moderate deficiency of erythrocyte GSH-Px activity have been described in adults, children and newborn infants (Boivin et al 1969, Necheles et al 1969). Despite these reports, however, recent observations suggest that moderate GSH-Px deficiency may not be a cause of haemolysis or other haematological problems. First of all, many healthy normal individuals, particularly those of Jewish or Mediterranean ancestry, have reduced GSH-Px activity without evidence of haemolysis (Beutler & Matsumoto 1975).

Secondly, low GSH-Px activity, in the absence of haemolysis, has also been observed in normal people from New Zealand with Selenium (Se) deficiency (Se is an integral part of GSH-Px) (Thomson et al 1977). In view of these observations, the putative role of GSH-Px deficiency as a cause of haemolysis is currently being questioned. It has been suggested that reported cases of haemolysis and partial GSH-Px deficiency are not causally related, but rather may reflect the coincidence of an unknown cause of haemolysis with a common benign enzyme variant (Beutler 1979). A partial explanation of these observations is that GSH-Px is only one of the cellular mechanisms available to detoxify peroxides. Under physiological conditions, catalase and non-enzymatic reduction of oxidants by GSH may also be important factors regulating the rate of H_2O_2 detoxification.

Of all the reported cases suggesting a relationship between haemolysis and GSH-Px deficiency, one of the most persuasive is that of a 9-month-old Japanese girl with chronic non-spherocytic haemolytic anaemia (Nishimura et al 1972). This patient's erythrocyte GSH-Px activity was 17% of control activity, while her haematologically normal parents had 51–66% control enzyme activity. In addition, incubation of the patient's RBCs with acetylphenylhydrazine revealed slightly increased Heinz body formation. Whether this specific enzyme defect was responsible for the patient's chronic haemolytic anaemia, however, is not known. In any event, because of the controversial role of GSH-Px as a cause of haemolysis, any patient with haemolytic anaemia and reduced GSH-Px activity should have an extensive evaluation to look for the presence of another enzymopathy.

Deficiencies of glutathione synthetic enzymes

Glutathione is actively synthesized in RBCs and has an intracellular half-life of only four days due, in part, to cellular efflux of oxidased glutathione (GSSG) (Srivastava & Beutler 1969). RBCs are capable of de novo GSH synthesis and this is accomplished by two critical enzymes (Fig. 79.1). Gamma-glutamyl-cysteine synthetase (gamma GCSynth) catalyzes the first step in GSH synthesis, the formation of gamma-glutamyl-cysteine from glutamic acid and cysteine. Glutathione synthetase (GSHSynth) catalyzes the formation of GSH from glutamyl-cysteine and glycine. In many tissues, but not RBCs, these two enzymes are part of the gamma glutamyl cycle, which is involved with the synthesis and degradation of GSH and is also thought to have a role in amino acid transport across cell membranes (Meister 1974). Hereditary haemolytic anaemia, characterized by reduced GSH content, has been reported in patients with deficiencies of both gamma GCSynth and GSHSynth activity. The clinical effects of these disorders depend on the severity of enzyme deficiency and whether the gamma glutamyl cycle in non-erythroid tissues is affected.

Gamma-Glutamyl-Cysteine Synthetase Deficiency is a rare haemolytic anaemia which has only been described in two adults who were brother and sister (Konrad et al 1972a). Both of these patients had a life-long history of anaemia, intermittent jaundice, cholelithiasis and splenomegaly. In addition, they also manifested severe neurological dysfunction (Richards et al 1974), a generalized aminoaciduria and low gamma GCSynth activity and GSH content in their leucocytes and muscle cells. This disorder appears to be an autosomal recessive condition and, in the one family studied, presumed carriers had reduced gamma GCSynth activity, although erythrocyte GSH levels were normal. Haemolytic anaemia is seen only in the homozygous state where erythrocyte GSH levels are approximately 5% of normal, and there is markedly reduced gamma GCSynth activity. There is no specific therapy for GCSynth deficiency although it would seem prudent to obtain periodic gallbladder ultrasound examinations since both affected patients had cholecystectomies.

Glutathione Synthetase Deficiency had been described in association with several cases of haemolysis. These fall into two distinct clinical syndromes, dependent upon whether the enzymatic defect is limited to RBCs or also affects other tissues. In cases limited to deficiency of erythrocyte GSHSynth, the major manifestations are splenomegaly, intermittent jaundice and compensated haemolytic anaemia (Boivin et al 1966, Mohler et al 1970). In contrast, in those cases where GSHSynth deficiency is generalized to other tissues, clinical problems include haemolytic anaemia, persistent metabolic acidosis presenting in the newborn period, overproduction of 5-oxoproline with oxoproluria, organic neurological defects and mental retardation (Jellum et al 1970, Marstein et al 1976). In these cases with a generalized absence of GSHSynth, a variety of feed-back mechanisms of the gamma glutamyl cycle lead to the accelerated synthesis of 5-oxoproline and thereby oxoprolinaemia, oxoproluria, and metabolic acidosis. Deficiency of GSH synthetase appears to be an autosomal recessive disorder. Relatives of affected patients have reduced enzyme activity, but erythrocyte GSH content is normal and there are no haematological problems. There are no unique haematological or morphological manifestations associated with this disorder and the diagnosis is suspected in patients with haemolytic anaemia and markedly reduced red blood cell GSH content. Virtually no GSHSynth activity is detected in homozygous-deficient individuals. In at least one case, splenectomy was efficacious in modifying the anaemia, although haemolysis continued as manifested by persistent reticulocytosis (Mohler et al 1970). In those individuals with GSHSynth deficiency and oxoprolinaemia, oral bicarbonate administration is necessary to control the acidosis.

Haemolysis associated with glycolytic enzyme abnormalities

General considerations

In mature red blood cells which lack mitochondria, glycolysis is the only metabolic pathway capable of adenosine triphosphate (ATP) synthesis (Fig. 79.1). The cause of haemolysis in RBC glycolytic defects, as in all other haemolytic anaemias, is invariably due to abnormal membrane function, leading to decreased red blood cell deformability. Which vital ATP-dependent membrane reactions are impaired, however, is not known.

Haemolytic anaemias due to glycolytic enzymopathies are relatively rare, affecting only a few thousand individuals in the world. Abnormalities in virtually every glycolytic enzyme have been described, although over 90% of all cases associated with haemolysis are due to pyruvate kinase (PK) deficiency (Valentine et al 1983, Mentzer 1987). In some of these disorders the enzyme deficiency is not limited to red blood cells, but also includes leucocytes, platelets, muscle and/or neural tissue. Most glycolytic enzymopathies manifest an autosomal recessive pattern of inheritance with haemolysis seen in the homozygous state. Heterozygotes are haematologically normal, although their red blood cells contain less than normal levels of enzyme activity. Clinical manifestations of haemolysis include chronic anaemia, reticulocytosis and some degree of hyperbilirubinaemia. The magnitude of anaemia is frequently increased during viral infections and this can be due to increased haemolysis, or transient aplastic crises associated with viral infections. Most children with red blood cell glycolytic defects have a history of neonatal jaundice, many require an exchange transfusion, and, rarely, kernicterus has been reported. There are no specific morphological abnormalities to suggest an RBC glycolytic enzymopathy, although anisocytosis and poikilocytosis are common. The possibility of a glycolytic enzymopathy is usually suggested when chronic haemolytic anaemia cannot be explained by the more common causes of haemolysis (i.e. hereditary spherocytosis or haemoglobinopathies). A major problem in the diagnosis of glycolytic enzymopathies is the fact that most severely affected cells are usually removed in vivo (i.e. haemolyzed) and are thus unavailable for analysis in vitro. In these cases, it is often necessary to examine parents for the presumed heterozygous state of the enzyme deficiency. Therapy for red blood cell glycolytic defects is similar to that for other chronic haemolytic anaemias. Folic acid supplementation is given to meet the requirements of accelerated erythropoiesis, and RBC transfusions are given to those patients demonstrating significant cardiovascular compromise. Severely anaemic patients often benefit from splenectomy, since this organ is usually responsible for destruction of enzymatically abnormal cells. However, the response to splenectomy is only partial and, in most cases, haemolysis usually continues, although RBC transfusion requirements decrease. Cholelithiasis is a constant problem and all patients with glycolytic enzymopathies should have periodic gallbladder ultrasound examinations. The most common of these rare disorders are summarized in the following paragraphs.

Pyruvate kinase (PK) deficiency

Pyruvate kinase catalyzes one of the two glycolytic reactions responsible for ATP production, and thus it is not surprising that PK deficiency leads to abnormal RBC function. The degree of haemolysis in PK deficiency varies greatly and is often severe enough to require frequent red blood cell transfusions. Almost all affected patients demonstrate a beneficial response to splenectomy because the 'splenic environment' is particularly damaging to PK-deficient reticulocytes (Mentzer et al 1971). Anaemia usually improves following splenectomy, although the reticulocyte count also increases to levels of 50–70%. This paradoxical reticulocytosis occurs because reticulocyte survival is increased once the adverse metabolic environment of the spleen is removed. The anaemia that persists following splenectomy is generally well tolerated and transfusions are rarely needed. In part this occurs because the enzymatic defect is distal to the

site of 2,3-DPG production, and thus there is a two- to three-fold increase in red cell 2,3-DPG content (i.e. an accumulation of metabolic intermediates proximal to the enzymatic lesion). This metabolic effect minimizes the adverse effects of anaemia since the increased 2,3,-DPG content enhances oxygen release from haemoglobin. The importance of this effect was clearly demonstrated in a study which compared two patients, one deficient in erythrocyte pyruvate kinase and the other deficient in erythrocyte hexokinase, a proximal glycolytic defect with low levels of red cell 2,3-DPG (Oski & Delivoria-Papadopoulous 1970). Both patients had the same degree of anaemia and reticulocytosis; they differed only in their red blood cell content of 2,3-DPG. The patient with PK deficiency tolerated the anaemia much better. Objectively, the PK-deficient individual also had a smaller increase in cardiac output and an increased arteriovenous oxygen difference in response to exercise stress.

Glucose phosphate isomerase (GPI) deficiency

This enzyme deficiency, first reported by Baughan et al (1968), is now recognized as the second most common glycolytic enzymopathy associated with haemolysis. In most cases, this defect is due to an unstable enzyme (Paglia & Valentine 1974). The activity of GPI is frequently reduced in leucocytes, and platelets too, but this is not associated with increased infections or bleeding problems in these patients. Usually there is a partial response to splenectomy.

Hexokinase (HK) deficiency

This is a rare glycolytic enzymopathy which was first identified several years ago (Valentine et al 1967) but has now been identified in 20 different individuals. Splenectomy ameliorates but does not cure the haemolytic process. As discussed above (see PK deficiency), HK deficiency leads to impaired 2,3-DPG production and these patients tolerate anaemia poorly.

Phosphoglycerate kinase (PGK) deficiency

The genetics of this disorder is unique amongst glycolytic enzymopathies in that it is X-linked (Valentine et al 1968). Haemolysis has been reported in at least 10 males with PGK deficiency. Leucocyte PGK activity is also low but there is no evidence that these individuals have leucocyte dysfunction or increased infections. Of interest, however, is the most severely PGK-deficient patients, haemolysis is associated with neurological abnormalities (i.e. seizures, mental retardation, aphasia and/or movement disorders) (Konrad et al 1972b).

Phosphofructokinase (PFK) deficiency

Phosphofructokinase in RBCs is a complex protein made up of two types of subunit: muscle or M type subunits, and liver or L type subunits (Kahn et al 1979). The clinical manifestations of this enzyme deficiency relate to the specific type of structural enzyme abnormality in PFK. In all cases associated with haemolysis, red cells show partial PFK deficiency, with about 50% normal enzyme activity although there is a profound enzyme deficiency in muscle and this is associated with a severe myopathy (Tarui et al 1965). In these cases of PFK deficiency, RBCs lack M subunits although the L subunits are present (Vora et al 1980). Haemolysis is thought to occur because tetramers of L type PFK subunits are unstable and their enzymatic function is inhibited under normal intracellular conditions. Interestingly, a second syndrome is recognized in which the degree of PFK deficiency is similar, but there is little, if any, haemolysis and no muscle disease. This latter condition is due to a deficiency in the L subunits.

Triose phosphate isomerase (TPI) deficiency

At least 15 cases of TPI deficiency with haemolytic anaemia have been described. However, the most unique feature of this enzymopathy is an associated severe neurological disorder characterized by spasticity, motor retardation and hypotonia (Schneider et al 1968). These neurological abnormalities usually become manifest after 6 months of age, and most affected patients die before they are 5 years old. Interestingly, the frequency of the heterozygous state for TPI deficiency is relatively high (0.1–0.5% in Caucasians, 5.5% in Blacks) (Mohrenweiser & Fielek 1982). The rare occurrence of homozygous TPI deficiency may reflect early fetal losses.

Abnormalities of purine and pyrimidine metabolism associated with haemolysis

Many of the enzymes utilized for purine and pyrimidine synthesis are present in erythrocytes (Fig. 79.1), although mature RBCs do not synthesize DNA and are incapable of de novo purine or pyrimidine synthesis. Abnormal activity of these erythrocyte enzymes, however, is often observed with inborn errors of metabolism (see Megaloblastic Anaemias and RBCs as a biopsy tool). In a few of these metabolic disorders there may be an associated haemolytic anaemia. In particular, hereditary haemolytic anaemias have been reported in association with three enzymes: pyrimidine nucleotidase, adenosine deaminase and adenylate kinase.

Pyrimidine 5′ nucleotidase (P5′N) deficiency

Pyrimidine 5′ nucleotidase is an enzyme which degrades pyrimidine nucleotides to inorganic phosphate and the corresponding pyrimidine nucleoside (Paglia & Valentine 1981). Deficiency of this enzyme is now recognized as one of the more common hereditary enzymopathies associated with haemolysis. At least 24 separate kindreds have been identified and it is found throughout the world, although there may be a predilection for individuals of Mediterranean and African ancestry. It is generally agreed that P5′N deficiency is inherited as an autosomal recessive disorder. Family members are haematologically normal, although they may manifest reduced P5′N activity consistent with heterozygosity. In many families of affected patients, there is a history of consanguinity, thus suggesting homozygosity for the enzyme defect. In almost all cases the disorder is characterized by mild to moderate anaemia, reticulocytosis and hyperbilirubinaemia. RBC morphology is unique, in that marked basophilic stippling is present. Splenomegaly is usually observed and occasionally there is hepatomegaly. There are no enzymatic abnormalities in platelets or leucocytes. The most reasonable explanation for haemolysis in P5′N deficiency is that retained aggregates of ribosomes may produce direct membrane injury, akin to that observed with Heinz bodies. Basophilic stippling of RBCs is the morphological equivalent of partially degraded ribosomes (Valentine et al 1974). The enzyme activity in affected patients is less than 5% of that detected in normal RBCs of comparable age. Treatment for this disorder is supportive and RBC transfusions are rarely required. Splenectomy has not proved to be particularly effective. However, since cholelithiasis is common, patients should have periodic ultrasound examinations for gallstones.

It is interesting that the normal P5′N enzyme is readily inactivated by heavy metals such as lead, and it has been proposed that the basophilic stippling in lead poisoning is secondary to acquired P5′N deficiency (Valentine et al 1976). In vitro studies support the hypothesis that a consequence of mild lead intoxication is acquired P5′N inhibition (Paglia et al 1975). Moreover, cases of acute lead poisoning associated with haemolytic anaemia are associated with basophilic stippling, decreased P5′N activity and increased pyrimidine nucleotides, all characteristics of hereditary P5′N deficiency.

Adenosine deaminase (ADA) excess

In contrast to all other enzyme disorders that cause haemolytic anaemia, abnormalities of adenosine deaminase that lead to haemolysis are due not to enzyme deficiency, but rather a 60–100-fold excess of enzyme activity. Also, in contrast to other enzymopathies, this haemolytic disorder due to ADA excess is inherited in an autosomal dominant pattern (Valentine et al 1977, Paglia & Valentine 1981). This is a rare cause of congenital haemolytic disease which has now been described in several members of three different families. Clinical features include mild to moderate anaemia, reticulocytosis and hyperbilirubinaemia. No other tissues share the enzyme excess and there are no other systemic effects. In contrast to these rare patients with a marked excess of enzyme activity and haemolytic anaemia, a much smaller increase in enzyme activity (2–4-fold) has been observed in Diamond-Blackfan anaemia (See Congenital Hypoplastic Anaemia).

In patients with haemolytic anaemia and marked ADA excess, the purified enzyme exhibits normal biochemical properties and the defect appears to be due to excess production of a structurally normal enzyme (Fujii et al 1982). The function of this enzyme is to catalyze the irreversible deamination of adenosine to inosine, a critical step in the purine salvage pathway. In patients with markedly increased ADA activity, erythrocyte ATP content is reduced, presumably because increased adenosine deaminase activity effectively competes with other adenosine-dependent reactions. There are no distinguishing clinical, haematological or morphological features to aid in the diagnosis of this disease. The specific diagnosis can be suspected if red cell ATP levels are low and confirmed by demonstrating increased ADA activity in a haemolysate. Usually no specific therapy is indicated since most patients have very mild anaemia.

Adenylate kinase (AK) deficiency

Adenylate kinase reversibly catalyzes the interconversion of adenine nucleotides (ATP + AMP $\overset{\leftrightarrow}{AK}$ 2 ADP) and thereby salvages AMP generated in a variety of RBC reactions (Fig. 79.1). Hereditary nonspherocytic haemolytic anaemia has been reported in a few families with erythrocyte AK deficiency, but it is not clear that this enzyme abnormality is causally related to haemolysis in these individuals (Szeinberg et al 1969, Miwa et al 1983). In a most interesting report, there was congenital haemolytic anaemia and a marked reduction of erythrocyte AK activity in one patient, although the proband's brother, who was haematologically normal, also had no detectable erythrocyte AK activity (Beutler et al 1983). On the basis of current information, it is not clear that deficiency of AK is necessarily associated with haemolysis and it is

possible that erythrocyte AK deficiency is only of significance when present in conjunction with another RBC enzyme abnormality. In view of the uncertainty regarding the pathophysiological significance of this enzyme, documentation of adenylate kinase deficiency in an individual with haemolysis should prompt a vigorous search for other enzymatic abnormalities.

HAEMOLYSIS ASSOCIATED WITH HEREDITARY RBC MEMBRANE DISORDERS

In virtually all haemolytic anaemias, shortened RBC survival is a consequence of some membrane-induced injury which secondarily leads to decreased RBC deformability, stagnation of erythrocytes in the microcirculation and removal of RBCs from the circulation by reticuloendothelial cells. However, in the hereditary RBC membrane disorders, the primary defect is in membrane structure or function. The most common inherited abnormality is hereditary spherocytosis, although hereditary elliptocytosis and certain membrane permeability defects are also associated with haemolytic anaemia.

Hereditary spherocytosis (HS)

This common haemolytic anaemia is an autosomal dominant disorder which affects about 1 per 5000 individuals of Northern European extraction. It is the most common hereditary haemolytic anaemia occurring in Caucasians. The major physiological abnormality in HS is due to RBC membrane instability, leading to membrane fragmentation (reviewed extensively in Lux 1987). Erythrocytes leave the bone marrow as normal biconcave discs, but once in the circulation, membranes undergo fragmentation and the resultant loss in surface area leads to spherocyte formation. These spherocytes are preferentially destroyed by macrophages in the splenic microcirculation. In addition, however, the adverse environment of the spleen (haemoconcentration, acidosis, hypoglycaemia) also accelerates membrane loss from HS erythrocytes, thereby furthering spherocyte formation. Thus, the spleen is the major organ of spherocyte destruction, as well as a site which accelerates spherocyte formation. The basic defect leading to membrane instability and spherocyte formation is currently an area of active research investigation. It is known that HS red cells lose membrane protein and membrane lipids (cholesterol and phospholipids) in approximately equivalent amounts. However, the primary lesion responsible for membrane instability is thought to be a deficiency of spectrin, a major protein of the RBC cytoskeleton (Agre et al 1986). In at least 75% of cases, HS is clearly an autosomal dominant disorder and one parent usually has the disease. Of the remaining 25%, some are considered to be autosomal dominant disorders with decreased penetrance, some are thought to represent new mutations, and a few are considered to be autosomal recessive conditions. The most severe RBC spectrin deficiency has been observed in these rare autosomal recessive cases, and these individuals have severe haemolysis.

Laboratory features of HS include mild to moderate anaemia, reticulocytosis, hyperbilirubinaemia and the presence of spherocytes (i.e. small RBCs with no central pallor) in the peripheral smear (Fig. 79.4). In a large majority of cases, the loss of membrane fragments leads to some degree of RBC dehydration as manifested by an elevated mean corpuscular haemoglobin concentration (MCHC) greater than 36%. A most useful procedure for diagnosing HS is the osmotic fragility test which indirectly detects spherocytes by measuring RBC lysis in sodium chloride solutions of varying concentration. In fresh blood samples from HS patients there is usually a small population of osmotically-sensitive RBCs which reflect those spherocytes formed after passing through the spleen (Fig. 79.5). More importantly, however, after HS red cells are incubated for 24 hours at 37°C (a procedure which accelerates membrane instability of these cells), the entire RBC population is osmotically fragile, thereby increasing the diagnostic utility of this test.

Common clinical features include neonatal hyperbilirubinaemia and exacerbations of anaemia due to haemolytic or aplastic crises associated with infections. Aside from these crises, symptoms of anaemia are uncommon. Excessive bilirubin production due to RBC destruction is often associated with the development of gallstones, but this complication is unusual before 10 years of age. However, in non-splenectomized patients the incidence of cholelithiasis increases markedly in the second and third decades of life (Bates & Brown 1952). Of those HS patients who develop gallstones, approximately 50% will develop symptomatic gallbladder disease.

Definitive therapy for this disorder is splenectomy, which removes the site of RBC destruction. Following splenectomy, the haemoglobin concentration almost always increases, reticulocytes decrease, bilirubin levels return to normal and RBCs have a relatively normal survival in the circulation. The one exception to this favourable response to splenectomy is seen in patients with the autosomal recessive form of HS, who may continue to haemolyze. It is interesting, since the intrinsic RBC defect in HS persists following splenectomy, that spherocyte formation continues and there may be more spherocytes present after the spleen is removed (i.e. in the absence of a spleen, spherocytes that form have a relatively normal survival in the circulation). In almost all HS patients, removal of the spleen virtually eliminates haemolysis (and thereby increased bilirubin production). Most haematologists, therefore, now recommend that HS

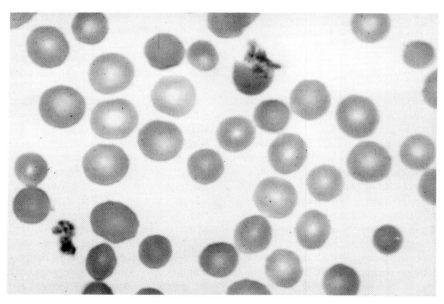

Fig. 79.4   Peripheral smear (Wright stain) of blood from patient with hereditary spherocytosis. Note that HS erythrocytes are smaller than normal and appear to have a more dense haemoglobin concentration with a relatively reduced area of central pallor.

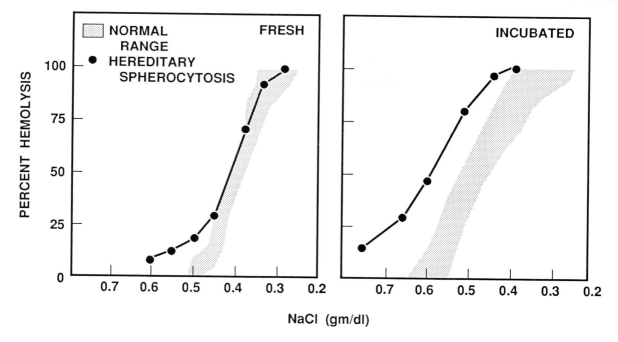

Fig. 79.5 Osmotic fragility (as manifested by percent haemolysis) of normal and hereditary spherocytosis erythrocytes following incubation in salt solutions of varying tonicity. In fresh HS erythrocytes, note the 'tail' of cells with increased sensitivity due to splenic conditioning (left). In the incubated RBC, note that the entire HS population of RBCs is more osmotically sensitive (right).

patients with moderate degrees of haemolysis should have a splenectomy after 5–10 years of age. If patients have not developed gallstones before splenectomy, it is unlikely they will develop bilirubin stones at a later date. Splenectomy is not generally indicated prior to age 5 years, since it is now recognized that a functioning spleen is important in young children for protection against severe infection due to encapsulated organisms. Splenectomized children are given pneumococcal vaccine and placed on prophylactic penicillin therapy until at least 12 years of age.

Hereditary elliptocytosis (HE)

Hereditary elliptocytosis is an autosomal dominant disorder which occurs in 1 per 2500 persons of Northern European extraction. At least 30% of the patients' RBCs have an elliptical shape (Fig. 79.6A), however, haemolysis is either absent or mild, with only slight anaemia and reticulocytosis. In a small fraction of patients, there may be significant chronic haemolysis, and this subset of patients is considered to have one of several haemolytic HE syndromes (reviewed in Lux 1987). In these patients with significant haemolysis, the blood smear is charac-

terized by poikilocytes, red cell fragments and microelliptocytes (Fig. 79.6B). The specific membrane abnormality in HE is unknown, but is presumed to be due to a defect in the spectrin-actin cytoskeleton, since ghosts (i.e. reconstituted RBC membranes devoid of haemoglobin and other cytoplasmic content) retain the elliptocytic or poikilocytic shape (Tomaselli et al 1981). In patients with haemolysis, RBCs have many of the features of HS red cells (i.e. increased osmotic fragility and membrane fragmentation) and these patients may also benefit from splenectomy. In contrast to HS, however, the response to splenectomy in haemolytic HE is usually incomplete and haemolysis persists. Cholelithiasis is a long-term complication and patients should receive periodic ultrasound examinations for gallstones.

Hereditary disorders of cation permeability and hydration

The RBC is freely permeable to water and controls its volume primarily through regulation of its monovalent cation content. Small passive cation leaks are normally balanced by the active outward transport of sodium (3 mEq per litre of red cells per hour) and inward transport

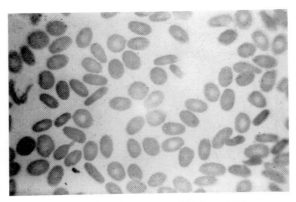

Fig. 79.6A   Peripheral blood smear (Wright stain) from an individual with the non-haemolytic variant of hereditary elliptocytosis.

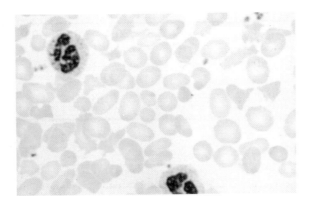

Fig. 79.6B   Peripheral blood smear (Wright stain) seen in a case of haemolytic hereditary elliptocytosis. This morphology is distinct from that seen in cases of non-haemolytic HE. In addition to elliptocytes, many distorted and fragmented RBCs are also present.

of potassium (2 mEq per litre per hour). These cation 'pumps' are linked, require ATP, and are dependent on the membrane enzyme Na-K ATPase. If the membrane permeability leak increases, cation pumps have limited compensatory ability and, if this capacity is exceeded, red cell volume changes in parallel with the total cation change. Red cells swell when the inward sodium leak exceeds the potassium leak out; and red cells shrink when the potassium leak out exceeds the sodium leak in. Two rare but intriguing haemolytic anaemias have been reported in association with increased membrane cation permeability. The identification of these membrane permeability abnormalities is made by observing an abnormal RBC monovalent cation content with correspondingly abnormal sodium-potassium transport studies.

Hereditary Hydrocytosis (Stomatocytosis) is characterized by an RBC permeability defect in which sodium leak into cells is greater than potassium loss and red cells thus accumulate sodium, gain water and swell (Zarkowsky et al 1968, Oski et al 1969). The RBCs usually have an increased mean cell volume (MCV) and a decreased mean cell haemoglobin concentration (MCHC), both due to increased intracellular water content. Blood smears reveal many stomatocytes (i.e. red cells with a mouth-like band of pallor across the centre of the stained cell) (Fig. 79.7A). In the few cases of haemolytic hereditary hydrocytosis described to date, the disorder appears to be an autosomal recessive condition, but an autosomal dominant pattern has also been described with very minimal haemolysis. Splenectomy has been beneficial in those cases associated with haemolytic anaemia.

Hereditary Xerocytosis (Desiccytosis) is a rare haemolytic anaemia in which the major physiological abnormality is a potassium leak which exceeds sodium gain. The red cells consequently have a decreased total monovalent cation and water content (Glader et al 1974). The cellular dehydration is also manifested by an increased mean cell haemoglobin concentration (MCHC). The peripheral blood smear contains many shrunken spiculated RBCs and cells where haemoglobin appears puddled within the cell (Fig. 79.7B). In the few reported cases of this disorder, the genetics suggests an autosomal dominant abnormality. In contrast to hereditary hydrocytosis, this disorder does not appear to benefit from splenectomy.

HEREDITARY HYPOPLASTIC ANAEMIAS

Congenital hypoplastic anaemia (Diamond-Blackfan anaemia)

This congenital red cell aplasia, also known as Diamond-Blackfan anaemia (DBA), was first recognized 50 years ago (Joseph 1936, Diamond & Blackfan 1938). This disorder is a consequence of impaired differentiation of developing erythroblasts (Lipton et al 1986). Several hundred individuals have been identified in the world's literature and these cases have been extensively analyzed (Alter 1987). The disorder is characterized by a life-long anaemia which usually presents in the first months of life, although a few patients may not present until after 1 year of age, and, rarely, an individual may not be diagnosed until adulthood. It occurs equally in both sexes and has been identified in all ethnic groups although the majority of reported cases have been in Caucasians. An intriguing feature of Diamond-Blackfan anaemia is that as many as 25% of affected children manifest physical abnormalities. The most common abnormality is short stature which is often apparent at the time of diagnosis. Many DBA patients also have thumb abnormalities which include

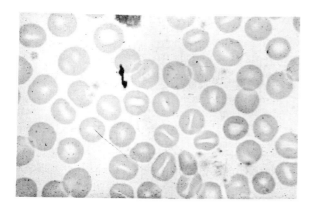

Fig. 79.7A Peripheral blood smear (Wright stain) from a patient with hereditary hydrocytosis. Note the characteristic RBCs have a mouth-like appearance, hence the term stomatocytosis.

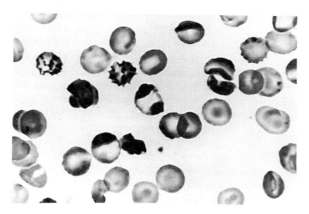

Fig. 79.7B Peripheral blood smear (Wright stain) from a patient with hereditary xerocytosis showing dense, abnormal RBC forms where haemoglobin appears puddled at the periphery.

triphalangeal thumbs, bifid thumbs and malformed thumbs (Alter 1978). Other physical abnormalities include a short webbed neck, cleft palate, high-arched palate, congenital heart disease, hypertelorism, strabismus, and structural abnormalities of the kidney. It is noteworthy that many of these same congenital abnormalitites seen in Diamond-Blackfan anaemia are also seen in children with Fanconi aplastic anaemia, a disorder characterized by pancytopenia and progressive bone marrow failure (see below). In contrast to Fanconi aplastic anaemia, however, only RBC production is impaired in Diamond-Blackfan anaemia. Also, chromosome studies in DBA patients are generally normal, without evidence of the increased breakage characteristic of Fanconi hypoplastic anaemia.

Although most DBA cases are sporadic, it is generally thought that this is a genetic disorder since 10–15% of cases occur in kindreds which have had more than one affected family member (Alter 1987). It has been observed in cousins, identical twins, full sibs, and, in several instances, DBA has occurred in half-sibs where the father or mother has had a different mate. It has also been observed to occur in a parent and child. Both autosomal dominant and autosomal recessive modes of inheritance have been postulated, although the precise genetics of this disease remains to be defined.

The diagnosis of Diamond-Blackfan anaemia is suggested by an anaemia with reticulocytopenia presenting in infancy. In almost all cases, the bone marrow reveals decreased erythroid precursors while myelopoiesis and megakaryopoiesis are normal. The peripheral white blood cell count is generally normal to slightly reduced, although the platelet count is commonly somewhat elevated. An intriguing aspect of this disorder is that circulating RBCs have many fetal-like characteristics and these abnormal erythrocyte features persist throughout life, independent of the patient's therapy or clinical state (Diamond et al 1976). Unique characteristics of these RBCs are that they are macrocytic relative to the patient's age, the fetal haemoglobin concentration is usually elevated, the fetal 'i' antigen is retained, and the activity of glycolytic and hexosemonophosphate shunt enzymes reveals a fetal-like pattern. However, the RBC enzyme pattern in DBA is not entirely 'fetal' since almost all patients have increased erythroid activity of adenosine deaminase (ADA), a purine salvage pathway enzyme whose activity is not increased in fetal or cord blood erythrocytes (Glader et al 1983). In young children it is often necessary to differentiate DBA from transient erythroblastopenia of childhood (TEC), a relatively benign erythroid hypoplasia occurring in otherwise normal children (6 months – 4 years of age). In TEC, however, there are no associated congenital abnormalities and RBCs have none of the abnormal characteristics described above for DBA erythrocytes.

Corticosteroids represent the one form of therapy which has been documented to be effective for over two-thirds of patients with this disorder (Allen & Diamond 1961, Alter 1987). In many patients a trivial prednisone dose is needed to sustain a clinical remission, and a few patients may remain in remission without steroid therapy. Patients who fail steroids usually do not respond to other pharmacological agents and most of these individuals have a life-time requirement for RBC transfusions. In these transfusion-dependent DBA patients, iron overload is an additional clinical problem and chelation therapy with desferoxamine should be instituted once transfusion dependency is established. Another therapeutic modality which has been used is bone marrow transplantation, but this is reserved for those DBA children who have an absolute dependence on RBC transfusions. Several DBA patients have now received a bone marrow transplant and most are alive and free of their anaemia. Justification for bone marrow transplantation is based upon the general consensus that the risks of this procedure are probably less than the risks of death from haemosiderosis.

The prognosis for the majority of Diamond-Blackfan anaemia patients who respond to steroids is generally quite good. Affected women are known to have become pregnant and delivered normal infants. Of concern, however, is that acute leukaemia may be a delayed complication of this disorder, and at least three DBA patients have been reported to develop this malignancy (see Alter 1987). In view of the relative rarity of Diamond-Blackfan anaemia these cases of leukaemia seem like more than a chance event. The outcome for transfusion-dependent patients is also ominous and several deaths due to iron overload have occurred.

Constitutional hypoplastic anaemia (Fanconi anaemia)

Aplastic anaemia is characterized by anaemia, thrombocytopenia and leucopenia (i.e. pancytopenia) with reduced or absent haemopoietic precursor cells in the bone marrow. Most commonly, this is an acquired disorder occurring in previously healthy individuals. In the majority of cases there is no specific aetiology. There is also a rare constitutional form of aplasia, known as Fanconi aplastic anaemia, which is recognised as an autosomal recessive disorder. In this constitutional hypoplastic anaemia the onset of pancytopenia usually occurs between 4 and 11 years of age, although it may appear earlier or later. The manifestations of this disease begin insidiously with thrombocytopenia and/or leucopenia which evolves into mild pancytopenia, and gradually becomes more severe over months to years. The anaemia characteristically is macrocytic and the fetal haemoglobin concentration is increased. In addition to these haematological features, this disorder is characterized by a variety of physical abnormalities (Fanconi 1967). Commonly associated congenital abnormalities include skin hyperpigmentation and/or increased café-au-lait spots, growth retardation, skeletal abnormalities (particularly of the thumb), renal anomalies, micro-ophthalmia, ear abnormalities (with and without deafness) and, rarely, congenital heart disease (Alter 1987). It is interesting that, in families with one member having Fanconi aplastic anaemia, pancytopenia does not necessarily evolve in other family members who manifest congenital abnormalities and, conversely, family members without congenital abnormalities may develop pancytopenia. In

suspected cases of Fanconi hypoplastic anaemia, the following studies should be obtained: complete blood counts, fetal haemoglobin measurements, skeletal X-rays particularly of the hand and forearm, renal ultrasound examination or an intravenous pyelogram and chromosomal studies (see below).

The cellular defect in Fanconi aplastic anaemia appears to be an increased sensitivity to agents which damage DNA. A characteristic feature is that increased chromosomal breaks are seen in cultured skin fibroblasts and peripheral blood lymphocytes after in vitro stimulation by phytohaemaggluttinin (Bloom et al 1966). These chromosomal abnormalities are not usually seen in fresh bone marrow cells, presumably because these cells divide slower than normal and/or die within the marrow. Cells from Fanconi aplastic anaemia patients are particularly sensitive to certain alkylating agents which damage DNA and produce significant numbers of chromosomal abnormalities and this is the basis of current laboratory tests used to diagnose the disorder (Latt et al 1975, Auerback & Wolman 1976). The reason for this increased susceptibility of DNA to injury is unknown. It has been estimated that the heterozygous state for Fanconi anaemia may have a frequency of 1 in 300 individuals. A prenatal diagnostic test is available which assesses the spontaneous and diepoxybutane-induced breaks in cultured amniotic fluid cells (Auerbach et al 1981). Some mothers of patients with Fanconi anaemia have had an unusual number of miscarriages and, in some cases, the examined fetuses have had related physical abnormalities.

In a majority of children with Fanconi aplastic anaemia, there is a beneficial response to androgen therapy (i.e. oxymetholone) and most children who respond require only small doses of androgens to maintain a remission. In months to years, however, refractoriness to androgen therapy usually develops, leading to progressive bone marrow failure and death from bleeding or infectious complications. In approximately 15% of known cases, acute leukaemia or other malignancies complicate the late course of this disease (Alter 1987). Most haematologists now believe that a child with Fanconi aplastic anaemia, who has an HLA compatible donor, should receive a bone marrow transplant. However, since it is thought that this may be an autosomal recessive disorder, it is important to check potential marrow donors for the possibility that they too may have Fanconi hypoplastic anaemia. This testing should include a complete blood count, fetal haemoglobin concentration, and a specific test to assess for increased chromosomal breaks after exposure to diepoxybutane. The appropriate time to perform a bone marrow transplant is not clear. Certainly it should be done before the child reaches the stage where

RBC and platelet transfusions are needed and HLA sensitization might occur. This time may be heralded by the observation of resistance to oxymetholone therapy. A major problem with bone marrow transplantation in children with Fanconi aplastic anaemia is severe graft versus host disease.

MEGALOBLASTIC ANAEMIAS

Megaloblastic anaemias refer to a group of disorders in which there is abnormal differentiation of bone marrow erythroblasts and the morphological appearance of the nucleus is immature compared to the degree of cytoplasmic maturation (i.e. the extent of haemoglobinization). In addition, however, megaloblastic erythropoiesis is often accompanied by dyserythropoiesis in which marrow RBC precursors are abnormal, as manifested by erythroblasts with two or more nuclei and/or abnormal nuclear fragmentation. Since there is a disparity between increased marrow erythroid activity (i.e. hyperplasia of erythroblasts) and what appears in the circulation (i.e. anaemia), the anaemia in megaloblastic disorders is felt to be largely due to 'ineffective erythropoiesis', a term which suggests intramedullary destruction of developing erythroblasts. The peripheral smear in megaloblastic anaemias is characterized by macrocytic RBCs with a variety of abnormal forms including ovalocytes and tear drop cells. The dysynchronous maturation of the nucleus and cytoplasm, however, is not limited to erythroblasts and is also seen in developing myeloid cells which have large, young-appearing nuclei for the degree of cytoplasmic granulation. Moreover, the anaemia is occasionally accompanied by thrombocytopenia and leucopenia; and peripheral blood leucocytes almost always manifest hypersegmentation (i.e. many neutrophils with more than five lobes). In all cases, megaloblastic erythropoiesis is a consequence of impaired DNA synthesis, the causes of which include abnormalities of vitamin B_{12} metabolism, disorders of folate metabolism and miscellaneous inborn errors of metabolism.

Disorders of vitamin B_{12} metabolism

General considerations

In order to appreciate the genetic disorders of B_{12} metabolism, it is necessary to understand the normal physiology of this vitamin. Dietary vitamin B_{12} (cobalamin), which is found in eggs, milk products, meats and vegetables, is released from complexed food forms by proteolytic enzymes in the stomach. However, once in the duodenum, vitamin B_{12} binds to intrinsic factor (IF), a protein secreted by gastric parietal cells. Subsequently,

the IF-B_{12} complex binds to specific receptors in the distal part of the ileum, IF is split off, and B_{12} is transported into intestinal cells. Following this, B_{12} binds to a transport protein, transcobalamin II (TC-II), which carries B_{12} to the liver, bone marrow and other tissue storage sites. Serum also contains two other B_{12} binding proteins, transcobalamin I and III (TC-I and TC-III). These latter two forms of transcobalamin have no specific transport role but are known to reflect vitamin B_{12} tissue stores. In fact, almost all B_{12} in plasma is bound to TC-I and TC-III and thus the measurement of serum B_{12} concentration reflects the storage of this vitamin. The metabolic importance of vitamin B_{12} and its derivatives is very complex and not fully understood. One important metabolic function known to be impaired in human B_{12} deficiency is methylmalonyl CoA isomerization, the conversion of methylmalonyl CoA to succinyl CoA, an important reaction in propionic and fatty acid metabolism. When this reaction is impaired, there is both methylmalonic acidaemia and methylmalonic aciduria, and testing for the latter is a good screening test for B_{12} deficiency. Increased excretion of methylmalonic acid is also associated with hereditary deficiency of methylmalonyl CoA mutase, a disorder seen in young infants characterized by severe acidosis, ketonuria and developmental retardation, but generally there is no anaemia (Rosenberg et al 1968). A second important reaction requiring B_{12} is homocysteine: methyltetrahydrofolate methyltransferase. In this reaction a methyl group from methyltetrahydrofolate is transferred to homocysteine, with the formation of methionine and tetrahydrofolate. The latter is a required co-factor for thymidine synthesis, partially explaining why DNA synthesis is defective in vitamin B_{12} deficiency. It should be noted that this is also one of the important reactions where folic acid is required for DNA synthesis (See Disorders of folate metabolism, below).

Megaloblastic anaemia due to vitamin B_{12} deficiency can occur because of an abnormality in any one of the steps in B_{12} absorption, transport or metabolism. Dietary insufficiency causing cobalamin deficiency is extremely rare, occurring almost exclusively in pure vegans, and takes years to develop in individuals who start with normal B_{12} stores. Acquired abnormalities due to previous surgery can occur because of loss of IF following gastrectomy or loss of B_{12} absorptive sites after extensive ileal resection. Moreover, tapeworm infestation or intestinal bacterial overgrowth (from broad spectrum antibiotic therapy) can also lead to megaloblastic anaemia because of competition for intestinal cobalamin.

The remainder of this section focuses on those megaloblastic anaemia conditions, due to B_{12} deficiency, which are considered genetic disorders. For more details the reader is referred to an excellent review by Lanz-kowsky (1987b).

Classical pernicious anaemia (PA)

This disorder is characterized by severe macrocytic anaemia and neurological disease. It is the most common form of B_{12} deficiency and usually occurs in middle aged to elderly adults. Previously, in the absence of appropriate therapy, most patients died, hence the designation pernicious anaemia. The cause of PA is impaired IF production and is associated with gastric atrophy, achlorhydria and antibodies to both gastric parietal cells and intrinsic factor. The disorder is diagnosed by low serum vitamin B_{12} levels and an abnormal Schilling test which measures B_{12} absorption with and without added intrinsic factor. Therapy consists of monthly injections with vitamin B_{12} throughout life. There may be an ethnic predisposition to develop PA for Northern Europeans, in particular Scandinavians, however the disorder is known to occur world-wide in many different ethnic groups. It is not clear that this is a genetic disease, although 20% of PA patients have an affected relative with the same disease.

Juvenile pernicious anaemia

This type of childhood PA resembles that seen in adults and is characterized by gastric atrophy, achlorhydria, absent IF and antibodies to intrinsic factor (McIntyre et al 1965). In these cases, however, onset of megaloblastic anaemia is usually after 10 years of age. Affected children often manifest antibodies to a variety of tissues and may have associated endocrinopathies or immunodeficiency. Whether juvenile PA per se is a genetic disease is not clear, although there are familial clusters with an increased incidence of megaloblastic anaemia in some family members, while others have a tendency to form autoantibodies to other tissues.

Congenital pernicious anaemia

This megaloblastic anaemia has its onset in the first two months of life. It is due to a congenital absence of IF production but there are none of the other gastric abnormalities or other antibody features of classic PA (Miller et al 1966). Infants may also manifest failure to thrive and, occasionally, abnormal neurological findings. The occurrence of multiple affected sibs suggests the possibility of autosomal recessive inheritance; no abnormalities have been found in parents or other relatives. Treatment is parenteral vitamin B_{12} for life.

Impaired vitamin B_{12} absorption

Imerslund (1960) and Grasbeck et al (1960) first described children with familial malabsorption of vitamin B_{12} due to impaired ileal uptake of cobalamin, presumably due to an abnormality of the receptor for B_{12} absorption. There are no gastric abnormalities and intrinsic factor production is normal. More than 80 cases of this syndrome have been reported and it is known to be transmitted as an autosomal recessive disorder. Clinically these children show marked failure to thrive and the diagnosis is usually made in the first two years of life. Characteristically there is a megaloblastic anaemia with low serum B_{12} levels. It is interesting, however, that mild proteinuria (mainly albumin) is present in nearly all patients. Therapy is monthly parenteral B_{12} given for life.

Transcobalamin II deficiency

This autosomal recessive disorder is due to a deficiency of the major transport protein for vitamin B_{12} (Hakami et al 1971). However, serum vitamin B_{12} levels are normal since TC-I and TC-III are not affected. Generally, this disorder manifests itself in the first weeks of life. Characteristically there is a failure to thrive, diarrhoea, vomiting, glossitis, neurological abnormalities and megaloblastic anaemia. The diagnosis of this disorder is suggested by the presence of severe megaloblastic anaemia with normal serum B_{12} and folate levels with no evidence of any other inborn errors of metabolism. The therapy for this disorder is large parenteral doses of vitamin B_{12} given twice a week for life. These frequent and large doses of cobalamin appear to overcome the transport deficiency. Most children with this disorder die if not treated in infancy.

Disorders of folate metabolism

Folic acid (pteroyl monoglutamic acid) is an essential nutrient for humans which is derived from microorganisms and plants (i.e. leafy green vegetables). In contrast to cobalamin, folate stores are relatively limited and signs of deficiency appear within three months on a folate-free diet. The reduced forms of folic acid, a variety of tetrahydrofolates, are the active compounds necessary for biological function. One of the most important reactions involving folate is the conversion of the deoxyuridine monophosphate (dUMP), to deoxythymidine monophosphate (dTMP), a critical reaction for DNA synthesis catalyzed by thymidylate synthetase. Most cases of megaloblastic anaemia due to folate deficiency are caused by an inadequate diet, decreased absorption secondary to various malabsorption syndromes, increased folate utilization (pregnancy, haemolysis), drug-induced inhibition of dietary folate absorption (dilantin, phenobarbital) or drugs which impair normal folate metabolism (methotrexate). Several rare inborn defects of folate metabolism have been described in association with severe neurological disease, and occasionally there is an associated megaloblastic anaemia (Lanzkowsky 1987a). Genetic disorders associated with megaloblastic anaemia are as follows.

Congenital malabsorption of folate, a syndrome which has been described in at least five patients, is characterized by an isolated defect of intestinal folate absorption. Clinical features of this syndrome include megaloblastic anaemia, ataxia, mental retardation and convulsions (Luhby et al 1961). The folate transport abnormality is also seen in spinal cord membranes. Responses to treatment have generally been unsatisfactory, and large doses of oral or parenteral folic acid are usually required.

Dihydrofolate reductase deficiency has been described in a few children, probably as a recessively inherited trait. This enzyme is responsible for converting folate to its active form (i.e. tetrahydrofolate). In one child with this disorder who had megaloblastic anaemia there was a poor response to folic acid therapy, but a satisfactory response to folinic acid (5-formyl tetrahydrofolate) (Walters 1967).

Formiminotransferase deficiency was the first reported inborn error of folate metabolism (Arakawa 1970). This enzyme is important in the catabolism of histidine and in its absence there is impaired conversion of formiminoglutamate acid to glutamate. This is an extremely heterogeneous disorder which may be asymptomatic, or may be associated with mental retardation, increased urinary formiminoglutamic acid (FIGLU) excretion, and rarely megaloblastic anaemia.

Homocysteine: methyltetrahydrofolate methyltransferase is a critical enzyme in methionine synthesis and, as noted above, vitamin B_{12} is a necessary co-factor for this reaction. Hereditary absence of this methyltransferase has been described in a patient with megaloblastic anaemia, mental retardation and dilated cerebral ventricles (Arakawa 1970). In this patient, serum folate levels were markedly elevated. The therapeutic response to large doses of folic acid was less than satisfactory.

Hereditary orotic aciduria

This autosomal recessive disorder usually appears in the first year of life and is characterized by growth failure, developmental retardation, megaloblastic anaemia and increased urinary excretion of orotic acid. This defect, the most common metabolic error in the de novo synthesis of pyrimidines, therefore affects nucleic acid synthesis. The usual form of hereditary orotic aciduria is caused by a deficiency (in all body tissues) of both orotidate phosphoribosyl transferase (OPT) and orotidine-5-phosphate decarboxylase (ODC), two sequential enzymatic steps in pyrimidine nucleotide synthesis. Affected individuals are 'starved' of pyrimidines, but generally there is a good response to supplementation with large doses of pyrimidine nucleosides such as uridine (Kelley & Smith 1978). The diagnosis of this disorder is suggested by the presence of severe megaloblastic anaemia with normal serum B_{12} and folate levels, and no evidence of TC-II deficiency. A presumptive diagnosis is made by finding increased urinary orotic acid. Confirmation of the diagnosis, however, requires assay of the transferase and decarboxylase enzymes in the patient's erythrocytes. The heterozygous state is characterized by intermediate levels of enzyme activity in otherwise asymptomatic individuals.

Lesch-Nyhan syndrome

This is an X-linked recessive disorder characterized by mental retardation, spasticity, choreoathetosis, self-mutilation and increased uric acid production. Such individuals manifest a near complete absence of hypoxanthine-guanine phosphoribosyl transferase (HPRT) in almost all tissues. The diagnosis of this disorder, however, is most easily made by assaying erythrocyte HPRT activity (Nyhan 1973). The only haematological defect associated with Lesch-Nyhan syndrome is mild megaloblastic anaemia related to a low serum folate concentration. Reduced folate levels reflect excessive folic acid utilization associated with enhanced de novo purine synthesis (Fox & Kelley 1971).

DYSERYTHROPOIETIC ANAEMIAS

As discussed in the section on megaloblastic anaemia, dyserythropoiesis occurs to some extent in a variety of anaemias where there is a severe 'erythroid stress'. However, in congenital dyserythropoietic anaemias (CDA), these unique features of marrow erythroblasts (multinuclearity, abnormal nuclear fragments, intrachromatin bridges between cells) are the predominant abnormality noted (Lewis & Verwilghen 1977). A variety of nuclear and cytoplasmic membrane abnormalities have been described in CDA but, to date, there is no consensus regarding the underlying defect. It is of interest that when CDA erythroid progenitors are cultured in vitro, erythroblasts manifest multinuclearity. There are no known chromosomal abnormalities. Clinically these disorders are characterized by variable degrees of anaemia, often with a reticulocyte count less than expected for the anaemia, despite the fact that there is increased marrow erythroid activity (i.e. ineffective erythropoiesis). Heimpel & Wendt (1968) have defined three major types of CDA (Types I, II and III).

Type I dyserythropoietic anaemia

This is a very rare autosomal recessive disorder in which the onset of anaemia and/or jaundice may be noted at any age. Affected patients manifest slight icterus, moderate splenomegaly, and there is a mild to moderate macrocytic anaemia. The reticulocyte count is less than expected for the degree of anaemia. Peripheral RBC morphology is characterized by anisocytosis and poikilocytosis. White blood cells and platelets are normal. Indirect bilirubin levels are slightly elevated, haptoglobin levels are low, and transferrin is saturated with iron (serum iron level approximates the TIBC concentration). Bone marrow aspiration reveals erythroid hyperplasia with megaloblastic erythroblasts in the absence of vitamin B_{12} or folate deficiency. A small number of erythroblasts manifest dyserythropoietic features, in particular interchromatin bridges between cells. In contrast to Type II CDA, there are no serological features of this dyserythropoietic anaemia (see below). Treatment of this disorder has been unsuccessful with the usual haematinics, including all types of vitamins, metals and steroids. Splenomegaly is common, although splenectomy has not been helpful. Gallstones have been a problem in some patients. The most important long-term complication may be haemosiderosis caused by increased intestinal absorption of iron and ineffective erythropoiesis, combined with mild haemolysis.

Type II dyserythropoietic anaemia

This is the most common variant of CDA and over 100 cases of this autosomal recessive disorder have been reported. Most of the clinical and laboratory features are similar to those seen in Type I CDA. However, one difference is that the severity of anaemia in Type II CDA is usually greater, and RBC transfusions are often necessary. Also, in contrast to Type I CDA, many more late marrow erythroblasts (up to 50%) may be abnormal, as manifested by binuclearity, multinuclearity and abnormal lobulation (Fig. 79.8). The pathognomonic findings in CDA Type II are serological in that the patient's red cells are lysed by acidified sera from many normal individuals, but not by the patient's own acidified serum. The combination of erythroblast multinuclearity and the sensitivity of circulating RBCs to lysis by acidified normal

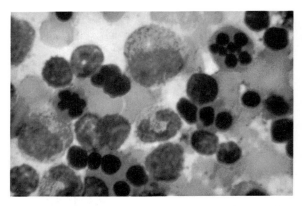

Fig. 79.8 Bone marrow aspirate (Wright stain) from a patient with HEMPAS showing erythroid hyperplasia and multinucleated erythroblasts.

serum are the reasons that Type II CDA is now known by the acronym HEMPAS (*H*ereditary *E*rythroblastic *M*ultinuclearity with a *P*ositive *A*cidified *S*erum test) (Crookston et al 1969). In contrast to paroxysmal nocturnal haemoglobinuria (PNH) which is characterized by RBC lysis in acidified serum and also in isotonic sucrose, HEMPAS red cells do not lyse in sucrose solution. HEMPAS red cells show increased strength of the 'i' antigen (which is usually a marker of fetal erythropoiesis) and are strongly agglutinated by anti-i serum. Moreover, HEMPAS erythrocytes are also strongly agglutinated by cold anti-I serum.

Patients with severe anaemia usually require blood transfusions. Splenectomy is occasionally helpful, as manifested by a decreased need for transfusions. Iron overload occurs from both transfusions and increased intestinal absorption (even in untransfused patients), and in select patients iron chelation therapy should be considered.

Type III dyserythropoietic anaemia

Approximately 30 patients have been reported to have Type III CDA. These patients have macrocytosis and a mild-to-moderate degree of anaemia. In contrast to CDA Types I and II, this disorder is inherited as an autosomal dominant defect. Bone marrow examination shows erythroid hyperplasia, with many multinucleated erythroblasts with up to 12 nuclei. Type III CDA erythrocytes resemble HEMPAS red cells in that they are strongly agglutinated by anti-i and anti-I sera. In contrast, however, Type III CDA erythrocytes are not lysed by acidified serum.

SIDEROBLASTIC ANAEMIAS

Sideroblastic anaemias are due to hereditary and acquired disorders of haem synthesis (reviewed in Valentine 1983, Robinson & Glass 1987). These disorders are characterized by a variable population of hypochromic RBCs similar to that seen in iron deficiency anaemia, but the serum iron concentration is usually normal. The defect in sideroblastic anaemias appears to be due to an abnormality in mitochondrial haem synthesis. The initial and final reactions of haem synthesis occur in mitochondria, while the intermediate reactions occur in the cytoplasm. In some patients with sideroblastic anaemia there is decreased activity of ALA synthetase, the enzyme used for the first rate-limiting reaction in mitochondrial haem synthesis. In all cases of sideroblastic anaemia, regardless of the specific aetiology, impaired haem synthesis leads to retention of iron within the mitochondria. Morphologically, this is seen in marrow aspirates which reveal many nucleated red cells with iron granules (i.e. aggregates of iron in mitochrondia) that have a perinuclear distribution. These unusual cells, known as 'ringed sideroblasts', are found only in pathological states, and are distinct from the sideroblasts in the marrows of normal subjects (i.e. RBC precursors that contain diffuse cytoplasmic ferritin granules).

Both acquired and hereditary sideroblastic anaemias occur. The most common forms are those acquired in later life, usually without an obvious cause and thus representing cases of primary or idiopathic acquired sideroblastic anaemia. In some of these acquired cases, this disorder represents a pre-leukaemic state and 20–30% of affected individuals go on to develop acute myelogenous leukaemia. The hereditary types of sideroblastic anaemia are much less common. In most cases, these conform to an X-linked pattern of inheritance and are usually seen in males. However, a few cases have been described where the pattern of inheritance appears to be that of an autosomal recessive trait. A unique variant of congenital sideroblastic anaemia has been reported which is characterized by the early onset of transfusion-dependent anaemia, neutropenia and thrombocytopenia (Pearson et al 1979). In addition to the usual marrow abnormalities of sideroblastic anaemia these children also had degenerative vacuolization of RBC and myeloid precursors, a macrocytic anaemia and pancreatic fibrosis (seen in two children who died before 3 years of age).

The clinical manifestations of hereditary and acquired forms of sideroblastic anaemia are similar. The hereditary disorders usually become apparent after the first decade of life, and patients present with pallor, icterus, moderate splenomegaly and/or hepatomegaly. In addition, there may be evidence of haemochromatosis including signs of diabetes mellitus, liver dysfunction, cardiac abnormalities and bronzing of the skin. The severity of the anaemia varies, such that some patients require no therapy, while others need regular RBC transfusions. There is a subgroup of patients, with both acquired and hereditary sideroblastic anaemia, who are 'pyridoxine-responsive', i.e. they have haematological responses to pharmacological doses of pyridoxine (2–4 mg/kg/24 hours). It is interesting that pyridoxal phosphate (the active form of pyridoxine) is a co-factor for the ALA synthetase reaction.

The peripheral blood contains hypochromic microcytic RBCs, poikilocytes, target cells, cells with basophilic stippling, and Pappenheimer bodies (RBCs with iron inclusions) and occasionally nucleated red cells. The white blood cell count and the platelet count are usually normal but may be depressed. The bone marrow reveals erythroid hyperplasia which appears normoblastic or occasionally megaloblastic. Most importantly, the bone marrow also contains increased storage iron and ringed sideroblasts. Despite the marked erythroid marrow hyperplasia, the reticulocyte count is usually low or minimally elevated for the degree of anaemia. In addition, these patients often have mild, unconjugated hyperbilirubinaemia. This constellation of features reflects ineffective erythropoiesis. Characteristically, serum iron concentration is elevated and the total iron binding capacity is mildly decreased. Free erythrocyte protoporphyrin is usually lower than normal.

METHAEMOGLOBINAEMIA

Methaemoglobin (MHb) is an oxidized derivative of haemoglobin in which iron (normally Fe^{++}) is in the oxidized or ferric (Fe^{+++}) state. The problem with methaemoglobin is that it does not complex with oxygen and, thus, increased MHb levels reduce blood oxygen capacity and transport. Under normal physiological conditions, small amounts of haemoglobin are continually being oxidized by endogenous agents including oxygen itself (auto-oxidation). Usually, however, MHb levels are less than 1% of the total haemoglobin because RBCs contain NADH-methaemoglobin reductase (also known as cytochrome b_5 reductase), an enzyme that catalyzes reduction of MHb. The cardinal clinical manifestation of methaemoglobinaemia is cyanosis without evidence of cardiac or respiratory disease (normal physical examination, chest X-ray, ECG and arterial PO_2). Blood appears dark in colour but, in contrast to deoxygenated blood, mixing with air does not change the colour to bright red. This is the basis of a simple screening test to detect methaemoglobin. A drop of blood is placed on filter paper and then allowed to dry while the filter paper is waved in air. Blood that is not saturated with oxygen turns red, while methaemoglobin remains brown. Cyanosis is apparent at MHb levels of 1.5 g/100 ml (10% of total haemoglobin), but symptoms due to decreased oxygen transport are generally not apparent until 30–40% of haemoglobin is oxidized to methaemoglobin. Levels greater than 70% are incompatible with life. Methaemoglobinaemia is not usually associated with anaemia, haemolysis or other haematological abnormalities.

An increased methaemoglobin concentration is caused by disruption of the delicate balance between oxidation and reduction of haemoglobin iron. Two forms of methaemoglobinaemia are seen: acquired or toxic methaemoglobinaemia (common), and hereditary methaemoglobinaemia (rare). Acquired methaemoglobinaemia occurs in normal individuals exposed to increased concentrations of chemicals that oxidize haemoglobin iron. Hereditary methaemoglobinaemia is due to inherited haemoglobin M disorders or deficiency of NADH-methaemoglobin reductase (Schwartz et al 1983).

Haemoglobin M disorders

These are rare autosomal dominant defects due to amino acid substitutions in the normal globin chain. As a result of these substitutions, haem iron is more stable in the ferric than the ferrous state, and RBC methaemoglobin reductive capacity cannot compensate for this instability of ferrous haem. In those rare M haemoglobin disorders due to gamma chain mutations, methaemoglobinaemia disappears as infants begin to make beta globin chains. Conversely, M haemoglobin disorders due to beta chain mutations do not usually appear until 3–5 months of age when beta chain synthesis predominates. Heterozygotes for haemoglobin M disorders have increased MHb levels and some degree of cyanosis but are otherwise asymptomatic. No therapy is indicated and none is possible. The homozygous state is incompatible with life. The presence of M haemoglobins can be detected by electrophoresis of a haemolysate in which the haemoglobin is converted to methaemoglobin (by potassium ferricyanide).

NADH-methaemoglobin (cytochrome b_5) reductase deficiency

This is an autosomal recessive disorder in which the rate of ferrihaemoglobin reduction is markedly reduced. Heterozygotes are asymptomatic and do not have methaemoglobinaemia unless challenged by toxic agents. Homozygous-deficient patients often have 15–40% methaemoglobin levels and these patients are cyanotic but otherwise asymptomatic. The diagnosis of NADH-methaemoglobin reductase deficiency requires an enzyme assay. Most individuals with this deficiency usually require no treatment. Occasionally, therapy is given for cosmetic reasons to decrease cyanosis. This is readily accomplished with daily oral administration of methylene blue or ascorbic acid. Methylene blue, the more effective of the two, will produce blue urine, but this is harmless. In NADH-MHb reductase deficient patients who are symptomatic (i.e. more than 25% methaemoglobin), intravenous methylene blue (4 mg/kg as a 1% solution) can be given for prompt relief.

Erythrocytes contain a second enzyme, NADPH-methaemoglobin reductase, which by itself is unable to reduce methaemoglobin and individuals lacking this enzyme do not have methaemoglobinaemia. In the presence of certain redox compounds (e.g. methylene blue), however, NADPH methaemoglobin reductase rapidly reduces MHb to ferrohaemoglobin. Thus, this enzyme is important in the treatment of methaemoglobinaemia with methylene blue as described above. The response to methylene blue is both therapeutic and diagnostic. A rapid decrease in methaemoglobin occurs within 1–2 hours if the cause of methaemoglobin is due to an acquired toxic agent or a deficiency of NADH-methaemoglobin reductase. Failure to note improvement following methylene blue suggests one of the M haemoglobins. It should be pointed out that G6PD deficiency per se is not a cause of methaemoglobinaemia, but rather it may cause a poor response to methylene blue because it is the primary source of NADPH.

THE RED BLOOD CELL AS A BIOPSY TOOL FOR NON-ERYTHROCYTE DISORDERS

Biochemical analysis of RBCs is obviously useful in the evaluation of intrinsic erythrocyte disorders. In addition, however, RBCs can also be used as biopsy material to diagnose conditions in which the erythrocyte is not primarily involved, or is only one of many affected tissues. The use of RBC as 'biopsy tissue' is advantageous for two reasons: (1) large numbers of cells can be readily obtained without major discomfort to patients; and (2) erythrocytes can be easily prepared and separated from contaminating cells. In some cases, these enzymes have no apparent function in mature RBCs and their presence is merely a vestige of the earlier more complex metabolism of developing erythroblasts. Some of the diseases diagnosed by studying RBCs are described below. These disorders are discussed more extensively elsewhere in this text.

Partial deficiency of hypoxanthine-guanine phosphoribosyltransferase (HPRT)

Complete deficiency of this enzyme in all tissues leads to the Lesch-Nyhan syndrome (see Megaloblastic Anaemia). However, partial HPRT deficiency (less than 30% normal activity) is associated with elevated levels of phosphoribosyl pyrophosphate (PRPP), hypoxanthine and guanine. The elevated purines lead to increased uric acid production and gouty arthritis (Kelley et al 1967).

Increased activity of PRPP synthetase (Ribosephosphate pyrophosphokinase)

Another group of patients with gout reportedly have elevated PRPP levels due to increased erythrocyte PRPP synthetase activity (Becker et al 1973). In this group, elevated PRPP levels are due to increased synthesis rather than decreased utilization, as is seen in HPRT deficiency. Elevated PRPP is a direct stimulus for de novo purine synthesis and thereby uric acid formation (Fox & Kelley 1971). This disorder can also be diagnosed by measuring erythrocyte PRPP synthetase activity.

Adenine phosphoribosyltransferase (APRT) deficiency

In a related disorder, urolithiasis without joint involvement has been described in a patient with adenine phosphoribosyl transferase (APRT) deficiency (Van Acker et al 1977). This enzyme is analogous to HPRT in that it catalyzes the reaction of adenine and PRPP to form adenylic acid (AMP) and pyrophosphate, the 'salvage pathway of adenine'. Deficiency of APRT is an autosomal recessive disorder. Heterozygotes have no clinical manifestations while homozygotes accumulate adenine. The only pathway for further metabolism of adenine is oxidation to 2,8-dihydroxyadenine, a very insoluble compound which forms renal stones. Individuals with APRT deficiency are identified by increased urinary adenine levels and absence of erythrocyte APRT activity.

Adenosine deaminase deficiency

Severe combined immune deficiency syndrome (SCIDS) is a congenital deficiency involving both humoral and cell-mediated immunity. Children with this disorder have severe infections early in life, which generally run a progressive downhill course leading to an early demise. Severe combined immune deficiency syndrome can be inherited as either an X-linked or an autosomal recessive disorder. The autosomal recessive form of this disease is frequently associated with lymphocyte deficiency of the enzyme adenosine deaminase (ADA) (Giblett et al 1972). In the absence of ADA, lymphocytes accumulate deoxy-ATP, a potent inhibitor of ribonucleotide reductase, thereby leading to impaired lymphocyte proliferation. Activity of ADA is also reduced in erythrocytes and this can be used for diagnosis.

Nucleoside phosphorylase deficiency

In another group of immune-deficient patients, lymphocytes are deficient in nucleoside phosphorylase, the enzyme that catalyzes the phosphorylytic cleavage of inosine to hypoxanthine and ribose phosphate (Giblett et al 1975). Individuals with this disorder have recurrent infections and megaloblastic anaemia. Progressive T-cell dysfunction also occurs, although B-cell function and humoral immunity remain intact. Just as in ADA deficiency, reduced nucleoside phosphorylase activity is detected in erythrocytes. Asymptomatic heterozygotes have intermediate levels of enzyme activity.

In a fascinating series of experiments, it has been demonstrated that the red blood cell is not only useful in the diagnosis of these immune disorders, but may actually have a role in therapy as well. In one patient with ADA deficiency (Polmar 1980), regular transfusions with normal irradiated RBCs resulted in the appearance of functional T-lymphocytes, a prolonged infection-free interval, and the appearance of a thymus shadow on chest X-ray. Similar results have been reported in a patient with nucleoside phosphorylase deficiency (Staal et al 1980) in whom this transfusion regimen resulted in increased urinary uric acid excretion and the appearance of functional T-lymphocytes. It is thought that these beneficial changes are due to donor RBC metabolism of circulating toxic intermediates of nucleoside metabolism which accumulate as a consequence of defective purine degradation.

Galactosaemia

Galactosaemia is an autosomal recessive disorder due to deficiency of either galactose-1-phosphate uridyl transferase or galactokinase, two major enzymes involved in the metabolism of galactose. The most common form of galactosaemia is associated with deficiency of galactose-1-phosphate uridyl transferase (Isselbacher et al 1956). Affected infants develop diarrhoea and vomiting shortly after their first milk feeding, and with continued exposure to dietary lactose (and therefore galactose), they develop cataracts, mental retardation and eventually progressive fatal liver failure. The second, but less common, form of galactosaemia is associated with deficiency of galactokinase, the enzyme which phosphorylates galactose to galactose-1-phosphate (Gitzelmann 1965). These patients classically manifest cataracts. A presumptive diagnosis of galactosaemia can be made by detection of urinary reducing substance in the absence of glucose. The specific diagnosis is confirmed by assay of galactokinase and galactose-1-phosphate uridyl transferase activity in the patient's erythrocytes. Heterozygotes are asymptomatic but have half-normal levels of enzymes.

Acatalasia (Takahara disease)

Acatalasia is an autosomal recessive disorder in which all tissues of the body lack catalase, an enzyme which degrades hydrogen peroxide into water and oxygen. Clinical manifestations occur in only about half of affected patients, and consist of periodontal ulceration, sometimes progressing to gangrene of the oral soft tissues and alveolar bone (Takahara 1952). The absence of more severe symptomatology in acatalasia may reflect the presence of other oxidant detoxifying systems (e.g. glutathione). The specific diagnosis can be made by assaying any one of several tissues, including erythrocytes.

Abetalipoproteinaemia

This disorder is a rare autosomal recessive trait which results in a total or partial failure of synthesis of very low density lipoproteins (VLDL) and low density lipoproteins (LDL). Clinical features include cerebellar ataxia, retinitis pigmentosa and fat malabsorption. In addition, at least 50% of the RBCs of homozygous-affected patients appear as acanthocytes (i.e. RBCs with long irregular spicules projecting from the membrane) and these changes are very useful in suggesting this diagnosis (Bassen & Kornzweig 1950). This RBC membrane abnormality (Fig. 79.9) develops as erythrocytes age in the circulation. It is due to an acquired loss of phosphatidylcholine with a corresponding increase in sphingomyelin, both reflecting abnormalities in the distribution of plasma phospholipids. In children, but usually not in adults, the resultant changes in RBC lipid content are associated with mild haemolysis.

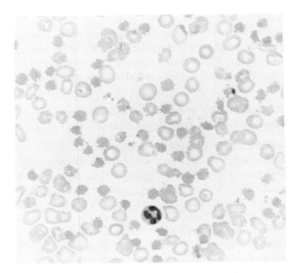

Fig. 79.9 Peripheral blood smear (Wright stain) from an individual with abetalipoproteinaemia. The characteristic feature is the increased number of acanthocytes (i.e.RBCs with thorny projections).

ACKNOWLEDGEMENTS

I wish to thank J. Lawrence Naiman, M.D., Stephen Hunger, M.D. and Karen Backer, M.T. for their critical comments in reviewing this manuscript. In addition, I would like to thank Luella Walter for secretarial assistance in preparing this chapter.

REFERENCES

Agre P, Asimos A, James B S, Casella J F, McMillan C 1986 Inheritance pattern and clinical response to splenectomy as a reflection of erythrocyte spectrin deficiency in hereditary spherocytosis. New England Journal of Medicine 315: 1579–1583

Allen D M, Diamond L K 1961 Congenital erythroid hypoplastic anaemia: Cortisone treated. American Journal of Diseases of Children 102: 416–423

Alter B P 1978 Thumbs and anaemias. Pediatrics 62: 613–614

Alter B P 1987 The bone marrow failure syndromes. In: Nathan D G, Oski F A (eds) Hematology of Infancy and Childhood, 3rd edn. W B Saunders, Philadelphia, p 159–241

Arakawa T 1970 Congenital defects in folate utilization. American Journal of Medicine 48: 594–598

Auerbach A D, Wolman S R 1976 Susceptibility of Fanconi's anaemia fibroblasts to chromosome damage by carcinogens. Nature 261: 494–496

Auerbach A D, Adler B, Chaganti R S K 1981 Prenatal and postnatal diagnosis and carrier detection of Fanconi anaemia by a cytogenetic method. Pediatrics 67: 128–135

Baehner R L, Nathan D G, Castle W B 1971 Oxidant injury of Caucasian glucose-6-phosphate dehydrogenase deficient red blood cells caused by phagocytosing leukocytes during infection. Journal of Clinical Investigation 50: 2466–2473

Bassen F A, Kornzweig A L 1950 Malformation of the erythrocytes in a case of atypical retinitis pigmentosa. Blood 5: 381–387

Bates G C, Brown C H 1952 Incidence of gallbladder disease in chronic hemolytic anaemia (spherocytosis). Gastroenterology 21: 104–109

Baughan M A, Valentine W N, Paglia D E, Ways P O, Simons E R, DeMarsh Q 1968 Hereditary hemolytic anaemia associated with glucose-phosphate isomerase (GPI) deficiency — a new enzyme defect of human erythrocytes. Blood 32: 236–249

Becker M A, Kostel P J, Meyer L J, Seegmiller J E 1973 Human phosphoribosyl pyrophosphate synthetase: increased enzyme specific activity in a family with gout and excessive purine synthesis. Proceedings of the National Academy of Sciences USA 70: 2749–2752

Beutler E 1969 Effect of flavin compounds on glutathione reductase activity: In vivo and in vitro studies. Journal of Clinical Investigation 48: 1957–1966

Beutler E 1979 Red cell enzyme defects as nondiseases and diseases. Blood 54: 1–7

Beutler E 1983 Glucose-6-phosphate dehydrogenase deficiency. In: Stanbury J B, Wyngaarden J B, Fredrickson D S, Goldstein J L, Brown M S (eds) The Metabolic Basis of Inherited Disease, 5th edn. McGraw Hill, New York, p 1629–1653

Beutler E, Matsumoto F 1975 Ethnic variation in red cell glutathione peroxidase activity. Blood 46: 103–110

Beutler E, Carson D, Dannawi H, Forman L, Kuhl H, West C, Westwood B 1983 Metabolic compensation for profound erythrocyte adenylate kinase deficiency. Journal of Clinical Investigation 72: 648–655

Bloom G E, Warner S, Gerald P S, Diamond L K 1966 Chromosome abnormalities in constitutional aplastic anaemia. New England Journal of Medicine 274: 8–14

Boivin P, Galand C, Andre R, Debray J 1966 Anemies hemolytiques congenitales avec deficit isole en glutathion reduit par deficit en glutathion synthetase. Nouvelle Revue Francaise D Hematologie (Heidelberg) 6: 859–866

Boivin P, Galand C, Hakim J, Roge J, Gueroult N 1969 Anemie hemolytique avec deficit en glutathion-peroxydase chez un adulte. Enzymologia Biologica et Clinica (Basel) 10: 68–80

Boyer S H, Porter I H, Weilbacher R G 1962 Electrophoretic heterogeneity of glucose-6-phosphate dehydrogenase and its relationship to enzyme deficiency in man. Proceedings of the National Academy of Sciences USA 48: 1868–1876

Carson P E, Flanagan D L, Ickes C E, Alving A S 1956 Enzymatic deficiency in primaquine-sensitive erythrocytes. Science 124: 484–485

Chevion M, Navok T, Glaser G, Mager J 1982 The chemistry of favism-inducing compounds. The properties of isouramil and divicine and their reaction with glutathione. European Journal of Biochemistry 127: 405–409

Childs B, Zinkham W, Browne E A, Kimbro E L, Torbert J V 1958 A genetic study of a defect in glutathione metabolism of the erythrocyte. Johns Hopkins Medical Journal 102: 21–37

Cotton H B, Harris J W 1962 Familial pyridoxine-responsive anaemia. Journal of Clinical Investigation 41: 1352

Crookston J H, Crookston M C, Burnie K L, Francombe W H 1969 Hereditary erythroblastic multinuclearity associated with a positive acidified serum test: a type of congenital dyserythropoietic anaemia. British Journal of Haematology 17: 11–26

Diamond L K, Blackfan K D 1938 Hypoplastic Anemia. American Journal of Diseases of Children 56: 464–467

Diamond L K, Wang W C, Alter B P 1976 Congenital hypoplastic anaemia. Advances in Pediatrics 22: 349–378

Eshaghpour E, Oski F A, Williams M 1967 The relationship of erythrocyte glucose-6-phosphate dehydrogenase deficiency to hyperbilirubinemia in Negro premature infants. Journal of Pediatrics 70: 595–601

Fanconi G 1967 Familial constitutional panmelocytopathy, Fanconi's Anaemia (F.A.) I. Clinical aspects. Seminars in Hematology 4: 233–240

Fox I H, Kelley W N 1971 Phosphoribosylpyrophosphate in man: biochemical and clinical significance. Annals of Internal Medicine 74: 424–433

Fujii H, Miwa S, Tani K, Fujiami N, Asano H 1982 Overproduction of structurally normal enzyme in man: Hereditary haemolytic anaemia with increased red cell adenosine deaminase activity. British Journal of Haematology 51: 427–430

Giblett E R, Anderson J E, Cohen F, Pollara B, Meuwissen H J 1972 Adenosine deaminase deficiency in two patients with severely impaired cellular immunity and normal B-cellular immunity. Lancet 2: 1067–1069

Giblett E R, Ammann A J, Wara D W, Sandman R, Diamond L K 1975 Nucleoside phosphorylase deficiency in a child with severely defective T-cell immunity. Lancet 1: 1010–1013

Gitzelmann R 1965 Deficiency of erythrocyte galactokinase in a patient with galactose diabetes. Lancet 2: 670–671

Glader B E 1976 Evaluation of the hemolytic role of aspirin in glucose-6-phosphate dehydrogenase deficiency. Journal of Pediatrics 89: 1027–1028

Glader B E, Fortier N, Albala M, Nathan D G 1974 Congenital hemolytic anemia associated with dehydrated erythrocytes and increased potassium loss. New England Journal of Medicine 291: 491–496

Glader B E, Backer K, Diamond L K 1983 Elevated erythrocyte adenosine deaminase activity in congenital hypoplastic anemia. New England Journal of Medicine 309: 1486–1490

Grasbeck R, Gordin R, Kantero I, Kuhlback B 1960 Selective vitamin B_{12} malabsorption and proteinuria in young people. Acta Medica Scandinavica 167: 289–296

Gray G R, Klebanoff S J, Stamatoyannopoulos G et al 1973 Neutrophil dysfunction, chronic granulomatous disease, and non-spherocytic haemolytic anaemia caused by complete deficiency of glucose-6-phosphate dehydrogenase. Lancet 2: 530–534

Hakami N, Neiman P E, Canellos G P, Lazerson J 1971 Neonatal megaloblastic anaemia due to inherited transcobalamin II deficiency in two siblings. New England Journal of Medicine 285: 1163–1170

Heimpel H, Wendt F 1968 Congenital dyserythropoietic anemia with karyorrhexis and multinuclearity of erythroblasts. Helvetica Medica Acta 34: 103–115

Imerslund O 1960 Idiopathic chronic megaloblastic anaemia in children. Acta Paediatrica Scandinavica (suppl 119) 1–115

Isselbacher K J, Anderson E P, Kurahashi K, Kalckar H M 1956 Congenital galactosemia, a single enzymatic block in galactose metabolism. Science 123: 635–636

Jellum E, Kluge T, Borresen H D, Stokke O, Eldjarn L 1970 Pyroglutamic aciduria: A new inborn error of metabolism. Scandinavian Journal of Clinical and Laboratory Investigation 26: 327–335

Johnson G J, Allen D W, Cadman S, Fairbanks V F, White J G, Lampkin B C, Kaplan M E 1979 Red-cell-membrane polypeptide aggregates in glucose-6-phosphate dehydrogenase mutants with chronic hemolytic disease. New England Journal of Medicine 301: 522–527

Joseph H W 1936 Anaemia of infancy and early childhood. Medicine 15: 307–451

Kahn A, Meinhoffer M-C, Cottreau D, LaGrange J-L, Dreyfus J-C 1979 Phosphofructokinase (PFK) isozymes in man. Human Genetics 48: 93–108

Kelley W N, Smith L H Jr. 1978 Hereditary orotic aciduria. In: Stanbury J B, Wyngaarden J B, Fredrickson D S (eds) The Metabolic Basis of Inherited Disease, 4th edn. McGraw-Hill, New York, p 1045–1071

Kelley W N, Rosenbloom F M, Henderson J F, Seegmiller J E 1967 A specific enzyme defect in gout associated with overproduction of uric acid. Proceedings of the National Academy of Sciences USA 57: 1735–1739

Konrad P N, Richards F, Valentine W N, Paglia D E 1972a Gamma glutamyl-cysteine synthetase deficiency: A cause of hereditary hemolytic anemia. New England Journal of

Medicine 286: 557–561

Konrad P N, McCarthy D J, Mauer A M, Valentine W N, Paglia D E 1972b Erythrocyte and leukocyte phosphoglycerate kinase deficiency with neurologic disease. Journal of Pediatrics 82: 456–460

Kosower N S, Kosower E M 1970 Molecular basis for selective advantage of glucose-6-phosphate dehydrogenase deficient subjects. Lancet 2: 1343–1344

Lanzkowsky P 1987a Disorders of erythrocyte production. II. Clinical, pathogenetic, and diagnostic considerations in folate deficiency. In: Nathan D G, Oski F A (eds) Hematology of Infancy and Childhood, 3rd edn. W B Saunders, Philadelphia, p 321–338

Lanzkowsky P 1987b Disorders of erythrocyte production. II. Clinical, pathogenetic, and diagnostic considerations of vitamin B_{12} (cobalamin) deficiency and other congenital and acquired disorders. In: Nathan D G, Oski F A (eds) Hematology of Infancy and Childhood, 3rd edn. W B Saunders, Philadelphia, p 344–362

Latt S A, Stetten G, Juergens L A, Buchanan G R, Gerald P S 1975 Induction by alkylating agents of sister chromatid exchanges and chromatid breaks in Fanconi's anemia. Proceedings of the National Academy of Sciences USA 72: 4066–4070

Lewis S M, Verwilghen R L 1977 Dyserythropoiesis. Academic Press, London

Lipton J M, Kudisch M, Gross R, Nathan D G 1986 Defective erythroid progenitor differentiation system in congenital hypoplastic (Diamond-Blackfan) anemia. Blood 67: 962–968

Loos H, Roos D, Weening R, Houwerzijl J 1976 Familial deficiency of glutathione reductase in human blood cells. Blood 48: 53–62

Luhby A L, Eagle F J, Roth E, Cooperman J M 1961 Relapsing megaloblastic anemia in an infant due to a specific defect in gastrointestinal absorption of folic acid. American Journal of Diseases of Children 102: 482–483

Lux S 1987 Disorders of the red cell membrane. In: Nathan D G, Oski F A (eds) Hematology of Infancy and Childhood, 3rd edn. W B Saunders, Philadelphia, p 443–544

Luzzatto L 1975 Inherited haemolytic states: Glucose-6-phosphate dehydrogenase deficiency. Clinics in Haematology 4: 83–108

Luzzatto L, Usanga E A, Reddy S 1969 Glucose-6-phosphate dehydrogenase deficient red cells: Resistance to infection by malarial parasites. Science 164: 839–842

Lyon M F 1961 Gene action in the X-chromosome of the mouse (mus musculus L). Nature 190: 372–373

McIntyre O R, Sullivan L W, Jeffries G H, Silver R H 1965 Pernicious anemia in childhood. New England Journal of Medicine 272: 981–986

Marstein S, Jellum E, Halpern B, Eldjarn L, Perry T L 1976 Biochemical studies of erythrocytes in a patient with pyroglutamic acidemia (5-oxoprolinemia). New England Journal of Medicine 295: 406–412

Meister A 1974 The gamma-glutamyl cycle. Diseases associated with specific enzyme deficiencies. Annals of Internal Medicine 81: 247–253

Mentzer W C Jr. 1987 Pyruvate kinase deficiency and disorders of glycolysis. In: Nathan D G, Oski F A (eds) Hematology of Infancy and Childhood, 3rd edn. W B Saunders, Philadelphia, p 545–582

Mentzer W C Jr., Collier E 1975 Hydrops fetalis associated with erythrocyte G6PD deficiency and maternal ingestion

of fava beans and ascorbic acid. Journal of Pediatrics 86: 565–567

Mentzer W C Jr., Baehner R L, Schmidt-Schoenbein H, Robinson S H, Nathan D G 1971 Selective reticulocyte destruction in erythrocyte pyruvate kinase deficiency. Journal of Clinical Investigation 50: 688–699

Miller D R, Bloom G E, Strieff R R, LoBuglio A F, Diamond L K 1966 Juvenile "congenital" pernicious anemia. New England Journal of Medicine 275: 978–983

Miwa S, Fujii H, Tani K, Takahashi K, Takizawa T, Igarashi T 1983 Red cell adenylate kinase deficiency associated with hereditary nonspherocytic hemolytic anemia: Clinical and biochemical studies. American Journal of Hematology 14: 325–333

Mohler D N, Majerus P W, Minnich V, Hess C E, Garrick M D 1970 Glutathione synthetase deficiency as a cause of hereditary hemolytic disease. New England Journal of Medicine 283: 1253–1257

Mohrenweiser H W, Fielek S 1982 Elevated frequency of carriers for triosephosphate isomerase deficiency in newborn infants. Pediatric Research 16: 960–963

Motulsky A G 1960 Metabolic polymorphisms and the role of infectious diseases in human evolution. Human Biology 32: 28–62

Necheles T F, Maldonado N, Barquet-Chediak A, Allen D M 1969 Homozygous erythrocyte glutathione-peroxidase deficiency: Clinical and biochemical studies. Blood 33: 164–169

Nishimura Y, Chida N, Hayashi T, Arakawa T 1972 Homozygous glutathione-peroxidase deficiency of erythrocytes and leukocytes. Tohoku Journal of Experimental Medicine 108: 207–217

Nyhan W L 1973 The Lesch-Nyhan syndrome. Annual Review of Medicine 24: 41–60

O'Flynn M E, Hsia D Y-Y 1963 Serum bilirubin levels and glucose-6-phosphate dehydrogenase activity in newborn American Negroes. Journal of Pediatrics 63: 160–161

Oski F A, Deli002ia-Papadopoulous M 1970 The red cell 2,3, diphosphoglycerate and tissue oxygen release. Journal of Pediatrics 77: 941–956

Oski F A, Naiman J L, Blum S F et al 1969 Congenital hemolytic anemia with high-sodium, low-potassium red cells: studies of three generations of a family with a new variant. New England Journal of Medicine 280: 909–916

Paglia D E, Valentine W N 1974 Hereditary glucosephosphate isomerase deficiency, a review. American Journal of Clinical Pathology 62: 740–751

Paglia D E, Valentine W N 1981 Haemolytic anaemia associated with disorders of the purine and pyrimidine salvage pathways. Clinics in Haematology 10: 81–98

Paglia D E, Valentine W N, Dahlgren J G 1975 Effects of low-level lead exposure on pyrimidine 5'-nucleotidase and other erythrocyte enzymes. Possible role of pyrimidine 5'-nucleotidase deficiency and intracellular accumulation of pyrimidine nucleotides. Journal of Clinical Investigation 56: 1164–1169

Pearson H A, Lobel J S, Kocoshis S A et al 1979 A new syndrome of refractory sideroblastic anemia with vacuolization of marrow precursors and exocrine pancreatic dysfunction. Journal of Pediatrics 95: 976–984

Piomelli S, Corash L M, Davenport D D, Miraglia J, Amorosi E L 1968 In vivo lability of glucose-6-phosphate dehydrogenase in Gd^{A-} and Gd^{Mediterranean} deficiency. Journal of Clinical Investigation 47: 940–948

Polmar S H 1980 Metabolic aspects of immunodeficiency

disease. Seminars in Hematology 17: 30–43

Richards R, Cooper M R, Pearce L A, Cowan R J, Spurr C L 1974 Familial spinocerebellar degeneration, hemolytic anemia and glutathione deficiency. Archives of Internal Medicine 134: 534–537

Robinson S H, Glass J 1987 Disorders of heme metabolism: Sideroblastic anemia and the porphyrias. In: Nathan D G, Oski F A (eds) Hematology of Infancy and Childhood, 3rd edn. W B Saunders, Philadelphia, p 363–388

Rosenberg L E, Lilljeqvist A C, Hsia Y–E 1968 Methylmalonic aciduria: metabolic block localization and vitamin B_{12} dependency. Science 162: 805–807

Schneider A S, Valentine W N, Baughan M A, Paglia D E, Shore N A, Heins H L Jr. 1968 Triosphosphate isomerase deficiency. A. A multi-system inherited enzyme disorder. Clinical and genetic aspects. In: Beutler E (ed) Hereditary Disorders of Erythrocyte Metabolism. Grune & Stratton, New York, p 265–272

Schwartz J M, Reiss A L, Jaffe E R 1983 Hereditary methemoglobinemia with deficiency of NADH cytochrome b5 reductase. In: Stanbury J B, Wyngaarden J B, Fredrickson D S, Goldstein J L, Brown M S (eds) The Metabolic Basis of Inherited Disease, 5th edn. McGraw Hill, New York, p 1654–1665

Srivastava S K, Beutler E 1969 The transport of oxidized glutathione from human erythrocytes. Journal of Biological Chemistry 244: 9–16

Staal G E, Stoop J W, Zegers B J M, Siegenbeek-van Heukelom L H, Van der Vlist M J M, Wadmon S K, Martin D W 1980 Erythrocyte metabolism in purine nucleoside phosphorylase deficiency after enzyme replacement therapy by infusion of erythrocytes. Journal of Clinical Investigation 65: 103–108

Stamatoyannopoulos G, Fraser G R, Motulsky A G, Fessas Ph, Akrivakis A, Papayannopoulou Th 1966 On the familial predisposition to favism. American Journal of Human Genetics 18: 253–263

Szeinberg A, Gavendo S, Cahane D 1969 Erythrocyte adenylate-kinase deficiency. Lancet 1: 315–316

Takahara S 1952 Progressive oral gangrene probably due to lack of catalase in the blood (acatalasemia) Lancet 2: 1101–1104

Tarui S, Okuno G, Ikura Y, Tanaka T, Suda M, Nishikawa M 1965 Phosphofructokinase deficiency in skeletal muscle. A new type of glycogenesis. Biochemical and Biophysical Research Communications 19: 517–523

Thomson C D, Rea H M, Doesburg V M, Robinson M D 1977 Selenium concentrations and glutathione peroxidase activities in whole blood of New Zealand residents. British Journal of Nutrition 37: 457–460

Tomaselli M B, John K M, Lux S E 1981 Elliptical erythrocyte membrane skeletons and heat-sensitive spectrin in hereditary elliptocytosis. Proceedings of the National Academy of Sciences USA 78: 1911–1915

Valaes T, Karaklis A, Stravrakakis D, Bavela-Stravrakakis K, Perakis A, Doxiadis S A 1969 Incidence and mechanism of neonatal jaundice related to glucose-6-phosphate dehydrogenase deficiency. Pediatric Research 3: 448–458

Valentine W N 1983 Sideroblastic anemias. In: Williams W J, Beutler E, Erslev A, Lichtman M A (eds) Hematology, 3rd edn. McGraw-Hill, New York, p 537–546

Valentine W N, Oski F A, Paglia D E, Baughan M A 1967 Hereditary hemolytic anemia with hexokinase deficiency. New England Journal of Medicine 276: 1–11

Valentine W N, Hsieh H–S, Paglia D E, Anderson H M, Baughan M A 1968 The hereditary hemolytic anemias associated with phosphoglycerate kinase deficiency in erythrocytes and leukocytes. Transactions of the Association of American Physicians 81: 49

Valentine W N, Fink K, Paglia D E, Harris S R, Adams W S 1974 Hereditary hemolytic anemia with human erythrocyte pyrimidine-5'-nucleotidase deficiency. Journal of Clinical Investigation 54: 866–879

Valentine W N, Paglia D E, Fink K, Modokoro G 1976 Lead Poisoning. Association with hemolytic anemia, basophilic stippling, erythrocyte pyrimidine 5'-nucleotidase deficiency and intraerythrocyte accumulation of pyrimidines. Journal of Clinical Investigation 58: 926–932

Valentine W N, Paglia D E, Tartaglia A P, Gilsanz F 1977 Hereditary hemolytic anemia with increased red cell adenosine deaminase (45- to 70-fold) and decreased adenosine triphosphate. Science 195: 783–785

Valentine W N, Tanaka K R, Paglia D E 1983 Pyruvate kinase and other enzyme deficiency disorders of the erythrocyte. In: Stanbury J B, Wyngaarden J B, Fredrickson D S, Goldstein J L, Brown M S (eds) The Metabolic Basis of Inherited Disease, 5th edn. McGraw Hill, New York, p 1606–1628

Van Acker K J, Simmonds H A, Potter C, Cameron J S 1977 Complete deficiency of adenine phosphoribosyltransferase. Report of a family. New England Journal of Medicine 297: 127–132

Vora S, Corash L, Engel W K, Durhma S, Seaman C, Piomeli S 1980 The molecular mechanism of the inherited phosphofructokinase deficiency associated with hemolysis and myopathy. Blood 55: 629–635

Walters T 1967 Congenital megaloblastic anemia responsive to N^5-formyl tetrahydrofolic acid administration. Journal of Pediatrics 70: 686–687

Yoshida A 1967 A single amino acid substitution (asparagine to aspartic acid) between normal (B^+) and the common Negro variant (A^+) of human glucose-6-phosphate dehydrogenase. Proceedings of the National Academy of Sciences USA 57: 835–840

Yoshida A 1973 Hemolytic anemia and G6PD deficiency. Science 179: 532–537

Yoshida A, Stamatoyannopoulos G, Motulsky A G 1967 Negro variant of glucose-6-phosphate dehydrogenase deficiency (A^-) in man. Science 155: 97–99

Zarkowsky H S, Oski F A, Sha'afi R, Shohet S B, Nathan D G 1968 Congenital hemolytic anemia with high sodium, low potassium red cells. I. Studies of membrane permeability. New England Journal of Medicine 278: 573–581

80. Congenital disorders of haemostasis

C. A. Ludlam

HAEMOSTASIS

Haemostasis is maintained by a complex sequence of interactions between endothelial cells, platelets and a series of plasma proteins (Colman et al 1987). The intact endothelium is non-thrombogenic, due, in part, to its production of a variety of substances that inhibit thrombosis, e.g. prostacyclin and tissue plasminogen activator. Trauma to a vessel results in damage to the endothelium and exposure of the subendothelial matrix which contains collagen fibres. Von Willebrand factor binds platelets to this damaged area (Fig. 80.1). Activation of the platelets causes the release of a variety of substances, e.g. ADP, which activate further platelets and induce them to aggregate to form a haemostatic plug resulting in arrest of haemorrhage. Other factors released from platelets, e.g. factor V and fibrinogen, promote coagulation on the platelet surface.

The coagulation system is activated by the conversion of factor XII to XIIa and this initiates the intrinsic coagulation pathway. Tissue thromboplastin from damaged cells promotes the activation of factor VII and the extrinsic coagulation system. Both these systems converge to activate factor X, which in turn promotes the final stages, or common pathway, resulting in fibrin generation. Many individual reactions of the coagulation cascade occur most efficiently when the components are spacially arranged on the platelet surface where the reaction rates may be magnified many thousands of times.

A series of endothelial, platelet and plasma derived proteins inhibit excessive activation of the coagulation cascade and platelet aggregation at the sites of injury. Once formed, fibrin can be enzymically degraded by plasmin, resulting in lysis of the clot.

Platelets

These small, anucleate cells are essential for maintaining vascular integrity and normal haemostasis. Following release from the bone marrow megakaryocytes they survive in the circulation for 10 days. Their complex structure enables a prompt response to any breach of vascular integrity (Crawford & Scrutton 1987, White 1987). The surface membrane contains several glycoproteins which act as receptors both for proteins released from granules within the platelets and for circulating plasma proteins. Glycoprotein IIb/IIIa, for example, acts as a receptor for fibrinogen, von Willebrand factor, thrombomodulin and fibronectin (Fig. 80.1).

Three types of granules can be observed in platelets: delta granules which store low molecular weight chemicals, e.g. calcium and ADP; alpha granules, which contain a variety of proteins, e.g. fibrinogen and factor V; and lysosomal granules containing acid hydrolases (Table 80.1). Many of these constituents promote further platelet activation or coagulation. Activation of platelets results in a series of complex reactions culminating in an increase in cytosolic calcium ion concentration. This in turn activates a kinase which phosphorylates the light chain of myosin. Another activation pathway is by the release of arachidonic acid from membrane phospholipid by the action of phospholipase C. The arachidonic acid is converted by cyclo-oxygenase to endoperoxides which are channelled by the action of thromboxane synthetase to thromboxane A_2 and to a lesser extent PGD_2. Thromboxane A_2 releases calcium from intracellular stores. Continued activation of the platelets is suppressed by stimulation of adenylate cyclase by PGD_2; the increased intracellular concentration of cAMP stimulates a calcium/magnesium ATP dependent pump which restores cytosolic calcium to its storage site. Other proteins also reduce platelet recruitment, e.g. endothelium derived ADPase and thrombomodulin which inactivates thrombin, thus preventing further platelet stimulation. Coagulation is further promoted by the release of coagulation factors, e.g. fibrinogen and factor V, which bind to further specific receptors. The surface bound factor V acts as a nidus for the binding of Xa which in the presence of calcium converts prothrombin to thrombin.

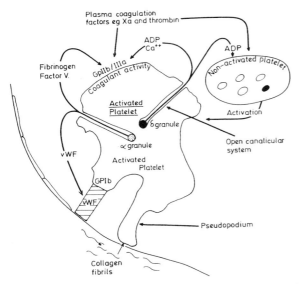

Fig. 80.1 Interaction of damaged vessel wall, von Willebrand factor, platelet and coagulation system during platelet adhesion and activation to form haemostatic plug.

This enzyme converts fibrinogen to fibrin and activates factors V and VIII.

A deficiency of platelet number, i.e. thrombocytopenia, or function, i.e. thrombopathy, which may be congenital or acquired, will result in characteristic bleeding. This is predominantly observed from mucocutaneous surfaces with purpura and echymosis on the skin, epistaxis, gastrointestinal haemorrhage and menorrhagia.

Table 80.1 Platelet granule constituents

Alpha granules
    Factor V
    von Willebrand factor
    Fibrinogen
    Fibronectin
    β-thromboglobulin
    Platelet factor 4
    Platelet derived growth factor
    α_2 antiplasmin
    β_2 macroglobulin
    Histidine rich glycoprotein
    Thrombospondin
Delta granules
    ATP
    ADP
    Ca^{++}
    Mg^{++}
    Serotonin
Lysosomes
    Acid hydrolases

Coagulation system

The coagulation cascade (Fig. 80.2) consists of a series of inactive zymogens each of which when activated in turn activates the next member of the clotting cascade (Davie & Ratnoff 1964, Macfarlane 1964). The components have been numbered factors I to XIII (Table 80.2) and activated proteins are designated with a lower case 'a', e.g. factor II is activated to factor IIa. When a factor is assayed by assessing its ability to promote coagulation this is designated as the coagulant activity, e.g. factor IIC, whereas if the protein is measured immunologically it is expressed as an antigen level, e.g. factor IIAg. Deficiencies of coagulation factors can be divided broadly into those in which there is a reduced concentration of an apparently normal molecule (Type I) and others in which the molecule is functionally defective (Type II). The latter are usually detected by finding a reduced activity, e.g. factor IXC, in the presence of a near normal antigen concentration, e.g. factor IXAg. For many coagulation factors, however, there is a broad range of different molecular variants in which both activity and antigen are reduced, often with the former being lower than the latter.

The intrinsic coagulation cascade is initiated by conversion of factor XII to XIIa by negatively charged surfaces, and this in turn activates prekallikrein and factor XI (Fig. 80.2). The resultant kallikrein causes the release of bradykinin from high molecular weight kininogen (HMWK), and conversion of factor XI to XIa. This in turn brings about the activation of factor IX to IXa. It is of interest to note that, whereas deficiencies of all other components of the coagulation sequence result in a bleeding diathesis, a deficiency of factor XII, prekallikrein or high molecular weight kininogen are not associated with bleeding. There is evidence that activated platelets may promote the conversion of factor XI to XIa, thus bypassing factor XII initiation of the intrinsic system. Factor IXa, along with factor XIII and calcium, promote the conversion of factor X to Xa on the platelet surface. Factor Xa, in the presence of factor Va and calcium, promotes the conversion of prothrombin to thrombin. This enzyme causes the release of fibrinopeptides A and B from fibrinogen and the resultant fibrin monomers polymerise and become crosslinked by factor XIII, a transcarboxylase. Thrombin also activates factors XIII, V, VIII and platelets. It therefore has a potent role in promoting haemostasis. Excessive thrombin activity is inhibited by several plasma proteins, e.g. antithrombin III and heparin cofactor II, as well as thrombomodulin on the endothelial cell surface.

Dissolution of fibrin clots is promoted by tissue plasminogen activator released from endothelial cells.

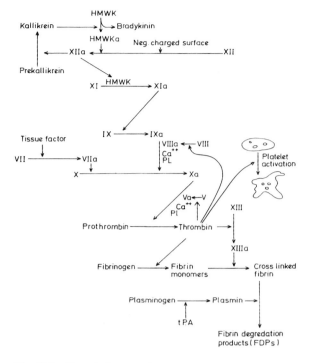

Fig. 80.2 Coagulation cascade.

Table 80.2 Nomenclature and inheritance of blood coagulation factors

Factor	Synonym	Inheritance
I	Fibrinogen	Autosomal
II	Prothrombin	Autosomal
III	Tissue thromboplastin	
IV	Calcium	
V	Proaccelerin	Autosomal
VII	Proconvertin	Autosomal
VIII	Antihaemophilic globulin(AHG)	X-linked recessive
IX	Christmas factor	X-linked recessive
X	Stuart Prower factor	Autosomal
XI	Plasma thromboplastin antecedent	Autosomal
XII	Hageman factor	Autosomal
XIII	Fibrin stabilising factor	Autosomal

This promotes the conversion of fibrin bound plasminogen to plasmin, which digests the fibrin to fibrin degradation products. Plasmin itself is inactivated by a_2 antiplasmin and the plasminogen activator by another endothelially derived protein, plasminogen activator inhibitor.

CONGENITAL DISORDERS OF THE COAGULATION SYSTEM

Congenital disorders of haemostasis are characterised clinically by haemarthroses, muscle haematoma and excessive bleeding following trauma and surgery. In general those with the most severe forms of these disorders usually have very low levels (<2% normal) of the deficient factor and they suffer from apparently 'spontaneous bleeds'. Individuals with more than 5% of the deficient factor usually only bleed after surgery or trauma.

Investigation of coagulation disorders

Screening tests of the coagulation cascade include the activated partial thromboplastin time (APTT) (intrinsic system), prothrombin time (extrinsic system), fibrinogen

concentration and thrombin time (dysfibrinogenaemias). If an abnormality in any of these tests is observed assay of appropriate coagulation factors should be undertaken. It should be noted that these screening tests may be insensitive to a mild deficiency. If, therefore, there is a strong clinical suspicion of a coagulation disorder, assay of individual factors may be appropriate even in the presence of a normal prothrombin time and activated partial thromboplastin time.

The haemophilias

The term haemophilia is used to include haemophilia A (factor VIIIC deficiency); haemophilia B or Christmas disease (factor IXC deficiency); and von Willebrand's disease, where the primary abnormality is a defect in the synthesis of von Willebrand factor (Bloom 1987a). While haemophilia A and B are X-linked recessive disorders, von Willebrand disease is autosomally inherited. Haemophilia A and B are clinically indistinguishable and can only be separately diagnosed by specific assays for factors VIIIC and IXC. Bleeding occurs principally into large joints, e.g. knees and elbows, muscles and following trauma or surgery. In von Willebrand disease the pattern of bleeding is quite different, presenting predominantly with bruising, gastrointestinal haemorrhage or menorrhagia. These three disorders are considered separately below.

Haemophilia A

This occurs with a frequency of approximately 1:10 000 of the population and is therefore the most common of the severe congenital bleeding disorders. The gene for factor VIIIC is close to the tip of the X chromosome (Xq28) in proximity to the genes for glucose-6-phosphate dehydrogenase variants (Boyer & Graham 1965), deutan colour blindness (Whittaker et al 1962), and X-linked persistence of fetal haemoglobin (Miyoshi et al 1978).

The activity of factor VIII can be measured by a functional, or coagulant assay, when it is termed factor VIIIC. The protein can be quantitated immunologically, when it is referred to as factor VIIIAg. In most individuals with haemophilia A there is a good correlation between factor VIIIC and factor VIIIAg. In a few a functionally defective protein is produced. Prior to the development of immunoradioactive assays for factor VIIIAg, such individuals were said to be haemophilia A+ variants or to have 'cross reacting material' (CRM+) in their plasma. This was detected by neutralisation of antifactor VIII alloantibody when this was added in vitro (Denson et al 1969, Peake et al 1979). The factor VIII gene has been cloned and is 186 kb long, having 26 exons coding for a native protein of 2332 amino acids (Gitschier et al 1984, Toole et al 1984). A large variety of molecular defects in the gene have been described, leading to a reduction in the plasma level of factor VIIIC. The defects include base substitutions leading to creation of stop codons, or changes in amino acids or gene deletions, either partial or total (Antonarakis et al 1987, Antonarakis 1988, Arai et al 1989, Inaba et al 1989, Patterson et al 1989).

The plasma factor VIIIC level in normal individuals ranges from 0.50–1.50 iu/ml. The severity of the clinical symptoms is related to the plasma factor VIIIC level: individuals with less than 0.02 iu/ml have severe haemophilia, those with 0.02–0.05 iu/ml moderate, and those with greater than 0.05 iu/ml mild disease.

In severe haemophilia 'spontaneous' recurrent haemarthroses occur into knees, elbows, ankles, shoulders and hip joints. Such bleeds may arise 2–4 times per month. Bleeds usually start to occur about the age of 6 months, when the baby becomes mobile. Untreated haemarthroses result in persistent severe pain lasting for many days and, because of their recurrent nature, lead to loss of cartilage and secondary osteoarthrosis (Fig. 80.3, Table 80.3). Early treatment with therapeutic factor VIII concentrates promptly arrests bleeding and substantially delays the development of chronic haemophilic arthropathy. Deep muscle haematoma, e.g. into calf or psoas, is also observed (Fig. 80.4). Frank haematuria is not uncommonly observed, but despite the presence of minor radiographic abnormalities kidney function is generally well preserved. Spontaneous intracranial bleeds occur suddenly, without warning and, particularly in adults, are severe and often fatal. Children have a remarkable ability to recover from a large intracranial haemorrhage provided factor VIII therapy is given early.

Table 80.3 Common complications of haemophilia

1. Due to recurrent bleeds
    Chronic arthropathy
    Muscle fibrosis
    Pseudotumours
    Entrapment neuropathies
2. Arising from factor VIII concentrates
    Antifactor VIII inhibitors
    Chronic liver disease (Hepatitis B virus, Non-A, Non-B virus)
    HIV infection and AIDS
    Allergic reactions to factor VIII infusions
    Immune modulation, e.g. depressed cell mediated immunity
    Anti-Gm and Fc antibodies
    Haemolysis (anti A and B) — only with large doses

Individuals with moderate haemophilia usually bleed following minor trauma, often with only 1–5 such bleeds per year. In mild haemophilia bleeding will only be observed after severe trauma or surgery. Because of the mild nature of the bleeding disorder many such patients may not present with haemorrhagic symptoms until adult life and therefore diagnosis is often delayed.

Diagnosis of haemophilia is dependant on finding a reduced plasma factor VIIIC with a normal vWFAg, ristocetin cofactor and bleeding time. In the UK, treatment of individuals with haemophilia and other congenital haemostatic disorders is given at Haemophilia Centres. These not only offer treatment for acute bleeds and arrange home therapy but offer a wide variety of other functions (Table 80.4) essential to provide a comprehensive care service. The aim of treatment of acute bleeds is to increase the plasma factor VIIIC level. In severe and moderate haemophilia this is best achieved by infusion of cryoprecipitate or factor VIII concentrate. In general, factor VIII concentrates are usually the treatment of choice but these are prepared from plasma pools that may be derived from 5–25 000 individual plasma donations. It will be apparent that if a few donations contain transmissible viruses this can potentially render the whole batch of factor VIII concentrate infectious, resulting in clinical disease in many recipients.

Transmission by factor VIII concentrates of hepatitis B and delta viruses (HBV and HDV), non-A non-B virus(es), HIV and parvovirus have all been observed. Despite screening individual plasma donations for HBsAg, factor VIII concentrates still transmit this virus and it is therefore prudent to vaccinate all potential recipients against HBV. The prevalence of non-A non-B virus(es) in donors remains uncertain because no diagnostic tests are available, but all bottles of factor VIII

Table 80.4 Functions of haemophilia centres

Diagnosis of congenital haemostatic disorders
Detection and counselling of carriers
Hospital treatment of bleeds
Provision of specialised nursing
Physiotherapy
Arrangements for self therapy at home
Regular medical assessment of patients
Liaison with:
       Paediatrician
       Orthopaedic surgeon
       Dentist
       Psychiatrist
       Psychologist
Social work support/counselling
Arrange for provision of appropriate blood products

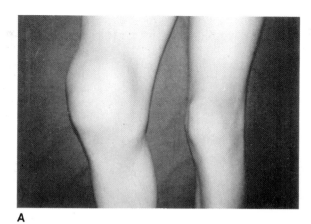

A

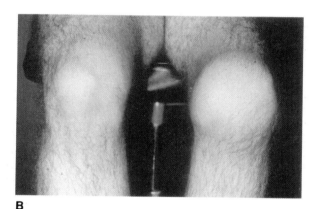

B

concentrate probably contain the virus(es). Almost all patients who receive even a single injection of concentrate develop hepatitis and evidence is accumulating that this results in serious chronic progressive liver disease, e.g. chronic active hepatitis or cirrhosis with portal hypertension and oesophageal varices (Hay et al 1985, Kernoff et al 1985). Contamination of the plasma pool by HIV has led to many haemophiliacs becoming infected. In the UK 59% of severe haemophiliacs are anti-HIV positive, while in moderate and mild disease this is only 23% and 9% respectively. The pattern of infection reflects the frequency with which factor VIII concentrates are infused; severe haemophiliacs receive many more injections of factor VIII. Not only are increasing numbers of haemophiliacs developing clinical stigmata of HIV infection, including persistent generalised lymphadenopathy and AIDS related complex, but more patients are now dying from AIDS than from intracranial haemorrhage, previously the most common cause of death. Furthermore, because the virus is sexually transmissible by heterosexuals, female partners may become infected. The wives therefore face not only the prospect of developing AIDS but also of passing HIV through pregnancy to offspring. This prospect has produced enormous tensions and strains between couples and within families.

In an attempt to reduce HIV infection all potential donors who belong to certain risk groups with a high incidence of infection, e.g. homosexuals and i.v. drug abusers, are asked to refrain from donating blood. All individual donations are screened for anti-HIV, and the factor VIII concentrates are heated to inactivate the virus. These three measures have greatly reduced the HIV infectivity of factor VIII concentrates but, as yet, not enough is known about the optimum heat treatment regimes to be certain that they are completely safe. Heat

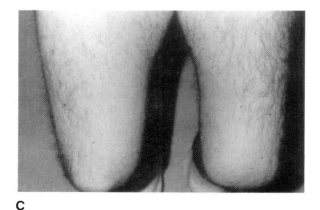

C

Fig. 80.3 Acute haemarthrosis – see page 1376.

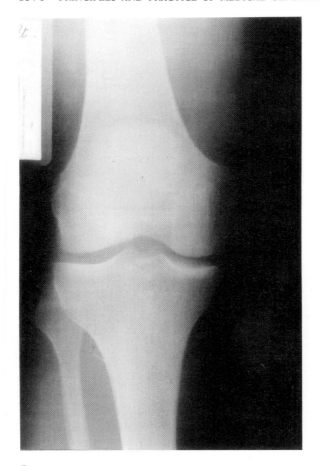

D

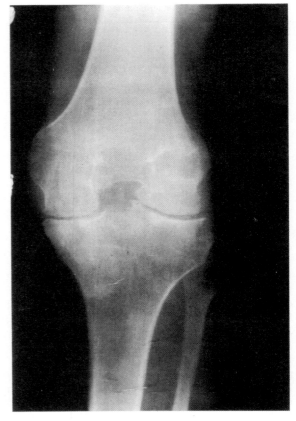

E

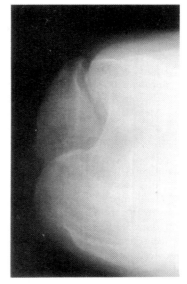

F

Fig. 80.3 Acute haemarthrosis **A**. Chronic haemophilic arthropathy particularly of left knee demonstrating enlargement of femoral condyles **B** with associated quadriceps wasting **C**. Radiographs of right **D** and left **E** knees of the same individual illustrating rarefaction, enlargement of condyles and intercondylar notch and loss of cartilage along with degeneration of the patello-femoral surface **F**.

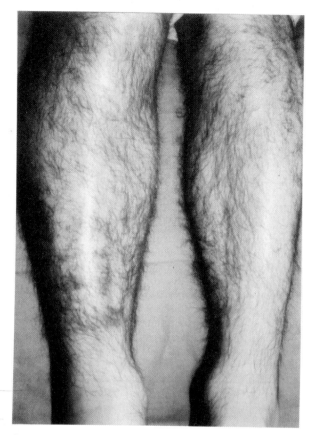

A

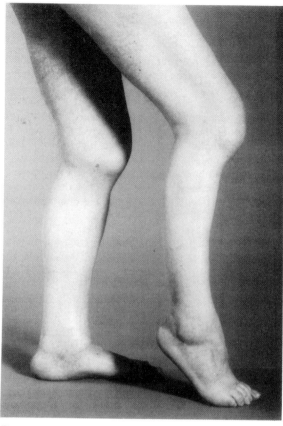

B

Fig. 80.4 Haematoma in calf **A**. If inadequately treated, ischaemic necrosis and subsequent fibrosis will ensue to give equinus deformity **B**.

also inactivates hepatitis viruses and much effort is currently being expended in developing either heat or chemical treatments that will inactivate all harmful viruses.

Between 5–10% of individuals develop antifactor VIIIC alloantibodies in response to transfusion of factor VIII concentrates. As a result subsequent factor VIII infusions are rendered much less effective, because its coagulant activity is quickly neutralised by the antifactor VIII antibody and consequently haemostasis is harder to achieve. There are other ways in which bleeding can be arrested, including the use of high dose factor VIII regimes to neutralise the inhibitor, possibly in combination with plasmapheresis to reduce the concentration of the inhibitor (Bloom 1987b). Both conventional factor IX concentrates as well as activated ones, e.g. FEIBA, have a role in treating patients, particularly those with high titre inhibitors. Porcine factor VIII is also available as a therapeutic product and may promote haemostasis.

This is often successful because the antifactor VIII antibody which develops in response to transfused human factor VIII only has limited cross reactivity with porcine factor VIII (Kernoff et al 1984).

Identification of carriers

To be able to offer genetic counselling it is first necessary to assess the likelihood that the potential woman counsellee is a carrier of the haemophilia gene. This is carried out in four separate stages. The assignment of carriership has been reviewed by Bulletin of the World Health Organisation (WHO 1977) Barrai and Cann (1982) and Graham (1987).

Verification of diagnosis Because the term 'haemophilia' is used sometimes rather loosely in connection with an individual with any congenital bleeding disorder, it is necessary to obtain a full history of the bleeding episodes of affected members of the family. Particular attention should be paid to the type of bleeding to ascertain whether it is characteristic of haemophilia, e.g. into large joints and muscles. An indication of its severity can often be obtained from the history, e.g. whether bleeding is 'spontaneous' or post-traumatic. It is essential to have documentary evidence that affected family members have haemophilia A and not some other congenital bleeding disorder. In severe haemophilia it may be reasonable to accept that absence of bleeding in a male family member implies he does not have haemophilia. In moderate and mild haemophilia it is highly desirable to test as many male family members as possible, as some may be affected by haemophilia but remain asymptomatic. It is also important to be certain of the degree of severity as this will greatly influence the desire for prenatal diagnosis.

Pedigree A full family tree should be carefully drawn up showing known affected individuals as well as those who have been tested and shown to be normal. In approximately one third of families there is no preceding affected male. This may arise either because the mutant gene has passed through females only for several generations, or because the mother is a new mutant. If a new mutant all her cells may be heterozygous for the haemophilia gene (true carrier), or only the ovum which gave rise to the affected son may have carried the mutation (mother not a carrier). It has been estimated that the spontaneous mutation rate is quite high, $1.3–4.2 \times 10^{-5}$ (Barrai et al 1968).

In the pedigree it is useful first to identify obligate carriers of the haemophilia gene. An obligate carrier can be defined as a woman who has:

1. two sons with haemophilia (provided they are not identical twins!); or
2. one son and a maternal male relative with haemophilia; or
3. father with haemophilia.

If the counsellee is not an obligate carrier the likelihood of her being a carrier can be calculated on the basis of established carriers having a 50% chance of a son being affected and a 50% chance of a daughter being a carrier. The prior probability that a female may be a carrier may be modified depending upon whether she has one or more normal sons, and this can be quantitated with Bayes theorem (Barrai & Cann 1972). For example, if a counsellee has had six normal sons without haemophilia it is very unlikely that she is a carrier!

Phenotype studies A female carrier is heterozygous for the haemophilia gene and on average her factor VIIIC level will be 50% of normal. (It is important to remember that there are other causes of reduced factor VIIIC levels (Table 80.5).) During embryogenesis random inactiva-

Table 80.5 Congenital causes of reduced plasma factor VIIIC levels

Haemophilia A
Carrier of haemophilia A
von Willebrand disease
Combined factor V and VIII deficiency
Deletions, inversions, translocations of X chromosome
    (Samama et al 1977)
Phenotypic females possessing a single X chromosome
which contains the haemophilia gene:
    Mosaicism (46,XX/45,X) (Gilchrist et al 1965)
    Turner syndrome (45,X) only reported to date for
    haemophilia B (Bithell et al 1970)

tion of one of each pair of X chromosomes occurs (Lyonisation). If in a particular female carrier by chance inactivation occurs of more of the X chromosomes carrying the normal gene then her factor VIIIC level will be further reduced. Although it is possible to give a probability of carriership using the factor VIIIC level alone it is much more informative to express it as a ratio to the vWFAg concentration. To do this it is first necessary to assess factor VIIIC:vWFAg ratios in a population of obligate carriers and normal females and this should be carried out for each centre offering genetic counselling (Fig. 80.5) (Zimmerman et al 1971, Peake et al 1981). The probability of carriership estimated from the phenotypic studies can be combined with that from the prior probability derived from the family tree to give an overall assessment of the likelihood of carriership. It should be noted that a normal factor VIIIC:vWFAg ratio does not exclude carriership. Additionally, a carrier may have a substantially reduced factor VIIIC level and may as a consequence have a mild bleeding disorder. Treatment with factor VIII concentrate, or preferably DDVP, may be required to cover operative surgery.

Genotype studies Haemophilia A and B were the first common congenital disorders for which gene probes became available to help with carrier assignment and prenatal diagnosis. Haemophilia A is a very heterogeneous disorder with many different genetic mutations resulting in a reduction in the plasma factor VIIIC level. If haemophilia were due to a single uniform gene defect, as in sickle-cell disease, it would be possible to use a specific oligonucleotide probe to track the haemophilia gene within all families. To date many different individual gene mutations have been reported. In some of these it is possible to use probes which detect a base change or deletion, but this requires prior knowledge of the individual genetic defect in the particular family. As this is not available for the majority of families use must be made of

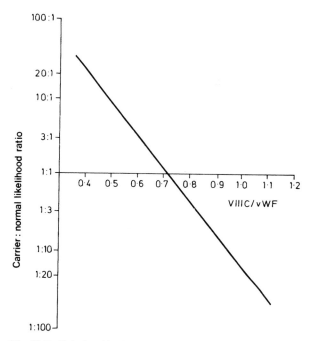

Fig 80.5 Relationship between factor VIIIC:vWF ratio and likelihood of carriership in haemophilia A (adapted from Peake et al 1981, with permission).

Genotype assignment

A 'final' probability that the counsellee is a carrier is calculated from knowledge of the prior probability derived from the pedigree, the phenotypic data using factor VIIIC:vWFAg and gene tracking with the aid of RFLPs either using linked or genomic probes.

With the knowledge of the final probability the counsellor is in a position to inform the counsellee of this information, along with appropriate interpretation. It is necessary to give a slow clear explanation of the situation, and of the possible options open to the woman if she has a high probability of being a carrier. In most instances it is appropriate to offer prenatal diagnosis for individuals with severe haemophilia, as moderate and mild disease do not result in great hardship to the affected individuals. One of the added advantages of using gene probes, particularly those that are intragenic, is that it may be possible to state with a high degree of certainty that a counsellee is not a carrier. Prior to the introduction of gene probes it was often not possible to give such firm reassurance. Such information is not only very acceptable to the woman but it avoids the necessity for prenatal diagnosis.

Prenatal diagnosis

A woman with a high probability of being a carrier may wish to consider the possibility of prenatal diagnosis. Until gene probes became available, this was undertaken as a two stage process. The fetal sex was determined by amniocentesis at about 16 weeks' gestation. If male, a fetal blood sample could be procured at about 19–20 weeks, and the factor VIIIC or VIIIAg measured to ascertain whether it was affected by haemophilia. Although this method for prenatal diagnosis is reliable and safe it may result in a therapeutic termination half-way through the pregnancy, a situation which is distressing to the woman and her family (Firshein et al 1979, Mibashan et al 1980, Ljung et al 1982, Mibashan et al 1982).

The introduction of gene probes has brought forward the time of diagnosis to about 10 weeks' gestation. Between 8 and 9 weeks a chorionic villus sample is obtained under ultrasound control. Following extraction of the fetal DNA a sample is digested by an appropriate endonuclease and Southern blotted with an appropriate probe. It is essential to choose an RFLP for which the mother is heterozygous and which has been informative in other appropriate family members. As before it is clearly more reliable to use an intragenic probe than a linked one because of the inherent 5–10% recombination rate. This technique of prenatal chorionic villus sampling is proving to be reliable and safe in skilled hands.

restriction fragment length polymorphisms (RFLPs). These are polymorphic changes in DNA which affect the fragment pattern seen after digestion of DNA with a particular restriction enzyme (endonuclease) and probing with a suitable DNA probe (Table 80.6). A polymorphic site can be situated either within the haemophilia gene (intragenic) or adjacent (linked or extragenic). If a linked probe is used there is a risk of recombination during meiosis between the RFLP site and the haemophilia gene, resulting in misclassification of the individual or fetus. The use, therefore, of an intragenic probe gives a more reliable result.

Although it is desirable to use intragenic probes these are only informative for a particular woman if she is heterozygous for the RFLP, i.e. the haemophilia gene can be associated with one of the alleles; most RFLPs are simple two allelic systems. If a woman is homozygous for an intragenic allelic site then it will be necessary to use a probe linked to the haemophilia gene provided this site is heterozygous. Of the available linked probes DX13 and ST14 have been most extensively studied. A recombination rate of approximately 5% between the allelic site and the haemophilia gene has been observed; thus these probes will give a false result on approximately 1 in 20 occasions.

Table 80.6 Factor VIII and IX intragenic and extragenic polymorphisms

	Endonuclease	Allelic fragments	Ref.
Factor VIII			
Intragenic			
Probe C	Bgl 1	20/5	Antonarakis et al 1985b
p114.12	Bcl 1	1.2/0.9	Gitschier et al 1985
p486.2	Xba 1	6.2/4.8	Wion et al 1986
		6.2/1.4	
F8-e16/19	Hind III	2.6/2.7	Ahrens et al 1987
Extragenic			
DX13	Bgl II	5.8/2.8	Harper et al 1984
ST14	Taq 1	Multiple	Oberle et al 1985
p625.5	Msp 1	7.5/4.3 & 2.3	Youssoufian et al 1987
Factor IX			
Intragenic			
Probe VIII	Taq 1	1.8/1.3	Giannelli et al 1984
Probe VIII	Xmn 1	11.5/6.5	Winship et al 1984
Probe XIII	Dde 1	1.75/1.7	Winship et al 1984
	Msp 1		Camerino et al 1985
	BamH1	25/23	Hay et al 1986
Extragenic			
DXS99	Pst 1	5.4/3.4	Mulligan et al 1985

Haemophilia B

Haemophilia B is an X-linked recessive disorder distinct from haemophilia A. Its prevalence is approximately one fifth that of haemophilia A. Haemophilia B is due to a deficiency of factor IXC, a vitamin K dependent coagulation factor synthesised by the liver (Bertina & Veltkamp 1987). It forms part of the intrinsic system in the coagulation cascade where it is activated by factor XIa. Factor IXa interacts with thrombin activated factor VIII, platelet membrane or phospholipid and calcium to activate factor X. A larger proportion of patients with Christmas disease than haemophilia A have circulating factor IXAg levels significantly in excess of factor IXC activity. The molecular abnormalities have been subdivided into several subgroups depending upon the activity/antigen ratio and function of the defective molecules (Brownlee 1987). One subgroup, Leyden variant, is of particular interest because as children the factor IXC level is <0.01 iu/ml but after puberty this rises by 0.04–0.05 iu/ml per annum (Veltkamp et al 1970, Briet et al 1982). Other variants have been studied in great detail and the structural and functional abnormalities defined (Bertina & Veltkamp 1987).

The factor IX gene is located on the X chromosome some distance from the factor VIII locus. It has been well characterised and consists of 34 kb and 8 exons (Anson et al 1984). A wide variety of different mutations have been described ranging from single base changes to extensive deletions.

Bleeding episodes are treated with fresh frozen plasma or, more usually, factor IX concentrate. This is prepared using cryoprecipitate supernatant from which the vitamin K dependent clotting factors are absorbed. Like factor VIII therapeutic products, this concentrate transmits viral infections, although HIV seems not to be transmitted so effectively since a lower proportion of individuals are infected with the virus. The development of antifactor IX antibodies is rare, being much less common than in haemophilia A.

Carrier assignment

On average the factor IXC level in carriers of haemophilia B is 0.5 iu/ml but because of the large variation in normal and carrier plasma factor IX concentrations this measurement alone is of limited value in assigning carriership. Use of the factor IXC:IXAg ratio does not offer any advantage in discriminating between normals and carriers. This is because in haemophilia B approximately half the patients have a parallel reduction in activity and antigen and hence the ratio will be similar in carriers and normals (Graham et al 1979).

Detection of carriers and prenatal diagnosis can be undertaken with much greater confidence using RFLPs (Table 80.6), probes that detect substantial deletions (Peake et al 1984), or methods that otherwise uniquely identify the abnormal gene (Bottema et al 1989).

Von Willebrand's disease

This condition was first described by von Willebrand in 1926 when he reported a clinical syndrome of excessive mucous membrane bleeding and prolonged bleeding times in the inhabitants of the Aland Islands at the mouth of the gulf of Bosnia (Coller 1987). The disease is due to a deficiency of a protein now known as the von Willebrand factor (vWF) which is synthesised by vascular endothelial cells and megakaryocytes. The gene coding for the protein is located on chromosome 12. The protein is synthesised as a pre-pro-von Willebrand factor. After removal of the pre or signal peptide the pro-von Willebrand factor forms dimers by interchain disulphide bonds at the carboxy terminal ends. The pro (or von Willebrand antigen II) peptide allows the dimers to polymerise by interchain disulphide bonds at the amino terminal end to form a series of multimers, after which the pro-peptides are removed and either secreted or stored in the endothelial cell Weibel-Palade bodies for later release induced by appropriate stimuli. vWF possesses receptors for factor VIII, platelet glycoprotein Ib and IIb/IIIa, collagen and heparin. It therefore acts as a carrier protein for factor VIII, to which it is bound non-covalently, as well as a bridge between activated platelets and subendothelial structures to promote adhesion of platelets to damaged vessel walls. Furthermore, in vitro, it supports ristocetin induced platelet aggregation, a useful test for the diagnosis and classification of the vWD variants. These variants have been classified in a number of different ways and the reader is referred to detailed descriptions elsewhere (Ruggeri 1987).

In summary, Type I variants are dominantly inherited and all molecular weight multimers are present in the plasma, although the largest ones may occur in reduced amounts. In Type II vWD there is a lack of high molecular weight multimers and most forms are dominantly inherited. Two of these variants are of particular interest. In Type IIB the platelets are unusually sensitive to aggregation by ristocetin, due to binding of the abnormal high molecular weight multimers to platelets. These platelets are cleared prematurely from the circulation resulting in thrombocytopenia. DDAVP infusion, which preferentially releases large molecular weight multimers from endothelial cells, may be followed by thrombocytopenia. A similar condition known as platelet type, or pseudo-von Willebrand's disease, has been reported. In this disorder the platelets are abnormal, having an increased affinity for high molecular weight vWF multimers. These platelets are also more sensitive to ristocetin induced aggregation and some individuals may be thrombocytopenic. Type III von Willebrand disease is autosomal recessive and both the factor VIII and vWF are

very low. Such individuals may have haemophilic type bleeding with haemarthroses as well as bruising and the usual vWD type mucosal haemorrhage. Parents are usually symptomless, although they may have slightly reduced vWFAg levels. Some of these individuals may in fact be double heterozygotes.

Factor V deficiency

Factor V, after activation by thrombin, acts as a cofactor in the conversion of prothrombin to thrombin by factor Xa in the presence of platelets and calcium. It is also stored in platelet granules from which it is liberated during the release reaction, becoming attached to a specific cell surface receptor where it interacts with other components of the coagulation cascade. There is structural and functional homology between factors V and VIII.

The deficiency is rare and is inherited as an autosomal recessive disorder (Owren 1947). Homozygous patients have haemorrhagic symptoms and occasionally heterozygotes may have mild symptoms if the factor V level is below the normal range (Mittersteiler et al 1978). Study of this deficiency has been hampered by lack of precipitating anti-sera to the protein but using neutralising antibodies some patients appear to have protein concentration in excess of activity. Clinically patients experience bruising, expistaxis and menorrhagia, but muscle haematoma and haemarthroses are rare. Some families have a combined deficiency of factors V and VIII (see below under Combined deficiencies).

Prothrombin deficiency

Prothrombin is converted to thrombin by factor Xa in the presence of factor Va, calcium and platelets. The thrombin formed not only converts fibrinogen to fibrin but also activates factor XIII (which crosslinks and stabilises fibrin), factors V and VIII and is a potent aggregator of platelets. It thus has multiple procoagulant activities.

Deficiencies of prothrombin are probably the most rare of all coagulation disorders (Owen et al 1978), about half are hypoprothrombinaemias and half dysprothrombinaemias. The normal prothrombin molecule may be present in a number of allelic forms, all with equivalent function (Board et al 1982). Diagnosis of a prothrombin deficiency is usually suspected in an individual with a long prothrombin time in which the other components of the extrinsic system are normal. The prothrombin activity can be quantitated either using a one stage assay with prothrombin deficient plasma or with a prothrombin converting snake venom (Jobin & Esnouf 1966). The protein can be measured immunologically, and the integrity of the carboxyglutamyl residues assessed by binding to inorganic absorbants. One interesting feature of some of the variants is that each parent appears to have a different abnormal molecule, and the proband is therefore a double heterozygote (Girolami et al 1978).

Clinically only homozygotes, or double heterozygotes, experience bleeding with excessive bruising, mucous membrane bleeding and menorrhagia. Haemarthroses do not occur.

Factor X deficiency

Factor X is at the convergent point for the intrinsic and extrinsic pathways. It is activated by factors IXa, VIIIa, calcium and platelets (intrinsic system) and factor VIIa (extrinsic system). Deficiencies are very uncommon and poorly characterised (Eastman et al 1983). Some cases arise from consanguineous parents and are therefore presumed homozygotes. Heterozygotes are usually symptomless but homozygotes may develop haemarthroses and spontaneous intracranial and intraspinal haemorrhage.

Factor VII deficiency

Factor VII is activated by tissue thromboplastin but this can also be brought about by factors Xa and XIIa as well as kallikrein. Factor VIIa, as well as activating factor X, will also activate factor IX. Thus the concept of separate intrinsic and extrinsic parts of the cascade is an over-simplification of the overall mechanism. Like factor X abnormalities, deficiencies of factor VII are poorly characterised (Mariani & Mazzucconi 1983). Homozygous patients may have a life-long bleeding disorder, although some individuals do not present until early adult life. Haemorrhagic symptoms may appear in the neonatal period with intracranial bleeds. There is a poor relationship between factor VII levels and the haemorrhagic state.

Combined deficiencies

The vitamin K dependent clotting factors II, VII, IX and X all have homology and glutamylcarboxyl residues. Apart from factor IX they are autosomally inherited.

Combined deficiencies of factors have been reported, e.g. factor VII and IX (Girolami et al 1980). A deficiency of all four factors has occurred but this may have resulted from a defect in the glutamylcarboxylation reaction (Johnson et al 1980). Combined deficiencies of factor V and VIII have been described and both are transmitted autosomally together in affected family members. Controversy surrounds the mechanism, and also the nature of the factor VIII deficiency and whether it is

combined with an equivalent reduction in vWFAg (Giddings et al 1977, Graham 1980).

Fibrinogen

Fibrinogen is a glycoprotein of molecular weight 340 000 daltons consisting of three pairs of homologous poly-peptide chains covalently linked through disulphide bonds (Doolittle 1984). Fibrinogen and fibrin interact with many plasma proteins at specific binding sites. The proteins include thrombin, plasminogen, α_2 antiplasmin, tissue plasminogen activator, factor XIII as well as activated platelets where the receptor is glycoprotein IIb/IIIa.

The conversion of fibrinogen to fibrin proceeds by a complex series of reactions initiated by thrombin, which cleaves fibrinopeptide A from the A chain and fibrino-peptide B from the B chain. The resultant fibrin mon-omers polymerise, and in the presence of the transglutaminase activity of thrombin activated factor XIII adjacent lysine and glutamate residues are covalently linked. This crosslinking of the monomers gives considerable strength to the fibrin clot and this is protected from lysis by the binding of α_2 antiplasmin to fibrin by factor XIIIa. The deposited fibrinogen is further strengthened by the adhesion of platelets in which the fibrinogen binds to glycoprotein IIb/IIIa and also by fibronectin which crosslinks with fibrin in the presence of factor XIIIa.

Plasma fibrinogen is synthesised in the liver and megakaryocytes and is present in platelet granules. It remains uncertain whether this is under the same genetic control as plasma fibrinogen with which it does not exchange. Fibrinogen is an acute phase reactant as its plasma concentration rises from its normal level of 1.5–4 g/dl in response to inflammation, trauma and pregnancy. In liver disease, especially with cirrhosis or hepatoma, the sialic acid content is greater and this may impair its function.

To date more than 150 different abnormalities of fibrinogen have been reported, ranging from simple amino acid substitutions to deletions and insertions. It is likely, as fibrinogen is a large protein, that there are many silent mutations that do not modify its function. A plethora of terms has developed to describe the type of fibrinogen abnormality based on its function and plasma concentration. The apparent concentration may depend upon whether this is measured by a functional or immunological assay. It is probably most appropriate to refer to all variants as congenital dysfibrinogenaemia even when the molecule is apparently normal but merely present in reduced concentration.

Amino acid substitutions within the first 16 residues of the A chain are particularly likely to produce clinical symptoms because the release of fibrinopeptide A by thrombin is delayed, e.g. fibrogen Rouen (A Gly_{12}-Val) or Bice +ve (A Arg_{16}-His), this being at the cleavage site with thrombin, resulting in delayed FpA release.

Others have abnormalities resulting in impaired interaction with other plasma proteins. In fibrinogen New York I (B 9–72 deletion) neither thrombin nor plasminogen bind well, resulting in both decreased release of FpA and fibrinolysis. Most congenital dysfibrinogenaemias are associated with delayed FpA release and fibrin monomer polymerisation and some are associated with recurrent thrombosis. An interesting exception is fibrinogen Oslo I in which the thrombin time is short due to faster than normal fibrin monomer polymerisation (and platelet aggregation to ADP is also enhanced).

The majority of patients are heterozygotes, having both a normal and abnormal molecule present in the plasma, and hence haemorrhagic symptoms are not severe; these usually only appear when the fibrinogen concentration falls below 1 g/dl. In fibrinogen Detroit, homozygotes bleed easily whereas heterozygotes are asymptomatic. Clinical manifestations are similar to factor XIII deficiency and include prolonged bleeding of the umbilical stump, intracranial haemorrhage and recurrent spontaneous abortions.

Diagnosis of a dysfibrinogenaemia is usually suspected in a patient with long thrombin or reptilase time, with or without a discrepancy between fibrinogen concentration assayed functionally or immunologically.

Factor XIII

Polymerisation of fibrin monomers is brought about by the transglutaminase action of factor XIII which links lysine and arginine residues on adjacent chains of fibrin (McDonagh 1987). This crosslinking enhances the mechanical strength of the clot as well as making it more resistant to digestion by plasmin. Factor XIII consists of a tetramer comprising two A and two B chains; thrombin activates the A peptide and this subunit possesses the catalytic site for the transglutaminase reaction. As well as crosslinking fibrin monomers, factor XIII will crosslink fibrinogen, but at a much slower rate, as well as fibronectin to both fibrin and collagen, thus increasing the binding of the developing clot to the vessel wall. Platelet cytosol contains factor XIII and this may serve to crosslink fibrin to the platelet contractile proteins actin and myosin.

In factor XIII deficiency there is an almost complete deficiency of A subunits with B subunits being reduced in concentration in the plasma. In some individuals platelet factor XIII is also reduced. The disorder is inherited as a recessive, with consanguinity being common. Bleeding can be moderate to severe with delayed healing being

characteristic. This arises because clots do not become mechanically strong through lack of crosslinking not only with fibrin but also with fibrinonectin, collagen and possibly platelets. Following trauma, bleeding may stop, only to restart after 24–36 hours; this results in poor wound healing and subsequent scarring. Bleeding within the central nervous system and spontaneous abortions are common. Soft tissue haematoma and joint haemarthrosis do occur but usually only after trauma. Homozygous females may suffer from recurrent abortions. Treatment can be with plasma, cryoprecipitate or factor XIII concentrates – this being heat treated to reduce the possibility of transmitting hepatitis or HIV. Because of its long half life of 8 days and because symptoms are rare over 5% normal plasma level, many patients can be successfully managed by monthly prophylactic injections.

Disorders of contact activation (Factors XII, XI, Prekallikrein, High Molecular Weight Kininogen)

A complex sequence of reactions between the components of the contact system may not only initiate the coagulation cascade but may also result in activation of the complement system, fibrinolysis and modification of blood pressure and tissue permeability by release of bradykinin (Schmaier et al 1987).

Factor XII, after binding to negatively charged surfaces, probably including subendothelial vessel wall components, is autocatalytically activated to a serine protease (Tang 1987). This in turn activates factor XI and prekallikrein, particularly when these are bound to high molecular weight kininogen (HMWK). The factor XI-HMWF-prekallikrein complexes bind tightly to negatively charged surfaces after HMWK has been activated by factor XIIa (Mannhalter 1987). Hence activated factor XII can interact with factor XI to give factor XIa, prekallikrein to produce kallikrein, as well as activate factor VII and the first component of complement. Although it would appear that these four factors are apparently pivotal in initiating coagulation, complement and fibrinolytic systems, deficiencies of factor XII, prekallikrein and HMWK are asymptomatic, while only a lack of factor XI results in a bleeding disorder. These activated components of the contact system are inhibited principally by CI-inhibitor, although antithrombin III, β_2 macroglobulin and α_1 antitrypsin also inhibit.

Factor XII (Hageman factor)

Autoactivation of this single chain polypeptide is observed when it binds to negatively charged surfaces; in vivo this may be to subendothelial components and in vitro by kaolin. A series of activation peptides are produced that catalytically activate prekallikrein to kallikrein, factor XI to XIa, and factor VII to VIIa. CI-inhibitor inhibits the factor XII activation peptide, as does antithrombin III.

A deficiency of factor XII may be asymptomatic, although Mr Hageman died of a pulmonary embolus and patients have been described with myocardial infarction. Deficient patients have no clinical stigmata of a haemorrhagic diathesis nor defective complement or fibrinolytic systems.

Factor XII deficiency is inherited as a recessive disorder. Heterozygotes, however, have a bimodal distribution of factor XII levels suggesting the presence of two alleles controlling the production of the factor (Veltkamp et al 1965). In the majority of patients there is a parallel reduction in activity and protein concentration although a few patients have been described with a non-functional protein.

Factor XI

In plasma most factor XI is bound to HMWK to give a bimolecular complex and can be activated by factor XIIa. Furthermore, as well as the HMWK bringing factor XI into close proximity with XIIa, it also protects it from inactivation by α_1 antitrypsin and antithrombin IIi.

In congenital deficiency of factor XI the majority of patients have an equivalent reduction in protein and activity levels. A bleeding state may be observed, but its clinical severity is not closely related to plasma concentration; many individuals are asymptomatic and in some the symptoms vary over a period of time (Rimon et al 1976).

It is probably recessively inherited as an incompletely recessive autosomal gene. Homozygotes have factor XI levels of <20% normal and may have haemorrhagic symptoms (Rapaport et al 1961). Heterozygotes are asymptomatic. The disorder is found most commonly in Ashkenazi Jews, where a homozygosity rate of 0.1–0.3% has been observed.

Prekallikrein (Fletcher factor)

Like factor XI, prekallikrein circulates bound to HMWK and is activated by factor XIIa to kallikrein. This, in turn, releases bradykinin from HMWK and plasmin from plasminogen, although in quantitative terms it is only a weak activator of the fibrinolytic system. Its activity is inhibited by CI-inhibitor and to a lesser extent β_2 macroglobulin and antithrombin III.

In most deficiencies detected by finding a prolonged APTT, the activity of the prekallikrein is less than the protein concentration, suggesting the presence of an inactive molecule (Hathaway et al 1965). Affected individuals, in whom it is inherited as a recessive disorder, have no symptoms referable to their haemostatic or fibrinolytic systems or inflammatory responses.

High molecular weight kininogen (HMWK) (Fitzgerald factor)

High molecular weight kininogen acts as a carrier for factor XI and prekallikrein. When acted upon by factor XIIa it binds tightly to negatively charged surfaces (Schmaier et al 1987). By this mechanism it brings factor XIIa, factor XI and prekallikrein into close proximity and so enhances their rate of activation. Prekallikrein is converted to kallikrein, which in turn liberates bradykinin from HMWK. This may increase tissue permeability resulting in extravasation of fluids.

Individuals who are deficient in HMWK are asymptomatic and are only detected because they have prolonged APTTs. It is inherited as a recessive disorder.

CI-inhibitor

This is an important inhibitor of activated products of the contact system, particularly kallikrein. A lack of this protein results in episodic severe oedema: of pharynx or larynx producing dyspnoea; of gastrointestinal tract causing severe abdominal pain and vomiting; or of skin causing periorbital oedema. Increased permeability is caused by excess activity of kallikrein releasing bradykinin from HMWK. Treatment of the acute attacks is with fresh frozen plasma; anabolic steroids or cyclokapron may be taken prophylactically to prevent attacks. It is dominantly inherited.

PLATELET DISORDERS

The mechanisms by which platelets promote haemostasis have been outlined in the introduction to this chapter. Congenital disorders of membrane glycoproteins, both alpha and delta storage granules (and release of their contents) as well as enzymopathies in the pathway leading from archidonate to thromboxane A_2 have all been described (Rao & Holmsen 1986). The severity of the resultant clinical manifestations is variable even within an apparently single disorder. For example, in Glanzmann thrombasthenia some individuals have only minimal bruising whilst others have spontaneous chronic persistent and recurrent bleeds which can be life threatening.

With increasingly sensitive techniques for studying the biochemistry of platelets it is becoming clear that at the molecular level there may be heterogeneity of the basic underlying biochemical defect. Congenital thrombocytopenias, both with and without platelet biochemical or structural abnormalities have been described, again these are a very heterogeneous group of disorders with variable clinical presentations and modes of inheritance.

Investigation of a patient with a possible platelet disorder usually begins with a whole blood platelet count, blood film, and exclusion of a coagulation disorder, particularly von Willebrand's disease (see above). The template bleeding time is a useful measure of the overall effectiveness of the platelet-vWF-vessel wall interaction in vivo and, if prolonged in the presence of a normal platelet count, usually indicates the presence of a platelet disorder or von Willebrand's disease. Platelets can be separated from red cells by differential centrifugation, and their ability to aggregate in response to ADP, adrenaline, collagen, ristocetin and arachidonate assessed. The response is usually described as occurring in two sequential phases, primary aggregation in which platelets clump together, and secondary aggregation which follows the release of proaggregatory granule constituents, e.g. ADP, into the surrounding milieu. Further investigation is determined by the results of the aggregation tracings but may include analysis of membrane glycoproteins, measurement of granule constituents and their release and metabolism of archidonic acid.

Clinical symptomatology

Bleeding occurs predominantly onto mucocutaneous surfaces, e.g. superficial bruising, gastrointestinal haemorrhage, epistaxis or menorrhagia. Some patients will have persistent chronic recurrent bleeds, but others will have minimal or no symptoms except after surgery.

Disorders of membrane glycoproteins

Thrombasthenia

Originally described in 1918 by Glanzmann, thrombasthenia is a heterogenous group of disorders with varying degrees of deficiency of the glycoprotein IIb/IIIa on the platelet surface (Nurden & Caen 1974, Nurden et al 1985). These glycoproteins act as receptors for fibrinogen, vWF, thrombospondin and fibronectin, the former three being actively secreted by the platelet during the release reaction. Platelet count and morphology are normal but the platelets fail to aggregate to ADP, adrenaline, collagen and thrombin, but do so in response to ristocetin.

The condition is an autosomal recessive disorder; consanguinity among parents of reported cases is common, suggesting that affected individuals are homozygous for the genetic abnormality. Heterozygotes have reduced membrane glycoprotein IIb/IIIa concentration but are usually asymptomatic.

Bernard-Soulier syndrome

The initial description was of a 5-month-old infant with severe bleeding from mucous membranes whose older sister had died from haemorrhage at 2 years of age (Bernard & Soulier 1948). The disorder is characterised by thrombocytopenia with abnormally large platelets on the blood film and a prolonged bleeding time. Aggregation is normal except to ristocetin. The initial reports of the glycoproteins demonstrated a lack of Ib but more recent studies suggest deficiencies also of glycoprotein V and IX (Clemetson et al 1982).

The condition is inherited as an autosomal recessive; glycoprotein abnormalities may be detectable in the parents of an affected individual.

Disorders of granule contents and their release

The alpha and delta storage granules may either have reduced levels of their constituents (storage pool disorder) or be unable to release their contents (release or aspirin like defect) (Weiss 1987). These abnormalities may occur as the only congenital abnormality or as part of a much more extensive congenital condition, e.g. thrombocytopenia with absent radius (TAR) syndrome (Table 80.7). Acquired disorders of the granules can also be observed during cardiopulmonary bypass and in leukaemias. Bleeding characteristic of a platelet disorder is observed but in most instances this is not severe and is usually only troublesome after trauma or surgery.

Treatment of congenital platelet disorders

The essence of treating individuals with congenital platelet disorders is to avoid, as far as possible, the use of platelet transfusions. This is because multiply transfused patients develop anti-HLA alloantibodies which may render subsequent therapy less effective. Furthermore, if a membrane glycoprotein is missing, e.g. in Bernard-Soulier syndrome or thrombasthenia, alloimmunisation to the absent glycoprotein may occur, again greatly reducing the value of subsequent platelet therapy (Levy-Toledano et al 1978). Therefore platelet transfusion should be avoided if at all possible. Other ways of preventing excessive bleeding include good preventive dental care to avoid the necessity for extractions and careful attention to haemostasis during surgery. For external surgery, e.g. dental or lymph node biopsy, a

Table 80.7 Platelet storage pool and release disorders

Granule disorders	Inheritance	Other features
Familial	Dominant	May be associated with granule deficiency.
Hermansky-Pudlak	Recessive	Tyrosine positive occulocutaneous albinism. Pigment accumulation in macrophages.
Chediak-Higashi	Recessive	Occulocutaneous albinism. Recurrent pyogenic infections. Large abnormal granules in polymorphs.
Wiscott-Aldrich	Recessive	Small platelets. Thrombocytopenia IgM deficiency. Recurrent infections. Eczema.
TAR Syndrome	Recessive	Thrombocytopenia. Absent radii.
Gray platelet	Recessive	Large amorphous platelets. Fibrosis in marrow.

fibrinolytic inhibitor may be useful. Menorrhagia may be controlled by the contraceptive pill. Recent reports have demonstrated that cryoprecipitate or even DDAVP may be valuable.

CONGENITAL PLASMA ABNORMALITIES PREDISPOSING TO THROMBOSIS

Congenital deficiencies of inhibitors of the coagulation cascade, e.g. antithrombin III and protein C, predispose to venous thrombosis. Elevated levels of certain coagulation factors, e.g. fibrinogen and factor VII, predispose to arterial thrombosis and the concentrations of these components of the cascade are genetically controlled. Other congenital disorders, not related to abnormalities of plasma proteins may be associated with recurrent thrombosis, e.g. homocysteinuria, in which there is a vessel wall abnormality.

Antithrombin III

Antithrombin III inhibits the activity of factors XIIa, XIa, IXa, Xa and IIa; heparin greatly potentiates its neutralisation of the latter three proteins. A modest deficiency, 40–70% of normal levels, predisposes to venous thrombosis (Egeberg 1965). In most subjects there is a parallel reduction in both activity and antigen but in some variants, e.g. ATIII Budapest (Sas et al 1975), the protein is present in normal concentrations but with reduced activity. Major venous thrombosis is rare before the age of 20 but by the age of 50 years about 50% of affected individuals will have developed symptoms. Thrombosis may first present during pregnancy or in relation to illness or trauma. Treatment is with oral anticogulants in individuals who have had a thrombotic episode. During early pregnancy it is prudent to avoid warfarin because of its teratogenic effects. Therapeutic concentrates of antithrombin III are available to treat individuals at times when they may be particularly vulnerable to thrombosis, e.g. late pregnancy and during delivery. The condition is transmitted as an autosomal dominant disorder.

Proteins C and S

Both protein C and S are vitamin K dependent factors, synthesised by the liver, which have gamma glutamylcarboxyl residues similar to factors II, VII, IX and X. These acidic residues are essential for the proteins to bind, via calcium bridges, to negatively charged surfaces, e.g. platelets, maximising the enzymic interaction with other haemostatic factors. Oral anticoagulation inhibits gamma glutamylcarboxylation and the resultant molecule is functionally inert.

Protein C is activated by thrombin; the reaction being considerably further enhanced by thrombin activated thrombomodulin which is found on endothelial cell membranes.

Clinically, protein C deficiency (Griffin et al 1981) is similar to ATIII deficiency except that in addition a number of cases of neonatal purpura fulmanans and warfarin induced skin necrosis have been reported. Treatment of symptomatic individuals is with long-term warfarin, although this should be introduced very gradually to avoid skin necrosis. The disorder is dominantly inherited.

Protein S deficiency (Comp & Esmon 1984) is clinically similar to protein C and antithrombin III deficiency except that only patients with deficiencies in the range 15–40% of normal are symptomatic. Treatment is by judicious oral anticoagulation.

REFERENCES

Ahrens P, Kruse T A, Schwartz M, Rosmussen P B, Din N 1987 A new Hind III restriction fragment length polymorphism in the haemophilia A locus. Human Genetics 76: 127–128

Anson D S, Choo K H, Rees D J G et al 1984 The gene structure of human anti-haemophilic factor IX. EMBO Journal 3: 1053

Antonarakis S T 1988 The molecular genetics of hemophilia A and B in man. Factor VIII and factor IX deficiency. Advances in Human Genetics 1: 27–59

Antonarakis S E, Waber P G, Kittur S D et al 1985a Haemophilia A: Detection of molecular defects and of carriers by DNA analysis. New England Journal of Medicine 313(14): 842–848

Antonarakis S E, Copeland K L, Carpenter R J Jr et al 1985b Prenatal diagnosis of haemophilia A by factor VIII gene analysis. Lancet 1: 1403

Antonarakis S E, Youssoufian H, Kazazian H H 1987 Molecular genetics of haemophilia A in man. Molecular Biology and Medicine 4: 81–94

Arai M, Inaba H, Higuchi M, Antonarakis S T, Kazazian H H Jr., Fujimaki M, Hoyer L W 1989 Direct characterization of factor VIII in plasma: detection of a mutation altering a thrombin cleavage site (arginine-3/2—histidine). Proceedings of the National Academy of Sciences USA 86: 4277–4281

Barrai I, Cann H M 1972 Inherited Clotting Disorders. World Health Organization Technical Report Series 504. WHO, Geneva

Barrai I, Cann H M, Cavall-Sforza L L, De Nicola P 1968 The effect of prenatal age on rate of mutation for haemophilia and evidence for differing mutation rates for hemophilia A and B. American Journal of Human Genetics 20: 175–196

Bernard J, Soulier J P 1948 Sur une nouvelle variete de dystrophie thrombocytaire hemorragipare congenitale. Semaine des Hopitaux de Paris 24: 3217

Bertina R M, Veltkamp J J 1987 Physiology and biochemistry of factor IX. In: Bloom A L, Thomas D P (eds) Haemostatsis and Thrombosis. Churchill Livingstone, Edinburgh, p 116–131

Bithell T C, Pizzaro A, Macdiarmid W B 1970 Variant of factor IX deficiency in females with 45X Turners Syndrome. Blood 36: 169–179

Bloom A L 1987a Inherited disorders of blood coagulation In: Bloom A L, Thomas D P (eds) Haemostasis and Thrombosis Churchill Livingstone, Edinburgh, p 393–437

Bloom A L 1987b Treatment of antifactor VIII inhibitors. In: Verstraete M et al (eds) Thrombosis and haemostasis. Leuven University Press p 447

Board P G, Coggan M, Pidock M E 1982 Genetic heterogeneity of human prothrombin. Annals of Human Genetics 46: 1–9

Bottema C D K, Koeberl D D, Sommer S S 1989 Direct carrier testing in 14 families with haemophilia B. Lancet 2: 526–528

Boyer S H, Graham J B 1965 Linkage between the X-chromosome loci for glucose-6 phosphate dehydrogenase electrophoretic variation and hemophilia A. American Journal of Human Genetics 17: 320–324

Briet E, Bertina R M, Tilburg N H van, Veltkamp J J 1982 Haemophilia B Leyden. A sex-linked hereditary disorder that improves after puberty. New England Journal of Medicine 306: 788–790

Brownlee G G 1987 The molecular pathology of haemophilia B. Biochemical Society Transactions 15: 1

Camerino G, Oberle I, Drayna D, Mandel J L 1985 A new Msp1 restriction fragment length polymorphism in the haemophilia B locus. Human Genetics 71: 79–81

Clemetson K J, McGregor J L, James E et al 1982 Characterisation of the platelet membrane glycoprotein abnormalities in Bernard-Soulier syndrome and comparison with normal by surface-labelling techniques and high-resolution two-dimensional gel electrophoresis. Journal of Clinical Investigation 70: 304

Coller B S 1987 von Willebrand Disease. In: Colman R W,

Hirsh J, Marder V J, Salzman E W (eds) Haemostasis and Thrombosis Lippincott Co, p 60–97

Colman R W, Marder V J, Salzman E W, Hirsh H 1987 Overview of Haemostasis. In: Colman R W, Hirsh J, Marder V J, Salzman E W (eds) Haemostasis and Thrombosis Lippincott, p 3–17

Comp P C, Esmon C T 1984 Recurrent venous thromboemoblism in patients with partial deficiency of Protein S. New England Journal of Medicine 311: 1525–1528

Crawford N, Scrutton M C 1987 Biochemistry of the blood platelet In: Bloom A L, Thomas D P (eds) Haemostasis and Thrombosis Churchill Livingstone, Edinburgh, p 47–77

Davie E W, Ratnoff O D 1964 Waterfall sequence for intrinsic blood clotting. Science 145: 1310–1311

Denson K W E, Biggs R, Haddon M E, Borrett R, Cobb K 1969 Two types of haemophilia (A^+ and A^-). A study of 48 cases. British Journal of Haematology 17: 163–171

Din N, Schwartz M, Kruse T et al 1985 Factor VIII gene-specific probe for prenatal diagnosis of haemophilia A. Lancet 1: 1446

Doolittle R F 1984 Fibrinogen and fibrin. Annual Review of Biochemistry 54: 195

Eastman J R Triplett D A, Nowakowski A R 1983 Inherited factor X deficiency. Presentation of a case with etiologic and treatment considerations. Oral Surgery 56: 461–466

Egeberg O 1965 Inherited antithrombin deficiency causing thrombophilia. Thrombosis Diathesis Haemorrhagica 13: 516

Firshein S I, Hoyer L W, Lazarchick J et al 1979 Prenatal diagnosis of classic haemophilia. New England Journal of Medicine 300: 937

Giannelli F, Choo K H, Winship P R et al 1984 Characterisation and use of an intragenic polymorphic marker for detection of carriers of haemophilia B. Lancet 1: 239–241

Giddings J C, Seligsohn U, Bloom A L 1977 Immunological studies in combined factor V and factor VIII. British Journal of Haematology 37: 257–264

Gilchrist G S, Hammond D, Mecnyk J 1965 Haemophilia A in a phenotypically normal female with XX/XO mosaicism. New England Journal of Medicine 273: 1402–1406

Girolami A, Coccheri S, Palareti G, Poggi I, Burul A, Cappellato G 1978 Prothrombin Molise: a 'new' congenital dysprothrombinemia, double heterozygosis with an abnormal prothrombin and 'true' prothrombin deficiency. Blood 52: 115–125

Girolami A, Dal B O, Zanon R, De Marco L, Cappellato G 1980 Haemophilia B with associated factor VII deficiency. A distinct variant of haemophilia B with low factor VII activity and normal factor VII antigen. Blut 40: 267–273

Gitschier J, Wood W I, Goralka T M et al 1984 Characterisation of the human factor VIII gene. Nature 312: 326

Gitschier J, Lawn R M, Rofblat F, Goldman E, Tuddenham E G D 1985 Antenatal diagnosis and carrier detection of haemophilia A using factor VIII gene probe. Lancet 1: 1093–1094

Graham J B 1980 Genetic control of factor VIII. Lancet I: 340–342

Graham J B 1987 Genetics of haemostasis In: Bloom A L, Thomas D P (eds) Haemostasis and Thrombosis. Churchill Livingstone, Edinburgh, p 494–510

Graham J B, Flyer P, Elston R C, Kasper C K 1979 Statistical study of genotype assignment (carrier detection) in hemophilia B. Thrombosis Research 15: 69–78

Griffin J H, Evatt B, Zimmerman T S et al 1981 Deficiency of protein C in congenital thrombotic disease. Journal of Clinical Investigation 68: 1370–1373

Harper K, Winter R M, Pembrey M E, Hartley D, Davies K E, Tuddenham E G D 1984 A clinically useful DNA probe closely linked to Haemophilia A. Lancet ii: 6

Hathaway W E, Belahnson L P, Hathaway H S 1965 Evidence for a new thromboplastin factor. Case report, coagulation studies and physicochemical studies Blood 26: 521

Hay C R M, Preston F E, Trigger D R, Underwood J C F 1985 Progressive liver disease in haemophilia: An understated problem. Lancet i: 1495–1498

Hay C W, Robertson K A, Young S L, Thompson A R, Grave G M, MacGillivray R T A 1986 Use of a BamH1 polymorphism in the factor IX gene for the determination of Haemophilia B carrier status. Blood 67(5): 1508–1511

Inaba H, Fujimaki M, Kazazian H H Jr., Antonarakis S T 1989 Mild hemophilia A resulting from Arg-to-Leu substitution in exon 26 of the factor VIII gene. Genetics 81: 335–338

Jobin F, Esnouf M P 1966 Coagulant activity of tiger snake (Notechis scutatus scutatus) venom. Nature 211: 873–875

Johnson C A, Chung K S, McGrath K M, Bean P E, Roberts H R 1980 Characterisation of variant prothrombin in a patient deficient in factors II, VII, IX and X. British Journal of Haematology 44: 461–469

Kernoff P B A, Thomas N D, Lilley P A, Mathews K B, Goldman E, Tuddenham E G D 1984 Porcine VIII. Blood 63: 31–41

Kernoff P B A, Lee C A, Karayiannis P, Thomas H C 1985 High risk of Non-A Non-B hepatitis after first exposure to volunteer or commercial clotting factor concentrates: effects of prophylactic immune serum globulin. British Journal of Haematology 60: 469–479

Levy-Toledano S, Tobelem G, Legrand C et al 1978 An acquired IgG antibody occurring in a thrombasthenic patient, its effect on human platelet function. Blood 51: 1065–1071

Ljung R, Holmberg L, Gustavii B, Philip J, Bang J 1982 Haemophilia A and B - two years experience of genetic counselling and prenatal diagnosis. Clinical Genetics 22: 70

McDonagh J 1987 Structure and function of factor XIII. In: Coleman R W, Hirch J, Marder V J, Salzman E W (eds) Haemostasis and Thrombosis Lippincott, p 289–300

Macfarlane R G 1964 An enzyme cascade in the blood clotting mechanism and its function as a biochemical amplifier. Nature 202: 498–499

Mannhalter C H 1987 Biochemical and functional properties of factor XI and prekallikrein. Seminars in Thrombosis and Haemostasis 13: 15–27

Mariani G, Mazzucconi M G 1983 Factor VII congenital deficiency: Clinical picture and classification of the variants. Haemostasis 13: 169–177

Mibasham R S, Rodeck C H, Furlong R A et al 1980 Dual diagnosis of prenatal haemophilia A by measurement of fetal factor VIIIC and VIIIC antigen (VIIICAg). Lancet ii: 994

Mibasham R S, Rodeck C H, Thumpston J K 1982 Prenatal diagnosis of the haemophiliacs. In: Bloom A L (ed) The Haemophilias. Churchill Livingstone, Edinburgh p 176–196

Mittersteiler G, Muller W, Geir W 1978 Congenital factor V deficiency. A family study. Scandinavian Journal of Haematology 21: 9–13

Miyoshi K, Sasaki N, Shirakami A et al 1978 Hereditary persistence of fetal haemoglobin and Xg blood group in haemophilia and von Willebrand's disease. Japanese Journal of Human Genetics 23: 268

Mulligan L M, Phillips M A, Foster-Gibson C J et al 1985 Genetic mapping of DNA segments relative to the locus for the fragile X syndrome at Xq 27.3. American Journal of Human Genetics 37: 463

Nurden A T, Caen J P 1974 An abnormal platelet glycoprotein pattern in three cases of Glanzmann's thrombasthenia. British Journal of Haematolgoy 28: 253

Nurden A T, Didry D, Kieffer N, McEver R P 1985 Residual amounts of glycoproteins IIb and IIIa may be present in the platelets of most patients with Glanzmann's thromboasthenia. Blood 65: 1021

Oberle I, Camerino G, Heilig R et al 1985 Genetic screening for haemophilia A (classic haemophilia) with a polymorphic probe. New England Journal of Medicine 312(11): 682–686

Owen C A, Henriksen R A, McDuffie F C, Mann K G 1978 Prothrombin Quick: a newly identified dysprothrombinemia. Mayo Clinic Proceedings 53: 29–33

Owren P A 1947 Parahaemophilia, haemorrhagic diathesis due to absence of a previously unknown clotting factor. Lancet 1: 446–448

Patterson M, Gitschier J, Bloomfield J et al 1989 An intronic region within the human factor VIII gene is duplicated within Xq28 and is homologous to the polymorphic locus DXS11S (767). American Journal of Human Genetics 44: 679–685

Peake I R, Bloom A L, Giddings J C, Ludlam C A 1979 An immunoradiometric assay for procoagulant factor VIII antigen: results in haemophilia, von Willebrand's disease and fetal plasma and serum. British Journal of Haematology 42: 269–281

Peake I R, Newcombe R C, Davies B L, Furlong R A, Ludlam C A, Bloom A L 1981 Carrier detection in haemophilia A by immunological measurement of factor VIII related antigen (VIII RAg) and factor VIII clotting antigen (VIII CAg). British Journal of Haematolgoy 48: 651–660

Peake I R, Furlong B L, Bloom A L 1984 Carrier detection by direct gene analysis in a family with haemophilia B (factor IX deficiency). Lancet i: 242

Rao A K, Holmsen H 1986 Congenital disorders of platelets. Seminars in Haematology 23: 102

Rapaport S I, Proctor R R, Patch M J, Yettra M 1961 The mode of inheritance of PTA deficiency. Evidence for the existence of major PTA deficiency and minor PTA deficiency. Blood 18: 149

Rimon A, Schiffman S, Feinstein D I Rapaport S I 1976 Factor XI activity and factor XI antigen in homozygous and heterozygous factor XI deficiency. Blood 48: 165

Ruggeri Z M 1987 Classification of von Willebrand Disease. In: Verstraete M et al (eds), Thrombosis and Haemostasis Leuven University Press, p 419

Samama M, Perrotez C, Houssa R, Hafsia A, Seger J 1977 Hamophile a feminine avec deletion d'une partie du bras long d'un chromosome X. Pathologie-Biologie 25, Suppl 10

Sas G, Pepper D S, Cash J D 1975 Further investigations on antithrombin III in the plasmas of patients with the abnormality of "antithrombin III-Budapest". Thrombosis Diathesis Haemorrhagica 33: 564

Schmaier A H, Silverberg M, Kaplan A P, Colman R W 1987 Contact Activation and its abnormalities. In: Colman R W, Hirsh J, Marder V J, Salzman E W (eds) Haemostosis and

Thrombosis. Lippincott, p 18–38

Tang G 1987 Structural and functional characterisation of factor XII. Seminars in Thrombosis and Haemostasis 13: 1–14

Toole J J, Kopf J L, Wozney J M et al 1984 Molecular cloning of a cDNA encoding human antihaemophilic factor. Nature 312: 342

Veltkamp J M, Demler H C, Loeliger E A 1965 Detection of heterozygotes for factors VIII, IX and XII deficiency. Thrombosis Diathesia Haemorrhagica (Suppl) 17: 181

Veltkamp J J, Meilof J, Remmelts H G, van der Vlerke D, Loeliger E A 1970 Another genetic variant of haemophilia B: haemophilia B Leyden. Scandinavian Journal of Haematology 7: 82–90

Weiss H J 1987 Inherited Disorders of Platelet Secretion In: Colman R W, Hirsh J, Marder V J, Salzman E W (eds) Haemostasis and Thrombosis Lippincott p 741–750

White J G 1987 Platelet Ultrastructure. In: Bloom A L, Thomas D P (eds) Haemostasis and Thrombosis. Churchill Livingstone, Edinburgh, p 20–47

Whittaker D L, Copeland D L, Graham J B 1962 Linkage of colour blindness to hemophilias A and B. American Journal of Human Genetics 14: 149–158

Winship P R, Anson D S, Rizza C R, Brownlee G G 1984 Carrier detection in Haemophilia B using two further intragenic RFLPs. Nucleic Acid Research 12: 8861

Wion K L, Tuddenham E G D, Lawn R M 1986 A new polymorphism in the factor VIII gene for prenatal diagnosis of haemophilia A. Nucleic Acid Research 14(11): 4535–4542

World Health Organization 1977 Methods for the detection of haemophilia carriers. A memorandum. Bulletin of the World Health Organization 55: 675–702

Youssoufian H, Phillips D G, Kazazian H M, Antonarakis S E Jr. 1987 Msp1 polymorphism in the 3′ flanking region of the human FVIII gene. Nucleic Acid Research 15(15): 6312–6313

Zimmerman T S, Ratnoff O D, Littell A S 1971 Detection of carriers of classic hemophilia using an immunologic assay for antihemophilic factor (factor VIII). Journal of Clinical Investigation 50: 255–258

81. Leukaemias, lymphomas and related disorders

Janet D. Rowley

INTRODUCTION

The close association of specific chromosome abnormalities with particular types of human leukaemia and lymphoma has been established by a number of investigators during the past decade. A few of the genes involved in consistent chromosome rearrangements, notably translocations, have already been identified, and it is likely that the identity of most of the genes affected by these aberrations will be determined within the next decade. Moreover, for several of the rearrangements, some of the changes in gene structure and function have been defined. Therefore, some general principles that may be applicable to all chromosome rearrangements in human malignant disease are beginning to emerge.

Much of the detailed information regarding the relevant chromosome rearrangements is contained in a number of recent reviews, and only a general summary will be presented here (Rowley & Testa 1983, Bloomfield et al 1987, Heim & Mitelman 1987, Mitelman 1988, Rowley 1988). Although carcinomas account for the largest proportion of malignant disease they represent only about 15% of the karyotypic data; the majority of karyotypic information applies to leukaemia and lymphoma. Only data obtained on untreated patients will be considered here.

It has been clear from the beginning of the cytogenetic analysis of human malignant disease that virtually all solids tumours, including the non-Hodgkin lymphomas, had an abnormal karyotype and that some of these abnormalities are limited to a given tumour. With regard to the leukaemias, it appeared from studies in the 1960s and early 1970s, that only about 50% had an abnormal karyotype. With improved culture techniques, and with the development of processing methods that resulted in longer chromosomes with a larger number of more clearly defined bands, Yunis and associates have provided evidence that a karyotypic abnormality can also be detected in virtually all leukaemias (Bloomfield et al 1987). Some malignant diseases, such as Hodgkin disease

or multiple myeloma, continue to show a high frequency of normal karyotypes. These diseases are characterized by malignant cells with a low mitotic index, and therefore it is likely that the dividing cells represent normal rather than malignant cells. This discussion will be restricted to clonal abnormalities, which are defined as at least two cells with the same extra chromosome or structural rearrangement (identified with banding) or three cells with the same missing chromosome (Rowley & Potter 1976). As can be seen from Table 81.1, with the exception of the t(9;22), the chromosome abnormalities in the myeloid leukaemias differ from those in the lymphoid leukaemias and lymphomas. Molecular analysis of the 9;22 translocation junction has revealed that the break in chromosome 22 may be different in chronic myeloid and acute lymphoblastic leukaemia.

Different chromosome changes have been observed in neoplastic cells, and these often occur in combination. The simplest change is either a gain or a loss of a whole chromosome. Common structural alterations are translocations, which involve the exchange of material between two or more chromosomes, and deletions, which involve loss of DNA from a chromosome and thus from the affected cell. Chromosome inversions have been observed; in this rearrangement, a single chromosome is broken in two places, and the central portion is inverted and rejoined to the ends of the chromosome. A number of international meetings over the last 25 years have led to the establishment of a universally accepted system for chromosome nomenclature; that standard nomenclature will be used here. Each chromosome band is numbered (ISCN 1981). The total chromosome number is followed by the sex chromosomes, and gains and losses of whole chromosomes are identified by a '+' or '−' before the chromosome number. A gain or loss of part of a chromosome is identified by a '+' or a '−' after the chromosome number; p and q represent the short and long arm respectively. Translocations are indicated by t; the chromosomes involved are noted in the first set of brackets and the breakpoints in the second set of brackets.

Table 81.1 Common chromosome changes in leukaemia

Type	Gains	Losses	Rearrangements
		Myeloid leukaemia	
CML			
Chronic phase			t(9;22)(q34;q11)
Blast crisis	+8,+Ph[1]	Rare; −7	t(9;22),i(17q)
ANLL			
AML(M2)	+8	−7;less −5	t(8;21)(q22;q22)
APL(M3)			(15;17)(q22;q11−12)
AMMoL(M4) (abn. eosinophils)	+22,+8	−7	inv(16)(p13q22), t(16;16)
AMoL(M5)			t(9;11)(p22;q23), (t11q), del(11q)
M2/M4(incr. basophils)			t(6;9)(p23;q34)
M4(incr. platelets)			t(3;3)(q21;q26), inv(3)
		Lymphoid leukaemia	
CLL			
B-cell	+12	−	14q+(q32);t(14;19)(q32;q13)
T-cell			t(8;14)(q24;q11)
			inv(14)(q11q32)
ALL			
Early B-precursor			t(4;11)(q21;q23)
Common	+21,+6	rare	t(9;22),del(6q)(q15−q21), near haploid
pre B			t(1;19)(q23;p13)
B-cell			t(8;14)(q24;q32)
			t(2;8)(p12;q24)
			t(8;22)(q24;q11)
Early T-precursor			t(9p), del(9p)(21−22)
T-cell			t(11;14)(p13;q11),
			t(8;14)(q24;q11)
			inv(14)(q11q32)
*CALLA-			

* CALLA-(Common acute lymphoblastic leukaemia antigen)

Other abnormalities will be defined when they are first described. To be relevant to the malignant disease, chromosomes for analysis must be obtained from the tumour cells. Thus, for leukaemia, bone marrow cells processed directly or after 1–3 day culture are used; lymph nodes or solid tumours are minced to yield a single cell suspension that can be harvested immediately or cultured for a short period of time. The cells are exposed to a hypotonic solution, fixed, and stained according to a variety of protocols (Testa & Rowley 1981, Le Beau 1984).

GENETIC AETIOLOGY AND SUSCEPTIBILITY

The major emphasis in this chapter is on acquired nonrandom cytogenetic aberrations that characterize human haematological malignancies and provide compelling evidence for the somatic mutation theory of carcinogenesis. However, the possible role of host genetic factors in the aetiology of human cancer has also long been recognized and has recently been the subject of several comprehensive reviews (Lynch 1976, Li &

Fraumeni 1982, Knudson 1983, Mulvihill 1984, Schneider et al 1986). For leukaemia and lymphoma, these investigations of genetic susceptibility have usually centred on retrospective studies and on studies of twins and pedigrees (Anderson 1975). Additional evidence for genetic predisposition to leukaemia has been derived from studies of patients with certain syndromes that are associated with constitutional aneuploidy or chromosomal instability and an increased risk of malignancy.

Family and twin studies

Retrospective studies have been used in comparisons of the morbidity and/or mortality rates in first-degree relatives of cancer patients with the rates in control relatives. In one such investigation (Vidabaek 1947), 17 of 209 patients with leukaemia (8.1%) were found to have at least one leukaemic relative, compared to only one such case among 200 controls (0.5%). Under-reporting of leukaemia in the control group and other methodological deficiencies make the results of such studies questionable, and indeed similar subsequent studies have shown little or only moderately increased familial incidence of leukaemia and lymphoma (Heath 1976, Marchetto et al 1978). Most instances of familial leukaemia/lymphoma have involved pairs of cases in individual families, although occasional pedigrees with as many as six related cases have been described (Zuelzer & Cox 1969, Heath 1976). Concordance, or at least similarity, of cell types tends to prevail within each family, again perhaps suggesting the operation of underlying genetic factors. A study in Japan compared the degree of consanguinity among parents of sib leukaemia patients and nonfamilial cases (Kurita et al 1974). In 20 families with familial leukaemia, 20% of the patients were found to be first cousins, and 10% were first cousins once removed or second cousins. In contrast, only 4.5% of the parents in 200 nonfamilial cases were first cousins.

Twin studies are usually considered to be a powerful means to assess the relative importance of genetic and nongenetic factors in a given disease. Reports that concordance rates among monozygotic (MZ) twins for childhood acute leukaemia far exceed random expectation (MacMahon & Levy 1964, Miller 1971) are complicated by the fact that shared placental circulation makes many MZ twins haematopoietic chimaeras. As a result, the observed high concordance rates (reported to be 17–25%) might simply reflect a single postzygotic prenatal oncogenic event and would not necessarily imply an inherited predisposition to leukaemia (Clarkson & Boyse 1971). Cytogenetic evidence has, in fact, been presented to support a single intrauterine origin of acute leukaemia in at least one pair of MZ twins (Chaganti et al 1979).

Constitutional chromosome abnormalities

The increased risk of leukaemia in patients with Down syndrome (47,+21) has been well substantiated in a number of surveys and appears to extend to all age groups (Krivit & Good 1957, Miller 1970); these patients do not appear to have an increased risk of solid lymphoreticular tumours (Miller 1970). Lymphoblastic leukaemia has been found to predominate in children with Down syndrome, as in the general pediatric population (Rosner & Lee 1972), although a recent review of the literature suggested that acute nonlymphocytic leukaemia may predominate (Kaneko et al 1981). The age peak for leukaemia in Down syndrome occurs somewhat earlier than in childhood leukaemia in general (Miller 1970), although the greater incidence of transient leukaemoid reactions in Down syndrome babies could mimic congenital leukaemia and lead to an exaggerated risk estimate in younger children (Rosner & Lee 1972). A gain of chromosome 21 is the most common change that occurs in childhood acute lymphoblastic leukaemia, with 30 of 98 children having +21 in their leukaemic cells; it is also common, but much less so, in acute nonlymphocytic leukaemia (4 of 60 children). These data suggested that the presence of +21 in patients with Down syndrome might, in itself, predispose to leukaemic transformation (Rowley 1981). This proposal is not universally accepted (Hecht 1982).

Leukaemia has also been reported in patients with other constitutional aneuploidies, including several with Klinefelter syndrome (47,XXY and mosaics), Turner syndrome (45,X), trisomy 13 (47,+13) or other D-group trisomies (Heath 1976). Most of these associations have been documented as single case reports only, making an accurate risk assessment very difficult. The various Workshops in Leukaemia provide some evidence that constitutional abnormalities may increase the incidence of leukaemia. For acute lymphoblastic leukaemia, 330 patients were included in the Third International Workshop (1981); 157 children and 173 adults. Five children had constitutional aberrations, Down syndrome in four and Klinefelter syndrome in one; two adults had balanced translocations. The overall incidence of 2.1% (3.2% in children and 1.2% in adults) is considerably higher than 0.73% constitutional abnormalities detected in a large newborn survey (Buckton et al 1980).

Chromosome instability diseases

Three rare genetic diseases (Bloom syndrome, Fanconi anaemia, ataxia telangiectasia) are characterized by increased rates of chromosome breakage and a predisposition to malignancies of the lymphoreticular system (German 1972, McCaw & Hecht 1983). All are inherited as autosomal recessive conditions, and each has a distinctive clinical course and phenotype as well as particular types of chromosome aberrations.

In Bloom Syndrome (BS), the cytogenetic hallmark is the quadriradial configuration, usually symmetrical and involving homologous chromosomes. It is seen in lymphocytes and fibroblasts, along with other types of chromosome breakage and an elevated spontaneous rate of sister chromatid exchange (Chaganti et al 1974, German 1983). Patients with Fanconi anaemia (FA) show an increased frequency of chromosome breakage and rearrangement in bone marrow and cultured lymphocytes, with no tendency for symmetrical quadriradial formation (Schroeder & German 1974). Cells from patients with ataxia telangiectasia (AT) also show increased levels of chromosome breakage, which may fluctuate over time; pseudodiploid clones containing a marker chromosome 14 are another common feature of AT lymphocytes (Cohen et al 1975, McCaw et al 1975).

Aurias and his co-workers have reported on chromosome studies in a large series of AT patients. They support the observations of earlier workers that the recurring re-arrangements in clonal cells affect 7p14, 7q35, 14q11, and 14q32; the breakpoints on chromosome 7 occur in bands containing the gamma and beta chain genes for the T cell receptor whereas those on chromosome 14 are the locations of the alpha chain for the T cell receptor (*TCRA*) and the immunoglobulin heavy chain genes respectively (Aurias & Dutrillaux 1986). With the use of in situ chromosome hybridization they have shown that the breakpoint in 14q11 splits *TCRA* in three AT patients, each with a karyotypically different clone (Stern et al 1988). In several AT patients who developed leukaemia, the chromosomally abnormal clone has become predominant (McCaw et al 1975, Saxon et al 1979).

The autosomal recessive mode of transmission suggests an inherited biochemical (enzymatic) defect, possibly involving DNA metabolism or repair, as in the case of xeroderma pigmentosum, another genetic disorder ex-hibiting cancer predisposition (basal cell and squamous cell carcinomas, malignant melanomas) and abnormal levels of chromosome damage following exposure to ultraviolet irradiation or alkylating agents (Friedberg et al 1979). Specific DNA repair defects have, in fact, been demonstrated in AT and FA cells, although there is evidence for genetic heterogeneity within each disease (Chaganti 1985). In any case, these syndromes remain valuable models for examining the inter-relations of genetic background, chromosome abnormalities, and cancer development.

MYELOID LEUKAEMIAS

Chronic myeloid leukaemia

The subtype of leukaemia termed chronic myeloid leukaemia (CML) is important because the first consist-ent chromosome abnormality in any malignant disease was identified in CML. The abnormality is the Philadel-phia or Ph[1] chromosome (Nowell & Hungerford 1960), which was shown with banding to involve chromosome 22 (22q-). The defect was shown to be a translocation involving chromosomes 9 and 22; this was the first consistent translocation specifically associated with any human or animal disease (Fig. 81.1) (Rowley 1973a). The reciprocal nature of the translocation was established only recently, when the Abelson proto-oncogene, *ABL*, normally on chromosome 9, was identified on the Ph[1] chromosome (de Klein et al 1982). Other studies with fluorescent markers or chromosome polymorphisms have

shown that, in a particular patient, the same chromo-somes 9 and 22 are involved in each cell. The karyotypes of many Ph[1]+ patients with CML have been examined with banding techniques by a number of investigators; in a recent review of 1129 Ph[1] patients, the 9;22 trans-location was identified in 1036 (92%) (Rowley & Testa 1983). Variant translocations have been discovered, however, in addition to the typical t(9;22). Until very recently, these were thought to be of two kinds; one appeared to be a simple translocation involving chromo-some 22 and some chromosome other than 9 (about 4%), and the other was a complex translocation involving three or more different chromosomes, two of which were 9 and 22 (about 4%). Recent data clearly demonstrate that chromosome 9 is affected in the simple as well as the complex translocations, and that its involvement had been overlooked (de Klein & Hagemeijer 1984). Virtually all chromosomes have been involved in these variant translocations, but chromosome 17 is affected more often than other chromosomes. The genetic consequences of the standard t(9;22) or the complex translocation invol-ving at least three chromosomes is to move the *ABL* proto-oncogene on chromosome 9 next to a gene on chromosome 22 called *BCR*, whose function is currently unknown (Fig. 81.2).

When patients with CML enter the terminal acute phase, about 10–20% appear to retain the 46, Ph[1]+ cell line unchanged, whereas most patients show additional chromosome abnormalities resulting in cells with modal chromosome numbers of 47 to 50 (Rowley & Testa 1983). During the acute phase of CML different abnormal chromosomes occur singly or in combination in a distinctly nonrandom pattern. In patients who have only a single new chromosome change, this most commonly involves a second Ph[1], an isochromosome for the long arm of chromosome 17 [i(17q)], or a +8, in descending order of frequency. Chromosome loss occurs only rarely; that most often seen is −7, which occurs in 3% of patients.

Early cases of acute leukaemia in which the Ph[1] chromosome was present were classified as CML pre-senting in blast transformation; at present, patients who have no prior history suggestive of CML are classified as Ph[1]+ acute leukaemia. In fact, as discussed in the section on Ph[1]+ ALL, some of these patients have a different breakpoint in *BCR*. In CML patients, the Ph[1] chromo-some is present in granulocytic, erythroid, and mega-karyocytic cells, in some B cells, and probably in a few T cells. In blast crisis, some blasts have intracytoplasmic IgM, which is characteristic of pre-B cells, and these cells have an immunoglobulin gene rearrangement (Bakhshi et al 1983).

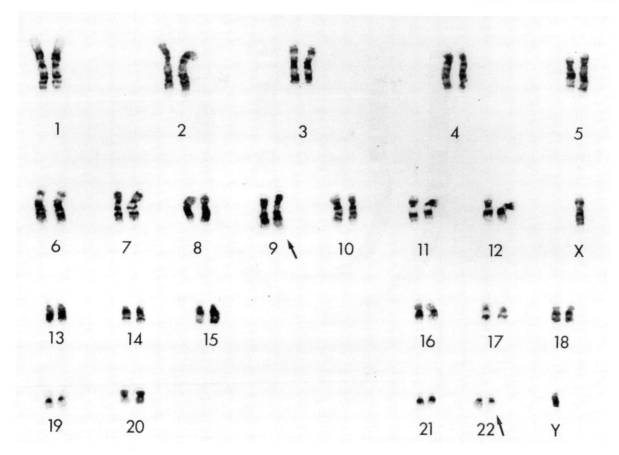

Fig. 81.1 Trypsin-Giemsa stained karyotype of a metaphase cell from a bone marrow aspirate obtained from an untreated male with chronic myeloid leukaemia illustrating the t(9;22)(q34;q11). The Philadelphia chromosome (Ph¹) is the chromosome on the right in pair 22 (arrow). The material missing from the long arm of this chromosome (22q-) is translocated to the long arm of chromosome 9 (9q+) (arrow), and is the additional pale band that is not present on the normal chromosome 9.

Marrow cells from some patients have appeared to lack a Ph¹ chromosome. The majority of these patients had a normal karyotype. Somewhat surprisingly, the survival of these patients was substantially shorter than those whose cells were Ph¹+ (Whang-Peng et al 1968). Our recent review of the histology of 25 Ph¹− patients showed that most of them did not have CML but they had some type of myelodysplasia, most commonly chronic myelomonocytic leukaemia or refractory anaemia with excess blasts. (Pugh et al 1985). However, the situation has become more complex because it has been shown recently (Morris et al 1986, Bartram 1988) that some patients with clinically typical CML who lack a Ph¹ chromosome cytogenetically, have evidence of the insertion of *ABL*

sequences into the *BCR* gene. Thus it can be proposed that the sine qua non of CML is the juxtaposition of *BCR* and *ABL*.

Acute nonlymphocytic leukaemia (ANLL) de novo

With initial banding analyses clonal chromosome abnormalities were detected in about 50% of patients with ANLL. This percentage has increased with improved banding and culture techniques; many laboratories are currently finding that at least 80% of patients have an abnormal karyotype. The most frequent abnormalities are a gain of chromosome 8 and a loss of chromosome 7, which are seen in most subtypes of ANLL (Rowley

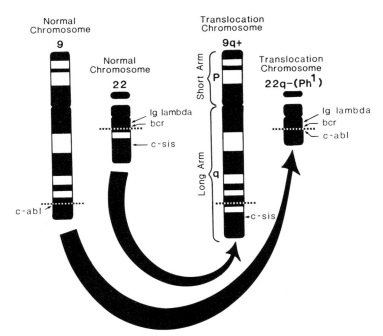

Fig. 81.2 Schematic drawing of chromosomes 9 and 22 illustrating the translocation that produces the 9q+ and 22q- (Ph¹) chromosomes. One proto–oncogene, *ABL*, is moved to 22 adjacent to a gene of unknown function called *BCR*; the break in 22 is distal to the IG lambda locus which is not involved in the translocation. The *SIS* proto–oncogene is moved to the 9q+ chromosome. It is located at some distance from the breakpoint on 22 and there is no evidence that it is altered as the result of the translocation.

& Testa 1983, Fourth International Workshop 1984, Mitelman 1988). Specific rearrangements are closely associated with a particular subtype of ANLL as defined by the French-American-British Cooperative Group [FAB classification] (Bennett et al 1976). The chromosome abnormalities associated with each subtype are illustrated in Figure 81.3.

A translocation between chromosomes 8 and 21 [t(8;21)(q22;q22)] was first identified in 1973 (Rowley 1973b). The frequency with which this translocation is detected varies from one laboratory to another; it accounted for 10% (25/249) of the abnormal cases reviewed by Rowley and Testa (1983), and 12% of the patients with an abnormal karyotype reviewed at the Fourth International Workshop on Chromosomes in Leukaemia (1984). The t(8;21) is the most frequent abnormality in children with ANLL, being reported in 17% (10 of 60) of karyotypically abnormal cases (Rowley & Testa 1983). The abnormality initially appeared to be restricted to patients with a diagnosis of M2 (AML or acute myeloblastic leukaemia with maturation), according to the FAB classification. However 7% of t(8;21) patients analyzed at the Fourth Workshop had a diagnosis

of M4 (AMMoL or acute myelomonocytic leukaemia).

The 8;21 translocation is of interest for three other reasons. First, chromosomes 8 and 21 can participate in three-way rearrangements similar to those involving chromosomes 9 and 22 in CML. Second, the t(8;21) is often accompanied by the loss of a sex chromosome; among the cases reviewed at the Fourth Workshop, 28 of 33 (85%) males were −Y and 8 of 12 (67%) females were −X. This association is particularly noteworthy because sex chromosome abnormalities are otherwise rarely observed in ANLL. Third, this translocation has never been reported as a constitutional abnormality or observed in other malignant diseases (Rowley, unpublished observations).

A structural rearrangement involving chromosomes 15 and 17 in acute promyelocytic leukaemia (APL or M3) was first recognized in 1977 (Rowley et al 1977). 43 patients (70%) analyzed at the Fourth Workshop had a t(15;17), 3 had other abnormalities, and only 15 of 61 (25%) patients had a normal karyotype. This rearrangement is unique to APL. In our recent review, all 44 APL patients had a t(15;17) (Rowley 1988).

The close association of translocations, or less often

deletions, of 11q and acute monoblastic leukaemia (AMoL or M5) was first observed by Berger et al (1982). Abnormalities of 11q occurred most frequently in children with monoblastic leukaemia (type *a*) (6 of 8); adults with monoblastic leukaemia had the next highest incidence (5 of 16). The incidence in monocytic, type *b*, leukaemia was low (1 of 3 children and 0 of 7 adults). At the Fourth Workshop 33 patients had some structural rearrangement involving 11q; 21 of the 33 (63.6%) were classified as M5, 5 as M4, and 3 were M2. Of the 21 patients with M5, 15 were of monoblastic type, 3 were monocytic, and slides from 3 could not be subclassified. Five of the patients were less than 1 year of age, and 7 others were less than 20 years old. When all patients with M5 leukaemia were considered, about 22% had an aberration involving 11q.

Aberrations of 11q differ from the t(8;22) and t(15;17) in two ways. First, the breakpoint in 11q involves band 11q23–24 in about two thirds of patients, but it can also occur in 11q13–14. Second, although translocations are more common (21 of 33 Fourth Workshop patients), 11 patients appeared to have what was identified as a

terminal deletion of 11q. Although the other chromosome involved in the translocation is variable, a t(9;11) (p22;q23) is common (Hagemeijer et al 1982).

Another clinical-cytogenetic association recently identified involves acute myelomonocytic (AMMoL or M4) leukaemia with abnormal eosinophils. Arthur and Bloomfield (1983) described 5 cases with M2 or M4 in which the bone marrow contained an excess of eosinophils (8–54%); all 5 patients had a deleted chromosome 16 [del(16)(q22)]. Our group has reported on a related entity, first in 18 patients and then in a larger series of 33 patients (Larson et al 1986). Most of these patients had M4 leukaemia with eosinophils that showed unique morphological changes, including large and irregular basophilic granules; one third lacked increased eosinophils because the marrow had fewer than 5% eosinophils. 27 patients had an inversion of chromosome 16, inv(16)(p13q22), and 6 had t(16;16)(p13;q22). The strong correlation between abnormal eosinophils and structural rearrangements of chromosome 16 was confirmed at the Fourth Workshop (1984). In fact, the morphological features of the eosinophils are so specific that our

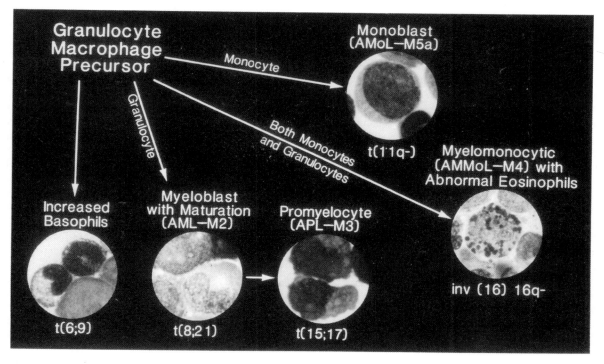

Fig. 81.3 Relationship of the subtypes of ANLL and the particular chromosome abnormality associated with each subtype. Each circle contains a photomicrograph illustrating the special features of the leukaemic cells from the bone marrow of untreated patients; the particular chromosome rearrangements associated with that type of leukaemia are listed under the photomicrograph.

pathologists can accurately classify patients as inv(16) or t(16;16) by examining the bone marrow aspirate. It appears that this relatively common (25% of our AMMoL patients) but subtle chromosome aberration was undetected in the past, in part, because of poor morphology. This chromosome abnormality has clinical implications as well. Among 32 treated patients, 78% achieved a complete remission compared with 36% of 58 other AMMoL patients. The median survival time was more than 65 weeks for patients with an abnormal chromosome 16 compared with 29 weeks for those with a normal chromosome 16 (Larson et al 1986). In fact, at the Fourth Workshop it was clearly shown that the type rather than the presence of a chromosome abnormality had prognostic importance. Thus, although the projected median survival for all patients was 8 months, those with a t(8;21) had the longest median survival (13 months), while those with abnormalities of chromosomes 5 and 7, t(15;17), or hyperdiploidy had the shortest survivals (3–4 months).

Acute nonlymphocytic leukaemia and myelodysplastic syndrome associated with prior cytotoxic treatment

A distinctive disorder of bone marrow morphology and function that terminates in myelodysplastic syndrome (MDS) or in ANLL has been recognized as a late complication of cytotoxic therapy used in the treatment of both malignant and non-malignant diseases (Le Beau et al 1986a). These conditions are termed t-MDS and t-ANLL, and characteristic nonrandom chromosome abnormalities are commonly observed in bone marrow cells of such patients. The abnormalities differ in their type and frequency from those noted in ANLL developing de novo. We reported previously that part or all of chromosome 5 and/or 7 was lost in cells from 23 of 26 (88%) t-MDS/t-ANLL patients. More recently, 61 of 63 patients had an abnormal karyotype and 55 of these had an abnormality of one or both chromosomes 5 and 7 (Le Beau et al 1986a). These observations have been confirmed by others (Arthur & Bloomfield 1984, Pedersen-Bjergaard et al 1984). We were able to analyze the data from 17 patients with a deletion of the long arm of chromosome 5 and to identify a region, namely 5q23 to 5q32, that was consistently missing in every patient. In contrast, only about 16% of patients with ANLL de novo have a similar abnormality of chromosomes 5 or 7 or both (Larson et al 1983). Moreover, the latter patients have frequently had significant occupational exposure to potential environmental carcinogens, such as chemicals, solvents, or pesticides (Mitelman et al 1981, Golomb et al 1982). Furthermore, one seldom finds the specific rearrangements in t-ANLL which are closely associated

with the distinct morphological subsets of ANLL de novo, such as t(8;21), t(15;17), or inv(16).

A number of growth factors or growth factor receptors have been mapped to the region 5q23–32 that is consistently deleted; whether any of them play a role in mutagen-associated leukaemia is unknown (Le Beau et al 1986b).

MALIGNANT DISEASES AFFECTING LYMPHOCYTES

The chromosome abnormalities in lymphoid disorders, especially in the non-Hodgkin lymphomas, have been reviewed in considerable detail. This section will review the consistent translocations seen in Burkitt lymphoma and in some cases of B-cell acute lymphoblastic leukaemia (ALL), and the other aberrations in ALL and in some T-cell disorders.

Lymphoma

Manolov and Manolova (1972) discovered that cells of Burkitt lymphomas had an additional band at the end of the long arm of one chromosome 14 (14q+). Zech and co-workers (1976) first observed that the end of one chromosome 8 was consistently absent, and they suggested that the missing part was translocated to chromosome 14 [t(8;14)(q24;q32)]. The t(8;14) has also been observed in non-endemic Burkitt tumours from America, Europe and Japan that are Epstein-Barr virus negative; thus it is a highly characteristic chromosome anomaly in Burkitt tumours. This translocation has also been observed in other lymphomas, particularly those of the diffuse large cell type. Two other related translocations were later identified in Burkitt tumours. All three translocations involved chromosome 8 with a break in the same band, 8q24. One variant translocation involved chromosome 2 with a break in the short arm [t(2;8)(p12;q24)], and the other involved chromosome 22 with a break in the long arm in the band (22q11) that is affected in CML. All these translocations have been identified in patients with B-cell ALL.

The data on Burkitt lymphoma indicate that chromosome 8 is consistently involved. When the karyotypic aberrations seen in lymphoid diseases as a whole are considered, a break at 14q32, with translocation of material from elsewhere to the breakpoint, is the single most common change. The only other recurring translocation, the t(14;18)(q32;q21), is, in fact, the most common translocation in lymphoma. This was first identified by Fukuhara and co-workers (1979) in 6 of 9 patients with poorly differentiated lymphocytic lymphoma, now called 'malignant lymphoma, follicular, predominantly small cleaved cell' (FSC) (Working Formulation 1982). This finding has been confirmed by many others (Bloomfield et al 1983, Fifth International Workshop 1987). The correlation between karyotype and histology in 260 patients reviewed at the Fifth International Workshop on Chromosomes in Leukaemia and Lymphoma (1987) is summarized in Figure 81.4. Among the 260 Workshop patients 15% had a normal karyotype. The karyotypic pattern varied greatly among the different subgroups. The t(14;18) was common in follicular lymphomas, whereas the t(8;14) was common in small noncleaved cell lymphoma.

What are the implications of the t(14;18) in tumours with a large cell or diffuse morphology? Analysis of the karyotypic pattern in these tumours shows that certain additional chromosomal changes, especially a gain of chromosome 7 or a deletion of the long arm of chromosome 6 [(del)6q] appear to correlate with a more malignant phenotype (Koduru et al 1987, Yunis et al 1987).

The translocation junction has been cloned and a gene on chromosome 18 called *BCL2* (the second B cell leukaemia gene to be cloned) has been identified (Tsujimoto et al 1984). Breakpoints cluster in at least two sites on the gene; the major cluster is in the 3' untranslated region of the second exon. In the lymphoma cells, the expression of the normal gene is suppressed and an abnormal chimaeric *BCL2-IGH* messenger RNA (mRNA) is expressed. This leads to inappropriate expression of a structurally normal protein whose function is unknown (Cleary & Sklar 1986).

The karyotype in chronic lymphocytic leukaemia

Chronic lymphocytic leukaemia (CLL) is the most common leukaemia in the United States and Europe, accounting for about 30% of all leukaemias. It is considered to be a monoclonal neoplastic proliferation of small lymphocytes which are of B cell origin in 95% of cases. The early studies of the cytogenetic pattern in CLL showed a normal karyotype in most samples. As better culture and banding methods have been applied to these studies, nonrandom clonal abnormalities have been detected. These include translocations involving 14q32, observed in 20–30% of patients, and trisomy for chromosome 12 in about 40% of patients with abnormal karyotypes (Robert et al 1982, Han et al 1984, Mitelman 1988, Bird et al 1989). There are somewhat conflicting reports about the prognostic significance of these abnormalities.

The karyotype in acute lymphoblastic leukaemia; clinical correlations

While the correlation of cytogenetic changes with morphology in ANLL led to the identification of the specific associations described in a previous section, this correlation was not useful in ALL, except for the t(8;14) and its variants in L3, B cell ALL. However, with the widespread use of precise immunophenotyping, the correlation of certain chromosome rearrangements with specific immunological subsets of ALL has been established (Table 81.1).

ALL is the most frequent leukaemia in children.

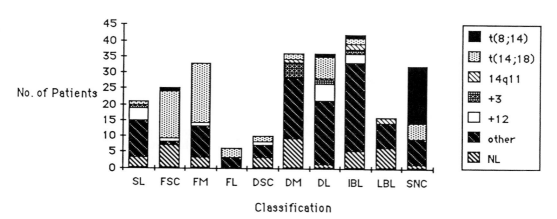

Fig. 81.4 Histogram showing the most common chromosome changes that were identified in 260 lymphomas studied prior to treatment and reviewed at the Fifth International Workshop on Chromosomes in Leukaemia/Lymphoma; each tumour was classified according to the Working Formulation.

Small lymphocytic (SL); Follicular small cleaved (FSC); Follicular mixed (FM); Follicular large (FL); Diffuse small cleaved (DSC); Diffuse mixed (DM); Diffuse large (DL); Immunoblastic (IBL); Lymphoblastic (LBL); Small noncleaved (SNC)

Patients who are between 3 and 7 years of age, with a WBC count of less than 10 000/mm^3, and whose leukaemic cells have non-T, non-B surface membrane, have the best prognosis. For many years metaphase chromosomes from ALL patients had poor morphology with indistinct bands making an accurate analysis difficult, and there have been fewer reports of chromosome patterns in ALL than in ANLL. Recent improvements permit the correlation of the karyotype with other recognized prognostic factors. It was rigorously demonstrated for the first time at the Third International Workshop on Chromosomes in Leukaemia (1981) that the karyotype is an important independent prognostic factor in ALL. Of 330 patients reviewed at the Third Workshop, 112 appeared to have a normal karyotype; the largest group (39 patients) with a well defined abnormality had a Ph^1 chromosome. Eighteen patients had a t(4;11), 16 had a t(8;14), and 15 had an abnormality of chromosome 14 not involving chromosome 8. Other patients with abnormalities were classified by the modal chromosome number.

The Ph^1 chromosome is the most frequent rearrangement comprising 17.3% of adult ALL. At the cytogenetic level the breakpoints appear identical to those in CML; recent molecular analysis suggests that the breakpoint in the *BCR* gene on chromosome 22 may be more proximal in some patients with Ph^1+ ALL than in those with CML. In the Workshop, the children with a Ph^1 chromosome had the second highest median leucocyte count (75 000/mm^3); all were non-B, non-T ALL, and they had a poor median survival of only 15 months. By identifying this chromosomal abnormality, one can therefore detect individuals who have a poor prognosis.

Of 216 Workshop patients with chromosomal abnormalities, 18 (8.3%) had a t(4;11)(q21;q23) rearrangement. Half of the patients were children, most of whom were less than 1 year old. The association of the t(4;11) with neonatal or early-childhood ALL is particularly interesting in view of the low incidence of ALL in this age group; acute leukaemias in this age group are usually of the myeloid type. Children with a t(4;11) had very high leucocyte counts (median WBC, 214 000/mm^3), which is a poor prognostic factor. Both children and adults had a short median survival, 9 and 7 months respectively. Only patients with abnormalities involving 8q24 or 14q32 had shorter survivals. Although the morphology of some cells often appears lymphoid, other features are more suggestive of a monocytic leukaemia. A t(4;11) cell line showed rearranged heavy and light chain (k) genes although cells lacked cytoplasmic immunoglobulin and thus were probably in a very early stage of B-cell differentiation (Stong et al 1986). However when cultured with the phorbol ester, TPA, a monocytic-like phenotype was induced. Thus these cells appear to be very early precursor cells that have dual lineage capabilities.

Another recurring chromosome abnormality is the t(1;19)(q21;p13) which has been identified in about 25% of patients with a pre-pre B phenotype, that is they have cytoplasmic immunoglobulin and are CALLA+ (Carroll et al 1984, Michael et al 1984, Williams et al 1984).

The leukaemic cells of some patients with ALL are characterized by a gain of many chromosomes and fewer structural abnormalities (Secker-Walker et al 1982, Williams et al 1982). Chromosome numbers usually range from 50–60, and a few patients have up to 65 chromosomes. Although identical karyotypes are unusual, certain additional chromosomes are commonly seen. Among 31 hyperdiploid Third Workshop patients (14% of patients with abnormalities) +21, +6, +18, +14, +4, and +10 in decreasing frequency were seen in 10–33% of patients. It is interesting that some of these chromosomes, particularly 10, 18 and 21, are also seen as additional chromosomes in patients with near-haploidy, with chromosome numbers of 26–36 (median, 28). The median age of the 22 children with this abnormality was 3 years, and that of all 31 patients was 5 years, which was less than that of patients with other abnormalities. The WBC count was low (median of 6000/mm^3). Thus, these patients have all the previously recognized factors, including age between 3 and 7 years, low WBC count, and non-T, non-B markers, that indicate a good prognosis.

In a follow-up study of the Third Workshop patients, the complete remission rate for children was 95%, with a median remission duration that will be greater than five years (Bloomfield et al 1986). The median survival of the children with hyperdiploidy is longer than those with a normal karyotype; for adults the median survival for the two groups is comparable. Chromosome losses were less frequent and involved Nos 9, 7, 13, 20 or 8 in that order. The three translocations seen in B-cell ALL were described under Burkitt lymphoma. With regard to karyotype and age, patients with a deletion of 6q and a modal chromosome number greater than 50 were younger, and those with a Ph^1 chromosome or a 14q+ were older than patients with other abnormalities. In summary, the highest remission rates were in patients with a normal karyotype and a modal number greater than 50; the lowest were seen in patients with a Ph^1 chromosome, a 14q+ chromosome, a t(8;14) or a t(4;11).

T-cell disorders

Although fewer leukaemias of T-cell origin have been studied, a distinct pattern of nonrandom karyotypic abnormalities is emerging. Rearrangements involving the proximal bands of chromosome 14 (14q11–13) are relatively common, and those involving two regions of chromosome 7 (7q35–36 and 7p15) also occur in T-cell malignancies, but have been observed in non-malignant T-cell disorders as well; breaks involving these regions are very rare in other malignant diseases. One recurring rearrangement in T-cell neoplasia, particularly CLL, is a paracentric inversion of chromosome 14 with a proximal breakpoint at q11 and a distal breakpoint at q32 (Ueshima et al 1984, Zech et al 1984). A closely related rearrangement, t(14;14)(q11;q32), is seen in T-cell neoplasia (Ueshima et al 1984, Kaiser-McCaw et al 1975) and in phytohaemagglutinin-stimulated lymphocytes from patients with ataxia telangiectasia (A-T) as well as in the leukaemic cells of A-T patients in whom this disease evolved (Kaiser-McCaw et al 1975, Aurias 1981). A number of reports from Japan have described the frequent occurrence of 14q11 breaks in adult T-cell leukaemia-lymphoma patients (Miyamoto et al 1984, Sadamori et al 1986); far fewer such patients have been described from Western countries, and 14q11 breaks are much less common (Rowley et al 1984, Whang-Peng et al 1985). Williams and her associates have described a t(11;14)(p13;q13) in the leukaemic cells of 4 of 16 patients with T-cell acute lymphoblastic leukaemia (Williams et al 1984). Thus in some of these T-cell diseases breaks occur in either 14q11 or 14q32, or in both bands in the same patient; in B-cell disorders, however, breaks occur essentially only in 14q32 and they rarely involve 14q11 (Ueshima et al 1984). The data confirm the observation made some time ago that the proximal region of chromosome 14 was important in T-cell neoplasia (Kaiser-McCaw et al 1975). More detailed analysis of rearrangements of 7q in T-cell disorders has revealed that a few patients have breaks at 7q32 to 7q36, the location of the B chain for the T-cell receptor (Ueshima et al 1984, Raimondi et al 1987).

Tumours originating in embryonic cells

These tumours are of particular interest to both the geneticist and cytogeneticist because some of them occur in patients who have specific *constitutional* chromosome abnormalities. In all preceding sections, the karyotypic changes were somatic mutations in malignant cells and they were not present in other unaffected cells. In contrast, some patients at risk of developing retinoblastoma have a variable deletion of chromosome 13 that always includes 13q14, whereas other patients with a deletion of chromosome 11 (band 11p13) are at risk of developing Wilms tumour. In general, these deletions are

also associated with various phenotypic abnormalities (Francke 1983). Relatively few tumours have been analyzed and deletions of chromosome 13 or, much less often, of chromosome 11 have been observed in tumour cells from some retinoblastomas or Wilms tumours respectively. The most common change that we have observed in Wilms tumours is trisomy for the long arm of chromosome 1 (+1q) (Kondo et al 1984). Both of these tumours have two patterns of inheritance, one as an autosomal dominant and one as a sporadic mutation.

The age at tumour detection as well as other observations led Knudson to propose the two-mutation hypothesis (Knudson 1971). According to this hypothesis, in patients who inherited the predisposing gene only one other change was needed for transformation of retinal cells to tumour cells and, in these individuals, multiple tumours were diagnosed at a very early age. In sporadic cases two independent mutations had to affect the same cell for transformation to occur; since this event was relatively uncommon, the tumours were unifocal and developed at an older age. Based on the consistent loss of chromosome band 13q14, this band was thought to be the location of the retinoblastoma or *RB* gene.

Studies confirming that chromosome 13 was the critical chromosome included the discovery that tumour cells were frequently homozygous for DNA markers on chromosome 13 that were heterozygous in cells of non-tumour tissue from the same patient (Cavenee et al 1983). Using probes cloned from 13q14, Dryja discovered that copies of one of the probes had been deleted from both chromosomes in one of 20 tumours; DNA probes from this region detected mRNA in a retinal cell line which was absent in some retinoblastomas (Dryja et al 1984). By making a DNA copy of this mRNA, they identified deletions or mutations in about 30% of retinoblastoma tumours or cell lines (Friend et al 1986). Others have identified mRNA abnormalities in each of six retinoblastomas (Lee et al 1987).

More recent data indicate that RB is a DNA binding protein that can complex with proteins of tumour producing viruses (Whyte et al 1988). The current assumption is that the RB gene, and the genes that will be identified in the deleted chromosome segments in other tumour cells, function as tumour suppressors or 'anti-oncogenes'. Presumably these genes inhibit the function of genes stimulating cell proliferation and their loss allows the growth promoting genes to function without modulation (Murphree & Benedict 1984).

Recurring chromosomes abnormalities, limited to the malignant cells, have also been observed in other childhood tumours; for example, a deletion of much of the long arm of chromosome 1 (1p−) has been noted in neuroblastomas (Brodeur et al 1981). Neuroblastomas

Table 81.2 Recurring chromosome abnormalities in solid tumours

A. *Involving embryonic cells*	
Neuroblastoma	Deletion of chromosome 1(p13–p36)
Ewing sarcoma/peripheral neuroepithelioma	t(11;22)(q24;q12)
Wilms tumour	Deletion of chromosome 11(p13) # Trisomy 1q
Retinoblastoma	Deletion of chromosome 13(q14) # Trisomy 1q
Testicular tumours	i(12p)
B. *Adult cancers*	
Malignant melanoma	Deletion of chromosome 1(p11–p22)
Small cell lung carcinoma	Deletion of chromosome 3(p14–p23)
Renal carcinoma	Deletion of chromosome 3(p11–p22)
Liposarcoma	t(12;16)(q13;p11)
Synovial sarcoma	t(X;18)(p11.2;q11.2)
Rhabdomyosarcoma (alveolar)	t(2;13)(q37;q14)
C. *Benign tumours*	
Pleomorphic adenoma	t(3;8)(p21;q12); t(9;12)(p13–22; q13–15)
Meningioma	Loss of chromosome 22 or deletion (q11)
Lipoma	t(3;12)(q27–q28;q13–q14)

Observed as a constitutional abnormality as well as in some tumours.

are also of interest because of their proclivity to undergo gene amplification which is manifested chromosomally as hundreds or thousands of small discrete pieces of chromosomes called double minutes, or long unbanded regions on chromosomes called homogeneously staining regions or HSR (Biedler & Spengler 1976). In some cell lines, these have been shown to represent amplification of *NMYC* (Schwab et al 1983). *NMYC* amplification has also been identified in tumour samples; it is highly correlated with advanced stage (III and IV) and with a poor survival of these patients (Brodeur et al 1984). Recurring chromosomal abnormalities in solid tumours are summarized in Table 81.2.

MOLECULAR ANALYSIS OF CONSISTENT CHROMOSOME ABNORMALITIES, PARTICULARLY TRANSLOCATIONS

How and when consistent translocations occur

We do not know how consistent structural rearrangements occur, but there are at least two possibilities

(Rowley 1984). The rearrangements may be random, but selection may act to eliminate the vast majority that do not provide the cell with a proliferative advantage. Alternatively, certain changes may occur preferentially and thus be the ones we see. Some tantalizing data show an association of chromosome rearrangements in tumour cells from patients with fragile sites affecting one of the chromosome bands broken in the tumour cells (Yunis & Soreng 1984, Sutherland & Hecht 1985, Le Beau 1988). However, much more research is required to clarify the role of fragile sites as a predisposing factor to malignant transformation.

Croce and his co-workers (Finger et al 1986) have proposed that many of the chromosome rearrangements in B- and T-cell tumours involve sequences used in the normal recombination of the V-D-J segments of the immunoglobulin and T-cell receptor genes. The presence of heptamer and nanomer sequences on the non-immunoglobulin gene involved in the translocation, namely *MYC* and *BCL2*, has been reported. We have no indication at present that the genes involved in the translocations in myeloid leukaemias undergo similar DNA rearrangements.

An equally important question is, when in the multistage process of malignant transformation of a particular cell do translocation or other chromosome aberrations occur? Some chromosome changes occur as part of the further evolution of the malignant phenotype, e.g. blast crisis of CML, and they are, therefore, relatively late events. But what about the occurrence of the t(9;22) in CML, for example? Does the Ph¹ occur in a single normal cell which becomes the progenitor of the leukaemia clone, or is there expansion of a clone, possibly a leukaemic one, in which a translocation occurs in one of these already abnormal cells? Fialkow and Singer (1985) have presented detailed evidence supporting the latter proposal.

More recently, Adams et al (1985) have constructed transgenic mice whose cells all have a vector containing the *myc/IgH* junction from a murine plasmacytoma. All cells contain this construct; however the B cell tumours that occurred in every animal were clonal, indicating that one or more additional changes occurred in the progenitor cell.

Chromosome location of proto-oncogenes

One of the most surprising revelations in the recent past has involved the cellular oncogenes and their chromosome location (Fig. 81.5). Much of the excitement derives from the observation that many proto-oncogenes are located in the bands that are involved in consistent translocation (Leder et al 1983, Rowley 1984, Klein &

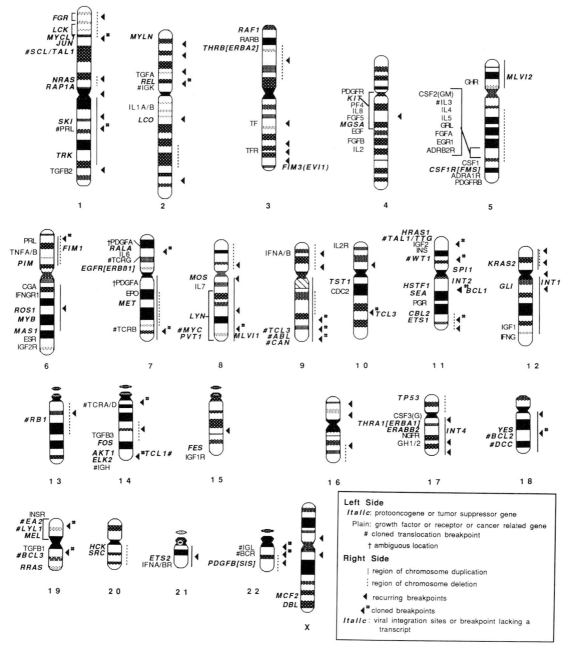

Fig. 81.5 Map of the chromosome location of protooncogenes or of genes that appear to be important in malignant transformation and the breakpoints observed in recurring chromosome abnormalities in human leukemia, lymphoma, and solid tumors. Known protooncogenes are indicated in bold italics and other cancer related genes are listed in standard type. The protooncogenes and their locations are placed to the left of the appropriate chromosome band or region (indicated by a bracket). The breakpoints in recurring translocations, inversions, etc., are indicated with an arrow head to the right of the affected chromosome band. The solid vertical lines on the right indicate regions frequently present in triplicate; the dashed lines indicate recurring deletions. Recurring viral integration sites and cloned translocation breakpoints with no identified transcripts are indicated to the right of the appropriate band. Genes or recurring breakpoints that have been cloned are identified by #. The locations of the cancer-specific breakpoints are based on the Report of the Committee on Structural Chromosome Changes in Neoplasia, Human Gene Mapping 10 (Trent et al 1989). [Author's note. Any map of this sort involves selection as to the genes that should or should not be included; I have been relatively conservative. Also for recurring breakpoints and deletions, I have included only those listed as Status I or II in HGM10. This figure was prepared by Michelle S. Rebelsky.] Reprinted with permission from Cancer Research 50: 3816–3825, 1990.

Trent J M, Kaneko Y, Mitelman F 1989 10: Report of the committee on structural chromosome changes in neoplasia. Cytogenet Cell Genet 51: 533–562

Klein 1986, Bishop 1987, Duesberg 1987). The evidence in Burkitt lymphoma and in CML clearly points the way for future research in this area. The gene for the proto-oncogene *MYC* (the cellular homologue of the avian myelocytomatosis virus) is on chromosome 8(q24). The immunoglobulin genes (heavy chain, and kappa and lambda light chain genes) are located at the breakpoints on the three chromosomes, other than 8, that are involved in the translocations in Burkitt lymphoma, 14q23, 2p12 and 22q11 respectively. These translocations result in the aberrant juxtaposition of *MYC* and one of the immunoglobulin genes; this in turn leads to abnormal regulation of *MYC* expression, although the precise nature of the derangement is not presently understood (Leder et al 1983, Klein & Klein 1986). Comparable chromosome translocations and gene rearrangements have been observed in mouse plasmacytomas (Klein 1983).

An analogous chromosome abnormality has been defined recently in T-cell leukaemia. In this translocation the breakpoint also involves *MYC* at 8q24, but the other gene is the alpha chain for the T-cell receptor (*TCRA*) which is located at 14q11 (Caccia et al 1985, Croce et al 1985). In SKW3, we, and others, have shown that the break in *MYC* is 3' of the 3rd exon and *MYC* remains on chromosome 8; in *TCRA* the break is just 5' of a J segment (J α D) (Mathieu-Mahul et al 1985, Shima et al 1986). This translocation is similar to those involving the immunoglobulin light chain genes in which *MYC* also remains on chromosome 8. *TCRA* is also involved with translocations affecting 14q32 and the heavy chain gene in the inv(14) (Baer et al 1985).

Investigators are now in the process of unravelling the mystery of the Ph[1] translocation in CML and ALL. In the t(9;22) in CML and ALL, the Abelson proto-oncogene (*ABL*) is translocated to the Ph[1] chromosome (de Klein et al 1982). This was an important observation because *ABL* was the first gene known to be on chromosome 9 that was shown to translocate to chromosome 22, thus establishing the fact that the translocation was reciprocal. The *ABL* gene was first identified because of its homology to the viral oncogene that had been isolated from a mouse pre B-cell leukaemia. The breakpoint junction in CML was cloned and the site on the Ph[1] was called bcr, for breakpoint cluster region, (Groffen et al 1984) since the majority of breaks cluster in a small 5.8 kilobase (kb) region. In contrast, the breaks on chromosome 9 occur over an incredible distance of more than 200 kb. We have used pulse field gel electrophoresis (PFGE) to great advantage in the study of the *ABL* proto-oncogene. Southern blotting with standard gel electrophoresis leads to separation of DNA fragments in the size range of 2 to about 25 kb. Since the *ABL* gene is larger than 200 kb,

mapping it in 10- to 20-kb pieces is a formidable task. In contrast, by using PFGE one can separate fragments more than 1000 kb in size, and this technique is also very effective in the 100–600 kb range. A normal chromosome band contains roughly 3000–5000 kb and thus several very large, overlapping fragments could contain a single band. Using many probes for *ABL* provided by various investigators Westbrook and Rubin have constructed a map of the normal *ABL* gene (Westbrook et al 1988). This is a very complex gene that normally uses one of two alternative beginnings, exon Ia or Ib. During transcription either of these can be spliced at the same point on the remainder of the gene, which is called the common splice acceptor site or exon II. One of their first discoveries was that the type Ib exon mapped more than 200 kb upstream from exon II. As a result, a very large segment of the RNA transcript is removed or spliced out to form the mature mRNA. This is a remarkable feat, not identified before in biological systems. The breakpoints in the chromosomes of various CML patients and cell lines occur in many locations upstream (5') of exon II. However, the same size (8.5 kb) mRNA is found in all CML patients; this occurs because the bcr exons are spliced to *ABL* exon II resulting in a chimaeric mRNA which is translated into a chimaeric protein (p210[BCR-ABL]) (Konopka et al 1984, Shtivelman et al 1985).

With regard to Ph[1]-positive ALL, it has always been an enigma why the typical Ph[1] translocation is seen in ALL and in fact is the most common translocation in adults with ALL (Third International Workshop 1981). One relatively trivial explanation would be that the patients really had CML in lymphoid blast crisis with an undiagnosed chronic phase; this may occur in some patients. However, analysis of DNA from some Ph[1]-positive ALL cells indicates that the breakpoint in chromosome 22 is outside the bcr region. In one study, the majority of adult patients (13 of 17) appeared to have the bcr rearrangement that is seen in CML, whereas it was not found in any of 7 children, who presumably had a more 5' breakpoint in the *BCR* gene (de Klein et al 1986).

Data from our laboratory, as well as others, indicate that the breakpoints on chromosome 22 are greater than 50 kb proximal to the CML break, but that they still are within the *BCR* gene (Rubin et al 1988). The breakpoints on chromosome 9 are similar to those in CML. In our studies, 4 of 6 Ph[1]+ (bcr negative) ALL patients have a rearrangement of *BCR* detected on PFGE. Several investigators have shown that these Ph[1]+ ALL patients have an abnormal sized chimaeric BCR-ABL mRNA (7.0–7.4 kb) and ABL protein (p185[BCR-ABL]) (Chan et al 1987, Clark et al 1987). It should be possible to use several DNA probes from the *BCR* gene and PFGE to distinguish the CML from the ALL breakpoint. In the future, we will understand the role of the BCR and ABL proteins in normal cells and that of the two different chimaeric BCR-ABL proteins in CML and in ALL. Thus the genetic analysis of what appeared to be a simple chromosome change, namely the 9;22 translocation, has revealed unexpected complexity. In the future an understanding of the altered function of the ABL protein will be central to the development of more specific and more effective forms of therapy.

Specificity of chromosome rearrangements

The evidence presented in this chapter clearly demonstrates the remarkable specificity of certain chromosome rearrangements for particular subtypes of tumours, especially leukaemia or lymphoma. The mechanism or mechanisms by which this specificity is achieved are unknown. However, a number of investigators have shown that certain proteins required for promotion of gene expression are synthesized in a very cell-type specific manner (Nomiyama et al 1987). These proteins are only present in the appropriate cell type and therefore the particular gene is activated only in that cell type. The chromosome rearrangements affecting *MYC* in B-cell and T-cell tumours strongly support the interpretation that the specificity resides in the gene that is uniquely active in a particular cell type. Thus the immunoglobulin genes are highly regulated in B cells and can therefore serve as the switch or activator mechanism for *MYC* in B-cells; on the other hand *TCRA* is an active gene in T-cells with a strong enhancer/promotor and it is clearly an activator for *MYC* in T-cells. A reasonable paradigm is that translocations bring together in an inappropriate manner a growth factor or growth factor receptor gene (the proto-oncogene in the examples defined to date) adjacent to an active cell specific gene. It should be emphasized that many of the proto-oncogenes were identified in viruses that cause tumours. However these genes have not been conserved through evolution from yeast and *Drosophila* to the chicken, mouse and man only to cause cancer! Where we have any insight into the function of these genes in normal cells they are growth

factors or growth factor receptors. It is not unexpected that the genes which a virus might co-opt if it developed into a tumour-producing virus would be genes that control proliferation, genes which, under viral regulation, would function abnormally with regard to cell growth. Further support for the concept that oncogenes are growth factors gone wrong is provided by studies at the Hall Institute in Melbourne. There, investigators inserted the cloned gene for granulocyte-macrophage colony stimulating factor into a viral vector, transfected mouse myeloid cells with this gene, and then injected the cells into mice which developed leukaemia (Lang et al 1985). The term 'oncogene' is too short and easy for it to be discarded, but it really refers to respectable genes for growth factors or their receptors.

The analysis of various tumours for alterations in proto-oncogenes has revealed that a number are abnormal as a result of translocations, amplification or mutations. In some situations the relationship of the change in the proto-oncogene to the multistage process of malignant transformation is unclear (Duesberg 1987). Such ambiguity is not a problem with chromosome translocations; the evidence is overwhelming that the t(8;14) in Burkitt lymphoma and the t(9;22) in CML is each an integral component of the cascade of events leading to the transformation of a normal to a malignant cell. The ever-increasing number of translocations reviewed in this chapter provide a potential goldmine for identifying new genes that are unequivocally related to the malignant phenotype of the affected cell. The challenge is to isolate these translocation breakpoint junctions, to identify the genes that are located at these breakpoints, and then to determine the change in gene function that occurs as a consequence of the translocation. The ultimate measure of success, however, will be in the application of these new insights in the development of new, more effective treatments for cancer. In the future, each particular subtype of tumour will be treated in a uniquely defined way that is most appropriate for the specific genetic defect present in that tumour. This should lead to a new era of cancer therapy that is both more effective and less toxic.

REFERENCES

Adams J M, Harris A W, Pinkert C A et al 1985 The c-myc oncogene driven by immunoglobulin in enhancers induces lymphoid malignancy in transgenic mice. Nature 318: 533–538
Anderson D E 1975 Familial susceptibility. In: Fraumeni J F Jr (ed) Persons at high risk of cancer. Academic Press, New York
Arthur D C, Bloomfield C D 1983 Partial deletion of the long

arm of chromosome 16 and bone marrow eosinophilia in acute nonlymphocytic leukemia: A new association. Blood 61: 944–998
Arthur D C, Bloomfield C D 1984 Banded chromosome analysis in patients with treatment-associated acute non-lymphocytic leukemia. Cancer Genetics and Cytogenetics 12: 189–199
Aurias A 1981 Analyse cytogenetique de 21 cas d'ataxie-telangiectasie. Journal de Génétique Humaine 29: 235–247
Aurias A, Dutrilleaux B 1986 Probable involvement of

immunoglobulin superfamily genes in most recurrent rearrangements from ataxia telangiectasia. Human Genetics 72: 210–214

Baer R, Chen K-C, Smith S D et al 1985 Fusion of an immunoglobulin variable gene and a T cell receptor constant gene in the chromosome 14 inversion associated with T cell tumours. Cell 44: 705–713

Bakhshi A, Minowada J, Arnold A et al 1983 Lymphoid blast crises of chronic myelogenous leukaemia represent stages in the development of B-cell precursors. New England Journal of Medicine 309: 826–831

Bartram C R 1988 Molecular genetic analyses of chronic myelocytic leukemia. In: Huhn D, Hellriegel P, Niederle N (eds) Chronic Myelocytic Leukemia and Interferon. Springer Verlag, New York

Bennett J M, Catovsky D, Daniel M-T et al 1976 Proposals for the classification of the acute leukemias: French-American-British (FAB) Co-operative Group. British Journal of Haematology 33: 451–458

Berger R, Bernheim A, Sigaux F et al 1982 Acute monocytic leukemia chromosome studies. Leukemia Research 6: 17–26

Biedler J L, Spengler B A 1976 Metaphase chromosome anomaly: Association with drug resistance and cell-specific products. Science 191: 185–187

Bird M L, Ueshima Y, Rowley J D et al 1989 Chromosome abnormalities in B-cell chronic lymphocytic leukaemia and their clinical correlations. Leukemia 3: 182–191

Bishop J M 1987 The molecular genetics of cancer. Science 235: 305–311

Bloomfield C D, Arthur D C, Frizzera G et al 1983 Nonrandom chromosome abnormalities in lymphoma. Cancer Research 43: 2975–2984

Bloomfield C D, Goldman A I, Alimena G et al 1986 Chromosomal abnormalities identify high-risk and low-risk patients with acute lymphoblastic leukemia. Blood 67: 415–420

Bloomfield C D, Trent J M, van den Berghe H 1987 Report of the committee on structural chromosome changes in neoplasia. Human gene mapping 9. Cytogenetics and Cell Genetics 46: 344–366

Brodeur G M, Green A A, Hayes F A et al 1981 Cytogenetic features of human neuroblastomas and cell lines. Cancer Research 41: 4678–4686

Brodeur G M, Seeger R L, Schwab M 1984 Amplification of N-myc in untreated neuroblastoma correlates with advanced disease stage. Science 224: 1121–1124

Buckton K E, O'Riordan M L, Ratcliffe S et al 1980 A G-banded study of chromosomes in liveborn infants. Annals of Human Genetics 43: 227–239

Caccia N, Bruns G A, Kirsch I R et al 1985 T-cell receptor α-chain genes are located on chromosome 14 at 14q11–14q12 in humans. Journal of Experimental Medicine 161: 1255–1260

Carroll A J, Crist W M, Parmley R T et al 1984 Pre-B cell leukemia associated with chromosome translocation 1;19. Blood 63: 721–724

Cavenee W K, Dryja T P, Phillips R A et al 1983 Expression of recessive alleles by chromosomal mechanisms in retinoblastoma. Nature 305: 779–784

Chaganti R S K 1985 Genetic indicators of cancer predisposition. In: Chaganti R S K, German J (eds) Genetics in Clinical Oncology. Oxford University Press, Oxford, p 149–158

Chaganti R S K, Schonberg S, German J 1974 A manyfold increase in sister chromatid exchange in Bloom's syndrome lymphocytes. Proceedings of the National Academy of Sciences, USA 71: 4508–4512

Chaganti R S K, Miller D R, Meyers P A, German J 1979 Cytogenetic evidence of the intrauterine origin of acute leukaemia in monozygotic twins. New England Journal of Medicine 30: 1032–1034

Chan L C, Karhi K K, Rayter S I et al 1987 A novel abl protein expressed in Philadelphia chromosome positive acute lymphoblastic leukaemia. Nature 325: 635–637

Clark S S, McLaughlin J, Crist W M et al 1987 Unique forms of the abl tyrosine kinase distinguish Ph^1- positive CML from Ph^1- positive ALL. Science 235: 85–88

Clarkson B D, Boyse E A 1971 Possible explanation of the high concordance for acute leukaemia in monozygotic twins (letter to editor) Lancet i: 699–701

Cleary M L, Sklar J 1986 Cloning and structural analysis of cDNA's for bcl-2 and a hybrid bcl-2/immunoglobulin transcript resulting from the t(14;18) translocation. Cell 47: 19–28

Cohen M M, Chaham M, Dagen J, Shmueli E, Kohn G 1975 Cytogenetic investigations in families with ataxia-telangiectasia. Cytogenetics and Cell Genetics 15: 338–356

Croce C M, Isobe M, Palumbo A et al 1985 Gene for α-chain of human T-cell receptor: Location on chromosome 14 region involved in T-cell neoplasms. Science 227: 1044–1047

de Klein A, Hagemeijer A 1984 Cytogenetic and molecular analysis of the Ph^1 translocation in chronic myeloid leukemia. Cancer Surveys 3: 515–529

de Klein A, van Kessel A G, Grosveld G et al 1982 A cellular oncogene is translocated to the Philadelphia chromosome in chronic myelocytic leukemia. Nature 300: 765–767

de Klein A, Hagemeijer A, Bartram C R et al 1986 Rearrangement and translocation of the c-abl oncogene in Philadelphia positive acute lymphoblastic leukemia. Blood 68: 1369–1375

Dryja T P, Cavenee W K, White R et al 1984 Homozygosity of chromosome 13 in retinoblastma. New England Journal of Medicine 310: 550–553

Duesberg P H 1987 Retroviruses as carcinogens and pathogens: expectations and reality. Cancer Research 47: 1199–1220

Fialkow P J, Singer J W 1985 Tracing development and cell lineages in human hemopoietic neoplasia. In: Weissman I L (ed) Leukemia. Dahlem Konferenzen. Springer-Verlag, Berlin p203–222

Fifth International Workshop on Chromosomes in Leukemia-Lymphoma 1987 Correlation of chromosome abnormalities with histologic and immunologic characteristics in non-Hodgkin's lymphoma and adult T-cell leukemia-lymphoma. Blood, 70: 1554–1564

Finger L R, Harvey R C, Moore R C A, Shaw L C, Croce C M 1986 A common mechanism of chromosomal translocation in T and B-cell neoplasia. Science 234: 982–985

Fourth International Workshop on Chromosomes in Leukemia 1984 Cancer Genetics and Cytogenetics 11: 249–360

Francke U 1983 Specific chromosome changes in the human heritable tumours retinoblastoma and nephroblastoma. In: Rowley J D, Ultmann J E (eds) Chromosomes and Cancer,

Bristol-Myers Symposia Series vol. 5. Academic Press, New York, p99–115

Friedberg E C, Ehmann U K, Williams J I 1979 Human diseases associated with defective DNA repair. Advances in Radiation Biology 8: 85–174

Friend S H, Bernards R, Rogelj S et al 1986 A human DNA segment with properties of the gene that predisposes to retinoblastoma. Nature 323: 643–646

Fukuhara S, Rowley J D, Variakojis D et al 1979 Chromosome abnormalities in poorly differentiated lymphocytic lymphoma. Cancer Research 39: 3119–3128

German J 1972 Genes which increase chromosomal instability in somatic cells and predispose to cancer. Progress in Medical Genetics 8: 61–101

German J 1983 Bloom's syndrome. X. The cancer proneness points to chromosome mutation as a crucial event in human neoplasia. In: German J (ed) Chromosome Mutation and Neoplasia. Alan Liss, New York p347–357

Golomb H M, Alimena G, Rowley J D et al 1982 Correlation of occupation and karyotype in adults with acute nonlymphocytic leukemia. Blood 60: 404–411

Groffen J, Stevenson J R, Heisterkamp N et al 1984 Philadelphia chromosomal breakpoints are clustered within a limited region, bcr, on chromosome 22. Cell 36: 93–99

Hagemeijer A, Hahlen K, Sizoo W et al 1982 Translocation (9;11)(p21;q23) in three cases of acute monoblastic leukemia. Cancer Genetics and Cytogenetics 5: 95–105

Han T, Ozer H, Sadamori N et al 1984 Prognostic importance of cytogenetic abnormalities in patients with chronic lymphocytic leukemia. New England Journal of Medicine 310: 288–292

Heath C W 1976 Hereditary factors in leukemia and lymphoma. In: Lynch H T (ed) Cancer Genetics. C C Thomas, Springfield

Hecht F 1982 Leukaemia and chromosome 21. Lancet i: 286–287

Heim S, Mitelman F 1987 Cancer cytogenetics. Alan R Liss, New York

ISCN (1981) 1981 An international system for human cytogenetic nomenclature-high resolution banding. Cytogenetics and Cell Genetics 31: 1–23

Kaiser-McCaw B, Hecht F, Harnden D G et al 1975 Somatic rearrangement of chromosome 14 in human lymphocytes. Proceedings of the National Academy of Sciences 72: 2071–2075

Kaneko Y, Rowley J D, Variakojis D, Chilcote R R, Moohr J W, Patel D 1981 Chromosome abnormalities in Down's syndrome patients with acute leukemia. Blood 58: 459–466

Klein G 1983 Specific chromosomal translocations and the genesis of B-cell derived tumours in mice and men. Cell 32: 311–315

Klein G, Klein E 1986 Conditioned tumorigenicity of activated oncogenes. Cancer Research 46: 3211–3224

Knudson A G 1971 Mutation and cancer: Statistical study of retinoblastoma. Proceedings of the National Academy of Sciences USA 68: 800–823

Knudson A G Jr 1983 Hereditary cancers of man. Cancer Investigations 1: 187–193

Koduru P R K, Filippa D A, Richardson M E et al 1987 Cytogenetic and histologic correlations in malignant lymphomas. Blood 69: 102

Kondo K, Chilcote R R, Maurer H S et al 1984 Chromosome abnormalities in tumor cells from patients with sporadic Wilms' tumor. Cancer Research 44: 5376–5381

Konopka J B, Watanabe S M, Witte O N 1984 An alteration of the human c-abl protein in K562 leukemia cells unmasks associate tyrosine kinase activity. Cell 37: 1035–1042

Krivit W, Good R A 1957 Simultaneous occurrence of mongolism and leukemia. Report of a nationwide survey. American Journal of Diseases of Children 94: 289–293

Kurita S, Kamei Y, Ota K 1974 Genetic studies on familial leukemia. Cancer 34: 1048–1101

Lang R A, Metcalf D, Gough N M et al 1985 Expression of a hemapoietic growth factor cDNA in a factor-dependent cell line results in autonomous growth and tumorigenicity. Cell 43: 531–542

Larson R A, Le Beau M M, Vardiman J W et al 1983 The predictive value of initial cytogenetic studies in 148 adults with acute nonlymphocytic leukemia. Cancer Genetics and Cytogenetics 10: 219–236

Larson R A, Williams S F, Le Beau M M et al 1986 Acute myelomonocytic leukemia with abnormal eosinophils and inv(16) or t(16;16) has a favourable prognosis. Blood 68: 1242–1249

Le Beau M M 1984 Cytogenetic analysis of hematologic malignancies. In: Wahrenburg G (ed) Association of Cytogenetic Technologists, Cytogenetics Laboratory Manual, p1–93

Le Beau M M 1988 Chromosomal fragile sites and cancer-specific rearrangements — a moderating view. Cancer Genetics and Cytogenetics 35: 55–61

Le Beau M M, Albain K S, Larson R A et al 1986a Clinical and cytogenetic correlations in 63 patients with therapy-related myelodysplastic syndromes and acute nonlymphocytic leukemia: Further evidence for characteristic abnormalities of chromosomes No 5 and 7. Journal of Clinical Oncology 4: 325–345

Le Beau M M, Pettenati M J, Lemons R S et al 1986b Assignment of the GM-CSF, CSF-1 and FMS genes to human chromosome 5 provides evidence for linkage of a family of genes regulating hematopoiesis and for their involvement in the deletion (5q) in myeloid disorders. Molecular Biology of Homo Sapiens, Cold Spring Harbor Symposium, vol 51: 899–909

Leder P, Battey J, Lenoir G et al 1983 Translocations among antibody genes in human cancer. Science 222: 765–771

Lee W-H, Bookstein R, Hong F et al 1987 Human retinoblastoma susceptibility gene: Cloning, identification, and sequence. Science 235: 1394–1399

Li F P, Fraumeni J F Jr 1982 Prospective study of a family cancer syndrome. Journal of the American Medical Association 247: 2692–2694

Lynch H T (ed) 1976 Cancer Genetics. C C Thomas, Springfield

McCaw B K, Hecht F 1983 The interrelationships in ataxia-telangiectasia of immune deficiency, chromosome instability and cancer. In: German J (ed) Chromosome mutation and neoplasia. Alan Liss, New York, p193–202

McCaw B K, Hecht F, Harnden D G, Teplitz R L 1975 Somatic rearrangement of chromosome 14 in human lymphocytes. Proceedings of the National Academy of Sciences 72: 2071–2075

MacMahon B, Levy M 1964 Prenatal origin of childhood leukemia: evidence from twins. New England Journal of Medicine 270: 1082–1085

Manolov G, Manolova Y 1972 Marker band in one chromosome 14 from Burkitt lymphomas. Nature 237: 33–34

Marchetto D J, Li F P, Meadows A T 1978 Cancer in parents of children with leukemia. Journal of Pediatrics 93: 537

Mathieu-Mahul D, Caubet J F, Bernheim A 1985 Molecular cloning of a DNA fragment from human chromosome 14(14q11) involved in T cell malignancies. EMBO Journal 4: 3427–3433

Michael P M, Levin M D, Garson O M et al 1984 Translocation 1;19-a new cytogenetic abnormality in acute lymphocytic leukemia. Cancer Genetics and Cytogenetics 12: 333–341

Miller R W 1970 Neoplasia and Down's syndrome. Annals of the New York Academy of Sciences 171: 637–644

Miller R W 1971 Deaths from childhood leukaemia and solid tumors among twins and other sibs in the United States, 1960-67. Journal of the National Cancer Institute 46: 203–209

Mitelman F 1988 Catalog of chromosome aberrations in Cancer. Alan Liss, New York

Mitelman F, Nilsson P G, Brandt C et al: 1981 Chromosome pattern, occupation and clinical features in patients with acute nonlymphocytic leukaemia. Cancer Genetics and Cytogenetics 4: 187–214

Miyamoto K, Tomita N, Ishii A et al 1984 Chromosome abnormalities of leukemia cells in adult patients with T-cell leukemia. Journal of the National Cancer Institute 73: 353–362

Morris C M, Reeve A E, Fitzgerald P H et al 1986 Genomic diversity correlates with clinical variation in Ph[1]− negative chronic myeloid leukemia. Nature 320: 281–283

Mulvihill J J 1984 Clinical ecogenetics of human cancer. In: Bishop J M, Rowley J D, Greaves M (eds) Genes and Cancer. Alan Liss, New York p19–36

Murphree A L, Benedict W F 1984 Retinoblastoma: Clues to human oncogenesis. Science 219: 1028–1033

Nomiyama H, Fromental C, Xiao J H et al 1987 Cell-specific activity of the constituent elements of the simian virus 40 enhancer. Proceedings of the National Academy of Sciences USA 84: 7881–7885

Nowell P C, Hungerford D A 1960 A minute chromosome in human granulocytic leukemia. Science 132: 1497

Pedersen-Bjergaard J, Philip P, Pederson N T, Hou-Jensen K, Svejgaard A, Jensen G, Nissen N I 1984 Acute nonlymphocytic leukemia, preleukemia, and acute myeloproliferative syndrome secondary to treatment of other malignant diseases. Cancer 54: 452–462

Pugh W C, Pearson M, Vardiman J W et al 1985 Philadelphia chromosome-negative chronic myelogenous leukaemia: A morphologic reassessment. British Journal of Haematology 60: 457–467

Raimondi S C, Pui C-H, Behm F G et al 1987 7q32–q36 translocations in childhood T cell leukemia: cytogenetic evidence for involvement of the T cell receptor β-chain gene. Blood 69: 131–134

Robert K-H, Gahrton G, Friberg K et al 1982 Extra chromosome 12 and prognosis in chronic lymphocytic leukemia. Scandinavian Journal of Haematology 28: 163–168

Rosner F, Lee S L 1972 Down's syndrome and acute leukaemia: myeloblastic or lymphoblastic? Report of forty-three cases and review of the literature. American Journal of Medicine 53: 203–218

Rowley J D 1973a A new consistent chromosomal abnormality in chronic myelogenous leukemia. Nature: 243: 290–293

Rowley J D 1973b Identification of a translocation with quinacrine fluorescence in a patient with acute leukemia. Annals de Génétique 16: 109–112

Rowley J D 1981 Down syndrome and acute leukemia: Increased risk may be due to trisomy 21. The Lancet ii 1020–1022

Rowley J D 1984 The biological implications of consistent chromosome rearrangements. Cancer Research 44: 3159–3165

Rowley J D 1988 Chromosome abnormalities in leukemia. Journal of Clinical Oncology 6: 194–202

Rowley J D, Potter D 1976 Chromosomal banding patterns in acute nonlymphocytic leukemia. Blood 47: 705–721

Rowley J D, Testa J R 1983 Chromosome abnormalities in malignant hematologic diseases. In: Advances in Cancer Research. Academic Press, New York, p 103–148

Rowley J D, Golomb H M, Vardiman J et al 1977 Further evidence for a nonrandom chromosomal abnormality in acute promyelocytic leukemia. International Journal of Cancer 20: 869–872

Rowley J D, Haren J M, Wong-Staal F et al 1984 Chromosome pattern in cells from patients positive for human T-cell leukemia virus In: Gallo R C, Essex M E, Gross L (eds): Human T-Cell Leukemia-Lymphoma Viruses. Cold Spring Harbor Laboratory, Cold Spring Harbor, NY, p 85–89

Rubin C M, Carrino J J, Dickler M N et al 1988 Heterogeneity of genomic fusion of BCR and ABL in Philadelphia chromosome-positive acute lymphoblastic leukemia. Proceedings of the National Academy of Sciences USA 85: 2795–2799

Sadamori N, Nishino K, Kusano M et al 1986 Significance of chromosome 14 anomaly at band q11 in Japanese patients with adult T-cell leukemia. Cancer 58: 2244–2250

Saxon A, Stevens R H, Golde D W 1979 Helper and suppressor T-lymphocyte leukemia in ataxia telangiectasia. New England Journal of Medicine 30: 700–704

Schneider N R, Williams W R, Chaganti R S K 1986 Genetic epidemiology of familial aggregation of cancer. In: Advances in Cancer Research. Academic Press, New York, p1–36

Schroeder T M, German J 1974 Bloom's syndrome and Fanconi's anemia: demonstration of two distinctive patterns of chromosome disruption and rearrangement. Humangenetik 25: 299–306

Schwab M, Alitalo K, Klempnauer K-H et al 1983 Amplified DNA with limited homology to myc cellular oncogene is shared by human neuroblastoma cell lines and a neuroblastoma tumour. Nature 305: 245–248

Secker-Walker L M, Swansbury G J, Hardisty R M et al 1982 Cytogenetics of acute lymphoblastic leukemia in children as a factor in the prediction of long-survival. British Journal of Haematology 52: 389–399

Shima E A, Le Beau M M, McKeithan T W et al 1986 T-cell receptor-chain genes move immediately downstream of c-myc in a chromosomal 8;14 translocation in a cell line from a human T-cell leukemia. Proceedings of the National Academy of Sciences USA 83: 3439–3443

Shtivelman E, Lifshitz B, Robert P et al 1985 Fused transcript of abl and bcr genes in chronic myelogenous leukaemia. Nature 315: 550–554

Stern M H, Zhang F, Griscelli C, Thomas G, Aurias A 1988 Molecular characterization of different ataxia telangiectasia T-cell clones. Human Genetics 78: 33–36

Stong R C, Korsmeyer S J, Parkin J L et al 1986 Human acute leukemia cell line with the t(4;11) chromosomal rearrangement exhibits B-lineage and monocytic characteristics. Blood 67: 391–397

Sutherland G R, Hecht F 1985 Fragile sites on human chromosomes. Oxford University Press, New York

Testa J R, Rowley J D 1981 Chromosomes in leukemia and lymphoma with special emphasis on methodology. In: Catovsky D (ed) The Leukemic Cell, Churchill Livingstone, Edinburgh, p184–202

Third International Workshop on Chromosomes in Leukemia. 1981 Cancer Genetics and Cytogenetics 4: 95–142

Tsujimoto Y, Finger L R, Yunis J J et al 1984 Cloning of the chromosome breakpoint of neoplastic B cells with the t(14;18) chromosome translocation. Science 226: 1098–1099

Ueshima Y, Rowley J D, Variakojis D et al 1984 Cytogenetic studies on patients with chronic T cell leukemia/lymphoma. Blood 63: 1028–1038

Vidabaek A 1947 Heredity in human leukemia and its relation to cancer. Munksgaard, Copenhagen

Westbrook C A, Rubin C M, Carrino J J et al 1988 Long range mapping of the Philadelphia chromosome by pulsed-field gel electrophoresis. Blood 71: 697–702

Whang-Peng J, Canellos G P, Carbone P P, Tjio J H 1968 Clinical implications of cytogenetic variants in chronic myelocytic leukemia (CML). Blood 32: 755–766

Whang-Peng J, Bunn P A, Knutsen T et al 1985 Cytogenetic studies in human T-cell lymphoma virus (HTLV)-positive leukemia-lymphoma in the United States. Journal of the National Cancer Institute 74: 357–369

Whyte P, Buchkovich K J, Horowitz J M et al 1988 Association between an oncogene and an antioncogene: the adenovirus EIA proteins bind to the retinoblastoma gene product. Nature 334: 124–129

Williams D L, Tsiatis A, Brodeur G M G et al 1982 Prognostic importance of chromosome number in 136 untreated children with acute lymphoblastic leukemia. Blood 60: 864–871

Williams D L, Look A T, Melvin S L et al 1984 New chromosomal translocations correlate with specific immunophenotypes of childhood acute lymphoblastic leukemia. Cell 36: 101–109

Working formulation for clinical usage 1982 National Cancer Institute sponsored study of classification of non-Hodgkin's lymphomas. Cancer 49: 2112–2135

Yunis J J, Soreng A L 1984 Constitutive fragile sites and cancer. Science 226: 1199–1204

Yunis J J, Frizzera G, Oken M M et al 1987 Multiple recurrent genomic defects in follicular lymphoma; a possible model for cancer. New England Journal of Medicine 316: 79–84

Zech L, Haglund U, Nilsson K, Klein G 1976 Characteristic chromosomal abnormalities in biopsies and lymphoid-cell lines from patients with Burkitt and non-Burkitt lymphomas. International Journal of Cancer 17: 47–56

Zech L, Gahrton G, Hammarstrom L et al 1984 Inversion of chromosome 14 marks human T-cell chronic lymphocytic leukemia. Nature 308: 858–860

Zuelzer W W, Cox D E 1969 Genetic aspects of leukemia. Seminars in Hematology 6: 228–249

82. Immunodeficiency disorders

R. Hirschhorn   K. Hirschhorn

INTRODUCTION

The immune deficiency diseases are part of a spectrum of conditions involving defects in host defence against infections. Adequate host defence is dependent upon the interaction between phagocytic cells, immunocompetent cells and their products, and the complement system. Diseases involving disorders of phagocytes and deficiencies of complement components will be discussed in subsequent chapters. Here we will concern ourselves with disorders of the immune system, including cellular and humoral immunity, both of which play a central role in our ability to resist infection. It is of course the occurrence of unusual types or frequency of infection which draws our attention to the possibility that a patient may be suffering from a host defence disorder.

The immune system, as opposed to the other components of host defence, is specific. Normal immunologic defences are dependent upon memory of cells which recognise foreign antigens and are capable of appropriate responses, either by producing cytotoxic lymphocytes or releasing circulating antibodies specifically directed against the invading antigen. One other component of host defence which is specific involves the ability of lymphocytes to recognize infected cells, a process which is partly mediated by products of the major histocompatibility complex, another topic to be discussed in a subsequent chapter. Derangements of the immune system not only lead to deficient or abnormal responses to foreign antigens, such as invading organisms, but can also lead to abnormalities of another property of the immune system, that of non-response to antigens of the host or recognition of self. This difficulty in appropriate recognition mechanisms leads in a number of immune deficiency diseases to a state of autoimmunity, either against specific antigens on cells of the host or against multiple organs. Therefore the discovery of autoimmune phenomena along with infection represents another clue leading to suspicion of the presence of an immune deficiency disease.

Immunodeficiency disorders are usually classified as if they represent arrests at different stages of differentiation from a common stem cell along a pathway leading to two different major classes of immunologically competent cells (Fig. 82.1). This developmental approach, although not truly satisfactory, is currently the commonly used framework for diagnosis and classification (World Health Organization Technical Report 1978).

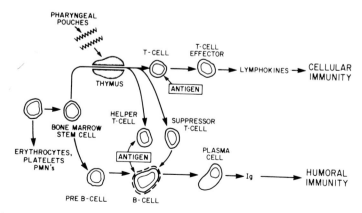

Fig. 82.1   Development of the immune system.

Several excellent text books and reviews exist which give detailed descriptions of the fields of immunodeficiency and basic and clinical immunology (Soothill et al 1983, Hood et al 1984, Paul 1984, Rosen et al 1984, Rosen et al 1986, Rosen & Colten 1987, Nossal 1987, Roitt 1988). In order to lay a groundwork for our description of specific immunodeficiency disorders, we will briefly sketch some of the basic principles.

A pluripotent haematopoietic stem cell is thought to be the progenitor for both a lymphoid stem cell and a stem cell which gives rise to all of the other formed elements of the blood. The lymphoid stem cell can then further differentiate into two developmentally divergent but functionally interacting families of lymphocytes termed T- and B-cells. These two families of cells are respectively responsible for cellular and humoral immunity (Fig. 82.1).

CELLULAR IMMUNITY (T-Cells) (Table 82.1)

Under the influence of the thymus epithelium the lymphoid stem cell differentiates into cells expressing T-cell characteristics, and which account for over 65% of peripheral blood lymphocytes in man. Further differentiation occurs following migration to peripheral tissues and is influenced by thymic humoral factors. This group of thymus-dependent or 'T'-cells can be recognized by its characteristic cell surface receptors. Differentiated T-cells in man carry receptors for sheep erythrocytes and can be identified, enumerated and separated by use of the rosettes which sheep erythrocytes form around these T-cells. It is now apparent that this group of cells is not homogeneous, but contains several functionally and probably developmentally different classes of T-cells which exert helper, suppressor and/or cytotoxic effects. More recently, monoclonal antibodies have been developed which have the potential to recognize either all T-cells, the various different funtionally distinct subsets of T-cells, or T-cell precursors. Many of these monoclonal antibodies are now commercially available and have replaced the sheep erythrocyte method for T-cell identification. It can be expected that new insights will develop as such reagents are more widely used in the study of immunodeficient patients. Mature T-cells also carry receptors for specific antigens. These receptors, whose genes have been cloned, are members of the immuno-globulin-like gene family, which derives most of its specificity by internal gene rearrangements (Royer & Reinherz 1987).

T-cells can be assessed functionally as well as enumerated and, in some immunodeficiency disorders, there is a dissociation of T-cell function and number. In vivo, abnormalities of cellular immune function usually result in infections with intracellular organisms which are then not limited in course by the normal host defences. Patients classically have moniliasis, pneumocystis carinii, generalized vaccinia and varicella, or other similar infections. Normal T-cell function is also required for delayed type skin reactions to common 'recall' antigens such as candida, streptokinase-streptodornase, tetanus and tuberculin. However, negative tests often occur in normal children under one year of age. De novo sensitization with DNCB tests the ability both to mount and to recall a delayed hypersensitivity skin reaction. However, because of the intense reaction which occurs in normal individuals, this test is usually utilized only if in vitro tests reveal a profound defect of cellular immune function.

Initial assessment of cellular immune function can therefore be provided by determination of the peripheral lymphocyte count, enumeration of T-cells, skin testing, routine chest X-ray in order to visualize the thymic shadow and a careful clinical history of types and frequencies of infections, as well as a family history.

In vitro, T-cells respond to several different stimuli including 'polyclonal activators', specific antigens and allogeneic cells. As a result of interaction with these stimuli, lymphocytes increase their rates of synthesis of RNA, protein and DNA and then divide. This proliferative response is most commonly measured by determining the incorporation of radio-labelled thymidine into DNA, although mitotic rate can be used as a rough estimate. Virtually all T-cells respond to a group of substances including plant lectins such as PHA, which are therefore termed 'polyclonal activators'. Only a subclass of 'antigen specific' T lymphocytes initially respond to antigens or foreign molecules. This 'antigen specific' response is only detected (under the standard in vitro conditions) if the donor of the lymphocytes has been previously exposed in vivo to the antigen. Finally, a subclass of T lymphocytes responds to alloantigens on cell surfaces, primarily to antigens coded for by the Ia-like or 'D' region of the histocompatibility complex, and present on surfaces of B lymphocytes. This response to allogeneic determinants is termed the 'mixed lymphocyte reaction', or MLR, since lymphocytes from two different individuals are mixed to elicit the response. The MLR is usually measured in such a fashion that the response of cells from only one of the individuals is measured (one way MLR). It is now clear that many of these stimuli also activate T-cells which can then either suppress or help the reaction of other T-cells and modulate the reactions of B-cells.

T-cells function either directly, by means of cell to cell contact, or by releasing soluble mediators. Thus, activated T-cells release a number of factors or 'lymphokines' which modulate the activity, not only of other lymphoid cells, but also of eosinophils, polymorphonuclear leucocytes and macrophages. The nature of these factors and their role in regulating the immune response is reviewed in the texts cited above. Immunodeficient patients may show a dissociation of ability to release soluble mediators and ability to respond to various stimuli. T lymphocytes when activated can also exhibit both non-specific and specific cytotoxicity.

HUMORAL IMMUNITY (B-CELLS) (Table 82.1)

The second major pathway of lymphoid development results in a terminally differentiated B-cell secreting immunoglobulins (antibodies) which have recognition sites for specific antigens (Cooper 1987). Immunoglobulins are a group of related glycoproteins containing two 'heavy' polypeptide chains and two 'light' polypeptide chains (Fig. 82.2). The prototypic four chain molecule can be broken into two major fragments: the Fab portion consisting of the light chains, linked to the N–terminal half of the heavy chains; and the Fc portion, consisting of the carboxy terminal half of the two heavy chains. The Fab portion contains the antigen binding site while the Fc portion contains sites for activation of complement and for binding of immunoglobulin to diverse cell types via cell membrane Fc receptors. The area of the heavy chains which joins the Fc and Fab portions is the hinge region, and the two heavy chains are joined at this site by several disulphide bonds. The Fab portion can be further subdivided into an N-terminal region which is variable in amino acid sequence in both the heavy and light chains and which determines antibody specificity, and a constant region (C_H1 and C_L) which is constant in

amino acid sequence for a given class or subclass of heavy or light chains. There are five different types of heavy chains, gamma, alpha, mu, delta and epsilon, which differ from each other in the amino acid sequence of their constant regions. There are only two different classes of light chains, kappa and lambda, which differ from each other as to their constant regions. Both kappa and lambda light chains combine with all the different classes of heavy chains, but a single immunoglobulin molecule contains only one class of light chain and one class of heavy chain. The combination of heavy and light chains results in five different classes of immunoglobulins in man: IgG; IgA; IgM; IgD and IgE. IgG is the most abundant serum immunoglobulin and is also the only immunoglobulin transferred across the placenta. There are four different isotypes of IgG, termed IgG_1, IgG_2, IgG_3 and IgG_4. IgA is the primary immunoglobulin in secretions, where it is associated as a dimer with a 'secretory component'. IgM is the next most abundant serum immunoglobulin, usually exists as a 17S pentamer and rises first after a primary response to antigenic challenge. Elevation of IgM in neonates usually indicates intrauterine infection. IgD concentrations in serum are minute but IgD is present on B-cell surfaces. IgE is lowest in concentration in serum, and is responsible for immediate hypersensitivity or allergic reactions and release of mediators such as histamine from basophils and mast cells. Normal values of all the immunoglobulins vary with age and environment and diminished concentrations may reflect increased rates of degradation as well as decreased rates of synthesis.

Genetic polymorphisms have been described for the

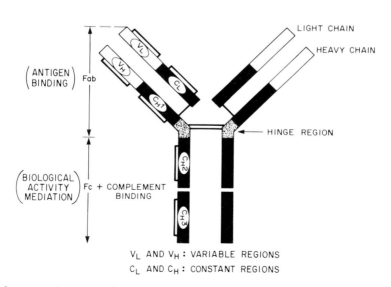

Fig. 82.2 Diagram of a prototypic immunoglobulin molecule.

kappa light chain (Inv), for gamma heavy chain (Gm), and for the alpha heavy chain (Am). The heavy chain for immunoglobulin of IgG, IgA and IgM, IgD and IgE are located on the fourteenth human chromosome (Croce et al 1979, Smith et al 1981). The gene for the kappa light chain has been mapped to chromosome two (McBride et al 1982), and that for the lambda light chain to chromosome twenty two (Erickson et al 1981). The molecular genetics of immunoglobulin synthesis has proven to be a complex process, so far unique for genes related to the immune response, including T-cell receptors. In brief, the genes for the variable and hinge regions are combined with different constant regions by a series of translocations and deletions. As a result, the same variable region can be expressed by immunoglobulin molecules of several different classes.

The development of the terminally differentiated immunoglobulin secreting plasma cell from the primary stem cell occurs in several steps, probably beginning first in fetal liver and then in the bone marrow. The first stage in the differentiation of the stem cell is the appearance of small amounts of cytoplasmic immunoglobulin of the IgM class and possibly only of mu heavy chains. These cells subsequently develop surface immunoglobulin, initially of the IgM class, later of the IgD, IgG and IgA classes. During this stage, B-cells develop receptors for EBV virus, C3 complement components and the Fc portion of aggregated immunoglobulin. By this stage of maturation, the B-cell secretes as well as synthesizes immunoglobulins. The next stage of B-cell differentiation is antigen specific, in that the B-cells secrete antibodies which are specifically directed against an immunising antigen. In some disorders, there is a marked dissociation between the ability to synthesize immunoglobulins and that to synthesize specific antibodies in response to immunisation with antigens. It is also clear that T-cell function is required for the synthesis of certain antibodies and that T-cell function markedly modulates the ability of B-cells both to synthesize immunoglobulins and specific antibodies.

Humoral immune function can be evaluated in vivo and in vitro. In vivo, severely defective humoral immunity is usually associated with recurrent pyogenic infections such as pneumococcal pneumonia, haemophilus influenza meningitis, otitis media, etc. With more prolonged defective humoral immunity (i.e. late onset and/or treated infantile agammaglobulinaemia), the effects of chronic pulmonary disease, diarrhoeal disorders, 'autoimmune phenomena' and infections with viruses which follow an unusual 'slow virus' type of course, are more prominent. In vivo assessment includes quantitative determination of serum IgG, IgM, IgA and IgE by radial immunodiffusion, and/or radioimmunoassay, iso-

haemagglutinins for evaluation of functional IgM, and if still available, Schick test. Specific antibodies are assessed both by reimmunising and/or actively immunising with a variety of protein and polysaccharide antigens (never as live agents) such as diphtheria, tetanus, killed poliomyelitis vaccine, pneumococcal vaccine, etc. and determining the presence and/or the rise of specific antibody titre.

In vitro studies include enumeration of B-cells by virtue of cell surface and intracytoplasmic immunoglobulins (complement and Fc receptors are also found on other cell types and are therefore less useful for initial screening) and newer B-cell specific monoclonal antibodies. In vitro functional assays are performed by stimulating peripheral blood lymphocytes with B-cell mitogens such as pokeweed mitogen, (although the mitogen is not totally B-cell specific) and measuring rates of immunoglobulin synthesis.

OTHER LYMPHOID CELLS

The last class of lymphocytes are the so-called null cells which derived their name from the fact that they bear neither the sheep E rosette receptor characteristic of T-cells, nor the immunoglobulins characteristic of B-cells. This null cell population is truly a heterogeneous population and includes within it the so-called natural killer (NK) cell. Studies of natural cytotoxicity or NK activity are currently an active area of research.

SPECIFIC INHERITED IMMUNODEFICIENCY DISORDERS (Table 82.2)

Combined cellular and humoral immune defects

Severe combined immunodeficiency disease

Severe combined immunodeficiency disease (SCID) is characterized by profound defects of both cellular and humoral immunity and is the most rapidly progressive and devastating of the primary immunodeficiency syndromes. SCID may be inherited as an autosomal or an X-linked recessive. These cannot be differentiated at this time either clinically or by standard immunological tests. This syndrome was originally called 'essential lymphocytophthisis', thymic alymphoplasia or Swiss type agammaglobulinaemia, depending upon the parameters which could be measured at the time. Patients present within the first few months of life with recurrent, persistent infections due to bacterial, viral and fungal pathogens. Candida infection is almost universal and chronic pneumonitis due to infection with *pneumocystis carinii* or other organisms is extremely common. Chronic watery diarrhoea, associated with various organisms, was almost universal in the past. A morbilliform exanthematous rash or exfoliative dermatitis may develop, the latter usually following blood transfusion and probably representing *graft versus host disease* (GVH) due to transfusion of foreign lymphocytes. Chimaerism and GVH can also result from transplacental passage of maternal lymphocytes, and in either case the occurrence of GVH with attendant hepatosplenomegaly and eosinophilia can obscure the diagnosis of SCID. Only irradiated blood should be transfused. Immunisation with live viruses (e.g. polio) can have disastrous consequences and should not be performed. The course of SCID, even without iatrogenic complications, is rapidly progressive, associated with wasting and runting and, if untreated, is fatal by 2 years of age.

Virtually all parameters of cellular and humoral immunity (Table 82.1) are abnormal. Patients usually have absent tonsils, small or absent lymph nodes; absent thymic shadow, are lymphopenic and have markedly diminished numbers of T–cells. Lymphopenia may wax and wane, but in vitro responses are absent or reduced. Immunoglobulins are usually absent, although passively transferred maternal immunoglobulin of the IgG class can be present during the first six months of life. Gm typing can indicate if IgG is maternally derived. Failure of development of serum IgA and/or IgM (which do not cross the placenta) can often provide a sensitive marker for immunoglobulin abnormality early in life. B–cells may be present. Pathologically, there is a lack of normal lymph node architecture and a small, dysplastic or fetal thymus.

The clinical picture of recently reported cases of SCID would appear to be slightly less severe at initial diagnosis (Hitzig & Kenny 1978). This may reflect earlier diagnosis due to the development and wider availability of more sensitive and easily applied in vitro diagnostic tests for evaluation of both cellular immunity and quantitation of immunoglobulins. Additionally, development and widespread and vigorous use of effective antibacterial, antifungal and antiprotozoal agents, as well as parenteral immunoglobulin, may have altered the rapidity of the clinical course and immunologic attrition. For example, the incidence of diarrhoea has declined from 80% in 1968 to only 47% in 1976. Lymphopenia was found in 90% of cases in 1968 compared to 50% in 1976, but in all cases response to PHA was absent or markedly diminished. Further immunologic attrition would appear to account for the fact that all untreated children, independent of their status at diagnosis, still die early in life.

It is now clear that some patients may initially have relatively normal amounts of immunoglobulins, albeit usually of restricted heterogeneity, and that further immunologic attrition then occurs over time. Such patients, previously classified as Nezelof syndrome, are considered to represent part of the spectrum of SCID (see ADA deficiency as an example).

Table 82.1 Cellular and humoral immunity

Lymphoid cells	Cell markers	In vitro functions	In vivo functions
T-cells (Cellular immunity)	1. Sheep erythrocyte ('E') rosettes 2. T-cell specific antigens defined by monoclonal antibodies	1. Proliferation responses to soluble and cell surface antigens or polyclonal activators (e.g. PHA) 2. Mediator production 3. Cytotoxic responses (CML) 4. Regulatory functions	1. 80% of peripheral blood lymphocytes 2. Delayed type skin responses to antigens 3. Defense against intracellular fungi, parasites, viruses 4. Graft rejection 5. Graft vs. Host Disease (GVH)
B-Cells (Humoral immunity)	1. C_3 receptors 2. E_c receptors 3. EBV receptors 4. Surface Ig 5. Intracellular Ig 6. B-cell specific antigens	1. Immunoglobulin synthesis 2. Proliferation responses to EBV, some polyclonal activators and T-cell factors	1. Serum immunoglobulin (IgG, IgA, IgM, IgE, IgD) 2. Specific antibodies 3. Defense against extracellular bacteria and viruses
Null Cells	1. No 'E' or surface Ig 2. Heterogeneous for C_3 and F_c receptors and I_a antigens	1. Precursors T, B myeloid and erythroid cells 2. Natural killer (NK) activity 3. Antibody dependent cellular cytotoxicity (ADCC)	1. ? Defence against tumour cells

Autosomal recessive SCID and adenosine deaminase (ADA) deficiency

In 1972, Giblett and co-workers described two children who presented with autosomal recessive combined immunodeficiency, who both also had autosomal recessive inherited absence of the enzyme adenosine deaminase (ADA). This represented the first molecular defect defined in immunodeficiency disorders (Ciba Foundation Symposium 1979, Hirschhorn 1986, Kredich & Hershfield 1989).

ADA deficiency has been estimated to account for SCID in 1/3–1/2 of families where the mode of inheritance is not clearly X-linked. In a small sample of definitely autosomal recessively inherited SCID (as defined by the occurrence of an affected female), the incidence of ADA deficiency has been found to be 57%, with 95% confidence limits of 18–90%. Therefore a substantial proportion of autosomal recessive SCID appears to be due to deficiency of ADA. These estimates are consistent with the results of an informal survey of 130 patients with SCID (both autosomal recessive and X-linked) which revealed 22% with ADA deficiency. Approximately 80–90% of ADA deficient SCID patients are indistinguishble clinically, as well as by in vitro tests of immune function, from other patients with SCID. Normal numbers of lymphocytes and T lymphocytes, as

Table 82.2 Primary immunodeficiency disorders

	Mode of inheritance	
	X-linked	AR
1. *Combined humoral (B-Cell) and cellular (T-Cell) immune defects*		
Severe combined immunodeficiency (SCID)		+
Adenosine deaminase deficiency	−	+
Other SCID	+	+
With leucopenia (reticular dysgenesis)	−	+
Bare lymphocyte syndrome	−	+
Cellular immunodeficiency with abnormal immunoglobulins (? Nezelof)	?	?
SCID with growth hormone deficiency	−	+
2. *Humoral (B-Cell) immune defects*		
Infantile agammaglobulinaemia	+	(rare)
Immunodeficiency with hyper IgM	+	?
Common variable hypogammaglobulinaemia	?	?
Lymphoproliferative syndrome	+	?
Selective IgA deficiency	−	+ (? AD)
Selective IgM deficiency	?	?
Selective IgG subclass deficiency	−	+
Hyper IgE, eczema and recurrent infections	−	+ (? AD)
3. *Cellular (T-Cell) immune defects*		
Thymic hypoplasia (DiGeorge syndrome)	−	+
Purine nucleoside phosphorylase deficiency	−	+
Chronic mucocutaneous candidiasis (with or without endocrinopathy)	−	+
Nezelof sydnrome	?	?
4. *Specific syndromes involving other organ systems with immunodeficiency as a significant manifestation*		
Wiskott-Aldrich syndrome	+	−
Ataxia telangiectasia	−	+
Short limbed dwarfism with cartilage hair hypoplasia and cellular immunodeficiency	−	+
With SCID	?	+
With antibody deficiency	−	+
Transcobalamin II deficiency	−	+
Multiple carboxylase deficiency		
Chromosome 18 abnormalities		
Down syndrome		
Chromosome instability syndromes	−	+
5. *Metabolic disorders with suspected immunodeficiency*		
Orotic aciduria	−	+
Methylmalonic aciduria	−	+
Storage disorders	+	+

AR = autosomal recessive; AD = autosomal dominant; X-linked = X-linked recessive well as some degree of response to PHA, may be found at birth and the diagnosis can be made in a family at risk, most reliably at birth by determination of ADA activity in the red cells. The disease is progressive and any residual T–cell function found at birth rapidly disappears. In 10–15% of the cases, onset of disease may occur later than 3–6 months. For example, one of the first reported patients, followed closely because of the prior death of a sib, was apparently immunocompetent and healthy until over 2 years of age. The outstanding feature in this late onset group is the persistence of immunoglobulins and even the presence of specific antibody. These patients were undoubtedly originally classified as having Nezelof syndrome. However immunoglobulin levels eventually fall, and in one case there was a preterminal monoclonal IgG. Unless treated, death has occurred by 3 years of age and usually earlier.

While genetic heterogeneity may contribute to the phenotypic diversity, this degree of differences in clinical manifestations has been found between sibs, probably indicating influence of environmental factors, although interaction with other genetic loci has not been ruled out.

Bony abnormalities, originally appreciated radiologically and subsequently studied pathologically, occur frequently in patients with ADA deficient SCID. This bony abnormality (8 of 13 families) was evident on physical examination as prominence of the costocondral rib junctions, similar to a rachitic rosary. On X–ray, cupping and flaring of the costochondral junctions was seen as well as a dysplastic pelvis. However, these changes are not pathognomonic and similar radiological changes can be observed in non-immunodeficient, severely malnourished patients as well as ADA-normal immunodeficient patients. Although the radiological changes may not be specific, these bony alterations have served to alert physicians to the possibility of ADA-deficient SCID. Thymic pathology is also proposed to differ in the ADA deficient cases, with the retention of some Hassall's corpuscles suggesting secondary atrophy of a previously differentiated thymus. However, on a practical level, examination of thymic pathology in patients from seven kindreds with and without ADA deficiency did not allow for consistent correlation between the type of thymic pathology and the presence or absence of ADA deficiency.

Currently, numerous investigators are attempting to define the precise pathophysiological mechanisms responsible for the relatively specific toxicity for the immune system. Whatever the mechanism, it is clear that affected children accumulate the substrates of the deficient enzyme, adenosine and deoxyadenosine, that they excrete massive amounts of deoxyadenosine in urine and

that they accumulate massive amounts of the phosphorylated compound deoxy ATP in their cells. The most probable toxic metabolite is deoxy ATP, a potent allosteric inhibitor of ribonucleotide reductase and therefore of DNA synthesis. Other compounds, such as methylated adenine derivatives, have been found to accumulate, but their significance is speculative.

The gene for ADA, which has been mapped to 20q13.1, has been cloned and sequenced from cDNA and genomic DNA. Most patients show point mutations, but some deletions have been described.

ADA deficiency with late onset or no immunodeficiency At least three individuals have been described who lack ADA in their erythrocytes and who show late onset immunodeficiency (after age 4), primarily involving T–cells. A number of children have been found who lack RBC ADA, but show sufficient residual activity in their lymphocytes to sustain normal immune function.

Other Forms of SCID with Unusual Characteristics

Dissociation of quantitative measures and function Normal numbers of lymphocytes with markers characteristic of T– and B–cells, plasma cells and normal quantities of immunoglobulin have been reported in two male offspring of a consanguineous family (Gelfand et al 1979). However, all functional parameters (Table 82.1) were markedly abnormal. A defect in the mobility of Con A receptors was found in the patients' lymphoid cells. It can be expected that more cases of SCID with dissociation of quantitative and functional parameters (with or without a Con A capping defect) will be described, as the appropriate functional assays are applied more widely. At least one such patient without a capping defect has been described (Fontán et al 1988).

Bare lymphocyte syndrome At least 30 patients have been described in which lymphocytes and platelets from affected children lack Class I HLA (A, B and C) determinants as well as the associated subunit, beta$_2$-microglobulin (Touraine et al 1985). Other patients lack Class II (D, DR, DQ and DP) determinants, while yet others lack both classes. Class I antigens are present in normal amounts on other cell types. In the Class II negative patients, the defect appears to be a trans-acting regulatory gene (DNA-binding protein) that controls the expression of Class II genes (de Préval et al 1988), even that induced by gamma-interferon in fibroblasts. This opens the possibility for prenatal diagnosis. The clinical picture has ranged from classical SCID, albeit with some retention of parameters of cellular and humoral immunity, to a less rapidly progressive clinical picture and a less complete absence of HLA antigens to cases resembling agammaglobulinaemia. The inheritance appears to be autosomal recessive.

Reticular dysgenesis or SCID with granulocytopenia

Six cases in five families have been reported of this rare disorder characterized by virtually complete loss of granulocytes and lymphocytes, a small thymus, but normal erythrocytes and platelets. In some cases, the diminution in lymphocyte and granulocyte numbers may initially be less profound, and in one case, although response of cord blood lymphocytes to PHA was absent, the percentage of T lymphocytes was normal (Ownby et al 1976). All reported patients died of infections by 4 months of age, which is not surprising in view of the deficit in two major host defense systems. The disorder appears to be autosomally recessively inherited. Some patients with SCID have shown eosinophilia (Omenn syndrome) apparently not due to GVH disease.

Therapy

Complete immunologic reconstitution (as well as clearing of abnormal metabolites in ADA deficiency) can be obtained by bone marrow transplantation if a histocompatible sib (or other family member in a consanguineous family) is available (Bortin & Rimm 1977). However, there is only a 1/4 chance for a normal sib to be histocompatible. Glven a reasonable probability of two normal living sibs, the probability of finding a compatible sib donor is less than half (7/16). However, if a patient is the offspring of a first cousin marriage, not only will there be a higher probability of finding a compatible sib donor, but there is a small but significant chance (3/64) that one of the parents will be compatible. In addition, the search for compatible donors in such consanguineous families should extend at least to aunts and uncles, since even they have a reasonable, although smaller, chance of being compatible. These are important considerations because there is an increased rate of consanguinity in the parents of children with rare recessive disorders. GVH reactions can occur even when current 'typing' procedures predict a successful transplant. Currently no equally effective and safe alternative therapy is available, but newer methods of depleting donor marrow of T(GVH) cells allows attempts at transplantation with haploidentical marrow from a parent or sib.

In ADA deficient SCID, multiple partial exchange transfusions with normal irradiated packed erythrocytes (which contain both the deficient enzyme and transport sites for the accumulated substrates) has resulted in marked diminution of abnormal metabolites, increased growth rate and length of survival and partial restoration of immunological function. However, it is now apparent that such therapy provides only temporary and/or partial amelioration in the hope that in the interim, more permanent therapy will become available. Recently, a modified preparation of ADA coupled to polyethylene glycol has been injected into several ADA deficient patients, resulting in sufficiently high circulating enzyme levels to more completely reduce toxic metabolites and restore immunofunction (Hershfield et al 1987). While promising, this therapy must still be evaluated on a long-term basis.

Genetics

The syndrome of SCID is genetically heterogeneous. The incidence of SCID has been estimated as between 1/100 000 and 1/500 000 live births, but the diagnosis is often missed and this may be a gross under-estimate of the incidence of this disorder. Both X-linked and autosomal recessive modes of inheritance as well as 'sporadic' cases have been found. The ratio of affected males to females in the whole group is approximately 3:1, suggesting that half of all cases are X-linked and that a majority of families with a single affected child who is male will be carrying an X-linked gene for SCID. A more accurate estimate in a particular family can be calculated by the use of Bayesian mathematics. The *gene* frequency for the X-linked gene is half the incidence of SCID in the population. The *gene* frequency of the autosomal recessive would be markedly greater (the square root of half the population incidence), if all autosomal cases were caused by the same abnormal gene. Since, however, there are at least two, and probably more, different loci responsible for autosomal recessive SCID (see below), the combined frequencies of genes responsible for autosomal recessive SCID is even higher. Based upon newborn screening, the incidence of complete ADA deficiency in the population would appear to be less than one in a million and the incidence of heterozygous carriers would then be less than one in 500. ADA deficient SCID can be diagnosed prenatally by assay of amniotic fluid fibroblasts for ADA activity or by chorionic villus sampling (Dooley et al 1987, Perignon et al 1987). Other forms of SCID have been diagnosed prenatally by testing in vitro responses of fetal blood lymphocytes obtained by fetoscopy to polyclonal activators as well as by use of monoclonal antibodies to T-cells. In X-linked SCID females will be unaffected, but it must be emphasized that occurrence of multiple male affected children does not establish X-linkage. For example, even in a family with three affected males, there is approximately a 12.5% risk of autosomal recessive inheritance. Therefore, except in cases of clear, well documented X-linkage, all cases of SCID should be tested for ADA deficiency, since this is currently the only form of SCID which can be easily diagnosed prenatally.

Detection of heterozygous carriers of SCID is currently feasible for ADA deficiency. Using quantitative determination of erythrocyte ADA, there is an approximately 10% overlap between carriers and normals. All living family members should be phenotyped for the normal genetic polymorphism of ADA (codominant expression of two common alleles) since anomalous inheritance of the polymorphism can demonstrate that a 'null' allele is segregating in the family. Based upon the gene frequency of the polymorphic forms of ADA, this approach can be diagnostic in approximately 30% of families if grandparents, uncles, aunts, etc. are tested. Heterozygote detection has recently become feasible for X–linked SCID, based on the finding that all T–cells of carrier females express only the genes of the X chromosome not carrying the mutant gene. Such lack of normal mosaicism can be detected by two methods. One of these (Puck et al 1987) is performed by fusing isolated T–cells with HPRT deficient rodent fibroblasts. Hybrid clones which have lost the inactive X after selection for the active X are examined for DNA polymorphisms for which the female in question is known to be heterozygous. If the clones all show the same allele, the female is a carrier. A less tedious, but presently a less generally applicable method (Fearon et al 1987, applied to X–linked SCID by Goodship et al 1988) uses the observation that certain genes on the inactive X are hypermethylated. If the female tested is heterozygous for a DNA polymorphism on the X chromosome, detectable by both a methylation sensitive and insensitive endonuclease, the methylation pattern of the polymorphic gene can be determined. If the T–cells are monomorphic for the methylation pattern, the same allele must be active in all T–cells, and the female is a carrier. Incidentally, the gene for X–linked SCID has been mapped to Xq11–13 (de Saint Basile et al 1987), but has not been cloned or identified as to function.

Primary B–cell deficiencies: humoral immune defects

Disorders of humoral immunity or antibody deficiency disorders can be of infantile or late onset, involve absence of all classes, or only specific classes, of immunoglobulins, with or without absence of B–cells of different maturational stages. In rare cases, quantitatively normal but functionally inactive immunoglobulins can occur. The primary clinical manifestation in all of these disorders is recurrent, invasive, severe infection with common pyogenic bacteria such as *haemophilus influenza* and *streptococcus pneumoniae*. The infections usually re-

spond to vigorous antibiotic therapy, but recur. The response to most viral, fungal or mycobacterial infections is normal, reflecting the retention of normal T–cell immunity. In the later onset form, diarrhoeal disorders, chronic pulmonary disease and autoimmune phenomena are more prominent features and variable degrees of cellular immune defects may become apparent.

Infantile agammaglobulinaemia

Infantile X–linked aggammaglobulinaemia (Bruton disease) is the classical example of an isolated B–cell defect (Rosen 1980). The clinical course of these patients is such that they are usually healthy during the first months of life, probably reflecting the presence of adequate amounts of placentally transferred maternal IgG. They then begin to suffer from multiple recurrent infections, usually with pyogenic organisms, while infections with viruses and gram negative bacteria are not strikingly increased. The infections are most prominent at sites of initial contact with pathogens and include infections of the upper and lower respiratory tract and skin and eventually complications of sepsis such as meningitis. Although the use of antibiotics has lessened mortality from acute infections, without more specific therapy these patients will go on to develop chronic pulmonary disease, bronchiectasis and respiratory failure. These children are more susceptible to infection with hepatitis virus and enteroviruses, particularly ECHO and poliomyelitis viruses. Paralytic polio can follow administration of live polio vaccine and a dermatomyositis–like syndrome apparently due to ECHO virus can evolve, even in patients treated with gammaglobulin. These patients also often develop rheumatoid-like arthritis which improves with therapy. Haemolytic anaemia and asthma are also seen.

The diagnosis is made by demonstrating a severe deficiency of IgG, IgM and IgA by immunoelectrophoresis or quantitative determination of immunoglobulins. The diagnosis is often suggested by the presence of hypoplastic tonsils; lymph nodes may appear to be present, but biopsy reveals hyperplasia of reticular cells. As expected, B–cells are lacking in over 90% of patients with X–linked agammaglobulinaemia, although pre-B–cells can be detected and isolated from bone marrow by special techniques. There may be some degree of intrafamilial variation as to the completeness of absence of B–cells. In rare cases of X–linked agammaglobulinaemia, B–cells are present, although these probably represent less mature B–cells. T–cell immunity is normal in affected children and childhood exanthems are handled normally. Standard therapy consists of 0.6 ml/kg immunoglobulin (100mg/kg) every month by deep IM injection, preceded by three loading doses, but a newly developed intravenous preparation has become the treatment of choice. Almost all cases of agammaglobulinaemia are X-linked, in that there is no male to male transmission, the healthy sisters of affected patients have affected male children and maternal uncles are affected.

Infantile agammaglobulinaemia must be differentiated from transient hypogammaglobulinaemia of infancy in which there is a prolongation of the normal physiological decline in IgG. Normally, after birth, the total IgG initially falls precipitously, then slowly begins to rise after a nadir at 5–6 months of age, reflecting the catabolism of maternal IgG counterbalanced by the slow increase in the child's own synthesis of IgG. Simultaneously, IgA and IgM concentrations begin to increase. In transient hypogammaglobulinaemia the expected rises can be delayed until 3 years of age. Sequential measurements demonstrating increases in IgA and IgM, as well as determination of B-cell numbers, help to differentiate this temporary disorder from X-linked agammaglobulinaemia. When present, a family history of maternal male relatives or previous male sibs with persistent agammaglobulinaemia (IgG less than 200 mg percent, and virtually absent IgM, IgA, IgD and IgE) aids in diagnosis.

Genetics Inheritance is that of a classical X-linked disorder. As in any lethal X-linked disorder, one third of patients should reflect new mutations and therefore a family history may not be obtained. The X-linkage indicates that the defect is not at the level of the structural genes for immunoglobulins which are located on autosomal chromosomes (number 14 for the heavy chains). The X-linked locus has recently been mapped to Xq21.3–22 (Kwan et al 1986, Malcolm et al 1987), but the gene has not been cloned or identified as to function. A rarer variant of X-linked agammaglobulinaemia has been shown to be due to abnormal variable chain gene rearrangement resulting in truncated heavy chains (Schwaber & Chen 1988). Prenatal diagnosis for the common form of the disease may become possible by B-cell analysis in fetal blood or by linkage analysis with closely linked RFLPs. Heterozygote detection is possible by the two methods described for X-linked SCID and has been achieved (Fearon et al 1987, Conley & Puck 1988) but with the use of B-cells rather than T-cells.

There is a familial incidence of transient hypogammaglobulinaemia but the formal genetics of this undoubtedly heterogeneous disorder has not been delineated. There is a high incidence of transient hypogammaglobulinaemia in sibs of children with immunodeficiency disorders but definitive studies to demonstrate that the increased incidence does not simply reflect more frequent determinations of immunogloblins in these children do not exist. In a small population of patients with transient hypogammaglobulinaemia we could not detect any heterozygotes for ADA deficiency, although transient hypogammaglobulinaemia has been observed in heterozygous sibs of ADA deficient patients. The bulk of transient hypogammaglobulinaemia would appear to be unassociated with a familial incidence of immunodeficiency.

Autosomal recessive infantile agammaglobulinaemia

Rare cases have been described of females affected with infantile agammaglobulinaemia, clinically indistinguishable from the X-linked form. They are unlikely to represent cases of an X-linked recessive mutant gene which is expressed in females because of extreme Lyonisation, since more than one affected female in a family has been reported, and patients have appeared in families without a history of the X-linked disorder.

X-linked agammaglobulinaemia and isolated growth hormone deficiency

A kindred with X-linked agammaglobulinaemia and isolated growth hormone deficiency has been reported (Fleisher et al 1980).

Late onset or common variable hypogammaglobulinaemia

Common variable hypogammaglobulinaemia is essentially a wastebasket diagnosis and encompasses a majority of patients with humoral immune defects. This group of disorders has unfortunately been previously termed 'acquired agammaglobulinaemia'. This term should not be used in view of the common occurrence of genetic disorders which are not phenotypically manifest until adult life, and genetic disorders such as alpha-1-antitrypsin deficiency which require as yet poorly defined environmental challenges to result in disease. This is a clinical entity characterized by late-onset panhypogammaglobulinaemia, although IgE production may be unaffected. A significant proportion of patients also have defects in some parameters of cell mediated immunity. Men and women are equally affected and the disorder can begin at any age. The clinical manifestations (Hermans et al 1976) include recurrent sinobronchopulmonary infections, chronic diarrhoea with malabsorption, giardiasis and small bowel abnormalities, including nodular lymphoid hyperplasia. In addition, other phenomena including pernicious anaemia, abnormalities of complement, cholelithiasis, thyroid abnormalities and neoplasia occur in a significant proportion of patients. Lymphadenopathy and splenomegaly due to reticular cell hyperplasia is common.

This group of disorders is also heterogeneous when examined at the cellular level. Patients may have no B–cells, as in the X–linked infantile syndrome, but more often B–cells are normal or even increased in number. B–cells from a small subset of patients synthesize but do not secrete immunoglobulin in vitro. Some of these latter patients appear to be unable to glycosylate immunoglobulin normally and their B–cells either lack or have markedly diminished EBV receptors (Schwaber et al 1980). In some cases, increased T–cell suppression of B–cell function is found (Waldmann et al 1976).

The possible role of heredity in this heterogeneous group is presently basically undefined. Several investigators have documented an increased incidence of serologic abnormalities or impairment of leucocyte function and autoimmunity in family members. Unfortunately, many of these studies do not have a carefully age matched control population. Familial constellations, with manifestations among sibs ranging from agammaglobulinaemia to selective immunoglobulin deficiency, have been described. Although some of these disorders may well represent primarily the effects of environmental factors, it is highly likely that further dissection and discovery of specific molecular defects will reveal a strong genetic component for these disorders.

Hyper IgM with hypogammaglobulinaemia

Hypogammaglobulinaemia with raised IgM is a group of disorders characterized by the presence of increased amounts of IgM and usually also IgD with a decrease in the other immunoglobulins. Clinically, patients show increased susceptibility to recurrent pyogenic infections, to autoimmune disease associated with IgM antibodies and to malignant lymphoproliferation of IgM producing B-cells (Geha et al 1979). B-cells are normal in number but qualitatively abnormal in that they either spontaneously secrete or can be driven to secrete IgM in vitro but cannot be induced in vivo to secrete IgG. The disease is often seen as an X-linked form, but autosomal recessive, sporadic early or later onset forms have also been reported. In one family with the X-linked form, the gene has been tentatively mapped to Xq24-27 (Mensink et al 1987).

X-linked lymphoproliferative syndrome

The relationship of the X-linked lymphoproliferative syndrome (Duncan Disease) to common variable hypo-

gammaglobulinaemia and/or hyper IgM is not clear. This syndrome could illustrate the marked variation in phenotype which can be expected in the immunodeficiency disorders because of the dependence upon interaction with environment for expression. An X–linked recessive lymphoproliferative syndrome has been described in several large kindreds (Purtilo et al 1977). The phenotypes described in a single family are of two major types, a proliferative phenotype including fatal infectious mononucleosis, Burkitt lymphoma or plasmacytoma and an aproliferative phenotype including late onset agammaglobulinaemia, agranulocytosis or aplastic anaemia. (Other abnormalities were described in a large kindred but may reflect some degree of earlier inbreeding, suggested by the marriages of three sisters to three brothers in the kindred.) What is clear is that there appears to be an X–linked recessive disorder which results in an inability to contain infection with EB virus. Affected male children at some time in the course may develop hyper IgM, agammaglobulinaemia, aplastic anaemia or lymphoid malignancies. The gene has been preliminary mapped to Xq24-27 (Skare et al 1987) in one family, but other studies do not agree.

Selective IgA deficiency

Selective IgA deficiency is the most commonly observed immunodeficiency with an incidence of 0.1-0.2% in normal blood donors. There is a 14-fold increase in incidence of IgA deficiency among the first-degree relatives of these normal individuals (Koistinen 1976, Ammann & Hong 1980). In most such individuals this deficiency is not associated with any disease. However, normal blood donors are by definition healthy adults and therefore individuals with an increased predisposition to infection beginning in childhood would not be included. A prospective study with matched controls beginning at an early age would be required to determine more critically the significance of IgA deficiency in the general population. Familial occurrence of IgA deficiency has been reported on numerous occasions, with patterns of inheritance consistent with both an autosomal dominant and autosomal recessive mode of inheritance and associated with increased infections, primarily sinopulmonary in nature. Discordance of IgA deficiency in identical twins has been described, indicating a strong environmental component for the determination of serum IgA. A high incidence of IgA deficiency has also been reported in patients with recurrent infections, autoimmune disorders such as rheumatoid arthritis, systemic lupus erythematosus, malabsorption syndrome, sometimes with gluten sensitivity, childhood asthma and other atopic disease. The possible aetiologic relationship of IgA deficiency and the disease are difficult to evaluate since most studies involve correlating types of disease with IgA deficiency in a population referred because of frequent infections, atopy, etc.

IgA deficiency is also found in one third to one half of individuals with a wide variety of chromosome 18 abnormalities; is associated with ataxia telangiectasia (see below); and can presage development of hypogammaglobulinaemia. Clearly, the IgA deficiency associated with defects in either the short or long arm of chromosome 18 does not involve the structural gene for IgA heavy chain which is on chromosome 14. As a note of warning, IgA deficient individuals often have antibodies to IgA and can have a severe transfusion reaction when given normal whole blood, plasma, or gamma-globulin.

Selective IgM deficiency

Selective IgM deficiency, in contrast to selective IgA deficiency, is rare. It has been reported in two patients with septicaemia, meningococcal meningitis, malabsorption, haemolytic anaemia and eczema. Familial aggregation has been noted and the deficiency has been described in sibs. A study in Great Britain reported fairly high frequency of isolated deficiency of IgM. Approximately 20% of subjects were asymptomatic while 60% had severe recurrent infections, often with bacteraemia. The condition was frequently familial and was four times more common in males than females (Hobbs 1975).

Selective IgG subclass deficiency

Selective deficiency of specific IgG subclasses either due to regulatory or structural mutations could, in theory, lead to inability to cope with a limited spectrum of infectious agents. This hypothesis is based upon the observation that certain antibody activities occur largely within specific subclasses of IgG. Various abnormalities in subclass distribution and an apparent structural gene defect in a family have been reported in patients examined because of immunodeficiency (Yount et al 1970). Here again, cause and effect relationships are unclear and possibly must await dissection at the level of the DNA. Alternatively, these variants may reflect primary imbalance of T-cell subsets.

Hyper IgE and recurrent infections

The hyper IgE syndrome would appear to encompass at least two or more different syndromes which are often confused. The first is a rare syndrome described by Buckley (Buckley 1980) characterized by recurrent staphylococcal abscesses, markedly elevated serum IgE,

coarsened facies and a history of pruritic dermatitis. The severe recurrent staphylococcal abscesses often begin in infancy and involve skin, lungs, joints and other sites, with virtually universal development of pneumatocoeles. The abscesses are tender and warm although systemic toxicity is less than expected. Infections with other bacterial and fungal agents can occur. All patients at some time have a pruritic dermatitis, but the distribution and characteristics of the lesion are said to be different from classical atopic dermatitis. Eosinophilia has been a consistent finding. A neutrophil or monocyte chemotactic defect is *not* a necessary part of this syndrome and is an inconstant finding. Variable abnormalities in cellular immunity are seen, manifested usually as skin test anergy and diminished proliferation in vitro to antigens and allogeneic cells.

Several patients have been described under the eponym of Job syndrome. The original patients were fair-skinned, red-headed girls with eczema and recurrent 'cold' staphylococcal abscesses of the skin, subcutaneous tissue, lymph nodes, lung, liver and abdominal cavity. There were systemic signs of infection but little local inflammatory reaction. These patients were subsequently found to have hyper IgE and a chemotactic defect.

Additional patients have been described with neutrophil chemotactic defects, hyper IgE, severe weeping atopic dermatitis, cellulitis and recurrent staphylococcal abscesses. The exact relationship of the various syndromes remains to be elucidated.

Genetics In the Buckley syndrome, both males and females have been affected with equal frequency and members of succeeding generations have also been affected, suggesting an autosomal dominant mode of inheritance with incomplete penetrance.

Cellular (T-cell) immune defects

Thymic hypoplasia (DiGeorge syndrome)

Until recently, the DiGeorge syndrome (thymic hypoplasia) had been considered the classic prototype example of an isolated T-cell defect. The DiGeorge syndrome is usually a congenital sporadic disorder in which there are abnormalities of structures derived from the third and fourth pharyngeal pouches, including the thymus and parathyroids. The absence of the parathyroid glands often results in neonatal tetany. Patients have a characteristic facies with micrognathia, low set malformed 'pixie' ears, cleft palate, short philtrum of the lip and anti-mongoloid slant of the eyes. There are often associated abnormalities of the aortic arch (commonly truncus arteriosus communis) and the cardiac manifestations may overshadow the other features of this disorder. Although the thymic shadow is absent radiographically, some ectopic thymic tissue may be identified at autopsy. This variability in the degree of thymic hypoplasia presumably explains the variability in the extent of the T-cell defect in different patients. Patients are not usually profoundly lymphopenic but cellular immune function is usually absent or markedly diminished with severely reduced, to absent, T-cells as determined by cell surface markers and absence of response to mitogens or antigens. These patients classically have multiple candida and viral infections, while antibody function is usually normal. B-cell percentages are elevated. These abnormalities can be explained by a lack of thymic factors needed to differentiate T-cell precursors into mature mitogen and antigen responsive T-cells. The immune defect appears to respond to implantation of fetal thymus. Therapy is difficult to evaluate critically since, in some patients, immune function gradually improves, presumably reflecting growth of thymic remnants.

Genetics The incidence is not known, and less than 100 cases have been reported in the literature (Conley et al 1979, Raatikka et al 1981). The diagnosis is often made at autopsy, suggesting that the syndrome is often missed. Almost all cases have been solitary, but three families with familial pharyngeal pouch syndrome have been reported. In these families, the findings were consistent with autosomal recessive inheritance, although dominant inheritance has been reported.

In the past few years, many cases of DiGeorge syndrome have been reported to show a deletion of 22q11 (de la Chapelle et al 1981, Cannizzaro & Emanuel 1985), either sporadic or as a result of an unbalanced translocation, often familial.

Purine nucleoside phosphorylase deficiency

Genetic deficiency of purine nucleoside phosphorylase (PNP) results in an isolated defect of cellular immunity and was the second specific genetic molecular defect described which results in immunodeficiency, it is rarer than ADA deficiency. The disorder was initially discovered in a 5-year-old girl with a history of recurrent infections. At least nine children with PNP deficiency in six families have been found to date (Ciba Foundation Symposium 1979, Kredich & Hershfield 1983, Hirschhorn 1986). It is apparent that all the patients have had severe T-cell dysfunction, as measured by marked reduction in T-cell numbers, reduced response to mitogens and allogeneic cells, and severe recurrent fungal and viral infections. The latter infections are often fatal. In marked contrast to ADA deficiency, humoral immunity has been quantitatively normal or increased as measured by normal numbers of B-cells in the blood, and of plasma cells in lymphoid tissue; normal to elevated immunoglobulin concentration in vivo, and normal antibody production. Several patients have had abnormally excessive antibody production, usually with concurrent viral infections. These abnormalities have included Coombs positive haemolytic anaemia, positive ANA, rheumatoid factor and monoclonal gammopathy, all suggesting abnormalities in T suppressor function.

In several patients, the disease has shown a course of immunologic attrition. Clinical onset of disease has varied from 6 months to 6 years of age. Non-immunologic abnormalities have included anaemia in five patients (four of the six families). Three patients (two families) have had neurological abnormalities of spastic tetraplegia or ataxia and tremor, reminiscent of the abnormalities seen in a few ADA deficient patients.

Purine nucleoside phosphorylase (PNP) reversibly catalyzes the phosphorylysis of the purine nucleosides guanosine, inosine, deoxyguanosine and deoxyinosine, and is thus the next enzyme in the purine salvage pathway following adenosine deaminase. Although the equilibrium of the reaction in vitro favours nucleoside synthesis, in vivo the direction is towards the generation of the free purine base from the corresponding nucleoside. Patients with PNP deficiency therefore accumulate large amounts of all four nucleoside substrates (inosine, guanosine, deoxyinosine and deoxyguanosine) in their urine. Because the block is near the terminal portion of the major common pathway to uric acid, patients with complete PNP deficiency have low serum uric acid and excrete diminished amounts of uric acid. However, excretion of total purine precursors of uric acid is increased, indicating purine overproduction. Of the four substrates, only deoxyguanosine has been reported to be directly phosphorylated without prior conversion to hypoxanthine or guanine, a reaction which is blocked in PNP deficiency. It is therefore not surprising that deoxy GTP is the major phosphorylated metabolite accumulated by PNP deficient children. Deoxy GTP like deoxy ATP is also an allosteric inhibitor of ribonucleotide reductase, albeit not as potent or all-encompassing. It has been hypothesized that accumulation of deoxy GTP accounts for the lymphospecific and T-cell specific effects of PNP deficiency. In vitro enzymatic and metabolic studies, similar to those described for deoxy ATP, also support this hypothesis.

PNP deficiency would appear to be a rarer disorder than ADA deficiency. It is inherited in an autosomal recessive mode, and obligate heterozygotes have usually been found to have half normal PNP activity in their red cells. The disorder is clearly genetically heterogeneous, with several different mutant alleles at the PNP locus. Thus, in one of the families (Toronto) the two affected brothers have detectable residual PNP activity but with an abnormal K_m. Correlated with the presence of residual enzyme activity, the two brothers are the oldest survivors, at over ten years of age. One of the brothers also had the latest age of onset. The two brothers, who are products of a non-consanguineous mating, would appear to be doubly heterozygous for two different mutant PNP alleles. Thus, the father has an electrophoretically abnormal PNP which is also detectable with anti PNP antibodies as excess cross reacting material, while the mother has reduced enzyme and reduced CRM and no electrophoretic aberrations of the enzyme molecule. Another patient has been demonstrated to have yet another mutation, resulting in an electrophoretically altered enzyme but different from that seen in the brothers mentioned above.

Prenatal diagnosis has been reported for PNP deficiency by assay of chorionic villi (Perignon et al 1987) and should be feasible in amniotic fluid cells, since they express PNP. Bone marrow transplantation has been successful. Partial exchange transfusions, as in ADA deficiency, have also been utilized, with marked metabolic clearing and some signs of clinical improvement. Complete immunological reconstitution has not resulted.

The gene for PNP has been cloned and sequenced, and has been mapped to chromosome 14q13.1.

Chronic mucocutaneous candidiasis

Chronic mucocutaneous candidiasis is a syndrome characterized by persistent Candida infection of the mucous membranes, scalp, skin and nails. It is often associated with an endocrinopathy. The defect appears to involve the cellular immune response only to Candida since susceptibility to other infectious agents is uncommon. Cutaneous anergy to Candida and often other antigens is observed. Following in vitro challenge with Candida, there is usually a diminished proliferative response and diminished release of the lymphokine MIF. Antibody to Candida as well as to other antigens is usually present. Other variable immunological abnormalities have been described.

The syndrome can be classified into four types (Lehrer et al 1978). The first form is early onset, severe disease in which associated endocrinopathy, usually hypothyroidism, is common and granulomas are seen. Survival past the third decade is unusual. The late onset type is the mildest and its only manifestations may be paranychia or involvement of the buccal mucosa. These two forms are usually sporadic. The two familial forms

of the syndrome essentially differ as to the presence or absence of endocrinopathies. The juvenile onset form is associated with polyendocrinopathies, most commonly hypoparathyroidism. The endocrine disorder can precede the candidiasis by several years. In other families, endocrinopathy rarely occurs. In both types inheritance is consistent with an autosomal recessive mode.

Specific syndromes involving other organ systems with immunodeficiency as a significant manifestation

Some of these disorders have conventionally not been listed as primary immunodeficiency diseases. However, as testing of immune function becomes more widespread, immunological abnormalities are likely to be detected in a variety of syndromes (e.g. TC II deficiency). We have therefore segregated immunodeficiencies which are associated with specific clinical syndromes, generally detected by virtue of their non-immunological manifestations.

Wiskott-Aldrich syndrome

The Wiskott-Aldrich syndrome is a rare X-linked recessive disorder characterized by thrombocytopenia, eczema and recurrent infections, usually with polysaccharide containing pyogenic bacteria, but also with other bacteria, viruses and fungi. Affected males have a median survival to 6 years and approximately 70% are dead by age 14 (Perry et al 1980). The major cause of death is infection, commonly of the respiratory system, followed by bleeding, most often into the CNS. Lymphoid malignancies occur frequently (over 12% of patients). Thrombocytopenia is usually observed at birth and is often exacerbated during periods of infection.

Platelets are small in size, respond abnormally to aggregating agents and have a diminished half life. Splenectomy usually results in increase in platelet number and size, a normal half life of autologous platelets and a normal aggregating response to epinephrine (Lum et al 1980). These observations suggest that the diminished half life, decreased size and abnormalities of aggregation may not be intrinsic defects but are alterations requiring splenic processing of abnormal platelets for expression. Following splenectomy, episodes of profound thrombocytopenia, possibly of an autoimmune nature, still occur. While splenectomy reduces the incidence of bleeding, there is an increased incidence of overwhelming sepsis which increases mortality unless antibiotics are administered prophylactically.

The eczema usually appears by one year of age and may be superinfected. The recurrent infections are associated with variable defects in humoral and cellular immunity. Immunoglobulins are both catabolised and synthesized more rapidly than normal and the most common resulting pattern of serum immunoglobulin is elevated serum IgA and IgE with low IgM. Serum iso-haemagglutinins are absent or very low. Patients are unable to mount an antibody response to polysaccharide antigens (e.g. pneumococcal vaccine) but can generate relatively normal antibody responses to protein antigens. B-cells are normal but in vitro synthesis of Ig is variably abnormal, depending on the stimulant utilized. Cellular immunity can also be abnormal. Patients are generally anergic to skin test antigens including DNCB, and cells do not proliferate normally in vitro in response to antigens or allogeneic cells. However, proliferation response to polyclonal activators (non-specific mitogens), lymphocyte count and number of T-cells are usually normal early in the course. Hepatosplenomegaly and autoimmune phenomena (e.g. haemolytic anaemia) are seen.

Genetics Wiskott-Aldrich syndrome has a crude incidence of approximately four per million male births. There is no widely accepted method for detection of heterozygous carriers. Although platelet abnormalities have been described in obligate heterozygotes, these observations are not consistent with reports that there is selection against platelets and lymphocytes expressing the X chromosome which bears the Wiskott-Aldrich mutation (as detected by clonal expression in G6PD heterozygotes). Heterozygote detection may be possible by studies similar to those outlined for other X-linked immunodeficiencies above, by detection of nonrandom X-inactivation. A population of small platelets has reportedly not been detected in obligate carriers. Recombination between the G6PD locus and the Wiskott-Aldrich gene (Gealy et al 1980), indicates that linkage between G6PD and Wiskott–Aldrich is not likely to provide accurate prenatal diagnosis. The gene has been mapped to the pericentric region of the X chromosome (Peacock & Siminovitch 1987). Absence of glycoproteins on the surface of T–cell and platelets has been reported (Rosen et al 1984). A defect of glycosylation has been postulated.

Prenatal detection (other than the 50% risk for a male) is not currently feasible. It has not been determined if affected fetuses have small abnormally functioning platelets and/or thrombocytopenia in utero. Recently, several children have been successfully engrafted with histocompatible bone marrow with return of platelet function to normal. This manoeuvre must be preceded by measures to extirpate the patient's own marrow, but it remains to be determined if such measures will result in a markedly increased incidence of malignancy in these patients who already have increased susceptibility to lymphoid malignancies.

Ataxia telangiectasia

Ataxia telangiectasia is characterized clinically by the occurrence of progressive cerebellar ataxia, ocular and cutaneous telangiectases, frequent and severe sinopulmonary infections, a very high incidence of neoplasia and variable abnormalities of both cellular and humoral immunity (McFarlin et al 1972, Gatti & Swift 1985). More recent investigations indicate that this is a genetically and clinically heterogeneous group of disorders with between five and nine complementation groups (see Gatti & Swift 1985).

The disease is usually first recognized as the child attempts to walk. The ataxia and dysarthria are progressive and additional neurological abnormalities develop, including choreoathetosis, myoclonic jerks, nystagmus, and oculomotor apraxia. Increased infections become evident during the first year of life but are not usually prominent until 3–8 years of age. The telangiectases usually appear between 2 and 8 years of age. Progeric changes develop in the adult and include premature greying of the hair, early loss of subcutaneous tissue, sclerodermoid changes, vitiligo and café-au-lait spots.

The most prominent and consistent immunological abnormality is absent or deficient serum and secretory IgA and serum IgE and the presence of a low molecular weight IgM. The latter may result in factitiously high IgM measurements by radial immunodiffusion. Autoantibodies are common. Diminished in vitro cellular immune responses are also common and the thymus often has a fetal-like histological pattern. Endocrine abnormalities involving several organs, are also frequent. Some patients have hyperinsulinism, insulin resistance and hyperglycaemia. Many patients show hypogonadism with absent or hypoplastic ovaries in females. Hepatic abnormalities also occur and elevated alphafetoprotein is common. Patients usually die before early adulthood as a result of the recurrent respiratory infections or a lymphoproliferative neoplasm.

Ataxia telangiectasia is one of the chromosome instability syndromes (Cohen & Levy 1989) and patients' cells develop chromosome abnormalities at high frequency. The chromosome abnormalities typically involve the translocation of the long arm of chromosome 14 with the breakpoint at 14q11-12 and 14q32, as well as chromosome 7 (7p13 and 7q35). These positions correspond to the loci for immunoglobulin heavy chains and the various genes for the T-cell receptor (Royer & Reinherz 1987). In addition to showing an increased rate of 'spontaneous' chromosome rearrangements, cells from patients with ataxia telangiectasia are also more sensitive to ionizing radiation and radiomimetic chemicals. In vivo, patients react adversely to standard radiotherapy and may die in the course of treatment. Studies of gamma induced radiation repair suggest that there are multiple complementation groups and a 'variant' group (Paterson 1979).

Genetics Ataxia telangiectasia has an incidence of approximately 25 per million and appears to be inherited as an autosomal recessive. The disorder occurs in higher frequency among Moroccan Jews. Obligate heterozygotes have been reported to be at increased risk for development of neoplasia. Definitive detection of heterozygotes is not available, although autoimmunity and oculocutaneous telangiectases have been reported in some heterozygotes. Prenatal diagnosis has recently been reported, based upon the ability of the amniotic fluid to induce chromosome aberrations in normal cells. Bone marrow transplantation has been attempted, but there was no evidence for permanent successful engraftment.

Other chromosome breakage syndromes

Immune defects have also been reported in Bloom syndrome (Cohen & Levy 1989), where increased rate of infection, decreased IgM and diminished delayed hypersensitivity have been described. Another chromosome breakage syndrome associated with microcephaly and immunodeficiency (absent IgA, impaired in vitro cellular lymphocyte response and infections) has been reported (Jaspers et al 1988). Another syndrome has been described with severe combined immunodeficiency associated with instability of the centromeric heterochromatin of chromosomes 1, 9 and 16 (Carpenter et al 1988). All these syndromes are inherited as autosomal recessives.

Short limbed dwarfism (SLD) with immunodeficiency

Short limbed dwarfism is associated with at least three distinct forms of immunodeficiency and appears to encompass at least three different disorders (Ammann et al 1974). McKusick (McKusick et al 1965) described the phenotype of 77 Amish children in 53 sibships affected with a form of short limbed dwarfism associated with cartilage hair hypoplasia. In addition to the cartilage and hair abnormalities, affected individuals typically could not fully extend their elbows, had hyperextensibility of fingers and wrists and often had a marked sternal deformity. The authors very astutely noted that two of the 77 died of chicken pox and at least three others had virulent varicella. They therefore suggested that increased susceptibility to viral infections, as well as intestinal abnormalities, could be part of the syndrome. Subsequent studies have indeed demonstrated in vitro-immune defects limited to cellular immune function. Although the in vitro defect is general, increased susceptibility to infection appears to be limited to vaccinia and varicella, while candida infections are notably absent. A similar disorder has been described in high frequency in the Finnish population (Virolainen et al 1978). The Finnish group appears to have a very mild defect in cellular immunity and an increased susceptibility to viral infections has not been noted. However the number of individuals examined was smaller (28). Chronic noncyclic neutropenia has been described in a non-Amish affected girl (Lux et al 1970) and congenital hypoplastic anaemia in an affected Amish boy (Harris et al 1981).

The second form of SLD is much rarer and fewer than 10 patients have been described. The clinical course and prognosis are indistinguishable from severe combined immunodeficiency. Redundant skin folds, scaly skin and variably progressive hair loss can be seen. Aplastic anaemia has been reported in at least one case and we have seen an additional case with marked anaemia. The inheritance appears to be autosomal recessive. Because of the bony abnormalities, we have tested two of these children and found normal erythrocyte ADA. Prenatal diagnosis has allowed exclusion by studies of fetal lymphocytes. At least one patient has had a successful bone marrow transplant. The disorder is otherwise fatal.

The last form of SLD is rare and is associated only with defective humoral immunity and apparently without cartilage hair hypoplasia. The reported male and female sibs of gypsy extraction had a prominent nose, high forehead and large ears, but it is not clear if the facies are typical for the syndrome or for the family.

Inheritance in all three types is compatible with an autosomal recessive mode. The disorder is frequently misdiagnosed during infancy as achondroplasia, an autosomal dominant disorder, and thus may lead to inaccurate counselling. In the Amish group, the frequency is 1–2 per 1000 live births and the inheritance is compatible with an autosomal recessive mode. If, as suggested, there is reduced (70%) penetrance, the estimated gene frequency among the Amish is 0.05.

Transcobalamin II deficiency

Inherited deficiency of transcobalamin II (the vitamin B_{12} binding protein necessary for transport of vitamin B_{12} into cells) is characterized by infantile megaloblastic anaemia, leukopenia, thrombocytopenia, infections and failure to gain weight. In several cases of transcobalamin II deficiency, agammaglobulinaemia has been detected. The various abnormalities are correctable by pharmacological doses of vitamin B_{12}. Interestingly, this deficiency appears to result in a block of clonal expansion and maturation of plasma cells, as well as of synthesis of antibodies, but not in the differentiation of antigen specific memory cells. Thus, following vitamin B_{12} therapy, an affected child synthesized specific antibodies to antigens with which he had been immunized several months previously during the unresponsive state (Hitzig 1979).

This is a rare disorder. Transcobalamin II is a genetically polymorphic protein and null alleles can thus be detected by anomalous inheritance of the polymorphic markers. Obligate heterozygotes have had half normal amounts of transcobalamin II and in at least one family an electrophoretically abnormal protein has been detected. Prenatal diagnosis is possible. Partial deficiency of transcobalamin II with only megaloblastic anaemia as a manifestation has also been reported. Therapy is provided by administration of pharmacological doses of vitamin B_{12}.

Biotin responsive multiple carboxylase deficiency

Two sibs have been reported with biotin responsive multiple carboxylase deficiency (Cowan et al 1979) who, in addition to seizures, alopecia and intermittent ataxia, also both had clinically significant candidiasis and an in vitro defective response to Candida antigen. The alopecia, organic aciduria and candidiasis cleared following therapy with biotin. However, the abnormal response to Candida remained and there were still several brief episodes of ataxia, suggesting that the biotin therapy was not totally effective. It remains to be determined if the organic acids which are accumulated in this disorder are toxic for immune function, or if biotin is also a cofactor for yet another enzyme crucial for immune function.

We have not attempted to cover all metabolic disorders in which patients have had multiple infections with unusual pathogens and/or died of varicella, vaccina, etc. It is very likely that children with many of the inherited metabolic defects which have severe global manifestations will exhibit measurable abnormalities in immune function. Such abnormalities are likely to be less informative than, and should be differentiated from, the yet to be discovered additional metabolic defects which primarily result in abnormalities of the immune system. Investigations of the purine pathway have been fruitful to date and there are indeed several immunodeficiency syndromes where the association of bony abnormalities and neurological abnormalities with immunodeficiency suggest that investigations of this pathway may still be rewarding. However, one must remember that the initial discovery of the importance of the purine pathway was serendipitous and totally unexpected, and unrelated metabolic pathways may subsequently be found to be important for normal immune function.

CONCLUSION

It should be clear from the descriptions above that, as in other genetic diseases, there is a great deal of heterogeneity in the immunodeficiency disorders. Such heterogeneity can be due to different alleles at the same locus or mutations at different loci resulting in similar phenotypes. Not only is there this expected genetic heterogeneity within each general phenotype, but due to the dependence of many of the symptoms upon chance exposure to environmental agents, there is superimposed a significant degree of non-genetic individual variation. In fact, a number of individuals demonstrating immunodeficiency, sometimes indistinguishable from the genetic diseases, develop their conditions as a result of such non-genetic problems as severe viral infections, malignancies, acquired immunodeficiency (e.g. AIDS), or therapy with immunosuppressive and cytotoxic agents. Additionally, a number of inborn errors of metabolism, including storage diseases, urea cycle defects and organic and amino-acidurias, as well as several chromosomal disorders, such as those involving chromosome 18 as well as Down syndrome, demonstrate a variety of immunological defects leading to increased susceptibility to infection. In great part, the difficulty of accurate classification, with a few notable exceptions, is due to our general lack of understanding of the fundamental molecular defects responsible for most of these conditions. In addition, the dependence of current classification systems upon the developmental model of stem cell, B-cell or T-cell defects, while initially highly useful, has become somewhat naive and therefore constricting. The continuous advance in our understanding of the interaction and interdependence of the components of the immune system with each other, and with even more cells and molecules, makes it clear that many modifications of the definitions of immunodeficiencies will come about. No doubt these discoveries, especially when they become understood on a molecular basis, will bring about the definition of many new defects associated with host defence problems.

One example of a fascinating puzzle to be solved is the role of genes on the X chromosome, which seem to be responsible for so many defects involving hematopoietic cells. Among the diseases covered in this chapter are X-linked agammaglobulinaemia, the Wiskott-Aldrich syndrome, most of the hyper IgM states, a proportion of SCID and the X-linked lymphoproliferative syndrome. Other X-linked diseases involving bone marrow elements include agranulocytosis and a form of thrombocytopenia. It may well be that a set of related genes on the X chromosome determine the orderly differentiation from primitive stem cells to the various functional elements and that different mutations result in one or other of these abnormalities.

It is not only our hope but our sincere conviction that the increased application of modern biochemical and molecular methodology and thought will, over the next few years, lead to a clearer understanding of the genetics and fundamental defects of primary immunodeficiency. It is only with such understanding that more rational counselling and therapy can develop. As so often true in the past for other fields, a dissection of these genetic defects will inevitably help to take the field of clinical and cellular immunology from its current state of descriptive phenomenology into the realm of a proper science, such as has already become the case in our understanding of the immunoglobulins and antibody diversity, as well as the specificity of T-cells.

REFFERENCES

Ammann A J, Sutliff W, Millinchick E 1974 Antibody mediated immunodeficiency in short-limbed dwarfism. Journal of Pediatrics 84: 200–203

Ammann A J, Hong R 1980 Disorders of the IgA system. In: Stiehm E R, Fulginiti V A (eds) Immunologic disorders in infants and children. W B Saunders, Philadelphia, ch 14, p 260–273

Baehner R L 1980 Lymphocytes. In: Miller D R, Pearson H A (Eds) Blood diseases in infancy and childhood. Mosby St. Louis, ch 20, p 557–572

Bortin M M, Rimm A A 1977 Severe combined immunodeficiency disease – characterization of the disease and results of transplantation – report of the advisory committee of the international bone marrow transplant registry. Journal of the American Medical Association 238: 591–600

Buckley R H 1980 Disorders of the IgE system. In: Stiehm E R, Fulginiti V A (eds) Immunologic disorders in infants and children. W B Saunders, Philadelphia, ch 15, p 274–285

Cannizzaro L A, Emanuel B S 1985 In situ hybridization and translocation breakpoint mapping III DiGeorge syndrome with partial monosomy of chromosome 22. Cytogenetics and Cell Genetics 39: 179–183

Carpenter N J et al 1988 Variable immunodeficiency with abnormal condensation of the heterochromatin of chromosomes 1, 9 and 16. Journal of Pediatrics 112:757–760

Ciba Foundation symposium 68 1979 Enzyme defects and immune dysfunction. Excerpta Medica, Amsterdam, p 1–279

Cohen M M, Levy H P 1989 Chromosome instability syndromes. In: Harris H, Hirschhorn K (eds) Advances in Human Genetics, vol. 18, p 43–149

Conley M E, Beckwith J B, Mancer J F K, Tenckhoff L 1979 The spectrum of the DiGeorge syndrome. Journal of Pediatrics 94: 883–890

Conley M E, Puck J M 1988 Carrier detection in typical and atypical X–linked agammaglobulinemia. Journal of Pediatrics 112: 688–694

Cooper M D 1987 B lymphocytes: normal development and function. New England Journal of Medicine 317: 1452–1456

Cowan M J, Packman S, Wara D W, Ammann A J, Yoshimo M, Sweetman L, Nyhan W 1979 Multiple biotin-dependent carboxylase deficiencies associated with defects in T–cell and B–cell immunity. Lancet I: 115–118

Croce C M, Shander M, Martinis J, Cicurel L, D'Ancona G, Dolby T, Koprowski H 1979 Chromosomal location of the genes for human immunoglobulin heavy chains. Proceedings of the National Academy of Sciences USA 76: 3416–3419

Davis M M, Kim S K, Hood L E 1980 DNA sequences mediating class switching in α-immunoglobulin. Science 209: 1353–1359

de la Chapelle A, Herva R, Koivista M, Aula P 1981 A deletion in chromosome 22 can cause diGeorge syndrome. Human Genetics 57: 253–256

de Préval C, Hadam M R, Mach B 1988 Regulation of genes for HLA class II antigens in cell lines from patients with severe combined immunodeficiency. New England Journal of Medicine 318: 1295–1300

de Saint Basile G et al 1987 Close linkage of the locus for X chromosome-linked severe combined immunodeficiency to polymorphic DNA markers on Xq11–q13. Proceedings of the National Academy of Sciences USA 84: 7576–7579

Dooley T et al 1987 First trimester diagnosis of adenosine deaminase deficiency. Prenatal Diagnosis 7: 561–565

Erickson J, Marituis J, Croce C M 1981 Assignment of the genes for human λ immunoglobulin chains to chromosome 22. Nature 294: 173–175

Fearon E R, Winkelstein J A, Civin C I, Pardoll D M, Vogelstein B 1987 Carrier detection in X–linked agammaglobulinaemia by analysis of X-chromosome inactivation. New England Journal of Medicine 316: 427–431

Fleisher T A, White R M, Broder S, Nissley S P, Blaese R M, Mulvihill J J, Olive G, Waldmann T A 1980 X-linked hypogammaglobulinemia and isolated growth hormone deficiency. New England Journal of Medicine 302: 1429–1434

Fontán G, Garcia Rodriguez M C, Carrasco S, Zabay J M de la Concha E G 1988 Severe combined immunodeficiency with T lymphocytes retaining functional activity. Clinical Immunology and Immunopathology 46: 432–441

Gatti R A, Swift M (eds) 1985 Ataxia telangectasia. Genetics, neuropathology and immunology of a degenerative disease of childhood. Liss, New York

Gealy W J, Dwyer J M, Harley J B 1980 Allelic exclusion of glucose-6-phosphate dehydrogenase in platelets and T lymphocytes from a Wiskott-Aldrich syndrome carrier. Lancet I: 63–65

Geha R S, Hyslop N, Alami S, Farah F, Schneeberger E E, Rosen F S 1979 Hyper immunoglobulin M immunodeficiency (dysgammaglobulinemia). Journal of Clinical Investigation 64: 385–391

Gelfand E W, Oliver J M, Shuurman R K, Matheson D S, Dosch H–M 1979 Abnormal lymphocyte capping in a patient with severe combined immunodeficiency disease. New England Journal of Medicine 301: 1245–1249

Giblett E R, Anderson J E, Cohen F, Pollara B, Meuwissen H J 1972 Adenosine deaminase deficiency in two patients with severely impaired cellular immunity. Lancet II: 1067–1069

Goodship J, Malcolm S, Lau Y L, Pembrey M E, Levinsky R J 1988 Use of X chromosome inactivation analysis to establish carrier status for X–linked severe combined immunodeficiency. Lancet I: 729–732

Harris R E, Baehner R L, Gleiser S, Weaver D D, Hodes M E 1981 Cartilage-hair hypoplasia, defective T–cell function and Diamond-Blackfan anemia in an Amish child. American Journal of Medical Genetics 8: 291–297

Hermans P E, Diaz-Buxo J A, Stobo J D 1976 Idiopathic late-onset immunoglobulin deficiency. American Journal of Medicine 61: 221–237

Hershfield M S et al 1987 Treatment of adenosine deaminase deficiency with polyethylene glycol-modified adenosine deaminase. New England Journal of Medicine 310: 589–596

Hirschhorn R 1986 Inherited enzyme deficiencies and immunodeficiency: adenosine deaminase (ADA) and purine nucleoside phosphorylase (PNP) deficiencies. Clinical Immunology and Immunopathology 40: 157–165

Hitzig W H 1979 Immunodeficiency due to transcobalamin II deficiency. In: Ciba foundation symposium 68, enzyme defects and immune dysfunction. Excerpta Medica, Amsterdam

Hitzig W H, Kenny A B 1978 Inheritance, incidence and epidemiology of severe combined immunodeficiency syndromes. In: Japan medical research foundation (ed) Immunodeficiency. Its nature and etiological significance in human disease. University of Tokyo Press, Tokyo, p 257–270

Hobbs J R 1975 IgM deficiency. In: Bergsma D, Good R A, Finstad J (eds) Immunodeficiency in man and animals - Birth Defects: Original Article Series, vol XI, 1, Sinauer Press, Sunderland, MA, p 112–117

Hood L E, Weissmann I L, Wood W B, Wilson J H (eds) 1984 Immunology. Benjamin/Cummings, Menlo Park, CA

Jaspers N G J, Taalman RDFM, Baan C 1988 Patients with an inherited syndrome characterized by immunodeficiency, microcephaly and chromosomal instability: genetic relationship to ataxia telangiectasia. American Journal of Human Genetics 42: 66–73

Koistinen J 1976 Familial clustering of selective IgA deficiency. Vox Sanguinis 30: 181–190

Kredich N M, Hershfield M S 1989 Immunodeficiency diseases caused by adenosine deaminase deficiency and purine nucleoside phosphorylase deficiency. In: Scriver C R, Beaudet A L, Sly W S, Valle D S (eds) The metabolic basis of inherited disease 6th edn. McGraw Hill, New York, p 1045–1076

Kwan S-P, Kunkel L, Bruns G, Wedgwood R J, Latt S, Rosen F S 1986 Mapping of the X-linked agammaglobulinemia locus by use of restriction fragment-length polymorphism. Journal of Clinical Investigation 77: 649–652

Lehrer R I, Stiehm E R, Fischer T J, Young L S 1978 Severe candidal infections: clinical perspective, immune defense mechanisms and current concepts of therapy. Annals of Internal Medicine 89: 91–106

Lum L G, Tubergen D G, Corash L, Blaese R M 1980 Splenectomy in the management of the thrombocytopenia of the Wiskott-Aldrich syndrome. New England Journal of Medicine 302: 892–896

Lux S E, Johnston R B Jr, August C S, Say B, Penchaszadeh V B, Rosen F S, McKusick V A 1970 Chronic neutropenia and abnormal cellular immunity in cartilage-hair hypoplasia. New England Journal of Medicine 282: 231–236

McBride O W, Hieter P A, Hollis G F, Swan D, Otey M C, Leder P 1982 Chromosomal location of human kappa and lambda immunoglobulin light chain constant region genes. Journal of Experimental Medicine 155: 1480–1490

McFarlin D, Strober W, Waldmann T A 1972 Ataxia-telangiectasia. Medicine 51: 281–314

McKusick V A, Eldridge R, Hostetler J A, Ruangwit U, Egeland J A 1965 Dwarfism in the Amish II: cartilage hair hypoplasia. Bulletin of Johns Hopkins Hospital 116: 285–326

Maki R, Kearney J, Paige C, Tonegawa S 1980 Immunoglobulin gene rearrangements in immature B cells. Science 290: 1360–1365

Malcolm S et al 1987 Close linkage of random DNA fragments from Xq21.3–22 to X-linked agammaglobulinemia. Human Genetics 77: 172–174

Mensink EJBM et al 1987 X-linked immunodeficiency with hyperimmunoglobulinaemia M appears to be linked to the DXS42 restriction fragment length polymorphism locus. Human Genetics 76: 96–99

Nossal G J V 1987 Immunology: the basic components of the immune system. New England Journal of Medicine 316: 1319–1325

Ownby D R, Pizzo S, Blackmon L, Gall S A, Buckley R H 1976 Severe combined immunodeficiency with leukopenia (reticular dysgenesis): Immunologic and histopathologic findings. Journal of Pediatrics 89: 382–387

Paterson M C 1979 Environmental carcinogenesis and imperfect repair of damaged DNA in *Homo Sapiens*: causal relation revealed by rare hereditary disorders. In: Griffin A C, Shaw C R (eds) Carcinogens: identification and mechanisms of action. Raven Press, New York, p 251-276

Paul W E (ed) 1984 Immunogenetics. Raven, New York

Peacock M, Siminovitch K A 1987 Linkage of the Wiskott-Aldrich Syndrome with polymorphic DNA sequences from the human X chromosome. Proceedings of the National Academy of Sciences, USA 84: 3430-3433

Perignon J L et al 1987 Early prenatal diagnosis of inherited severe immunodeficiencies linked to enzyme deficiencies. Journal of Pediatrics 111: 595-598

Perry G S III, Spector B D, Schuman L M et al 1980 The Wiskott-Aldrich syndrome in the United States and Canada (1892-1979). Journal of Pediatrics 97: 72-78

Puck J M, Nussbaum R L, Conley M E 1987 Carrier detection in X-linked severe combined immunodeficiency based on patterns of X chromosome inactivation. Journal of Clinical Investigation 79: 1395-1400

Purtilo D T, DeFlorio D, Hutt L M, Bhawan J, Yang J P S, Otto R, Edwards W 1977 Variable phenotypic expression of an X-linked recessive lymphoproliferative syndrome. New England Journal of Medicine 297: 1077-1081

Raatikka M, Rapola J, Tuuteri L, Louhimo I, Savilahti E 1981 Familial third and fourth pharyngeal pouch syndrome with Truncus Arteriosus: DiGeorge syndrome. Pediatrics, 67: 173-175

Race R R, Sanger R 1975 Blood groups in man. Blackwell Scientific, Oxford, p 606

Roitt I 1988 Essential Immunology. Blackwell, Oxford

Rosen F S, Colten H R 1987 Primary immunodeficiencies and serum complement defects. In: Nathan D G, Oski F A (eds) Hematology of infancy and childhood, 3rd edn. Saunders, Philadelphia, p 878-899

Rosen F S, Merler E 1978 Genetic defects in gamma globulin synthesis. In: Stanbury J B, Wyngaarden J B, Fredrickson D S (eds) The metabolic basis of inherited disease, 4th edn McGraw Hill, New York, p 1726-1737

Rosen F S, Cooper M D, Wedgwood R J P 1984 The primary immunodeficiencies. New England Journal of Medicine 311: 235-242, 300-309

Rosen F S, Wedgwood R J, Eibl M 1986 Primary immunodeficiency diseases: report of a World Health Organization Scientific Group. Clinical Immunology and Immunopathology 40: 166-196

Royer H D, Reinherz E L 1987 T lymphocytes: ontogeny, function, and relevance to clinical disorders. New England Journal of Medicine 317: 1136-1142

Schwaber J, Chen R H 1988 Premature termination of variable gene rearrangement in B lymphocytes from X-linked agammaglobulinemia. Journal of Clinical Investigation 81: 2004-2009

Schwaber J F, Klein G, Ernberg I, Rosen A, Lazarus H, Rosen F S 1980 Deficiency of Epstein-Barr virus (EBV) receptors on B lymphocytes from certain patients with common varied agammaglobulinemia. Journal of Immunology 124: 2191-2196

Shaham M, 1981 Personal communication

Skare J C, Milunsky A, Byron K S, Sullivan J L 1987 Mapping the X-linked lymphoproliferative syndrome. Proceedings of the National Academy of Sciences, USA 84: 2015-2018

Smith M, Krinsky A M, Arrendondo V F, Wang A-L, Hirschhorn K 1981 Confirmation of the assignment of genes for human immunoglobulin heavy chains to chromosome 14 by analyses of Ig synthesis by man-mouse hybridomas. European Journal of Immunology 11: 852-855

Soothill J F, Hayward A R, Wood C B S (eds) 1983 Pediatric Immunology. Blackwell, Oxford

Touraine J L, Marseglia G-L, Betuel H 1985 Thirty international cases of bare lymphocyte syndrome. Biological significance of HLA antigens. Experimental Hematology (Supplement 17) 13: 86-87

Virolainen M, Savilahti E, Kaitila I, Perheentupa J 1978 Cellular and humoral immunity in cartilage hair hypoplasia. Pediatric Research 12: 961-966

Waldmann T A, Broder S, Krakauer R, MacDermott R P, Durm M, Goldman C, Meade B 1976 The role of suppressor cells in the pathogenesis of common variable hypogammaglobulinemia and in the immunodeficiency associated with myeloma. Federation Proceedings 35: 2067-2072

World Health Organization 1978 Immunodeficiency; technical report series 630, Geneva

Yount W S, Hong R, Seligmann M, Good R A, Kunkel H G 1970 Imbalances of gamma globulin subgroups and gene defects in patients with primary hypogammaglobulinemia. Journal of Clinical Investigation 49: 1957-1966.

83. Complement defects

F. S. Rosen   C. A. Alper

INTRODUCTION

The complement system is a formidably complex system of interacting plasma proteins, strongly conserved in vertebrate evolution, which functions as the principal effector system for antibody-mediated immune reactions. Three types of genetic variation in complement components have been discovered:

1. Polymorphism of individual components based on differences in electric charge. Such polymorphisms are well studied for C3, Factor B, C4 and C6 where there are at least two high frequency alleles and also for C2, C7 and C8 where the frequency of the second most common allele is less.

One of the more interesting results from this work is the discovery that the genes for Factor B, C2 and C4 are coded within HLA in close proximity to the HLA-B locus. The gene for C6 is closely linked to that for C7, but the locus for C6–C7 is so far unassigned.

2. Genes contolling the level of certain components of which the s gene in the mouse is the best known.

3. The isolated deficiencies which are dealt with elsewhere.

THE COMPLEMENT REACTION PATHWAYS

From a functional point of view the complement activation sequence occurs in two overlapping but distinct parts.

The first of these is a triggered enzyme cascade culminating in the cleavage and fixation of C3. This is, in quantitative terms, the major reaction of complement fixation and the fixation of C3 at complement fixation sites is probably the system's most important activity. Bound C3 reacts with the various receptors on phagocytic cells, platelets, erythrocytes (in primates) and certain lymphocytes. The retention of cells at complement fixation sites contributes largely to the phlogistic activity of the complement system.

The cleavage of C3 is brought about by two distinct pathways known for historical reasons as the 'classical' and 'alternative' pathways. It is possible to picture these as homologues of each other and this is shown in Figure 83.1. Here it can be seen that the C3 cleaving enzyme of the classical pathway C4b,2a is generated from a complex between C4b and C2a in the presence of magnesium ions by proteolytic cleavage by C1. Similarly, in the alternative pathway, a complex C3b,Bb is formed between C3b and Factor B cleaved by Factor D in the presence of magnesium ions. There are sufficient physico-chemical resemblances between C4b and C3b on the one hand, and C2 and Factor B on the other to suggest that the similarities at this level are not fanciful and that indeed one may be looking at the results of a duplicated enzyme system. The significant difference between the two pathways is that in the alternative pathway it is C3b itself which is the essential component of the C3 splitting enzyme, and this enables the alternative pathway to act as

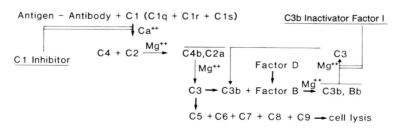

Fig. 83.1 Pathways of C3 cleavage.

a positive feedback amplification loop for C3 activation no matter how C3 cleavage is originally produced. Thus, this pathway can amplify not only immunologically-induced C3 activation, but also that produced by other enzymes as, for example, plasmin or leucocyte proteases, which may occur at inflammation sites even if this is not primarily of immunological origin. The initial activating steps of the alternative pathway are not fully understood. Properdin is now believed to act as a stabilizing factor for the alternative pathway C3 coverting enzyme, C3bBb, rather than as an initiating factor. It seems probable that the alternative pathway may 'tick over' continuously and that the triggering of the system by activators is a consequence of the stabilization of feedback enzyme. It has recently been suggested that C3b bound to activating particles may be more resistant to C3b inactivator, which would be sufficient to account for the triggering role (Müller-Eberhard 1975).

COMPLEMENT DEFECTS

Hereditary angioneurotic oedema

Hereditary angioneurotic oedema was recognized during the last century, but the molecular basis of the disease, a genetically determined deficiency of the $C\bar{1}$ inhibitor, was not defined until 1963. The defect is transmitted as an autosomal dominant. The serum of most affected patients contains between 5 and 30% of the normal concentration of C1 inhibitor (Donaldson & Evans 1963, Rosen et al 1971).

Patients with this disease are prone to recurrent episodes of swelling. The oedema fluid accumulates rapidly in the affected part, which becomes tense but not discoloured; no itching, no pain, and no redness are associated with the oedema. Laryngeal oedema may be fatal because of airway obstruction and consequent pulmonary oedema. If the intestinal tract is involved, most often the jejunum, severe abdominal cramps and bilious vomiting ensue. Diarrhoea, which is clear and watery in character occurs when the colon is affected. The attacks last 48–72 hours. Although they are often unheralded, attacks may occur subsequent to trauma, menses, excessive fatigue, and mental stress. Attacks of angio-oedema are infrequent in early childhood; the disease intensifies during adolescence and tends to subside in the sixth decade of life. In children especially, a mottling of the skin reminiscent of erythema marginatum may be frequently noticed not necessarily associated with attacks of angio-oedema.

The pathophysiology of hereditary angioneurotic oedema is directly related to the diminished activity of the $C\bar{1}$ inhibitor in the plasma of affected persons. The latter leads to increased 'spontaneous' activation of C1 and attack on C4 and C2, the natural substrates of the $C\bar{1}$, resulting in a marked lowering of the serum concentrations of these proteins, particularly during attacks. The swelling that is the essential clinical feature of hereditary angioneurotic oedema appears to result from the action of the C2-kinin, a low molecular weight fragment of C2, modified by plasmin, on the postcapillary venule.

The autosomal dominant inheritance of hereditary angioneurotic oedema presents an interesting puzzle. Obviously, affected individuals are heterozygous for the abnormality but despite this, their serum contains very little $C\bar{1}$ inhibitor (average 17% of normal). Liver biopsy specimens can be shown to contain no hepatic parenchymal cells detectably engaged in synthesis of $C\bar{1}$ inhibitor, whereas 3–5% of normal hepatic cells give positive fluorescence with a fluorescein-labelled antibody to $C\bar{1}$ inhibitor.

In 15% of affected kindreds, sera of patients contain normal or elevated concentrations of an immunochemically cross-reacting (CRM+), nonfunctional protein. The CRM+, nonfunctional $C\bar{1}$ inhibitors differ from kindred to kindred with respect to electrophoretic mobility, ability to bind to activated $C\bar{1}$ esterase, and ability to inhibit the cleavage of certain synthetic esters by $C\bar{1}$ esterase. However, all CRM+ $C\bar{1}$ inhibitors fail to inhibit destruction of C4 by $C\bar{1}$. The clinical expression of hereditary angioneurotic oedema is the same in CRM+ and CRM- patients, and the CRM+ proteins are inherited as autosomal dominant traits. Little normal $C\bar{1}$ inhibitor is detectable in serum from patients with CRM+ proteins.

Approximately 50% of patients with hereditary angioneurotic oedema will have a complete cessation of symptoms by taking androgen daily. Recent studies with synthetic androgens have shown striking suppression of attacks and, remarkably, a rise in $C\bar{1}$ inhibitor serum levels in deficient patients. In those patients with increased levels of dysfunctional protein, the latter have fallen in concentration with the appearance of normal $C\bar{1}$ inhibitor. C4 and C2 levels in serum of patients under treatment have increased towards normal. Epsilon-aminocaproic acid and its analogue, tranexamic acid, are also effective as prophylactic therapy. It is now known that plasmin is required for the production of the C2-kinin, and this fact explains the efficacy of plasminogen inhibitors in the therapy of this disease. Although plasma infusions have been attempted in the therapy of acute attacks of angio-oedema, this procedure has no merit in light of present knowledge, and may in fact be dangerous, in that substrate for C$\bar{1}$ is being infused along with inhibitor (Gelfand et al 1976).

Factor I deficiency

Patients with Factor I deficiency have lifelong histories of severe infections with such organisms as *Diplococcus pneumoniae*, *Haemophilus influenzae*, *Neisseria meningitidis*, and β-haemolytic streptococci. The infections have included septicaemia, pneumonia, meningitis and otitis media (Alper et al 1970a, Alper et al 1970b). The serum of all affected persons shows the same complement protein and functional abnormalities. The primary defect in each case is an absence, detected both immunochemically and functionally, of Factor I (Alper et al 1972b). Because of this absence, there is spontaneous activation of the alternative pathway of complement activation with continuous conversion and consumption in vivo of C3 and Factor B. Native C3 concentration is about 5% of normal, and C3b is present in the patients' circulating plasma in moderately high concentration (20–25 mg/dl). No Factor B is detectable but the conversion products Bb and Ba are present in trace amounts. Factor B added to the patients' serum is immediately cleaved. The classical pathway proteins C1, C4 and C2 are entirely normal in concentration, there is only a slight decrease in C5 concentration, and C6–9 are at normal levels. Almost all complement-mediated functions such as bactericidal activity for smooth Gram-negative organisms, opsonization of pneumococci and endotoxin particles, haemolytic activity for antibody-sensitized sheep red cells, and the like, are markedly diminished or absent in their serum. The functional abnormalities in vitro can be reversed only by the addition of Factor I, C3 and B to the serum but not by any single protein. Partial normalization in vivo, on the other hand, can be achieved by the infusion of whole plasma or purified Factor I. This partial normalization lasts for two weeks (Ziegler et al 1975).

In family studies of Factor I deficiency, heterozygotes are detected with 50% normal levels. These carriers have no abnormalities in C3 or Factor B levels or in complement-mediated functions. Factor I is controlled by a locus on chromosome 4.

Factor H deficiency

Factor H is a necessary cofactor for Factor I in the inhibition of the alternative pathway C3 cleaving enzyme, C3bBb. Factor H deficiency has the same pathophysiological consequences as Factor I deficiency. Heterozygotes are detected with 50% normal levels but have no clinical abnormalities (Thompson & Winterborn 1981).

C1q deficiency

C1q deficiency results from absence of C1q or presence of mutant C1q that is not functional. Cases of C1q deficiency have immune complex disease with skin lesions, glomerulonephritis and a lupus-like disease. Absent haemolytic activity can be restored by addition of purified C1q. The gene for C1q is on the short arm of chromosome 1 (Reed 1989).

C1r deficiency

Seven patients in three families have inherited deficiency of C1r. All other components of complement are in normal concentration except for C1s, which is reduced to about half of normal. One patient at 16 years of age had a lupus-like syndrome with malar rash, arthralgia, and subacute focal membranous glomerulitis, but negative lupus erythematosus (LE) cell test. His 24-year-old sister had recurrent fever, arthralgia, and a malar rash. An unrelated 11-year-old girl had chronic glomerulonephritis. The last two cases were of young adult siblings with severe discoid LE, recurrent fevers, and polyarthritis, one with antinuclear antibody, one without, but both with positive latex fixation tests. These two patients had two affected but healthy siblings. In all patients, C1r was absent by both immunochemical and functional assay of the serum. Obligatory heterozygotes sometimes had normal C1r levels, but not invariably (De Bracco et al 1974). The genes for C1r and C1s are linked on the short arm of chromosome 12.

C4 deficiency

The serum of an 18-year-old girl with a lupus-like syndrome was found to be totally deficient in C4 by functional and immunochemical criteria. Although she had a typical malar rash and arthralgia, her LE cell test was negative. The serum of the patient's mother contained half-normal levels of C4. Other family members were possible heterozygotes (Hauptmann et al 1974).

A second C4-patient subject has been identified. This patient was a 5-year-old boy with typical systemic lupus erythematosus (SLE). He had fever, myalgia, arthritis, and, more recently, nephrotic syndrome. Renal biopsy showed diffuse proliferative glomerulonephritis. He has since died with clear-cut severe SLE. As pointed out above, the identification of carriers for C4 deficiency of this sort is difficult, if not impossible. By determining C4 haplotypes in the second family, it was possible to demonstrate that the proband had inherited a 'double deletion' haplotype C4AQO C4BQO (Ochs et al 1977).

19 cases of C4 deficiency are known. They have almost all died of immune complex disease.

C2 deficiency

Inherited deficency of C2 is probably the most common of genetic complement deficiency states (Klemperer et al 1966). One healthy C2–deficient blood donor was found in a survey of 10 000 blood donors in Manchester, England. Glass and co-workers found 1.2% of random individuals to be heterozygous for C2 deficiency, in approximate keeping with the Manchester findings.

Many reports of individuals homozygous for C2 deficiency have appeared in the literature. The defect is transmitted as an autosomal recessive trait, but heterozygotes are usually detected by their half-normal serum C2 concentration as determined by functional or immunochemical measurements.

The probands in the first four kindreds discovered to have C2 deficiency and four homozygous affected siblings were all found to be healthy individuals. In fact, in two cases the discovery was made in immunologists whose blood was being used for routine haemolytic or immune adherence tests. Subsequently, four more kindreds were discovered because the probands presented with SLE. The probands in three further kindreds presented with Schönlein-Henoch purpura, and yet another with polymyositis. These findings suggested the C2 deficiency may be associated with a high incidence of connective tissue disease. This subject is dealt with in more detail below.

Serum from homozygotes for C2 deficiency lacks certain complement-mediated functions: haemolytic activity, bactericidal activity, and immune adherence. The deficiency gene for C2 is an allele of the structural locus for this protein and occurs in the extended haplotype HLA-B18, HLA-DR2, complotype SO42.

C3 deficiency

Hereditary deficiency of C3 was first detected in heterozygotes who had approximately 50% of the normal level of this protein (Alper et al 1969). Affected persons were entirely healthy, although minor defects in complement-mediated functions could be detected in their serum. Serum haemolytic complement was variably slightly reduced, and the enhancement of phagocytosis of antibody-sensitized pneumococci was subnormal.

Analysis of the inheritance patterns of partial C3 deficiency revealed that affected persons had inherited a silent C3 gene, C3–, that produced no detectable protein. This gene was allelic to the common structural genes, and it has been shown that some C3 is produced in homozygous-deficient subjects. This C3 is normal in molecular weight, subunit composition and surface charge (Alper et al 1972a, Alper et al 1976).

Subsequently, five unrelated patients homozygous for C3 deficiency have been identified. Four of them have had numerous episodes of infection by pyogenic bacteria, including pneumonia, septicaemia, otitis media and meningitis. The fifth patient was a 3-year-old with no history of severe infections who had an episode of fever, rash, and arthralgia, which suddenly terminated with the infusion of normal plasma. In two of the C3-deficient patients there was no leucocytosis or a blunted response in connection with systemic infection with Gram-positive organisms. This may relate to a known role for C3, and specifically the C3e fragment, in leucocyte mobilization (Ballow et al 1975, Davis et al 1977).

Studies in vitro of serum from homozygous C3–deficient subjects have uniformly revealed marked depression or absence of most complement-mediated functions such as haemolytic activity for antibody-sensitized sheep red cells, chemotactic activity, opsonization of endotoxin particles, and bactericidal activity. Purified C3 corrected these abnormalities. In contrast to these severe deficits, immune adherences was near normal, consistent with the requirement only for the first two complement components, C1 and C4, for this function.

C5 deficiency

Inherited deficiency of the fifth component of complement has been studied in detail in at least three families. Most heterozygotes for the deficiency had about half-normal levels of C5 and inheritance is Mendelian. One of five homozygous deficient persons had SLE, two had disseminated gonococcal sepsis, and one had recurrent N. meningitidis meningitis.

Serum from deficient subjects showed decreased or absent total haemolytic complement, bactericidal activity and chemotactic activity. Opsonization for endotoxin particles and a variety of microorganims, including Baker's yeast, was entirely normal. The abnormalities in vitro in C5-deficient serum were corrected by the addition of purified C5 (Rosefeld et al 1976, Snyderman et al 1979).

C6 deficiency

Four patients homozygous for C6 deficiency have been studied in detail. All have had repeated episodes of neisserial sepsis involving either meningococcaemia or gonococcaemia. As with other complement component deficiencies, the gene for the deficiency state appears to be a null or blank allele at the structural locus for the protein, and severely deficient patients are homozygous for this blank allele.

The only defects in complement function detectable in C6-deficient serum in vitro are absent haemolytic and bactericidal activities. In particular, opsonization and chemotaxis induction are normal (Leddy et al 1974, Lim et al 1976).

C7 deficiency

There are at least seven unrelated individuals homozygous for C7 deficiency. C7 levels are undetectable to 10% of normal in these sera. One patient had SLE and a second had renal disease with recurrent urinary tract infection, but most of the remaining patients have had recurrent neisserial infections (Wellek & Opferkuch 1975).

Of all the complement-mediated functions tested, only haemolytic and bactericidal activities were reduced to absent in C7-deficient serum. Inheritance is autosomal recessive and carriers have about half-normal C7 concentrations.

A single family has been reported with a healthy proband whose serum had low but detectable levels of both C6 (1%) and C7 (8%). This combined defect was inherited as a single trait, reflecting the close linkage of the genetic loci for C6 and C7. The specific nature of this combined defect is unknown but is complicated since the small amount of C6 present is smaller in size than, and antigenically deficient compared with, normal C6.

C8 deficiency

Homozygous C8 deficiency has been reported in a number of individuals with a variety of clinical disorders, including lupus, xeroderma pigmentosum (which was clearly fortuitous) and several cases with severe neisserial infection. The homozygotes for C8 deficiency in these families had no detectable C8, heterozygotes often, but not always, had reduced C8 levels, and of the complement-mediated functions, only haemolytic and bactericidal activity were affected (Petersen et al 1976, Jasin 1977, Matthews et al 1980).

There are, in addition to these families with straightforward C8 deficiency, four families with individuals who apparently have dysfunctional C8 molecules which are antigenically deficient compared with the normal molecule. No C8 function or total complement haemolytic activity was detected in the serum of the probands, some of whom had recurrent neisserial infections.

C8 is composed of three polypeptide chains: α, β and γ. In Blacks C8α,C8γ deficiency is common, whereas in Caucasians C8β deficiency is common (Tedesco et al 1983).

C9 deficiency

Two unrelated elderly healthy men were found to have no C9 in both functional and immunochemical tests. The only abnormalities of complement-mediated functions in these sera were slower haemolysis of antibody-sensitised sheep red blood cells and bacteriolysis than that produced by normal serum. Both haemolytic and bacteriocidal activity approached normal with longer incubation times (Lint et al 1978). One in 40 normal Japanese is heterozygous for C9 deficiency.

BIOLOGICAL SIGNIFICANCE OF COMPLEMENT DEFICIENCY STATES IN HUMANS

In general, persons deficient in specific complement proteins have one or more kinds of disorder (if they have symptoms at all): 'allergic' vascular, increasing susceptibility to bacterial infections, and collagen vascular. These associations are dealt with separately (Lachmann & Rosen 1978).

'Allergic' vascular manifestations

Persons with hereditary angio-oedema (C1 inhibitor deficiency) and Factor I deficiency have clear-cut vascular permeability changes related to their basic genetic abnormalities. In these disorders there is unbridled activation of complement, either through the classical or the alternative pathway.

As mentioned above, the uninhibited action of C1 on C4 and C2 is attended by cleavage of these substrates, and the elaboration of a vasoactive peptide that has been isolated from patients' plasma and partly characterized. Recently, this material has been generated in vitro from mixtures of purified C1, C4, C2, and plasmin. With sufficient input of C2, C4 can be eliminated, providing further evidence for the earlier conclusion that the vasoactive peptide is derived from C2. The requirement for plasmin in the in vitro generation system is almost certainly important in vivo, because C1 inhibitor inhibits plasmin, and synthetic inhibitors of plasminogen activation, such as ε-aminocaproic acid or tranexamic acid, can provide effective prophylaxis against attacks of angio-oedema in this disease. Although patients with hereditary angio-oedema have hyperhistaminuria, perhaps from some elaboration of C3a in vivo, they do not have urticaria.

In contrast, there is massive histaminuria in Factor I deficiency, and the first patient to be described with this disorder had intermittent urticaria, particularly after a shower or when given normal plasma (and hence C3 as substrate). It is reasonable to attribute these abnormalities to the elaboration in vivo of large amounts of C3a from uninhibited alternative pathway activation with attendant C3 cleavage.

Increased susceptibility to infection

There appear to be two groups of complement-deficient patients with undue susceptibility to infection: those with deficits of C3 directly, or of C3 and Factor B secondary to Factor I or Factor 4 deficiency; and those with deficiencies of later-acting, or common pathway proteins, particularly C6 and C8. The organisms involved in C3 deficient patients are chiefly the pyogens: the streptococcus, the pneumococcus, the meningococcus and *H. influenzae*. These bacteria are much the same as those that afflict agammaglobulinaemics. Although severe deficits in most complement-mediated functions can be demonstrated in serum from these patients, it appears that a deficit in opsonization is central to their reduced host resistance. It is dangerous to be too simplistic, however, inasmuch as one C3-deficient subject had had no serious infections by the age of 4 years, and an 11-year-old with Factor I deficiency has also been infection free. Clearly other factors, including environment, play their part in any specific instance.

Deficiency of the late-acting complement components, C5 through C8, is associated in over half the propositi with *N. meningitides* and *N. gonorrhoeae* systemic infections. There is some ascertainment bias in assessing the incidence of such infections in these subjects since the incidence in homozygous deficient sibs of index cases is only 14%. Of patients with recurrent meningococcal meningitis, it is estimated that about 10% have a deficiency of a late acting complement component. The mechanism for this increased susceptibility is presumably a defective bactericidal capacity for *Neisseria*.

Collagen vascular disease

There is a striking incidence of SLE, 'lupus-like' disease, and a variety of phenomena, probably not the same, but all suspected of having an immunological basis, among all patients with complement deficiencies, including hereditary angio-oedema. These associations are with deficiencies of late-acting components of complement as well as of early components. Because C2 deficiency is so common, most attention has been directed to this deficiency. Of 38 homozygous C2-deficient subjects, 23 have disease, chiefly of suspected immunological type. 14 had systemic lupus erythematosus or discoid lupus erythematosus, and of these the female/male ratio was 6:1, whereas the overall female/male ratio in the non-SLE C2 deficient subjects was nearly 1:1.

This association between lupus and C2 deficiency may have one or more of several explanations. The gene for C2 deficiency (and the structural locus for C2) is on the sixth human chromosome, closely linked with the HLA regions. The C2 locus is very close to HLA-B and probably even closer to the HLA-D region. In other words, the genes at the C2 locus are inherited together with those for HLA with only minimal recombination. Furthermore, there is marked linkage disequilibrium between the C2 deficiency gene (C2D) and HLA A10 B18, and even more striking linkage disequilibrium between C2D and HLA DR2 and Bf^s. Thus, among random, apparently unrelated individuals, C2D is found linked to specific nearby genes. This disequilibrium could be the result of selective pressure keeping them together, or could result because the C2 deficiency mutation occurred fairly recently in human evolution. That the latter is the case is suggested by the fact that all the cases of C2 deficiency uncovered to date have been in white people. In contrast, many of the homozygotes for deficiency of later-acting components, such as C5, C6 or C8 are in Black people.

In any event, it is possible that an unusual immune response gene linked with C2D is somehow involved in an increased incidence of lupus in C2-deficient subjects. This possibility is enhanced by the evidence that lupus may result from viral infection. Further evidence for this hypothesis was obtained in a study of C2-deficient heterozygotes wherein it was found that although the incidence among normal individuals was 1.2%, the incidence in patients with lupus was significantly greater (two or three times).

Homozygous deficiency of complement proteins, particularly early-acting components, may predispose to lupus because of the deficiency per se. A possible mechanism is the requirement for complement in the solubilization of immune complexes. This would help explain the observed high incidence of lupus in C4 deficiency, hereditary angio-oedema, and C1r deficiency. Because the system only through C3 appears to participate in this function, it cannot be invoked to explain lupus in association with deficiencies of C5 and C8.

Finally, there is the problem of bias in the ascertainment and reporting of cases of complement deficiencies that favours a higher incidence of disease in general and collagen vascular disease in particular. Total haemolytic complement was measured initially only in specialised laboratories, so that it is not surprising that the first few cases of C2 deficiency were found among immunologists. As the test became a relatively common routine procedure, those tested tended to have or be suspected of having, 'immunological disease' and, in particular, lupus. The association may therefore reflect the incidence of these diseases in the tested population.

That there is a real association is suggested by the studies in heterozygous deficient subjects mentioned above. It is also suggested by a brief consideration of numbers. Assuming that the incidence of lupus (both systemic and discoid varieties) is between 1 and 0.1% of the general population in the United States, and the incidence of homozygous C2 deficiency is 1 in 10 000, there are approximately 20 000 homozygous for C2

deficiency in the United States, of whom 20-200 would be expected to have lupus by chance alone. To have already identified many subjects suggests that the number who have both C2 deficiency and lupus is much greater than the random association would predict. Thus, it appears likely that C4 and C2 deficiency (and perhaps other complement deficiencies) predispose to lupus, but the exact relationship and possible explanations need further exploration.

REFERENCES

Alper C A 1980 Complement and the MHC. In: Dorf M E (ed) The role of the major histocompatibility complex in immunobiology. Garland Press, New York p 173–200

Alper C A, Propp R P, Klemperer R, Rosen F S 1969 Inherited deficiency of the third component of human complement (C3). Journal of the Clinical Investigation 48: 553–557

Alper C A, Abramson N, Johnston R B Jr, Jandl J H, Rosen F S 1970a Increased susceptibility to infection associated with abnormalities of complement-mediated functions and of the third component of complement (C3). New England Journal of Medicine 282: 349–354

Alper C A, Abramson N, Johnston R B Jr, Jandl J H, Rosen F S 1970b Studies in vivo and in vitro on an abnormality in the metabolism of C3 in a patient with increased susceptibility to infection. Journal of Clinical Investigation 49: 1975–1985

Alper C A, Colten H R, Rosen F S, Rabson A R, Macnab G M, Gear J S S 1972a Homozygous deficiency of C3 in a patient with repeated infections. Lancet 2: 1170–1181

Alper C A, Rosen F S, Lachmann P J 1972b Inactivator of the third component of complement as an inhibitor in the properdin pathway. Proceedings of the National Academy of Sciences, USA 69: 2910–2913

Alper C A, Colten H R, Gear J S S, Rabson A R, Rosen F S 1976 Homozygous human C3 deficiency. The role of C3 in antibody production, C1s-induced vasopermeability, and cobra venom-induced passive hemolysis. Journal of Clinical Investigation 57: 222–229

Ballow M, Shira J E, Harden L, Yang S Y, Day N K 1975 Complete absence of the third component of complement in man. Journal of Clinical Investigation 56: 703–710

Davis A E III, Davis J S IV, Rabson A R, Osofsky S G, Colten H R, Rosen F S, Alper C A 1977 Homozygous C3 deficiency: Detection of C3 by radioimmunoassay. Clinical Immunology and Immunopathology 8: 543–550

De Bracco M M E, Windhorst D, Stroud M, Moncada B 1974 The autosomal recessive mode of inheritance of C1r deficiency in a large Puerto Rican family. Clinical and Experimental Immunology 16: 183–188

Donaldson V H, Evans R R 1963 A biochemical abnormality in hereditary angioneurotic edema. Absence of serum inhibitor of C1 esterase. American Journal of Medicine 35: 35–45

Gelfand J A, Sherins R J, Alling D W, Frank M M 1976 Treatment of hereditary angioneurotic edema with Danazol. Reversal of clinical and biochemical abnormalities. New England Journal of Medicine 295: 1444–1448

Hauptmann G, Grosshans E, Heid E, Mayer S, Basset A 1974 Lupus erythemateux aigu avec deficit complet de la fraction C4 du complement. Nouveau Presse de Medicine 3: 881–882

Jasin H E 1977 Absence of the eighth component of complement in association with systemic lupus erthematosis-like disease. Journal of Clinical Investigation 60: 709–715

Klemperer M R, Woodworth H C, Rosen F S, Austen K F 1966 Hereditary deficiency of the second component of complement in man. Journal of Clinical Investigation 45: 880–890

Lachmann P J, Rosen F S 1978 Genetic defects of complement in man. Seminars in Immunopathology 1: 339–353

Leddy J P, Frank M M, Gaither T, Baum J, Klemperer M R 1974 Hereditary deficiency of the sixth component of complement in man. I. Immunochemical, biologic, and family studies. Journal of Clinical Investigation 53: 544–553

Lim D, Gewurz A, Lint T F, Ghaze M, Sepheri B, Gewurz H 1976 Absence of the sixth component of complement in a patient with repeated episodes of meningococcal meningitis. Journal of Pediatrics 89: 42–47

Lint T F, Zeitz H J, Scott D, Malkinson J R, Gewurz H 1978 Hereditary deficiency of the ninth component of complement (C) in man (abstract). Clinical Research 26: 714

Matthews N, Stark J M, Harper P S, Doran J, Jones D M 1980 Recurrent meningococcal infections associated with a functional deficiency of the C8 component of human complement. Clinical and Experimental Immunology 39: 53–59

Müller-Eberhard H J 1975 Complement. Annual Review of Biochemistry 44: 697–724

Ochs H D, Rosenfeld S I, Thomas E D et al 1977 Linkage between the gene (or genes) controlling synthesis of the fourth component of complement and the major histocompatibility complex. New England Journal of Medicine 296: 470–475

Petersen B H, Graham J A, Brooks G F 1976 Human deficiency of the eighth component of complement. The requirement of C8 for serum *Neisseria gonnorrhoeae* bactericidal activity. Journal of Clinical Investigation 57: 283–290

Reed K B M 1989 Deficiency of the first component of human complement. Immunodeficiency Reviews 1: 297

Rosen F S, Alper C A, Pensky J, Klemperer M R, Donaldson V H 1971 Genetically determined heterogeneity of the C1 estrase inhibitor in patients with hereditary angioneurotic edema. Journal of Clinical Investigation 50: 2143–2149

Rosenfeld S J, Kelly M E, Leddy J P 1976 Hereditary deficiency of the fifth component of complement in man. I.

Clinical, immunochemical, and family studies. Journal of Clinical Investigation 57: 1626–1634

Synderman R, Durack D J, McCarthy G A, Ward F E, Meadows L 1979 Deficiency of the fifth component of complement in human subjects. American Journal of Medicine 67: 638–645

Tedesco F, Densen P, Villa M A, Peterson B H, Siirchia G 1983 Two types of dysfunctional eighth component of complement (C8) molecules in C8 deficiency in man. Reconstitution of normal C8 from the mixture of the two abnormal C8 molecules. Journal of Clinical Investigation 71: 183–191

Thompson R A, Winterborn M H 1981

Hypocomplementaemnia due to a genetic deficiency of beta-1H globulin. Clinical and Experimental Immunology 46: 110–119

Willek B, Opferkuch W 1975 A case of deficiency of the seventh component of complement in man. Biological properties of a C7-deficient serum and description of a C7-inactivating principle. Clinical and Experimental Immunology 19: 223–235

Ziegler J B, Alper C A, Rosen F S, Lachmann P J, Sherington L 1975 Restoration by purified C3b inactivator of complement-mediated function in vivo in a patient with C3b inactivator deficiency. Journal of Clinical Investigation 55: 668–672

84. Disorders of leucocyte function

M. E. Miller   H. R. Hill

Over the past 20 years, the field of phagocytic disorders has attained major clinical and biological significance. Despite this relatively short period of time much literature has accumulated on these disorders, which are frequently hereditary. Recently, due to the development of exciting new techniques in molecular biology, it has been possible to identify the genetic mechanisms involved in at least some of these disorders. Moreover, through recombinant DNA technology we have begun to find means to augment abnormal leucocyte function and at least partially correct genetic defects in cellular physiology.

HISTORICAL BACKGROUND

Two major observations, one basic and one clinical, set the foundation for current knowledge of this field. In the late 1800s Elie Metchnikoff (1893) established that 'the essential and primary element in typical inflammation consists in a reaction of the phagocyte *against* a harmful agent.' Prior to this it was believed that phagocytes were harmful to the host, and that they contributed to the untoward consequences of bacterial infection. However, once Metchnikoff had established that phagocytes were helpful rather than harmful to the human host, he predicted that defects in phagocyte function might predispose the host to increased numbers and toxicity of infections with foreign micro-organisms. The last 20 years of clinical recognition of phagocyte disorders have proven his hypothesis to be true.

Holmes and co-workers (1966) provided the first evidence of an inborn error of phagocyte function. They studied patients with chronic granulomatous disease (CGD), a disorder characterized by indolent, granulomatous type infections. The disease most frequently occurs in an X-linked pattern.

In in vitro experiments it was shown that polymorphonuclear leucocytes (PMNs) from the afflicted children were able to ingest bacteria normally, but were unable to kill the ingested organisms. This was in sharp contrast to normal PMNs which effectively killed the same organisms intracellularly. Of additional interest was the observation that PMNs from the mothers (presumed carriers in an X-linked disorder) were intermediate in their killing capacity. Not only did these observations establish the first intrinsic defect of PMN function, but the intermediate bactericidal defect in maternal PMNs was consistent with the Lyon hypothesis.

Baehner and Nathan (1968) demonstrated a primary metabolic abnormality in PMNs from CGD patients by utilizing a colourless dye – nitroblue tetrazolium (NBT) – which turns to blue formazan in the reduced state. It was shown that normal PMNs stimulated to ingest and kill bacteria reduced the dye, but similarly stimulated PMNs from the children with CGD were unable to reduce the dye. Again, maternal PMNs were found to be intermediate in dye reduction. This suggested a biochemical lesion under genetic control as the underlying basis for the bactericidal defect.

On a broader scale, the observation that dysfunction of one PMN activity, i.e. bactericidal mechanisms, could lead to a clinically recognizable syndrome suggested that other PMN functions such as movement and/or ingestion could also, if deficient, lead to recurrent infections. Further, the observation that one of these defects was genetically determined suggested that other disorders of PMN function might also have a hereditary basis.

Over the past 20 years, these hypotheses have been proven true. An entire spectrum of disorders of PMN, and more recently monocyte-macrophage (MNL) functions, have been recognized, many of which are genetically determined. More recently still, the abnormal or missing components in the phagocytes of some of these patients have been specifically identified, and the genetic loci responsible for the abnormality pinpointed. In this chapter, we will summarize the current status of this exciting field. To grasp the subject better, it will be helpful first to review three basic mechanisms of normal phagocytic cells – movement, ingestion and bactericidal activities. This review is intended only to provide the reader with the necessary background to interpret the clinical findings. More comprehensive reviews of each function are cited in the appropriate sections (Mills & Quie 1980, Roberts & Gallin 1983, Boxer & Morganroth 1987, Hill 1987).

BASIC PHAGOCYTIC ACTIVITIES

Polymorphonuclear leucocytes (PMNs)

Movement

Mobilization of phagocytic cells from the bone marrow and other storage sites of the body requires active movement. The mechanisms by which phagocytes move have been the focus of extensive recent laboratory interest.

A major advance in the ability to study movement of PMNs was provided by the development of an in vitro filter assay by Stephen Boyden (1962). Prior to that time, it was commonly held that there was little, if any, biological significance to the movement of phagocytic cells. In principle, the Boyden assay consists of measuring the migration of cells through a small-pored filter towards a chemotactically active gradient. Such a gradient can be generated by a variety of methods, but is usually derived by activation of complement following exposure of fresh serum to endotoxin or antigen-antibody complexes. Such activated sera contain a variety of chemotactically active materials, including C5a. Additional substances found to have chemotactic activity include: serum factors; coagulation-derived factors; bacterial metabolites; secretory products of sensitized lymphocytes and PMNs; denatured proteins; and synthetic chemotactic factors such as the N-formylmethionyl peptides (Gallin & Quie 1978, Ackerman & Douglas 1979). Also, lipoxygenases in a variety of mammalian cells transform arachidonic acid to stable mono-hydroxyeicosatetraenoic (HETE) products. Various endogenously produced HETE products are chemotactic for PMNs (Goetzl & Sun 1979).

The precise mechanisms by which a PMN initiates and sustains movement following exposure to chemotactically active material are surrounded by controversy. A number of potentially important steps have, however, been identified.

Initially, a brief but rapid membrane depolarization occurs. This is coincident with calcium and/or sodium influx, and is followed by a prolonged hyperpolarization associated with increased potassium permeability (Gallin et al 1978).

Subsequent events include: increased levels of cyclic guanosine monophosphate (cGMP) (Hill 1978); lysosomal enzyme release (Becker & Showell 1974); increased

glycolysis and hexosemonophosphate shunt activity (Goetzl & Austen 1974); cell swelling (Becker 1976); increased numbers of microtubules (Stossel 1978); and probable activation of contractile proteins (Boxer et al 1974, Hill 1987).

While considerable information on overall cell movement has been gained from filter, i.e. Boyden-type assays, such techniques yield little information on the process(es) of cell movement. In other words, cells are placed on one side of a filter and counted on the opposite side. How they got there, however, is anyone's guess. Such information is obviously critical if we are to understand and diagnose individual disorders of PMN movement.

Partial answers to these questions have been provided by the development of assays which permit observations of single and/or small numbers of cells during movement. These include the visual assay system of Zigmond (1978) in which cells are observed under phase microscopy on a bridge across which a gradient of chemotactic factor is established; deformability of PMNs by the technique of cell elastimetry (Miller & Myers 1975); and cinemicrography and videotape analysis of PMNs subjected to a chemotactic gradient (Cheung & Miller 1980). Such techniques have now been applied not only to normal PMNs but to PMNs from patients with various defects of movement. Since data so derived will be of significance in the following clinical discussion, the results will be briefly summarized.

(a) Deformability. Deformability is measured by the technique of cell elastimetry, which measures the amount of negative pressure required to aspirate a cell into a micropipette. In 1970, Lichtman utilized this technique in the study of human bone marrow granulocytes and found that less negative pressure was required for aspiration as cells matured. In other words, myeloblasts and promyelocytes were relatively resistant to deformation, while myelocytes were more easily deformed. Mature PMNs were highly deformable, and it was postulated that increasing deformability of PMNs correlated with the ability of granulocytes to leave the bone marrow. Miller and Myers (1975) adapted the technique to the study of human peripheral blood PMNs and demonstrated a correlation between deformability and cell motility. Deformability of PMNs from patients with PMN movement disorders provides one means of demonstrating heterogeneity of the group (Miller 1979).

(b) Visual assays. Several visual techniques have been applied to the study of motile PMNs. Early assays employed time-lapse photography and demonstrated that motile PMNs were able to turn in response to a chemotactic stimulus. Zigmond utilized an improved technique for studying the nature and mechanisms responsible for the turning (1978). Basically, the system consisted of a

microscope slide with a bridge separated by a shadow well on either side. A chemotactic gradient could be established by placing a chemoattractant in one well and a suitable buffer in the other well. A suspension of PMNs was then deposited on the bridge and the cells observed microscopically. Cells appeared to orient or turn towards the chemotactic stimulus, and once oriented, retained their direction and moved towards the chemotactic stimulus. These observations led to a new terminology for PMN movement. Formerly, the term 'chemotaxis' was applied to the general phenomenon of PMNs moving towards a chemical gradient (as measured in a Boyden or filter type assay). The more current terminology, however, designates the turning or orientation phase as *chemotaxis*, and the increased rate of locomotion of motile cells as *chemokinesis* (Gallin & Quie 1978). These new terms are important in understanding disorders of human PMN movement, as some of the defects appear to be ones of abnormal chemotaxis and some of abnormal chemokinesis.

More recent studies have described the use of high speed cinemicrography and videotape analysis in the study of motile human PMNs (Cheung & Miller 1980). Such studies suggest that the concept of PMNs turning towards the chemotactic stimulus may not be correct. Although human PMNs oriented towards a chemotactic gradient move steadily towards the gradient in terms of net activity, individual cells constantly oscillate and reorient during the process. This is accomplished not by turning in any one direction, but rather by extending one or more pseudopodia from any area of the cell surface. A primary requirement of the PMN in order to move effectively is a highly deformable membrane (see above).

Phagocytosis

Ingestion of foreign substances of particulate nature (phagocytosis) or soluble nature (pinocytosis) involves two distinct phases – recognition and ingestion. The recognition phase involves specific receptors on the cell membrane. Several PMN membrane receptors which have been identified include a receptor for the Fc fragments of immunoglobulin molecules and receptors for several activation products of complement (C3b, iC3b and C5a) (Henson 1976, Gordan et al 1986). These receptors presumably play a significant role in increasing efficiency of the ingestion process by fixing opsonised particles to the cell surface.

Following adherence, particles are then actually ingested. This involves many of the same cellular functions and activities as in movement, and some investigators feel that the two activities are part of the same overall process. Ingestion involves the flow of cytoplasmic hyaline pseu-

dopods around the phagocytosed particle (Stossel 1975). Formation of these pseudopods probably involves active participation of the actin-myosin filament system of the PMN (Stossel 1975, Stossel & Hartwig 1976, Hill 1987). The pseudopods surround and fuse about the attached particle in forming a phagosome. The internalized phagosome is then merged with lysosomes and degranulation occurs, with ultimate discharge of lysosomal contents into the phagosome, i.e. phagolysosome.

Bactericidal activity

An immense literature has accumulated on the characterization of bactericidal mechanisms of human PMNs. A comprehensive review of this topic is obviously outside the scope of this chapter, and we will, therefore, summarize those points which are relevant to the following clinical discussion.

A sophisticated array of biochemical processes are available to the human PMN in the killing of ingested micro-organisms. Bactericidal activity of human PMNs is associated with oxidative activity, although the precise relationships are not yet known. Upon contact with the PMN membrane by a foreign particle, and coincident with ingestion and onset of killing, a sequence of metabolic events occurs, This is known as the 'respiratory burst' and includes increased oxygen consumption, oxidation of glucose via the hexosemonophosphate shunt, and the generation of hydrogen peroxide (Johnston & Newman 1977).

A group of potentially bactericidal products is generated during this process. The reaction is initiated by contact of the cell surface with a foreign particle or microbe. This presumably activates an enzyme closely related to the cell surface, NADPH oxidase. Activation of the oxidase results in the transfer of a single electron to oxygen, thereby forming an unstable radical known as superoxide anion (O_2^-). The oxidase is a multicomponent complex which includes a cytochrome b_{-245} responsible for electron transfer. Two superoxide radicals can form hydrogen peroxide (H_2O_2) when they spontaneously interact. The continuing reaction between H_2O_2 and O_2^- yields free hydroxyl radical (OH), a potent oxidizing agent. Transfer of energy from O_2^- to an unstable, excited species called singlet oxygen may result in a burst of energy which can be measured as emitted light in the chemiluminescence assay. Transfer of 'extra' electrons from superoxide anions may be responsible for NBT dye reduction.

Each of these oxidation products – superoxide anion, hydrogen peroxide, hydroxyl radicals and singlet oxygen – possess potent bactericidal activities. While the extent to which any one shares in normal PMN bactericidal activity has not yet been determined, it seems likely that some, if not all, are of clinical significance. Additional microbicidal activities result from the release of PMN lysosomal materials such as myeloperoxidase, lysozyme, phagocytin and other cationic proteins.

Monocytes and macrophages

These cells subserve many of the same functions as PMNs, including movement, ingestion and microbicidal activities. In addition, a major role in modulating the immune response has been demonstrated. The macrophage is involved in the enhancement of antibody responses and cell-mediated immunity, particularly towards T cell-dependent antigens. This topic is reviewed in detail elsewhere (Cohn 1978, Karnovsky & Lazdins 1978, North 1978).

The importance of macrophages in the inflammatory response was first suggested by Metchnikoff (1893), who noted from his observations of tubercle bacilli that:

The polynuclear cells engulf the tubercle bacilli readily but perish after a short time, and then with the microbes they contain, are eaten up by various mononuclear phagocytes which may be classed together under the term of macrophages. These latter cells have a much greater power of resistance, and in some cases are even capable of destroying the tubercle bacilli.

The relationship between macrophages and the circulating monocytes has not been conclusively determined. It is generally believed, however, that blood monocytes evolve into macrophages (histiocytes) in various anatomic sites, including the peritoneal cavity, lung, bone marrow, spleen, lymph nodes and liver. Increasing evidence suggests that subpopulations of macrophages from different, and even the same, tissues exist. For example, alveolar and peritoneal macrophages differ metabolically and functionally.

Mackaness (1962) immensely heightened interest in the role of the macrophage in the immune-inflammatory response when he demonstrated that macrophages which had been infected with the intracellular pathogen, *Listeria monocytogenes*, were able to significantly inhibit the growth and infectivity of other intracellular organisms (which normal macrophages cannot do).

Thus was born the concept of the 'activated macrophage' (Cohn 1978, Karnovsky & Lazdins 1978, North 1978). These cells are larger, and adhere and spread more on glass than normal macrophages. A number of functional and biochemical activities are enhanced in activated macrophages over those seen in normal macrophages. Phagocytosis of some (but not all) materials is increased. Glucose utilization through the hexosemonophosphate shunt is increased. Membrane enzymes such as adenylate cyclase, and cytoplasmic enzymes such as lactic

dehydrogenase, show increased activities. Increased numbers of lysosomes and enhanced release of lysosomal enzymes – e.g. collagenase – are also seen. Monocytes and macrophages also produce 'monokines' that are critically important in regulating several aspects of inflammation. These include interleukin 1 (IL 1) and tumour necrosis factor (TNF). IL 1, or endogenous pyrogen as it used to be known, is responsible for generation of the febrile response, elevation of the acute phase proteins and enhancement of the acute inflammatory response. Tumour necrosis factor, which can cause necrosis of some malignant cell lines, acts in concert with IL 1 to affect inflammation profoundly. This monokine is felt to mediate the biological effects of endotoxin.

The major effects which have been noted in activated macrophages are enhanced bactericidal activities and increased tumour inhibition and killing. These two activities do not, however, consistently correlate. In other words, macrophages which have been 'activated' in enhanced killing may not always show increased tumouricidal activities, and vice versa.

It is not yet known whether all clinical disorders of phagocyte function involve both PMNs and MNLs, or whether there are entities which only involve one or the other cell line. To the extent that data is available, comparative studies will be noted in the following clinical discussion.

CLINICAL DISORDERS OF PHAGOCYTE FUNCTION

DISORDERS OF BACTERICIDAL FUNCTION

Chronic granulomatous disease

The CGD syndrome is characterized by recurrent, purulent infections of the skin, reticulo-endothelial organs and lungs, associated with an inability of the patient's phagocytes to kill intracellular, catalase positive, non-hydrogen peroxide producing bacteria. Onset of symptoms usually occurs within the first year of life, although cases have been reported where the initial infections occurred as late as 12 years of age. Although common signs and symptoms may affect virtually any part of the body, suppurative, indolent lymphadenitis, pneumonitis, dermatitis, hepatomegaly, splenomegaly and osteomyelitis are particularly frequent findings. Table 84.1 summarizes the relative frequency of clinical findings in CGD. The dermatologic involvement may be in the form of low grade abscesses, or frequently as a perioral eczematoid lesion.

A unique group of bacteria is associated with CGD. This includes primarily catalase-positive, non-hydrogen peroxide producing organisms. As shown in Table 84.2,

Table 84.1 Signs and symptoms in 168 patients with chronic granulomatous disease (Johnston & Newman 1977)

Findings	Number of patients involved
Marked lymphadenopathy	137
Pneumonitis	134
Dermatitis	120
Hepatomegaly	114
Onset by one year	109
Suppuration of nodes	104
Splenomegaly	95
Hepatic-periphepatic abscess	69
Osteomyelitis	54
Onset with dermatitis	42
Onset with lymphadenitis	38
Facial periorificial dermatitis	35
Persistent diarrhoea	34
Septicaemia or meningitis	29
Perianal abscess	28
Conjunctivitis	27
Death from pneumonitis	26
Persistent rhinitis	26
Ulcerative stomatitis	26

Staphylococcus aureus and enteric organisms predominate. Of additional significance is the relatively high frequency of the enteric organisms *Klebsiella-Aerobacter* and *Serratia marcescens*. In many of the earlier case descriptions, postmortem examinations yielded these organisms, but those interpreting the findings tended to discard them as insignificant. Notably absent from the list of common pathogens in patients with CGD are *Haemo-*

Table 84.2 Micro-organisms cultured from blood, cerebrospinal fluid, or purulent foci (Johnston & Newman 1977)

Organism	Number of patients involved*
Staphylococcus aureus	87
Klebsiella-Aerobacter organisms	29
E. coli	26
Serratia marcescens	16
Pseudomonas organisms	15
Staphylococcus albus	13
Aspergillus organisms	13
Candida albicans	12
Salmonella organisms	10
Proteus organisms	9
Streptococci	9
Nocardia organisms	4
Mycobacteria	4
Paracolobactrum organisms	4
Actinomyces organisms	2
Other enteric bacteria	9

* Refers to number of different patients from whom that organism was cultured.

philus influenzae, streptococci and pneumococci. This correlates with the ability of the patients' phagocytes to kill these catalase-negative, peroxide-producing organisms in vivo (Mandell & Hook 1969, Johnston & Newman 1977). In addition to bacterial organisms, the fungi Aspergillus and Candida are relatively frequent pathogens.

An additional laboratory finding in CGD is an almost constant neutrophilia, even during periods when the patient does not appear to be acutely infected. As we shall later describe, this contrasts with the neutropenia of some patients with chemotactic defects.

Laboratory diagnosis

Two procedures are generally performed in the confirmation of a diagnosis of CGD. The first is a screening technique which measures the ability of the patient's PMNs to reduce nitroblue tetrazolium dye (NBT). Reduction converts the colourless oxidized NBT to blue formazan, which can be measured qualitatively or spectrophotometrically (Johnston & Baehner 1971). Normal PMNs reduce NBT as a consequence of metabolic products generated during the bactericidal process. PMNs from patients with CGD fail, however, to reduce the dye. Decreased total dye reduction could result if all the PMNS were working at diminished capacity or if two populations of PMNs – one normal and one defective – were present. This is important as the carrier state would more readily fit the Lyon hypothesis if two populations were present. Histochemical techniques (Ochs & Igo 1973) have confirmed the presence of two populations. In these techniques, the PMNs of the patients and controls are allowed to attach to glass coverslips and are then stimulated with endotoxin or the protein kinase C activator, phorbol myristate acetate (PMA). This results in maximal enhancement of the respiratory burst in normal PMNs so that over 90% of the cells reduce the dye to a black intracellular deposit. In the classical X–linked form of CGD, none of the PMNs of the patients reduce the dye. An intermediate number (30–50%) of the carrier female's PMNs are NBT positive. Employing fetal blood samples, this test has been used successfully in the prenatal diagnosis of CGD in known carrier mothers (Newburger et al 1979).

Regardless of the results from an NBT test, specific diagnosis of CGD should be confirmed by an in vitro bactericidal assay (Holmes et al 1966). Ideally this should be performed with isolates of the patient's infecting organism, but if not available, staphylococci or E. coli can be used.

Modifications of the chemiluminescence assay by the addition of luminol have increased its sensitivity and utility in the study of patients and carriers with CGD (Mills et al 1980). It remains to be proven, however, that this relatively new assay can be relied upon in lieu of a specific bactericidal test. Studies of monocytes from CGD patients have yielded essentially the same results as PMNs.

Recently, techniques have been devised to detect the absence of the critical cytochrome b_{-245} in patients with X-linked CGD (Segal et al 1983, Lutter et al 1984). The gene for the heavy chain of this cytochrome, which is missing in these patients, has now been identified and cloned (Royer-Pokora et al 1986, Dinauer et al 1987) so that probes can be made to assess levels of mRNA transcripts for this protein in the leucocytes of suspected patients (Ezekowitz et al 1988).

Mechanisms of CGD

The CGD sydnrome probably reflects a number of related, yet specific, underlying molecular abnormalities. Until each molecular defect is precisely identified, however, separation of the cases into specific entities is not always possible. Despite this limitation, much has been learned of the probable mechanisms. The basic molecular defect is deficient activity of an enzyme responsible for conversion of oxygen to bactericidal species. Membrane associated NADPH oxidase is a multicomponent complex which includes the cytochrome b_{-245} responsible for electron transfer and generation of superoxide anion (O_2^-) from molecular oxygen during the respiratory burst. Segel and associates (1983) have reported that the vast majority of patients with X-linked CGD lack this cytochrome, while those with apparently autosomal recessive disease have an abnormal, nonfunctioning cytochrome. The cytochrome is a heterodimer consisting of a 91 kD heavy chain and a 22 kD light chain. The heavy chain appears to be missing in the classical X-linked patients (Royer-Pokora et al 1986, Dinauer et al 1987). Variant CGD patients with low levels of NBT dye reduction following stimulation with endotoxin or PMA (3–20%), low levels of superoxide production and decreased cytochrome b heavy chain message have been described (Ezekowitz et al 1988). These patients have onset at a later age, in general, and usually have a milder clinical course.

In the absence of oxidase activation, the events associated with the normal respiratory burst fail to occur. PMNs from patients with CGD fail to show a phagocytosis-associated increase in oxygen consumption, generation of superoxide and hydrogen peroxide. As a consequence, NBT reduction and chemiluminescence responses fail to occur. Decreased bactericidal activity presumably reflects the absence of these potent bactericidal oxidation products of normal PMN respiration.

Genetics of CGD

X-linked recessive inheritance has been established in the majority of males with CGD. In reported cases a male:female ratio of 6:1 further supports this mode of inheritance as the most frequent (Johnston & Newman 1977). In familial studies, the use of the histochemical NBT test has supported X-linked transmission and provided confirmation of the Lyon hypothesis. In this test, over 90% (usually in excess of 98%) of PMNs from normal individuals will reduce the dye upon appropriate stimulation. Virtually none of the patients' mothers, sisters or female maternal relatives who are presumed carriers of the disease generally have a mixture of normal and abnormal PMNs (35–65% of PMNs will reduce the dye). If inactivation of one X chromosome is, as required by the Lyon hypothesis, a completely random event, then one might expect to occasionally find a female carrier with wide deviation from 50% normal PMNs. Such has been reported by Repine et al (1975) who found that PMNs from one sister of a boy with CGD had only 20% normal cells by NBT reduction.

Much controversy surrounds the question of other modes of inheritance of CGD. The two most widely cited occurrences are case reports of CGD in females (Baehner & Nathan 1968, Quie et al 1968, Azimi et al 1968, Ochs & Igo 1973, Wilson et al 1974, Biggar et al 1976, Carruthers & Greaves 1976, McPhail et al 1977, Clark & Klebanoff 1978, Segal et al 1978), and in boys without demonstrable leucocyte defects in either parent (Kontras & Bass 1969, Dupree et al 1972, Repine et al 1975).

The mode of inheritance in females with CGD is unknown. Data yielded by the NBT and bactericidal assays has generally failed to demonstrate PMN defects in either parent. This inability to detect the carrier state in families of females with chronic granulomatous disease has been interpreted as suggesting a non-X-linked inheritance in these patients. Recently, however, Mills et al (1980) applied the luminol-dependent chemiluminescence assay to detect subtle abnormalities in PMN oxygen metabolism in females with CGD. PMNs from three of four CGD females showed extremely low chemiluminescence production. Their asymptomatic mothers' PMNs had intermediate values, and PMNs from the fathers were normal. PMNs from two affected males in these kinships also generated virtually no chemiluminescence. All unaffected males showed normal PMN chemiluminescence, but two of seven female relatives had intermediate values. PMNs in three of the families were also studied by NBT reduction. In each family, two populations of PMNs were demonstrated for the female patients and/or their mothers. The authors suggested that these findings support an X-linked inheritance in at least these families of females with CGD, based upon: (a) the wide phenotypic variability for clinical disease; (b) evidence of two PMN populations in the patients or their mothers and; (c) low but detectable chemiluminescence in PMNs from the affected females.

In reports of boys with CGD whose parents have lacked demonstrable PMN abnormalities, transmission by an autosomal recessive gene or, in some cases, the possibility of spontaneous mutation has been postulated. Study of these kindreds with sensitive assays such as the luminol enhanced chemiluminescence have not yet been reported but may help shed light on the problem.

Variants of CGD

Most reported 'variants' of CGD have provided relatively indirect evidence, such as apparent selectivity of bacterial strains to which the patient was susceptible or the presence of PMN defects in addition to the bactericidal defect. Such case reports are difficult to interpret.

Several probable variants have, however, been reported. A brother and sister with clinical CGD were described whose PMNs could ingest but not kill, staphylococci (Van Der Meer et al 1975, Weening et al 1976). As expected, PMNs from either patient demonstrated defective oxygen consumption, O_2^- production, hexose monophosphate shunt activation and iodination of ingested particles upon in vitro ingestion of serum-opsonized zymosan or latex. Upon ingestion of latex particles heavily coated with IgG or IgG aggregates, however, the same PMNs demonstrated normal oxidative, 'respiratory burst' activities. It thus appeared that the patients' PMNs possessed normal oxidative metabolic activities, but had an abnormal trigger or activating mechanism. Six other patients (three boys and three girls) with CGD studied by the authors failed to demonstrate this finding.

Clark and Klebanoff (1978) described a brother and sister, ages 24 and 20, who had classical clinical and laboratory findings of CGD and also marked impairment in the chemotactic responses of their PMNs and in the level of chemotactic activities generated in their serums by activation of the complement system. Impaired leucocyte migration has not generally been found in patients with CGD. As noted by the authors, however:

It remains to be determined what the relationship between the leukocyte bactericidal and chemotactic defects is, what their relative contributions to increased susceptibility to infections are, and whether similar impairment of chemotaxis is present in other patients with chronic granulomatous disease.

Giblett et al (1971) observed that patients with the X-linked form of CGD carried the very rare null Kell blood group phenotype K_0, in which all antigenic products of the Kell locus are absent. Marsh and co-workers (1975, 1977) found K_0 phenotypes in five boys with X-linked CGD, while 50 normal individuals possessed a Kell group antigen, designated K_x. In the brother and sister with CGD (presumably not X-linked) described by Clark and Klebanoff (1978), both patients were K_x. Although these findings support an association between K_0 phenotype and the X-linked form of CGD, more recent evidence suggests that the correlation is not always present.

Glucose-6-phosphate dehydrogenase (G6PD) deficiency

Patients with severe leucocyte G6PD deficiency (generally 5% or less of normal G6PD levels) have a clinical syndrome which mimics CGD, although infections are usually somewhat milder. Oxidative metabolic defects are also similar to CGD, with the exception that methylene blue stimulates glucose-C-1 oxidation by the PMNs of CGD patients, but not always of G6PD deficient subjects (Holmes et al 1967). The actual existence of functionally significant intrinsic leucocyte G6PD deficiency has been questioned. An increased lability of G6PD in PMNs of CGD patients has been described (Bellanti et al 1970) which may be due to a deficiency in a stabilizing factor (Erickson et al 1972). It should be emphasized that the vast majority of subjects with erythrocyte G6PD deficiency have normal leucocyte G6PD activity (Marks et al 1959, Klebanoff & Clark 1978).

Clinical management

Specific therapy for CGD must await definite identification and replacement of primary molecular deficiencies. Despite this, significant improvements have occurred in management and long-term prognosis. Prolonged antimicrobial therapy with an agent as specific as possible for the infecting organism is the treatment of choice. When possible, one should select antimicrobial agents which penetrate the cell adequately such as clindamycin, rifampin and trimethoprim-sulphamethoxazole. This means that the treating physician must be alert to the most subtle signs of infection in these compromised hosts and take seriously the results of appropriate cultures. In particular, organisms such as *Klebsiella aerobacter* or *Serratia marcescens* must be regarded as pathogens in patients with CGD.

Long-term administration of sulphonamides or trimethoprim-sulphamethoxazole has been utilized with some success. These agents may exert an effect upon intracellular PMN microbicidal mechanisms (Johnston & Newman 1977). Other reported therapeutic trials include bone marrow transplantation (Delmas et al 1975) and repeated granulocyte transfusions (Quie 1969, Raubitschek et al 1973). These measures are of doubtful benefit.

Exciting new clinical and laboratory data suggest that interferon gamma may have a beneficial effect in patients with CGD (Ezekowitz et al 1988). Interferon gamma has been reported to enhance the respiratory burst of monocytes and macrophages and to improve bacterial killing by these cells. Ezekowitz et al (1987) have shown that interferon gamma can enhance the respiratory burst activity of both PMNs and monocyte/macrophages from CGD patients in vitro. Incubation of the patient's cells with this agent also increased the very low level of cytochrome b heavy chain gene expression. Subsequently, this group reported that two consecutive daily doses of interferon gamma significantly improve respiratory burst activity, superoxide production, bacterial killing and the levels of phagocyte cytochrome b in CGD patients. Additional unpublished anecdotal data suggest a beneficial effect of interferon gamma on the clinical course of some CGD patients. A controlled trial of its effect in CGD is currently in progress.

Glutathione synthetase deficiency

Glutathione synthetase deficiency occurs in two forms – with or without associated 5-oxoprolinuria. GSD without 5-oxoprolinuria is usually limited in clinical findings to haemolytic anaemia and acidosis (Mohler et al 1970). GSD with associated 5-oxoprolinuria may be of broader clinical significance with the additional findings of CNS dysfunction cataracts (at least in experimental animals), increased susceptibility to infections and PMN bactericidal defects (Spielberg et al 1977, Boxer et al 1979).

Mechanism of GSD

We will concentrate the discussion on GSD with 5-oxoprolinuria. The basic defect is presumed to result from negative effects of superoxide and hydrogen peroxide. Although, as previously discussed, these metabolites are important contributors to normal PMN bactericidal activities, they are also highly reactive waste products which must eventually be eliminated by the phagocyte. This elimination is accomplished by: (a) superoxide dismutase which converts superoxide to hydrogen peroxide; and (b) catalase and the glutathione peroxidase-glutathione reductase system which convert hydrogen peroxide to water and molecular oxygen. In the absence of these enzymes, significant auto-oxidative damage occurs to the phagocytic cells (Oliver et al 1976).

PMNs from a patient with GSD with 5-oxoprolinuria were studied for oxidant damage (Boxer et al 1979). Compared with normal PMNs, GSD PMNs released 60% more hydrogen peroxide, iodinated 20–25% as many ingested particles, showed markedly decreased bactericidal activity towards ingested *S. aureus* 502A, and failed to assemble microtubules during phagocytosis.

Genetics of GSD

Genetic heterogeneity has been demonstrated in GSD. In GSD without 5-oxoprolinuria, Mohler et al (1970) demonstrated an autosomal recessive pattern. Erythrocytes from their patient (a 32-year-old male) lacked glutathione synthetase, while erythrocytes from each of his parents and his four children had intermediate levels. Spielberg et al (1977) demonstrated that GSD without associated 5-oxoprolinuria resulted from an unstable mutant enzyme. Nucleated cells such as PMNs and fibroblasts maintained adequate levels of GS and glutathione, but erythrocytes did not.

GSD with 5-oxoprolinuria is also inherited as an autosomal recessive disorder (Spielberg et al 1977). Almost undetectable levels of GS were found in cell lines from two patients, and intermediate levels in each of the parents studied. Unlike the erythrocyte defect, however, deficient GS activity was found in erythrocytes, PMNs and cultured skin fibroblasts. Further genetic heterogeneity was suggested by the finding of different enzyme kinetics for the mutant glutathione synthetases of the two patients studied. More studies will be necessary before concluding that different forms of GSD with oxoprolinuria exist.

Clinical management of GSD

Boxer et al (1979) reported successful treatment of a patient with GSD and 5-oxoprolinuria with alpha-tocopherol (vitamin E) therapy. The patient was placed on 400 IU of alpha-tocopherol per day for three months. Normalization of PMN defects occurred including improved microtubule assembly during phagocytosis. The mechanism of this response is unclear. Despite the improvement in PMN functions, glutathione levels remained at 25% normal levels. The authors suggested that vitamin E might have hastened the destruction of excess peroxide within the PMNs during phagocytosis.

Congenital myeloperoxidase deficiency

In congenital myeloperoxidase deficiency (MPOD), there is a complete absence of MPO from PMNs and

MNLs. The eosinophil peroxidase differs in several respects from the PMN enzyme and is present in normal amounts (Archer et al 1965, Desser et al 1972). The clinical picture in hereditary MPOD is considerably less severe than that of CGD, and a number of the patients have been in reasonably good health (Klebanoff & Clark 1978). In addition to occasional difficulty with the same spectrum of bacteria as encountered in CGD, several of these patients have encountered severe difficulty with *C. albicans* (Lehrer & Cline 1969, Moosmann & Bojanovsky 1975). Mills and Quie (1980) indicated that 4 of the 15 patients with hereditary deficiency of myeloperoxidase have suffered serious and prolonged candida infections.

Mechanism of MPOD

Peroxidases do not exert direct antimicrobial activities, but may catalyze the conversion of a substance from a weak to a strong antimicrobial agent. The mechanism of the MPO-mediated antimicrobial activity in human PMNs is complex. Hydrogen peroxide reacts with the iron of the haem prosthetic groups of MPO to form an enzyme-substrate complex or complexes with strong oxidative capacity. The oxidizable cofactors are presumably halides. The oxidation of a halide by MPO and hydrogen peroxide results in the formation of (a) strong antimicrobial agent(s) (iodine>bromine>chlorine) (Klebanoff & Clark 1978)

Diagnosis of MPOD

MPOD is diagnosed by the complete absence of peroxidase-positive granules in the cytoplasm of PMNs and MNLs. Eosinophils stain normally for peroxidase. A more accurate quantitative MPO assay from lysed PMNs has been described (Lehrer & Cline 1969, Stendahl & Lindgren 1976, Rosen & Klebanoff 1976).

Genetics of MPOD

Of the 12 reported cases, six were female and 12 were male. Three pairs of siblings were found within this relatively small group, suggesting an hereditary basis. In at least one family with MPOD, autosomal recessive inheritance has been proposed (Lehrer & Cline 1969). Quantitative MPO assays of the patient's four sons each yielded MPO levels in their PMNs from 22–38% of the mean control value.

Chediak-Higashi syndrome

Chediak-Higashi Syndrome (CHS) is characterized by increased susceptibility to bacterial infections, oculocutaneous albinism, peripheral granulocytopaenia and giant azurophil lysosomes in PMNs (Blume & Wolff 1972). The majority of patients succumb at an early age to recurrent pyogenic infections. PMNs from the affected patients have impaired chemotaxis, poor degranulation and kill bacteria inefficiently (Boxer et al 1976). Occasionally, patients develop lymphoreticular infiltration in the liver, spleen, lymph nodes and bone marrow, which bear many similarities to malignant lymphoma. This pattern of CHS is known as the 'accelerated phase' (Kritzler et al 1964). Animal models of CHS occur in mink, cattle, mice, killer whales and cats.

The upper and lower respiratory tract and the skin are among the most frequent sites of involvement. Pneumonitis, bronchitis, otitis, pharyngitis and sinusitis are also regularly encountered in CHS (Blume & Wolff 1972). The causative agents in the CHS infections are the usual pyogenic bacteria.

Mechanism of CHS

An abnormality of microtubule assembly has been demonstrated in CHS (Boxer et al 1976). Normal PMNs demonstrate aggregation, or 'capping' of the lectin, concanavalin A (con A) following treatment with colchicine. PMNs from patients with CHS, however, cap spontaneously upon con A treatment in the absence of colchicine (Boxer et al 1976). This functional defect has been linked to abnormal levels of cyclic nucleotides in CHS PMNs, in turn leading to impaired function of cytoplasmic microtubules. Con A treatment of normal PMNs results in polymerization of cytoplasmic microtubules. This does not occur in CHS PMNs. Impaired lysosomal degranulation with consequent bactericidal deficiency may result from the generalized impairment of microtubule structural support. Nath et al (1980) have demonstrated abnormal tyrosylation of the alpha chain of tubulin in two brothers with the disorder who had decreased centriole-associated microtubules. This finding presents direct evidence that the functional defect may lie in abnormal microtubule function.

Diagnosis of CHS

This is probably the easiest of the phagocyte disorders to diagnose. A history of recurrent pyogenic infections and at least some manifestations of partial oculocutaneous albinism are usually present. Additional findings such as lymphadenopathy, hepatosplenomegaly and neurologic dysfunction may be noted if the patient is in the accelerated phase. Confirmation of the diagnosis is made by examination of an ordinary Wright's stained peripheral blood smear. Up to 100% of the PMNs contain one or more 2-4μ azurophilic, peroxidase-positive cytoplasmic granules.

Genetics of CHS

This is a well established, simple autosomal recessive disorder. In the first reported family, the parents were consanguineous and four of the 13 sibs were affected. Consanguinity has been reported in approximately half of the published cases (Blume & Wolff 1972). Breeding experiments in various animal models of CHS have also demonstrated an autosomal pattern of inheritance in the various involved species. Detection of heterozygotes has had limited success, perhaps due to the paucity of homozygotes. Heterozygotes are usually healthy and lack albinoid features. Controversy exists over published reports of subtle PMN granule abnormalities (Klebanoff & Clark 1978). Tanaka (1980) has reported a marked decrease in lysosomal enzymes of PMNs from patients with CHS.

Surprisingly, PMNs from heterozygous family members showed significantly elevated levels of different lysosomal enzymes. Tanaka suggested that CHS heterozygotes could, therefore, be detected by the altered PMN granule enzyme levels. Confirmation of this observation and explanation for the decreased levels in CHS patients and increased levels of different enzymes in the heterozygotes are necessary.

Clinical management of CHS

Treatment of CHS remains largely symptomatic, with vigorous treatment of infections with appropriate antibiotics. Although the accelerated phase has been treated with corticosteroids and chemotherapeutic agents such as vincristine, their success is questionable. Boxer et al (1976) exposed PMNs from patients with CHS to ascorbic acid, both in vitro and in vivo. Cyclic AMP levels were reduced to near normal, PMN functions were corrected and normal numbers of microtubules were restored. Improvement in clinical course of the patients, however, has not yet been conclusively demonstrated. Subsequently, other investigators have not found a uniform response to ascorbic acid in animals or humans with the disorder (Gallin et al 1979).

DISORDERS OF PHAGOCYTIC FUNCTION

No intrinsic, isolated abnormalities of PMN or MNL phagocytosis have been described. Boxer et al (1974) have described an 8-month-old infant with pyogenic infections from birth whose PMNs were deficient in chemotaxis,

bactericidal activity and phagocytosis. Cytoplasmic actin isolated from the patient's PMNs was quantitatively equal to that extracted from PMNs of a normal 8 month old. In vitro polymerization of the patient's actin was markedly decreased, however, in comparison to polymerization of the normal actin. No comment was made on the potential genetic implications.

Numerous phagocytic dysfunction syndromes resulting from deficiencies of various opsonins have been recognized. These have been extensively reviewed elsewhere (Miller 1975, Johnston & Stroud 1977, Spitzer 1977) and are also discussed in another chapter.

DISORDERS OF PHAGOCYTE MOVEMENT

Disorders of PMN and MNL movement constitute a large and important group of functional phagocyte deficiency states. As reviewed in the section of this chapter dealing with normal phagocyte movement, a number of mechanisms are involved and are, therefore, potential sites for clinically significant perturbations. To date, few of these disorders have been positively shown to be genetically determined. It should be stressed, however, that improvements in methodology of study of individual steps in PMN and MNL movement make it highly likely that some of these deficiencies will turn out to have a hereditary basis. In order to prepare the reader for these future developments, several general points should be stressed:

(a) Extensive heterogeneity exists among these disorders (Miller 1975, Klebanoff & Clark 1978). No single clinical or laboratory finding is consistently abnormal within this group of disorders. Assays such as the Boyden chamber reflect a number of individual steps in the overall movement process.

(b) Four basic types of movement defects have been recognized (Miller 1975): (1) intrinsic defects of only phagocyte movement; (2) intrinsic defects of phagocyte movement with the addition of at least one other deficiency of phagocyte function such as phagocytosis or bactericidal activity; (3) disorders of phagocyte movement secondary to deficiencies of humoral chemotactic agents, such as in primary disorders of the complement system; (4) disorders of phagocyte movement secondary to the effects of a humoral inhibitor. Inhibitors may be directed either towards the phagocyte, or towards a humoral chemotactic factor which in turn results in deficient stimulation of phagocyte movement.

(c) At least one primary disorder of phagocyte movement appears to have a hereditary basis (Miller et al 1973). Three children – a girl in one family, a brother and sister in another family – presented with a symptom complex of congenital ichthyosis and *Trichophyton rubrum* infections. Movement of PMNs from each of the patients was abnormal in filter movement, but normal in undirected, or random movement (as measured in a capillary tube assay). On examination of PMNs from the two sets of parents, each of the fathers' PMNs showed an identical pattern of abnormalities in vitro. Upon further questioning, it was found that each father had been troubled intermittently throughout life by low-grade cutaneous fungal infections. These clinical and laboratory findings supported the suggestion of a familial chemotactic defect.

Hyperimmunoglobulinaemia E and recurrent infections

Although considerable controversy exists about the many subtle immunological abnormalities described in patients with extreme elevation of IgE and recurrent infections (Job syndrome), a number of investigators have reported a defect in PMN chemotaxis (Clark et al 1973, Hill & Quie 1974, Hill et al 1974, Hill 1982, Donabedian & Gallin 1983). The defect is an intermittent one that most likely results from the release, by the patient's cells, of inflammatory mediators or monokines that affect PMN chemotaxis. Although a variety of defects have been described in these patients, including abnormalities in suppressor cell activity (Geha et al 1981), increased levels of IgE directed against staphylococci and candida (Schopfer et al 1979), absence of IgA to staphylococci (Dreskin et al 1985) and even IgG subclass deficiencies (Leung et al 1988), none of these defects adequately explain the large staphylococcal abscesses which they suffer, especially since no investigator has demonstrated any abnormality in opsonic activity to staphylococci in the serum of these patients. The intermittent PMN chemotactic defect might also have some role in the chronic candida infections that these patients suffer, since host defense against this organism is also at least partially dependent upon PMNs. Familial occurrence of the syndrome was first reported by Van Scoy et al (1975). In the affected family, a 20-year-old female and her 1-year-old daughter had marked elevation of IgE and recurrent and often severe staphyloccocal and candida infections. Elevated IgE and depressed PMN chemotactic responses were also found in the mother's brother, father and 87-year-old paternal grandfather, along with an history of recurrent infections. Jacobs & Norman (1977) also reported a familial occurrence of the disease in both parents and three of four children in a family. Moreover, each of the affected family members was positive for HLA-B12 while the unaffected child was not. The disease has also been reported in association with bone abnormalities, including osteogenesis imperfecta (Hill 1982). Clearly more work needs to be carried out to define the exact pathophysiology and mode of inheritance of this fascinating syndrome.

LEUCOCYTE ADHERENCE DEFECT (LAD)

A fascinating new inherited disorder of leucocyte function has recently been defined. The abnormality is due to the deficiency of a family of adherence glycoproteins of the CD18 complex. The CD18 glycoproteins are heterodimers found on the surface of some leucocytes that share a common beta chain. The heterodimers consist of three distinct alpha subunits connected to the beta chain. These are termed leucocyte function antigen 1 (LFA-1-alpha), Mac-1-alpha, and p150,95 alpha. Deficiency of the common beta subunit leads to a disease characterized by delayed separation of the umbilical cord, recurrent bacterial and fungal infections, and periodontal disease (Crowley et al 1980, Anderson et al 1985, Schmalstieg 1988). The most common infections include recurrent otitis, abscesses, periodontitis and spreading necrotizing skin lesions (Schmastieg 1988). The CD18 glycoproteins appear to be critical in adherence related phenomena including chemotaxis, phagocytosis, natural killer cell activity and antibody dependent cellular cytotoxicity. The genetic defect in these patients has been studied in several families and appears to be autosomal recessive. There are at least five categories of defect at the RNA level resulting in moderate to severe phenotypes (Anderson et al 1985, Schmalstieg 1988). Therapy is supportive in most cases, although successful marrow transplantation has been performed on several patients.

REFERENCES

Ackerman S K, Douglas S D 1979 Pepstatin A – a human leukocyte chemoattractant. Clinical Immunology and Immunopathology 14: 244–250

Anderson D C, Schmalstieg F C Finegold M J et al 1985 The severe and moderate phenotypes of heritable Mac-1, LFA-1 deficiency: Their quantitative definition and relation to leukocyte dysfunction and clinical features. Journal of Infectious Diseases 152: 668–689

Archer G T, Air G, Jackas M, Morell D B 1965 Studies on rat eosinophil peroxidase. Biochimica et Biophysica Acta 99: 96–101

Azimi P H, Bobenbender J G, Hintz R L, Kontras S B 1968 Chronic granulomatous disease in three female siblings. Journal of the American Medical Association 206: 2865–2870

Baehner R L, Nathan D G 1968 Quantitative nitro-blue tetrazolium test in chronic granulomatous disease. New England Journal of Medicine 278: 971–976

Becker E L 1976 Some interrelations among chemotaxis, lysosomal enzyme secretion and phagocytosis by neutrophils. In: Johansson S G O, Strandberg K, Uvnas B (eds) Molecular and Biological aspects of the acute allergic reaction. Plenum, New York, p353–370

Becker E L, Showell H J 1974 The ability of chemotactic factors to induce lysosomal enzyme release. II. The mechanism of release. Journal of Immunology 112: 2055–2062

Bellanti J A, Cantz B E, Schlegel R J 1970 Accelerated decay of glucose-6-phosphate dehydrogenase activity in chronic granulomatous disease. Pediatric Research 4: 405–411

Biggar W D, Buron S, Holmes B 1976 Chronic granulomatous disease in an adult male: a proposed X-linked defect. Journal of Pediatrics 88: 63–70

Blume R S, Wolff S M 1972 The Chediak-Higashi syndrome Studies in four patients and a review of the literature. Medicine 51: 247–280

Boxer L A, Morganroth M L 1987 Neutrophil function disorders. Disease Month 33: 681–780

Boxer L A, Hedley-Whyte E T, Stossel T P 1974 Neutrophil actin dysfunction and abnormal neutrophil behavior. New England Journal of Medicine 291: 1093–1099

Boxer L A, Watanabe A M, Rister M, Besch H R Jr, Allen J, Baehner R L 1976 Correction of leukocyte function in Chediak-Higashi syndrome by ascorbate. New England Journal of Medicine 295: 1041–1045

Boxer L A, Oliver J M, Spielberg S P, Allen J M, Schulman J D 1979 Protection of granulocytes by vitamin E in glutathione synthetase deficiency. New England Journal of Medicine 301: 901–905

Boyden S V 1962 The chemotactic effect of mixtures of antibody and antigen on polymorphonuclear leukocytes. Journal of Experimental Medicine 115: 453–466

Carruthers J A, Greaves M W 1976 Chronic granulomatous disease. British Journal of Dermatology (Supplement) 14: 72–74

Cheung A T W, Miller M E 1980 Movement of human polymorphonuclear leukocytes: a videotape analysis. Journal of the Reticuloendothelial Society 31: 193–205

Clark R A, Klebanoff S J 1978 Chronic granulomatous disease. Studies of a family with impaired neutrophil chemotactic, metabolic and bactericidal function. American Journal of Medicine 65: 941–948

Clark R A, Root R K, Kimball H R et al 1973 Defective neutrophil chemotaxis and cellular immunity in a child with recurrent infections. Annals of Internal Medicine 78: 515–519

Cohn A A 1978 The activation of mononuclear phagocytes: Fact, fancy and future. Journal of Immunology 121: 813–816

Cross A R, Higson F K, Jones O T G, Harper A M, Segal A W 1982 The enzyme reduction and kinetics of oxidation of cytochrome b_{-245} of neutrophils. Biochemical Journal 204: 479–85

Crowley C A, Curnutte J T, Rosin R E et al 1980 An inherited abnormality of neutrophil adhesion: Its genetic transmission and its association with a missing protein. New England Journal of Medicine 302: 1163–1168

Delmas Y, Goudemand J, Ferriaux J P 1975 La granulomatose familiale chronique: Traitment per greffe de moelle (une observation). Nouvelle Presse Medicale 4: 2334

Desser R K, Himmelhoch S R, Evans W H, Januska M, Mage M, Shelton E 1972 Guinea pig heterophil and eosinophil peroxidase. Archives of Biochemistry 148: 452–465

Dinauer M C, Orkin S H, Brown R, Jesaitis A J, Parkos C A 1987 The glycoprotein encoded by the X-linked chronic granulomatous disease locus is a component of the neutrophil cytochrome b complex. Nature 327: 717–720

Donabedian H, Gallin J I 1983 The hyperimmunoglobulin E recurrent-infection (Job's) syndrome: A review of the NIH experience and the literature. Medicine 63: 195–208

Dreskin S C, Goldsmith P K, Gallin J I 1985 Immunoglobulins in the hyperimmunoglobulin E and recurrent infection (Job's) syndrome. Deficiency of anti-Staphylococcus aureus immunoglobulin A. Journal of Clinical Investigation 75: 26–34

Dupree E, Smith C W, Taylor-MacDougall N L 1972 Undetected carrier state in chronic granulomatous disease. Journal of Pediatrics 81: 770–774

Erickson R P, Stites D P, Fudenberg H H, Epstein C J 1972 Altered levels of glucose-6-phosphate dehydrogenase stabilizing factors in X-linked chronic granulomatous disease. Journal of Laboratory and Clinical Medicine 80: 644–653

Ezekowitz R A B, Orkin S H, Newburger P E 1987 Recombinant interferon gamma augments phagocyte superoxide production and X-chronic granulomatous disease gene expression in X-linked variant chronic granulomatous disease. Journal of Clinical Investigation 80: 1009–1016

Ezekowitz R A B, Dinauer M C, Jaffe H S, Orkin S H, Newburger P E 1988 Partial correction of the phagocyte defect in patients with X-linked chronic granulomatous disease by subcutaneous interferon gamma. New England Journal of Medicine 319: 146–151

Gallin J I, Quie P G (eds) 1978 Leukocyte chemotaxis: Methods, physiology, and clinical implications. Raven Press, New York

Gallin J I, Gallin E K, Malech H L, Cramer E B 1978 Structural and ionic events during leukocyte chemotaxis. In: Gallin J I, Quie P G (eds) Leukocyte chemotaxis. Raven Press, New York p123–141

Gallin J I, Hin R J, Hubert R T, Fauci A S, Kaliner M A, Wolff S M 1979 Efficacy of ascorbic acid in Chediak-Higashi syndrome (CHS): Studies in humans and mice. Blood 53: 226

Geha R S, Reinherz E, Leung D, McKee K T Jr, Schlossman S, Rosen F S 1981 Deficiency of suppressor T cells in the hyperimmunoglobulin E syndrome. Journal of Clinical Investigation 68: 783–791

Giblett E R, Klebanoff S J, Pincus S H, Swanson J, Park B H, McCullough J 1971 Kell phenotypes in chronic granulomatous disease: A potential transfusion hazard. Lancet I: 1235–1236

Goetzl E J, Austen K F 1974 Stimulation of human neutrophil leukocyte aerobic glucose metabolism by purified chemotactic factors. Journal of Clinical Investigation 53: 591–599

Goetzl E J, Sun F F 1979 Generation of unique monohydroxyeicosatetraenoic acids from arachinoid acid by human neutrophils. Journal of Experimental Medicine 150: 406–411

Gordan D L, Johnson G M, Hostetter M K 1986 Ligand-receptor interactions in the phagocytosis of virulent

Streptococcus pneumoniae by polymorphonuclear leukocytes. Journal of Infectious Diseases 154: 619–626

Henson P M 1976 Membrane receptors on neutrophils. Immunology Communication 5: 757–775

Hill H R 1978 Cyclic nucleotides as modulators of leukocyte chemotaxis. In: Gallin J I, Quie P G (eds) Leukocyte chemotaxis. Raven Press, New York, p179–193

Hill H R 1982 The syndrome of hyperimmunoglobulinemia E and recurrent infections. American Journal of Diseases of Children 136: 767–771

Hill H R 1987 Biochemical, structural and functional abnormalities of polymorphonuclear leukocytes in the neonate. Pediatric Research 22: 375–382

Hill H R, Quie P G 1974 Raised serum IgE levels and defective neutrophil chemotaxis in three children with eczema and recurrent bacterial infections. Lancet 1: 183–187

Hill H R, Ochs H D, Quie P G et al 1974 Defect in neutrophil granulocyte chemotaxis in Job's syndrome of recurrent 'cold' staphylococcal abscesses. Lancet 2: 614–619

Holmes B, Quie P G, Windhorst D B, Good R A 1966 Fatal granulomatous disease of childhood: An inborn abnormality of phagocytic function. Lancet I: 1225–1228

Holmes B, Page A R, Good R A 1967 Studies of the metabolic activity of leukocytes from patients with a genetic abnormality of phagocytic function. Journal of Clinical Investigation 46: 1422–1432

Jacobs J C, Norman M E 1977 A familial defect of neutrophil chemotaxis with asthma, eczema, and recurrent skin infections. Pediatric Research 11: 732–736

Johnston R B Jr, Baehner R L 1971 Chronic granulomatous disease: Correlation between pathogenesis and clinical findings. Pediatrics 48: 730–739

Johnston R B Jr, Newman S L 1977 Chronic granulomatous disease. Pediatric Clinics of North America 24: 365–376

Johnston R B Jr, Stroud R M 1977 Complement and host defense against infection. Journal of Pediatrics 90: 169–179

Karnovsky M L, Lazdins J K 1978 Biochemical criteria for activated macrophages. Journal of Immunology 121: 809–813

Klebanoff S J, Clark R A 1978 The Neutrophil: Function and Clinical Disorders. North-Holland Publishing Company, New York

Kontras S B, Bass J C 1969 Chronic granulomatous disease. Lancet II: 646–647

Kritzler R A, Terner J Y, Lindenbaum J, Magidson J, Williams R, Preisig R, Phillips G B 1964 Chediak-Higashi syndrome. Cytologic and serum lipid observations in a case and family. American Journal of Medicine 36: 583–594

Lehrer R I, Cline M J 1969 Leukocyte myeloperoxidase deficiency and disseminated candidiasis: The role of myeloperoxidase in resistance to Candida infection. Journal of Clinical Investigation 48: 1478–1488

Le J, Vilcek J 1987 Biology of disease. Tumour necrosis factor and interleukin 1: Cytokines with multiple overlapping biological activities. Laboratory Investigation 56: 234–248

Leung D Y M, Ambrosino D M, Arbeit R D, Newton J L, Geha R S 1988 Impaired antibody responses in the hyperimmunoglobulin E syndrome. Journal of Allergy and Clinical Immunology 81: 1082–1087

Lichtman M A 1970 Cellular deformability during

maturation of the myeloblast: Possible role in marrow egress. New England Journal of Medicine 283: 493–498

Lutter R, van Zwieten R, Weening R S, Hamers M N, Roos D 1984 Cytochrome b. flavins, and ubiquinone-50 in enucleated human neutrophils (polymorphonuclear leukocyte cytoplasts). Journal of Biological Chemistry 259: 9603–9606

Mackaness G B 1962 Cellular resistance to infection. Journal of Experimental Medicine 116: 381–406

McPhail L C, DeChatelet L R, Shirley P S, Wilfert C, Johnston R B Jr, McCall C E 1977 Deficiency of NADPH oxidase activity in chronic granulomatous disease. Journal of Pediatrics 90: 213–217

Mandell G L, Hook E W 1969 Leukocyte bactericidal activity in chronic granulomatous disease: Correlation of bacterial hydrogen peroxide production and susceptibility to intracellular killing. Journal of Bacteriology 100: 531–532

Marks P A, Gross R T, Hurwitz R E 1959 Gene action in erythrocyte deficiency of glucose-6-phosphate dehydro-genase: Tissue enzyme levels. Nature 183: 1266–1267

Marsh W L 1977 The Kell blood group, K_x antigen, and chronic granulomatous disease. Mayo Clinic Proceedings 52: 150–152

Marsh W L, Uretsky S C, Douglas S D 1975 Antigens of the Kell blood group system on neutrophils and monocytes: Their relation to chronic granulomatous disease. Journal of Pediatrics 87: 1117–1120

Metchnikoff E 1893 Lectures on the comparative pathology of inflammation. Kegan, Paul & Co., London

Miller M E 1975 Pathology of chemotaxis and random mobility. Seminars in Hematology 12: 59–82

Miller M E 1979 Cell elastimetry in the study of normal and abnormal movement of human neutrophils. Clinical Immunology and Immunopathology 14: 502–510

Miller M E, Myers K A 1975 Cellular deformability of human peripheral blood polymorphonuclear leukocyte: Method of study, normal variation, and effects of physical and chemical alterations. Journal of the Reticuloendothelial Society 18: 337–345

Miller M E, Norman M E, Koblenzer P J, Schonauer T 1973 A new familial defect neutrophil movement. Journal of Laboratory and Clinical Medicine 82: 1–8

Mills E L, Quie P G 1980 Congenital disorders of the functions of polymorphonuclear neutrophils. Reviews of Infectious Diseases 2: 505–517

Mills E L, Rholl K S, Quie P G 1980 X-linked inheritance in females with chronic granulomatous disease. Journal of Clinical Investigation 66: 332–340

Mohler D N, Majerus P W, Minnich V, Hess C E, Garrick M D 1970 Glutathione synthetase deficiency as a cause of hereditary hemolytic disease. New England Journal of Medicine 283: 1253–1257

Moosmann K, Bojanovsky A 1975 Rezidivierende candidosis bei myeloperoxidase-mangel. Mschr. Kinderheilkunde 123: 408–409

Nath J, Flain M, Gallin J I 1980 Tubulin tyrosylation in normal and Chediak-Higashi syndrome neutrophils. Journal of Cell Biology 87: 1952

Newburger P E, Cohen H J, Rothchild S B, Hobbins J C, Malawista S E, Mahoney M J 1979 Prenatal diagnosis of chronic granulomatous disease. New England Journal of Medicine 300: 178–181

North R J 1978 The concept of the activated macrophage. Journal of Immunology 121: 806–809

Ochs H D, Igo R P 1973 The NBT slide test: a simple screening method for detecting chronic granulomatous disease and female carriers. Journal of Pediatrics 83: 77–82

Oliver J M, Albertini D F, Berlin R D 1976 Effects of Glutathione-oxidizing agents on microtubule assembly and microtubule-dependent surface properties of human neutrophils. Journal of Cell Biology 71: 921–932

Quie P G 1969 Chronic granulomatous disease of childhood. Advances in Pediatrics 16: 287–300

Quie P G, Kaplan E L, Page A R, Gruskay F L, Malawista S E 1968 Defective polymorphonuclear leukocyte function and chronic granulomatous disease in two female children. New England Journal of Medicine 289: 976–980

Raubitschek A A, Levin A S, Stites D P, Shaw E B, Fudenberg H H 1973 Normal granulotype infusion therapy for aspergillosis in chronic granulomatous disease. Pediatrics 51: 230–233

Repine J E, Clawson C C, White J G, Holmes B 1975 Spectrum of function of neutrophils from carriers of sex-linked chronic granulomatous disease. Journal of Pediatrics 87: 901–907

Roberts R, Gallin J I 1983 The phagocytic cell and its disorders. Annals of Allergy 51: 330–343

Rosen H, Klebanoff S J 1976 Chemiluminescence and superoxide production by myeloperoxidase-deficient leukocytes. Journal of Clinical Investigation 58: 50–60

Royer-Pokora B, Kunkel L M, Monaco A P et al 1986 Cloning the gene for an inherited disorder – chronic granulomatous disease – on the basis of its chromosomal location. Nature 322: 32–38

Schmalstieg F C 1988 Leukocyte adherence defect. Pediatric Infectious Disease 7: 867–872

Schopfer K, Baerlocher K, Price P, Krech U, Quie P G, Douglas S D 1979 Staphylococcal IgE antibodies, hyperimmunoglobulinemia E and Staphylococcus aureus infections. New England Journal of Medicine 300: 835–838

Schulman J D, Mudd S H, Schneider J A, Spielberg S P, Boxer L, Oliver J, Corash L, Sheetz M 1980 Genetic disorders of glutathione and sulfur amino-acid metabolism. Annals of Internal Medicine 93: 330–346

Segal A Q, Jones O T G, Webster D, Allison A C 1978 Absence of a newly described cytochrome b from neutrophils of patients with chronic granulomatous disease. Lancet II: 446–449

Segal A W, Cross A R, Garcia R C et al 1983 Absence of cytochrome b$_{-245}$ in chronic granulomatous disease: a multicenter European evaluation of its incidence and relevance. New England Journal of Medicine 308: 245–251

Spielberg S P, Kramer L I, Goodman S I, Butler J, Tietze F, Quinn P, Shulman J D 1977 5-Oxoprolinuria: Biochemical observations and case report. Journal of Pediatrics 91: 237–241

Spitzer R E 1977 The complement system. Pediatric Clinics of North America 24: 341–364

Stendahl O, Lindgren S 1976 Function of granulocytes with deficient myeloperoxidase-mediated iodination in a patient with generalized pustular psoriasis. Scandinavian Journal of Haematology 16: 144–153

Stossel T P 1975 Phagocytosis: Recognition and ingestion. Seminars in Hematology 12: 83–116

Stossel T P 1978 The mechanism of leukocyte locomotion. In: Gallin J I, Quie P G (eds) Leukocyte chemotaxis. Raven Press, New York, p143–160

Stossel T P, Hartwig J H 1976 Interaction of actin, myosin, and a new actin-binding protein of rabbit pulmonary macrophage. II. Role in cytoplasmic movement and phagocytosis. Journal of Cell Biology 68: 602–619

Tanaka T 1980 Chediak-Higashi syndrome: Abnormal lysosomal enzyme levels in granulocytes of patient and family members. Pediatric Research 14: 901–904

van der Meer J W M, van Zwet T L, van Furth R, Weemaes C M R 1975 New familial defect in microbicidal function of polymorphonuclear leucocytes. Lancet ii: 630–632

Van Scoy R E, Hill H R, Ritts R E, Quie P G 1975 Familial neutrophil chemotaxis defect, recurrent bacterial infections, mucocutaneous candidiasis, and hyperimmunoglobulinemia E. Annals of Internal Medicine 82: 766–771

Weening R S, Roos D, Weemaes C M R, Homan-Müller J W T, vanSchaik M L J 1976 Defective initiation of the metabolic stimulation in phagocytizing granulocytes: A new congenital defect. Journal of Laboratory and Clinical Medicine 88: 757–768

Zigmond S H 1978 Chemotaxis of polymorphonuclear leucocytes. Journal of Cell Biology 77: 269

85. The HLA system

T. Strachan   R. Harris

INTRODUCTION

The HLA story began more than three decades ago when the serum of multiply transfused patients was found to contain antibodies which, while unable to agglutinate the donor's leucocytes (or those of an identical twin), did agglutinate those of some other individuals. However the relevance of the Human Leucocyte Antigens system (HLA) to human organ transplantation (Morris et al 1987) and to disease susceptibility (Batchelor & McMichael 1987) was a major incentive for intensive research.

HLA antigens have been shown to be controlled by several closely linked genetic loci, the HLA complex or major histocompatibility complex (MHC), in man which map to the short arm of chromosome 6 at position 6p21.3. Even when confined to serological and mixed lymphocyte response (MLR) tests a very high degree of polymorphism of individual HLA loci was discerned (Table 85.1) and more recent work, including recombinant DNA methods (see below), has suggested even greater polymorphism. Molecular biological approaches have permitted extensive characterization of HLA structural genes and have also revealed several neighbouring DNA sequences with high sequence homology to HLA genes, but which appear to be defective regarding gene expression (pseudogenes). In addition to genes which encode HLA antigens, the HLA complex contains a number of other genes and the complex has been envisaged to include three major chromosomal regions (Fig. 85.1):

Class I: includes genes encoding the heavy chains of Class I HLA antigens and probably unrelated genes including the uncharacterized idiopathic haemochromatosis gene;

Class II: includes genes encoding the class II HLA antigens;

Class III: includes genes specifying complement components C2, C4 and factor B, and also steroid 21-hydroxylase.

BIOCHEMISTRY OF THE HLA COMPLEX
(Strominger 1987)

Class I HLA antigens

Class I HLA antigens are cell surface antigens which are distributed over a wide variety of tissues. They are principally involved in guiding the recognition by cytotoxic T lymphocytes of alien antigen on host cell surfaces. Such foreign antigens may arise from invasion by foreign antigen (virus infection, organ transplantation) or alteration of host antigen (e.g. tumorigenesis). Class I antigens are constituted by a non-covalent association between two chains: a polymorphic heavy chain (mol. wt. $= 44\,000$ daltons $= 44$ kDa) which is encoded at loci in the HLA complex, notably HLA-A, HLA-B and HLA-C; and an invariant light chain, β_2-microglobulin (12 kDa) which is encoded at a single locus which maps outside the MHC on chromosome 15. The heavy chain is a transmembrane glycoprotein of about 340 amino acids, including three large extracellular domains, $\alpha_1, \alpha_2, \alpha_3$ of about 90 amino acids each. Of these, α_1 and α_2 are highly polymorphic while α_3 is highly conserved and is predominantly associated with a fourth extracellular domain provided by the light chain, β_2-microglobulin.

The detailed structure of the extracellular component of a class I antigen, HLA-A2, has recently (Bjorkman et al 1987) been determined by X-ray crystallography (Fig. 85.2). The relatively conserved membrane-proximal extracellular domains, α_3 and β_2-microglobulin have tertiary structures resembling antibody domains. The polymorphic membrane-distal domains, α_1 and α_2, are nearly identical in structure (but are not similar to either constant or variable immunoglobulin domains) and together comprise a platform of eight anti-parallel β-strands which support outwardly-directed α-helices, with the α-helices forming a site for processed foreign antigens.

Table 85.1 HLA specificities defined by serological and MLR testing as recognized by the 10th International Histocompatibility Workshop, New York, 1987 (Dupont 1988)

A	B		C	D	DR	DQ	DP
A1	B5	Bw50 (21)	Cw1	Dw1	DR1	DQw1	DPw1
A2	B7	B51 (5)	Cw2	Dw2	DR2	DQw2	DPw2
A3	B8	Bw52 (5)	Cw3	Dw3	DR3	DQw3	DPw3
A9	B12	Bw53	Cw4	Dw4	DR4	DQw4	DPw4
A10	B13	Bw54 (w22)	Cw5	Dw5	DR5	DQw5 (w1)	DPw5
A11	B14	Bw55 (w22)	Cw6	Dw6	DRw6	DQw6 (w1)	DPw6
Aw19	B15	Bw56 (w22)	Cw7	Dw7	DR7	DQw7 (w3)	
A23 (9)	B16	Bw57 (17)	Cw8	Dw8	DRw8	DQw8 (w3)	
A24 (9)	B17	Bw58 (17)	Cw9 (w3)	Dw9	DR9	DQw9 (w3)	
A25 (10)	B18	Bw59	Cw10 (w3)	Dw10	DRw10		
A26 (10)	B21	Bw60 (w40)	Cw11	Cw11 (w7)	DRw11(5)		
A28 (10)	Bw22	Bw61 (w40)		Dw12	DRw12		
A29 (W19)	B27	Bw62 (15)		Dw13	DRw13 (w6)		
A30 (w19)	B35	Bw63 (15)		Dw14	DRw14 (w6)		
A31 (w19)	B37	Bw64 (14)		Dw15	DRw15 (2)		
A32 (w19)	B38 (16)	Bw65 (14)		Dw16	DRw16 (2)		
Aw33 (w19)	B39 (16)	Bw67		Dw17 (w7)	DRw17 (3)		
Aw34 (10)	B40	Bw70		Dw18 (w6)	DRw18 (3)		
Aw36	Bw41	Bw71 (w70)		Dw19 (w6)			
Aw43	Bw42	Bw72 (w70)		Dw20	DRw52		
Aw66 (10)	B44 (12)	Bw73		Dw21			
Aw68 (28)	B45 (12)	Bw75 (15)		Dw22	DRw53		
Aw69 (28)	Bw46	Bw76 (15)		Dw23			
Aw74 (w19)	Bw47	Bw77 (15)		Dw24			
	Bw48			Dw25			
	B49 (21)	Bw4		Dw26			
		Bw6					

HLA-A, -B, -C loci are defined by the microlymphocytotoxic test employing specific antisera and peripheral blood lymphocytes. HLA-DR typing is by a similar test but enriched with B-lymphocytes. HLA-D is defined by the mixed lymphocyte response and defines antigens that are closely related but not identical to the DR antigens. The letter 'w' (Workshop) denotes an antigen whose definition is still provisional. Antigens followed by bracketed numbers denote splits of parent specificities which are represented in the brackets. HLA-Bw4 and Bw6 are supertypic specificities that divide the HLA-B series into two complex cross-reacting families.

THE HLA COMPLEX (~3,500 kb)

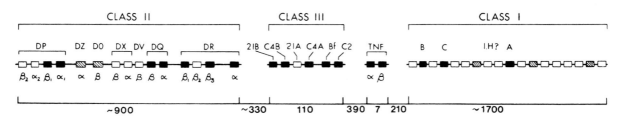

Fig. 85.1 Gene organization of the HLA complex. Numbers at bottom represent distance in kilobases between indicated markers. Genes are represented schematically as boxes: closed boxes – functional genes whose products have been well characterized; hatched boxes – genes that are capable of being expressed but whose products have not been well characterized; open boxes – genes whose expression is considered to be defective (pseudogenes). The precise order and number of the genes in the class I region is unknown and in addition to about 20 class I HLA genes is expected to include at least some other genes such as the, as yet unidentified, idiopathic haemochromatosis (I.H) gene.

Class II HLA antigens

Class II HLA antigens are cell surface antigens evolutionarily related to class I HLA antigens and, like them, are considered to be members of the immunoglobulin superfamily. Class II antigens have a limited distribution to B lymphocytes, macrophages and certain other cells. They serve to modulate immune responses by mediating interactions between different functional subclasses of T-cells and between T-cells and B-cells. They are constituted by a non-covalent association between two chains: a heavy chain, α (34 kDa); and a light chain, β (29 kDA). Both chains are transmembrane polypeptides containing about 235 amino acids with two large extracellular domains of about 90 amino acids in length. The membrane proximal extracellular domains, α_2 and β_2, show sequence homology with immunoglobulin constant region domains and are less polymorphic than the membrane-distal domains, α_1 and β_1. Both chains are independently encoded at several loci in the HLA complex, including HLA-DP, HLA-DQ, and HLA-DR. The β chains are all highly polymorphic, especially DQ_β and DR_β whereas the α chains may be polymorphic, as with DP_α and DQ_α, or may be non-polymorphic as with DR_α. Although the predominant associations between class II heavy and light chains are cis-associations between α and β chains of one locus, certain trans-associations may occur, e.g. DQ_α and DQ_β products from different haplotypes may associate.

Class III products

Class III region products include steroid 21-hydroxylase, two components of the classical complement pathway, C2 and C4, and one of the alternative pathway components, factor B. Whereas factor B and C2 are single-chain glycoproteins of 90 kDa and 102 kDa respectively, C4 is a triple chain glycoprotein consisting of alpha (95 kDa), beta (75 kDa) and gamma (30 kDa) subunits. Unlike factor B and C2, each of which is encoded at a single locus, the C4 molecule is synthesized initially as a single long chain by two loci, C4A and C4B. While the C4 protein is highly polymorphic, factor B and C2 are only moderately so.

MOLECULAR GENETICS OF HLA

The HLA complex encompasses about 3500 kilobases of DNA (approximately 1/1000 of the haploid DNA content) including more than 40 genes. Genes in the HLA complex which encode functionally similar products are clustered such that the functional subdivision largely correlates with a physical subdivision into the three regions described above (Fig. 85.1). Class III HLA genes are flanked centromerically by the class II HLA region and telomerically by the class I HLA region. Considerable portions of the HLA complex have been defined by overlapping genomic DNA clones and many of the genes have been intensely characterized at the level of DNA sequencing.

Class I HLA genes (Strachan 1987)

Although only three major allelic series of class I antigens have been defined at the serological level, HLA-A, HLA-B and HLA-C, the genes which encode the class I heavy chain belong to a multigene family of about 20 genes which are highly homologous in DNA sequence and are thought to share a close evolutionary relationship. DNA sequence analysis of the genes suggests that a considerable proportion of them may be pseudogenes, or gene fragments which lack several of the eight exons that are normally associated with functional class I HLA genes. However, in addition to the three genes which encode the heavy chain of the classical antigens, HLA-A, B and C, at least three of the non-classical class I genes are also capable of being expressed. At present the functions of the non-classical class I genes are unknown.

Class II HLA genes (Trowsdale 1987)

There are approximately 15 class II HLA genes within a span of about 900 kb of DNA, although minor differences in the organization of the class II multigene family have been recorded in different haplotypes. Of these, at least seven are functional, comprising three genes which encode classical DP_α, DQ_α and DR_α chains and four genes which encode classical class II beta chains, of which one encodes DP_β, one DQ_β and two DR_β. The expression of two functional DR_β genes lead to two types of DR antigen, one which correlates with the serologically defined specificities DR1 to DR14, and one which is associated with the DRw52 or DRw53 specificities. Of the remaining genes, some are capable of being expressed, while others are thought to be pseudogenes (Fig. 85.1).

Genes of the Class III HLA region (Campbell 1987, Carroll & Alper 1987)

Genes in the class III HLA region are contained within a stretch of about 100 kb of DNA and appear to be organized as three pairs of related genes: C2 and factor B; C4A and C4B; and the two steroid 21-hydroxylase genes, 21-OHA and 21-OHB. Of these, there is a very high degree of sequence homology between the two C4 genes and also between the two 21-hydroxylase genes. The physical distribution of these genes suggests previous duplication of an ancestral 21-hydroxylase + C4 gene unit to give the existing arrangement of 21-OHB – C4B – 21-OHA – C4A. A consequence of the tandem duplication of this pair of genes is the frequent occurrence of haplotypes containing three (21-OH + C4) units or one (21-OH + C4) unit, as a result of unequal crossing-over. As DNA sequencing and other studies strongly suggest that there is only one functional 21-hydroxylase gene, 21-OHB, while the 21-OHA gene appears to be a pseudo-gene, haplotypes with deletions of the 21-OHB gene are strongly associated with congenital adrenal hyperplasia (CAH) due to 21-hydroxylase deficiency (see below).

Other genes mapping in the HLA complex

These include the two tumour necrosis factor genes TNF_α and TNF_β which map approximately 200 kb centromeric to HLA-B and about 390 kb telomeric to C2 (Fig. 85.1). Also, the most recent recombinational data suggest a location for the idiopathic haemochromatosis gene between HLA-B and HLA-A, and most probably in the vicinity of the HLA-A locus. The relatively large regions between the HLA-DR locus and the 21-OHB locus, and between the C2 locus and HLA-B await detailed investigations, and several as yet unidentified genes are expected to be located in these regions.

FUNCTIONAL SIGNIFICANCE OF HLA ANTIGENS

The degree of genetic polymorphism of HLA antigens is considerably greater than that of any other known human genetic system. DNA sequencing studies of genomic DNA clones have verified that, in most cases, serologically defined HLA specificities represent true alleles. However, the degree of HLA polymorphism estimated by serological approaches may be a considerable underestimate, as shown by recent 'splitting' of serologically defined specificities on the basis of differential functional responses (e.g. cytotoxic T lymphocyte recognition), biochemical investigations (e.g. isoelectric focusing) and DNA studies (RFLP typing and DNA sequencing). Explanations for the existence of such a high degree of polymorphism in this region of the human genome has largely proceeded from the assumption that heterozygosity at the HLA loci is selectively advantageous. The increased repertoire of HLA antigens would be expected to provide an individual with a more flexible, and

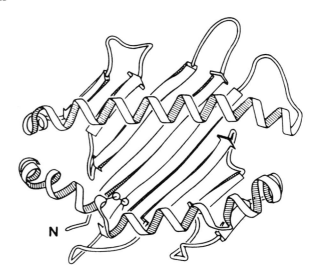

Fig. 85.2 Schematic representation of the structure of the membrane-distal region of HLA–A2. The amino terminus of α_1 is denoted by the letter N. A platform of eight anti-parallel β-strands (broad arrows) is topped by α-helices. A large groove between the α-helices provides a binding site for processed foreign antigens. Reproduced from Bjorkman et al (1987) with permission.

consequently more protective, immune response to the challenge posed by antigen variation in pathogens.

The predominant function of HLA antigens is to bind selected antigens and present them in a form that can be recognized by T lymphocytes. The recognition by T-cell receptors of foreign antigen is generally 'restricted' by the requirement for concomitant recognition of self–HLA antigen. Class I antigens act in this way with cytotoxic T lymphocytes leading to the destruction of cells expressing both HLA and foreign antigen. Class II antigens perform an analogous role in relations between different cell types, typically initiating and regulating immune recognition and subsequent responses. Recent evidence has strongly supported the concept of a single T-cell receptor which recognizes a complex HLA antigen bound to foreign antigen. The definition, by X-ray crystallography, of the structure of the HLA-A2 antigen (Fig. 85.2) suggests a single binding site on HLA antigens for foreign antigens, only large enough to accommodate peptides of about 8–20 amino acids in length. This is consistent with the observation that the epitopes recognized by class I restricted T-cells can be defined with short peptides, as is also generally the case with class II restricted T-cells.

APPLICATION OF HLA

HLA and disease associations (Tiwari & Terasaki 1985)

By 1985 there were more than 4000 references describing associations between HLA antigens and a wide variety of diseases. These showed that groups of patients may have quite different HLA antigen frequencies from the general population. These differences are conveniently described by 'Relative Risk' which compares the increased (or decreased) likelihood of disease in individuals with various HLA antigens. The statistical means used to establish and validate disease associations are described by Emery (1986).

Mechanisms of HLA-disease associations

No single mechanism can be responsible for all HLA associations (Table 85.2). The strongest association (100%) involves narcolepsy and is of unknown aetiology. In contrast, some associations are known to be the consequence of close genetic linkage between Mendelian disease genes and HLA. Thus there is a strong association between 21-hydroxylase deficiency and the normally rare HLA-Bw47 antigen, while approximately 75% of idiopathic haemochromatosis patients possess the HLA-A3 antigen as opposed to about 28% of controls. In these instances there is *linkage disequilibrium* between specific HLA antigens and the relevant diseases, e.g. the frequency of haplotypes possessing both an HLA-Bw47

Table 85.2 Examples of HLA related diseases

Disease	Marker	Relative risk	Proposed mechanism
A. Not due to autoimmunity			
21-Hydroxylase deficiency	Bw47	15	Linkage disequilibrium: autosomal recessive in class III region
Idiopathic haemochromatosis	A3	8	Linkage disequilibrium: autosomal recessive in class I region
B. Autoimmune disease			
Ankylosing spondylitis	B27	90-350	Cytotoxic T lymphocytes specific for *Klebsiella* bacterial protein, and restricted by HLA-B27 contribute to disease process
Rheumatoid arthritis	DR4/DRw4	4-6	Association with specific DQ beta RFLP has relative risk of 78
Coeliac disease	B8/DR3/DQw2	8-11	Immune response to peptide sequence shared by alpha gliadin and an adenovirus
Insulin-dependent diabetes mellitus	B8/DR3/DQw2 B15/DR4/DQw3 B7/DR2	3-6 2-3 0.5-0.25	Insulitis induced by virus infection (e.g. coxsackie or congenital rubella), progresses to insulin deficiency via MHC mediated autoimmune process. B7/DR2 'protective'. Strongest association is with DQ beta and has been localised to specific amino acid at position 57 on the DQ beta chain
Multiple sclerosis			Possibly shared peptide sequence in myelin and virus
Caucasoids	B7/DR2/DQw1	2-5	
Jordanians	DR4	13	
Cedar pollenosis	DQw3		Absence of T suppressor cells that suppress IgE response to cedar pollen, a possible example of the direct influence of HLA polymorphism on immune response
Grave disease	DR (variable)		Thyroid epithelium inappropriately expresses class II antigen after virus infection and interferon-gamma release
Systemic lupus erythematosus and	DR3 C4 Nul C4A*6		Partial deficiency of complement action, leading to tissue damage due to failure to localize, clear or limit size of immune complexes
Hydralazine induced lupus	DR3 C4 Nul C4A*6		Commonest in females The drug Hydralazine is a precipitant in slow acetylators
C. Unknown aetiology			
Narcolepsy	DR2	100% association	

Adapted, with modifications, from Batchelor & McMichael (1987). Diseases selected to illustrate some of the proposed pathogenic mechanisms. For more complete list of associations see Tiwari & Tiwari & Terasaki (1985).

allele and a 21-hydroxylase deficiency allele is considerably greater than the product of the population frequencies of the HLA-Bw47 and the 21–hydroxylase deficiency alleles.

Abnormalities of class I or II antigen-restricted immune responses and reduced or inappropriate complement activity are responsible for other associations. This category of HLA-disease associations is represented by autoimmune diseases such as juvenile insulin-dependent diabetes mellitus (IDDM) and rheumatoid arthritis (RA). About 95% of IDDM patients possess either HLA-DR3 or HLA-DR4 (or both) compared to 45–54% of the normal population. The underlying basis of HLA associations with autoimmune diseases is believed to be linkage disequilibrium of HLA genes, notably HLA-DR genes, with immune response genes for high or low immune responsiveness and responses to specific but generally unknown antigens.

In addition drugs, viruses and other environmental agents are known to precipitate disease preferentially in individuals of certain HLA phenotypes.

New polymorphisms

As indicated earlier, the combined use of serological, cellular, biochemical and molecular techniques is revealing significantly greater polymorphism of HLA. Some of the 'new' polymorphisms are proving to be very strongly associated with disease, and there is reason therefore to believe that many of the 'real' disease genes are in the process of being uncovered.

Recently, DNA studies have permitted considerable clarification of these associations. Thus, a specific HLA-DQ_β RFLP has recently been shown to be strongly associated with rheumatoid arthritis (relative risk = 78, Singal et al 1987). In insulin-dependent diabetes mellitus, DNA sequence studies of the four major expressed polymorphic class II HLA gene products ($DR_{\beta1}$, $DR_{\beta3}$, DQ_α and DQ_β) in three patients and several controls showed that the DQ_β chain amino acid sequence is directly correlated with predisposition. In this case, the DQ_β related susceptibility has been shown to be largely determined by the identity of a specific amino acid at position 57 on the DQ_β chain (Todd et al 1987).

HLA AND GENETIC COUNSELLING

Paradoxically, HLA is used in counselling for a few of the many diseases with which it is associated. The reasons for this are:
1. The relevant diseases are relatively uncommon amongst referrals for genetic counselling compared with diseases like muscular dystrophy, Huntington chorea and cystic fibrosis.

2. HLA associated diseases are generally of rather late onset, reduced penetrance and variable severity, and most can be treated.
3. HLA associated diseases rarely justify termination of pregnancy, with the exception of 21-OH deficiency.

Linkage with 21-hydroxylase deficiency (CAH)

Because genes encoding steroid 21-hydroxylase (21-OH) have been shown to map within the HLA complex, disease due to inherited deficiency in expression of 21-OH is associated with HLA specificities. The inheritance of disease-associated haplotypes may be monitored in individual families by using linkage to serologically-based HLA protein polymorphisms or to DNA RFLPs. In such indirect methods there is a requirement to type an affected child in a family in order to identify parental haplotypes and permit prenatal diagnosis, where appropriate, in subsequent pregnancies. As recombination rates are generally low in the HLA complex (e.g. 1.5% between HLA-DR and HLA-B), the error rate due to misdiagnosis through recombination between the disease allele and linked HLA markers is normally very low. However, several cases have been reported of 21-hydroxylase deficiency families where there is marked discordance in clinical features between HLA-identical sibs.

Because of close linkage to class II genes and C4, carriers (heterozygotes) and symptomless homozygotes can be detected in families with 21–OH deficiency. Prenatal diagnosis of 21-hydroxylase deficiency may become particularly important if present work confirms that treating the mother with dexamethasone prevents virilisation of female fetuses diagnosed by chorion villus sampling (CVS). The methods used for diagnosis include:
1. HLA antigens and haplotypes, now mainly limited to postnatal tests as HLA typing of CVS is not easy at the serological level and amniocentesis at 16 weeks leads to very late abortions and does not allow prospective treatment.
2. DNA RFLPs, which can be used for any tissue including chorion villus for early prenatal diagnosis. Intragenic RFLPs detected by 21-hydroxylase gene probes and closely linked RFLPs detected by C4, HLA-B and HLA-DR DNA probes allow over 90% of families to be informative, while close linkage and flanking probes largely obviate recombinational errors (Strachan et al 1987)
3. Direct detection of homozygotes with deletions of the 21-OH gene is possible, allowing precise diagnosis in about 20% of affected fetuses. Measuring gene dosage also permits the identification of heterozygotes for deletions.

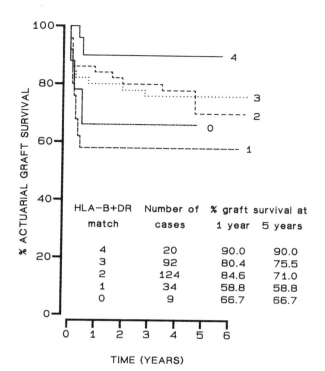

Fig. 85.3 Graft survival and HLA antigen matching between cadaver donors and first graft recipients treated with cyclosporin. Numbers at top right illustrate graft survival for the indicated number of HLA-B + HLA-DR matches between donor and recipient tissue. Trend for beneficial effect of matching, $p = 0.03$, log rank statistic (updated from Dyer et al 1985).

HLA-B+DR match	Number of cases	% graft survival at 1 year	% graft survival at 5 years
4	20	90.0	90.0
3	92	80.4	75.5
2	124	84.6	71.0
1	34	58.8	58.8
0	9	66.7	66.7

Linkage with haemochromatosis

Putative homozygotes and heterozygote carriers of haemochromatosis can be identified within families by using HLA and RFLPs markers of haplotypes shown to be carrying the haemochromatosis gene in the family under study. This may be important in geographical areas where the gene is believed to be very common, when carriers in known families frequently ask for their spouses to be screened biochemically so they can be alerted to a 25% risk of a homozygous offspring. HLA studies are complementary to iron transport investigations for homozygote detection. The greatest interest at present is the molecular search for the haemachromatosis gene using HLA probes.

Strong associations between HLA and disease

Few associations are so strong that they are of use in genetic counselling, but the absence of an antigen may be useful in helping to *exclude* disease, even when the presence of the antigen is not a reliable guide to disease. For example, effectively all patients with narcolepsy are HLA-DR2 positive and the absence of DR2 confirms that narcolepsy is not present. However, most people who do have DR2 do not suffer from this disorder. Molecular analysis of cloned HLA-DR2 genes from individuals with narcolepsy and from normal individuals do not reveal any differences that are specifically associated with narcolepsy. Similarly the absence of B27 in the son of a B27 man with ankylosing spondylitis is a strong indication that the son is unlikely to develop the disease. The probability of disease in a B27 positive son is unlikely to much exceed 10%, although this is considerably greater than the population risk of less than 1%. As with narcolepsy and HLA-DR2 direct molecular analysis of the HLA-B27 gene sequences from normal individuals and ankylosing spondylitis patients reveals no difference that can be correlated with disease. The strong association between HLA-B27 and various arthropathies such as ankylosing spondylitis may consequently reflect linkage disequilibrium between HLA-B27 and alleles of closely linked genes such as the tumour necrosis factor genes whose biological properties are consistent with a role in the destruction of cartilage.

Insulin-dependent diabetes mellitus

Juvenile onset insulin dependent diabetes mellitus (IDDM) presents a special challenge to medical geneticists. HLA identical siblings of IDDM patients are at maximum risk, at least 15% in some families, compared with less than 1% for sibs who share no HLA antigens with the proband. It is very likely that IDDM will prove to be a preventable disease, and thus be an important ecogenetic paradigm in which HLA led molecular studies will uncover the process converting genetic susceptibility to frank disease, perhaps by preventable viral action. Recent studies of class II HLA antigen sequences, referred to earlier, strongly imply that susceptibility is concentrated in specific amino-acid sequences in the HLA-DQ$_\beta$ chain. If this is fully substantiated, and is consistent, it will be possible to seek analogous viral sequences and plan possible preventive strategies. These will initially be concentrated on sibs with the appropriate class II susceptibility genes in families with one or more affected children.

TISSUE-TYPING FOR ORGAN TRANSPLANTATION (Morris et al 1987)

Two different discoveries changed kidney allotransplantation from a difficult and dangerous experimental procedure to a routine and highly successful treatment of choice for end stage renal failure. The first was the use of immunosuppressive drugs (most recently and successfully Cyclosporin A) which dampen down the recipient's immunological rejection of the kidney graft. The second was the application of tissue-typing to select, from a panel of renal patients, recipients closely HLA matched to donor kidneys and lacking damaging pre-formed antibodies (negative cross-match).

Not every transplant surgeon believes that the advantages of tissue-typing outweigh the potential delay and administrative challenge of national or international kidney exchange schemes. However our 20-year experience in Manchester confirms that sophisticated cross-matching and HLA class II antigen identity are associated with very significant improvements in kidney graft survival (Fig. 85.3).

REFFERENCES

Batchelor R J, McMichael A J 1987 Progress in understanding HLA and disease associations. British Medical Bulletin 43: 156–183

Bjorkman P J, Saper M A, Samraoui B, Bennett W S, Strominger J L, Wiley D C 1987 Structure of the human class I histocompatibility antigen, HLA-A2. Nature 329: 506–512

Campbell R D 1987 The molecular genetics and polymorphism of C2 and factor B. British Medical Bulletin 43: 37–49

Carroll M C, Alper C 1987 Polymorphism and molecular genetics of human C4. British Medical Bulletin 43: 50–65

Dupont B (ed) 1988 Immunobiology of HLA, vols 1 & 2, Proceedings of the 10th International Histocompatibility Workshop. Springer-Verlag, New York

Dyer P A, Johnson R W G, Bakran A et al 1985 HLA matching is important for cadaver renal transplant recipients treated with cyclosporin, Lancet ii: 212–213

Emery A E H 1986 Methodology in Medical Genetics, 2nd edn. Churchill Livingstone, Edinburgh

Morris P J, Fuggle S V, Ting A, Wood K J 1987 HLA and Organ Transplantation. British Medical Bulletin 43: 184–202

Singal D P, D'Souza M, Reid B, Bensen W G, Kassam Y B, Adachi J D 1987 HLA-DQ Beta-chain polymorphism in HLA-DR4 haplotypes associated with rheumatoid arthritis. Lancet ii: 1118–1120

Strachan T 1987 Molecular genetics and polymorphism of class I HLA antigens. British Medical Bulletin 43: 1–14

Strachan T, Sinnott P J, Smeaton I, Dyer P A, Harris R 1987 Prenatal diagnosis of congenital adrenal hyperplasia. Lancet ii: 1272–1273

Strominger J L 1987 Structure of class I and class II HLA antigens. British Medical Bulletin 43: 81–93

Tiwari J L, Terasaki P I 1985 HLA and Disease Associations. Springer-Verlag, New York

Todd J A, Bell J I, McDevitt H O 1987 HLA-DQ gene contributes to susceptibility and resistance to insulin-dependent diabetes mellitus. Nature 329: 599–604

Trowsdale J 1987 Genetics and polymorphism: Class II HLA antigens. British Medical Bulletin 43: 15–36

86. Genetic disorders of the pituitary gland

D. L. Rimoin

The pituitary gland is composed of two embryologically morphologically and functionally distinct units – the *anterior pituitary* (adenohypophysis) and *posterior pituitary* (neurohypophysis). Disease processes usually involve only one of the units unless the disease affects both glands because of their anatomical proximity or because of hypothalamic involvement. Thus disorders of anterior and posterior pituitary function will be discussed separately in this chapter.

DISORDERS OF THE ANTERIOR PITUITARY

The anterior pituitary is derived from an epithelial invagination of the roof of the posterior pharynx, known as Rathke's pouch (Daughaday 1985). This mass of cells migrates upwards towards the base of the brain to meet an out-pouching of the third ventricle – the future posterior pituitary. The pituitary gland comes to lie in a bony cavity of the sphenoid bone known as the sella turcica. It is separated from the brain superiorly by the diaphragma sella, an extension of the dura mater. The pituitary stalk, composed primarily of neurohypophyseal tissue surrounded by nerves and blood vessels, passes through the diaphragma sella, connecting the gland with the hypothalamus. It is this intimate vascular connection between the hypothalamus and pituitary which allows for the sensitive hypothalamic control of pituitary function. The anterior pituitary gland contains a number of distinct cell types responsible for the secretion of the seven or more pituitary hormones: growth hormone (hGH), thyrotropic hormone (TSH), adrenocorticotropic hormone (ACTH), luteinizing hormone (LH), follicle stimulating hormone (FSH), prolactin (Pr) and melanocyte stimulating hormone (MSH). The secretion of each of these pituitary hormones is under the direct control of the hypothalamus. This hypothalamic control of pituitary secretion is mediated by a variety of hypothalamic releasing hormones, which stimulate the secretion of the specific pituitary hormones (e.g. TRH stimulates TSH secretion) and hypothalamic inhibitory hormones, which inhibit the secretion of the specific pituitary hormones (e.g. somatostatin which inhibits hGH secretion). It is the interplay between the specific releasing and inhibitory hormones that directly controls the secretion of each of the pituitary hormones. In turn, the secretion of the hypothalamic inhibitory and releasing hormones by the hypothalamus is modulated by a variety of humoral and central nervous system factors. The pituitary hormones, once released into the plasma, exert their effects on a variety of specific target organs, either a specific endocrine gland (e.g. thyroid, adrenal gland) or a variety of end organs. Human growth hormone (hGH) is unique in that it affects receptors in a variety of tissues including the liver; stimulation of the hepatic receptors results in the release of the somatomedins (insulin-like growth factors: IGF I & II) a class of peptide hormones which stimulate growth and anabolism in a variety of other tissues (Underwood & van Wyk 1985). Because of the complexity of this hypothalamic-pituitary axis, a wide variety of pathogenetic mechanisms can operate at each level of the system, resulting in a widely heterogeneous group of disorders with similar symptoms of pituitary insufficiency (Fig. 86.1).

hGH consists of a single polypeptide chain of 191 amino acid residues. Two other proteins, chorionic somatomammotropin (hCS, placental lactogen) and prolactin (hPRL), are similar in structure to hGH and probably evolved through gene duplication (Miller & Eberhardt 1983). The hGH gene has been mapped to 17q22–24 (Phillips 1989). It lies in the so-called 'hGH gene cluster' which consists of five loci – two hGH, two hCS and one hCS-like genes. One hGH gene (GH1) encodes the known protein sequence, while GH2 encodes a protein differing in 13 amino acid residues. The prolactin gene lies on 6p23–q12. The IGF I and II genes have been mapped to 12q22–q24.1 and 11p15.5, respectively. The growth hormone releasing factor gene (somotocrinin) has been mapped to 20p and the somatostatin gene to 3q28.

1461

Hereditary disorders of both pituitary hypofunction and hyperfunction have been described. Similar to genetic disorders of the other endocrine glands, diseases involving the hormonal deficiency states are much more common and better delineated than hereditary forms of hyperpituitarism. Pituitary deficiency disorders may involve a single tropic hormone (monotropic deficiency) or a combination of two or more pituitary hormones (multitropic hormone deficiency) and may result from disturbances in any part of the hypothalamic-hypophyseal-target organ complex (Rimoin et al 1986). Theoretically, a syndrome of pituitary hormonal insufficiency might result from developmental degenerative or receptor lesions of the hypothalamus, deficiencies of the hypothalamic releasing hormones or their receptors, developmental or degenerative lesions of the pituitary gland, deficiencies or structural abnormalities of the pituitary hormones, or defects in target organ responsiveness to hormonal action. Each of these mechanisms has now been described in patients with pituitary insuffi-

ciency, resulting in the marked genetic heterogeneity that has been observed in pituitary dwarfism.

Hereditary forms of growth hormone deficiency

Proportionate dwarfism may result from a wide variety of endocrinological, metabolic, nutritional, emotional, and genetic disorders. Pituitary deficiency has long been recognised as a cause of proportionate short stature and it is now apparent that pituitary dwarfism represents a heterogeneous group of disorders secondary to a variety of genetic and acquired defects in human growth hormone (hGH) secretion or action (Rimoin 1976, Rimoin & Schimke 1971, Phillips 1989). Indeed, defects at all levels of the hypothalamic-pituitary-somatomedin-chondroosseous end organ axis have now been described in proportionate dwarfs (Fig. 86.1). Delineation of the distinct disorder in each pituitary dwarf has obvious implications for genetic counselling; as growth hormone releasing hormone becomes generally available for treatment an exact diagnosis will also have great therapeutic significance.

The various types of pituitary dwarfism can be classified on the basis of: (1) the level of the defect in the hypothalamic-pituitary axis; (2) whether it is a genetic or acquired disorder and, if genetic, on the mode of inheritance; (3) whether or not there is an obvious developmental or degenerative disease of the hypothalamus or pituitary; (4) whether the pituitary deficiency is monotropic (isolated growth hormone deficiency) or multitropic (panhypopituitary dwarfism); and (5) in those cases due to a defect in growth hormone action, as to whether somatomedin generation and responsiveness is normal or defective.

Although the pathogenesis of the growth hormone deficiency is unknown in most forms of pituitary dwarfism, a number of developmental anomalies of the hypo-

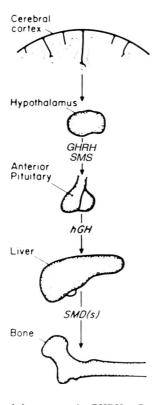

Fig. 86.1 Growth hormone axis. GHRH – Growth hormone releasing hormone; SMS – somatostatin; hGH – human growth hormone; SMD(s) – somatomedin(s). Defects at each of the steps of the axis have now been described which result in proportionate dwarfism.

Table 86.1 Developmental anomalies of the pituitary and hypothalamus

Congenital absence of the pituitary
Pituitary dwarfism with abnormal sella
Familial hypopituitarism with large sella
Anencephaly
Holoprosencephaly
Trans-sphenoidal encephalocele
Empty sella syndrome
Septo-optic dysplasia
Cleft lip and palate with pituitary insufficiency
Solitary central maxillary incisor
Pallister-Hall syndrome
CHARGE association
18p- syndrome
20p- syndrome

Table 86.2 Genetic syndromes associated with hypopituitarism

Aarskog syndrome*
Achondroplasia with obstructive sleep apnoea
Borjeson-Forssman-Lehmann syndrome
EEC (ectrodactyly-ectoderma dysplasia-clefting) syndrome*
Fanconi pancytopenia syndrome
Gonadal dysgenesis
Haemochromatosis
Haemoglobinopathies
Histiocytosis X
Neurofibromatosis
Orocraniodigital syndrome
Rieger syndrome (iris-dental dysplasia)
Sensorineural deafness
Weaver syndrome*

* Only isolated cases reported with hypopituitarism.

thalamus and pituitary (Table 86.1) and complex genetic syndromes associated with hypopituitarism (Table 86.2) have been described which result in growth hormone deficiency with or without other tropic hormone deficiencies.

Developmental anomalies

Congenital absence of the pituitary Complete absence of the anterior pituitary gland results in severe neonatal adrenal insufficiency, hypothyroidism and hypoglycaemia and, if untreated, usually results in neonatal death (Steiner & Boggs 1965, Sadeghi-Nejad & Senior 1974a). This syndrome probably goes unrecognised in the majority of cases, unless the adrenal insufficiency is diagnosed early and pituitary function is then studied, or postmortem examination includes detailed examination of the pituitary fossa. The sella turcica is usually small and no trace of anterior pituitary tissue is found at autopsy. Posterior pituitary tissue may be present or absent. There is atrophy of the adrenals with absence of the fetal zone, presumably secondary to ACTH deficiency.

Clinical features include early lethargy, cyanosis, convulsions, circulatory collapse and hypoglycaemia. Neonatal jaundice has been documented in most patients and Herman et al (1975) have pointed out that hyperbilirubinaemia may be associated with most forms of neonatal hypopituitarism (Moncrieff et al 1972). The thyroid and gonads may be hypoplastic and the penis is usually minute. Survival past the neonatal period will result in severe dwarfism, hypogonadism, and cretinism, but early total hormone replacement therapy should result in complete phenotypic reversal.

This disorder has been described in at least three sets of sibs and there is an increased prevalence of consanguinity, suggesting autosomal recessive inheritance (Steiner &

Boggs 1965, Willard 1973, Sadeghi-Nejad & Senior 1974a). The adrenal atrophy leads to a deficiency in maternal urinary oestriol excretion and thus urinary oestriol levels may provide a means of prenatal diagnosis, as might studies of fetal thyroid function.

Lovinger et al (1975) have described a syndrome of congenital hypopituitarism with severe hypoglycaemia and microphallus which resembles congenital absence of the pituitary clinically. Plasma prolactin was normal or elevated and there was a TSH rise following TRH administration, indicative of hypothalamic defect. All these cases were sporadic.

Hypoplasia or ectopia of the pituitary gland has also been described with pituitary insufficiency (Mosier 1957, Ehrlich 1957). It is impossible to state whether these latter disorders are simply less complete forms of pituitary agenesis or secondary to distinct pathogenetic mechanisms.

Familial pituitary dwarfism with abnormal sella turcica Ferrier and Stone (1969) described two sisters who had severe growth failure, hypoglycaemia, and mental retardation, and manifested evidence of relative growth hormone, thyrotropin and ACTH deficiency. These individuals differed from the usual form of hereditary panhypopituitary dwarfism in that both had a very small sella turcica located in a morphologically abnormal sphenoid bone. They postulated that the association of panhypopituitary dwarfism, mental retardation and abnormal sella turcica may represent a distinct syndrome inherited as an autosomal recessive trait. Two sisters with a similar syndrome of panhypopituitarism with a poorly developed sella turcica were later described by Sipponen et al (1978). On autopsy, no pituitary gland could be found in one child and a rudimentary, partly ectopic pituitary in the other. Thus there is some question as to whether this represents a distinct syndrome or is simply a less severe form of congenital absence of the pituitary. Stoll et al (1978) have shown that amniotic fluid prolactin levels may be useful for prenatal diagnosis.

Familial hypopituitarism with large sella turcica Parks et al (1978) have described three sibs from a nonconsanguineous mating who had short stature, growth hormone deficiency and thyrotropin deficiency. Skull X-rays demonstrated abnormally large sella turcicas (3.7–5.9 standard deviations above age specific means). Computed tomography and pneumoencephalography showed full sellae without suprasellar extension and a normal ventricular system ruling out the 'empty sella syndrome'. ACTH reserve and prolactin appeared normal. The $18\frac{1}{2}$-year-old sister had lack of pubertal development and the 10-year-old brother had extremely small testes, suggesting gonadotropin deficiency. Although their gonadotropin levels were normal for skeletal age, the latter was markedly retarded and true gonadotropin deficiency is likely. The authors postulate that this syndrome is secondary to a pituitary tumour or a regulatory defect, but elucidation of the pathogenesis will probably require direct visualization of pituitary tissue. This probably represents a distinct syndrome inherited as an autosomal recessive trait. It must be differentiated from the empty sella syndrome, which has been described in sibs, associated with short stature, unusual facies, spinal anomalies and delayed sexual maturation (Merle et al 1979).

Anencephaly Anencephaly is associated with the complete absence of a normal hypothalamus, absence or severe hypoplasia of the posterior pituitary and variable degree of anterior pituitary hypoplasia (Angevine 1938, Naeye & Blanc 1971). These infants have hypoplastic adrenals and often die from adrenal insufficiency. Plasma hGH levels have been found to vary from low normal to deficient in anencephalics (Grunt & Reynolds 1970, Hayek et al 1973). Basal thyrotropin levels were low, and plasma prolactin levels normal. Hayek et al (1973) found that the intravenous insulin tolerance test failed to evoke elevations in plasma growth hormone in anencephalics. Administration of lysine-vasopressin caused an active growth hormone release, however, and there was a large increase in serum thyrotropin releasing hormone. Thus, the anterior pituitary appears to be capable of releasing growth hormone and thyrotropin when directly stimulated, but anterior pituitary function mediated by hypothalamic releasing hormones appears to be totally deficient. The normal prolactin values presumably reflect the absence of the hypothalamic prolactin inhibitory hormone, the major factor controlling prolactin secretion from the pituitary. These endocrinological data are supported by the morphological observation of thyrotropin, gonadotropin, and somatotropin secreting cells in the pituitary of these infants.

Holoprosencephaly The holoprosencephalies form a spectrum of developmental anomalies associated with impaired midline cleavage of the embryonic forebrain, aplasia of the olfactory bulbs and tracts, and midline dysplasia of the face, ranging from cyclopia to cleft lip and palate with hypotelorism. Anomalies of the pituitary gland have been described in all forms of holoprosencephaly, ranging from malformation of the gland to its complete absence (Edmonds 1950, Haworth et al 1961, Gorlin et al 1968). In individuals with absence of the pituitary, the adrenals are also hypoplastic and there may or may not be thyroid hypoplasia as well. Hypoplastic or aplastic pancreas, testes and ovaries have also been described (Cohen et al 1971). ACTH deficiency and vasopressin-sensitive diabetes insipidus have been documented (Hintz et al 1968). All degrees of insufficiency may occur in the holoprosencephalies and the degree of pituitary dysfunction appears to be unrelated to the severity of the facial deformity. The pituitary insufficiency is presumably secondary to a developmental anomaly of the hypothalamus. Romshe and Sotos (1973) have described growth hormone deficiency in a sib of two sisters with classic holoprosencephaly. This dwarfed brother had normal facies other than for mild hypotelorism. The holoprosencephalies are a genetically heterogeneous group of disorders associated with trisomy 13, deletion of the short arm of chromsome 18, simple autosomal dominant and recessive inheritance and a variety of unusual chromosomal anomalies (Rimoin & Schimke 1971, Benke & Cohen 1983).

Thus holoprosencephaly can be caused by a wide variety of aetiological factors and is an integral part of a number of different syndromes, all of which may be associated with pituitary insufficiency. Many of the specific developmental anomalies included in this section are associated with holoprosencephaly (Table 86.1)

Trans-sphenoidal encephalocele A number of cases of trans-sphenoidal encephalocele associated with variable degrees of hypothalamic-pituitary dysfunction have been reported (Lieblich et al 1978, Ellyin et al 1980). In trans-sphenoidal encephalocele, a defect exists in the sphenoid bone, and the encephalocele usually extends into the epipharynx. Associated features include an epipharyngeal or nasopharyngeal mass, hypertelorism midfacial or midline craniocerebral anomalies and optic nerve abnormalities. The facies is characterized by a broad nasal root, increased interpupillary distance and a wide bitemporal diameter. A wide variety of pituitary hormonal deficiencies have been reported in these patients, indicating hGH, TSH, ACTH, LH, FSH, prolactin and ADH deficiencies. In individual patients, pituitary function has ranged from normal, to a single hormonal deficiency, to multitropic hormone deficiencies (Yagnik et al 1973, Lieblich et al 1978, Ellyin et al 1980). In one proband autopsied, degeneration of the hypothalamus and agenesis of the supraoptic nuclei were found (Pollock et al 1968). Duplication of the pituitary and agenesis of the corpus callosum have also been described (Bale & Reye 1976). Double pituitary glands have been described with a variety of craniofacial malformations (Bagherian et al 1984). Diagnosis of this syndrome is important, as iatrogenic hypopituitarism had been described following extirpation of a nasopharyngeal mass containing anterior and posterior pituitary tissue, whose sphenoidal defect was not recognized preoperatively (Weber et al 1977). Although the majority of cases of trans-sphenoidal encephalocele are sporadic, two sibs with trans-sphenoidal pituitary herniation, midfacial anomalies and multitropic hormonal deficiencies, who were the offspring of a consanguineous mating, have been described, suggestive of autosomal recessive inheritance (Ellyin et al 1980).

Empty sella syndrome Primary empty sella usually occurs in obese, middle-aged women who have normal pituitary function. It is due to defect in the diaphragma sella with extension of the subarachnoid space into the sella turcica, resulting in a diffusely enlarged sella. When it occurs in children, it can be familial and associated with other anomalies, as well as short stature and pituitary deficiency (Lehman et al 1977, Merle et al 1979).

Septo-optic dysplasia The association of hypoplasia of the optic discs with absence of the septum pellucidum was described by de Morsier in 1956. In 1970, Hoyt et al described nine dwarfed children with this developmental anomaly in whom they documented growth hormone deficiency, with or without other tropic hormone deficiencies. Septo-optic dysplasia is a rare malformation of anterior midline structures of the brain, including agenesis of the septum pellucidum, primitive optic ventricle and hypoplasia of the chiasma, optic nerves and infundibulum. Severely affected neonates may present with hypotonia, seizures, microphallus, hypoglycaemia and prolonged jaundice, progressing to a young infant with defective vision, behavioural delay, hypotonia and seizures (Harris & Haas 1972, Patel et al 1975, Morishima & Aranoff 1986). In mildly affected cases, the children may simply present with proportionate short stature and pendular nystagmus, with or without amblyopia. Ophthalmological examination reveals bilateral hypoplasia of the optic nerves, with small optic discs and irregular field defects. Brain imaging can reveal absence of the septum pellucidum, but it has been shown that agenesis of the septum pellucidum is inconstant and not essential for diagnosis (Patel et al 1975, Manelfe & Rochicciolo 1979, Margalith et al 1985, Morishima & Aranoff 1986).

Indeed, any or all of the three major defects (brain, optic tract, pituitary) may be present (Acers 1981). Morishima and Aranoff (1986) concluded that only 30% of fully evaluated patients had evidence of all three components. Intelligence may be normal or mild to moderately subnormal. The sella turcica and suprasellar cisterns have been normal. The pituitary insufficiency, which may vary from isolated growth hormone deficiency to panhypopituitarism is probably secondary to a diencephalic malformation resulting in deficiency of one or more of the hypothalamic releasing hormones (Toublanc et al 1976, Benoit-Gonin et al 1978). Sexual precocity has been described as has other tropic hormone hypersecretion including hGH, ACTH and prolactin (Huseman et al 1978, Stewart et al 1983, Margalith et al 1985). Autopsy has shown absence of the posterior pituitary and diffuse lesions of the hypothalamus, optic nerves, corpus callosum and olfactory tract as well as defects in the cerebral cortex (Patel et al 1975, Morishima & Aranoff 1986). A variety of other anomalies, including hand and facial defects, have occasionally been described (Pagon & Stephan 1984). This syndrome should be considered in any child with pituitary dwarfism who has nystagmus or abnormalities of the optic disc. All but one of the cases described to date with septo-optic dysplasia and growth retardation have been sporadic, with no evidence of ocular anomalies or dwarfism in their parents or sibs. The exception was a girl with septo-optic dysplasia, whose maternal first cousin had hypopituitarism without obvious optic defects; brain imaging was not done in this cousin.

Simple cleft lip and palate associated with pituitary insufficiency Functional pituitary insufficiency has been described in a number of individuals with cleft lip and palate who did not have other facial or neurological abnormalities (Frances et al 1966, Laron et al 1969, Roitmen & Laron 1978, Rudman et al 1978). Pituitary insufficiency may vary from complete panhypopituitarism associated with congenital aplasia of the pituitary to isolated growth hormone deficiency. Rudman et al (1978) studied 200 children with isolated clefts and found 4% with hGH deficiency: 40 times higher than the frequency in children without clefts. Short children with cleft lip and palate and growth retardation should thus be subjected to a complete pituitary evaluation. One can speculate that this disorder is simply the mild end of the spectrum of the holoprosencephaly-septo-optic dysplasia range of hypothalamic anomalies associated with pituitary insufficiency. Thus any individual with cleft lip and palate and hypopituitarism deserves brain imaging.

Solitary maxillary central incisor Rappaport et al (1977) described seven patients with a single maxillary central incisor in both deciduous and permanent dentition and short stature. Five of the patients had documented hGH deficiency and the two who were treated had good growth response to growth hormone therapy. No other pituitary hormone deficiencies were found. All had normal skull radiographs except for one patient with a 'small J-shaped sella'. Their patients had normal facies or only mild midline facial anomalies and there was no evidence of hypothalamic or optic defects.

A number of other cases of single central maxillary incisor, with and without short stature have since been reported (Wesley et al 1978, Vanelli et al 1980). Boudailliez et al (1983) reported a child with hypopituitarism, mental retardation, dysmorphia and solitary central maxillary incisor who had a deletion of 18p. This observation suggests that the cause of the pituitary insufficiency in other cases of 18p- and pituitary dwarfism may be secondary to midline brain and hypothalamic defects.

A number of families have been reported in which

single central maxillary incisor has occurred among the relatives of patients with holoprosencephaly (Lowry 1974, Berry et al 1984, Hattori et al 1987, Fryns & van den Berghe 1988). Affected individuals within these families have had a wide range of defects from full blown holoprosencephaly and midline facial clefts, to midline cleft lip, to isolated single maxillary central incisor. Thus the dental anomaly may be the mildest manifestation of autosomal dominant holoprosencephaly.

Single central maxillary incisor has also been described in association with precocious puberty and a hypothalamic hamartoma (Winter et al 1982) and in a dominant ectodermal dysplasia syndrome consisting of mild short stature, sparse scalp hair, skin pigmentation $+/-$ hypoplastic thumbs (Winter et al 1988). Thus this dental defect should alert one to the possibility of midline CNS defects and pituitary deficiency.

Pallister-Hall syndrome (Congenital hypothalamic hamartoblastoma, hypopituitarism, imperforate anus, postaxial polydactyly syndrome) Hall et al (1980) have described a neonatally lethal malformation syndrome consisting of hypothalamic hamartoblastoma, hypopituitarism, postaxial polydactyly and imperforate anus. Variable features include laryngeal cleft, abnormal lung lobulation, renal agenesis and/or renal dysplasia, short 4th metacarpals, nail dysplasia, multiple buccal frenula, hypoadrenalism, microphallus, congenital heart defect and intrauterine growth retardation. The hypothalamic tumour was apparent on the inferior surface of the cerebrum and extended from the optic chiasma to the interpeduncular fossa (Claren et al 1980). The tumour replaced the hypothalamus and other nuclei which originate in the embryonic hypothalamic plate. It was principally composed of cells resembling primitive undifferentiated germinal cells. The olfactory bulbs and tracts were short and thick, suggesting a relationship to the holoprosencephaly syndromes. An anterior pituitary gland was absent in all cases. The posterior pituitary was absent in the majority. The adrenal hypoplasia, small thyroid and microphallus are presumably secondary to pituitary insufficiency.

Most infants die in infancy, probably as a result of the secondary adrenal insufficiency. Graham et al (1986) reported the survival of one child past infancy who was promptly treated for pituitary insufficiency in infancy and then had a hypothalamic tumour surgically resected at one year of age. Thus, medical and surgical treatment of this syndrome is possible. Prenatal diagnosis of this syndrome may also be accomplished by measurement of decreased levels of maternal oestriol, prenatal ultrasonography for the fetal adrenal, renal or brain abnormalities and measurement of amniotic fluid disaccharides, which would be decreased with an imperforate anus.

All of the patients reported to date have been sporadic, except for one case, in which a maternal aunt with polydactyly, microglossia and flat nasal bridge died at age 17 (Graham et al 1986).

CHARGE association CHARGE is an acronym that was coined to describe a non-random association of anomalies by Pagon et al (1981): C – coloboma of the eye; H – heart disease; A – atresia of the choanae; R – retarded growth, development and/or CNS anomalies; G – genital hypoplasia; and E – ear anomalies or deafness. Other prominent features include facial palsy, micrognathia, cleft palate, swallowing difficulties, tracheo-oesophageal fistula and a 'wedge-shaped' audiogram (Davenport et al 1986).

Growth retardation, which is usually of postnatal onset, and hypogonadism are prominent features of this syndrome which may well be due to hypothalamic defects. August et al (1983) documented growth hormone and gonadotropin deficiencies in a girl with the association, who also had a delayed peak TSH response to TRF. Davenport et al (1986) found hGH borderline responses to arginine and insulin in one patient and prepubertal levels of FSH in three young women with no signs of pubertal development. Boys may have cryptorchidism, microphallus and/or hypospadias. Adult males were also reported to have genital hypoplasia and no secondary sexual characteristics. Arrhinencephaly and holoprosencephaly have been reported, suggesting a hypothalamic cause for the pituitary deficiencies. Zuppinger et al (1971) described an unusual patient with coloboma of the right choroid and optic nerve, cleft lip, hGH deficiency, diabetes insipidus and secondary type hypothyroidism. None of the other features of the CHARGE association were present.

The aetiology of the CHARGE association is unknown and may well be heterogeneous. Although most cases are sporadic, a few familial occurrences suggestive of both dominant and recessive inheritance have been reported (Pagon et al 1981, Davenport et al 1986, Metlay et al 1987).

Chromosomal syndromes Growth hormone deficiency has been described with 18p- and 20p- chromosomal deletions (Leisti et al 1973, Korenberg J, personal communication). In addition, molecular detection of deletions of 17q (i.e. the hGH gene cluster region) has been documented in isolated hGH deficiency type IA (see below). Since the gene for growth hormone releasing hormone (GHRH) has been mapped to 20p, the hGH deficiency in 20p- could result from either the deletion of the GHRH gene or a developmental anomaly of the hypothalamus (Mitrakou et al 1985, Riddell et al 1985). The deletion in one such 20p- patient, however, did not include the GHRH locus (Shohat et al 1990). A patient with 18p- has been reported with hypopituitarism and solitary central maxillary incisor, suggesting that the pituitary insufficiency in 18p- may be due to a structural malformation of the hypothalamus (Boudailliez et al 1983).

Complex genetic syndromes

Achondroplasia with obstructive sleep apnoea Achondroplasia is a common skeletal dysplasia in which the dwarfism is due to an abnormality in endochondral ossification. Up to 10% of patients with achondroplasia have been reported to have serious respiratory complications secondary to such factors as abnormal thorax, upper airway obstruction, neurological factors, such as brain stem compression at the level of the foramen magnum and hydrocephalus, as well as coincidental chronic respiratory disease (Stokes et al 1983). Obstructive sleep apnoea has been reported in a number of these cases, in whom symptoms have been markedly improved by tracheostomy (Larsen et al 1983, Goldstein et al 1987). Goldstein et al (1987) studied a 9-year-old boy with achondroplasia and obstructive sleep apnoea who had low growth hormone secretion during sleep. Following tracheostomy his hGH secretion during sleep normalized and his growth rate almost doubled. Thus short patients with craniofacial syndromes which can lead to obstructive sleep apnoea may have diminished sleep entrained growth hormone secretion as a contributing cause to their growth retardation.

Borjeson-Forssman-Lehmann syndrome This X-linked syndrome is characterized by short stature, hypogonadism, hypotonia, severe mental deficiency, coarse facial appearance with a prominent brow ridge and large ears in affected males (Borjeson et al 1962, Robinson et al 1983, Ardinger et al 1984). Carrier females show a wide range of expression. A variety of other ocular and skeletal anomalies may also occur. Although Weber et al (1978) reported normal stimulated hGH secretion in one patient, Robinson et al (1983) documented markedly deficient hGH responses to arginine and L-Dopa, as well as low somatomedin C levels in a severely affected male and two of his mildly affected twin sisters. The growth deceleration in this syndrome, however, may not begin until age 8–10 years, and therefore the pituitary deficiency may be progressive. Indeed, the associated hypogonadism has been reported to be both primary and secondary, and may also evolve with age. Thus further endocrine studies over a wide age range are indicated in this disorder.

Fanconi anaemia The Fanconi syndrome is an autosomal recessive disorder characterized by chronic pancytopenia with bone marrow hypoplasia, abnormal pigmentation, upper limb malformations, kidney anomalies, growth retardation, small genitalia and increased frequency of chromosomal breaks in cultured lymphocytes. Nilsson (1960) found that 38 of 68 published cases of Fanconi anaemia had stunted growth and 24 had genital anomalies. In 1965, Cussen reported a child with Fanconi anaemia who appeared to be a pituitary dwarf and pointed out that small pituitary glands, adrenocortical atrophy and atrophic testis have been described in this syndrome. A number of investigators have now documented hGH deficiency in patients with Fanconi anaemia, in most of whom other endocrine function was normal (Pochedly et al 1971, Zachman et al 1972, Costin et al 1972, Clarke & Weldon 1975). Administration of hGH resulted in excellent short-term and long-term responses in most of these patients, but Gleadhill et al (1975) were unable to find evidence of growth acceleration in response to long-term hGH treatment in their patients. In view of the intrauterine growth retardation commonly associated with this syndrome, it appears that both cellular factors and growth hormone deficiency probably contribute to the short stature.

Gonadal dysgenesis Although growth hormone secretion has been reported to be normal, or paradoxically increased, following glucose in most patients with gonadal dysgenesis, pituitary insufficiency has now been reported in several patients. Faggiano et al (1975) described two women with XO/XX mosaicism who showed absent hGH response to arginine and insulin induced hypoglycaemia, low levels of gonadotropins and limited ACTH reserve. In addition, Kauli et al (1979) described a girl with XY gonadal dysgenesis who was deficient in both growth hormone and gonadotropin secretion. Although the most likely explanation for these cases is chance association, a hypothalamic disturbance in gonadal dysgenesis has been postulated.

Ross et al (1985) studied growth hormone secretion in 30 patients with Turner syndrome and found no differences in mean hGH concentration or peak amplitudes throughout the day and night between patients less than 8 years of age and controls. Patients over 9 years of age had lower mean hGH levels and peak amplitudes. Reduced plasma somatomedin C levels and delayed bone age were found in patients of all ages. Laczui et al (1979) found diminished hGH reserve in adolescent and adult Turner patients with increased oestrogen therapy. These abnormalities in growth hormone secretion in Turner syndrome are probably secondary to the absence of sex hormones during adolescence.

Haemochromatosis Male hypogonadism and pituitary haemosiderosis have long been considered integral features of idiopathic haemochromatosis (Walsh et al 1976, Bezwoda et al 1977, Charbonnel et al 1981, McNeil et al

1983). Abnormalities of gonadotropin, cortisol, hGH, prolactin and TSH secretion have all been reported. Stocks and Martin (1968) demonstrated that functional pituitary insufficiency of varying degree occurs in 60% of patients with haemochromatosis. Signs and symptoms of gonadal dysfunction included depressed sexual function, testicular atrophy, absent urinary gonadotropins, decreased plasma levels of LH, and low plasma testosterone levels, indicating that the hypogonadism in haemochromatosis is secondary to a deficiency of pituitary gonadotropin. In seven of their 15 patients there was no plasma hGH response to hypoglycaemia, six had an absent or decreased plasma cortisol response to hypoglycaemia, and two were hypothyroid. The degree of pituitary insufficiency was not related to the severity of the liver disease or to the degree of abnormality in either iron or oestrogen metabolism.

This pituitary deficiency state appears to be secondary to iron deposition in the anterior pituitary (Althausen & Kerr 1933, MacDonald & Mallory 1960, Peillon & Racadot 1969). The testes of hypogonadal haemochromatotics usually show evidence of secondary atrophy without iron deposition, documenting the hypogonadotropic nature of the hypogonadism in this disease (MacDonald & Mallory 1960, Stocks & Martin 1968). Most studies have reported testicular atrophy with low levels of gonadotropins, and unresponsive to gonadotropin releasing hormone. However, in a 78-year-old man with haemosiderosis, secondary to sideroblastic anaemia and multiple transfusions, Williams and Frohman (1985) documented hypothyroidism and hypogonadism that was hypothalamic in origin. Haemochromatosis is an autosomal recessive trait tightly linked to the HLA loci.

Haemoglobinopathies There have been well-documented cases of acquired pituitary insufficiency occurring in adults with haemoglobinopathies, presumably secondary to infarction of the gland. In one instance, a 41-year-old American Black with sickle-cell trait (haemoglobin SA) developed fatigue, weight loss, decreased libido, impotence, polyuria and polydypsia a few months after a prolonged high altitude flight (Pastore et al 1969). Endocrinological evaluation revealed evidence of both anterior and posterior pituitary insufficiency. Suprasellar calcification was present radiographically, but an exploratory craniotomy was unrevealing. Another case was a 32-year-old Nigerian female with haemoglobin SC disease who developed both aseptic necrosis of the femoral neck and hypopituitarism (amenorrhoea, hypothyroidism, adrenal insufficiency, and insulin hypersensitivity) following delivery of a stillborn infant (Adadevoch 1968). This case was interpreted as an instance of the Sheehan syndrome (postpartum pituitary necrosis) caused by pitui-

tary infarction associated with an SC haemoglobin crisis. The author postulated that the relatively frequent occurrence of the Sheehan syndrome in Nigeria may be caused by the high prevalence of haemoglobinopathies in this population. Among 130 autopsied cases of sickle trait (SA), McCormick (1961) found two instances of pituitary infarction. Eunuchoid habitus and male hypogonadism have long been known to be associated with sickle-cell anaemia; pituitary insufficiency had been suggested as the cause of these symptoms. Further endocrine evaluation of such cases will be required to establish this association, but it is apparent that anterior and posterior pituitary insufficiency may result from pituitary infarction, secondary to erythrocyte sickling in haemoglobinopathies such as sickle-cell trait.

Short stature and delayed adolescence are common problems in the haemoglobinopathies. Phebus et al (1984) studied a large series of patients with sickle-cell disease and found a drop off in their mean heights by two years of age. The height deficit increased with age, especially in adolescence, associated with their delayed puberty. Borgna-Pignatti et al (1985) studied 250 adolescents with transfusion-dependent beta thalassaemia and found the majority to have growth retardation and delayed or absent puberty. These symptoms may well be due to a haemosiderotic deposition of iron in the pituitary and decreased IGF I synthesis in the affected liver.

Histiocytosis X (Letterer-Siwe disease, Hand-Schuller-Christian disease, eosinophilic granuloma) Histiocytosis X is characterized by foamy histiocyte infiltration in many areas of the body, including the hypothalamus. When the histiocytic infiltration involves the hypothalamus, prepubertal growth retardation associated with growth hormone deficiency and diabetes insipidus frequently occur (Braunstein & Kohler 1972, Latorre et al 1974). Delayed puberty and hypogonadism are also frequent accompaniments of this syndrome. Autopsy reports in adults with histiocytosis X suggest that the pituitary insufficiency is secondary to hypothalamic destruction. Diabetes insipidus and growth hormone deficiency frequently occur together, but either endocrine abnormality may exist alone. In contrast to a previous suggestion of hGH unresponsiveness, Braunstein et al (1975) documented a significant increment in growth rate in response to growth hormone therapy in these individuals.

Neurofibromatosis A variety of endocrine disturbances have been reported in patients with neurofibromatosis (Saxena 1970). The most common associated endocrine disorder in children is sexual precocity, while phaeochromocytoma is the most common in adults. Marked growth retardation, unrelated to skeletal anomalies, has also been reported. Andler et al (1979) have documented a variety of pituitary dysfunctions in affected children, including hGH deficiency, both diminished and elevated TSH response to TRH, and hyperprolactinaemia. All of their patients with neurofibromatosis and pituitary dysfunction had a suprasellar tumour.

Orocraniodigital syndrome (Juberg-Hayward syndrome) Juberg and Hayward (1969) described a large sibship in which five of six sibs had oral (cleft lip and palate), cranial (microcephaly) and various digital (thumbs and toes) abnormalities. Kingston et al (1982) described a single case with short stature and growth hormone deficiency and a normal sella turcica. Nevin et al (1981) reported an affected female who had short stature and absence of the pituitary fossa with flat anterior and posterior clinoid processes. Although Nevin et al (1981) stated that there was no evidence of endocrine dysfunction, hGH secretion was apparently not assessed.

Rieger syndrome (iris-dental dysplasia) The Rieger syndrome is an autosomal dominant disorder associated with malformation of the iris, with pupillary anomalies and hypoplasia of the teeth, with or without maxillary hypoplasia (Feingold et al 1969). Sadeghi-Nejad and Senior (1974b) reported a large family in which three and possibly five individuals had both Rieger syndrome and isolated growth hormone deficiency. Sibs of the proband had Rieger syndrome with normal pituitary function, but a deficiency of growth hormone was not present in any member of the family who did not have Rieger syndrome. Affected individuals had insulin hypersensitivity, but normal plasma insulin responses to arginine and glucose. One subject who was treated with growth hormone exhibited substantial enhancement of his rate of growth. It is postulated that the basic pathogenetic mechanism in this autosomal dominant disorder is maldevelopment of the neural crest, resulting in ocular, dental and hypothalamic abnormalities.

Primary empty sella with normal pituitary function has also been reported in association with dominantly inherited Rieger syndrome in multiple members of a large kindred (Kleinmann et al 1981). Gorlin et al (1975) have described an apparently distinct syndrome in two brothers, consisting of Rieger anomaly, growth retardation, normal pituitary function, joint hypermobility, inguinal hernia, delayed dentition, and megalocornea. Definition of this syndrome must await the recognition of other similarly affected patients.

The Rieger eye malformation sequence is a structural defect of the anterior chamber of the eye with iris hypoplasia and adhesion (Jones 1988).

Pituitary dwarfism associated with sensorineural deafness Winkelmann et al (1972) described two sisters, offspring of a nonconsanguineous mating, who had pituitary dwarfism, primary amenorrhoea and sensori-neural deafness. Deficiency of human growth hormone and gonadotropins was documented, and thyroid and adrenal function were normal. It was postulated that the combination of sensorineural deafness with pituitary insufficiency could represent a simple autosomal recessive trait. Further families with this combination of abnormalities will have to be described before it can be accepted as a distinct syndrome.

Syndromes in which pituitary deficiency has been occasionally reported

Aarskog syndrome The Aarskog syndrome is characterized by mild to moderate short stature, hypertelorism and peculiar facies, digital anomalies and a shawl scrotum. Isolated growth hormone deficiency has been described in one case of this syndrome, but has not been generally well documented (Kodama et al 1981). Further endocrine studies should be pursued in this X-linked syndrome.

EEC syndrome One patient with the EEC syndrome (ectrodactyly-ectodermal dysplasia-clefting) associated with growth hormone deficiency has been described by Knudtzon and Aarskog (1987). Significant short stature is not a common feature of this syndrome and thus this observation may be coincidental.

Polydactyly Culler and Jones (1984) described an association between postaxial polydactyly and hypopituitarism in four patients. However, one of them had the Pallister-Hall syndrome and one had the single central maxillary incisor syndrome. It is quite possible that the hypopituitarism in the other two cases was unrelated to their familial polydactyly.

Weaver syndrome A mother and son were described as having the Weaver syndrome (accelerated growth and osseous maturation, dysmorphic features, camptodactyly, developmental retardation and widened distal femora) (Stoll et al 1985). The boy did not respond with a rise in plasma hGH to any stimuli; however somatomedin C and all other pituitary hormones were normal. His mother had postpartum amenorrhoea and galactorrhoea with hyperprolactinaemia and did not have a rise in plasma hGH following stimulation. All other patients described with the Weaver syndrome, however, have had normal pituitary function when studied.

Genetic nonsyndromic forms of pituitary dwarfism

Hereditary forms of pituitary insufficiency unassociated with apparent anatomical defects of the CNS, hypothalamus or pituitary represent a genetically heterogeneous group of disorders that can result from interruptions at any point in the hypothalamic pituitary-somatomedin-peripheral tissue axis. The various types of pituitary dwarfism can be classified on the basis of the level of the defect; on its mode of inheritance; whether the pituitary deficiency is monotropic (isolated hGH deficiency) or multitropic (panhypopituitarism); whether the hormone is totally absent, deficient or abnormal; and, in those patients with a defect in growth hormone action, whether somatomedin generation is normal or defective and whether hGH or IGF receptors are normal or defective (Table 86.3).

Familial panhypopituitary dwarfism (multitropic hormone deficiency) Panhypopituitary dwarfism is associated with hGH deficiency and a deficiency of one or more of the other pituitary tropic hormones. Although the great majority of cases of panhypopituitary dwarfism are sporadic, at least two distinct genetic types of the disease have been described (Rimoin 1976). Numerous kindreds with multiple affected family members have been described, the majority of which have occurred in inbred communities. The occurrence of affected sibs of both sexes, the high frequency of consanguinity and a segregation ratio of close to 25% in familial cases indicate that one form of panhypopituitary dwarfism is inherited as an autosomal recessive trait (Rimoin et al 1968) (Fig. 86.2). Schimke et al (1971), Phelan et al (1971) and Zipf et al (1977) have reported pedigrees in which panhypopituitary dwarfism appears to be inherited as an X-linked recessive trait, and review of the older reported pedigrees reveals several families with only male sibs affected, compatible with either autosomal or X-linked recessive inheritance. Thus, there appear to be at least two distinct forms of hereditary

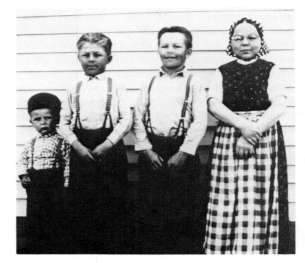

Fig. 86.2 Autosomal recessive multitropic pituitary hormone deficiency. Three affected Hutterite sibs on the right and their cousin on the left.

panhypopituitary dwarfism, one inherited as an autosomal recessive and one as an X-linked recessive trait. Unfortunately, there are no clinical or endocrinological differences between the two genetic disorders and the more common acquired disease, and thus in a sporadic case or in a family in which only male sibs are affected, accurate genetic counselling is impossible.

The non-genetic form of the disease was well docu-

Table 86.3 Genetic forms of pituitary dwarfism

Type	Panhypopituitary Dwarfism		Isolated Growth Hormone Deficiency (IGHD)				Bioinactive hGH	Laron Dwarfism	IGF-1 Resistance
	I	II	1-A	1-B	II	III			
Defect	Hypothalamus or pituitary	?	Gene deletion	Hypothalamus	hGH	?	hGH gene mutation?	hGH receptor	? IGF-1 receptor
Inheritance	AR	X-linked	AR	AR	AD	X-linked	?	AR	?
Plasma GH	↓	↓	-O-	↓	↓	↓	N	↑	N/↑
IGF before/ after hGH	↓/N	↓/N	↓/N	↓/N	↓/N	↓/N	↓/N	↓/↓	↑/↑
Insulin	↓	↓	↓	↓	↑	↓	↓	↓	↓
Response to GH treatment	+	+	±	+	+	+	+	−	−

AD = autosomal dominant; AR = autosomal recessive; GH = growth hormone; hGH = human growth hormone; IGF = insulin-like growth factor; N = normal; O = zero; ↓ = decreased; ↑ = increased.

mented by the report of discordant MZ twins (Rosenfield et al 1967).

The clinical features of hereditary panhypopituitary dwarfism are identical to those of the nongenetic forms of the disease and are dependent upon which of the tropic hormones are deficient. The most frequently associated hormonal deficiency is that of gonadotropin, followed in order of frequency by ACTH and TSH deficiency. Deficiency of hGH results in proportionate dwarfism, increased subcutaneous adipose tissue and characteristic high-pitched voice and wrinkled skin. Gonadotropin deficiency results in sexual immaturity with primary amenorrhoea and lack of secondary sexual characteristics in the female, and small testes and phallus and lack of beard in the male. Epiphyses remain open throughout life. TSH deficiency, when it occurs, does not often result in severe thyroid deficiency, but in certain instances definite signs of hypothyroidism can occur with myxoedematous facies, slow reflexes, hypometabolism and epiphyseal dysplasia. ACTH deficiency may contribute to severe hypoglycaemia in infancy and childhood. There is both inter- and intrafamilial variability in the associated hormonal deficiencies; in certain families one individual may lack only hGH and gonadotropin. In families with multitropic deficiencies, however, at least both hGH and gonadotropin deficiencies occur in all affected members, there being no familial crossovers between panhypopituitary dwarfism and isolated hGH deficiency yet reported.

McArthur et al (1985) restudied the Hutterite family illustrated in Figure 86.2. They demonstrated that the tropic hormone loss was sequential. In one sibship hGH and gonadotropin deficiency occurred in the first decade, with subsequent loss of TSH and, finally, ACTH deficiency in the third decade. In a related sibship TSH loss also occurred in the first decade.

In hereditary panhypopituitary dwarfism, it would be difficult to visualize a metabolic defect or structural gene mutation resulting in the deficiency of two or more tropic hormones which lack a common subunit; thus, it is quite likely that a structural, degenerative, or secretory defect in the pituitary or hypothalamus exists in these disorders. McArthur et al (1985) demonstrated a lack of close linkage between the Hutterite autosomal recessive form of the disease and both the hGH gene (17q) and the HLA region (6p). Studies with TRH and LHRH in sporadic panhypopituitary dwarfs have demonstrated that the basic defect in the majority of cases lies in the hypothalamus, rather than in the pituitary, since TRH and LHRH administration resulted in TSH and LH secretion, respectively, in approximately two thirds of the patients (Costom et al 1971, Folley et al 1972, Medeiros-Neto et al 1973, Rogol et al 1985). In those patients with a positive response to the hypothalamic releasing hormone, the pituitary is capable of synthesizing and secreting the tropic hormone, indicating that the basic defect lies in the hypothalamus. In those cases who do not respond to TRH or LHRH a defect located in the pituitary itself would be more likely, unless the pituitary atrophied or became non-responsive over time. There was virtually no response to provocative testing in all five of the Hutterites who received releasing hormones, suggesting a primary pituitary defect (McArthur et al 1985).

Isolated human growth hormone deficiency (IGHD) An isolated deficiency of hGH with otherwise normal pituitary function results in proportionate dwarfism with normal sexual development and a fairly typical physical appearance and characteristic metabolic abnormalities. It is now apparent that on the basis of clinical, genetic, and metabolic variability, IGHD is a heterogeneous group of disorders.

Type IA IGHD. Illig (1970) described a type of growth hormone deficiency which she called Type A, that was felt to be distinct from Type I, on the basis of the appearance of high concentration of hGH antibodies following hGH therapy. This syndrome is inherited as an autosomal recessive trait and results in shortness at birth and even more severe dwarfism and exaggerated pinched facies than the more common forms of hGH deficiency. Nitrogen retention following exogenous hGH was also greater. The major distinguishing features, however, are an absence of immunoreactive hGH and the development of hGH antibodies in high concentration, which suppress the growth promoting effects of hGH. She postulated that these children have an hereditary complete deficiency of hGH, which is present before birth and which causes a lack of immune tolerance to homologous hGH.

Phillips et al (1981) studied the growth hormone genes in Illig's original family using restriction endonuclease techniques. All affected children in this family were found to be homozygous for a deletion in their growth hormone gene, whereas their parents and two thirds of their unaffected sibs appeared to be heterozygous for the deletion.

A number of families with IGHD Type IA from diverse ethnic backgrounds have now been documented to have homozygous deletions of the GH1 gene (Nishi et al 1984, Rivarola et al 1984, Laron et al 1985, Goossens et al 1986, Frisch & Phillips 1986, Braga et al 1986) (Fig. 86.3). The Swiss, Argentinian, Japanese and Austrian patients all had deletions of approximately 6.7 kb, while the Italian and Western Spanish patients studied had larger deletions of 7.6 kb (Phillips 1989) (Fig. 86.4). Affected individuals from different families and ethnic backgrounds with the 6.7 kb deletion had different RFLP haplotypes, suggesting that the deletions occurred inde-

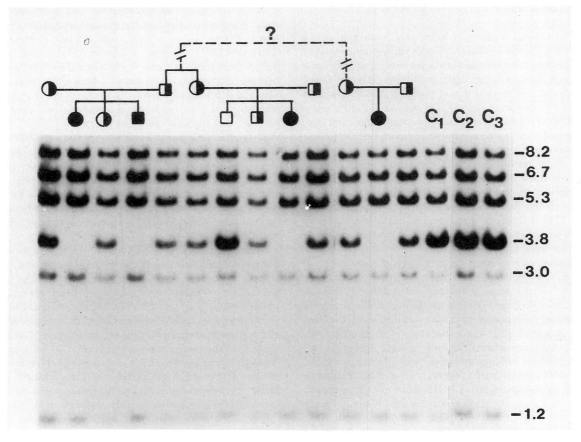

Fig. 86.3   Type IA isolated growth hormone deficiency. Autoradiogram patterns of DNA from three Swiss families and three controls (from Phillips et al 1981).

pendently (Phillips 1985, 1989). In each of these families described with 6.7 kb and 7.6 kb deletions, only the GH1 locus was deleted and the remaining components of the cluster remained intact (Vrencak-Jones et al 1988). Goossens et al (1986) reported two sibs who were homozygous for a double deletion in which the only component of the GH gene cluster remaining was the CHSP1 pseudogene. Homozygosity for deletions encompassing the genes for CSH1 or CSH1-GH2-CSH2 has also been reported in phenotypically normal individuals (Wurzel et al 1982, Parks et al 1985). These various deletions probably occurred because of unequal recombinational events through chromosome misalignment.

These patients have extremely low to absent levels of immunoreactive hGH before and after provocative testing. High titres of anti-hGH antibodies occur in about two thirds of the patients following hGH therapy. Although most patients do not have good growth re-

sponses to hGH over time, a number of patients have now been described who achieved normal adult height (Laron et al 1985, Braga et al 1986). Heterozygosity for these deletions results in lowered hGH responses to provocative testing, but normal IGF I levels and normal growth.

Thus type IA IGHD is the result of a variety of deletions in the hGH gene resulting in the congenital absence of normal hGH and a lack of immunotolerance to homologous hGH. This would explain the total absence of immunoreactive plasma hGH and the high antibody titres following hGH administration.

Type IB IGHD. The most common form of IGHD, Type IB, is inherited as an autosomal recessive trait and is associated with proportionate dwarfism, increased subcutaneous fat, typical pinched facies with high forehead, wrinkled skin and high-pitched voice (Royer et al 1970, Rimoin & Schimke 1971, Rimoin 1976, Donaldson et al 1980) (Fig. 86.5).

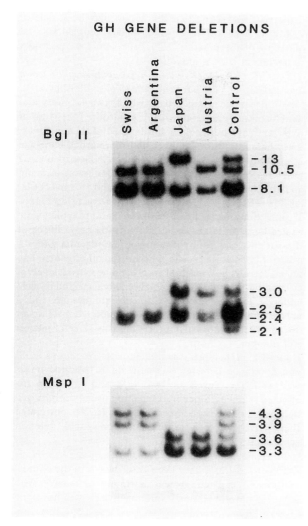

Fig. 86.4 Isolated growth hormone deficiency Type 1A – different RFLP haplotypes occurring on chromosomes from patients from different ethnic groups that have growth hormone gene deletions (from Phillips et al 1986).

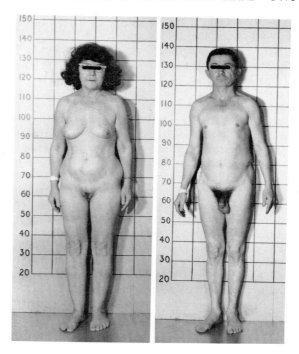

Fig. 86.5 Autosomal recessive type 1B isolated growth hormone deficiency in two sibs who are the offspring of a consanguineous mating.

Plasma hGH is deficient, but clearly detectable after provocative stimuli. Deficient growth velocity responds quickly and consistently to hGH therapy and patients do not develop high titres of blocking antibodies. They may have spontaneous hypoglycaemic episodes in infancy, but spontaneous hypoglycaemia is not a problem after early childhood, although they maintain hypersensitivity to exogenous insulin into adulthood. As adults, abnormal glucose tolerance associated with insulinopenia is a characteristic feature, both of these quickly revert to normal following hGH therapy. Puberty occurs spontan-

eously, but is frequently delayed to the late teens or early twenties. Puberty frequently appears abruptly during the first few months of hGH therapy. Thus, in the prepubertal individual, IGHD cannot be clinically distinguished from a combined deficiency of hGH and gonadotropins until at least the early twenties. LHRH stimulation studies can distinguish between these two disorders.

Autopsy studies in three cases of IGHD Type IB have all revealed the presence of typical somatotropic cells in the pituitary and, in the one case assayed, the presence of significant amounts of immunoreactive growth hormone (Hewer 1944, Rimoin & Schechter 1973, Merimee et al 1975). Though the relative number of somatotropic cells in the pituitary differed between the three cases studied, they clearly demonstrate the pituitary's capability of synthesizing growth hormone. Administration of GHRH to two sibs with IGHD Type IB resulted in a significant rise in plasma hGH levels (Rogol et al 1985). Sporadic cases of IGHD have been found to be heterogeneous in regard to their response to GHRH (Grossman et al 1983, Borges et al 1983, Mitrakou et al 1985), suggesting that IGHD can occur secondarily to either hypothalamic or pituitary defects. To date, the GH1 gene has been present in all individuals with this syndrome who have been studied (Phillips et al 1982, Rogol et al 1985). Phillips et al (1982) found that in the majority of families with IGHD Type IB, the disease did not cosegregate with RFLPs at the GH gene cluster. Thus, the defect in Type IB IGHD would appear to be a deficiency of growth hormone releasing hormone synthesis or secretion. Further heterogeneity must be excluded.

Type II IGHD. Merimee et al (1969) described a distinct form of hGH deficiency, apparently inherited as an autosomal dominant trait, which they called Type II IGHD. These individuals did not have the wrinkled skin or characteristic voice seen in other pituitary dwarfs. They had glucose intolerance, but an increased rather than decreased insulin response to both glucose ingestion and arginine infusion. Furthermore, they were relatively resistant to exogenous insulin and to the metabolic effects of exogenous hGH. It is clear that there must be further heterogeneity in the IGHD syndromes, since there have also been families reported with apparent dominant inheritance who have the metabolic features of the recessive form of the disease. For example, Poskitt and Rayner (1974) have described two families with a father and son with IGHD, suggestive of autosomal dominant inheritance. These individuals had wrinkled skin, spontaneous hypoglycaemia of infancy, hyper-responsiveness to exogenous insulin and a marked increase in growth velocity following hGH therapy, all features of the 'recessive' form of the disease. Sheikholislam and Stempfel (1972) have described a family in which a father and four of his seven children had IGHD, again suggestive of autosomal dominant inheritance. These individuals had the typical features of IGHD Type IB with high pitched voice, infantile facies, delayed onset of puberty and marked growth acceleration following hGH therapy, but they had glucose intolerance with relative hyperinsulinism, which increased even further following hGH administration. On the other hand Bierich (1973) described two sibs with normal insulin sensitivity, but plasma hyperinsulinism in response to an intravenous glucose load. Unfortunately, they did not mention whether or not a parent was affected, so it is impossible to state whether the syndrome is dominantly or recessively inherited in this family. Rogol et al (1985) and Tani et al (1987) found little or no hGH release following GHRH administration in two large families with autosomal dominant inheritance of IGHD, suggesting a pituitary rather than a hypothalamic defect. Furthermore, cerebral CT of the Japanese family showed empty sellas. The GH1 gene was present in the latter family, but by Southern analysis, they could not find evidence of a mutation. Phillips (1989) studied a large dominant family in whom the GH1 gene present in the affected members cosegregated with a particular RFLP

haplotype, suggesting that this lesion may be associated with a mutant allele. Further linkage studies and sequencing of the putative GH1 gene would be necessary to document such a mutation.

Type III IGHD (X-linked hypogammaglobulinaemia and isolated growth hormone deficiency). Fleisher et al (1980) described a kindred in which two brothers and their two maternal uncles had a syndrome consisting of hypogammaglobulinaemia and isolated hGH deficiency. They had proportionate short stature, retarded bone age in childhood, delayed onset of puberty, lack of plasma hGH response to insulin-arginine stimulation, low bio and immunoassayable somatomedin and normal TSH, ACTH, FSH and LH secretion. Recurrent sinopulmonary infections were a problem in two patients, which were abated by parenteral gamma globulin therapy. Three of the patients had panhypogammaglobulinaemia and absence of circulating B cells, whereas the other patient had normal serum IgA and IgM levels and decreased levels of circulating B cells. All had an absence of specific in vitro antibody production after antigenic stimulation and a failure of in vitro immunoglobulin production. Two of the patients had normal appearing tonsils. T-cell function and number was normal.

One of the patients was treated with exogenous hGH and developed detectable circulating B lymphocytes as well as higher levels of IgA, IgM and IgE than his affected relatives. Since hGH therapy usually results in a decrease in B lymphocytes, Phillips (1989) postulated that IGHD III may represent a contiguous deletion syndrome.

Pituitary dwarfism with biologically inactive hGH. A number of patients have been described with the clinical features of isolated growth hormone deficiency who achieved normal plasma immunoactive growth hormone levels following stimulation, but low levels of somatomedin (Kowarski et al 1978, Hayek et al 1978, Rudman et al 1980, 1981, Frazer et al 1982, Bright et al 1983). Less hGH was detected by radioreceptor assay than by radioimmunoassay. Following hGH administration, however, they generated normal somatomedin levels, and had a significant increase in their growth rates. TSH and ACTH secretion were normal. In view of their clinical syndrome of isolated growth hormone deficiency, normal plasma hGH, low basal somatomedin levels, and their normal response to exogenous hGH, they appear to secrete a biologically inert growth hormone. Since their endogenous growth hormone reacted normally in the immunoassay, this appears to represent a CRM (cross-reactive-material) positive mutation.

Valenta et al (1985) reported a similar patient with short stature, normal levels of immunoreactive hGH, but decreased radioreceptor activity. This patient responded well to exogenous hGH, but his plasma somatomedin level was normal. When analyzed by column chromatography, his growth hormone exhibited unusual patterns, with most of it migrating as large tetramers or dimers. However, there is a question as to whether his growth failure occurred before age 8–9 years.

Molecular documentation of a mutation has not yet been accomplished in any of these patients. Phillips (1985) has postulated that these patients have a defect in their hGH receptor rather than in hGH itself, since some have been found to have a deletion on chromosome 13 and not 17, where the GH gene is located.

In contrast, a number of patients have been described with 'invisible growth hormone', i.e. individuals with normal growth, deficient hGH secretion as measured by radioimmunoassay, but normal growth hormone concentrations as measured by radioreceptor assay (Geffner et al 1986, Bistritzer et al 1988). Thus, these individuals appear to secrete a mutant molecule with normal biological activity which is 'invisible' to hGH radio-immunoassay. Bistritzer et al (1988) postulated that this unusual molecule could be expressed from the GHV gene.

Laron dwarfism Laron et al (1966) described a syndrome with the clinical features of pituitary dwarfism, associated with high plasma concentration of immunoreactive hGH (Fig. 86.6). Although their patients were all oriental Jews, this autosomal recessive syndrome has since been described in numerous other ethnic groups (Van Gemund et al 1969, Najjar et al 1971, Van den Brande et al 1974, Saldanha & Toledo 1981). These individuals have the clinical appearance of patients with IGHD to an exaggerated extent, with severe growth retardation, severely pinched facies, high-pitched voices and small male genitalia (Laron 1974). Males have delayed puberty. Birthweight is normal but birth length may be retarded. Motor development may be delayed and some are mildly retarded. Teething and fontanelle closure are delayed. Their hands and feet are small and, like pituitary dwarfs, they are obese and their body proportions are childlike. They may have spontaneous hypoglycaemic episodes in infancy and usually have insulinopenia in response to glucose and arginine. ACTH, TSH, gonadotropin and vasopressin secretion are normal. Fasting plasma hGH concentrations are usually elevated, but may fluctuate from normal levels to over 100 ng/ml in the same patient. There is further elevation of plasma immunoreactive growth hormone concentration following insulin induced hypoglycaemia and arginine infusion. Plasma somatomedin levels are low, and unlike those in hGH deficient patients, do not respond to hGH administration (Laron et al 1971). Furthermore, they are relatively unresponsive to metabolic and growth promoting effects of growth hormone. Laron et al (1966)

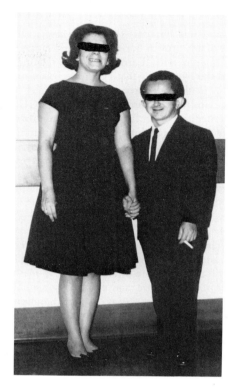

Fig. 86.6 A woman with isolated growth hormone deficiency and her husband with Laron dwarfism.

first postulated that this disorder was due to the synthesis of a structurally altered hGH molecule which was immunologically active but biologically inert. Several groups of investigators, however, have been unable to distinguish between plasma hGH of Laron dwarfs and normal individuals on the basis of serial immunoassay dilutions, electrofocusing and molecular size distribution (Eshet et al 1973, Bala & Beck 1973, Elders et al 1973, Van den Brande et al 1974, Pierson et al 1978). Furthermore, substantial quantities of receptor active hGH have been found in their sera by a hepatic radioreceptor assay (Jacobs et al 1976). Golde et al (1980) have directly demonstrated specific cellular resistance of hGH in Laron dwarfs, utilizing an in vitro erythroid progenitor technique.

Eshet et al (1984) could find no binding of hGH to liver pellets from patients with Laron dwarfism, demonstrating a defect in the liver hGH receptors which would account for the lack of somatomedin generation. Their liver samples, however, actively bound insulin, demonstrating the specificity of the defect to the hGH receptor. Plasma growth hormone binding protein is thought to represent a soluble form of the hGH membrane receptor. Daughaday and Trivedi (1987) have demonstrated the absence of any growth hormone binding in the serum of three children with Laron dwarfism, adding further proof to the hypothesis that Laron dwarfism is due to a mutation in the hGH receptor. Amselem et al (1989) have demonstrated a point mutation in the hGH receptor gene in Mediterranean families with Laron dwarfism.

While thyroid progenitor cells and transformed T-cell lines from patients with Laron dwarfism do not respond to hGH, Geffner et al (1987) found a normal response to IGF I. Furthermore, Laron et al (1988) found a rapid in vivo response of hypoglycaemia and a fall in plasma insulin to the administration of exogenous IGF I in these patients, suggesting that long-term IGF I therapy may stimulate their growth.

Pituitary dwarfism with somatomedin unresponsiveness Lanes et al (1980) have described an adolescent male with proportionate dwarfism, normal plasma hGH response to stimulation and elevated somatomedin by bioassay, radioreceptor assay and radioimmunoassay. Bone age was clinically retarded, but by age 15 years his sexual development was well established. 24 hour growth hormone secretion was normal, as were his ACTH, TSH and gonadotropin functions. In view of his elevated somatomedin and clinical hypopituitarism, peripheral unresponsiveness to somatomedin at either the receptor or postreceptor level was postulated. Cultured fibroblasts from such a patient had a 50% decrease in IGF binding compared to controls.

The African Pygmies Peripheral unresponsiveness to human growth hormone administration, in the presence of normal concentrations of immunoreactive plasma hGH and normal bioassayable somatomedin activity, has been documented in the African Pygmies (Rimoin et al 1969, Merimee et al 1972). This population, who inhabit the rain forests of equatorial Africa, resemble pituitary dwarfs in size and skeletal proportions, but do not have the truncal obesity, peculiar facies and wrinkled skin of pituitary dwarfism. Following insulin induced hypoglycaemia and arginine infusion, plasma hGH levels are normal, but like Type I IGHD, they are insulinopenic and hypersensitive to the effects of exogenous insulin. They are completely unresponsive to the lipolytic, insulinotropic and nitrogen retaining properties of hGH. Merimee et al (1981) have reported a deficiency of insulin-like growth factor I with normal IGF II in these pygmies.

Merimee et al (1987) studied IGF I and II levels as well as testosterone in a different group of pygmies in Zaire. They found that prepubertal pygmy children and controls did not differ in linear growth or in serum concentrations of IGF I or II. Adolescent pygmies, however, had a significant reduction in IGF I as compared to control adolescents, whereas IGF II and testosterone levels were comparable. Pubertal growth acceleration was blunted or absent in the pygmy adolescents. Furthermore, low plasma levels of high affinity growth hormone binding protein have been found in the pygmies (Baumann et al 1989). This may indicate a reduced number of GH receptors in their tissues.

Isolated deficiencies of TSH, ACTH, LH and FSH

Isolated deficiencies of each of these pituitary hormones have been reported. Since the clinical symptoms produced are the result of the target organ hormonal deficiency (e.g. hypothyroidism, hypoadrenalism or hypogonadism), they are discussed in the corresponding endocrine organ chapters.

Disorders of pituitary hypersecretion and/or neoplasia

Genetic disorders of pituitary hyperfunction are far less common than those of pituitary insufficiency. Furthermore, except in instances of multiple endocrine adenomatosis or in patients who have a positive family history of pituitary hyperfunction, it is impossible to denote which of the sporadic cases have a genetic form of pituitary disease. The most common form of hereditary pituitary neoplasia is the multiple endocrine adenomatosis syndrome, Type I. Although multiple cases of familial acromegaly and of the amenorrhoea-galactorrhoea syndrome have been described in certain kindreds with no evidence of other endocrine involvement, these disorders may well represent limited forms of the multiple endocrine adenomatosis syndrome.

Acromegaly Hypersecretion of human growth hormone by a pituitary neoplasm leads to the classic syndromes of acromegaly and gigantism, depending upon the age of onset of the disorder. The clinical features and diagnostic criteria of acromegaly have been well reviewed in the endocrinological literature and will not be discussed here (Daughaday 1985). The diagnosis can be made readily on the basis of high fasting plasma concentrations of human growth hormone, which usually do not fall following oral glucose ingestion.

Although the majority of cases of acromegaly are sporadic, many families have been reported in which multiple members are said to be affected (Koch & Tiwisina 1959, Rimoin & Schimke 1971). This literature must be regarded with caution, however, as very few of the familial cases have been anatomically confirmed or had high hGH levels documented by radioimmunoassay. Indeed, a number of the families described in the older literature as hereditary acromegaly represent instead cases of pachydermoperiostosis, a dominantly inherited disorder (Rimoin & Schimke 1971). In other reports of familial acromegaly, the affected relatives are said to be 'acromegaloid', rather than acromegalic, that is, they are of tall stature but have no evidence of pituitary dysfunction (Lehmann 1964). Another syndrome that might be confused with acromegaly is cerebral gigantism, in which increased growth rate occurs from infancy but no abnormalities in hGH secretion are found (Hook & Reynolds 1967, Jones 1988). In spite of these reservations, pathological and radiographic documentation of pituitary adenomas have been described in successive generations in several families, strongly suggesting autosomal dominant inheritance. Two cousins from a highly inbred family have also been described with 'acromegaly', suggesting autosomal recessive inheritance (Leva 1915). Objective evidence for the disease was obtained in only one of these cousins. Levin et al (1974) reported two brothers with acromegaly, acanthosis nigricans, pituitary tumours and elevated plasma hGH levels. It would be of great value to study hGH secretion in the 'acromegaloid' relatives of documented acromegalic cases to see if minor abnormalities of hGH secretion do exist. Many of the familial cases of acromegaly may represent partial expression of the multiple endocrine adenomatosis syndrome.

Familial amenorrhoea-galactorrhoea (Chiari-Frommel syndrome, Forbes-Albright syndrome) The association of secondary amenorrhoea and galactorrhoea is generally thought to occur in two distinct syndromes – the Forbes-Albright syndrome, in which amenorrhoea and galactorrhoea are accompanied by a pituitary tumour, with or without prior pregnancy, and the Chiari-Frommel syndrome, in which the amenorrhoea and galactorrhoea commence following pregnancy, unassociated with a pituitary neoplasm (Young et al 1967). This distinction may be artificial, however, as the pituitary adenomas may be too small to recognize; progression from the benign Chiari-Frommel syndrome to the neoplastic Forbes-Albright syndrome had been documented. Linquette and associates (1967) have described a family in which both mother and daughter developed amenorrhoea and galactorrhoea associated with pituitary adenomas. The mother first developed the clinical signs of this syndrome following a pregnancy, whereas the daughter was never pregnant and amenorrhoea ensued following emotional trauma. Both patients had a large sella turcica radiographically and were found on craniotomy to have pituitary adenomas. Histologically, the tumours resembled chromophobe adenomas, but there was fine eosinophilic granulation on tetrachrome staining, indicative of prolactin secreting cells. Hyperprolactinaemia may result in galactorrhoea, gynaecomastia, hypogonadism and even precocious puberty. Cases of isolated hyperprolac-

tinaemia have been well documented. The amenorrhoea-galactorrhoea syndrome has also been described as a part of the multiple endocrine neoplasia (MEN) I syndrome, associated with gastric ulcers, islet cell adenomas, and hyperparathyroidism. It is impossible to state whether or not the family reported by Linquette represents a distinct entity or whether both mother and daughter had partial forms of the MEN syndrome. In any case, the pituitary adenomas in this syndrome, like most other hereditary tumours, are inherited as dominant traits.

Multiple endocrine neoplasia Type I (MEN Type I, Wermer syndrome) Multiple endocrine adenomatosis is a familial disorder characterized by multiple tumours or hyperplasia of the endocrine glands and a high incidence of multifocal, unremitting peptic ulcer disease (Zollinger-Ellison syndrome) (Ballard et al 1964). The clinical manifestations of pituitary disease are dependent upon the predominating cell type. Chromophobe adenoma is the most common lesion and results in symptoms of pituitary insufficiency, especially hypogonadism and/or headache and visual disturbances secondary to mechanical pressure. Acromegaly is associated with eosinophilic adenoma and does not differ clinically from acquired cases of this disease. Pituitary involvement has been found without other apparent endocrine disease in certain patients whose relatives have the full-blown syndrome, but it may occur in combination with any or all of the other manifestations of the disorder. On histopathological examination, the pituitary may show simple hyperplasia, benign adenoma, or invasive neoplasm.

LeBriggs and Powell (1969) described a woman with the MEN I syndrome who developed the amenorrhoea-galactorrhoea syndrome following parturition. Although there was no clinical evidence of a pituitary neoplasm, pituitary gonadotropins were absent in the urine and she may well have had a small prolactin secreting adenoma. It is impossible to state whether or not the familial cases of 'pure' amenorrhoea-galactorrhoea syndrome and acromegaly are all part of the MEN I syndrome or whether they represent distinct entities. In any patient with a pituitary neoplasm, however, an effort should be made to rule out involvement of the other endocrine organs, in both the patient and his close relatives.

The MEN I syndrome is inherited as an autosomal dominant trait, with marked intrafamilial variability.

POSTERIOR PITUITARY

The posterior pituitary gland (neurohypophysis), which is derived from an invagination of the hypothalamus, is embryologically and functionally distinct from the anterior pituitary. The primary function of the neurohypophysis is the storage and secretion of two octapeptide hormones: antidiuretic hormone (ADH, vasopressin, ADP) and oxytocin. These hormones are synthesized by neurones in the supraoptic and paraventricular nuclei of the hypothalamus. They are bound to a carrier protein (neurophysin) and transported down the neuronal axons (supraopticoneurohypophyseal tracts) to the posterior pituitary, in vesicular form. The hormones are stored in the posterior pituitary and released into the circulation following appropriate stimuli (Culpepper et al 1985).

Genetic disorders of vasopressin deficiency

Hereditary vasopressin-sensitive diabetes insipidus is a syndrome characterized by polyuria, polydipsia, and dehydration secondary to a deficiency of antidiuretic hormone. This syndrome is characterized by acute thirst, especially for cold water, enormous daily urinary output (3000 to 15 000 ml per day), and persistent nocturia. If water is withheld, the patient rapidly loses weight and develops hypertonic dehydration. A variety of acquired lesions of the hypothalamus, such as neoplasia, basilar skull fractures, granulomatous diseases, vascular lesions, meningitis, and encephalitis can result in ADH deficiency (Culpepper et al 1985). In approximately 50% of the cases of diabetes insipidus, however, no obvious primary lesion can be found and the disease is termed 'idiopathic'. It is quite likely that many of the idiopathic cases of diabetes insipidus represent sporadic cases of the genetic form of the disease.

In 1841, Lacombe was the first to document a familial form of diabetes insipidus; he described excessive thirst and polyuria in five males and three females in two generations of a family. Numerous other families with multiple affected members have since been described (Blotner 1942, Walker & Rance 1954, Blackett et al 1983, Toth et al 1984, Pedersen et al 1985). Both males and females have been affected in successive generations, and male-to-male transmission has been documented on numerous occasions, indicating that vasopressin-sensitive diabetes insipidus can be inherited as an autosomal dominant trait. The signs and symptoms of this autosomal dominant disorder are quite similar to those of the acquired forms of diabetes insipidus. There is, however, a great deal of intrafamilial variability in the clinical severity and age of onset of the disease. Pender and Fraser (1953) reported a large family in which urinary output varied from 3–4 quarts per day to 15–20 quarts per day among affected relatives. Some, but not all, affected individuals have an increase in fluid requirements during febrile episodes, exercise, or pregnancy. In most cases the onset of the disease occurs in infancy, but symptoms may

not occur until late childhood or adolescence. Abatement of symptoms may occur in old age (Martin 1959). In many of the affected families, the condition is regarded as an unpleasant family habit, rather than a disease. Apart from drinking enormous quantities of water, the disease did not impair health or well being. Imaging studies of brain and sella have been normal (Pedersen et al 1985).

If all forms of hereditary diabetes insipidus were inherited as an autosomal dominant trait, one would expect an equal number of affected males and females. A deficiency of female affected individuals was noted by several authors who assembled previously reported kindreds with this disease (Martin 1959). Forssman (1945) has documented an X-linked recessive form of vasopressin-sensitive diabetes insipidus in several families and suggested that the previously reported unequal sex ratio was caused by inclusion of families with the X-linked form of the disease. He described several large kindreds in which a number of males were affected with vasopressin-sensitive diabetes insipidus, the disease apparently being transmitted through females, who were either completely unaffected or only minimally affected Thus both autosomal dominant and X-linked recessive varieties of vasopressin-sensitive diabetes insipidus exist, but affected males of either type are clinically indistinguishable.

Hereditary vasopressin-sensitive diabetes insipidus is caused by a marked deficiency of vasopressin. Plasma levels of AVP have been found to be very low or undetectable in these cases (Kaplowitz et al 1982, Blackett et al 1983, Toth et al 1984, Pedersen et al 1985). Plasma ADH was found to rise following furosemide administration, suggesting a hypothalamic osmoreceptor defect, but with a normal response to volume change (Toth et al 1984). Selective involvement of osmoreceptors has also been proposed in a patient with histiocytosis (DeRobertis et al 1971). Autopsy studies of individuals with the hereditary, autosomal dominant or sporadic idiopathic forms of the disease found a severe reduction in the number of neurosecretory neurons in both the supraoptic and paraventricular nuclei of the hypothalamus (Gaupp 1941, Green et al 1967). There is associated gliosis, and in the paraventricular nucleus, the small to medium-sized neurons may be normal or reduced in number. The posterior pituitary gland has been found to be normal in size or small in these cases, but no neurosecretory material was observed on special staining. Thus the vasopressin deficiency appears to be secondary to aplasia or degeneration of the neurosecretory neurons of the hypothalamus. Although these individuals appear to have no neurosecretory neurons in their hypothalamic nuclei and have all the signs and symptoms of ADH deficiency, oxytocin secretion appears to be normal in most. Several females with the dominantly inherited form of vasopressin-sensitive diabetes, including one in whom a marked deficiency of neurosecretory cells was documented, have undergone normal pregnancies and deliveries and have successfully nursed their children. Thus they appear to secrete oxytocin, despite the deficiency of neurosecretory neurons. Although a small number of secretory cells remain in the paraventricular nuclei of these patients, Green and associates (1967) suggested that oxytocin might also be produced by cells located outside these areas. Several patients with diabetes insipidus have been reported, however, who have had difficulty in expelling the fetus and placenta during labour and/or inability to secrete milk (Blackett et al 1983), suggesting that oxytocin deficiency might also exist. In one such family plasma levels of oxytocin and its carrier protein were normal, but did not increase normally following oestrogen administration.

Nagai et al (1984) reported a family with hereditary diabetes insipidus that they considered to be autosomal dominant with reduced penetrance. The pedigree, however, could be better interpreted as X-linked with occasional expression in females, as the majority of affected individuals were male. There were several instances of transmission through unaffected females, and there was no male-to-male transmission. At autopsy, one affected male demonstrated no atrophy of the supraoptic and paraventricular nuclei, similar to the findings of Forssman (1945) in another X-linked case. Immunohistochemical studies revealed that the paraventricular nucleus scarcely had any vasopressin-positive cells, in contrast to an autopsy control. This would suggest that the basic defect in the X-linked form of this disease may be a genetic defect in ADH synthesis. Circulating antibodies to arginine-vasopressin containing hypothalamic cells have been found in patients with histiocytosis X and diabetes insipidus, suggesting that they may be a marker of hypothalamic invasion (Scherbaum et al 1985). Antibodies to vasopressin itself, however, are usually only found after AVP therapy, and may result in secondary resistance to its antidiuretic effect (Vokes et al 1988).

Diabetes insipidus of the vasopressin-sensitive variety has been reported to be an autosomal recessive trait in the Brattleboro strain of rat (Valtin 1969). Although these animals have an absolute deficiency of antidiuretic hormone in their hypothalamic and posterior pituitaries, unlike the human disease, there is hypertrophy of the hypothalamo-pituitary system. The neurons in the supraoptic nucleus are extremely well developed although they lack neurosecretory granules (Valtin 1976). Similar, but less marked changes, are seen in the paraventricular nuclei, and the posterior lobe of the pituitary is three to four times heavier than normal.

Heterozygous animals have a reduced concentration of vasopressin in the hypothalamus and pituitary and have deficient secretion and release of the hormone. In vivo vasopressin and its neurophysin carrier are absent (Sokol & Valtin 1982). However, detectable, although markedly reduced, levels of vasopressin mRNA are present in the hypothalamus (Majzoub et al 1984). The molecular defect in the Brattleboro rat has now been found to be a single deletion of a G residue in the region of the vasopressin gene which codes for the neurophysin carrier protein (Schmale & Richter 1984). The basic defect in the autosomal recessive variety of diabetes insipidus in the rat is decreased synthesis of active hormone with compensatory hypertrophy of the secretory neurons. The differences in the genetics and pathogenesis of diabetes insipidus between humans and rats support the general rule of recessive inheritance of peptide hormone deficiency syndromes. In the rat, the basic defect is in the synthesis of the peptide hormone, and the disease is inherited as an autosomal dominant trait, but the primary defect appears to involve a degenerative or developmental disorder of the hypothalamus, rather than a primary defect in peptide synthesis.

Vasopressin deficiency associated with complex genetic syndromes

A variety of developmental malformations may result in both anterior and posterior pituitary deficiency (see previous discussion of congenital absence of pituitary, anencephaly, holoprosencephaly, trans-sphenoidal encephalocele, septo-optic dysplasia and histiocytosis X).

The diabetes mellitus-optic atrophy, diabetes insipidus-deafness syndrome (DIDMOAD syndrome, Wolfram syndrome).

This autosomal recessive syndrome consists of diabetes mellitus, optic atrophy, diabetes insipidus and neurosensory deafness. (Gunn et al 1976, Fraser & Gunn 1977, Fishman & Ehrlich 1986, Blasi et al 1986). The optic atrophy is of the primary variety and is characterized by white discs and, in some instances, peripheral retinal pigmentation as well. The diabetes mellitus is of the severe juvenile onset variety and frequently precedes the other symptoms. Bilateral neurosensory deafness is an integral component of this syndrome; it begins as a high frequency hearing loss and may remain quite mild. Indeed, in many affected patients, the hearing loss was not suspected until audiograms were performed.

A number of other associated abnormalities have been described in certain families, including ataxia, autonomic dysfunction with a neurogenic bladder, sideroblastic anaemia, and hyperalaninuria (Jarnerot 1973). In view of the progression with time of simple optic atrophy and diabetes mellitus to the full-blown syndrome with neuro-sensory hearing loss, atonic bladder and ataxia in the original family by Wolfram (Wolfram 1938, Turnbridge & Paley 1956), all of these anomalies appear to be the result of a single pleiotropic mutant gene and represent one distinct syndrome.

Vasopressin sensitive diabetes insipidus occurs in over one third of the patients with this syndrome (Bretz et al 1970). Several families have been reported in which several members have the full blown syndrome while others have the diabetes mellitus and optic atrophy, without the diabetes insipidus (Gossain et al 1975, Richardson & Hamilton 1977). Thus it is clear that the diabetes insipidus is simply another pleiotropic effect of a single mutant gene. ADH deficiency had been documented in affected patients following a hypermolar stimulus; normal free water resorption resumes following DDAVP administration (Richardson & Hamilton 1977, Wit et al 1986). Postmortem examination of two sibs with this syndrome revealed degeneration of the hypothalamic nuclei, more severe in the paraventricular than supraoptic nuclei, and atrophy of the posterior lobe of the pituitary, adrenal cortex, pons and substantia nigra (Carson et al 1972).

Reduction of the dilatation of the urinary tract and normalization of bladder function following long-term DDAVP administration suggest that the urinary tract anomalies in this syndrome are secondary to the polyuria (Aragona et al 1983, Wit et al 1986).

Peripheral resistance to vasopressin

Nephrogenic diabetes insipidus Type I

Nephrogenic diabetes insipidus is characterized by polyuria, polydipsia, and hyposthenuria, resistant to vasopressin. In the typical X-linked form of the disease there is renal unresponsiveness to vasopressin, biologically active antidiuretic hormone has been found to be present in the serum and urine of affected individuals and there is deficient cyclic AMP excretion in the urine following ADH administration (Bell et al 1974).

These individuals have severe polyuria and polydipsia. A concentrating defect has been demonstrated within six days of birth. Polyuria and polydipsia, however, may be overlooked in the early days of life. Several patients have been described who have an absence of thirst. The infants are usually irritable, eager to suck, and vomit milk soon after ingestion. They show a distinct preference for water over milk in early life. They often have constipation, unexplained fever, and failure to gain weight. Episodes of hypernatraemic dehydration may result in seizures and

death. Mental retardation was first thought to be one of the inherited features of the disease, but it is now known to result from the acute episodes of severe hypertonic dehydration in infancy (Hillman et al 1958). These children are constantly preoccupied with drinking, ingest a hypocaloric diet, and have little opportunity for prolonged sleep. It is this preoccupation with drinking which is thought to result in the hypocaloric dwarfism and retardation of mental and emotional development. A large urinary volume and an effort to avoid urinary frequency and enuresis may result in distension and trabeculation of the bladder, with dilated ureters and calyces, which can mimic lower urinary tract obstruction. Chronic renal insufficiency may occur in late childhood. The renal lesion appears to be limited to vasopressin resistance, but associated generalized aminoaciduria and cysthioninuria have been occasionally described (Perry et al 1967).

Nephrogenic diabetes insipidus must be differentiated from the various forms of vasopressin-sensitive diabetes insipidus, as well as from a number of other renal lesions that result in an inability to reabsorb adequate amounts of filtered water. These renal disorders include glomerulonephritis, chronic pyelonephritis, obstructive uropathy, multiple myeloma, amyloidosis, hypokalaemic and hypercalcaemic nephropathy, and unilateral renal artery occlusion (Leaf & Coggins 1974). Several complex genetic disorders also result in the syndrome of vasopressin-resistant diabetes insipidus, these include sickle-cell anaemia, hereditary renal retinal dysplasia, juvenile nephronophthisis, and medullary cystic disease. The diagnosis of nephrogenic diabetes insipidus can be made only after excluding other renal and nonrenal involvement.

Bell et al (1974) demonstrated a defect in the formation of cAMP in X-linked nephrogenic diabetes insipidus, as ADH administration did not increase cyclic AMP excretion into the urine. In contrast, patients with nephrogenic diabetes insipidus have been described who increase urinary cAMP in response to ADH, and they have been referred to as nephrogenic diabetes insipidus type II (see below). A patient with nephrogenic diabetes insipidus has been described in a family with autosomal dominant hypoparathyroidism (Hunter et al 1981). Moses and Coulson (1982) documented an absence of overlapping resistance to ADH and PTH in patients with nephrogenic diabetes insipidus and pseudohypoparathyroidism, demonstrating the specificity of the renal abnormalities involved in patients with these two hormone-resistant states.

The majority of families described with nephrogenic diabetes insipidus suggest X-linked recessive inheritance (Forssman 1945, Waring et al 1945). Families with nephrogenic diabetes insipidus have been described who did not fit X-linked inheritance (Dancis et al 1948, Cannon 1955, Robinson & Kaplan 1960). The majority of these families probably represent examples of the autosomal dominant type II disease (Ohzeki et al 1984) or families in which the putative male-to-male transmission was not documented (Cannon 1955). Bode and Crawford (1969) have illustrated the unreliability of a family history for diagnostic purposes in this disease. They studied one large pedigree extending over nine generations in which male-to-male transmission was suggested by history in six instances. In three of these males concentrating ability was shown to be normal, and in the remaining three, consanguinity of the parents was documented. The great majority of heterozygous females manifest partial concentrating defects and are unable to excrete urine with a specific gravity greater than 1.018 (Bode & Crawford 1969). Discrimination by this test, however, is not perfect, as obligate heterozygotes have been reported who have normal concentrating capabilities (Feigin et al 1970). A severely affected girl was found to have a deletion of one X chromosome (Bode & Crawford 1969). A linkage study using X chromosome marker RFLPs has mapped the gene to Xq28 (Kambouris et al 1988).

Bode and Crawford (1969) have traced a large number of kindreds with this disorder to a group of Ulster Scotsmen who settled in Nova Scotia. These settlers arrived in Halifax in 1761 aboard the ship Hopewell, and the authors postulate that most, if not all, of the persons with nephrogenic diabetes insipidus in this country originated from these original settlers. At least three families with X-linked nephrogenic diabetes insipidus have been described in Blacks, and there has been a report of this disease in a large family of Samoan descent (Rimoin & Schimke 1971). Thus, although the great majority of patients with this disorder may originally have inherited their mutant gene from a common ancestor, the infrequent occurrence of new mutations is quite likely.

Nephrogenic diabetes insipidus type II

In contrast to the typical X-linked variety of nephrogenic diabetes insipidus (Type I), in which cyclic AMP excretion in the urine does not increase following ADH administration, a number of the patients with ADH unresponsive diabetes insipidus have been reported who significantly increase their AMP excretion following ADH (Zimmerman & Green 1975, Monn et al 1976, Ohzeki et al 1984). A large family with nephrogenic diabetes insipidus demonstrating autosomal dominant inheritance has been described in whom affected individuals had a six-fold increase in urinary cAMP excretion following DDAVP, but there was no significant elevation of osmolarity (Ohzeki et al 1984). Thus, the basic defect in nephrogenic diabetes insipidus type II appears to be a defect in the reception of the cAMP signal, i.e., a post receptor defect.

REFERENCES

Acers T E 1981 Optic nerve hypoplasia: septooptic dysplasia syndrome: Transactions of the American Ophthalmological Society 79: 425

Adadevoh B K 1968 Haemoglobin sickle cell disease and Sheehan's syndrome. British Journal of Clinical Practice 22: 442

Althausen T L, Kerr W J 1933 Hemochromatosis II. A report of three cases with endocrine disturbances and notes on a previously reported case; discussion of etiology. Endocrinology 17: 621

Amselem S, Duquernoy P, Attree O, Novelli G, Bousnina S, Pastel-Vinay M, Goosens M 1989 Laron dwarfism and mutations of the growth hormone receptor gene. New England Journal of Medicine 321: 989

Andler W, Roosen K, Kohns U, Stolecke H 1979 Endokrine Storungen bei Kindern mit Neurofibromatose von Recklinghausen. Monatsschrift fur Kinderheilkunde 127: 135

Angevine D M 1938 Pathologic anatomy of hypophysis and adrenals in anencephaly. Archives of Pathology 26: 507

Aragona F, Garat J, Martinez E 1983 Urological aspects of Wolfram's syndrome. European Urology 9: 75

Ardinger H, Hanson J, Zellweger H 1984 Borjeson-Forssman-Lehmann syndrome. American Journal of Medical Genetics 19: 653

August G, Rosenbaum K, Friendly D, Hung W 1983 Hypopituitarism and the CHARGE association. Journal of Pediatrics 103: 424

Bagherian V, Graham M, Gerson L P, Armstrong D L 1984 Double pituitary-glands with partial duplication of facial and fore brain structures with hydrocephalus. Computerized Radiology 8: 203

Bala R M, Beck J C 1973 Fractionation studies on plasma of normals and patients with Laron dwarfism and hypopituitary gigantism. Canadian Journal of Physiology and Pharmacology 51: 845

Bale P M, Reye R D K 1976 Epignathus, double pituitary and agenesis of corpus callosum. Journal of Pathology 120: 161

Ballard H S, Frame B, Hartsock R J 1964 Familial multiple endocrine adenomapeptic ulcer complex. Medicine 43: 481

Baumann G, Shaw M, Merimee T 1989 Low levels of high affinity growth hormone-binding protein in African pygmies. New England Journal of Medicine 320: 1705

Bell N H, Clark C M Jr., Avery S, Sinha T, Trygstad C W, Allen D O 1974 Demonstration of a defect in the formation of adenosine 3-prime, 5-prime monophosphate in vasopressin-resistant diabetes insipidus. Pediatric Research 8: 223

Benke P J, Cohen M M 1983 Recurrence of holoprosencephaly in families with a positive history. Clinical Genetics 24: 324

Benoit-Gonin J J, David M, Feit J P, Bourgeois J, Chopard A, Kopp N, Jeune M 1978 La dysplasie septo-optique avec deficit en hormone antidiuretique et insuffisance surrenal centrale. Nouvelle Presse Medicale 37: 3327

Berry S, Pierpont M, Gorlin R 1984 Single control incisor in familial holoprosencephaly. Journal of Pediatrics 104: 877

Bezwoda W R, Bothwell T H, Van Der Walt L A, Kronheim S, Pimstone B L 1977 An investigation into gonadal dysfunction in patients with idiopathic haemochromatosis. Clinical Endocrinology 6: 377

Bierich J R 1973 On the aetiology of hypopituitary dwarfism. 'Proceedings of the International Congress of Endocrinology.' Excerpta Medica, Amsterdam, p 408

Bistritzer T, Chalew S, Lovchik J, Kowarski A 1988 Growth without growth hormone – The "invisible" GH syndrome. Lancet I: 321

Blackett P R, Seif S M, Altmiller D H, Robinson A G 1983 Familial central diabetes insipidus: vasopressin and nicotine stimulated neurophysin deficiency with subnormal oxytocin and estrogen stimulated neurophysin. American Journal of Medical Sciences 286: 42

Blasi C, Pierelli F, Rispoli E, Soponara M, Vingola E, Andreani D 1986 Wolfram's syndrome: a clinical, diagnostic and interpretive contribution. Diabetes Care 9: 521

Blotner H 1942 The inheritance of diabetes insipidus. American Journal of Medical Science 204: 261

Bode H H, Crawford J D 1969 Nephrogenic diabetes insipidus in North America-the Hopewell hypothesis. New England Journal of Medicine 280: 750

Bode H H, Miettinen O S 1970 Nephrogenic diabetes insipidus: absence of close linkage with Xg. American Journal of Human Genetics 22: 221

Borges J, Blizzard R, Gelato M et al 1983 Effects of human pancreatic tumor growth hormone releasing factor on growth hormone and somatomedin C with levels in patients with ideopathic growth hormone deficiency. Lancet II: 119

Borgna-Pignatti C, DeStefano P, Zonta L et al 1985 Growth and sexual maturation in thalassemia major. Journal of Pediatrics 106: 150

Borjeson M, Forssman H, Lehmann O 1962 An X-linked, recessively inherited syndrome characterized by grave mental deficiency, epilepsy and endocrine disorders. Acta Medica Scandinavica 171: 13

Boudailliez B, Morichon-Delvallez N, Goldfarb A, Pautard J C 1983 Solitary upper incisor, hypopituitarism and monsomy 18p chromosome aberration. Journal Genetique Humaine 31: 239

Braga S, Phillips J A III, Joss E, Schwarz H, Zuppinger K 1986 Familial growth hormone deficiency resulting from a 7.6 kb deletion within the growth hormone gene cluster. American Journal of Medical Genetics 25: 443

Braunstein G D, Kohler P P 1972 Pituitary function in Hand-Schuller-Christian disease: Evidence for deficient growth-hormone release in patients with short stature. New England Journal of Medicine 286: 1225

Braunstein G D, Raiti S, Hansen J W, Kohler P O 1975 Response of growth-retarded patients with Hand-Schuller-Christian disease to growth hormone therapy. New England Journal of Medicine 292: 332

Bretz G W, Baghdassarin A, Graher J D, Zacherle B J, Norum R A, Blizzard R M 1970 Coexistence of diabetes mellitus and insipidus and optic atrophy in two male siblings. American Journal of Medicine 48: 398

Bright G, Rogol A, Johanson A, Blizzard R 1983 Short stature associated with normal growth hormone and decreased somatomedin-C concentrations. Pediatrics 71: 576

Cannon J F 1955 Diabetes insipidus: clinical and experimental studies with consideration of genetic relationship. Archives of Internal Medicine 96: 215

Carson M J, Slager U T, Steinberg R M 1972 Occurrence of diabetes insipidus, simultaneous and optic atrophy in a brother and sister. American Journal of Diseases of Children 131: 1382

Charbonnel B, Chupin M, LeGrand A, Guillon J 1981 Pituitary function in idiopathic hemochromatosis: hormonal study in 36 male patients. Acta Endocrinologica 98: 178–183

Clarke W L, Weldon V V 1975 Growth hormone deficiency and Fanconi anaemia. Journal of Pediatrics 86: 814

Clarren S K, Alvord E C, Hall J G 1980 Congenital hypothalamic hamartoblastoma, hypopituitarism imperforate anus and postaxial polydactyl – a new syndrome? Part II. American Journal of Medical Genetics 7: 75

Cohen M M, Jirasek J E, Guzman R T, Gorlin R J, Peterson M Q 1971 Holoprosencephaly and facial dysmorphia. Birth Defects: Original Article Series 7(7): 125

Costin G, Kogut M D, Hyman C B, Ortega J 1972 Fanconi's anaemia associated with isolated growth hormone (GH) deficiency. Clinical Research 20: 253

Costom B H, Grumbach M M, Kaplan S L 1971 Effect of thyrotropin-releasing factor on serum thyroid stimulating hormone. Journal of Clinical Investigation 50: 2219

Crawford J D, Bode H H 1975 Disorders of the posterior pituitary in children. In: Gardner L I (ed) Endocrine and Genetic Diseases of Childhood. W B Saunders, Philadelphia p 126

Culler F, Jones K 1984 Hypopituitarism in association with post-axial polydactyly. Journal of Pediatrics 104: 881

Culpepper R, Hebert S, Andreoli T 1985 The posterior pituitary and water metabolism. In: Wilson J, Foster D (eds) Williams textbook of endocrinology, 7th edn. Saunders, Philadelphia, p 155

Cussen L J 1965 Primary hypopituitary dwarfism with Fanconi's hypoplastic anaemia syndrome, renal hypertension and phycomycosis: Report of a case. Medical Journal of Australia 2: 367

Dancis J, Birmingham J R, Leslie S H 1948 Congenital diabetes insipidus resistant to treatment with pitressin. American Journal of Diseases of Children 75: 316

Daughaday W H 1985 The anterior pituitary. In: Wilson J, Foster D (eds) Williams textbook of endocrinology, 7th edn. Saunders, Philadelphia

Daughaday W, Trivedi B 1987 Absence of serum growth hormone binding protein in patients with growth hormone receptor deficiency (Laron dwarfism). Proceedings of the National Academy of Sciences 84: 4636

Davenport S, Hefner M, Mitchell J 1986 The spectrum of clinical features of CHARGE syndrome. Clinical Genetics 29: 298

de Morsier G 1956 Etudes sur les dysraphies cranio-encephaliques. III. Agenesie du septum lucidum avec malformation du tractus optique: La dysplasie septo-optique. Schweitzer Archiv fur Neurologie, Neurochirurgie und Psychiatrie 77: 267

DeRobertis F, Michelis N, Bells N et al 1971 "Essential" hypernatremia due to ineffective osmotic and intact volume regulation of vasopressin secretion. Journal of Clinical Investigation 50: 97

Donaldson M D C, Tucker S M, Grant D B 1980 Recessively inherited growth hormone deficiency in a family from Iraq. Journal of Medical Genetics 17: 288

Edmonds H W 1950 Pituitary, adrenal and thyroid in cyclopia. Archives of Pathology 50: 727

Ehrlich R M 1957 Ectopic and hypoplastic pituitary with adrenal hypoplasia. Journal of Pediatrics 51: 377

Elders M J, Garland J T, Daughaday W A, Fisher D A, Whitney J E, Hughes E R 1973 Laron's dwarfism: studies on the nature of the defect. Journal of Pediatrics 83: 253

Ellyin F, Khatir A H, Singh S P 1980 Hypothalamic – pituitary functions in patients with transsphenoidal encephalocoele and midfacial anomalies. Journal of Clinical Endocrinology 51: 854

Eshet R, Laron Z, Brown M, Arnon R 1973 Immunoreactive properties of the plasma hGH from patients with the syndrome of familial dwarfism and high plasma IR-hGH. Journal of Clinical Endocrinology and Metabolism 37: 819

Eshet R, Laron Z, Pertzelon A, Arnon R, Dintzman M 1984 Defect of human growth hormone receptors in the liver of two patients with Laron type dwarfism. Israel Journal of Medical Sciences 20: 8

Faggiano M, Minozzi M, Lombardi G, Carella C, Criscoulo T 1975 Two cases of the chromatin positive variety of ovarian dysgenesis (XO/XX mosaicism) associated with hGH deficiency and marginal impairment of other hypothalamic-pituitary functions. Clinical Genetics 8: 324

Feigin R D, Rimoin D L, Kaufman R L 1970 Nephrogenic diabetes insipidus in a Negro kindred. American Journal of Diseases of Children 120: 64

Feingold M, Shiere F, Fogels H R, Donaldson D 1969 Rieger's syndrome. Pediatrics 44: 564

Ferrier P E, Stone E F 1969 Familial pituitary dwarfism associated with an abnormal sella turcica. Pediatrics 43: 858

Fishman L, Ehrlich R 1986 Wolfram syndrome: report of four new cases and a review of the literature. Diabetes Care 9: 405

Fleisher T A, White R M, Broder S et al 1980 X-linked hypogammaglobulinemia and isolated growth hormone deficiency. New England Journal of Medicine 302: 1429

Folley T P, Owings J, Hayford J T, Blizzard R M 1972 Serum thyrotropin responses to synthetic thyrotropin-releasing hormone in normal children and hypopituitary patients. Journal of Clinical Investigation 51: 431

Forssman H 1945 On hereditary diabetes insipidus. With special reference to a sex-linked form. Acta Medica Scandinavica 121: 1

Frances J M, Knorr D, Martinez R, Neuhauser G 1966 Hypophysarer Zwergwuchs bei Lippen-Kiefer-Spalte. Helvetica Paediatrica Acta 21: 315

Fraser F C, Gunn T 1977 Diabetes mellitus, diabetes insipidus, and optic atrophy. An autosomal recessive syndrome? Journal of Medical Genetics 14: 190

Frazer T, Gavin J R, Daughaday W H, Hillman R E,

Weldon V 1982 Growth hormone-dependent growth failure. Journal of Pediatrics 101: 12

Frisch H, Phillips J A III 1986 Growth hormone deficiency due to GH-N gene deletion in an Austrian family. Acta Endocrinologica 113: 107

Fryns J, Van den Berghe H 1988 Single central maxillary incisor and holoprosencephaly. American Journal of Medical Genetics 30: 943

Gaupp R 1941 Ueber den Diabetes Insipidus, Zentralblatt fur die gesamte Neurologie und Psychiatrie 171: 514

Geffner M, Bersch N, Kaplan S et al 1986 Growth without growth hormone: evidence for a patient circulating human growth factor. Lancet I: 343

Geffner M, Golde D, Lippe B, Kaplan S, Bersch N, Li C 1987 Tissues of the Laron dwarf are sensitive to insulin-like growth factor I but not to growth hormone. Journal of Clinical Endocrinology and Metabolism 64: 1042

Gleadhill V, Bridges J M, Hadden D R 1975 Fanconi's aplastic anaemia with short stature. Absence of response to human growth hormone. Archives of Disease in Childhood 50: 318

Golde D W, Bersch N, Kaplan S, Rimoin D L, Li C H 1980 Peripheral unresponsiveness to human growth hormone in Laron dwarfism. New England Journal of Medicine 303: 1156

Goldstein S, Wu R, Thorpy M, Shprintzen R, Marion R, Saarger P 1987 Reversibility of deficient sleep entrained growth hormone secretion in a boy with achondroplasia and obstructive sleep apnea. Acta Endocrinologica 116: 95

Goossens M, Brauner R, Czernichow P, Duquesnoy P, Rappaport R 1986 Isolated growth hormone (GH) deficiency type IA associated with a double deletion in the human GH gene cluster. Journal of Clinical Endocrinology and Metabolism 62: 712

Gorlin R, Yunis J, Anderson V 1968 Short arm deletion of chromosome 18 in cebocephaly. American Journal of Diseases of Children 115: 473

Gorlin R J, Cervenka J, Moller K, Horrobin M, Witkop C J 1975 A selected miscellany. Birth Defects Original Article Series XI(2): 39

Gossain V V, Sugawara M, Hagen G A 1975 Co-existent diabetes mellitus and diabetes insipidus, a familial disease. Journal of Clinical Endocrinology and Metabolism 41: 1020

Graham J, Saunders R, Fratkin J, Spiegel P, Harris M, Klein R 1986 A cluster of Pallister-Hall syndrome cases. American Journal of Medical Genetics Supplement 2: 53

Green J R, Buchan G C, Alvard E J Jr., Savonson A G 1967 Hereditary and idiopathic types of diabetes insipidus. Brain 90: 707

Grossman A, Savage M, Wass J, Lytras N, Sueiras-Diaz J, Coy D, Besser G 1983 Growth hormone-releasing factor in growth hormone deficiency: demonstration of a hypothalamic defect in growth hormone release. Lancet II: 137

Grunt J A, Reynolds D W 1970 Insulin, blood sugar and growth hormone levels in anencephalic infant before and after intravenous administration of glucose. Journal of Pediatrics 76: 112

Gunn T, Bortolussi R, Little J M, Andermann F, Fraser F C, Belmonte M M 1976 Juvenile diabetes, optic atrophy, sensory nerve deafness, and diabetes insipidus – a syndrome. Journal of Pediatrics 89: 565

Hall J G, Pallister P D, Clarren S K et al 1980 Congenital hypothalamic hamartoblastoma, hypopituitarism, imperforate anus and postaxial polydactyly – a new syndrome? Part 1. American Journal of Medical Genetics 7: 47

Harris R J, Haas L 1972 Septo-optic dysplasia with growth hormone deficiency (de Morsier syndrome). Archives of Disease in Childhood 47: 973

Hattori H, Okuno T, Momoi T, Kataoka K, Mikawa H, Shiota K 1987 Single central maxillary incisor and holoprosencephaly. American Journal of Medical Genetics 28: 483

Haworth J C, Medovy H, Lewis A J 1961 Cebocephaly with endocrine dysgenesis. Journal of Pediatrics 59: 726

Hayek A, Driscoll S G, Warshaw J B 1973 Endocrine studies in anencephaly. Journal of Clinical Investigation 52: 636

Hayek A, Peake G T, Greenberg R E 1978 A new syndrome of short stature due to biologically inactive growth hormone. Pediatric Research 12: 413

Herman S P, Baggenstoss A H, Cloutier M D 1975 Liver dysfunction and histologic abnormalities in neonatal hypopituitarism. Journal of Pediatrics 87: 892

Hewer T F 1944 Ateliotic dwarfism with normal sexual function: A result of hypopituitarism. Journal of Endocrinology 3: 397

Hillman D A, Neyzi O, Porter P, Cushman A, Talbot N B 1958 Renal (vasopressin resistant) diabetes insipidus: definition of the effects of a homeostatic limitation in capacity to conserve water on the physical, intellectual and emotional development of a child. Pediatrics 21: 430

Hintz R L, Menking M, Sotos J T 1968 Familial holoprosencephaly with endocrine dysgenesis. Journal of Pediatrics 72: 81

Hook E B, Reynolds J W 1967 Cerebral gigantism: endocrinological and clinical observations of six patients including a congenital giant, concordant monozygotic twins and a child who achieved adult gigantic size. Journal of Pediatrics 70: 900

Hoyt W F, Kaplan S L, Grumbach M M et al 1970 Septo-optic dysplasia with pituitary dwarfism. Lancet 1: 893

Hunter W, Heick H, Poznanski W, McLaine J 1981 Autosomal dominant hypoparathyroidism: a proband with concurrent nephrogenic diabetes insipidus. Journal of Medical Genetics 18: 431

Huseman C, Kelch R, Hopwood N, Zipf W 1978 Sexual precocity in association with septo-optic dysplasia and hypothalamic hypopituitarism. Journal of Pediatrics 92: 748

Illig R 1970 Growth hormone antibodies in patients treated with different preparations of human growth hormone (HGH). Journal of Clinical Endocrinology 42: 403

Jacobs L S, Sneid D S, Garland J T, Laron Z, Daughaday W A 1976 Receptoractive growth hormone in Laron dwarfism. Journal of Clinical Endocrinology 42: 403

Jarnerot G 1973 Diabetes mellitus with optic atrophy-thalassemia-like sideroblastic anemia and weak isoagglutinins – a new genetic syndrome. Acta Medica Scandinavica 193: 359

Jones K 1988 Smith's Recognizable Patterns of Human Malformation, 4th edn. Saunders, Philadelphia

Juberg R, Hayward J 1969 A new familial syndrome of oral, cranial and digital anomalies. Journal of Pediatrics 74: 755

Kambouris M, Bledlouhy S R, Trofatter J A, Conneally P M, Hodes M E 1988 Location of the gene for X-linked nephrogenic diabetes insipidus to X-q 28. American Journal of Medical Genetics 29: 239

Kaplowitz P, D'Ercole J, Robertson G 1982 Radioimmunoassay of vasopressin in familial central diabetes insipidus. Journal of Pediatrics 100: 76

Kauli R, Pertzelan A, Prager-Lewin R, Maimon Z, Ovadia J, Laron Z 1979 XY gonadal dysgenesis associated with hGH and gonadotrophin deficiencies. Clinical Genetics 15: 369

Kingston H, Hughes I, Harper P 1982 Orocraniodigital (Juberg-Hayward) syndrome with growth hormone deficiency. Archives of Disease in Childhood 57: 790

Kleinmann R E, Kazarian E L, Raptopoulos V, Braverman L E 1981 Primary empty sella and Rieger's anomaly of the anterior chamber of the eye. New England Journal of Medicine 304: 90

Knudtzon J, Aarskog D 1987 Growth hormone deficiency associated with the ectrodactyly-ectodermal dysplasia-clefting syndrome and isolated absent septum pellucidum. Pediatrics 79: 410

Koch G, Tiwisina T 1959 Beitrag Zur Erblichkeit der Akromegalie und der Hyperostosis Generalisata mit Pachydermie. Arzneimittel-Forschung 13: 489

Kodama M, Fujimoto S, Namikawa T, Matsuda J 1981 Aarskog syndrome with isolated growth hormone deficiency. European Journal of Pediatrics 135: 273

Kowarski A A, Schneider J, Ben-Galim E, Weldon V V, Daughaday W H 1978 Growth failure with normal serum RIA-GH and low somatomedin activity: somatomedin restoration and growth acceleration after exogenous GH. Journal of Clinical Endocrinology 47: 461

Lacombe L U 1941 De la polydipsia. L'experience 7: 309

Laczi F, Julesz J, Janaky T, Lazlo F 1979 Growth hormone reserve capacity in Turner's syndrome. Hormone and Metabolic Research 11: 664

Lanes R, Plotnick L P, Spencer E M, Daughaday W A, Kowarski A A 1980 Dwarfism associated with normal serum growth hormone and increased bioassayable, receptorassayable, and immunoassayable somatomedin. Journal of Clinical Endocrinology 50: 485

Laron Z 1974 Syndrome of familial dwarfism and high plasma immunoreactive growth hormone. Israel Journal of Medical Science 10: 1247

Laron Z, Pertzelan A, Karp M 1966 Pituitary dwarfism with high serum concentration of human growth hormone – A new inborn error in metabolism? Israel Journal of Medical Science 2: 152

Laron Z, Taube E, Kaplan I 1969 Pituitary growth hormone insufficiency associated with cleft lip and palate. An embryonal developmental defect. Helvetica Paediatrica Acta 24: 576

Laron Z, Pertzelan A, Karp M, Kowaldo-Silbergeld A, Daughaday W H 1971 Administration of growth hormone to patients with familial dwarfism with high plasma immunoreactive growth hormone. Journal of Clinical Endocrinology 33: 332

Laron Z, Kelijman M, Pertzelan A, Keret R, Shoffner J M, Parks J S 1985 Human growth hormone gene deletion without antibody formation or growth arrest during treatment – a new disease entity. Israel Journal of Medical Science 21: 999

Laron Z, Klinger B, Erster B, Anin S 1988 Effect of acute administration of insulin-like growth factor in patients with Laron-type dwarfism. Lancet II: 1170

Larsen P, Snyder E, Matsuo F, Watanabe S, Johnson L 1983 Achondroplasia associated with obstructive sleep apnea. Archives of Neurology 40: 769

Latorre H, Kenney F M, Lahey M E, Drash A 1974 Short stature and growth hormone deficiency in histiocytosis X. Journal of Pediatrics 85: 813

Leaf A, Coggins C H 1974 The Neurohypophysis: In: William R H (ed) Textbook of Endocrinology, 5th edn. Saunders, Philadelphia

LeBriggs R, Powell J R 1969 Chiari-Frommel syndrome as part of the Zollinger-Ellison multiple endocrine adenomatosis complex. California Medicine 111: 92

Lehman R A W, Stears J C, Wesenberg R L, Nusbaum E D 1977 Familial osteosclerosis with abnormalities of the nervous system and meninges. Journal of Pediatrics 90: 49

Lehmann V W 1964 Krankheiten der Drusen mit innerer Sekretion. In: Becker P E (ed) Humangenetik. Verlang, Stuttgart

Leisti J, Leiti S, Perheentupa J, Savilahti E, Aula P 1973 Absence of IgA and growth hormone deficiency associated with short arm deletion of chromosome 18. Archives of Disease in Childhood 48:320

Leva J 1915 Uber familiare Akromegalie. Medicine Klink 11: 1266

Levin S R, Hafeldt F D, Becker N, Wilson C B, Seymour R, Forsham P H 1974 Hypersomatotropism and acanthosis nigricans in two brothers. Archives of Internal Medicine 134: 365

Lieblich J M, Rosen S W, Guyda H, Reardan J, Schaaf M 1978 The syndrome of basal encephalocoele and hypothalamic-pituitary dysfunction. Annals of Internal Medicine 89: 910

Linquette M, Herlant M, Laine E, Fossati P, Dupont-Lecompte M 1967 Adenome a prolactine chez une jeune fille dont la mére etait porteuse adénome hypophysaire avec fille dont la mére etait porteuse adénome hypophysaire avec aménorrhée. Annals of Endocrinology (Paris) 28: 773

Lovinger R D, Kaplan S L, Grumbach M M 1975 Congenital hypopituitarism associated with neonatal hypoglycaemia. Journal of Pediatrics 87: 1171

Lowry R B 1974 Holoprosencephaly. American Journal of Diseases of Children 128: 887

McArthur R G, Morgan K, Phillips J A III, Bala M, Klassen J 1985 The natural history of familial hypopituitarism. American Journal of Medical Genetics 22: 553

McCormick W F 1961 Abnormal hemoglobins II. The pathology of sickle cell trait. American Journal of Medical Sciences 91: 329

MacDonald R A, Mallory G K 1960 Hemochromatosis and hemosiderosis. Study of 11 autopsied cases. Archives of Internal Medicine 105: 686

McNeil L W, McKee L C, Lorber D, Rabin D 1983 The endocrine manifestations of hemochromatosis. American Journal of Medical Sciences 285: 7

Majzoub J, Pappey A, Burg R, Habener J 1984 Vasopressin gene is expressed at low levels in the hypothalamus of the Brattleboro rat. Proceedings of the National Academy of Sciences 81: 5296

Manelfe C, Rochicciolo P 1979 CT of septo-optic dysplasia. American Journal of Roentgenology 133: 1157

Margalith D, Tzo W J, Jan N E 1985 Congenital optic nerve hypoplasia with hypothalamic-pituitary dysplasia. American Journal of Diseases of Children 139: 361

Martin F I R 1959 Familial diabetes insipidus. Quarterly Journal of Medicine 28: 573

Medeiros-Neto G A, Toledo S P A, Pupo A A et al 1973 Characterization of the LH response to luteinizing hormone-releasing hormone (LH-RH) in isolated and multiple tropic hormone deficiencies. Journal of Clinical Endocrinology and Metabolism 37: 972

Merimee T J, Rimoin D L, Hall J D, McKusick V A 1969 A metabolic and hormonal basis for classifying ateliotic dwarfs. Lancet 1: 963

Merimee T J, Rimoin D L, Penetti E, Cavalli-Sforza L L 1972 Growth retardation in the African pygmy. Journal of Clinical Investigation 51: 395

Merimee T J, Ostrow P, Aisner S C 1975 Clinical and pathological studies in a growth hormone-deficient dwarf. Johns Hopkins Medical Journal 136: 150

Merimee T J, Zapf J, Froesch E R 1981 Dwarfism in the pygmy. An isolated deficiency of insulin-like growth factor I. New England Journal of Medicine 305:965

Merimee T, Zapf J, Hewett B, Cavalli-Sforza L 1987 Insulin-like growth factors in pygmies. The role of puberty in determining final stature. New England Journal of Medicine 316: 906

Merle P, Georget A M, Goumy P, Jarlot D 1979 Primary empty sella turcica in children: report of two familial cases. Pediatric Radiology 8: 209

Metlay L, Smythe P, Miller M 1987 Familial CHARGE syndrome. American Journal of Medical Genetics 26: 577

Miller W L, Eberhardt N L 1983 Structure and evolution of the growth hormone gene family. Endocrine Reviews 4: 97

Mitrakou A, Hadiidakis D, Raptis S, Bartsocas C S, Souvatzoglou A 1985 Heterogeneity of growth hormone deficiency. Lancet I: 399

Moncrieff M W, Hill D S, Archer J, Arthur L J H 1972 Congenital absence of pituitary gland and adrenal hypoplasia. Archives of Disease in Childhood 47: 136

Monn E, Osnes J, Oye I 1976 Basal and hormone-induced urinary cyclic AMP in children with renal disorders. Acta Paediatrica Scandinavica 65: 739

Morishima A, Aranoff G S 1986 Syndrome of septo-optic dysplasia: the clinical spectrum. Brain and Development 8: 233

Moses A, Coulson B 1982 Absence of overlapping resistance to vasopressin and parathyroid hormone in patients with nephrogenic diabetes insipidus and pseudohypoparathyroidism. Journal of Clinical Endocrinology and Metabolism 55: 699

Mosier H D 1957 Hypoplasia of the pituitary and adrenal cortex: Report of occurrence in twin siblings and autopsy findings. Journal of Pediatrics 51: 377

Naeye R L, Blanc W A 1971 Organ and body growth in anencephaly. Archives of Pathology 91: 140

Nagai I, Li C H, Hsieh S M, Kizaki T, Urano Y 1984 Two cases of hereditary diabetes insipidus, with an autopsy finding in one. Acta Endocrinologica 105: 318

Najjar S S, Khachadurian A K, Ilbawi M N, Blizzard R M 1971 Dwarfism with elevated levels of plasma growth hormone. New England Journal of Medicine 284: 809

Nevin N, Henry P, Thomas P 1981 A case of the orocraniodigital (Juberg-Hayward) syndrome. Journal of Medical Genetics 18: 478

Nilsson L R 1960 Chronic pancytopenia with multiple congenital abnormalities. Acta Paediatrica 49: 518

Nishi Y, Aihara K, Usui T, Phillips J A III, Mallonee R L, Migeon C J 1984 Isolated growth hormone deficiency type IA in a Japanese family. Journal of Pediatrics 104: 885

Ohzeki T, Igarashi T, Okamoto A 1984 Familial cases of congenital nephrogenic diabetes insipidus type II: remarkable increment of urinary adenosine 3-prime, 5-prime-monophosphate in response to antidiuretic hormone. Journal of Pediatrics 104: 593

Pagon R A, Stephan M J 1984 Septo-optic dysplasia with digital anomalies. Journal of Pediatrics 105: 966

Pagon R A, Graham J, Zonara J, Young S L 1981 Coloboma, congenital heart disease and choanal atresia with multiple anomalies: CHARGE association. Journal of Pediatrics 99: 223

Parks J S, Tenore A, Bongiovanni A M, Kirkland R T 1978 Familial hypopituitarism with large sella turcica. New England Journal of Medicine 298: 698

Parks J S, Nielsen P V, Sexton L A, Jorgensen E H 1985 An effect of gene dosage on production of human chorionic sommatomammotropin. Journal of Clinical Endocrinology and Metabolism 60: 944

Pastore R A, Anderson J W, Herman R H 1969 Anterior and posterior hypopituitarism associated with sickle cell trait. Annals of Internal Medicine 71: 593

Patel H, Tze J W, Crichton J U et al 1975 Optic nerve hypoplasia with hypopituitarism. American Journal of Diseases of Children 129: 175

Pedersen E B, Lamm L U, Albertsen K et al 1985 Familial cranial diabetes insipidus: a report of five families: genetic, diagnostic and therapeutic aspects. Quarterly Journal of Medicine 57: 883

Peillon F, Racadot J 1969 Modifications histopatholoques de l'hypophyse dans six cas d'hemochromatose. Annales Endocrinologie (Paris) 30: 800

Pender C B, Fraser F C 1953 Dominant inheritance of diabetes insipidus. Pediatrics 11: 246

Perry T L, Robinson G C, Teasdale J M, Hansen S 1967 Cystathioninuria, nephrogenic diabetes insipidus and anemia. New England Journal of Medicine 276: 721

Phebus C, Gloninger M, Maciak B 1984 Growth patterns by age and sex in children with sickle cell disease. Journal of Pediatrics 105: 28

Phelan P D, Connelly J, Martin F I R, Wettenhall H N B 1971 X-linked recessive hypopituitarism. In: The Endocrine System, Birth Defects: Original Article Series vol VII, no. 6. Williams and Wilkins, Baltimore, for The National Foundation – March of Dimes, Part X, p 21

Phillips J A III 1985 Genetic diagnosis: differentiating growth disorders. Hospital Practice 20: 85

Phillips J A 1989 Inherited defects in growth hormone synthesis and action. In: Stanbury J, Wyngaarden J B, Fredrickson D S, Goldstein J L, Brown M S (eds) The metabolic basis of inherited disease, 6th edn. McGraw-Hill, New York

Phillips J A, Hjelle B L, Seeburg P H, Zachmann M 1981 Molecular basis of familial isolated growth hormone deficiency. Proceedings of the National Academy of Sciences USA 78: 6372

Phillips J A III, Parks J S, Hjelle B L, Herk J E, Plotnick L P, Migeon C J, Seeberg P H 1982 Genetic analysis of familial isolated growth hormone deficiency, Type I. Journal of Clinical Investigation 70: 489

Phillips J A III, Ferrandez A, Frisch H, Illig R, Zuppinger K 1986 Defects of GH genes: clinical syndromes. In: Raiti S, Tolman R (eds) Human growth hormone. Plenum, New York, p 221–226

Pierson M, Malaprade D, Fortier G, Belleville F, Lasbennes A, Wuilbreq L 1978 Le nanisme familial de type Laron, deficit genetique primaire en somatomedine. Archives Francais Pediatrics 35: 151

Pochedly C, Collip P J, Wolman S R et al 1971 Fanconi's anemia with growth hormone deficiency. Journal of Pediatrics 79: 93

Pollock J A, Newton T H, Hoyt W 1968 Transsphenoidal and transethmoidal encephaloceles. Radiology 90: 442

Poskitt E M E, Rayner P H W 1974 Isolated growth hormone deficiency. Two families with autosomal dominant inheritance. Archives of Disease in Childhood 49: 55

Rappaport E B, Ulstrom R A, Gorlin R J, Lucky A W, Colle E, Miser J 1977 Solitary maxillary central incisor and short stature. Journal of Pediatrics 91: 924

Richardson J E, Hamilton W 1977 Diabetes insipidus, diabetes mellitus, optic atrophy and deafness. Archives of Disease in Childhood 52: 796

Riddell D C, Mallonee R, Phillips J A, Parks J S, Sexton L A, Hamerton J L 1985 Chromosomal assignments of human sequences encoding arginine vasopressin-neurophysin II and growth hormone releasing factor. Somatic Cell Molecular Genetics 11: 189

Rimoin D L 1976 Hereditary forms of growth hormone deficiency and resistance. Birth Defects: Original Article Series 12(6): 15

Rimoin D L, Schechter J E 1973 Histological and ultrastructural studies in isolated growth hormone deficiency. Journal of Clinical Endocrinology and Metabolism 37: 725

Rimoin D L, Schimke R N 1971 Genetic disorders of the endocrine glands. Mosby, St Louis

Rimoin D L, Merimee T J, Rabinowitz D, McKusick V A 1968 Genetic aspects of clinical endocrinology. Recent Progress in Hormone Research 24: 365

Rimoin D L, Merimee T J, Rabinowitz D et al 1969 Peripheral subresponsiveness of human growth hormone in the African pygmies. New England Journal of Medicine 281: 1383

Rimoin D L, Borochowitz Z, Horton W A 1986 Short stature-physiology and pathology. Western Journal of Medicine 144: 710

Rivarola M A, Phillips J A III, Migeon C J, Heinrich J J, Hjelle B J 1984 Phenotypic heterogeneity in familial isolated growth hormone deficiency (IGHD) Type A. Journal of Clinical Endocrinology and Metabolism 59: 34

Robinson L, Jones K, Culler F, Nyhan W, Sakati N 1983 The Borjeson-Forssman-Lehmann syndrome. American Journal of Medical Genetics 15: 457

Robinson M G, Kaplan S A 1960 Inheritance of vasopressin resistant ('nephrogenic') diabetes insipidus. American Journal of Diseases of Children 99: 164

Rogol A, Blizzard R, Foley T, Furlanetto R, Selden R, Mayo K, Thorner M 1985 Growth hormone releasing hormone and growth hormone: genetic studies in familial growth hormone deficiency. Pediatric Research 19: 489

Roitman A, Laron Z 1978 Hypothalamic-pituitary hormone insufficiency associated with cleft lip and palate. Archives of Disease in Childhood 53: 952

Romshe C A, Sotos J F 1973 Hypothalamic-pituitary dysfunction in siblings of patients with holoprosencephaly. Journal of Pediatrics 83: 1088

Rosenfield R L, Root A W, Bongiovanni A M, Eberlein W R 1967 Idiopathic anterior hypopituitarism in one of monozygotic twins. Journal of Pediatrics 70: 114–117

Ross J, Long L, Loriaux D, Cutler G 1985 Growth

hormone secretory dynamics in Turner syndrome. Journal of Pediatrics 106:202

Royer P, Rappaport R, Gabilan J C, Canet J, Bonnici F 1970 Manifestations hypoglycemiques initials dans une forme familiale de defaut isole en somathormone. Annales de Pediatrie 17: 828

Rudman D, Davis G T, Priest J H Patterson J H, Kutner M H, Heymsfield S B, Bethel R A 1978 Prevalence of growth hormone deficiency with cleft lip or palate. Journal of Pediatrics 93: 378

Rudman D, Kutner M H, Goldsmith M A, Kenny J, Jennings H, Bain R P 1980 Further observations on four subgroups of normal variant short stature. Journal of Clinical Endocrinology and Metabolism 51: 1378

Rudman D, Kutner M H, Blackston R D, Cushman R A, Bain R P, Patterson J H 1981 Children with normal variant short stature: Treatment with human growth hormone for six months. New England Journal of Medicine 305: 123

Sadeghi-Nejad A, Senior B 1974a A familial syndrome of isolated 'aplasia' of the anterior pituitary. Journal of Pediatrics 84: 79

Sadeghi-Nejad A, Senior B 1974b Autosomal dominant transmission of isolated growth hormone deficiency in iris-dental dysplasia (Rieger's syndrome). Journal of Pediatrics 85: 644

Saldanha P, Toledo S 1981 Familial dwarfism with high IR-GH: Report of two affected siblings with genetic and epidemiologic considerations. Human Genetics 59: 367

Saxena K M 1970 Endocrine manifestations of neurofibromatosis in children. American Journal of Diseases of Children 120: 265

Scherbaum W, Czernichow G, Bottazzo G, Doniach D 1985 Diabetes insipidus in children: IV. A possible autoimmune type with vasopressin cell antibodies. Journal of Pediatrics 107: 922

Schimke R N, Spaulding J J, Hollowell J G 1971 X-linked congenital panhypopituitarism. In: Bergsma D (ed) The Endocrine System, Birth Defects: Original Article Series 7(6): 21. Williams and Wilkins, Baltimore, for The National Foundation – March of Dimes, Part X

Schmale H, Richter D 1984 Single base deletion in the vasopressin gene is the cause of diabetes insipidus in Brattleboro rats. Nature 308: 705

Schweiger M, Auer B, Burtscher H J, Hirsch-Kauffmann M, Klocker H, Schneider R 1987 DNA repair in human cells: biochemistry of the hereditary diseases Fanconi's anaemia and Cockayne syndrome. European Journal of Biochemistry 165: 235

Sheikholislam B M, Stempfel R S 1972 Hereditary isolated somatotropin deficiency: Effects of human growth hormone administration. Pediatrics 49: 362

Shohat M, Hermon V, Melmed S et al 1990 Deletion of 20p 11.23→pter with growth hormone neurosecretory disorder but normal growth hormone releasing hormone genes. American Journal of Medical Genetics (in press)

Sipponen P, Simila S, Collan Y, Autere T, Herva R 1978 Familial syndrome with panhypopituitarism, hypoplasia of the hypophysis, and poorly developed sella turcica. Archives of Disease in Childhood 53: 664

Sokol H, Valtin H 1982 The Brattleboro rat: Proceedings of the International Symposium. Annals of the New York Academy of Science 394: 1

Stanley C A, Spielman R S, Zmijewski C M, Baker L 1979 Wolfram syndrome not HLA linked. New England Journal of Medicine 301: 1398

Steiner M M, Boggs J D 1965 Absence of pituitary gland, hypothyroidism, hypoadrenalism and hypogonadism in a 17-year-old dwarf. Journal of Clinical Endocrinology and Metabolism 25: 1591

Stewart C, Castro-Magana M, Sherman J, Angulo M, Collipp P 1983 Septo-optic dysplasia and median cleft face syndrome in a patient with isolated growth hormone deficiency and hyperprolactinemia. American Journal of Diseases of Children 137: 484

Stocks A E, Martin F I R 1968 Pituitary function in haemochromatosis. American Journal of Medicine 45: 839

Stokes D, Phillips J, Leonard C, Dorst J, Kopits S, Trojack J, Brown D 1983 Respiratory complications of achondroplasia. Journal of Pediatrics 102: 534

Stoll C, Willard D, Czornichow P, Boue J 1978 Prenatal diagnosis of primary pituitary dysgenesis. Lancet 1: 932

Stoll C, Talon P, Mengus L, Roth M, Dott B 1985 A Weaver-like syndrome with endocrinological abnormalities in a boy and his mother. Clinical Genetics 28: 255

Tani N, Kaneko K, Mornotsu et al 1987 A family case with autosomal dominantly-inherited pituitary dwarfism. Tohoku Journal of Experimental Medicine 152: 319

Toth E L, Bowen P A, Crockford P M 1984 Hereditary central diabetes insipidus: plasma levels of antidiuretic hormone in a family with a possible osmoreceptor defect. Canadian Medical Association Journal 131: 1237

Toublanc J E, Chaussain J L, Lejeune D, dePaillerets F, Job J C 1976 Hypopituitarisme avec hypoplasie des nerfs optiques. Archives Francais Pediatrie 33: 67

Turnbridge R E, Paley R G 1956 Primary optic atrophy in diabetes mellitus. Diabetes 2: 295

Underwood L E, Van Wyk J J 1985 Normal and aberrant growth. In Wilson J, Foster E (eds), Williams textbook of endocrinology, 7th edn. Saunders, Philadelphia, p155

Valenta L, Siegel M, Lesniak M, Elias M, Lewis U, Friesen H, Kershnar A 1985 Pituitary dwarfism in a patient with circulating abnormal growth hormone polymers. New England Journal of Medicine 312: 214

Valtin H 1969 Hereditary diabetes insipidus – lessons learned from animal models. Excerpta Medica International Congress 184: 321

Valtin H 1976 Hereditary hypothalamic diabetes insipidus. American Journal of Pathology 83: 633

Van den Brande J L, Du Caju M V L, Visser H K A et al 1974 Primary somatomedin deficiency. Archives of Disease in Childhood 49: 297

Vanelli M, Bernasconi S, Balestrazzi P 1980 Solitary maxillary central incisor with growth hormone deficiency. Archives Francais Pediatrie 37: 321

Van Gemund J J, de Angulo M S L, Van Gelderen H H 1969 Familial prenatal dwarfism with elevated serum immunoreactive growth hormone levels and end-organ unresponsiveness. Maandsch, Kindergeneesk 37: 372

Vokes T, Gaskill M, Robertson G 1988 Antibodies to vasopressin in patients with diabetes insipidus. Annals of Internal Medicine 108: 190

Vrencak-Jones C, Phillips J, Chen E, Seeburg P 1988 Molecular basis of human growth hormone gene deletions. Proceedings of the National Academy of Sciences 85: 5615

Walker N F, Rance C P 1954 Inheritance of diabetes insipidus. American Journal of Human Genetics 6:354

Walsh C H, Wright A D, Williams J W, Holder G 1976 A study of pituitary function in patients with idiopathic hemochromatosis. Journal of Clinical Endocrinology and Metabolism 43: 866

Waring A J, Kajdi L, Tappan V 1945 A congenital defect of water metabolism. American Journal of Diseases of Children 69: 323

Weber F T, Donnelly W H, Bejar R L 1977 Hypopituitarism following extirpation of a pharyngeal pituitary. American Journal of Diseases of Children 131: 525

Weber F, Frias J, Julius R, Felman A 1978 Primary hypogonadism in the Borjeson-Forssman-Lehmann syndrome. Journal of Medical Genetics 15: 63

Wesley R, Hoffman W, Perrin J, Delaney J 1978 Solitary maxillary control incisor and normal stature. Oral Surgery 46: 837

Willard D 1973 Primary pituitary dysgenesis. Journal of Pediatrics 73: 586

Williams T, Frohman L 1985 Hypothalamic dysfunction associated with hemochromatosis. Annals of Internal Medicine 103: 550

Winkelmann W, Solbach H G, Wiegelmann W et al 1972 Hypothalamo-hypophysarer Minderwuchs mit Innenhorschwerhorigkeit bei zwei Schwestern. Internist (Berlin) 13: 52

Winter R, MacDermot K, Hill F 1988 Sparse hair, short stature, hypoplastic thumbs, single upper central incisor and abnormal skin pigmentation. American Journal of Medical Genetics 29: 209

Winter W, Rosenbloom A, MacLaren N, Mickle P 1982 Solitary central maxillary incisor associated with precocious puberty and hypothalamic hamartoma. Journal of Pediatrics 101: 965

Wit J, Donckerwolcke M, Schulpen T, Deutman A 1986 Documented vasopressin deficiency in a child with Wolfram's syndrome. Journal of Pediatrics 109: 493

Wolfram D J 1938 Diabetes mellitus and simple optic atrophy among siblings: report of four cases. Mayo Clinic Proceedings 13: 715

Wurzel J M, Parks J S, Herd J E, Nielsen P V 1982 A gene deletion is responsible for absence of human choronic somatomammotropin. DNA 1: 251

Yagnik R, Reber R M, Katz R, Root R 1973 Anterior pituitary function in neonate with craniofacial dysraphia. Journal of Pediatrics 83: 1090

Young R L, Bradley E M, Goldzieher J W, Myers P W, Lecocq F R 1967 Spectrum of nonpuerperal galactorrhea: report of two cases evolving through the various syndromes. Journal of Clinical Endocrinology 27: 461

Zachman I M, Illig R, Prader A 1972 Fanconi's anemia with isolated growth hormone deficiency. Journal of Pediatrics 80: 159

Zimmerman D, Green O 1975 Nephrogenic diabetes insipidus Type II: defect distal to the adenylate cyclase step. Pediatric Research 9: 381

Zipf W B, Kelch R P, Bacon G E 1977 Variable X-linked recessive hypopituitarism with evidence of gonadotropin deficiency in two pre-pubertal males. Clinical Genetics 11: 249

Zuppinger K, Sutter M, Zurbrugg R, Joss E, Detliker D 1971 Cleft lip and choroideal coloboma associated with multiple hypothalamo-pituitary dysfunctions. Journal of Clinical Endocrinology and Metabolism 33: 934

87. Thyroid disorders

D. A. Fisher

INTRODUCTION

The mammalian thyroid gland, a derivative of the primitive gut, evolved from an iodine-concentrating gland in lower vertebrates to an endocrine gland capable of storing and secreting iodothyronines in higher vertebrate species (Gorbman 1986). The active iodothyronines, tetraiodothyronine (thyroxine or T4) and 3,5,3' – triiodothyronine (T3) are amino acids bearing, respectively, four and three iodine atoms per molecule. They are synthesized within the thyroid gland follicular cells from tyrosine and iodine substrates. Efficient synthesis requires an optimal dietary iodine intake and appropriate pituitary thyroid stimulating hormone (TSH) stimulation (Taurog 1986). TSH synthesis and secretion by the anterior pituitary thyrotroph cell is, in turn, stimulated by hypothalamic thyrotropin-releasing factor (TRF or TRH) and inhibited by circulating thyroid hormone via a classic endocrine negative feedback control system. TSH is secreted directly into blood where, via thyroid perfusion, it has access to TSH receptors on the thyroid follicular cell. TSH binding to plasma membrane receptors activates a membrane bound adenyl cyclase-cyclic AMP second messenger system and stimulates iodine uptake and organification, thyroglobulin degradation and thyroid hormone secretion. T4 (and to a lesser extent T3), like TSH, is secreted directly into peripheral blood but, unlike TSH, T4 is stored in plasma and in extracellular fluids tightly bound to one of three carrier protein species, thyroxine-binding globulin (TBG), thyroxine-binding prealbumin (TBPA), or albumin. The saturation of thyroid-hormone binding protein sites on TBG is regulated by the pituitary TSH negative feedback control system to adjust circulating free (or unbound) T4 concentrations within narrow limits (Fisher 1987).

Circulating free T4 diffuses into peripheral tissue cells where it is enzymatically monodeiodinated to a triiodothyronine. A beta ring monodeiodinase converts T4 to T3, an analogue with 3–4 times the metabolic potency of T4. An alpha ring monodeiodinase converts T4 to reverse T3 (rT3), an inactive iodothyronine analogue (Engler & Burger 1984). The triiodothyronines then diffuse back into circulating blood where they, too, are bound to TBG, although less avidly than T4 is bound. T4 beta ring monodeiodinase activity and T4 to T3 conversion are minimal in the fetus, so that fetal serum T3 levels are low; alpha ring monodeiodination does occur and fetal serum rT3 levels are elevated. T4 to T3 conversion and serum T3 levels increase markedly after birth. After birth, a variety of circumstances are known to inhibit T4 to T3 conversion, including undernutrition, starvation, severe illness, adrenal corticosteroids, propylthiouracil, propranalol, and some iodine-containing radiographic contrast agents.

Thyroid hormone effects on tissue are mediated via binding to specific nuclear receptors in thyroid responsive tissues (Oppenheimer et al 1976). These receptors have a predominant affinity for T3; T4 binds with only one tenth the affinity of T3. It is possible that T4 may bind directly to nuclear chromosomal receptors and mediate thyroid hormone action, but the most active hormone at the tissue level is T3. The metabolic effects of thyroid hormone are largely mediated by T3 from three sources: (1) circulating T3 derived from T4 tissues and released into blood; (2) circulating T3 secreted by the thyroid gland; and (3) intracellular T3 derived directly from intracellular monodeiodination of T4.

Optimal thyroid function and tissue metabolism are dependent on integrity of the entire hypothalamic-pituitary-thyroid tissue axis; and a variety of congenital anomalies, environmental factors and inborn defects are known to alter thyroid function parameters in the newborn; some may result in congenital hypothyroidism (Fisher 1980). These defects may occur at four levels, the hypothalamus, the pituitary, the thyroid gland, or the peripheral tissue levels. A listing of possible abnormalities is shown in Table 87.1.

Table 87.1 Congenital disorders of thyroid function

I Hypothalamus
  A. Hypothalamic dysplasia
  B. TRH deficiency
II Pituitary gland
  A. Pituitary aplasia or hypoplasia
  B. TSH deficiency
III Thyroid gland
  A. Dysgenesis
    Agenesis, hypoplasia or ectopy
  B. Dyshormonogenesis
    (1) Iodide concentrating defect
    (2) Organification defects
    (3) Iodotyrosine deiodinase deficiency
    (4) Defects in thyroglobulin synthesis
  C. TSH unresponsiveness
  D. Goitrogen exposure in utero
  E. Abnormal thyroid stimulator (neonatal Graves disease)
  F. Maternal TSH receptor antibody
IV Peripheral thyroid metabolism
  A. Disorders of thyroid hormone transport
    (1) Abnormalities of TBG concentration
    (2) Abnormalities of TBPA or TBPA-like protein
    (3) Abnormalities of albumin
  B. Decreased tissue response to thyroid hormones

HYPOTHALAMIC-PITUITARY HYPOTHYROIDISM

Hypothalamic-pituitary disorders associated with hypothalamic-pituitary anomalies and with panhypopituitarism are reviewed in another chapter and recently published reviews are available (Friedman & Fialkow 1986, Dumont et al 1989).

Familial isolated TSH deficiency

Miyai and colleagues (1971) first reported familial isolated TSH deficiency in 1971. Two sisters aged 12 and 14 years with nongoitrous cretinism were described. Both had low serum T4 and TSH concentrations and were markedly retarded with IQ values of 28 and 49. Pituitary growth hormone, ACTH and gonadotropin secretion were intact. The thyroid gland responded to exogenous TSH but there was no TSH response to TRH. The sisters were products of a consanguineous marriage. One other sib was retarded and died at age 3 years. Later studies indicated detectable levels of circulating TRH, normal prolactin responses to TRH (Miyai et al 1976), normal LH and FSH reponses to gonadotropin-releasing hormone (GnRH), normal GH responses to insulin hypoglycaemia and normal urinary 17 OHCS responses to metyrapone (normal ACTH reserve). These patients appear to have an inherited isolated defect in pituitary capacity to synthesize or release TSH. An abnormal TSH

is a less likely possibility because of the absence of TSH-like immunoreactivity in serum.

THYROID DYSGENESIS

The major cause for congenital hypothyroidism in nonendemic areas is thyroid dysgenesis due to abnormal thyroid gland embryogenesis (Fisher & Klein 1981). The aetiology of thyroid dysgenesis is not clear; a variety of mechanisms may be represented including single gene defects and familial autoimmune factors but these familial causes are rare and remain to be characterized. The majority of cases represent sporadic nonfamilial embryological defects. A high risk population has not been identified. There is a marked female predominance in reported series (female to male ratio is 5:2), and a seasonal variation has been reported in Japan, Australia and Canada (Miyai et al 1984). Thyroid aplasia or hypoplasia as well as thyroid ectopia have been described. Ectopic tissue may occur at the base of the tongue or in the midline along the line of descent of the thyroid gland during embryogenesis. The relative prevalence of thyroid aplasia, thyroid ectopy, and thyroid hypoplasia may vary geographically; estimate for North America was 40%, 40% and 20% respectively, of the total cases of thyroid dysgenesis (La Franchi et al 1985).

Although in the usual case only one affected infant occurs in a sibship, familial instances have been reported, and nongoitrous hypothyroidism has been reported both in identical and non-identical twins (Greig et al 1966). The mechanism is not clear. The McKusick (1988) catalogue lists these as ectopic thyroid with hypothyroidism (22525) and Kocher-Debre-Semelaigne syndrome – athyreotic cretinism with myotonia and muscular pseudohypertrophy (21870).

GOITROUS HYPOTHYROIDISM (FAMILIAL GOITRE)

Patients with inborn defects in thyroid metabolism are often referred to as having goitrous hypothyroidism or familial goitre (Stanbury 1986, Stanbury & Dumont 1983, Stanbury et al 1979). The events in thyroid hormone synthesis and release by thyroid follicular cells and the sites of identified or postulated defects in patients with goitrous hypothyroidism are illustrated in Figure 87.1. These defects include: (1) absence or malfunction of the cell membrane mechanism for trapping and transporting iodide from blood; (2) absence or inefficiency of the mechanisms for oxidizing iodide and 'organifying' or covalently binding the iodide to tyrosine, possibly including an inefficient 'coupling' of iodotyrosines to form thyroid hormones; (3) absent or defective

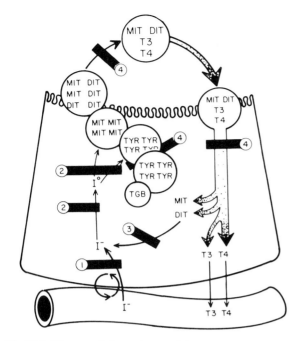

Fig. 87.1 Diagram of the pathways of thyroid hormone synthesis and release by the thyroid follicular cell. Iodine is transported across the plasma membrane and oxidized to a reactive state. Thyroglobulin (TGB) is synthesized by the cell and transported to the apical cell membrane where the incorporated tyrosine residues react with the reactive iodine, first to form monoiodotyrosine (MIT) and then diiodotyrosine (DIT). The iodinated tyrosine (TYR) residues spatially oriented for coupling combine to form the iodothyronines: DIT + DIT = T4 and MIT + DIT = T3. TGB stored in colloid re-enters the cell via endocytosis and is digested under the influence of lysosomal enzymes to release the iodotyrosines as well as T4 and T3. The MIT and DIT are deiodinated and the released iodine reutilized. The T3 and T4 are secreted. Numbers indicate sites of possible abnormality. See text for details. (Reproduced with permission from Pediatrics in Review 2: 70, 1980.)

enzymes for deiodinating iodotyrosines released into thyroid follicular cell cytoplasm in the process of thyroglobulin hydrolysis and thyroid hormone release; and (4) abnormalities in thyroglobulin synthesis, storage or release. All appear to be transmitted as autosomal recessive traits, and all may be associated with congenital hypothyroidism.

Except for the familial incidence and tendency for affected individuals to develop large goitres, the clinical manifestations of congenital hypothyroidism due to a biochemical defect are similar to those arising from an embryological error in development. Thyroid enlargement may appear at birth but in some patients the goitre

is delayed for months and may be small. Presumably, similar but less severe errors in synthesis may produce goitres that first make their appearance in later childhood or adulthood; such patients may remain euthyroid or may develop only mild hypothyroidism.

Failure to concentrate iodide

The transport of iodide across the thyroid follicular cell membrane from plasma to cytosol is the first step in thyroid hormone biosynthesis (Tauroq 1986). Under normal circumstances the thyroid cell membrane iodide pump generates a thyroid/serum (T/S ratio) concentration gradient in excess of 20–30; this gradient can reach several hundredfold when the thyroid gland is stimulated by a low-iodine diet, by thyroid stimulating hormone (TSH), by a variety of thyroid-stimulating immunoglobulins in Graves disease, or by drugs that impair the efficiency of hormone synthesis. Other tissues such as the salivary glands, gastric mucosa, mammary glands, ciliary body, choroid plexus and placenta are also capable of concentrating iodide against a gradient. However, these tissues are not capable of organifying inorganic iodide.

TSH stimulates iodide transport through a sequence of increased cyclic AMP formation and RNA and protein synthesis. Certain anions that are themselves accumulated by the thyroid are capable of competitively inhibiting iodide transport. These, in order of increasing potency, include bromide (Br^-), nitrite (NO_2^-), thiocyanate (SCN^-), selenocyanate ($SeCN^-$), fluoroborate (BF_4^-), and perchlorate (ClO_4^-). Thiocyanate and perchlorate have been utilized clinically to block iodide transport.

Several patients have been described with hyperplastic thyroid glands but only minimal uptake of radioactive iodide at 24 hours (Federman et al 1958, Gilboa et al 1963, Wolff et al 1964, Wolff 1983, Dumont et al 1989). The thyroid glands in these patients are enlarged twofold to fourfold and the patients are usually hypothyroid cretins. Other iodine-concentrating tissues (salivary glands, gastric mucosa) also fail to concentrate iodide from the circulation. Lugol solution ameliorates the hypothyroidism by increasing the serum iodide to high levels and increasing the intrathyroidal inorganic iodide concentration via diffusion. The molecular defect in this disorder is not known.

Several patients have been reported with a partial defect in iodide trapping also manifest in thyroid, salivary and gastric tissues (Papadopoulos et al 1970, Medeiros-Neto et al 1972, Wolff 1983). Thyroid radioiodine uptake was decreased but not absent in these patients and did not respond to TSH. The salivary/plasma ratio of radioiodine also was reduced but not entirely absent. Nonetheless the patients were hypothyroid with mental retardation.

Peroxidase system defects (organification defects)

Normally, iodide concentrated by the thyroid follicular cell is rapidly oxidized and bound in organic form (organified); less than 1% of the total thyroidal iodine is present as inorganic iodide (Lever et al 1983, Dumont et al 1989). Organification of iodide involves two processes: oxidation of iodide and iodination of thyroglobulin-bound tyrosine. First, iodide is oxidized to an active intermediate (perhaps $I°$ or I^+) followed by iodination of thyroglobulin-bound tyrosyl residues to form the iodotyrosines MIT and DIT. These processes are very rapid; the half-time of incorporation of iodide into protein approximates two minutes. Two DIT residues are 'coupled' to form T4, and MIT and DIT couple to form T3. The coupling reaction however is relatively slow. Both tyrosyl iodination and 'coupling' are catalyzed by a thyroid peroxidase enzyme system. Thyroid peroxidase is a membrane-bound haem protein that requires peroxide and an acceptor, which in the normal thyroid gland is thyroglobulin, but can be albumin or other proteins or peptides. The hydrogen peroxide may be provided by one or more of several flavoprotein enzyme systems.

Deficient thyroid peroxidase

The first of the iodide organification defects described by Stanbury was attributed to an absence or deficiency of the peroxidase enzyme(s) necessary to oxidize thyroidal iodide to iodine (Stanbury & Hedge 1950). Patients with the defect presented as goitrous cretins. The administration of thiocyanate or perchlorate to a patient with such a defect within two hours after administration of a test dose of radioiodine is followed by a precipitous fall in thyroid radioactivity. This 'perchlorate (or thiocyanate) discharge' indicates an organification defect, assuming the patient has no other reason for defective iodination, such as antithyroid drugs, high iodine intake or Hashimoto thyroiditis. The diagnosis of the specific defect is confirmed by measuring low or absent levels of thyroid peroxidase activity in thyroid tissue obtained at the time of biopsy (Stanbury & Hedge 1950, Hagen et al 1971, Niepomniszcze et al 1973, Valenta et al 1973, Pommier et al 1974, Mederios-Neto 1980, Lever et al 1983).

Abnormal thyroid peroxidase

More recently, two patients have been described who were euthyroid or mildly hypothyroid but manifested goitre and partial discharge of radioiodine following perchlorate administration. In these patients the thyroid gland was found to contain no peroxidase activity, but such activity could be restored by adding haematin, the noncovalently bound prosthetic group of the peroxidase (Niepomniszcze et al 1972, 1975, Lever et al 1983). This suggests an abnormal peroxidase apoenzyme deficient in binding to its haem moiety.

Deficient H_2O_2 generation

An adult woman presenting with euthyroidism and a non-toxic goitre in association with a positive perchlorate discharge was reported by Kusakabe in 1975. In vitro iodination in thyroid homogenates was reduced in tissue obtained from thyroidectomy. However, iodination capacity was restored by addition of riboflavin, FMN, oxidized cytochrome b_2, cytochrome C, NADH or NADPH. Microsomal NADH-cytochrome b_2 reductase activity was low and restored by addition to flavine-adenine dinucleotide (FAD); FAD, 250 mg/24 hours, administered prior to thyroidectomy decreased goitre size, serum TSH and thyroid radioiodine uptake, whereas treatment with riboflavin, a precursor of FAD, was without effect. A defect in thyroid H_2O_2 generation was postulated due to a defect in biosynthesis of FAD from riboflavin. Niepomniszcze et al (1987) reported a 71-year-old male with a large goitre and an organification defect with a positive perchlorate discharge test, but normal peroxidase activity. Iodine binding to thyroid proteins was impaired and addition of a source of H_2O_2 to the thyroid slices in vitro restored iodine organification to normal.

Pendred syndrome

A large group of patients with familial goitre and congenital eighth nerve deafness has been described. These patients are referred to as having Pendred syndrome. Pendred in 1896 described two sisters with deafness and goitre living in a nonendemic goitre area (Pendred 1896). Subsequently many such patients have been described (Fraser et al 1960, Nilsson et al 1964, Fraser 1969, Medeiros-Neto 1980, Lever et al 1983, Dumont et al 1989). The prevalence is estimated to be 1.5–3 cases per 100,000 school children. One in 60 persons has one abnormal Pendred gene and is a carrier; about 1 in 14,000 persons has the autosomal recessive clinical disease (Fraser 1969, Friedman & Fialkow 1986). The syndrome includes high tone or complete congenital deafness, goitre of variable degree appearing in middle or late childhood and euthyroidism or mild hypothyroidism. Perhaps a third of patients have the complete syndrome; others present without hearing loss or with mild goitre (Medeiros-Neto 1980). Most patients have a positive perchlorate discharge test, but atypical patients without an abnormal perchlorate discharge have been described (Cave & Dunn 1975, Medeiros-Neto 1980). The biochemical defect in these patients is not clear; thyroid peroxidase activity is normal (Burrow et al 1973, Ljunggren et al 1973, Cave & Dunn 1975). The cause of deafness is not known, a cochlear defect due to hypothyroidism in utero and a defect common to the thyroid and cochlea have been postulated. If the former, a variety of thyroid defects could produce the same phenotype.

Coupling defect

An abnormality of the thyroid peroxidase system can lead to an apparent inability of the thyroid to couple iodotyrosines to form thyroid hormones (Lever et al 1983, Dumont et al 1989). It now seems clear that 'coupling' of iodotyrosines is also catalyzed by thyroid peroxidase. Pommier et al (1974) reported a patient with a euthyroid familial goitre, a positive perchlorate discharge test, and a high level of thyroid peroxidase activity. After solubilization, thyroid peroxidase enzyme activity was found to be abnormal; it catalyzed iodide peroxidation similarly to a control hog peroxidase but catalyzed hormone synthesis 3–6 times less efficiently than the hog peroxidase. A structural defect in the thyroid peroxidase was postulated; the defective enzyme showed little iodide peroxidation activity, but retained 'coupling' activity (Pommier et al 1974).

Iodotyrosine deiodinase defect

Deficiency of the iodotyrosine dehalogenase enzyme can produce an hereditary defect causing either congenital hypothyroidism or a less severe form of familial goitre. Failure to deiodinate thyroid MIT and DIT as they are released from thyroglobulin leads to severe iodine wastage, since these non-deiodinated iodotyrosines diffuse out of the thyroid and are excreted in urine. As a result the iodine is lost rather than being recycled within the thyroid gland. Iodotyrosine deiodinases are present in both thyroid cells and peripheral tissues, and abnormalities involving both deiodinase systems have been described.

The patients originally described were cretinous and hypothyroid with goitres presenting at birth or shortly thereafter (Lever et al 1983, Dumont et al 1989). Detailed studies of three patients by Stanbury and colleagues (Stanbury et al 1956) showed early rapid thyroid radioiodine uptake and rapid spontaneous discharge; by 48 hours most of the thyroidal radioiodine had been discharged. After administration of a test dose of radioiodine, the serum of these patients contained high concentrations of labelled iodotyrosines. Moreover, these patients excreted essentially all of an intravenous dose of labelled iodotyrosine directly into urine, whereas normal subjects excrete the label almost entirely as free iodide. Thyroid tissue, when examined, also failed to deiodinate labelled diiodotyrosine to iodide. Administration of thyroid hormone or iodide induced remission (Dumont et al 1989).

Kusakabe and Miyake (1963, 1964) have reported patients with euthyroid goitre and partial defects in deiodination of iodotyrosine: (a) in both thyroid and peripheral tissues; (b) in peripheral tissues only; or (c) in thyroid tissue only. Three sibs with goitre and mild hypothyroidism and selective thyroidal iodotyrosine deiodinase deficiency were also reported by Ismail-Beigi and Rahimifar (1977).

Defects in thyroglobulin synthesis

Thyroglobulin is an essential substrate for organification and is the major protein component of thyroid colloid. It is an iodinated glycoprotein with a molecular weight approximating 650 000 daltons and a sedimentation coefficient of 19.7 (19S) (Edelhoch & Robbins 1986). It is composed of two 12S subunits, each of which is composed of two to four peptide chains. The iodine content of thyroglobulin depends on dietary iodine intake varying from negligible amounts in areas of severe iodine deficiency to 40% in areas of iodine excess. MIT, DIT, T3 and T4 (and to a lesser extent rT3) are present within the protein molecule as iodoaminoacyl residues that can be cleaved by proteolytic enzymes. The tyrosine residues, which are the iodine acceptors of thyroglobulin, comprise about 3% of the weight of the protein, and perhaps one third of these residues are spatially oriented to be susceptible to iodination.

Thyroglobulin synthetic defects probably comprise a spectrum of related abnormalities. Coupling of iodotyrosines is a complex chemical transformation that requires the presence of normal thyroglobulin. A number of possible defects may lead to similar functional abnormalities, so that the defects are difficult to distinguish. A coupling defect could be caused by absent or abnormal thyroglobulin. In this instance alternative protein substrates for the organification reactions would result in release of increased quantities of iodoalbumin or other iodoproteins. An abnormal perchlorate discharge also might occur, as well as abnormal ratios of iodotyrosines to iodothyronines within the gland. A structural abnormality of thyroglobulin could be so minimal that only the spatial orientation of the tyrosyl residues is altered or the postulated receptor for the peroxidase enzyme could be altered.

Impaired thyroglobulin synthesis

A number of patients have been described with findings suggestive of impaired thyroglobulin synthesis. These patients present with familial congenital hypothyroidism of variable degree associated with goitre and circulating non-thyroglobulin iodoprotein. The latter is detected as butanol insoluble iodoprotein or radioiodoprotein. Little or no thyroglobulin is detectable in thyroid tissue by radioimmunoassay (Cabrer et al 1986). Some patients have a positive perchlorate discharge test (Lissitzky et al 1973, Savoie et al 1973, Desai et al 1974, Bernal & Abregon 1974). Interestingly these patients tend to excrete abnormal quantities of iodohistidine, presumably as a degradation product of the iodinated iodoalbumin (Savoie et al 1973, Cabrer et al 1986). Study of thyroid tissue in two sibs by Cabrer et al (1986) revealed normal amounts of thyroglobulin mRNA. Defective translation or abnormal routing of the translation product was postulated.

Thyroglobulin transport defect

Lissitzky and colleagues in 1975 reported two brothers with an apparent defect in thyroglobulin transport as well as synthesis. The boys presented with congenital goitre and hypothyroidism, circulating non-thyroxine iodoprotein, and decreased thyroidal thyroglobulin. Further evaluation revealed partially immunoreactive carbohydrate deficient thyroglobulin associated with intracytoplasmic membranes. The immunoreactive thyroglobulin chains were synthesized and discharged into the intracisternal cisternae, but not into the colloid spaces.

Structurally abnormal thyroglobulin

Kusakabe (1972) reported a woman with a euthyroid goitre and positive thiocyanate discharge with normal thyroid peroxidase, catalase, transaminase and protease and a normal thyroglobulin content. However, assessment of absorbance as a function of pH and susceptibility to iodination or acetylation suggested that two thirds of the tyrosyl residues were buried within the molecule, and Kusakabe postulated an abnormal stereostructure of the thyroglobulin in this patient.

TSH UNRESPONSIVENESS

The thyroid follicular cell response to TSH involves a series of coordinated steps including TSH binding to a receptor in the plasma membrane, activation of adenyl cyclase, synthesis of cyclic AMP, activation of protein kinase(s), phosphorylation of receptor protein(s), and stimulation of the several intracellular events of thyroid hormone synthesis and release. A defect at one of several sites could, therefore, lead to an abnormality in thyroid responsiveness to TSH.

To date only a few such patients have been reported. The first, reported by Stanbury et al (1968) was an 8-year-old male with severe growth and mental retardation. His parents were consanguineous and his thyroid was not enlarged in spite of the fact that his serum TSH level was markedly increased. Thyroid slices in vitro failed to respond to TSH.

Codaccioni et al (1980) reported a 12-year-old boy with a history of congenital hypothyroidism diagnosed at 18 months. The boy's grandparents were first cousins, but there was no family history of thyroid disease. His serum thyroxine was low and TSH markedly increased. Thyroid radioiodine uptake increased significantly in response to dibutyryl cAMP but not in response to TSH. The thyroid follicles, histologically, were devoid of colloid. Studies of thyroid TSH receptors on thyroid membrane preparations showed normal TSH receptor binding and normal fluoride-stimulated TSH receptor adenylate cyclase system activity. TSH stimulation of the TSH receptor-adenylate cyclase system was markedly reduced, suggesting a TSH receptor-adenylate cyclase coupling abnormality (Codaccioni et al 1980). Medeiros-Neto et al (1979) reported a 19-year-old hypothyroid male without goitre development, with increased serum levels of bioactive TSH and normal radioactive iodine uptake unresponsive to TSH. The thyroid gland contained no thyroglobulin and there was no increase in cyclic AMP levels in thyroid tissue in response to TSH. Impaired generation of cyclic AMP was postulated. Job and colleagues in 1969 reported an infant with hypothyroidism and a normal radioiodine uptake unresponsive to TSH. The child did not have a goitre and in vitro studies were not conducted.

DECREASED PERIPHERAL RESPONSIVENESS TO THYROID HORMONES

Refetoff and associates in 1967 first described a familial syndrome in three sibs with deaf-mutism, stippled epiphyses, retarded skeletal age, goitre, and greatly elevated levels of serum free T4 and free T3, but normal plasma TSH concentrations. Growth rate, metabolic rate and intelligence were normal. Kinetic studies indicated that the thyroid glands were secreting about five times the normal amount of T4 daily. Administration of 1000 μg/24 hours of T4 or 375 μg/24 hours of T3 produced little or no metabolic effects. As the patients matured, the plasma T4 tended to return to normal levels, the epiphyses closed, and the goitre disappeared (Refetoff et al 1967,

1972b). Recent studies of the youngest affected sib show a normal TSH response to TRH despite 3-fold elevated serum free T4 and free T3 levels (Refetoff et al 1980). Administration of T3 produced paradoxical enhancement of the TSH response to TRH whereas administration of glucocorticoid produced a normal suppression of the TSH and prolactin reponses to TRH. These results indicate that the pituitary shares the TSH resistance.

Several other patients have been described with variable degrees of thyroid hormone unresponsiveness and goitre (Bode et al 1973a, Schneider et al 1975, Elewaut et al 1976, Lamberg et al 1978, Seif et al 1978). Both single (Bode et al 1973a, Schneider et al 1975, Seif et al 1978) and familial cases (Elewaut et al 1976, Lamberg et al 1978) were included. The family of Refetoff et al (1967, 1972b) manifest consanguinity and presumed autosomal recessive inheritance. The families reported by Elewaut et al (1976) and Lamberg et al (1978), in contrast, seemed most consistent with a dominant inheritance pattern.

Although there have been many attempts to identify a defect in thyroid hormone nuclear receptor binding in patients with thyroid resistance, such studies have been inconclusive (Eil et al 1982, Ceccarelli et al 1987). Reduced affinity has been observed in a few patients from different families, and reduced maximal binding capacity in others. However, the majority demonstrate normal thyroid hormone receptor binding. Thus, an as yet unidentified post-receptor defect or defects is postulated. A reduced response of patient fibroblasts to T3-induced suppression of fibronectin synthesis has been proposed for the tissue diagnosis of thyroid hormone resistance (Ceccarelli et al 1987).

cDNA probes for at least two thyroid hormone receptor proteins, alpha and beta, have been cloned. Restriction fragment length polymorphism (RFLP) studies in a few families with thyroid hormone resistance have shown intragenic polymorphism for the beta gene in one family (Usala et al 1988). This supports the view that thyroid resistance is due, at least in some instances, to genetic abnormalities of the receptor protein.

DISORDERS OF THYROID HORMONE TRANSPORT

Several presumably genetic abnormalities of iodothyronine-binding serum proteins have been described. These include: (1) absent TBG; (2) decreased (low) TBG; (3) excess TBG; (4) increased TBPA; (5) an increased TBPA-like protein; and (6) analbuminaemia.

TBG deficiency

Tanaka and Starr in 1959 first reported TBG deficiency in a euthyroid male. Since that time many reports of a familial TBG deficiency syndrome have appeared (Robbins 1973, Stanbury et al 1979). The prevalence of TBG deficiency varies from 1 in 5000 to 1 in 12 000 newborn infants; this prevalence estimate includes infants with partial TBG deficiency (low TBG) (Mori et al 1988). The disorder seems to be transmitted as a X-linked trait; serum TBG levels measured either by immunoassay or T4 binding capacity are very low in affected males and approximately half normal in carrier females. Serum T4 levels vary similarly, but affected subjects are euthyroid with normal serum free T4 concentrations, normal serum TSH levels and normal serum TSH responses to exogenous TRH. Male to male transmission has not been observed and there is invariable transmission of the trait from affected males to female offspring (Stanbury et al 1979). An abnormality in hepatic TBG synthesis rate has been postulated on the basis of TBG production rate measurements; variations in TBG production rates have been shown to correlate highly with variations in TBG concentrations (Refetoff et al 1976). Recent RFLP analysis in six families failed to reveal differences in fragment size in the affected subjects (Mori et al 1988). Thus large deletions, insertions or rearrangements of the TBG gene are not common mechanisms accounting for complete TBG deficiency in man.

Low TBG

A second disorder has been described, characterized by diminished but not absent TBG. A number of families have been reported (Levy et al 1971, Refetoff et al 1972b, 1976, Bode et al 1973b, Stanbury & Dumont 1983, Takamatsu et al 1987). Careful studies indicate that in these families, as in those with very low serum TBG levels, serum free T4 and TSH levels are normal. The TBG levels are diminished in affected males and there is a tendency to decreased concentrations in carrier females. However, the carrier state in females is sometimes difficult to identify because of overlap with affected males or normals; Bode et al (1973b) were able to characterize more definitively the genotype of 15–16 families tested by utilizing the product of the T4 concentration and the T4 binding capacity of TBG. This abnormality also seems to be transmitted as an X-linked trait (Refetoff et al 1972a, Bode et al 1973b, Takamatsu et al 1987). More recently, TBG levels have been assessed directly by radioimmunoassay (Levy et al 1971). Kinetic studies using purified TBG in these patients have shown that the total daily degradation rate of TBG is proportional to the serum concentration of the protein, indicating that the abnormality, like the absent TBG abnormality, is due to altered TBG production (Refetoff et al 1976).

Recent studies have indicated that partial TBG deficiency with low measured TBG concentrations by RIA is often due to the presence of a defective TBG molecule with reduced stability; a single base substitution in the TBG coding sequence has been defined in one family (Takamatsu et al 1987, Mori et al 1988). The demonstration of mutation sites and characterization of the extent of the heterogeneity in TBG deficiency must await the cloning and sequencing of the abnormal genes.

High TBG

Subjects with increased levels of TBG have increased total serum T4 concentrations with normal free T4 and TSH levels; thus they are euthyroid (Robbins 1973, Refetoff et al 1976). Studies in these subjects, as in those with low TBG concentrations, have shown correlation between TBG production rates and serum levels, suggesting that the mechanism for the high TBG concentrations is increased production, presumably by the liver (Refetoff et al 1976). TBG levels are increased up to 4.5 times normal in affected individuals, and carrier females have serum concentrations intermediate between normal values and the high levels in affected males (Robbins 1973, Stanbury et al 1979). Early reports suggested a dominant mode of inheritance (Beierwaltes et al 1961, Florsheim et al 1962), but subsequent studies and review of the earlier data are compatible with an X–linked mode of inheritance (Refetoff et al 1972a, Robbins 1973, Stanbury et al 1979). Refetoff and colleagues (1972a) have proposed that the several TBG concentration abnormalities reflect mutations at a single X–linked gene locus involved in the control of TBG synthesis.

High TBPA

Moses et al (1982) reported a 52-year-old euthyroid male with an elevated serum T4 not corrected by the use of a free T4 index, but with normal free T4, normal total serum T3 and TSH concentrations, and normal TSH and T3 responses to TRH. Serum TBG and albumin levels were normal, but the serum TBPA concentration measured by radioimmunoelectrophoresis was 2.5-3.0 times greater than the level in a normal human serum pool. Moreover 70% of the serum T4 was selectively removed by an anti-TBPA immunoglobulin affinity column. One of the subject's three children had a similar abnormality, but the mode of inheritance was not clearly defined.

Familial dysalbuminaemic hyperthyroxinaemia

This binding protein abnormality was described recently by several investigators who characterized euthyroid subjects with increased serum T4 concentrations not corrected by the use of the free T4 index correction and with normal free T4, total serum T3 and TSH levels (Lee et al 1979, Hennemann et al 1979, Barlow et al 1980). Thus, thyroid function parameters in these subjects resemble those in the patients with high TBPA reported by Moses et al (1982). Serum thyroxine in affected subjects migrates with albumin by conventional polyacrylamide electrophoresis (Lee et al 1979, Henneman et al 1979, Stockigt et al 1981), and the patients of Barlow et al (1980) had normal TBPA levels on the basis of saturation-binding studies in vitro. The disorder seems to be transmitted as an autosomal dominant trait (Ruiz et al 1982). There is male to male transmission and an affected to unaffected ratio of one or greater in first-degree relatives.

Analbuminaemia

Analbuminaemia is a rare autosomal recessive trait associated with serum albumin concentrations less than 100mg/ml. Serum albumin levels in heterozygotes are within the normal range (Bennhold et al 1954-55, Bennhold and Kallee 1959, Stanbury et al 1979). There is little clinical disability. Since albumin normally binds a significant proportion of circulating thyroid hormones, the distribution of T4 and T3 binding to serum proteins in these patients is abnormal (Hollander et al 1968). In association with essentially absent iodothyronine binding to albumin, both serum TBG and T4 binding prealbumin (TBPA) binding capacities are increased, perhaps due to increased levels of these binding proteins (Hollander et al 1968). After long-term infusion of albumin, TBG and TBPA binding return to normal. Free T4 and free T3 concentrations are normal and the patients are euthyroid.

FAMILIAL GRAVES DISEASE AND HASHIMOTO THYROIDITIS

Graves disease and Hashimoto thyroiditis are now recognized to be autoimmune thyroid disorders associated with circulating autoantibodies to thyroid and other tissues as well as cell mediated immunity directed against one or more thyroid antigens (Weetman & McGregor 1984). Graves disease comprises a constellation of hyperthyroidism, ophthalmopathy and dermopathy; Hashimoto thyroiditis is usually characterized by progressive lymphoid infiltrate of the thyroid gland with a gradual progression to hypothyroidism. The hyperthyroidism in Graves disease is believed to be due to the production by sensitized lymphocytes of one or more circulating thyroid stimulating immunoglobulins. Hashimoto thyroiditis is thought to be caused by progressive destruction of thyroid follicular cells by sensitized lymphocytes.

The familial incidence of Graves disease and Hashimoto thyroiditis are well documented. Both disorders tend to aggregate in families and both may occur in the same family (Weetman & McGregor 1984, Friedman & Fialkow 1986). In a recent study nearly half of the first-degree relatives of patients with Graves disease or Hashimoto thyroiditis were found to have some evidence of thyroid autoimmunity, with or without evidence of thyroid dysfunction (Chopra et al 1977). In another report, 36% of children of parents with Graves disease had one or more physical, functional or autoimmune markers of thyroid dysfunction as compared to 24% of control children (Carey et al 1980). During a three year follow-up of these children of Graves disease patients, one child out of 129 developed thyrotoxicosis, one developed Hashimoto thyroiditis, one manifested vitiligo and one exopthalmos (Carey et al 1980).

Age specific incidence rates for Graves disease and Hashimoto thyroiditis show an increasing rate of onset through the fifth decade and a decline thereafter (Volpe et al 1973, Volpe 1978). This has been interpreted as suggesting the existence of a subpopulation of subjects with genetic predisposition who develop thyroid autoimmune disease with increasing exposure to some environmental factor(s). Ultimately the unaffected portion of the sub-population becomes so small that age specific incidence rates for the entire population fall with increasing age (Volpe et al 1973, Volpe 1978). A genetic predisposition to thyroid autoimmunity is also suggested by observations in twins. There is an approximately 50% concordance for Graves disease in monozygotic twins, as contrasted with a 5% concordance rate in fraternal twins (Volpe 1978). Moreover there are several reports of monozygotic twins pairs in which one twin manifested Graves disease and the other Hashimoto thyroiditis (Jayson et al 1967, Chertov et al 1973).

Graves disease may occur in the newborn, usually as a result of transplacental passage of maternal thyroid stimulating immunoglobulins (Fisher 1987, Smallridge et al 1978). In this instance neonatal Graves disease is transient, abating as the maternal thyroid stimulator degrades in the newborn. There is, however, a group of newborns with more prolonged or recurrent disease (Hollingsworth & Mabry 1972). These patients are usually born into families with a high prevalence of Graves disease and may represent familial hyperthyroidism with fetal-neonatal onset.

The mechanism of thyroid autoimmunity in Graves disease and Hashimoto thyroiditis remains unclear. Recent studies have documented an increased incidence of HLA-B8 and HLA-DR3 transplantation antigens in Caucasian patients with Graves disease, HLA-Bw35 antigen in Japanese patients and HLA-B46 in Chinese patients with the disorder (Grumet et al 1974, Chan et al 1978, Allannic et al 1980, Farid et al 1980, Weetman & McGregor 1984, Friedman & Fialkow 1986). An increased risk for Hashimoto thyroiditis in subjects with an HLA-DR3 or HLA-DR5 haplotype has been reported. These studies suggest that the risk of thyroid autoimmune disease, particularly Graves disease, may be conditioned by an unidentified antigen stimulus governed by immune response gene(s) in linkage disequilibrium with the HLA loci on chromosome 6. Genes outside the major histocompatibility complex are probably also involved. Thus a familial predisposition to autoimmune thyroid disease is clear and genetic factors are pathogenetically involved. However, the mechanism(s) and mode of transmission remain unresolved.

MULTIPLE ENDOCRINE DEFICIENCY DISEASE

Many case reports have connected Hashimoto (lymphocytic) thyroiditis with other diseases suspected to include immune features. An increased incidence of Hashimoto disease or hypothyroidism has been documented in patients with multiple endocrine deficiency syndromes involving the thyroid gland, the adrenal glands, the gonads, the parathyroid glands and the pancreas (Carpenter et al 1964, Blizzard et al 1966, Irvine 1968, Spinner et al 1968, Edmonds et al 1973, Winter & Green 1976, Faber et al 1979). There also have been reports of an association between diabetes mellitus and hyperthyroidism (Hung et al 1978). In addition, many such patients have gastric mucosal involvement, vitiligo and/or candidosis. The syndromes involve deficiency of glandular or tissue function associated with the presence of organ-specific antibodies (Blizzard et al 1966, 1967, Spinner et al 1968). Thus, syndromes in which Hashimoto thyroiditis occurs in association with idiopathic Addison disease, idiopathic hypoparathyroidism, hypogonadism, diabetes mellitus, pernicious anaemia and/or candidosis are believed to result from an autoimmune process. Perhaps the most common clinical entity is Schmidt syndrome, the combination of Hashimoto thyroiditis, adrenal insufficiency and, more recently, diabetes mellitus. Deficiency syndromes involving any two of the three glands are being recognized more frequently. The familial nature of the syndromes (Spinner et al 1968, Friedman & Fialkow 1986) suggests a genetic predisposition and a degree of homogeneity. However, genetic heterogeneity has been invoked to explain the wide variety of manifestations, differences among families and varying age of onset.

THYROID DISEASE AND CHROMOSOMAL DISORDERS

Hashimoto (lymphocytic) thyroiditis has been reported with increased frequency in patients with Turner syndrome, Down syndrome and Klinefelter syndrome

(Sparkes & Motulsky 1963, Williams et al 1964, Vallotton & Forbes 1967, Fialkow et al 1971, Pai et al 1977). Patients with Noonan syndrome who have phenotypic features of Turner syndrome without a chromosomal disorder have also been reported with thyroid disease (Vesterhus & Aarskog 1973). Thus, there seems to be an increased prevalence of thyroid autoimmunity among patients with chromosomal disorders. However, there is no specific chromosomal disorder associated with lymphocytic thyroiditis or with the production of thyroid autoantibodies. Families of these patients also have an increased incidence of thyroid autoantibodies, as well as thyroid autoimmune disease, so that the association may be coincidental.

MEDULLARY THYROID CARCINOMA

In addition to thyroid hormone secreting cells within the thyroid gland, there are parafollicular 'C' cells which secrete calcitonin. These cells usually lie between the follicular cells and the basement membrane and form small nests of cells in an apparent interfollicular location. Hazard et al in 1959 recognized that medullary carcinoma of the thyroid is a tumour derived from the 'C' cells

and is a separate entity from other thyroid tumours (Hazard et al 1959, Williams 1979). Since that time medullary carcinoma has been reported as a feature of a variety of genetically conditioned syndromes. An association between familial phaeochromocytoma and medullary thyroid carcinoma has been reported (Sipple 1961, Schimke & Hartmann 1965, Williams 1979). Medullary carcinoma can also be inherited alone or in association with multiple mucosal neuromas, phaeochromocytomas, ganglioneuromas of the intestinal tract and other anomalies (Williams & Pollock 1966, Nankin et al 1970, Melvin et al 1972, Williams 1979, Melvin 1986). It is of interest that parathyroid hyperplasia or clinical hyperparathyroidism with hypercalcaemia may occur in any patient with medullary thyroid carcinoma (Melvin et al 1972, Williams 1979). Moreover, elevated serum levels of parathyroid hormone are commonly seen (Melvin et al 1972, Williams 1979). The mechanism is not clear.

These three familial syndromes account for some 20% of all cases of medullary thyroid carcinoma (Williams 1979). All three are separately heritable and appear to be transmitted as autosomal dominant traits with high penetrance (Williams 1979, Melvin 1986). The combina-

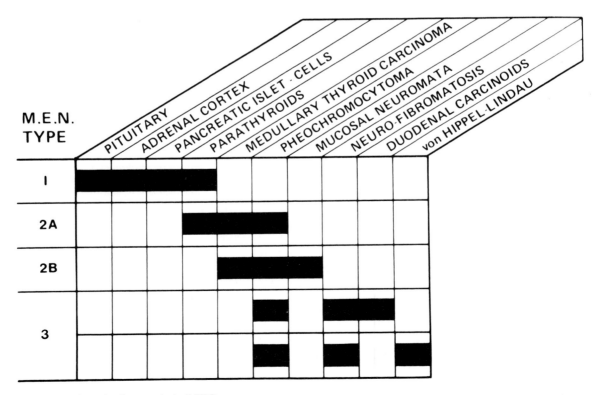

Fig. 87.2 Multiple endocrine neoplasia (MEN) types.

tion of medullary carcinoma and phaeochromocytoma has been referred to as Sipple syndrome. The term multiple endocrine neoplasia (MEN) has also been utilized and a classification of MEN 1, 2A, 2B and MEN 3 have been proposed to designate the combination syndromes as shown in Figure 87.2. MEN types 1 and 3 are not associated with medullary thyroid carcinoma.

The medullary carcinomas found in MEN 2A and 2B are often bilateral and may appear during childhood or later; the average age of presentation ranges from 19-36 years (Williams 1979, Melvin 1986). The phaeochromocytomas are usually bilateral and may be multiple. Either medullary thyroid carcinoma or phaeochromocytomas

may be the presenting abnormality. There is suggestive evidence that the incidence of malignancy is greater in these syndromes than with sporadic phaeochromocytomas (Williams 1979). In MEN 2B, the mucosal neuromas occur in the eyelid, lip and tongue. Medullated nerves are sometimes visible in the cornea (Williams 1979, Melvin 1986). The ganglioneuromas of the gastrointestinal tract involve enlargement of Auerbach's plexus and may extend from the oesophagus to the rectum. These patients may also manifest a marfanoid habitus, muscular weakness, pes cavus, and a high arched palate, as well as other less frequent anomalies (Melvin et al 1972, Williams 1979, Melvin 1986).

REFERENCES

Allannic H, Fouchet R, Lorey Y, Heim J, Gueguen M, Leguerrier A M, Genetet B 1980 HLA and Graves disease: an association with HLA DRW3. Journal of Clinical Endocrinology and Metabolism 51: 863

Barlow J W, Topliss D J, White E L, Hurley D M, Funder J W, Stockigt J R 1980 Familial euthyroid thyroxine excess due to increased prealbumin-like binding in plasma. In: Stockigt J R and Nagataki S (eds) Thyroid Research VIII. Australian Academy of Science, Canberra, p 509–512

Beierwaltes W H, Carr E A Jr, Hunter R L 1961 Hereditary increase in the thyroxine binding in the serum alpha globulin. Transactions of the Association of American Physicians 74: 170

Bennhold H, Kallee E 1959 Comparative studies of the half-life of I[131]- labelled albumins and nonradioactive human serum albumin in a case of analbuminemia. Journal of Clinical Investigation 38: 863

Bennhold H, Peters H, Roth E 1954–55 Ueber einen fall von kompletter analbuminaemie ohne wesentliche klinische krankheitszeichen. Verhandlungen der Deutschen Gesellschaft für innere medizin 4: 72

Bernal J, Abregon M J 1974 Thyroglobulin-like antigens in a goitre with impaired thyroglobulin synthesis. Journal of Clinical Endocrinology and Metabolism 39: 592

Bernal J, Refetoff S, DeGroot L J 1978 Abnormalities of triiodothyronine binding to lymphocyte and fibroblast nuclei from a patient with peripheral resistance to thyroid hormone action. Journal of Clinical Endocrinology and Metabolism 47: 1266

Blizzard R M, Chee D, Davis W 1966 The incidence of parathyroid and other antibodies in the sera of patients with idiopathic hypoparathyroidism. Clinical and Experimental Immunology 1: 119

Blizzard R M, Chee D, Davis W 1967 The incidence of adrenal and other antibodies in the sera of patients with idiopathic adrenal insufficiency (Addison's disease). Journal of Experimental Immunology 2: 119

Block M A, Horn R C Jr, Miller J M, Barrett J L, Brush B E 1967 Familial medullary carcinoma of the thyroid. Annals of Surgery 166: 403

Bode H H, Danon M, Weintraub B D 1973a Partial target organ resistance to thyroid hormone. Journal of Clinical Investigation 52: 776

Bode H H, Rothman K J, Danon M 1973b Linkage of thyroxine binding globulin deficiency to other X-chromosome loci. Journal of Clinical Endocrinology and Metabolism 37: 25

Burrow G N, Spaulding S W, Alexander N M, Bower B F 1973 Normal peroxidase activity in Pendred's syndrome. Journal of Clinical Endocrinology and Metabolism 36: 522

Cabrer B, Brocas H, Perez-Castillo A et al 1986 Normal level of thyroglobulin messenger ribonucleic acid in a human congenital goitre with thyroglobulin deficiency. Journal of Clinical Endocrinology and Metabolism 63: 931

Carey C, Skosey C, Pinnamaneni K M, Barsano C P, DeGroot L J 1980 Thyroid abnormalities in children of parents who have Graves' disease: possible pre-Graves' disease. Metabolism 29: 369

Carpenter C C J, Solomon N, Silverberg S G, Bledsoe T, Northcutt R C, Klinenberg J R, Bennett L I Jr, Harvey A M 1964 Schmidt's syndrome (thyroid and adrenal insufficiency): a review of the literature and a report of fifteen new cases including ten instances of coexistant diabetes mellitus. Medicine 43: 153

Cave W T Jr., Dunn J T 1975 Studies on the thyroidal defect in an atypical form of Pendred's syndrome. Journal of Clinical Endocrinology and Metabolism 41: 590

Ceccarelli P, Refetoff S, Muratay 1987 Resistance to thyroid hormone diagnosed by the reduced response of fibroblasts to the triiodothyronine-induced suppression of fibronectin synthesis. Journal of Clinical Endocrinology and Metabolism 65: 242

Chan S H, Yeo P P B, Lui K F, Wee G B, Woo K T, Pin L, Cheak J S 1978 HLA and thyrotoxicosis (Graves disease) in Chinese. Tissue Antigens 12: 109

Chertov B S, Fidler W J, Fariss B L 1973 Graves disease and Hashimoto's thyroiditis in monozygotic twins. Acta Endocrinologica 72: 18

Chopra I J, Solomon D H, Chopra U, Yoshihara E, Terasaki P I, Smith F 1977 Abnormalities in thyroid function in relatives of patients with Graves' disease and Hashimoto's thyroiditis: Lack of correlation with inheritance of HLA-B8. Journal of Clinical Endocrinology and Metabolism 45: 45

Codaccioni J L, Carayon P, Michel-Becket M, Foucault F, Lefort G, Pierron H 1980 Congenital hypothyroidism associated with thyrotropin unresponsiveness and thyroid cell membrane alterations. Journal of Clinical Endocrinology and Metabolism 50: 932

DeLange F, Beckers C, Hofer R 1979 Screening for congenital hypothyroidism in Europe. Acta Endocrinol Suppl 223, 90: 1

Desai K B, Mehta M N, Patel M C, Sharma S M, Ramana L, Ganatra R D 1974 Familial goitre with absence of thyroglobulin and synthesis of thyroid hormones from thyroidal albumin. Journal of Endocrinology 60: 389

Dumont J, Vassart G, Refetoff S 1989 Thyroid disorders. In: Scriver C R et al (eds) The metabolic basis of inherited disease, 6th edn. McGraw Hill, New York, p 1843–1879

Dussault J H, Letarte J, Guyda H, Laberge C 1977 Serum thyroid hormone and TSH concentrations in newborn infants with congenital absence of thyroxine-binding globulin. Journal of Pediatrics 90: 264

Edelhoch H, Robbins J 1986 Thyroglobulin chemistry and biosynthesis. In: Ingbar S H, Braverman L E (eds) The Thyroid, 5th edn. Lippincott, Philadelphia, p 98–115

Edmonds M, Lamki L, Killinger D W, Volpe R 1973 Autoimmune thyroiditis, adrenalitis and oophoritis. American Journal of Medicine 54: 782

Eil C, Fein H G, Smith T J, Furlanetto R W, Bourgeois M, Stelling M W, Weintraub B O 1982 Nuclear binding of triiodothyronine to dispersed cultured skin fibroblasts from patients with resistance to thyroid hormones. Journal of Clinical Endocrinology and Metabolism 55: 502

Elewaut A, Mussche M, Vermeulen A 1976 Familial partial target organ resistance to thyroid hormones. Journal of Clinical Endocrinology and Metabolism 43: 575

Engler D, Burger A G 1984 The deiodination of the iodothyronines and their derivatives in man. Endocrine Reviews 5: 151

Faber J, Colin D, Kirkegaard C, Christy M, Siersback-Nielsen K, Friis T, Nerup J 1979 Subclinical hypothyroidism in Addison's disease. Acta Endocrinologica 91: 674

Farid N R, Moens H, Larsen B, Payne R, Saltman K, Fifield F, Ingram D W 1980 HLA haplotypes in familial Graves disease. Tissue Antigens 15: 492

Federman D, Robbins J, Rall J E 1958 Some observations on cretinism and its treatment. New England Journal of Medicine 259: 610

Fialkow P J, Thuline H C, Hecht F, Bryant J 1971 Familial predisposition to thyroid disease in Down's syndrome: controlled immunoclinical studies. American Journal of Human Genetics 23: 67

Fisher D A 1980 Hypothyroidism in childhood. Pediatrics in Review 2: 67

Fisher D A 1987 The thyroid. In: Rudolph A, Hoffman J I E (eds) Pediatrics, 18th edn. Appleton & Lange, New York, p 1504-1526

Fisher D A, Klein A H 1981 Thyroid development and disorders of thyroid function in the newborn. New England Journal of Medicine 304: 702

Fisher D A, Dussault J H, Foley T P Jr et al 1979 Screening for congenital hypothyroidism: results of screening 1 million North American infants. Journal of Pediatrics 94: 700

Florsheim W II, Dowling J T, Meister L, Bodfish R E 1962 Familial elevation of serum thyroxine-binding capacity. Journal of Clinical Endocrinology and Metabolism 22: 735

Fraser G R 1969 The genetics of thyroid disease. In: Steinberg A G and Bearn A G (eds) Progress in medical genetics, vol VI. Grune and Stratton, New York, p 89–115

Fraser G R, Morgans M E, Trotter W R 1960 The syndrome of sporadic goitre and congenital deafness. Quarterly Journal of Medicine 53: 279

Friedman J M, Fialkow P J 1978 The genetics of Graves' disease. Journal of Clinical Endocrinology and Metabolism 7: 47

Friedman J M, Fialkow P J 1986 Genetic factors in thyroid disease. In: Ingbar S H, Braverman L E (eds) The Thyroid, 5th edn. Lippincott, Philadelphia, p 634–650

Gilboa Y, Ber A, Lewitus Z and Hasenfratz J 1963 Goitrous myxedema due to iodide trapping defect. Archives of Internal Medicine 112: 110

Gorbman A 1986 Comparative anatomy and physiology. In: Ingbar S H, Braverman L E (eds) The Thyroid 5th edn. Lippincott, Philadelphia, p 43–52

Greig W R, Henderson A S, Boyle J A, McGirr E M, Hutchison J H 1966 Thyroid dysgenesis in two pairs of monozygotic twins and in a mother and child. Journal of Clinical Endocrinology and Metabolism 26: 1309

Grumet F C, Payne R O, Konishi J, Kriss J P 1974 HLA antigens as marker for disease susceptibility and autoimmunity in Graves disease. Journal of Clinical Endocrinology and Metabolism 39: 115

Hagen G A, Niepomniszcze H, Haibach H et al 1971 Peroxidase deficiency in familial goiter with iodide organification defect. New England Journal of Medicine 285: 1394

Hazard J B, Hawk W A, Crile G Jr 1959 Medullary (solid) carcinoma of the thyroid — a clinicopathologic entity. Journal of Clinical Endocrinology and Metabolism 19: 152

Henneman G, Doctor R, Krenning E P, Box G, Otten M, Visser T J 1979 Raised total thyroxine and free thyroxine index but normal free thyroxine. Lancet 1: 639

Hollander C S, Bernstein G, Oppenheimer J H 1968 Abnormalities of thyroxine binding in analbuminemia. Journal of Clinical Endocrinology and Metabolism 28: 1064

Hollingsworth D R, Mabry C 1972 Hereditary aspects of Graves disease in infancy and childhood. Journal of Pediatrics 81: 446

Hung W, August G P, Glasgow A M 1978 Hyperthyroidism in juvenile diabetes mellitus. Pediatrics 61: 583

Ingbar S H, Woeber K A 1974 The thyroid gland. In: Williams R H (ed) Textbook of endocrinology, 5th edn. W B Saunders Philadelphia, p 95–227

Irvine W J 1968 Clinical and immunological associations in adrenal disorders. Proceedings of the Royal Society of Medicine 61: 271

Ismail-Beigi F, Rahimifar M 1977 A variant of iodotyrosine dehalogenase deficiency. Journal of Clinical Endocrinology and Metabolism 44: 499

Jayson M I V, Doniach D, Benhamour-Glynn N 1967 Thyrotoxicosis and Hashimoto goitre in a pair of monozygotic twins with long acting thyroid stimulator. Lancet 2: 15

Job J C, Canlorbe P, Thomassin N et al 1969 L'hypothyroidie infantile a debut precoce avec glande en place, fixation faible de radio-iode et default de response a la thyreostimuliue. Annales d'endocrinologie (Paris) 80: 696

Kusakabe T 1972 A goitrous subject with structural abnormality of thyroglobulin. Journal of Clinical Endocrinology and Metabolism 35: 785

Kusakabe T 1975 Deficient cytochrome b5 reductase activity in nontoxic goiter with iodide organification defect. Metabolism 24: 1103

Kusakabe T, Miyake T 1963 Defective deiodination of I^{131}-labeled 1-diiodotyrosine in patients with simple goiter.

Journal of Clinical Endocrinology and Metabolism 23: 132

Kusakabe T, Miyake T 1964 Thyroidal deiodination defect in three sisters with simple goiter. Journal of Clinical Endocrinology and Metabolism 24: 456

LaFranchi S H, Hanna C E, Krainz P L, Skeels M R, Miyahira R S, Sesser D E 1985 Screening for congenital hypothyroidism with specimen collection at two time periods: results of the Northwest Regional Screening Program. Pediatrics 76: 734

Lamberg B A, Rosengard S, Liewendahl K, Saarinen P, Evered D C 1978 Familial partial peripheral resistance to thyroid hormones. Acta Endocrinologica 87: 303

Lee W N P, Golden M P, Van Herle A J, Lippe B M, Kaplan S A 1979 Inherited abnormal thyroid hormone-binding protein causing selective increase in total serum thyroxine. Journal of Clinical Endocrinology and Metabolism 49: 292

Lever E G, Medeiros-Neto G A, DeGroot L J 1983 Inherited disorders of thyroid metabolism. Endocrine Reviews 4: 213

Levy R P, Marshall J S, Velayo N L 1971 Radioimmunoassay of human thyroxine binding globulin. Journal of Clinical Endocrinology and Metabolism 32: 372

Lissitzky S, Bismuth J, Jaquet P et al 1973 Congenital goiter with impaired thyroglobulin synthesis. Journal of Clinical Endocrinology and Metabolism 36: 17

Lissitzky S, Torresani J, Burrow G N, Bouchilloux S, Chabaud O 1975 Defective thyroglobulin export as a cause of congenital goiter. Clinical Endocrinology 4: 363

Ljunggren J G, Linstrom H, Hjern B 1973 The concentration of peroxidase in normal and adenomatous human thyroid tissue with special reference to patients with Pendred's syndrome. Acta Endocrinologica 72: 272

McKusick V A 1988 Mendelian Inheritance in Man. 8th edn. Johns Hopkins University Press, Baltimore

Medeiros-Neto G A, Bloise W, Ulhoa Cintra A G 1972 Parital defect of iodide trapping mechanism in two siblings with congenital goiter and hypothyroidism. Journal of Clinical Endocrinology and Metabolism 35: 370

Meideros-Neto G A, Knobel M, Bronstein M D, Simonetti J, Filho F F, Mattar E 1979 Impaired cyclic-AMP response to thyrotropin in congenital hypothyroidism with thyroglobulin deficiency. Acta Endocrinologica 92: 62

Medeiros-Neto G A 1980 Inherited disorders of intrathyroidal metabolism. In: Stockigt J R, Nogataki S (eds) Thyroid Research VIII, Australian Academy of Sciences, Canberra p 101–108

Melvin K E W 1986 Medullary carcinoma of the thyroid. In: Ingbar S H, Braverman L E (eds) The Thyroid, 5th edn. Lippincott, Philadelphia, p 1349–1362

Melvin K E W, Tashjian A H Jr., Miller H H 1972 Studies in familial (medullary) thyroid carcinoma. Recent Progress in Hormone Research 28: 399

Miyai K, Azukizawa M, Kumahara Y 1971 Familial isolated thyrotropin deficiency with cretinism. New England Journal of Medicine 285: 1043

Miyai K, Azukizawa M, Onishi T, Hashimoto T, Sawazaki N, Nishi K, Kumahara Y 1976 Familial isolated thyrotropin deficiency. In: James V H T (ed) Excerpta Medica International Congress Series No 403, Endocrinology, p 345–349

Miyai K, Connelly J F, Foley T P et al 1984 An analysis of the variation of incidence of congenital dysgenetic hypothyroidism in various countries Endocrinol Japan 31: 77

Moens H, Farid N R 1978 Hashimoto's thyroiditis is associated with HLA DRW3. New England Journal of Medicine 299: 133

Mori Y, Refetoff S, Flink I L et al 1988 Detection of the thyroxine binding globulin gene in six unrelated families with complete TBG deficiency. Journal of Clinical Endocrinology and Metabolism 67: 727

Moses A A C, Lawlor J F, Haddow J E, Jackson I M D 1982 Familial euthyroid hyperthyroxinemia resulting from increased immunoreactive thyroxine-binding prealbumin (TBPA) New England Journal of Medicine 306: 366

Nankin H, Hydovitz J, Sapira J 1970 Normal chromosomes in mucosal neuroma variant of medullary thyroid carcinoma syndrome. Journal of Medical Genetics 7: 374

Niepomniszcze H, DeGroot L J, Hagen G A 1972 Abnormal thyroid peroxidase causing iodide organification defect. Journal of Clinical Endocrinology and Metabolism 34: 607

Neipomniszcze H, Castells S, DeGroot L J, Refetoff S, Kim O S, Rapoport B, Hati R 1973 Peroxidase defect in congenital goiter with complete organification block. Journal of Clinical Endocrinology and Metabolism 36: 347

Niepomniszcze H, Rosenbloom A L, DeGroot L J, Shimaoka K, Refetoff S, Yamamoto K 1975 Differentiaton of two abnormalities in thyroid peroxidase causing organification defect and goitrous hypothyroidism. Metabolism 24: 57

Niepomniszcze H, Targovnik H M, Gluzman B E, Curutchet P 1987 Abnormal H_2O_2 supply in the thyroid of a patient with goiter and iodine organification defect. Journal of Clinical Endocrinology and Metabolism 65: 344

Nilsson L R, Borgfors N, Gamstrop I, Holst H E, Liden G 1964 Nonendemic goitre and deafness. Acta Paediatrica 53: 117

Oppenheimer J H, Schwartz H L, Surks M I, Koerner D, Dillman W H 1976 Nuclear receptors and the initiation of thyroid hormone action. Recent Progress in Hormone Research 32: 529

Pai G S, Leach D C, Weiss L, Wolf C, Van Dyke D L 1977 Thyroid abnormalities in 20 children with Turner's syndrome. Journal of Paediatrics 91: 267

Papadopoulos S N, Vagenakis A G, Maschos A, Koutras D A, Matsaniotis N, Malamos B 1970 A case of a partial defect of the iodide trapping mechanism. Journal of Clinical Endocrinology and Metabolism 30: 302

Pendred V 1896 Deaf-mutism and goitre. Lancet 2: 532

Pommier J, Tourniaire J, Deme D, Chalendar P, Bornet H, Nunez J 1974 A defective thyroid peroxidase solubilized from a familial goiter with iodine organification defect. Journal of Clinical Endocrinology and Metabolism 39: 69

Refetoff S, DeWind L T, DeGroot L J 1967 Familial syndrome combining deaf-mutism, stippled epiphyses, goiter and abnormally high PBI: possible target organ refractoriness to thyroid hormone. Journal of Clinical Endocrinology and Metabolism 27: 279

Refetoff S, Robin N I, Alper C A 1972a Study of four new kindreds with inherited thyroxine binding globulin abnormalities. Journal of Clinical Investigation 51: 848

Refetoff S, DeGroot L J, Bernard B, DeWind L T 1972b Studies of a sibship with apparent hereditary resistance to the intracellular action of thyroid hormone. Metabolism 21: 723

Refetoff S, Fang V S, Marshall J S, Robin N I 1976 Metabolism of thyroxine-binding globulin (TBG) in man: abnormal rate of synthesis in inherited TBG deficiency and excess. Journal of Clinical Investigation 57: 485

Refetoff S, DeGroot L J, Barsano C P 1980 Defective thyroid

hormone feedback regulation in the syndrome of peripheral resistance to thyroid hormone. Journal of Clinical Endocrinology and Metabolism 51: 41

Robbins J 1973 Inherited variations in thyroxine transport. Mount Sinai Journal of Medicine NY 40: 511

Ruiz M, Rajatanavin R, Young R A, Taylor C, Brown R, Braverman L E, Ingbar S H 1982 Familial dysalbuminemic hyperthyroxinemia. New England Journal of Medicine 306: 635

Savoie J C, Massin J P, Savoie F 1973 Studies on mono and diiodohistidine. II congenital goitrous hypothyroidism with thyroglobulin defect and iodohistidine-rich iodoalbumin production. Journal of Clinical Investigation 52: 116

Schimke R N, Hartmann W H 1965 Familial amyloid producing medullary thyroid carcinoma and pheochromocytoma. Annals of Internal Medicine 63: 1027

Schneider G, Keiser H R, Bardin C W 1975 Peripheral resistance to thyroxine: a cause of short stature in a boy without goiter. Clinical Endocrinology 4: 111

Seif F J, Sherbaum W, Klinger W 1978 Syndrome of elevated thyroid hormone and TSH blood levels: a case report. Acta Endocrinologica 87 Suppl 215: 81

Sipple J H 1961 The association of pheochromocytoma with carcinoma of the thyroid gland. American Journal of Medicine 31: 163

Smallridge R C, Wartofsky L, Chopra I J, Morinelli P V, Broughton R E, Dimond R C, Burman K D 1978 Neonatal thyrotoxicosis: alterations in serum concentrations of LATS-protector, T4, T3, reverse T3 and 3,3'T2. Journal of Pediatrics 93: 118

Sparkes R S, Motulsky A G 1963 Hashimoto's disease in Turner's syndrome with isochromosome X. Lancet 1: 947

Spinner M W, Blizzard R M, Childs B 1968 Clinical and genetic heterogeneity in idiopathic Addison's disease and hypoparathyroidism. Journal of Clinical Endocrinology and Metabolism 28: 795

Stanbury J B 1986 Inherited metabolic disorders of the thyroid system. In: Ingbar S H, Braverman L E (eds) The Thyroid, 5th edn. Lippincott, Philadelphia, p687–695

Stanbury J B, Hedge A M 1950 A study of a family of goitrous cretins. Journal of Clinical Endocrinology and Metabolism 10: 1471

Stanbury J B, Meijer J W A, Kassenaar A A H 1956 The metabolism of iodotyrosines I The fate of mono and diiodotyrosine in certain patients with familial goiter. Journal of Clinical Endocrinology and Metabolism 16: 735

Stanbury J B, Rocmans P, Buhler U K, Ochi Y 1968 Congenital hypothyroidism with impaired thyroid response to thyrotropin. New England Journal of Medicine 279: 1132

Stanbury J B, Aiginger P, Harbison M D 1979 Familial goiter and related disorders. In: DeGroot L J, Cahill G F Jr., Martini L, Nelson D H, Odell W D, Potts J T Jr., Steinberger E, Winegrad A I (eds) Endocrinology. Grune Stratton, New York, p 523–539

Stockigt J R, Topliss O J, Barlow J W, White E L, Hurley D M, Taft P 1981 Familial euthyroid thyroxine excess. An appropriate response to abnormal thyroxine binding associated with albumin. Journal of Clinical Endocrinology and Metabolism 53: 353

Takamatsu J, Refetoff S, Charbonneau M, Dussault J H 1987 Two new inherited defects of the thyroxine-binding globulin (TBG) molecule presenting as partial TBG deficiency. Journal of Clinical Investigation 79: 833

Tanaka S, Starr P 1959 A euthyroid man without thyroxine binding globulin. Journal of Clinical Endocrinology and Metabolism 19: 485

Taurog A 1986 Hormone synthesis: thyroid iodine metabolism In: Ingbar S H, Braverman L E (eds) The Thyroid 5th edn. Lippincott, Philadelphia, p 53–97

Usala S J, Bale A E, Gesundheit N, Weinberger C, Henezes-Ferreira M, Lash R W, Weintraub B D 1988 The role of human C-ERB-α and C-ERB-β receptor genes in generalized thyroid hormone resistance. Proceedings of the Endocrine Society, Abst 33, p 29

Valenta L J, Bode H, Vickery A L, Caufield J B, Maloof F 1973 Lack of thyroid peroxidase activity as the cause of congenital goitrous hypothyroidism. Journal of Clinical Endocrinology and Metabolism 36: 830

Vallotton M B, Forbes A P 1967 Autoimmunity in gonadal dysgenesis and Klinefelter's syndrome. Lancet 1: 648

Vesterhus P, Aarskog D 1973 Noonan's syndrome and autoimmune thyroiditis. Journal of Pediatrics 83: 237

Volpe R 1978 The genetics and immunology of Graves and Hashimoto's diseases. In: Rose N, Bigazzi P E, Warner N L (eds) Genetic control of autoimmune disease. Elsevier/North Holland, New York, p 43–56

Volpe R, Clarke P V, Row V V 1973 Relationship of age-specific incidence rates to immunologic aspects of Hashimoto's thyroiditis. Canadian Medical Association Journal 109: 898

Weetman A P, McGregor A M 1984 Autoimmune thyroid disease: Developments in our understanding. Endocrine Reviews 5: 309

Williams E D 1979 Medullary carcinoma of the thyroid. In: DeGroot L J, Cahill G F Jr., Martini L, Nelson D H, Odell W D, Potts J T Jr., Steinberger E, Winegrad A I (eds) Endocrinology. Grune Stratton, New York, p 777–792

Williams E D & Pollock D J 1966 Multiple mucosal neuromata with endocrine tumours: a syndrome allied to von Recklinghausen's disease. Journal of Pathology and Bacteriology 91: 71

Williams E D, Engel E, Forbes A P 1964 Thyroiditis and gonadal dysgenesis. New England Journal of Medicine 270: 805

Winter R J, Green O C 1976 Carbohydrate homeostasis in chronic lymphocytic thyroiditis: increased incidence of diabetes mellitus. Journal of Pediatrics 89: 401

Wolff J, Thompson R H, Robbins J 1964 Congenital goitrous cretinism due to absence of iodide-concentrating ability. Journal of Clinical Endocrinology and Metabolism 24: 699

Wolff J 1983 Congenital goiter with defective iodine transport. Endocrine Reviews 4: 240

88. Parathyroid disorders

C. E. Jackson

INTRODUCTION

This chapter is concerned with the genetic aspects of clinical disorders of the parathyroid glands. The topics will be discussed under the main headings of primary hyperparathyroidism, primary hypoparathyroidism (or hormone deficiency) and pseudohypoparathyroidism (or end organ unresponsiveness). Genetic factors are important to a variable extent in each of these three heterogeneous conditions. Knowledge of parathyroid conditions has considerable practical importance not only in genetic counselling but also in their treatment potential.

PRIMARY HYPERPARATHYROIDISM

Clinical description and pathogenesis

Primary hyperparathyroidism is a generalized disorder of calcium and phosphate metabolism resulting from an increased production of parathyroid hormone (PTH) by the parathyroid glands without identifiable cause. In secondary hyperparathyroidism the increased PTH production is most often secondary to chronic renal disease or intestinal malabsorption, and the exact mechanism of the parathyroid hyperplasia is not well understood. Primary hyperparathyroidism was initially recognized most frequently by the development of severe bone disease, osteitis fibrosa cystica. Later, the association with nephrolithiasis and kidney stones led to the diagnosis of this entity. Since the reports of the detection of hyperparathyroidism by elevated serum calcium determinations on routine analysis (Boonstra & Jackson 1962) and the advent of the almost universal clinical use of multiphasic biochemical screening procedures, this condition has become recognized with increasing frequency.

It is estimated that 1 per 800–1000 patients seen in a general medical clinic will have this condition (Boonstra & Jackson 1965, 1971). The disease is no longer thought of as being one of just 'bones and stones' but one also of 'abdominal groans and psychic moans with fatigue overtones'. At times it is almost completely asymptomatic and evident only by an elevated serum calcium value obtained as a routine screening procedure. Primary hyperparathyroidism is generally related to the presence of an adenoma of one of the four parathyroid glands in the neck (Fig. 88.1). However some cases (about 15–20%) are related to an adenoma of more than one gland, or to diffuse hyperplasia of all glands. Thorough family studies of patients with primary hyperparathyroidism have revealed that 1/6–1/8 of the cases have other family members affected with hyperparathyroidism alone or with one of the hereditary multiple endocrine neoplasia syndromes (Jackson et al 1977).

The pathological differentiation of adenoma from hyperplasia is difficult, if not impossible. Glucose-6-phosphate-dehydrogenase studies of parathyroid 'adenomas' have disclosed that those studied are of multicellular origin, as one would expect of hyperplastic lesions (Fialkow et al 1977). Although these findings would not have been unexpected in hereditary hyperparathyroidism, multicellular origin in sporadic cases suggests that unknown factors are stimulating many cells in the parathyroid glands to become hyperplastic, instead of some neoplastic change occurring as a mutation originating in one cell only. Molecular biological studies by Arnold et al (1988) and by Friedman et al (1989) have suggested that some parathyroid tumours are of clonal origin.

Natural history and complications

The natural history of primary hyperparathyroidism is quite variable, at times being asymptomatic into old age and at other times causing symptoms in early adulthood (or in infancy, as in familial neonatal hyperparathyroidism). The symptoms may involve different organ systems such as the bones, gastrointestinal tract, kidneys or central nervous system, and are thought to represent generally the effect of hypercalcaemia on those particular systems. The age of onset is usually considerably earlier in the hereditary syndromes associated with hyperparathyroidism, although onset is rarely before puberty. Hyperparathyroidism is rarely detected by symptomatic bone disease at the present time. Nephrolithiasis and kidney stones often lead to diagnosis as do the gastrointestinal complications of ulcer, pancreatitis or nonspecific nausea and vomiting. The complications of other organ involvement associated with the hereditary multiple endocrine neoplasia syndromes will be discussed under those topics.

Differential diagnosis

The differential diagnosis of primary hyperparathyroidism from other conditions causing hypercalcaemia has become increasingly important with the frequent detection of hypercalcaemia in biochemical screening programmes. Non-parathyroid hypercalcaemia occurs with vitamin D intoxication, the milk-alkali syndrome, sarcoidosis and hyperthyroidism. However, the most frequent, and often the most difficult, differential diagnosis lies between primary hyperparathyroidism and the hypercalcaemia of malignancy related to multiple myeloma, bony metastases or the ectopic production of substances which elevate the serum calcium. This differentiation requires a thorough study of the patient for tumours of those organs (lungs, kidneys, ovaries or breasts) which are most likely to cause hypercalcaemia. Another important differential diagnosis is the determination of the type of genetic disease present in those 1/6–1/8 of all cases of hyperparathyroidism which present hereditary conditions. It is felt that studies of the relatives of patients with hypercalcaemia can contribute greatly to the establishment of the correct diagnosis. The finding of another relative with hypercalcaemia provides evidence for primary hyperparathyroidism being the correct diagnosis if hereditary hypocalciuric hypercalcae-mia is excluded by calcium:creatinine clearance studies. The finding of a hypercalcaemic relative also requires investigation of the patient for manifestations of the multiple endocrine neoplasia (MEN) syndromes. The important associated conditions are pancreatic islet cell adenoma or carcinoma (causing hyperinsulinism, or more commonly the Zollinger-Ellison syndrome with peptic ulceration) and pituitary tumours of the MEN-1 syndrome (Marx et al 1986); or, rarely, the phaeochromocytoma or medullary thyroid carcinoma of the MEN-2 syndrome.

Therapy

The treatment of primary hyperparathyroidism is still surgical, with the excision of all hyperfunctioning parathyroid tissue by a competent neck surgeon. Those patients with hereditary hyperparathyroidism, whether from hereditary hyperparathyroidism alone or associated with MEN-1 or MEN-2, are much more likely to have multiple parathyroid gland involvement or generalized

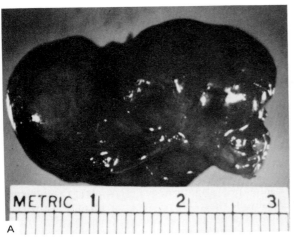

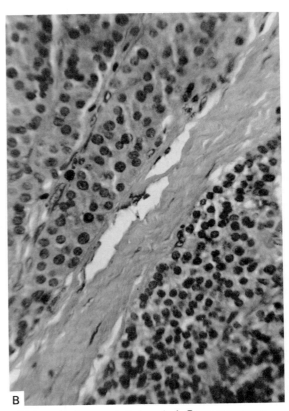

Fig. 88.1 Extremely large parathyroid adenoma from patient with multiple endocrine neoplasia type 1. **A** Gross appearance; **B** Microscopic appearance (H & E stain) showing hyperplasia of two different cell types.

hyperplasia of all parathyroid glands which may require subtotal (usually 3½ gland removal) parathyroidectomy. It is the policy of some surgeons (Block et al 1975), however, to do a selective parathyroidectomy in MEN-2 removing only those glands which are enlarged. In hereditary hyperparathyroidism, Jackson and Boonstra (1967) found the frequency of multiple parathyroid involvement to be 40%, with selective parathyroid excision being carried out in these cases. Some surgeons have advocated subtotal parathyroidectomy in all cases with the hereditary types of hyperparathyroidism, and Wells et al (1976) have recommended total parathyroidectomy and autotransplantation of parathyroid tissue into forearm muscle in patients with parathyroid hyperplasia. Clearly the apparent increasing prevalence of hyperparathyroidism (what has been termed the epidemic of hyperparathyroidism) suggests the need for effective medical treatment which would preclude surgery, although the prospects for this possibility are bleak at present.

The heterogeneity of hereditary conditions causing hyperparathyroidism

Several hereditary entities are known at the present time to cause hyperparathyroidism. These include neonatal primary hyperparathyroidism, hereditary hyperparathyroidism, multiple endocrine neoplasia type 1 (MEN-1), and multiple endocrine neoplasia type 2A (or MEN-2A) (Table 88.1). Each of these is a distinct entity and will be discussed separately. Although not truly hereditary hyperparathyroidism, hereditary hypocalciuric hypercalcaemia will be included in this discussion because it is associated with parathyroid hyperplasia and is an important condition to be differentiated from the various entities causing hereditary hyperparathyroidism.

Hereditary hypocalciuric hypercalcaemia

This entity was described by Marx et al (1977) in a report of family studies of patients with parathyroid hyperplasia. They found a high failure rate in parathyroid exploration in two kindreds with a syndrome which they termed familial hypocalciuric hypercalcaemia (FHH). The name was derived from the fact that this appeared to be an autosomal dominant condition of high penetrance of the hypercalcaemia, with the hypocalciuria being the distinctive characteristic. They emphasized that this condition could be distinguished from primary hyperparathyroidism by the low ratio of urinary calcium clearance to creatinine clearance and that this distinction was important, not only because of the high failure rate of

Table 88.1 Heterogeneity of hereditary conditions causing hyperparathyroidism

	Mode of inheritance	Age of onset	Pathology	Main ass'd conditions	Surgical treatment
Hereditary hypocalciuric hypercalcaemia	Autosomal dominant	Birth	Parathyroid hyperplasia	None	Not true hyperparathyroidism – surgery not indicated
Neonatal hyperparathyroidism	Autosomal recessive	Birth	Parathyroid hyperplasia	None	Early surgery with subtotal parathyroidectomy
Hereditary hyperparathyroidism	Autosomal dominant	About puberty	Parathyroid hyperplasia, single or multiple adenomas	None	Selective parathyroidectomy
Multiple endocrine neoplasia type 1	Autosomal dominant	About puberty	Generally parathyroid hyperplasia	Pancreatic islet cell adenoma or carcinoma; pituitary tumours	Subtotal parathyroidectomy. Surgery for pancreatic neoplasm may be the first treatment with total gastrectomy
Multiple endocrine neoplasia type 2 (or 2a)	Autosomal dominant	Childhood	Parathyroid hyperplasia	Phaeochromocytomas; medullary thyroid carcinoma	Phaeochromocytoma removal first. Total thyroidectomy and selective parathyroidectomy
Multiple endocrine neoplasia type 2b (or 3)	Autosomal dominant	Childhood	Parathyroids generally *not* affected	Mucosal neuromas, phaeochromocytoma; medullary thyroid carcinoma	Phaeochromocytoma removal first. Total thyroidectomy

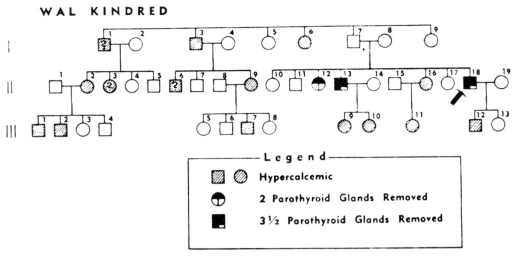

Fig. 88.2   Pedigree of family with hereditary hypocalciuric hypercalcaemia originally reported by Jackson & Boonstra (1967) as hereditary hyperparathyroidism.

parathyroid surgery for correcting the hypercalcaemia. In a subsequent article Marx et al (1980b) have emphasized that this condition was of sufficient prevalence to account for 9% of a large group of patients referred after unsuccessful parathyroidectomy. Following the description of this entity by Marx's group (1977, 1980b) we have reinvestigated a large family which we reported earlier as hereditary hyperparathyroidism (Jackson & Boonstra 1967). This family had 19 members (Fig. 88.2) with hypercalcaemia in an autosomal dominant type of inheritance pattern with failure to correct the hypercalcaemia in three members having surgery (2, 3¼ and 3½ parathyroid glands removed). It was recognized (Jackson & Boonstra 1966) that this condition was a separate entity from hereditary hyperparathyroidism but it was not until the work of Marx et al (1977) that the distinguishing characterisitcs became evident. Further studies have revealed calcium: creatinine clearance ratios in this family consistent with the diagnosis of this entity (Fig. 88.3). The findings in this family (Jackson & Kleerekoper 1981) have re-emphasized the benign nature of this condition – one member was still alive at 82, having been asymptomatic his entire life, and several known affected members died in their 70s without ever having had symptoms.

This condition is characterized by the presence of hypercalcaemia in the neonatal period and throughout childhood which contrasts with hereditary hyperparathyroidism or the hyperparathyroidism associated with the multiple endocrine neoplasia syndromes in which hypercalcaemia generally does not occur until late childhood, and mostly after puberty. The early age of hypercalcae-

mia would therefore most resemble that occurring with neonatal primary hyperparathyroidism from which it should be distinguished. Marx et al (1980a) stated that the principle differences appear to be the higher degree of hypercalcaemia seen in the reported cases of neonatal primary hyperparathyroidism and its apparent autosomal

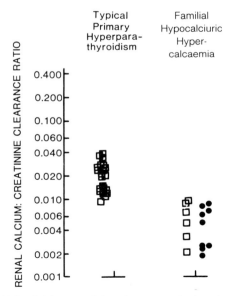

Fig. 88.3   Calcium:creatinine clearance ratios in primary hyperparathyroidism and hypocalciuric hypercalcaemia from Marx et al (1980a) indicated by the open squares and from individuals in Figure 88.2 indicated by closed circles.

recessive mode versus the autosomal dominant mode of inheritance of FHH.

Familial hypocalciuric hypercalcaemia should probably have been termed hereditary hypocalciuric hypercalcaemia since the hereditary nature has been established. Law and Heath (1985) have chosen to use the term 'familial benign hypercalcaemia' because of the priority in the literature for this term being used in the 1972 description of the entity by Foley et al. It should not actually be listed under the heading of primary hyperparathyroidism since it is not associated with an increased production of parathyroid hormone. The entity deserves much emphasis because of the prognostic and treatment implications apparent in its diagnosis and differentiation from true hereditary primary hyperparathyroidism. The aetiological mechanisms causing FHH have not been elucidated, but their study may contribute much to our understanding of calcium homeostasis.

An apparent excess of affected offspring from affected parents (Marx 1987) is interesting, especially considering its potential evolutionary effects (Jackson 1990). It has been emphasized that the families of hypercalcaemic patients should be studied prior to surgery since the finding of an affected relative tends to support the diagnosis, and provides further incentive to the surgeon to investigate all parathyroid glands because of the greater likelihood of multiple involvement. (It is at this time also that maximum co-operation can be obtained from family members for such studies). The differentiation of the entity of FHH from primary hyperparathyroidism provides an important additional reason for thoroughly studying the families of all patients with hypercalcaemia prior to surgery.

Neonatal primary hyperparathyroidism

Hypercalcaemia in the neonatal period is extremely rare. It may be related to familial hypocalciuric hypercalcaemia (FHH) (Marx et al 1982, 1985) or to neonatal primary hyperparathyroidism. In FHH surgery is not indicated but in the latter condition the disease is very serious and often fatal without surgery (Goldbloom et al 1972, Marx et al 1980b) making the differential diagnosis crucial. The hereditary cases of neonatal primary hyperparathyroidism appear to be autosomal recessively inherited. Besides the necessity to differentiate this condition from FHH, it is important to differentiate it from the hypercalcaemia seen in infants of hypoparathyroid mothers, and from a syndrome known as idiopathic hypercalcaemia of infancy, in neither of which surgery is indicated. Here again study of the parents and other family members is sometimes critical in the differential diagnosis.

Hereditary hyperparathyroidism

Hereditary hyperparathyroidism without features of the multiple endocrine neoplasia syndromes may occur as a separate dominantly inherited entity. It has been postulated however (Jackson & Boonstra 1967) that most cases thought to be this entity are part of the MEN-1 syndrome in which the family has not been followed long enough or thoroughly enough to note the other endocrine involvement. Figure 88.4 shows the affected members in the pedigree of the family of hereditary hyperparathyroidism first observed in association with pancreatitis by Jackson (1958). Most affected members were found by performing serum calcium tests on asymptomatic members of the family. It was the finding of these cases of hyperparathyroidism in this family which led to the performance of serum calcium screening (Boonstra & Jackson 1962, 1965, 1971) which has become routine almost throughout the world and which has led to the recognition of the remarkably high prevalence of a disease previously thought to be somewhat rare.

Study of the families of all cases of hyperparathyroidism has disclosed that 12–18% of all cases have other family members affected (Jackson & Boonstra 1967, 1971, Jackson et al 1977), some with hyperparathyroidism alone and others with other associated endocrine tumours. Hereditary hyperparathyroidism has the same spectrum of manifestation as does sporadic or non-hereditary hyperparathyroidism. However, the age of onset tends to be much earlier, even excluding those cases found by family studies. It may be that affected individuals have an increased risk of parathyroid carcinoma,

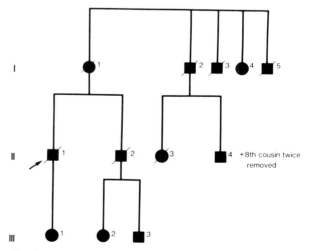

Fig. 88.4 Abbreviated pedigree indicating only the affected individuals with hyperparathyroidism in the family reported by Jackson (1958).

as is discussed under familial parathyroid carcinoma (Jackson 1985).

Multiple endocrine neoplasia type 1 (MEN-1)

The term multiple endocrine neoplasia was emphasized by Steiner et al (1968) for those syndromes rather than the previously used term of multiple endocrine adenomatosis (MEA) originally proposed by Wermer (1954). The change in terminology has a solid basis since the lesions are known to be neoplastic with carcinoma occurring frequently. Ptak and Kirsner (1970) emphasized that 50% of the pancreatic islet cell lesions of the Zollinger-Ellison syndrome are malignant. Reports of parathyroid carcinoma occuring in hereditary hyperparathyroidism and MEN-1 are reviewed later in this chapter. In the autosomal dominantly inherited type 1 syndrome, the parathyroid glands are the endocrine glands involved most frequently (Ballard et al 1964) with pancreatic islet

cell and pituitary gland involvement also frequent (88%, 81% and 65% respectively of 85 cases). Other studies have suggested parathyroid gland involvement in nearly 100% of MEN-1 families (Lamers & Froeling 1979, Shepherd 1985, Marx et al 1986). Thorough study of the families of patients with hereditary hyperparathyroidism has disclosed that often affected members have other endocrine involvement (Jackson & Boonstra 1967, Boey et al 1975, Jackson et al 1977). Pancreatic islet cell manifestations may involve tumours producing gastrin (Zollinger-Ellison sydnrome) insulin (insulinomas) or glucagon (glucagonomas). The literature reports of the MEN-1 syndrome are voluminous and will not be reviewed in detail here. They generally reveal an autosomal dominant type of inheritance with variable expressivity which sometimes appears to represent decreased penetrance (Fig. 88.5).

Although the MEN syndromes have generally been thought to be distinct clinical and genetic entities, with

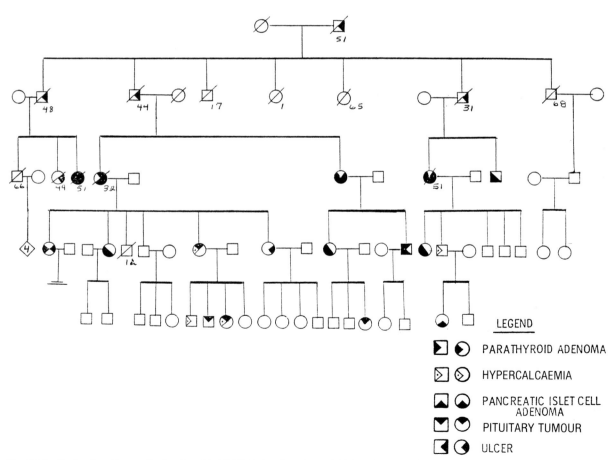

LEGEND

PARATHYROID ADENOMA

HYPERCALCAEMIA

PANCREATIC ISLET CELL ADENOMA

PITUITARY TUMOUR

ULCER

Fig. 88.5 Updated pedigree of a family with MEN-1 showing the variability of evident involvement (modified from 1975 article by Majewski and Wilson by the addition of subsequent clinical data).

parathyroid tumours being shared by each (Schimke & Hartmann 1965), overlap situations have been reported. Phaeochromocytomas are reported to occur in the same patients and the same families with pancreatic islet cell neoplasms (Carney et al 1980). The overlap families reviewed and others (including one with glucagonomas, medullary thyroid cancer and phaeochromocytoma reported by Boden & Owen 1977) suggest that a mechanism may be present resulting in a wider spectrum of endocrine involvement than was originally anticipated (Table 88.2). It is probable that in the future other hereditary endocrine neoplasia syndromes will be identified which may be separable from those recognized at present. These may be separated from each other by clinical findings, genetic linkage investigations or chromosomal studies. The gene for MEN–1 has been linked to DNA markers on the proximal long arm of chromosome 11 (Nakamura et al 1989). MEN–1 parathyroid tumours have been found to have allelic deletions on this same region of chromosome 11 (Thakker et al 1989).

Multiple endocrine neoplasia type 2 (MEN–2)

Although the syndrome of medullary thyroid carcinoma with phaeochromocytoma was identified earlier by Sipple (1961), Steiner et al (1968), in reporting a large kindred, originated the term multiple endocrine neoplasia type 2. This has appropriately come to be the accepted terminology for the autosomal dominant syndrome which also includes parathyroid gland involvement.

The 1970 report by Tashjian et al on radioimmunoassay for calcitonin in patients with medullary thyroid cancer has provided the tool, not only for the early detection of this cancer in families, but also for a greater understanding of the mechanisms of neoplasia. The value of calcitonin assay for detection of medullary thyroid cancer has been established in many other studies (Jackson et al 1973, Keiser et al 1973, Samaan et al 1973, Gagel et al 1975, Wells et al 1975, Sizemore et al 1977, Saad et al 1984 and many others). The provocative test used initially was a 4 hour calcium infusion (Fig. 88.6). Pentagastrin (Hennessy et al 1974) has largely replaced the 4 hour calcium infusion as the stimulating agent because of convenience (requiring only a rapid injection and measurements of calcitonin at 2, 5 and 10 minutes) and generally increased sensitivity. Wells et al (1978) have utilized the combination of calcium infusion (2 mg/kg) and pentagastrin (0.5 µg/kg) to obtain what they feel is the optimum stimulus to create the most sensitive test. The utilization of calcitonin radioimmunoassay in such studies for the early detection of medullary thyroid cancer in families has provided one of the best examples of the practical application of genetic studies.

Parathyroid gland involvement in this syndrome is quite variable from family to family and also within families. Within the group of families with MEN-2 studied at Henry Ford Hospital, some have been noted (Block et al 1980, Talpos et al 1983) to have the entire spectrum of medullary thyroid cancer, phaeochromocytomas and parathyroid tumours (Fig. 88.7), whereas

Table 88.2 Endocrine neoplasia overlap

Gland involvement	Adrenal cortex	Pituitary	Pancreas	Parathyroid	Medullary thyroid cancer	Adrenal medulla (Phaeochromocytoma)	Mucosal neuroma
Typical MEN-1		+	+	+	+		
Typical MEN-2 or -2a				+	+	+	
Typical MEN-2b or -3					+	+	+
Boden & Owen (1977)			+		+	+	
Cameron & Spiro (1978)			+	+		+	
Heikkinen & Åkerblom (1977)			+	+		+	
Block et al (1980)			+		+		
			+		+		
			+		+		
Carney et al (1980)			+			+	
Alberts et al (1980)	+		+	+		+	
Janson et al (1978)		+	+			+	
Hansen et al (1976)	+			+	+		
Tateishi et al (1978)			+			+	

Other combinations have been reported in association with von Hippel-Lindau disease.

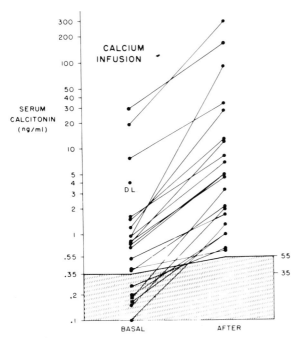

Fig. 88.6 Calcitonin responses to 4 hour calcium infusion in patients with medullary thyroid carcinoma (from Jackson et al 1973). Note that several individuals had normal basal levels of calcitonin and were identified as being affected only by the rise with calcium stimulation. Presently pentagastrin is generally used as a provocative agent at 0.5 μg/kg.

SMI KINDRED

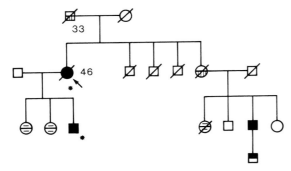

Fig. 88.7 Pedigree of family with multiple endocrine neoplasia (MEN) type 2 with medullary thyroid cancer, phaeochromocytoma and parathyroid tumours. The 46–year–old woman in generation II also had the Cushing syndrome secondary to ACTH production by the thyroid cancer.

■	●	Medullary thyroid carcinoma
▣	◔	Pheochromocytoma
▤	◉	Negative calcitonin test
▤	◉	Negative catecholamines
▥	⊕	Probable pheochromocytoma
	*	Parathyroid adenoma

others have had only medullary thyroid cancer and parathyroid tumours (Fig. 88.8), and others only the medullary thyroid cancers. The treatment of patients with this syndrome involves a thorough study of patients for their particular gland involvement. If a phaeochromocytoma can be identified as being present, surgery for this serious and potentially fatal condition should be performed first. Because of the high frequency of bilateral and multicentric involvement and because of the presence of adrenal medullary hyperplasia in these hereditary cases (Carney et al 1976, DeLellis et al 1976), bilateral adrenalectomy is generally performed. Since urinary and plasma catecholamine determinations do not permit as early a diagnosis as is possible in medullary thyroid carcinoma with provocative calcitonin testing, plasma catecholamine determination after submaximal exercise has been suggested as a provocative test (Telenius–Berg et al 1987). Computerized tomography and MIBG isotope scans of the adrenal have come to be helpful in patients with suspected phaeochromocytomas (Sisson et al 1984). Generally, patients with this syndrome have their thyroid condition detected and treated and need to be followed periodically for the development of phaeochromocytomas. They also need to be followed periodically by the sensitive provocative calcitonin procedures in order to detect recurrences of medullary thyroid carcinoma. Block et al (1978) have suggested a conservative approach in those patients with elevated calcitonin levels who do not have palpable nodes postoperative to total thyroidectomy.

For the medullary thyroid cancer, total thyroidectomy is advised, along with lymphatic node dissection as indicated. For the parathyroid involvement some surgeons have advocated subtotal parathyroidectomy whereas others (Block et al 1975) have advocated selective parathyroidectomy of any enlarged parathyroid glands.

The following of young patients at risk of inheriting medullary thyroid carcinoma has permitted the construction of curves which have proved useful in genetic counselling for this autosomal dominant condition. The curve provided from data on 38 patients whose provocative calcitonin tests had converted from negative to positive is illustrated in Figure 88.9 (Gagel et al 1982). For example, an individual in the 50% risk category at birth and a normal calcitonin level following either pentagastrin or calcium infusion at age 25 has only a 10% chance of subsequently developing this tumour.

Approximately 25% of all medullary thyroid cancers are hereditary (Block et al 1980). Comparison of the clinical and pathological characteristics have provided evidence for distinctive differences important not only in prognosis but also in therapy (Table 88.3). These findings are also of potential significance in the aetiology of

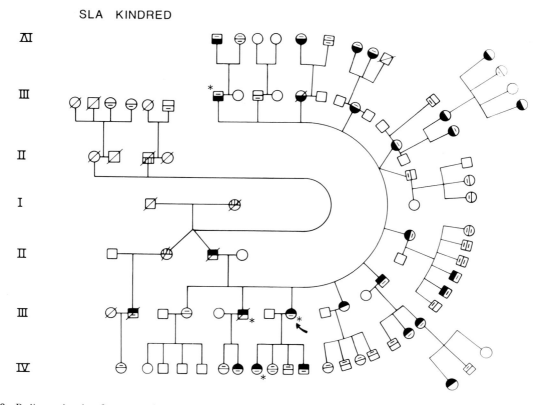

SLA KINDRED

Fig. 88.8 Pedigree showing five generations of a family affected with MEN-2 with medullary thyroid cancer and parathyroid tumours without phaeochromocytomas being present in any member (key as in Fig. 88.7).

cancer. Reports in 1973 of the new entity of C-cell hyperplasia of the thyroid (Jackson et al and Wolfe et al) postulated this condition to be the expression of the initial genetic mutation in Knudson's (1971) two-mutational-event theory on the initiation of cancer. Age of onset curves for palpable hereditary medullary carcinoma of the thyroid (MCT) (Fig. 88.10), when compared with those of sporadic MCT, are similar to those obtained by Knudson with retinoblastoma, and what is predictable on a one-hit occurrence for the hereditary tumours and two-hit occurrence for the sporadic type (Jackson et al 1979). Data from Gagel et al (1982) on the age of detectability of hereditary cases by provocative calcitonin testing (38 cases with conversion from negative to positive tests) also provide evidence for this theory.

C-cell hyperplasia (CCH) peripheral to the cancers has been observed (Jackson et al 1979) invariably in the thyroid glands of patinets with the hereditary type, but not in those of patients with the sporadic type. This is predictable if CCH is actually the manifestation of the first or genetic mutation in Knudson's theory. This

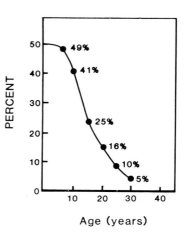

Fig. 88.9 Probability of subsequently developing the autosomal dominantly inherited medullary carcinoma of the thyroid (MCT) for individuals who have a negative stimulated calcitonin (CT) procedure at the stated age, even though they have a 50% risk at birth (based on data of Gagel et al 1982).

Table 88.3 Comparison of hereditary and sporadic medullary thyroid carcinoma (from Block et al 1980)

	Hereditary	Sporadic
Others in family	Yes, autosomal dominant pattern	No
Pathology	Bilateral, associated C-cell hyperplasia	Unilateral, no C-cell hyperplasia
Other endocrine involvement	Adrenal medulla & parathyroid glands as part of MEN-2 syndrome	Not part of MEN-2
Age of onset of palpable lesions	Average 36 years	Average 50 years
Curability by surgery based on calcitonin assay	Almost 100% of non-palpable tumours detected by calcitonin studies within families; 17% of palpable tumours	45% (all palpable)
Average life expectancy	Age about 50 (average for palpable tumours)	Age about 66

finding also has practical value in enabling the pathologist to indicate which patients are most likely to have the hereditary type of tumour so that more concentrated studies can be performed on the families of such patients. G6PD studies showing the clonal origin of medullary thyroid cancer by Baylin et al (1978) also provide evidence for the concept that these cancers occur as a change in a cell genetically predisposed by the first mutation to cancer formation. In their paper tumours of one origin in one thyroid lobe were reported with tumours of another origin in the other lobe, suggesting that the second mutation had occurred in different cells predisposed by prior mutations.

Two tumours, retinoblastoma (Yunis & Ramsay 1978) and Wilms tumour (Francke et al 1979) have forms associated with specific chromosomal deletions. Using the prometaphase culture techniques of Yunis et al (1978), Babu et al (1984, 1987) reported a deletion in the short arm of chromosome 20 in members of several kindreds with MEN-2. Although the deletion in MEN-2 was confirmed by Butler et al (1987), studies of MEN-2A families utilizing restriction fragment length polymorphism (RFLP) linkage markers have established that the

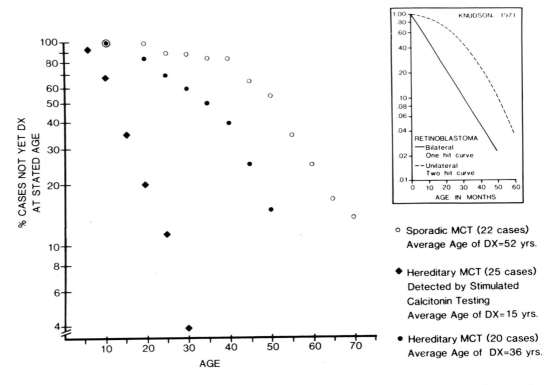

○ Sporadic MCT (22 cases)
Average Age of DX=52 yrs.

◆ Hereditary MCT (25 cases)
Detected by Stimulated
Calcitonin Testing
Average Age of DX=15 yrs.

● Hereditary MCT (20 cases)
Average Age of DX=36 yrs.

Fig. 88.10 Comparison of the proportion of cases of medullary cancer of the thyroid not yet detected at various ages for palpable sporadic cases and palpable hereditary cases (from Jackson et al 1979) and nonpalpable hereditary cases detected in family studies by calcitonin testing (Gagel et al 1982).

gene for MEN–2A lies near the centromere of chromosome 10 (Mathew et al 1987, Simpson et al 1987). Even though cytogenetic studies have not revealed visible deletions in chromosome 10 (Flejter et al 1988), a deletion of variable length must still be considered as an attractive aetiological hypothesis for MEN–2. Knudson (1980) suggested that cancer may develop when a heterozygous cell becomes homozygously defective by a mutation at a specific chromosomal site, resulting in a loss of growth control of a particular cell type. One could postulate in the MEN–2 syndrome that a chromosomal deletion results in C–cell hyperplasia (described by Wolfe et al 1973), the adrenal medullary hyperplasia (described by DeLellis et al 1976 and Carney et al 1976) and also parathyroid hyperplasia. If a second mutagenic event occurs at the allelic site on the homologous chromosome of one of the cells in these endocrine tissues, that cell becomes a malignant cell with all the potential associated with such cells. Evidence for this hypothesis has been obtained in molecular biological studies of retinoblastoma by Cavenee et al (1983). The multiple endocrine neoplasia syndromes have an importance far beyond their population prevalence because they may provide understanding of the pathogenesis not only of hereditary cancers, but also of neoplasia in general (Schimke 1986).

The syndrome of mucosal neuromas, medullary thyroid carcinoma and phaeochromocytoma was recognized as a separate syndrome by Schimke et al (1968) and Gorlin et al (1968). It has been termed MEN–2B by the Mayo Clinic group (Chong et al 1975) and MEN–3 by Khairi et al (1975). In this distinct entity, which also includes the marfanoid habitus, parathyroid involvement is rarely observed. The inheritance is autosomal dominant with MEN–2B resulting frequently from mutation and the thyroid cancers having an earlier age of onset and a more aggressive course (Jackson et al 1984). The gene for MEN–2B has also been linked to DNA markers on chromosome 10 (Jackson et al 1988).

Familial parathyroid carcinoma

Parathyroid carcinoma is a rare disease, considered on the basis of autopsy findings to represent about 3–4% of all cases of primary hyperparathyroidism (Schantz & Castleman 1973). The increasingly frequent detection of hyperparathyroidism by automated chemical screening suggests that 3–4% is likely to be an overestimate. Eight cases of parathyroid carcinoma have been reported in five families with hereditary hyperparathyroidism (Fig. 88.11). The presence of so many cases of the rarely occurring parathyroid cancer in families with hereditary hyperparathyroidism suggests that those individuals with hereditary parathyroid tumours are at greater risk of malignancy (Jackson 1985) with their parathyroid hyper-

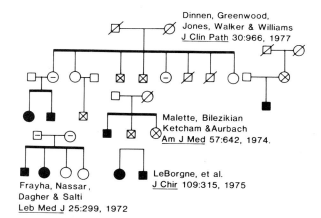

Fig. 88.11 Pedigrees from the literature showing eight cases of parathyroid cancer within five families with hereditary hyperparathyroidism (from Jackson et al 1982).
■● Parathyroid carcinoma
⊠⊗ Hyperparathyroidism

plasia occurring as a manifestation of the first or genetic event in the two-mutational-event theory on the initiation of cancer of Knudson (1971). The younger ages of onset of the eight cases of parathyroid cancer reported in hereditary hyperparathyroidism are also compatible with this theory (Table 88.4).

Genetic counselling

Genetic counselling in hyperparathyroidism is clearly dependent on the establishment of the correct diagnosis

Table 88.4 Comparison of ages of onset of sporadic and hereditary parathyroid cancer (from Jackson et al 1982)

	Cases	Average age
Parathyroid carcinoma		
Schantz & Castleman (MGH) 1973	64	44.3
Van Heerden et al (Mayo) 1979	14	50.6
	78	45.3
Hereditary cases		
LeBorgne et al 1975	1	35
	1	38
Frayha et al 1972	1	25
	1	33
Mallette et al 1974	1	51
Dinnen et al 1977	1	33
(2 families)	1	35
	1	32
	8	35.2

of the aetiology of the particular entity involved. Although most conditions are inherited as autosomal dominant diseases, autosomal recessive inheritance has been reported in one family (Law et al 1983). The age of onset is variable, as are the ramifications and the seriousness of the various conditions. Prenatal diagnosis is not possible at present in any of the conditions. Establishment of the specific diagnosis and the provision of risk figures will allow recommendations to be given to individuals as to the procedures available for the early diagnosis and treatment possible in most of the entities. The rapid advances being made in molecular biology will soon allow diagnoses to be made by linkage investigations utilizing DNA RFLP markers (Sobol et al 1989).

PRIMARY HYPOPARATHYROIDISM

Primary hypoparathyroidism is caused by a group of heterogeneous conditions associated with a deficiency of parathyroid hormone production. These are characterized by hypocalcaemia and consequent neuromuscular symptoms. As in hyperparathyroidism, hypoparathyroidism is important clinically because it is generally related to conditions for which adequate and effective treatment is available, making the need for recognition of the condition critical to the health of the individuals. Excellent classifications of hypoparathyroidism disease states have been presented by Bronsky in 1970 and by Nusynowitz et al in 1976. The latter authors separated these into two major categories – hormonopenic hypoparathyroidism and hormonoplethoric hypoparathyroidism. The hormonoplethoric states will be discussed in this chapter under the heading of pseudohypoparathyroidism (or hormone resistance states). An excellent discussion of the genetic disorders of parathyroid hormone deficiency is found in Rimoin and Schimke's book (1971) on genetic disorders of the endocrine glands.

Hypoparathyroidism is most commonly non-genetic and surgically acquired (with the excision of parathyroids or damage to the glands or their blood supply with thyroid or parathyroid surgery). Hypoparathyroidism may occur rarely following ^{131}I therapy for hyperthyroidism. Neonatal hypoparathyroidism may occur due to maternal hyperparathyroidism and subsequent suppression of the fetal parathyroid glands by maternal hypercalcaemia. This is usually transient, although it may be associated with convulsions. Hypocalcaemia may also occur secondary to hypomagnesaemia neonatally (Friedman et al 1967) – these cases would be expected to respond to magnesium therapy, but not to calcium alone.

Hypoparathyroidism can also occur neonatally as part of the third and fourth branchial arch syndrome reported by DiGeorge (1965). This condition is associated with congenital aplasia of the parathyroid glands and thymus and can be associated with an abnormality of chromosome 22 (de la Chapelle et al 1981). The patients with this syndrome have a characteristic appearance with low-set ears. It is apparently sporadic, although Steele et al (1972) have reported a girl, her maternal half-brother and possibly their mother as being affected by a condition resembling this syndrome. Although hypoparathyroidism has been reported to be related to bioinactive hormone production (Nusynowitz & Klein 1973), later studies did not confirm this possibility (Ahn et al 1986). Idiopathic hypoparathyroidism has been reported as an X–linked recessive trait (Peden 1960) with the distribution of cases within other families suggesting autosomal recessive and autosomal dominant transmission as discussed in Rimoin and Schimke's book (1971) and in McKusick's catalogue (1988).

Hypoparathyroidism occurs in association with adrenal cortical insufficiency (Addison disease) in a group of conditions which are clinically and genetically heterogeneous (Spinner et al 1968). Hypoparathyroidism and Addison disease in association with moniliasis has been termed autoimmune polyglandular syndrome type I (Neufeld et al 1980), the inheritance pattern of which seems to be most consistent with that of an autosomal recessive condition. This syndrome should be distinguished from Schmidt syndrome in which Addison disease is associated with autoimmune thyroid disease. Knowledge of the variable characteristics of these syndromes will allow physicians to screen the individuals and members of their families for other associated diseases.

Therapy

Therapy for hypoparathyroidism (and also for pseudohypoparathyroidism) involves the correction of the hypocalcaemia with oral calcium supplementation and with the addition of a proper dose of vitamin D, or one of its more potent analogues or metabolites, with attention also being directed towards any associated conditions.

PSEUDOHYPOPARATHYROIDISM (or end-organ unresponsiveness)

Pseudohypoparathyroidism (PHP) is a heterogeneous group of disorders characterized by end-organ unresponsiveness to parathyroid hormone. These disorders may occur with or without the typical skeletal or somatic abnormalities of Albright osteodystrophy. Fuller Albright et al (1942) described patients with the clinical picture of hypoparathyroidism in whom the cause was a lack of response to parathyroid hormone instead of being related to insufficient hormone production. The biochemical findings are hypocalcaemia, hyperphosphataemia and elevated parathyroid hormone levels.

PHP has been classified into 2 types: PHP type 1 with no increase in urinary cyclic AMP (cAMP) levels after parathyroid extract (PTE) infusion; and PHP type 2 with an increase in cAMP after PTE (Drezner et al 1973). The clinical picture is one of convulsions and tetany and other evidence of neuromuscular irritability similar to that seen in patients with primary or post-surgical hypoparathyroidism. Additionally, some patients with PHP show characteristic somatic abnormalities of short stature and shortened fingers and toes (Fig. 88.12 and Table 88.5). The diagnosis of PHP depends on demonstrating resistance to PTH by the lack of increase in urinary excretion of phosphate or cAMP following PTH administration. The serum PTH level is elevated in PHP, accounting for the term 'hormonoplethoric' type of hypoparathyroidism, used by Nusynowitz et al (1976). Farfel et al (1980) described a generalized deficiency of the N protein component of adenyl cyclase in some patients with PHP type 1, which was measurable at about 50% of normal levels in erythrocyte membranes. Levine et al (1980, 1986) termed this receptor-cyclase coupling G protein. Farfel et al (1980) described the classic PHP-1 phenotype (with brachydactyly, short stature and deficiency of erythrocyte N protein) as following a pattern suggestive of an autosomal dominant mode of inheritance and reported some families in which PHP-1 was not associated with abnormalities of receptor-cyclase coupling protein. Another family reported by this group (Bourne et al 1981) have the erythrocyte defect in a pattern of affected individuals suggesting autosomal recessive inheritance.

The application of the knowledge of a deficiency of erythrocyte G or N protein to the study of families should make it possible to elucidate the genetic mechanisms in particular kindreds and to delineate specific types of PHP-1. It should also allow the early detection and treatment of some cases. It will be very important to determine which types are associated with mental retardation and whether or not such early detection and treatment will prevent the mental retardation which is so troublesomely and unpredictably associated with pseudohypoparathyroidism.

Pseudo-pseudohypoparathyroidism (PPHP) is a condition described by Albright et al (1952) to indicate those patients who have the skeletal or somatic defects of pseudohypoparathyroidism (Fig. 88.12) with normal calcium values (a false PHP). Instances in which PPHP and PHP exist in the same individuals at different stages (Palubinskas & Davies 1959) and PPHP and PHP exist in different members of the same families (Mann et al 1962, Williams et al 1977) suggest that these conditions may represent variable expression of one genetic disease entity.

Genetics

Pseudohypoparathyroidism has in the past been considered to be inherited by an X-linked mechanism as discussed in McKusick's catalogue (1988) and the problems of attributing PHP to this genetic mechanism are discussed by him. These problems have become more obvious as the result of an increasing appreciation of the variability in the biochemical defects in a syndrome in which the heterogeneity is so evident.

Genetic counselling

Genetic counselling in pseudohypoparathyroidism is extremely difficult and will continue to be so until we have a more firm biochemical understanding of the heterogeneous entities which comprise this condition. The mental retardation which is associated at times is of great concern to the counsellor, even in those families in which it has not been evident in known affected individuals. At present genetic counselling in PHP must be individualized and must depend on thorough pedigree-taking within the family of that individual and the delineation of the manifestations in those affected within that kindred. This requires the utilization in those family studies of all the biochemical parameters available at the time. In the many instances in which the cases appear to be sporadic or to be a part of only a limited number of affected individuals in a kindred, the genetic counsellor must express to the patients and their families the difficulties of providing accurate predictions of risk in the state of knowledge of the condition at that particular time.

Table 88.5 Signs and symptoms in pseudohypoparathyroidism type 1 (from Drezner & Neelon 1983)

Hypocalcaemia	96% of 175 cases
Short stature (<16 inches, age 16 or older)	80%
Round face	92%
Short metacarpals	68%
Short metatarsals	43%
Mental retardation	75%
Seizures	59%

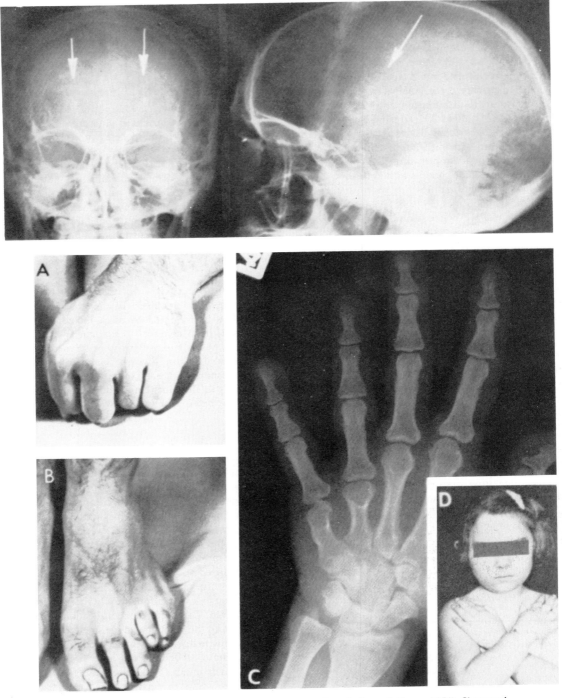

Fig. 88.12 Illustration of somatic features of pseudohypoparathyroidism (from Jackson & Frame 1972). Shortened metacarpal bones are illustrated in **A** & **C** and the shortened metatarsals are shown in **B**. The rounded face in a girl who has short stature is shown in **D**. Basal ganglia calcification seen on skull X-ray is shown in the top illustration.

REFERENCES

Ahn T G, Antonarakis S E, Kronenberg H M, Igaraski T, Levine M A 1986 Familial isolated hypoparathyroidism: A molecular genetic analysis of 8 families with 23 affected persons. Medicine (Baltimore) 65: 73–81

Alberts W M, McMeekin J O, George J M 1980 Mixed multiple endocrine neoplasia syndromes. Journal of the American Medical Association 244: 1236–1237

Albright F, Burnett C H, Smith P H, Parson W 1942 Pseudohypoparathyroidism of 'Seabright-Bantam Syndrome'. Endocrinology 30: 922–932

Albright F, Forbes A P, Henneman P H 1952 Pseudo-pseudohypoparathyroidism. Transactions of the Association of American Physicians 65: 337–350

Arnold A, Staunton C E, Kim H G, Gaz R D, Kronenberg H M 1988 Monoclonality and abnormal parathyroid hormone genes in parathyroid adenomas. New England Journal of Medicine 318: 658–662

Babu V R, Van Dyke D L, Jackson C E 1984 Chromosome 20 deletion in human multiple endocrine neoplasia types 2A and 2B: a double blind study. Proceedings of the National Academy of Sciences USA 81: 2525–2528

Babu V R, Van Dyke D L, Flejter W L, Jackson C E 1987 Chromosome 20 deletion in multiple endocrine neoplasia type 2: Expanded double-blind studies. American Journal of Medical Genetics 28: 738–748

Ballard H S, Frame B, Hartsock R J 1964 Familial multiple endocrine adenoma – peptic ulcer complex. Medicine (Baltimore) 43: 481–515

Baylin S B, Hsu S H, Gann D S, Smallridge R C, Wells S A Jr. 1978 Inherited medullary thyroid carcinoma: a final monoclonal mutation in one of multiple clones of susceptible cells. Science 199: 429–431

Block M A, Jackson C E, Tashjian A H Jr. 1975 Management of parathyroid glands in surgery for medullary thyroid carcinoma. Archives of Surgery 110: 617–624

Block M A, Jackson C E, Tashjian A H Jr. 1978 Management of occult medullary thyroid carcinoma: evidenced only by serum calcitonin elevations after apparently adequate neck operations. Archives of Surgery 113: 368–372

Block M A, Jackson C E, Greenawald K A, Yott J B, Tashjian A H Jr. 1980 Clinical characteristics distinguishing hereditary from sporadic medullary thyroid carcinoma. Archives of Surgery 115: 142–148

Boden G, Owen O E 1977 Familial hyperglucagonemia – an autosomal dominant disorder. New England Journal of Medicine 296: 534–538

Boey J H, Cooke T J C, Gilbert J M, Sweeney E C, Taylor S 1975 Occurrence of other endocrine tumours in primary hyperparathyroidism. Lancet 2: 781–784

Boonstra C E, Jackson C E 1962 The clinical value of routine serum calcium analysis. Annals of Internal Medicine 57: 963–969

Boonstra C E, Jackson C E 1965 Hyperparathyroidism detected by routine serum calcium analysis: prevalence in a clinic population. Annals of Internal Medicine 63: 468–474

Boonstra C E, Jackson C E 1971 Serum calcium survey for hyperparathyroidism: results in 50,000 clinic patients. American Journal of Clinical Pathology 55: 523–526

Bourne H R, Farfel Z, Brickman A S 1981 Pseudo-hypoparathyroidism: an inherited disorder of adenylate cyclase. Advances in Cyclic Nucleotide Research 14: 43–49

Bronsky D 1970 Hyperparathyroidism with Albright's osteodystrophy: Case report and a proposed new classification of parathyroid disease. Journal of Clinical Endocrinology and Metabolism 31: 271–276

Butler M G, Rames L J, Joseph G M 1987 Cytogenetic studies of individuals from four kindreds with multiple endocrine neoplasia type II. Cancer Genetics and Cytogenetics 28: 253–280

Cameron D, Spiro H M 1978 Zollinger-Ellison Syndrome with multiple endocrine adenomatosis type II. New England Journal of Medicine 299: 152–153

Carney J A, Sizemore G W, Sheps S G 1976 Adrenal medullary disease in multiple endocrine neoplasia, type 2: Phaeochromocytoma and its precursors. American Journal of Clinical Pathology 66: 279–290

Carney J A, Go V L W, Gordon H, Northcutt R C, Pearse A G E, Sheps S 1980 Familial phaeochromocytoma and islet cell tumour of the pancreas. American Journal of Medicine 68: 515–521

Cavenee W K, Dryja T P, Phillips R A et al 1983 Expression of recessive alleles by chromosomal mechanisms in retinoblastoma. Nature 305: 779–784

Chong G C, Beahrs O H, Sizemore G W, Woolner L H 1975 Medullary carcinoma of the thyroid gland. Cancer 35: 695–704

de la Chapelle A, Herva R, Loivisto M, Aula P 1981 A deletion in chromosome 22 can cause DiGeorge syndrome. Human Genetics 57: 253–256

DeLellis R A, Wolfe H G, Gagel R F 1976 Adrenal medullary hyperplasia: a morphometric analysis in patients with familial medullary thyroid carcinoma. American Journal of Pathology 83: 177–196

DiGeorge A M 1965 Discussions on a new concept of the cellular basis of immunity. Journal of Pediatrics 67: 907–908

Dinnen J S, Greenwood R H, Jones J H, Walker D A, Williams E D 1977 Parathyroid carcinoma in familial hyperparathyroidism. Journal of Clinical Pathology 30: 966–975

Drezner M K, Neelon F A 1983 Pseudohypoparathyroidism. In: Stanbury J B, Wyngaarden J B, Fredrickson D S, Goldstein J L, Brown M S (eds) The Metabolic Basis of Inherited Disease. McGraw-Hill, New York, p 1508–1527

Drezner M, Neelon F A, Lebovitz H E 1973 Pseudohypoparathyroidism type II: a possible defect in the reception of the cyclic AMP signal. New England Journal of Medicine 289: 1056–1060

Farfel Z, Brickman A S, Kaslow H R, Brothers V M, Bourne H R 1980 Defect of receptor – cyclase coupling protein in pseudohypoparathyroidism. New England Journal of Medicine 303: 237–242

Fialkow P J, Jackson C E, Block M A, Greenawald K A 1977 Multicellular origin of parathyroid adenomas. New England Journal of Medicine 297: 696–698

Flejter W L, Babu V R, Van Dyke D L, Jackson C E 1988 High resolution studies of chromosome 10 in 23 MEN-2 families. Cancer Genetics and Cytogenetics 32: 301–303

Foley T P Jr., Harrison H C, Arnaud C D, Harrison H E 1972 Familial benign hypercalcemia. Journal of Pediatrics 81: 1060–1067

Francke U, Holmes L B, Atkins L 1979 Aniridia – Wilm's tumor association: evidence for specific deletion of 11p13. Cytogenetics and Cell Genetics 24: 183–192

Frayha R A, Nassar V H, Dagher F, Salti I S 1972 Familial

parathyroid carcinoma. Lebanese Medical Journal 25: 299-309

Friedman E, Sakaguchi K, Bale A E et al 1989 Clonality of parathyroid tumors in familial multiple neoplasia type 1. New England Journal of Medicine 321: 213-218

Friedman M, Hatcher G, Watson I 1967 Primary hypomagnesemia with secondary hypocalcemia in an infant. Lancet 1: 703-705

Gagel R F, Melvin K E W, Tashjian A H Jr. et al 1975 Natural history of the familial medullary thyroid carcinoma – phaeochromocytoma syndrome and the identification of preneoplastic stages by screening studies, a five year report. Transactions of the Association of American Physicians 88: 177-191

Gagel R F, Jackson C E, Block M A, Feldman Z T, Reichlin S, Hamilton B P, Tashjian A H Jr. 1982 Age-related risk of development of hereditary medullary thyroid carcinoma. Journal of Pediatrics 101: 941-946

Goldbloom R B, Gillis D A, Prasad M 1972 Hereditary parathyroid hyperplasia: a surgical emergency of early infancy. Pediatrics 49: 514-523

Gorlin R J, Sedano H O, Vickers R A, Cervenka J 1968 Multiple mucosal neuromas, phaeochromocytoma and medullary carcinoma of the thyroid – a syndrome. Cancer 22: 293-299

Hansen O P, Hansen M, Hansen H H, Rose B 1976 Multiple endocrine adenomatosis of mixed type. Acta Medica Scandinavica 200: 327-331

Heikkinen E S, Akerblom H K 1977 Diagnostic and operative problems in multiple pheochromocytomas. Journal of Pediatric Surgery 12: 157-163

Hennessy J F, Wells S A Jr., Ontjes D A, Cooper C W 1974 A comparison of pentagastrin injection and calcium infusion as provocative agents for the detection of medullary carcinoma of the thyroid. Journal of Clinical Endocrinology and Metabolism 39: 487-500

Jackson C E 1958 Hereditary hyperparathyroidism associated with recurrent pancreatitis. Annals of Internal Medicine 49: 829-836

Jackson C E 1985 The two-hit theory of neoplasia: implications for the pathogenesis of hyperparathyroidism. Cancer Genetics and Cytogenetics 14: 175-178

Jackson C E 1990 Parathyroid Disease. In: King R A, Rotter J I, Motulsky A G (eds) The Genetic Basis of Common Disease. Oxford University Press, Oxford, (in press)

Jackson C E, Boonstra C E 1966 Hereditary hypercalcemia and parathyroid hyperplasia without definite hyperparathyroidism. Journal of Laboratory and Clinical Medicine 68: 883

Jackson C E, Boonstra C E 1967 The relationship of hereditary hyperparathyroidism to multiple endocrine adenomatosis. American Journal of Medicine 43: 727-734

Jackson C E, Frame B 1972 Diagnosis and management of parathyroid disorders. Orthopedic Clinics of North America 3: 699-712

Jackson C E, Kleerekoper M 1981 Hereditary hypocalciuric hypercalcemia is benign in 15 year followup. Clinical Research 29: 409A

Jackson C E, Tashjian A H Jr., Block M A 1973 Detection of medullary thyroid cancer by calcitonin assay in families. Annals of Internal Medicine 78: 845-852

Jackson C E, Frame B, Block M A 1977 Prevalence of endocrine neoplasia syndromes in genetic studies of parathyroid tumours. In: Mulvihill J J, Miller R W,

Fraumini J F Jr. (eds) Genetics of Human Cancer. Raven Press, New York, p 205-208

Jackson C E, Block M A, Greenawald K A, Tashjian A H Jr. 1979 The two-mutational-event theory in medullary thyroid cancer. American Journal of Human Genetics 31: 704-710

Jackson C E, Cerny J P, Block M A, Fialkow P J 1982 Probable clonal origin of aldosteronomas vs the multiple cell origin of parathyroid 'adenomas'. Surgery 92: 875-879

Jackson C E, Talpos G B, Block M A, Norum R A, Lloyd R V, Tashjian A H Jr. 1984 Clinical value of tumour doubling estimations in multiple endocrine neoplasia type II (MEN-II). Surgery 96: 981-986

Jackson C E, Norum R A, O'Neal L W, Nikolai T F, Delaney J P 1988 Linkage between MEN2B and chromosome 10 markers linked to MEN2A. American Journal of Human Genetics 43: A147

Janson K L, Roberts J A, Varela M 1978 Multiple endocrine adenomatosis: in support of the common origin theories. Journal of Urology 119: 161-165

Keiser H R, Beaven M A, Doppman J, Wells S Jr., Buja L M 1973 Sipple's syndrome: medullary thyroid carcinoma, pheochromocytomas, and parathyroid disease. Annals of Internal Medicine 78: 561-579

Khairi M R A, Dexter R B M, Burzynski N J, Johnston C C Jr 1975 Mucosal neuroma, pheochromocytoma and medullary thyroid carcinoma: multiple endocrine neoplasia type 3. Medicine (Baltimore) 54: 89-112

Knudson A G Jr 1971 Mutation and cancer: statistical study of retinoblastoma. Proceedings of the National Academy of Sciences USA 78: 820-823

Knudson A G Jr. 1980 Genetics and Cancer. American Journal of Medicine 69: 1-3

Lamers C B H W, Froeling P G A M 1979 Clinical significance of hyperparathyroidism in familial multiple endocrine adenomatosis type 1 (MEA 1). American Journal of Medicine 66: 422-424

Law W M Jr., Heath H 1985 Familial benign hypercalcemia (hypocalciuric hypercalcemia). Clinical and pathogenetic studies in 21 families. Annals of Internal Medicine 201: 511-519

Law W M Jr., Hodgson S F, Heath H III 1983 Autosomal recessive inheritance of familial hyperparathyroidism. New England Journal of Medicine 309: 650-653

LeBorgne J, Le Neel J-C, Buzelin F, Malvy P 1975 Cancer familial des parathyroides. Journal de Chirurgie (Paris) 109: 315-326

Levine M A, Downs R W Jr., Singer M, Marx S J, Aurbach G D, Spiegel A M 1980 Deficient activity of guanine nucleotide regulatory protein in erythrocytes from patients with pseudohypoparathyroidism. Biochemical and Biophysical Research Communications 94: 1319-1324

Levine M A, Jap T S, Mauseth R S, Downs R W, Spiegel A M 1986 Activity of the stimulatory guanine nucleotide-binding protein is reduced in erythrocytes from patients with pseudohypoparathyroidism and pseudo-pseudohypoparathyroidism: biochemical, endocrine and genetic analysis of Albright's hereditary osteodystrophy in six kindreds. Journal of Clinical Endocrinology and Metabolism 62: 497-502

McKusick V A 1988 Mendelian inheritance in man: catalogs of autosomal dominant, autosomal recessive and X-linked phenotypes, 8th edn. The Johns Hopkins University Press, Baltimore

Majewski T J, Wilson S D 1975 The MEA-I syndrome: an all

for none phenomenon? Surgery 86: 475–84

Mallette L E, Bilezikian J P, Ketcham A S, Aurbach G D 1974 Parathyroid carcinoma in familial hyperparathyroidism. American Journal of Medicine 57: 642–648

Mann J B, Alteman S, Hill A G 1962 Albright's hereditary osteodystrophy comprising pseudohypoparathyroidism with and pseudo-pseudohypoparathyroidism with report of two cases representing the complete syndrome occurring in successive generations. Annals of Internal Medicine 56: 315–342

Marx S J, Spiegel A M, Brown E M, Aurbach G D 1977 Family studies in patients with primary parathyroid hyperplasia. American Journal of Medicine 62: 698–706

Marx S J, Spiegel A M, Brown E M, Gardner D G, Downs R W, Attie M, Aurbach G D 1980a Familial hypocalciuric hypercalcemia. In: DeLuca H F, Anast C C (eds) Pediatric Diseases Related to Calcium. Elsevier North Holland, New York, p 413–431

Marx S J, Stock J L, Attie M F et al 1980b Familial hypocalciuric hypercalcemia: recognition among patients referred after unsuccessful parathyroid exploration. Annals of Internal Medicine 92: 351–356

Marx S J, Attie M F, Spiegel A M, Levine M A, Lasker R D, Fox M 1982 An association between neonatal severe primary hyperparathyroidism and familial hypocalciuric hypercalcemia. New England Journal of Medicine 306: 257–264

Marx S J, Fraser D, Rapaport A 1985 Familial hypocalciuric hypercalcemia. Mild expression of the gene in heterozygotes and severe expression in homozygotes. American Journal of Medicine 78: 15–22

Marx S J, Vinik A I, Santen R J, Floyd J C Jr., Mills J L, Green J III 1986 Multiple endocrine neoplasia type I: Assessment of laboratory tests to screen for the gene in a large kindred. Medicine (Baltimore) 65: 226–238

Mathew C G P, Chin K S, Easton D F et al 1987 A linked genetic marker for multiple endocrine neoplasia type 2A on chromosome 10. Nature 328: 527–528

Nakamura Y, Larsson C, Julier C et al 1989 Localization of the genetic defect in multiple endocrine neoplasia type 1 within a small region of chromosome 11. American Journal of Human Genetics 44: 751–755

Neufeld M, Maclaren N, Blizzard R 1980 Autoimmune polyglandular syndromes. Pediatric Annals 9: 154–162

Nusynowitz M L, Klein M H 1973 Pseudoidiopathic hypoparathyroidism. Hypoparathyroidism with ineffective parathyroid hormone. American Journal of Medicine 55: 677–686

Nusynowitz M L, Frame B, Kolb F O 1976 The spectrum of the hypoparathyroid states: a classification based on physiologic principles. Medicine (Baltimore) 55: 105–119

Palubinskas A J, Davies H 1959 Calcification of the basal ganglia of the brain. American Journal of Roentgenology 82: 806–822

Peden V H 1960 True idiopathic hypo-parathyroidism as a sex-linked recessive trait. American Journal of Human Genetics 12: 323–337

Ptak T, Kirsner J B 1970 The Zollinger-Ellison Syndrome, polyendocrine adenomatosis and other endocrine associations with peptic ulcer. Advances in Internal Medicine 16: 213–242

Rimoin D L, Schimke R N 1971 Genetic disorders of the endocrine glands. Mosby, St Louis, p 79–112

Saad M F, Ordonez N G, Rashid R K, Guido J J, Hill C S Jr., Hickey R C, Samaan N A 1984 Medullary carcinoma of the thyroid: a study of the clinical features and prognostic factors in 161 patients. Medicine (Baltimore) 63: 319–342

Samaan N A, Hill C S Jr., Beceiro J R, Schultz P N 1973 Immunoreactive calcitonin in medullary carcinoma of the thyroid and in maternal and cord serum. Journal of Laboratory and Clinical Medicine 81: 671–681

Schantz A, Castleman B 1973 Parathyroid carcinoma: a study of 70 cases. Cancer 31: 600–605

Schimke R N 1986 Multiple endocrine neoplasia: Search for the oncogenic trigger. New England Journal of Medicine 314: 1315–1316

Schimke R N, Hartmann W H 1965 Familial amyloid-producing medullary thyroid carcinoma and pheochromocytoma: a distinct genetic entity. Annals of Internal Medicine 63: 1027–1039

Schimke R N, Hartmann W H, Prout T E, Rimoin D L 1968 Syndrome of bilateral pheochromocytoma, medullary thyroid carcinoma and multiple neuromas. New England Journal of Medicine 279: 1–7

Shepherd J J 1985 Latent familial multiple endocrine neoplasia in Tasmania. The Medical Journal of Australia 142: 395–397

Simpson N E, Kidd, Goodfellow P J et al 1987 Assignment of multiple endocrine neoplasia type 2A to chromosome 10 by linkage. Nature 328: 528–530

Sipple J H 1961 The association of pheochromocytoma with carcinoma of the thyroid gland. American Journal of Medicine 31: 163–166

Sisson J C, Shapiro B, Bierwaltes W H 1984 Scintigraphy with I[131] MIBG as an aid to the treatment of pheochromocytomas in patients with the multiple endocrine neoplasia type 2 syndromes. Henry Ford Hospital Medical Journal 32: 254–261

Sizemore G W, Carney J A, Heath H 1977 Epidemiology of medullary carcinoma of the thyroid gland: a 5 year experience (1971–1976). Surgical Clinics of North America 57: 633–645

Sobol H, Narod S A, Nakamura Y et al 1989 The screening for multiple endocrine neoplasia type 2A by DNA polymorphism analysis. New England Journal of Medicine 321: 996–1001

Spinner M W, Blizzard R M, Childs B 1968 Clinical and genetic heterogeneity in idiopathic Addison's disease and hypoparathyroidism. Journal of Clinical Endocrinology and Metabolism 28: 795–804

Steele R W, Limas C, Thurman G B, Schuelein M, Bauer H, Bellanti J A 1972 Familial thymic aplasia. New England Journal of Medicine 287: 787–791

Steiner A L, Goodman A D, Powers S R 1968 Study of a kindred with pheochromocytoma, medullary thyroid carcinoma, hyperparathyroidism and Cushing's disease: multiple endocrine neoplasia type 2. Medicine (Baltimore) 47: 371–409

Talpos G B, Jackson C E, Yott J B, Van Dyke D L 1983 Phenotype mapping of the multiple endocrine type II syndrome. Surgery 94: 650–654

Tashjian A H Jr., Howland B G, Melvin K E W 1970 Immunoassay of human calcitonin. Clinical measurement, relation to serum calcium and studies in patients with medullary carcinoma. New England Journal of Medicine 283: 890–895

Tateishi R, Wada A, Ishigura S et al 1978 Coexistence of

bilateral pheochromocytoma and pancreatic islet cell tumour: report of a case and review of the literature. Cancer 42: 2928–2934

Telenius-Berg M, Berg B, Hamberger B, Tibblin S 1987 Screening for early asymptomatic pheochromocytoma in MEN-2. Henry Ford Hospital Medical Journal 35: 110–114

Thakker R V, Bouloux P, Wooding C et al 1989 Association of parathyroid tumours in multiple endocrine neoplasia type 1 with loss of alleles on chromosome 11. New England Journal of Medicine 321: 218–224

Van Heerden J A, Weiland L H, ReMine W H, Walls J T, Purnell D C 1979 Cancer of the parathyroid glands. Archives of Surgery 114: 475–480

Wells S A Jr., Ontjes D A, Cooper C W, Hennessy J F, Ellis G J, McPherson H T, Sabiston D C 1975 The early diagnosis of medullary carcinoma of the thyroid gland in patients with multiple endocrine neoplasia type II. Annals of Surgery 182: 362–370

Wells S A Jr., Ellis G J, Gunnells J C, Schneider A B, Sherwood L M 1976 Parathyroid autotransplantation in primary parathyroid hyperplasia. New England Journal of Medicine 295: 57–62

Wells S A Jr., Baylin S B, Linehan W M, Farrel R E, Cox E B, Cooper C W 1978 Provocative agents and the diagnosis of medullary carcinoma of the thyroid gland. Annals of Surgery 188: 139–141

Wermer P 1954 Genetic aspects of adenomatosis of the endocrine glands. American Journal of Medicine 16: 363–371

Williams A J, Wilkinson J L, Taylor W H 1977 Pesudohypoparathyroidism: variable manifestations within a family. Archives of Disease of Childhood 52: 798–800

Wolfe H J, Melvin K E W, Cervi-Skinner S J, Al Saadi A A, Juliar J F, Jackson C E, Tashjian A H Jr. 1973 C-cell hyperplasia preceding medullary thyroid carcinoma. New England Journal of Medicine 289: 437–441

Yunis J J, Ramsay N 1978 Retinoblastoma and sub band deletion of chromosome 13. American Journal of Diseases of Children 132: 161–163

Yunis J J, Sawyer J R, Ball D W 1978 The characterization of high-resolution G-banded chromosomes of man. Chromosoma (Berlin) 67: 293–307

89. Diabetes mellitus

C. M. Vadheim   D. L. Rimoin   J. I. Rotter

INTRODUCTION

Diabetes mellitus is a diagnostic term for a group of disorders characterized by abnormalities in glucose homeostasis, i.e. elevated blood sugar. Its manifestations can range from asymptomatic glucose intolerance (i.e. higher than normal blood glucose levels in response to an administered glucose load), to an acute medical emergency (diabetic ketoacidosis), to chronic complications such as nephropathy, neuropathy, retinopathy, or accelerated atherosclerosis. It is among the most common of chronic disorders, affecting up to 5–10% of the adult population of the Western world. Its prevalence varies over the globe with certain populations, such as certain American Indian tribes and the inhabitants of Micronesia and Polynesia having extremely high rates of disease (West 1978, Zimmet 1979, Knowler et al 1981).

It has been clearly established that diabetes mellitus is not a single disease but a genetically heterogeneous group of disorders that share a common factor of glucose intolerance (Creutzfeldt et al 1976, Rotter et al 1978, Fajans et al 1978, Friedman & Fialkow 1980, Rotter & Rimoin 1981a,b, Kobberling & Tattersall 1982, Rotter et al 1984, Rotter et al 1990). The concept of genetic heterogeneity, i.e. that different genetic and/or environmental aetiological factors can result in similar phenotypes, has significantly altered the genetic analysis of this common disorder. It is now apparent that diabetes and glucose intolerance are not diagnostic terms but, like anaemia, are simply a symptom complex and a laboratory abnormality respectively which can result from a number of distinct aetiological factors.

Until 1979 there were no generally accepted uniform criteria for diagnosing diabetes worldwide, making both clinical diagnosis and epidemiological comparisons difficult (West 1975, Bennett 1979, Stern 1988). Now two sets of closely related diagnostic criteria are widely accepted: one suggested by the US National Institutes of Health (NIH) National Diabetes Data Group (NDDG), and the other by the World Health Organization (WHO) (NDDG 1979, WHO 1980, Nelson 1988). Another set of diagnostic criteria, outlined by the European Association for the Study of Diabetes, is roughly comparable to the WHO criteria (Keen et al 1979). Although the NDDG and WHO criteria are similar, there are some significant differences, particularly in the classification of persons with borderline glucose values. Several authors have recently compared and discussed the differences between these two diagnostic systems, and the current consensus is to favour the WHO criteria because of their greater simplicity and worldwide acceptance (Agner et al 1982, Massari et al 1983, Haffner et al 1984, Harris et al 1985, Riccardi et al 1985, Stern 1988).

Diabetes mellitus is currently classified into 'idiopathic diabetes mellitus' and 'diabetes or glucose intolerance associated with genetic syndromes and other conditions'. The majority of cases of diabetes mellitus currently are placed into the idiopathic category, and the exact prevalence of the latter category is unknown. The idiopathic category is subdivided into two major groups: (1) an insulin dependent type (IDDM or type I; previously referred to as juvenile onset) and; (2) a non-insulin dependent type (NIDDM or type II; previously referred to as maturity onset). Even these major categories can be further subdivided. The subclassification of disease is of major importance, because it is only through the delineation of clinical and aetiological heterogeneity that distinct disease entities will be identified. To be meaningful, pathophysiological studies, genetic analysis, prospective epidemiological studies, delineation of risk factors, and creation of risk tables for genetic counselling, must be independently performed on each of the specific disease entities constituting the diabetic phenotype.

DIFFICULTIES IN GENETIC STUDIES OF DIABETES

The geneticist is confronted with a number of obstacles in his or her attempts to unravel the genetics of diabetes, including differences in the definition of affected individuals, modification of the expression of the diabetic genotype by environmental factors, and variability in the age of onset of the disease. One of the major sources of confusion in the study of diabetes mellitus has been the definition of an 'affected' individual. Some investigators have called an individual 'diabetic' only if he or she has clinical symptoms of the disease, while others have accepted a mildly abnormal glucose tolerance test. There is still some argument as to whether diabetes mellitus, or at least some forms of diabetes, are a distinct disease or simply the tail-end of the normal distribution of blood sugar concentrations.

Another problem in the definition of affected individuals is the marked clinical variability of diabetes. The phenotypic expression of the diabetes genotype appears to be modified by a variety of environmental factors, including diet, obesity, infection, and physical activity, as well as sex and parity. Obese non-insulin dependent diabetics may lose all signs of the disorder, clinical as well as chemical, if their weight returns to normal. Because of the marked variability in the age of onset of the disease, only a fraction of those individuals possessing the diabetic genotype may be recognized. Therefore, it is impossible to say at any given point in time whether a clinically unaffected individual carries the diabetic genotype. Thus, longitudinal studies are required to detect genetically affected family members who may eventually manifest clinical disease.

The high prevalence of diabetes in the population presents additional difficulties for the geneticist. Are a given pair of relatives affected because they have the same genotype, because they share the same environment, or do they have different types of diabetes altogether? The diabetic syndromes are sufficiently common for different forms to occasionally occur in the same family by chance alone.

The most important impediment to genetic analysis has been a lack of knowledge concerning the basic defect(s) in each of the disorders leading to diabetes. Because of this, there is no certain method for detecting all individuals with the mutant genotype prior to its clinical manifestations, that is, individuals who possess the diabetic genotype but have no signs of abnormal carbohydrate metabolism.

Nevertheless, despite all these obstacles major strides have been made in delineating the genetic basis of the diabetic syndromes. This progress has come through an increasing recognition of the genetic heterogeneity of diabetes, and its delineation by a variety of lines of evidence as discussed below.

DIABETES IN FAMILIES AND TWINS

Familial aggregation of diabetes

Clinical heterogeneity and the importance of genetic factors have long been recognized in diabetes. For example, the Hindu physicians Charaka and Sushruta, over 2000 years ago, commented on 'honey urine' of two causes — genetic, i.e. passed from one generation to another in 'the seed', and environmental, i.e. injudicious diet. They also discussed the existence of two types of disease: one associated with emaciation, dehydration, polyuria and lassitude; the other associated with stout build, gluttony, obesity, and sleepiness (Simpson, 1976, Cahill 1979a).

Many authors have shown that diabetics have an 'increased family history' of the disease (Rimoin & Schimke 1971). In most reports the frequency of diabetics with positive family histories of the disease ranges from 25–50%. Since the frequency of non-diabetic individuals with a positive family history of diabetes has usually been found to be below 15%, this family history information has been used to support the hypothesis that diabetes mellitus is an hereditary disorder. These types of data, however, are not very powerful. A more accurate method of assessing familial aggregation is by comparing the diabetes prevalence in specific relatives of affected individuals to that found among similar relatives of non-diabetic controls. Pincus and White (1933) were the first to use this method in the study of diabetes, when they established the increased prevalence of the disease among the relatives of diabetics statistically. These findings have since been confirmed by many other investigators (Table 89.1). Using more sensitive markers of the diabetic phenotype, such as oral, intravenous, and cortisone-induced glucose tolerance tests, the prevalence of affected individuals among the relatives of diabetics is even higher (usually ranging between 10–30% of the parents, sibs, or close relatives, compared to a prevalence of 1–6% of the relatives of nondiabetic individuals). Thus, the prevalence of both clinical diabetes and abnormal glucose tolerance is significantly greater among the close relatives of diabetics than among similar relatives of nondiabetic individuals.

Early twin studies

Familial aggregation of a trait may be caused by either genetic or environmental factors. Twin studies represent one approach to resolving this question. The frequency of concordance (both members of the twin pair affected) of monozygotic (identical) twins is compared with that of dizygotic (fraternal) twins. Monozygotic twins share all genes, and thus theoretically should be concordant for disorders with purely genetic aetiology. Dizygotic twins share only half their genes and are thus no more alike genetically than any pair of sibs.

Twin studies have confirmed the importance of genetic factors in the aetiology of diabetes (Table 89.2). Using clinical diabetes as the criterion for being affected,

Table 89.1 Prevalence of diabetes and glucose intolerance among the relatives of diabetic and control patients

Authors	Relatives studied	Criteria	Percentage affected[†] Diabetic	Control
Keen & Track (1968)*	Parents	Clinical	4.0–9.7	1.1–2.9
Working Party College of Practitioners (1965)*	Parents	Clinical	4.2–9.2	1.5–3.1
Levit & Pessikova (1934)	Parents	Clinical	4.3	
Simpson (1964)	Parents	Clinical	4.8	
Harris (1950)	Parents	Clinical	5.0	
Thompson & Watson (1952)	Parents	Clinical	7.1	
Pincus & White (1933)	Parents	Clinical	8.3	2.0
Bartels (1953)	Parents	Clinical	9.0	
Hunter & McKay (1967)**	Parents	IV GTT	24.0	
Braunsteiner et al (1966)	Parents	IV GTT	76.0	
Working Party College of Practitioners (1965)	Sibs	Clinical	2.4–4.8	0.2–2.1
Keen & Track (1968)*	Sibs	Clinical	3.3–3.5	0.5–0.8
Levit & Pessikova (1934)	Sibs	Clinical	3.6	
Harris (1950)	Sibs	Clinical	4.3	
Pincus & White (1933)	Sibs	Clinical	5.9	0.6
Thompson & Watson (1952)	Sibs	Clinical	9.0	
Kobberling (1969)**	Sibs	Clinical	10.9	
Bartels (1953)**	Sibs	Clinical	11.7	
Burkeholder et al (1967)**	Sibs	Oral GTT	18.0	
Sisk (1968)**	Sibs	Oral GTT	23.0	
Pickens (1964)**	Sibs	Oral GTT	29.0	
Kobberling et al (1969)	Sibs	Oral GTT	38.9	
Hanhart (1951)	Close relatives	Clinical	5.3	1.2
Lambert et al (1961)	Relatives	Oral GTT	6.0	3.0
Notelovitz (1969)	Close relatives	Oral GTT	12.3	6.0
Jakobson & Nikkila (1969)	Close relatives	Oral GTT	13.7	
Joslin et al (1959)	Close relatives	Random Sugar	14.0	2.0
Conn & Fajans (1961)	Close relatives	Oral GTT	18.0	<1
Joslin et al (1959)	Close relatives	Oral GTT	25.0	2.0
Lambert et al (1961)	Relatives	Cortisone GTT	23.0	6.0
Conn & Fajans (1961)	Close relatives	Cortisone GTT	26.0	4.0

* Depending on age of proband.
[†] Figures rounded off to one decimal place.
** Probands are all juvenile diabetics.

most investigators have found the concordance rate for monozygotic twins to vary from 45–96% and that for dizygotic twins to range between 3–37%. With NIDDM, when glucose tolerance tests are performed in the 'non-diabetic' monozygotic co-twins, the concordance rate is usually above 70%. Thus, the concordance of diabetes mellitus in monozygotic twins is significantly greater than in dizygotic twins. Furthermore, the concordance for older monozygotic twins approaches 100%, and concordance increases with more sensitive markers for the diabetic genotype (Pyke 1979, Barnett et al 1981a,b). As discussed below, the monozygotic concordance rates are very different for IDDM and NIDDM. Since concordance is not complete among younger monozygotic twins or when clinical criteria alone are used, it is obvious that environmental factors are important for the phenotypic expression of the diabetic genotype.

GENETIC HETEROGENEITY IN DIABETES

Although the evidence from studies of familial aggregation and twins leaves no doubt as to the importance of genetic factors in the aetiology of diabetes, for many years there was little agreement as to the nature of the genetic factors involved and every possible mode of genetic transmission was proposed. This confusion can, in large part, be explained by the genetic heterogeneity which we now know prevails in diabetes. Indeed, the evidence marshalled for the concept of heterogeneity within diabetes is now overwhelming (Creutzfeldt et al 1976, Rotter et al 1978, Fajans et al 1978, Friedman & Fialkow 1980, Rotter & Rimoin 1981a,b, Kobberling & Tattersall 1982, Rotter et al 1984, 1990). In 1966, the hypothesis of genetic heterogeneity was proposed, based on several lines of evidence, as reviewed below (Rimoin

Table 89.2 Concordance of diabetes and glucose intolerance in twins

Authors	Criteria	Age of patients	Percentage concordant	
			Monozygotic	Dizygotic
White (1965)	Clinical		48.0	3.0
Werner (1936)	Clinical		75.0	10.0
Lemser (in Mimura & Miyao 1962)	Clinical		85.5	29.2
Verschuer (in Mimura & Miyao 1962)	Clinical		84.0	37.0
Steiner (1936)	Clinical		96.6	9.1
Harvald & Hauge (1963, 1965)	Clinical		47.0	9.5
Harvald & Hauge (1963, 1965)	Clinical	>70 years	73.0	32.0
Harvald & Hauge (1963)	GTT		57.0	9.0
Gottlieb & Root (1968)	Clinical	<40 years	10.0	3.1
Gottlieb & Root (1968)	Clinical	>40 years	70.0	3.5
Gottlieb & Root (1968)	GTT		14.0	35.0
Then Berg (1939)	GTT		65.0	22.0
Then Berg (1939)	GTT	>43 years	100.0	39.0
Pyke & Taylor (1967)	GTT		78.0	
Cerasi & Luft (1967)	Glucose infusion		92.0	
Mimura & Miyao (1962)	Combined data		80.5	28.0
Tattersal & Pyke (1972)	Clinical & GTT (96 pairs)	<40 years	52.5	
		>40 years	91.9	
Pyke & Nelson (1976)	Clinical & GTT (106 pairs)	<40 years	50.0	
		>40 years	92.9	
Pyke (1978)	Clinical & GTT (150 pairs)	<45 years	50.9	
		>45 years	88.6	
Pyke (1979)	Clinical & GTT (185 pairs)	Insulin dependent	55.3	
		Noninsulin dependent*	88.6	
Barnett et al (1981b)	Clinical & GTT (200 pairs)	Insulin dependent	54.4	
		Noninsulin dependent	90.6	

* In the NIDDM discordant pairs, the index twin was ascertained only within 5 years of time of examination.

1967). Indirect evidence included: (1) the existence of distinct, mostly rare genetic disorders (now numbering over 60), that have glucose intolerance as one of their features; (2) genetic heterogeneity in diabetic animal models; (3) ethnic variability in prevalence and clinical features; (4) clinical variability between the thin, ketosis prone, insulin dependent, juvenile onset diabetic versus the obese, nonketotic, insulin resistant, adult onset diabetic; and (5) physiological variability — the demonstration of decreased plasma insulin in juvenile, versus the relative hyperinsulinism of maturity onset diabetics. In addition, some direct evidence for heterogeneity came from clinical genetic studies which suggested that juvenile and adult onset diabetes differ genetically (Simpson 1976, Rotter et al 1978).

Genetic syndromes associated with glucose intolerance

There are over 60 distinct genetic disorders associated with glucose intolerance and, in some cases, clinical diabetes (see Table 89.3) (Rotter & Rimoin 1981a,

Rimoin & Rotter 1982). Although individually rare, these syndromes demonstrate that mutations at many different loci can produce glucose intolerance. Furthermore, they illustrate the wide variety of pathogenetic mechanisms which can result in glucose intolerance. These pathogenetic mechanisms include: absolute insulin deficiency due to pancreatic degeneration, in such disorders as hereditary relapsing pancreatitis, cystic fibrosis, and polyendocrine deficiency disease; relative insulinopenia in the growth hormone deficiency syndromes; inhibition of insulin secretion in the hereditary phaeochromocytoma syndromes associated with elevated catecholamines; various deficits in the interaction of insulin and its receptor in the nonketotic insulin resistant states such as myotonic dystrophy and the lipoatrophic diabetes syndromes; and relative insulin resistance in the hereditary syndromes associated with obesity. Even within these individual categories further division can be made, either by mechanism or by genetic criteria. For example, the lipoatrophic syndromes – characterized by the total or partial absence of adipose tissue, hyperlipidaemia, insulin resistance, nonketotic diabetes mellitus, increased basal metabolic rate, and hepatomegaly – can be further subdivided into a recessive, several dominant, and non-genetic forms (Kobberling 1976b, Rimoin & Rotter 1982). There are a variety of syndromes which are characterized by marked insulin resistance. The patho-physiology of the resistance of many of these disorders has been defined by studies of the insulin receptor and its interactions, with some disorders characterized by de-creased receptor number, others by decreased receptor affinity, and still others by humoral antagonists to the receptor (Flier et al 1979, Rimoin & Rotter 1982). Several distinct molecular defects in the insulin receptor gene have been described in leprechaunism and in Type A acanthosis nigricans syndrome (Kadowaki et al 1988, Yoshimasa et al 1988, Kahn & Goldstein 1989). Even within what is currently felt to be one genetic entity, multiple endocrine neoplasia syndrome type I, an auto-somal dominant disorder characterized by pituitary, para-thyroid and pancreatic adenomas, a variety of different hormonal mechanisms can result in insulin antagonism; e.g. eosinophilic adenomas of the pituitary may secrete growth hormone, adenomas of the adrenal gland can secrete cortisol, and nonbeta islet cells of the pancreas can produce glucagon. Each of the hormones individually is an insulin antagonist and its excess can lead to marked glucose intolerance. Thus, there are many different genetic diseases capable of resulting in carbohydrate intolerance, through a variety of different pathogenetic mechanisms. These rare syndromes clearly suggest that a similar degree of heterogeneity, both genetic and patho-genetic, may exist in 'idiopathic' diabetes mellitus.

Animal models of heterogeneity

Animal models also support the concept of genetic heterogeneity in diabetes. For example, genetic hetero-geneity for glucose intolerance has been well documen-ted in the rodent (Coleman 1982, Leiter et al 1986, Jackson 1988). A number of distinct single gene mutants have been found to result in glucose intolerance in the mouse. Coleman's studies have not only documented clear genetic heterogeneity for glucose intolerance in the mouse, but have also shown that the phenotypic expression of the mutant gene is greatly influenced by the total genotype of the animal. Important components of this genetic background appear to be the H2 locus (the major histocompatibility complex of the mouse) and sex (Leiter et al 1981a). Thus, the overall genetic constitu-tion of the individual can clearly influence the pheno-typic expression of the mutant diabetogenic gene. Similarly, differences in the genetic background of humans could result in differences in clinical expression

of diabetes in different ethnic groups. It has also been shown that dietary composition can influence the occurrence of islet-cell necrosis (Leiter et al 1981b). By analogy, diet might modify the expression of diabetes in those humans genetically predisposed. In addition to the single gene mutations, a number of genetic forms of glucose intolerance have been described whose mode of inheritance is not fully elucidated. Immunological factors appear to be important in the pathogenesis of the diabetes in several of these animal models, such as the BB rat and the NOD mouse (Jackson 1988). These two animal disorders are considered potential models of IDDM in man (see below). It is of interest that evidence suggests that up to three different independent genetic loci are involved in providing susceptibility in these animals, only one of which is the major histocompatibi-lity complex (Colle et al 1981, 1983, Leiter et al 1983, Jackson et al 1984, Prochazka et al 1987). Because of the indirect implication of viruses in the aetiology of human insulin-dependent diabetes, there is a great deal of interest in the diabetic syndrome following encephalo-myocarditis (EMC) and other infections in certain strains of mice (Craighead 1981) (see below). A single genetic locus, unrelated to the major histocompatibility complex, appears to influence mouse susceptibility to the diabeto-genic effects of the EMC virus (Onodera et al 1978). In summary, it is apparent that a large number of different genetic and environmental factors can produce glucose intolerance in the rodent, supporting the concept of heterogeneity in the idiopathic forms of diabetes in man.

Ethnic variability

Marked ethnic variability in the prevalence and clinical features of diabetes mellitus has also been well docu-mented (Rimoin 1969, Rimoin & Schimke 1971, West 1978). Variability in the prevalence and pattern of disease among ethnic groups can be secondary to both genetic and environmental modifying factors, but may also indicate the presence of genetic heterogeneity. Epide-miological surveys have revealed significant differences in the prevalence of diabetes among different populations (West 1978). For non-insulin dependent forms of diabetes there appears to be a general correlation between overnutrition and the prevalence of diabetes. In certain populations, such as the Kurdish and Yemenite Jews in Israel, the prevalence of diabetes has increased markedly, following their migration to Israel and their subsequent change in diet (Cohen 1961). A similar increase in diabetes prevalence has occurred in the Pima Indians of the American Southwest (Knowler et al 1981, Melish et al 1982, Rotter et al 1990).

Table 89.3 Genetic syndromes associated with glucose intolerance and diabetes mellitus

Syndromes	Types of DM	Associated clinical findings	Pattern of inheritance
Syndromes associated with pancreatic degeneration			
Congenital absence of the pancreas	IDDM (congenital)	IUGR, poor adipose and muscle malabsorption, dehydration	?AR
Congenital absence of the islets of Langerhans	IDDM (congenital)	IUGR, dehydration	?AR or XR
Congenital pancreatic hypoplasia	IDDM (infancy)	IUGR, pancreatic exocrine deficiency	?AR
Renal-hepatic-pancreatic dysplasia	IDDM	Renal cystic dysplasia, biliary dysgenesis, pancreatic fibrosis and cysts. ± polysplenia	AD
Hereditary relapsing pancreatitis	IGT → IDDM	Abdominal pain, chronic pancreatitis	AD
Cystic fibrosis	IGT → IDDM	Malabsorption, chronic respiratory disease	AR
Polyendocrine deficiency disease (Schmidt syndrome)	IDDM	Autoimmune endocrine disease, hypothyroidism, hypoadrenalism	?AR, AD
IgA deficiency, malabsorption and diabetes	IDDM	IgA deficiency, malabsorption	?AD
Haemochromatosis	NIDDM	Hepatic, pancreatic, skin, cardiac, and endocrine complications of iron storage	AR
Thalassaemia	IGT → NIDDM	Anaemia, iron overload	AR
Alpha-1-antitrypsin deficiency	IGT	Emphysema, cirrhosis	AR
Hereditary endocrine disorders with glucose intolerance			
Isolated growth hormone deficiency	NIDDM	Proportionate dwarfism	AR, AD
Hereditary panhypopituitary dwarfism	NIDDM	Proportionate dwarfism hypogonadism ± TSH and ACTH deficiency	AR, XR
Laron dwarfism	NIDDM	Proportionate dwarfism	AR
Phaeochromocytoma	IGT	Hypertension, tremor, paroxysmal sweating	AD
Multiple endocrine adenomatosis	IGT	Pituitary (acromegaly), parathyroid (renal stones), pancreatic adenomas (peptic ulcer)	AD
Inborn errors of metabolism with glucose intolerance			
Alaninuria	IDDM (infancy)	Mental retardation, microcephaly IUGR, dwarfism, enamel hypoplasia, high blood pyruvate, lactate and alanine	?AR
Glycogen storage disease type I (von Gierke disease)	IGT	Hepatomegaly, early hypoglycaemia	AR
Acute intermittent porphyria	IGT	Paroxysmal abdominal pain, hypertension	AD
Hyperlipidaemias	NIDDM	Hyperlipidaemia, coronary artery disease	AD
Fanconi syndrome-hypophosphataemia	NIDDM	Renal tubular dysfunction, metabolic bone disease	AR

Table 89.3 Genetic syndromes associated with glucose intolerance and diabetes mellitus (*contd.*)

Syndromes	Types of DM	Associated clinical findings	Pattern of inheritance
Thiamine responsive megaloblastic anaemia	IGT, IDDM	Megaloblastic anaemia, deafness	AR
Syndromes with non-ketotic insulin resistant early onset diabetes mellitus Ataxia telangiectasia	Insulin resistant	Ataxia, telangiectasia, IgA deficiency	AR
Myotonic dystrophy	Insulin resistant	Myotonia cataracts, balding, testicular atrophy	AD
Lipoatrophic diabetes syndromes Seip-Berardinelli syndrome	Insulin resistant	Hepatomegaly, acanthosis nigricans, elevated BMR, polycystic ovaries, clitoral hypertrophy	AR
Brunzell syndrome	Insulin resistant	Same as Seip-Berardinelli with cystic angiomatosis of soft tissues and bone (?same syndrome)	AR
Familial partial lipodystrophy (Kobberling-Dunnegan syndrome) Type A: confined to limbs, sparing face and trunk Type B: Trunk also affected with exception of vulva	Insulin resistant	Hyperlipidaemia, xanthomata, acanthosis nigricans	?AD, XLD
Partial lipodystrophy with Reiger anomaly	IGT → NIDDM	Reiger anomaly, mid face hypoplasia, short stature, hypotrichosis	AD
Aredlyd syndrome (Acrorenal and ectodermal dysplasia)	Insulin resistant	IUGR and growth retardation, lipoatrophy, hepatosplenomegaly, unusual facies, hypotrichosis, dental abnormalities, scoliosis, hyperostosis of cranial vault, hand malformations, hypoplasia of breasts, genital abnormalities, ectodermal dysplasia	AR
Alstrom syndrome	Insulin resistant	Pigmentary retinopathy, nerve deafness, obesity	AR
Edwards syndrome	Insulin resistant	Mental retardation, deafness, retinitis pigmentosa, obesity, hypogonadism, ± acanthosis nigricans	AR
Leprechaunism (point mutations in insulin receptor gene)	Insulin resistant	IUGR and growth retardation, large hands, feet and genitals, acanthosis nigricans, decreased subcutaneous fat, hirsutism	AR
Rabson-Mendenhall syndrome	Insulin resistant	Unusual facies, enlarged genitals, precocious puberty, acanthosis nigricans, hirsutism, pineal hyperplasia	AR
Acanthosis nigricans insulin resistant diabetes syndromes Type A	Insulin resistant decreased receptors	Acanthosis nigricans, ovarian hirsutism, accelerated growth	?AD
Type A with acral hypertrophy and cramps	Insulin resistant (post receptor defect)	Large hands, acanthosis nigricans, muscle cramps, enlarged kidneys, polycystic ovaries	?AR

Table 89.3 Genetic syndromes associated with glucose intolerance and diabetes mellitus (*contd.*)

Syndromes	Types of DM	Associated clinical findings	Pattern of inheritance
Type A with bradydactyly, dental anomalies	Insulin resistant	Acanthosis nigricans, bitemporal narrowing, acral hypertrophy, decreased body fat, bradydactyly, dental anomalies	?AR
Type A with muscle cramps and coarse facies	Insulin resistant (post receptor defect)	Coarse facies, muscular women, acanthosis nigricans, headaches, muscle cramps, hyperprolactinaemia, no ovarian dysfunction	AD
Type B	Insulin resistant (circulating inhibitor)	Acanthosis nigricans, immunological disease	?
Hereditary neuromuscular disorders associated with glucose intolerance Anosmia-hypogonadism syndrome	IGT or IDDM	Anosmia, hypogonadotropic, hypogonadism, hearing loss, ± cleft lip and palate	?AR
Muscular dystrophies	IGT → NIDDM	Muscular dystrophy	AD, AR, XR
Late onset proximal myopathy	IGT → NIDDM	Myopathy, cataracts	?AR
Huntington disease	IGT → NIDDM	Chorea, dementia	AD
Machado disease	NIDDM	Ataxia	AD
Herrman syndrome	NIDDM	Photomyoclonus, deafness, nephropathy, dementia	AD
Diabetes mellitus-optic atrophy-diabetes insipidus-deafness syndrome (Wolfram, DIDMOAD syndrome)	IDDM	Optic atrophy, diabetes insipidus, deafness, neurological symptoms	AR
Friedreich ataxia	IDDM or NIDDM	Spinocerebellar degeneration	AR
Pseudo-Refsum syndrome	NIDDM	Muscle atrophy, ataxia, retinitis pigmentosa	?AD
Stiff man syndrome	IDDM	Fluctuating muscle rigidity with painful spasm, characteristic EMG, autoimmune disease of nervous and endocrine systems	?AD (most sporadic)
Roussy-Levy syndrome	NIDDM	Ataxia, areflexia with amyotrophy	AD
Progeroid syndromes associated with glucose intolerance Cockayne syndrome	IGT	Dwarfism, progeria, MR, deafness, blindness	AR
Metageria	NIDDM	Early atherosclerosis, tall and thin, bird-like facies and aged appearance, normal sexual development, atrophic mottled skin, telangiectasia, little subcutaneous fat	?
Werner syndrome	NIDDM	Premature ageing, cataracts, arteriosclerosis	AR
Syndromes with glucose intolerance secondary to obesity Achondroplasia	IGT	Disproportionate dwarfism, relative obesity	AD

Table 89.3 Genetic syndromes associated with glucose intolerance and diabetes mellitus (*contd.*)

Syndromes	Types of DM	Associated clinical findings	Pattern of inheritance
Bardet-Biedl syndrome	IGT → NIDDM	Mental retardation, pigmentation retinopathy, polydactyly, hypogonadism and obesity	AR
Prader-Willi syndrome	NIDDM	Obesity, short stature, acromicria, MR, disproportionate dwarfism	15q abnormality
Miscellaneous syndromes associated with glucose intolerance Christian syndrome	IGT → NIDDM	Short stature, ridged metopic suture, mental retardation, fusion of cervical vertebrae, thoracic hemivertebrae, scoliosis, sacral hypoplasia, abducens palsy, carrier females may have NIDDM or IGT	XR or SLAD
Steroid-induced ocular hypertension	IGT	Steroid-induced ocular hypertension	AD
Epiphyseal dysplasia and infantile onset diabetes mellitus	IDDM (congenital)	Epiphyseal dysplasia, tooth and skin defects	AR
Progessive cone dystrophy, degenerative liver disease, endocrine dysfunction, hearing defect	MODY	Colour blindness, liver disease, deafness, hypogonadism	AR
Symmetrical lipomatosis	IGT → NIDDM	Diffuse symmetrical lipomas of neck and trunk, stiff skin, muscle cramps, decreased sensation, hearing loss, urolithiasis, hypertension, peptic ulcers	AD
Woodhouse-Sakati syndrome	NIDDM	Unusual facies, hypogonadism, absent breast tissue, sparse hair, mental retardation, sensorineural deafness and ECG abnormalities	AR
Cytogenetic disorders associated with glucose intolerance Down syndrome	IGT	MR, short stature, typical facies	Trisomy 21
Klinefelter syndrome	IGT → NIDDM	Hypogonadism, tall stature, MR	47,XXY
Turner syndrome	IGT → NIDDM	Short stature, gonadal dysgenesis, web neck	45,X

IDDM	– Insulin dependent diabetes mellitus (Type I)
NIDDM	– Noninsulin dependent diabetes mellitus (Type II)
IGT	– Impaired glucose tolerance
AR	– Autosomal recessive
AD	– Autosomal dominant
SLAD	– Sex limited autosomal dominant
XR	– X-linked recessive
IUGR	– Intrauterine growth retardation
MR	– Mental retardation
MODY	– Maturity onset type diabetes of the young.

Nevertheless, there are clear differences in the clinical phenotype of diabetes between different ethnic groups that do not appear to be totally the result of environmental differences (Rimoin 1969, West 1978). For example, there are different ethnic groups with low fat/high carbohydrate diets, some of which have common vascular complications and rare ketosis; while in other ethnic groups with similar diets, ketosis is the usual presenting symptom and vascular complications are rare (Rimoin & Schimke 1971). There are even types of diabetes frequent in tropical countries, namely type J and pancreatic diabetes, that do not appear to occur in temperate zones (West 1978) (see below).

Heterogeneity between type I (IDDM) and type II (NIDDM) disease

As summarized in Table 89.4, a number of lines of clinical and genetic evidence led to the eventual separation of type I and type II diabetes as clearly distinct groups of disorders. Clinical differences which tended to run true in families provided some of the first evidence (Cammidge 1928, 1934, Harris 1949, 1950, Simpson 1962, 1968, Working Party 1965, Kobberling 1969, Lestradet et al 1972, MacDonald 1974, Irvine et al 1977a, Cudworth 1978, Degnbol & Green 1978). In addition, the extensive monozygotic twin studies by Pyke and his co-workers in England strongly supported the separation of juvenile insulin dependent and maturity non-insulin dependent diabetes (Pyke 1979). Among 200 pairs of monozygotic (identical) twins, concordance for diabetes was shown to be less than 50% for type I, but close to

100% for type II diabetes. This suggests that there may be a large group of individuals with type I diabetes in whom non-genetic as well as genetic factors play a role in the development of clinical disease.

Physiological studies further support the separation of type I and type II diabetes. The absolute insulinopenic response of the juvenile-onset diabetic and the relative hyperinsulinaemic response of the maturity-onset diabetic parallel therapeutic observations of the absolute insulin requirement of the juvenile (insulin dependent) diabetic in contrast to adult cases, most of whom can be managed with oral hypoglycaemics and/or diet (non-insulin dependent).

Immunological studies pinpointed the importance of immune mechanisms in the aetiology of type I, but not type II diabetes. Direct evidence for an autoimmune role in the pathogenesis of insulin dependent diabetes came from the discovery of organ specific cell-mediated immunity to pancreatic islets, and then of antibodies to the islet cells of the pancreas (Bottazzo et al 1974, MacCuish et al 1974, Cahill & McDevitt 1981). While these antibodies were first detected only in insulin dependent diabetics with coexistent autoimmune endocrine disease, it soon became apparent that they were common (60–80%) in newly diagnosed juvenile diabetics. Islet cell antibody studies supported the differentiation of insulin dependent from non-insulin dependent diabetes, as autoantibodies were present in 30–40% of the former group (even after onset), as opposed to 5–8% of the latter. It is interesting that many (possibly the majority) of the 'non-insulin dependent' yet antibody positive patients appear to become insulin dependent with time. They also

Table 89.4 Separation of IDDM from NIDDM

Evidence	IDDM Type I (juvenile onset type)	NIDDM Type II (maturity onset type)
Clinical	Thin	Obese
	Ketosis prone	Ketosis resistant
	Insulin required for survival	Often treatable by diet or drugs
	Onset predominantly in childhood and early adulthood	Onset predominantly after 40
Family studies	Increased prevalence of juvenile or Type I	Increased prevalence of maturity or Type II
Twin studies	<50% concordance in monozygotic twins	Close to 100% concordance in monzygotic twins
Insulin response to a glucose blood	Flat	Variable
Associated with other autoimmune endocrine diseases and antibodies	Yes	No
Islet cell antibodies and pancreatic cell mediated immunity	Yes	No
HLA associations and linkage	Yes	No
Association with DNA variable near the insulin gene	Yes (small inserts)	No
Mutant insulins	No	Rare cause

have flat insulin responses to a glucose load. This has suggested that aetiologically these cases belong in the insulin-dependent category, although they are not yet totally insulin dependent (Irvine et al 1977b, Wilson et al 1985, Kilvert et al 1986).

Finally, the clear and consistent association of juvenile insulin dependent, but not maturity onset non-insulin dependent diabetes, with HLA antigens B8 and B15 became a major argument for aetiological differences between these two disorders (Nerup et al 1977, Cudworth 1978, Rotter & Rimoin 1981a, Cahill & McDevitt 1981). These HLA associations are even stronger for antigens DR3 and DR4 of the HLA D locus; approximately 95% of IDDM patients have DR3 or DR4 or both, and B7 and DR2 are decreased in frequency in IDDM (Platz et al 1981, Rotter et al 1983, Wolf et al 1983, Maclaren et al 1988). These HLA alleles are believed to serve as markers for closely linked, but as yet untypable, 'diabetogenic' genes which may be immune response genes that are

directly responsible for the individual's susceptibility to IDDM (see below).

Based in large part on the evidence reviewed above, both the NDDG and the WHO systems currently classify diabetes mellitus into four major sub-categories: Type I diabetes (insulin dependent diabetes), Type II diabetes (non-insulin dependent diabetes), gestational diabetes, and diabetes secondary to other medical conditions. The major characteristics of each of these categories are summarized in Table 89.5.

A few cautions are in order. Just because we are able to separate the bulk of patients and families into insulin dependent and non-insulin dependent types does not mean this phenotypic distinction is absolute. There is at least some evidence that families of either type also have more of the other type of diabetes than do families in the general population (Cahill 1979b, Gottlieb 1980). Part of this overlap may be attributed to the insulin independent phase of the insulin dependent type (the frequency of

Table 89.5 Classification of the types of diabetes

Class name	Former terminology	Characteristics
Insulin-dependent diabetes mellitus (IDDM, Type I)	Juvenile diabetes Juvenile-onset diabetes (JOD) Ketosis-prone diabetes Brittle diabetes	Low or absent levels of circulating endogenous insulin; dependent on injected insulin to prevent ketosis and sustain life Onset predominantly in youth but can occur at any age Associated with HLA DR3 and DR4 Islet cell antibodies are frequently present prior to and at diagnosis
Noninsulin-dependent diabetes mellitus (NIDDM, Type II) Subtype obese Subtype nonobese	Adult-onset diabetes Maturity-onset diabetes (MOD) Ketosis-resistant diabetes Stable diabetes	Insulin levels may be normal, elevated or depressed Not insulin-dependent or ketosis-prone under normal circumstances, but may use insulin for treatment of hyperglycaemia or during stress conditions Onset predominantly after age 40, but can occur at any age Approximately 60% of patients are obese Hyperinsulinaemia and insulin resistance characterize some patients Includes MODY patients and those with mutant insulins
Gestational diabetes (GDM)	Gestational diabetes	Glucose intolerance that has its onset during pregnancy; virtually all patients return to normal glucose tolerance following parturition Conveys increased risk for progression to diabetes
Other types of diabetes, including or secondary to those associated with: Pancreatic disease Hormonal disease Drugs or chemical exposure Insulin receptor abnormalities Certain genetic syndromes	Secondary diabetes	In addition to the presence of the specific condition, hyperglycaemia at a level diagnostic of diabetes is also present (See Table 89.3 for further list of conditions with which hyperglycaemia is associated)

Adapted from: National Diabetes Data Group 1979.

which is still being defined) (Irvine et al 1977a, 1979, Wilson et al 1985, Kilvert et al 1986). However, this observation may also be the result of even further aetiological heterogeneity (see below). Furthermore, while the distinction between insulin dependence and independence provides the primary basis for dividing the two subtypes of diabetes, age of onset and other clinical differences should not be dismissed summarily. For example, a distinct form of non-insulin dependent diabetes has been termed 'maturity onset diabetes of the young' (MODY) (Tattersall 1974, Tattersall & Fajans 1975) (to be discussed below). The delineation of this entity clearly demonstrates that age of onset is a useful clinical criterion for classification purposes. Similarly, there is evidence that B15 and DR4 appear to be more prominently increased in younger insulin dependent diabetics, suggesting heterogeneity within IDDM (Svejgaard et al 1982, Anderson et al 1983).

INSULIN DEPENDENT DIABETES MELLITUS (IDDM, TYPE I)

As reviewed in Table 89.5, insulin dependent diabetes mellitus is characterized by low levels or absence of endogeneous insulin production. In the majority of cases this is secondary to destruction of the insulin producing beta cells of the pancreas, and is the single characteristic which most decisively separates type I and type II diabetes. It is estimated that 5–10% of all US diabetics are type I diabetics (Herman et al 1984) and the estimated U S incidence in children of 0 to 16 years is in the range 12–14/100 000 (Palumbo et al 1976, Fishbein et al 1982, Melton et al 1983, LaPorte & Cruikshanks 1985, Tajima et al 1985). The incidence appears to vary dramatically worldwide, from less than 1/100 000 children in Japan, to greater than 25/100 000 in Scandinavia (DERI 1988).

Difficulties in genetic analysis

The discovery of the HLA antigen associations with IDDM raised the expectation that the use of these disease marker associations in appropriate studies might fully clarify the genetics of IDDM. While these associations have provided a useful tool to further investigate the genetics and pathogenesis of IDDM and have identified the genetic region that provides the major (but not only) genetic susceptibility to IDDM, the genetics of this group of disorders remains an area of some controversy, with many different modes of inheritance being proposed (Rotter 1981a, Rotter et al 1983, 1984, 1990). There are several major difficulties that confound any attempt to analyze the genetics of IDDM. These include the reduced penetrance of the disorder, the confounding of

linkage and association, and heterogeneity within the disorder.

The first problem is reduced penetrance of the IDDM diabetic genotype. When the mode of inheritance is unclear, the only estimate we have for penetrance is identical twin concordance data. The largest twin data set is that of the British diabetic twin study, which reports concordance for IDDM of some 50% (Pyke 1979, Barnett et al 1981a). However it is clear that this sample is a biased one, with only a fraction of the twins in the British Isles identified, and thus a presumed bias toward concordant pairs (Pyke 1978). Reports from less biased but much smaller samples report concordances of 20% (Gottlieb & Root 1968, Cahill 1979b). The reduced penetrance, whatever its true value, indicates that what is inherited in IDDM is disease susceptibility; other factors, presumably environmental, are required to convert genetic susceptibility into clinical disease. This view is supported both by the observations that the onset of IDDM clusters in families (Gamble 1980b) and the epidemiological, experimental animal, and clinical evidence for viral infections as a supervening factor in at least some cases (Craighead 1981, Rayfield & Seto 1981) (see below).

Genes in the HLA region appear to be associated with IDDM in the population at large, as well as in families. Disease association studies examine the prevalence of a well defined genetic marker, such as blood groups or serum enzyme polymorphisms, among individuals with and without the disease of interest. If the disease occurs more commonly with a particular allele of a well defined genetic locus (e.g. increased duodenal ulcer among blood group O individuals), i.e. there is positive association, then the pathogenesis of the disorder can be considered to have a genetic component (Rotter & Rimoin 1979, 1981c). Linkage refers to the relative proximity of gene loci on the chromosome map. If two genes are linked, they tend to accompany one another through meiosis and therefore travel together vertically down a pedigree. But because of crossing-over or recombination, specific alleles at the linked loci are not associated throughout a population. Thus, linkage is usually demonstrable within families but not across populations, whereas association is a phenomenon in the population, and not necessarily in families. For many years, most mathematical techniques for linkage detection included the assumption that there was no population association between the disease (phenotype) under study and the genetic marker alleles. However, the genetics of the HLA region violates these general rules because alleles at various HLA loci are in linkage disequilibrium. The HLA region has several well defined loci — three serologically defined Class II loci (A, B, and C), the Class II genes (defined serologically, by mixed lymphocyte culture, and molecularly) which consist of at least three different subgroups (DP, DQ, and DR) and the class III loci including several components of the complement series. Each of these loci has multiple alleles or antigens. These genes are located close to one another on chromosome 6, and thus are linked. However, certain pairs of HLA antigens are found together in the population in greater frequency than would be expected by chance and are consequently said to be in 'linkage disequilibrium'. The most popular explanation for linkage disequilibrium is that selective forces exist that tend to select for certain advantageous combinations of antigens. One of the major speculations regarding the aetiology of various autoimmune diseases is that we are seeing today the residual effect of the selective advantage of these antigenic associations against the infectious diseases that our species was exposed to in the past (Svejgaard et al 1975, McMichael & McDevitt 1977). While methods to deal with the problem of linkage disequilibrium are being developed, and the biases inherent in linkage analysis under conditions of linkage disequilibrium are currently being explored, the analytical situation remains extremely complex (Morton & Lalouel 1981, Clerget-Darpoux 1982, Clerget-Darpoux et al 1988, Thomson et al 1988).

The HLA region and IDDM

A large number of studies have consistently found an increased frequency of HLA antigens B8 and B15, and more prominently DR3 and DR4, among Caucasian IDDM patients. These population associations, initially reported by Singal and Blajchman (1973), Nerup et al (1974), and Cudworth and Woodrow (1975), are now well established. The IDDM association is unusual among HLA disease associations, because the association involves two antigens, HLA DR3 and DR4. In addition, the relative risk for IDDM in individuals who have both DR3 and DR4 (compound heterozygotes) is greater than those homozygous for either DR3 or DR4 (Platz et al 1981, Rotter et al 1983, Wolf et al 1983). This finding of the increased risk of the DR3/DR4 (initially B8/B15) heterozygote was the first suggestion that more than one gene predisposes to IDDM, and was thus the first evidence for heterogeneity within IDDM using HLA data (Svejgaard et al 1975, Rotter et al 1978).

Approximately 95% of all IDDMs (in Caucasian populations) have HLA-DR3, DR4 or both, compared to about 50% of individuals in the non-diabetic population (Platz et al 1981, Rotter et al 1983, Wolf et al 1983, Maclaren et al 1988). There are also more subtle relative increases in HLA-DR1 (especially among those who have only DR3 and DR4), and DR2 and DR5 are decreased in individuals with IDDM (Ludwig et al 1976, Ilonen et al 1978, Maclaren et al 1988, Thomson et al 1988).

HLA-DR3 and DR4 (as defined serologically) are not pathognomonic of IDDM; nearly half the US population has DR3 or DR4 (only 1–3% have both), yet IDDM will develop in only a small percentage (about 0.5%) of this group of the population. However, if one's sib has IDDM, the chance of a DR3 or DR4 individual developing IDDM rises sharply (12–24%). Such findings are consistent with two possibilities. The diabetogenic gene(s) may lie very close to the DR locus and, by chance or selection, be in linkage disequilibrium with the DR3 and DR4 alleles. If present, the diabetogenic gene(s) would then be inherited along with these specific DR alleles. Alternatively, certain variants of the DR3 and DR4 alleles may themselves be diabetogenic or, possibly, whole haplotypes may be diabetogenic. A better understanding of the role of HLA in IDDM susceptibility is likely to come from studies at the molecular genetic level.

The serologically defined HLA-DR types are actually broad specificities which are found on a number of different class II gene products. The HLA class II region consists of at least three genetic loci — DR, DQ, and DP — each of which codes for a slightly different glycoprotein consisting of two peptide chains, alpha and beta. The complexity of the class II region allows for a far greater diversity in class II region haplotypes than was previously suspected. Thus, individuals who type as HLA-DR4 actually have one of at least seven distinct haplotypes, defined by variation in the DR beta and DQ beta regions. Studies of restriction fragment length polymorphisms in the HLA-D (class II) region suggest that there are differences at the DNA level between diabetics and non-diabetics, even when they share the same serological type. The best evidence to date suggests that variation in the DQ beta region may be more strongly associated with risk for IDDM than is variation in the DR region, at least as regards the HLA-DR4 associated susceptibility. Several groups have reported a variant of HLA-DR4, defined by variation in the DQ beta region, which occurs with increased frequency in IDDMs (Owerbach et al 1983, Bohme et al 1986, Festenstein et al 1986, Nepom et al 1986, Monos et al 1987, Todd et al 1987). This variant, called the DQw3.2 allele, occurs in as many as 90–95% of those IDDMs who carry the HLA-DR4 allele and in about 60–75% of DR4-carrying non-diabetic controls. Whether HLA-DR3 can be similarly split into high and low-risk haplotypes is currently unclear (Stetler et al 1985). Todd et al (1987), in molecular studies focused on the DQ-beta region, noted a difference between haplotypes which are and are not associated with increased risk for IDDM; those haplotypes which are not associated with increased risk all coded for the amino acid residue aspartic acid (Asp) at position 57 of the DQ beta chain. The 'high risk' haplotypes, including DR4/DQ-beta w3.2, DR3/DQ-beta w2, DR1/DQ-beta w1.1 and DR2/DQ-beta w1.AZH, were all associated with residues other than Asp at position 57. They concluded that this was the principal determinant for IDDM. However, others have challenged the universality of this single residue as being totally responsible for HLA linked IDDM susceptibility; for example Owerbach et al (1988) found that other amino acid residues (other than residue 57 of the DQ beta chain) are important for IDDM susceptibility. Their data suggest that the DQ-alpha gene also plays a role in diabetes susceptibility. They and others have suggested that the DR3/4 heterozygote excess in IDDM may be the result of transallelic complementation of the DQ-alpha and DQ-beta loci (Nepom et al 1987, Owerbach et al 1988).

Although these observations appear to increase the specificity of the HLA-DR IDDM associations, calculations of the absolute risk for IDDM suggest that the specific diabetes susceptibility genes have not yet been identified. If the 'diabetogenic gene(s)' in the HLA region were identified, they should be nearly as predictive of disease risk in random individuals as in sibs of a diabetic (i.e. a risk as high as 1 in 4 or 5 for the highest combinations). There are currently no markers, molecular or serological, which are this sensitive and specific for IDDM susceptibility at the population level (as contrasted with the specificities of the haplotypes in families).

Aetiological heterogeneity within IDDM

Even IDDM now appears to represent a heterogenous group of disorders. Immunological studies have suggested that some forms of insulin dependent diabetes are associated with thyrogastric autoimmunity while others are not. This aggregation of autoimmunity appears to be consistent within families (Nissley et al 1973, Fialkow et al 1975, Bottazzo et al 1978). Based on the additive risk of B8 and B15, it was suggested that more than one gene in the HLA complex might affect the susceptibility to insulin dependent diabetes (Svejgaard et al 1975). Subsequently, Bottazzo and Doniach (1976) and Irvine (1977) proposed that insulin dependent diabetes could be subdivided into autoimmune and viral-induced types. After analysing published immunological and metabolic data, Rotter and Rimoin (1978) proposed further heterogeneity among the juvenile insulin dependent form of diabetes and postulated that the HLA B8-DR3 and the B15-DR4 associated forms of diabetes were distinct diseases: B8-DR3 (an autoimmune form) and B15-DR4

(an insulin antibody responder type) (Rotter & Rimoin 1978).

The evidence supporting the existence of genetic heterogeneity within typical insulin dependent juvenile onset type of diabetes is summarized in Table 89.6. One line of evidence is the increased risk for the compound heterozygote, i.e. the individual with two HLA-associated alleles, both DR3 and DR4. This is true whether one uses the standard relative risks, odds ratio (Svejgaard & Ryder 1981), or simple counting methods (Rotter et al 1983). The most direct proof has come from the British monozygotic twin studies. They have shown an increased concordance rate for IDDM in those twins who are DR3/DR4 versus those with other genotypes (Johnston et al 1983). Thus, by direct inference, an individual with both DR3 and DR4 has a more penetrant genotype. This is also supported by data from sibs sharing both HLA haplotypes with the diabetic proband; those sibs with DR3/DR4 have a higher risk (i.e. are more penetrant) than those other HLA genotypes (Rotter et al 1986, Thomson et al 1988).

A second line of evidence for heterogeneity is the phenotypic differences accompanying the HLA associations (Rotter 1981a, Schernthaner 1982, Ludvigsson & Lindblom 1984, Knip et al 1986, Ludvigsson et al 1986). The HLA-DR3 form of the disease (autoimmune form) is characterized by an increased persistence of pancreatic islet cell antibodies and antipancreatic cell-mediated immunity, and lack of antibody response to exogenous insulin. This form apparently has onset throughout life and probably accounts for a significant fraction of older-onset IDDM, which in the older age groups may be treatable without insulin for a significant period, but in whom the presence of islet-cell antibodies presages eventual insulin dependence (Wilson et al 1985, Kilvert et al 1986). The second form of IDDM is associated with HLA-DR4. While not as strongly associated with autoimmune disease or islet cell antibodies, this form is accompanied by an increased antibody response to exogenous insulin (Rotter 1981a, Sklenar et al 1982). Some individuals with the highest insulin antibody titres had only been treated with insulin for less than five years; thus, duration of treatment is not the cause of the high insulin immune response (Anderson et al 1983). HLA-DR4 is also associated with the insulin antibodies that occur prior to disease onset (Srikanta et al 1986, Karjalainen et al 1986). This disorder also appears to have an earlier age of onset, exhibit seasonality, and may be related to viral infections. A direct relationship between persistent islet cell antibodies and lower insulin antibody levels has been shown, thus directly confirming the differential immunologic features of the two forms (Irvine et al 1978b, Schernthaner 1982).

Table 89.6 Heterogeneity within insulin-dependent diabetes mellitus

Evidence	DR3	DR4	Combined form (DR3/DR4)
Linkage disequilibrium	A1,B8	B15, DQw3.2	↑ penetrance in MZ twins ↑ risk to sibs
Insulin antibodies	Nonresponder (low antibody titres)	High responder (high antibody titres)	↑ occurrence in familial cases
Islet cell antibodies	Persistent	Transient	
Insulin autoantibodies	Less frequent	Increased frequency	Highest titres
Antipancreatic cell-mediated immunity	Increased	Not increased	
Thyroid autoimmunity in IDDM	Yes	Less frequent	
Associated with other autoimmune endocrine diseases	Yes	No	
IgA deficiency in IDDM	Increased	Not increased	
Age of onset	Any age	Younger age	Youngest
Ketoacidosis at clinical onset	Lesser frequency	Greater frequency	
Levels of C-peptide	Preserved longer	Absent after shorter duration	Lowest

There is good evidence for even further heterogeneity within insulin dependent diabetes. The compound DR3/DR4 heterozygote may be considered a distinct form, characterized by an increased relative risk, an increased prevalence among concordant twins and familial cases and a increased risk to sibs for diabetes (Rotter 1981a, Johnston et al 1983, Rotter et al 1986, Thomson et al 1988). It also appears to have the earliest age of onset (Anderson et al 1983). It is of interest that the youngest onset cases have the highest titres of insulin antibodies prior to diagnosis (Srikanta et al 1986). The DR3/DR4 group may also have greater islet cell damage, as indicated by the lowest levels of measurable C peptide (Ludvigsson et al 1977). The BfF1-IDDM association may identify a fourth type of IDDM, one associated with the BfF1-B18-DR3 haplotype (Bertrams 1982).

Not all investigators have concluded that these observations indicate genetic heterogeneity. Some have argued that the phenotypic heterogeneity only reflects other linked (in disequilibrium) immune reactivity in the HLA complex; reactivity that may be unrelated to diabetes pathogenesis per se. For this and other reasons, they favoured the simple recessive hypothesis (Curie-Cohen 1981, Rubinstein et al 1981). A third line of evidence for heterogeneity, and one of which tends to refute these explanations, has been the ability of mathematical models based on the heterogeneity hypothesis to make accurate population predictions.

We have proposed that the DR3 and DR4 associated diabetic genetic susceptibilities act through different pathogenetic mechanisms (Rotter & Rimoin 1983, Rotter et al 1984). If an individual has both alleles, the effect of both mechanisms was proposed to be synergistic, thereby leading to the increased penetrance/susceptibility of the compound DR3/DR4 heterozygote. An alternative explanation of this synergism is that the DR3/DR4 heterozygote forms a hybrid antigen that has an increased susceptibility to IDDM; the existence of such a hybrid molecule has indeed been shown (Nepom et al 1987). There is, however, no direct evidence that this molecule has different or distinctive immunogenicity. In contrast, the observation of the association of persistent pancreatic autoimmunity with B8-DR3 and insulin-immune reactivity with B15-DR4 has been repeatedly confirmed (Rotter 1981a, Rotter et al 1984). The authors have proposed that these phenotypic differences are clues to the underlying pathophysiological mechanisms. We proposed a model in which the B8-DR3 axis predisposes to autoimmunity against a class of antigens shared by several endocrine glands, and the B15-DR4 axis predisposes to autoimmunity against a precursor form of insulin found only in the pancreatic beta cell. When this precursor form of insulin, normally sequestered from the immune system, is revealed as a result of pancreatic beta cell damage, the result could be rapid destruction of the beta cell mass in susceptible individuals. The tendency to form high insulin antibody levels can then be seen as a pleiotropic manifestation of B15-DR4 susceptibility. Damage to the beta cell, whether by viruses or autoimmunity, would allow this mechanism to operate. This model explains the synergistic effect of the B8-DR3 and the B15-DR4 axes, as well as the clinical differences between DR3 and DR4-associated forms of IDDM. The model has gained increased support from the discovery of anti-insulin autoantibodies that precede clinical disease and insulin therapy (Palmer et al 1983, Karjalainen et al 1986, Srikanta et al 1986). Thus, this pathophysiological model can provide an explanation as to how the phenotypic heterogeneity may reflect the underlying genetic heterogeneity.

Modes of inheritance of IDDM

The mode of inheritance of IDDM remains an area of some debate. Based on population studies of HLA antigens and family studies of HLA haplotypes, susceptibility to IDDM has been variously proposed, at various times, to be inherited as a single autosomal dominant, a single autosomal recessive, a mixture of recessive and dominant forms, via an intermediate gene dosage model, in a heterogeneous three allele or two-HLA loci model, and as a two-locus disorder (Rotter 1981a). Because of this debate one important line of investigation has been the development of mathematical genetic models that incorporate heterogeneity at the HLA complex, and models and methods of analysis for two-locus disorders (Hodge et al 1980, Thomson et al 1988). The current consensus is that among models, the three allele heterogeneity model provides the best fit to the available data (Bauer 1986, Louis & Thomson 1986, Rotter et al 1986, Thomson et al 1988).

In families with more than one IDDM offspring, sibs who are affected with IDDM share both HLA haplotypes more often than is expected by chance alone. If there were no linkage between the HLA region and the IDDM gene(s), affected pairs of sibs would be expected to share two haplotypes, one haplotype, and zero haplotypes in a ratio of 25% to 50% to 25%. Instead, the aggregate of a very large amount of data indicates that pairs of diabetic sibs share two haplotypes approximately 55–60% of the time, share one haplotype approximately 40%, and share zero haplotypes in only a few cases (Svejgaard et al 1980, Anderson et al 1983). The distribution of haplotype sharing falls between that expected for simple autosomal recessive inheritance (for rare disorders) and that expected for a rare autosomal dominant. This increased sharing is seen even for haplotypes that do not contain the IDDM-associated DR3 and DR4 (Rubinstein et al 1981), and provides additional evidence that genes in the HLA region play a central role in IDDM susceptibility.

Autosomal dominant inheritance has been proposed by MacDonald (1980), who demonstrated that such a model was consistent with US Black/Caucasian differences in the frequency of IDDM. The simple dominant model can be rejected, however, given that 55–60% of affected sib pairs have been found to share both HLA haplotypes (Svejgaard et al 1980). Analysing family data under a simple dominant model, no more than 50% of affected sib pairs can share HLA haplotypes (Thomson & Bodmer 1977). The autosomal recessive model can only explain the sib pair haplotype data and to do so would require a

gene frequency for the diabetes susceptibility allele of 0.2 to 0.3 or higher (Rubinstein et al 1981). This would necessitate the population disease prevalence to be at least tenfold higher than actually observed (Platz et al 1981). Thus substantially different penetrances for familial and non-familial cases must be invoked and, while this is theoretically possible, it is certainly quite suspect. The gene dosage model, by invoking a higher penetrance for an individual with two doses of the susceptibility allele, can resolve both the prevalence and sib pair data (Spielman et al 1980). However, neither the gene dosage model, nor its simpler extremes (dominant or recessive) can account for the consistent excess of DR3/DR4 heterozygotes observed (Svejgaard & Ryder 1981, Rotter et al 1983). Thus, a simple gene dosage model is also an inadequate explanation.

The accumulated evidence for heterogeneity, plus the observations regarding the compound DR3/DR4 individual, make the simple autosomal recessive and autosomal dominant hypotheses unfavourable. A more restricted hypothesis would be that at least some forms of juvenile diabetes are due to inheritance of recessive or dominant susceptibility. Barbosa et al ascertained their patients in order to select two sets of families: those with horizontal and those with vertical aggregation. For the purpose of linkage analysis, they then assumed recessive inheritance for the first set and dominant for the second (Barbosa et al 1978a, 1980a). While this is an intriguing hypothesis, it now appears that these different aggregation patterns did not reflect true differences in mode of inheritance but rather differential ascertainment of families with an aggregation of diabetes susceptibility genes (Suarez & Van Eerdewegh 1981).

For the most part, these simple genetic models ignore the increasingly well documented immunogenetic heterogeneity within IDDM reviewed above. A three-allele model was developed for a diabetic susceptibility locus tightly linked to the HLA complex (Hodge et al 1980). This model has made numerous predictions which have been confirmed by subsequent observations (Rotter & Hodge 1980, Rotter et al 1984, 1986, Bauer 1986, Louis & Thomson 1986, Rotter & Vadheim 1986, Thomson et al 1988). This three-allele heterogeneity model postulates a susceptibility locus for IDDM tightly linked to the HLA complex, with two different susceptibility alleles and one normal allele (Hodge et al 1980). There would thus be three forms of the disease: form 1, a B8-DR3 associated autoimmune form; form 2, a B15-DR4 insulin antibody responder form; and a compound form 3 due to occurrence of both alleles in the same individual. The predicted relative proportions of the three forms among all juvenile diabetics in the Caucasian population were 10%, 60% and 30%, for forms 1, 2 and 3, respectively. This prediction is consistent with various reported immunological studies. The reason why form 3 is so frequent among diabetics is its high penetrance, despite the fact that it has a low genotype frequency in comparison to the other two forms. Due to the higher penetrance of form 3, the distribution of the forms of the disease should differ in families with single and multiple-affected members. In fact, approximately 30% of all affected individuals are predicted to have form 3, but almost 50% of all affected sib pairs will have this form. Families with more affected individuals should have an even greater aggregation of high-risk genes, and more individuals of the form 3 genotype (Rotter et al 1986, Rotter & Vadheim 1986).

This model has had remarkable success in making population predictions which have been subsequently confirmed. Given the racial differences and estimated gene admixture proposed by MacDonald (1980) and subsequently supported by studies of Reitnauer et al (1982), use of this model predicted that the frequency of autoimmunity in US IDDM Blacks would be half that in US Caucasian IDDM patients (Rotter & Hodge 1980). This was confirmed both qualitatively and quantitatively (Neufeld et al 1980, Maclaren 1983). In addition, the model predicted that form 2, the DR4 association, would be more prominent in US Black IDDM patients, and this was confirmed (Maclaren et al 1982).

Some investigators claimed that linkage analysis assuming recessive inheritance revealed tight linkage for the DR3/DR4 pairs (equivalent to the proposed form 3), but loose linkage for the other pairs (Dunsworth et al 1982, Green et al 1982). In fact, the three allele heterogeneity model predicts that sibs pairs with DR3/DR4 share HLA haplotypes more often than sib pairs with other genotypes (Anderson et al 1983, Rotter et al 1986). As a result, the various reports of linkage heterogeneity, which were interpreted first as linkage heterogeneity (Dunsworth et al 1982, Green et al 1982), then as evidence for pseudolinkage, i.e. the involvement of other, non-HLA loci (Morton et al 1983), can be interpreted as a predictable consequence of the two different HLA susceptibilities (Rotter & Vadheim 1986). This three allele model has received further support from two recent international modelling efforts which concluded that it provided the best fit to the available data (Bauer 1986, Thomson et al 1988).

There is, however, evidence for further genetic complexity in IDDM. In calculating HLA-related risks for IDDM (Maclaren et al 1984), use of family-based data results in risk estimates that are higher by an order of magnitude than those calculated from population data. This suggests that it is unlikely that HLA DR3 and DR4 provide all the genetic susceptibility. At least three factors

probably contribute in part to this discrepancy. First, we may not yet have identified the specific contributory HLA genes and/or defined the DR specificities adequately. Thus, there may be more specific susceptibility genes, one associated with DR3, the other with DR4. Alternatively, there may be ways to subdivide the DR alleles into more specific diabetes-related types of DR3 and DR4. As reviewed above, molecular techniques have been successful in subdividing the DR4 associated susceptibility. The magnitude of this effect, however, can account for only a twofold difference in the population risks estimated above, and thus is not a sufficient explanation. Another possibility is that not only do genes at single HLA loci predispose to IDDM, but the entire HLA haplotype contributes susceptibility (Bertrams 1982, Contu et al 1982). This concept is supported by another HLA-associated disease, gluten-sensitive enteropathy (primarily associated with HLA DR3), in which evidence implicates the direct role of B8 as well (Strober 1980), supporting the concept that the different functional alleles of the genes in the major histocompatibility complex could, as a group, predispose to disease susceptibility. A third possibility is that non-HLA, non-chromosome 6 genes also predispose to IDDM (Rotter 1981a). There are suggestions that there may be contributions to IDDM from genes on several chromosomes, namely associations with the Kidd blood group on chromosome 18, Gm on chromosome 14, the DNA region flanking the insulin gene on chromosome 11, and the T-cell receptor beta chain gene on chromosome 7 (Hodge et al 1981, Nakao et al 1981, Barbosa et al 1982, Bell et al 1984, Field et al 1984, 1986, Rich et al 1986, Millward et al 1987, Field 1988). By comparing the risks of HLA identical sibs to that of MZ twins, it has been estimated that HLA provides approximately 60–70% of the overall genetic susceptibility to IDDM (Rotter & Landaw 1984).

Pathophysiology of IDDM

It is now apparent that IDDM is a chronic autoimmune disorder that gradually develops over many years. A variety of abnormalities in immune function and insulin release precede the 'abrupt' development of the diabetic syndrome in patients genetically predisposed to diabetes (Gorsuch et al 1981, Atkinson et al 1986, Eisenbarth 1986, Maclaren 1988). Eisenbarth (1986) has proposed dividing the development of Type I diabetes into six stages: (1) genetic susceptibility; (2) triggering events; (3) active autoimmunity; (4) gradual loss of glucose-stimulated insulin secretion; (5) appearance of overt diabetes, with some residual insulin secretion; (6) complete beta cell destruction. At the onset of Type I diabetes as few as 10% of the beta cells remain, and within several years essentially all beta cells are destroyed. Thus, if interventional therapy is to be effective it must be started well before the onset of the acute diabetic syndrome (see below).

Non-obese diabetes (NOD) mice and Biobreeding (BB) rats appear to be excellent models of the auto-immune form of diabetes (Eisenbarth 1986, Jackson 1988). It has been suggested that Class II genes within the major histocompatibility complex and T-lymphocytes are both important in the pathogenesis of islet cell destruction (Rossini et al 1984, Mordes et al 1987). Indeed, activated T-lymphocytes from acute-diabetic BB rats can transfer diabetes to other animals (Koevary et al 1983).

Similar evidence for the interaction of the MHC region and T-lymphocytes in human diabetes comes from the studies of pancreatic transplantation between identical twins (Sutherland et al 1984, 1989). When pancreases are transplanted from a non-diabetic twin to his diabetic monozygotic co-twin without immuno-suppression, islet cell destruction with massive T-cell infiltration, and relapse of the diabetes, occurs within weeks. Thus, the basic defect in Type I diabetes appears to be extrinsic to the pancreas and related to the activation of T-lymphocytes, which then mediate the destruction of the islets.

Uncovering the basis of MZ twin discordance in IDDM will be important in understanding the relationship of the basic underlying genetic defect in this disease to the subsequent immunological derangements and clinical disease. MZ twins, who are identical genotypically, can differ phenotypically by a variety of different mechanisms including; environmental exposure, Lyonization in the case of females, somatic mutation, activation of normally unexpressed genes, and gene rearrangement, as in the immunoglobulin and T-cell receptor genes (Rimoin & Rotter 1985, Eisenbarth 1987). T-cell activation through gene rearrangement may well be the proximal step in the development of IDDM in an individual who is genetically predisposed to the disease through his or her HLA type and other genes. The various environmental agents discussed below may well operate in triggering or selecting the appropriate T-cell receptor rearrangement and the specific HLA type may be necessary to present these activated T-cells and islet cell antibodies to the pancreas.

The role of environmental factors in IDDM

The monozygotic twin data, which show an IDDM concordance of approximately 30–40%, suggest that there are important environmental components to the aetiology of IDDM, although immunological gene arrangements could also provide an explanation for such a reduced penetrance (Rimoin & Rotter 1985, Eisenbarth 1987). As the pathogenetic processes which lead to IDDM appear to be complex, and may take years from initiation to completion, environmental agents could play one of several roles (Gamble 1980a,b, Bosi et al 1987). Environmental agents might function as initiating factors, i.e. factors which begin or continue the aetiological processes which eventually terminate in IDDM. If environmental factors function in this role, then more than one agent (for example, several different viruses, or viruses and chemical agents) might be involved in the aetiology. Alternatively, environmental factors could act mainly as precipitating factors — factors which convert preclinical diabetes into clinical disease. Several classes of environmental agents have been implicated in the aetiology of IDDM.

Infectious agents

A viral aetiology for diabetes has been suggested for many years, with case reports of diabetes following an episode of an infectious disease dating back to the 1800s (Gunderson 1927, McCrae 1963, Craighead 1978, Peig et al 1981). The current evidence for a role of viral agents comes from several sources, including case reports, epidemiological studies, clinical studies, and evidence from animal and human models.

Anecdotally, a 'viral-like illness' is known to precede the onset of many cases of IDDM (Craighead 1978, Gamble 1980b). Several lines of epidemiological evidence are also consistent with an infectious aetiology. For example, it has been noted that trends in age at onset of diabetes are consistent with a viral aetiology (Gamble 1980b). These data are most consistent with infectious agents playing a precipitating role in IDDM. Another suggestion that environmental agents play a role in the aetiology of IDDM comes from studies of time of onset in pairs of sibs with IDDM. At least one study suggests that sib pairs are more likely to have the onset of diabetes within a year of one another than would be expected by chance (Gamble 1980b).

There is also limited evidence for a viral influence (e.g. mumps, Coxsackie) from seroepidemiological studies, i.e. studies which compare viral and bacterial antibody titres in Type I diabetics and non-diabetic controls. (Gamble et al 1969, Champsaur et al 1982, King et al 1983a,b, Banatvala et al 1985, Schernthaner et al 1985). Other studies have found no evidence of increased titres to Coxsackie B viruses in new onset cases (Orchard et al 1983) while others have suggested that Coxsackie B3 and B4 titres are actually decreased in IDDM (Palmer et al 1982). Detection of the human cytomegalovirus genes by molecular hybridization with a human CMV specific probe has been observed in 22% of IDDM patients, compared to 2.6% of controls (Pak et al 1988). There was a strong correlation between the CMV gene and islet cell antibodies in the diabetic patients, suggesting that persistent CMV infection may be relevant to pathogenesis in some cases of type I diabetes.

Evidence from clinical studies also suggests a role for infectious agents in IDDM. The insulitis which has been noted in early IDDM could be consistent with viral infection of the pancreas, and autopsy studies have clearly documented pancreatic beta cell damage in children dying from overwhelming viral infections (Jenson et al 1980). Coxsackie B-specific antigens have specifically been found in the islets of Langerhans, and the Coxsackie B4 virus itself has been isolated from the pancreas of a child dying of acute onset IDDM (Yoon et al 1979). Several types of virus are known to be capable of infecting human pancreatic beta cells in vitro, suggesting that Coxsackie virus B groups, rubella virus and possibly cytomegalovirus (CMV) are capable of producing pathological beta cell changes in vivo.

Evidence from animal studies is strongly suggestive of a viral component to the aetiology of IDDM. The first evidence came from the discovery that the M strain of the encephalomyocarditis (EMC) virus infects pancreatic beta cells, and produces a diabetes-like disease in some strains of mice (Yoon & Notkins 1976, Rayfield & Ishimura 1987). This model has been widely studied, and it is now clear that the EMC-D variant (but not the EMC-B variant of the M strain) causes direct viral destruction of the beta cells in certain genetically susceptible (SJL/JH; C3H/HeJ) mouse lines (Boucher & Notkins 1973, Hayashi et al 1974, Craighead & Higgins 1974, Onodera et al 1978, Yoon et al 1980, 1982, 1983, Iwo et al 1983, Gould et al 1984, 1985). In addition, in other mouse strains (for example BALB/CBy), EMC-M strains appear to initiate an immunologically-mediated form of diabetes (Huber et at 1985, Jordan & Cohen 1987), suggesting that the same virus can have multiple effects, depending on the genetic predisposition of the host. Diabetes in SJL/J mice can be be prevented by vaccinating animals with live-attenuated EMC vaccine (Yoon & Notkins 1983, Yoon & Ray 1984). Several other promising animal models of infectious agents and diabetes have been developed (Rayfield & Ishimura 1987).

Only some strains of mice are susceptible to virally-induced diabetes, and this suggests a genetic component to disease susceptibility. The fact that only certain strains of virus are capable of inducing diabetes in specific animal models indicates that genetic factors in the agent are also important. The genetic/strain specificity of the agent may be particularly important in viruses which change rapidly in the population, and may explain several puzzling aspects of IDDM epidemiology; specifically, the possible changing incidence of IDDM over time, as well as the interesting observation that the proportion of complicated mumps cases who were ICA + decreased rapidly from the late 1970s to the mid-1980s (Helmke et al 1986).

The animal models suggest that infectious agents can cause diabetes or diabetes-like syndromes by at least four different mechanisms: (1) by acute infection of the beta cell, leading to necrosis (EMC and reovirus models); (2) through autoimmune mechanisms (rubella model); (3) through persistent infection, leading to decreased growth and lifespan of the beta cell (LCB model); and (4) through biochemical alterations in the cell or cell membrane which lead to decreased insulin synthesis/release (VE model) (Rayfield & Ishimura 1987). While our knowledge of infectious agents in human diabetes is less advanced, it is possible that all four mechanisms also occur in human diabetes.

The animal models have also raised the hope that vaccination against promoting or initiating viral agents may protect genetically susceptible individuals against Type I diabetes. Vaccination against EMC virus in SJL/J mice and pertussis (whole cell vaccine) in CD-1 mice with streptozotocin-induced diabetes suggests that beta cell destruction can either be prevented or halted in at least some mouse models (Yoon & Notkins 1983, Huang et al 1984).

The best human models of infectious agents in IDDM come from studies of individuals with the congenital rubella syndrome and from serial studies of children with viral infections who subsequently develop IDDM. The incidence of IDDM and other autoimmune diseases among children and young adults with the congenital rubella syndrome is markedly increased over that in the general population, and may be as high as 15–40%. Those cases of congenital rubella with IDDM have an increased frequency of HLA-DR3 and DR4 and a decreased frequency of HLA-DR2, much as in non-rubella IDDM cases (Rubinstein et al 1982). A significant proportion of patients with congenital rubella syndrome have T-cell sub-set abnormalities, and a variety of autoimmune antibodies, including anti-thyroid microsomal, anti-thyroglobulin, and anti-islet cell and islet-cell surface antibodies, suggesting an autoimmune aetiology for their IDDM (Rubinstein et al 1982, Rabinowe et al 1986). Rubella virus has been isolated from the pancreas of several cases with congenital rubella syndrome (De Prins et al 1978), and at least one case of insulitis and beta cell destruction is known in an infant with congenital rubella infection who died of acute diabetes (Patterson et al 1981). This evidence suggests that rubella can indeeed infect and damage the beta cell, and that the diabetes seen in congenital rubella syndrome could be due either to initiation of an immune process by the rubella virus or directly to persistent pancreatic rubella infection.

Chemical agents

Several chemical agents are known to cause an insulin-dependent diabetes in animals and in humans. In the rat, streptozotocin and alloxan are classic diabetogenic agents, although the mechanism through which these beta cell toxins cause diabetes is still not entirely understood. In humans, several agents are known to cause diabetes upon ingestion. The best documented is the rodenticide N-3-pyridylmethyl-N'-p-nitrophenylurea (RH-787; 'Vacor') (Karam et al 1980).

Genetic counselling in Type I diabetes

At the current time, the recommendations for genetic counselling are based on empirically derived recurrence risks, i.e. the actual recurrence risks seen in relatives of large series of patients (Table 89.7). These recurrence risks are frequently reassuring to many families, as the risk to the sib of an IDDM diabetic is of the order of

5–10%, and the risk to the offspring of an IDDM diabetic is of the order of 2–5%. These recurrence risks are lower than many families expect. Table 89.8 gives the risk for IDDM for various classes of individuals. Several studies have shown that the risk to offspring of IDDM fathers (4–6%) is approximately double that to offspring of IDDM mothers (2–3%) (Warram et al 1984). It is also clear that HLA typing can further refine the risk for sibs, since those sharing both HLA haplotypes are at greatest risk; this is especially so when the index case has both HLA DR3 and DR4 (Rotter et al 1986, Thomson et al 1988).

Screening and prevention of Type I diabetes

The decision to undertake screening for a disease (or risk for a disease) should not be taken lightly. Such a decision should be based on clearly established criteria such as the frequency and severity of the disease, the availability of a safe, accurate, cost-effective screening test, and the ability to sucessfully intervene in preventing or ameliorating the disease or its complications.

It has been estimated that as much as 60% of the overall genetic susceptibility to IDDM is contributed by HLA region genes. Thus, an accurate marker for the

Table 89.7 Empiric recurrence risks for insulin dependent diabetes

Reference	Proband	Risk to sibs %	Risk to offspring %	Comments
Harris (1950)	<30	4.1		Interview
			1.4	Predicted by age 40
Working Party College of Practitioners (1965)	<30	4.8		Interview
Simpson (1962)	<20	5.7	0.9	Interview
Simpson (1968)	<20	2.4	1.8	Mailed questionnaire
Kobberling (1969)	<25	10.9 ± 3.9		Predicted by age 25
Darlow & Smith (1973)	<25	4.7–7.6		Predicted by age 25
Tattersal & Fajans (1975)	<25	11		Interview and GTT
Nerup et al (1974)	juvenile	9.7		HLA typed
Degnbol & Green (1978)	<20	6.2 ± 1.3	5.4 ± 2.9*	Questionnaire interview-predicted by age 35
West et al (1979)	<17	4.1		Medical record review
Gottlieb (1980)	<20	4.5	3.1	Mailed questionnaire of proband and relatives
Gamble (1980a)	<16	5.6		Observed by age 16, mailed questionnaire of families
Kobberling & Bruggeboes (1980)	insulin treated since diagnosis		2.4	Medical questionnaire, includes both parents affected
			1.5	Only mother affected
Wagener et al (1982)	<17	3.3–6 10.5^+		+ If parents also affected
Chern et al (1982)	insulin treated	$4.6 \pm 0.8 + +$		$+ +$ If probands diagnosed > 10 yrs of age
	since diagnosis	8.5 ± 2.0**		** If probands diagnosed ≤ 10 yrs of age

* Actual observed recurrence 2.8%.

HLA-linked genetic susceptibility would allow us to identify the majority of those individuals genetically at increased risk to develop IDDM. It should be noted, however, that even an identical twin of a person with Type I diabetes, who is genetically at the highest risk for diabetes, has only a 30–40% chance of becoming diabetic. Thus other factors, presumably environmental, but also possibly due to random variation in the immune system, are needed to convert the genetic susceptibility into clinically manifest diabetes.

There are two ways in which HLA might be used in screening: (1) to test for 'high-risk' HLA types in random samples of the population; (2) to test for genetic risk in sibs, offspring and other relatives of IDDM index cases. Approximately 50% of the non-diabetic population have the same DR types as patients with IDDM. Thus, at least 98% of the people with HLA-DR3 or DR4 will never develop IDDM. For every 1000 persons with HLA-DR3 or DR4 in the population, only 2–4 will develop IDDM in their lifetime (Table 89.8). Population genetic screening using currently available HLA typing will result in many more 'false' positives than 'true' positives in terms of genetic risk. Identification of other genetic markers, such as the DQ alpha and beta molecular markers, may result in more specific identification of people at risk for the development of IDDM (Owerbach et al 1988). At the current time, however, they do not provide sufficient specificity dramatically to improve population screening.

The individuals at highest risk of developing IDDM, other than identical twins, are the sibs of Type I diabetic patients who have an overall 5–10% risk of developing IDDM. HLA testing can be used to refine these risks within families (Table 89.8). The sib of an IDDM patient who shares all HLA types is at greatest risk (12–24%) for developing IDDM. A sib who is HLA haplo-identical (one HLA haplotype in common) has a risk in the range of 4–7%; whereas a sib who shares no HLA types has a risk in the range of only 1–2%. While these risks are higher than those for population screening, 75% or more of the identified sibs will never develop IDDM and would represent false positives.

Until we can prevent IDDM, HLA typing is probably best used as a research tool to better understand how diabetes develops. Other premorbid markers of IDDM, such as islet cell antibodies and activated T-cells might be used to screen for pre-clinical IDDM in those HLA-susceptible individuals, either within families or in the population (Eisenbarth 1986, 1987, Maclaren 1988). As discussed above, islet cell antibodies are detectable at onset of clinical diabetes in about 80% of all IDDMs and have been shown to precede clinically detectable diabetes by months and even years in some cases.

Immunosuppressive therapy has been successful in modulating the progression of the diabetes in newly diagnosed IDDM patients (Stiller et al 1984). However, since only a few percent of the islet cells remain intact at the onset of the diabetic syndrome, initiation of this therapy closer to the onset of T-cell activation or islet cell antibody development may well be more effective. The side-effects of the immunosuppressive therapy, however, have precluded widespread use of these agents in clinically normal individuals. Identification of the specific diabetes susceptibility HLA subtypes by molecular techniques and screening only genetically predisposed individuals for T-cell activation or islet cell antibody formation should allow for the more timely onset of such therapy, once relatively safe methods of immunosuppression become available.

Screening and prevention for other autoimmune diseases

In addition to diabetes, patients with IDDM and their relatives are known to have increased risks for other autoimmune diseases such as autoimmune thyroid disease (Hashimoto thyroiditis, Graves disease), Addison disease, pernicious anaemia, vitiligo and myasthenia gravis (Eisenbarth et al 1978, Bottazzo et al 1978, Riley et al 1981). In a series of Type I diabetics and their families who were screened for clinical and latent (antibody positive) autoimmune disease, 21% of the diabetics and 22% of their first-degree relatives were found to have evidence of autoimmune disease (Betterle et al 1984). Among patients who had persistent islet cell antibodies

Table 89.8 Risks for IDDM

Population risks	Overall — 1/500
	HLA-DR related
	No high risk allele — 1/5000
	1 high risk allele — 1/400
	HLA-DR3/3 or DR4/4 — 1/150
	HLA-DR3/4 — 1/40
	HLA-DR4 subset defined by molecular techniques — 1/300
Risks in relatives	
Sibs	Overall — 1/14
	HLA haplotypes shared with diabetic sib
	0 haplotypes shared — 1/100
	1 haplotypes shared — 1/20
	2 haplotypes shared — 1/6
	2 haplotypes shared and DR3/4 — 1/5 to 1/4
Offspring	Overall — 1/25
	Offspring of affected female — 1/50 to 1/40
	Offspring of affected male — 1/20
Monozygotic twin of diabetic — 1/3	

(>3 years after diagnosis of diabetes) the percentage with other autoimmune manifestations was 57%, compared to 15% in those who did not have persistent ICAs (Betterle et al 1984). As 75% of the autoimmune disease in family members occurred in families with a proband with autoimmune disease (Betterle et al 1984), this may be of use in deciding which family members to screen for autoimmunity.

Autoimmune thyroid disease is the most common form of autoimmune disease occurring in families with IDDM (Gorsuch et al 1980). The proportion of IDDM patients with clinical or subclinical thyroid disease is thought to be in the range of 15–20%, although in a series of adult IDDM patients the proportion was 35% (Fialkow et al 1975, Riley et al 1981, Betterle et al 1984). Among 771 children and young adults with Type I diabetes who were screened using thyroid microsomal antibodies (TMA) and thyroid function tests, 17% were TMA-positive; of these, 1% were clinically hyperthyroid, 7% hypothyroid, and 92% clinically euthyroid (Riley et al 1981). The prevalence of thyroid autoimmunity among non-diabetic Caucasians, in contrast, was less than 4.5% in this age group (Riley et al 1981). Among first-degree relatives of Type I diabetics, the prevalence of clinical or latent thyroid disease is in the range of 15–25%, with the prevalence increasing with increasing age (Fialkow et al 1975, Betterle et al 1984). As with autoimmune thyroid disease in the general population, females have higher rates of thyroid and gastric autoimmunity than do males (Gorsuch et al 1980).

Pernicious anaemia or gastric parietal cell autoantibodies are found in 5–12% of Type I diabetics and perhaps half that in their first-degree relatives (Fialkow et al 1975, Riley et al 1982, Betterle et al 1984).

The prevalence of Addison disease, while elevated over rates for non-diabetics, is much lower than for autoimmune thyroid or gastric disease. Among 466 Type I diabetics screened for adrenal antibodies, 1.5% were found to be positive (1.9% of Caucasian IDDM patients) (Riley et al 1980). This is consistent with results from other studies, in which the prevalence of adrenal autoantibodies ranged between 1–3% in Type I diabetic cases and 0.0–0.6% among non-diabetic controls (Riley et al 1980, Betterle et al 1984).

The results of family studies strongly suggest that autoimmune disease occurs frequently enough in certain Type I diabetics and their first-degree relatives to warrant some level of screening. The presence of thyrogastric autoimmunity and/or persistent islet cell antibodies in a diabetic proband indicates a family which merits closest attention, since 60–65% of families with autoimmune disease will have a diabetic proband who also has evidence of autoimmune disease (Bottazzo et al 1978,

Betterle et al 1984). Perhaps 40% of all families which include a Type I proband will include another family member with latent or clinical autoimmune disease (Betterle et al 1984). This suggests that screening for thyroid disease and perhaps also for pernicious anaemia/atrophic gastritis may become standard parts of family follow-up.

Because of the increased risk of clinical autoimmune disease in IDDM diabetics and their family members, a reasonable case can be made for routine periodic screening of patients and their relatives for those disorders easily and non-invasively detected by such a screening process. This includes testing for thyroid dysfunction, both hypo and hyperthyroidism, using standard tests such as T4 and TSH levels; and testing for the B12 deficiency of pernicious anaemia-atrophic gastritis and, possibly in the future, testing for the early atrophic gastritis itself by the pepsinogen I/pepsinogen II ratio which appears to be a sensitive and non-invasive test for atrophic gastritis (Samloff et al 1982).

NON-INSULIN DEPENDENT DIABETES (NIDDM) (TYPE II)

Type II diabetes, also known as non-insulin dependent diabetes (NIDDM), and previously referred to as maturity-onset or adult-onset diabetes, is characterized by a relative disparity between endogenous insulin production and insulin requirements, leading to an elevated blood glucose. In contrast to Type I diabetes, there is always some endogenous insulin production in Type II diabetes; many Type II patients have normal or even elevated blood insulin levels. The disease usually occurs in persons over the age of 40, and the onset may be insidious, or even clinically unapparent. The hyperglycaemia of Type II diabetes can often be controlled by diet or oral hypoglycaemic agents, although exogenous insulin may be required to control hyperglycaemia.

Genetic predisposition and heterogeneity

Monozygotic twin studies demonstrate almost complete concordance for NIDDM in identical twins (Pyke 1979, Barnett et al 1981a); yet the familial aggregation of clinical disease or glucose levels is not consistent with a single, simple mode of inheritance (Rotter & Rimoin 1981a). Genetic heterogeneity would seem the most likely explanation. In addition, population studies have shown a marked increase in the frequency of NIDDM when primitive populations migrate to more urban and affluent environments (Cohen 1961, Zimmet et al 1982) demonstrating that environmental factors are also important. The identical twin data, with close to 100%

concordance in MZ twins, suggest that in the urbanized Western world, the environment is sufficiently constant (and diabetogenic) for genetic susceptibility to be the primary determinant for development of NIDDM.

Clinical genetic studies have suggested heterogeneity within NIDDM. When Kobberling (1971) divided his adult-onset probands into low, moderate, and markedly overweight categories, he found a significantly higher frequency of affected sibs in the light-proband category (38%) and a significantly lower frequency in the heavy-proband category (10%). Irvine et al (1977b) also suggested a difference between the non-obese and obese insulin-dependent probands. They observed a different clinical range of diabetes in the relatives of the non-obese and obese probands.

Fajans (1976) and co-workers have demonstrated metabolic heterogeneity in non-obese latent diabetes. These investigators were able to divide their latent diabetic patients into two broad groups: those with an insulinopenic form of glucose intolerance, and those with high levels of plasma-immunoreactive insulin. The high responders and low responders have remained consistent and distinct over many years of follow-up, suggesting that they represented different metabolic disorders.

Subclinical and genetic markers in NIDDM

One group of investigators has observed antibodies to specific endocrine cells of the gut (glucose insulinotropic peptide or GIP cells), in 15–20% of NIDDM patients (Mirakian et al 1980, Bottazzo et al 1982). This hormone plays a role in the modulation of insulin secretion. It is conceivable that these antibodies identify an autoimmune form of NIDDM, due to destruction of the gut endocrine influences on glucose homeostasis. Some IDDM patients were also found to have these anti-GIP cell antibodies. This would be one possible explanation for the overlap of NIDDM and IDDM seen in some families. Further support for an autoimmune connection in some forms of NIDDM is the report of an HLA association in Fiji NIDDM patients of Indian origin (Serjeantson et al 1981). This sub-group could well occur in other populations, as the association is with HLA antigen Bw61, a split of the B40 antigen, which has been reported to be associated with juvenile-onset (but not necessarily IDDM) diabetes in Caucasian populations (Cudworth 1978).

In the early 1980s, several groups reported an association of NIDDM with a DNA restriction fragment length polymorphism (RFLP) of the insulin gene. Owerbach et al (1981) localized the insulin gene to the short arm of chromosome 11, using nucleic acid hybridization techniques. Extending this work, two groups examined RFLPs of the insulin gene in NIDDM and IDDM patients, and found a greater frequency of the large DNA restriction fragments (i.e. inserts) in NIDDM patients and controls (Rotwein et al 1983, Owerbach & Nerup 1981). These RFLPs are not in the coding portion of the insulin gene, but are due to insertions in the 5'-flanking region of the gene. However, subsequent observations have been unable to confirm these initial findings. Conversely Bell et al (1984), in the largest series, found an association between small inserts of this DNA polymorphism and IDDM, but no relationship with NIDDM. The localization of this insertional polymorphism to a potential promoter region of the gene suggests it may play a role in insulin gene expression. How this might relate to either IDDM or NIDDM pathogenesis remains speculative.

There appears to be heterogeneity in the pathogenetic mechanisms operative in NIDDM, with some forms due to impaired insulin secretion and others to impaired insulin responsiveness (O'Rahilly et al 1986). For example, abnormalities in the amount and temporal organization of insulin secretion have been found in NIDDM patients (Polonsky et al 1988) and impaired pulsatile secretion of insulin in their first-degree relatives (O'Rahilly et al 1988). On the other hand, studies of Pima Indians before and after the development of NIDDM indicate that their impaired glucose tolerance is primarily due to impaired insulin action (Lillioja et al 1987). Molecular defects in the insulin receptor gene have now been documented in several of the rare insulin resistance syndromes and it is possible that molecular defects in the insulin receptor gene will be uncovered in patients with non-syndromal forms of NIDDM.

Diabetes caused by mutant insulins

Molecular biological studies have provided the most exciting evidence concerning the genetics of NIDDM. A number of patients have now been described with discrete point mutations in the insulin gene who present with hyperglycaemia, hyperinsulinaemia, and yet have a normal responsiveness to exogenous insulin. Abnormal insulins of markedly reduced biological potency are produced. The syndrome is inherited as an autosomal dominant trait. Three well-characterized mutations are the so-called Insulin Chicago, Insulin Los Angeles, and Insulin Wakayama. Insulin Chicago is due to the substitution of a leucine for phenylalanine residue at position 25 of the B chain, as a result of single nucleotide change (TTC to TTG) (Kwok et al 1983). Insulin Los Angeles is due to the substitution of a serine for a phenylalanine residue at position 24 of the B chain and is also the result of a single nucleotide change (TTC to

TCC) (Haneda et al 1984). The third mutant insulin, Insulin Wakayama, described in three Japanese families, is due to a leucine for valine substitution at position 3 of the insulin A chain. (Nanjo et al 1987, Awata et al 1988).

These mutant insulins can be detected in serum by means of variant migration on high pressure liquid chromatography (HPLC) and in DNA by alterations in restriction enzyme cleave sites (Given et al 1980, Shoelson et al 1983, Haneda et al 1984, Tager 1984, Seino et al 1985). In addition, several patients have been described with point mutations at the cleavage site of the C peptide, resulting in hyperproinsulinaemia (Gruppuso et al 1984, Elbein et al 1985). It is likely that additional mutations will be found which alter the structure or processing of the insulin molecule. While it is apparent that many more such point mutations will be described (in patients with and without glucose intolerance), it is important to note that in a population of NIDDMs screened for mutant insulins, less than 0.5% were found to have such mutations (Sanz et al 1986). Definitive identification of each mutation has been obtained by cloning both alleles of the insulin gene from the affected individual and analysing the nucleotide sequences. Miyano et al (1988) have described a simple sensitive and accurate screening test for these mutations, using polymerase chain reaction (PCR) DNA amplification coupled with dot blot hybridization, which should prove useful for screening larger diabetic populations to detect base substitutions in the insulin gene that lead to altered insulin or proinsulin structure and/or insulin production.

Maturity onset diabetes of the young (MODY)

MODY diabetes has also been called Mason-type diabetes, non-insulin dependent diabetes of the young (NIDDY) and maturity-onset type hyperglycaemia of the young (MOHY) (Tattersall & Fajans 1975, Johansen & Gregersen 1977). In addition to the criteria for the diagnosis of diabetes, the MODY diabetic must meet the following additional criteria: (1) age of onset for at least one family member under 25 years; (2) correction of fasting hyperglycaemia for at least two years without insulin; and (3) non-ketotic diabetes (Tattersall 1982). Using these criteria, a number of families with clearly dominant inheritance have been established. However, the considerable clinical and genetic heterogeneity among diabetics currently classified as MODY/NIDDY is just beginning to be appreciated. The early descriptions of Caucasian families with MODY suggested considerable homogeneity of a mild, early-onset, relatively complication-free diabetes inherited as an autosomal dominant. As more families were described, particularly in non-European populations, the wide diversity of early-onset, 'Type-II-like' diabetes became apparent. It is unclear whether some types of diabetes (NIDDY in Asian Indians; 'Type II diabetes of early onset' in Black African and other non-Caucasian populations) should be included within MODY.

While MODY was first reported to be inherited as an autosomal dominant disorder, it is now clear that there is considerable genetic heterogeneity within this type of diabetes (Tattersall 1982). An autosomal dominant form of MODY occurs in some families, with an estimated penetrance ranging from 36% to almost 100% (Barbosa et al 1978b, Serjeantson & Zimmet 1982). Among Asian Indians, who have a high rate of positive family history, perhaps 25% have unequivocal autosomal dominant inheritance, another 50% have possible dominant inheritance, and 25% appear to be sporadic (Mohan et al 1985a). Among a series of German MODY patients, 75% had an affected parent, 30% reported three-generational vertical transmission, 14% had an affected sib and 18% had no known affected relative (Panzram & Adolph 1981).

Despite the large numbers of affected individuals in particular pedigrees, the search for genetic markers has thus far met with little success. A number of studies in widely divergent populations have found no evidence for association with HLA antigens (Nelson & Pyke 1976, Panzram & Adolph 1981, Platz et al 1982, Serjeantson & Zimmett 1982, Tattersall 1982, Arnaiz-Villena et al 1983, Barbosa 1983, Deschamps et al 1983, Naidoo et al 1986, Elbein et al 1987). In addition, there is no evidence for an association with insulin gene polymorphisms on chromosome 11 (Bell et al 1983, Owerbach et al 1983, Johnston et al 1984, Andreone et al 1985, Elbein et al 1987) or the insulin receptor gene on chromosome 9 (Elbein et al 1987, O'Rahilly & Turner 1988). Studies of common genetic polymorphic markers in MODY are rare; however, two studies suggest that MODY is not linked to the acid phosphatase, glyoxylase, glutamic pyruvic transaminase (GPT), properdin factor B (Bf), complement components C6 and C7, immunoglobulin heavy chain allotypes (Gm), haptoglobulin, or group-specific component (Gc) loci (Serjeantson & Zimmet 1982). Chlorpropamide alcohol-induced flushing, once suggested as a physiological marker for MODY (and for much of NIDDM) has not been found to be useful in most MODY pedigrees (Kobberling et al 1980, Fajans 1981, Panzram & Adolph 1981, Jialal & Joubert 1984, Johnston et al 1984).

In terms of disease aetiology, MODY will almost certainly be found to be heterogenous. Both hypo- and hyper-insulinism has been reported in MODY patients (Fajans 1982, Mohan et al 1985b), although a number of studies suggest that C-peptide levels are often below normal even in non-obese MODY patients and in the clinically normal offspring of MODY diabetics (Mohan et al 1985b). Studies in several ethnic groups have documented a low insulin response to intravenous glucose, particularly a loss of the first phase insulin response (Tattersall 1974, Fajans 1976, Barbosa et al 1978b, Naidoo et al 1986, Sandler 1986). In studies of Asian Indians, the first phase insulin response is attenuated, but still present, in response to intravenous glucagon and tolbutamide, suggesting that MODY diabetes may be due to decreased glucose recognition by the beta cells (Naidoo et al 1986). At least one study suggests that peripheral insulin binding and insulin action are not impaired in MODY diabetics when compared to non-diabetic family members (Gelenter et al 1981).

While early studies suggested clinical homogeneity within individual families, it is now clear that there can be considerable variability, even within families. Early reports suggested that MODY diabetes was a mild form of the disease, with a low incidence of long-term diabetic complications (Tattersall 1974, Barbosa et al 1978b). Others have suggested that low rates of complications occur only in those families with an autosomal dominant form of inheritance (Tattersall 1982, Mohan et al 1985a). In Asian Indians from the south of India, it has been suggested that proliferative retinopathy and nephropathy rates may be lower in long-duration MODY diabetics with an autosomal dominant form of disease (Mohan et al 1985a). Other studies suggest that rates of complications in MODY may be similar to those seen in Type II diabetes (Fajans et al 1978, Fajans 1982).

O'Rahilly et al (1987) have suggested that those islet cell antibody-negative patients with NIDDM occurring before age 40 and with microvascular complications have a disease which is distinct from MODY: they called this 'Type II diabetes of early onset'. On the basis of their finding that 90% of the parents and 69% of the sibs had diabetes or an abnormal glucose infusion test, they postulated that this syndrome is the result of homozygosity for the gene responsible for late-onset NIDDM in the heterozygous state.

Winter et al (1987) have described an atypical form of diabetes among American Blacks which has an acute insulin-dependent presentation, followed by non-insulin dependence months to years later. It is non-progressive, non-immune, and dominantly inherited. They believe it may account for 10% of all cases of youth-onset diabetes in Black Americans.

Genetic counselling for type II diabetes

For the most part, we must depend on empiric recurrence risks for genetic counselling. For relatives of an NIDDM diabetic, the empiric recurrence risk to first-degree relatives is of the order of 10–15% for clinical diabetes and 20–30% for an abnormal glucose tolerance test (impaired glucose tolerance). For many MODY diabetics, i.e. those in whom it is an autosomal dominant disorder, the risk to sibs and offspring is 50%.

Screening and prevention in type II diabetes

Screening of first-degree relatives of NIDDM diabetics can be accomplished by periodic glucose tolerance testing. Those relatives with impaired glucose tolerance should be advised to attain ideal body weight. This should be encouraged strongly, with the goals being to reverse the glucose intolerance, delay or prevent progression to frank diabetes, and minimize the cardiovascular risks associated with impaired glucose intolerance.

OTHER FORMS OF DIABETES MELLITUS

The separation of idiopathic diabetes into IDDM and NIDDM by no means exhausts the potential heterogeneity within the diabetic phenotype. There could well be genetically distinct forms of diabetes whose phenotypic presentation could include either IDDM or NIDDM. The atypical form of diabetes among American Blacks reported by Winter et al (1987) may be an example. There is ample precedent for this phenomenon in other common diseases: examples include combined gastric and duodenal ulcer, which appears to be a separate disorder from either solitary duodenal ulcer or solitary gastric ulcer (Rotter 1981b), and familial combined hyperlipidaemia, where a given individual in a family can present with either an elevated cholesterol, an elevated triglyceride, or both (Motulsky 1976). Evidence for 'overlap' phenotypes in diabetes include suggestions of too high a frequency of either type in family members of the other type compared to the general population, and reports that NIDDM in parents of IDDM patients increases the risk to other sibs for IDDM (Cahill 1979b, Chern et al 1982, Wagener et al 1982). Some of this may be due to the occurrence of an NIDDM-like phase of IDDM in patients with a more protracted natural history, as discussed earlier, but it quite possibly reflects further heterogeneity. In addition, it has been reported that in some non-Caucasian populations, i.e. South African, Indian, and Black diabetics, regardless of the type of diabetes in the proband, there was an increase in NIDDM in first-degree relatives (Omar & Asmal 1983). In addition, low order of magnitude HLA associations have been reported with HLA antigen Bw61 in diabetics from the Indian subcontinent (Serjeantson et al 1981), and with HLA antigen A2 in Pima Indian diabetics (Williams et al 1981). The genetic-aetiological relationship of these HLA associations with diabetes in these non-Caucasian populations would seem fundamentally different from that of HLA and IDDM in Caucasian populations. Since there is no evidence for the role of immunological factors in these NIDDM types of diabetes, these HLA associations may have a polygenic background role more analogous to that of the mouse H2 locus and the effect of strain differences. Essentially, there are whole groups or classes of diabetes for which our knowledge of aetiology, genetics, and nosology is minimal. This includes not only most forms of diabetes in the developing world, but also gestational diabetes in general; the latter was separated in the National Diabetes Data Group (1979) classification for essentially counting and diagnostic purposes, not because of special knowledge regarding its genetics or aetiology.

Tropical forms of diabetes

Several types of diabetes are seen only in the tropical areas of the world. These forms of diabetes, grouped by a WHO Study Group (1985) under the category 'Malnutritional-Related Diabetes Mellitus' are characterized by onset in early adult life, under-weight, and/or a history of malnutrition, relative insulin resistance (at least at the time of diagnosis), and high insulin requirements to control hyperglycaemia. In some patients, usually with a history of abdominal pain, fibrocalculus lesions of the pancreatic ducts are seen on X-ray or ultrasound.

A familial predisposition has been suggested and some researchers suggest that tropical pancreatitis may play a role in tropical/malnutritional diabetes (Narendranatham 1981). However, the few studies which have specifically considered the genetics of tropical/malnutritional diabetes suggest that a negative family history for diabetes is characteristic, and that islet cell antibodies and increased frequencies of HLA DR3 and DR4 are not seen in these patients (Rao et al 1983, Ahuja 1985, Abu-Bakare et al 1986). More research is needed before a genetic predisposition can be ruled out; however, the currently available data suggest that environmental factors may play a more important role.

Gestational diabetes

Gestational diabetes is defined as 'carbohydrate intolerance of variable severity, with onset or first recognition during the present pregnancy'. Thus, gestational diabetes is a term which covers: (1) women who are carbohydrate intolerant only during pregnancy; (2) women who remain carbohydrate intolerant postpartum; and (3) women who were carbohydrate intolerant prior to pregnancy but whose diagnosis is made during pregnancy.

While once thought to represent 'pre-type II diabetes', gestational diabetes is probably a highly heterogeneous disorder, including individuals who have Type I diabetes (or pre-Type I diabetes), Type II diabetes, and other as yet undelineated forms of diabetes. As a large proportion (50–75%) of individuals with gestational diabetes eventually become clinically diabetic outside pregnancy, an understanding of the aetiologies of this disorder would be useful for both primary and secondary prevention.

HLA-DR3 and DR4 have been reported to be increased in gestational diabetics compared to non-diabetics, and the HLA-DR types of those who become insulin dependent (with low C-peptide levels) within a year postpartum appear to be the same as in Type I diabetics (Freinkel & Metzger 1985, Freinkel et al 1985). The frequency of the molecularly defined diabetogenic HLA-DQ-beta gene marker also appears to be increased in gestational diabetics (Owerbach et al 1988). In addition, gestational diabetics have 10–20 times the population frequency of circulating serum islet cell antibodies, and many with such antibodies are found to have abnormal postpartum GTTs (Metzger et al 1985). These data suggest that a fraction of the gestational diabetics have a genetic and physiological profile consistent with Type I diabetes.

PREGNANCY IN DIABETES

Diabetes is one of the most common chronic conditions complicating pregnancy. With improvements in the management of mothers with insulin dependent, non-insulin dependent, and gestational diabetes, the morbidity and mortality (both for mother and child) have been markedly improved (Gyves et al 1977). The earliest classification system categorizing mothers as to severity of diabetes (age of onset, duration of illness, and presence of complications) was the grouping according to White (White 1978). In general, the more severe the diabetes, the worse the outcome, particularly in the presence of vascular disease (Gabbe et al 1977). Besides the status of the mother when she entered pregnancy, degree of control of the mother's disease during pregnancy appeared to be related to outcome. If the mean blood sugar level was less than 100 mg/dl in the third trimester, perinatal mortality was 3.8%, compared with a perinatal mortality of 23.6% with a mean blood sugar greater than 150 mg/dl (Karlsson & Kjellmer 1972). Similar improvement was seen in morbidity, although third-trimester management did not affect the incidence of congenital malformations.

The infant of a diabetic mother is more likely to have a major congenital malformation than the infant of a woman without diabetes. The risk appears to be related to the severity of diabetes; women with IDDM are at the highest risk, those with NIDDM next, and women with gestational diabetes appear to be at the least increased risk compared to non-diabetics. IDDM women are at approximately 5–6 times the risk of having an infant with congenital malformations compared to the general population.

A wide range of malformations involving multiple organ systems have been associated with diabetes (Table 89.9). Cardiovascular, renal, skeletal, and central nervous system anomalies are prominent. The malformations most closely associated with diabetes originate before the seventh week of gestation, and there is preliminary evidence suggesting that poor diabetic control increases the risk of congenital malformations, since high first trimester haemoglobin A_{1c} values have been associated with high malformation rates.

Attempts at prevention thus require identification of patients and therapy prior to conception, as organogenesis occurs before most women would come to medical attention. Normoglycaemia appears to be the goal of therapy but care must be taken to avoid frequent episodes of hypoglycaemia, as this may also damage the developing fetus.

Genetic counselling of the female diabetic (IDDM or NIDDM) should thus include a discussion of the risk of having an infant with a congenital malformation and the postulated benefits of achieving good control prior to becoming pregnant and throughout the pregnancy. Because of the increased risk of abnormalities, including neural tube defects, which can be diagnosed prenatally, prenatal diagnosis, including serial ultrasound and maternal serum alpha fetoprotein (MSAFP), should be considered in all pregnancies of diabetic women. Since maternal serum AFP levels are altered in diabetic women, tables specific to diabetic mothers should be used in interpreting MSAFP levels in pregnant diabetics.

CONCLUSIONS

Heterogeneity within both the insulin dependent and non-insulin dependent types appears extensive. An important question thus arises from the population genetic viewpoint. These diabetic disorders, whose susceptibility appears to be primarily genetically determined, are deleterious, and thus reproductive fitness should be impaired. How then did these genes become so frequent? As regards NIDDM, a possible explanation is the concept of a 'thrifty' genotype, as first proposed by Neel (1962). He proposed that the diabetic genotype somehow allowed more efficient utilization of foodstuffs by the body in periods of famine to which primitive man was often exposed. Such a 'thrifty' gene would therefore have a selective survival advantage and would tend to increase in frequency. However, in the modern Western world, with its continuous abundance of calories, such a gene would lead to diabetes and obesity. Neel's hypothesis has received support by observations in both man and animals. The extremely high frequency of diabetes and obesity in populations such as the Pima Indians (Knowler et al 1981) and Pacific Islanders (Zimmet 1979), and its apparent increase with modernization and urbanization, are entirely consistent with the thrifty genotype hypothesis. Direct support comes from studies which have shown that heterozygotes for rodent diabetes-obesity genes exhibit a much better ability to survive fasting than normal rodents (Coleman 1979).

What might be the selective advantage of the genes that predispose to IDDM? Since IDDM is a disorder in which autoimmunity and immune response genes seem implicated, a possible role in the resistance to infectious agents has been proposed. However, one should realize that the problem of the selective advantage of IDDM is much greater than for NIDDM. Before the onset of insulin therapy, IDDM usually conferred zero fitness through failure to reproduce. This occurred both because of its severity, and because its onset was usually at such an age that reproduction would have been prevented altogether, or at least severely impaired. Also, since the susceptibility seems to be provided even by single HLA-linked susceptibility genes, negative selection should be much greater than for recessive disorders such as sickle-cell anaemia or Tay-Sachs disease, where selection operates only on those homozygous for the disease genes.

Table 89.9 Congenital malformations in infants of diabetic mothers

Anomaly	Ratio of incidences*
Caudal regression	252
Spina bifida, hydrocephalus, and other CNS defects	2
Anencephaly	3
Heart anomalies	4
Transposition of great vessels	
Ventricular septal defect	
Atrial septal defect	
Anal/rectal atresia	3
Renal anomalies	5
Agenesis	6
Cystic kidney	4
Ureter duplex	23
Situs inversus	84

* In diabetic versus nondiabetic pregnancies.
 Adapted from Mills et al 1979.

Thus, one would suppose the positive selective advantage would of necessity be dramatic. The positive selection should have continued into modern human history. Otherwise, the incidence of the disorder would have been decreasing dramatically prior to the advent of insulin therapy. Yet no such positive selective advantage has been discerned, at least postnatally.

Evidence has now accumulated that suggests a potential selective advantage mechanism for IDDM and at the same time provides at least a partial explanation for the recently recognised fact that the risk for IDDM appears to be higher to offspring of males with IDDM than to offspring of females with IDDM (at least in the first 20 years of life) (Degnbol & Green 1978, Kobberling & Bruggeboes 1980, Warram et al 1984), through the preferential transmission of diabetogenic HLA haplotypes, not only to affected offspring but to unaffected offspring as well (Vadheim et al 1986, Thivolet et al 1988). While this occurs for both high-risk (DR3 or DR4) diabetic alleles/haplotypes in fathers, it has been reported to occur for only DR3-associated haplotypes in mothers, providing an explanation for the increased paternal risk effect. Furthermore, the available evidence suggests that this possibly occurs via in-utero selection. These data thus provide an explanation for the maintenance of the high population frequency of this disease. In addition, the suggestion that prenatal selection could occur via immunologically mediated events raises the theoretical possibility that an additional consequence of these events, in fetuses that survive, might be immune changes that presage the eventual development of IDDM.

Given these recent advances in our knowledge of the genetics and heterogeneity of the diabetic syndrome, what genetic counselling can we provide for our diabetic patients at this time? First, as in all genetic counselling, an accurate diagnosis must be made. On clinical grounds one can distinguish between juvenile insulin dependent type diabetes, maturity-onset non-insulin dependent type diabetes, and maturity-onset diabetes of the young. In being able to distinguish between these phenotypes, one already has important counselling information. As discussed above, in a given family the increased risk for diabetes over the general population is only for the specific type of diabetes that has already occurred in the family, not for all diabetes. Thus, if the proband presenting for counselling is a juvenile insulin-dependent diabetic, the increased risk for that patient's relatives is for insulin dependent diabetes. If the proband is a non-insulin-dependent diabetic, the increased risk for the patient's relatives is, for the most part, for non-insulin dependent diabetes only. Associated abnormalities or diseases may suggest the rare genetic syndromes that include diabetes – each of which has its own risk of recurrence (see Table 89.3).

Once we have accurately characterized the clinical phenotype of the patient, how do we then proceed? At this stage, we must fall back on empiric recurrence risks derived from a large number of families. Even these empiric recurrence risks have limitations, since for the most part they have been reported only from Caucasian populations. The most reassuring aspect of the data is the overall low absolute risk for the development of clinical diabetes in first-degree relatives, especially for insulin dependent diabetes.

The heterogeneity that has so far been discovered among typical diabetes mellitus probably only represents the tip of the iceberg. But even this currently demonstrable heterogeneity has immediate relevance to current research efforts into the pathogenesis and therapy of the diabetic state. The susceptibility to a given environmental agent may very well depend on the heterogeneity elucidated by these studies. The long-standing debate on the efficacy of tight versus loose control in preventing vascular complications might very well be answered when this heterogeneity is taken into account in appropriately designed studies – i.e. there may be forms of diabetes where control is vital, and others where it is less so, subgroups with inexorable complications, and others which are complication-free (Barbosa 1980, Rimoin & Rotter 1981).

Delineation of genetic heterogeneity and the search for genetic markers should have profound implications not only for understanding the genetics and aetiology of diabetes, but also for its vascular complications. Only when each of the many disorders resulting in diabetes mellitus and/or glucose intolerance are delineated will specific prognostication and therapy be possible for all diabetic patients.

ACKNOWLEDGEMENT

This work was supported in part by a grant from the Stuart Foundation.

REFERENCES

Abu-Bakare A, Taylor R, Gill G V, Alberti K G M M 1986 Tropical or malnutrition-related diabetes — a real syndrome? Lancet i: 1135–1138

Agner E, Thorsteinsson B, Eriksen M 1982 Impaired glucose tolerance and diabetes mellitus in the elderly. Diabetes Care 5: 600–604

Ahuja M M 1985 Heterogeneity in tropical diabetes mellitus. Diabetologia 28: 708

Anderson C E, Hodge S E, Rubin R, Rotter J L, Terasaki P I, Irvine W J, Rimoin D L 1983 A search for heterogeneity in insulin-dependent diabetes mellitus (IDDM): HLA and autoimmune studies in simplex, multiplex, and multigenerational families. Metabolism 32: 471–477

Andreone T, Fajans S, Rotwein P, Skolnick M, Permutt M A 1985 Insulin gene analysis in a family with maturity-onset diabetes of the young. Diabetes 34: 108–114

Arnaiz-Villena A, Castellanos R B, Oliver J A, Blanco M A 1983 HLA and maturity onset diabetes of the young. Diabetologia 24: 460

Atkinson M A, Maclaren N K, Riley W J, Winter W E, Fisk D D, Spillar R P 1986 Are insulin autoantibodies markers for insulin-dependent diabetes mellitus? Diabetes 35: 894–898

Awata T, Iwamoto Y, Matsuda I A, Kuzuya T 1988 Identification of nucleotide substitution in gene encoding (Leu^{A3}) insulin in third Japanese family. Diabetes 37: 1068

Banatvala J E, Bryant J, Schernthaner G et al 1985 Coxsackie B, mumps, rubella and cytomegalovirus-specific IgM responses in patients with juvenile-onset, insulin-dependent diabetes mellitus in Britain, Austria and Australia. Lancet 1: 1409–1412

Barbosa J 1980 Nature and nurture: the genetics of diabetic microangiopathy. In: Podolsky S, Viswanathan M (eds) Secondary diabetes, the spectrum of the diabetic syndromes. Raven Press, New York, p 67–74

Barbosa J 1983 No linkage between HLA and maturity-onset hyperglycemia in the young. Diabetologia 24: 137 (1-page ref.)

Barbosa J, Chern M M, Noreen H, Anderson V E 1978a Analysis of linkage between the major histocompatibility system and juvenile insulin dependent diabetes in multiplex families: reanalysis of data. Journal of Clinical Investigation 62: 492–495

Barbosa J, King R, Goetz F C, Noreen H, Yunis E J 1978b HLA in maturity-onset type of hyperglycemia in the young. Archives of Internal Medicine 138: 90–93

Barbosa J, Chern M M, Anderson V E et al 1980a Linkage analysis between the major histocompatability system and insulin-dependent diabetes in families with patients in two consecutive generations. Journal of Clinical Investigation 65: 592–601

Barbosa J, Cohen R A, Chavers B et al 1980b Muscle extracellular membrane immunofluorescence and HLA as possible markers of prediabetes. Lancet ii: 330–333

Barbosa J, Rich S S, Dunsworth T, Swanson J 1982 Linkage disequilibrium between insulin-dependent diabetes and the Kidd blood group Jkb allele. Journal of Clinical Endocrinology and Metabolism 55: 193–195

Barnett A H, Eff C, Leslie R D G, Pyke D A 1981a Diabetes in identical twins: a study of 200 pairs. Diabetologia 20: 87–93

Barnett A H, Spiliopoulos A J, Pyke D A, Stubbs W A, Burrin J, Alberti K G M M 1981b Metabolic studies in unaffected co-twins of non-insulin dependent diabetes. British Medical Journal ii: 1656–1658

Bartels E D 1953 Endocrine disorders. In: Sorsby A (ed) Clinical genetics, 2nd edn. Mosby, St Louis

Bauer M G 1986 Genetic analysis work IV: insulin-dependent diabetes mellitus summary. Genetic Epidemiology 3 (supplement 1): 299

Bell G I, Horita S, Karam J H 1984 A polymorphic locus near the human insulin gene is associated with insulin-dependent diabetes mellitus. Diabetes 33: 176

Bell J I, Wainscoat J S, Old J M, Chlouverakis C, Keen H,

Turner R C, Weatherall D J 1983 Maturity-onset diabetes of the young is not linked to the insulin gene. British Journal of Medicine 286: 590–592

Bennett P H 1979 Recommendations on the standardization of methods and reporting of tests for diabetes and its microvascular complications in epidemiologic studies. Diabetes Care 2: 98–104

Bertrams J 1982 Non HLA markers for type I diabetes on chromosome 6. In: Kobberling J, Tattersall R (eds) Genetics of diabetes mellitus. Academic Press, London p 91–98

Betterle C, Zanette F, Pedini B, Presotto F, Rapp L B, Monsciotti C M, Rigon F 1984 Clinical and subclinical organ-specific autoimmune manifestations in type 1 (insulin-dependent) diabetic patients and their first-degree relatives. Diabetologia 26: 431–436

Bohme J, Carlsson B, Wallin J, Moller E, Persson B, Peterson P A, Rask L 1986 Only one DQ-beta restriction fragment pattern of each DR specificity is associated with insulin-dependent diabetes. Journal of Immunology 137: 941–947

Bosi E, Todd I, Pujol-Borrell R, Bottazzo G F 1987 Mechanisms of autoimmunity: Relevance to the pathogenesis of Type I (insulin-dependent) diabetes mellitus. Diabetes/Metabolism Reviews 3(4): 893–924

Bottazzo G F, Doniach D 1976 Pancreatic autoimmunity and HLA antigens. Lancet ii: 800

Bottazzo G F, Florin-Christensen A, Doniach D 1974 Islet-cell antibodies in diabetes mellitus with autoimmune polyendocrine deficiences. Lancet ii: 1279–1282

Bottazzo G F, Mann J I, Thorogood M, Baum J D, Doniach D 1978 Autoimmunity in juvenile diabetics and their families. British Medical Journal ii: 165–168

Bottazzo G F, Mirakian R, Dean B M, McNally J M, Doniach D 1982 How immunology helps to define heterogeneity in diabetes mellitus. In: Kobberling J, Tattersall R (eds) Genetics of diabetes mellitus. Academic Press, London p 79–90

Boucher D W, Notkins A L 1973 Virus-induced diabetes mellitus. I. Hyperglycemia and hypoinsulinemia in mice infected with encephalomyocarditis virus. Journal of Experimental Medicine 137: 1226–1239

Braunsteiner H, Hansen W, Jung A, Sailer S 1966 Latent diabetes in parents of juvenile diabetics. German Medical Monthly 11: 227–232

Burkeholder J N, Pickens J M, Womack W N 1967 Oral glucose tolerance test in siblings of children with diabetes mellitus. Diabetes 16: 156–160

Cahill C F Jr. 1979a Diabetes mellitus In: Beeson P B, McDermott W, Wyngaarden J B (eds) Cecil textbook of medicine. Saunders, Philadelphia, p 1969–1989

Cahill C F Jr. 1979b Current concepts of diabetic complications with emphasis on hereditary factors: a brief review. In: Sing C F, Skolnick M H (eds) Genetic analysis of common diseases: Applications to predictive factors in coronary heart disease. Liss, New York p 113–129

Cahill G F Jr., McDevitt H O 1981 Insulin-dependent diabetes mellitus: The initial lesion. New England Journal of Medicine 304: 1454–1464

Cammidge P J 1928 Diabetes mellitus and heredity. British Journal of Medicine ii: 738–741

Cammidge P J 1934 Heredity as a factor in the aetiology of diabetes mellitus. Lancet i: 393–395

Cerasi F, Luft R 1967 Insulin response to glucose infusion in diabetic and nondiabetic monozygotic twin pairs – genetic control of insulin response? Acta Endocrinologia 55: 330

Champsaur H F, Bottazzo G F, Bertrams J, Assan R, Bach C 1982 Virologic, immunologic, and genetic factors in insulin-dependent diabetes mellitus. Journal of Pediatrics 100: 15–20

Chern M M, Anderson V E, Barbosa J 1982 Empirical risk for insulin-dependent diabetes (IDD) in sibs. Further definition of genetic heterogeneity. Diabetes 31: 1115–1118

Christy M, Green A, Christau B et al 1979 Studies of the HLA system and insulin-dependent diabetes mellitus. Diabetes Care 2: 209–214

Clerget-Darpoux F 1982 Bias of the estimated recombination fraction and lod score due to an association between a disease gene and a marker gene. Annals of Human Genetics 46: 363–372

Clerget-Darpoux F, Babron M C, Prum B, Lathrop G M, Deschamps I, Hors J 1988 A new method to test genetic models in HLA-associated diseases: the MASC method. Annals of Human Genetics 52: 247–258

Cohen A M 1961 Prevalence of diabetes among different ethnic Jewish groups in Israel. Metabolism 10: 50–58

Coleman D L 1979 Obesity genes: beneficial effects in heterozygous mice. Science 203: 663–644

Coleman D L 1982 The genetics of diabetes in rodents. In: Kobberling J, Tattersall R (eds) Genetics of diabetes mellitus. Academic Press, London p 183–193

Colle E, Guttmann R D, Seemayer T 1981 Spontaneous diabetes mellitus syndrome in the rat. I. Association with the major histocompatibility complex. Journal of Experimental Medicine 154: 1237

Colle E, Guttmann R D, Seemayer T A, Michel F 1983 Spontaneous diabetes mellitus syndrome in the rat. IV. Immunogenetic interactions of MHC and non-MHC components of the syndrome. Metabolism 32 (suppl. 1): 54–61

Conn J W, Fajans S S 1961 The prediabetic state. American Journal of Medicine 31: 839–850

Contu L, Deschamps I, Lestradet H et al 1982 HLA haplotype data for risk assessment and estimation of genetic contribution of the HLA genes to IDDM. Diabetes 32: 275a

Craighead J E 1978 Current views on the etiology of insulin-dependent diabetes mellitus. New England Journal of Medicine 299: 1439–1445

Craighead J E 1981 Viral diabetes mellitus in man and experimental animals. American Journal of Medicine 70: 127–133

Craighead J E, Higgins D A 1974 Genetic influences affecting the occurrence of a diabetes mellitus-like disease in mice infected with the encephalomyocarditis virus. Journal of Experimental Medicine 139: 414–426

Creutzfeldt W, Kobbering J, Neel J V (eds) 1976 The genetics of diabetes mellitus. Springer-Verlag, Berlin

Cudworth A G 1978 Type I diabetes mellitus. Diabetologia 14: 281–291

Cudworth A G, Woodrow J C 1975 Evidence for HLA linked genes in juvenile diabetes mellitus. British Medical Journal ii: 133–135

Curie-Cohen M 1981 HLA antigens and susceptibility to juvenile diabetes: Do additive relative risks imply genetic heterogeneity? Tissue Antigens 17: 136–148

Darlow J M, Smith C 1973 A statistical and genetical study of diabetes III. Empiric risks to relatives. Annals of Human Genetics 37: 157–174

Degnbol B, Green A 1978 Diabetes mellitus among first and second-degree relatives of early onset diabetics. Annals of Human Genetics 42: 25–34

DePrins F, Van Assche F A, Desmyter J 1978 Congenital rubella and diabetes mellitus. Lancet 1: 439

Deschamps I, Lestradet H, Demenais F, Feingold N, Schmid M, Hors J 1983 A linkage study of HLA and maturity-onset type diabetes of the young (MODY). Tissue Antigens 21: 391–396

Diabetes Epidemiology Research International Group 1988 Geographic patterns of childhood insulin and dependent diabetes mellitus. Diabetes 37: 1113–1119

Dunsworth T S, Rich S S, Morton N E, Barbosa J 1982 Heterogeneity of insulin-dependent diabetes — new evidence. Clinical Genetics 21: 233–236

Eisenbarth G 1986 Type I diabetes mellitus: a chronic autoimmune disease. New England Journal of Medicine 314: 1360

Eisenbarth G S 1987 Genes, generator of diversity, glycoconjugates, and autoimmune B-cell insufficiency in Type I diabetes. Diabetes 36: 355

Eisenbarth S, Wilson P, Ward F, Lebovitz H E 1978 HLA type and occurrence of disease in familial polyglandular failure. New England Journal of Medicine 298: 92–94

Elbein S C, Gruppuso P, Schwartz R, Skolnick M, Permutt, M A 1985 Hyperproinsulinemia in a family with proposed defect in conversion is linked to the insulin gene. Diabetes 34: 821–824

Elbein S C, Borecki I, Corsetti L et al 1987 Linkage analysis of the human insulin receptor gene and maturity-onset diabetes of the young. Diabetologia 30: 641–647

Fajans S S 1976 The natural history of idiopathic diabetes mellitus. Heterogeneity in insulin responses in latent diabetes. In: Creutzfeldt W, Kobberling J, Neel J V (eds) The genetics of diabetes mellitus. Springer Verlag, Berlin p 64–78

Fajans S S 1981 Etiologic aspects of types of diabetes. Diabetes Care 4: 69

Fajans S S 1982 Heterogeneity between various families with noninsulin-dependent diabetes of the MODY type. In: Kobberling J, Tattersall R (eds) Genetics of diabetes mellitus. Academic Press, London, p 251–260

Fajans S S, Cloutier M C, Crowther R L 1978 Clinical and etiologic heterogeneity of idiopathic diabetes mellitus. Diabetes 27: 1112–1125

Festenstein H, Awad J, Hitman G A et al 1986 New HLA DNA polymorphisms associated with autoimmune diseases. Nature 322: 64–67

Fialkow P J, Zavala C, Nielsen R 1975 Thyroid autoimmunity: increased frequency in relatives of insulin dependent diabetes patients. Annals of Internal Medicine 83: 170–176

Field L L 1988 Insulin-dependent diabetes mellitus: a model for the study of multifactorial disorders (invited editorial). American Journal of Human Genetics 43: 793–798

Field L L, Anderson C E, Neiswanger K, Hodge S E, Spence M A, Rotter J I 1984 Interaction of HLA and immunoglobulin antigens in Type I (insulin-dependent) diabetes. Diabetologia 27: 504–508

Field L L, Dozier M H, Anderson C E, Spence M A, Rotter J I 1986 HLA-dependent Gm effects in insulin-dependent diabetes — evidence from affected pairs of siblings. American Journal of Human Genetics 39: 640–647

Fishbein H A, Faich G A, Ellis S E 1982 Incidence and hospitalization patterns of insulin-dependent diabetes mellitus. Diabetes Care 5: 630–633

Flier J S, Kahn C R, Roth J 1979 Receptors, antireceptor antibodies and mechanisms of insulin resistance. New England Journal of Medicine 300: 413–419

Freinkel N, Metzger B E 1985 Gestational diabetes: problems in classification and implications for long-range prognosis. In: Vranic M, Hollenberg C H, Steiner G (eds) Comparison of Type I and II diabetes: similarities and dissimilarities in etiology, pathogenesis and complications. Plenum, New York

Freinkel N, Metzger B E, Phelps R L, Dooley S L, Ogata E S, Radvany R M, Belton A 1985 Gestational diabetes mellitus: Heterogeneity of maternal age, weight, insulin secretion, HLA antigens, and islet cell antibodies and the impact of maternal metabolism on pancreatic b-cell and somatic development in the offspring. Diabetes 34(suppl.2): 1–7

Friedman J M, Fialkow P J 1980 The genetics of diabetes mellitus In: Steinberg A G, Bearn A G, Motulsky A G, Childs B (eds) Progress in medical genetics vol. IV. Saunders, Philadelphia, p 199–232

Gabbe S G, Mestman J H, Freeman R K et al 1977 Management and outcome of pregnancy in diabetes mellitus, Classes B to R. American Journal of Obstetrics and Gynecology 129: 723–729

Gamble D R 1980a An epidemiological study of childhood diabetes affecting two or more siblings. Diabetologia 19: 341–344

Gamble D R 1980b The epidemiology of insulin-dependent diabetes, with particular reference to the relationship of viral infections to its etiology. Epidemiologic Reviews 2: 49

Gamble D R, Kinsley M L, Fitzgerald M G, Bolton R, Taylor K W 1969 Viral antibodies in diabetes mellitus. British Medical Journal 3: 627

Gelenter T, Dilworth V, Valka B, McDonald R, Schorry E 1981 Insulin binding and insulin action in fibroblasts from patients with maturity-onset diabetes of the young. Diabetes 30: 940

Given B D, Mako M E, Tager H S et al 1980 Diabetes due to secretion of an abnormal insulin. New England Journal of Medicine 302: 129–135

Gorsuch A N, Dean B M, Bottazzo G F, Lister J, Cudworth A G 1980 Evidence that type I diabetes and thyrogastric autoimmunity have different genetic determinants. British Medical Journal i: 145–147

Gorsuch A N, Spencer K M, Lister J 1981 Evidence for a long pre-diabetic period in Type I (insulin-dependent) diabetes mellitus. Lancet 2: 1363–1365

Gottlieb M S 1980 Diabetes in offspring and siblings of juvenile and maturity-onset type diabetes. Journal of Chronic Diseases 33: 331–339

Gottlieb M S, Root H F 1968 Diabetes mellitus in twins. Diabetes 17: 693–704

Gould C L, Trombley M L, Bigley N J, McMannama K G, Giron D J 1984 Replication of diabetogenic and non-diabetogenic variants of encephalomyocarditis (EMC) virus in ICR Swiss mice (41819). Proceedings of the Society for Experimental Biology and Medicine 175: 449–453

Gould C L, McMannama K G, Bigley N J K, Giron D J 1985 Virus-induced murine diabetes: Enhancement by immunosuppression. Diabetes 34(12): 1217–1221

Green A, Morton N E, Iselius L, Svejgaard A, Platz P, Ryder L P, Hauge M 1982 Genetic studies of insulin-dependent diabetes: segregation and linkage analysis. Tissue Antigens 19: 213–221

Gruppuso P A, Gorden P, Kahn C R, Cornblath M, Zeller W P, Schwartz R 1984 Familial hyperproinsulinemia due to a proposed defect in conversion of proinsulin to insulin. New England Journal of Medicine 311: 629–634

Gunderson E 1927 Is diabetes of infectious origin? Journal of Infectious Diseases 41: 197–202

Gyves M T, Rodman H, Little A B, Fanaroff A A, Merkatz I R 1977 A modern approach to management of pregnant diabetics: two-year analysis of perinatal outcome. American Journal of Obstetrics and Gynecology 128: 606

Haffner S M, Rosenthal M, Hazuda H P, Stern M P, Franco L J 1984 Evaluation of three potential screening tests for diabetes mellitus in a biethnic population. Diabetes Care 7: 247–353

Haneda M, Polonsky K S, Bergenstil R M et al 1984 Familial hyperinsulinemia due to a structural abnormal insulin, definition of an emerging new clinical syndrome. New England Journal of Medicine 310: 1288–1294

Hanhart E 1951 Zur Vererbung des diabetes mellitus. Schweizerische Medizinische Wochenschrift 81: 1127–1131

Harris H 1949 The incidence of parental consanguinity in diabetes mellitus. Annals of Eugenics 14: 293–300

Harris H 1950 The familial distribution of diabetes mellitus: a study of the relatives of 1241 diabetic propositi. Annals of Eugenics 15: 95–110

Harris M I, Hadden W C, Knowler W C, Bennett P H 1985 International criteria for the diagnosis of diabetes and impaired glucose tolerance. Diabetes Care 8: 562

Harvald B, Hauge M 1963 Selection in diabetes in modern society. Acta Medica Scandinavica 173: 459–465

Harvald B, Hauge M 1965 Heredity factors elucidated by twin studies. In: Neel J V, Shaw M W, Schull W J (eds) Genetics and the epidemiology of chronic diseases. Public Health Service Publication No. 1163, p 61–76

Hayashi K, Boucher D W, Notkins A L 1974 Virus-induced diabetes mellitus. II. Relationship between beta cell damage and hyperglycemia in mice infected with the encephalomyocarditis virus. American Journal of Pathology 75: 91–102

Helmke K, Otten A, Willems W R et al 1986 Islet cell antibodies and the development of diabetes mellitus in relation to mumps infection and mumps vaccination. Diabetologia 29: 30–33

Herman W H, Sinnock P, Brenner E et al 1984 An epidemiologic model for diabetes mellitus: Incidence, prevalence and mortality. Diabetes 7: 367–371

Hodge S E, Spence M A 1981 Some epistatic two-locus models of disease II: The confounding of linkage and association. American Journal of Human Genetics 33: 396–406

Hodge S E, Rotter J I, Lange K L 1980 A three-allele model for heterogeneity of juvenile onset dependent diabetes. Annals of Human Genetics 43: 399–412

Hodge S E, Anderson C E, Neiswanger K et al 1981 Close linkage between IDDM and the Kidd blood group. Lancet ii: 893–895

Huang S W, Taylor G, Basid A 1984 The effect of pertussis vaccine on the insulin-dependent diabetes induced by streptozotocin in mice. Pediatric Research 18(2): 221–226

Huber S A, Babu G, Craighead J E 1985 Genetic influences on the immunologic pathogenesis of encephalomyocarditis (EMC) virus-induced diabetes mellitus. Diabetes 34: 1186–1190

Hunter S, McKay E 1967 Intravenous glucose tolerance test in parents of diabetic children. Lancet i: 1017–1019

Ilonen J, Herva E, Tiilikainen A, Akerblom H K, Koivukangas T, Kouvalainen K 1978 HLA-Dw2 as a marker of resistance against juvenile diabetes mellitus. Tissue Antigens 11: 144–146

Irvine W J 1977 Classification of idiopathic diabetes. Lancet i: 638–642

Irvine W J, Toft A D, Holton D E, Prescott R J, Clar B F, Duncan L J P 1977a Familial studies of Type I and Type II idiopathic diabetes mellitus. Lancet ii: 325–328

Irvine W J, Gray R S, McCallus C J, Duncan L J P 1977b Clinical and pathogenic significance of pancreatic islet cell antibodies in diabetics treated with oral hypoglycemic agents. Lancet i: 1025–1027

Irvine W J, Mario U D, Feek C M, Gray R S, Ting A, Morris P J, Duncan L J P 1978a Autoimmunity and HLA antigens in insulin-dependent (type I) diabetes. Journal of Clinical and Laboratory Immunology 1: 107–110

Irvine W J, Mario U D, Feek C M, Ting A, Morris P J, Gray R S, Duncan L P J 1978b Insulin antibodies in relation to islet cell antibodies and HLA antigens in insulin-dependent (type I) diabetes. Journal of Clinical and Laboratory Immunology 1: 111–114

Irvine W J, Sawen J S A, Prescott R J, Duncan L J P 1979 The value of islet cell antibody in predicting secondary failure of oral hypoglycemic agent therapy in diabetes mellitus. Journal of Clinical and Laboratory Immunology 2: 23–26

Iwo K, Bellomo S C, Mukai N, Craighead J E 1983 Encephalomyocarditis virus-induced diabetes mellitus in mice: long-term changes in the structure and function of islets of Langerhans. Diabetologia 25: 39–44

Jackson R 1988 Animal models of diabetes. In: Farid N R (ed) Immunogenetics of endocrine disorders. Liss, New York, p 89–110

Jackson R A, Buse J B, Rifai R et al 1984 Two genes required for diabetes in BB rats. Evidence from cyclical intercrosses and backcrosses. Journal of Experimental Medicine 159: 1629–1636

Jakobson T, Nikkila E A 1969 Serum lipid levels and response of plasma insulin to the oral administration of glucose in first-degree relatives of diabetic patients. Diabetologia 5: 427

Jenson A B, Rosenberg H S, Notkins A L 1980 Virus-induced diabetes mellitus. Pancreatic islet cell damage in children with fatal virus infections. Lancet i: 892

Jialal I, Joubert S M 1984 Obesity does not modulate insulin secretion in Indian parents with non-insulin dependent diabetes in the young. Diabetes Care 7: 404

Johansen K, Gregersen G 1977 A family with dominantly inherited mild juvenile diabetes. Acta Medica Scandinavica 201: 567–570

Johnston C, Pyke D A, Cudworth A G, Wolf E 1983 HLA-DR typing in identical twins with insulin-dependent diabetes: a difference between concordant and discordant pairs. British Medical Journal 286: 253

Johnston C, Owerbach D, Leslie R D G, Pyke D A, Nerup J 1984 Mason type diabetes and DNA insertion polymorphism. Lancet i: 280

Jordan G W, Cohen S H 1987 Encephalomyocarditis virus-induced diabetes mellitus in mice: model of viral pathogenesis. Reviews of Infectious Diseases 9: 917–924

Joslin E P, Root F H, White P, Marble A 1959 In: The treatment of diabetes mellitus, 10th edn. Lea & Febiger, Philadelphia p 47–98

Kadowaki T, Bevins E, Cama A et al 1988 Two mutant alleles of the insulin receptor gene in a patient with extreme insulin resistance. Science 240: 787

Kahn C R, Goldstein B J 1989 Molecular defects in insulin action. Science 245: 13

Karam J H, Lewitt P A, Young C W et al 1980 Insulinopenic diabetes after rodenticide (Vacor) ingestion. Diabetes 29: 971–978

Karjalainen J, Knip M, Mustonen A, Illonen J, Akerblom H K 1986 Relation between insulin antibody and complement-fixing islet cell antibody at clinical diagnosis of IDDM. Diabetes 35: 620–622

Karlsson K, Kjellmer I 1972 The outcome of diabetic pregnancies in relation to the mother's blood sugar level. American Journal of Obstetrics and Gynecology 112: 213

Keen H, Track N S 1968 Age of onset and inheritance of diabetes: the importance of examining relatives. Diabetologia 4: 317–321

Keen H, Jarrett R J, Alberti K G M 1979 Diabetes mellitus: a new look at diagnostic criteria. Diabetologia 16: 283–285

Kilvert A, Fitzgerald M G, Wright A D, Nattrass M 1986 Clinical characteristics and etiological classification of insulin-dependent diabetes in the elderly. Quarterly Journal of Medicine 60: 865

King M L, Bidwell D, Voller A, Bryant J, Banatvala J E 1983a Coxsackie B viruses in insulin-dependent diabetes mellitus. Lancet 2: 915–916

King M L, Shaikh A, Bidwell D, Voller A, Banatvala J E 1983b Coxsackie B virus-specific IgM responses in children with insulin-dependent (juvenile-onset; Type I) diabetes mellitus. Lancet 1: 1397–1399

Knip M, Illonen J, Mustonen A, Akerblom H K 1986 Evidence of an accelerated b-cell destruction in HLA-Dw3/Dw4 heterozygous children with Type 1 (insulin-dependent) diabetes. Diabetologia 29: 347–351

Knowler W C, Pettitt D J, Savage P J, Bennett P H 1981 Diabetes incidence in Pima Indians: Contributions of obesity and parental diabetes. American Journal of Epidemiology 113: 144–156

Kobberling J 1969 Untersuchungen zur Genetik des Diabetes Mellitus. Eine Geeignete Methode zur Durchfuhrung von Alterskorrekturen. Diabetologia 5: 392–396

Kobberling J 1971 Studies on the genetic heterogeneity of diabetes mellitus. Diabetologia 7: 46–49

Kobberling J 1976a Genetic heterogeneities within idiopathic diabetes. In: Creutzfeldt W, Kobberling J H, Neel J V (eds) The genetics of diabetes mellitus. Springer-Verlag, Berlin, p 79–87

Kobberling J 1976b Genetic syndromes associated with lipatrophic diabetes. In: Creutzfeldt W, Kobberling J, Neel

J V (eds) The genetic of diabetes mellitus. Springer-Verlag, Berlin, p 147–154

Kobberling J, Bruggeboes B 1980 Prevalence of diabetes among children of insulin-dependent diabetic mothers. Diabetologia 18: 459–462

Kobberling J, Tattersall R 1982 The genetics of diabetes mellitus. Proceedings of the Serono Symposia (vol. 47), Academic Press, London

Kobberling J, Appels A, Kobberling G, Creutzfeldt W 1969 Glucose tolerance test: 727 first-degree relatives of maturity-onset diabetics. German Medical Monthly 14: 290–294

Kobberling J, Bengsch N, Bruggeboes B, Schwarch H, Tillil H, Weber M 1980 The chlorpropamide alcohol flush — Lack of specificity for familial non-insulin dependent diabetes. Diabetologia 19: 359–363

Koevary S B, Williams D E, Williams R M, Chick W L 1983 Passive transfer of diabetes from BB/W to Wistar-Furth rats. Journal of Clinical Investigation 75: 1904–1907

Kwok S C M, Steiner D F, Rubenstein A H, Tager H S 1983 Identification of a point mutation in the human insulin gene giving rise to a structurally abnormal insulin (Insulin Chicago). Diabetes 32: 872–875

Laakso M, Pyorala K 1985 Age of onset and type of diabetes. Diabetes Care 8: 114–117

Lambert T H, Johnson R B, Geoffrey P R 1961 Glucose and cortisone-glucose tolerance in normal and prediabetic humans. Annals of Internal Medicine 54: 916

LaPorte R E, Cruikshanks K J 1985 Incidence and risk factors for insulin-dependent diabetes. In: Diabetes in America, National Diabetes Data Group, U.S. Department of Health and Human Services. NIH Publication No. 85-1468, p III.1–12

Leiter E H, Coleman D L, Hummel K P 1981a The influence of genetic background on the expression of mutations at the diabetes locus in the mouse. III. Effect of H-2 haplotype and sex. Diabetes 30: 1029–1034

Leiter E H, Coleman D L, Eisenstein A B, Strack I 1981b Dietary control of pathogenesis in C57BL/KsJ db/db mice. Metabolism 30: 544–562

Leiter E H, Coleman D L, Ingram D K, Reynolds M A 1983 Influence of dietary carbohydrate on the induction of diabetes in C57BL/KsJ-db/db diabetes mice. Journal of Nutrition; 113: 184–195

Leiter E H, Prochazka M, Coleman D L, Serreze D V, Schultz L D 1986 Genetic factors predisposing to diabetes susceptibility in mice. In: Jaworsky M A, Molnar G D, Rojolfe R V, Singh B (eds) The immunology of diabetes mellitus. Elsevier, Amsterdam, p 29–36

Lestradet H, Battistelli J, Ledoux M 1972 L'heredite dans le diabete infantile. Le Diabete 2: 17–21

Levit S G, Pessikova L N 1934 The genetics of diabetes mellitus. Proc Maxim Gorky Medico Biol Institute 3: 132

Lillioja S, Mott D M, Zawadzki J K et al 1987 In vivo insulin action is familial characteristic in non-diabetic Pima Indians. Diabetes 35: 1329–1335

Louis E J, Thomson G 1986 Three-allele synergistic mixed model for insulin-dependent diabetes mellitus. Diabetes 35: 958

Ludvigsson J, Lindblom B 1984 Human lymphocyte antigen DR types in relation to early clinical manifestations in diabetic children. Pediatric Research 18(12): 1239

Ludvigsson J, Safwenberg K, Heding L G 1977 HLA-types, C-peptide and insulin antibodies in juvenile diabetes. Diabetologia 13: 13

Ludvigsson J, Samuelsson U, Beauforts C 1986 HLA-DR 3 is associated with a more slowly progressive form of Type 1 (insulin-dependent) diabetes. Diabetologia 29: 207

Ludwig H, Schernthaner G, Mayr W R 1976 Is HLA-B7 a marker associated with a protective gene in juvenile-onset diabetes mellitus? New England Journal of Medicine 294: 1066

McCrae W M 1963 Diabetes mellitus following mumps. Lancet 1: 1300

MacCuish A C, Barnes E E W, Irvine W J, Duncan L J P 1974 Antibodies to pancreatic islet cells in insulin-dependent diabetics with coexistent autoimmune disease. Lancet ii: 1529–1531

MacDonald M J 1974 Equal incidence of adult-onset diabetes among ancestors of juvenile diabetics and non diabetics. Diabetologia 10: 767

MacDonald M J 1980 Hypothesis: the frequencies of juvenile diabetes in American Blacks and Caucasians are consistent with dominant inheritance. Diabetes 29: 110–114

Maclaren N K 1983 personal communication

Maclaren N K 1988 How, when and why to predict IDDM. Diabetes 37: 1591

Maclaren N, Riley W, Rosenbloom E, Elder M, Spillar R, Cuddeback J 1982 The heterogeneity of Black insulin-dependent diabetes. Diabetes 31: 257a

Maclaren N, Rotter J, Riley W, Vadheim C, Winter W, Beckwith D, Henson V 1984 HLA DR phenotypes and the absolute risks of insulin-dependent diabetes. Proceedings of the American Society for Histocompatibility

Maclaren N, Riley W, Skordis N et al 1988 Inherited susceptibility to insulin-dependent diabetes is associated with HLA-DR1 (and DR3 and DR4) while DR5 (and DR2) are protective. Autoimmunity 1: 197–205

McMichael A, McDevitt H 1977 The association between the HLA system and disease. In: Steinberg A G, Motulsky A G, Child B (eds) Progress in medical genetics, vol. II. Saunders, Philadelphia, p 39–100

Massari V, Eschwege E, Valleron A J 1983 Imprecision of new criteria for the oral glucose tolerance test. Diabetologia 24: 100

Melish J S, Hanna J, Baba S (eds) 1982 Genetic environmental interactions in diabetes mellitus. Excerpta Medica, Amsterdam

Melton L J, Ochi J W, Palumbo P J, Chu C P 1983 Sources of disparity in the spectrum of diabetes mellitus at incidence and prevalence. Diabetes Care 6: 427

Metzger B E, Bybee D E, Freinkel N, Phelps R L, Radvany R M, Vaisrub N 1985 Gestational diabetes mellitus: Correlations between the phenotypic and genotypic characteristics of the mother and abnormal glucose tolerance during the first year postpartum. Diabetes 34(2): 111

Mills J L, Baker L, Goldman A S 1979 Malformations in infants of diabetic mothers occur before the seventh gestational week. Diabetes Care 28: 292–293

Millward B A, Welsh K I, Leslie R D G, Pyke D A, Demaine A G 1987 T cell receptor beta chain polymorphisms are associated with insulin-dependent diabetes. Clinical and Experimental Immunology 70: 152–157

Mimura G, Miyao S 1962 Heredity and constitutions of diabetes mellitus. Bulletin Research Institute Diabetic Medicine Kumamoto University 12: 1

Mirakian R, Bottazzo G F, Doniach D 1980 Autoantibodies to duodenal gastric-inhibitory peptide (GIP) cells and to secretin (S) cells in patients with coeliac disease, tropical sprue and maturity onset diabetes. Clinical and Experimental Immunology 41: 33–42

Miyano M, Nanjo K, Chan S J, Sanke T, Kondo M, Steiner D F 1988 Use of in vitro DNA amplification to screen family members for an insulin gene mutation. Diabetes 37: 862

Mohan V, Ramachandran A, Snehalatha C, Mohan R, Bharani G, Viswanathan M 1985a High prevalence of maturity-onset diabetes of the young (MODY) among Indians. Diabetes Care 8: 371–374

Mohan V, Snehalatha C, Ramachandran A, Jayashree R, Viswanathan M 1985b C-peptide responses to glucose load in maturity-onset diabetes of the young. Diabetes Care 8: 69

Monos D S, Spielman R S, Gogolin K J, Radka S F, Baker L, Zimjenski C M, Kamoun M 1987 HLA-DRw3.2 allele of the DR4 haplotype is associated with insulin-dependent diabetes: correlation between DQ beta restriction fragments and DQ beta chain variation. Immunogenetics 26: 299–303

Mordes J P, Desemone J, Rossini A A 1987 The BB rat. Diabetes Metabolism Reviews 3(3): 725–750

Morton N E, Lalouel J M 1981 Resolution of linkage for irregular phenotype systems. Human Heredity 31: 3–7

Morton N E, Green A, Dunsworth T et al 1983 Heterozygous expression of insulin-dependent diabetes mellitus (IDDM) determinants. American Journal of Human Genetics 35: 201

Motulsky A G 1976 The genetic hyperlipidemias. New England Journal of Medicine 294: 823

Naidoo C, Jialal I, Hammond M G, Omar M A K, Joubert S M 1986 HLA and NIDDM in the young. Diabetes Care 9: 436–438

Nakao Y, Matsumoto H, Miyazaki T et al 1981 IgG heavy chain (Gm) allotypes and immune response to insulin in insulin-requiring diabetes mellitus. New England Journal of Medicine 304: 407

Nanjo K, Miyano M, Kondo M et al 1987 Insulin Wakayama: Familial mutant insulin syndrome in Japan. Diabetologia 30: 87–92

Narendranatham M 1981 Chronic calcific pancreatitis of the tropics. Tropic Gastroenterology 2: 40–45

National Diabetes Data Group International Workgroup 1979 Classification of diabetes mellitus and other categories of glucose intolerance. Diabetes 28: 1039

Neel J V 1962 Diabetes mellitus: a "thrifty" genotype rendered detrimental by "progress"? American Journal of Human Genetics 14: 353–362

Nelson P G, Pyke D A 1976 Genetic diabetes not linked to the HLA locus. British Medical Journal i: 196

Nelson R L 1988 Oral glucose tolerance test: Indications and limitations. Mayo Clinic Proceedings 63: 263

Nepom B D, Palmer J, Kim S J, Hansen J A, Holbeck S L, Nepom G T 1986 Specific genomic markers for the HLA-DQ subregion discriminate between DR4+ insulin-

dependent diabetes mellitus and DR4+ seropositive juvenile rheumatoid arthritis. Journal of Experimental Medicine 164: 1–6

Nepom B S, Schwarz D, Palmer J P, Nepom G T 1987 Transcomplementation of HLA genes in IDDM: HLA-DQ alpha and beta-chains produce hybrid molecules in DR3/4 heterozygotes. Diabetes 36: 114–117

Nerup J, Platz P, Ortved-Anderson O et al 1974 HLA antigens and diabetes mellitus. Lancet ii: 864–866

Nerup J, Cathelineau C, Seignalet J, Thomssen M 1977 HLA and endocrine diseases. In: Dausset J, Svejgaard A (eds) HLA and disease. Munksgaard, Copenhagen, p 149–161

Neufeld M, Maclaren N K, Riley W J et al 1980 Islet cell and other organ-specific antibodies in U.S. Caucasians and Blacks with insulin-dependent diabetes mellitus. Diabetes 29: 589–592

Nissley P S, Drash A L, Blizzard R M, Sperling M, Childs B 1973 Comparison of juvenile diabetes with positive and negative organ specific antibody titres: evidence for genetic heterogeneity. Diabetes 22: 63–65

Notelovitz M 1969 Genetics and the Natal Indian diabetic. South African Medical Journal 43: 1245–1247

Omar M A K, Asmal A C 1983 Family histories of diabetes mellitus in young African and Indian diabetics. British Medical Journal 286: 1786

Onodera T, Yoon J, Brown K, Notkins A L 1978 Evidence for a single locus controlling susceptibility to virus-induced diabetes mellitus. Nature 276: 693

O'Rahilly S, Turner R C 1988 Linkage analysis of the receptor gene and MODY. Diabetologia 34: 185

O'Rahilly S P, Nugent Z, Rudenski A S, Hosker J P, Burnett M A, Darling P, Turner R C 1986 Beta-cell dysfunction, rather than insulin insensitivity, is the primary defect in familial type 2 diabetes. Lancet 2: 360–364

O'Rahilly S, Holman R R, Turner R C 1987 Maturity-onset diabetes in young Black Americans. New England Journal of Medicine 317: 381

O'Rahilly S P, Turner R C, Matthews D R 1988 Impaired pulsatile secretion of insulin in relatives of patients with non-insulin-dependent diabetes. New England Journal of Medicine 318: 1225–1230

Orchard T J, Atchison R W, Becker D et al 1983 Coxsackie infection and diabetes. Lancet 2: 631

Owerbach D, Nerup J 1981 Restriction fragment length polymorphism of the insulin gene in diabetic individuals. Diabetologia 21: 311

Owerbach D, Bell G I, Rutter W J, Brown J A, Shows T B 1981 The insulin gene is located on the short arm of chromosome 11 in humans. Diabetes 30: 267

Owerbach D, Lernmark A, Platz P, Ryder L P, Rask L, Peterson P A, Ludvigsson J 1983 HLA-DR beta chain DNA endonuclease fragments differ between healthy and insulin-dependent diabetic individuals. Nature 303: 815–817

Owerbach D, Gunn S, Ty G, Wible L, Gabbay K H 1988 Oligonucleotide probes for HLA-DQA and DQB genes define susceptibility to Type I (insulin-dependent) diabetes mellitus. Diabetologia 31: 751–757

Pak C Y, Eun H M, McArthur R G, Yoon J W 1988 Association of cytomegalovirus infection with autoimmune type 1 diabetes. Lancet ii: 1–4

Palmer J P, Cooney M K, Ward R H et al 1982 Reduced Coxsackie antibodies titres in Type 1 (insulin-dependent) diabetic patients presenting during an outbreak of Coxsackie B3 and B4 infection. Diabetologia 22: 426–429

Palmer J P, Asplin C M, Clemons P, Lyen K, Tatpati O, Raghu P K, Paquette T L 1983 Insulin antibodies in insulin-dependent diabetics before insulin treatment. Science 222: 1337–1339

Palumbo P J, Elveback L R, Chu C P, Conolly D C, Kurland L T 1976 Diabetes mellitus: incidence, prevalence, survivorship, and causes of death in Rochester, Minnesota, 1945–1970. Diabetes 25: 566–573

Panzram G, Adolph W 1981 Heterogeneity of maturity-onset diabetes at young age (MODY). Lancet ii: 986

Patterson K, Chandra R S, Jenson A B 1981 Congenital rubella, insulitis and diabetes mellitus in an infant. Lancet ii: 1048

Peig M, Ercilla G, Milian M, Gomis R 1981 Post-mumps diabetes mellitus. Lancet 1: 1007

Pickens J M 1964 The pre-diabetic state in siblings of known juvenile diabetic children. 51st Ross Conference on Pediatric Research, p 64

Pincus G, White P 1933 On the inheritance of diabetes mellitus. I. An analysis of 675 family histories. American Journal of Medical Science 186: 1

Platz P, Jakobsen B D, Morling N et al 1981 HLA-D and DR antigens in genetic analysis of insulin-dependent diabetes mellitus. Diabetologia 21: 108–115

Platz P, Jacobsen B K, Svejgaard A, Thomsen B S, Jensen J B, Henningsen K, Lamm L V 1982 No evidence for linkage between HLA and maturity-onset type of diabetes in young people. Diabetologia 23: 16–18

Polonsky K S, Given B D, Hirsch L J et al 1988 Abnormal patterns of insulin secretion in non-insulin dependent diabetes mellitus. New England Journal of Medicine 318: 1231–1239

Prochazka M, Leiter E, Serreze D V, Cokman D L 1987 Three recessive loci required for insulin dependent diabetes in monobed mice. Science 237: 280–284

Pyke D A 1978 Twin studies in diabetes. In: Nance W E, Allen G, Parisi P (eds) Twin research, Part C, Clinical Studies. Liss, New York, p 1

Pyke D A 1979 Diabetes: the genetic connections. Diabetologia 17: 333–343

Pyke D A, Nelson P G 1976 Diabetes mellitus in identical twins. In: Creutzfeldt W, Kobberling J, Neel J V (eds) The genetics of diabetes mellitus. Springer-Verlag, Berlin p 194

Pyke D A, Taylor K W 1967 Glucose tolerance and serum insulin in unaffected identical twin of diabetics. British Medical Journal ii: 21

Rabinowe S L, George K L, Loughlin R, Soeldner J S, Eisenbarth G S 1986 Congenital Rubella: Monoclonal antibody-defined T-cell abnormalities in young adults. The American Journal of Medicine 81: 779–782

Rao R H, Vigg B L, Rao K S J 1983 Suppressible glucagon secretion in young ketosis-resistant, Type J diabetic patients in India. Diabetes 32: 1168

Rayfield E J, Ishimura K 1987 Environmental factors and insulin-dependent diabetes mellitus. Diabetes/Metabolism Reviews 3(4): 925

Rayfield F J, Seto Y 1981 Etiology: viruses. In: Brownlee M (ed) Handbook of diabetes mellitus. Garland STPM

Press, vol. 1: 95–120

Reitnauer P J, Go R C P, Acton R T, Murphy C C, Budowle B, Barger B O, Roseman J M 1982 Evidence for genetic admixture as a determinant in the occurrence of insulin-dependent diabetes mellitus in U.S. Blacks. Diabetes 31: 532–537

Riccardi G, Vaccaro O, Rivellese A, Pignalosa S, Tutino L, Mancini M 1985 Reproducibility of the new diagnostic criteria for impaired glucose tolerance. American Journal of Epidemiology 121: 422–429

Rich S S, Weitkamp L R, Guttormsen S, Barbosa J 1986 Gm, Km and HLA in insulin-dependent diabetes mellitus. A log-linear analysis of association. Diabetes 35: 927–932

Riley W J, Maclaren N K, Neufeld M 1980 Adrenal autoantibodies and Addison's disease in insulin-dependent diabetes mellitus. Journal of Pediatrics 97: 191

Riley W J, Maclaren N K, Lezotte D C, Spillar R P, Rosenbloom A L 1981 Thyroid autoimmunity in insulin-dependent diabetes mellitus: the case for routine screening. Journal of Pediatrics 98: 350

Riley W J, Toskes P P, Maclaren N K, Silverstein J H 1982 Predictive value of gastric parietal cell autoantibodies as a marker for gastric and hematologic abnormalities associated with insulin-dependent diabetes. Diabetes 31: 1051

Rimoin D L 1967 Genetics of diabetes mellitus. Diabetes 16: 346–351

Rimoin D L 1969 Ethnic variability in glucose tolerance and insulin secretion. Archives of Internal Medicine 124: 695–700

Rimoin D L 1976 Genetic syndromes associated with glucose intolerance. In: Creutzfeldt W, Kobberling J, Neel J V (eds) The genetics of diabetes mellitus. Springer-Verlag, Berlin, p 43–63

Rimoin D, Rotter J I 1981 Genetic heterogeneity in diabetes mellitus and diabetic microangiopathy. Hormone and Metabolic Research, supplement ii: 63–72

Rimoin D L, Rotter J I 1982 Genetic syndromes associated with diabetes mellitus and glucose intolerance. In: Kobberling J, Tatterall R (eds) Genetics of diabetes mellitus. Academic Press, London, p 149–181

Rimoin D L, Rotter J I 1985 Progress in understanding the genetics of diabetes mellitus in genetic disorders. In: Berg K (ed) Medical genetics: past, present and future. Liss, New York, p 393

Rimoin D L, Schimke R N 1971 Endocrine pancreas. In: Genetic disorders of the endocrine glands. Mosby, St. Louis, p 150–216

Rossini A A, Slavin S, Woda B A, Geisberg M, Like A A, Mordes J P 1984 Total lymphoid irradiation prevents diabetes mellitus in the bio-breeding/Worcester (BB/W) rat. Diabetes 33: 543–547

Rotter J I 1981a The modes of inheritance of insulin-dependent diabetes. American Journal of Human Genetics 33: 835–851

Rotter J I 1981b Gastric and duodenal ulcer are each different diseases. Digestive Diseases and Sciences 26: 154

Rotter J L, Hodge S E 1980 Racial differences in diabetes are consistent with more than one mode of inheritance. Diabetes 29: 115–118

Rotter J I, Landaw E M 1984 Measuring the genetic contribution of a single locus to a multilocus disease. Clinical Genetics 26: 529–542

Rotter J I, Rimoin D L 1978 Heterogeneity in diabetes mellitus—update 1978: Evidence for further genetic heterogeneity within juvenile onset insulin-dependent diabetes mellitus. Diabetes 27: 599–608

Rotter J I, Rimoin D L 1979 Diabetes mellitus: the search for genetic markers. Diabetes Care 2: 215–226

Rotter J I, Rimoin D L 1981a Etiology genetics. In: Brownlee M (ed) Handbook of diabetes mellitus. Garland STPM Press, New York, Vol. 1: 3

Rotter J I, Rimoin D L 1981b The genetics of the glucose intolerance disorders. American Journal of Medicine 70: 116

Rotter J I, Rimoin D L 1981c The genetics of insulin-dependent diabetes. In: Martin J M, Ehrlich R M, Holland F J (eds) Etiology and pathogenesis of insulin-dependent diabetes mellitus. Raven Press, New York, p 37

Rotter J I, Rimoin D L 1983 Genetics of type I diabetes. Acta Endocrinologica 103 (Supplement 256): 26

Rotter J I, Vadheim C M 1986 Differential HLA haplotype sharing conditional on proband genotype is likely a necessary consequence of all three allele heterogeneity models: a rebuttal. Genetic Epidemiology (suppl)1: 359–362

Rotter J I, Rimoin D L, Samloff I M 1978 Genetic heterogeneity in diabetes mellitus and peptic ulcer. In: Morton N E, Chung C S (eds) Genetic epidemiology. Academic Press, New York, p 381–414

Rotter J I, Anderson C E, Rubin R, Congleton J E, Terasaki P I, Rimoin D L 1983 HLA genotype study of insulin-dependent diabetes, the excess of DR3/DR4 heterozygotes allows rejection of the recessive hypothesis. Diabetes 32: 169

Rotter J I, Vadheim C M, Raffel L J, Rimoin D L 1984 Genetics, diabetes mellitus heterogeneity, and coronary heart disease. In: Rao D C, Elston R C Kuller L H (eds) Genetic epidemiology of coronary heart disease: past, present and future. Liss, New York, p 445–470

Rotter J I, Vadheim C M, Petersen G M, Cantor R M, Riley W J, Maclaren N K 1986 HLA haplotypes sharing and proband genotype in IDDM. Genetic Epidemiology 3 (supplement 1): 327

Rotter J I, Vadheim C M, Rimoin D L 1990 Diabetes mellitus. In: King R A, Rotter, J I, Motulsky A G (eds) The genetic basis of common diseases. Oxford University Press, New York, in press

Rotwein P S, Chirgwin J, Province M et al 1983 Polymorphism in the 5'-flanking region of the human insulin gene: a genetic marker for noninsulin-dependent diabetes. New England Journal of Medicine 308: 65–71

Rubinstein P, Ginsberg-Fellner F, Falk C 1981 Genetics of Type I diabetes mellitus: a single, recessive predispositon gene mapping between HLA-B and GLO. American Journal of Human Genetics 33: 865–882

Rubinstein P, Walker M E, Fedun B, Witt M E, Cooper L Z, Ginsberg-Feliner F 1982 The HLA system in congenital rubella patients with and without diabetes. Diabetes 31: 1088

Samloff I M, Varis K, Ihamaki T, Siurala M, Rotter J I 1982 Relationships among serum pepsinogen I, serum pepsinogen II, and gastric mucosal histology, a study in relatives of patients with pernicious anemia. Gastroenterology 83: 204

Sandler M 1986 Insulin secretion and erythrocyte insulin binding in Cape coloured non-obese, non-insulin dependent diabetes in the young: effects of sulphonylurea therapy. Diabetes Research Clinical Practice 2: 9–14

Sanz N, Karam J H, Horita S, Bell G I 1986 Prevalence of insulin-gene mutations in non-insulin dependent diabetes mellitus. New England Journal of Medicine 314: 1322

Schernthaner G 1982 The relation between clinical, immunological and genetic factors in insulin-dependent diabetes mellitus. In: Kobberling J, Tattersall R B (eds) The genetics of diabetes mellitus. Academic Press, London, p 99–114

Schernthaner G, Banatvala J E, Scherbaum W, Bryant J, Borkenstein M, Schober E, Mayr W R 1985 Coxsackie B virus specific IgM responses, complement-fixing islet cell antibodies, HLA DR antigens and C-peptide secretion in insulin-dependent diabetes mellitus. Lancet 2: 630–632

Schopfer K, Matter L, Flueler U, Werder E 1982 Diabetes mellitus, endocrine auto-antibodies and prenatal rubella infection. Lancet 2: 159

Seino S, Funakoshi A, Fu Z Z, Vinik A 1985 Identification of insulin variants in patients with hyperinsulinemia by reversed-phase, high-performance liquid chromatography. Diabetes 34: 1–7

Serjeantson S W, Zimmet P 1982 Analysis of linkage relationships in maturity-onset diabetes of young people and independent segregation of C-6 and HLA. Human Genetics 62: 214

Serjeantson S W, Ryan D P, Zimmet P 1981 HLA and non-insulin dependent diabetes in Fiji Indians. Medical Journal of Australia i: 462

Shoelson S, Haneda M, Blix P et al 1983 Three mutant insulins in man. Nature 302: 540–543

Simpson N E 1962 The genetics of diabetes: a study of 233 families of juvenile diabetics. Annals of Human Genetics 26: 1

Simpson N E 1964 A multifactorial inheritance: a possible hypothesis for diabetes. Diabetes 13: 462

Simpson N E 1968 Diabetes in the families of diabetics. Canadian Medical Association Journal 98: 427

Simpson N E 1976 A review of family data. In: Creutzfeldt W, Kobberling J, Neel J V (eds) The genetics of diabetes mellitus. Springer-Verlag, Berlin, p 12–20

Singal D P, Blajchman M A 1973 Histocompatibility (HL-A) antigens, lymphocytotoxic antibodies and tissue antibodies in patients with diabetes mellitus. Diabetes 22: 429–432

Sisk C W 1968 Application of a one hour glucose tolerance test to genetic studies of diabetes in children. Lancet i: 262

Sklenar I, Nerit M, Berger W 1982 Association of specific immune responses to pork and beef insulin with certain HLA-DR antigens in Type I diabetes. British Medical Journal 285: 1451

Spielman R S, Baker L, Zmijewski C M 1980 Gene dosage and susceptibility to insulin-dependent diabetes. Annals of Human Genetics 44: 135

Srikanta S, Ricker A T, McCulloch D R, Soeldner J S, Eisenbarth G S, Palmer J P 1986 Autoimmunity to insulin, beta cell dysfunction and development of insulin-dependent diabetes mellitus. Diabetes 35: 139

Steiner F 1936 Untersuchungen zur Frage der Erblichkeit des diabetes mellitus. Deutches Archiv fur Klinische Medezin 178: 497

Stern M P 1988 Type 2 diabetes mellitus: interface between clinical and epidemiological investigation. Diabetes

Care 11: 119–126

Stetler D, Grumet F C, Erlich H A 1985 Polymorphic restriction of endonuclease sites linked to the HLA-DRalpha gene: Localization and use as genetic markers of insulin-dependent diabetes. Proceedings of the National Academy of Sciences USA 82: 8100–8104

Stiller C R, Dupre J, Gent M et al 1984 Effects of cyclosporine immunosuppression in insulin-dependent diabetes mellitus of recent onset. Science 223: 1362–1367

Strober W 1980 Genetic factors in gluten-sensitive enteropathy. In: Rotter J I, Samloff I M, Rimoin D L (eds) The genetics and heterogeneity of common gastrointestinal disorders. Academic Press, San Francisco, p 243

Suarez B K, van Eerdewegh P 1981 Type I (insulin-dependent) diabetes mellitus. Is there strong evidence for a non-HLA linked gene? Diabetologia 20: 524

Sutherland D E R, Sibley R K, Za X Z et al 1984 Twin-to-twin pancreas transplantation reversal and reenactment of the pathogenesis of Type I diabetes. Transactions of the Association of American Physicians 97: 80–87

Sutherland D E R, Goetz F C, Sibley R K 1989 Recurrence of disease in pancreas transplants. Diabetes 38 (supplement 1): 85

Svejgaard A, Ryder L P 1979 HLA markers and disease. In: Sing C F, Skolnick M (eds) Genetic analysis of common diseases: Applictions to predictive factors in coronary heart disease. Liss, New York, p 523

Svejgaard A, Ryder L P 1981 HLA genotype distribution and genetic models of insulin-dependent diabetes mellitus. Annals of Human Genetics 45: 293–298

Svejgaard A, Platz P, Ryder L P, Staub-Nielsen L, Thomsen M 1975 HLA and disease association — a survey. Transplantation Reviews 22: 3

Svejgaard A, Platz P, Ryder L P 1980 Insulin-dependent diabetes mellitus. In: Terasaki P I (ed) Histocompatibility testing 1980. UCLA Tissue Typing Laboratory, Los Angeles, p 638–656

Svejgaard A, Jakobsen B K, Morling N, Platz P, Ryder L P, Thomsen M 1982 Genetics of the HLA system. In: Kobberling J, Tattersall R B (eds) Genetics of diabetes mellitus. Academic Press, London, p 27

Tager H S 1984 Abnormal products of the human insulin gene. Diabetes 33: 693–699

Tajima N, LaPorte R E, Hibi I, Kitagawa T, Fujita H, Drash A L 1985 A comparison of the epidemiology of youth-onset insulin-dependent diabetes mellitus between Japan and the United States (Allegheny County, Pennsylvania). Diabetes Care 8(Suppl.1): 17–23

Tattersall R B 1974 Mild familial diabetes with dominant inheritance. Quarterly Journal of Medicine 43: 339–357

Tattersall R B 1982 The present status of maturity-onset type of diabetes mellitus. In: Kobberling J, Tattersall R B (eds) Genetics of diabetes mellitus. Academic Press, New York, p 261

Tattersall R B, Fajans S S 1975 A difference between the inheritance of classical juvenile onset and maturity onset type diabetes of young people. Diabetes 24: 44–53

Tattersall R B, Pyke D A 1972 Diabetes in identical twins. Lancet ii: 1120

Then Berg H 1939 The genetic aspect of diabetes mellitus. Journal of the American Medical Association 112: 1091

Thivolet C H, Beaufrere B, Betuel H et al 1988 Islet cell and insulin autoantibodies in subjects at high risk for development of Type I (insulin-dependent) diabetes mellitus: the Lyon family study. Diabetologia 31: 741–746

Thompson M W, Watson E M 1952 The inheritance of diabetes mellitus: an analysis of the family histories of 1631 diabetics. Diabetes 1: 268

Thomson G, Bodmer W 1977 The genetic analysis of HLA and disease associations. In: Dausset J, Svejgaard A (eds) HLA and disease. Munksgaard, Copenhagen, p 84

Thomson G, Robinson W P, Kuhner M K et al 1988 Genetic heterogeneity, modes of inheritance, and risk estimates for a joint study of Caucasians with insulin-dependent diabetes mellitus. American Journal of Human Genetics 43: 799–816

Todd J A, Bell J I, McDevitt H O 1987 HLA-DQ beta gene contributes to susceptibility and resistance to insulin-dependent diabetes mellitus. Nature 329: 599

Vadheim C M, Rotter J I, Maclaren N K, Riley W J, Anderson C E 1986 Preferential transmission of diabetic alleles within the HLA gene complex. New England Journal of Medicine 315: 1314–1318

Wagener D K, Sacks J M, LaPorte R E, MacGregor J M 1982 The Pittsburg study of insulin-dependent diabetes mellitus. Diabetes 31: 136–144

Walker A, Cudworth A G 1980 Type I (insulin-dependent) diabetic multiplex families, mode of genetic transmission. Diabetes 29: 1036–1039

Warram J H, Krolewski A S, Gottlieb M S, Kahn R C 1984 Differences in risk of insulin-dependent diabetes in offspring of diabetic mothers and fathers. New England Journal of Medicine 311: 149

Werner N 1936 Blutzuckerregulation und Erbanlage. Deutches Archiv Fur Klinische Medezin 178: 308

West K M 1975 Substantial differences in the diagnostic criteria used by diabetes experts. Diabetes 24: 541–644

West K M 1978 Epidemiology of diabetes and vascular lesions. Elsevier North Holland, Amsterdam, p 19–126

West R, Belmonte M M, Colle E, Crepeau P, Wilkins P, Poirier R 1979 Epidemiologic survey of juvenile-onset diabetes in Montreal. Diabetes 28: 690–693

White P 1965 The inheritance of diabetes. Medical Clinics of North America 49: 857–863

White P 1978 Classification of obstetric diabetes. American Journal of Obstetrics and Gynecology 130: 228

WHO Expert Committee on Diabetes Mellitus 1980 Second report on diabetes mellitus. Technical Report Series 646, Geneva, Switzerland, WHO

WHO Study Group Technical Report 1985 Malnutritional-related diabetes mellitus. WHO, Geneva

Williams R C, Knowler W C, Butler W J et al 1981 HLA-A2 and Type 2 (insulin-independent) diabetes mellitus in Pima Indians: An association of allele frequency with age. Diabetologia 21: 460–463

Wilson R M, van Der Minne P, Deverill I, Heller S R, Gelsthorpe K, Reeves W G, Tattersall R 1985 Insulin dependence: problems with the classification of 100 consecutive patients. Diabetic Medicine 2: 167–172

Winter W E, MacLaren N K, Riley W J, Clarke D W, Kappy M S, Spillar R P 1987 Maturity-onset diabetes of youth in Black America. New England Journal of Medicine 316: 285–291

Wolf E, Spencer K M, Cudworth A G 1983 The genetic

susceptibility to Type 1 (insulin-dependent) diabetes: analysis of the HLA-DR association. Diabetologia 24: 224

Working Party, College of General Practitioners 1965 Family history of diabetes. British Medical Journal i: 960–962

Yoon J W, Notkins A L 1976 Virus-induced diabetes mellitus. VI. Genetically determined host differences in the replication of encephalomyocarditis virus in pancreatic beta cells. Journal of Experimental Medicine 143: 1170

Yoon J W, Notkins A L 1983 Virus-induced diabetes in mice. Metabolism 32(7): 37

Yoon J W, Ray U R 1985 Perspectives on the role of viruses in insulin-dependent diabetes. Diabetes 8(supplement 1): 39

Yoon J W, Austin M, Onodera T, Notkins A L 1979 Virus-induced diabetes mellitus: isolation of a virus from the pancreas of a child with diabetic ketoacidosis. New England Journal of Medicine 300: 1173

Yoon J W, McClintock P R, Onodera T, Notkins A L 1980 Virus-induced diabetes mellitus. XVIII. Inhibition by a non-diabetogenic variant of encephalomyocarditis virus. Journal of Experimental Medicine 152: 878–882

Yoon J W, Rodriques M M, Currier C, Notkins A L 1982 Long-term complications of virus-induced diabetes mellitus in mice. Nature 296: 566

Yoon J W, Cha C Y, Jordan G W 1983 The role of interferon in virus-induced diabetes. Journal of Infectious Diseases 147: 155

Yoshimasa Y, Seino S, Whittaker J et al 1988 Insulin-resistant diabetes due to a point mutation that prevents insulin proreceptor processing. Science 240: 784

Zimmet P 1979 Epidemiology of diabetes and its macrovascular manifestations in Pacific populations — the medical effects of social progress. Diabetes Care 2: 144–153

Zimmet P, Kirk R, Serjeantson S, Whitehouse S, Taylor R 1982 Diabetes and environmental interactions. In: Genetic environmental interactions in diabetes mellitus. Excerpta Medica, Amsterdam, p 9

90. Congenital adrenal hyperplasia

Maria I. New   Perrin C. White   Phyllis W. Speiser
Christopher Crawford   Bo Dupont

CLINICAL ASPECTS (A): NORMAL AND ABNORMAL ADRENAL FUNCTION

Endocrine functions of the adrenal cortex

The adrenal cortex produces numerous steroids, secreted in widely varying amounts and each with different potency of hormonal action (Fig. 90.1). According to

their primary effect, these are classified as mineralocorticoids (MC), glucocorticoids (GC), or sex steroids.

Aldosterone is the end-product of the mineralocorticoid pathway and is the most potent steroid affecting active transport of sodium ions across membranes and thus in maintaining electrolyte balance. The primary site of action of aldosterone is at the distal and collecting

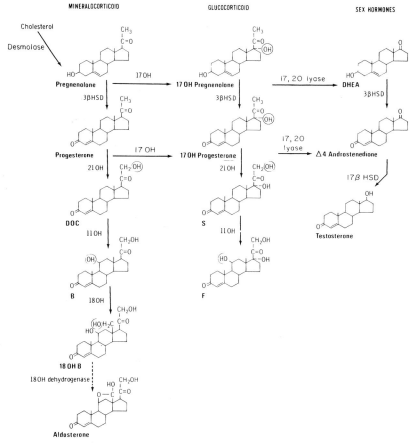

Fig. 90.1 Simplified scheme for adrenal steroidogenesis. Each hydroxylation step is indicated and the newly added hydroxyl group is circled. (Adapted from New M I, Levine L S 1973. Advances in Human Genetics 4:251, with permission).

tubule where it promotes reabsorption of the crucial final 2% of sodium to be regained from the renal filtrate.

Cortisol, the principal glucocorticoid in man and most mammalian species (Nussdorfer 1986), is the main secretory product of the adrenal cortex and is indispensable for proper carbohydrate metabolism and in ensuring systemic capacity to withstand events of stress such as infection and trauma. New studies are starting to define important mediating roles for glucocorticoids in the functioning of the immune response.

The major sex steroids secreted by the adrenal cortex are the weak androgen dehydroepiandrosterone (DHEA) and its sulphate; the more highly androgenic steroids (and oestrogens) are normally very minor products. In late childhood there is a significant rise in adrenal sex steroid production, termed the adrenarche, leading to further complex interactions with the hypothalamus-pituitary and the gonads in preparation for puberty and the transition to sexual maturity. This remains probably the least understood aspect of the function of the adrenal cortex.

Regulation of steroid synthesis

The adrenal cortex divides histologically into three regions: the outer zona glomerulosa, the wide middle zona fasciculata, and the more compact inner zona reticularis adjoining the adrenal medulla. Differences in production of mineralocorticoids, glucocorticoids, and sex steroids by the adrenal cortex are determined by local activities of certain adrenal enzymes, which correspond in large part with this zonation (Hornsby 1987, Hyatt 1987). Synthesis of the mineralocorticoid aldosterone is dependent on an enzyme activity limited to the zona glomerulosa, while production of cortisol and androgens requires an enzyme found in the middle and inner zones, the fasciculata-reticularis.

Adrenal steroid synthesis depends on the trophic effects of the anterior pituitary peptide, corticotrophin (ACTH). ACTH exercises acute and chronic effects on adrenocortical cell processes (Waterman & Simpson 1985). The acute ACTH response produces up to 10-fold amplification of the rate of steroidogenesis within 2–6 minutes.

The most direct result of the intracellular changes induced by ACTH in the adrenal cortex is increased availability of cholesterol as substrate to cholesterol desmolase, the first and rate-limiting enzyme in steroid synthesis. Maximum rates require the mediation of ACTH-sensitive protein factors affecting intramitochondrial transfer and binding of cholesterol (Pedersen 1985). Cholesterol for steroid biosynthesis is provided by the cytoplasmic pool of free cholesterol, which is supplied primarily by the action of the kinase-dependent enzyme cholesteryl ester hydrolase (CEH), which hydrolyses cholesterol from cholesteryl esters in cytoplasmic lipid droplet stores. Continued adrenal steroid demand depletes this intracellular source, at which stage uptake of plasma lipoprotein (LDL) provides further quantities of cholesterol, and after prolonged stimulation cholesterol biosynthesis within the cell becomes significant.

Continued elevation of ACTH also produces progressively wider effects within the cell, increasing mRNA transcription and protein translation rates for each of the enzymes in the cortisol synthetic pathway, the enzymes governing lipoprotein endocytosis and intracellular movement of cholesterol (with upregulation of the cell-surface lipoprotein receptor), and, given sufficiently prolonged stimulation, for the enzymes of cholesterol synthesis (Boggaram et al 1985, Voutilainen & Miller 1987).

Cortisol and ACTH The synthesis of cortisol is modulated directly by the net circulating levels of ACTH. ACTH, a peptide with a relatively short plasma half-life, is one of a group of trophic hormones cleaved from a large molecular weight-precursor, pro-opiomelanocortin (POMC). ACTH is stored in the corticotroph cells of the anterior pituitary. Pulsatile release of ACTH from this cell population is in turn modulated by corticotrophin releasing factor (CRF) originating in the hypothalamus (Ganong 1963, Guillemin & Schally 1963, Ganong et al 1974, Ganong 1980, Rivier & Plotsky 1986). The hypothalamic-pituitary-adrenal axis forms a regulated system (Fig. 90.2) Negative feedback control is exerted by cortisol, and the central nervous system determines the hypothalamic setpoint for the expected plasma cortisol

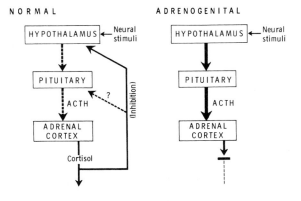

Fig. 90.2 The regulation of cortisol secretion in normal subjects and in patients with congenital adrenal hyperplasia. (From New M I, Levine L S 1973. Advances in Human Genetics 4:251, with permission).

level. Net ACTH release has basal, diurnal and stress-induced components. Plasma cortisol levels lower than the hypothalamic-pituitary setpoint will increase the rate and intensity of ACTH secretory pulses. Adrenal enzyme deficiencies causing impaired synthesis and decreased secretion of cortisol thus lead to chronic elevations of ACTH with overstimulation and consequent hyperplasia of the adrenal cortex.

Aldosterone and renin-angiotensin The primary regulation of aldosterone synthesis is via the renin-angiotensin system (Davis 1974), which is responsive to the state of electrolyte balance and plasma volume. The enzyme renin, which arises from the renal juxtaglomerular apparatus, cleaves the decapeptide angiotensin I from angiotensinogen, a plasma α_2-globulin. Angiotensin I is then further converted enzymatically by passage through the lungs to the octapeptide angiotensin II. Angiotensin II is a potent vasoconstrictor and directly stimulates aldosterone secretion by the zona glomerulosa (Laragh 1971). Aldosterone secretion is also stimulated directly by high serum K^+ concentration, less sensitively by low serum Na^+ concentration, and by ACTH (Reid & Ganong 1977). ACTH has a permissive role through its general effect on adrenocortical function, but in addition to this the zona glomerulosa is transiently very sensitive to ACTH, especially when the late aldosterone synthetic stages specific to this zone have been potentiated by chronic angiotensin II stimulation or electrolyte imbalance (K^+ loading/Na^+ restriction) (Ganong 1984, Koushanpour & Kriz 1986). Other mediators have been named, but their physiological significance remains unconfirmed. Thus the four major factors affecting aldosterone synthesis by the zona glomerulosa are angiotensin II, K^+, Na^+ and ACTH (Fig. 90.3).

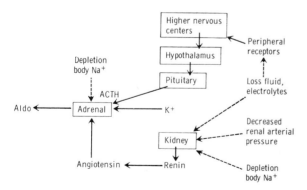

Fig. 90.3 Regulation of aldosterone production by the four major factors, angiotensin II, corticotropin (ACTH), potassium (K^+) and sodium (Na^+). (From New M I, Petersen R E 1966. Pediatric Clinics of North America. 13:43, with permission).

The adrenal cortex as two glands According to the view of adrenocortical zonation proposed by New and Seaman (1970), the zona glomerulosa and the zona fasciculata are not merely histologically distinct cell populations but behave hormonally and biochemically as two separate glands with respect to regulation and secretion, steroidogenesis in the fasciculata being regulated primarily by ACTH, and in the glomerulosa primarily by the renin-angiotensin system such that: (1) ACTH stimulates secretion of cortisol, deoxycorticosterone, corticosterone and androgens by the zona fasciculata and zona reticularis and; (2) angiotensin stimulates aldosterone secretion by the glomerulosa, with ACTH presumably exerting only a secondary influence in this zone on secretion of aldosterone (Fig. 90.4). Whereas the zona fasciculata does not exhibit the enzyme activity necessary for the terminal step of aldosterone synthesis, the zona glomerulosa lacks the 17α-hydroxylase activity required for the production of 17-hydroxycorticoids and androgens.

Adrenal steroids in development

Normal male genital differentiation in embryonic and fetal life is dependent on two functions of the fetal testes (Jost 1953, 1966, 1971): first, the secretion of sufficient quantities of testosterone to direct the formation of the internal male genital structures – the epididymides, vasa deferentia, seminal vesicles, and ejaculatory ducts – from the wolffian (mesonephric) ducts, and second the secretion of a nonsteroidal factor to suppress development of the Müllerian ducts into the female internal structures, i.e. the fallopian tubes, uterus, cervix and upper vagina (Fig. 90.5). This factor, anti-Müllerian hormone (AMH), also termed Müllerian-inhibiting substance (MIS) or factor (MIF), is a glycoprotein dimer (Picard et al 1986) first synthesized by differentiating Sertoli cells (Josso 1986) between 6 and 7 weeks of fetal life, and thus precedes testosterone secretion by the Leydig cells which starts at about the 8th week. Since there is no anomalous production of AMH in females suffering even the most extreme virilization from androgen excess, the internal genital structures are fully normal. The rescue of childbearing capacity in these gonadally intact patients is thus a prime goal of treatment in congenital adrenal hyperplasia.

Testosterone is also required for suppression of the breast anlage and, indirectly, for normal formation of the male external genitalia. In order to act on the tissues of the external genital primordium, testosterone must first undergo peripheral conversion to dihydrotestosterone (DHT). The differentiation promoted by DHT includes formation of the scrotum from the genital swellings, midline closure of the genital folds and elongation into the body of the phallus, and extension of the urogenital sinus by fusion along the ventral groove to form a penile urethra (Peterson et al 1977, Wilson et al 1983). Pertaining to the virilizing forms of congenital adrenal hyperplasia, progressive differentiation towards the male type in genetic females has been given a five-stage classification by Prader (Prader 1958a). Raised androgen levels from abnormal fetal adrenal function (virilizing adrenal hyperplasia) or from the mother (an androgen-producing tumour or exogenous androgen administration during pregnancy) do not affect genital development in the male fetus because of the already high levels of androgens produced by the gonads, but are high enough to cause significant masculinization of the external genitalia in females (New et al 1983a). In pregnancies at risk for a female child affected with virilizing adrenal hyperplasia, suppression of fetal adrenal androgen production has been attempted by giving the mother glucocorticoids that are able to cross the placental barrier.

Pathogenesis of congenital adrenal hyperplasia

Congenital adrenal hyperlasia (CAH) refers to the histological alterations consequent to elevated ACTH and chronic glandular overactivity resulting from the inability of the adrenal cortex to achieve normal plasma

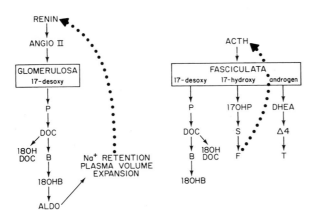

Fig. 90.4 Regulation of adrenocortical steroidogenesis considering the fasciculata and glomerulosa as two separate glands. Dotted arrows indicate negative feedback. Symbols: P, progesterone; DOC, 11-deoxycorticosterone; B, corticosterone; 17-OHP, 17α-hydroxyprogesterone; S, 11-deoxycortisol; F, cortisol; Δ4, Δ⁴-androstenedione; DHEA, dehydroepiandrosterone; T, testosterone; 18ODOC, 18-hydroxydeoxycorticosterone; 18OHB, 18-hydroxycorticosterone; ALDO, aldosterone. (From New et al 1983a, with permission).

cortisol levels in response to (normal) ACTH stimulation (Fig. 90.2). This arises biochemically from reduced or absent enzymatic activity at one of the stages of steroid synthesis. Each enzyme deficiency produces characteristically abnormal adrenal hormone and precursor levels, the varying patterns of imbalance giving rise to a wide range of clinical effects manifest in metabolic disturbances and also in developmental abnormalities (New et al 1989b). (See Table 90.1).

The following enzymatic defects of steroidogenesis and their associated clinical syndromes have been described (New et al 1983a, White et al 1987):

1. 21-hydroxylase deficiency (salt-wasting [classical], simple virilizing [classical] and nonclassical);
2. 11β-hydroxylase deficiency (hypertensive CAH) with corticosterone methyl oxidase (CMO) type I and II (salt-wasting);
3. 3β-ol dehydrogenase deficiency (classical and nonclassical);
4. 17α-hydroxylase deficiency with 17,20-lyase deficiency;
5. cholesterol desmolase deficiency (lipoid hyperplasia).

The 21- and 11β-hydroxylase deficiencies, occurring distal to the common precursor stages, cause channelling of these precursor steroids into the androgen pathway, resulting in virilization of females and hyperandrogenic effects in both sexes. Blocked conversion of precursors to C_{19}/C_{18} steroids in the 17α-hydroxylase deficiency causes pseudohermaphroditism in males and sexual infantilism in females. In the 3β-ol dehydrogenase defect there is production only of the relatively inactive Δ^5 steroids. While severe lack of Δ^4 androgens produces pseudovaginal hypospadias in the male, enormously high levels of the weak androgen DHEA may cause clitoral enlargement in females. Cholesterol desmolase deficiency (lipoid adrenal hyperplasia) blocks all steroid production, and accordingly, among its very serious effects, results in pseudohermaphroditism in genetic males. Sexual ambiguity is not a feature of 18-hydroxylase (CMO I) or 18-dehydrogenase (CMO II) deficiency, since these distal blocks have quantitatively small effects on the steroid economy and adrenal sex steroid secretion is thus unaffected.

Classical and nonclassical forms

Total or near-total blocks in the activity of these enzymes result in genital ambiguity and abnormalities of salt retention in 3/4 of cases (New et al 1989b). These comprise the classical forms of CAH. Improved biochemical assessment of adrenal function allows the identification now also of lesser enzyme defects which cause milder endocrine disturbance and absence of genital ambiguity. Called nonclassical forms, such partial defects have been confirmed for steroid 21-hydroxylase (Kohn et al 1982, New & Levine 1984), steroid 11β-hydroxylase (Rosler & Leiberman 1984),) and 3β-hydroxysteroid dehydrogenase (Bongiovanni 1984, Pang et al 1985a), and are presumed to exist for the other enzymes. As might be expected, nonclassical defects are much more common than occurrences of the corresponding classical defects. Epidemiological studies have shown that nonclassical 21-hydroxylase deficiency is in fact the most common autosomal recessive disorder in man (Speiser et al 1985).

CLINICAL ASPECTS (B): THE SPECIFIC ENZYME DEFECTS

21-Hydroxylase deficiency

Decreased cortisol synthesis owing to impaired 21-hydroxylation is the most common biochemical cause of congenital adrenal hyperplasia. The decreased plasma cortisol induces ACTH secretion into the blood (Sydnor et al 1953, Binoux et al 1972), causing elevated adrenal production both of cortisol/androgen precursors, and of androgens, which do not require 21-hydroxylase for their biosynthesis. Early clinical studies showed increased amounts of pregnanetriol, the principal metabolite of

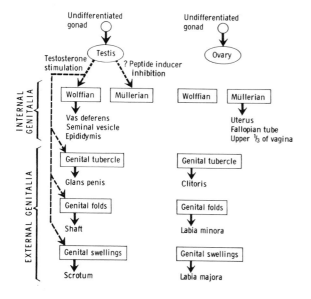

Fig. 90.5 Fetal sex differentiation (From New M I, Levine L S 1973. Advances in Human Genetics 4:251, with permission).

17α-hydroxyprogesterone (17-OHP) (Butler & Marrian 1937), and also of 17-ketosteroids (17-KS; 17-oxosteroids), resulting from the metabolism of DHEA, Δ⁴-androstenedione and testosterone, present in the urine of patients with 21-hydroxylase deficiency (Mason & Kepler 1945). Radioimmunoassay-based laboratory procedures for the determination of hormone levels in serum are simple and reliable and allow more accurate diagnosis (New et al 1983b) than could be provided formerly by methods assessing urinary hormone and metabolite levels.

Simple virilizing form

The prominent feature of 21-hydroxylase deficiency is progressive virilism with advanced somatic development. The classical disorder is of the simple virilizing type in about one in four cases. Developmental genital anomalies are manifest in females as varying degrees of genital ambiguity, which should flag the diagnosis in the female. Because genital formation in males is normal, the syndrome often goes unrecognized in the male until signs of androgen excess such as accelerated height and precocious sexual hair appear later in childhood.

Adrenocortical cell differentiation and the formation of the fetal zone occur early in embryogenesis, and although the biochemical schedule of steroid synthesis has not been completely elucidated, it is clear that genital development in the fetus takes place under the influence of active adrenal steroid synthesis. Thus, in the female, the extent of masculinization of the external genitalia ranges from mild clitoral enlargement, through varying degrees of fusion of the labio-scrotal folds (posterior to anterior), to the profound morphological anomaly of a penile urethra.

Genetic sex, gonadal differentiation and internal genital morphogenesis are normal in 21-hydroxylase deficiency. Since there is no anomalous secretion of AMH (anti-Müllerian hormone), the Müllerian ducts in the female develop normally into uterus and fallopian tubes. Wolffian duct stabilization and differentiation proceeds under the control of high intraluminal levels of gonadal androgens in the male; this process appears to be unaffected by elevated adrenal androgens and there is no observable wolffian development in females with 21-hydroxylase deficiency congenital adrenal hyperplasia.

21-Hydroxylase deficiency is the most common cause of ambiguous genitalia in the newborn female, and because affected females have the capacity for an entirely normal female sex role, including childbearing, it is very important to recognize this disorder in newborns with ambiguous genitalia. Although the male is not jeopardized by inappropriate sex assignment, premature mascu-

Table 90.1 The forms of adrenal hyperplasia: clinical and hormonal aspects

Deficiency (syndrome)	Genital ambiguity	Postnatal viriliz-ation	Salt meta-bolism	Steroid pattern increased	decreased
Cholesterol desmolase (lipoid hyperplasia)	M	No	salt wasting	none	all
3β-ol dehydrogenase a. classical	M	Yes	salt wasting	17-OH-pregnenolone dehydroepiandro-sterone (DHEA)	aldosterone (aldo) cortisol testosterone (TT)
b. nonclassical	No	Yes	normal	17-OH-pregnenolone DHEA	–
17α-hydroxylase	M	No	salt re-tention	deoxycortico-sterone (DOC) corticosterone (B)	cortisol, T
17,20-lyase	M	No	normal	none	DHEA, T, andro-stenedione (Δ⁴-A)
21-hydroxylase a. classical salt-wasting	F	Yes	salt wasting	17-OH-progesterone (17-OHP), Δ⁴-A	aldo, cortisol
simple viriziling	F	Yes	normal (↑renin)	17-OHP, Δ⁴-A	cortisol
b. nonclassical (symptomatic and asymptomatic)	No	Yes	normal	17-OHP, Δ⁴-A	–
11β-hydroxylase a. classical (hypertensive CAH)	F	Yes	salt re-tention	DOC, 11-deoxy-cortisol (S)	cortisol ± aldo
b. nonclassical	No	Yes	normal	S ± DOC	
corticosterone methyl oxidase type II	No	No	salt wasting	18-OH-cortico-sterone	aldo

linization and accelerated physical development cause problems of adjustment. In addition, continued adrenal androgen excess may suppress the pituitary-gonadal axis, preventing maturation of the testes and resulting in infertility. In both sexes there is early fusion of the epiphyses with resulting short stature.

Salt-wasting form

In three quarters of classical cases (i.e. presenting at birth) of 21-hydroxylase deficiency there is renal salt wasting from deficient aldosterone synthesis; this is defined by hyponatraemia and hyperkalaemia, inappropriately high urinary sodium, and low serum and urinary aldosterone with concomitantly high plasma renin activity (PRA). The increase in the proportion of salt-wasting cases in recent years can be attributed to better case identification and patient survival. In addition to inadequate secretion of aldosterone or other salt-retaining steroids, other precursors with natriuretic action produced in excess may counter the marginally competent sodium-conserving mechanism of the im-

mature newborn renal tubule (Prader et al 1955, Klein 1960, Kowarski et al 1965, Kuhnle et al 1986). The loss of salt in infancy from an aldosterone biosynthesis defect may improve with age (Luetscher 1956, Stoner et al 1986), and possible adjustments in sodium intake and mineralocorticoid replacement in patients labelled neo-natally as salt wasters can be made on the basis of careful monitoring of PRA.

Although correlation of the severity of salt wasting with the extent of virilization has been claimed (Verkauf & Jones 1970), the degree of genital ambiguity in a female newborn does not indicate the form. In the paper most frequently quoted to demonstrate that severe 21-hydroxylase deficiency and hence salt wasting is correlated with the degree of masculinization, the patient described was no longer a salt-waster by 4 years of age (Prader 1958a). Thus even mildly virilized newborn females with 21-hydroxylase deficiency should be observed carefully for signs of adrenal insufficiency in the first weeks of life.

With few exceptions (Rosenbloom & Smith 1966a), the literature has indicated that the presence or absence of salt wasting in 21-hydroxylase deficiency is seen consistently within a family, and subsequent affected offspring have thus been predicted to have the same form of the disease as the index case. A recent report, however, has identified discordance for salt wasting and aldosterone synthetic capacity in several families among sibs who in addition carried identical markers (HLA-B antigen alleles; see HLA and molecular genetics below) for the genetic defect (Stoner et al 1986). Distinct zonal defects in the two classical forms of 21-hydroxylase deficiency have been clinically investigated (Kuhnle et al 1981).

Nonclassical 21-hydroxylase deficiency

An attenuated, late-onset form of adrenal hyperplasia was first suspected in the early 1950s by gynaecologists in clinical practice who used glucocorticoids for the treatment of women with physical signs of hyperandrogenism, including infertility (Jones & Jones 1954, Jeffries et al 1958). The first documentation of suppression of 21-hydroxylase precursors in the urine of such individuals after glucocorticoid therapy was by Baulieu and co-workers in 1957 (Decourt et al 1957). During the next two decades, the empirical use of glucocorticoids for the treatment of virilized women became commonplace, as it was assumed that adrenal androgens were often elevated in those patients. Diagnosis of a 21-hydroxylase defect by serum measurement became possible in the early 1970s with the development of a radioimmunoassay specific for 17-hydroxyprogesterone (17-OHP) (Abraham et al 1971). Based on this radioimmunoassay, findings of family members with serum elevations of 17-OHP, the enzyme substrate in the 17-deoxy pathway, led to the erroneous speculation that these individuals were 'expressing heterozygotes' of a severe 21-hydroxylase deficiency gene (Zachmann & Prader 1978, 1979). Many family studies on classical 21-hydroxylase deficiency followed the initial report by Dupont et al (1977) of genetic linkage of CAH (21-hydroxylase deficiency) with HLA (see HLA Linkage below). Through such studies it became apparent that the nonclassical 21-hydroxylase deficiency was also genetically transmitted as an autosomal recessive (Rosenwaks et al 1979, Levine et al 1980a, Kohn et al 1982). Linkage of nonclassical 21-hydroxylase deficiency to HLA was established (Laron et al 1980, Pollack et al 1981), confirming that this disorder was allelic with the classical defect (Levine et al 1980a, 1981). The HLA associations for the nonclassical defect (Blankstein et al 1980a, Migeon et al 1980, Pollack et al 1981) are distinct from those found in the classical forms (see HLA Linkage below) and differ by ethnicity (Laron et al 1980, Speiser et al 1985).

Clinical symptomatology of nonclassical 21-hydroxy-lase deficiency is variable, and may present at any age (Fig. 90.6). Nonclassical 21-hydroxylase deficiency can result in premature development of pubic hair in children; to our knowledge, the youngest such patient was noted to have pubic hair at 6 months of age (Kohn et al 1982). In a review of 23 cases presenting to The New York Hospital-Cornell Medical Center for evaluation of premature pubarche, 7 children demonstrated a 17-OHP response to ACTH stimulation consistent with the diagnosis of nonclassical 21-hydroxylase deficiency, a prevalence of 30% in this pre-selected group of pediatric patients at high risk (Temeck et al 1987). Other investigators found only one of 15 children with premature adrenarche demonstrating an ACTH-stimulated 17-OHP response greater than that of obligate heterozygote carriers of the 21-hydroxylase deficiency gene (Granoff et al 1985). Elevated adrenal androgens promote the early fusion of epiphyseal growth plates, and children with this disorder commonly have advanced bone age and accelerated linear growth velocity, and ultimately are shorter than the final height prediction based on mid-parental height and on linear growth percentiles before the apparent onset of excess androgen secretion.

Severe cystic acne refractory to oral antibiotics and retinoic acid has been attributed to nonclassical 21-hydroxylase deficiency. In one study comparing the responses of 11 female patients with acne and 8 (female) control subjects to a 24-hour infusion of ACTH, elevated urinary excretion of pregnanetriol suggestive of a partial 21-hydroxylase deficiency was found in 6 patients (Rose et al 1976). In another study of 31 young female patients with acne and/or hirsutism tested with low dose ACTH stimulation after overnight dexamethasone suppression, no cases of 21-hydroxylase deficiency were found (Lucky et al 1986). Male-pattern baldness has been noted in other cases as the sole presenting symptom in young women with nonclassical 21-hydroxylase deficiency.

Menarche in females may be normal or delayed, and secondary amenorrhoea is a frequent occurrence. A sector of female nonclassical 21-hydroxylase deficiency patients represents a subgroup of women affected with polycystic ovarian disease. An initial-phase adrenal sex-steroid excess, disrupting the usual cyclicity of gonadotropin release and/or with direct effects on the ovary, is probable in the pathophysiology of this syndrome, leading ultimately to the formation of ovarian cysts, which may then continue autonomously to produce androgens.

In retrospective analysis it was revealed that 16 of 108 (14%) of women presenting to this institution (NYH-CMC) for evaluation of hirsutism and oligomenorrhoea demonstrated a partial 21-hydroxylase defect (Pang et al 1985a). The prevalence of nonclassical 21-hydroxylase deficiency as an aetiology of these endocrine complaints in women in other published series ranges from 1.2–30% (Child et al 1980, Gibson et al 1980, Lobo & Goebelsmann 1980, Chrousos et al 1982, Chetkowski et al 1984, Kuttenn et al 1986). The wide range of frequencies in these reports may relate to differences in ethnic make-up of the groups studied since the disease frequency is ethnic group specific.

Although the androgen profiles in serum and urine in either the basal or ACTH-stimulated state may not be markedly different overall from those demonstrated by women with the syndrome of polycystic ovaries from other causes, the serum 17-OHP response on ACTH stimulation clearly differentiates patients with an adrenal 21-hydroxylase defect (New et al 1983b, Pang et al 1985a). In six women with nonclassical 21-hydroxylase deficiency who underwent sonography or laparoscopic visualization of the ovaries, four had polycystic ovaries (Pang et al 1985a). Thus even sonograms of the ovary do not distinguish women with excess androgens due to polycystic ovarian disease from those with nonclassical 21-hydroxylase deficiency. ACTH tests are required for the differential diagnosis. The response of the hypothalamic-pituitary-gonadal axis to LHRH has

been observed to be variably abnormal in virilized women with nonclassical 21-hydroxylase deficiency (Gangemi et al 1983, Speiser et al 1987). Similarly, ACTH tests are necessary to differentiate polycystic ovarian disease from nonclassical 21-hydroxylase deficiency after LHRH testing of pituitary gonadotropin secretion.

In boys, early beard growth, acne and growth spurt may be detected. In cases of pubic hair growth and enlarged phallus from an androgen excess condition in boys, a reliable indication of an adrenal (as opposed to testicular) source of androgens is the proportionately small size of the testes that results from suppression of the hypothalamic-pituitary-gonadal axis. In men, signs of androgen excess are difficult to appreciate, and the manifestations of adrenal androgen excess may be limited to short stature or oligospermia and diminished fertility from this same adrenal sex-steroid induced gonadal suppression.

Certain individuals – males and females – affected with nonclassical 21-hydroxylase deficiency have no overt symptoms of disease while demonstrating biochemical abnormalities comparable with patients. Longitudinal follow-up of these cases (usually detected as part of a

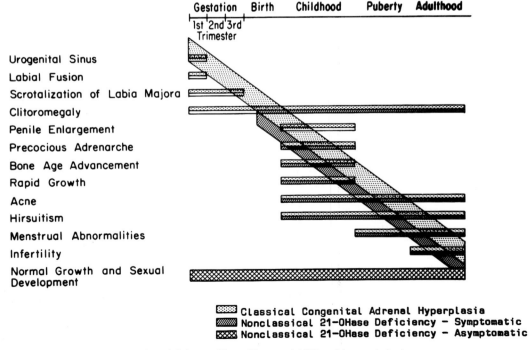

Fig. 90.6 Clinical spectrum of 21-hydroxylase deficiency. (From New et al 1983a with permission).

family study) often shows that signs of hyperandrogenism wax and wane with time.

3β-ol Dehydrogenase deficiency

The enzyme 3β-hydroxysteroid dehydrogenase (3β-HSD), or 3β-ol dehydrogenase, is necessary for the synthesis of all adrenal and gonadal steroids beyond the relatively inactive 3β-ol Δ^5 precursors. First described in 1962 by Bongiovanni, 3β-HSD deficiency has seemed most likely to have a monogenic autosomal recessive mode of transmission based on pedigree analysis (Bongiovanni 1962, Kenny et al 1971, Pang et al 1983).

As gonadal 3β-HSD enzyme activity is reduced also (though not always equally with the adrenal defect), gonadal androgen production is deficient. In genetic males incomplete genital development results in recognizable ambiguity at birth. In affected females on the other hand, the very high levels of circulating DHEA – and perhaps some peripheral conversion of DHEA to more potent androgens – may produce a limited androgen effect (restricted to clitoral enlargement).

A high ratio of Δ^5 to Δ^4 steroids, characterized specifically by elevated serum levels of the Δ^5 steroids prenenolone, 17-hydroxypregnenolone and DHEA, and increased excretion of the Δ^5 metabolites pregnenetriol and 16-pregnenetriol in the urine, is diagnostic for this enzyme disorder.

Deficient aldosterone production in cases of a complete or near-complete 3β-HSD enzyme block results in salt wasting; in other cases the ability to conserve sodium has been intact (Bongiovanni 1962, Hamilton & Brush 1964, Cathro et al 1965, Kogut 1965, Janne et al 1970, Kenny et al 1971, Parks et al 1971, Zachmann et al 1970, Schneider et al 1975, de Peretti et al 1980). Zonal function has been studied with regard to salt wasting (Pang et al 1983). Thus, in 3β-HSD deficiency, as in 21-hydroxylase and 11β-hydroxylase deficiency (see following), the other common forms of congenital adrenal hyperplasia, there is a phenotypic spectrum for each clinical feature. As with the other two common defects, it is not possible to judge the degree of severity of the 3β-HSD enzyme defect based on the appearance of the external genitalia at birth.

Nonclassical 3β-HSD deficiency As with 21-hydroxylase, nonclassical 3β-HSD is an attenuated enzyme defect with no major developmental abnormalities (Pang et al 1985a). With post-adrenarchal or peripubertal onset (Rosenfield et al 1980), it appears to affect the fasciculata-reticularis zones, the spared functioning of the glomerulosa ensuring adequate salt retention (Pang et al 1983). Signs of virilization in females appearing postnatally are similar to those in a 21-hydroxylase defect. 60-minute

ACTH testing (serum sampling at 0' and 60' after administration of cortrosyn (synthetic $ACTH_{1-24}$) 0.25 mg IV) will reveal a 3β-HSD defect when serum Δ^5-17-hydroxypregnenolone (Δ^5-17P) and DHEA levels, and serum ratios Δ^5-17P:17-OHP and Δ^5-17P:F are all more than 2 SD above the normal mean values (Pang et al 1983).

11β-Hydroxylase deficiency

Abnormal adrenal steroid secretion attributable specifically to impeded 11β-hydroxylation was first reported by Eberlein & Bongiovanni (1955). The characteristic steroid profile of 11β-hydroxylase deficiency shows elevated 11-deoxycortisol (compound S) and deoxycorticosterone (DOC) in the serum, with marked urinary elevation of the corresponding tetrahydro metabolites, THS and THDOC, and complete absence of any 11-oxygenated C_{19} or C_{21} steroids in the blood or urine (Eberlein & Bongiovanni 1956).

Hypertension with hypokalaemic alkalosis is the single clinical feature distinguishing 11β-hydroxylase from 21-hydroxylase deficiency, yet is not uniformly present. DOC has been thought to be the causative agent of hypertension (Eberlein & Bongiovanni 1956, New & Levine 1973) but this is not certain. While it has moderately potent mineralocorticoid effects, causing sodium retention, plasma volume expansion and suppression of PRA, DOC may be elevated in 11β-hydroxylase deficiency patients who are normotensive (Gandy et al 1960, Blunck 1968) and normal or only mildly elevated in hypertensive patients (Green et al 1960, Glenthoj et al 1980). In addition, intravenous DOC infusion does not uniformly induce hypertension in control subjects (Ferrebee et al 1939, Perera et al 1944) nor does suppression of DOC always cause remission of hypertension in 11β-hydroxylase deficiency patients (Rosler et al 1982). Mineralocorticoid excess and hypertension is not necessarily proportional to the degree of hypokalaemia (Rosler et al 1982) and two cases even showing lack of suppression of PRA, considered a hallmark of this defect, have now been noted (New et al 1989a). More recently, the role of DOC metabolites such as 18-hydroxy-DOC has been considered, but the specific adrenocortical factor – if any – operative in the hypertension seen in this disorder remains to be established (Ulick 1976, Rosler et al 1982).

As in 21-hydroxylase deficiency, excess fetal androgen production causes prenatal virilization of females, resulting in ambiguous external genitalia with normal female internal reproductive organs. In newborn males with 11β-hydroxylase deficiency the external genitalia may be normal, but in either sex virilization ensues postnatally if the disorder is untreated. There is no direct correlation between the degree of virilization and hypertension (Rosler et al 1982).

Nonclassical 11β-hydroxylase deficiency Mild, late-onset and even cryptic forms of 11β-hydroxylase deficiency have been reported (Gabrilove et al 1965, Newmark et al 1977, Cathelineau et al 1980, Birnbaum & Rose 1984, Rosler & Leiberman 1984, Hurwitz et al 1985). As in 21-hydroxylase deficiency, this clinical variability may represent allelism at the 11β-hydroxylase structural gene locus, but investigations so far have not demonstrated a consistent measurable biochemical defect in obligate heterozygote parents either in the baseline state or with ACTH stimulation, some, but not all, showing an elevated 17-OHP:cortisol or 11-deoxycortisol:cortisol ratio (Pang et al 1980b). It is possible that the group with incomplete penetrance or late-onset of clinical symptoms may represent compound heterozygotes for one severe and one mild 11β-hydroxylase gene defect. However, just as the heterozygote states for severe and mild defects in 21-hydroxylase deficiency, for example, produce the same range of hormonal values, heterozygotes for a mild 11β-hydroxylase deficiency may not be biochemically distinguishable from normals.

CMO II deficiency Since recent biochemical studies of Hall and his group indicate that the enzymatic activities of 11β-hydroxylase and corticosterone methyl oxidase type I (CMO I; 18-hydroxylase) and type II (CMO II; 18-dehydrogenase or aldosterone synthetase) activities all reside in one protein (Yanagibashi et al 1986), it is possible that patients with CMO II deficiency may represent allelic variants of the 11β-hydroxylase deficiency. Previous studies had indicated that the 18-hydroxylase enzyme was defective in patients with the 11β-hydroxylase deficiency (Levine et al 1980b, Rosler & Leiberman 1984). CMO II deficiency presents at birth with hyponatraemic hyperkalaemia and dehydration. The disorder was first described by Royer et al (1961) and Russell et al (1963) and is reviewed by Ulick (1984). Diagnosis is established by raised precursor:product ratios of 18-hydroxytetrahydro-11-dehydrocorticoster-one (18OH-THA) to tetrahydroaldosterone (THaldo) measured in urine, or 18-hydroxycortic-osterone (18-OHB) to aldosterone in serum. A cluster of cases amongst Jews of Iranian origin was described by Rosler et al (1977b) but American pedigrees have been described as well (Veldhuis et al 1980, Lee et al 1986).

17α-Hydroxylase/17,20-lyase deficiency

17α-Hydroxylase deficiency: A 17α-hydroxylase defect reduces conversion of steroid precursors to 17-hydroxy (C_{21}) and consequently 17-keto (C_{19}) steroids; adrenal secretion of glucocorticoid and sex steroids is thus diminished, and there is overproduction of 17-deoxysteroids. Plasma DOC and especially corticosterone are elevated. The defect was first identified by Biglieri et al (1966) in a female, and first reported in a male by New (1970); additional cases have since been documented in males and females (Mantero et al 1971, Madan & Shoemaker 1980, Dean et al 1984, Scaroni et al 1986). About forty patients have been reported to date.

Corticosterone secreted in significant excess (producing plasma levels up to 60 times normal) appears to provide marginally sufficient glucocorticoid activity for survival. The hypertension and hypokalaemia are attributed to chronically elevated DOC and corticosterone. Untreated 17α-hydroxylase deficiency in females at pubertal age results in primary amenorrhoea and lack of development of secondary sex characteristics. Male pseudohermaphroditism is evident at birth and includes incomplete wolffian duct development (while Müllerian structures are absent due to normal testicular production of AMH). Lack of androgens embryonically also fails to suppress the breast anlage in males, and gynaecomastia is a prominent feature at puberty. Plasma gonadotrophins are very high in both sexes postpubertally.

While studies have shown renin levels to rise soon after glucocorticoid treatment has begun, and DOC levels to fall, it may take many months for normal aldosterone levels and proper glomerulosa function to be established (Scaroni et al 1986).

17,20-Lyase deficiency 17,20-Lyase activity resides in the same protein as 17α-hydroxylase (Kominami et al 1982). Deficiency of 17,20-lyase causes an isolated defect in the synthesis of C_{19} sex steroids (Zachmann et al 1972, 1982). Urinary pregnanetriolone, a metabolite of 17-hydroprogesterone, is increased, and increases further after ACTH and hCG stimulation, the latter observation indicating concordance for the gene defect in both adrenal gland and testes (Forest et al 1980). Testosterone or DHEA excretion does not rise appreciably. Seven patients in a total of three different kindreds with this disorder have been reported (Goebelsmann et al 1976, Forest et al 1980, Zachmann & Prader 1984). All seven patients were genetic males.

Cholesterol desmolase deficiency

This enzyme defect is extremely rare. Deficient enzymatic conversion of cholesterol to pregnenolone leads to profoundly impaired synthesis of all steroids. The condition was first described by Prader (Prader & Gurtner 1955, Prader & Siebenmann 1957) who termed it lipoid adrenal hyperplasia because of the characteristic appearance of the cholesterol-laden adrenocortical tissue. It is also known as Prader syndrome. Gonadal hypogenesis or agenesis, severe fluid and electrolyte disturbances, susceptibility to infection and addisonian pigmentation are seen, and affected individuals often do not survive beyond infancy. Further reports include histological examinations (Dhom 1958, Sasano et al 1963, Roidot et al 1964) and clinical descriptions (O'Doherty 1964, Camacho et al 1968) including one instance of a less severe deficiency (Kirkland et al 1973). A recent case report also reviewing 32 known cases in the literature describes a patient diagnosed in the newborn period who was successfully treated for 18 years (Hauffa et al 1985).

One in vitro study on specific enzymatic reaction intermediates using adrenal tissue (Degenhart et al 1972) sought to clarify the biochemical basis of the defect. This crucial initial step in steroid synthesis, which involves three distinct reactions (Hochberg et al 1974), is now known to be catalyzed by a single mitochondrial cytochrome P450 (Takikawa et al 1978).

TREATMENT

Endocrine therapy

The fundamental aim of endocrine therapy in CAH is to provide replacement of the deficient hormones. Since 1949, when Wilkins et al (1950) and Bartter et al (1951) discovered the efficacy of cortisone therapy for CAH due to 21-hydroxylase deficiency, glucocorticoid therapy has been the keystone of treatment for this disorder. Glucocorticoid administration both replaces the deficient cortisol and reduces ACTH release and overstimulation of the adrenal cortex, suppressing excessive adrenal androgen production. Proper glucocorticoid replacement therapy in 21- and 11β-hydroxylase deficiency ameliorates the noxious effects of oversecreted adrenal androgens, averting further virilization, slowing accelerated growth and bone age advancement to a more normal rate, and allowing a normal onset of puberty. Glucocorticoid treatment also leads to remission of hypertension in 11β and 17α-hydroxylase deficiencies, by diminishing oversecretion of hormonal precursors with mineralocorticoid activity. Excessive glucocorticoid administration should be avoided since this produces cushingoid facies, growth retardation, and inhibition of epiphyseal maturation. In the enzyme deficiencies impairing mineralocorticoid synthesis, the inclusion of a salt-retaining steroid in the replacement therapy is required to maintain adequate sodium balance.

Hydrocortisone (cortisol) is most often used; it is the physiological hormone and does not introduce the complication of adjustment for potency, biological half-life or altered profile of steroid action. Oral administration is the preferred and usual mode of treatment; it has conventionally been believed that better suppression of adrenal androgen production is achieved with divided doses, although this has been questioned (Winterer et al 1985); 10–20 mg/m^2 hydrocortisone divided equally in two daily doses by tablet is adequate for the otherwise healthy child. In non-life-threatening illness or stress, increased dosage of 2–3 times the maintenance regimen is indicated for a few days. Each family must be given injection kits of hydrocortisone (50 mg for young children; 100 mg for older patients) for emergency use. In the event of a surgical procedure, a total of 5–10 times the daily maintenance dose (depending on the nature of the operative procedure) may be required over the first 24 hours and can be rapidly tapered.

If there is poor response to hydrocortisone at the standard dose, dosage may be increased to 20–30 mg/m^2/d or the regimen may be changed to either one of the hormone analogues prednisone (17α,21-dihydroxypregna-1,4-diene-3,11,20-trione) or dexamethasone (9α-fluoro-16α-methylprednisolone). These agents are more potent and are longer-acting, although their relative glucocorticoid and mineralocorticoid effects differ and the smaller amounts used make dosage adjustment more critical. Because of differences in hepatic metabolism and variability in the plasma half-life of 11-oxosteroids, prednisolone (11β-hydroxyprednisone) is found in some patients to be more effective than prednisone in the replacement of cortisol function. Classical 21-hydroxylase patients with salt losing additionally require mineralocorticoid replacement. The cortisol analogue (21-acetyloxy)-9α-fluorohydrocortisone (Florinef; 9α-FF), is used for its potent mineralocorticoid activity. In an adrenal crisis a patient unable to ingest medication or take fluids is administered parenteral DOC along with liberal infusions of isotonic saline.

Increasing attention has been focused on the role of the renin-angiotensin system in 21-hydroxylase deficiency CAH. Although aldosterone levels may not be deficient in simple virilizing cases, it is well known that PRA is elevated in non-salt-wasting as well as salt-wasting 21-hydroxylase deficiency (Rosler et al 1977a, Kuhnle et al 1983). In spite of this observation, it has not been customary to attempt to correct PRA in the therapeutic management of non-salt-wasting 21-hydroxylase deficiency. Rosler et al (1977a) demonstrated that the inclusion of a salt-retaining steroid in the steroid regimen for non-salt-wasting patients with elevated PRA does in fact improve hormonal control. Rosler showed that the PRA in 21-hydroxylase deficiency patients was closely correlated to the ACTH level. Thus, when PRA was normalized by the administration of 9α-FF, the ACTH level fell and excessive adrenal androgen secretion diminished. In addition, it was found in these patients that the glucocorticoid dose could often be decreased, and that normalization of PRA often resulted in improved statural growth, a finding that has been borne out in subsequent reports (Kuhnle et al 1983).

The newly developed steroid radioimmunoassays have been useful, not only for the initial diagnosis of CAH, but also for improved monitoring of hormonal control once therapy has been instituted. Serum 17-OHP and Δ^4-androstenedione levels provide a sensitive index of biochemical control in 21-hydroxylase deficiency (Golden et al 1978, Winter 1980, Korth-Schutz et al 1978). In females and prepubertal males, but not in newborn and pubertal males, the serum testosterone level is also a useful index (Golden et al 1978). The combined determinations of PRA, 17-OHP, and serum androgens, as well as the clinical assessment of growth and pubertal status, must all be considered in adjusting the dose of glucocorticoid and salt-retaining steroid for optimal therapeutic control. Both in our clinic and in others, combinations of hydrocortisone and 9α-FF have proved to be highly effective (Winter 1980).

Measurement of PRA can be used to monitor efficacy of treatment not only in 21-hydroxylase deficiency but also in other salt-losing forms of CAH (cholesterol desmolase and 3β-HSD deficiencies). It is also useful as a therapeutic index in those forms of CAH with mineralocorticoid excess and suppressed PRA (11β-hydroxylase and 17α-hydroxylase deficiencies). In poor control, PRA is elevated in the salt-losing forms and suppressed in the mineralocorticoid excess forms.

Fertility in nonclassical 21-hydroxylase deficiency Treatment with glucocorticoids is effective in suppressing adrenal androgen production, and with time clinical signs of androgen excess show improvement. Given the 9-month life expectancy of established hair follicles, remission of hirsutism generally takes at least one or two years. Since the presumptive identification of the first nonclassical patients some 30 years ago it has been recognized that infertility in women may be reversed during glucocorticoid therapy (Jones & Jones 1954, Decourt et al 1957, Jeffries et al 1958, Birnbaum & Rose 1979). An exact timetable to regression of each clinical sign has yet to be established, but Riddick & Hammond (1975) reported that five patients with postmenarchal onset of 21-hydroxylase deficiency resumed regular menses and demonstrated adequate suppression of 17-ketosteroids and pregnanetriol within 2 months of beginning therapy with glucocorticoids alone. Birnbaum & Rose (1979) found that of 18 infertile women with acne and/or facial hirsutism and hormonal criteria consistent with 21-hydroxylase deficiency, five conceived after two months and one after seven months of prednisone

treatment alone; four more women conceived within two months of the addition of clomiphene to the therapeutic regimen. Hormonal profiles after initiation of therapy were not reported in this study. Oligospermia and subfertility have been reported in men with non-classical 21-hydroxylase deficiency (Chrousos et al 1981, Wischusen et al 1981) and reversal of infertility with glucocorticoid treatment in two men (Ojeifo et al 1984, Bonaccorsi et al 1987). In the only published study of response to ACTH stimulation in a population of men with infertility and idiopathic oligospermia, none of the 50 subjects tested by Ojeifo and colleagues demonstrated a 17-OHP response consistent with the diagnosis of nonclassical 21-hydroxylase deficiency (Ojeifo et al 1984). It is again conceivable that variations in reported disease frequency when small populations are studied are attributable to sampling error in this disorder which is more prevalent in selected ethnic groups.

Sex assignment

Sexual ambiguity at birth characteristic of male or female pseudohermaphrodism is a common presenting sign of CAH (Table 90.1). In such cases, a rational and judicious choice of sex assignment is a critical aspect of treatment, since the decision of sex assignment has obvious lifelong implications. Determination of genetic sex by karyotype or buccal smear and the accurate diagnosis of the specific underlying enzymatic defect are essential in assessing a patient's potential for future sexual activity and fertility.

In cases of female pseudohermaphrodism due to 21- or 11β-hydroxylase deficiency, a female sex assigment is appropriate. When medical treatment is begun early in life, the initially large and prominent clitoris shrinks slightly and, as the surrounding structures grow normally, it becomes much less prominent, so that surgery may not be required. When the clitoris is conspicuously enlarged or when the abnormal genitalia interfere with parent-child bonding, surgical revision to correct the appearance of the clitoris should be carried out. Definitive vaginoplasty should, in general, be performed later in childhood or in early adolescence by an experienced gynaecological surgeon (Nihoul-Fekete 1981). Because of the normal internal genitalia, gonadal structure and karyotype in these patients, normal puberty, fertility, and child-bearing are possible when there is early therapeutic intervention. In view of this potential for normal female sexual development it is unfortunate when, as a result of a hasty delivery room examination of the virilized external genitalia, affected females are improperly assigned and reared as males.

In cases of male pseudohermaphrodism due to enzyme deficiencies impairing androgen synthesis, a sex assignment consistent with the genetic sex – i.e. a male sex assignment – is not always optimal. Virilization of the genitalia in these children is frequently so extremely and irrevocably incomplete that the anatomy precludes normal male functioning. There are certain physiological capacities which we consider integral to 'normal' male sexual development: a capacity for urinating in a standing position in prepuberty, and a capacity for relatively normal, albeit infertile sexual activity and sexual development. In cases of impaired androgen synthesis, administration of sex steroids is usually required to induce development of appropriate sex characteristics at puberty – either oestrogens if the patient is to be reared as a female or androgens if reared as a male.

Society sees phenotype, not genotype. Accordingly, the genetic sex is of less consideration in the assigning of a sex of rearing for a male or female pseudohermaphrodite infant than the physiological and anatomical character of the genitalia and their potential for development and function. Because of the wide individual variability in the presentation of ambiguous genitalia, there are no all-inclusive rules for sex assignment of these patients solely on the basis of genetic sex or type of enzyme deficiency.

Psychoendocrine treatment Psychologists and psychiatrists well acquainted with these endocrine disorders provide a vital component of the treatment regimen as one of the major goals of therapy is to ensure that gender role, gender behaviour and gender identity are isosexual with the sex of assignment (Money & Ehrhardt 1972, Baker 1981).

GENETICS

Epidemiology

21-Hydroxylase deficiency The incidence of classical 21-hydroxylase deficiency as reported by several investigators in the past 30 years shows considerable variation (see Table 90.2). The highest incidence (specifically of the salt-wasting form) is found among the Yup'ik Eskimos of southwestern Alaska (Hirshfeld & Fleshman 1969); possible selective advantage maintaining an extremely high gene frequency has been proposed (Petersen et al 1984). European case survey studies give incidences ranging from 1 in 26 000 to 1 in 5041 live births (see Table 90.2); the disparity in incidence of over 3.6 to 1 between two studies in Switzerland (Prader 1958b, Prader et al 1962) in the same approximate period was attributed to better case identification in a metropolitan area (Prader et al 1962). The very low incidence in the early Maryland study (Childs et al 1956) is also probably due to incomplete case identification as well as imprecision in estimates of the study population size.

Other regional studies in the more heterogeneous North American population reported figures of 1:26 292 for salt-wasting only in one (Qazi & Thompson 1972) and 1:15 000 confirmed – but suggested closer to 1:10 000 – in a second (Rosenbloom & Smith 1966b). Results of a case survey study in Japan (Suwa et al 1981) indicate a somewhat lower frequency (1:43 674) than in Caucasian populations.

3β-ol dehydrogenase deficiency The assumption that the same gene or closely associated genes encode for both the adrenal and gonadal enzymes has recently been confirmed (Stalvey et al 1987). The separation of congenital and late-onset forms of the disease most probably results from allelism at the structural gene locus. As in the case of 21-hydroxylase deficiency, the attenuated or late-onset form of 3β-HSD deficiency is much more common than the severe deficiency form (Bongiovanni 1984, Pang et al 1985b). Although it has been claimed that the 3β-HSD deficiency is the second most common steroidogenic defect (Bongiovanni 1986), no epidemiological studies to date have verified the true frequency. There have been no reports of geographical clusters of 3β-HSD deficiency, nor is there a recognized ethnic predominance.

11β-Hydroxylase deficiency This enzyme defect accounts for approximately 5% of all cases of CAH (Wilkins 1965, Bongiovanni 1978, Werder et al 1980). The mode of genetic transmission is autosomal recessive. Linkage studies showed that 11β-hydroxylase deficiency is not linked to the HLA complex (Brautbar et al 1979, Glenthoj et al 1979, Pang et al 1980b). More recently, the gene for 11β-hydroxylase has been assigned to chromosome 8 (Chua et al 1987) (see Molecular Genetics below). While 11β-hydroxylase deficiency accounts for approximately 5% of the worldwide cases of CAH, a retrospective survey in Israel (1957-1973) revealed that 20% of that country's CAH population comprised 11β-hydroxylase deficiency patients (Porter et al 1977). There was one 11β-hydroxylase deficiency patient per 60 000 live births with a corresponding heterozygote frequency of 1/123. This unexpected clustering of cases was traced to families of North African origin, particularly Morocco and Tunisia where Jews had settled before the destruction of the Second Temple in Jerusalem by the Romans in A.D. 70, and where inbreeding had occurred until the mid-20th century. Turkish Jews have also been found to carry the 11β-hydroxylase deficiency gene in high frequency (Blunck & Bierich 1968, Rosler et al 1982, Zachmann et al 1983).

Nonclassical 21-hydroxylase deficiency Population genetic techniques were utilized to determine the frequency of nonclassical 21-hydroxylase deficiency (Speiser et al 1985) in an analysis carried out for each of a number of ethnic groups. (See also section under HLA linkage

Table 90.2   Incidence of classical CAH by case survey

Geographical area	Population	Incidence	Study	Year
Baltimore, MD, USA	heterogeneous	1:67 000	Childs et al	1956
Switzerland	Caucasian	1:18 445	Prader	1958b
Zurich, Switzerland	Caucasian	1:5041	Prader et al	1962
Wisconsin, USA	heterogenous	1:15 000	Rosenbloom & Smith	1966b
Birmingham, UK	Caucasian	1:7255	Hubble	1966
Alaska, USA	Yup'ik Eskimo	1:490	Hirschfeld &	1969
Alaska, USA	native Alaskan	1:1481	Fleshman (both)	1969
Toronto, Canada	heterogenous	1:26 292	Qazi & Thompson	1972
Munich, W Germany	Caucasian	1:9831	Mauthe et al	1977
Tyrol, Austria	Caucasian	1:8991	Muller et al	1979
Switzerland	Caucasian	1:15 472	Werder et al	1980
Wales	Caucasian	1:12 099	Murtaza et al	1980
Japan	Asiatic	1:43 674	Suwa et al	1981
France (metropolitan)	Caucasian	1:23 044	Bois et al	1985
Republic of Ireland	Caucasian	1:21 000	McKiernan	1985
Scotland	Caucasian	1:20 907	Wallace et al	1986

below). The frequencies found have more recently been confirmed in a computer-aided study using the method of commingling distributions (Sherman et al 1988). The gene frequency for nonclassical 21-hydroxylase deficiency was highest in Ashkenazi Jews and was also high in Hispanics, Yugoslavs and Italians. Disease frequencies were .037 (1/27) for Ashkenazi Jews, 0.19 (1/53) for Hispanics, .016 (1/63) for Yugoslavs, .003 (1/333) for Italians, and .001 (1/1000) for other Caucasians (Fig. 90.7). Thus nonclassical 21-hydroxylase deficiency is the most frequent autosomal recessive disease in man.

HLA and 21-hydroxylase deficiency

The human major histocompatibility complex (MHC), or HLA, is an extended genetic segment of approximately 3500 kb located on the short arm of chromosome 6 (between subregions 6p21.1 and 6p21.3). This assembly contains the genes for the cell-surface antigens that are the major barriers for allogenic transplantation (hence the name MHC), and others providing a basis for control of the immune response in lymphocytes, but also a number of genes for factors with functions outside histocompatibility and immune responses including the genes encoding the adrenal cytochrome P450 specific for steroid 21-hydroxylation (Fig. 90.8).

Classical genetic analysis showed the HLA complex to span a recombination distance of approximately 3 cM (centiMorgans) (Baur et al 1984). During the period 1976–1982 the gene for 21-hydroxylase deficiency was mapped within HLA between HLA-B and HLA-DR (a distance of 0.8 cM), segregating more frequently with HLA-B (New 1988). Molecular genetic studies soon led to isolation and characterization of essentially all active genes within the MHC (Moller 1985a,b,c).

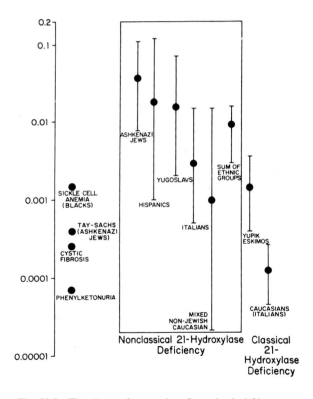

DISEASE FREQUENCY:

AUTOSOMAL RECESSIVE GENETIC DISORDERS

Fig. 90.7   The disease frequencies of nonclassical 21-hydroxylase deficiency and classical 21-hydroxylase deficiency relative to other common autosomal recessive disorders. Bars represent 95% confidence ranges. (From Speiser et al 1985, with permission).

A 1000 kb segment contains the loci for HLA antigens A, B and C (the main components of Class I), expressed on most somatic cell types, while HLA-D (Class II) antigens expressed by activated lymphocytes are coded for in a more proximally situated 800-1000 kb segment (Hardy et al 1986).

Approximately 20 genes have been identified occupying the Class I regions in addition to the well-characterized HLA-A, -B and -C genes; the presence of other Class I-like genes – some pseudogenes and some appearing to be expressed – is still puzzling. The class II region in man has been subdivided into three major subregions, DP, DQ and DR, each encoding both a and β chains (Bell et al 1985). Genomic cloning, clarifying the original serological determinations, has led to the identification of as many as 15 different Class II genes per HLA haplotype. Cloning from DNA libraries has identified seven expressed genes per haplotype: one DR-a and two DR-β genes, one DQ-a and one DQ-β gene, one DP-a and one DP-β gene. In addition, RNA has been found in some cell lines for genes termed DO-β and DZ-a.

Class III is situated between Class I and II. In this region are found the gene loci for the second and fourth components of serum complement (C2, C4A and C4B) and properdin factor B (Bf), and for adrenal steroid 21-hydroxylase, OH21A and OH21B (Moller 1985c). The genes encoding tumour necrosis factors, cachectin (TNF-α) and lymphotoxin (TNF-β), have now also been mapped to Class III of the MHC in both mouse (Nedospasov et al 1986) and man (Spies et al 1986). From a recently prepared restriction map of the MHC, a length of about 3500 kb has been established and the entire region is presumed to contain at least 50 genes (Caroll et al 1987) (Fig. 90.8.).

HLA linkage

Linkage between HLA and 21-hydroxylase deficiency was first shown by Dupont et al (1977). Reports from the same group (Levine et al 1978) and other groups soon after (New 1988) confirmed linkage with HLA. Compiled data on intra-HLA recombinations strongly indicated a gene locus for 21-hydroxylase between HLA-B and – DR (Dupont et al 1981). The more recent molecular studies have confirmed this location in Class III. Steriod 21-hydroxylase deficiency is a monogenic trait, and the close genetic linkage of the 21-hydroxylase gene to HLA is utilized for genotyping sibs in pedigrees with an affected index case; thus a sib sharing both HLA haplotypes with the index case is predicted to be affected, one who shares a single haplotype is predicted to be a heterozygote, and one who shares no HLA haplotype is predicted to be unaffected.

Linkage disequilibrium The study by Dupont et al (1977) first showing linkage between HLA and the gene for 21-hydroxylase deficiency obtained a total maximum lod score of 3.394 (recombinant fraction $\theta = 0.00$) with data from six families. The most recent calculated lod scores are in excess of 22 ($\theta = 0.00$). In addition to linkage of the 21-hydroxylase locus with the neighbouring HLA-B and -DR antigen loci, 21-hydroxylase deficiency alleles are found in linkage disequilibrium with HLA antigen genes or haplotypic combinations that may include specific alleles of complement component C4 (Awdeh et al 1983). The salt-wasting form of 21-hydroxylase deficiency shows increased association with HLA-Bw60(40) and with HLA-Bw47 within the extended haplotype HLA-A3,Bw47,DR7, which also carries a null allele at C4B (Klouda et al 1978, Dupont et al 1984). Simple

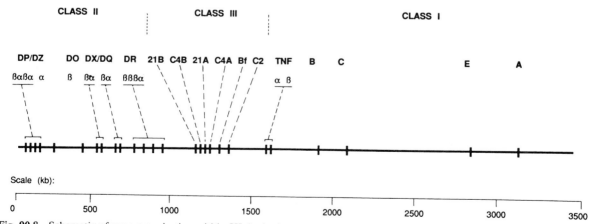

Fig. 90.8 Schematic of gene organization within HLA, the human major histocompatibility complex (after Carroll et al 1987. PNAS 84:8535) Order and spacing determined from restriction map prepared from results of pulsed-field gel electrophoresis and Southern blot analysis using five different restriction endonucleases (NotI, NruI, MluI, SalI and BssHI) and DNA probes (11 cDNA probes and 6 genomic DNA probes; sites not shown). (Pulse f 1/60 to 1/30 sec^{-1}. Limit of resolution : 50 kb fragments).

virilizing disease is associated with HLA-Bw51(5) in selected ethnic groups (Dupont et al 1984). Nonclassical disease is associated with the partial haplotype HLA-B14,DR1 which has been shown to have a duplicated C4 isotype (O'Neill et al 1982, Fleischnick et al 1983, Raum et al 1984). The nonclassical association with HLA-B14;DR1 has been observed in all ethnic groups examined except the Yugoslav population (Kastelan et al 1985, Speiser et al 1985). Negative association with 21-hydroxylase deficiency has been noted for the haplotype HLA-A1,B8,DR3, which carries a null allele at C4A; this haplotype occurs with somewhat greater frequency in certain autoimmune disorders.

Population genetics of nonclassical 21-hydroxylase deficiency Nonclassical 21-hydroxylase deficiency (NC21-OHD) cannot be reliably detected by random measurement of serum 17-OHP concentrations, as values obtained outside the early morning diurnal peak may not differ from normal. The frequency of occurrence of NC21-OHD has been studied using known HLA-B associations in conjunction with ACTH testing in families (Speiser et al 1985). Affected status in the parents was determined by ACTH testing using criteria provided by reference hormone data (New et al 1983b). By counting the incidence of nonclassical deficiency genes relative to the presumed normal genes among allowed parental haplotypes, the frequency of nonclassical 21-hydroxylase deficiency was calculated. Thus, for example, from among the Ashkenazi Jewish families in the named study:

1. There were 94 parental haplotypes, of which 47 were obligate 21-hydroxylase deficiency haplotypes and the other 47 represented, a priori, a random sample of (normal and 21-OH deficiency) haplotypes in the population.
2. Of the parents, nine were found on hormonal testing to be nonclassical patients rather than heterozygotes.
3. The gene frequency, q, for the nonclassical 21-hydroxylase gene is estimated as:

$$\frac{9 \text{ (nonclassical genes)}}{47 \text{ (random genes)}} = 0.191 \text{ or } 1/5$$

(95% confidence limits: 0.092 to 0.333)

4. By the Hardy-Weinberg law for a population at equilibrium (Cavalli-Sforza & Bodmer 1971), the heterozygote frequency ($2pq$) is:

$$2(0.191)(0.809) = 0.309$$

or approximately 1/3; and

5. therefore the nonclassical disease frequency (q^2) is:

0.037 or 1/27

(95% confidence limits: 0.008 to 0.111, or 1/125 to 1/9).

This analysis was carried out for each ethnic group studied. The gene frequency for NC21-OHD was highest in Ashkenazi Jews (19.1%) and was also high in Hispanics (13.6%), Yugoslavs (12.5%) and Italians (5.8%). In other Caucasians, 41% of whom had some Anglo-Saxon ancestry, the gene frequency was 3.2%. Corresponding heterozygote frequencies were: 1/3 for Ashkenazi Jews; 1/4 for Hispanics; 1/5 for Yugoslavs; 1/9 for Italians; 1/14 for other Caucasians. Disease frequencies were: 1/27 for Ashkenazi Jews, 1/53 for Hispanics, 1/63 for Yugoslavs, 1/333 for Italians, and 1/1000 for other Caucasians (see Table 90.3). Confirmation of this approach was obtained by the affected sib pair method of Thomson & Bodmer (1977). These overall gene and disease frequencies and ethnic specificities were independently confirmed in a more recent computer-aided study analyzing family data by the method of commingling distributions (Sherman et al 1988).

MOLECULAR GENETICS

Steroid 21-hydroxylase

The initial molecular genetic analysis of 21-hydroxylase deficiency made use of the known associations between this disorder, specific HLA antigens and alleles of HLA linked complement loci. In particular, salt-wasting 21-hydroxylase deficiency is often (15–20% of all alleles) associated with an extended HLA haplotype A3,Bw47, DR7. This haplotype carries a null allele at one of the C4 loci encoding the fourth component of serum complement (O'Neill et al 1982, Fleischnick et al 1983, Raum et al 1984). Because 21-hydroxylase and C4 loci are both affected on this haplotype, it was hypothesized that a single major DNA deletion or arrangement had affected both loci. Therefore, to determine if the HLA-linked defect in 21-hydroxylase deficiency involved a structural gene for the P450c21, a bovine cDNA clone encoding part of this enzyme was hybridized with Southern blots of DNA samples obtained from normal individuals and from patients with 21-hydroxylase deficiency who carried the Bw47 haplotype. It was found that normal DNA samples after digestion with several restriction endonucleases yielded two fragments hybridizing with the probe at equal intensity. After analysis in this manner, DNA from an HLA-Bw47 homozygous patient showed total absence of one of these bands, consistent

Table 90.3 Nonclassical 21-hydroxylase (NC21-OHD) gene and disease frequencies (Part A)

A. Hormonal criteria[a]

| Ethnic group[b] | Total | Parental Haplotypes | | Gene frequency (q) | Disease frequency (q²) | Heterozygotes frequency (2q.(1-q)) |
| | | Random | | | | |
		Total	Affected[c]			
Ashkenazi Jewish	94	47	9	0.191 (0.089–0.308)	0.037 (0.0079–0.099)	0.309 (0.162–0.431)
Hispanic	44	22	3	0.136 (0.015–0.302)	0.019 (0.0002–0.091)	0.235 (0.085–0.421)
Yugoslav	80	40	5	0.125 (0.035–0.240)	0.016 (0.0001–0.058)	0.219 (0.061–0.366)
Italian	208	104	6	0.058 (0.018–0.108)	0.003 (0.0003–0.012)	0.109 (0.034–0.195)
Other Caucasians[b]	112	56	2	0.036[d] (<0.001–0.094)	0.001 (<0.0001–0.008)	0.069 (<0.001–0.163)
Black American	14	7	0	–[d]	–	–
American Indian	4	2	0	–[d]	–	–
Sum of all groups	556	278	25	0.090 (0.058–0.125)	0.009 (0.003–0.016)	0.164 (0.104–0.221)

B. Sib pair analyses

Ethnic group[b]	Total haplotypes	Sib pairs sharing one HLA haplotype	Gene frequency (q)	Disease frequency (q²)	Heterozygotes frequency (2q·(1-q))
Mixed ethnic group[e]	18	3 (0.401–6.601)	0.100 (0.050–0.300)	0.010 (0.0025–0.090)	0.180 (0.095–0.421)

a – Only parents who had undergone ACTH testing were included.
b – Ethnic background was homogeneous in each category except 'Other Caucasians' which includes non-Jewish persons of German, French, Polish, Russian, Hungarian, Greek, Anglo-Saxon and Nordic origin.
c – As revealed by ACTH testing
d – Because of low disease frequency in these ethnic groups, more families must be studied.
e – Including Ashkenazi Jews, Anglo-Saxons, Italians, Hispanics, Germans and American Indians.

with a deletion of one of two P450c21 (i.e. steroid 21-hydroxylase) genes (White et al 1984a,b) (Fig. 90.9A,E).

From the probable extent of a single deletion on the HLA-Bw47 haplotype encompassing the 21-hydroxylase and null C4 gene loci, it appeared that these genes were very closely situated. Their precise arrangement was determined by examination of long (40 kb) cosmid clones originally isolated for study of C4 (White et al 1985, Carroll et al 1985a,b).

There are two 21-hydroxylase genes, A and B, each adjacent to one of the C4 genes; all four genes of this tandem arrangement are transcribed in the same direction (White et al 1985) (Fig. 90.10). The position of the class III genes relative to the direction of transcription has been known for some time. It has recently been shown that the entire class III segment is oriented on the chromosome in the opposite direction from that presumed formerly; thus the gene order of class III is (distal. . .B-) C2-Bf-C4A-21A-C4B-21B (-DR. . .centromere) (Dunham et al 1987, Carroll et al 1987) (Fig. 90.9). The current nomenclature is CYP21 (B gene) and

CYP21P (A pseudogene) (formerly CYP21A and CYP21B); other names in the literature are OH21A/OH21B (White et al 1987), P450C21A/P450C21B (Nebert & Gonzales 1987) and CA21H-A/CA21H-B (McKusick 1986).

The functional roles of these genes were deduced by comparing Southern blots of cosmid DNA with blots of uncloned DNA from patients with 21-hydroxylase deficiency and from selected normal individuals (White et al 1985). The restriction endonuclease Taq I excises a 3.2 kb genomic fragment within the CYP21P gene, while the CYP21 gene carries a 3.7 kb Taq I fragment; both fragments hybridize with a 21-hydroxylase cDNA probe. The 3.7 kb Taq 1 fragment was not found in DNA from individuals with the Bw47/Bw47 genotype, the presence of severe salt-wasting disease in these patients suggesting that expression of the CYP21 gene product is necessary for steroid 21-hydroxylation. By contrast, no 3.2 kb fragment was observed in the Taq I digest of DNA from hormonally normal individuals homozygous for HLA-AI;B8;DR3 (this haplotype is itself negatively associated with 21-hydroxylase deficiency), and thus absence of CYP21P is without clinical effect (White et al 1985, Garlepp et al 1986) (Fig. 90.9B,D). The boundaries of these deletions have been determined by detailed mapping of restriction endonuclease recognition sites and by using cloned cDNA encoding C4. The HLA-

A1,B8,DR3 haplotype carries a deletion of both C4A and CYP21P, consistent with the null allele for C4A which is known to occur on this haplotype (Carroll et al 1985b, Donohoue et al 1986a, Garlepp et al 1986). This haplotype occurs in about 5% of all normal chromosomes (Dupont et al 1981). In contrast, the A3,Bw47,DR7

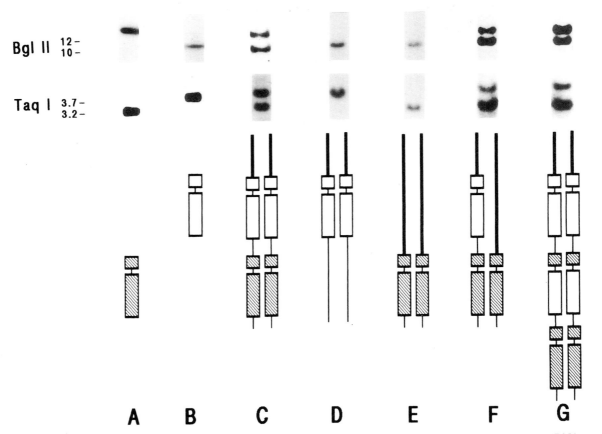

Fig. 90.9 Analysis of 21-hydroxylase deficiency of genomic blot hybridization. Samples of cloned and uncloned human DNA were digested with restriction endonucleases Taq I or Bgl II, subjected to agarose gel electrophoresis, blotted to nitrocellulose and hybridized with a radioactive probe encoding 21-hydroxylase (P450c21). Hybridizing fragments of 3.7 or 3.2 kb (Taq I) or 10 or 12 kb (Bgl II) were observed. These respectively correspond to the CYP21B or CYP21 (unfilled bar) and CYP21A or CYP21P (filled bar) genes in normal DNA (see previous figure). The C4A and C4B genes are also shown.
A: cloned CYP21A gene. **B:** cloned CYP21B gene. **C:** DNA from a normal individual. Each of the subject's two chromosomes 6 has an A and a B gene, yielding a pattern with two fragments of equal intensity for both digests. **D:** hormonally normal individual homozygous for the HLA haplotype A1;B8;DR3. The absence of the CY21A pseudogene has no apparent clinical effect. **E:** patient with 21-hydroxylase deficiency, homozygous for HLA-A3;Bw47;DR7. The CYP21B gene is deleted. Note that Bgl II digests for this and D above (deletion of CYP21A) are identical. **F:** patient with 21-hydroxylase deficiency, heterozygous for HLA-A3;Bw47;DR7. Such a patient has a total of two A genes and one B gene, and so the 3.7 kb Taq I band is less intense than the 3.2 kb band, and the 12 kb Bgl II band is also decreased in intensity. The non-deleted CYP21B gene presumably has a small mutation not detectable with these techniques. **G:** patient with nonclassical 21-hydroxylase deficiency, homozygous for HLA-B14;DR1. This patient has a total of four A genes and two B genes, so that the hybridization pattern after Taq I digestion is indistinguishable from that of the patient with a heterozygous deletion (i.e., a 2:1 ratio of intensity of the 3.2 and 3.7 kb Taq I bands). However, the Bgl II pattern has increased intensity of the 21 kb band, reflecting the extra CYP21A genes (From New et al 1989b, The metabolic basis of inherited disease, 6th edn., Chap 74, McGraw-Hill, with permission.)

haplotype has C4B deleted as well as CYP21, explaining the null C4B allele on this haplotype (Awdeh et al 1983). This latter deletion 'splices' the chromosomal region 3' of the CYP21 gene onto the CYP21P gene, causing the CYP21P gene to migrate like a CYP21 gene on electrophoresis after DNA is digested with certain restriction endonucleases. Accurate identification of deletions is difficult in such cases (Mornet et al 1986a) and may lead to errors of interpretation of Southern blots (Matteson et al 1987) (Fig. 90.9).

The apparent lack of function of the CYP21P gene has been explained by nucleotide sequence analysis (White et al 1986, Higashi et al 1986). The A and B genes are about 98% homologous in their coding regions. A nearly full-length cDNA clone derived from human fetal adrenal glands is identical with the reading sequence of CYP21, while the exonic sequence of the CYP21P gene shows significant small differences: there are two shifts of reading frame, from an 8 base-pair (bp) deletion and a single bp insertion, a nonsense mutation, and several non-conservative amino acid substitutions. As the frameshift and nonsense mutations prevent an active protein from being synthesized, it was concluded that the OHA21A gene is a pseudogene. The C4 and 21-hy-

droxylase gene arrangement probably arose by tandem duplication of a single set of these genes at some time in the past. While both C4 genes have remained active in man, only one 21-hydroxylase gene was necessary for normal steroidogenesis, so the extra gene accumulated deleterious mutations with no apparent ill-effects on the organism.

The tandemly duplicated C4 and 21-hydroxylase gene arrangement creates the possibility of misalignment and unequal crossing-over between chromatids during meiosis, resulting in chromosomes containing one or three sets of C4 and 21-hydroxylase genes (Fig. 90.11). This mechanism presumably created the rearrangements observed in the HLA-A1,B8,DR3 and A3,Bw47,DR7 haplotypes, on which the C4A-CYP21P and C4B-CYP21 gene pairs respectively have been deleted (Carroll et al 1985b). In the HLA-B14,DR1 haplotype associated with nonclassical 21-hydroxylase deficiency a third C4 gene was suggested by electrophoretic separation of the C4 proteins (Raum et al 1984), and analysis of DNA from individuals carrying this haplotype has identified a third set of genes, consisting of an extra C4B gene (Carroll et al 1984) and an extra CYP21P or CYP21P-like gene, based on the sizes of the extra restriction enzyme fragments

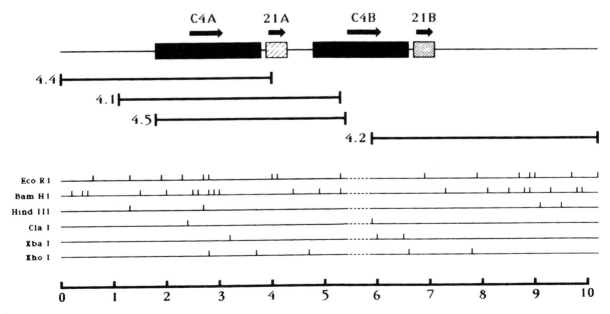

Fig. 90.10 Map showing the extents of four C4/21-hydroxylase cosmid clones and recognition sites for six endonuclease enzymes within a length of 100 kb. Dotted lines mark segment with no overlapping of cosmids. Direction of transcription of the 21-hydroxylase genes was deduced by determining lengths of BamHI/EcoRI double digest fragments hybridizing to 5'- and 3'- end probes, and fitting these to the restriction sites. Limits and orientation of the C4 genes taken from published data (Carroll M C et al 1984. Philosophical Transactions of the Royal Society of London B306:379). Size and position of 21-hydroxylase A and B is that of the Taq I fragment carrying most of the gene in each case (From White et al 1985).

(Garlepp et al 1986, Werkmeister et al 1986). If the extra CYP21P gene is a pseudogene like the normally present CYP21P gene, it should not contribute to the development of the nonclassical 21-hydroxylase deficiency phenotype, instead merely signalling the causative lesion, presumably an associated CYP21 gene mutation.

While the HLA-B14,DR1 haplotype and nonclassical 21-hydroxylase deficiency are very common, the HLA-A3,Bw47,DR7 haplotype is extremely rare in the normal population and only comprises perhaps 20% of classical 21-hydroxylase deficiency alleles. Additional patients with nonclassical 21-hydroxylase deficiency who do not carry the HLA-Bw47 haplotype have been examined by hybridization analysis using 21-hydroxylase and/or C4 probes (Rumsby et al 1986, Werkmeister et al 1986). Approximately one quarter of the alleles in these patients have deletions of the CYP21 gene; the majority of such alleles also have a deletion of C4B. In one family, on one chromosome a second CYP21P gene has been substituted for CYP21 (Donohoue et al 1986b). All patients with homozygous deletions of the CYP21 gene have salt-wasting 21-hydroxylase deficiency.

The remaining three quarters of classical alleles do not have associated restriction fragment polymorphisms and cannot be detected by Southern blot hybridization. Small exchanges of sequences between homologous genes, termed gene conversions, could cause many of these alleles by transfering one of the deleterious mutations from the CYP21P pseudogene to the CYP21 gene. Gene conversion has been previously documented in other cytochrome P450 genes (Atchison & Adesnik 1986). Thus far, a number of gene conversions have been documented in mutant CYP21 genes (Rodrigues et al 1987, Amor et al 1988, Globerman et al 1988, Higashi et al 1988, Speiser et al 1988). One of these transfers the point mutation producing a stop codon (nonsense mutation) at position 318 from the CYP21P gene into CYP21 (Globerman et al 1988), while another changes isoleucine-172 to asparagine (Amor et al 1988), possibly affecting interactions between the P450 protein and the membrane of the endoplasmic reticulum. Each of these mutations was noted in three of 20 patients with classical 21-hydroxylase deficiency. All patients with the nonsense mutation have salt-wasting disease, whereas the patients

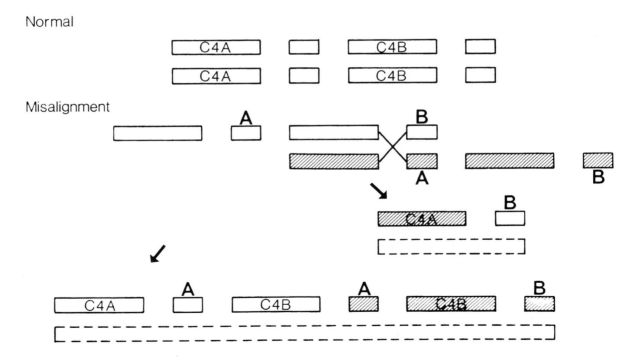

Fig. 90.11 Schematic showing normal aligment of the C4A-A-C4B-B chromosomal segments, and misalignment with crossing over during meiosis. This unequal exchange between the non-sister homologues results in one set of C4 and 21-hydroxylase genes on one chromatid and three sets on the other. Haplotypes such as HLA-B8;DR3 carry a single such set, while the triplicate arrangement seen here occurs on haplotype HLA-B14;DR1 associated with nonclassical 21-hydroxylase deficiency. (From New et al 1989c Recent Advances in Endocrinology 3, Churchill Livingstone, with permission).

with the asparagine-172 mutation have retained the ability to synthesize aldosterone (two have simple virilizing disease, while one has an elevated plasma renin:aldosterone ratio without clinical salt-wasting). One patient with salt-wasting disease carries a larger rearrangement involving exons 3–6 that transfers an 8 bp deletion from CYP21P to CYP21, shifting the reading frame of translation and preventing synthesis of a functional protein (Rodrigues et al 1987).

These data suggest that gene conversions are about as common as deletions as a cause of 21-hydroxylase deficiency alleles. However, one report (Matteson et al 1987) suggesting that most deletions of CYP21 are instead gene conversions is incorrect, containing misinterpretations of data (in particular, confusion between deletions of CYP21P and CYP21).

Other alleles may carry point mutations affecting transcription of the gene or processing of RNA, or that result in amino acid substitutions altering enzymatic function. One mutant gene from an individual with salt-wasting 21-hydroxylase deficiency has two mutations: serine-269 is changed to threonine, and asparagine-494 is changed to serine. However, neither of these residues is conserved in P450c21 from other species, and so the functional significance of these mutations is unclear.

In general, the molecular genetic characterization of patients with different forms of 21-hydroxylase deficiency suggests that clinical severity is roughly correlated with the severity of each mutation. Thus, deletions, nonsense mutations, frameshifts and presumably some amino acid substitutions result in salt-wasting alleles, one non-conservative substitution causes a simple-virilizing allele, and a conservative substitution is associated with a nonclassical allele. It should be pointed out that the distinctions between these diagnostic categories are not absolute; some males diagnosed as having simple virilizing 21-hydroxylase deficiency by hormonal testing in fact carry the presumed nonclassical allele associated with HLA-B14,DR1. Conversely, some patients with documented episodes of salt-wasting in infancy develop the ability to synthesize adequate amounts of aldosterone later in life. This recovery might result from increased expression of a poorly active P450c21, or from individual variations in level of some other P450 enzyme, distinct from P450c21, with some 21-hydroxylase activity (Tukey et al 1985, Muller-Eberhard et al 1985).

Steroid 11β-hydroxylase and the other enzymes (see Table 90.4)

Steroid 11β-hydroxylase If this disorder follows the model of 21-hydroxylase deficiency (the first CAH disorder in which a mutation in the structural gene has been correlated with disease) then presumably mutations in the structural gene for the 11β-hydroxylase/CMO-I/II enzyme complex can reproduce the spectrum of clinical symptoms from hypertension and virilism to salt wasting without virilism. As no mutations causing any of the clinical syndromes of 11β-hydroxylase or CMO I or II deficiency have yet been identified, it remains for future studies to elucidate whether the clinical polymorphism results from genetic allelism.

A cDNA clone encoding human P450c11 has been isolated and used to locate the corresponding structural gene on the long arm of chromosome 8 (Chua et al 1987). Mutually confirmatory results were obtained by hybridization in situ to metaphase spreads of human chromosomes, and hybridization to a panel of human-rodent somatic cell hybrids of known chromosomal composition (Chua et al 1987). Other genes of interest in this chromosomal region include the MYC and MOS cellular oncogenes, glutamic-pyruvate transaminase, thyroglobulin and the DNA polymerase β polypeptide. Further studies will be required to establish a linkage map of the structural gene in relation to other genes. It has been determined (Mornet et al 1989) that there are two closely linked homologues; these are termed CYP11B1 and CYP11B2.

3β-ol dehydrogenase In contrast with the other adrenal steroidogenic enzymes, the 3β-ol dehydrogenase enzyme, a dehydrogenase typically requiring NAD^+ as a cofactor, is not a cytochrome P450. Closely associated with 3β-ol dehydrogenase is the enzyme activity 3-ketosteroid Δ^{5-4} isomerase, which requires NAD^+ or NADH. In mammalian species these two functions appear to reside within the same protein, but the enzyme generally has not been well characterized. Purified rat adrenal and testicular 3β-ol dehydrogenase/Δ^{5-4} isomerase enzymes exhibited the same molecular weight (46.5 kDa) and similar catalytic activities (Ishii-Ohba et al 1987).

The gene encoding 3β-ol dehydrogenase/Δ^{5-4} isomerase has not been cloned. Deficiency of 3β-ol dehydrogenase is not linked to the HLA complex (Pang et al 1983). A recent study showed in several strains of mouse that 3β-ol dehydrogenase is encoded by the same structural gene in the adrenals and gonads, and is under separate regulatory control genetically in these two tissues (Stalvey et al 1987).

17α-Hydroxylase Earlier, family studies showed no HLA association with this enzyme defect (Mantero et al 1980, D'Armiento et al 1983). The P450c17 structural gene (CYP17) has now been located on chromosome 10 (Matteson et al 1986a), but thus far has not been regionally localized. Apparently the same gene is expressed in both the adrenal and the testis (Chung et al 1987). Other genes have been reported but not mapped

Table 90.4 The forms of adrenal hyperplasia: molecular genetic aspects

Deficiency (syndrome)	Enzyme	Chromosomal location	Frequency	Gene	Gene cloned
Cholesterol desmolase (lipoid hyperplasia)	P450scc	15	rare	CYP11A (tentative)	yes
3β-ol dehydrogenase					
a. classical	3β-HSD/$\Delta^{5\text{-}4}$SI	–	rare	–	no
b. nonclassical	3β-HSD/$\Delta^{5\text{-}4}$SI	–	frequent (?)	–	no
17α-hydroxylase	P450c17	10	rare	CYP17	yes
17,20-lyase	P450c17	10	rare	CYP17	yes
21-hydroxylase					
a. classical	P450c21	6p	1/12 000	CYP21B	yes
salt wasting		(HLA-B40; HLA-Bw47,DR7)	75%		
simple virilizing		(HLA-B51(5))	25%		
b. nonclassical (symptomatic and asymptomatic)	P450c21	6p (HLA-B14;DR1)	0.1–1% (3% in European Jews)	CYP21B	–
11β-hydroxylase					
a. classical (hypertensive CAH)	P450c11	8q	1/100 000	CYP11B1	yes
b. nonclassical	P450c11	8q	frequent (?)	CYP11B1	–
CMO-II (corticosterone methyl oxidase type II)	P450c11	8q (?)	rare (except in Iranian Jews)	CYP11B11 or CYP11B2	–

(Voutilainen & Miller 1987). Hybridization studies of DNA samples from patients with 17α-hydroxylase deficiency have not demonstrated gross deletions or rearrangements of this gene (Bradshaw et al 1987), and the disease is sufficiently rare for linkage studies to be difficult to perform.

Cholesterol desmolase (P450scc) The gene for this mitochondrial P450 enzyme (tentatively CYP11A) has been isolated, cloned, and localized to chromosome 15 (Chung et al 1986). Mutation of the structural gene has not yet been identified in lipoid adrenal hyperplasia (Matteson et al 1986b); remote lesions, affecting other cellular components fundamental to early steroidogenesis could have similar effects.

PRENATAL DIAGNOSIS

Amniocentesis

Since the report by Jeffcoate et al (1965) of the successful identification of an affected fetus by elevated concentrations of 17-ketosteroids and pregnanetriol in the amniotic fluid, several investigators have undertaken prenatal diagnosis for congenital adrenal hyperplasia by similar measurements of hormone levels in pregnancy (New & Levine 1973, Levine 1986). The most specific hormonal diagnostic test for 21-hydroxylase deficiency is amniotic fluid 17-OHP (Frasier et al 1975, Nagamani et al 1978, Hughes & Laurence 1979, Pang et al 1980a, Hughes &

Laurence 1982); Δ^4-androstenedione may be employed as an adjunctive diagnostic assay (Pang et al 1980a). It has been suggested that elevated amniotic fluid 21-deoxycortisol may also be a marker for 21-hydroxylase deficiency (Blankstein et al 1980b). Amniotic fluid testosterone levels may not be outside the normal range in the case of an affected male (Frasier et al 1974, Pang et al 1980b).

HLA genotyping of a fetus in a family with an affected sib provides an additional method for prenatal diagnosis of 21-hydroxylase deficiency (Couillin et al 1979, Pollack et al 1979). Fetal HLA typing is done by standard serological testing of cells cultured from the amniotic fluid. Whether or not the fetus is affected is determined by comparison with the HLA genotypes of the parents and affected sib(s) as in family studies. Exceptions are found in cases of intra-HLA recombination. Because Class II (HLA-DR) antigens are not expressed in these cell cultures, recombination on either fetal haplotype occuring in the B to DR segment and possibly including the 21-hydroxylase locus will not be detected. Possible homozygosity at the HLA-B locus in either parent and antigen sharing between parents are factors limiting categorization of the fetal 21-hydroxylase genotype by this method.

Amniotic fluid assay for 17-OHP should thus still be performed, since anomalous hormone levels may in some cases call into question the HLA result. Forest et al (1981), in evaluating 17 pregnancies at risk for CAH, found in two cases in which HLA-A and B typing of amniotic cell cultures predicted an affected fetus, that amniotic fluid hormone levels were normal. These pregnancies were terminated, and while the inconsistency of test results could have been due to recombination between HLA-B and DR, the authors postulated that there may also have been an enzyme defect not expressed in mid-gestation. Pang et al (1985b) have reported normal amniotic fluid 17-OHP and Δ^4-A levels in affected cases. In one case, where the infant proved postnatally to have simple virilizing 21-hydroxylase deficiency, the fetus was haploidentical (maternal) with the affected older sib, and was predicted to be a carrier. Because of a paternal recombination, HLA typing-hampered also in this case by antigen sharing between the parents – failed to identify inheritance of the second 21-hydroxylase deficiency allele prenatally. (The recombination was revealed postnatally by peripheral blood leucocyte HLA typing.) In a second case, normal amniotic fluid hormone levels did not contribute to the diagnosis for a nonclassically affected fetus, and the HLA identical index case, also affected with nonclassical deficiency, had earlier been miscategorized as a classical patient. These were the only two negative results in a total of 32 pregnancies at risk for 21-hydroxylase deficiency. A third diagnostic error in this series resulted from the HLA identity of a normal fetus (with normal hormone values) with the index case, thought to be classically affected; the diagnosis of both sibs was later corrected to normal.

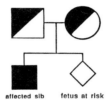

affected sib   fetus at risk

1. Pre-pregnancy:

a) Hybridization analysis using HLA class I and II cDNA probes in genomic DNA digests from father. mother and affected sib (*RFLPs)

b) Serologic testing for HLA class I and II antigens

c) ACTH (adrenocorticotropin) stimulation testing

2. In pregnancy:

FETAL AGE	DIAGNOSTIC TEST	RESULT	THERAPY
a) 8-10 days	Pregnancy test (β-hCG assay)	positive	dexamethasone
b) 8-11 weeks	Chorionic villus biopsy		
	i) Ascertain sex of fetus (karyotype cultured cells)	M / F	stop dexamethasone / continue dexamethasone
	ii) Hybridization analysis comparing fetal RFLPs with those of proband	affected F	continue dexamethasone
	iii) HLA serotypes of cultured villus cells	unaffected F	stop dexamethasone
c) 16 weeks	Amniocentesis (if CVB risk unacceptable or if CVB results equivocal)		
	i) sex	(as above)	(as above)
	ii) HLA serotype of cultured amniotic cells	(as above)	(as above)
	iii) +17-OHP level in amniotic fluid (RIA)		

* - RFLPs: restriction fragment length polymorphisms

+ - not useful if mother is on dexamethasone

Fig. 90.12 Algorithm depicting prenatal management of pregnancy in families at risk for a fetus affected with 21-hydroxylase deficiency. Current dosage recommendation for dexamethasone to the mother is 20 μg/kg per 24 hours, divided 2 (or 3) times, orally.

Chorionic villus biopsy

With the advent of chorionic villus biopsy (CVB), evaluation of the fetus at risk is now possible in the first trimester at 8–11 weeks' gestation. As normative standards for hormonal levels measurable at this early stage remain to be established, CVB diagnosis at present depends on HLA typing of the chorionic tissue. A new option is HLA typing by molecular genetic techniques, which indentifies HLA polymorphisms in the genes for antigens of both Class I (HLA-A, B, C) and Class II (HLA-DR) with the aid of specific probes (Mornet et al 1986b). This technique is more exact (it has already begun to resolve subgroups of the standard serological specificities), and the availability of Class II probes makes possible the identification of B/DR recombinations. It is interesting to note that in the French experience, amniotic fluid 17-OHP was clearly elevated even at 10–13 weeks' gestation in three affected pregnancies; there was no discordance between hormonal results and restriction fragment length polymorphism-based diagnostic prediction in seven families studied (Mornet et al 1986b). An algorithm for diagnostic management of potentially affected pregnancies is given in Figure 90.12.

It is currently estimated that 25% of classical 21-hydroxylase deficiency alleles carry a deletion of the active 21-hydroxylase B gene (Werkmeister et al 1986). Identification of the presumed sequence aberrations occurring in the remaining 80% of cases will depend on the appearance of characteristic RFLPs in digests of genomic DNA samples. It is hoped that, with the characterization of specific non-deletional mutations, a growing panel of oligonucleotide probes informative in the resolution of 21-OHD genotypes may be used in prenatal diagnosis.

Prenatal treatment

Treatment with dexamethasone has recently been employed in pregnancies at risk for 21-hydroxylase deficiency (Evans et al 1985, Dorr et al 1986, Forest et al 1987). In pregnancies at risk for 21-hydroxylase deficiency where treatment was begun at 3–10 weeks' gestation (dexamethasone orally) all had complete suppression of adrenocortical hormones at amniocentesis. Only when dexamethasone therapy was discontinued for 5–7 days before amniotic fluid sampling, were the amniotic fluid hormone levels elevated. Masculinization

of genitalia was completely prevented in one of three affected female fetuses and partially prevented in another female. In the third case where treatment failed, the mother had begun dexamethasone at 10 weeks and terminated therapy at 28 weeks. No congenital malformations were found in any of the 21 treated fetuses (Forest et al 1987). The failure of one group of investigators to find evidence of suppression of the fetal pituitary-adrenal axis after acute administration of dexamethasone at midterm (Charnvises et al 1985) is not necessarily reflective of the situation in which sustained therapy is begun in the first trimester. German investigators (Dorr et al 1986) also found high amniotic fluid 17-OHP levels in two pregnancies at risk for CAH treatment with dexamethasone from the 10th to the 17th week, although therapy was stopped 5 days before the amniocentesis. The latter group postulated increased metabolic clearance of dexamethasone, or inadequate dosage.

Theoretically, institution of such therapy at 6–7 weeks of gestation – before onset of adrenal androgen secretion – should effectively suppress adrenal androgen production, and allow normal separation of the vaginal and urethral orifices in addition to preventing clitoromegaly. Current recommendation is dexamethasone 20 µg/kg per 24 hours divided b.i.d. Obviously, if dexamethasone is to be administered at such an early date, treatment is blind to the status of the fetus. Following HLA and/or hormonal diagnosis by either chorionic villus biopsy or amniocentesis, cessation of prenatal therapy may be considered if the fetus is male, or if it is an unaffected female (Fig. 90.12).

To date, no fetus of a mother treated with dexamethasone in low doses has been found to have any congenital malformation. Specifically, no cases have been reported of cleft palate, or of placental degeneration, intrauterine growth retardation or fetal death, which have been observed in a rodent model of in utero exposure to high-dose glucocorticoids (Goldman et al 1978).

ACKNOWLEDGEMENTS

Support is acknowledged from the National Institutes of Health under USPHS grants HD00072, AM07029, DK37867, CA22507 and CA08748, and grant RR47 from the General Clinical Research Centers Program. Support is also acknowledged from the Horace Goldsmith Foundation and the Harold and Juliet Kalikow Foundation.

REFERENCES

Abraham G E, Swerdloff R S, Tulchinsky D, Hopper K, Odell W D 1971 Radioimmunoassay of plasma 17-

hydroxyprogesterone. Journal of Clinical Endocrinology and Metabolism 33: 42

Amor M, Parker K L, Globerman H, New M I, White P C 1988 Mutation in the CYP21B gene (Ile-172→Asn) causes steroid 21-hydroxylase deficiency. Proceedings of the National Academy of Sciences USA 85: 1600

Atchison M, Adesnik M 1986 Gene conversion in a cytochrome P450 gene family. Proceedings of the National Academy of Sciences USA 83: 2300

Awdeh Z L, Raum D, Yunis E J, Alper C A 1983 Extended HLA complement allele haplotypes: evidence for T/t-like complex in man. Proceedings of the National Academy of Sciences USA 80: 259

Baker S W 1981 Psychological management of intersex children. In: Josso N (ed) The Intersex Child (Pediatr Adolesc Endocrinol, vol 8), Karger, Basel, p 261

Bartter F C, Albright F, Forbes A P, Leaf A, Dempsey E, Carroll E 1951 The effects of adrenocorticotropic hormone and cortisone in the adrenogenital syndrome associated with congenital adrenal hyperplasia: an attempt to explain and correct its disordered hormone pattern. Journal of Clinical Investigation 30: 237

Baur M P, Sigmund S, Sigmund M, Rittner C 1984 Analysis of MHC recombinant families. In: Albert E D, Baur M P, Mayr W R (eds) Histocompatibility Testing 1984. Springer-Verlag, Berlin, p 324.

Bell J I, Denney D W, McDevitt H O 1985 Structure and polymorphism of murine and human class II major histocompatibility antigens. Immunological Reviews 84: 51.

Biglieri E G, Herron M A, Brust N 1966 17α-Hydroxylation deficiency in man. Journal of Clinical Investigation 45: 1946.

Binoux M, Pham-Huu-Trung M T, Gourmelen M, Girard F, Canlorbe P 1972 Plasma ACTH in adrenogenital syndrome. Acta Paediatrica Scandinavica 61: 269.

Birnbaum M D, Rose L I 1979 The partial adrenocortical hydroxylase deficiency syndrome in infertile women. Fertility and Sterility 32: 536.

Birnbaum M D, Rose L I 1984 Late onset adrenocortical hydroxylase deficiencies associated with menstrual dysfunction. Obstetrics and Gynecology 63: 445

Blankstein J, Faiman C, Reyes F I, Schroeder M L, Winter J S D 1980a Adult-onset familial adrenal 21-hydroxylase deficiency. American Journal of Medicine 68: 441.

Blankstein J, Fujieda K, Reyes F I, Faiman C, Winter J S D 1980b Cortisol 11-deoxycortisol concentrations in amniotic fluid during normal pregnancy. American Journal of Obstetrics and Gynecology 137: 781.

Blunck W 1968 Die α-ketolischen Cortisol-und Corticosteronmetaboliten sowie die 11-Oxy und 11-Desoxy 17-ketosteroide im Urin von Kindern. Acta Endocrinologica (vol 59) Suppl. 134: 9.

Blunck W, Bierich W R 1968 CAH with 11β-hydroxylase deficiency. A case report and contribution to diagnosis. Acta Paediatrica Scandinavica 57: 157.

Boggaram V, Funkenstein B, Waterman M R, Simpson E R 1985 Lipoproteins and the regulation of adrenal steroidogenesis. Endocrine Research 10: 387

Bois E, Mornet E, Chompret A, Feingold J, Hochez J, Goulet V 1985 Population genetics of congenital adrenal-hyperplasia (21-OH) in France. Archives Francaises de Pediatrie 42: 175

Bonaccorsi A C, Adler I, Figueiredo J G 1987 Male infertility due to congenital adrenal hyperplasia: testicular biopsy findings, hormonal evaluation, and therapeutic results in three patients. Fertility and Sterility 47: 664.

Bondy P W 1980 The adrenal cortex. In: Bondy P K, Rosenberg L E (eds) Metabolic Control and Disease, 8th

edn. Saunders, Philadelphia, p 1482.

Bongiovanni A M 1953 Detection of pregnanediol and pregnanetriol in urine of patients with adrenal hyperplasia: suppression with cortisone (preliminary report). Bulletin of Johns Hopkins Hospital 92: 244.

Bongiovanni A M 1962 The adrenogenital syndrome with deficiency of 3β-hydroxysteroid dehydrogenase. Journal of Clinical Investigation 41: 2086.

Bongiovanni A M 1978 Congenital adrenal hyperplasia and related conditions. In: Stanbury J B, Wyngaarden J B, Fredickson D S (eds). The Metabolic Basis of Inherited Disease, 4th edn. McGraw-Hill, New York, p 868.

Bongiovanni A M 1984 Congenital adrenal hyplasia due to 3β-hydroxysteroid dehydrogenase deficiency. In: New M I, Levine L S (eds) Adrenal Disease in Childhood (Pediatr Adolesc Endocrinol, vol 13). Karger, Basel, p 72.

Bongiovanni A M 1986 Late-onset adrenal hyperplasia (letter). New England Journal of Medicine 314: 450.

Bongiovanni A M, Eberlein W R 1958 Adrenogenital syndrome: uncomplicated and hypertensive forms. Pediatrics 21: 661.

Bongiovanni A M, Eberlein W R, Cara J 1954 Studies on metabolism of adrenal steroids in adrenogenital syndrome. Journal of Clinical Endocrinology and Metabolism 14: 409.

Bradshaw K D, Waterman M R, Couch R T, Simpson E R, Zuber M X 1987 Characterization of complementary deoxyribonucleic acid for human adrenocortical 17α-hydroxylase: a probe for analysis of 17-hydroxylase deficiency. Molecular and Cellular Endocrinology 1: 348.

Brautbar C, Rosler A, Landau H et al 1979 No linkage between HLA and congenital adrenal hyperlasia due to 11β-hydroxylase deficiency. New England Journal of Medicine 300: 205.

Butler G C, Marrian G F 1937 Isolation of pregnane-3,17,20-triol from urine of women showing adrenogenital syndrome. Journal of Biological Chemistry. 119: 565.

Camacho A M, Kowarski A, Migeon C J, Brough A J 1968 Congenital adrenal hyperplasia due to a deficiency of one of the enzymes involved in the biosynthesis of pregnenolone. Journal of Clinical Endocrinology and Metabolism 28: 153.

Carroll M C, Campbell R D, Bentley D R, Porter R 1984 A molecular map of the major histocompatibility complex class III region linking the complement genes C4, C2 and factor B. Nature 307: 237.

Carroll M C, Campbell R D, Porter R R 1985a The mapping of steroid 21-hydroxylase genes adjacent to complement component C4 genes in HLA, the major histocompatibility complex in man. Proceedings of the National Academy of Sciences USA 82: 521.

Carroll M C, Palsdottir A, Belt W F, Porter R R 1985b Deletion of complement of C4 and steroid 21-hydroxylase genes in the HLA class III region. Embo Journal 4: 2547.

Carroll M C, Katzman P, Alicot E M et al 1987 Linkage map of the human major histocompatibility complex including the tumor necrosis factor genes. Proceedings of the National Academy of Sciences USA 84: 8535.

Cathelineau G, Brerault J L, Fiet W, Julien R, Dreux C, Canivet J 1980 Adrenocortical 11β-hydroxylation defect in adult women with postmenarchial onset of symptoms. Journal of Clinical Endocrinology and Metabolism 51: 287.

Cathro D M, Birchall K, Mitchell F L, Forsyth C C 1965 3β, 21-Dihydroxypregn-5-ene-20-one in urine of normal human infants and in third day urine of child with deficiency of 3β-hydroxysteroid-dehydrogenase. Archives of

Disease in Childhood 40: 251.

Cavalli-Sforza L L, Bodmer W R 1971 The Genetics of Human Populations. Freeman, San Francisco.

Charnvises S, Fencl MdeM, Osathanondh R, Zhu M-G, Underwood R, Tulchinsky W 1985 Adrenal steroids in maternal and cord blood after dexamethasone administration at midterm. Journal of Clinical Endocrinology and Metabolism 61: 1220

Chetkowski R, DeFazio J, Shamonki I et al 1984 The incidence of late-onset congenital adrenal hyperplasia due to 21-hydroxylase deficiency among hirsute women. Journal of Clinical Endocrinology and Metabolism 58: 595.

Child D R, Bu'lock D E, Anderson D E 1980 Adrenal steroidogenesis in hirsute women. Clinical Endocrinology 12: 595.

Childs B, Grumbach M M, Van Wyk W J 1956 Virilizing adrenal hyperplasia: a genetic and hormonal study. Journal of Clinical Investigation 35: 213.

Chrousos G P, Loriaux D L, Sherins R J, Cutler G B 1981 Bilateral testicular enlargement resulting from inapparent 21-hydroxylase deficiency. Journal of Urology 126: 127

Chrousos G P, Loriaux D L, Mann D L, Cutler G B 1982 Late-onset 21-hydroxylase deficiency mimicking idiopathic hirsutism or polycystic ovarian disease. An allelic variant of congenital virilizing adrenal hyperplasia with a milder enzymatic defect. Annals of Internal Medicine. 96: 143.

Chua S C, Szabo P, Vitek A, Grzeschik K-H, John M, White P C 1987 Cloning of cDNA encoding steroid 11β-hydroxylase (P450cII). Proceedings of the National Academy of Sciences USA 84: 7193.

Chung B C, Matteson K J, Voutilainen R, Mohandas T K, Miller W M 1986 Cloning and sequence of cDNA for the human cholesterol side-chain cleavage enzyme, P450scc (20,22-desmolase), and location of its gene on chromosome 15. Proceedings of the National Academy of Sciences USA 83: 8962.

Chung B C, Picado-Leonard J, Haniu M, Bienkowski M, Hall P F, Shively J E, Miller W M 1987 Cytochrome P450c17(steroid 17β-hydroxylase/17,20-lyase): cloning of human adrenal testis cDNA indicates the same gene is expressed in both tissues. Proceedings of the National Academy of Sciences USA 84: 407.

Couillin P, Nicolas H, Boue J, Boue A 1979 HLA typing of amniotic-fluid cells applied to prenatal diagnosis of congenital adrenal hyperplasia. Lancet 1: 1076

D'Armiento M, Reda G, Bisignani G, Tabolli S, Cappellaci S, Lulli P 1983 No linkage between HLA and congenital adrenal hyperplasia due to 17α-hydroxylase deficiency. New England Journal of Medicine 308: 970

Davis J O 1974 The renin-angiotensin system in the control of aldosterone secretion In: Page I H, Bumpus F M (eds) Handbook of Experimental Pharmacology, vol 37. Springer-Verlag, New York p 322.

Dean H J, Shackelton C H L, Winter J S D 1984 Diagnosis and natural history of 17-hydroxylase deficiency in a newborn male. Journal of Clinical Endocrinology and Metabolism. 59: 513.

Decourt M J, Jayle M F, Baulieu 1957 Virilisme cliniquement tardif avec excretion de pregnanetriol et insuffisance de la production du cortisol. Annales d'Endocrinologie (Paris) 18: 416.

Degenhart H L, Visser H K A, Boon H, O'Doherty N J 1972 Evidence for deficient 20α-cholesterol-hydroxylase activity in adrenal tissue of a patient with lipoidadrenal hyperplasia.

Acta Endocrinologica 71: 512.

De Peretti E, Forest M G, Feut J P, David M 1980 Endocrine studies in two children with male pseudohermaphroditism due to 3β-hydroxysteroid dehydrogenase defect. In: Genazzani A R, Thijssen J H H, Siiteri P K (eds) Adrenal Androgens. Raven Press, New York, p 141.

Dhom G 1958 Zur Morphologie und Genese der kongenitalen Nebennieren-rindenhyperplasie beim mannlichen Scheinzwitter. Zentralblatt fur allgemeine Pathologie und Pathologische Anatomie 97: 346.

Dillon M J, Rynes J 1975 Plasma renin activity and aldosterone concentrations in children: results in salt-wasting states. Archives of Disease in Childhood. 50: 330.

Donohoue P, Jospe N, Migeon C J, McLean R H, Bias W B, White P C, Van Dop C 1986a Restriction maps and restriction fragment length polymorphisms of the human 21-hydroxylase genes. Biochemical and Biophysical Research Communications 136: 722.

Donohoue P A, Van Dop C, McLean R H, White P C, Jospe N, Migeon C J 1986b Gene conversion in salt-losing congenital adrenal hyperplasia with absent complement C4 protein. Journal of Clinical Endocrinology and Metabolism 62: 9951

Dorr H G, Sippel W G, Haack D, Bidlingmaier F, Knorr D 1986 Pitfalls of prenatal treatment of congenital adrenal hyperplasia (CAH) due to 21-hydroxylase deficiency. Prog and Abstr, 25th Annual Meeting of the European Society for Paediatric Endocrinology, August 1986, Zurich

Dunham I, Sargent C A, Trowsdale J, Campbell R D 1987 Molecular mapping of the human major histocompatibility complex by pulsed-field gel electrophoresis. Proceedings of the National Academy of Sciences USA 84: 7237

Dupont B, Oberfield S E, Smithwick E M, Lee T D, Levine L S 1977 Close genetic linkage between HLA and congenital adrenal hyperplasia (21-hydroxylase deficiency). Lancet 2: 1309

Dupont B, Pollack M S, Levine L S, O'Neill G J, Hawkins B R, New M I 1981 Congenital adrenal hyperplasia and HLA: joint report from the Eighth International Histocompatibility Workshop. In: Terasaki P I (ed) Histocompatibility Testing 1980. HLA Tissue Typing Laboratory Los Angeles, p 693

Dupont B, Virdis R, Lerner A K, Nelson C, Pollack M S, New M I 1984 Distinct HLA-B antigen associations for the salt-wasting and simple virilizing forms of congenital adrenal hyperplasia due to 21-hydroxylase deficiency. In: Albert E D, Baur M P, Mayr W R (eds) Histocompatibility Testing 1984. Springer-Verlag, Berlin, p 660

Eberlein W R, Bongiovanni A M 1955 Congenital adrenal hyperplasia with hypertension: unusual steroid pattern in blood and urine (letter) Journal of Clinical Endocrinology and Metabolism 15: 1531

Eberlein W R, Bongiovanni A M 1956 Plasma and urinary corticosteroids in the hypertensive form of congenital adrenal hyperplasia. Journal of Biological Chemistry 223: 85

Edwin C, Lanes R, Migeon C J, Lee P A, Plotnick L P, Kowarski A A 1979 Persistence of the enzymatic block in aldolescent patients with salt-losing congenital adrenal hyperplasia. Journal of Pediatrics 95: 534

Evans M I, Chrousos G P, Mann D W et al 1985 Pharmacologic suppression of the fetal adrenal gland in utero. Journal of the American Medical Association 253: 1015

Federman D D 1968 Disorders of fetal endocrinology: female pseudohermaphroditism. In: Abnormal Sexual Development, W B Saunders, Philadelphia, p 121

Ferrebee J W, Ragan C, Atchley D W, Loeb R F 1939 Deoxycorticosterone esters. Certain effects in the treatment of Addison's disease. Journal of the American Medical Association 113: 1725

Finkelstein M, Schaeffer J M 1979 Inborn errors of steroid biosynthesis. Physiological Reviews 59: 353

Fleischnick E, Raum D, Alosco S M et al 1983 Extended MHC haplotypes in 21-hydroxylase deficiency congenital adrenal hyperplasia. Lancet 1: 152

Forest M G, Lecornu M, DePeretti E 1980 Familial male pseudohermaphroditism due to 17,20-desmolase deficiency. I. *In vivo* endocrine studies. Journal of Clinical Endocrinology and Metabolism 50: 826

Forest M G, Betuel H, Couillin P et al 1981 Prenatal diagnosis of congenital adrenal hyperplasia (CAH) due to 21-hydroxylase deficiency by steroid analysis in the amniotic fluid of mid-pregnancy: comparison with HLA typing in 17 pregnancies at risk for CAH. Prenatal Diagnosis 1: 197

Forest M G, Betuel H, David M 1987 Traitement antenatal de l'hyperplasie-congenitale des surrenales par deficit en 21-hydroxylase: etude multicentrique Annnales d'Endocrinologie (Paris) 48: 31

Frasier S D, Weiss B A, Horton R 1974 Amniotic fluid testosterone: implications for the prenatal diagnosis of congenital adrenal hyperplasia. Journal of Pediatrics 84: 738

Frasier S D, Thorneycroft I H, Weill B A, Horton R 1975 Elevated amniotic fluid concentration of 17-hydroxyprogesterone in congenital adrenal hyperplasia. Journal of Pediatrics 86: 310

Gabrilove J L, Sharma D C, Dorfman R I 1965 Adrenocortical 11β-hydroxylase deficiency and virilism first manifest in the adult woman. New England Journal of Medicine 272: 1189

Gandy H L M, Keutmann E H, Isso A J 1960 Characterization of urinary steroids in adrenal hyperplasia: isolation of metabolites of cortisol, compound S, and deoxycorticosterone from a normotensive patient with adrenogenital syndrome. Journal of Clinical Investigation 39: 364

Gangemi M, Benato M, Guacci A M, Menghetti G 1983 Stimulation tests in adrenogenital syndrome induced by 21-hydroxylase deficit. Clinical and Experimental Obstetrics and Gynecology 10: 127

Ganong W F 1963 The central nervous system and the synthesis and release of adrenocorticotropic hormone. In: Nalbandov A V (ed) Advances in Neuroendocrinology. University of Illinois Press, Urbana IL, p 92

Ganong W F 1980 Neurotransmitters and pituitary function: regulation of ACTH secretion. Federation Proceedings 39: 2923

Ganong W F 1984 Cortisol of aldosterone secretion. In: Martini L, Gordan G S, Sciarra F (eds) Steroid modulation of neuroendocrine function, Sterols steroids and bone metabolism. Elsevier, New York, p 111

Ganong W F, Alpert L C, Lee T C 1974 ACTH and the regulation of adrenocortical secretion. New England Journal of Medicine 290: 1006

Garlepp M J, Wilton A N, Dawkins R L, White P C 1986 Rearrangement of 21-hydroxylase genes in disease-associated MHC supratypes. Immunogenetics 23: 100

Gibson M, Lackritz R, Schiff I, Tulchinsky D 1980 Abnormal adrenal responses to adrenocorticotropic hormone in hyperandrogenic women. Fertility and Sterility 33: 43

Glenthoj A, Neilsen M D, Starup J, Svejjaard A 1979 HLA and congenital adrenal hyperplasia due to 11-hydroxylase deficiency. Tissue Antigens 14: 181

Glenthoj A, Nielsen M D, Starup J 1980 Congenital adrenal hyperplasia due to 11-β hydroxylase deficiency: final diagnosis in adult age in three patients. Acta Endocrinologica 93: 94

Globerman H, Amor M, New M I, White P C 1988 Nonsense mutation causing steroid 21-hydroxylase deficiency in man. Journal of Clinical Investigation 82: 139

Godard C, Riondel A M, Veyrat R, Megevand A, Muller A F 1968 Plasma renin activity and aldosterone in congenital adrenal hyperplasia. Pediatrics 41: 883

Goebelsmann U, Zachmann M, Davajan V et al 1976 Male pseudohermaphroditism consistent with 17–20 desmolase deficiency. Gynecological and Obstetric Investigation 7: 138

Golden M P, Lippe B M, Kaplan S A, Lavin N, Slavin J 1978 Management of congenital adrenal hyperplasia using serum dehydroepiandrosterone sulfate and 17-hydroxyprogesterone concentrations. Pediatrics 61: 867

Goldman A S, Sharpior B H, Katsumata M 1978 Human foetal placental corticoid receptors and teratogens for cleft palate. Nature 272: 464

Granoff A B, Chasalow F I, Blethen S L 1985 17-Hydroxyprogesterone responses to adrenocorticotrophin in children with premature adrenarche. Journal of Clinical Endocrinology and Metabolism 60: 409

Green O C, Migeon C J, Wilkins L 1960 Urinary steroids in the hypertensive form of congenital adrenal hyperplasia. Journal of Clinical Endocrinology and Metabolism 20: 929

Gregory T, Gardner L I 1976 Hypertensive virilizing adrenal hyperplasia with minimal impairment of synthetic route to cortisol. Journal of Clinical Endocrinology and Metabolism. 43: 769

Guillemin R, Schally A V 1963 Recent advances in the chemistry of neuroendocrine mediators originating in the central nervous system. In: Nalbandov A V (ed) Advances in Neuroendocrinology. University of Illinois Press, Urbana IL, p 314

Hamilton W, Brush M G 1964 Four clinical variants of congenital adrenal hyperplasia. Archives of Disease in Childhood 39: 66

Hardy D A, Bell J I, Long E O, Lindsten T, McDevitt H O 1986 Genomic organization of the HLA Class II region genes. Nature 323: 453

Hauffa B P, Miller W L, Grumbach M M et al 1985 Congenital adrenal hyperplasia due to deficient cholesterol side-chain cleavage activity (20, 22 desmolase) in a patient treated for 18 years. Clinical Endocrinology 23: 481

Higashi Y, Yoshioka H, Yamane M, Gotoh O, Fujii-Kuriyama Y 1986 Complete nucleotide sequence of two steroid 21-hydroxylase genes tandemly arranged in [the] human genome. Proceeding of the National Academy of Sciences USA 83: 2841

Higashi Y, Tanae A, Inoue H, Hiromasa T, Fujii-Kuriyama Y 1988 Aberrant splicing and missense mutations cause steroid 21-hydroxylase [P-450(C21)] deficiency in humans: possible gene conversion products. Proceedings of the National Academy of Sciences USA 85: 7486

Hirschfeld A G, Fleshman J K 1969 An unusually high incidence of congenital adrenal hyperplasia in the Alaskan Eskimo. Journal of Pediatrics 75: 492

Hochberg R B, McDonald P D, Feldman M, Lieberman S 1974 Studies on the biosynthetic conversion of cholesterol into pregnenolone. Journal of Biological Chemistry 249: 1277

Hornsby P J 1987 Physiological and pathological effects of steroids on the function of the adrenal cortex. Journal of Steroid Biochemistry 27: 1161

Hubble D 1966 Congenital adrenal hyperplasia. In: Holt K S, Raine D N (eds) Basic concepts of inborn errors and defects of steroid biosynthesis. Proceeding of the Third Symposium of the Society for the Study of Inborn Errors of Metabolism. Churchill Livingstone, Edinburgh, p 68–74

Hughes I A, Laurence K 1979 Antenatal diagnosis of congenital adrenal hyperplasia. Lancet 2: 7

Hughes I A, Laurence K M W 1982 Prenatal diagnosis of congenital adrenal hyperplasia due to 21-hydroxylase deficiencies: amniotic fluid steroid analyses. Prenatal Diagnosis 2: 97

Hughes I A, Winter J S D 1976 The application of a serum 17OH-progesterone radioimmunoassay to the diagnosis and management of congenital adrenal hyperplasia. Journal of Pediatrics 88: 766

Hurwitz A, Brautbar C, Milwidsky A, Vecsei P, Milewicz A, Navot D, Rosler A 1985 Combined 21-and 11β-hydroxylase deficiency in familial congenital adrenal hyperplasia. Journal of Clinical Endocrinology and Metabolism 60: 631–638

Hyatt P J 1987 Functional significance of the adrenal zones. In: D'Agata R, Chrousos G P (eds) Recent Advances in Adrenal Regulation and Function (Serono Sym. Publ. vol 40). Raven Press, New York, p 35

Ishii-Ohba H, Inano N, Tamaoki B-I 1987 Testicular and adrenal 3β-hydroxy-5-ene-steroid dehydrogenase and 5-ene-4-ene isomerase. Journal of Steroid Biochemistry 27: 775

Janne O, Perheentupa J, Vihko R 1970 Plasma and urinary steroids in an eight year old boy with 3β-hydroxysteroid-dehydrogenase deficiency. Journal of Clinical Endocrinology and Metabolism 31: 162

Janoski A H 1977 Naturally occurring adrenal steroids with salt-losing properties: Relationship to congenital adrenal hyperplasia. In: Lee P A, Plotnick L P, Kowarski A A, Migeon C J (eds) Congenital Adrenal Hyperplasia. University Park Press, Baltimore M D, p99

Jeffcoate T N A, Fleigner J R H, Russell S H, Davis J C Wade A P 1985 Diagnosis of the adrenogenital syndrome before birth. Lancet 2: 553

Jeffries W M, Weir W C, Weir D R, Prouty R L 1958 The use of cortisone and related steroids in infertility. Fertility and Sterility 9: 145

Jones H W, Jones G E S 1954 The gynecological aspects of adrenal hyperplasia and allied disorders. American Journal of Obstetrics and Gynecology 68: 1330

Josso N 1986 AntiMullerian hormone: new perspective for a sexist molecule. Endocrine Reviews 6: 421

Jost A 1953 Problems of fetal endocrinology: the gonadal and hypophyseal hormones. Recent Progress in Hormone Research 8: 379

Jost A 1966 Steroids and sex differentiation of the mammalian foetus. Excerpta Medica International Congress Series 132: 74

Jost A 1971 Embryonic sexual differentiation. In: Jones H W,

Scott W W (eds) Hermaphroditism, Genital Anomalies and Related Endocrine Disorders, 2nd edn. Williams & Wilkins, Baltimore MD, p 16

Kastelan A, Brkjacic-Surkalovic L J, Dumic M 1985 The HLA associations in congenital adrenal hyperplasia due to 21-hydroxylase deficiency in a Yugoslav population. Annals of the New York Academy of Sciences 458: 36

Kenny F M, Reynolds J W, Green O C 1971 Partial 3β-hydroxysteroid dehydrogenase (-3β-HSD) deficiency in a family with congenital adrenal hyperplasia: evidence for increasing 3β-HSD activity with age. Pediatrics 48: 756

Kirkland R T, Kirkland J L, Johnson C M, Horning M G, Librik L, Clayton G W 1973 Congenital lipoid adrenal hyperplasia in an eight-year-old phenotypic female. Journal of Clinical Endocrinology and Metabolism 36: 48

Klein R 1960 Evidence for and evidence against the existence of a salt-losing hormone. Journal of Pediatrics 57: 452

Klouda P T, Harris R, Price D A 1978 HLA and congenital adrenal hyperplasia. Lancet 2: 1046

Kogut M D 1965 Adrenogenital syndrome. American Journal of Diseases of Children 110: 562

Kohn B, Levine L S, Pollack M S et al 1982 Late-onset steroid 21-hydroxylase deficiency: a variant of classical congenital adrenal hyperplasia. Journal of Clinical Endocrinology and Metabolism 55: 817

Kominami S, Ochi H, Kobayashi Y, Takemori S 1980 Studies on the steroid hydroxylation system in adrenal cortex microsomes. Journal of Biological Chemistry 255: 3386

Kominami S, Shinzawa K, Takemori S 1982 Purification and some properties of cytochrome P-450 specific for steroid 17α-hydroxylation and CI7-C20 bond cleavage from guinea pig adrenal microsomes. Biochemical and Biophysical Research Communications 109: 916

Korth-Schutz S, Levine L S, New M I 1976 Serum androgens in normal prepubertal and pubertal children and in children with precocious adrenarche. Journal of Clinical Endocrinology and Metabolism 42: 117

Korth-Schutz S, Virdis R, Saenger P, Chow D Levine L S, New M I 1978 Serum androgens as a continuing index of adequacy of treatment of congenital adrenal hyperplasia. Journal of Clinical Endocrinology and Metabolism 46: 452

Koushanpour E, Kriz W 1986 In: Renal Physiology: Principles, Structure, and Function, 2nd edn. Springer-Verlag, New York, p 196

Kowarski A A, Finkelstein J W, Spaulding J S, Holman G S, Migeon C J 1965 Aldosterone secretion rate in congenital adrenal hyperplasia. A discussion of the theories of the pathogenesis of the salt-losing form of the syndrome. Journal of Clinical Investigation 44: 1505

Kuhnle U, Chow D, Rapaport R, Pang S, Levine L S, New M I 1981 The activity of the 21-hydroxylase (21-OH) enzyme in the glomerulosa and fasciculata of the adrenal cortex in congenital adrenal hyperplasia (CAH). Journal of Clinical Endocrinology and Metabolism 52: 534

Kuhnle U, Rosler A, Pareira J A, Gunczler P, Levine L S, New M I 1983 The effects of long term normalization of sodium balance on linear growth in disorders with aldosterone deficiency. Acta Endocrinologica 102: 577

Kuhnle U, Land M, Ulick S 1986 Evidence for the secretion of an antimineralocorticoid in congenital adrenal hyperplasia. Journal of Clinical Endocrinology and Metabolism 62: 934

Kuttenn F, Couillin P, Girard F et al 1986 Late-onset adrenal hyperplasia in hirsutism. New England Journal of Medicine 313: 224

Lambeth J D, Stevens V L 1985 Cytochrome P-450scc: enzymology, and the regulation of intramitochondrial cholesterol delivery to the enzyme. Endocrine Research 10: 283

Laragh J H 1971 Aldosteronism in man: factors controlling secretion of the hormone. In: Christy N P (ed) The Human Adrenal Cortex. Harper & Row, New York, p 483

Laron Z, Pollack M S, Zamir R et al 1980 Late onset 21-hydroxylase deficiency and HLA in the Ashkenazi population; a new allele at the 21-hydroxylase locus. Human Immunology 1: 55

Lee P D K, Patterson B D, Hintz R L, Rosenfeld R G 1986 Biochemical diagnosis and management of corticosterone methyl oxidase type II deficiency. Journal of Clinical Endocrinology and Metabolism 62: 225

Levine L S 1986 Prenatal detection of congenital adrenal hyperplasia. In: Milunsky A (ed) Genetic Disorders and the Fetus. Plenum Press, New York, pp 369–385

Levine L S, Zachmann M, New M W et al 1978 Genetic mapping of the 21-hydroxylase deficiency gene within the HLA linkage group. New England Journal of Medicine 299: 911

Levine L S, Dupont B, Lorenzen F et al 1980a Cryptic 21-hydroxylase deficiency in families of patients with classical congenital adrenal hyperplasia. Journal of Clinical Endocrinology and Metabolism 51: 1316

Levine L S, Rauh W, Gottesdiener K et al 1980b. New studies of the 11β-hydroxylase and 18-hydroxylase enzymes in the hypertensive form of congenital adrenal hyperplasia. Journal of Clinical Endocrinology and Metabolism 50: 258

Levine L S, Dupont B, Lorenzen F et al 1981 Genetic and hormonal characterization of cryptic 21-hydroxylase deficiency. Journal of Clinical Endocrinology and Metabolism 53: 1193

Lobo R A, Goebelsmann U 1980 Adult manifestion of congenital adrenal hyperplasia due to incomplete 21-hydroxylase deficiency mimicking polycystic ovarian disease. American Journal of Obstetrics and Gynecology 138: 720

Lucky A W, Rosenfield R L, McGuire J, Rudy S, Helke J 1986 Adrenal androgen hyperresponsiveness to adrenocorticotropin in women with acne and/or hirsutism: adrenal enzyme defects and exaggerated adrenarche. Journal of Clinical Endocrinology and Metabolism 62: 840

Luetscher J A 1956 Studies of aldosterone in relation to water and electrolyte balance in man. Recent Progress in Hormone Research 12: 175

McKiernan J 1985 Congenital adrenal hyperplasia in the Republic of Ireland, 1966–1982. Irish Medical Journal 78: 6–7

McKusick V A 1973 Phenotypic diversity of human diseases resulting from allelic series. American Journal of Human Genetics 25: 446

McKusick V A 1986 The human gene map 15 April 1986. Clinical Genetics 29: 545

Madan K, Shoemaker J 1980 XY females with enzyme deficiencies of steroid metabolism: a brief review. Human Genetics 53: 291

Mantero F, Busnardo B, Riondel A, Vayrat R, Austoni M 1971 Hypertension arterielle, alcalose hypokaliemique et pseudohermaphroditisme male par deficit en 17α-hydroxylase. Schweizerische Medizinische Wochenschrift 101: 38

Mantero F, Scaroni C, Pasini C V, Fagiolo U 1980 No linkage between HLA and congenital adrenal hyperplasia

due to a 17α-hydroxylase deficiency. New England Journal of Medicine 303: 530

Mason H L, Kepler E J 1945 Isolation of steroids from urine of patients with adrenal cortical tumors and adrenal cortical hyperplasia: new 17-ketosteroid, androstane-3α, 11-diol-17-one. Journal of Biological Chemistry 161: 235

Matteson K J, Picado-Leonard J, Chung B-C, Mohandas T K, Miller W L 1986a Assignment of the gene for adrenal P450c17 (steroid 17α-hydroxylase/17,20-lyase) to human chromosome 10. Journal of Clinical Endocrinology and Metabolism 63: 789

Matteson K J, Chung B-C, Urdea M S, Miller W L 1986b Study of cholesterol side-chain cleavage (20,22-desmolase) deficiency causing congenital lipoid adrenal hyperplasia using bovine-sequence p450scc oligodeoxyribonucleotide probes. Endocrinology 118: 1296

Matteson K J, Phillips J A III, Miller W L et al 1987 P450XXI (steroid 21-hydroxylase) gene deletions are not found in family studies of congenital adrenal hyperplasia. Proceedings of the National Academy of Sciences. 84: 5858

Mauthe I, Lapse H, Knorr D 1977 The frequency of congenital adrenal hyperplasia in Munich. Klinische Padiatrie 189: 172–176

Migeon C J 1979 Diagnosis and treatment of adrenogenital disorders. In: Degroot L J, Cahill G F, Odell W D, Martini L, Potts J T Jr, Nelson W H, Steinberger E, Winegard A I (eds) Endocrinology, Grune and Stratton, New York, p 1204

Migeon C J, Rosenwaks Z, Lee P A, Urban M D, Bias W B 1980 The attenuated form of congenital adrenal hyperplasia as an allelic form of 21-hydroxylase deficiency. Journal of Clinical Endocrinology and Metabolism 51: 647

Mininberg D T, Levine L S, New M I 1979 Current concepts in congenital adrenal hyperplasia. Investigative Urology 17: 169

Moller G (ed) 1985a Molecular genetics of class I and II MHC antigens 1. Immunological Reviews 84: 1–143

Moller G (ed) 1985b Molecular genetics of class I and II MHC antigens 2. Immunological Reviews 85: 1–168

Moller G (ed) 1985c Molecular genetics of class III MHC antigens. Immunological Reviews 87: 1–208

Money J, Ehrhardt A A 1972 In: Man and Woman, Boy and Girl. Differentiation and Dimorphism of Gender Identity. Johns Hopkins University Press, Baltimore

Mornet E, Couillin P, Kuttenn F et al 1986a Associations between restriction fragment length polymorphisms detected with a probe for human 21-hydroxylase (21-OH) and two clinical forms of 21-hydroxylase deficiency. Human Genetics 74: 402

Mornet E, Boue J, Raux-Demay M et al 1986b. First trimester prenatal diagnosis of 21-hydroxylase deficiency by linkage analysis of HLA-DNA probes and by 17-hydroprogesterone determination. Human Genetics 73: 358

Mornet E, Dupont J, Vitck A, White P C 1989 Characterization of two genes encoding human steroid 11β-hydroxylase (P450c11). Journal of Biological Chemistry 264: 20961–20967

Müller W, Prader M, Kofler J, Glatzl J, Geir W 1979 Frequency of congenital adrenal hyperplasia. Paediatrie und Paedologie 14: 151

Muller-Eberhard U, Ghizzoni L, Liem H H, New M I, Finlayson M, Johnson E F 1985 Evidence that variation among untreated rabbits in hepatic progesterone 21-hydroxylase activity is indicative of enzyme heterogeneity rather than a transient inductive effect. Annals of the New York Academy of Sciences. 458: 225

Murtaza L, Sibert J R, Hughes I, Balfour I C 1980 Congenital adrenal hyperplasia — a clinical and genetic survey. Archives of Disease in Childhood 55: 622

Nagamani M, McDonough P G, Ellegood J O, Mahesh M B 1978 Maternal and amniotic fluid 17-hydroxyprogesterone levels during pregnancy: diagnosis of congenital adrenal hyperplasia in utero. American Journal of Obstetrics and Gynecology 130: 791

Natoli G, Moschini L, Acconcia P et al 1981 Newborn screening for 21-hydroxylase deficiency. Radioimmunoassay (RIA) 17α-hydroxyprogesterone by microfilter paper method (abstract). In: 2nd Intl Symp in Recent Progress in Pediatric Endocrinology (Serono), Milan Oct 22–23, 1981. Raven Press, New York, p 33

Nebert D W, Gonzalez F J 1987 P450 genes: structure, evolution and regulation. Annual Review of Biochemistry 56: 945

Nedospasov S A, Hirt B, Shakhov A N, Dobrynin V N, Kawashima E, Accolla R S, Jongeneel C V 1986 The genes for tumor necrosis factor (TNF-α) and lymphotoxin (TNF-β) are tandemly arranged on chromosome 17 of the mouse. Nucleic Acids Research 14: 7713

New M I 1970 Male pseudohermaphroditism due to 17α-hydroxylase deficiency. Journal of Clinical Investigation 49: 1930

New M I 1988 HLA and adrenal disease. In: Farid N (ed) The Immunogenetics of Endocrine Disorders, 2nd edn. Alan Liss, New York, p 309

New M I, Levine L S 1973 Congenital adrenal hyperplasia. In: Harris H Hirschhorn K (eds) Advances in Human Genetics, vol 4, Plenum Press, New York, p 251

New M I, Levine L S 1984 Steroid 21-hydroxylase deficiency. In: New M I, Levine L S (eds) Adrenal Diseases in Childhood (Pediatr Adolesc Endocrinol vol. 13). Karger, Basel, p 9

New M I, Peterson R E 1966 Disorders of aldosterone secretion in childhood. Pediatric Clinics of North America 13: 43

New M I, Seaman M P 1970 Secretion rates of cortisol and aldosterone precursors in various forms of congenital adrenal hyperplasia. Journal of Clinical Endocrinology and Metabolism 30: 361

New M I, Lorenzen F, Pang S, Gunczler P, Dupont B, Pollack M S, Levine L S 1979 'Acquired' adrenal hyperplasia with 21-hydroxylase deficiency is not the same genetic disorder as congenital adrenal hyperplasia. Journal of Clinical Endocrinology and Metabolism 48: 356

New M I, Dupont B, Pang S, Pollack M S, Levine L S 1981 An update of congenital adrenal hyperplasia. Recent Progress in Hormone Research 37: 105

New M I, Dupont B, Grumbach K, Levine L S 1983a Congenital adrenal hyperplasia and related conditions. In: Stanbury J B, Wyngaarden J B, Fredrickson D S, Goldstein J L Brown M S (eds) The Metabolic Basis of Inherited Disease, 5th edn. McGraw-Hill New York, p 973

New M I, Lorenzen F, Lerner A J et al 1983b Genotyping steroid 21-hydroxylase deficiency: hormonal reference data. Journal of Clinical Endocrinology and Metabolism 57: 320

New M I, Nemery R L, Chow D M et al 1989a Low-renin hypertension of childhood. In: Mantero F, Takeda R, Scoggins B A, Biglieri E G, Funder J W (eds) The adrenal and hypertension: from cloning to clinic. Ares-Serona

Symposium, Tokyo, July 15–26, 1988. Raven Press, New York Vol. 57: 323–343

New M I, White P C, Pang S, Dupont B, Speiser P W 1989b The adrenal hyperplasias. In: Scriver C R, Beaudet A L, Sly W S, Valle D (eds) The Metabolic Basis of Inherited Disease, 6th edn. McGraw-Hill, New York, p 1881

New M I, White P C, Speiser P, Crawford C, Dupont B 1989c Congenital adrenal hyperplasia. In: Edwards C R W, Lincoln D W (eds) Recent advances in endocrinology and metabolism, vol 3. Churchill Livingstone, Edinburgh

Newmark D, Dluhy R G, Williams G H, Pochi P, Rose L I 1977 Partial 11- and 21-hydroxylase deficiencies in hirsute women. American Journal of Obstetrics and Gynecology 127: 594

Nihoul-Fekete C 1981 Feminizing genitoplasty in the intersex child. In: Josso N (ed) The Intersex Child (Pediatr Adolesc Endrocrinol, vol 8) Karger, Basel, p 247

Nussdorfer G G 1986 Cytophysiology of the Adrenal Cortex (Intl Rev Cytol vol 98). Academic Press, New York

O'Doherty N J 1964 Lipoid adrenal hyperplasia. Guys Hospital Reports 113: 364

Ojeifo J O, Winters S J, Troen P 1984 Basal and ACTH-stimulated serum 17α-hydroxyprogesterone in men with idiopathic infertility. Fertility and Sterility 42: 97

O'Neill G J, Dupont B, Pollack M S, Levine L S, New M I 1982 Complement C4 allotypes in congenital adrenal hyperplasia due to 21-hydroxylase deficiency. Clinical Immunology and Immunopathology 23: 312

Pang S, Levine L S, Chow D, Faiman C, New M I 1979 Serum androgen concentrations in neonates and young infants with congenital adrenal hyperplasia due to 21-hydroxylase deficiency. Clinical Endocrinology 11: 575

Pang S, Levine L S, Cederqvist L L et al 1980a Amniotic fluid concentration of Δ5 and Δ4 steroids in fetuses with congenital adrenal hyperplasia due to 21-hydroxylase deficiency and in anencephalic fetuses. Journal of Clinical Endocrinology and Metabolism 51: 223

Pang S, Levine L S, Lorenzen F et al 1980b Hormonal studies in obligate heterozygotes and siblings of patients with 11β-hydroxylase deficiency congenital adrenal hyperplasia. Journal of Clinical Endocrinology and Metabolism. 50: 586

Pang S, Levine L S, Stoner E, Opitz J M, New M I 1983 Nonsalt-losing congenital adrenal hyperplasia due to 3β-hydroxysteroid dehydrogenase deficiency with normal glomerulosa function. Journal of Clinical Endocrinology and Metabolism 56: 808

Pang S, Lerner A J, Stoner E, Levine L S, Oberfield S E, New M I 1985a Late onset adrenal steroid 3β-hydroxysteroid dehydrogenase. A cause of hirsutism in pubertal and postpubertal women. Journal of Clinical Endocrinology and Metabolism 60: 428

Pang S, Pollack M S, Loo M, Green O, Nussbaum R, Clayton G, Dupont B, New M I 1985b Pitfalls of prenatal diagnosis of 21-hydroxylase deficiency congenital adrenal hyperplasia. Journal of Clinical Endocrinology and Metabolism 61: 89

Parks G A, Bermudez J A, Anast C S, Bongiovanni A M, New M I 1971 Pubertal boy with the 3β-hydroxysteroid dehydrogenase defect. Journal of Clinical Endocrinology and Metabolism 33: 269

Pedersen R C 1985 Polypeptide activators of cholesterol side-chain cleavage. Endocrine Research 10: 533

Perera G A, Knowlton A I, Lowell A, Loeb R F 1944 Effect of deoxycorticosterone acetate on the blood pressure of man. Journal of the American Medical Association 125: 1030

Petersen G, Rotter J, MacCracken J 1984 Selective advantage of the 21-hydroxylase deficiency (21-OH DEF) gene in Alaskan Eskimos: use of a linked marker to identify heterozygotes (abstract). American Journal of Human Genetics 36: 177S

Peterson R E, Imperato-McGinley J, Gautier T et al 1977 Male pseudohermaphroditism due to steroid 5α-reductase deficiency. American Journal of Medicine 62: 170

Picard J Y, Goulut C, Bourillon R, Josso N 1986 Biochemical analysis of bovine testicular anti-Mullerian hormone. FEBS Letters 195: 73

Pollack M S, Levine L S, Pang S et al 1979 Prenatal diagnosis of congenital adrenal hyperplasia (21-hydroxylase deficiency) by HLA typing. Lancet 1: 1107

Pollack M S, Levine L S, O'Neill G J et al 1981 HLA linkage and B14, DR1, BfS haplotype association with the genes for late onset and cryptic 21-hydroxylase deficiency. American Journal of Human Genetics 33: 540

Porter B, Finzi M, Leiberman E, Moses S 1977 The syndrome of congenital adrenal hyperplasia in Israel. Pediatrician 6: 100

Prader A 1958a Vollkommen mannliche auszere Genitalentwicklung und Salzverlustsyndrom bei Madchen mit kongenitalem adrenogenitalem Syndrom. Helvetica Paediatrica Acta 13: 231

Prader A 1958b Die Haufigkeit des kongenitalen adrenogenitalen Syndroms. Helvetica Paediatrica Acta 13: 426

Prader A, Gurtner H P 1955 Das Syndrom des Pseudohermaphroditismus masculinus bei kongenitaler Nebennierenrinden-Hyperplasia ohne Androgenuberproduktion (adrenaler Pseudoherm. masc.) Helvetica Paediatrica Acta 10: 397

Prader A, Siebenmann R E 1957 Nebennereninsuffiziens bei kongenitaler Lipoid-hyperplasie der Nebennieren. Helvetica Paediatrica Acta 12: 569

Prader A, Spahr A, Neher R 1955 Erhohte Aldosteronausscheidung beim kongenitalen adrenogenitalen Syndrom. Schweizerische Medizinische Wochenschrift 85: 45

Prader A, Anders G J P A, Habich H 1962 Zur Genetik des kongenitalen adrenogenitalen Syndroms. (virilisierende Nebennierenhyperplasie). Helvetica Paediatrica Acta 17: 271

Qazi Q H, Thompson M W 1972 Incidence of salt-wasting form of congenital adrenal hyperplasia. Archives of Disease in Childhood 47: 302

Raum D L, Awdeh Z L, Anderson J et al 1984 Human C4 haplotypes with duplicated C4A or C4B. American Journal of Human Genetics 36: 72

Reid I A, Ganong W F 1977 Control of aldosterone secretion. In: Genest J, Koiw E, Kuchel O (eds) Hypertension: Physiopathology and Treatment. McGraw Hill, New York, p 265

Riddick D H, Hammond C B 1975 Adrenal virilism due to 21-hydroxylase deficiency in the postmenarchial female. Obstetrics and Gynecology 45: 21

Rivier C L, Plotsky P M 1986 Mediation by corticotrophin releasing factor (CRF) of adrenohypophyseal hormone secretion. Annual Review of Physiology 48: 475

Rodrigues N R, Dunham I, Yu C-Y et al 1987 Molecular characterization of the HLA-linked steroid 21-hydroxylase B gene from an individual with congenital adrenal hyperplasia. Embo Journal 6: 1653

Roidot M, Menuel M-C, Coiffard N et al 1964 Hyperplasie lipoidique cerebriforme congenitale des surrenales. Etude anatomo-clinique de la premiere observation francaise du syndrome de Prader. Annales d'Anatomie Pathologique 9: 363

Rose L I, Newmark S R, Strauss W S, Pochi P E 1976 Adrenocortical hydroxylase deficiencies in acne vulgaris. Journal of Investigative Dermatology 66: 324

Rosenbloom A L, Smith D W 1966a Varying expression for salt losing in related patients with congenital adrenal hyperplasia. Pediatrics 38: 215

Rosenbloom A L, Smith D W 1966b Congenital adrenal hyperplasia (letter). Lancet 1: 660

Rosenfield R L, Rich B H, Wolfsdorf J L et al 1980 Pubertal presentation of congenital Δ5-3β-hydroxysteroid dehydrogenase deficiency. Journal of Clinical Endocrinology and Metabolism 51: 345

Rosenwaks Z, Lee P A, Jones G S et al 1979 An attenuated form of congenital virilizing adrenal hyperplasia. Journal of Clinical Endocrinology and Metabolism 49: 335

Rosler A, Leiberman E 1984 Enzymatic defects of steroidogenesis: 11β-hydroxylase-deficiency congenital adrenal hyperplasia. In: New M I, Levine L S (eds) Adrenal Diseases in Childhood (Pediatr Adolesc Endocrinol vol 13). Karger, Basel, p 47

Rosler A, Levine L S, Schneider B, Novogroder M, New M I 1977a The interrelationship of sodium balance, plasma renin activity and ACTH in congenital adrenal hyperplasia. Journal of Clinical Endocrinology and Metabolism 45: 500

Rosler A, Rabinowitz D, Theodor R et al 1977b The nature of the defect in a salt-wasting disorder in Jews of Iran. Journal of Clinical Endocrinology and Metabolism 44: 279

Rosler A, Leiberman E, Sack J, Landau H, Benderly A, Moses S W, Cohen T 1982 Clinical variability of congenital adrenal hyperplasia due to 11β-hydroxylase deficiency. Hormone Research 16: 133

Royer P, Lesteradet H, DeMenibus C I H, Vermeil G 1961 Hypoaldosteronisme familial chronique a debut neonatal. Annales de Pediatrie (Paris) 8: 133

Rumsby G, Carroll M C, Porter R R, Grant D B, Hjelm M 1986 Deletion of the steroid 21-hydroxylase and complement C4 in congenital adrenal hyperplasia. Journal of Medical Genetics 23: 204

Russell A, Levin B, Sinclair L, Oberholzer V G 1963 A reversible salt-wasting syndrome of the newborn and infant: possible infantile hypoaldosteronism. Archives of Disease in Childhood 38: 313

Sasano N, Furuyama M, Yamazaki M 1963 Congenital adrenal hyperplasia associated with gonadal agenesis. Endocrinologica Japonica 10: 215

Scaroni C, Opocher G, Mantero F 1986 Renin-angiotensin-aldosterone system: a long-term follow-up study in 17α-hydroxylase deficiency syndrome (17OHD). Hypertension (Clin Exper-Theory Prac) 8: 773

Schneider G, Genel M, Bongiovanni A M, Goldman A S, Rosenfield R L 1975 Persistant testicular Δ5-isomerase-3β-hydroxysteroid dehydrogenase (Δ5-3β-HSD) deficiency in the Δ5M-3β-HSD form of congenital adrenal hyperplasia. Journal of Clinical Investigation 55: 681

Sherman S L, Aston C E, Morton N E, Speiser P W, Dupont B, New M I 1988 A segregation and linkage study of classical and nonclassical 21-hydroxylase deficiency. American Journal of Human Genetics 42: 830

Simopoulos A P, Marshall J R, Delea C S, Bartter F C 1971 Studies on the deficiency of 21-hydroxylation in patients with congenital adrenal hyperplasia. Journal of Clinical

Endocrinology and Metabolism 32: 438

Speiser P W, Dupont B, Rubinstein P, Piazza A, Kastelan A, New M I 1985 High frequency of nonclassical steroid 21-hydroxylase deficiency. American Journal of Human Genetics 37: 650

Speiser P W, Drucker S, New M I 1987 Hypothalamic-pituitary-gonadal axis in nonclassical 21-hydroxylase deficiency (abstract). Endocrinology 120(S): 171

Speiser P W, New M I, White P C 1988 Molecular genetic analysis of nonclassic 21-hydroxylase deficiency associated with HLA-B14;DR1. New England Journal of Medicine 319: 19

Spies T, Morton C C, Neodospasov S A, Fiers W, Pius D, Strominger J L 1986 Genes for the tumor necrosis factors alpha and beta are linked to the human major histocompatibility complex. Proceedings of the National Academy of Sciences USA 83: 8699

Stalvey J R D, Meisler M H, Payne A H 1987 Evidence that the same structural gene encodes testicular and adrenal 3β-hydroxysteroid dehydrogenase-isomerase. Biochemical Genetics 25: 181

Stoner E, DiMartino J, Kuhnle U, Levine L S, Oberfield S E, New M I 1986 Is salt wasting in congenital adrenal hyperplasia genetic? Clinical Endocrinology 24: 9

Strickland A L, Kotchen T A 1972 A study of the renin-aldosterone system in congenital adrenal hyperplasia. Journal of Pediatrics 81: 962

Suwa S Y, Igarashi I, Kato K, Kusunoki T, Tanae A, Niimi K, Yata J 1981 A case survey study for congenital adrenal hyperplasia in Japan. 1. Study for incidence. Acta Paediatrica Japonica 85: 204

Sydnor K L, Kelley V C, Raile R B et al 1953 Blood adrenocorticotrophin in children with congenital adrenal hyperplasia. Proceedings of the Society for Experimental Biology and Medicine 82: 695

Takikawa O, Gomi T, Suhara K, Itagaki E, Takemori S, Katagiri M 1978 Properties of an adrenal cytochrome P450 (P450scc) for the side chain cleavage of cholesterol. Archives of Biochemistry and Biophysics 190: 300

Temeck J, Pang S, Nelson C, New M I 1987 Genetic defects of steroidogenesis in premature pubarche. Journal of Clinical Endocrinology and Metabolism 64: 609

Thompson G, Bodmer W 1977 The genetic analysis of HLA and disease associations. In: Dausset J, Svejgaard A (eds) HLA and Disease. Williams & Wikins, Baltimore MD, p 84

Tukey R H, Okino S, Barnes H, Griffin K J, Johnson E F 1985 Multiple gene-linked sequences related to the rabbit hepatic progesterone 21-hydroxylase cytochrome P-450 1. Journal of Biological Chemistry 260: 13347

Ulick S 1976 Adrenocortical factors in hypertension. 1. Significance of 18-hydroxy-11-deoxycorticosterone. American Journal of Cardiology 38: 814

Ulick S 1984 Selective defects in the biosynthesis of aldosterone. In: New M I, Levine L S (eds): Adrenal Disease in Childhood (Pediatr Adolesc Endocrinol. vol 13). Karger, Basel, P 145

Veldhuis J D, Kulin H K, Santen R J, Wilson T E, Melby J C 1980 Inborn error in the terminal step of aldosterone biosynthesis. Corticosterone methyl oxidase type II deficiency in a North American pedigree. New England Journal of Medicine 303: 117

Verkauf B S, Jones H W 1970 Masculinization of the female genitalia in congenital adrenal hyperplasia: relationship to the salt-losing variety of the disease. Southern Medical Journal 63: 634

Voutilainen R, Miller W R 1987 Hormonal regulation of genes for steroidogenic enzymes. In: D'Agata R, Chrousos G P (eds) Recent Advances in Adrenal Regulation and Function (Serono Symp. vol 40). Raven Press, New York, p23

Wallace A M, Beastall G H, Cook B, Currie A J, Ross A M, Kennedy R, Girdwood R W A 1986 Neontal screening for congenital adrenal hyperplasia: a programme based on a novel direct radioimmunoassay for 17-hydroxyprogesterone in blood spots. Journal of Endocrinology 108: 299

Waterman M R, Simpson E R 1985 Cellular mechanisms involved in the acute and chronic actions of ACTH. In: Anderson D C, Winter J S D (eds) Adrenal Cortex. Butterworths, London, p 57

Werder E A, Siebenmann R E, Knorr-Murset W et al 1980 The incidence of congenital adrenal hyperplasia in Switzerland – a survey of patients in 1960 to 1974. Helvetica Paediatrica Acta 35: 5

Werkmeister J W, New M I, Dupont B, White P C 1986 Frequent deletion and duplication of the steroid 21-hydroxylase genes. American Journal of Human Genetics 39: 461

White P C, Chaplin D D, Weis J H, Dupont B, New M I, Seidman J G 1984a Two steroid 21-hydroxylase genes located in the murine S region. Nature 312: 465

White P C, New M I, Dupont B 1984b HLA linked congenital adrenal hyperplasia results from a defective gene encoding a cytochrome P-450 specific for steroid 21-hydroxylation. Proceedings of the National Academy of Sciences USA 81: 7505

White P C, Grossberger D, Onufer B J, New M I, Dupont B, Strominger J L 1985 Two genes encoding steroid 21-hydroxylase are located near the genes encoding the fourth component of complement in man. Proceedings of the National Academy of Sciences USA 82: 1089

White P C, New M I, Dupont B 1986 Structure of human steroid 21-hydroxylase genes. Proceedings of the National Academy of Sciences USA 83: 5111

White P C, New M I, Dupont B 1987 Congenital adrenal hyperplasia. New England Journal of Medicine 316: 1519, 1580

Wilkins L 1965 The diagnosis and treatment of endocrine disorders in childhood and adolescence, 3rd edn. Chas C. Thomas, Springfield

Wilkins L, Lewis R A, Klein R, Rosemberg E 1950 The suppression of androgen secretion by cortisone in a case of congenital adrenal hyperplasia. Bulletin of Johns Hopkins Hospital 86: 249

Wilson J D, Griffin J E, George F W, Leshin M 1983 The endocrine control of male phenotypic development. Australian Journal of Biological Sciences 36: 101

Winter J S D 1980 Current approaches to the treatment of congenital adrenal hyperplasia. Pediatrics 97: 81

Winterer J, Chrousos G P, Loriaux D L, Cutler G B 1985 Effect of hydrocortisone dose schedule on adrenal steroid secretion in congenital adrenal hyperplasia. Journal of Pediatrics 106: 137

Wischusen J, Baker H W G, Hudson B 1981 Reversible male infertility due to congenital adrenal hyperplasia. Clinical Endocrinology 14: 571

Yanagibashi K, Haniu M, Shively J E, Shen W H, Hall P

1986 The synthesis of aldosterone by the adrenal cortex. Journal of Biological Chemistry 261: 3556

Zachmann M, Prader A 1978 Unusual heterozygotes of congenital adrenal hyperplasia due to 21-hydroxylase deficiency. Acta Endocrinologica (Kbh) 87: 557

Zachmann M, Prader A 1979 Unusual heterozygotes of congenital adrenal hyperplasia due to 21-hydroxylase deficiency confirmed by HLA tissue typing. Acta Endocrinologica (Kbh) 92: 542

Zachmann M, Prader A 1984 17,20-Desmolase deficiency. In: New M I, Levine L S (eds): Adrenal Disease in Childhood (Pediatr Adolesc Endocrinol. vol 13). Karger, Basel, p 95

Zachmann M, Vollmin J A, Murset G, Curtius H-C, Prader A 1970 An unusual type of congenital adrenal hyperplasia probably due to deficiency of 3β-hydroxysteroid dehydrogenase. Case report of a surviving girl and steroid studies. Journal of Clinical Endocrinology and Metabolism 30: 719

Zachmann M, Vollmin W A, New M I, Curtius H-C, Prader A 1971 Congenital adrenal hyperplasia due to deficiency of 11β-hydroxylation of 17α-hydroxylated steroids. Journal of Clinical Endocrinology and Metabolism 33: 501

Zachmann M, Vollmin W A, Hamilton W, Prader A 1972 Steroid 17,20-desmolase deficiency: a new cause of male pseudohermaphroditism. Clinical Endocrinology 1: 369

Zachmann M, Werder E A, Prader A 1982 Two types of male pseudohermaphroditism due to 17,20-desmolase deficiency. Journal of Clinical Endocrinology and Metabolism 55: 487

Zachmann M, Tassinari D, Prader A 1983 Clinical and biochemical variability of congenital adrenal hyperplasia due to 11β-OHD. A study of 25 patients. Journal of Clinical Endocrinology and Metabolism 56: 222

91. Disorders of gonads and internal reproductive ducts

Joe Leigh Simpson

Genetic advances have greatly facilitated the delineation of disorders of sexual differentiation. In this chapter we shall discuss those disorders of gonadal differentiation that result from mutant genes. Abnormalities involving sex chromosomes are alluded to only briefly. Both Mendelian and cytogenetic disorders of sex differentiation have been discussed elsewhere by this author (Simpson 1976, 1987a,b, 1988a,b) in publications that this review inevitably reflects.

GENETIC CONTROL OF SEX DIFFERENTIATION

Both sex chromosomes (X and Y) as well as autosomes contain loci that must remain intact for normal sexual development. Location of these loci is important for clinical management. That autosomal factors influence sexual development means, as an example, that autosomal translocations may be associated with genital abnormalities. Before formally considering the various disorders, it is therefore helpful to review current knowledge concerning the genetic control of human sex differentiation.

Testicular development

That 46, X, i(Yq) individuals were female in appearance led, over 20 years ago, to the assumption that the major testicular determinants (now called TDF, or testis determining factor) were localized to the Y short arm (Yp). Later, the most distal portion of the Y short arm was excluded because non-mosaic ring Y individuals proved to be male. Such observations were also consistent with the existence of an obligatory pairing region between Xp and Yp, presumed for decades but only later proved (Andersson et al 1986). (Because a pairing region is presumed to be pseudoautosomal, one would not expect it to contain sex determining genes.) Conversely, other studies indicated that TDF was not located immediately near the centromere. A del(Yp) individual proved female

(Magenis et al 1984). XX males rarely showed heteromorphic X chromosomes (Evans et al 1977), indicating that X–Y interchange involves only a small portion of Yp.

Localizing TDF further in region Yp11.2 required molecular technology. Investigations utilizing cloned DNA sequences initially allowed TDF to be localized to a relatively distal portion of Yp11.2, near sequence DXYS5 (Vergnaud et al 1986). This strategy is illustrated in Table 91.1, with the result illustrated in Figure 91.1. Because sequence DXYS5 does not correspond to TDF (Table 91.1), strategies for 'walking the gene' were next applied to localized TDF. Later Page et al (1987) localized TDF to a 140 kb sequence. The region contains several unique sequences homologous to those on Xp, and shows sequences reminiscent of those defining zinc finger proteins. The latter finding suggests that TDF is a DNA binding protein.

In addition to genes on the Y chromosome, it is clear that testicular differentiation requires loci on the X and

Table 91.1 An early study illustrating the principle of localizing TDF by analysis of presence or absence of selected cloned DNA sequences in XX males and XY males.
Interval 3 is never present without interval 2, nor is 2 present without 1. Thus, TDF lies closer to interval 1 than to other intervals. However, none of these clones correspond to TDF because some XX males lack all clones tested. (Data of Vergnaud et al 1986.) Later, TDF was localized to a small (140 kb) portion of interval 1 [Interval 1B] (Page et al 1987).

| Diagnosis | N | DNA Sequences (Probe) | | | | Interval (Vergnaud) |
		DXYS5 (47)	DXYS7 (13d)	DYS8 (118)	DXYS1 (DP34)	
XX Male	7	−	−	−	−	
XX Male	1	+	−	−	−	1
XX Male	6	+	+	−	−	2
XY Male	5	+	+	+	−	3
XY Male	5	+	+	+	+	4

+ = present; − = absent

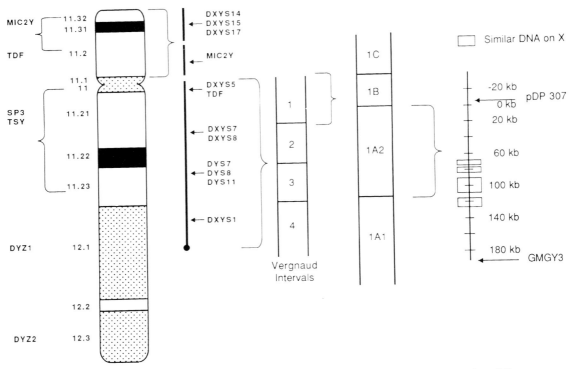

Fig. 91.1 Location of Testis Determining Factor (TDF) and other loci on the Y chromosome. The region of Yp most likely to contain TDF is interval 1 (Vergnaud et al 1986), as defined by DNA sequence DXYS5. Page et al (1987) further subdivided region 1 into sub-intervals, one of which (interval 1B) localized TDF within a 140 kb fragment.

on the autosomes. The importance of genes on the X is evidenced by the X–linked recessive form of XY gonadal dysgenesis (Simpson et al 1971a, German et al 1978). In addition, we shall discuss below the occurrence of agonadia in sibs (de Grouchy et al 1985), and the occurrence of rudimentary testes syndrome in sibs (Najjar et al 1974). Autosomal factors are also capable of causing germ cell hypoplasia in both males (germinal cell aplasia) and females (streak gonads) (Hamet et al 1973, Smith et al 1979, Granat et al 1983, Al–Awadi et al 1985, Mikati et al 1985).

In mice it can be proved even more definitively that atuosomal loci are integral for testicular differentiation. Eicher et al (1982) crossed C57BL females to *Mus posciavinus* males. The F1 males were then back–crossed to C57 females, placing the *Mus posciavinus* Y on a predominantly C57 autosomal background. The Y sometimes proved incapable of directing testicular differentiation, demonstrating capacity of murine autosomes to affect male differentiation. The autosomal region responsible for this perturbation was localized to mouse chromosome 17 (Washburn & Eicher 1983). Interestingly,

mouse 17 may be homologous to human chromosome 6 because each chromosome contains the major histocompatibility complex (MHC) for its species (H–2 in mice, HLA in man). That a structural gene for serological H–Y antigen may be localized to human chromosome 6 (Lau 1989) is even more intriguing.

Isolating the DNA responsible for male differentiation will allow some fundamental questions concerning TDF to be answered. In particular, we will be able to determine the relationship between testicular differentiation, spermatogenesis and H–Y antigen. Circumstantial data implicating H–Y as pivotal for testicular differentiation is well referenced by Wachtel (1983), namely the invariable correlation between testes and H–Y antigen. (XX males and XX true hermaphrodites are H–Y positive.) Antibodies against H–Y antigen also prevent reaggregation of disrupted testicular cells, which are then directed into follicular-like rather than tubular-like structures (Zenzes et al 1978). On the other hand, E Simpson et al (1984) recovered H–Y positive female mice carrying Sxr (Sex–reversal) (X/X^{Sxr}), and McLaren et al (1984) observed testicular differentiation in X/X^{Sxr} mice lacking H–Y.

Those groups believe that H–Y is necessary for spermatogenesis (Burgoyne et al 1986), but not testicular differentiation.

Additional support for H–Y not being synonymous with TDF are derived from studies in which DNA sequence DXYS5 was absent in 46,XY phenotypic females who showed H–Y antigen (Page 1986, E Simpson et al 1987). If governed by the Y, the locus for H–Y antigen must then exist in a region other than interval 1 (Fig. 91.1), which contains TDF.

Related genes on the Y long arm (Yq)

In addition to a locus integral for H–Y, the Y long arm (Yq) may contain several other genes. These include: (1) a region that if deleted protects against neoplasia; (2) a region essential for spermatogenesis (so–called AZO or SP3); (3) a region exerting a positive effect on stature (cell growth (CGY); and (4) a region exerting a positive effect on tooth size (TSY). Unanswered is whether all these regions (loci) truly exist and, if so, what their relationship is?

The most solid data for a locus on Yq controlling morbid anatomical traits are those relating to growth. Yq has plausibly been said to contain factors exerting a positive effect on height (cell growth Y chromosome) (CGY) (Smith et al 1985) and tooth size (TSY) (Alvesalo & de la Chapelle 1981). Such loci have been postulated on the basis of comparison of normal and abnormal individuals, including XY males with androgen insensitivity. That a single locus (region) is responsible for both traits (CGY and TSY) also seems plausible (Simpson 1988).

A locus on Yq important for azoospermia (AZO, azoospermia, or SP3, so–called spermatogenesis Factor 3) has been postulated on the basis of: (1) infertile males showing deletions of Yq; and (2) infertile males showing nonfluorescent Y chromosomes deficient for Yq (Tiepolo & Zuffardi 1976). However, several potential pitfalls preclude readily accepting such a hypothesis. First, male infertility and even azoospermia are relatively common conditions; thus, detection of sex chromosomal abnormalities in azoospermic men may have been merely coincidental. Second, alternative cytogenetic interpretations are possible. In particular, nonfluorescent Y chromosomes are ususally dicentric, an aberration invariably accompanied by monosomic lines because of the inherent instability of dicentric chromosomes (breakage-fusion-bridge cycle).

Finally, loss of the fluorescent (and presumably contiguous nonfluorescent) portion of Yq was observed by Lukusa et al (1986) to exert a protective effect against germ cell neoplasia. Page (1988) refers to this locus as GBY (gonadoblastoma Y), and postulated that its wild type function concerns spermatogenesis. The various Yq loci for somatic traits are certainly not necessarily mutually exclusive. In addition to the thoughts of Page (1987), Simpson (1988) wondered whether CGY, TSY and GBY were synonymous.

Ovarian development

In the absence of a Y chromosome, the indifferent gonad develops into an ovary. Germ cells exist in 45,X human fetuses (Jirásek 1976) and 39,X mice (Burgoyne & Baker 1987); thus, the pathogenesis of germ cell failure involves increased germ cell attrition. If two intact X chromosomes are not present, 45,X ovarian follicles usually degenerate by birth. The second X chromosome is therefore responsible for *ovarian maintenance*, rather than ovarian differentiation. Further supporting constitutive ovarian differentiation are observations that oocyte development occurs in infants with XY gonadal dysgenesis (Cussen & McMahon 1979) or genito-palato-cardiac syndrome (Greenberg et al 1987). As already noted, oocyte development in the presence of a Y chromosome is well documented in mice (Evans et al 1977).

For years efforts have been directed towards localizing those regions of the X chromosome important for ovarian maintenance. Reviewed elsewhere by this author (Simpson 1987a,b, 1988a), ovarian maintenance determinants can be deduced (phenotypic-karyotypic correlations) to exist on both the X short arm and the X long arm. Each arm probably has at least two regions of importance for ovarian development.

With respect to the short arm, 11 of 24 reported terminal del(X)(p11.2–11.4) cases (45.8%) showed primary amenorrhoea (Simpson 1987a,b) (Fig. 91.2). The 13 other individuals showed secondary amenorrhoea, and pregnancy was rare. A locus in regions Xp11.2–11.4 is thus clearly important for ovarian maintenance. More telomeric terminal deletions [del(X)(p21)] can be deduced to be less deleterious because all reported women have menstruated. However, five of the 10 reported del(X)(p21) women were infertile, manifesting secondary amenorrhoea. Thus, there must exist a second region on Xp important for ovarian maintenance, albeit less important than region Xp11.2–11.4.

Similar topography appears to exist on the X long arm (Xq) (Fig. 91.2). Deletions involving Xq11.3 or proximal Xq21 are usually (10 of 11 reported cases) associated with complete ovarian failure (Simpson 1987a,b, 1988a). However, region Xq25 or Xq26 also seems necessary. An interstitial deletion involving this region resulted in secondary amenorrhoea in a mother and her daughters

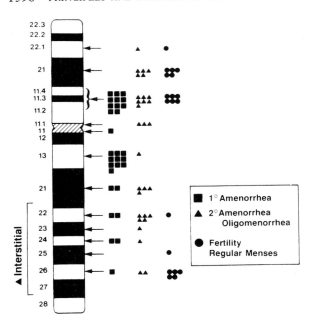

Fig. 91.2 Schematic diagram of X chromosome, showing ovarian function as function of terminal deletion. The bracketed area to the left connotes the interstitial deletion reported by Krauss et al (1987). From Simpson (1988a).

(Krauss et al 1987). Familial terminal deletions of Xq25 (Simpson 1987a) and Xq26 (Fitch et al 1982) yield similar phenotypes. Thus, two or more regions on Xq must play roles in ovarian maintenance, with the two regions differing in importance.

In addition to these regions on the X chromosome, autosomal loci are essential for normal ovarian development. An autosomal recessive gene causes gonadal dysgenesis in XX individuals (Simpson et al 1971a) with several distinct entities having been identified (genetic heterogeneity) (Simpson 1979). In addition, we have already noted the existence of families in which autosomal genes cause germ cell failure in both male and female sibs.

X–Y homologies

Regions on the X and Y chromosome have long been suspected of showing homologies. In addition to pseudoautosomal regions (Xp and Yp), homologies have been demonstrated for Yp and Xq, Yq and Xq, and Yq and Xp.

Existence of these homologies led this author to propose a novel mechanism for control of sex differentiation. Perhaps gonadal determinants on the X and Y were identical (Simpson 1987a). If so, sex determinants could be controlled by X-inactivation, males having twice the gene product as females because the Y chromosome is not inactivated. For other reasons Chandra (1985) had earlier proposed X-inactivation as a mechanism for sex determination. Although the Xq–Yp homologies proposed by Simpson (1987a) differ from the Yp–Xp homologies found by Page et al (1987), there is increasing overall interest in the possible relationship between gonadal determinants on the X and on the Y. Discussion is provided by Simpson (1987a), Page et al (1987) and German (1988).

Genital and ductal development

Although the precise nature of gonadal determinants on the X and Y is uncertain, genital and ductal differentiation proceed predictably after gonadal development is established.

After having differentiated from the indifferent gonad, the developing testes secrete two hormones (Fig. 91.3). Fetal *Leydig* cells produce an androgen, probably testosterone, that stabilizes the Wolffian ducts and permits differentiation of vasa deferentia, epididymides and seminal vesicles. After conversion by 5α-reductase to dihydrotestosterone, the external genitalia are virilized. These actions can be mimicked by the administration of testosterone to female or castrated male embryos, as demonstrated clinically by the existence of teratogenic forms of female pseudohermaphroditism (Carson & Simpson 1984). Fetal *Sertoli* cells produce a different hormone, a glycoprotein of high molecular weight that diffuses locally to cause regression of Mullerian derivatives (uterus and Fallopian tubes). This gene product – anti-Mullerian hormone (AMH) – has not only been isolated (Cates et al 1986) but the gene has also been localized to chromosome 19 (Cohen-Haguenauer et al 1987). Sertoli cells are also the first cells to become evident in testicular differentiation, organizing surrounding cells into tubules. Both Leydig cells (Patsavoudi et al 1985) and Sertoli cells (Magre & Jost 1984) function in dissociation from testicular morphogenesis, consistent with their having directed gonadal development.

In the absence of AMH and testosterone, internal genitalia develop along female lines. Mullerian ducts develop into uterus and Fallopian tubes; Wolffian ducts regress. External genitalia also develop along female lines. These changes, first shown decades ago in rabbits (Jost 1947), also occur in 46,XX embryos and in castrated 46,XY embryos.

MALE PSEUDOHERMAPHRODITISM

Male pseudohermaphrodites are individuals with a Y chromosome whose external genitalia fail to develop as

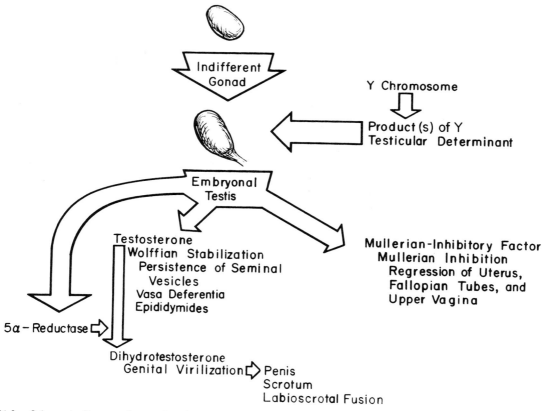

Fig. 91.3 Schematic diagram of normal male differentiation.

expected for normal males. Some authors apply the appellation only to those whose external genitalia are ambiguous enough to confuse the sex of rearing; however, applying the term more liberally seems more useful clinically. Disorders not strictly fulfilling the above definition but usually considered with male pseudohermaphrodites include persistence of Mullerian derivatives in males, and the syndrome of rudimentary testes. In addition, cytogenetic forms of male pseudohermaphroditism (45,X/46,XY and variants) are discussed here in order to contrast their phenotype with those of genetic male pseudohermaphroditism.

Cytogenetic forms: 45,X/46,XY and variants

These individuals have both a 45,X cell line and at least one cell line containing a Y chromosome. They may manifest a variety of phenotypes, ranging from almost normal males with cryptochidism or penile hypospadias to females indistinguishable from those with the 45,X Turner syndrome (Simpson 1976, McDonough & Tho 1983, Rosenberg et al 1987). The different phenotypes

presumably reflect different tissue distributions of the various cell lines. Not infrequently a structurally abnormal Y chromosome is present. 45,X/46,XY individuals may be grouped clinically into one of three categories, namely, individuals with: (a) unambiguous female external genitalia; (b) ambiguous external genitalia, i.e., the sex of rearing is in doubt; or (c) almost normal male external genitalia.

Female external genitalia

These patients may have the Turner stigmata and thus be clinically indistinguishable from 45,X individuals. These 45,X/46,XY individuals are usually normal in stature and show no somatic anomalies. As in any type of gonadal dysgenesis, the external genitalia, vagina, and Mullerian derivatives remain unstimulated because of the lack of sex steroids. Breasts fail to develop, and little pubic or axillary hair develops. If breast development occurs in a 45,X/46,XY individual, in fact, one should suspect an oestrogen-secreting tumour like a gonadoblastoma or dysgerminoma (Verp & Simpson 1987). Occasionally virilization may result from gonadotropin stimulation of streak gonads (Bosze et al 1986)

Although the streak gonads of 45,X/46,XY individuals are usually histologically indistinguishable from the streak gonads of individuals with 45,X gonadal dysgenesis, gonadoblastomas or dysgerminomas develop in about 15–20% of 45,X/46,XY individuals. In contrast to the syndrome of androgen insensitivity, neoplasia may develop in the first or second decade. As already mentioned, Lukusa et al (1986) observed that germ cell neoplasia was uncommon in 45,X/46,XY individuals having a nonfluorescent Y chromosome. That is, loss of a region (locus) seemed to confer a protective effect, suggesting existence of a cancer–predisposing region on the long arm (Yq). The locus is presumed localized in distal nonfluorescent Yq, a region often lost in formation of a dicentric chromosome. Gonadal extirpation is recommended for all 45,X/46,XY individuals with female external genitalia.

Ambiguous genitalia

The term asymmetrical or mixed gonadal dysgenesis is applied to individuals with one streak gonad and one dysgenetic testis. Such individuals usually have ambiguous external genitalia and a 45,X/46,XY complement. Occasionally only 45,X or only 46,XY cells are demonstrable. Many investigators believe that the phenotype is invariably associated with 45,X/46,XY mosaicism, ostensibly nonmosaic cases merely reflecting the inability to sample appropriate tissues.

One important clinical observation is that 45,X/46,XY individuals with ambiguous external genitalia usually have Mullerian derivatives (e.g. a uterus). Presence of a uterus is diagnostically helpful because that organ is absent in almost all genetic (Mendelian) forms of male pseudohermaphroditism (see below). If an individual has ambiguous external genitalia, bilateral testes, and a uterus, it is therefore reasonable to infer that such an individual has 45,X/46,XY mosaicism, regardless of whether both lines can be demonstrated cytogenetically. Occasionally the uterus is rudimentary, or a Fallopian tube may fail to develop ipsilateral to a testis.

Almost normal male genitalia

Occasionally 45,X/46,XY mosaicism is detected in individuals with almost normal male external genitalia. A uterus is less likely to be present than in 45,X/46,XY individuals with ambiguous or female external genitalia. 45,X/46,XY individuals with almost normal male external genitalia do not seem to develop neoplasia as often as 45,X/46,XY individuals with female or frankly ambi-

guous genitalia. Gonadal extirpation is probably not necessary if a male sex-of-rearing is chosen, provided gonads can periodically be palpated within the scrotum or assessed by ultrasound studies.

45,X/47,XXY;45,X/46,XY/47,XYY.

These complements are rarer than 45,X/46,XY, but associated with the same phenotypic spectrum. Of particular interest is one family in which two and possibly three sibs with 45,X/46,XY/47,XYY mosaicism were products of a second cousin marriage (Hsu et al 1970). Recessive factors influencing nondisjunction may thus exist.

Hypospadias without other defects

This is the first of many genetic forms of male pseudohermaphroditism that we shall discuss. In hypospadias, the urinary meatus terminates on the ventral aspect of the penis, proximal to its usual site at the tip of the glans penis. Hypospadias is classified according to the site of the urethral meatus: glans penis, penile shaft, penoscrotal junction, or perineum. Sometimes testicular hypoplasia coexists, especially with penoscrotal or perineal hypospadias. More often testes are normal.

The pathogenesis of uncomplicated hypospadias is not known. Decreased fetal testosterone is plausible but unproved. Partial androgen receptor deficiency has been postulated, but this mechanism probably does not explain all cases. A relationship to maternal progestin exposure seems unlikely (Simpson 1985).

Both multiple affected sibs as well as affected individuals in more than one generation have been reported to have uncomplicated hypospadias. After the birth of one affected child, the recurrence risk for subsequent male progeny is 6–10% (Sweet el al 1974). These risks are higher than those usually associated with multifactorial/polygenic inheritance, suggesting genetic heterogeneity with failure to identify clinically indistinguishable autosomal recessive forms. In fact, hypospadias is not infrequently observed as one of several components of a multiple malformation pattern whose aetiology involves an autosomal recessive gene. Presence of other anomalies should, therefore, be excluded before offering the recurrence risks cited above.

Persistence of Mullerian derivatives in otherwise normal males

The uterus and Fallopian tubes (Mullerian derivatives) may persist in ostensibly normal males. The external genitalia, Wolffian (mesonephric) derivatives and testes develop as expected; virilization occurs at puberty. However, infertility is common, and about 5% of reported individuals develop a seminoma or other germ cell tumour. The disorder is sometimes ascertained because uterus and Fallopian tubes prolapse into an inguinal hernia, hence the appellation 'uterine hernia inguinalis'.

Multiple affected sibs and concordant monozygotic twins have been reported (Brook et al 1973). In one family, maternal half sibs were affected (Sloan & Walsh 1976), indicating X–linked recessive inheritance. Failure of Mullerian duct regression could theoretically result either from end-organ (uterus) insensitivity to anti-Mullerian hormone (AMH) or from failure of Sertoli cells to synthesize or secrete AMH. It is of relevance that the gene coding for anti-Mullerian hormone (AMH) has been isolated (Cates et al 1986) and localized to chromosome 19 (Cohen-Haguenauer et al 1987). If the aetiology is truly an X–linked recessive gene, the pathogenesis would not seem likely to involve the structural locus for AMH. Rather, a regulatory mutation or receptor abnormality might be more plausible.

Disorders with multiple malformation patterns

Genital ambiguity may occur in individuals with multiple malformation patterns due to mutant genes. Long recognized is the association of genital ambiguity with the Meckel syndrome, the Smith-Lemli-Opitz (type I) syndrome, the brachio-skeletal-genital syndrome (Elsahy & Waters 1971) and the oesophageal-facial-genital syndrome (Opitz & Howe 1969). These disorders are inherited in autosomal recessive or X–linked recessive fashion. A host of other syndromes are characterized by simple hypospadias or cyptorchidism; however, in these conditions the sex of rearing is not in doubt.

Several newly recognized conditions deserve comment. Drash syndrome is the term now applied to individuals with Wilms tumour, aniridia and male pseudohermaphroditism (Eddy & Mauer 1985, Habib et al 1985).

Because Wilms tumour is associated with deletion of chromosome 11p13, its association with the Drash syndrome localizes an autosomal region integral for male development. Smith-Lemli-Opitz syndrome, type II, is an autosomal recessive condition in which 46,XY individuals show genital abnormalities extending beyond the hypospadias of Smith-Lemli-Opitz, type I, to female external genitalia (sex-reversal) (Curry et al 1987). In the genito-palatal-cardiac (Gardner-Silengo-Wachtel) syndrome, 46,XY individuals not only show variability in external genitalia but also in gonads (Greenberg et al 1987); sex-reversal can occur, 46,XY individuals showing ovaries (Greenberg et al 1987). Ieshima et al (1986) reported two sibs with peculiar facies, deafness, cleft palate, growth retardation, mental retardation and male pseudohermaphroditism.

Enzyme deficiencies in testosterone biosynthetic pathways

An enzyme deficiency should be suspected if testosterone or its metabolities are decreased. Although diagnosis of the conditions to be discussed is not difficult in older children, detection is more difficult in infancy because baseline testosterone levels are normally low. Provocative tests (hCG) are usually recommended to facilitate diagnosis.

Male pseudohermaphroditism may result from deficiencies of 17α-hydroxylase, 3β-ol-dehydrogenase, 17-ketosteroid reductase, 17–20 desmolase or one of the enzymes required to convert cholesterol to pregnenolone (congenital adrenal lipoid hyperplasia) (Fig. 91.4). Deficiencies of 21- or 11β-hydroxylase, the most common causes of female pseudohermaphroditism, do not cause male pseudohermaphroditism. Indeed, androgen secretion is increased in these two conditions. However, males with 21-hydroxylase deficiency may lose sodium whereas those with 11β-hydroxylase deficiencies may retain sodium. The latter leads to hypervolaemia and hence hypertension. Inheritance is autosomal recessive in most deficiencies. In 17–20 desmolase deficiency, X–linked recessive inheritance is possible. In 17–ketosteroid reductase deficiency, only affected males have been reported.

Congenital adrenal lipoid hyperplasia

In this condition male pseudohermaphrodites show ambiguous or female-like external genitalia, severe salt wasting and adrenals characterized by foamy appearing cells filled with cholesterol. Approximately 30 cases have been described (Degenhart 1984, Frydman et al 1986). Accumulation of cholesterol indicates that this compound cannot be converted to pregnenolone (Fig. 91.4). The enzyme responsible for this defect could be any of the three required to convert cholesterol to pregnenolone: 20α–hydroxylase, 20,22–desmolase, 22α–hydroxylase. Probably genetic heterogeneity will eventually be demonstrated. Inheritance is autosomal recessive, based upon increased parental consanguinity.

3β-ol-dehydrogenase deficiency

Deficiency of 3β-ol-dehydrogenase, an autosomal recessive disorder, results in decreased synthesis of both androgens and oestrogens (Fig. 91.4). In 1985 Perrone et

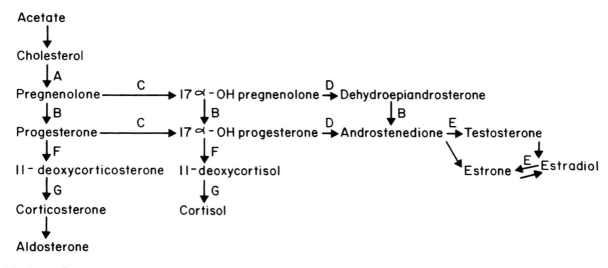

Fig. 91.4   Important adrenal and gonadal biosynthetic pathways. Letters designate enzymes required for the appropriate conversions. From Simpson (1976)

A = 20α-hydroxylase, 22α-hydroxylase, and 20,22-desmolase
B = 3β-ol-dehydrogenase
C = 17α-hydroxylase
D = 17,20-desmolase

E = 17-ketosteroid reductase
F = 21-hydroxylase
G = 11β-hydroxylase

al (1985) collected 27 cases. The major androgen produced is dehydroepiandrosterone (DHEA), a weaker androgen than testosterone. Diagnosis is usually made on the basis of elevated 16-hydroxypregnenolone. In addition to genital abnormalities, 3β-ol-dehydrogenase deficiency is often associated with severe salt wasting because of decreased levels of aldosterone and cortisol.

The incompletely developed external genitalia of 3β-ol-dehydrogenase deficiency is clinically similar to the external genitalia of most other male pseudohermaphrodites: small phallus, urethra opening proximally on the penis, incomplete labioscrotal fusion. Testes and Wolffian ducts differentiate normally. Affected females (46,XX) also show genital ambiguity, 3β-ol-dehydrogenase thus being the only enzyme that, when deficient, produces male pseudohermaphroditism in males and female pseudohermaphroditism in females.

Partial defects may cause hirsutism but no other abnormalities in females (Rosenfield et al 1980, Pang et al 1985), and less severe forms of hypospadias in males (Bongiovanni 1979). These disorders indicate genetic heterogeneity, as further illustrated by an isozyme variant reported by Cravioto et al (1986).

17α-hydroxylase deficiency

Males with deficiency of 17α-hydroxylase usually show ambiguous external genitalia, normal Wolffian duct development, and normal testicular differentiation. Some severely affected males show female external genitalia (Heremans et al 1976). Unlike females deficient for 17α-hydroxylase, males usually display normal blood pressure. Affected females have normal genitalia; however, they fail to undergo normal secondary sexual development. Their oocytes appear incapable of reaching diameters greater than 2.5 mm (Araki et al 1987). Autosomal recessive inheritance is accepted.

17,20-desmolase deficiency

Zachmann et al (1972) reported a family in which two maternal cousins had genital ambiguity, bilateral testes, and no Mullerian derivatives. A maternal 'aunt' was said to have abnormal external genitalia and bilateral testes. The deficient enzyme was deduced to be 17,20-desmolase deficiency on the basis of both cousins showing low plasma testosterone, low dehydroepiandrosterone (DHEA) and normal urinary excretion of pregnanediol, pregnanetriol, and 17-hydroxycorticoids. Incubation of testicular tissue demonstrated that testosterone could be synthesized from androstenedione or dehydroepiandrosterone, excluding 17-ketosteroid reductase and thus suggesting deficiency of 17,20-desmolase. A few other cases have been described, but it remains unclear whether this disorder is autosomal recessive or X–linked recessive.

Deficiency of 17-ketosteroid reductase

Inability to convert dehydroepiandrosterone to testosterone is the result of deficiency of 17-ketosteroid reductase (Fig. 91.4). Approximately 25 cases have been reported (Balducci et al 1985). Plasma testosterone is usually decreased; androstenedione and dehydroepiandrosterone are increased. Affected males show ambiguous external genitalia, bilateral testes, and no Mullerian derivatives. Breast development may or may not be present, apparently reflecting the oestrogen/testosterone ratio (Imperato-McGinley et al 1979). Pubertal virilization is greater than in some other enzyme deficiencies, with gynaecomastia sometimes not even being evident (Caufriez 1986). This is well illustrated by a report in which the sex of rearing of an affected individual was changed from female to male after puberty (Imperato-McGinley et al 1979). The disorder is either autosomal recessive or X-linked recessive. That affected females have not been reported dictates consideration of the latter.

Instability of multiple P–450 enzymes

After studying a 6-month-old 46,XY infant with genital ambiguity and multiple enzyme defects (17α-hydroxylase, 21-hydroxylase, 17,20-desmolase), Peterson et al (1985) proposed a new form of male pseudohermaphroditism. The multiple adrenal biosynthetic abnormalities raised the possibility of an abnormality involving cytochrome P–450. [Adrenal biosynthetic enzymes are usually P–450 enzymes, either mitochondrial or cytoplasmic (Miller & Levine 1987).] Additional data are necessary to be certain that some of the enzyme defects did not merely arise secondarily. No information concerning heritability could be deduced.

Complete androgen insensitivity (complete testicular feminization).

In complete androgen insensitivity (complete testicular feminization), 46,XY individuals have bilateral testes, female external genitalia, blindly-ending vagina, and no Mullerian derivatives. Affected individuals undergo breast development and pubertal feminization.

Despite pubertal feminization, some individuals with androgen insensitivity show clitoral enlargement and labioscrotal fusion; the term incomplete (partial) androgen insensitivity (incomplete testicular feminization) is applied to these patients. Both complete and incomplete (partial) androgen insensitivity are inherited in X-linked recessive fashion. Not only are the two disorders genetically distinct, but heterogeneity exists in each. The gene for complete androgen insensitivity has been localized to the X long arm (Brown & Migeon 1986).

Clinical features of complete androgen sensitivity are well-known, and need not be repeated in detail. Affected individuals may be quite attractive and show excellent breast development, but most are similar in appearance to unaffected females in the general population. Breasts contain normal ductal and glandular tissue, but the areolae are often pale and underdeveloped. Pubic and axillary hair are usually sparse but scalp hair is normal. The vagina terminates blindly. Sometimes the length is shorter than usual, presumably because Mullerian ducts fail to contribute to formation of the vagina. Rarely, the vagina is only 1–2 cm long or represented merely by a dimple.

Neither a uterus nor Fallopian tubes are ordinarily present. Occasionally one detects fibromuscular remnants, rudimentary Fallopian tubes or rarely even a uterus (Ulloa-Aguirre et al 1986). The absence of Mullerian derivatives is not unexpected because the anti-Mullerian hormone (AMH) secreted by the fetal Sertoli cells is not an androgen; therefore Mullerian regression would be expected to occur in males with androgen sensitivity, just as in normal males. The only other condition in which a uterus is absent in a phenotypic female is Mullerian aplasia, readily distinguishable on the basis of pubic hair and a 46,XX complement.

Testes are usually normal in size, located in the abdomen, inguinal canal or labia, i.e. anywhere along the path of embryonic testicular descent. If present in the inguinal canal, testes may produce inguinal hernias. One-half of all individuals with testicular feminization developed inguinal hernias. It is therefore worthwhile to determine cytogenetic status of prepubertal girls with inguinal hernias, although most will be 46,XX. Height is slightly increased over that of normal women, but unremarkable compared to 46,XY males. Presumably the increased height reflects influence of the Y chromosome. Likewise, many clinicians have the impression that hands and feet are relatively large.

The frequency of gonadal neoplasia is increased, but the exact magnitude is uncertain. In one frequently cited publication, Morris and Mahesh (1963) tabulated that 22% of affected patients had neoplasia. However, the actual risk is probably no greater than 5% (Simpson & Photopulos 1976, Verp & Simpson 1987). Most investigators agree that the risk of neoplasia is low before 25–30 years of age, increasing thereafter. Benign tubular adenomas (Pick adenomas) are especially common in postpubertal patients, probably as the result of increased secretion of LH. For all the above reasons orchiectomy is eventually necessary. It is acceptable to leave the testes in situ until after pubertal feminization, but most surgeons would perform orchiectomies if herniorrhaphies prove necessary before puberty. There may also be psychological benefit in prepubertal orchiectomies.

The pathogenesis of complete androgen insensitivity clearly involves end-organ insensitivity to androgens. This has long been deduced on the basis of baseline plasma testosterone being normal, yet patients neither virilizing nor retaining nitrogen after administration of androgen (testosterone or dehydrotestosterone). In addition, hyperplastic Leydig cells and elevated LH levels suggest abnormal gonadal-hypothalamic feed back.

Genetic heterogeneity clearly exists. In perhaps 60–70% of cases androgen receptors are not present (receptor negative). In 30–40% receptors are present (receptor positive). In the latter, a defect at a more distal step in androgen action is presumed to exist. Receptor positive and receptor negative cases are clinically indistinguishable. Pinsky et al (1985) have exhaustively reviewed the tissue of androgen receptors.

Incomplete (partial) androgen sensitivity (incomplete testicular feminization and the Reifenstein syndrome)

At puberty we have already noted that certain 46,XY individuals feminize (show breast development) despite having external genitalia that are characterized by phallic enlargement and partial labioscrotal fusion. Such individuals are said to have incomplete or partial androgen insensitivity (incomplete testicular feminization). Both incomplete and complete androgen insensitivity share the following features: bilateral testes with similar histological findings; no Mullerian derivatives: pubertal breast development; lack of pubertal virilization; normal (male) plasma testosterone; and failure to respond to androgen. The pathogenesis of partial androgen insensitivity, a topic considered in detail by Pinsky et al (1985), appears to involve decreased numbers or qualitative defects of androgen receptors (Griffin et al 1986, Sultan 1986, Pinsky et al 1987).

Incomplete (partial) androgen insensitivity is an X-linked recessive condition that encompasses several entities once considered separate: Lubs syndrome, Gilbert–Dreyfus syndrome, Reifenstein syndrome. Traditionally, the appellation 'Reifenstein syndrome' was applied to males whose phallic development was more nearly normal than that of males with traditionally defined incomplete androgen insensitivity. In the Reifenstein phenotype there was no vagina-like perineal orifice, and testes were small (Reifenstein 1947). On the basis of the latter, decreased virilization was logically deduced to result from inadequate testosterone secretion. The Lubs phenotype (Lubs et al 1959) was considered intermediate between the Reifenstein phenotype and traditional incomplete androgen insensitivity.

Later, males with small testes and elevated gonadotropin levels were shown capable of displaying partial androgen insensitivity (Amrhein et al 1977). Wilson et al (1974) first demonstrated the occurrence in a single kindred of the Reifenstein phenotype and traditionally defined incomplete androgen insensitivity. The same group later confirmed partial androgen receptor deficiency in two individuals with Lubs syndrome phenotype (Wilson et al 1984). In contrast to the usual trend towards genetic heterogeneity, it thus appears that the traditional separation of Reifenstein syndrome, Lubs syndrome and incomplete androgen insensitivity as defined above was not valid. These disorders merely represent different ranges in the spectrum of a single X-linked recessive disorder (Wilson et al 1974) preferably called incomplete (partial) androgen insensitivity. Although genetic heterogeneity may still exist, the basis should not be considered to be differences in clinical appearance.

The clinical significance of incomplete (partial) androgen insensitivity is that this disorder must be excluded before a male sex of rearing is assigned. Presence of androgen receptors and demonstration of a response to exogenous androgen is necessary to exclude androgen insensitivity.

5α-reductase deficiency (pseudovaginal perineoscrotal hypospadias)

For over 20 years it has been recognized that some genetic males show ambiguous external genitalia at birth, yet at puberty virilize like normal males. They undergo phallic enlargement, increased facial hair, muscular hypertrophy, voice deepening, and no breast development. Their external genitalia consist of a phallus that resembles a clitoris more than a penis, a perineal urethral orifice, and usually a separate blindly ending perineal orifice that resembles a vagina (pseudovagina) (Fig. 91.5). Testes are relatively normal in size and secrete testosterone in normal amounts.

By 1971–1972 colleagues and I had shown conclusively that this trait, then called pseudovaginal perineoscrotal hypospadias (PPSH), was inherited in autosomal recessive fashion (Simpson et al 1971b, Opitz et al 1972). Later, the disorder was shown to result from deficiency of 5α-reductase (Imperato-McGinley et al 1974, Walsh et al 1974, Peterson et al 1977, Fisher et al 1978). This enzyme converts testosterone to dihydrotestosterone. That intracellular 5α-reductase deficiency results in the PPSH phenotype is consistent with observations that virilization of the external genitalia during embryogenesis requires dihydrotestosterone, whereas Wolffian differentiation requires only testosterone. Pubertal virilization can be accomplished by testosterone alone.

Studies in the Dominican Republic verified that 5α–

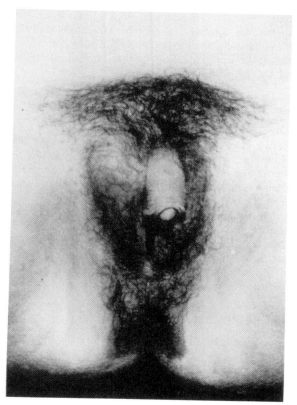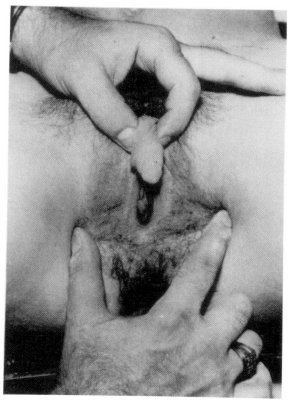

Fig. 91.5 External genitalia of one of three 46,XY sibs with the pseudovaginal perineoscrotal hypospadias (PPSH) phenotye. Many if not all individuals with this phenotype have deficiences of 5α-reductase. Patient of the author reported in Opitz et al (1972).

reductase deficiency is autosomal recessive (Imperato-McGinley et al 1974). Familial aggregates (sibships) of 5α-R (PPSH phenotype) have also been observed in United States black and white populations, in Northern Europe, in Turkey (Akgun et al 1986) and elsewhere. There is evidence for genetic heterogeneity, based upon enzyme kinetic studies (Leshin et al 1978).

Diagnosis of 5α–reductase deficiency is most easily made on the basis of an elevated testosterone(T)/dihydro-testosterone(DHT) ratio after administration of hCG or testosterone propionate (Greene et al 1987). The ratio of the respective urinary metabolites of T and DHT (i.e. etiocholanolone/androsterone) is also elevated.

5α–reductase (5α–R) activity is higher in genital tissue than in cultured fibroblasts, fibroblast homogenates or tissue homogenates. For this reason, it is preferable to assay cells derived from genital tissue (e.g. foreskin). There is, however, considerable variability in 5α-R activity among control genital tissue, with near overlap

between controls and individuals recognized on other grounds to be deficient for 5α-R. Thus, presence of 5α-R in cultured genital fibroblasts excludes 5α-R deficiency, but absence of 5α-R does not necessarily confirm the diagnosis of 5α-R deficiency. This is especially true if genital tissues cannot be studied.

In infants, baseline levels of testosterone and dihydro-testosterone are so low that distinguishing normal from affected individuals may be difficult. Imperato-McGinley et al (1986) have suggested elevated urinary tetrahydro-cortisol/5α-tetrahydrocortisol ratio as the basis for diagnosis, utilizing gas chromatography/mass spectrometry.

Syndrome of rudimentary testes

Bergada et al (1962) were the first to report males who, despite well-formed testes less than 1 cm in greatest diameter, had small penises. Testes consisted of a few

Leydig cells, small tubules containing Sertoli cells, and an occasional spermatogonium. Wolffian derivatives were present; Mullerian derivatives were absent. Relatively few individuals with the rudimentary testes syndrome have been described, and probably the phenotype is very heterogeneous. Nonetheless, Najjar et al (1974) described five affected sibs of consanguineous parents, suggesting that at least one form of this entity is genetic.

The pathogenesis is unclear, for such small testes seem incapable of directing normal male development. Perhaps testes were initially normal during embryogenesis, only later decreasing in size. The aetiology might thus be analogous to that of anorchia (see below), albeit with retention of some testicular tissue.

Agonadia (Testicular Regression Syndrome)

In agonadia the gonads are absent, the external genitalia abnormal, and all but rudimentary Mullerian or Wolffian derivatives absent. External genitalia usually consist of a phallus about the size of a clitoris, underdeveloped labia majora, and nearly complete fusion of labioscrotal folds. A persistent urogenital sinus is often present. By definition, gonads cannot be detected. Neither normal Mullerian derivatives nor normal Wolffian derivatives are ordinarily present; however, rudimentary structures may be present along the lateral pelvic wall. A distinctive feature is coexistence of somatic anomalies – craniofacial and vertebral – and mental retardation (Sarto & Opitz 1973).

Any pathogenic explanation for agonadia must take into account not only absence of gonads, but also abnormal external genitalia and lack of normal internal ducts. At least two explanations seem plausible: (1) fetal testes functioned sufficiently long to inhibit Mullerian development, yet not sufficiently long to complete male differentiation (hence the appellation 'testicular regression syndrome', preferred by some); (2) alternatively, the gonadal, ductal and genital systems all developed abnormally as a result of either defective anlagen, defective connective tissue, or action of a teratogen. Given both heritable tendencies (see below) and the frequent coexistence of somatic anomalies, existence of defective connective tissue is an especially plausible hypothesis.

Among the approximately 30 reported cases are several sibships of affected males (de Grouchy et al 1985). Autosomal recessive inheritance seems likely, but X–linked recessive inheritance cannot be excluded. H–Y antigen is present (Wachtel 1983), indicating that pathogenesis does not involve perturbation of that system.

Several other observations concerning agonadia are unexplained. Josso and Briard (1980) reported an interesting family. Of two 46,XY sibs, one had agonadia and the other anorchia. In addition, 46,XX individuals have shown the agonadia phenotype (Duck et al 1975). Whether the phenomena observed in these two reports reflect the same mutant gene that causes more typical 46,XY agonadia is unknown.

Leydig cell agenesis

Several 46,XY patients have shown complete absence of Leydig cells (Brown et al 1976, Lee et al 1981). The phenotype consists of female external genitalia, no uterus, and bilateral testes devoid of Leydig cells; epididymides and vasa deferentia are present. Predictably, LH is elevated.

Affected sibs have been recognized (Perez-Palacios et al 1982, Saldanha et al 1987), and parental consanguinity observed (Schwartz et al 1981, Saldanha et al 1987). In addition to the autosomal recessive condition described above Toledo et al (1985) described a milder phenotype in three brothers whose parents were consanguineous.

TRUE HERMAPHRODITISM

True hermaphrodites display both ovarian and testicular tissue. They may have a separate ovary and a separate testis, or, more often, one or more ovotestes. Most true hermaphrodites have a 46,XX chromosomal complement; however, others have 46,XX/46,XY; 46,XY; 46,XX/47,XXY, or other complements (Simpson 1978). There are suggestions that phenotype depends upon karyotype (Simpson 1978, Van Niekerk & Retief 1981), but it is preferable here to generalize about the phenotype of all true hermaphrodites.

Phenotype

About two-thirds of true hermaphrodites are raised as males, although their external genitalia may be frankly ambiguous or predominantly female. Breast development usually occurs at puberty even with predominantly male external genitalia.

Gonadal tissue may be located in the ovarian, inguinal or labioscrotal regions. A testis or an ovotestis is more likely to be present on the right than the left. Spermatozoa are rarely present (Aaronsen 1985); however, apparently normal oocytes are often present, even in ovotestes (Fig. 91.6). The greater the proportion of testicular tissue in an ovotestis, the greater the likelihood of gonadal descent. In 80% of ovotestes, testicular and ovarian components are juxtaposed in end-to-end fashion (Van Niekerk 1974); thus, an ovotestis can usually be detected by inspection or possibly by palpation because testicular tissue is softer and darker than ovarian tissue. Ultrasound

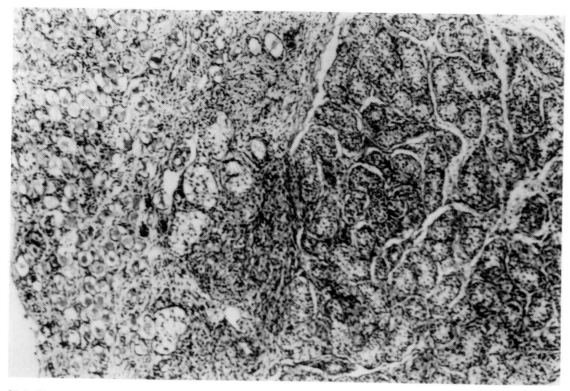

Fig. 91.6 Photomicrograph of the left ovotestis of patient No. 2 of Van Niekerk (1974). The patient had a 46,XX complement. Numerous primordial follicles are present in the smaller left portion; infantile testicular tissue is evident on the right.

evaluation may also be useful in determining gonadal status. Accurate identification is particulary necessary if one wishes to extirpate the inappropriate portion of an ovotestis.

A uterus is usually present, albeit sometimes bicornuate or unicornuate. Absence of a uterine horn usually indicates an ipsilateral testis or ovotestis. The fimbriated end of the Fallopian tube may be occluded ipsilateral to an ovotestis, and squamous metaplasia of the endocervix may occur (Van Niekerk 1974). Menstruation is not uncommon, occasionally manifested as cyclic haematuria (Raspa et al 1986).

The diagnosis is usually made after excluding male and female pseudohermaphroditism. If a female sex of rearing is chosen, less extensive surgery may be necessary. If a male sex of rearing is chosen, genital reconstruction and selective gonadal extirpation is invariably indicated. Five 46,XX true hermaphrodites have become pregnant (Tegenkamp et al 1979, Minowada et al 1984), usually but not always after removal of testicular tissue.

Gonadal neoplasia has been reported, as has carcinoma of the breast (Simpson 1978, Verp & Simpson 1987).

Aetiology

The aetiology of true hermaphroditism is heterogeneous. The most common complement is 46,XX, but other complements also exist. Aetiologies probably differ according to chromosomal complement. 46,XX/46,XY cases presumably result from chimaerism (the presence in a single individual of two or more cell lines, each derived from different zygotes). On the other hand, 46,XX/46,XY humans do not always show true hermaphroditism. 46,XX/47,XXY cases may result from either chimaerism or mitotic nondisjunction. This author has also suggested that most 46,XY cases are unrecognized chimaeras (Simpson 1978).

A few 46,XX true hermaphrodites doubtless result from undetected chimaerism, but undetected chimaerism cannot explain all 46,XX true hermaphrodites. The presence of testicular tissue in 46,XX individuals is ostensibly perplexing because the testis determining factor (TDF) is localized to the Y chromosome, specifically to the short arm (see above). Possible explanations for the presence of testes in individuals who ostensibly lack a Y include: (1) translocation of the testis determining factor (TDF) from the Y to an X; (2) translocation of testicular determinants(s) from the Y to an autosome; (3) undetected mosaicism or chimaerism; and (4) sex-reversal genes.

That the first or second hypothesis was correct was suggested by presence of the H–Y antigen in almost all 46,XX true hermaphrodites (Wachtel 1983). Especially impressive is the detection of H–Y antigen in 46,XX true hermaphrodite sibs (Fraccaro et al 1979). On the other hand, 46,XX true hermaphrodites fail to show DNA sequences from their father's Y (Mueller 1988, Ramsay et al 1988). By contrast, most 46,XX males show DNA sequences derived from their father's Y (Petit et al 1987), verifying translocation of a portion of the paternal Y to Xp. Paternal Y sequences are presumably accompanied by TDF.

That genetic factors, perhaps autosomal factors, play a role in true hermaphroditism is suggested by several familial aggregates. Sibships with XX true hermaphroditism have been reported (Clayton et al 1958, Mori &

Mitzutani 1968, Armendares et al 1975, Fraccaro et al 1979). Perhaps different genetic factors are responsible for the occurrence of 46,XX males and 46,XX true hermaphrodites in the same kindred (Berger et al 1970, Kasdan et al 1978, Skordis et al 1987). Three such kindreds are shown in Figure 91.7; in two of these the disorder was present in more than one generation.

Familial true hermaphroditism is more likely to be characterized by bilateral ovotestes and uterine absence than nonfamilial cases (Simpson 1978). Given the existence of autosomal genes causing sex-reversal in mice (Washburn & Eicher 1983), it is tempting to postulate that perturbation of an ordinarily dormant autosomal gene induces inappropriate sex-reversal. The mechanism could be reminiscent for oncogene induction of neoplasia, i.e. the induced gene is possibly normally responsible for directing testicular development in 46,XY males.

46,XX MALES (SEX-REVERSAL)

46,XX (sex-reversed) males are phenotypic males with bilateral testes (de la Chapelle 1972, 1981).

Phenotype

Affected individuals show small testes and signs of androgen deficiency (Klinefelter phenotype). Facial and

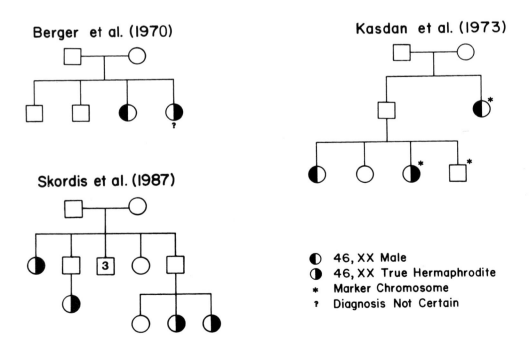

Fig. 91.7 Partial pedigrees of families in which 46,XX males and 46,XX true hermaphroditism occurred in a single kindred.

body hair are decreased, and pubic hair may be distributed in the pattern characteristic of females. About one-third have gynaecomastia. The penis and scrotum are small but traditionally considered to be well differentiated. By definition, the sex of rearing is not in doubt (de la Chapelle 1972). Wolffian derivatives are normal. The predominant pathological findings involve seminiferous tubules that are decreased in number and size. Peritubular and interstitial fibrosis is present, Leydig cells are hyperplastic, and spermatogonia are not usually detectable. Occasionally immature spermatogonia are detected, and sometimes the ejaculate contains spermatozoa.

Aetiology

As already noted, both 46,XX males and 46,XX true hermaphrodites have testes, contrary to expectations that the Y chromosome is required for testicular differentiation; several explanations for this are possible.

In XX males the likely aetiology is an abnormal cytological exchange involving Xp and Yp. The interchange is initiated proximal to the testis determining factor (TDF) on Yp, and extends to the Y telomere to include the pseudoautosomal region. The length of X–Y interchange varies, an observation that was exploited to localize TDF to a small region on Yp (Vergnaud et al 1986, Page et al 1987). In the few cases in which paternal Y sequences are not observed (Petit et al 1987), one can postulate other mechanisms, such as mosaicism or a mutant gene. In fact, familial aggregates of 46,XX males are known (de la Chapelle et al 1975), and we have already mentioned the occurrence of both 46,XX males and 46,XX true hermaphrodites in a single kindred (Berger et al 1970, Kasdan et al 1978, Skordis et al 1987). (Fig. 91.7).

GENETIC FORMS OF GONADAL DYSGENESIS:

Gonadal dysgenesis is usually associated with monosomy for the X chromosome (45,X) or structural abnormalities of sex chromosomes. This topic is discussed elsewhere in this volume. Here we restrict our comments to individuals with apparently normal male (46,XY) or female (46,XX) chromosomal complements.

XX gonadal dysgenesis

Gonadal dysgenesis histologically similar to that detected in individuals with an abnormal sex chromosomal complement has been observed repeatedly in 46,XX individuals in whom mosaicism is reasonably excluded. The term XX gonadal dysgenesis is applied to affected individuals (Simpson et al 1971a, Simpson 1979).

External genitalia and streak gonads of affected individuals are indistinguishable from those of individuals who have gonadal dsygenesis due to an abnormal chromosomal complement. Likewise, both endocrine findings (elevated FSH and LH) and lack of secondary sexual development are similar to those of other individuals with streak gonads. Most individuals with XX gonadal dysgenesis are normal in stature (mean height 165 cm) (Simpson 1979), and the Turner stigmata are usually absent.

XX gonadal dysgenesis is inherited in autosomal recessive fashion. Of interest are families in which one affected sib had streak gonads, whereas another had primary amenorrhoea and extreme ovarian hypoplasia (presence of a few oocytes) (Boczkowski 1970, Simpson 1979, Portuondo et al 1987). These families suggest that the mutant gene responsible for XX gonadal dysgenesis is capable of exerting a more variable effect than originally supposed. It follows that the XX gonadal dysgenesis mutation may be responsible for some sporadic cases of premature ovarian failure.

XX gonadal dysgenesis may occur alone, or it may coexist with distinctive patterns of somatic anomalies. The combination of XX gonadal dysgenesis and neuro-sensory deafness (Perrault syndrome) has been observed in several sibships (Christakos et al 1969, Pallister & Opitz 1979, McCarthy & Opitz 1985). Other syndromes include XX gonadal dysgenesis and myopathy (Lundgren 1973); XX gonadal dysgenesis and cerebellar ataxia (Skre et al 1976); and XX gonadal dysgenesis, microcephaly and arachnodactyly (Maximilian et al 1970).

Gonadal dysgenesis in 46,XX individuals may also result from nongenetic causes (phenocopies). Plausible mechanisms include infections (e.g. mumps), infarctions, infiltrative processes (e.g. tuberculosis, tumours), and autoimmune phenomena (Verp 1983). Of note is a possible relationship between infection and XX gonadal dysgenesis in two sibs (Aleem 1981)

XY gonadal dysgenesis

Gonadal dysgenesis may occur in individuals with apparently normal male (46,XY) chromosomal complements. In at least some cases the gonads of these individuals appeared to have been ovaries during embryological development (Cussen & MacMahon 1979). As discussed above, these findings helped to suggest that ovarian development is constitutive. Loss of testicular tissue before 7–8 weeks' embryogenesis would produce a female phenotype, as shown by Jost (1953).

Individuals with XY gonadal dysgenesis show female external genitalia, a uterus and Fallopian tubes. At puberty secondary sexual development fails to occur. Height is normal and somatic anomalies are usually absent. However, a relationship between XY gonadal dysgenesis and renal failure of uncertain pathogenesis exists (Simpson et al 1981, 1982, Haning et al 1985).

Approximately 20–30% of XY gonadal dysgenesis patients develop a dysgerminoma or gonadoblastoma (Simpson & Photopulos 1976). Often the neoplasia arises in the first or second decade. About two-thirds of XY gonadal dysgenesis individuals are H–Y antigen positive. H–Y positive subjects are far more likely to develop neoplasia than H–Y negative individuals (Wachtel 1983). Because of the relatively high probability of undergoing neoplastic transformation, gonads should be extirpated from individuals with XY gonadal dysgenesis. The uterus and Fallopian tubes should not be removed, even though it is technically easier to remove all these organs than to extirpate only the streaks. Retention of the uterus allows pregnancy through donor oocytes or donor embryos.

At least one form of XY gonadal dysgenesis segregates in the fashion expected of an X–linked recessive (Simpson 1979, Simpson et al 1971a, 1981). In some X–linked kindreds, neoplasia and H–Y positivity has been observed (Mann et al 1983). An autosomal form of the disorder may also exist (Simpson et al 1981) and clinically indistinguishable cases may be due to deletion of TDF from Yp (Disteche et al 1986, Page 1986). The latter were verified by failure of DNA of affected individuals to hybridize to cloned sequences known to lie near TDF. Analysis of such cases allowed TDF to be localized to a small portion of Yp (Page et al 1987).

Additional evidence for genetic heterogeneity (Simpson et al 1981) is provided by the existence of at least three other syndromes: (a) XY gonadal dysgenesis and campomelic dwarfism (Bricarelli et al 1981, Puck et al 1981): (b) XY gonadal dysgenesis and ectodermal anomalies (Brosnan et al 1980); and (c) genito-palato-cardiac (Gardner-Silengo-Wachtel) syndrome (Greenberg et al 1987).

Germ cell failure in both sexes

In five sibships, male and female sibs have each shown germinal cell failure. Females showed streak gonads, whereas males showed germ cell aplasia (Sertoli-cell only syndrome or del Castillo phenotype) (see below). In two of the families parents were consanguineous, and in each no somatic anomalies coexisted (Smith et al 1979, Granat et al 1983). In three other families, characteristic patterns of somatic anomalies coexisted, suggesting distinct entities. Hamet et al (1973) reported germ cell failure, hypertension and deafness; Al-Awadi et al (1985) reported germ cell failure and alopecia; Mikati et al (1985) reported germ cell failure, microcephaly, short stature and minor anomalies.

These families demonstrate that several different autosomal genes are capable of affecting germ cell development in both sexes, presumably acting at a site common to early germ cell development. Elucidation of such genes could have profound implications for an understanding of normal developmental processes.

ANOMALIES LIMITED TO INTERNAL GENITAL DUCTS (MULLERIAN OR WOLFFIAN DERIVATIVES)

Many different developmental abnormalities affect the internal genital ducts. In this section only the most common disorders are discussed.

Transverse vaginal septa

Transverse vaginal septa may occur at several locations. Septa may be complete or incomplete. They are usually about 1 cm thick and located near the junction of the upper third and lower two-thirds of the vagina; however, they may be located in the middle or lower third of the vagina. If a perforation is not present, mucus and menstrual fluid lack egress; thus, hydrocolpos or hydrometrocolpos may develop. Other pelvic structures are usually normal, although occasionally the uterus is bicornuate.

Transverse vaginal septa presumably result from failure of urogenital sinus derivatives and Mullerian duct derivatives to fuse or canalize. An autosomal recessive gene is responsible for some cases, at least in the Amish (McKusick et al 1968). Some individuals with transverse vaginal septa also have polydactyly, in which case the term McKusick-Kaufman (Kaufman-McKusick) syndrome is often applied. These cases may or may not be aetiologically distinct from those without polydactyly.

Longitudinal septa

Longitudinal vaginal septa (sagittal or coronal) rarely produce clinical problems. They presumably result from abnormal mesodermal proliferation or from persisting epithelium. Occasionally longitudinal septa impede the second stage of labour. Heritable tendencies do not appear paramount in isolated cases. However, Edwards and Gale (1972) reported an autosomal dominant syndrome characterized by a longitudinal vaginal septum, hand anomalies and a possible bladder neck anomaly.

Vaginal atresia

In vaginal atresia the urogenital sinus fails to contribute to the caudal portion of the vagina. The lower 20–40% of the vagina is replaced by 2–3 cm of fibrous tissue, superior to which lie a well differentiated upper vagina, cervix, uterine corpus and Fallopian tubes. Vaginal atresia is a condition distinct from both transverse vaginal septa and Mullerian aplasia (see below). Rarer than the latter, only 10–20% of phenotypic females with 'absence of vagina' have vaginal atresia. More likely, Mullerian aplasia or complete androgen insensitivity will exist. Ultrasound may help confirm the pressure of a uterus in vaginal atresia (Bennet & Dewhurst 1983), but rectal examination alone usually verifies the diagnosis.

No familial aggregates of isolated vaginal atresia have been reported. On the other hand, Winter et al (1968) described four sibs with an apparent autosomal recessive syndrome characterized by vaginal atresia, renal hypoplasia or agenesis, and middle ear anomalies (malformed incus, fixation of the malleus and incus). Two other families have since been described, and one affected female became pregnant following surgical reconstruction (King et al 1987). Another malformation syndrome in which vaginal atresia occurs is the Fraser (1962) syndrome, characterized by cryptophthalmos and occasionally also gonadal absence (agonadia) (Greenberg et al 1986).

Mullerian aplasia

Aplasia of the Mullerian ducts leads to absence of the uterine corpus, absence of the uterine cervix, and absence of the upper portion of the vagina. A 1–2 cm vagina is present, presumably derived exclusively from invagination of the urogenital sinus. Ultrasound may be helpful (Rosenberg et al 1986), and laparoscopy is not always necessary to achieve diagnosis. Except for primary amenorrhoea, secondary sexual development is normal. Some investigators apply the appellation 'Rokitansky-Kustner-Hauser syndrome' to this condition, especially if rudimentary bands persist. The only disorder that ordinarily needs to be considered in the differential diagnosis is complete androgen insensitivity (complete testicular feminization). The latter can be excluded on the basis of chromosomal studies and gonadal composition. Pubertal patients with Mullerian aplasia show pubic hair, whereas those with complete androgen insensitivity usually do not (Griffin et al 1976, Simpson 1976).

Renal anomalies are detected in about 40% of individuals with Mullerian aplasia (Griffin et al 1976, Simpson 1976, Carson et al 1983). Pelvic kidney, renal ectopia and unilateral renal aplasia are most common. Parenthetically, some investigators believe that a mutant dominant gene causes an entity characterized by renal dysplasia and Mullerian aplasia (Opitz 1987). Vertebral anomalies are also relatively common in isolated Mullerian aplasia. Thus, urological and vertebral studies are obligatory in the evaluation of Mullerian aplasia.

Of interest is the report of Cramer et al (1987), who found galactase-1-phosphatidyl transferase deficiency or a variant in two unrelated individuals with Mullerian aplasia. The significance of this observation remains uncertain. The enzyme cited is known to be necessary for oogenesis (Hoefnagel et al 1978, Kaufman et al 1979), but germ cell differentiation need not parallel ductal differentiation. Actually, existence of a relationship would be unexpected because galactosaemic females ordinarily have a uterus.

Sibs with Mullerian aplasia have been reported on several occasions, as referenced by Carson et al (1983). Shokeir (1978) reported several kindreds in which the condition appeared to be inherited in sex-limited autosomal dominant fashion; however, in a study of 24 probands Carson et al (1983) found no affected sibs (0/30), paternal aunts (0/31), or maternal aunts (0/41). Possibly excepting the Canadian population studied by Shokeir (1978), the few reported familial aggregates seem most consistent with polygenic/multifactorial inheritance.

Incomplete Mullerian fusion

During embryogenesis the Mullerian ducts are originally paired organs. Fusion and canalization subsequently produce the upper vagina, uterus and Fallopian tubes. Failure of fusion results in two hemiuteri, each associated with no more than one Fallopian tube. In true Mullerian duplication, by contrast, each hemiuterus has two tubes. Thus, the common clinical practice of applying the term 'double uterus' to incomplete Mullerian fusion constitutes a misnomer. Sometimes one Mullerian duct fails to contribute to the definitive uterus, leading to a single rudimentary horn. Incomplete Mullerian fusion may be associated with fetal losses. Surgical reconstruction may be helpful, especially if a uterine septum exists.

Familial aggregates of isolated incomplete Mullerian fusion have been reported. There are reports of multiple affected sibs, as well as an affected mother and daughter (see Simpson 1988c). A proper study would be difficult, requiring invasive procedures to assess relatives. The one formal genetic study attempted has shown a low (1/37; 2.7%) recurrence risk in female sibs (Elias et al 1984). This rate is consistent with polygenic/multifactorial inheritance.

Incomplete Mullerian fusion may also be one component of a genetically determined malformation syndrome (see Verp et al 1983). Meckel syndrome, Fraser syndrome and Rudiger syndrome are examples. Especially noteworthy is the 'hand-foot-uterus' syndrome, an autosomal dominant disorder in which affected females have a bicornuate uterus and characteristic malformations of the hands and feet (Verp et al 1983). The skeletal anomalies are frequently unappreciated by gynaecologists, for which reason the condition is probably underdiagnosed. Longmuir et al (1986) recently discussed management of skeletal anomalies.

Wolffian aplasia

Absence of Wolffian derivatives (Wolffian aplasia) may or may not be associated with absence of the upper urinary tract. Absence of both Wolffian duct derivatives and the upper urinary tract implies total failure of the mesonephric development. By contrast, agenesis of Wolffian derivatives without upper urinary tract anomalies implies resorption of Wolffian elements after the Wolffian duct reached the cloaca. Even if absence of Wolffian derivatives is accompanied by abnormalities of the upper urinary tract, the gonads are only rarely involved. More frequently, the upper urinary tract is normal in individuals who lack an epididymis, ductus deferens and seminal vesicle. If Wolffian aplasia is bilateral, affected patients are of course infertile, due to azoospermia. If the defect is unilateral, patients are usually asymptomatic.

There are several reports of affected sibs (Schellen & von Straaten 1980, Budde et al 1984, Czeizel 1985). No formal genetic studies have been performed, but polygenic/multifactorial aetiology would not be unexpected.

Absence of the ductus deferens also occurs in cystic fibrosis.

Failure of fusion of epididymis and testis

Another relatively common urological defect is failure of the rete cords of the testis to fuse with the mesonephric tubules destined to form the ductuli efferentia (Simpson 1976). As result, spermatozoa cannot exit from the testis. If the defect is bilateral, infertility results. One or both testes may also fail to descend.

Fusion defects of this type occur in about 1% of cryptorchid and in about 1% of azoospermic men. No familial aggregates have been reported, to my knowledge.

MISCELLANEOUS DISORDERS

Germinal cell aplasia (Sertoli-cell only syndrome; Del Castillo syndrome).

Del Castillo et al (1947) described several normally virilized yet sterile males. Their seminiferous tubules lacked spermatogonia and their testes were slightly smaller than average. However Leydig cells appeared normal, explaining normal secondary sexual development. When assays later became available, FSH predict-

ably proved elevated; LH was normal. In contrast to the Klinefelter syndrome, tubular hyalinization and sclerosis rarely occur. Occasionally a few spermatozoa are even present, but affected individuals should be considered sterile. However, androgen therapy is unnecessary because secondary sexual development is normal.

Although occasionally familial (Edwards & Bannerman 1971), germinal cell aplasia is probably more often nongenetic – the end result of a variety of prenatal or postnatal testicular insults. However, the phenotype has been observed in a variety of circumstances in which somatic anomalies coexist, as alluded to earlier. In each of five reported families, male sibs showed germ cell aplasia and female sibs showed streak gonads.

Anorchia

Males (46,XY) with unilateral or bilateral anorchia have unambiguous male external genitalia, normal Wolffian derivatives, no Mullerian derivatives, and no detectable testes (Simpson 1976, Kogan et al 1986). Unilateral anorchia is asymptomatic and not extraordinarily rare. Bilateral anorchia is relatively rare. Somatic abnormalities are not ordinarily present.

Despite absence of testes, the phallus is well differentiated. Pathogenesis presumably involves atrophy of fetal testes after 12–16 weeks' gestation, by which time genital virilization has already been completed. Vasa deferentia terminate blindly, often in association with the spermatic vessels. The diagnosis should be applied only if testicular tissue is undetected in the scrotum, the inguinal canal or the entire path along which the testes descended during embryogenesis. Splenic-gonadal fusion can also occur, mimicking the disorder. Laparoscopy (Boddy et al 1985), ultrasound and magnetic resonance are newer diagnostic techniques helpful in confirming the diagnosis.

Heritable tendencies clearly exist (Hall et al 1975), but the occurrence of monozygotic twins discordant for bilateral anorchia (Simpson et al 1971c) indicates that genetic factors are not paramount in all cases. The heritable tendency could involve in utero torsion of the testicular artery. This explanation does not, however, explain the relationship between agonadia and anorchia observed by Josso and Briard (1980).

Accessory or malpositioned gonads

More than two ovaries and more than two testes (Case 1985) have been reported. Gonadal malposition also occurs and we have also previously alluded to splenic-gonadal fusion. No familial aggregates have been observed for any of these conditions.

Rudimentary ovary syndrome and unilateral streak ovary syndrome.

The 'rudimentary ovary syndrome' is a poorly defined entity of unknown aetiology, traditionally said to be characterized by ovaries containing decreased numbers of follicles. Analogous to the rudimentary testes syndrome, the rudimentary ovary syndrome is surely heterogeneous and probably not even a true entity. Many cases have been associated with sex chromosomal abnormalities, particulary 45,X/46,XX mosaicism. Similar statements apply also to individuals said to have the unilateral streak ovary syndrome.

Premature ovarian failure (POF)

The genetics of premature ovarian failure (POF) cannot be discussed succinctly because the heterogeneity is so great. As considered in detail elsewhere by this author (Simpson 1990), ovarian failure occurring before age 35 or 40 may be familial. Some familial aggregates result from terminal or interstitial deletions of the X long arm (Fitch et al 1982, Krauss et al 1987, Simpson 1987a). In other families partial expression of the XX autosomal recessive gonadal dysgenesis mutant is suspected (see above). In yet other kindreds, unexplained premature ovarian failure is transmitted in dominant fashion (Mattison et al 1984). Various genetic and nongenetic mechanisms could be postulated – meiotic abnormalities, diminished germ cell number, immune phenomena, or environmental toxins common to a household or region.

Polycystic ovarian disease (PCOD)

Polycystic ovarian disease is a common disorder characterized by obesity, oligomenorrhoea and virilization (hirsutism). Clinicians appreciate the great variability shown in PCOD, frequently a cause of female infertility. The LH/FSH ratio is increased; androstenedione and testosterone are elevated.

Elucidating the genetics is hindered by substantial genetic heterogeneity. For example, polycystic ovarian disease is associated with adult-onset 21-hydroxylase deficiencies (both heterozygotes and homozygotes) (Kutten et al 1985), 3-β-ol dehydrogenase (homozygotes) (Rosenfeld et al 1980, Pang et al 1985) and 11β-hydroxylase deficiencies (homozygotes) (Cathelineau et al 1980). Polycystic ovaries have also been associated with X–chromosomal abnormalities.

Despite the evident heterogeneity, PCOD in women not having adrenal hyperplasia is well recognized (Simpson 1990). Autosomal dominant or even X–linked dominant inheritance has been proposed (Cooper et al 1968, Cohen et al 1975, Ferriman & Purdue 1979). Dominant inheritance is most consistent with the variable expressivity, but recurrence risks for symptomatic relatives are far less than expected.

Mutant genes affecting meiosis

In plants and lower mammals meiosis is known to be under genetic control. Similar mechanisms presumably exist in humans. Mutation involving such genes must therefore exist, and are presumably deleterious for reproduction. One would expect clinical manifestations to be infertility in otherwise normal individuals.

Mutants causing desynapsis or asynapsis are already known (Chaganti et al 1980). Heritable sperm abnormalities have been described. An example is the large (4C) sperm described in an isolated case by German et al (1981) and in three sibs by Carson and Rao (1983). A further example is the sperm immobility characteristic of Kartagener syndrome, the result of axonemal abnormalities. Elucidation of male and female meiosis should uncover further evidence for the role of meiotic mutants in otherwise unexplained infertility.

REFFERENCES

Aaronson I A 1985 True hermaphroditism. A review of 41 cases with observations on testicular histology and function. British Journal of Urology 57: 775–779

Akgun S, Ertel N H, Imperato-McGinley J, Sayli B S, Shackleton C 1986 Familial male pseudohermaphroditism due to 5-alpha-reductase. American Journal of Medicine 81: 267–74

Al-Awadi S A, Farag T I, Geebie A S et al 1985 Primary hypergonadism and partial alopecia in three sibs with Mullerian hypoplasia in the affected females. American Journal of Medical Genetics 22: 619–622

Aleem F A 1981 Familial 46XX gonadal dysgenesis.

Fertility and Sterility 35: 317–320

Alvesalo L, de la Chapelle A 1981 Tooth size in two males with deletion of the long arm of the Y chromosome. Annals of Human Genetics 54: 49–54

Amrhein J A, Klingensmith G J, Walsh P C, McKusick V A, Migeon C J 1977 Partial androgen insensitivity. The Reifenstein syndrome revisited. New England Journal of Medicine 297: 350–356

Andersson M, Page D C, de la Chapelle A 1986 Chromosome Y-specific DNA is transferred to the short arm of X chromosome in humans. Science 233: 786–788

Araki S, Chikazawa K, Sekisuchi I, Yamauchi H, Motoyama M, Tamada T 1987 Arrest of follicular development in a patient with 17 alpha-hydroxylase deficiency: folliculogenesis in association with a lack of estrogen synthesis in the ovaries. Fertility and Sterility 47: 169–172

Armendares S, Salamanca F, Canty S D et al 1975 Familial true hermaphroditism in three siblings. Humangenetik 29: 99–109

Balducci R, Toscano V, Wright F et al 1985 Familial male pseudohermaphroditism with gynaecomastia due to 17β-hydroxysteroid dehydrogenase deficiency. A report of 3 cases. Clinical Endocrinology 23: 439–444

Bennet M J, Dewhurst J 1983 The use of ultrasound in the management of vaginal atresia. Pediatric and Adolescent Gynecology 1: 25–37

Bergada C, Cleveland W W, Jones H W, Wilkins L 1962 Variants of embryonic testicular dysgenesis: Bilateral anorchia and the syndrome of rudimentary testes. Acta Endocrinology 40: 521

Berger R, Abonyi D, Nodot A, Vialatte J, Lejeune J 1970 Hermaphroditism vrai et 'garcon XX' dans une fratrie. Revue Europeenne d'Etudes Clinique et Biologiques 15: 330–333

Boczkowski K 1970 Pure gonadal dysgenesis and ovarian dysplasia in sisters. American Journal of Obstetrics and Gynecology 106: 626–628

Boddy S A, Cockery J J, Gornall P 1985 the place of laparoscopy in the management of the impalpable testis. British Journal of Surgery 72: 918–919

Bongiovanni A M 1979 Further studies of congenital adrenal hyperplasia due to 3β-hydroxysteroid dehydrogenase deficiency. In: Vallet H L, Porter I H (eds) Genetic Mechanisms of Sexual Development. Academic Press, New York, NY, p 189–196

Bosze P, Szamel I, Molnar F, Laszlo J 1986 Nonneoplastic gonadal testosterone secretion as a cause of vaginal cell maturation in streak gonad syndrome. Gynecologic and Obstetric Investigation 22: 153–156

Bricarelli F D, Fraccaro M, Lindsten J et al 1981 Sex-reversed XY females with campomelic dysplasia are H-Y negative. Human Genetics 57: 15–22

Brook C G D, Wagner H, Zachman M et al 1973 Familial occurrence of persistent Mullerian structures in otherwise normal males. British Medical Journal 1: 771–773

Brosnan P C, Lewandowski R C, Toguri A G, Payer A F, Meyer W J 1980 A new familial syndrome of the 46,XY gonadal dysgenesis with anomalies of ectodermal and mesodermal structures. Journal of Pediatrics 97: 586–590

Brown D M, Markland C, Dehner L P 1976 Leydig cell hypoplasia: A case of male pseudohermaphroditism. Journal of Clinical Endocrinology and Metabolism 46: 1–7

Brown T F, Migeon C J 1986 Androgen receptors in normal and abnormal male sexual differentiation. Advances in Experimental Medicine and Biology 156: 227–255

Budde W J, Verjaal M, Hamerlynck J V, Bobrow M 1984 Familial occurrence of azoospermia and extreme oligozoospermia. Clinical Genetics 26: 555–562

Burgoyne P S, Baker T G 1987 Perinatal oocyte loss in XO mice and its implication for the etiology of gonadal dysgenesis in XO women. Journal of Reproductive Fertility 75: 633–645

Burgoyne P S, Levy E R, McLaren A 1986 Spermatogenic failure in male mice lacking H-Y antigen. Nature 320: 170–172

Carson S A, Rao R 1983 Mutant gene causing large sperm heads with multiple tails. Abstracts, Society for Gynecologic Investigation, Washington, D.C., March 1983, p 271

Carson S A, Simpson J L 1984 Virilization of female fetuses following maternal ingestion of progestional and androgenic steriods. In: Mahesh V B, Greenblatt R B (eds) Hirsutism and Virilization. PSG Publishing, Littleton, Mass., p 177–187

Carson S A, Simpson J L, Malinak L R et al 1983 Heritable aspects of uterine anomalies II: Genetic analysis of Mullerian aplasia. Fertility and Sterility 34: 86–90

Case W G 1985 Triorchidism. European Urology 11: 433–434

Cates R L, Mattaliano R J, Hession C et al 1986 Isolation of the bovine and human genes for Mullerian inhibiting substance and expression of the human gene in animal cell. Cell 45: 685–698

Cathelineau G, Brerault J L, Fiet J, Julien R, Dreux C, Canivet J 1980 Andrenocortical 11β-hydroxylation defect in adult women with postmenarchial onset of symptoms. Journal of Clinical Endocrinology and Metabolism 51: 287–291

Caufriez A 1986 Male pseudohermaphroditism due to 17-ketoreductase deficiency: Report of a case without gynecomastia and without vaginal pouch. American Journal of Obstetrics and Gynecology 154: 148–149

Chaganti R S K, Jhanwar S C, Ehrenbard L T, Kourides I A, Williams J J 1980 Genetically determined asynapsis, spermatogenic degeneration and infertility in man. American Journal of Human Genetics 32: 833–848

Chandra H S 1985: Is human X chromosome inactivation a sex determining device. Proceedings of the National Academy of Sciences USA 82: 6947–6949

Christakos A C, Simpson J L, Younger J B, Christian C D 1969 Gonadal dysgenesis as an autosomal recessive condition. American Journal of Obstetrics and Gynecology 104: 1027–1030

Clayton G W, Smith J D, Rosenberg H S 1958 Familial true hermaphroditism in pre- and postpuberal genetic females. Hormonal and morphologic studies. Journal of Clinical Endocrinology and Metabolism 18: 1349

Cohen P N, Givens J R, Wiser W L et al 1975 Polycystic ovarian disease, maturation arrest of spermatogenesis and Klinefelter's syndrome in siblings of a family with familial hirsutism. Fertility and Sterility 26: 1228–1238

Cohen-Haguenauer O, Picard J Y, Mattei M G et al 1987 Mapping of the gene for anti-mullerian hormone to the short arm of human chromosme 19. Cytogenetics and Cell Genetics 44: 2–6

Cooper H E, Spellacy W N, Prem K A, Cohen W D 1968 Hereditary factors in the Stein-Leventhal syndrome. American Journal of Obstetrics and Gynecology 100: 371–387

Cramer D W, Ravnikar V A, Craighill M, Ng W G, Goldstein D P, Reilly R 1987 Mullerian aplasia associated with maternal deficiency of galactose-1-phosphate uridyl transferase. Fertility and Sterility 47: 930–934

Cravioto M D, Ulloa-Agurire A, Bermudez J A et al 1986 A new inherited variant of the 3 beta-hydroxysteroid dehydrogenase-isomerase deficiency syndrome: evidence of existence of two isoenzymes. Journal of Clinical Endocrinology and Metabolism 63: 360–367

Curry C J R, Carey J C, Holland J S et al 1987 Smith-Lemli-Opitz syndrome: Type II: Multiple congenital anomalies with male pseudohermaphroditism and frequent early lethality. American Journal of Medical Genetics 26: 45–57

Cussen L K, McMahon R 1979 Germ cells and ova in

dysgenetic gonads of a 46,XY female dizygote twin. Archives of Diseases in Children 133: 373–375

Czeizel A 1985 Congenital aplasia of the vasa deferentia of autosomal recessive inheritance in two unrelated sib-pairs. Human Genetics 70: 288

Degenhart H J 1984 Prader's syndrome (congenital lipoid adrenal hyperplasia). In: Laron Z (ed) Adrenal Diseases in Childhood. Pediatric Adolescence Endocrinology, Vol 13. Karger, Basel, p 125–144

de la Chapelle A 1972 Analytical review: Nature and origin of males with XX sex chromosomes. American Journal of Human Genetics 24: 71–105

de la Chapelle A 1981 The etiology of maleness in XX men. Human Genetics 58: 105–116

de la Chapelle A, Koo G C, Wachtel S S 1975 Recessive sex-determining genes in human XX male syndrome. Cell 15: 837–842

de Grouchy J, Gompel A, Salmon-Bernard Y 1985 Embryonic testicular regression syndrome and severe mental retardation in sibs. Annales de Genetique 28: 154–160

Del Castillo E B, Trabucco A, De La Balze F A 1947 Syndrome produced by absence of the germinal epithelium without impairment of the Sertoli or Leydig cells. Journal of Clinical Endocrinology 7: 493–502

Disteche C M, Casanova M, Saal H et al 1986 Small deletions of the short arm of the Y chromosome in the 46,XY female. Proceedings of the National Academy of Sciences USA 83: 7841–7844

Duck S C, Sekkan G S, Wilbois R, Pagliara A S, Weldon V V 1975 Pseudohermaphroditism with testes and 46,XX karyotypes. Journal of Pediatrics 87: 58–62

Eddy A A, Mauer M 1985 Pseudohermaphroditism, glomerulopathy, and Wilms tumor (Drash syndrome): Frequency in end-stage renal failure. Journal of Pediatrics 106: 584–587

Edwards J A, Bannerman R M 1971 Familial gynecomastia. Birth Defects 7(6): 193–195

Edwards J A, Gale R P 1972 Camptobrachydactyly: A new autosomal dominant trait with two probable homozygotes. American Journal of Human Genetics 24: 464–474

Eicher E M, Washburn L L, Whitney J B III, Morrow K E 1982 Mus poschiavinus Y chromosome in C57BL/65 murine genome causes sex reversal. Science 217: 535–537

Elias S, Simpson J L, Carson S A, Malinak L R, Buttram V C Jr. 1984 Genetic studies in incomplete Mullerian fusion. Obstetrics and Gynecology 63: 276–279

Elsahy N I, Waters W R 1971 The brachio-skeleto-genital syndrome. Plastic and Reconstructive Surgery 48: 542–550

Evans E P, Ford C E, Lyon M F 1977 Direct evidence of the capacity of the XY germ cell in the mouse to become an oocyte. Nature 267: 430–431

Ferriman D, Purdue A W 1979 The inheritance of polycystic ovarian disease and possible relationship to premature balding. Clinical Endocrinology 11: 291–300

Fisher L K, Kogut M D, Moore R J et al 1978 Clinical, endocrinological, and enzymatic characterization of two patients with 5α-reduction of cortisol and testosterone. Journal of Clinical Endocrinology and Metabolism 47: 653–664

Fitch N, de Saint V J, Richer C L, Pinsky L, Sitahal S 1982 Premature menopause due to small deletion in long arm of the X chromosome: A report of three cases and a review. American Journal of Obstetrics and Gynecology 142: 968–972

Fraccaro M, Tiepolo L, Zuffardio-Chiumello G et al 1979 Familial XX true hermaphroditism and H–Y antigen. Human Genetics 48: 45–52

Fraser G R 1962 Our genetical 'load'. A review of some aspects of genetic malformations. Annals of Human Genetics 25: 387–415

Frydman M, Kauschansky A, Zamir R, Bonne-Tamir B 1986 Familial lipoid adrenal hyperplasia: genetic marker data and an approach to prenatal diagnosis. Amercian Journal of Medical Genetics 25: 319–325

German J 1988 Gonadal dismorphism explained as a dosage effect of a locus on the sex chromosomes, the gonad-differentiation locus (GDL). American Journal of Human Genetics 42: 414–421

German J, Simpson J L, McLemore G 1973 Abnormalities of human sex chromosomes. I. Abnormal human Y chromosome: 46,XYr. Annales de Genetique 16: 225–231

German J, Simpson J L, Chaganti R S K, Summitt R L, Reid L B, Markatz I R 1978 Genetically determined sex-reversal in 46,XY humans. Science 202: 53–56

German J, Rasch E M, Huang C Y, McLeod J, Imperato-McGinley J 1981 Human infertility due to production of multiple-tailed spermatozoa with excessive amounts of DNA. American Journal of Human Genetics 33: 64A

Granat M, Amar A, Mor-Yosef S, Brautbar C, Schenker J G 1983 Familial gonadal germinative failure: Endocrine and human leukocyte antigen studies. Fertility and Sterility 40: 215–219

Greenberg F, Keenan B, De Yanis V, Finegold M 1986 Gonadal dysgenesis and gonadoblastoma in situ in a female with Fraser (Cryptophthalmos) syndrome. Journal of Pediatrics 108: 952–954

Greenberg F, Gresik M W, Carpenter R J, Law S W, Hoffman L P, Ledbetter D H 1987 The Gardner-Silengo-Wachtel or Genito-Palato-Cardiac syndrome: Male pseudohermaphroditism with micrognathia, cleft palate, and conotruncal cardiac defects. American Journal of Medical Genetics 26: 59–64

Greene S, Zachmann M, Manella B et al 1987 Comparison of two tests to recognize or exclude 5 alpha-reductase deficiency in prepubertal children. Acta Endocrinology (Copenhagen) 114: 113–117

Griffin J E, Edwards C, Madden J D, Harrod M J, Wilson J D 1976 Congenital absence of the vagina. The Mayer-Rokitansky-Kuster-Hauser syndrome. Annals of Internal Medicine 85: 224–236

Habib R, Loirat C, Gubler M C et al 1985 The nephropathy associated with male pseudohermaphroditism and Wilms' tumor (Drash syndrome): a distinctive glomerular lesion – report of 10 cases. Clinical Nephrology 24: 269–278

Hall J G, Morgan A, Blizzard R M 1975 Familial congenital anorchia. Birth Defects 11(4): 115–119

Hamet P, Kuchel O, Nowacynski J M, Rojo Ortega J M, Sasaki C, Genest J 1973 Hypertension with adrenal, genital, renal defects, and deafness. Archives of Internal Medicine 131: 563–569

Haning R V Jr., Chesney R W, Moorthy A V, Gilbert E F 1985 A syndrome of chronic renal failure and XY gonadal dysgenesis in young phenotypic females without genital ambiguity. American Journal of Kidney Disease 6: 40–48

Heremans G F P, Moolenaar A J, Van Gelderen H M 1976 Female phenotype in a male child due to 17α-hydroxylase deficiency. Archives of Diseases in Children 51: 721–723

Hoefnagel D, Wurster-Hill D Y, Dupree W B Benirschke K 1978 Campomelic dwarfism associated with XY gonadal dysgenesis and chromosome anomalies. Clinical Genetics 13: 489–499

Hsu L Y F, Hirschhorn K, Goldstein A, Barcinski M A 1970 Familial chromosomal mosaicism, genetic aspects. Annals of Human Genetics 33: 343–349

Ieshima A, Koeda T, Inagaka M 1986 Peculiar face, deafness, cleft palate, male pseudohermaphroditism, and growth and pyschomotor retardation; a new autosomal recessive syndrome? Clinical Genetics 30: 136–141

Imperato-McGinley J, Guerrero L, Gauiter T, Peterson R E 1974 Steriod 5α–reductase deficiency: An inherited form of male pseudohermaphroditism. Science 186: 1213–1215

Imperato-McGinley J, Peterson R E, Stoller R, Goodwin W E 1979 Male pseudohermaphroditism secondary to 17α-hydroxysteroid dehydrogenase deficiency: Gender role with puberty. Journal of Clinical Endocrinology and Metabolism 49: 391– 395

Imperato-McGinley J, Gautier T, Pichardo M, Shackleton C 1986 The diagnosis of 5 alpha-reductase deficiency in infancy. Journal of Clinical Endocrinology and Metabolism 63: 1313–1318

Jirásek J 1976 Principles of reproductive embryology In: Simpson J L (ed) Disorders of Sexual Differentiation. Academic Press, New York, p 51–111

Josso N, Briard M I 1980 Embryonic testicular regression syndrome: Variable phenotypic expression in siblings. Journal of Pediatrics 97: 200–204

Jost A 1947 Recherches sur la differenciation sexuelle de l'embryon de lapin II. Action des androgenese de synthese sur l'histogenese genitale. Archives de Anatomie Microscopique et de Morphologie Experimentale 36: 242–270

Jost A 1953 Problems of fetal endocrinology: the gonadal and hypophyseal hormones. Recent Progress in Hormone Research 8: 379–383

Kasdan R, Nankin H R, Troen P, Wald S, Yanaihara T 1973 Paternal transmission of maleness in XX human beings. New England Journal of Medicine 288: 539–545

Kasdan R, Nankin H P, Troen P, Wald N, Pan S, Yanaihara T 1978 Paternal transmission of maleness in XX human beings. New England Journal of Medicine 288: 539–545

Kaufman F, Kogut M D, Donnell G N, Goebelsmann U 1979 Ovarian failure in galactosemia. Lancet 2: 737–738

King L A, Sanchez-Ramos L, Tallado O E, Reindollar R H 1987 Syndrome of genital, renal, and middle ear anomalies: A third family and report of pregnancy. Obstetrics and Gynecology 69: 491–493

Kogan S J, Gill B, Bennett B, Smey P, Reda E F, Levitta S B 1986 Human monorchism: A clinicopathological study of unilateral absent testes in 65 boys. Journal of Urology 135: 758–761

Krauss C M, Turkray R N, Atkins L, McLaughlin C, Brown L G, Page D C 1987 Familial premature ovarian failure due to interstitial deletion of the long arm of the X chromosome. New England Journal of Medicine 317: 125–131

Kutten F, Couillin P, Giraud F et al 1985 Late-onset andrenal hyperplasia in hirsutism. New England Journal of Medicine 313: 224–231

Lau Y C 1989 Are male enhanced antigens and serological H-Y antigen the same? In: Wachtel S S (ed) Evolutionary mechanisms in sex determination. CRC Press, Baton Rogue, LA, p 151–161

Lee P A, Rock J A, Brown T R, Fichman K M, Migeon C J, Jones H W Jr. 1981 Leydig cell hypofunction resulting in male pseudohermaphroditism. Fertility and Sterility 37: 675–679

Leshin M, Griffin J E, Wilson J D 1978 Hereditary male pseudohermaphroditism associated with unstable form of 5α-reductase. Journal of Clinical Investigation 62: 685–691

Longmuir G A, Conley R N, Nicholson D L, Whitehead M 1986 The hand-foot-uterus syndrome: A case study. Journal of Manipulative Physical Therapy 9: 213–217

Lubs H A Jr., Vilar O, Bergenstal D M 1959 Familial male pseudohermaphroditism of labial testes and partial feminization: Endocrine studies and genetic aspects. Journal of Clinical Endocrinology and Metabolism 19: 1110–1120

Lukusa T, Fryns J P, Van den Berge H 1986 Gonadoblastoma and Y-chromosome fluorescence. Clinical Genetics 29: 311–316

Lundgren P O 1973 Hereditary myopathy, oligophrenia, cataract, skeletal abnormalities and hypergonadotrophic hypogonadism: A new syndrome. European Neurology 10: 261–280

McCarthy D J, Opitz J M 1985 Perrault syndrome in sisters. American Journal of Medical Genetics 22: 629–631

McDonough P G, Tho P T 1983 The spectrum of 45,X/46,XY gonadal dysgenesis and its implications (A study of 19 patients). Pediatric and Adolescent Gynecology 1: 1–18

McKusick V A, Weilbaecher R G, Gregg C W 1968 Recessive inheritance of a congenital malformation syndrome. Journal of the American Medical Association 204: 113–118

McLaren A, Simpson E, Tomonari K, Chandler P, Hogg H 1984 Male sex differentiation in mice lacking H-Y antigen. Nature 312: 552–555

Magenis R E, Tochen M L, Holahan K P, Carey T, Allen L, Brown M G 1984 Turner syndrome resulting from partial deletion of Y chromosome short arm: localization of male determinants. Journal of Pediatrics 105: 916–919

Magre S, Jost A 1984 Dissociation between testicular morphogenesis and endocrine cytodifferentiation of Sertoli cells. Proceedings of the National Academy of Sciences USA 81: 7831

Mann J R, Corkery J J, Fisher H J W et al 1983 The X–linked recessive form of XY gonadal dysgenesis with high incidence of gonadal cell tumours: clinical and genetic studies. Journal of Medical Genetics 20: 264–270

Mattison D R, Evans M I, Schwinner W B, White B J, Jensen B, Schulman J D 1984 Familial ovarian failure. American Journal of Human Genetics 36: 1341–1348

Maximilian C, Ionescu B, Bucur A 1970 Deux soeurs avec dysgenesie gonadique majeure, hypotrophic staturale, microcephalie, arachondactylie et caryotype 46,XX. Journal de Genetique Humaine 18: 365–378

Mikati M A, Samir S N, Sahil I F 1985 Microcephaly, hypergonadotropic hypoganadism, short stature and minor anomalies. A new syndrome. American Journal of Medical Genetics 22: 599–608

Miller W L, Levine L S 1987 Molecular and clinical advances in congential adrenal hyperplasia. Journal of Pediatrics 11: 1–17

Minowada S, Fukutani K, Hara M et al 1984 Childbirth in

a true hermaphrodite. European Urology 10: 414–415

Mori V, Mitzutani S 1968 Familial hermaphroditism in genetic families. Japanese Journal of Urology 59: 857–864

Morris J M, Mahesh V B 1963 Further observations on the syndrome 'testicular feminization'. American Journal of Obstetrics and Gynecology 87: 731–748

Mueller U 1989 Molecular Biology of the human Y chromosome. In: Wachtel S S (ed) Evolutionary Mechanisms in Sex Determination. CRC Press, Baton Rogue, LA p 91–99

Najjar S S, Takla R J, Nassar V H 1974 The syndrome of rudimentary testes: Occurrence in five siblings. Journal of Pediatrics 84: 119–122

Opitz J M 1987 Vaginal atresia (von Mayer-Rokitansky-Kuster or MRK Anomaly) in hereditary renal adysplasia (HRP). American Journal of Medical Genetics 26: 873–876

Opitz J M, Howe J J 1969 The Meckel syndrome (dysencephalic splanchnocystica-the Gruber syndrome). Birth Defects Original Article Series 5(2): 167–172

Opitz J M, Simpson J L, Sarto G E, Summitt R L, New M, German J 1972 Pseudovaginal perineoscrotal hypospadias. Clinical Genetics 3: 1–26

Page D C 1986 Sex reversal: deletion mapping, the male determining function of the Y chromosome. Cold Spring Harbor Symposia on Quantitative Biology 51: 229–235

Page D C 1987 Hypothesis: A Y-chromosome gene causes gonadoblastoma in poorly differentiated gonads. Development 101 (Suppl): 151–155

Page D C, Mosher R, Simpson E M et al 1987 The sex-determining region of the human Y chromosome encodes a finger protein. Cell 51: 1091–1104

Pallister P D, Optiz J M 1979 The Perrault syndrome: Autosomal recessive ovarian dysgenesis with facultative, non sex-limited senorineural deafness. American Journal of Medical Genetics 4: 239–246

Pang S Y, Lerner A J, Stoner E et al 1985 Late-onset adrenal steroid 3 beta–hydroxysteroid dehydrogenase deficiency. I. A cause of hirsutism in pubertal and postpubertal women. Journal of Clinical Endocrinology and Metabolism 60: 428–439

Patsavoudi E, Magre S, Castinior M, Scholler R, Jost A 1985 Dissociation between testicular morphogenesis and functional differentiation of Leydig cells. Journal of Endocrinology 105: 235

Perez-Palacios G, Scaglia H E, Kofman-Afaro S et al 1982 Inherited male pseudohermaphroditism due to gonadotrophin unresponsiveness. Acta Endocrinologica 98: 148–155

Perrone L, Criscuolo T, Sinisi A A et al 1985 Male pseudohermaphroditism due to 3β-hydroxysteroid dehydrogenase–isomerase deficiency associated with atrial septal defect. Acta Endocrinologica 110: 532–539

Peterson R E, Imperato-McGinley J, Gautier T, Sturla E 1977 Male pseudohermaphroditism due to steroid 5α-reductase deficiency. American Journal of Medicine 62: 170–191

Peterson R E, Imperato-McGinley J, Gautier T, Shackleton C 1985 Male pseudohermaphroditism due to multiple defects in steroid-biosynthetic microsomal mixed-function oxidase. A new variant of congenital adrenal hyperplasia. New England Journal of Medicine 313: 1182–1192

Petit C, de la Chapelle A, Levilliers J, Castillo S, Noel B, Weissenback J 1987 An abnormal terminal X-Y interchange accounts for most but not all cases of human XX maleness. Cell 49: 595–602

Pinsky L, Kaufman M 1987 Genetics of steroid rec᎐ptors and their disorders. Advances in Human Genetics 16: 299–472

Pinsky L, Kaufman M, Chudley A E 1985 Reduced affinity of the androgen receptor for 5 alpha-dihydrotestosterone but not methyltrienolone in a form of partial androgen resistance. Studies on cultured genital skin fibroblasts. Journal of Clinical Investigation 15: 1291–1296

Pinsky L, Kaufman M, Levitsky L L 1987 Partial androgen resistance due to a distinctive qualitative defect of the androgen receptor. American Journal of Medical Genetics 27: 459–466

Portuondo J A, Neyro J L, Benito J A, de la Rios A, Barral A 1987 Familial 46,XX gonadal dysgenesis. International Journal of Fertility 32: 56–58

Puck S M, Haseltine F P, Francke U 1981 Absence of H-Y antigen in an XY female with compomelic dysplasia. Human Genetics 57: 23–27

Ramsay M, Bernstein R, Zwane E, Page D C, Jenkins T 1988 XX true hermaphroditism in Southern African blacks: an enigma of primary sexual differentiation. American Journal of Human Genetics 43: 4–13

Raspa R W, Subramaniam A P, Romas N A 1986 True hermaphroditism presents as intermittent hemituria and groin pain. Urology 28: 133–136

Reifenstein E C 1947 Hereditary familial hypogonadism. Clinical Research 3: 86

Rosenberg C, Frota-Pessoa O, Vianna-Morgante A M, Chu T H 1987 Phenotypic spectrum of 45,X/46,XY individuals. American Journal of Medical Genetics 27: 553–559

Rosenberg H K, Sherman N H, Tarry W F, Duckett J W, Snyder H Mc 1986 Mayer-Rokitansky-Kuster-Hauser syndrome: US aid to diagnosis. Radiology 161: 815–819

Rosenfield R L, Rich B H, Wolfsdorl J I et al 1980 Pubertal presentation of congenital Δ-3β- hydroxysteroid dehydrogenase deficiency. Journal of Clinical Endocrinology and Metabolism 51: 345–353

Saldanha P H, Arnhold I J P, Mendonca B B, Bloise W, Toledo S P A 1987 A clinico-genetic investigation of Leydig cell hypoplasia. American Journal of Medical Genetics 26: 337–344

Sarto G E, Opitz J M 1973 The XY gonadal agenesis syndrome. Journal of Medical Genetics 10: 288–293

Schellen T M, von Straaten A 1980 Autosomal recessive hereditary congenital aplasia of the vasa deferentia in four siblings. Fertility and Sterility 34: 401–404

Schwartz M, Imperato-McGinley J, Peterson R E et al 1981 Male pseudohermaphroditism secondary to an abnormality in Leydig cell differentiation. Journal of Clinical Endocrinology and Metabolism 53: 123–127

Shokeir M H K 1978 Aplasia of the Mullerian system: Evidence for probable sex-limited autosomal dominant inheritance. Birth Defects 14(6c): 147–165

Simpson E, McLaren A, Chandler P, Tomonari K 1984 Expression of H-Y antigen by female mice carrying SXR. Transplantation 37: 17–21

Simpson E, Chandler P, Goulmy E, Disteche C M, Ferguson-Smith M A, Page D C 1987 Separation of the genetic loci for the H–Y antigen and for testis determination on human Y chromosome. Nature 326: 876–878

Simpson J L 1976 Disorders of Sexual Differentiation: Etiology and Clinical Delineation. Academic Press, New York

Simpson J L 1978 True hermaphroditism. Etiology and phenotypic considerations. Birth Defects 14:(6C): 9–35

Simpson J L 1979 Gonadal dysgenesis and sex chromosome abnormalities. Phenotypic/karyotypic correlations In: Vallet H L, Porter I H (eds) Genetic Mechanisms of Sexual Development. Academic Press, New York, p 365–405

Simpson J L 1985 Relationship between congenital anomalies and contraception. Advances in Contraception 1: 3–30

Simpson J L 1987a Phenotypic-karyotypic correlations of gonadal determinants: Current status and relationship to molecular studies. In: Sperling K, Vogel F (eds) Proceedings 7th International Congress, Human Genetics (Berlin, 1986). Springer-Verlag, Heidelberg, p 224–232

Simpson J L 1987b Genetic control of sexual development. In: Ratnam S S, Teoh E S (eds) Proceedings 12th World Congress on Fertility and Sterility (Singapore 1986). Parthenon Press, Lancaster, UK, p 165–173

Simpson J L 1988 Genetics of sex determination: In: Iizuka R (ed) Proceedings of VIth World Congress on Human Reproduction (Tokyo 1987). Elsevier Scientific Publishing, Amsterdam p 19–33

Simpson J L 1989 Genetic heterogeneity in XY sex-reversal: potential pitfalls in isolating the Testes-Determining-Factor: TDF. In: Wachtel S S (ed) Evolutionary Mechanisms in Sex Determination. CRC Press, Baton Rouge, LA, p 265–277

Simpson J L 1990 Gynecologic disorders. In: King R A, Rotter J I, Motulsky A G (eds) The Genetic Basis of Common Disease. Oxford University Press, Oxford (in press)

Simpson J L, Photopulos G 1976 The relationship of neoplasia to disorders of abnormal sexual differentiation. Birth Defects 12(1): 15–50

Simpson J L, Christakos A C, Horwith M, Silverman F 1971a Gonadal dysgenesis associated with apparently chromosomal complements. Birth Defects 7(6): 215–218

Simpson J L, New M, Peterson R E, German J 1971b Pseudovaginal perineoscrotal hypospadias (PPSH) in sibs. Birth Defects 7(6): 140–144

Simpson J L, Horwith M, Morillo-Cucci G, McGovern J H, Levine M I German J 1971c Bilateral anorchia: Discordance in monozygotic twins. Birth Defects 7(6): 196–200

Simpson J L, Blagowidow N, Martin A O 1981 XY gonadal dysgenesis: Genetic heterogeneity based upon clinical observations. H–Y antigen status and segregation analysis. Human Genetics 58: 91–97

Simpson J L, Chaganti R S K, Mouradian J, German J 1982 Chronic renal disease myotonic dystrophy, and gonadoblastoma in an individual with XY gonadal dysgenesis. Journal of Medical Genetics 19: 73–76

Skordis N A, Stetka D G, MacGillivray M H, Greenfield S P 1987 Familial 46,XX coexisting with familial 46,XX true hermaphrodites in same pedigree. Journal of Pediatrics 110: 244–248

Skre H, Bassoe H H, Berg K, Frovig A G 1976 Cerebellar ataxia and hypergonadism in the two kindreds. Chance occurrence, pleiobokism or linkage? Clinical Genetics 9: 234–244

Sloan W R, Walsh P C 1976 Familial persistent Mullerian duct syndrome. Journal of Urology 115: 459–461

Smith A, Fraser I S, Noel M 1979 Three siblings with premature gonadal failure. Fertility and Sterility 32: 528–530

Smith W D, Marokus R, Graham J M Jr. 1985 Tentative evidence of Y-linked statural gene(s). Growth in the testicular feminization syndrome. Clinical Pediatrics 24: 189–192

Sultan C 1986 Androgen receptors and partial androgen insensitivity in male pseudohermaphroditism. Annales de Genetique 29: 5–10

Sweet R A, Schrott H G, Kurland R, Culp O S 1974 Study of the incidence of hypospadias in Rochester Minnesota, 1940–1970, and a case control comparison of possible etiologic factors. Mayo Clinic Proceedings 49: 52–58

Tegenkamp T R, Brazzel J W, Tegenkamp I, Labodi F 1979 Pregnancy without benefit of reconstructive surgery in a bisexually active true hermaphrodite. American Journal of Obstetrics and Gynecology 135: 427–432

Tiepolo L, Zuffardi O 1976 Localization of factors controlling spermatogenesis in the non-fluorescent portion of the human Y chromosome long arm. Human Genetics 34: 119–124

Toledo S P, Arnhold I J, Luthold W, Russo E M, Saldanha P H 1985 Leydig cell hypoplasia determining familial hypergonadotropic hypogonadism. Progress of Clinical Biology and Research 200: 311–314

Ulloa-Aguirre A, Mendez J P, Angeles A, del Castillo A F, Charez B, Perez-Palaccio G 1986 The presence of Mullerian remnants in the complete androgen insensitivity syndromes: A steroid hormone-mediated defect? Fertility and Sterility 45: 302–305

Van Niekerk W A 1974 True hermaphroditism. Harper & Row, New York

Van Niekerk W A, Retief A E 1981 The gonads of human true hermaphrodites. Human Genetics 58: 117–122

Vergnaud G, Page D C, Simmler M C et al 1986 A deletion map of the human Y based on DNA hybridization. American Journal of Human Genetics 38: 109–124

Verp M S 1983 Environmental causes of ovarian failure. Seminars in Reproductive Endocrinology 1: 101–111

Verp M S, Simpson J L 1987 Abnormal sexual differentiation and neoplasia. Cancer Genetics and Cytogenetics 25: 191–218

Verp M S, Simpson J L, Elias S, Carson S A, Sarto G E, Feingold M 1983 Heritable aspects of uterine anomalies. I. Three familial aggregates with Mullerian Fusion anomalies. Fertility and Sterility 34: 80–85

Wachtel S S 1983 H–Y antigen and the Biology of Sex Determination. Grune and Stratton, New York

Washburn L L, Eicher M E 1983 Sex reversal in XY mice caused by dominant mutation on Chromosome 17. Nature 303: 338–340

Wilson J D, Harrod M J, Goldstein J L, Hemsell D L, MacDonald P C 1974 Familial incomplete male pseudohermaphroditism, type I. New England Journal of Medicine 290: 1097–1103

Wilson J D, Carlson B R, Weaver D D, Kovacs·W J, Griffin J E 1984 Endocrine and genetic characterization of cousins with male pseudohermaphroditism: Evidence that the Lubs phenotype can result from a mutation that alters the structure of the androgen receptor. Clinical Genetics 26: 363–370

Winter J S D, Kohn G, Mellman W J, Wagner S 1968 A

familial syndrome of renal, genital and middle ear
anomalies. Journal of Pediatrics 71: 88–93
Zachmann M, Vollmin J A, Hamilton W, Prader A 1972
Steroid 17,20-desmolase deficiency: A new cause of male
pseudohermaphroditism. Clinical Endocrinology 1:
369–385
Zenzes M T, Wolf W, Gunther E 1978 Studies on the
function of H–Y antigen: Dissociation and reorganization
experiments on rat gonadal cells. Cytogenetics & Cell
Genetics 20: 365–372

92. Disorders of vitamin D metabolism or action

Stephen J. Marx

HISTORY

Rickets and osteomalacia were widespread problems until the discovery of the calciferols (Mellanby 1919). After this calciferols were used for prevention and treatment of these disorders. Some cases of rickets or osteomalacia did not respond to the usual doses of calciferols, and multiple genetic and other causes were subsequently recognized. In 1937 Albright reported detailed studies of a child with this problem and suggested an hereditary resistance to the actions of calciferols (Albright et al 1937). Rickets resistant to calciferols was subsequently recognized as a common cause of hereditary dwarfism. Most hereditary cases showed biochemical features different from calciferol nutritional deficiency and are now classified as phosphate diabetes or X–linked hypophosphataemia.

In 1961 Prader et al characterized a distinctive form of hereditary rickets, which they called pseudodeficiency rickets (Prader et al 1961). Features which clearly distinguished pseudodeficiency rickets from X–linked hypophosphataemia were hypocalcaemia, the potential for complete remission with high doses of calciferols, and an autosomal transmission pattern.

In 1971 $1\alpha,25(OH)_2D_3$ was shown to be the active metabolite of vitamin D_3 that accumulated in the nuclei of target tissues (Holick et al 1971, Lawson et al 1971, Norman et al 1971). This discovery led quickly to the development of methods to measure active metabolites in blood, characterization of defects in $1\alpha,25(OH)_2D$ synthesis and action, and an understanding of the roles of 1α hydroxylated and other analogues for therapy. Fraser and associates showed that pseudodeficiency rickets in one patient was corrected with physiological doses of $1\alpha,25(OH)_2D_3$; they suggested that this disorder represented a defect in $25OHD_3$ 1α hydroxylase enzyme (Fraser et al 1973). Subsequently Brooks and co-workers described a patient with similar clinical features but high serum levels of $1\alpha,25(OH)_2D$ before and during treatment; they suggested that pseudodeficiency rickets be classified as type 1 (deficient production of

$1\alpha,25(OH)_2D$) or type II (impaired end-organ response to $1\alpha,25(OH)_2D$) (Brooks et al 1978).

NORMAL PHYSIOLOGY OF CALCIFEROLS

Vitamin D sources

Cholecalciferol (vitamin D_3) (Aurbach et al 1985) is a seco-steroid produced via opening the B-ring of 7-dehydrocholesterol (Fig. 92.1). In man, this reaction is driven by ultraviolet radiation (from sunlight) in the basal layers of the epidermis (Holick et al 1980). Skin pigment can decrease the amount of cholecalciferol synthesized in response to UV radiation (Clemens et al 1982). Ergocalciferol (vitamin D_2) is produced via opening the B-ring of ergosterol, a sterol found in plants and fungi. Plants do not contain important amounts of ergocalciferol, but this

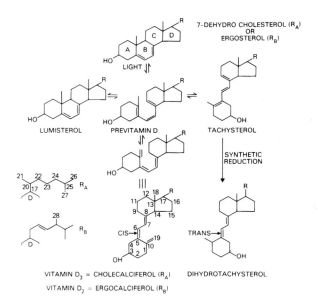

Fig. 92.1 Synthesis of cholecalciferol, ergocalciferol, and dihydrotachysterol (Aurbach et al 1985a).

1619

chemical is synthesized in bulk for use as a nutritional supplement. Man obtains calciferols either endogenously through metabolism of precursors in the skin, or exogenously as a dietary component or dietary supplement. The metabolism and actions of vitamin D_3 and vitamin D_2 are similar in man.

Vitamin D 25-hydroxylation

Cholecalciferol and ergocalciferol are inert when exposed directly to calciferol target tissues. They must be hydroxylated at positions 25- and 1α- to become maximally active (Fig. 92.2). The initial hydroxylation at carbon-25 is carried out only in the liver by a mitochondrial cytochrome P–450 mono–oxygenase (Saarem et al 1984). 25-hydroxylation of vitamin D is not highly regulated; the principal determinant of its rate is the circulating level of vitamin D.

1-Alpha hydroxylation

25(OH)D is 1α-hydroxylated to 1α,25(OH)$_2$D (Turner 1984) or 24-hydroxylated to 24,25(OH)$_2$D by enzyme systems in the kidney. 25(OH)D$_3$ 1α-hydroxylase activity is also found in the placenta, in certain cultured cells of diverse origin, and in certain pathological tissues (such as granulomas and malignant T–cells). Virtually all 1α,25(OH)$_2$D normally in blood comes from the kidney (Reeve et al 1983). The renal 1α-hydroxylase enzyme is stringently regulated. Parathyroid hormone activates it in

the renal proximal tubule through a cyclic AMP mediated pathway (Trechsel et al 1979). 1α,25(OH)$_2$D (perhaps through its receptor) and phosphate inhibit the renal 1-hydroxylation. The renal 25(OH)D$_3$ 1α-hydroxylase enzyme contains a cytochrome P–450 and renoredoxin (Hiwatashi et al 1982, Paulson & DeLuca 1985); dephosphorylation of the renoredoxin component may mediate activation of the 1α-hydroxylase by parathyroid hormone (Siegel et al 1986).

24-Hydroxylation

25(OH)D, 1α,25(OH)$_2$D, and other metabolites are substrates for 24-hydroxylation. Many similarities between the 1-hydroxylase and 24-hydroxylase systems suggest that they share certain components. Both are mitochondrial enzymes containing cytochrome P–450 (Burgos-Trinidad et al 1985). Both are modulated (though in opposing directions) by cAMP and by 1α,25(OH)$_2$D (Colston & Feldman 1982). Their normal anatomical distributions differ; the 1α-hydroxylase is confined to the proximal renal tubule, but the 24-hydroxylase is found in a wide range of tissues. The role of 24-hydroxylase has not been fully determined; it may be the only route to a group of calciferols with unique actions not obtainable with 1α,25(OH)$_2$D (see below), and it might be the most important step in 1α,25(OH)$_2$D removal. Induction of 24-hydroxylase by 1α,25(OH)$_2$D in target tissues (Colston & Feldman 1982) and preference of the 24-hydroxylase for 1α,25(OH)$_2$D rather than 25(OH)D as substrate suggest an important role in ending the action of 1α,25(OH)$_2$D.

5,6 Cis-trans isomerization

25(OH)D may also be converted to 5,6-trans-25(OH)D. This pathway has so far only been documented with plasma from rats that were treated with pharmacological amounts of vitamin D_3 (Kumar et al 1981). However, the pathway is of interest because it produces a metabolite analogous to 25(OH)-dihydrotachysterol (Fig. 92.3) (dihydrotachysterol is a synthetic calciferol analogue used in therapy). These metabolites have an A-ring rotated 180 degrees, bringing the 3-hydroxyl group into a pseudo 1α-hydroxyl position. This rotation increases the agonist potency versus that of the parent metabolite on the 1α,25(OH)$_2$D receptor. 5,6-trans metabolites might have important roles in states where the renal 1α hydroxylase enzyme is severely deficient.

Vitamin D binding protein in plasma

All calciferols are fat soluble and circulate principally bound to an alpha globulin of 58 000 daltons (Haddad

CALCIFEROL ACTIVATION

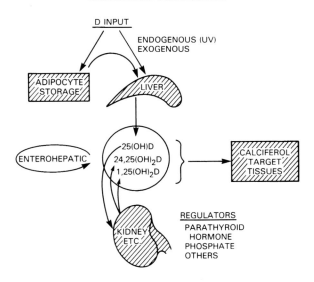

Fig. 92.2 Metabolic pathways for activation of cholecalciferol or ergocalciferol (Aurbach et al 1985a).

1984). It contains one high affinity sterol binding site with the following order of affinities: $25(OH)D_3$-26,23-lactone > $25(OH)D = 24,25(OH)_2D > 1\alpha,25(OH)_2D$ >> vitamin D. It is a major component of plasma protein (normal concentration 10^{-5} M) that has multiple isoforms (Coppenhaver et al 1983) extensively studied for their genetic diversity long before a function in calciferol transport was recognized. The messenger RNA for this vitamin D binding protein, also known as group-specific component, or Gc, has been sequenced and is homologous to that for albumin and alpha fetoprotein (Cooke 1985).

Calciferol turnover and requirements

Most of the body pool of vitamin D is in fat, compared to only a small fraction of the pools of $25(OH)D$ or $1\alpha,25(OH)_2D$ (Lawson et al 1986). In the circulation more than 99% of each metabolite is bound to proteins. Normal turnover of vitamin D is approximately 30 µg per day; most of this is cleared through catabolic pathways with only 1 µg per day being cleared as $1\alpha,25(OH)_2D$ (Table 92.1).

$1\alpha,25(OH)_2D$ receptors

$1\alpha,25(OH)_2D$ acts by binding to a high affinity receptor, analogous to the receptors for other steroid hormones (Haussler et al 1988). $1\alpha,25(OH)_2D$ is the most potent natural calciferol metabolite with an ED_{50} of approximately 1/1000 that of $25(OH)D$ in most test systems (Procsal et al 1975). Because of differing concentration ranges for metabolites (Table 92.1), the receptor may be activated in vivo by a mixture of agonists including $1\alpha,25(OH)_2D$, $25(OH)D$, and 5,6-trans-$25(OH)D$. The

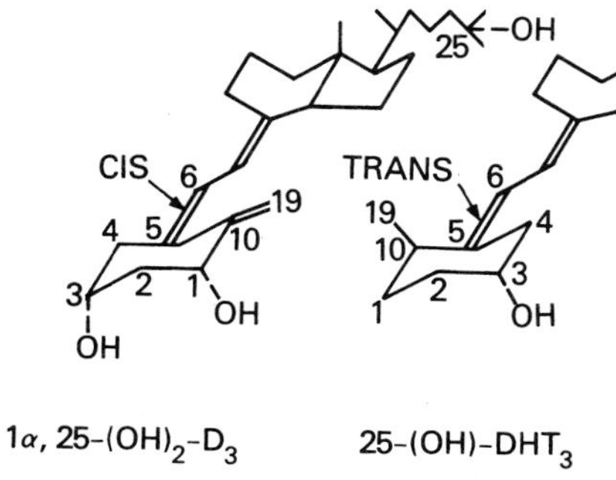

$1\alpha, 25\text{-}(OH)_2\text{-}D_3$ $25\text{-}(OH)\text{-}DHT_3$

Fig. 92.3 Steric conformation of two activated calciferol analogues. $1\alpha,25(OH)_2D_3$ has the 5–6 double bond in cis configuration. 25(OH)dihydrotachysterol$_3$ has the 5–6 double bond in trans configuration; the 180 degree rotation of the A ring (lowest ring in figure) brings the 3–β hydroxyl group into a pseudo–1α-configuration.

Table 92.1 Serum levels and body pools of calciferol metabolites in adults (Marx 1989)

Metabolite	Concentration in serum (ng/ml)	Half-time in serum (days)	Pool size in body (µg)	Turnover in body (µg/day)
D_3	10*	30	1000	30
$25(OH)D$	25	15	500	15
$1\alpha,25(OH)_2D$	0.03	0.2	0.5	1
$24,25(OH)_2D$	1	2	10	10

With the exception of serum concentrations, these numbers are based on limited data. * Typical summer mean in temperate climate; normal winter mean is below 0.5 ng/ml

$1\alpha,25(OH)_2D$ receptor is a 50–60 000 dalton peptide structurally homologous with a family of DNA-binding (McDonnell et al 1987) proteins that includes the receptors for other steroid hormones, the receptor for tri-iodothyronine, the receptor for retinoic acid, and a product of the v-ERB-A oncogene (Evans 1988, Evans & Hollenberg 1988). The $1\alpha,25(OH)_2D$ receptor is found in many tissues (Stumpf et al 1979) and can be induced by increased cell proliferation, by exposure to $1\alpha,25(OH)_2D$, and by ontogenetic state. For example, the receptor first appears in the rat intestine 14 days postnatally and correlates with the onset of $1\alpha,25(OH)_2D$-dependent calcium transport therein (Halloran & DeLuca 1981).

Transcriptional effects of $1\alpha,25(OH)_2D$

The specific molecules with which the $1\alpha,25(OH)_2D$ receptor interacts have not yet been established, but $1\alpha,25(OH)_2D$ directly or indirectly regulates mRNA levels for many different proteins. For example cholecalcin (see below) mRNA levels in duodenal mucosa (and in many other tissues) are increased (Perret et al 1985), osteocalcin (also termed bone gamma-carboxy glutamic acid-containing protein) mRNA rises in osteoblasts (Lian et al 1985), preprocollagen type I mRNA levels rise or fall in bone cultures (Rowe & Kream 1982), and preprarathyroid hormone mRNA levels fall in parathyroid cells (Cantley et al 1985) (see below for more details concerning the proteins encoded by some of these mRNAs).

Nongenomic effects of $1\alpha,25(OH)_2D$

$1\alpha,25(OH)_2D$ may have some cellular effects not mediated by the genomic pathway. Evidence for these mechanisms includes extremely rapid effects (Nemere et al 1984, Baran & Milne 1986) and dependency on normal receptor genes (Barsony & Marx 1988).

Cholecalcin and intestinal transport of calcium

The most important physiological action of $1\alpha,25(OH)_2D$ is stimulation of active calcium transport across the duodenum from lumen to bloodstream. Surprisingly, few details are known about the molecular basis of this process (Wasserman et al 1984). In particular the roles of cholecalcin (also called calbindin or vitamin D dependent calcium binding protein) are not known; this is despite the facts that it binds calcium with high affinity (the calcium-binding regions are homologous to those of the calmodulin family), it constitutes approximately 2% of duodenal mucosal cell protein in the D-replete state, and it is undetectable in duodenum in the D-deficient state. Cholecalcin in duodenum might act as a buffer of intracellular calcium (Feher 1983) or as a regulator of calcium ATPase (Morgan et al 1986). There are at least two cholecalcin genes in the rat; one codes for a 9 kD protein concentrated in the duodenum, the other for a homologous 28 kD protein concentrated in kidney, brain, and many other tissues.

A widespread tissue distribution of $1\alpha,25(OH)_2D$ receptors and of a family of cholecalcin proteins indicates that $1\alpha,25(OH)_2D$ may act directly in many tissues. Several potential target tissues outside the intestine are discussed here.

$1\alpha,25(OH)_2D$ actions on bone

Most of the antirachitic actions of calciferols are secondary to maintenance of calcium and phosphate concentrations in extracellular fluid adequate for bone mineralization (Underwood & DeLuca 1984, Weinstein et al 1984, Holtrop et al 1986). $1\alpha,25(OH)_2D$ inhibits proliferation and collagen synthesis in fetal bone and in fetal osteoblasts (Rowe & Kream 1982). In osteoblast-like cells from adult humans, however, $1\alpha,25(OH)_2D$ stimulates collagen synthesis (Beresford et al 1986). Differing effects on alkaline phosphatase have been reported in several systems; however, there is general agreement that in rapidly growing osteoblast-like cells alkaline phosphatase levels are low and that they rise in response to $1\alpha,25(OH)_2D$ (Majeska & Rodan 1982).

In vivo and in organ culture, $1\alpha,25(OH)_2D$ is a potent activator of osteoclasts. Isolated osteoclasts, however, show no response to $1\alpha,25(OH)_2D$ (Chambers et al 1985) and contain no receptors for $1\alpha,25(OH)_2D$ (Merke et al 1986). At least three mechanisms have been suggested for $1\alpha,25(OH)_2D$ activation of osteoclasts: first, $1\alpha,25(OH)_2D$ may stimulate differentiation of osteoclast precursors, related to monocytes and macrophages (Roodman et al 1985, Bar-Shavit et al 1986); second, $1\alpha,25(OH)_2D$ may stimulate fusion and metabolism of the immediate precursor of the multinucleated osteoclast (Abe et al 1984); and third, $1\alpha,25(OH)_2D$ might stimulate adjacent cells (McSheehy & Chambers 1987) such as osteoblasts to activate osteoclasts.

$1\alpha,25(OH)_2D$ actions on skin and hair

Receptors for $1\alpha,25(OH)_2D$ have been identified directly by in vivo autoradiography in basal layers of epidermis and in the outer root sheath cells of the rat hair follicle (Stumpf et al 1984). $1\alpha,25(OH)_2D$, moreover, stimulates differentiation of epidermal keratinocytes in tissue culture (Smith et al 1986).

$1\alpha,25(OH)_2D$ actions on the parathyroid gland

$1\alpha,25(OH)_2D$ inhibits parathyroid gland functions in vitro. In particular, it decreases transcription of mRNA for preproparathyroid hormone (Cantley et al 1985).

$1\alpha,25(OH)_2D$ actions on calciferol metabolism

$1\alpha,25(OH)_2D$ may regulate calciferol metabolism at several steps. It can increase the levels of 7,8-didehydrocholesterol in skin (Esvelt et al 1980), is a potent inhibitor of the renal $25(OH)D_3$ 1α-hydroxylase enzyme (Turner 1984) (see above), and activates the $25(OH)D_3$ 24-hydroxylase enzyme in kidney and in many other tissues (Colston & Feldman 1982). $1\alpha,25(OH)_2D$ stimulates the clearance of $25(OH)D$ and $1\alpha,25(OH)_2D$; this regulated clearance is a combination of 24-hydroxylation, 23-hydroxylation, and other less well defined processes (Engstrom et al 1986, Clements et al 1987).

Specific role of $24,25(OH)_2D_3$

It has been reported that $24,25(OH)_2D_3$ shows unique actions on cartilage from fetal or newborn animals, not reproduced by any dosage of $1\alpha,25(OH)_2D_3$ (Binderman & Somjen 1984, Somjen et al 1984). These actions include stimulation of proliferation and stimulation of creatine kinase BB isoenzyme. However, despite extensive experiments no important role for $24,25(OH)_2D_3$ has been proven in vivo (Brommage & DeLuca 1985). For example, rats have been raised for two generations without this metabolite, by raising them on a vitamin D_3 free diet supplemented with $24,24(Fl)_2-25(OH)D_3$, a metabolite that precludes formation of $24,25(OH)_2D_3$ (though it might not preclude formation of analogues of $24,25(OH)_2D_3$).

GENERAL FEATURES OF CALCIFEROL DEFICIENCY

Clinical presentation

The general features of vitamin D deficiency will be reviewed (Aurbach et al 1985b, Marel et al 1986) because almost all are shown in patients with hereditary defects in calciferol metabolism or action.

The clinical features of calciferol deficiency are weakness, bone pain, bone deformity and fracture. The most rapidly growing bones show the most striking abnormalities. In the first year of life the most rapidly growing bones are the skull, ribs and wrists. Calciferol deficiency at this time leads to widened cranial sutures, frontal bossing, posterior flattening of the skull, bulging of costo-chondral junctions, and enlargement of the wrists. The rib cage may be so deformed that it contributes to respiratory failure. Dental eruption is delayed, and teeth show enamel hypoplasia. Muscular weakness and hypotonia are severe and result in a protuberant abdomen. Muscular weakness may also contribute to respiratory failure. Linear growth may be adequate, but the child may be unable to walk without support. Tetany is unusual as the degree of hypocalcaemia is mild and its onset is slow. After age 1, deformities are most prominent in the legs because of their weight bearing function. Anaemia is common.

The clinical features of calciferol deficiency states depend principally on age of onset. Calcium and phosphate levels in fetal plasma are sustained by placental transport from maternal plasma, and this transport is probably not regulated by calciferols (Brommage & DeLuca 1984). A fetus with an hereditary abnormality in calciferol metabolism that develops in a mother with normal calciferol metabolism is presumed to have normal calcium and phosphate levels in plasma and bone until birth.

In children, mineralization defects cause abnormalities of diaphyses, metaphyses and epiphyses. In particular, deficient mineralization of the epiphyseal growth plate results in distorted (bulging) epiphyses and bone deformity.

Calciferol deficiency that begins after epiphyseal fusion causes less deformity. In the mature, remodelling skeleton less than 5% of the calcium is newly deposited per year. Thus a mineralization defect in an adult must exist for several years to be clinically manifest. The earliest symptom is bone pain, particularly low in the back. Proximal muscle weakness may be so prominent as to suggest a primary neurological disturbance.

Treatment

During the first 1–4 months of treatment, endogenous production of $1\alpha,25(OH)_2D$ is regulated at rates greater than normal (Papapoulos et al 1980, Stanbury et al 1981, Garabedian et al 1983, Venkataraman et al 1983). Successful initiation of therapy is evidenced by diminution of secondary hyperparathyroidism; i.e. PTH and urinary cAMP fall, serum phosphate rises, and alkaline phosphatase falls. In children, normal bone mass may be achieved after recovery from calciferol deficiency, but in adults bone mass may remain low (Parfitt et al 1985).

Pathophysiology

Virtually all the features of calciferol deficiency can be understood as direct or remote consequences of the effect of deficient calciferol on duodenal transport of calcium. Malabsorption of calcium causes hypocalcaemia. Hypocalcaemia (and perhaps also the effect of deficient calciferol on the parathyroid gland (Lopez-Hilker et al 1986)) leads to increased secretion of parathyroid hormone (i.e. secondary hyperparathyroidism). If this process continues for many months, the parathyroid glands develop hypertrophy and hyperplasia. Parathyroid hormone acts on the proximal renal tubule to decrease reabsorption of phosphate and bicarbonate, producing hypophosphataemia and hyperchloraemic acidosis. However, the phosphaturic effect of PTH is not uniform; severe and longstanding hypocalcaemia can paradoxically inhibit the phosphaturic effect of PTH. This can produce a confusing picture of secondary hyperparathyroidism with high urinary cyclic AMP but not hypophosphataemia (Rao et al 1985) (so called pseudo-hypoparathyroidism type II). In children, secondary hyperparathyroidism also causes generalized amino-aciduria. The combination of hypocalcaemia and hypophosphataemia reduces the rate of mineralization of bone matrix. Parathyroid hormone also acts directly on bone, where it increases osteoclastic reabsorption (but the release of calcium and phosphate from bone does not fully compensate for the hypocalcaemia or hypophosphataemia).

The principal goal of therapy is to provide enough calcium in extracellular fluid to allow normalization of bone mineralization and suppression of secondary hyperparathyroidism. Chronic deficiency of calciferol causes deficiency of calcium in the skeleton that can result in removal of calcium from plasma for many months during remineralization. During the early months of treatment with vitamin D or $25(OH)D_3$, serum contains low calcium, high PTH, low phosphate, and normal or high $25(OH)D$, all of which promote synthesis of $1\alpha,25(OH)_2D$.

HEREDITARY DEFECTS IN CALCIFEROL METABOLISM OR ACTION

Nomenclature

The calciferols traverse a metabolic pathway that could justify their being described as normal metabolites, vitamins (vitamin D is a dietary factor required in trace amounts in states of limited skin exposure to ultraviolet light), or hormones ($1\alpha,25(OH)_2D$ is secreted into the bloodstream at a regulated rate by the kidney and acts on the intestine and other targets). Prior nomenclature for calciferol deficiency states has been confusing because the terms evolved prior to detailed understanding of calciferol metabolism. Nomenclature in this chapter is based on our present understanding of calciferol metabolism (Marx 1989).

Deficiency of $1\alpha,25(OH)_2D$ could arise from deficiency of vitamin D or $25(OH)D$. With other causes both of these precursors can be normal. In this chapter the term 'selective' implies that a deficiency is associated with normal levels of the immediate precursor of the metabolite specified.

Several terms, related to the term deficiency, have been used. These include pseudo-deficiency, dependency, and resistance. The term 'vitamin D pseudo-deficiency' refers to a state with many features of vitamin D deficiency (i.e. calcium deficiency, secondary hyperparathyroidism, impaired skeletal mineralization) but no presumed deficiency in vitamin D levels or dietary calcium. Vitamin D pseudo-deficiency has been subdivided into type I (selective deficiency of $1\alpha,25(OH)_2D$) and type II (generalized resistance to $1\alpha,25(OH)_2D$). The term 'vitamin D dependency' has been used interchangeably with vitamin D pseudo-deficiency. This latter term is particularly confusing when applied to patients responding to high doses of $1\alpha,25(OH)_2D$ but not to vitamin D, or patients unresponsive to vitamin D or $1\alpha,25(OH)_2D$ but responsive to high doses of calcium.

Since defects in calciferol metabolism or action can be associated with, or even secondary to, defects in other pathways, nomenclature can be used to indicate if dysfunction extends to other pathways. In this chapter, 'simple' denotes an abnormality not associated with defects in other pathways and 'complex' implies the converse. Other important qualifying terms can indicate if a defect is hereditary or acquired, or if a defect is anatomically localized or generalized. Two hereditary defects, limited to metabolism or action of calciferols, have been recognized. The first is selective and simple deficiency of $1\alpha,25(OH)_2D$; further developments will probably justify reclassifying all cases in this category as simple deficiency of $25(OH)D_3$ 1α-hydroxylase. The second is generalized resistance to $1\alpha,25(OH)_2D$; it seems likely that all cases in this second category will ultimately be attributed to generalized deficiency of $1\alpha,25(OH)_2D$ receptor function.

HEREDITARY SELECTIVE AND SIMPLE DEFICIENCY OF $1\alpha,25(OH)_2D$

Clinical features

Deficiency of $1\alpha,25(OH)_2D$ develops in several hereditary disorders affecting the renal proximal tubule (X–linked hypophosphataemia, Fanconi syndromes), but selective and simple deficiency of $1\alpha,25(OH)_2D$ is a distinctive state, described below. This disorder (other terms used are hereditary vitamin D dependency type I, hereditary vitamin D pseudo-deficiency type I) is an unusual cause of hereditary rickets (Dommergues et al 1978, Karpouzas et al 1979, Bravo et al 1986). Patients appear normal at birth but dysfunction is recognizable at 2–24 months, suggesting lack of calciferol effect that began at the time of birth. Muscle weakness is prominent, radiographic features are striking, and response to calciferols is complete (see below).

Serum shows low calcium, high PTH, but low or even undetectable $1\alpha,25(OH)_2D$ (Scriver et al 1978, Garabedian et al 1981). The latter can be associated with normal or even modestly increased $25(OH)D$ (reflecting vitamin D supplementation and/or diminished clearance of $25(OH)D$). Therapy with $1\alpha(OH)D_3$ leads to normal concentrations of $1,25(OH)_2D$ in serum; therapy with $1\alpha,25(OH)_2D_3$ is equally effective; although random serum levels may be hard to interpret because of the rapid turnover of this drug. Serum calcium and phosphate in the partially treated patient can be difficult to interpret. With partial treatment, or early after discontinuation of treatment, mild secondary hyperparathyroidism can be associated with hypophosphataemia and normal serum calcium (Delvin et al 1981); this can cause confusion with X–linked hypophosphataemia, particularly because some patients with that disorder can also show secondary hyperparathyroidism.

Inheritance

Several sibships show features highly suggestive of autosomal recessive inheritance. There is a widespread assumption that this is the transmission mechanism in all cases. Very few families, however, have been evaluated in any detail with analyses of $1\alpha,25(OH)_2D$ in serum. Tests to recognize the heterozygous state have not yet been developed. The Saguenay population in Canada show a high incidence of this disorder, reflecting their descent from a small group of settlers (Bouchard et al 1985). Linkage analysis in this population revealed that the gene is on the long arm of chromosome 12 and supported the notion of a founder effect (Labuda et al 1989).

Treatment

Patients have been treated successfully with all widely available calciferol analogues (Delvin et al 1981, Balsan & Garabedian 1972, Balsan et al 1975, Reade et al 1975). Initially, (during the first 3–6 months of treatment) they should be given doses 2–5 times those expected for long-term maintenance (Table 92.2), since the undermineralized skeleton requires unusually large amounts of calcium. Long-term maintenance therapy is accomplished with any regimen that provides active metabolites in blood sufficient to activate normally receptors for $1\alpha,25(OH)_2D$ (Table 92.2). During successful treatment with vitamin D or $25(OH)D_3$, serum $25(OH)D$ levels are in the region of 250 ng/ml, but serum $1\alpha,25(OH)_2D$ may remain low or undetectable (Scriver et al 1978, Garabedian et al 1981). Successful therapy maintains fractional intestinal absorption of calcium near a constant value. Since fractional absorption of calcium from the gut is not regulated by endogenous mechanisms because of defective $1,25(OH)_2D$ synthesis, calcium homeostasis must be regulated by direct actions of PTH on kidney and/or bone. Thus these patients could show an unusually rapid fall of urine calcium or rise of urine calcium at times of calcium deficiency or excess respectively. Such fluctuations can be minimized by giving a fixed calcium supplement (1000 mg per 24 hours as elemental calcium). Treatment must be continued indefinitely.

Cellular defect

The presumption is that hereditary selective and simple deficiency of $1\alpha,25(OH)_2D$ is always attributable to defects in $25(OH)D_3$ 1α-hydroxylase. It seems inconceivable that accelerated clearance of $1\alpha,25(OH)_2D$ could produce this state. It is likely that the cause of the deficiency is heterogeneous, and that the degree of enzyme deficiency will also prove variable.

Animal models

Ploniat reported an autosomal recessive rachitic disorder in pigs (Ploniat 1962). More recent studies showed that the animals had hypocalcaemic rickets responsive to 'physiological' doses of $1\alpha,25(OH)_2D_3$ or $1\alpha(OH)D_3$ (Harmeyer et al 1981). A similar trait was transferred to miniature pigs for detailed study. Direct assay of renal homogenates taken from homozygotes of each strain established undetectable 1α-hydroxylase activity (Fox et al 1985, Winkler et al 1986). Both strains also exhibited low circulating $24,25(OH)_2D$ and undetectable renal 24-hydroxylase activity. This raised the possibility of associated hereditary deficiency of 24-hydroxylase or of low 24-hydroxylase activity secondary to $1\alpha,25(OH)_2D$ deficiency, hypocalcaemia, hypophosphataemia and secondary hyperparathyroidism.

Table 92.2 Calciferol doses for maintenance treatment of patients with hereditary defects in calciferol metabolism (Marx 1989). Dose requirements are uncorrected for body weight and are similar in children and adults

Calciferol analogue	Dosage in Deficient $25(OH)D$ 1α-hydroxylase (μg/24 hours)	Dosage in Generalized resistance to $1\alpha,25(OH)_2D$ (μg/24 hours)
Vitamin D_3 or D_2	500–3000	500–?*
$25(OH)D_3$	30–200	30–?*
$1\alpha,25(OH)_2D_3$	0.3–2	5–60**
$1\alpha(OH)D_3$	0.5–3	5–60**
Dihydrotachysterol	150–1000	2000–20 000**

* Patients with milder grades of resistance to $1\alpha,25(OH)_2D$ (usually with normal hair) can respond to analogues requiring 1-hydroxylation. Maximal useful doses have not been defined. Serum $1\alpha,25(OH)_2D$ must be maintained in the range of 200–1000 pg/ml.
** Maximal doses are limited only by cost and patient acceptance; some patients have shown no response to maximal doses tested.

Other deficiency states

In several hereditary or acquired disorders, $25(OH)D_3$ 1α-hydroxylase deficiency represents one component of a more complex disturbance. These disorders affecting the proximal renal tubule include X–linked hypophosphataemia (Lyles et al 1982, Harrell et al 1985, Read et al 1986), renal tubular acidosis (Brenner et al 1982, Kawashima et al 1982, Chesney et al 1984), Fanconi syndromes (Kitagawa et al 1980, Steinherz et al 1983, Baran & Marcy 1984), and tumour-associated osteomalacia (in which a humoral factor seems to cause impairment of 1α-hydroxylase and renal wasting of phosphate (Ryan & Reiss 1984). Replacement of $1\alpha,25(OH)_2D$ is an important component of the therapy of these disorders.

HEREDITARY GENERALIZED RESISTANCE TO $1\alpha,25(OH)_2D$

Clinical features

Hereditary generalized resistance to $1\alpha,25(OH)_2D$ (also called vitamin D dependency type II or vitamin D pseudo-deficiency type II) is a rare disorder, first recognized in a sporadic case (Brooks et al 1978). The clinical features are almost identical to those in hereditary selective and simple deficiency of $1\alpha,25(OH)_2D$, but in hereditary generalized resistance to $1\alpha,25(OH)_2D$, alopecia is found in about half the kindreds (Marx et al 1978, Rosen et al 1979, Marx et al 1984). Cases with hereditary generalized resistance to $1\alpha,25(OH)_2D$ appear normal at birth but generally develop the clinical and biochemical features of calciferol deficiency (see above) with hypocalcaemic rickets over the first 2–8 months of life. In many cases, hair is lost between the ages of 2–12 months. Alopecia may be complete or incomplete (Fig. 92.4); sometimes there is selective sparing of the eyelashes. Light microscopic examination of a scalp biopsy showed normal numbers and morphology of hair follicles in a patient with total alopecia (Hochberg et al 1985a). Alopecia occurs in patients with the most severe resistance to $1\alpha,25(OH)_2D$ (see below). Without therapy, this disorder leads to inanition, severe skeletal deformity, recurrent respiratory infections, and death by age 8. Other ectodermal defects have been reported in small numbers of cases and have an uncertain relation to the syndrome; these include oligodontia (Liberman et al 1980) and papular skin rash (Liberman et al 1980, Sakati et al 1986). All patients suffer from the consequences of intestinal malabsorption of calcium. Attempts to show $1\alpha,25(OH)_2D$ receptor-mediated dysfunctions outside the intestine in vivo have so far been inconclusive. Basal and stimulated concentrations of insulin, thyrotropin, prolactin, growth hormone, and testosterone have been

normal (aside from deficiencies in insulin stimulation attributable to hypocalcaemia) (Hochberg et al 1985b). Bone biopsies have shown normal or increased numbers of osteoclasts (Balsan et al 1986, Weisman et al 1987) (suggesting that $1\alpha,25(OH)_2D$ is not essential for osteoclast formation), but their resorptive activity was suggested to be impaired (Balsan et al 1986).

In several cases, neonatal development was apparently normal, and dysfunction was not evident until late in childhood (Kudoh et al 1981) or even in adulthood (Fujita et al 1980) (in the latter case, serum $1\alpha,25(OH)_2D$ was not measured, so alternative aetiologies for high calciferol dose, such as noncompliance, were not excluded). In each report the patient did not show alopecia, and each responded to high doses of calciferols, indicating a mild variant of the syndrome. Neither showed clear features of a genetic aetiology in that there was no parental consanguinity and no affected sib.

Measurement of calciferol metabolites in plasma usually provides the most useful information for diagnosis. Serum $1\alpha,25(OH)_2D$ is 50–1000 pg/ml (normal in children is 30–100 pg/ml) before treatment; during calciferol treatment typical concentrations are

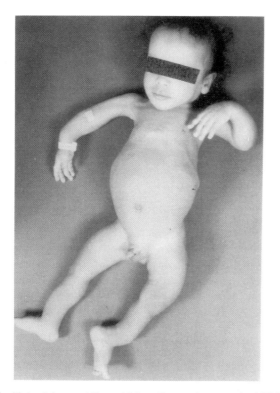

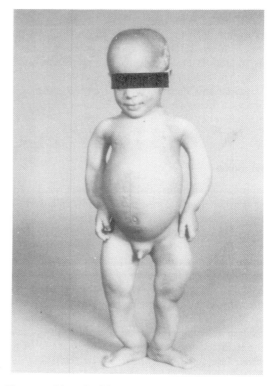

A   B

Fig. 92.4   A 5-year-old boy with hereditary resistance to $1\alpha,25(OH)_2D$. He was unable to sit without support at age 5 **A**. Though unresponsive to high doses of calciferols, he showed improvement two years later following treatment with high doses of calcium orally **B**. Though weakness and deformity improved, alopecia worsened during treatment (Sakati et al 1986).

200–10 000 pg/ml (Fig 92.5). High $1\alpha,25(OH)_2D$ in an affected female can allow a normal pregnancy (Marx et al 1980b); this is important because of concern that high $1\alpha,25(OH)_2D$ might disturb fetal tissues (see calciferol excess states below).

Inheritance

Approximately 30 kindreds have been reported (Marx et al 1986). There have usually been strong suggestions of autosomal recessive transmission (parental consanguinity, etc). Most cases have been recognized in a broad region centred about the Mediterranean Sea, and this may relate to the very high consanguinity rate in the populations with $1,25(OH)_2D$ receptor disease in this area (Al-Awadi et al 1985). No clinical abnormalities have been reported in obligate heterozygotes.

Treatment

Many cases show complete remission while receiving extraordinarily high doses of calciferols (Marx et al 1984) (Table 92.2). Alopecia is one simple predictor of potential for response to therapy (Marx et al 1986). Virtually all cases with normal hair can sustain remission when given high doses of analogue not requiring 1-hydroxylation. Among cases with alopecia, approximately half are resistant to the highest doses of calciferols achievable; the other half have shown a satisfactory calcaemic response,

but the dose requirement is typically 10-fold higher than in cases with normal hair (Fig. 92.5). Maintenance treatment is based upon four considerations; (a) some patients can be treated with calciferols (vitamin D_3, vitamin D_2, or $25(OH)D_3$) that provide substrate for a high renal secretion of $1\alpha,25(OH)_2D$; (b) others may respond only to high doses of analogues ($1\alpha,25(OH)_2D_3$, $1\alpha(OH)D_3$, dihydrotachysterol) that do not require 1α-hydroxylation by the kidney; (c) a minority may not respond to maximal doses of any calciferols; and (d) the role of calcium supplements is different in each of the prior three groups (see below).

Several patients have shown remissions while receiving high doses of vitamin D_2 or $25(OH)D_3$ (Brooks et al 1978, Marx et al 1978). In these cases tissue resistance is only moderate; sufficient $1\alpha,25(OH)_2D$ is produced endogenously in the presence of a high level of substrate for 1α-hydroxylation. In this group calcium supplements may have little or no role, as serum concentrations of PTH and $1\alpha,25(OH)_2D$ can compensate for fluctuations in calcium availability.

Patients unable to produce sufficient $1\alpha,25(OH)_2D$ endogenously (because of a requirement for particularly high $1\alpha,25(OH)_2D$ concentrations) may still respond to extraordinarily high doses of analogues not requiring 1α-hydroxylation (i.e. $1\alpha,25(OH)_2D_3$, $1\alpha(OH)D_3$, dihydrotachysterol). Patients in this group requiring therapy that bypasses 1α-hydroxylation should receive fixed calcium supplements (1000 mg per 24 hours elemental calcium)

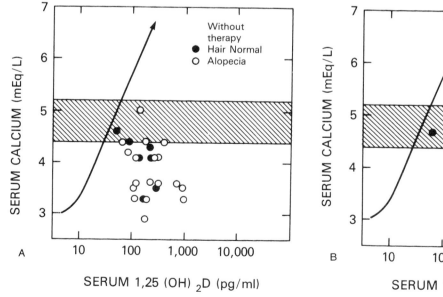
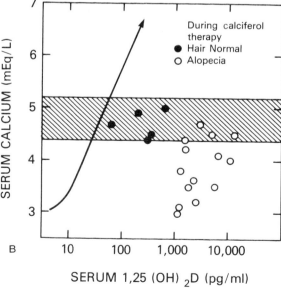

Fig. 92.5 Relationship between serum concentrations of calcium and $1\alpha,25(OH)_2D$. Hatched area is normal range for calcium. Solid curve is theoretical normal relationship between calcium and $1\alpha,25(OH)_2D$. **A** Without calciferol therapy; **B** during calciferol therapy (Marx et al 1986).

for the same reasons as patients with hereditary selective deficiency of $1\alpha,25(OH)_2D$.

Some patients show no response to maximal calciferol doses (Fig. 92.6) (Balsan et al 1983, Hochberg et al 1984, Balsan et al 1986). Patients with undetectable response to calciferols can still obtain substantial benefit if large amounts of calcium can be delivered to the bloodstream. The most effective way to accomplish this is by intravenous infusions (Balsan et al 1986, Weisman et al 1987, Bliziotes et al 1988); high calcium doses (1000 mg elemental calcium per 24 hours infused over 12 hours) can be tolerated even by young children with this disorder. Since normal positive calcium balance during childhood growth is approximately 300 mg/24 hours and deficits prior to treatment are large, such infusions must be given repeatedly over many months to accomplish significant results. This form of therapy requires methods similar to those used in hyperalimentation programmes. Another way to increase calcium input to the bloodstream is to increase net absorption independent of calciferols (Sakati et al 1986). Unfortunately the upper limit of tolerance to calcium by mouth is around 6000 mg per day and requires great co-operation; in the absence of calciferol bioeffect, the net calcium retention is approximately 10%. The utility of therapy with intravenous or oral calcium confirms the centrality of the intestine as a target tissue for $1\alpha,25(OH)_2D$.

As in the calciferol deficiency states, total body calcium requirements are highest at the onset of treatment. Thus the doses of calcium, the doses of calciferols, and the type of approach judged necessary to initiate therapy (for example, intravenous calcium) may not prove to be the same as those required for maintenance therapy.

Cellular defects

Cells from patients with hereditary generalized resistance to $1\alpha,25(OH)_2D$ have been used to characterize the defect presumed to exist in all target tissues. Because of the widespread expression of the $1\alpha,25(OH)_2D$ effector system in many tissues, these studies have been possible with skin fibroblasts (Eil et al 1981, Liberman et al 1983b), keratinocytes (Clemens et al 1983), bone cells

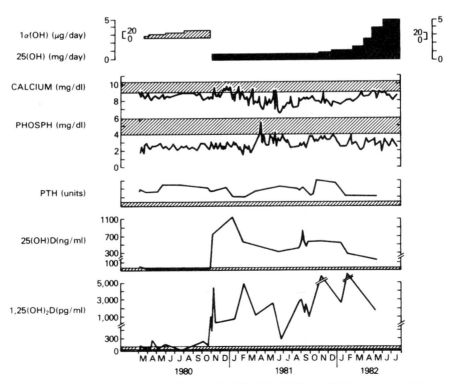

Fig. 92.6 Absent calcaemic response during a long therapeutic trial with calciferols. Calciferol therapy is in upper panel: $1\alpha(OH)$ refers to $1\alpha(OH)D_3$ or $1\alpha,25(OH)_2D_3$ and $25(OH)$ refers to $25(OH)D_3$. Hatched zones indicate normal ranges. Not only is hypocalcaemia persistent, but also secondary hyperparathyroidism persists (high parathyroid hormone and low phosphate), and very high serum levels of $1\alpha,25(OH)_2D$ are documented (Marx et al 1984).

(Liberman et al 1983a, Silve et al 1986), and peripheral lymphocytes (Koren et al 1985). Five categories of defect have been identified.

1. *Hormone-binding negative*. The commonest defect has been undetectable high affinity binding of $1\alpha,25(OH)_2D$ (Liberman et al 1983b, Chen et al 1984). Cell extracts from four hormone-binding negative kindreds were tested with a monoclonal antibody against the receptor for $1\alpha,25(OH)_2D$; cross reacting material was found in each, suggesting that the phenotype usually results not from absence of receptor protein but from mutations in the hormone-binding region (Pike et al 1984).

2. *Decreased maximal capacity of hormone-binding*. This abnormality has been reported in only one kindred (Balsan et al 1983). Cells extracts showed a hormone-binding capacity only 10% of normal but a hormone-binding affinity that was normal.

3. *Decreased affinity of hormone-binding*. A selective abnormality in hormone-binding affinity with normal hormone-binding capacity has been suggested, but not proven conclusively, in one kindred (Castells et al 1986).

4. *Normal hormone-binding but undetectable intranuclear retention*. Extracts of cells from two kindreds have shown normal capacity and affinity of hormone-binding; however, high affinity uptake of hormone into the nucleus was undetectable (Eil et al 1981, Liberman et al 1983b). The receptors from both kindreds showed a normal affinity for nonspecific DNA (Liberman et al 1986). The underlying nature of this interesting defect has not been fully determined.

5. *Nuclear localization positive*. Cells from five kindreds have shown nearly normal nuclear uptake of hormone (Griffin et al 1983, Hirst et al 1985, Liberman et al 1986, Hughes et al 1988); hormone binding to receptors was normal in capacity and affinity. With four kindreds the $1\alpha,25(OH)_2D$ receptor showed abnormal elution from nonspecific DNA (Hirst et al 1985, Liberman et al 1986, Hughes et al 1988). In each the receptor eluted at lower salt concentration than normal. Such findings can be classified as a DNA-binding defect of the receptor.

To summarize, no case has met strict criteria for a possible pre- or post-receptor defect. Only one case has so far showed no receptor defect (Griffin et al 1983), but DNA-binding studies with that receptor have not been reported. Wherever detailed testing of $1\alpha,25(OH)_2D$ receptor properties has been done, abnormalities have been found.

The class of defect has shown no correlation with

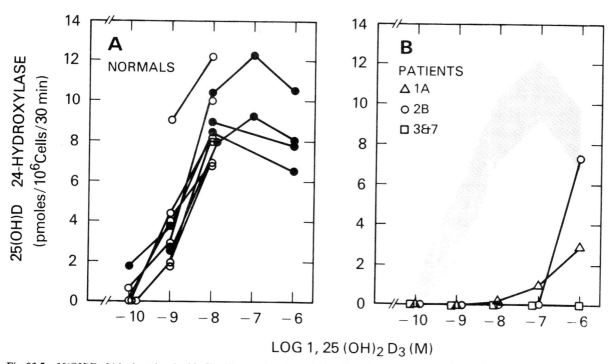

Fig. 92.7 $25(OH)D_3$ 24-hydroxylase in skin fibroblasts preincubated with indicated concentrations of $1\alpha,25(OH)_2D_3$. **A** Normal subjects; **B** patients with hereditary generalized resistance to $1\alpha,25(OH)_2D$. Patients 1A and 2B each showed a satisfactory calcaemic response to high doses of $1\alpha,25(OH)_2D_3$, but patients 3 and 7 showed no calcaemic response (Gamblin et al 1985).

clinical features. Rather, these cases seem to fit within a continuous spectrum of severity that correlates with indices of post-transcriptional actions of $1\alpha,25(OH)_2D$.

$1\alpha,25(OH)_2D_3$ actions in patients' cells

Post-transcriptional actions of $1\alpha,25(OH)_2D_3$ in cells from these patients have been evaluated. Each patients' cells have shown severely deficient actions. The most extensively tested response to $1\alpha,25(OH)_2D_3$ is induction of $25(OH)D_3$ 24-hydroxylase activity (Griffin et al 1983, Gamblin et al 1985). In general, patients with milder disease (normal hair, calcaemic response to high doses of calciferols) show inducible 24-hydroxylase with supraphysiological concentrations of $1\alpha,25(OH)_2D_3$ (Fig. 92.7) but patients with the severest disease (alopecia, no calcaemic response to maximal doses of calciferols) show no 24-hydroxylase response to maximal concentrations of $1\alpha,25(OH)_2D_3$. Five of six obligate heterozygotes showed no abnormality (Chen et al 1984); the sixth showed a 50% decrease in hormone-binding capacity and a similar decrease in maximal induction of 24-hydroxylase. Similar severe defects have been identified with analyses of inhibition of cell growth by $1\alpha25(OH)_2D$ (in cultured skin fibroblasts and keratinocytes (Clemens et al 1983) or in peripheral mononuclear cells (Koren et al 1985)) and stimulation of 24-hydroxylase and of osteocalcin secretion in osteoblast-like bone cells (Silve et al 1986).

Gene defects

The $1\alpha,25(OH)_2D_3$ receptor gene has been analyzed in members of two kindreds with DNA-binding defects (Hughes et al 1988). DNA from affected members of both kindreds showed a homozygous point mutation. In each case the mutation caused a major shift in electrostatic charge at the tip of one 'zinc finger' (Fig. 92.8). The 'zinc finger' is a domain present in two or more homologous copies in certain proteins thought to bind to DNA (Evans & Hollenberg 1988); the finger conformation is believed to be dependent upon zinc that is bound to four highly conserved residues (4 cysteines or 2 cysteines and 2 histidines).

Animal model

A state resembling hereditary generalized resistance to $1\alpha,25(OH)_2D$ is found in new world primates (marmosets and tamarins). These animals sometimes develop osteomalacia in captivity and are known to have high nutritional requirements for calciferols (Yamaguchi et al 1986). New world primates show high circulating concentrations of $1\alpha,25(OH)_2D$ (Adams et al 1985a). Intestinal and other cells from these animals have shown deficient hormone binding capacity (in comparison to cells from old world primates) (Adams et al 1985b, Liberman et al 1985, Takahashi et al 1985), and deficient

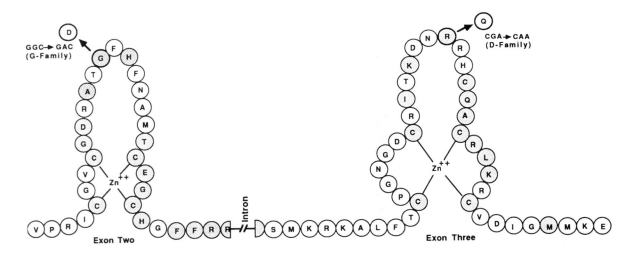

Fig. 92.8 Amino acid sequence and hypthetical structure of a portion of the receptor for $1\alpha,25(OH)_2D_3$ in normals and in affected members from two kindreds with hereditary generalized resistance to $1\alpha,25(OH)_2D_3$. Amino acids are represented by a single-letter code. For example, C depicts cysteine. The deduced amino acids from complementary DNA are shown as two potential zinc-finger arrays. The change in a triplet codon in exon 2 converts a glycine to aspartic acid in one kindred; the mutation in exon 3 converts an arginine to glutamine in another kindred (modified from Hughes et al 1988).

hormone-binding affinity (Liberman et al 1985). These new world primates also exhibit hereditary generalized resistance to several steroid hormones, including glucocorticoids, oestrogens and progestogens (Lipsett et al 1985). Thus their defects appear to involve elements shared by many of the nuclear-active steroids and secosteroids.

States resembling hereditary generalized resistance to $1\alpha,25(OH)_2D$

There are multiple forms of hereditary or acquired rickets or osteomalacia in which calciferol metabolism is normal or, if abnormal, only as an appropriate response to a primary disturbance in mineral flux. Rickets or osteomalacia with high circulating $1\alpha,25(OH)_2D$ is found in generalized resistance to $1\alpha,25(OH)_2D$ and in two additional states (calcium deficiency or phosphate deficiency).

Calcium deficiency

Severe deficiency of calcium has been recognized as a common dysfunction in Bantu adolescents, who consume a diet severely deficient in calcium (Pettifor et al 1981). Of course, calcium repletion cures all abnormalities. Osteopetrosis (marble-bones disease) is caused by several types of defect (usually hereditary) in osteoclast function. Both in humans and in animal models of this disease, serum $1\alpha,25(OH)_2D$ is increased and subtle histological changes of osteomalacia have been noted (Zerwekh et al 1987). At least one patient has been treated with a low calcium diet, plus high doses of $1\alpha,25(OH)_2D_3$ with apparent improvement in osteoclast function (Key et al 1984). Other cases of osteopetrosis have not responded to similar treatment, and at least one cellular defect (carbonic anhydrase II deficiency) unlikely to be overcome by $1\alpha,25(OH)_2D_3$ has been discovered (Sly et al 1985).

Phosphate deficiency

Severe deficiency of phosphate can cause rickets with high $1\alpha,25(OH)_2D$. In hereditary hypophosphataemic rickets with hypercalciuria, the primary renal loss of phosphate causes osteomalacia and activation of the renal 1α-hydroxylase (Tieder et al 1985, 1987). High $1\alpha,25(OH)_2D$ causes absorptive hypercalciuria; parathyroid function is suppressed, unlike in hereditary generalized resistance to $1\alpha,25(OH)_2D$.

Survivors of extreme prematurity can pass through a phase when their growing bones (deprived of the placental pump) are severely deficient in both calcium and phosphate, producing neonatal rickets with high serum $1\alpha,25(OH)_2D$ (Chesney et al 1981, Steichen et al 1981). In this group immaturity of intestinal responsiveness to $1\alpha,25(OH)_2D$ may contribute to the disturbance (Halloran & DeLuca 1981).

Deficient bone mineralization with normal calcium and phosphate in serum

There are several causes of deficient bone mineralization with otherwise normal calcium and phosphate fluxes. These include hypophosphatasia (Opshaug et al 1982), the chondrodystrophies (which can disturb epiphyseal function), and skeletal accumulation of aluminium, diphosphonates or fluoride (Aurbach et al 1985b). Since parathyroid hormone is not high or phosphate not low in serum, $1\alpha,25(OH)_2D$ is normal in serum.

OTHER HEREDITARY DEFECTS IN CALCIFEROL METABOLISM OR ACTION

Calciferol deficiency states

Though antigenic variation in vitamin D binding protein (Gc) is common, no differences in its function for calciferol transport have been identified in man (Kawakami et al 1979). However, in the chicken this protein shows 10-fold higher affinity for vitamin D_3 metabolites than for vitamin D_2 metabolites, and this seems to account for a higher requirement for vitamin D_2 than D_3 in this species (Belsey et al 1974).

Deficient 25-hydroxylation of vitamin D was suggested as an additional defect in one patient with hereditary generalized resistance to $1\alpha,25(OH)_2D$ (Zerwekh et al 1979). Increased clearance of 25(OH)D is an alternative mechanism for these observations.

Deficient 24-hydroxylation of 25(OH)D was suggested in another patient with hereditary generalized resistance to $1\alpha,25(OH)_2D$ (Liberman et al 1980). That patient showed low concentrations of $24,25(OH)_2D$ and showed partial remission of resistance when given $24,25(OH)_2D_3$. Those observations remain unexplained, but a persistent abnormality in DNA-binding of the $1\alpha,25(OH)_2D$ receptors has been documented in cells cultured from this patient (Liberman et al 1986), suggesting that the receptor defect is her primary problem. Decreased production of $24,25(OH)_2D$ could be secondary to the abnormality in $1\alpha,25(OH)_2D$ action, as one of its actions is induction of $25(OH)D_3$ 24-hydroxylase.

Calciferol excess states

Three groups (Lightwood 1952, Williams et al 1961, Beuren et al 1962) helped recognize a syndrome of infantile hypercalcaemia, elfin facies, mental retardation and supravalvular aortic stenosis (Williams syndrome).

The characteristic dysmorphology includes the following: wide slack mouth, malocclusion, prominent upper lip, underdeveloped mandible, depressed nasal bridge, hypertelorism, epicanthic folds, low-set ears, increased bone density, craniostenosis, and osteosclerosis especially of the base of the skull. Cases showing portions of the phenotype have sometimes been collected within this syndrome without implying identical pathophysiology for all cases (Jones & Smith 1975). Most cases have been sporadic, but some have had similarly affected siblings (Wiltse et al 1966), and autosomal dominant transmission was suggested in one kindred (Mehes et al 1975). Certain biochemical features suggest excess vitamin D effect; there is increased calcium absorption, hypercalciuria, and nephrocalcinosis. In some cases glucocorticoids have lessened the hypercalcaemia. Early studies suggested that calciferol bioactivity was increased in plasma (Fellers & Schwartz 1958), but recent assays of specific calciferol metabolites have not provided a consistent explanation of these findings. Taylor et al found that these patients and their phenotypically normal relatives show an abnormal accumulation of 25(OH)D when given a test dose of vitamin D_2 (Taylor et al 1982). Serum 25(OH)D_2 and 25(OH)D_3, however, have been normal in most other cases during the normocalcaemic or hypercalcaemic phase (Martin et al 1985). Serum 24,25(OH)$_2$D and 25,26(OH)$_2$D have also been normal (Martin et al 1985). Garabedian et al evaluated serum 1α,25(OH)$_2$D in four cases and found inappropriate increases (Garabedian et al 1985). Other cases have shown clear suppression of 1α,25(OH)$_2$D (Aarskog et al 1981, Chesney et al 1985, Martin et al 1985) suggesting more than one mechanism for the hypercalcaemia (Culler et al 1985). The implication of factors related to calciferols is strengthened by an animal model for this diorder. The offspring of rabbits with vitamin D intoxication show similar skeletal features (mandibular hypoplasia and characteristic dental abnormalities) (Friedman & Mills 1969) and typical supravavular aortic lesions (Friedman & Roberts 1966).

To summarize, it is unclear whether the syndrome of idiopathic hypercalcaemia with its associated abnormalities can result from a defect in calciferol metabolism or action.

REFFERENCES

Aarskog D, Aksnes L, Markestad T 1981 Vitamin D metabolism in idiopathic infantile hypercalcemia. American Journal of Diseases of Children 135: 1021-1024

Abe E, Shinna Y, Miyaura C et al 1984 Activation and fusion induced by 1α,25-dihydroxyvitamin D_3 and their relation in alveolar macrophages. Proceedings of the National Academy of Sciences USA 81: 7112-7116

Adams J S, Gacad M A, Baker A J, Gonzales B, Rude R K 1985a Serum concentrations of 1,25-dihydroxyvitamin D_3 in platyrrhini and catarrhini: a phylogenetic appraisal. American Journal of Primatology 9: 219-224

Adams J S, Gacad M A, Baker A J, Kheun G, Rude R K 1985b Diminished internalization and action of 1,25-dihydroxyvitamin D_3 in dermal fibroblasts cultured from New World primates. Endocrinology 116: 2523-2527

Al-Awadi S A, Moussa M A, Naguib K K, Farag T I, Teebi A S, El-Khalifa M, El-Dossary L 1985 Consanguinity among the Kuwaiti population. Clinical Genetics 27: 483-486

Albright F, Butler A M, Bloomberg E 1937 Rickets resistant to vitamin D therapy. American Journal of Diseases of Children 54: 531-547

Aurbach G D, Marx S J, Spiegel A M 1985a Parathyroid hormone, calcitonin, and the calciferols. In: Wilson J D, Foster D W (eds) Williams Textbook of Endocrinology, 7th edn., W B Saunders, Philadelphia p1137-1217

Aurbach G D, Marx S J, Spiegel A M 1985b Metabolic bone disease. In: Wilson J D, Foster D W (eds) Williams Textbook of Endocrinology, 7th edn., W B Saunders, Philadelphia p 1218-1255

Balsan S, Garabedian M 1972 25-Hydroxycholecalciferol: a comparative study in deficiency rickets and different types of resistant rickets. Journal of Clinical Investigation 51: 749-759

Balsan S, Garabedian M, Sorgniard R, Holick M F, DeLuca H F 1975 1,25-Dihydroxyvitamin D_3 and 1,a-hydroxyvitamin D_3 in children: biologic and therapeutic effects in nutritional rickets and different types of vitamin D resistance. Pediatric Research 9: 586-593

Balsan S, Garabedian M, Liberman U A et al 1983 Rickets and alopecia with resistance to 1,25-dihydroxyvitamin D: two different clinical courses with two different cellular defects. Journal of Clinical Endocrinology and Metabolism 57: 803-811

Balsan S, Garabedian M, Larchet M et al 1986 Long-term nocturnal calcium infusions can cure rickets and promote normal mineralization in hereditary resistance to 1,25-dihydroxyvitamin D. Journal of Clinical Investigation 77: 1661-1667

Baran D T, Marcy T W 1984 Evidence for a defect in vitamin D metabolism in a patient with incomplete Fanconi syndrome. Journal of Clinical Endocrinology and Metabolism 59: 998-1001

Baran D T, Milne M L 1986 1,25-Dihydroxyvitamin D increases hepatocyte cytosolic calcium levels: a potential regulator of vitamin D-25-hydroxylase. Journal of Clinical Investigation 77: 1622-1626

Bar-Shavit Z, Khan A J, Stone K R, Trial J, Hilliard T, Reitsma P H, Teitelbaum S L 1986 Reversibility of vitamin D-induced human leukemia cell-line maturation. Endocrinology 118: 679-686

Barsony J, Marx S J 1988 A receptor-mediated rapid action of 1α-dihydroxycholecalciferol: increase of intracellular cyclic GMP in human skin fibroblasts. Proceedings of the National Academy of Sciences USA 85: 1223-1226

Belsey R, DeLuca H F, Potts J T Jr. 1974 Selective binding properties of the vitamin D transport protein in chick plasma in vitro. Nature 247: 208

Beresford J N, Gallagher J A, Russel R G G 1986 1,25-Dihydroxyvitamin D_3 and human bone-derived cells in vitro: effects on alkaline phosphatase, type I collagen, and proliferation. Endocrinology 119: 1776–1785

Beuren A J, Apitz J, Harmjanz D 1962 Supravalvular aortic stenosis in association with mental retardation and a certain facial appearance. Circulation 26: 1235

Binderman I, Somjen D 1984 24,24-Dihydroxy-cholecalciferol induces the growth of chick cartilage in vitro. Endocrinology 115: 430–432

Bliziotes M, Yergey A, Nanes M 1988 Absent intestinal response to calciferols in hereditary resistance to 1,25-dihydroxyvitamin D: documentation and effective therapy with high dose intravenous calcium infusions. Journal of Clinical Endocrinology and Metabolism 66: 294–300

Bouchard G, Laberge C, Scriver C R 1985 La tyrosinemie hereditaire et le rachitisme vitamino-dependent au Saguenay: une approche genetique et demographique. Union Medicale du Canada 114: 633–636

Bravo H, Almeida S, Tato I G, Bustillo J M, Tojo R 1986 Early pseudo-deficiency or Prader's hypocalcemic familial type I rickets. Anales Espanoles de Pediatria 25: 121–124

Brenner R J, Spring D B, Sebastian A, McSherry E M, Genant H K, Palubinskas A J, Morris R C Jr. 1982 Incidence of radiographically evident bone disease, nephrocalcinosis, and nephrolithiasis in various types of renal tubular acidosis. New England Journal of Medicine 307: 217–221

Brommage R, DeLuca H F 1984 Placental transport of calcium and phosphate is not regulated by vitamin D. American Journal of Physiology 246: F526–F529

Brommage R, DeLuca H F 1985 Evidence that 1,25-dihydroxyvitamin D_3 is the physiologically active metabolite of vitamin D_3. Endocrine Reviews 6: 491–507

Brooks M H, Bell N H, Love L et al 1978 Vitamin-D-dependent rickets type II: resistance of target organs to 1,25-dihydroxyvitamin D. New England Journal of Medicine 298: 996–999

Burgos-Trinidad M, Brown A J, DeLuca H F 1985 Solubilization and reconstitution of chick renal mitochondrial 25-hydroxyvitamin D_3 24-hydroxylase. Biochemistry 25: 2692–2696

Cantley L K, Russel J, Lettieri D, Sherwood L M 1985 1,25-Dihydroxyvitamin D_3 suppresses parathyroid hormone secretion from bovine parathyroid cells in tissue culture. Endocrinology 117: 2114–2119

Castells S, Greig F, Fusi M et al 1986 Severely deficient binding of 1,25-dihydroxyvitamin D to its receptors in a patient responsive to high doses of this hormone. Journal of Clinical Endocrinology and Metabolism 63: 252–256

Chambers T J, McSheehy P M J, Thomson B M, Fuller K 1985 The effect of calcium-regulating hormones and prostaglandins on bone resorption by osteoclasts disaggregated from neonatal rabbit bones. Endocrinology 60: 234–239

Chen T L, Hirst M A, Cone C M, Hochberg Z, Tietze H-U, Feldman D 1984 1,25-Dihydroxyvitamin D resistance, rickets, and alopecia: analysis of receptors and bioresponse in cultured fibroblasts from patients and parents. Journal of Clinical Endocrinology and Metabolism 59: 383–388

Chesney R W, Hamstra A J, DeLuca H F 1981 Rickets of prematurity: supranormal levels of serum 1,25-dihydroxyvitamin D. American Journal of Diseases of Children 135: 24–37

Chesney R W, Kaplan B S, Phelps M, DeLuca H F 1984 Renal tubular acidosis does not alter circulating values of calcitriol. Journal of Pediatrics 104: 51–55

Chesney R W, DeLuca H F, Gertner J M, Genel M 1985 Increased plasma 1,25-dihydroxyvitamin D in infants with hypercalcemia and elfin facies. Letter to the editor. New England Journal of Medicine 313: 889

Clemens T L, Adams J S, Henderson S L, Holick M F 1982 Increased skin pigment reduces the capacity of skin to synthesise vitamin D_3. Lancet I: 74–76

Clemens T L, Adams J S, Horiuchi N et al 1983 Interaction of 1,25-hydroxyvitamin-D_3 with keratinocytes and fibroblasts from skin of normal subjects and a subject with vitamin-D-dependent rickets, type II: a model for study of the mode of action of 1,25-dihydroxyvitamin D_3. Journal of Clinical Endocrinology and Metabolism 56: 824–830

Clements M R, Johnson L, Fraser D R 1987 A new mechanism for induced vitamin D deficiency in calcium deprivation. Nature 325: 62–65

Colston K, Feldman D 1982 1,25-Dihydroxyvitamin D_3 receptors and functions in cultured pig kidney cells ($LLCPK_1$): regulation of 24,25-dihydroxyvitamin D_3. production. Journal of Biological Chemistry 257: 2504–2508

Cooke N E 1985 Rat vitamin D binding protein: determination of the full-length primary structure from cloned cDNA. Journal of Biological Chemistry 261: 3441–3450

Coppenhaver D H, Sollenne N P, Bowman B H 1983 Post-translational heterogeneity of the human vitamin-D-binding protein (group-specific component). Archives of Biochemistry and Biophysics 226: 218–223

Culler F L, Jones K L, Deftos L J 1985 Impaired calcitonin secretion in patients with Williams syndrome. Journal of Pediatrics 107: 720–723

Delvin E E, Glorieux F H, Marie P J, Pettifor M 1981 Vitamin D dependency: replacement therapy with calcitriol. Journal of Pediatrics 99: 26–34

Dommergues J-P, Garabedian M, Gueris J, LeDeunff M-J, Creignou L, Courtecuisse V, Balsan S 1978 Effets des principaux derive de la vitamine D: chez trois enfants d'une fratrie atteints de rachitisme 'pseudo-carentiel'. Archives Francaises de Pediatrie 35: 1050–1062

Eil C, Liberman U A, Rosen J F, Marx S J 1981 A cellular defect in hereditary vitamin-D-dependent rickets type II: defective nuclear uptake of 1,25-dihydroxyvitamin D in cultured skin fibroblasts. New England Journal of Medicine 304: 1588–1591

Engstrom G W, Reinhardt T A, Horst R L 1986 25-Hydroxyvitamin D_3-23-hydroxylase, a renal enzyme in several animal species. Archives of Biochemistry and Biophysics 250: 86–93

Esvelt R P, DeLuca H F, Wichman J K, Yoshizawa S, Zurcher J, Sar M, Stumpf W E 1980 1,25-dihydroxyvitamin D_3 stimulated increase of 7,8-didehydrocholesterol levels in rat skin. Biochemistry 19: 6158–6161

Evans R M 1988 The steroid and thyroid hormone receptor superfamily. Science 240: 889–894

Evans R M, Hollenberg S M 1988 Zinc fingers: gilt by association. Cell 52: 1–3

Feher J J 1983 Facilitated calcium diffusion by intestinal calcium-binding protein. American Journal of Physiology 244: C303

Fellers F X, Schwartz R 1958 Etiology of the severe form of idiopathic hypercalcemia of infancy. New England Journal of Medicine 259: 1050–1058

Fox J, Maunder E M W, Randall V R, Care A D 1985 Vitamin D-dependent rickets type I in pigs. Clinical Science 69: 541–548

Fraser D, Kooh S W, Kind H P, Holick M F, Tanaka Y, DeLuca H F 1973 Pathogenesis of hereditary vitamin-D-dependent rickets: an inborn error of vitamin D metabolism involving defective conversion of 25-hydroxyvitamin D to 1-a,25-dihydroxyvitamin D. New England Journal of Medicine 289: 817–822

Friedman W F, Mills L F 1969 The relationship between vitamin D and the craniofacial and dental anomalies of the supravalvular aortic stenosis syndrome. Pediatrics 43: 12–18

Friedman W F, Roberts W C 1966 Vitamin D and the supravalvular aortic stenosis syndrome. The transplacental effects of vitamin D on the aorta of the rabbit. Circulation 34: 77–86

Fujita T, Nomura M, Okajima S, Furuya H 1980 Adult-onset vitamin D-resistant osteomalacia with the unresponsiveness to parathyroid hormone. Journal of Endocrinology and Metabolism 50: 927–931

Gamblin G T, Liberman U A, Eil C, Downs R W Jr., DeGrange D A, Marx S J 1985 Vitamin D dependent rickets type II: defective induction of 25-hydroxyvitamin D_3-24-hydroxylase by 1,25-dihydroxyvitamin D_3 in cultured skin fibroblasts. Journal of Clinical Investigation 75: 954–960

Garabedian M, N'Guyen T M, Guillozo H, Grimberg R, Balsan S 1981 Mesure des taux circulants des metabolites actifs de la vitamine D chez l'enfant; interet et limites. Archives Francaises de Pediatrie 38: 857–865

Garabedian M, Vainsel M, Mallet E et al 1983 Circulating vitamin D metabolite concentrations in children with nutritional rickets. Journal of Pediatrics 103: 381–386

Garabedian M, Jacqz E, Guillozo H et al 1985 Elevated plasma 1,25-dihydroxyvitamin D concentrations in infants with hypercalcemia and an elfin facies. New England Journal of Medicine 312: 948–952

Griffin J E, Chandler J S, Haussler M R, Zerwekh J E 1983 Receptor-positive resistance to 1,25-dihydroxy vitamin D: a new cause of osteomalacia associated with impaired induction of 24-hydroxylase in fibroblasts. Journal of Clinical Investigation 72: 1190–1199

Haddad J G 1984 Nature and functions of the plasma binding protein for vitamin D and its metabolites. In: Kumar R (ed) Vitamin D: Basic and Clinical Aspects. Martinus Nijhoff Publishing, Boston, Mass. p 383–395

Halloran B P, DeLuca H F 1981 Appearance of the intestinal cytosolic receptor for 1,25-dihydroxyvitamin D_3 during neonatal development in the rat. Journal of Biological Chemistry 256: 7338–7342

Harmeyer J, Grabe V, Winkler I 1981 Vitamin D pseudo-deficiency rickets in pigs. An animal model for the study of familial vitamin D dependency. Experimental Biology and Medicine 7: 117–125

Harrell R M, Lyles K W, Harrelson J M, Friedman N E,

Drezner M K 1985 Healing of bone disease in X-linked hypophosphatemic rickets/osteomalacia: induction and maintenance with phosphate and calcitriol. Journal of Clinical Investigation 75: 1858–1868

Haussler M R, Mangelsdorf D J, Komm B S et al 1988 Molecular biology of the vitamin D hormone. Recent Progress in Hormone Research 44: 263–296

Hirst M, Hochman H, Feldman D 1985 Vitamin D resistance and alopecia: a kindred with normal 1–25-dihydroxyvitamin D binding, but decreased receptor affinity for deoxyribonucleic acid. Journal of Clinical Endocrinology and Metabolism 60: 490–495

Hiwatashi A, Nishii Y, Ichikawa Y 1982 Purification of cytochrome p-450 $_{D1\alpha}$(25-hydroxyvitamin D_3-1α-hydroxylase) of bovine kidney mitochondria. Biochemical and Biophysical Research Communications 105: 320–327

Hochberg Z, Benderli A, Levy J, Vardi P, Weisman Y, Chen T, Feldman D 1984 1,25-Dihydroxyvitamin D resistance, rickets, and alopecia. American Journal of Medicine 77: 805–811

Hochberg Z, Gilhar A, Haim S, Friedman-Birnbaum R, Levy J, Benderly A 1985a Calcitriol-resistant rickets with alopecia. Archives of Dermatology 121: 646–647

Hochberg Z, Borochowitz Z, Benderli A et al 1985b Does 1,25-dihydroxyvitamin D participate in the regulation of hormone release from endocrine glands. Journal of Clinical Endocrinology and Metabolism 60: 57–61

Holick M F, Schnoes H K, DeLuca H F 1971 Identification of 1,25-dihydroxycholecalciferol, a form of vitamin D_3 metabolically active in the intestine. Proceedings of the National Academy of Sciences USA 68: 803–804

Holick M F, MacLaughlin J A, Clark M B et al 1980 Photosynthesis of previtamin D_3 in human skin and the physiological consequences. Science 210: 203–205

Holtrop M E, Cox K A, Carnes D L, Holick M F 1986 Effects of serum calcium and phosphate on skeletal mineralization in vitamin D-deficient rats. American Journal of Physiology 251: E234–E240

Hughes M R, Malloy P J, Kieback D G, Kesterson R A, Pike J W, Feldman D, O'Malley B W 1988 Point mutations in the human vitamin D receptor gene associated with hypocalcemic rickets. Science 242: 1702–1705

Jones K L, Smith D W 1975 The Williams elfin facies syndrome: a new perspective. Journal of Pediatrics 86: 718–723

Karpouzas J, Papathanasiou-Klontza D, Xipolita-Zachariadu A, Benetos S, Matsaniotis N 1979 Pseudo-vitamin D deficiency rickets: report of a case. Helvetica Paediatrica Acta 34: 461–464

Kawakami M, Imawari M, Goodman D S 1979 Quantitative studies of the interaction of cholecalciferol (Vitamin D_3) and its metabolites with different genetic variants of the serum binding protein for these sterols. Biochemical Journal 179: 413–423

Kawashima H, Kraut J A, Kurokawa K 1982 Metabolic acidosis suppressed 25-hydroxyvitamin D_3-1α-hydroxylase in the rat kidney: distinct site and mechanism of action. Journal of Clinical Investigation 70: 135–140

Key L, Carnes D, Cole S et al 1984 Treatment of congenital osteopetrosis with high-dose calcitriol. New England Journal of Medicine 310: 409–415

Kitagawa T, Akatsuka A, Owada M, Mano T 1980 Biologic

and therapeutic effects of 1α-hydroxycholecalciferol in different types of Fanconi syndrome. Contributions to Nephrology 22: 107–119

Koren R, Ravid A, Liberman U A, Hochberg Z, Weisman Y, Novogrodsky A 1985 Defective binding and function of 1,25-dihydroxyvitamin D_3 receptors in peripheral mononuclear cells of patients with end-organ resistance to 1,25-dihydroxyvitamin D. Journal of Clinical Investigation 76: 2012–2015

Kudoh T, Kumagai T, Uetsuji N et al 1981 Vitamin D dependent rickets: decreased sensitivity to 1,25-dihydroxyvitamin D. European Journal of Pediatrics 137: 307–311

Kumar R, Nagubandi S, Jardine I, Londowski J M, Bollman S 1981 The isolation and identification of 5,6-trans-25-hydroxyvitamin D_3 from the plasma of rats dosed with vitamin D_3. Journal of Biological Chemistry 256: 9389–9392

Labuda M, Morgan K, Glorieux F H 1989 Mapping of the mutation causing vitamin D dependency type 1 to chromosome 12q by linkage analysis. Journal of Bone and Mineral Research 4 (Suppl.1): S253 (Abstract)

Lawson D E M, Fraser D R, Kodicek E, Morris H R, Williams D H 1971 Identification of 1,25-dihydroxycholecalciferol, a new kidney hormone controlling calcium metabolism. Nature 230: 228–230

Lawson D E M, Douglas J, Lean M, Sedrani S 1986 Estimation of 1,25 and 25-hydroxyvitamin D_3 in muscle and adipose tissue of rats and man. Clinica Chimica Acta 157: 175–182

Lian J B, Coutts M, Canalis E 1985 Studies of hormonal regulation of osteocalcin synthesis in cultured fetal rat calvariae. Journal of Biological Chemistry 260: 8706–8710

Liberman U A, Samuel R, Halabe A et al 1980 End-organ resistance to 1,25-dihydroxycholecalciferol. Lancet I: 504–507

Liberman U A, Eil C, Holst P, Rosen J F, Marx S J 1983a Hereditary resistance to 1,25-dihydroxyvitamin D: defective function of receptors for 1,25-dihydroxyvitamin D in cells cultured from bone. Journal of Clinical Endocrinology and Metabolism 57: 958–961

Liberman U A, Eil C, Marx S J 1983b Resistance to 1,25(OH)$_2$D: association with heterogeneous defects in cultured skin fibroblasts. Journal of Clinical Investigation 71: 192–200

Liberman U A, DeGrange D, Marx S J 1985 Low affinity of the receptor for 1α,25-dihydroxyvitamin D_3 in the marmoset, a new world monkey. FEBS Letters 182: 385–388

Liberman U A, Eil C, Marx S J 1986 Receptor positive hereditary resistance to 1,25-dihydroxyvitamin D: chromatography of hormone-receptor complexes on deoxyribonucleic acid-cellulose shows two classes of mutation. Journal of Clinical Endocrinology and Metabolism 62: 122–126

Lightwood R 1952 Idiopathic hypercalcemia with failure to thrive. Proceedings of the Royal Society of London 45: 401–410

Lipsett M B, Chrousos G P, Tomita M, Brandon D D, Loriaux D L 1985 The defective glucocorticoid receptor in man and nonhuman primates. Recent Progress in Hormone Research 41: 199–241

Majeska R J, Rodan G A 1982 The effect of 1,25(OH)$_2$D$_3$

on alkaline phosphatase in osteoblastic osteosarcoma cells. Journal of Biological Chemistry 257: 3362–3365

Marel G M, McKenna M J, Frame B 1986 Osteomalacia. In: Bone and Mineral Research/4. Elsevier, New York p335–412

Martin N D T, Snodgrass G J A I, Cohen R D, Porteous C E, Coldwell R D, Trafford D J H, Makin H L J 1985 Vitamin D metabolites in idiopathic infantile hypercalcemia. Archives of Disease in Childhood 60: 1140–1143

Marx S J 1989 Vitamin D and other calciferols. In: Scriver C R, Beaudet A L, Sly W S, Valle D (eds) The Metabolic Basis of Inherited Disease, 6th edn. McGraw Hill, New York, p 2029–2048

Marx S J, Spiegel A M, Brown E M et al 1978 A familial syndrome of decrease in sensitivity to 1,25-dihydroxyvitamin D. Journal of Endocrinology and Metabolism 47: 1303–1310

Marx S J, Swart E G Jr., Hamstra A J, DeLuca H F 1980 Normal intrauterine development of the fetus of a woman receiving extraordinarily high doses of 1,25-dihydroxyvitamin D_3. Journal of Clinical Endocrinology and Metabolism 51: 1138–1142

Marx S J, Liberman U A, Eil C, Gamblin G T, DeGrange D A, Balsan S 1984 Hereditary resistance to 1,25-dihydroxyvitamin D. Recent Progress in Hormone Research 40: 589–615

Marx S J, Bliziotes M M, Nanes M 1986 Analysis of the relation between alopecia and resistance to 1,25-dihydroxyvitamin D. Clinical Endocrinology 25: 373–381

Mehes K, Szelid Z, Toth P 1975 Possible dominant inheritance of the idiopathic hypercalcemic syndrome. Human Heredity 25: 30–34

Mellanby E 1919 An experimental investigation on rickets. Lancet I: 407–412

Merke J, Hugel U, Waldherr R, Ritz E 1986 No 1,25-dihydroxyvitamin D_3 receptors on osteoclasts of calcium-deficient chickens despite demonstrable receptors on circulating monocytes. Journal of Clinical Investigation 77: 312–324

Morgan D W, Welton A F, Heick A E, Christakos S 1986 Specific in vitro activation of Ca, Mg-ATPase by vitamin D-dependent rat renal calcium binding protein (Calbindin D_{28K}). Biochemical and Biophysical Research Communications 138: 547–553

Nemere I, Yoshimoto Y, Norman A W 1984 Calcium transport in perfused duodena from normal chicks: enhancement within fourteen minutes of exposure to 1,25-dihydroxyvitamin D_3. Endocrinology 115: 1476–1483

Nesbitt T, Lobaugh B, Drezner M 1987 Calcitonin stimulation of renal 25-hydroxyvitamin D-1α-hydroxylase activity in hypophosphatemic mice: evidence that regulation of calcitriol production is not universally abnormal in X-linked hypophosphatemia. Journal of Clinical Investigation 79: 15–19

Norman A W, Midgett R J, Myrtle J F, Nowicki H G, Williams W, Popjack G 1971 1,25-Dihydroxycholecalciferol: identification of the proposed active form of vitamin D_3 in the intestine. Science 173: 51

Opshaug O, Maurseth K, Howlid H, Aksnes L, Aarskog D 1982 Vitamin D metabolism in hypophosphatasia. Acta Paediatrica Scandinavica 71: 517–521

Papapoulos S E, Clemens T L, Fraher L J, Gleed J,

O'Riordan JLH 1980 Metabolites of vitamin D in human vitamin D deficiency: effect of vitamin D_3 or 1,25-dihydroxycholecalciferol. Lancet II: 612–615

Parfitt A M, Rao D S, Stanciu J, Villanueva A R, Kleerekoper M, Frame B 1985 Irreversible bone loss in osteomalacia: comparison of radial photon absorptiometry with iliac bone histomorphometry during treatment. Journal of Clinical Investigation 76: 2403–2412

Paulson S K, DeLuca H F 1985 Subcellular location and properties of rat renal 25-hydroxyvitamin D_3-1α-hydroxylase. Journal of Biological Chemistry 260: 11488–11492

Perret C, Desplan C, Brehier A, Thomasset M 1985 Characterisation of rat 9-kDa cholecalcin (CaBP) messenger RNA using a complimentary DNA. Absence of homology with 28-kDa cholecalcin mRNA. European Journal of Biochemistry 148: 61–66

Pettifor J M, Ross F P, Travers R, Glorieux F H, DeLuca H F 1981 Dietary calcium deficiency: a syndrome associated with bone deformities and elevated serum 1,25-dihydroxyvitamin D concentrations. Metabolic Bone Disease and Related Research 2: 301–305

Pike J W, Dokoh S, Haussler M R, Liberman U A, Marx S J, Eil C 1984 Vitamin D_3-resistant fibroblasts have immunoassayable 1,25-dihydroxyvitamin D_3 receptors. Science 224: 879–891

Ploniat H 1962 Klinische fragen der calciumstoff wechselstorungen beim schwein. Deutsche Tierarztliche Wochenschrift 69: 198–202

Prader V A, Illig R, Heidi E 1961 Eine besondere form der primaren vitamin-D-resintenten rachitis mit hypocalcamie und autosomal-dominantem erbgang: die hereditare pseudo-mangelrachitis. Helvetica Paediatrica Acta 5/6: 452–468

Procsal D A, Okamura W H, Norman A W 1975 Structural requirements for the interaction of 1α,25(OH)$_2$-vitamin D_3 with its chick intestinal receptor system. Journal of Biological Chemistry 250: 8382–8388

Rao D S, Parfitt A M, Kleerekoper M, Pumo B S, Frame B 1985 Dissociation between the effects of endogenous parathyroid hormone on adenosine 3', 5'-monophosphate generation and phosphate reabsorption in hypocalcemia due to vitamin D depletion: an acquired disorder resembling pseudo-hypoparathyroidism type II. Journal of Clinical Endocrinology and Metabolism 61: 285–290

Read A P, Thakker R V, Mountford R C et al 1986 Mapping of human X–linked hypophosphatemic rickets by multilocus linkage analysis. Human Genetics 73: 267–270

Reade T M, Scriver C R, Glorieux F H et al 1975 Response to crystalline 1α-hydroxyvitamin D_3 in vitamin D dependency. Pediatric Research 9: 593–599

Reeve L, Tanaka Y, DeLuca H F 1983 Studies on the site of 1,25-dihydroxyvitamin D_3 synthesis in vivo. Journal of Biological Chemistry 258: 3615–3617

Roodman G D, Ibbotson K J, MacDonald B R, Kuehl T J, Mundy G R 1985 1,25-Dihydroxyvitamin D_3 causes formation of multinucleated cells with several osteoclast characteristics in cultures of primate marrow. Proceedings of the National Academy of Sciences USA 82: 8213–8217

Rosen J F, Fleischman A R, Finberg L, Hamstra A, DeLuca H F 1979 Rickets with alopecia: an inborn error of vitamin D metabolism. Journal of Pediatrics 94: 729–735

Rowe D W, Kream B E 1982 Regulation of collagen synthesis in fetal rat calvaria by 1,25-dihydroxyvitamin D_3. Journal of Biological Chemistry 257: 8009–8015

Ryan E Q, Reiss E 1984 Oncogenous osteomalacia: a review of the world literature of 42 cases and report of two new cases. American Journal of Medicine 77: 501–512

Saarem K, Bergseth S, Oftebro H, Pedersen J I 1984 Subcellular localization of vitamin D_3 25-hydroxylase in human liver. Journal of Biological Chemistry 259: 10936–10940

Sakati N, Woodhouse N J Y, Niles N, Harfi H, de Grange D A, Marx S 1986 Hereditary resistance to 1,25-dihydroxyvitamin D: clinical and radiological improvement during high-dose oral calcium therapy. Hormone Research 24: 280–287

Scriver C R, Reade T M, DeLuca H F, Hamstra A J 1978 Serum 1,25-dihydroxyvitamin D levels in normal subjects and in patients with hereditary rickets or bone disease. New England Journal of Medicine 299: 976–979

Siegel N, Wongsurawat N, Armbrecht H J 1986 Parathyroid hormone stimulates dephosphorylation of the renoredoxin component of the 25-hydroxyvitamin D_3-1α-hydroxylase from rat renal cortex. Journal of Biological Chemistry 261: 16998–17003

Silve C, Grosse B, Tau C et al 1986 Response to parathyroid hormone and 1,25-dihydroxyvitamin D_3 of bone-derived cells isolated from normal children and children with abnormalities in skeletal development. Journal of Clinical Endocrinology and Metabolism 62: 583–590

Sly W S, Whyte M P, Sundaram V et al 1985 Carbonic anhydrase II deficiency in 12 families with the autosomal recessive syndrome of osteopetrosis with renal tubular acidosis and cerebral calcification. New England Journal of Medicine 313: 139–145

Smith E L, Walworth N C, Holick M F 1986 Effect of 1α,25-dihydroxyvitamin D_3 on the morphologic and biochemical differentiation of cultured human epidermal keratinocytes grown in serum-free conditions. Journal of Investigative Dermatology 86: 709–714

Somjen D, Kaye A M, Binderman I 1984 24R, 25-Dihydroxyvitamin D stimulates creatine kinase BB activity in chick cartilage cells in culture. FEBS Letters 167: 281–284

Stanbury S W, Taylor C M, Lumb G A, Mawer B A, Berry J, Hann J, Wallace J 1981 Formation of vitamin D metabolites following correction of human vitamin D deficiency. Mineral and Electrolyte Metabolism 5: 212–227

Steichen J J, Tsang R C, Greer F R, Ho M, Hug G 1981 Elevated serum 1,25-dihydroxyvitamin D concentrations in rickets of very low-birth-weight infants. Journal of Pediatrics 99: 293–297

Steinherz R, Chesney R W, Schulman J D, DeLuca H F, Phelps M 1983 Circulating vitamin D metabolites in nephropathic cystinosis. Journal of Pediatrics 102: 592–594

Stumpf W E, Sar M, Reid F A, Tanaka Y, DeLuca H F 1979 Target cells for 1,25-dihydroxyvitamin D_3 in intestinal tract, stomach, kidney, skin, pituitary, and parathyroid. Science 206: 1188–1190

Stumpf W E, Clark S A, Sar M, DeLuca H F 1984
Topographical and developmental studies on target sites of
$1,25(OH)_2$ vitamin D_3 in skin. Cell and Tissue Research
238: 489–496

Takahashi N, Suda S, Shinki T et al 1985 The mechanism
of end-organ resistance to $1\alpha,25$-dihydroxycholecalciferol in
the common marmoset. Biochemical Journal 227:
555–563

Taylor A B, Stern P H, Bell N H 1982 Abnormal
regulation of circulating 25-hydroxyvitamin D in the
Williams syndrome. New England Journal of Medicine
306: 972–975

Tieder M, Modai D, Samuel R et al 1985 Hereditary
hypophosphatemic rickets with hypercalciuria. New
England Journal of Medicine 312: 611–617

Tieder M, Modai D, Shaked U et al 1987 'Idiopathic'
hypercalciuria and hereditary hypophosphatemic rickets:
two phenotypical expressions of a common genetic
defect. New England Journal of Medicine 316: 125–129

Trechsel U, Bonjour J P, Fleisch H 1979 Regulation of the
metabolism of 25-hydroxyvitamin D_3 in primary cultures of
chick kidney cells. Journal of Clinical Investigation 64:
206–217

Turner R T 1984 Mammalian 25-hydroxyvitamin D-1α-
hydroxylase: measurement and regulation. In: Kumar R
(ed) Vitamin D: Basic and Clinical Aspects. Martinus
Nijhoff Publishing, Boston, Mass., p175–196

Underwood J L, DeLuca H F 1984 Vitamin D is not
directly necessary for bone growth and mineralization.
American Journal of Physiology 246: E493–E498

Venkataraman P S, Tsang R C, Buckley D B, Ho M,
Steichen J J 1983 Elevation of serum 1,25-
dihydroxyvitamin D in response to physiologic doses of
vitamin D in vitamin D-deficient infants. Journal of
Pediatrics 103: 416–419

Wasserman R H, Fullmer C S, Shimura F 1984 Calcium
absorption and the molecular effects of vitamin D_3. In:
Kumar R (ed) Vitamin D: Basic and Clinical Aspects.
Martinus Nijhoff Publishing, Boston, Mass., p233–257

Weinstein R S, Underwood J L, Hutson M S, DeLuca H F
1984 Bone histomorphometry in vitamin D-deficient rats
infused with calcium and phosphate. American Journal
of Physiology 246: E499–E505

Weisman Y, Bab I, Gazit D, Spirer Z, Jaffe M, Hochberg Z
1987 Long term intracaval calcium infusion therapy in end-
organ resistance to 1,25-dihydroxyvitamin D. American
Journal of Medicine 83: 984–990

Williams J C P, Barratt-Boyes B G, Lowe J B 1961
Supravalvular aortic stenosis. Circulation 24: 1311

Wiltse H E, Goldbloom R B, Antia A U, Ottesen O E,
Rowe R D, Cooke R E 1966 Infantile hypercalcemia
syndrome in twins. New England Journal of Medicine
275: 1157–1160

Winkler I, Schreiner F, Harmeyer J 1986 Absence of 25-
hydroxycholecalciferol-1-hydroxylase activity in a pig strain
with vitamin D-dependent rickets. Calcified Tissue
International 38: 87–94

Yamaguchi A, Kohno Y, Yamazaki T 1986 Bone in the
marmoset: a resemblance to vitamin D-dependent rickets,
type II. Calcified Tissue International 39: 22–27

Zerwekh J E, Glass K, Jowsey J, Pak C Y C 1979 An
unique form of osteomalacia associated with end organ
refractoriness to 1,25-dihydroxyvitamin D and apparent
defective synthesis of 25-hydroxyvitamin D. Journal of
Clinical Endocrinology and Metabolism 49: 171–175

Zerwekh J E, Marks S C Jr., McGuire J L 1987 Elevated
serum 1,25-dihydroxyvitamin D in osteopetrotic mutations
in three species. Bone and Mineral 2: 193–199

93. Disorders of amino acid metabolism

C. R. Scott S. D. Cederbaum

The inborn errors of amino acid metabolism are a family of genetic conditions in which an enzyme deficiency typically results in the accumulation of a ninhydrin-positive amino acid. They are conceptually identical to disorders caused by enzyme defects that result in accumulation of the organic acid intermediates. As our understanding of the dynamics of amino acid metabolism grows, simplistic notions of metabolic pathways being solely conduits for elimination of excess substrate have been abandoned. We now realize that most, if not all, of these reactions are highly regulated and integrated into the total fabric of metabolic homeostasis in which amino acids play an important role. Nevertheless, such considerations are largely beyond the scope of this concise overview and are covered more fully in Scriver et al (1989a) the standard reference work on these and other inborn errors of metabolism and one which explores the physiological interactions more fully.

In this chapter we will highlight the clinical, biochemical, and pathological features of the more frequent of these uncommon disorders. Although approached in a reductionist manner, providing quick reference for a geneticist with a patient carrying the diagnosis, we realize that in practice the undiagnosed patient presents to the physician with symptoms in search of an explanation. Based on the clinical features described below, the physician must decide whether or not specific diagnostic tests, plasma amino acids and ammonia for acutely ill patients, urinary amino acids for those with more insidious clinical symptoms, should be performed.

This revision includes improved therapeutic approaches and revised prognoses for some of the disorders and new information from recombinant DNA studies for many of the enzymes deficient in these diseases. Such approaches will change the field of inborn errors of amino acids in the next decade. To accommodate these new data, we have reluctantly decided to forego references to some original published studies, alluding instead to their distillation and summary in later, but definitive reviews.

DISORDERS OF PHENYLALANINE METABOLISM (Table 93.1)

The hyperphenylalaninaemias

Folling, a Norwegian chemist, first recognized the existence of a disorder of phenylalanine metabolism in 1934 (Folling 1934). He found phenylpyruvic acid and phenylacetic acid in the urine of mentally retarded patients in an institution for the retarded. This condition would eventually be called *phenylketonuria* and be a cornerstone of research in clinical and biochemical genetics (Scriver & Clow 1980). We now recognize several genetic entities that can cause an elevation of blood phenylalanine and mimic the clinical phenotype of phenylketonuria. Each disorder interferes with the conversion of phenylalanine to tyrosine by reducing the activity of phenylalanine hydroxylase. They each cause an elevation of phenylalanine concentration in the blood and are referred to as the 'hyperphenylalaninaemias'.

Phenylalanine hydroxylase reaction

Phenylalanine is hydroxylated to tyrosine by the enzyme *phenylalanine hydroxylase*. The reaction requires molecular oxygen, and tetrahydrobiopterin (BH_4) is the active cofactor (Kaufman 1976). The tetrahydrobiopterin is generated from dihydrobiopterin by the enzyme *dihydrofolate reductase*. The dihydrobiopterin is normally synthesized de novo in man (Fig. 93.1).

The products of the phenylalanine hydroxylase reaction are tyrosine and an oxidized biopterin, quinonoid-XH_2. The quinonoid-XH_2 may be regenerated to tetrahydrobiopterin by *dihydropteridine reductase* for conservation and reutilization. In humans the conversion of phenylalanine to tyrosine occurs primarily, if not entirely, in the soluble fraction of liver hepatocytes.

Deficiencies of phenylalanine hydroxylase

The range of residual enzymatic activity in individuals carrying two mutant phenylalanine hydroxylase alleles

Table 93.1   Disorders of phenylalanine metabolism – the hyperphenylalaninaemias

Disorder	Enzyme deficiency	Inheritance pattern	Heterozygote detection	Prenatal diagnosis	Gene cloned	Chromosome localization
Phenylketonuria (PKU)	Phenylalanine hydroxylase	AR	yes	yes	yes	12p
Benign hyperphenyl-alaninaemia	Phenylalanine hydroxylase	AR	possible	yes	yes	12p
Transient hyperphenyl-alaninaemia	Phenylalanine hydroxylase	AR	no	no	yes	12p
Dihydropteridine reductase deficiency	Dihydropteridine reductase	AR	yes	yes	yes	4p
Biopterin synthesis deficiency	GTP cyclohydrolase	AR	?	no	no	?
Biopterin synthesis deficiency	2,6-pyruvoyl-tetrahydro-pteridine reductase	AR	?	no	no	?

The information contained in this and subsequent tables was obtained from several sources, the most helpful being Erbe (1977) and Scriver & Clow (1980)

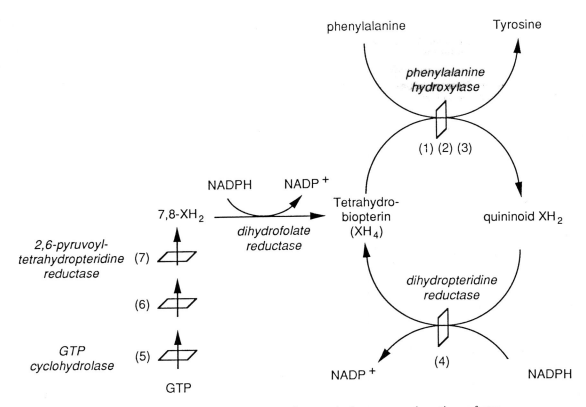

Fig. 93.1   The phenylalanine hydroxalation system and the reactions required to generate the active co-factor, tetrahydrobiopterin (XH_4). The known genetic defects are phenylketonuria (1), mild hyperphenylalaninaemia (2), transient hyperphenylalaninaemia (3), dihydropteridine reductase deficiency (4), and defects in biopterin synthesis (5) (6) (7).

should, and has been demonstrated to, vary continuously (Cederbaum 1984). Nevertheless, for operational purposes we will employ the historical and artificial convention and consider three distinct groups of phenylalanine hydroxylase deficient patients; those with 'classic' phenylketonuria, those with benign hyperphenylalaninaemia and those with transient phenylketonuria.

Classic phenylketonuria

Classic phenylketonuria (PKU) occurs when 5–10% or less of normal phenylalanine hydroxylase activity remains (Scriver & Clow 1980, Scriver et al 1989b). The enzyme deficiency was first documented by Jervis (1953) and subsequently by others. The application of immunological and molecular methods has revealed a full spectrum of genetic defects, ranging from partial gene deletion to point mutations resulting in immunologically normal amounts of inactive protein (Bartholome & Dresel 1982, Avigad et al 1987).

Patients affected with classic phenylketonuria will develop mental retardation, eczema, hypopigmentation and neurological symptoms if untreated. Knox (1972) has reviewed the intellectual results of untreated children and adults with phenylketonuria and concluded that the majority would have an IQ in the severely retarded range. Only 4% or less would have an IQ above 60. In screening approximately 250 000 blood samples submitted to the Massachusetts State Health Laboratory for syphilis testing Levy et al (1970) found only three persons with an elevated blood phenylalanine; each was retarded. Thus, normal intelligence is infrequently achieved in persons with phenylketonuria who remain untreated.

The characteristic 'mousey' odour that is present in untreated persons with phenylketonuria is from the excretion of phenylacetic acid. The hypopigmentation of the skin and hair occurs because of competitive inhibition of *tyrosine hydroxylase* by the increased concentration of phenylalanine. The inhibition of tyrosine hydroxylase activity prevents the conversion of tyrosine to DOPA and the subsequent formation of melanin. Thus, affected individuals have been described as having blue eyes, blond hair and pale skin.

Neurological symptoms in untreated persons with phenylketonuria include hypertonicity, irritability, agitated behaviour, tremors, hyperactivity and occasionally seizures; some were considered autistic. The exact mechanism that causes the neurological abnormalities and the mental retardation is unknown, but is believed to be related to interference in the functioning of metabolic pathways within the nervous system by phenylalanine and its accumulated by-products (Knox 1972).

Diagnosis   In most developed countries, infants are being screened for phenylketonuria by the measurement of blood phenylalanine during the newborn period, using either a fluorometric or a microbiological assay. Patients with classic phenylketonuria will eventually demonstrate a persistent elevation of phenylalanine in their blood of >1.0–1.2 mmoles/l while receiving a normal dietary intake of protein. Their plasma tyrosine will be in the normal range and ortho-hydroxyphenylacetic acid and phenylpyruvic acid will usually be detectable in the urine.

The majority of infants with an elevated blood phenylalanine detected through a screening programme do not have classic phenylketonuria but one of the other forms of hyperphenylalaninaemia; these are usually benign and do not require therapy (see below).

Genetics   Classic PKU is inherited in an autosomal recessive manner and occurs in approximately 1:10 000 births in populations of Western European origin. In these populations, the phenylalanine hydroxylase-deficient alleles can be considered as a polymorphism since their frequency (q) exceeds 0.01 and the heterozygote frequency is therefore approximately 0.02 (2pq). DiLella and Woo (1987) have shown that a few alleles account for 90% of the phenylalanine hydroxylase deficient genes in the Danish population, implying the possibility of positive selection for the heterozygote. The gene is located on the short arm of chromosome 12 (DiLella & Woo 1987).

A considerable difference in gene frequency exists among ethnic groups. The gene is most common in Ireland, Scotland, Belgium and West Germany; in other ethnic groups PKU is rare (Blacks, Asians, American Indians, Finns and Ashkenazi Jews).

Heterozygote detection utilizing plasma phenylalanine and tyrosine levels under standard conditions has been possible, but imprecise (Griffin & Elsas 1975). The situation is now radically improved with the availability of the complete cDNA for phenylalanine hydroxylase, the definition of restriction fragment length polymorphisms rendering more than 95% of families informative for linkage of the haplotype and the defective allele, and the increasing availability of oligonucleotide probes specific for the most common mutations in the Western European populations (DiLella & Woo 1987). These same recombinant DNA techniques render prenatal diagnosis practical in almost all nuclear families in which PKU has occurred, and in most families in which the first-degree relative of a PKU patient is a parent.

Therapy of phenylketonuria   Dietary therapy has been shown to be effective in preventing mental retardation in patients with PKU. In long-term studies in the United Kingdom, Canada and the United States, the restriction of dietary phenylalanine within 30 to 90 days of birth and continuing for 6–8 years has resulted in intelligence comparable to normal sibs (Scriver & Clow 1980, Koch et al 1984).

It is currently believed that a restriction of dietary phenylalanine should begin as soon after birth as possible and should continue throughout life (Holtzman et al 1986). Recent studies suggest a reversible diminution in performance in almost all PKU patients when plasma phenylalanine rises (Krause et al 1985). In some, permanent loss of intellectual achievement results from dietary termination (Cabalska et al 1977). The diet should be managed by a competent team consisting of a nutritionist, a physician and a person with skills in social work to assure dietary compliance. It has been established that blood levels of $100{-}600\ \mu M$ (2–10 mg %) of phenylalanine are satisfactory for achieving normal development in patients with PKU.

Maternal phenylketonuria   It has been recognized that children born to mothers with PKU have a high risk of having mental retardation or congenital defects. At least 90% of offspring will be affected with microcephaly, mental and growth retardation, or congenital heart or vascular problems (Lenke & Levy 1980). These intrauterine effects on development are believed to be a direct consequence of the elevated maternal phenylalanine on the developing fetus.

Reduced serum phenylalanine, especially when achieved prior to conception, may have a favourable effect on pregnancy outcome, but the magnitude of the risk in different circumstances is yet to be determined.

Benign hyperphenylalaninaemia

A large number of infants are detected with elevated levels of phenylalanine, but with values below the level seen in children with 'classic phenylketonuria'. Their plasma phenylalanine values are usually between $100{-}600\ \mu M$ (4–10 mg %) on a normal diet. They require no dietary intervention and do not develop neurological sequelae.

Sibs may be affected, lending credence to the genetic nature of the condition. A partial deficiency of phenylalanine hydroxylase has been measured in a few cases (Justice et al 1967, Kang et al 1970). Ledley et al (1986) and Güttler et al (1987) have shown specific haplotypes of the phenylalanine hydroxylase gene associated with this in two populations.

Transient phenylketonuria

Occasional infants are diagnosed as having phenylketonuria during infancy who eventually 'outgrow' their disorder, except when subject to great catabolic stress. They have been referred to as having 'transient phenylke-

tonuria'. The pathophysiology of this condition is poorly understood. It is believed to be due to a partial deficiency of phenylalanine hydroxylase (Justice et al 1967, Kang et al 1970).

Atypical phenylketonuria due to deficiency of reduced biopterin

Approximately 1% of infants ascertained with phenylalanine levels above $600\ \mu M$ (10 mg %) appear to suffer from neurological deterioration despite adequate and timely restriction of phenylalanine intake. Most of these children lack adequate levels of tetrahydrobiopterin, due either to a defect in dihydrobiopterin biosynthesis or the deficiency of dihydropteridine reductase (Fig. 93.1, Table 93.1) (Danks et al 1979). Tetrahydrobiopterin is an indispensable cofactor in the tyrosine and tryptophan hydroxylase reactions as well. Decreased activity of these two steps results in low levels of two important neurotransmitters in the brain, dopamine and serotonin (Koslow & Butler 1977, McInnes et al 1984) resulting in neurological damage, mental retardation and, in many instances, death.

Deficiencies of these enzymes are inherited as autosomal recessive conditions. The first deficiency described was that of dihydropteridine reductase, the enzyme responsible for the reduction of the dihydrobiopterin produced in the phenylalanine hydroxylase reaction (as well as by the tryptophan and tyrosine hydroxylases). This enzyme is measurable in amniocytes (and presumably chorionic villi) and prenatal diagnosis is possible. The gene has been cloned and is located on the short arm of chromosome 4 (MacDonald et al 1987).

BH_2 is synthesized by a series of reactions that are in the process of being characterized (Naylor et al 1987). Some patients appear to have a deficiency of the first enzyme in the pathway, whereas the majority appear to have a deficiency of the 'phosphate elimination enzyme', now called 2,6-pyruvoyl-tetrahydropteridine reductase (Niederwieser et al 1985). Others have defects which have yet to be defined. The enzymes appear to be confined to liver and their deficiencies do not lend themselves readily to prenatal diagnosis. The range and severity of BH_4 deficiencies have not been fully established and are expected to be particularly wide for the BH_2 biosynthetic deficiencies.

The discovery of BH_4 deficiency as a cause for hyperphenylalaninaemia has led to an alteration in the evaluation of the positive newborn screening test for phenylalanine. All infants with elevated levels, even those in the range of benign hyperphenylalaninaemia, should have, in addition to a tyrosine assay (to rule out elevated tyrosine as a cause for secondary hyperphenylalaninaemia) one or more of a number of studies to eliminate BH$_4$ deficiency as a cause. These studies may include measurement of plasma phenylalanine following BH$_4$ administration; measurement of dihydropteridine reductase in red blood cells (or in filter paper specimens from the newborn screening study); measurement of BH$_2$, BH$_4$ and their precursors in urine using a high performance liquid chromatographic system; and measurement of L-DOPA and 5-hydroxytryptophan metabolites in the urine (Naylor 1986).

5-hydroxytryptophan, L-DOPA and carbidopa, as well as biopterin derivatives, have been given to affected children in an attempt to replace these deficient compounds. Tentative reports have been encouraging in some patients (Naylor 1986).

DISORDERS OF TYROSINE METABOLISM
(Table 93.2)

Approximately half of the available tyrosine in man is formed from the oxidation of phenylalanine. Tyrosine is essential for the synthesis of thyroid hormones, the formation of pigment and the production of neurotransmitters. Tyrosine is metabolized through a series of oxidation steps to form acetic and fumaric acid (Fig. 93.2). Enzyme deficiencies within the catabolic pathway may cause an accumulation of tyrosine or a tyrosine product. The only common disorder of tyrosine metabolism is *neonatal tyrosinaemia*, a problem of delayed developmental synthesis or stability of a normal enzyme. The other known disorders are genetically determined and rare (Goldsmith & Laberge 1989).

Neonatal tyrosinaemia

It is estimated that 30% of premature infants and 10% of full term infants develop neonatal tyrosinaemia (Avery

et al 1967). Gestational age rather than birth weight is the most consistent predisposing factor. Neonatal tyrosinaemia, per se, is not believed to be associated with clinical symptomatology or to cause developmental problems (Avery et al 1967, Partington et al 1967). Menkes and co-workers (1972) have however suggested that small infants with tyrosine values greater than 1 mM may be at risk for mild mental retardation. This has not been proven.

The cause of tyrosinaemia in immature infants has been shown to be an impairment in the activity of *p-hydroxyphenylpyruvic acid (pHPPA) oxidase*. Kretchmer and co-workers (1956) showed that the development of adequate enzyme activity in the liver tissue of infants was related to gestational age. Thus, young infants may have insufficient pHPPA oxidase to metabolize the pHPPA formed from tyrosine. The enzyme pHPPA oxidase is synthesized more efficiently after birth, may be stabilized by ascorbic acid, and is inhibited by its substrate pHPPA. Each of these factors is used to assist in the clinical management of infants who may demonstrate tyrosinaemia. Lowering the dietary protein to 2 gm/kg/24 hours will decrease the formation of pHPPA from tyrosine, and administering 100 mg/24 hours of ascorbic acid will stabilize those enzyme molecules that have been synthesized. Most infants with neonatal tyrosinaemia will promptly lower their plasma tyrosine concentration to the normal range (<0.1 mM) with these two manoeuvres.

Neonatal tyrosinaemia is not believed to occur as the result of an abnormal allele. However, genetic factors may influence its incidence, since it is common in the Arctic Eskimo, with a frequency of 12% in term births (Clow et al 1975).

Hereditary tyrosinaemia

Inherited disorders leading to tyrosine elevation in the plasma are relatively rare; the frequency in most

Table 93.2 Disorders of tyrosine metabolism – the hypertyrosinaemias

Disorder	Enzyme deficiency	Inheritance pattern	Heterozygote detection	Prenatal diagnosis
Neonatal tyrosinaemia	p-OH-phenylpyruvic acid oxidase	Not inherited		
Hepatorenal tyrosinaemia	fumarylacetoacetate hydrolase	AR	no	yes
Oculocutaneous tyrosinaemia	tyrosine aminotransferase (cytoplasm)	AR	no	no
Tyrosinosis	?			
Alkaptonuria	homogentisic acid oxidase	AR	no	no

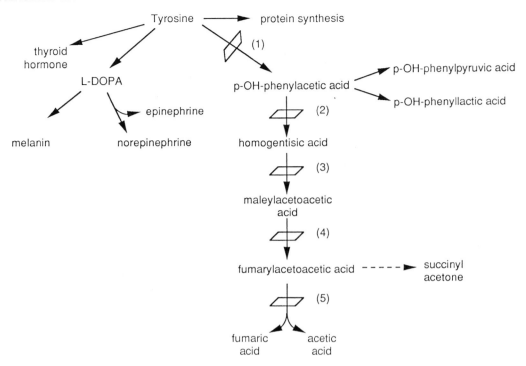

Fig. 93.2 The metabolic fate of tyrosine. The known defects of tyrosine metabolism include oculocutaneous tyrosinaemia (1), neonatal tyrosinaemia (2), alkaptonuria (3), and hepatorenal tyrosinaemia (5). Another form of hepatorenal tyrosinaemia has been implicated by a deficiency of *maleylacetoacetase isomerase* (4).

populations is less than 1 in 250 000. Two discrete disorders, both autosomal recessive, encompass most of the cases. They have been given a variety of names, but we believe they are best described as the hepatorenal and oculocutaneous forms of tyrosinaemia.

Hepatorenal tyrosinaemia

Hepatorenal tyrosinaemia is a rare and usually lethal inborn error of metabolism. It may occur either as an 'acute' infantile form associated with liver failure and early death or, at the other extreme, a more chronic form accompanied by growth failure, nodular cirrhosis with liver dysfunction and renal tubular nephropathy (Partington et al 1967). Both forms may be associated with hypoglycaemia and hyperplasia of the islets of Langerhans. Patients with the chronic form may also develop hypophosphataemic rickets from their kidney disease and are at high risk for hepatic carcinoma.

The observed biochemical abnormalities include the massive excretion of tyrosine metabolites, p-hydroxyphenylpyruvic and p-hydroxyphenyllactic acids. There is an increased concentration of tyrosine (2–3 times normal) and methionine in the plasma (Partington et al 1967). Serum α-fetoprotein has been noted to be increased during the postnatal period and has been recommended for use as a screening assay for the condition (Belanger et al 1973). Levels may be 1000 times normal or more. The diagnostic hallmark is the presence of succinylacetone in both blood and urine, under virtually all circumstances (Linblad et al 1977). Succinylacetone is formed as a consequence of the primary enzyme defect, deficiency of fumarylacetoacetate hydrolase, a distal enzyme in tyrosine catabolism (Linblad et al 1977, Kvittingen et al 1981). Succinylacetone is a highly toxic compound that is thought to cause the renal tubular and hepatic damage and lead secondarily to the para-hydroxy-phenylpyruvate oxidase deficiency previously implicated in the pathogenesis of the condition.

Restriction of dietary phenylalanine and tyrosine has caused a reduction in α-fetoprotein and liver disease in many affected patients and may delay the onset of growth failure, cirrhosis and carcinoma (Partington et al 1967).

During the acute stage of the illness, methionine restriction has also been of value. Some feel that maintenance of adequate nutrition and the suppression of catabolism may be of value. Orthotopic liver transplantation appears to cure the disease, at least in the short-term (Fisch et al 1978, Tuchman et al 1985, 1987). Small amounts of succinylacetone continue to be present in urine and suggest a synthetic source other than liver (Tuchman et al 1985, 1987).

Hereditary tyrosinaemia is inherited as an autosomal recessive condition. Both forms of the disease have been documented to occur in the same sibship (Partington et al 1967). The condition has been recognized in many ethnic groups. A particularly high incidence exists in a French Canadian isolate where the heterozygote frequency has been estimated to be 1 in 14 persons (Bergeron et al 1974). More recently, genocopies in which succinylacetone is absent in body fluids (Berger et al 1988) and phenocopies, possibly due to viral infection, have been recognized (Nyhan 1984). The accumulation of succinylacetone in the amniotic fluid of affected patients makes prenatal diagnosis in affected families (at least) possible. Mass screening for this disorder is possible (Grenier et al 1982).

Oculocutaneous tyrosinaemia

Between 20 and 30 patients have been reported with markedly elevated concentrations of tyrosine (1–2 mM or 10–20 times normal), but normal levels of methionine in their blood (Nyhan 1984, Goldsmith & Laberge 1989). They suffer from severe corneal ulceration which may lead to visual loss. Painful hyperkeratotic lesions of palms and soles and peculiar horizontal cracks of the tips of the fingers and toes are common clinical findings. Some patients are mentally retarded. They do not have any

hepatic or renal problems and are not at direct risk for a shortened life-span.

Patients with oculocutaneous tyrosinaemia excrete large quantities of p-hydroxyphenylpyruvic acid and smaller amount of p-hydroxyphenyllactic, p-hydroxyphenylacetic acids and p-tyramine in their urine. They are unresponsive to ascorbic acid therapy.

The enzymatic defect has been shown to be a deficiency of the cytosol form of hepatic tyrosine aminotransferase. The mitochondrial form of this enzyme has normal activity (Fellman et al 1972).

Dietary restriction of phenylalanine and tyrosine lowers the plasma tyrosine value in affected patients and decreases the urinary excretion of the tyrosyl products. Clinical improvement of the keratosis and corneal ulcers occurs with dietary therapy (Nyhan 1984).

The disorder is inherited as an autosomal recessive condition (Fois et al 1986). No information is available on heterozygote detection or prenatal diagnosis.

Tyrosinosis

A single patient was reported by Grace Medes in 1932 with a condition she called 'tyrosinosis'. Excretion of tyrosyl products in the urine led her to suggest this patient had a defect in para-hydroxyphenylpyruvic acid oxidase (Medes 1932). The precise defect remains undetermined. Additional information is not available to offer any genetic conclusions about the condition (Goldsmith & Laberge 1989).

DISORDERS OF GLYCINE METABOLISM
(Table 93.3)

Glycine is the smallest and the most ubiquitous of the naturally occurring amino acids. It is not an essential

Table 93.3 Disorder of glycine metabolism

Disorder	Enzyme deficiency	Inheritance pattern	Heterozygote detection	Prenatal diagnosis
Non-ketotic hyperglycinaemia	Glycine cleavage reaction	AR	no	possible
Sarcosinaemia	Sarcosine dehydrogenase	AR	possible	not indicated
Hyperoxaluria Type I	2-oxo-glutarate: glyoxylate carboligase (soluble)	AR	no	possible
Type II	D-glyceric acid dehydrogenase	?		

amino acid in either infants or adults. Its major synthetic sources are probably through the one-carbon metabolic pathway and recovery from protein catabolism. Glycine may account for 25% of the composition of many proteins, and is involved in the synthesis of creatine, glutathione, haem, and porphyrins. Glycine may also be used in the formation of glycogen and purine synthesis (Nyhan 1989).

The major reaction of glycine, however, is its reversible conversion to serine catalyzed by *serine hydroxymethyltransferase* (Fig. 93.3). This enzyme requires tetrahydrofolate as a co-factor and the energetics favour the formation of glycine (Nyhan 1989). An alternative, and major, route for the conversion of glycine to serine is via the glycine cleavage reaction. In this system, glycine reacts with tetrahydrofolate, is decarboxylated and deaminated to form an 'active' formaldehyde (Nyhan 1989). This active formaldehyde condenses with a second molecule of glycine to form serine and regenerate tetrahydrofolate. The glycine cleavage system takes place only in the mitochondria by a complex 4-protein system that is responsible for the decarboxylation. This 4-protein system is similar in structure to the pyruvate-dehydrogenase complex and contains: (1) a P-protein that is pyridoxal dependent, the glycine decarboxylase; (2) an H-protein that is lipoic acid-containing and is a hydrogen carrier protein; (3) a T-protein that is required for binding of tetrahydrofolate; and (4) an L-protein that is the lipoamide dehydrogenase. Mutational alterations in any of these four proteins can theoretically lead to the syndrome of non-ketotic hyperglycinaemia and two, and possibly three, of the four have been described (Tada 1987).

The hyperglycinaemias

Disorders of metabolism resulting in hyperglycinaemia were originally divided into two groups, 'ketotic' and 'non-ketotic'. The term 'ketotic' hyperglycinaemia was coined by Childs et al (1961) to describe infants with

metabolic acidosis, ketonuria, and hyperglycinaemia. It was subsequently determined that children with this syndrome have disorders of organic acid metabolism with secondary perturbations in glycine metabolism. These, principally, are children with propionic acidaemia, methylmalonic acidaemia, or isovaleric acidaemia. The recognition of 'non-ketotic' hyperglycinaemia occurred in a group of children who typically present with severe neurological symptoms soon after birth, absence of acidosis and organic acidaemia, and elevated concentrations of glycine in plasma, spinal fluid, and urine.

Non-ketotic hyperglycinaemia

The non-ketotic hyperglycinaemias represent several distinct genetic abnormalities that have similar clinical presentations. The classic infant with non-ketotic hyperglycinaemia appears normal at birth, but soon develops poor feeding, listlessness, lethargy and seizures. These symptoms typically occur prior to one week of age. The neurological progression is irreversible, and the children develop intractable seizures, hypertonicity and failure of intellectual development. The majority die from their neurological complications at less than a month of age or, if they survive, they die from infections before two years of age. Few live beyond this age (Tada 1987, Tada & Hayasaka 1987, Nyhan 1989).

Milder forms of non-ketotic hyperglycinaemia do exist. Some young children may present with mental retardation with slowly progressive neurological features. Some families have had children who have a clinical course most similar to a neuro-degenerative disease with its onset between six months and one year of age. Still older persons have been described who present in adolescence with weakness and spasticity which may be confused with Friedreich ataxia or even Charcot-Marie-Tooth disease (Bank & Morrow 1972). The critical finding in establishing these individuals as having a form of non-ketotic hyperglycinaemia is dependent on documentation of elevated glycine in plasma and spinal fluid.

The metabolic abnormality in non-ketotic hyperglycinaemia is a defect in the conversion of glycine to serine. The major route for this conversion is through the glycine cleavage reaction (Nyhan 1989). Liver tissue from patients with non-ketotic hyperglycinaemia is unable to cleave the C_1 carbon of the glycine molecule to form Co_2 in the presence of tetrahydrofolate (Tada 1987, Nyhan 1989). A deficiency of the glycine decarboxylase (P-protein) (Tada 1987), the amino acyl protein (H-protein) (Hiraga et al 1981, Tada & Hayasaka 1987), and T-protein deficiency in brain and liver (Tada 1987) have all been identified as separate mutations responsible for the clinical phentoype of the infantile form of non-

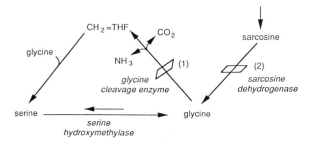

Fig. 93.3 Abbreviated pathway for some of the metabolic reactions related to glycine. The known genetic defects involve nonketotic hyperglycinaemia (1), and sarcosinaemia (2).

ketotic hyperglycinaemia. No defect has yet been identified in the lipoamide dehydrogenase (L-protein). Patients with a defect of the glycine cleavage reaction excrete massive quantities of glycine in the urine. This is associated with a 3–5-fold increase in plasma glycine and a 10–20-fold increase in glycine concentration in spinal fluid. Infants with hyperglycinaemia typically have CSF/plasma ratios of glycine concentration between 0.1 and 0.3, compared to normal values of 0.02. This ratio is of greater diagnostic importance than the actual concentration of glycine in either of the two fluids separately. Elevation of serum and spinal fluid glycine in the absence of ketosis and identified organic acidaemia is the diagnostic indicator for non-ketotic hyperglycinaemia.

No effective treatment is available to reverse the neurological damage that occurs in non-ketotic hyperglycinaemia. Low protein diets, sodium benzoate, folic acid, and benzodiazepines have not been effective (Tada & Hayasaka 1987). Strychnine has been given to a number of patients with reports of improvement in muscle tone, but no improvement has been documented in their neurological status (Tada & Hayasaka 1987). The use of large doses of diazepam, choline, and sodium benzoate led to cessation of seizure activity and increased responsiveness in two affected children (Matalon et al 1983).

Non-ketotic hyperglycinaemia is inherited as an autosomal recessive condition. Males and females are equally affected, and an increased incidence of consanquinity has been noted among parents. Genetic heterogeneity exists based on variation in clinical presentation, and known deficiencies of the P, H, and T enzymes of the glycine cleavage reaction. Heterozygote detection is not reliable. The glycine cleavage reaction is not detectable in normal white cells or fibroblasts. There is no detectable alteration in plasma glycine levels of obligate heterozygotes.

Prenatal diagnosis is unreliable. The glycine cleavage reaction is not expressed in cultured amniotic fluid cells and the usefulness of the concentration of glycine in amniotic fluid in the second trimester of pregnancy has led to conflicting reports (Garcia-Castro et al 1982, Mesavage et al 1983). Tada and Hayasaka (1987) have reported low activity in the placenta and liver of a fetus at risk for this disorder and speculate that prenatal diagnosis with chorionic villi may be possible. The gene for the H protein of the glycine cleavage system has recently been cloned (Hiraga et al 1988).

Sarcosinaemia

Sarcosine is an intermediate in one carbon metabolism and is a precursor of glycine. Sarcosine (N-methylglycine) is formed by the oxidative demethylation of N-dimethylglycine, and sarcosine undergoes further demethylation to form glycine. The enzyme responsible for this latter reaction is *sarcosine dehydrogenase*.

Sarcosinaemia, presumably due to a genetic deficiency, has been described in more than 16 people (Sewell et al 1986). High concentrations of sarcosine are found in the plasma and large quantities are excreted in the urine (Scott et al 1970).

Although originally suspected of being causally related in children with mental retardation, it is currently believed that sarcosinaemia is a benign condition, unrelated to clinical symptomatology (Gerritsen & Waisman 1966, Scott et al 1970a, Levy et al 1984).

Sarcosinaemia is inherited as an autosomal recessive condition. Heterozygote detection using oral loading studies of sarcosine is possible, but unreliable. Prenatal diagnosis is not feasible, since the enzyme is not expressed in cultured amniotic fluid cells, and undesirable, in view of the probability that the condition may not cause significant illness.

Hyperoxaluria

Two rare metabolic errors may result in primary hyperoxaluria. Both lead to the development of renal stones, which leads to renal failure. They are referred to as hyperoxaluria (or oxalosis) type I and type II.

Hyperoxaluria, type I Hyperoxaluria type I typically occurs in young children who have symptoms of renal colic and who develop calcium oxalate nephrolithiasis. The affected children may develop growth retardation, uraemia, and often succumb before the age of 20 years. A few patients have been reported who did not have symptoms in childhood and did not, in fact, develop symptoms until the third or fourth decade. Patients with hyperoxaluria type I excrete increased quantities of both oxalic acid and L-glycolic acid (Hillman 1989).

The primary defect in hyperoxaluria type I was defined as a deficiency of the soluble 2-oxo-glutarate: glyoxylate carboligase (Koch et al 1967), but has now been more specifically identified as the peroxisomal alanine: glyoxylate aminotransferase (Watts et al 1987).

Renal transplantation alone fails in these patients because oxalate stones reform in the donor kidney. Combined hepatic and renal transplantation is successful because oxalate metabolism is restored to normal (Watts et al 1987). Oxalate excretion may be moderately or nearly completely normalized by the administration of physiological or pharmacological doses of pyridoxine (Will & Bijvoet 1979, Yendt & Cohanim 1985).

Type I hyperoxaluria is inherited as an autosomal recessive condition. It has been reported in sibs, identical twins and in the offspring of consanguineous matings. The detection of heterozygotes is not reliable. Prenatal diagnosis by fetal liver biopsy appears to be possible (Danpure et al 1988).

Table 93.4 Disorders of sulphur amino acids

Disorder	Enzyme deficiency	Inheritance pattern	Heterozygote detection	Prenatal diagnosis
Hypermethioninaemia	Methionine adenosyltransferase	AR probable		
The homocystinurias (B$_6$ responsive)	Cystathionine β-synthase	AR	yes	possible
Homocystinuria (B$_6$ nonresponsive)	Cystathionine β-synthase	AR	yes	possible
Homocystinuria	N^{5,10}-methylene-tetrahydrofolate reductase	AR	probable	
Homocystinuria (Cobalamin defects) 'cbl C'	Synthesis of methyl-B$_{12}$ and adenosyl-B$_{12}$ (? cobalamin reductase)	AR		possible
'cbl D'	(Same as above, but less severe deficiency)	AR		possible
'cbl E'	?	AR	?	yes
'cbl G'	?	?	no	?
'cbl F'	?	?	no	?
Cystathioninuria (B$_6$ responsive)	γ-cystathionase	AR	yes	?
Cystathioninuria (B$_6$ nonresponsive)	γ-cystathionase	AR	yes	?
Sulphite oxidase deficiency	Sulphite oxidase	AR?	?	

Hyperoxaluria, type II A second rare form of hyperoxaluria has been reported to occur in children. The children suffer from L-glyceric aciduria and develop nephrocalcinosis, urolithiasis, and the consequences of renal disease with growth failure and uraemia.

Patients with type II hyperoxaluria excrete large amounts of oxalate and D-glyceric acid in the urine. Unfortunately this latter compound cannot be routinely or easily measured.

Affected patients have been shown to lack activity for the enzyme D-glyceric acid dehydrogenase when assayed in peripheral leucocytes (Hellman 1989).

Hyperoxaluria type II is probably inherited as an autosomal recessive condition, but confusion exists over its exact mode of inheritance. Shepard et al (1960) reported hyperoxaluria in at least two generations, and Hellman (1989) found decreased enzyme activity in the mothers of three patients but not in the fathers. Information on heterozygote detection will need to await clarification of the inheritance pattern.

DISORDERS OF SULPHUR AMINO ACIDS
(Table 93.4)

Recognized disorders of sulphur amino acids have so far involved methionine, homocysteine, cystathionine, and cysteine (Table 93.4). Secondary effects on the regulation of sulphur amino acid metabolism may occur from primary disorders in vitamin B$_{12}$ metabolism or from deficiencies of vitamin B$_6$.

Methionine is an essential amino acid that is converted to cysteine through a series of enzymatic reactions (Fig. 93.4) (Mudd et al 1989). Cysteine is not an essential amino acid in adults, but is required as a nutritional supplement to maintain adequate growth in infants (Sturman et al 1970). Methionine and cysteine alone amongst the four sulphur-containing amino acids are incorporated into protein. The metabolism of the sulphur amino acids is outlined in Figure 93.4.

Methionine forms S-adenosyl-L-methionine through the action of methionine adenosyl-transferase. Methionine and adenosylmethionine are the major methyl donors for mammalian metabolism. Methionine adenosyltransferase deficiency is known, but does not appear to be associated with clinical disease (Mudd et al 1989).

S-adenosylmethionine is converted to S-adenosylhomocysteine in the course of donating its methyl group. S-adenosylhomocysteine in turn serves as a product inhibitor of most methyl transfer reactions, thus regulating the rate of methylation reactions (Mudd et al 1989). S-adenosylhomocysteine is then hydrolyzed to homocysteine and adenosine, a reaction catalyzed by a specific hydrolase (Mudd et al 1989).

Homocysteine plays a central role in the transulphuration pathway. It undergoes three major enzymatically mediated conversions (Mudd et al 1989). Two of the reactions allow homocysteine to be recycled to methionine. Betaine-homocysteine methyltransferase uses betaine as a methyl donor to combine with homocysteine to synthesize methionine; and the enzyme N^5-methyltetrahydrofolate: homocysteine methyltransferase uses N^5-methylfolic acid as a methyl donor to recycle homocysteine to methionine. The latter reaction requires methyl B_{12} as a cofactor. The major catabolic reaction, however, is the conversion of homocysteine to cystath-

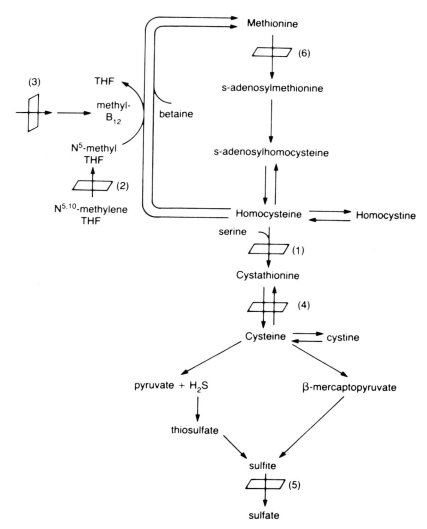

Fig. 93.4   Abbreviated diagram for the transulphuration pathway. The known genetic defects are those that cause homocystinuria from a deficiency of *cystathionine-β-synthase* (I), $N^{5,10}$ *methylene-tetrahydrofolate reductase* (2), or deficient synthesis of methyl-B_{12} (3). Other defects in the pathway are cystathioninaemia (4), sulfite oxidase deficiency (5), and hypermethioninaemia from *methionine adenosyl transferase deficiency* (6).

ionine. This conversion is catalyzed by cystathionine β-synthase. This step requires pyridoxal phosphate as a cofactor.

Cystathionine is cleaved by gamma-cystathionase to form cysteine and α-ketobutyrate. Cystathionine is not known to function in other reactions. This enzyme also requires pyridoxal phosphate as a cofactor. Cysteine may undergo a number of enzymatic reactions. It is an important amino acid in proteins, playing a key role in folding and stabilization; as noted, it may be an essential or a conditionally essential amino acid in the neonate (Sturman et al 1970). It is a component of glutathione, a compound important in the maintenance of the redox state of the cell and the stabilization of cell membranes. It also participates in the formation of coenzyme A and is metabolized to organic sulphate via sulphite. The most common and important genetic defects of the sulphur amino acids cause an accumulation of homocysteine. They are classified as the 'homocystinurias' and are the result of three different enzymatic defects: (1) a deficiency of cystathionine β-synthase; (2) a deficiency of $N^{5,10}$-methylenetetrahydrofolate reductase; and (3) a deficiency of the formation of methyl-B_{12}.

Cystathionine β-synthase deficiency

Clinical picture

Prior to the recognition of homocystinuria as a defined entity, affected patients were confused with those with the Marfan syndrome because of similarities in the clinical phenotype, including tall stature, scoliosis, pectus excavatum, dislocated lenses with myopia and, occasionally, some degree of arachnodactyly (Mudd et al 1989). A significant number have mental retardation. In 1962, and the immediate years thereafter, homocystinuria was recognized as a discrete entity and the enzymatic defect defined (Carson et al 1963, Gerritsen & Waisman 1964, Mudd et al 1964, Schimke et al 1965). The separation of homocystinuria from the Marfan syndrome represented one of the earliest and best clinical examples of the concept of genocopies (Schimke et al 1965).

The classic description of the patient with homocystinuria is the young teenager who is tall and slender, has scoliosis, long extremities, a high arched palate, light coloured and dry hair, pale skin with livedo reticularis, and bilateral dislocation of the lenses with myopia. X-rays of the skeletal system demonstrate osteoporosis. A mild to moderate degree of mental retardation may be present. The above description undoubtedly represents the extreme clinical phenotype, since most patients with homocystinuria do not fit this classic description. It is striking that the disorder was first described in a more severely mentally retarded population in which the classical phenotype was not noted (Carson et al 1963, Gerritsen & Waisman 1964).

Since the observation by Hooft et al in 1967 that some patients with cystathionine β-synthase deficiency may respond to vitamin B_6 therapy, two major subgroups have traditionally been defined; vitamin B_6 responsive homocystinuria, and vitamin B_6 nonresponsive homocystinuria. The clinical manifestations of the two groups are different, with those that are pyridoxal responsive tending to have a later onset, a milder phenotype and a better prognosis (Mudd et al 1985). Approximately 50% of all patients with the β-synthase deficiency respond to 25–500 mg/24 hours of pyridoxine by significantly lowering their plasma homocysteine concentration (Mudd et al 1985).

The most consistent clinical finding in β-synthase deficiency is ectopia lentis. 90% of patients have dislocated lenses and, in these patients, 90% of the lenses are dislocated downwards. The dislocated lens may be observed as early as two years of age, with at least half the patients having documented lens abnormalities by 6–10 years of age (Mudd et al 1985, 1989). Myopia always accompanies lens subluxation and, occasionally, secondary glaucoma occurs.

Mental retardation is a frequent observation in affected patients. The median IQ for pyridoxine responsive patients has been estimated at 78, compared with pyridoxine nonresponsive patients with a mean of 56 (Mudd et al 1985). Abnormal electroencephalograms and seizures may occasionally be noted, and there is an impression of significant psychiatric disturbances in approximately half of the patients (Mudd et al 1989). Personality and behaviour disorders tend to predominate in the latter group.

Osteoporosis can usually be documented by age 20 in at least 50% of patients. It has been suggested that the osteoporosis may be a contributing cause in those patients that develop scoliosis, and it certainly is contributory to those patients that demonstrate vertebral collapse.

The major life-threatening symptom in patients with classic homocystinuria is the propensity towards vascular thrombosis. 25% of patients will have had a thromboembolic event by the age of 15–20 years. Mudd and co-workers have estimated that the risk for a significant thromboembolic event in a young adult with untreated homocystinuria is approximately 4%/year (Mudd et al 1985).

Diagnosis

Patients may be suspected of having homocystinuria by their clinical phenotype, the presence of dislocated lenses in a child, or the occurrence of a thromboembolic phenomenon in a child or young adult. Some are found as a consequence of a metabolic evaluation of a retarded individual. Homocystine in the urine is most easily detected by a sensitive qualitative test for disulphide compounds. The urinary cyanide-nitroprusside reaction is sensitive and will give a pink to magenta colour in the presence of any disulphide compound in the urine (Mudd et al 1989). A positive test requires further confirmation of the presence of homocystine. This may be accomplished by the identification of homocystine in the urine by a number of chromatographic techniques, or a modification of the cyanide-nitroprusside reaction described by Spaeth and Barber (1967). Finally, confirmation of elevated methionine in the range of 500–2000 μM, and homocystine in the range of 50–200 μM in plasma is obtained. The documentation of elevated methionine concentration in plasma is necessary for the presumptive diagnosis of cystathionine β-synthase deficiency in the absence of a direct enzymatic assay.

Enzymatic assay to confirm the diagnosis of cystathionine β-synthase deficiency can be achieved by measuring the reaction in cultured skin fibroblasts (Mudd et al 1964, 1989), phytohaemagglutinin-stimulated lymphocytes (Goldstein et al 1972) or in liver biopsy specimens (Mudd et al 1989). These assays are usually not mandatory, however, for clinical management.

The finding of homocystinuria, or the documentation of homocystinaemia does not, however, confirm the diagnosis of cystathionine β-synthase deficiency. It must be distinguished from the other defects that may cause homocystinuria: a deficiency of N^5-methyltetrahydrofolate: homocystine methyltransferase; a deficiency of $N^{5,10}$-methylenetetrahydrofolate reductase; or a defect in cobalamin metabolism that results in a deficiency of methylcobalamin (Mudd et al 1989). These latter disorders typically have low or low normal plasma levels of methionine. Homocystine may also be seen in the urine of some patients with cystathioninuria, due to bacterial contamination and the synthesis of homocysteine from cystathionine. In contrast, some patients who have homocystinuria may be missed by urinary screening if they have been taking vitamin supplements containing pyridoxine that corrects their homocystinaemia.

Therapy

Therapy is available for patients with cystathionine β-synthase deficiency. 50% of patients can lower their homocystine concentration in blood to a significant degree by taking an oral dose of pyridoxine (50–100 mg/24 hours). Lowering plasma homocystine concentration may protect the majority of patients from thromboembolic events (Harker et al 1974). Clinical data would suggest that those patients with the lowest levels of plasma homocystine have the lowest incidence of thrombotic episodes. Folic acid may also be helpful in management. Folic acid depletion has been noted in a number of patients with β-synthase deficiency. Pyridoxine therapy has occasionally only been effective when supplemented with oral folate (Mudd et al 1989). This phenomenon may relate to the ability to recycle homocystine to methionine, a reaction that is both vitamin B_{12} and folate dependent. Betaine has been orally administered in some cases with beneficial results (Mudd et al 1989).

A low methionine diet has been used to prevent the accumulation of homocystine (Mudd et al 1985, 1989). This is most effective when utilized in young infants detected to have homocystinuria through newborn screening programmes or early diagnosis. Special low methionine formulas are available for dietary management. These formulas are supplemented with a small amount of milk and L-cysteine to meet the methionine and L-cysteine requirements and to maintain plasma methionine levels at a near-normal range. Preliminary evidence would indicate that methionine restricted diets are beneficial to children who are non-pyridoxine responsive. These children have IQs in the normal range (94 $\pm$ 4), delay in the development of lens dislocation, and no early evidence of thromboembolism or osteoporosis.

To assist in the prevention of thromboembolism in patients who have persistent homocystinaemia, dipyridamole (100 mg/24 hours) combined with aspirin (1 gm/24 hours) is recommended. While short of unequivocal statistical proof, the prevailing impression is that these drugs are helpful.

Genetics

Deficiency of cystathionine β-synthase is inherited as an autosomal recessive condition. The estimated incidence varies from 1/100 000 to 1/400 000 (Mudd et al 1989). The average estimate approaches 1/300 000 based on the screening of newborns for elevated methionine in blood or urine. The gene for cystathionine β-synthase is located on chromosome 21 between bands 21q21 and 21q22.1 (Chadefaux et al 1985, Kraus et al 1986).

Two clinical phenotypes of cystathionine β-synthase deficiency are recognized: pyridoxine responsive and pyridoxine nonresponsive. Sibs affected with homocystinuria share the clinical response to pyridoxine (Mudd et al 1989). Significant genetic heterogeneity is known to exist, based on : (1) variation in residual enzyme activity between unrelated patients; (2) variation in immunologically reacting protein to antiserum prepared against purified cystathionine β-synthase enzyme; (3) variation in thermal stability of residual enzyme activity; (4) variation in mRNA synthesis; and (5) variation in substrate and cofactor requirements for maximum enzyme activity (Mudd et al 1989). This biochemical evidence indicates multiple molecular lesions that await confirmation by more definitive analysis of gene structure.

Obligate heterozygotes have been documented to have less than normal activity when cystathionine β-synthase activity has been measured in extracts of cultured fibroblasts, stimulated lymphocytes, long-term cultured lymphocytes, and liver tissue (Goldstein et al 1973, Mudd et al 1989). In general, this activity has been less than 50% of the mean control specific activity observed in each tissue. It has been implied that the decrease of activity below 50% of normal is because of impaired activity of hybrid molecules when the normal subunits of the enzyme are combined with mutant subunits. Because of the rarity of the mutant gene in the population it would be difficult, using these enzymatic assays alone, to definitively assign any person as a heterozygote because of his or her enzymatic activity, even if it fell below the normal expected level of enzyme activity. Sardharwalla et al (1974) have reported a loading study using L-methionine under carefully controlled circumstances to measure the excretion of homocystine and other sulph-hydryl compounds in the urine and thus to distinguish heterozygotes from normal persons.

The hypothesis that heterozygotes for the β-synthase deficiency may be prone to vascular thromboses has been explored in several studies. Mudd et al (1981), using an historical survey of 203 families, could find no evidence for an increased incidence of vascular events in parents and grandparents of known homozygous individuals. Using methionine loading studies and fibroblast enzyme assays Wilcken and Wilcken (1976) and Boers et al (1985) have concluded that a significant number of younger individuals with premature occlusive vascular disease and without other known risk factors may be heterozygous for cystathionine β-synthase deficiency. In an accompanying editorial Mudd (1985) suggested that this population group be systematically tested for heterozygosity so that appropriate prophylactic measures could be taken.

Prenatal diagnosis of cystathionine β-synthase deficiency is feasible. The diagnosis has been excluded in several pregnancies at risk in which the enzyme has been assayed in cultured amniotic fluid cells, while two pregnancies at risk have been confirmed to carry affected fetuses by enzyme activity that has been measured from cells cultured from amniotic fluid (Fowler et al 1982) or chorionic villi (Mudd et al 1989). Apparently the catalytic activity of cystathionine β-synthase obtained in the direct assay from chorionic villus biopsy reveals insufficient activity to be of use (Mudd et al 1989).

$N^{5,10}$ Methylenetetrahydrofolate reductase deficiency

The active cofactor necessary for the conversion of homocystine to L-methionine is N^5-tetrahydrofolate. This cofactor is resynthesized from $N^{5,10}$-methylenetetra-hydrofolate by the enzyme $N^{5,10}$-methylenetetrahydrofo-late reductase. A small number of children have been reported with a deficiency of this enzyme (Freeman et al 1975, Mudd et al 1989). Patients deficient in the synthesis of $N^{5,10}$-methylenetetrahydrofolate accumulate homocys-teine and have a low plasma methionine.

Affected patients show a spectrum of clinical symp-toms. Older children have been identified with mental retardation, acute pyschosis, muscle weakness, ataxia, and spastic paraparesis. Some have shown improvement in symptoms when supplemented with pharmacological doses of folate. Young infants have been identified with more severe symptoms of hypotonia, failure to thrive, failure of neurological development and severe apnoea. Most have died at less than a year of age. Several infants have responded well to high protein intake, with or without additional vitamins.

The disorder is inherited as an autosomal recessive condition, with both males and females being affected. There is evidence that obligate heterozygotes can be distinguished by measurement of the enzyme (Wong et al 1977). Prenatal diagnosis has been accomplished in at least one case.

Homocystinuria from a deficiency of methylcobalamin

Methyl-B_{12} is the active cofactor for the conversion of homocysteine to L-methionine by the enzyme N^5-methylenetetrahydrofolate: homocysteine methyltrans-ferase. A deficiency of methyl-B_{12}, by any number of mechanisms, can result in homocystinuria, homocystin-aemia, hypomethioninaemia, and significant clinical symptoms. At least two groups of inherited defects of vitamin B_{12} metabolism have been identified with the above symptoms: cobalamin mutant classes C and D; and cobalamin mutant classes E and G. (For review see Cooper & Rosenblatt 1987, Fenton & Rosenberg 1989).

Cobalamin mutants C and D have a genetic deficiency in converting hydroxycobalamin to a further reduced form of methylcobalamin and 5′ deoxyadenosyl cobala-min. The failure to form the active methyl and 5′ deoxyadenosyl forms of vitamin B_{12} results in an accumulation of homocysteine and methylmalonic acid. The former occurs because of the failure of homocystine to recycle to methionine, and the latter because of the failure of converting methylmalonyl-CoA to succinyl-CoA.

Patients with an inability to form methyl-B_{12} have presented soon after birth with lethargy, failure to thrive, feeding difficulties and megaloblastic anaemia. A few older patients have been identified whose symptoms were psychiatric in nature, with developmental delay, microcephaly, seizures, spasticity, and retinal changes with perimacular pigmentation. Patients classified as having either cobalamin C or cobalamin D defects are classified on the basis of biochemical complementation by tissue culture studies. Most patients with cobalamin C or D mutations may improve with intramuscular injections of hydroxycobalamin (1 mg) administered daily or as infrequently as once per week.

Another group of patients characterized as having homocystinuria without methylmalonic aciduria and defective synthesis of methyl-B_{12} have been classified as cobalamin mutants E and G. This group of patients have a defect in synthesizing methyl-B_{12}, but form normal amounts of 5′ adenosyl-B_{12}. Whether a patient is subclassified as having mutant E or mutant G is based on complementation analysis in cultured cells. Clinical symptoms in these patients are similar to those previously listed; early presentation in childhood with megaloblastic anaemia, pancytopenia, failure to thrive, vomiting, failure of neurological development, and biochemical evidence of homocystinuria, homocystinaemia, and hypomethioninaemia. If identified early, these patients may respond to therapy consisting of intramuscular hydroxycobalamin, supplemental oral L-methionine, and folic acid.

No convenient assay is available for the detection of heterozygotes. One child with a defect of cobalamin E was identified in utero by assays performed on cultured cells from amniotic fluid (Rosenblatt et al 1985).

Other causes of homocystinuria

Homocystinuria can occur by any mechanism that causes severe vitamin B_{12} deficiency. Two children have been reported with an inherited form of vitamin B_{12} malabsorption (Hollowell et al 1969). These children excreted homocystine, methylmalonic acid and cystathionine in their urine. Homocystinuria has been identified in some infants with severe transcobalamin II deficiency and has been documented in subjects given 6-azauridine triacetate. This compound apparently interferes with pyridoxine metabolism, with the theoretical reduction of 5′ methyltetrahydrofolate and an inability to recycle homocysteine to methionine (Mudd et al 1989).

Cystathioninuria

Gamma-cystathionase cleaves L-cystathionine to cysteine and α-ketobutyrate. This reaction completes the transfer of sulphur from methionine to cysteine. Cystathionine is not normally detectable in the plasma, but with sensitive assays small amounts can be detected in the urine of most persons (Endres & Seibold 1978). Normal quantities may be as high as 150 μmol/gm creatinine. Modestly increased cystathioninuria may be detectable in premature infants and young newborns, and patients with neuroblastomas or hepatic tumours (Mudd et al 1989).

Deficiency of γ-cystathionase activity causes a massive excretion of cystathionine in the urine. Patients classified as having γ-cystathionase deficiency excrete cystathionine in amounts ranging from 1400 to 1600 μmoles/gm creatinine (Finkelstein et al 1966). The highest excretions are in younger children and may correlate with methionine intake. Approximately 50 patients have been identified with apparent γ-cystathionase deficiency (Mudd et al 1989).

The original patients reported with cystathioninuria had symptoms of mental retardation, convulsions, nephrogenic diabetes insipidus and diabetes mellitus. Subsequent reports have indicated that the condition can occur in normal individuals (Scott et al 1970b, Lyon et al 1971). The current belief is that a genetic deficiency of γ-cystathionase causing cystathioninuria is a benign condition that is not clinically deleterious, and is not related to the development of mental retardation.

Cystathioninuria is inherited as an autosomal recessive condition. Male and female sibs have been reported and increased cystathionine excretion can be detected in obligate heterozygotes (Mudd et al 1989). Deficient activity of γ-cystathionase has been documented in liver tissue, cultured skin fibroblasts, and PHA stimulated lymphocytes from patients and from the latter two tissues in heterozygotes. Obligate heterozygotes have demonstrated decreased activity of γ-cystathionase activity from PHA stimulated lymphocytes (Mudd et al 1989).

Genetic heterogeneity is obvious among patients with γ-cystathionase deficiency. The majority of patients respond to pyridoxal phosphate therapy (100 mg/24 hours) with a marked reduction in their excretion of cystathionine. 10–20% of patients will not respond to this therapy. There is intrafamilial concordance in pyridoxine responsiveness. Patients that are pyridoxine responsive have higher residual activity of γ-cystathionase in stimulated lymphocytes than patients who are nonresponsive. Variations in quantity of immunologically detectable protein, variation in enzyme kinetics, and variation in heat stability are evidence of heterogeneity at the molecular level (Mudd et al 1989).

The incidence of apparent γ-cystathionase deficiency from newborn screening programmes has varied between 1/68 000 in New England, to 1/300 000 in Australia (Mudd et al 1989). The gene for γ-cystathionase has been assigned presumptively to chromosome 16 by somatic cell genetic techniques (Donald et al 1982). Prenatal

Table 93.5 Disorders of the branched chain amino acids.

Disorder	Enzyme deficiency	Inheritance pattern	Heterozygote detection	Prenatal diagnosis
Branched chain ketoaciduria (maple syrup urine disease) Classic form	Branched chain α-ketoacid dehydrogenase (BCKD)	AR	difficult	yes
Intermediate and mild forms	Less severe deficiency of BCKD	AR	difficult	yes
Thiamine responsive forms	Thiamine binding/stabilization/activation of BCKD	AR?		
Hypervalinaemia	Branched chain aminotransferase	AR?		
Leucine-isoleucinaemia	Branched chain aminotransferase	AR?		

diagnosis has not been reported and is probably unnecessary, but presumably would be feasible by assay of the enzyme in cultured amniocytes or a chorionic villus biopsy.

Sulphite oxidase deficiency

Two families have been reported with an isolated deficiency of sulphite oxidase (Mudd et al 1967, Shih et al 1977). Infants in each family died with severe neurological abnormalities. A striking clinical feature was the presence of ectopia lentis, similar to that seen in patients with homocystinuria. The urine of these affected infants contained increased quantities of S-sulpho-L-cysteine, sulphite, and thiosulphate. No sulphate was detectable in the urine. An absence of sulphite oxidase was shown to exist in postmortem samples from liver, kidney, and brain. Intermediate levels of sulphite oxidase could be detected in cultured fibroblasts in the single family reported by Shih et al (1977).

A similar disorder occurs as a consequence of a deficiency of a novel pterin that binds molybdenum to sulphite oxidase and xanthine oxidase. These patients, in addition to the symptoms of sulphite oxidase deficiency, demonstrate hypouricaemia and xanthinuria as a consequence of their xanthine oxidase deficiency. Urinary xanthine stones may be identified in these children in association with severe neurological symptoms and dislocated ocular lenses (Roesel et al 1986, Johnson & Wadman 1989).

Each of the above disorders is believed to be inherited as an autosomal recessive condition. Little information is

available on disease frequency, heterozygote detection, or range of heterogeneity.

DISORDERS OF THE BRANCHED CHAIN AMINO ACIDS (Table 93.5)

Leucine, isoleucine, and valine are essential amino acids in man. Each is required for normal nutrition and growth in children and to maintain protein synthesis in adulthood. The term 'branched chain' is used because each contains a methyl group that branches from the main aliphatic carbon chain. These amino acids play an important regulatory role in body nitrogen, carbohydrate and ketone body homeostasis, but their fate is to be used primarily for protein synthesis; that quantity of amino acids not used for protein synthesis undergoes a series of irreversible oxidative steps to form organic acids that eventually enter the tricarboxylic cycle or are used for gluconeogenesis.

Two major groups of clinical disorders are associated with deficiencies in the steps of branched chain amino acid metabolism. One group of disorders in which there is accumulation of one or more of the amino acids includes (1) maple syrup urine disease; (2) hypervalinaemia; and (3) leucine-isoleucinaemia. Disorders more distal in the catabolic pathway are associated with the accumulation of organic acids and are termed the 'organic acidaemias'. The more common disorders of organic acid metabolism include: (1) isovaleric acidaemia; (2) methylmalonic acidaemia; and (3) propionic acidaemia. A significant number of other organic acidaemias exist within this catabolic pathway, and the entire group is reviewed elsewhere in this book.

Maple syrup urine disease (MSUD)

Enzymatic transamination and decarboxylation of branched-chain amino acids

The steps in the metabolism of leucine, isoleucine and valine are similar (Fig. 93.5). There is an initial transamination reaction with α-ketoglutarate serving as the amino group acceptor, forming respectively, α-ketoisocaproic acid, α-keto-β-methylvaleric acid and α-ketoisovaleric acid. Biochemical evidence indicates that a single transaminase is responsible for all of these conversions (Danner & Elsas 1989).

The second reaction is an oxidative decarboxylation of the branch chain α-keto-acids. It is likely from biochemical data and from the study of human mutants that a single branched chain decarboxylase is used by the branched chain α-keto acids for the reaction (Danner & Elsas 1989). Branched-chained ketoacid decarboxylase is a large multienzyme complex similar in both structure and reaction mechanism to the pyruvate and 12-oxoglutarate decarboxylases (Danner & Elsas 1989). It is located on the outer face of the inner mitochondrial membrane. It consists of four separate proteins: $E_{1\alpha}$ and $E_{1\beta}$ that form a decarboxylase, a transacylase (E_2), and a lipoamide oxidoreductase (E_3). The latter enzyme is identical in this complex and in those specific to pyruvate and 2-oxoglutarate dehydrogenases.

The decarboxylase component requires and is stabilized by thiamine (Danner & Elsas 1989). Maximum

activity of the entire complex is dependent upon lipoic acid, NAD, and coenzyme A. Phosphorylation of the decarboxylase regulates and inactivates the complex; it is reversed by the action of a phosphatase, and the two reactions interact to regulate the total complex. The complexity of the enzyme system allows for at least six separate genes at different loci to affect the integrity of the entire complex, at least three of which are unique. The potential exists for many mutational events to affect the activity of this reaction.

Clinical disorders

A genetic deficiency of the activity of the dehydrogenase complex prevents further oxidation of the α-keto acids that are formed from their respective amino acids. This deficiency is responsible for the clinical syndrome of 'maple syrup urine disease' one of the the earliest and best known of inborn errors of amino acid metabolism (Menkes et al 1954, Danner & Elsas 1989). Affected patients accumulate α-keto-isocaproic acid, α-keto-β-methylcaproic acid, and α-keto-isovaleric acid. These α-keto acids may be reversibly reaminated by transamination to again form their respective branched chain amino acids. Thus, patients with a dehydrogenase deficiency accumulate both the branched chain α-keto acids and leucine, isoleucine, and valine (and allo-isoleucine).

Infants affected with the 'classical' form of MSUD

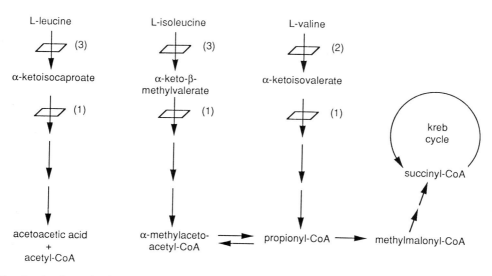

Fig. 93.5 Abbreviated pathway for the metabolism of the branched chain amino acids. The known enzyme defects affecting amino acid metabolism are *branched chain keto-acid decarboxylase* causing maple syrup urine disease (1), conformational changes in *branched chain transaminase* causing hypervalinaemia (2), and hyperisoleucine-leucinaemia (3).

have symptoms that occur within the first few days or weeks of life. This is associated with severe acidosis and hypoglycaemia. Affected infants appear normal at birth but soon demonstrate neurological deterioration manifest by flaccidity, a high-pitched cry, hypertonicity, and opisthotonic posturing. The odour of 'maple syrup' can usually be detected in the urine, scalp and skin of these affected infants. It is unusual for such infants to survive the newborn period, and those who do usually demonstrate residual neurological damage. Those in whom the onset is more indolent may have symptoms of poor feeding, vomiting, lethargy, coma and seizures. Prognosis for these individuals is improved if treated appropriately.

In addition to patients with the classical form of MSUD, there exist more mildly affected individuals. They are divided into two classes: an 'intermediate' form; and a 'mild' form of the disorder (Morris et al 1961, Dancis et al 1967a, Schulman et al 1970, Danner & Elsas 1989). A child responsive to thiamine therapy has also been identified and classified as a 'thiamine-responsive' variant (Scriver et al 1985). This child responded dramatically to 10 mg/24 hours of thiamine with improvement in her clinical course.

There probably exists a continuum of clinical heterogeneity for MSUD, varying from the severe classical form to quite mild forms of the illnesses. The degree of severity would be related to the residual enzyme activity of the dehydrogenase complex that exists under physiological conditions for the substrates (Danner & Elsas 1989). Abnormal enzyme kinetics have been documented in tissue obtained from patients with different degrees of severity of MSUD. Indo et al (1987) have shown some correspondence between the clinical phenotype and the kinetic parameters of the $E_{1\beta}$ subunit of the dehydrogenase complex. They also identified an E_2 subunit deficiency in a patient who would be classified as having an intermittent form of the disorder (Indo et al 1988). A similar defect in the E_2 component was originally documented by Danner et al (1985). These are summarized in Danner and Elsas (1989).

Diagnosis and biochemical abnormalities

Diagnosis of patients with the classic form of MSUD is not difficult. When symptomatic as infants, these patients have urines that give abnormal reactions to screening tests: a blue-grey colour when reacted with ferric chloride, and a yellow precipitate with the addition of 2-4-dinitrophenylhydrazine. Quantitation of amino acids in plasma document the marked increase in leucine, isoleucine and valine, and the presence of allo-isoleucine. Allo-isoleucine in plasma may be considered pathognomonic of MSUD. This unusual amino acid is formed through keto-enol tautomerization of the α-keto-β-methyl valerate. The identification of the specific keto acids associated with MSUD can be accomplished by a variety of chromatographic techniques, but add little to the diagnosis.

The milder forms of MSUD may be difficult to diagnose. The patients may only be clinically ill when affected with an intercurrent viral illness, or when exposed to a high protein intake. At such times, they may have symptoms of nausea, vomiting, lethargy and mild acidosis. Some of these patients will show a persistent elevation of branched chain amino acids and the presence of allo-isoleucine in their plasma; others may only demonstrate these changes when ill. The majority will only excrete abnormal quantities of α-keto acids when clinically symptomatic.

The branched-chain ketoacid dehydrogenase activity can be measured in peripheral monocytes, skin fibroblasts, amniotic fluid cells, chorionic villi, muscle and of course liver and other visceral organs. The measurement of the branched chain keto acid dehydrogenase may be of value in these mild cases where the diagnosis is difficult to establish by the measurement of plasma amino acids.

Treatment

Management of the child with the classic form of MSUD is frustrating. The majority have either died as infants or have significant neurological and intellectual impairment, in spite of special dietary intervention. Snyderman et al (1964) and Clow et al (1981) have summarized their experiences with the management of MSUD and are more enthusiastic than most clinicians.

The patients tend to do well between acute intercurrent illnesses, but are vulnerable to rapid deterioration when they become anorexic, dehydrated or are subject to severe endogenous protein catabolism. The onset of an acute febrile illness is hazardous; the patient who cannot sustain oral intake with high carbohydrate fluids and/or has a diminished state of consciousness must be brought to hospital immediately for intravenous nutritional support. Valine and isoleucine are important carbon sources for normal gluconeogenesis, a pathway that is compromised in these patients.

Therapy of the acute presentation or of an acute deterioration involves the exclusion of exogenous sources of protein and high glucose and high calorie intravenous solutions to minimize the hypoglycaemic drive to protein catabolism. Peritoneal dialysis may be necessary to remove very high levels of leucine, toxic to the central nervous system, and well reabsorbed by the kidneys. Early readdition to the diet of the 17 non-branched-chain amino acids may hasten protein synthesis and the return towards normal levels of the offending amino acids.

The longer term care of patients with MSUD involves the use of high calorie diets with limiting amounts of leucine, isoleucine and valine. Commercial products tailored to these requirements are available. The diets have been useful in maintaining lowered and near normal levels of amino acids. Thiamine (10–100 mg/24 hours or more) may be tried to help stabilize the dehydrogenase complex and allow greater branched chain amino acid dietary tolerance in patients who retain structurally identifiable $E_{1\alpha}$ and $E_{1\beta}$, but who are deficient in these activities (Danner & Elsas 1989).

The milder forms of MSUD can normally be successfully managed by dietary intervention, and uniformly excellent clinical results are achieved with this group of patients. Despite this the patients remain vulnerable to acute catabolic episodes, and instances of death during adolescence of otherwise normal individuals has been reported (Dancis et al 1967a).

Genetics

MSUD is inherited as an autosomal recessive condition. It is rare, with an incidence no greater than 1/100 000 live births. Neonatal screening programmes have detected an incidence between 1/120 000–1/300 000 (Danner & Elsas 1989). These estimates may be low because they rely on the detection of elevations of branched chain amino acids in blood or urine samples. At birth, patients with MSUD may have normal levels of branched chain amino acids. There is no apparent increased incidence of MSUD in specific ethnic groups. An increased incidence does exist, by founder effect, in the Amish population of Pennsylvania. Heterozygote detection is difficult (Langenbeck et al 1975). This can be appreciated because of the complexity of the enzymatic reaction, the clinical heterogeneity of affected patients, and documentation of different mutations within the dehydrogenase complex. A decreased rate of CO_2 production in leucocytes of obligate heterozygotes has been documented in some families, but not all. The dehydrogenase reaction is expressed in cultured amniotic fluid cells and chorionic villi; prenatal diagnosis can be reliably performed from these tissues (Danner & Elsas 1989). The concentration of amino acids or keto acids in amniotic fluid is unreliable for prenatal diagnosis, since the branched chain amino acid concentrations in fetal serum may not be significantly elevated.

cDNA clones for three of the four major proteins of the complex $E_{1\alpha}$, E_3 and the acetyltransferase have been isolated (Litwer & Danner 1985, Otulakowski & Robinson 1987, Zhang et al 1987, Danner & Elsas 1989) and may now be used, along with western immunoblotting, for genetic studies in some families.

Hypervalinaemia

Valine undergoes reversible deamination to form α-keto-isovaleric acid (Fig. 93.5). An infant from Japan has been reported to be missing activity for the branched chain amino acid transaminase responsible for the conversion of valine to its keto acid (Wada et al 1963, Dancis et al 1967b). The child was detected because of developmental delay, vomiting and lethargy. The infant is reported to have responded to a diet low in valine. The mode of inheritance is assumed to be autosomal recessive. An abnormality in valine metabolism could not be detected in the parents.

Hyperleucine-isoleucinaemia

A single family with two sibs has been reported with a deficiency of the enzyme which deaminates leucine and isoleucine to their respective α-keto acids (Fig. 93.5). These children were evaluated because of severe mental deficiency, seizures, deafness, and retinal degeneration (Jeune et al 1970). These children were also found to have hyperprolinaemia, type II. This hyperprolinaemia is an independent disorder and unrelated to the elevations of the branched chain amino acids.

It is presumed that the disorder is autosomal recessive, but no abnormalities in leucine or isoleucine deamination could be demonstrated in the parents.

The existence of hypervalinaemia and leucine-isoleucinaemia as separate entities raises the possibility of separate branched chain transaminases responsible for the metabolism of the branched chain amino acids. Careful evaluation supports the existence of only a single enzyme responsible for the conversion of all three amino acids to their respective α-keto acids (Goto et al 1977). Thus, hypervalinaemia and hyperisoleucinaemia probably represent conformational changes in the transaminase that alters substrate specificity.

DISORDERS OF HISTIDINE METABOLISM
(Table 93.6)

Histidine is an essential amino acid for human infants and probably for adults. The amino acid is necessary for protein synthesis and can be decarboxylated to form histamine. The major pathway of histamine metabolism, however, is degradation to eventually yield glutamic acid (Fig. 93.6). A minor pathway allows histidine to undergo transamination with the formation of imidazole pyruvic acid.

Histidinaemia

Patients with histidinaemia are unable to adequately convert histidine to urocanic acid. The enzyme respon-

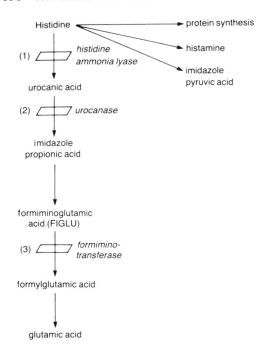

Fig. 93.6 The major metabolic reactions of histidine metabolism. The enzymatic blocks are for histidinaemia (1), urocanic aciduria (2), and formiminoglutamic aciduria (3).

sible for this reaction is *histidine ammonia lyase*, and it has been documented to be deficient in affected patients (La Du et al 1963, Zannoni & La Du 1963). Histidine is markedly increased in the urine, blood and CSF. The elevated blood histidine levels (>0.5 mM) cause an increased formation of imidazole pyruvic acid which is excreted in the urine. This compound reacts with ferric chloride solution to yield a green colour, similar to that observed in phenylketonuria. Histidine ammonia lyase may be assayed in stratum corneum or in liver tissue.

The diagnosis of histidinaemia is typically dependent upon the documentation of histidinuria, histidinaemia and a deficiency of enzyme activity in the stratum corneum.

A consistent clinical picture for patients with histidinaemia never evolved. Although the original patients had mental retardation (Woody et al 1965, Ghadimi & Partington 1967) this feature has certainly been stressed unduly because of ascertainment bias. Delayed speech development and defects in auditory perception have been present in some probands. When histidinaemia probands were detected prospectively, it was found to be a benign condition (Levy et al 1974).

Scriver, Levy and their collaborators undertook a comprehensive retrospective and prospective analysis of this condition and concluded that the disorder was not associated with demonstrable clinical consequences (Scriver & Levy 1983, Rosenmann et al 1983, Coulombe et al 1983).

Histidinaemia is inherited as an autosomal recessive trait. It has an incidence of 1:15 000 in live born infants (Levy et al 1972). Evidence for heterogeneity exists from variation in the expression of histidine ammonia lyase between liver and stratum corneum. The majority of patients are lacking this enzyme in both tissues, but at least one pedigree had activity of the enzyme in the stratum corneum (Woody et al 1965).

Heterozygotes cannot reliably be detected by fasting histidine concentrations in blood or by enzyme activity from skin samples. The most consistent test for discriminating heterozygotes from normals within a pedigree is the measurement of urinary FIGLU following an L-histidine load (Rosenblatt et al 1970).

Prenatal diagnosis has not been reported. The documentation of an affected fetus is unlikely since the enzyme is not expressed in cultured amniotic fluid cells.

Urocanic aciduria

Only two families have been reported with urocanic aciduria from a deficiency of urocanase. Insufficient data exist to reach any conclusions concerning the clinical symptomatology or genetic transmission of the disorder (Yoshida et al 1971, Kalafatic et al 1980).

Table 93.6 Disorders of histidine metabolism

Disorder	Enzyme deficiency	Inheritance pattern	Heterozygote detection	Prenatal diagnosis
Histidinaemia	Histidine ammonia lyase	AR	possible	not indicated
Urocanic aciduria	Urocanase	?		
Formiminoglutamic aciduria	Formiminotransferase	AR?		

Formiminoglutamic (FIGLU) aciduria

A small number of patients have been documented who excrete a marked excess of FIGLU and have a deficiency of *formiminotransferase*. Some patients have had symptoms of profound mental retardation, while others have been normal. The relationship of this enzyme deficiency to neurological symptoms remains unclear.

The pedigree information is consistent with an autosomal recessive trait. No information is available concerning the reliability of heterozygote detection or prenatal diagnosis.

DISORDERS OF LYSINE METABOLISM
(Table 93.7)

Those patients who present with an increased lysine concentration in the plasma and/or urine represent a confusing group of disorders. In many families the primary biochemical defect has not been clearly delineated and the relationship of the elevated plasma or urine lysine concentrations to the mental retardation syndrome precipitating the study is unclear. These problems cause considerable difficulty in offering precise genetic information to families who seek counselling and treatment.

The pathway of lysine degradation is outlined in Figure 93.7. There is now little question that the major degradative pathway for lysine is through saccharopine and α-aminoadipic acid (Cederbaum 1985). Further degradation through glutaric acid results in the formation of acetyl-CoA. A small fraction of lysine appears to be metabolized via pipicolic acid in the peroxisomes. Defects of most steps in these pathways are known. Those involving glutaric acid and more distal steps are discussed in the chapter on the organic acidemias, and pipicolic acidaemia in that on the peroxisomal disorders.

The first two major steps of lysine degradation appear

to be catalyzed by a single bifunctional enzyme resulting in the formation of α-aminoadipic acid (Hutzler & Dancis 1975, Dancis et al 1976, Markovitz et al 1984). The most clearly defined enzymatic deficiency in lysine

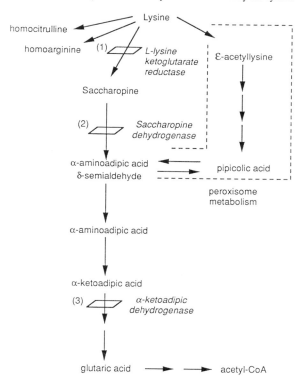

Fig. 93.7 Initial steps in the metabolism of lysine. The defects implicated in hyperlysinaemia are indicated by a deficiency of *L-lysine keto-glutarate reductase* (1), and in saccharopinuria by a deficiency of *saccharopine dehydrogenase* (2). These two reactions are believed to occur on the same bifunctional enzyme. A deficiency of *α-keto-adipic dehydrogenase* (3) is implicated for α-keto-adipic aciduria.

Table 93.7 Disorders of lysine metabolism

Disorder	Enzyme deficiency	Inheritance pattern	Heterozygote detection	Prenatal diagnosis
Hyperlysinaemia	Lysine-ketoglutarate reductase Saccharopine dehydrogenase	AR	probably	not indicated
Saccharopinuria	Saccharopine dehydrogenase	AR	probably	not indicated
Hyperlysinaemia with hyperammonaemia	Unknown	?	no	no
α-Aminoadipic aciduria	'α-ketoadipic acid dehydrogenase'	AR	no	not indicated
Lysinuric protein intolerance	'Diabasic amino acid transporter'	AR	?	no

degradation involves this complex and results in the accumulation of lysine and a number of secondary products in the body fluids (Cederbaum 1985). Based on the diversity of the clinical picture in probands, the normal clinical status of affected sibs and the normal outcome in infants ascertained at newborn screening, this enzyme deficiency appears to cause no clinical consequences (Dancis et al 1983, Cederbaum 1985). A single family has been reported in which saccharopine accumulated in excess of lysine. In this instance saccharopine dehydrogenase activity was more diminished than lysine-ketoglutarate reductase activity and probably reflected the particular mutation that was present in the structural gene (Fellows & Carson 1974, Cederbaum 1985).

This enzyme defect is inherited in an autosomal recessive manner and heterozygotes can be ascertained. Prenatal diagnosis is possible, but is not indicated.

A second clear-cut defect in this pathway occurs in α-ketoadipic dehydrogenase which leads to the accumulation of both α-ketoadipic and α-amino adipic acids (Cederbaum 1985). Like the defect in the first two steps in the catabolic pathway, no clinical symptoms can be ascribed to this enzyme deficiency. It too is inherited in an autosomal recessive manner (Cederbaum 1985).

Periodic hyperlysinaemia with hyperammonaemia has been described only twice and the basis for the disorder remains unelucidated (Colombo et al 1967, Sogawa et al 1977). In contrast to the apparently benign disorders whose biochemical basis we understand, this disorder seems more likely to be causally related to the severe neurological symptoms seen.

It is ironic that in three of the first four hyperlysinaemic patients described, no enzyme defect was either sought or described. Two of the three had normal levels of lysine-ketoglutarate reductase activity, only one had this defect and falls into the group already described. The precise defect in these patients may never be known and the relationship between the hyperlysinaemia and the retardation may never be proven or disproven (Cederbaum 1985).

Lysinuric protein intolerance is inherited as an autosomal recessive disorder and is a defect of diabasic amino acid absorption in the small intestine and reabsorption in the kidney (Simell 1989). It is particularly common in Finland (Simell 1989). The patients present with diarrhoea, vomiting, failure to thrive, hepatomegaly and cirrhosis. They have hyperammonia and excessive excretion of lysine, arginine and ornithine in the urine. The symptoms are exacerbated by higher protein intake. Oral citrulline therapy results in considerable improvement in many of these patients with increased protein tolerance and growth and improvement in gastrointestinal symptoms and hyperammonaemia (Rajanatie et al 1980, Carpenter et al 1985, Simell 1989).

A number of patients have been described with elevations of hydroxylysine in the plasma, and excretion of increased quantities of it in the urine (Goodman et al 1972). Although the patients were retarded, it is unclear whether the symptoms were related to the biochemical defect. The nature of the defect is unknown, but affected sibs and consanguinity in at least one family imply autosomal recessive inheritance.

DISORDERS OF PROLINE AND HYDROXYPROLINE (Table 93.8)

Proline and hydroxyproline are non-essential amino acids. Proline is synthesized from glutamic acid with a small quantity being formed from ornithine. Hydroxyproline is formed by the oxidation of proline that is bound in peptides, usually within collagen.

The synthesis of proline occurs through the intermediary Δ'-pyrroline-5-carboxylic acid (PC). The conversion of PC to proline is catalyzed by Δ'-pyrroline-5-carboxylic reductase. The intermediate in the reaction, PC, is in equilibrium with its isomer, glutamic-gamma-semialdehyde. The interconversion of PC and glutamic-gamma-semialdehyde occurs through a non-enzymatic rearrangement. The catabolism of proline is almost a reversal of its synthesis but is mediated by separate

Table 93.8 Disorders of proline and hydroxyproline

Disorder	Enzyme deficiency	Inheritance pattern	Heterozygote detection	Prenatal diagnosis
Prolinaemia, Type I	Proline oxidase	AR	possibly	not indicated
Prolinaemia, Type II	Δ'-pyrroline-5-carboxylic acid dehydrogenase	AR	yes	not indicated
Hyperhydroxy-prolinaemia	Hydroxyproline oxidase(?)	AR	possibly	not indicated

enzymes. Proline oxidase converts proline to PC, and PC dehydrogenase further oxidizes the glutamic-gamma-semialdehyde to glutamic acid. A small amount of glutamic-gamma-semialdehyde may be converted to ornithine via ornithine aminotransferase. These reactions are summarized in Figure 93.8 (Phang & Scriver 1989).

Genetic deficiencies of proline oxidase and PC dehydrogenase exist and are responsible for Type I and Type II hyperprolinaemia respectively. A deficiency of 'hydroxyproline oxidase' is believed to be responsible for hydroxyprolinaemia.

Hyperprolinaemia, Type I

Patients with Type I hyperprolinaemia have increased plasma concentrations of proline (approximately 1 mM) and excrete proline, hydroxyproline and glycine in the urine (Phang & Scriver 1989). At least 12 families have been identified with this disorder. A deficiency of proline oxidase was documented in liver tissue obtained from a postmortem specimen (Efron 1965, Phang & Scriver 1989). Proline oxidase is a mitochondrial-bound enzyme found only in kidney, liver, heart and brain, and is not detectable in cultured skin fibroblasts or blood leucocytes.

The original families with Type I hyperprolinaemia were ascertained because of kidney disease, deafness, and neurological disorders (Schafer et al 1962). Subsequent

families have been unaffected with clinical problems, and it is reasonable to assume that Type I hyperprolinaemia is a benign condition that is not associated with clinical illness (Phang & Scriver 1989).

Proline oxidase deficiency is inherited as an autosomal recessive condition. Heterozygotes may not have plasma proline values above the normal range. This feature of Type I hyperprolinaemia tends to confuse the interpretation of the inheritance pattern in some pedigrees (Phang & Scriver 1989). The chromosomal location of the gene coding for proline oxidase is unknown.

A mouse model exists for Type I hyperprolinaemia with proline oxidase deficiency in liver, brain and kidney tissue. It has been labeled Pro/Re, and has similar residual enzyme activity to that observed in human patients, and has no apparent developmental sequelae or clinical symptoms.

Hyperprolinaemia, Type II

Persons with Type II hyperprolinaemia have greatly elevated concentrations of proline in plasma (1.5 to 3.0 mM), and excrete substantial quantities of proline, hydroxyproline, glycine, and Δ'-pyrroline-5-carboxylic acid. The concentration of plasma proline is greater than that observed in Type I hyperprolinaemia and the excretion of PC in the urine is significant. These latter points distinguish the biochemical phenotype of Type II hyperprolinaemia from Type I (Applegarth et al 1974). The enzyme deficiency is in the second step of proline catabolism; a deficiency of Δ'-pyrroline-5-carboxylic acid dehydrogenase (Valle et al 1976).

There exists no specific clinical phenotype associated with hyperprolinaemia, Type II. The enzyme deficiency resulting in increased levels of proline is not associated with any abnormal clinical symptoms.

Type II hyperprolinaemia is inherited as an autosomal recessive condition. Heterozygotes are not detectable by increased plasma concentrations of proline, and do not excrete increased quantities of PC in the urine. Heterozygotes do show partial activity of the dehydrogenase in cultured fibroblasts and in blood leucocytes (Valle et al 1976). The chromosomal location of the gene encoding for Δ'-pyrroline-5-carboxylic dehydrogenase is unknown.

Hyperhydroxyprolinaemia

Hyperhydroxyprolinaemia is a rare disorder characterized by markedly elevated concentration of hydroxyproline in the plasma (0.15–0.5 mM; normal <0.01 mM). Free hydroxyproline may be much increased in the urine

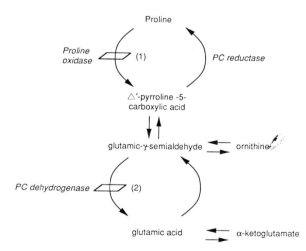

Fig. 93.8 Biosynthesis degradation of proline. *Proline oxidase* deficiency (1) and *PC dehydrogenase* deficiency (2) are responsible for Type I and Type II hyperprolinaemia respectively.

of affected persons, but such concentrations rarely reach a level that interferes with the renal imino-glycine transport system. Thus, the urinary phenotype of hyperhydroxyprolinaemia may not include an increased excretion of proline and glycine (Phang & Scriver 1989).

Similar to hyperprolinaemia, Types I and II, hyperhydroxyprolinaemia is considered a harmless condition. It was originally detected in a child with mental retardation, but subsequent persons have been identified who are mentally and physically normal. Hyperhydroxyprolinaemia has been detected in infants through newborn screening programmes and they are free of sympton on long-term follow-up (Pelkonen & Kivirikko 1970, Levy 1973).

Specific enzyme assays have not been performed to confirm the deficiency. Loading studies using oral hydroxyproline have implied that the enzymatic block is between hydroxyproline and Δ'-pyrroline-3-hydroxy-5-carboxylic acid (Efron et al 1965, Pelkonen & Kivirikko 1970). This step is catalyzed by hydroxyproline oxidase, an enzyme distinct from proline oxidase.

Pedigree data is consistent with hyperhydroxyprolinaemia being an autosomal recessive trait (Efron et al 1965, Rama Rao et al 1974). Heterozygotes do not have elevated levels of hydroxyproline in plasma, do not excrete increased quantities of hydroxyproline in the urine, but may be detectable after a hydroxyproline load (Phang & Scriver 1989). A homozygous female has had normal children (Pelkonen & Kivirikko 1970). The

Table 93.9 Genetic causes of hyperammonaemia

Disorders of the urea cycle (Table 93.10)
Hyperornithinaemia, hyperammonaemia, homocitrullinuria
Lysinuric protein intolerance
Hyperlysinaemia with hyperammonaemia
Various organic acidaemias

chromosomal location of the gene coding for hydroxyproline oxidase is unknown.

DISORDERS OF THE UREA CYCLE AND OF ORNITHINE (Tables 93.9 and 93.10)

The urea cycle is a five step pathway which results in the conversion of two molecules of ammonia and one of bicarbonate to urea. It is the only major metabolic pathway for the removal of waste nitrogen formed from protein turnover or ingestion and occurs primarily, if not exclusively, in the liver. High levels of ammonia in blood and tissue results in toxicity to the central nervous system. The primary effect of elevated ammonia appears to be the uptake of fluid into astrocytes causing cerebral oedema. Table 93.9 lists the disorders that are associated with hyperammonaemia; only those primarily involved in ammonia metabolism and the urea cycle will be discussed below and are detailed in Table 93.10.

Complete deficiency of any of enzymes 1–5 (Fig. 93.9) leads to severe hyperammonaemia in the neonatal period

Table 93.10 Disorders of the urea cycle and of ornithine

Enzyme defect	Inheritance pattern	Heterozygote detection	Prenatal diagnosis	Gene cloned	Chromosomal location
Acetylglutamate synthetase	uncertain	no	no	no	unknown
Carbamylphosphate synthetase	AR	no	yes	yes	7
Ornithine transcarbamylase	XL	yes	yes	yes	Xp21
Argininosuccinate synthetase	AR	no	yes	yes	9
Argininosuccinate lyase	AR	yes	yes	yes	12
Arginase I	AR	yes	yes	yes	6q23
'Ornithine transporter'?	AR	no	yes	no	unknown
Ornithine aminotransferase	AR	yes	yes	yes	10

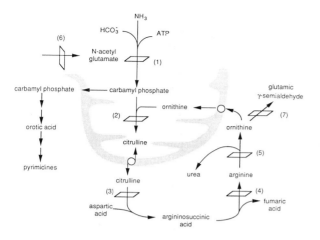

Fig. 93.9 Abbreviated pathway for the urea cycle and the degradation of ornithine. The genetic conditions that are known to cause hyperammonaemia are *carbamyl phosphate synthetase-I* deficiency (1), *ornithine transcarbamylase* deficiency (2), citrullinaemia (3), argininosuccinic aciduria (4), argininaemia (5), and *acetylglutamate synthetase* (6). The enzyme defect responsible for gyrate atrophy of the retina is a deficiency of *ornithine aminotransferase* (7).

with symptoms of lethargy, poor feeding, coma, and often death (Brusilow & Horwich 1989). Ammonia levels often exceed 1000 μM (normal <50). Less complete enzyme deficiencies may delay clinical symptoms until later in life and be associated with lower ammonia levels. The presentation could be indolent or occur as an acute catastrophic collapse in conjunction with some infectious event. Episodes of hyperammonaemia, nausea and vomiting may be the initial, or only, symptoms. Most symptomatic patients are developmentally retarded and have a variety of neurological abnormalities.

The enzymatic basis of hyperammonaemia can usually be inferred from determination of the plasma amino acid levels, acid base balance, urinary organic acids and urinary orotic acid (Brusilow & Horwich 1989). Specific confirmation by enzyme assays is desirable whenever possible. Therapy is both generic and specific and will be detailed below.

Acetylglutamate synthetase deficiency

Acetylglutamate is an obligatory allosteric activator of carbamylphosphate synthetase I and it is synthesized in liver mitochondria by acetylglutamate synthetase. Four patients with deficiency of this enzyme are known to us, two published (Bachmann et al 1982, 1988) and two unpublished (Julian Williams, M.D.).

The patients present with symptoms of hyperammonaemia, usually in the newborn period. Plasma amino acid changes are those typically associated with hyperammonaemia and include elevation of glutamine and alanine concentrations and low values for citrulline. Urinary orotic acid excretion is not increased. Acetylglutamate synthetase in liver tissue has been deficient, whereas levels of carbamylphosphate synthetase I have been normal (Bachmann et al 1988).

Of the four patients, one died in the neonatal period, one is mildly retarded, one moderately so, and one too young to judge. The brother of one patient died of 'hepatic failure' at 7 months and that of another in the neonatal period. All have recurrent episodes of hyperammonaemia. All patients have been male, but no specific pedigree evidence for sex-linked or autosomal recessive inheritance is available. Treatment is that for urea cycle disorders (see below). The usefulness of carbamylglutamate is being explored (Bachmann et al 1982).

Carbamylphosphate synthetase I deficiency (CPS-I)

CPS-I is the first enzyme in the urea cycle and forms carbamylphosphate from ammonium and bicarbonate ions with the energy provided by two ATP molecules. The enzyme uses magnesium as a cofactor and is dependent upon acetylglutamate as an allosteric activator. It is located in the liver mitochondrion and may constitute as much as 25% of the protein in that organelle (Brusilow & Horwich 1989).

CPS-I deficiency has been documented or inferred in a number of patients, some with acute neonatal hyperammonaemia and others with a more indolent presentation. Residual enzyme activity has varied from less than 1% of normal to 5–15% (Walser 1983). In at least one case enzyme protein was entirely absent (Graf et al 1984).

Hyperammonaemia with generalized amino acidaemia and relatively normal acid base balance is the typical biochemical presentation. When the enzyme deficit is severe, plasma citrulline levels are practically undetectable (Brusilow & Horwich 1989). It is distinguished in the acute presentation from ornithine transcarbamylase deficiency by normal or reduced levels of orotic acid in the urine.

The gene for carbamyl phosphate synthetase I has been cloned and mapped to chromosome 7. Reliable carrier testing (using either physiological or recombinant DNA approaches) is not available, and prenatal diagnosis techniques are limited to liver biopsy or to haplotype analysis in a minority of families (Adcock & O'Brien 1984, Fearon et al 1986).

Ornithine transcarbamylase deficiency

Ornithine transcarbamylase (OTC), an X–linked enzyme (Xp21) found in the mitochondrial matrix, is the second enzyme of the urea cycle. It is responsible for catalyzing the condensation of carbamylphosphate and ornithine to form citrulline (Brusilow & Horwich 1989).

Male infants with OTC deficiency usually have an intractable and lethal neonatal hyperammonaemic course. Blood ammonia levels always exceed 1000 μM. This is accompanied by generalized amino acidaemia and amino aciduria with particular elevations of glutamine, alanine and glutamate in the plasma. Citrulline concentration is reduced and may be undetectable. Partial enzyme deficiencies have been described; these lead to a more mild presentation than that outlined above.

Most female carriers of the gene are asymptomatic. A minority may have signs of chronic mild hyperammonaemia, intermittent acute hyperammonaemia, or both. As a consequence the IQ of this population may be reduced (Brusilow & Horwich 1989). Rarely, a female carrier presents in a manner similar to that of a severely affected male, presumably as an extreme example of disproportionate inactivation of the normal X chromosome. A deficiency of OTC in females may be one cause of aversion to protein and/or cyclic vomiting. At least one of our patients with arginase deficiency became hyperammonaemic at the time of her menstrual periods and a similar phenomenon in some female OTC carriers would not be unexpected.

In contrast to CPS-I deficiency, excretion of orotic acid in the urine of patients with OTC deficiency is markedly elevated, and is used to distinguish these two conditions (and presumably acetylglutamate synthetase deficiency as well). This occurs because the accumulation of carbamylphosphate is shunted to pyrimidine metabolism via CPS-II (Fig. 93.9). CPS-II is a different enzyme from CPS-I, is located in the cytoplasm, and requires glutamate as a cofactor. Patients with partial OTC deficiency and intermittent symptoms may have normal orotic acid excretion and plasma citrulline concentration.

OTC is found primarily in liver and is not detectable in cultured fibroblasts or leucocytes. In affected males the enzyme is virtually absent, with less than 1% of normal activity. In symptomatic females the enzyme activity has been shown to vary from 10% to 40% of normal.

The allele for OTC has been shown to be X–linked by pedigree data (Short et al 1973), the demonstration of two populations of hepatocytes in female carriers (Ricciuti et al 1976), and by genetic linkage and in situ hybridization using cloned cDNA (Brusilow & Horwich 1989). X–linkage explains the severe form of the disease in males and the more mild and variable expression in females. A number of techniques have been proposed to detect asymptomatic carrier females, but because of X-inactivation none will detect all carriers. The best is probably the allopurinol challenge proposed by Brusilow and his colleagues (Brusilow & Valle 1987). The drug inhibits orotidine metabolism and allows for orotic acid and orotidine to be detected in female carriers under standard conditions. OTC carriers will have higher levels than non-carriers. The test is distinguished by its safety, since no ammonia load is administered.

The assessment of RFLPs or deletions detected by the cloned OTC cDNA permits prenatal diagnosis in 80% or more of pregnancies of women who are known carriers of OTC (Brusilow & Horwich 1989).

Outcome in the acute form of this disease is uniformly poor. Those who survive the acute hyperammonaemia as newborns are usually left with severe neurological impairment and are subject to recurrent episodes of hyperammonaemia, one of which is usually fatal. More mild manifestations are more successfully managed by the methods outlined below.

Citrullinaemia

The condensation of citrulline (previously transported out of the mitochondrion) and aspartate to form argininosuccinic acid (ASA) is catalyzed by ASA synthetase (Fig. 93.9). Deficiency of this enzyme leads to citrullinaemia, citrullinuria, hyperammonaemia and orotic aciduria. The diagnosis of this deficiency is not difficult as massive amounts of citrulline are found in both plasma and urine. Confirmation of the enzyme deficiency may be carried out in fibroblast extracts. In practice this is not often done since ASA synthetase deficiency is the only known cause of massive citrulline elevation in plasma.

The clinical picture of patients with citrullinaemia varies in severity with residual enzyme activity; some patients have a course so benign that no disorder is suspected (Brusilow & Horwich 1989). Genetic heterogeneity for the disorder has been shown by variation in residual enzymatic activity in liver or cultured skin fibroblasts, by variation in the kinetic parameters of the residual enzymatic activity, and by examination of the structural gene and its messenger RNA using an ASA synthetase cDNA clone (Su et al 1983, Walser 1983, Brusilow & Horwich 1989).

The ASA synthetase locus is located on chromosome 9 and clinical deficiency of the enzyme is inherited in an autosomal recessive manner (Carritt et al 1977). Heterozygote detection by protein intolerance or enzymatic assay in fibroblasts is unreliable. Prenatal diagnosis is easy, since affected patients accumulate elevated levels of citrulline in the amniotic fluid at midtrimester. An indirect enzyme assay, measuring the rate of citrulline incorporation into protein as compared with leucine, is arduous and less reliable (Beaudet et al 1986).

Argininosuccinic aciduria

ASA is cleaved into two smaller molecules, arginine and fumarate, in an equilibrium reaction catalyzed by ASA lyase. The enzyme is active in liver, brain and kidney. In the latter organ, at least, working in concert with ASA synthetase, it is responsible for synthesizing most of the arginine used for biosynthetic purposes (Walser 1983, Brusilow & Horwich 1989). Deficiency of ASA lyase leads to marked elevations of ASA in plasma, urine and CSF, and a variety of tissues (Walser 1983, Brusilow & Horwich 1989). The enzyme is present in red cells and fibroblasts.

Symptoms associated with ASA lyase deficiency may vary from neonatal hyperammonaemic crises to mild mental retardation or aversion to protein. Some patients are asymptomatic. All patients appear to have at least some degree of trichorrhexis nodosa, a nodular condition of hair causing it to be friable.

ASA lyase has been cloned and mapped to chromosome 12 (O'Brien et al 1986). Its deficiency is inherited in an autosomal recessive manner. Heterozygote detection is possible, primarily by enzymatic means. Prenatal diagnosis is accomplished through ASA accumulation in amniotic fluid. The indirect assay of ASA lyase by measuring the conversion of radioactive citrulline to arginine and the incorporation of arginine into protein is considered to be less reliable than substrate accumulation, and therefore unnecessary (Fleisher et al 1979).

Sequencing of the ASA lyase cDNA has revealed its remarkable similarity to, if not identity with, the lens structural protein delta-crystallin (Piatigorsky et al 1988). Duck crystallin has ASA lyase activity. The significance of these provocative findings for both biochemistry and evolution remains to be determined.

Hyperargininaemia

Like the previous two disorders, a defect in arginase, the final enzyme in the urea cycle that catalyzes the hydrolysis of arginine to urea and ornithine, is named after the substrate that accumulates as a result of its deficiency. Arginase is most active in liver, but is expressed at lower levels in a variety of other tissues, including red blood cells. Red cells may be used to measure the enzyme for diagnosis (Walser 1983). A second isozyme of arginase, encoded by a separate gene, is localized to the mitochondrion and is more widely distributed than its more abundant namesake (Grody et al 1987).

Clinical symptoms of liver arginase deficiency are more subtle and occur at a later age than those of the other urea cycle defects. Recognized episodes of hyperammonaemia are the presenting symptoms in only a minority of patients. Most patients experience progressive spasticity beginning at age 2 or 3 years with obvious intellectual loss beginning somewhat later. It is the only urea cycle defect in which cortical and pyramidal tract signs predominate. More than 80% of reported patients are still alive, some are nearly 30 years of age. It seems likely that the mild clinical course in these patients is due to the presence of residual activity as a result of the existence of the second arginase isozyme, whose activity appears augmented as a consequence of hyperargininaemia (Grody et al 1987). Although most patients are severely retarded, therapy is beneficial and may largely prevent symptoms if begun early and pre-emptively.

An increased concentration of arginine is found in the plasma and CSF of all patients, but urinary amino acid excretion may be normal in some patients most of the time and in all patients some of the time. The pattern of urinary amino acid excretion may be confused with cystinuria.

Arginase deficiency is inherited in an autosomal recessive manner; parents have half normal arginase activity. A full-length cDNA for arginase has been obtained and the gene maps to 6q23 (Grody et al 1987). Prenatal diagnosis should be possible, since the affected enzyme is found in red blood cells at 16–20 weeks of gestation (Spector et al 1980). Arginase found in chorionic villi is of the mitochondrial type and cannot be used for prenatal diagnosis (unpublished observations). Two RFLPs found at the arginase locus are of too low a frequency to be generally useful for prenatal diagnosis or for linkage analysis (Brusilow & Horwich 1989).

Treatment of urea cycle disorders

The two linchpins of therapy for urea cycle disorders are the diminution of the amount of ammonia that must be detoxified, and the removal of the ammonia that is formed. Treatment can be divided into that for acute life-threatening hyperammonaemia, and that used between episodes to keep ammonia levels near normal values. Details of these approaches are well described (Brusilow 1985, Brusilow & Horwich 1989). Ammonia is derived from the amino acids of protein, either ingested or endogenously catabolized as part of normal turnover or breakdown and heightened by intercurrent events. Over the short term, increased catabolism presents a far greater threat and must be more feared than small variations in exogenous protein intake. Any more than 12–15 hours of anorexia and caloric deprivation is likely to trigger gluconeogenesis and hyperammonaemia.

When patients become ill, maintenance of fluid intake with sugared juices is essential. If unsuccessful, earlier, rather than later, intravenous intervention is recommended. Adequate calories will remove the hypoglycaemic stimulus to protein catabolism. Dietary intake of protein should be limited to 1–2 gm/kg/24 hours for infants and 0.5–1.0 gm/kg/24 hours for older children. The quality of the dietary protein may be enhanced by the use of an essential amino acid preparation if required. Surprising flexibility in protein intake is permitted, providing plasma levels of amino acids approximate the normal range and hypoaminoacidaemia is not permitted to function as a stimulus to endogenous protein catabolism.

A major breakthrough in the therapy of these disorders occurred when Brusilow and his colleagues devised a number of means to divert ammonia from urea production and reduce plasma ammonia. These involve the recognition that arginine may become an essential amino acid and that indirect removal of amino acids in the process of organic acid detoxification will divert nitrogen away from the urea cycle (Brusilow 1985, Brusilow & Horwich 1989).

The amino acid product of the first two steps of the urea cycle catalyzed by CPS-I and OTC is citrulline; the next two steps catalyzed by ASA synthetase and ASA lyase convert citrulline to arginine. Hydrolysis of arginine produces the ornithine needed to react with carbamyl phosphate, which carries the first of the two ammonia molecules destined to be excreted as urea. It seems that all patients with deficiencies of the first four enzymes of the urea cycle may be deficient in arginine, and arginine supplementation is an appropriate part of the therapy (Brusilow 1985, Brusilow & Horwich 1989). In patients with CPS-I or OTC deficiency, the substitution of citrulline for arginine is desirable; citrulline is efficiently converted to arginine and in the process removes another nitrogen molecule from the ammonia pool. In the case of ASA synthetase and ASA lyase deficiencies, higher amounts of arginine reduce blood and body ammonia levels, and promote their conversion into the more readily excreted compounds citrulline and argininosuccinate (Brusilow & Horwich 1989).

The organic anions benzoate and phenylacetate (or phenylbutyrate) are excreted respectively as benzoylglycine (hippurate) or phenylacetylglutamine. Resynthesis of glycine requires one molecule of ammonia and two of glutamine. Administration of either or both of these compounds in stoichiometric amounts diverts ammonia from the urea cycle and, in patients with urea cycle enzymopathies, reduces the accumulation of ammonia and other metabolites proximal to the enzymatic deficiency (Brusilow & Horwich 1989). Their use has greatly diminished the frequency and intensity of intercurrent hyperammonaemic episodes and has been associated with a markedly improved prognosis for patients with these disorders.

The hyperornithinaemias

Two inborn errors of metabolism cause elevated levels of plasma ornithine: (1) gyrate atrophy of the retina with hyperornithaemia; and (2) homocitrullinuria and hyperornithinaemia associated with hyperammonaemia.

Hyperornithinaemia with gyrate atrophy

Gyrate atrophy of the retina associated with a 10–20-fold elevation of plasma ornithine was described in the Finnish population in 1973. The disorder primarily affects vision with no associated problems in intellectual development (Valle & Simell 1989). Visual loss begins to occur during the second decade and is slowly progressive. The retinal atrophy begins in the periphery with loss of the pigment epithelium. The fundal picture is characterized by sharply defined margins of choroidal atrophy which slowly progress towards the posterior pole of the eye.

A deficiency of ornithine aminotransferase (OAT) in affected patients has been documented in cultured fibroblasts (Valle & Simell 1989). Clinical studies suggest that some patients may respond to pyridoxal phosphate by lowering their plasma ornithine concentration (Berson et al 1981, Weleber & Kennaway 1981). One study reported an improvement in vision following restriction of dietary ornithine (Kaiser-Kupfer et al 1981, Valle & Simell 1989).

The disorder is inherited as an autosomal recessive trait. The majority of reported patients have been of Finnish origin, although patients of other ethnic groups have been identified. Heterozygotes have been noted to have an abnormal response to ornithine loading and to have less than normal enzyme activity in cultured cells (Valle & Simell 1989). Prenatal diagnosis is feasible since the enzyme is expressed in cultured cells.

The cDNA for OAT has been cloned and the gene is located on chromosome 10 (Mitchell et al 1988b). A pseudogene is found on the short arm of the X chromosome. Mutations have been identified in a number of patients and two independent mutations have been found in the Finnish population (Mitchell et al 1988a, 1989).

Hyperornithinaemia-hyperammonaemia-homocitrullinuria syndrome

This syndrome is as infrequent as its name is uneuphonious. The name describes the three cardinal biochemical features of the disorder. Ornithine concentration in plasma is usually 2–4 times normal values (far lower than in gyrate atrophy) and ammonia is rarely greater than three times the upper limit of normal. Homocitrulline is always detectable in the urine and may be the predominant urinary amino acid.

The patients show the symptoms of moderate hyperammonaemia with anorexia, vomiting and episodes of lethargy and coma. Some neurological damage is quite general and most patients have had mental retardation, some relatively severe. The retinal changes of OAT deficiency are not seen (Valle & Simell 1989).

The primary defect has not been shown unambiguously, but is believed to reside in the uptake of ornithine by the mitochondrion (Fell et al 1974). Ornithine aminotransferase levels are normal. Shih et al have demonstrated defective ornithine metabolism in fibroblasts from patients with the disorder, but the basis for this is unknown (Shih et al 1981). The cause of homocitrullinuria is unknown, but homocitrulline has been reported in a number of other defects of ammonia metabolism, albeit with less regularity.

Treatment is symptomatic and involves limiting protein intake and diverting ammonia from the urea cycle with sodium benzoate and sodium phenylbutyrate.

REFERENCES

Adcock M W, O'Brien W E 1984 Molecular cloning of cDNA for rat and human carbamyl phosphate synthetase I. Journal of Biological Chemistry 259: 13471–13478

Applegarth D A, Ingram P, Kingston J, Hardwick D F 1974 Hyperprolinemia type II. Clinical Biochemistry 7: 14–22

Avery M E, Clow C L, Menkes J H, Ramos A, Scriver C R, Stern L, Wasserman B P 1967 Transient tyrosinemia of the newborn: dietary and clinical aspects. Pediatrics 39: 378–384

Avigad S, Cohen B E, Woo S L C, Shiloh Y 1987 A specific deletion within the phenylalanine hydroxylase gene is common to most Yemenite Jewish phenylketonuria patients. American Journal of Human Genetics 41: A205

Bachmann C, Colombo J P, Jaggi K 1982 N-acetylglutamate synthetase (NAGS) deficiency: diagnosis, clinical observations and treatment. In: Lowenthal A, Mori A, Marescau B (eds) Urea cycle diseases. Plenum, New York, p 39–45

Bachmann C, Brandis M, Weissenbarth-Riedel E, Burghard R, Colombo J P 1988 N-acetylglutamate synthetase deficiency, a second patient. Journal of Inherited Metabolic Disease 11: 191–193

Bank W J, Morrow G 1972 A familial spinal cord disorder with hyperglycinemia. Archives of Neurology 27: 136–148

Bartholome K, Dresel A 1982 Studies on the molecular defect in phenylketonuria and hyperphenylalaninemia using antibodies against phenylalanine hydroxylase. Journal of Inherited Metabolic Disease 5: 7–10

Beaudet A L, O'Brien W E, Bock H-G O, Freytag S O, Su T-S 1986 The human argininosuccinate synthetase locus and citrullinemia. In: Harris H, Hirschhorn K (eds) Advances in human genetics. Plenum, New York, vol. 15. p 161–195

Belanger L, Belanger M, Prive L, Larochelle J, Tremblay M, Aubin G 1973 Tyrosinemia hereditaire et α-1-foetoproteine, 1. Interet clinique de l'α-foeto-proteine dans la tyrosinemie hereditaire. Pathologie et Biologie 21: 449–455

Berger R, Michals K, Galbraeth J, Matalon R 1988 Tyrosinemia type Ib caused by maleylacetoacetase isomerase deficiency: a new enzyme defect. Pediatric Research 23: 328A

Bergeron P, Laberge C, Grenier A 1974 Hereditary tyrosinemia in the province of Quebec: prevalence at birth and geographic distribution. Clinical Genetics 5: 157–162

Berson E L, Shih V E, Sullivan P L 1981 Ocular findings in patients with gyrate atrophy on pyridoxine and low protein, low arginine diets. Ophthalmology 88: 311–315

Boers G H J, Smals A G H, Trijbels F J M et al 1985 Heterozygosity for homocystinuria in premature peripheral and cerebral occlusive arterial disease. New England Journal of Medicine 313: 709–715

Brusilow S W 1985 Inborn errors of urea synthesis. In: Lloyd J K, Scriver C R (eds) Genetic and metabolic disease in pediatrics. Butterworths, London, p 140–165

Brusilow S W, Horwich A L 1989 Urea cycle enzymes. In: Scriver C L, Beaudet A L, Sly W S, Valle D (eds) The metabolic basis of inherited disease, 6th edn. McGraw Hill, New York, p 629–663

Brusilow S, Valle D 1987 Allopurinol induced orotidinuria: a test of heterozygosity for ornithine transcarbamylase deficiency. Pediatric Research 21: 289A

Cabalska B, Duszynska N, Borzymowska J, Zorska K, Koslacz-Folga A, Bozkowa K 1977 Termination of dietary treatment in phenylketonuria. European Journal of Pediatrics 126: 253–260

Carpenter T O, Levy H L, Holtrop M E, Shih V E, Anast C S 1985 Lysinuric protein intolerance presenting as childhood osteoporosis: clinical and skeletal response to citrulline therapy. New England Journal of Medicine 312: 290–294

Carritt B, Goldfarb P S G, Hooper M L, Slack C 1977 Chromosome assignment of a human gene for argininosuccinate synthetase expression in Chinese hamster X human somatic cell hybrids. Experimental Cell Research 106: 71–78

Carson N A J, Cusworth D C, Dent C E, Field C M B, Neill D W, Westall R G 1963 Homocystinuria: a new inborn error of metabolism associated with mental deficiency. Archives of Disease in Childhood 38: 425–436

Cederbaum S D 1984 Phenylketonuria. In: Velazquez A, Bourges H (eds) Genetic factors in nutrition. Academic Press, San Diego, p 79–91

Cederbaum S D 1985 Disorders of lysine metabolism. In: Kelley V C (ed) Practice of pediatrics. Harper & Row, Philadelphia, chapter 61

Chadefaux B, Rethore M O, Raoul O, Ceballos I, Poissonier M, Gilgenkrantz S, Allard D 1985 Cystathionine beta synthase: gene dosage effect in trisomy 21. Biochemical and Biophysical Research Communications 128: 40–44

Childs B, Nyhan W L, Borden M, Bard L, Cooke R E 1961 Idiopathic hyperglycinuria: new disorder of amino acid metabolism I. Pediatrics 27: 522–538

Clow C L, Laberge C, Scriver C R 1975 Neonatal hypertyrosinemia and evidence for deficiency of ascorbic acid in Arctic and subarctic peoples. Canadian Medical Association Journal 113: 624–626

Clow C L, Reade T M, Scriver C R 1981 Outcome of early and long-term management of classical maple syrup urine disease. Pediatrics 68: 856–862

Colombo J P, Vasella F, Humbel R, Buergi W 1967 Lysine intolerance with periodic ammonia intoxication. American Journal of Diseases of Children 113: 138–141

Cooper B A, Rosenblatt D S 1987 Inherited defects of

vitamin B-12 metabolism. Annual Review of Nutrition 7: 291–320

Coulombe J T, Kammerer B L, Levy H L, Hirsch B Z, Scriver C R 1983 Histidinemia. Part III: Impact; a prospective study. Journal of Inherited Metabolic Disease 6: 58–61

Dancis J, Hutzler J, Rokkones T 1967a Intermittent branched-chain ketonuria: variant of maple syrup urine disease. New England Journal of Medicine 276: 84–89

Dancis J, Hutzler J, Tada K, Wada Y, Morikawa T, Arakawa T 1967b Hypervalinemia. A defect in valine transamination. Pediatrics 39: 813–817

Dancis J, Hutzler J, Woody N C, Cox R P 1976 Multiple enzyme defects in familial hyperlysinemia. Pediatric Research 10: 686–691

Dancis J, Hutzler J, Ampola M G, Shih V E, van Gelderen H H, Kirby L T, Woody N C 1983 The prognosis of hyperlysinemia: an interim report. American Journal of Human Genetics 35: 438–442

Danks D M, Bartholome K, Clayton B E et al 1979 Malignant hyperphenylalanenemia – current status (June 1977). Journal of Inherited Metabolic Disease 1: 49–53

Danner D J, Elsas L J 1989 Disorders of branched chain amino acid and acid metabolism. In: Scriver C R, Beaudet H L, Sly W S, Valle D (eds) The metabolic basis of inherited disease, 6th edn. McGraw-Hill, New York, p 671–692

Danner D J, Armstrong N, Heffelfinger S C, Sewell E T, Priest J H, Elsas L J 1985 Absence of branched chain acyl-transferase as a cause of maple syrup urine disease. Journal of Clinical Investigation 75: 858–860

Danpure C J, Jennings P R, Penketh R J, Wise P J, Rodeck C H 1988 Prenatal exclusion of primary hyperoxaluria type I. (Letter) Lancet 1: 367

DiLella A, Woo S L C 1987 Molecular basis of phenylketonuria and its clinical applications. Molecular Biology and Medicine 4: 183–192

Donald L J, Wang H S, Hamerton J L 1982 Assignment of the gene for cystathionase (CTH) to human chromosome 16. Cytogenetics and Cell Genetics 32: 368

Efron M L 1965 Familial hyperprolinemia: report of a second case, associated with congenital renal malformation, hereditary hematuria and mild mental retardation, with demonstration of enzyme defect. New England Journal of Medicine 22: 1243–1254

Efron M L, Bixby E M, Pryles C V 1965 Hydroxyprolinemia. II. A rare metabolic disease due to deficiency of enzyme 'hydroxyproline oxidase'. New England Journal of Medicine 272: 1299–1309

Endres W, Siebold H 1978 Renal excretion of cystathionine and creatinine in humans at different ages. Clinica Chimica Acta 87: 425–435

Erbe R W 1977 Prenatal diagnosis of inherited disease. In: Altman P L, Katz D D (eds) Biological handbooks II, human health and disease, FASEB, Bethesda, p 91–97

Fearon E R, Mallonee R L, Phillips, J A III, O'Brien W E, Brusilow S W, Adcock M W, Kirby L T 1986 Genetic analysis of carbamyl phosphate synthetase I deficiency. Human Genetics 70: 207–215

Fell V, Pollitt R, Sampson G A, Wright T 1974 Ornithinemia, hyperammonemia and homocitrullinuria. A disease associated with mental retardation and possibly caused by defective mitochondrial transport. American Journal of Diseases of Children 127: 752–759

Fellman J H, Buist N R M, Kennaway N G, Swanson R E 1972 The source of aromatic ketoacids in tyrosinemia and phenylketonuria. Clinica Chimica Acta 39: 243–246

Fellows F C I, Carson N A J 1974 Enzyme studies in a patient with saccharopinuria: a defect in lysine metabolism. Pediatric Research 8: 42–47

Fenton W A, Rosenberg L E 1989 Inherited disorders of cobalamin transport and metabolism. In: Scriver C R, Beaudet A L, Sly W S, Valle D (eds) The metabolic basis of inherited disease, 6th edn. McGraw-Hill, New York, p 2065–2082

Finkelstein J D, Mudd S H, Irreverre F, Laster L 1966 Deficiencies of cystathionase and serine dehydratase in cystathioninuria. Proceedings of the National Academy of Sciences USA 55: 865–874

Fisch R O, McCabe E R B, Doeden D, Koep L J, Kohlhoff J G, Silverman A, Starzl T E 1978 Homotransplantation of the liver in a patient with hepatoma and hereditary tyrosinemia. Journal of Pediatrics 93: 592–596

Fleisher L D, Rassin D K, Desnick R J, Saliven H R, Rogers P, Bean M, Gaull G E 1979 Argininosuccinic aciduria: prenatal studies in a family at risk. American Journal of Human Genetics 31: 439–445

Fois A, Borgogni P, Cioni M et al 1986 Presentation of the data of the Italian registry for oculocutaneous tyrosinemia. Journal of Inherited Metabolic Disease 9 (Supplement 2): 262–264

Folling A 1934 Uber ausscheidung von phenylbrenztraubensaure in den harn als stoffwechselanomalie in verbindung mit imbezillitat. Zeitschrift fur Physiologische Chemie 277: 169–176

Fowler B. Borresen A L, Boman N 1982 Prenatal diagnosis of homocystinuria. Lancet II: 875

Freeman J M, Finkelstein J D, Mudd S H 1975 Folate-responsive homocystinuria and 'schizophrenia': a defect in methylation due to deficiency 5,10-methylenetetrahydrofolate reductase activity. New England Journal of Medicine 292: 491–496

Garcia-Castro J M, Isales-Forsythe C M, Levy H L, Shih V E, Velez M, Gonzalez-Rios M, Terres C 1982 Prenatal diagnosis of non-ketotic hyperglycinemia. New England Journal of Medicine 306: 79–81

Gerritsen T, Waisman H A 1964 Homocystinuria; an error in the metabolism of methionine. Pediatrics 33: 413–421

Gerritsen T, Waisman H A 1966 Hypersarcosinemia: an inborn error of metabolism. New England Journal of Medicine 275: 66–69

Ghadimi H, Partington M W 1967 Salient features of histidinemia. American Journal of Diseases of Children 113: 83–87

Goldsmith L A, Laberge C 1989 Tyrosinemia and related disorders. In: Scriver C R, Beaudet A L, Sly W S, Valle D (eds) The metabolic basis of inherited disease, 6th edn. McGraw-Hill, New York, p 547–576

Goldstein J L, Campbell R K, Gartler S M 1972 Cystathionine synthetase activity in human lymphocytes: induction by phytohemagglutinin. Journal of Clinical Investigation 51: 1034–1037

Goldstein J L, Campbell R K, Gartler S M 1973 Homocystinuria: heterozygote detection using phytohemagglutinin-stimulated lymphocytes. Journal of Clinical Investigation 52: 218

Goodman S I, Browder J A, Hiles R A, Miles B S 1972 Hydroxylysinemia: a disorder due to a defect in the metabolism of free hydroxylysine. Biochemical Medicine 6: 344–354

Goto M, Shinno H, Ichihara A 1977 Isozyme patterns of branched chain amino acid transaminase in human tissues and tumors. Gann 68: 663–672

Graf L, McIntyre P, Hoogenraad N, Brown G, Haan E A 1984 A carbamylphosphate synthetase deficiency with no detectable immunoreactive enzyme and no translatable mRNA. Journal of Inherited Metabolic Disease 7: 104–106

Grenier A, Lescault A, Laberge C, Gagne R, Mamer O 1982 Detection of succinylacetone and the use of its measurement in mass screening of hereditary tyrosinemia. Clinica Chimica Acta 123: 93–99

Griffin R F, Elsas L J 1975 Classic phenylketonuria: diagnosis through heterozygote detection. Journal of Pediatrics 86: 512–517

Grody W W, Dizikes G J, Cederbaum S D 1987 Human arginase isozymes. In: Isozymes: current topics in biological and medical research. 13: 181–214

Güttler F, Ledley F D, Lidsky A S, DiLella A G, Sullivan S E, Woo S L C 1987 Correlation between polymorphic DNA haplotypes at the phenylalanine hydroxylase locus and clinical phenotype of phenylketonuria. Journal of Pediatrics 110: 68–71

Harker L A, Slichter S J, Scott C R, Ross R 1974 Homocystinemia: vascular injury and arterial thrombosis. New England Journal of Medicine 291: 537–544

Hillman R E 1989 Primary hyperoxalurias. In: Scriver C R, Beaudet A L, Sly W S, Valle D (eds) The metabolic basis of inherited disease, 6th edn. McGraw-Hill, New York, p 933–944

Hiraga K, Kochi H, Hayasaka K, Kikurchi G, Nyhan W L 1981 Defective glycine cleavage system in nonketotic hyperglycinemia: occurrence of a less active glycine decarboxylase and an abnormal aminomethyl carrier protein. Journal of Clinical Investigation 68: 525–534

Hiraga K, Kure S, Yamamoto M, Ishiguro Y, Suzuki T 1988 Cloning of cDNA encoding human H-protein, a constituent of the glycine cleavage system. Biochemical and Biophysical Research Communications 151: 758–762

Hollowell J G Jr., Hall W K, Coryell M E, McPherson J Jr., Hahn D A 1969 Homocystinuria and organic aciduria in a patient with vitamin B$_{12}$ deficiency. Lancet 2: 1428

Holtzman N A, Kronmal R A, van Doornick W, Azen C, Koch R 1986 Effect of age at loss of dietary control on intellectual performance and behaviour of children with phenylketonuria. New England Journal of Medicine 314: 593–598

Hooft C, Carton D, Somyn W 1967 Pyridoxine trreatment in homocystinuria. (Letter) Lancet I: 1384

Hutzler J, Dancis J 1975 Lysine-ketoglutarate reductase in human tissues. Biochimica et Biophysica Acta 377: 42–51

Indo Y, Kitano A, Endo F, Akaboshi I, Matsuda I 1987 Altered kinetic properties of the branched chain α-keto acid dehydrogenase complex due to mutation of the α subunit of the branched chain α-keto acid decarboxylase (E1) component in lymphoblastoid cells derived from patients with maple syrup urine disease. Journal of Clinical Investigation 80: 63–70

Indo Y, Akaboshi I, Nobukuni Y, Endo F, Matsuda I 1988 Maple syrup urine disease: a possible biochemical basis for the clinical heterogeneity. Human Genetics 80: 6–10

Jay D L, Wang H S, Hammerton J L 1982 Assignment of the gene for cystathionase (CTH) to human chromosome 16. Cytogenetics & Cell Genetics 32: 268

Jervis G A 1953 Phenylpyruvic oligophrenia: deficiency of phenylalanine oxidizing system. Proceedings of the Society for Experimental Biology and Medicine 82: 514–515

Jeune M, Collombel C, Michel M, David M, Guibault P, Guerrier G, Albert J 1970 Hyperleucinisoleucinemie par defaut partiel de transamination associee a une hyperprolinemie de type 2. Observation familiale d'une double aminoacidopathie. Semaine des Hopitaux de Paris (Annales de Pediatrie) 17: 85–99

Johnson J L, Wadman S K 1989 Molybdenum cofactor deficiency. In: Scriver C R, Beaudet A L, Sly W S, Valle D (eds) The metabolic basis of inherited disease, 6th edn. McGraw-Hill, New York, p 1463–1474

Justice P, O'Flynn M E, Hsia D Y 1967 Phenylalanine hydroxylase activity in hyperphenylalaninemia. Lancet 1: 928–930

Kaiser-Kupfer M I, De Monosterio F, Valle D, Walser M, Brusilow S W 1981 Visual results of a long-term trial of a low arginine diet in gyrate atrophy of the choroid and retina. Ophthalmology 88: 307–310

Kalafatic Z, Lipovac K, Jezerinac Z, Juretic D, Dumic M, Zurga B, Res L 1980 A liver urocanase deficiency. Metabolism 29: 1013–1019

Kang E S, Kaufman S, Gerald P S 1970 Clinical and biochemical observation of patients with atypical phenylketonuria. Pediatrics 45: 83–92

Kaufman S 1976 The phenylalanine hydroxylating system in phenylketonuria and its variants. Biochemical Medicine 15: 42–54

Knox W E 1972 Phenylketonuria. In: Stanbury J B, Wyngaarden J B, Fredrickson D S (eds) The metabolic basis of inherited disease, 3rd edn. McGraw-Hill, New York, p 266–295

Koch J, Stokstad E L R, Williams H E, Smith L H 1967 Deficiency of 2-oxo-glutarate glyoxylate carboligase activity in primary hyperoxaluria. Proceedings of the National Academy of Sciences USA 57: 1123–1129

Koch R, Azen C, Friedman E G, Williamson M L 1984 Paired comparisons between early treated PKU children and their matched sibling controls on intelligence and school achievement test results at eight years of age. Journal of Inherited Metabolic Disease 7: 86–90

Koslow S H, Butler I J 1977 Biogenic amine biosynthesis defect in dihydropteridine reductase deficiency. Science 198: 522–525

Kraus J P, Williamson C L, Figaira F A, Yang-Feng T L, Munke M, Francke U, Rosenberg L E 1986 Cloning and screening with nanogram amounts of immunopurified mRNAs: cDNA cloning and chromosome mapping of cystathionine beta synthase and the beta subunit of propionyl-CoA carboxylase. Proceedings of the National Academy of Sciences USA 83: 2047–2051

Krause W, Halminski M, McDonald M, Dembure P, Freides D, Elsas L 1985 Biochemical and neuropsychological effects of elevated plasma phenylalanine in patients with treated phenylketonuria. Journal of Clinical Investigation 75: 40–48

Kretchmer N, Levine S Z, McNamara H, Barnett H L 1956 Certain aspects of tyrosine metabolism in the young. I. The development of the tyrosine oxidizing system in human liver. Journal of Clinical Investigation 35: 236–244

Kvittingen E A, Jellum E, Stokke O 1981 Assay of fumaryl acetoacetate fumarylhydrolase in human liver: deficient activity in a case of hereditary tyrosinemia. Clinica Chimica Acta 115: 311–319

La Du B N, Howell R R, Jacoby G A et al 1963 Clinical and biochemical studies on two cases of histidinemia. Pediatrics 32: 216–227

Langenbeck U, Grimm T, Rudiger H W, Passarge E 1975 Heterozygote tests and genetic counselling in maple syrup urine disease. An application of Bayes' theorem. Humangenetik 27: 315–322

Ledley F D, Levy H L, Woo S L C 1986 Molecular analysis of the inheritance of phenylketonuria and mild hyperphenylalanininemia in families with both disorders. New England Journal of Medicine 314: 1276–1280

Lenke R R, Levy H L 1980 Maternal phenylketonuria and hyperphenylalaninemia. New England Journal of Medicine 303: 1202–1208

Levy H L 1973 Genetic screening. Advances in Human Genetics 4: 1–104

Levy H L, Karolkewicz V, Houghton S A, MacGready R A 1970 Screening of the 'normal' population in Massachusetts for phenylketonuria. New England Journal of Medicine 282: 1455–1458

Levy H L, Shih V E, MacCready R A (eds) 1972 Massachusetts metabolic disorders screening program. In: Early diagnosis of human genetic defects. M Harris, Washington DC, US Government Printing Office, p 47–66

Levy H L, Shih V E, Madigan P M 1974 Routine newborn screening for histidinemia. Clinical and biochemical results. New England Journal of Medicine 291: 1214–1219

Levy H L, Coulombe J T, Benjamin R 1984 Massachusetts metabolic screening program. III Sarcosinemia. Pediatrics 74: 509–513

Linblad B, Linstedt S, Steen G 1977 On the enzymatic defects in hereditary tyrosinemia. Proceedings of the National Academy of Sciences USA 74: 4641–4645

Litwer S, Danner D J 1985 Identification of a cDNA clone in lambda gt11 for the transacetylase component of branched chain ketoacid dehydrogenase. Biochemical and Biophysical Research Communications 131: 961–967

Lyon I C T, Procopis P G, Turner B 1971 Cystathioninuria in a well baby population. Acta Paediatrica Scandinavica 60: 324–328

MacDonald M E, Anderson M A, Lockyer J L et al 1987 Physical and genetic localization of quinonoid dihydropteridine reductase gene (QDPR) on short arm of chromosome 4. Somatic Cell and Molecular Genetics 13: 569–574

McInnes R, Kaufman S, Warsh J J et al 1984 Biopterin synthesis defect: treatment with L-dopa and 5-hydroxytryptophan compared with therapy with tetrahydrobiopterin. Journal of Clinical Investigation 73: 458–469

McKusick V A 1988 Mendelian inheritance in man, 8th edn. Johns Hopkins University Press, Baltimore

Markovitz P J, Chuang D T, Cox R P 1984 Familial hyperlysinemia: purification and characterization of the bifunctional aminoadipic semialdehyde synthase with lysine-ketoglutarate reductase and saccharopine dehydrogenase activities. Journal of Biological Chemistry 259: 11643–11646

Matalon R, Naidu S, Hughes J R, Michals K 1983 Non-ketotic hyperglycinemia: treatment with diazepam, a competitor of glycine receptors. Pediatrics 71: 581–584

Medes G 1932 A new error of tyrosine metabolism: tyrosinosis. The intermediary metabolism of tyrosine and phenylalanine. Biochemical Journal 26: 917–940

Menkes J H, Hurst P L, Craig J M 1954 A new syndrome: progressive familial infantile cerebral dysfunction associated with an unusual urinary substance. Pediatrics 14: 462–466

Menkes J H, Welcher D W, Levi H S, Dallas J, Gretsky N E 1972 Relationship of elevated blood tyrosine to the ultimate intellectual performance of premature infants. Pediatrics 49: 218–224

Mesavage C, Nance C S, Flannery D B, Weiner D L, Sucky S F, Wolf B 1983 Glycine-serine ratios in amniotic fluid: an unreliable indicator for the prenatal diagnosis of an NKH. Clinical Genetics 23: 354–358

Mitchell G A, Brody L C, Looney J et al 1988a An initiator codon mutation in ornithine-delta-aminotransferase causing gyrate atrophy of the choroid and retina. Journal of Clinical Investigation 81: 630–633

Mitchell G A, Looney J E, Brody L C et al 1988b Human ornithine-delta-aminotransferase: cDNA cloning and analysis of the structural gene. Journal of Biological Chemistry 263: 14288–14295

Mitchell G A, Brody L C, Sipila I et al 1989 At least two mutant alleles of ornithine-delta-aminotransferase cause gyrate atrophy of choroid and retina in Finns. Proceedings of the National Academy of Sciences USA 86: 197–201

Morris M D, Lewis B D, Doolan D D, Harper H A 1961 Clinical and biochemical observations on an apparently non-fatal variant of branched-chain ketoaciduria (maple syrup urine disease). Pediatrics 28: 918–923

Mudd S H 1985 Vascular disease and homocystine metabolism (editorial). New England Journal of Medicine 313: 751–753

Mudd S H, Finkelstein J D, Irreverre F, Laster L 1964 Homocystinuria: an enzymatic defect. Science 143: 1443–1445

Mudd S H, Irreverre F, Laster L 1967 Sulfite oxidase deficiency in man: demonstration of the enzymatic defect. Science 156: 1599–1601

Mudd S H, Havlik R, Levy H L, McKusick V A, Feinleib M 1981 A study of cardiovascular risk in heterozygotes for homocystinuria. American Journal of Human Genetics. 33: 883–893

Mudd S H, Skovby F, Levy H L et al 1985 The natural history of homocystinuria due to cystathionine β-synthase deficiency. American Journal of Human Genetics 37: 1–31

Mudd S H, Levy H L, Skovby F 1989 Disorders of transsulfuration. In: Scriver C L, Beaudet A L, Sly W S, Valle D (eds) The metabolic basis of inherited disease 6th edn. McGraw Hill, New York, p 693–734

Naylor E W 1986 Screening for PKU cofactor variants. In: Carter T (ed) Genetic disease. Screening and management. Liss, New York, p 211–230

Naylor E W, Ennis D, Davidson G F, Wong L T K, Applegarth D A, Niederwieser A 1987 Guanosine triphosphate cyclohydrolase deficiency: early diagnosis by routine pteridine screening. Pediatrics 79: 374–378

Niederwieser A, Lumbacher W, Curtius H-Ch, Ponzone A, Rey F, Leupold D 1985 Atypical phenylketonuria with "dihydrobiopterin synthesis" deficiency. Absence of phosphate eliminating activity demonstrated in liver. European Journal of Pediatrics 144: 13–16

Nyhan W L 1984 Abnormalities in amino acid metabolism in clinical medicine. Appleton-Century-Crofts, Norwalk p 161

Nyhan W L 1989 Nonketotic hyperglycinemia. In: Scriver C R, Beaudet A L, Sly W S, Valle D (eds) The metabolic basis of inherited disease, 6th edn. McGraw-Hill, New York, p 743–753

O'Brien W E, McInnes R, Kalumuck K, Adcock M 1986 Cloning and sequence anlaysis of cDNA for human arginiosuccinate lyase. Proceedings of the National Academy of Sciences USA 83: 7211–7215

Otulakowski G, Robinson B H 1987 Isolation and sequence determination of cDNA clones for porcine and human lipoamide dehydrogenase: homology to other disulfide oxidoreductases. Journal of Biological Chemistry 262: 17313–17318

Partington M W, Scriver C R, Sass-Kortsak E 1967 Conference on hereditary tyrosinemia. Canadian Medical Association Journal 97: 1045–1101

Pelkonen R, Kivirikko K I 1970 Hydroxyprolinemia. New England Journal of Medicine 283: 451–456

Phang J M, Scriver C R 1989 Disorders of proline and hydroxyproline metabolism. In: Scriver C R, Beaudet A L, Sly W S, Valle D (eds) The metabolic basis of inherited disease, 6th edn. McGraw-Hill, New York, p 577–597

Piatigorsky J, O'Brien W E, Norman B L et al 1988 Gene sharing by delta-crystallin and argininosuccinate lyase. Proceedings of the National Academy of Sciences USA 85: 3479–3483

Rajantie J, Simell O, Rapola J, Perheentupa J 1980 Lysinuric protein intolerance: a two year trial of dietary supplementation therapy with citrulline and lysine. Journal of Pediatrics 97: 927–932

Rama Rao B S, Subhash N M, Marayaman H S 1974 Hydroxyprolinemia: case report. Indian Pediatrics 11: 829–830

Ricciuti F C, Gelehrter T D, Rosenberg L E 1976 X chromosome inactivation in human liver: confirmation of X-linkage of ornithine transcarbamylase. American Journal of Human Genetics 28: 332–338

Roesel R A, Bowyer F, Blankenship R R, Hommes F A 1986 Combined xanthine and sulfite oxidase defect due to a deficiency of molybdenum cofactor. Journal of Inherited Metabolic Diseases 9: 343–347

Rosenblatt D, Mohyuddin F, Scriver C R 1970 Histidinemia discovered by urinary screening after renal transplantation. Pediatrics 46: 47–53

Rosenblatt D S, Cooper B A, Schmutz S M, Zaleski W A, Casey R E 1985 Prenatal vitamin B-12 therapy of a fetus with methylcobalamin deficiency (cobalamin E disease). Lancet I: 1127–1129

Rosenmann A, Scriver C R, Clow C L, Levy H L 1983 Histidinemia. Part II: Impact; a retrospective study. Journal of Inherited Metabolic Disease 6: 54–57

Sardharwalla I B, Fowler B, Robins A J, Komrower G M 1974 Detection of heterozygotes for homocystinuria: study of sulfur containing amino acids in plasma and urine after L-methionine loading. Archives of Disease in Childhood 49: 553–559

Schafer I A, Scriver C R, Efron M L 1962 Familial hyperprolinemia, cerebral dysfunction and renal anomalies occurring in a family with hereditary nephropathy and deafness. New England Journal of Medicine 267: 51–60

Schimke R N, McKusick V A, Huang T, Pollock A D 1965 Homocystinuria, a study of 38 cases in 20 families. Journal of the American Medical Association 193: 711–719

Schulman J D, Lustberg T J, Kennedy J L, Museles M, Seegmiller J E 1970 A new variant of maple syrup urine disease (branched chain ketoaciduria). American Journal of Medicine 49: 118–124

Scott C R, Dassell S E, Clark S H, Chang-Teng C, Swedberg K R 1970a Cystathioninemia: a benign genetic condition. Journal of Pediatrics 76: 571–577

Scott C R, Clark S H, Teng C C, Swedberg K R 1970b Clinical and cellular studies of sarcosinemia. Journal of Pediatrics 77: 805–811

Scriver C R, Clow C L 1980 Phenylketonuria: epitome of human biochemical genetics. New England Journal of Medicine 303: 1336–1342, 1394–1400

Scriver C R, Levy H L 1983 Histidinemia. Part I: reconciling retrospective and prospective findings. Journal of Inherited Metabolic Disease 6: 51–53

Scriver C R, Smith R J, Phang J M 1983 Disorders of proline and hydroxyproline metabolism. In: Stanbury J B, Wyngaarden J B, Fredrickson D S, Goldstein J L, Brown M S (eds) The metabolic basis of inherited disease, 5th edn. McGraw-Hill, New York, chapter 18, p 360–381

Scriver C R, Clow C L, George H 1985 So-called thiamin-responsive maple syrup urine disease: a fifteen year followup of the original patient. Journal of Pediatrics 107: 763–765

Scriver C R, Beaudet A L, Sly W S, Valle D (eds) 1989a The metabolic basis of inherited disease, 6th edn. McGraw Hill, New York

Scriver C R, Kaufman S, Woo S L C 1989b The hyperphenylalaninemias. In: Scriver C R, Beaudet A L, Sly W S, Valle D (eds) The metabolic basis of inherited disease, 6th edn. McGraw-Hill, New York, p 495–546

Sewell A C, Krille M, Wilhelm I 1986 Sarcosinemia in a retarded, amaurotic child. European Journal of Pediatrics 144: 508–510

Shepard T H, Lee L W, Krebs E G 1960 Primary hyperoxaluria II. Genetic studies in a family. Pediatrics 255: 869–871

Shih V E, Abrams J F, Johnson J L et al 1977 Sulfite oxidase deficiency: biochemical and clinical investigations of a hereditary metabolic disorder in sulfur metabolism. New England Journal of Medicine 297: 1022–1028

Shih V E, Mandell R, Herzfeld A 1981 Defective ornithine metabolism in the syndrome of hyperornithinemia, hyperammonemia and homocitrullinuria. Journal of Inherited Metabolic Disease 4: 95–96

Short E M, Conn H O, Snodgrass P J, Campbell A G M, Rosenberg L E 1973 Evidence for X-linked dominant inheritance of ornithine transcarbamylase deficiency. New England Journal of Medicine 288: 7–12

Simell O 1989 Lysinuric protein intolerance and other cationic aminoacidurias. In: Scriver C R, Beaudet A L, Sly W S, Valle D (eds) The metabolic basis of inherited disease, 6th edn. McGraw-Hill, New York, p 2497–2513

Skovby F, Krasslkoff N, Francke U 1984 Assignment of the gene for cystathionine β-synthase to human chromosome 21 in somatic cell hybrids. Human Genetics 65: 291

Snyderman S E, Norton P M, Roitman E, Halt L E Jr. 1964 Maple syrup urine disease, with particular reference to dietotherapy. Pediatrics 34: 454–472

Sogawa H, Oyanagi K, Nakao T 1977 Periodic hyperammonemia, hyperlysinemia and homocitrullinuria associated with decreased arginonosuccinate synthetase and

arginase activities. Pediatric Research 11: 949–953

Spaeth G L, Barber G W 1967 Prevalence of homocystinuria among the mentally retarded: evaluation of a specific screening test. Pediatrics 40: 586–589

Spector E B, Kiernan M, Bernard B, Cederbaum S D 1980 Properties of fetal and adult red blood cell arginase: a possible prenatal diagnostic test for arginase deficiency. American Journal of Human Genetics 32: 79–87

Sturman J A, Gaull G E, Raiha N C R 1970 Absence of cystathionase in human fetal liver: is cystine essential? Science 169: 74–78

Su T-S, Bock H-G O, Beaudet A L, O'Brien W E 1983 Abnormal nRNA for argininosuccinate synthetase in citrullinemia. Nature 301: 533–535

Tada K 1987 Nonketotic hyperglycinemia: clinical and metabolic aspects. Enzyme 38: 27–35

Tada K, Hayasaka K 1987 Non-ketotic hyperglycinemia: clinical and biochemical aspects. European Journal of Pediatrics 146: 221–227

Tuchman M, Freese D K, Sharp H L et al 1985 Persistent succinylacetone excretion after liver transplantation in a patient with hereditary tyrosinemia type I. Journal of Inherited Metabolic Disease 8: 21–24

Tuchman M, Freese D K, Sharp H L, Ramnaraine M L R, Ascher N, Bloomer J 1987 Contribution of extrahepatic tissues to biochemical abnormalities in hereditary tyrosinemia type I. Study of three patients following liver transplant. Journal of Pediatrics 110: 399–403

Valle D, Simell O 1989 The hyperornithinemias. In: Scriver C R, Beaudet A L, Sly W S, Valle D (eds) The metabolic basis of inherited disease, 6th edn. McGraw-Hill, New York, p 599–627

Valle D, Goodman S I, Applegarth D A, Shih V E, Phang J M 1976 Type II hyperprolinemia. Δ'-pyrroline-5-carboxylic acid dehydrogenase deficiency in cultured skin fibroblasts and circulating lymphocytes. Journal of Clinical Investigation 58: 598–603

Wada Y, Tada K, Minagawa A, Yoshida T, Morikawa T, Okamura T 1963 Idiopathic valinemia: probably a new entity of inborn error of valine metabolism. Tohoku Journal of Experimental Medicine 81: 46–55

Walser M 1983 Urea cycle disorders and other hereditary hyperammonemic syndromes. In: Stanbury J B, Wyngaarden J B, Fredrickson D S, Goldstein J L, Brown M S (eds) The metabolic basis of inherited disease. 5th edn. McGraw Hill, New York, p 402–438

Watts R W E, Calne R Y, Rolles K et al 1987 Successful treatment of primary hyperoxaluria type I by combined hepatic and renal transplantation (letter) Lancet II: 474–475

Weleber R G, Kennaway N G 1981 Clinical trial for B_6 for gyrate atrophy of the choroid and retina. Ophthalmology 88: 316–321

Wilcken D E, Wilcken B 1976 The pathogenesis of coronary artery disease: a possible role for methionine metabolism. Journal of Clinical Investigation 57: 1079–1082

Will E J, Bijvoet O L M 1979 Primary oxalosis: clinical and biochemical response to high dose pyridoxine therapy. Metabolism 28: 542–548

Williams H E, Smith L H Jr. 1978 Primary hyperoxaluria. In: Stanbury J B, Wyngaarden J B, Fredrickson D S (eds) The metabolic basis of inherited disease, 4th edn. McGraw-Hill, New York, p 182–204

Wong P W K, Justice P, Hruby M, Weiss E B, Diamond E

1977 Folic acid nonresponsive homocystinuria due to methylene-tetrahydrofolate reductase deficiency. Pediatrics 59: 749–756

Woody N C, Snyder C H, Harris J A 1965 Histidinemia. American Journal of Diseases of Children 110: 606–613

Yendt E R, Cohanim M 1985 Response to a physiologic dose of pyridoxine in type I primary hyperoxaluria. New England Journal of Medicine 312: 953–957

Yoshida T, Tada K, Honda Y, Arakaw T 1971 Urocanic aciduria: a defect in the urocanase activity in the liver of a mentally retarded. Tohoku Journal of Experimental Medicine 104: 305–312

Zannoni V G, La Du B N 1963 Determination of histidine-deaminase in human stratum corneum and its absence in histidinemia. Biochemical Journal 88: 160–162

Zhang B, Kuntz M J, Goodwin G W, Harris R A, Crabb D W 1987 Molecular cloning of cDNA for the $E_{1\alpha}$ subunit of rat liver branched chain α-ketoacid dehydrogenase. Journal of Biological Chemistry 262: 15220–15224

94. Disorders of carbohydrate metabolism

Won G. Ng   Thomas F. Roe   George N. Donnell

INTRODUCTION

Inborn errors of carbohydrate metabolism discussed in this chapter include disaccharidase deficiencies, disorders of monosaccharide metabolism, glycogen storage diseases and gluconeogenic disorders. Additional detailed information may be sought in *Inherited Disorders of Carbohydrate Metabolism* (Burman et al 1980) and *The Metabolic Basis of Inherited Disease* (Scriver et al 1989).

DISACCHARIDASE DEFICIENCIES

The major sources of dietary carbohydrate in man are starch and the disaccharides lactose and sucrose. In adults starch constitutes 60% of the carbohydrate ingested; however, in newborns and young infants the primary carbohydrate is lactose (milk sugar). Sucrose consumption varies widely with the choice of infant formula and other eating habits. The normal digestive process involves the splitting of disaccharides by intestinal hydrolytic enzymes (lactase, sucrase, isomaltase and maltase) into monosaccharides prior to absorption (Fig. 94.1). Defective intestinal absorption of dietary sugars leads to clinical manifestations, such as flatulence, abdominal cramps, diarrhoea, and perianal irritation. Levels of enzymes involved in the hydrolysis of disaccharides may be depressed on either a genetic or acquired basis. The latter situation results from damage to the brush border cells of the small intestine, consequent to infection or other injuries. When enzymatic hydrolysis is impaired, ingested disaccharide accumulates and provides a growth medium for intestinal bacteria which produce carbon dioxide, hydrogen and organic acids. The stools tend to be sour, foamy, loose and watery with an acidic pH. A diagnosis of disaccharidase deficiency may be suspected from the history of symptoms developing in association with the ingestion of a particular sugar and a laboratory finding of disaccharides in the urine. Direct confirmation may be obtained by measuring enzyme activity in intestinal mucosal cells removed on peroral small bowel biopsy. Indirect confirmation of the diagnosis can be made by a disaccharide tolerance test. Disaccharidase deficiency is suggested if the blood glucose curve is flat upon ingestion of the suspect disaccharide.

Lactase deficiency

Primary lactase deficiency is a rare disorder in infants and young children. The disorder is thought to be of genetic origin and inherited as an autosomal recessive trait

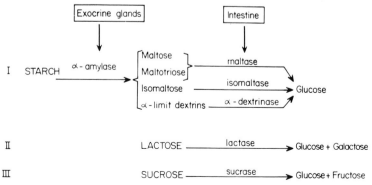

Fig. 94.1 Digestion of carbohydrates.

(Savilahti et al 1983). Another disorder, distinct from inherited lactase deficiency, has been described which begins in early infancy with vomiting and diarrhoea. Lactose, sucrose amd amino acids are excreted in the urine in increased amounts (Durand 1958). Death may result unless lactose is removed from the diet. Autopsy findings include atrophic enteritis and degenerative change in the renal tubule. The basic cause is unknown.

Late onset (adult type) lactase deficiency differs from that encountered in infants. Symptoms usually do not occur until adult life, but occasionally may start at an earlier age. This form of lactase deficiency is common in Mediterraneans, Blacks, Asians, American Indians and Eskimos. Some surveys indicate that more than 60% of adults in these racial groups may have a deficiency of the enzyme lactase. It is not known whether genetic predisposition leads to loss of lactase activity with increasing age or whether a post weaning decrease in intestinal lactase occurs because of dietary change. Thus, the term 'hypolactasia' has also been used to describe this condition (Schmidt & Schmidt 1979). Treatment for patients with lactase deficiency usually consists of a diet free of lactose. In infants, a lactose-free formula or lactose-hydrolyzed human milk have been used (Simila et al 1982). There is usually rapid clinical response.

Sucrase-isomaltase deficiency

The mode of inheritance of this condition appears to be autosomal recessive. An incidence of 0.2% has been reported for North Americans (Peterson & Herber 1967) and 10% for Greenland Eskimos (McNair et al 1972). Clinical manifestations described above tend to be more severe in the younger child and depend upon the amount of ingested sucrose which often comes from fruits and sweetened foods. Absence of sucrase activity is generally associated with absence of isomaltase activity in intestinal cells. Whereas sucrase-isomaltase occurs as an enzyme complex of two distinct subunits, each acting independently of its specific substrate (Conklin et al 1975), genetic deficiency usually results in the absence of cross-reacting material detected by radioimmunoassay, suggesting either a major structural alteration or lack of production of the enzyme molecule (Gray et al 1976). In a patient with the enzyme deficiency, a defect in processing of the oligosaccharide chain was demonstrated (Lloyd & Olsen 1987).

GLUCOSE-GALACTOSE MALABSORPTION

This is a rare disorder in which an acute, profuse, watery diarrhoea develops in newborn infants following initial feeding (Abraham et al 1967). Intestinal disaccharidase

activities are normal. Fructose is absorbed normally, but glucose and galactose are not. There is no significant rise in blood glucose levels following an oral glucose-galactose tolerance test. The stool usually contains large amounts of reducing sugars (>2 gm%). Diarrhoea may be decreased by the feeding of a diet composed of casein, butterfat and fructose. All patients have mild defects in renal tubular reabsorption of glucose. The basic defect is probably at the carrier-mediated transport process via mutarotase (Keston et al 1982). Four cases have been presented in detail (Burke & Danks 1966), and additional cases have been described later. Pedigree analysis of a consanguineous Swedish family going back ten generations suggested that the defect has an autosomal recessive mode of inheritance (Melin & Meeuwisse 1969).

DISORDERS OF GALACTOSE METABOLISM

Galactose metabolism

Galactose, a component of lactose, is an important nutrient for newborn infants and young children. In human breast milk the lactose content is about 7 gm/dl, and in cow's milk the concentration is approximately 5 gm/dl. In the newborn infant lactose may provide as much as 40% of the caloric intake, but only 3–4% in the adult because of lower milk intake. Galactose is also a constituent of many glycoproteins, glycolipids and mucopolysaccharides. The principal pathway for metabolism of galactose has been designated as the 'Leloir Pathway' (Fig. 94.2). Galactose is phosphorylated to galactose-1-phosphate by the enzyme galactokinase. Galactose-1-phosphate is exchanged for the glucose-1-phosphate moiety of uridine diphosphate glucose (UDPG) to form uridine diphosphate galactose (UDPGal) by galactose-1-phosphate uridyltransferase (transferase). The glucose-1-phosphate released leads into the glucose pathway. The UDPGal formed is converted to UDPG by the enzyme UDPGal-4-epimerase (epimerase). The sum of these three enzymatic reactions involving galactokinase, transferase, and epimerase is

Galactose + ATP = Glucose-1-phosphate + ADP

UDPGal is also utilized for synthesis of complex galactose-containing carbohydrates. A small amount of galactose is converted to galactitol by aldose reductase and to galactonic acid by galactose dehydrogenase.

All of the three galactose enzymes in the major pathway are widely distributed in tissues, including erythrocytes, leucocytes, skin fibroblasts, liver, kidney, brain and cultured amniotic fluid cells. The gene loci in man for galactokinase, transferase, and epimerase are on

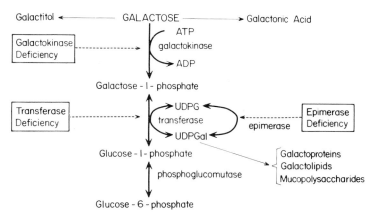

Fig. 94.2 Pathway of galactose metabolism.

chromosomes 17, 9 and 1, respectively (Orkwiszewski et al 1974, Mohandas et al 1977, Lin et al 1979).

Galactokinase deficiency

Clinical aspects

Galactokinase deficiency was first reported by Gitzelmann in 1965. The patient was a 42-year-old man originally described as having galactose diabetes at 9 years of age. Additional patients were reported subsequently. The major clinical manifestations are cataracts and pseudotumour cerebri, both appearing early in infancy. In contrast to the transferase defect, hepatomegaly, jaundice and mental retardation are not usually features of this disorder; yet isolated reports of one or more of these findings have been made in patients with galactokinase deficiency. Hyperbilirubinaemia was observed in one child (Cook et al 1971); and hepatosplenomegaly in another (Thalhammer et al 1968). Generalized seizures and mental deterioration in a 17-year-old patient (Pickering & Howell 1972) and severe mental retardation in two siblings have also been described (Segal et al 1979). How these manifestations relate to the basic enzymatic defect is still unclear.

Biochemical aspects

Ingestion of lactose will raise blood galactose concentrations to values as high as 100 mg/dl. As a consequence, galactose appears in the urine. Galactitol and galactonic acid are produced in increased amounts due to diversion of galactose into these secondary pathways; they also appear in the urine. It is thought that the accumulation of galactitol is the cause of cataract formation and cerebral oedema. In contrast to classical galactosaemia (transferase deficiency), amino aciduria and proteinuria are absent. The diagnosis of galactokinase deficiency can be confirmed by measurement of activity of the enzyme in erythrocytes. One should be aware that the activity is high in the blood of newborns and decreases with age (Ng et al 1965), and that the enzyme activity is not stable in stored erythrocytes.

Treatment

Early detection is important because the cataracts can be averted by removing lactose from the diet. Treatment is relatively simple and consists of exclusion of lactose and other sources of galactose from the diet.

Genetic aspects

Galactokinase deficiency is transmitted as an autosomal recessive trait. Parents of affected children exhibit intermediate values of erythrocyte galactokinase activity. Based upon results of newborn screening programmes, the frequency of occurrence has been estimated at about 1:250 000. This is in contrast to the findings of an apparent carrier frequency in the general population of approximately 1 in 100, giving an estimated incidence of 1:40 000 (Mayes & Guthrie 1968). A low activity galactokinase variant (Philadelphia) has been described among Blacks (Tedesco et al 1977). Galactokinase activity is present in cultured amniotic fluid cells; this provides a means for prenatal diagnosis. Families at risk should receive counselling, with the pregnant mother electing to go to term being advised to restrict intake of lactose to protect the affected fetus.

Galactose-1-phosphate uridyltransferase deficiency (galactosaemia)

Clinical aspects

Galactosaemia probably was first described in 1908 by von Reuss, but it was not until 1956 that Kalckar and his associates established the defect in activity of the enzyme galactose-1-phosphate uridyltransferase. Untreated patients show distinctive manifestations early in life. The infant appears normal at birth, and symptoms usually do not develop until milk feedings are given. Food may be refused; vomiting is common, and diarrhoea occurs occasionally. Other manifestations include lethargy, hypotonia, jaundice, hepatomegaly and susceptibility to infection with Gram-negative organisms. Later, in untreated patients, cataracts become evident, and physical and mental retardation occur. The clinical course of many infants is fulminant, and death occurs early from inanition, infection and hepatic failure. In some individuals the course is much milder and may even escape early detection. Late clinical manifestations have been reported in both untreated and treated galactosaemia patients. Hypergonadotrophic hypogonadism in nearly all females (Kaufman et al 1979), speech defects (Waisbren et al 1983), and neurological sequelae (Lo et al 1984) are the most important of these.

Biochemical aspects

Galactosaemia may be suspected on clinical grounds, but laboratory confirmation is essential. Many of the tests formerly used for diagnosis depended upon ingestion of galactose. This approach should not be employed because it may be hazardous to the patient. Direct enzyme assay in erythrocytes can be readily carried out to confirm the diagnosis. On a galactose-containing diet, affected individuals excrete large amounts of galactose, galactitol and galactonic acid in the urine. Gross generalized amino aciduria and proteinuria are also evident. The erythrocyte galactose-1-phosphate level is elevated. It is believed that this compound produces hepatic damage, whereas galactitol accounts for the formation of cataracts. Deficits of UDPGal have been observed in erythrocytes, cultured skin fibroblasts and liver autopsy samples of galactosaemia patients (Shin et al 1985, Ng et al 1987). How this finding may contribute to some of the late manifestations of the disease is still not known.

There are many reliable methods for measurement of erythrocyte transferase activity; affected individuals exhibit either little or no activity in their red blood cells. Blood transfusions in patients will interfere with or invalidate the interpretation of the test because transferase is present in the donor cells. Under this circumstance, studies on both parents to determine heterozygosity can be helpful in reaching a presumptive diagnosis. Neonatal screening has been initiated effectively in many countries. Methods depend upon the measurement of galactose and/or galactose-1-phosphate by microbiological assays (Guthrie 1968), or by galactose dehydrogenase (Misuma et al 1981), or measurement of transferase activity by a fluorometric technique (Beutler & Baluda 1966). The assays measuring galactose will detect both galactokinase and transferase defects, whereas the enzyme assay is limited to recognition of the transferase defect. Due to the high frequency of Duarte variants (described below), the Duarte-galactosaemia compond heterozygotes (D/G) are not infrequently picked up in neonatal programmes utilizing the Beutler fluorescent spot test. Infants who are D/G compound heterozygotes have 20–25% of normal activity and often show significant elevations of erythrocyte galactose-1-phosphate. Some of the values approximate to those found for affected galactosaemia patients. The children are asymptomatic, and the necessity for dietary treatment is not established.

Treatment

Treatment is directed towards minimizing the accumulation of galactose and its metabolites in body tissues by excluding milk and milk-containing products from the diet. Various milk substitutes are available (casein hydrolysates, soybean formulas). While a galactose-free diet is the basis of treatment, supplementary measures are often required in the neonate to correct secondary manifestations, such as hyperbilirubinaemia, hypoprothrombinaemia, sepsis with Gram-negative organisms and anaemia. The infections often respond poorly to antibiotic therapy unless restriction of galactose is also carried out. The immediate effects of dietary treatment are dramatic, with reversal of the acute manifestations. Galactose restriction is compatible with good general health and normal patterns of physical development. Treated patients, as a group, can achieve normal intelligence scores, but in spite of dietary restriction of lactose many patients still have significant problems in later life. Speech disorders and difficulties in school are frequently encountered. Galactosaemic men and women have had normal offspring but reports have been scarce. Many female patients develop ovarian hypofunction, while gonadal function in adult males appears to be normal.

Genetic aspects

Galactosaemia has been found in all races, but the incidence appears to be lower in Asians. The frequency of occurrence of galactosaemia based upon newborn screening is approximately 1:60 000. The disorder is transmitted as an autosomal recessive condition. Carriers can be identified and exhibit about half of normal erythrocyte tranferase activity. However, transferase polymorphism renders identification of carriers difficult unless electrophoretic analysis is carried out simultaneously with activity measurements.

Several biochemical variants of transferase have been described. Some are asymptomatic; others are associated with disease. The two most common variants are the Duarte (Beutler et al 1965) and the Los Angeles (Ng et al 1973) variants. These are not associated with any clinical symptoms of disease. Both variant enzymes can be distinguished from the normal by their banding pattern on electrophoresis. The Duarte variant is a low-activity variant; erythrocyte transferase activity in the homozygote is similar to that for the galactosaemia heterozygote, about half of normal. The Los Angeles variant has a slightly higher than normal activity. The frequencies of the occurrence of Duarte variant/normal heterozygotes and the Los Angeles/normal heterozygotes are 10–12% and 5% respectively. A third asymptomatic transferase variant designated as the 'Berne variant' exhibits decreased activity and slower electrophoretic mobility than normal (Scherz et al 1976).

Several transferase variants have been described which are associated with clinical manifestations similar to classical galactosaemia. These include the Negro (Segal 1969), Indiana (Chacko et al 1971), Rennes (Schapira & Kaplan 1969), Chicago (Chacko et al 1977); and atypical galactosaemia variants (Matz et al 1975, Lang et al 1980). Different physicochemical properties have been described for each variant enzyme, but no attempt has been made to compare one to another in the same study. Symptoms of the 'Rennes' and the 'Indiana' variants are said to be more severe than the 'Negro'. All of these very low activity variants can be identified upon neonatal screening (Ng et al 1978) but require special biochemical approaches to be differentiated from classical galactosaemia. The authors have studied a 6-month-old patient with bilateral lenticular cataracts suspected of galactokinase deficiency. The defect turned out to be a variant form of transferase deficiency (less than 5% of normal activity).

Prenatal diagnosis of galactosaemia is feasible and has been performed successfully in a number of instances (Ng et al 1977). Galactitol concentration in the amniotic fluid of an affected fetus was shown to be elevated (Allen et al 1980). Prenatal diagnosis in this disorder may have value in determining the need for dietary restriction of lactose during pregnancy.

Uridine diphosphate galactose-4-epimerase deficiency

Epimerase deficiency can be found in two forms: benign and severe. The benign form is more common and is not associated with any known clinical problem. The decrease in epimerase activity is confined to the red cells and is not manifest in nucleated cells, such as liver, cultured skin fibroblasts and lymphocytes (Gitzelmann et al 1976). The deficiency is attributed to the presence of an unstable variant enzyme requiring higher NAD concentration for maximum activity. The mode of inheritance is autosomal recessive, in which the heterozygote exhibits about half of normal erythrocyte epimerase activity. The erythrocyte galactose-1-phosphate concentration in early infancy may reach levels as high as 50 mg/dl, and affected individuals may be suspected of having galactosaemia on screening with the use of the microbiological assay. No treatment is required. One case with confirmed epimerase deficiency associated with severe clinical manifestations was reported (Holton et al 1981). The female patient presented on the fifth day of life with symptoms of classical galactosaemia. These include jaundice, weight loss, vomiting, hypotonia and hepatomegaly. Dietary treatment with limitation on galactose intake has been tried, but the outcome was uncertain (Henderson et al 1983). Developmental delay persisted.

DISORDERS OF FRUCTOSE METABOLISM

Fructose metabolism

Fructose is a monosaccharide found in honey, fruits and other plant tissues. In combination with glucose it forms the disaccharide sucrose. It also exists in a number of oligosaccharides, such as raffinose (a trisaccharide) and stachyose (a tetrasaccharide). The latter is found abundantly in legumes. Ingested sucrose is hydrolyzed by intestinal sucrase to glucose and fructose. The oligosaccharides raffinose and stachyose, which also contain galactose and glucose, are not digested in man.

The liver plays a dominant role in the metabolism of fructose; other organs metabolize fructose, but to a lesser extent (Fig. 94.3). The overall process results in conversion of the sugar to glycolytic intermediates leading to the formation either of glucose or lactic acid. In the liver, fructose is phosphorylated to fructose-1-phosphate (F-1-P) in the presence of fructokinase. The enzyme is also present in kidney and in intestinal mucosa. Fructokinase is not present in muscle, adipose tissue and blood cells, and in these tissues fructose is phosphorylated to fructose-6-phosphate by hexokinase (Herman & Zakim 1968). In the liver, F-1-P is further metabolized to D-glyceraldehyde and dihydroxyacetone phosphate by F-1-P aldolase or 'aldolase B'. Aldolase B differs from aldolases A and C in that the latter isozymes act principally on fructose-1,6-diphosphate. In the seminal vesicles, the lens of the eye, and peripheral nerves, fructose can be metabolized to sorbitol. In normal subjects, in vivo radioisotope studies have shown that

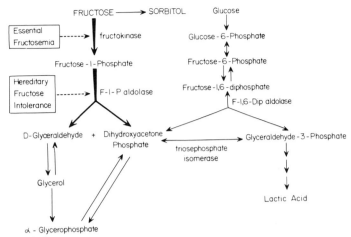

Fig. 94.3   Pathways of fructose metabolism.

fructose is converted to glucose solely by way of F-1-P (Landau et al 1971). Sorbitol does not appear to be an intermediate. In two patients with hereditary fructose intolerance due to F-1-P aldolase deficiency, it was estimated that 12–20% of fructose was metabolized by way of fructose-6-phosphate.

In man, deficiencies in hepatic fructokinase and F-1-P aldolase have been described. Inactivity of fructokinase is responsible for essential fructosuria (fructosaemia), whereas deficiency of F-1-P aldolase results in hereditary fructose intolerance. Fructose-1,6-diphosphatase deficiency is sometimes included among the disorders of fructose metabolism, but it seems more appropriate to list it as one of the gluconeogenic disorders described later in this chapter.

Essential fructosuria (fructosaemia)

The incidence of this benign condition is estimated as 1:130 000 in the general population (Froesch 1978). However, essential fructosuria usually causes no symptoms and the incidence may be somewhat higher. Transmission follows an autosomal recessive pattern. The genetic defect is a deficiency of hepatic fructokinase (Schapira et al 1961/62). Ingested fructose is not well metabolized by the liver and reaches to high levels in the blood with overflow into the urine. The presence of the sugar in the urine can readily be demonstrated. No treatment is necessary.

Hereditary fructose intolerance (HFI)

Clinical aspects

The clinical manifestations in individuals with HFI may vary with the age at which fructose is introduced into the diet and with the quantity of sugar ingested. In some individuals, symptoms are quite subtle. In infants, ingestion of fructose may produce findings, similar to those found in galactosaemia, e.g. failure to thrive, vomiting, hepatomegaly, oedema, hyperbilirubinaemia and seizures. Because many formulas contain sucrose, the opportunities of an affected infant for exposure to fructose are increased accordingly. In older children and in adults with HFI, ingestion of fructose causes abdominal pain and lowers the blood glucose level precipitously. Pallor, vomiting, sweating, and even coma may be manifest. It is typical for these individuals to develop a strong aversion for all sweets and to be free of dental caries.

Biochemical aspects

The biochemical defect in HFI is a deficiency of liver fructose-1-phosphate aldolase. Enzyme activity is usually less than 10% of normal when F-1-P is utilized as the assay substrate, and between 10 and 50% of normal when fructose-1,6-diphosphate is the substrate. The enzyme deficiency can also be demonstrated in intestinal mucosa. Blood cells cannot be utilized for diagnosis since the enzyme is not present in leucocytes or erythrocytes.

Whereas the diagnosis of HFI can be suspected on clinical grounds, laboratory confirmation is essential. Untreated patients ingesting fructose in their diet excrete large amounts of this sugar in their urine and also show a gross generalized amino aciduria. A fructose tolerance test is a useful first step in facilitating diagnosis before assay of the enzyme, which requires either a biopsy sample of liver or intestinal mucosa. Administration of fructose, either orally or parenterally, is followed by a fall in the blood glucose level and serum inorganic phosphate (presumably due to its utilization in the formation of fructose-1-phosphate). The uric acid level in blood rises from rapid degradation of purine nucleotides to uric acid. The hypoglycaemia is related to inhibition of glycogenolysis by F-1-P (van den Berghe et al 1973).

HFI may be confused biochemically with tyrosinosis in early infancy insofar as elevation of blood tyrosine and methionine levels have been observed in some cases, presumably because of liver damage (Grant et al 1970). The gross generalized amino aciduria is akin to that seen in galactosaemia patients and may result from toxic action of F-1-P on the proximal renal tubules. Observation of fructosuria, however, serves to distinguish HFI from galactosaemia or tyrosinosis.

Treatment

The clinical manifestations in young infants with HFI may be severe, and prompt elimination of fructose from the diet is important. Major sources of fructose include cane sugar, honey, fruits and formulas utilizing sucrose as the source of carbohydrate. The prognosis for treated patients is good. Liver and kidney damage is reversed, and neurological residuals are uncommon. The use of fructose infusion as a source of calories in hospitalized patients must be approached with caution until it is known that the patient does not have HFI.

Genetic aspects

The frequency of occurrence of HFI in the general population is not known because many patients with HFI may go unrecognized. An incidence of 1: 20 000 has been reported for Switzerland (Gitzelmann et al 1973). The defect is inherited as an autosomal recessive trait. Heterozygote detection has been complicated by relative inaccessibility of tissue for enzyme assay and the inability to differentiate normals from heterozygotes by parenteral loading with fructose (Beyreiss et al 1968). Biochemical studies of F-1-P aldolase from liver biopsies of five patients with HFI using antibody techniques suggest that genetic heterogeneity is probably common (Gitzelmann et al 1974). The gene for aldolase B was localized to chromosome 9q13-9q32 using a cDNA probe on rodent human somatic cell hybrids (Henry et al 1985). Restriction fragments were studied in 11 patients and compared with the normal pattern. No major deletions of the gene were observed (Gregori et al 1984).

ESSENTIAL PENTOSURIA

Essential pentosuria is a benign disorder encountered principally in Ashkenazi Jews and is inherited as an autosomal recessive trait. The urine contains L-xylulose which is excreted in increased amounts because of a block in the conversion of xylulose to xylitol due to xylitol dehydrogenase deficiency. The condition is usually discovered accidentally and no treatment is required.

GLYCOGEN STORAGE DISEASES

Glycogen metabolism

Glycogen is the principal storage form of carbohydrate in animal cells; it is present in virtually every type of tissue. Glycogen is a polymer composed of highly branched chains of glucose molecules. The glucose units are linked in the 1-4 positions, whereas the branch points are attached in 1-6 linkage. Glycogen molecules are relatively large, spherical structures, and their aggregations are easily recognizable by electron microscopy in cell cytoplasm. Liver has the highest glycogen content of all tissues, usually 3-5 gm/100gm. Skeletal muscle normally contains 1-1.5gm/100gm. The glycogen content of liver increases following carbohydrate-rich meals and decreases during periods of fasting. During a fast, liver glycogen is degraded to glucose which is released into the circulation to maintain glucose homoeostasis.

The regulation of glycogenolysis in the liver is complex (Fig. 94.4). The most clearly defined mechanism involves activation of the enzyme adenyl cyclase (AC) by the hormone glucagon or epinephrine. This increases the cyclic adenosine monophosphate (cAMP) level in the cytosol, which in turn activates protein kinase, phosphorylase kinase and phosphorylase (P'lase) in rapid sequence by phosphorylation of these enzymes (Hers 1976). P'lase

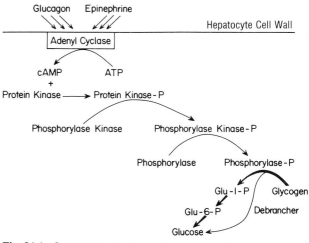

Fig. 94.4 Sequential activation of the enzymes in glycogenolysis.

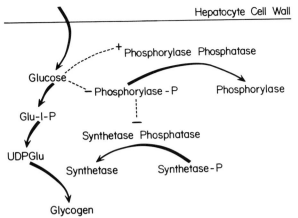

Fig. 94.5 Regulation of glycogen synthesis.

Glycogen synthesis involves the following steps:

1) Glu-1-P + UTP --------------------$>$UDPG + PP

(UDPG pyrophosphorylase)

2) UDPG + glycogen$_{(n)}$-------$>$glycogen$_{(n+1)}$+UDP

(glycogen synthetase)

Glycogen synthetase adds glucosyl units to the ends of the chains. Brancher enzyme adds new branch points and initiates the formation of additional branch chains.

The disorders of glycogen metabolism, generally named glycogen storage diseases (GSD), result from deficiencies of various enzymes in the catabolic pathways of glycogen metabolism. They can be divided into those disorders in which hepatomegaly is the dominant feature, and those in which muscle involvement is paramount. Glycogen storage diseases were originally identified numerically: from GSD type I (glucose-6-phosphatase deficiency) to GSD type VI (hepatic P'lase deficiency). The authors prefer to designate the disorders according to the enzyme deficiency.

GSD with marked hepatomegaly

Glucose-6-phosphatase deficiency (GSD type Ia, von Gierke disease)

Clinical aspects This disorder, described in 1929 by von Gierke, was the first abnormality of glycogen metabolism to be recognized. Clinical manifestations usually appear in the first 6 months of life. The infants are mildly obese and have abdominal distension due to hepatomegaly, but little or no splenomegaly. Brief periods of fasting (3–4 hours) produce irritability due to hypoglycaemia and acidosis, usually without convulsions. Perspiration is excessive and older children show heat intolerance. Epistaxis and easy bruising are common. Bowel movements tend to be loose. Renomegaly is characteristic, but renal function is normal during childhood. Some affected infants and children are prone to severe lactic acidosis during minor infections and, until recently, the mortality rate was high. In older untreated children growth is slow, and sexual development is incomplete.

Uric acid production is increased, and renal clearance is decreased. As a consequence hyperuricaemia and urinary tract stones are common, and gouty arthritis may occur. Hyperlipidaemia is invariably present and may cause cutaneous xanthoma. Hepatic adenomas are frequently demonstrable by adolescence (Howell et al 1976, Miller et al 1978). Haemorrhagic necrosis of the hepatic adenomas may cause severe acute abdominal pain. Several patients have died with hepatocellular carcinoma (Zangeneh et al 1969, Etsuro et al 1987), suggesting that the adenomas are premalignant lesions. Uric acid nephropathy and/or diffuse interstitial nephritis, focal glomer-

acts upon the terminal units of the glycogen chains liberating glucose-1-phosphate (Glu-1-P). Debrancher enzyme removes branch points and liberates free glucose. Approximately 7% of the glycosyl units are released as free glucose.

Several other factors have been shown to affect the activity of P'lase in addition to glucagon. Vasopressin (Keppens & de Wulf 1975) and angiotensin I (Keppens & de Wulf 1976) both activate P'lase without increasing cAMP. Ionic calcium enhances, and potassium ion inhibits P'lase activation. Insulin acts at several levels to inhibit P'lase activity (van de Werve et al 1977). An amylase is present in hepatocytes which removes oligosaccharide chains, 3–5 units long, from glycogen. Lysosomal acid maltase breaks down these oligosaccharides and provides an alternate pathway for glycogen catabolism. The rate of glycogen synthesis increases when the concentrations of glucose and insulin rise in the blood, and the glucagon level falls. When the concentration of glucose in the hepatocyte increases, binding to P'lase (Fig. 94.5) causes partial inactivation of that enzyme (Stalmans et al 1974). At the same time, binding of glucose to phosphorylase phosphatase enhances the conversion of P'lase to the inactive form. The decrease in active P'lase diminishes inhibition of glycogen synthetase phosphatase (Stalmans et al 1971), thereby promoting the conversion of glycogen synthetase to the active (dephosphorylated) form. Insulin stimulates the activation of glycogen synthetase, apparently through inactivation of P'lase (Witten & Avruch 1978). A fall in glucagon concentration in blood also leads to deactivation of P'lase and inhibition of glycogenolysis.

ulosclerosis, nephrotic syndrome and renal failure may occur during the second or third decade of life (Chen et al 1988). Other complication are osteoporosis (Soejima et al 1985), bone fractures, neurological deficits (apparently from hypoglycaemia) and seizures, pancreatitis and pulmonary hypertension. There is variability in the severity of manifestations in GSD Ia. A moderate number of individuals are mildly affected and some are discovered as adults with hepatomegaly and gout (Stamm & Webb 1975).

Biochemical aspects The production of glucose by glycogenolysis is impaired because of glucose-6-phosphatase deficiency in the liver and kidney (Fig. 94.6). Normal plasma glucose concentration cannot be maintained in the postprandial state. This results in inhibition of insulin and enhancement of glucagon secretion by the pancreas. This decrease in the insulin to glucagon ratio in blood stimulates glycogen breakdown in the liver but, in the absence of glucose-6-phosphatase, lactic acid and pyruvic acid are produced in excess, instead of glucose (Sadeghi-Nejad et al 1974).

The laboratory findings are characteristic in GSD type I. Blood obtained after a brief fasting period reveals hypoglycaemia (10–30 mg/dl) and elevated lactic acid levels (50–100 mg/dl). In this condition, lactate serves as an important substitute fuel for the brain (Fernandes et al 1984). Hyperlipidaemia (primary hypertriglyceridaemia) and hyperuricaemia are almost always present. Uric acid production is stimulated by the action of glucagon on the liver, causing the catabolism of ATP to uric acid (Roe & Kogut 1977, Cohen et al 1985). Glucagon administration causes little if any rise in blood glucose, but a marked rise

in blood lactate. Intravenous administration of galactose or fructose cause a rise in blood lactate but no rise in blood glucose. Other types of GSD, clinically similar to GSD type I (debrancher and phosphorylase system deficiencies), have normal blood lactate values in the fasting state.

Fructose-1,6-diphosphatase deficiency is similar clinically to GSD type I and fasting blood lactate levels are elevated. Glucagon administration causes a rise in blood glucose and no rise in lactate. As little as 0.25mg/kg of fructose, given intravenously, produces a rapid fall in blood glucose in fructose-1,6 diphosphatase deficiency, but not in GSD type I. Measurement of hepatic enzyme activity is a standard method of diagnosis of GSD. Since errors in handling of biopsy samples and in assay methods may occur, enzyme values are not always diagnostic. Carbohydrate test results are important in arriving at a correct diagnosis.

Histological findings in the liver in GSD type I include steatosis, glycogenosis and mild periportal fibrosis. Glucose-6-phosphatase activity is absent or markedly decreased in both liver and kidney. More than one enzyme deficiency has been reported in some patients (Service et al 1978); however it is not clear whether a double enzyme defect or adaptive inactivation of one of the enzymes is involved (Moses et al 1966).

Treatment Frequent feedings of carbohydrate during the daytime and the infusion of a concentrated glucose solution or high carbohydrate formula at night, via nasogastric tube or by gastrostomy (Greene et al 1976), are used to maintain euglycaemia and to suppress the levels of lactic acid and uric acid and lipids in the circulation. Limitation of the dietary intake of fructose and galactose is advocated.

Lactic acid production can be suppressed by administering glucose enterally at a rate of 8–9 mg/kg/minute (Schwenk & Haymond 1986). Feeding of cornstarch (approximately 1.5–2 g/kg/6 hours, day and night) has been very successful in maintaining euglycaemia, especially in older patients (Chen et al 1984). Feeding of pancreatic enzymes along with cornstarch has been recommended for infants (who may not adequately digest the starch). These treatment regimens produce a marked improvement in strength and growth (Greene et al 1979). Use of these regimens also appear to inhibit hepatoma formation (Roe et al 1979, Parker et al 1981). Allopurinol may be needed to control hyperuricaemia. For those with liver failure, liver transplantation can be life-saving and bring normal glucose homeostasis (Malatack et al 1983).

Genetic aspects Glucose-6-phosphatase deficiency is inherited as an autosomal recessive disease. The incidence is estimated to be in the order of 1: 200 000 births, but it may be higher in some population groups. A

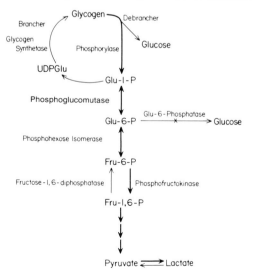

Fig. 94.6 Glycogen metabolism and enzyme deficiency (Glu-6-phosphatase) in GSD Type I.

method for prenatal diagnosis using enzyme assays has not been established. Glucose-6-phosphatase activity was reported in placenta (Matalon et al 1977) and in amniotic fluid epithelial cells (Negishi & Benke 1977); however these tissues have not proven useful for prenatal diagnosis. There are several reports of successful pregnancies in women with GSD type I.

Glycogen storage disease type Ib

Some individuals with all the clinical and biochemical manifestations of GSD type I have normal activity of glucose-6-phosphatase when their liver tissue is assayed after freezing. However, when the assay is done on fresh tissue, no enzyme activity is shown (Narisawa et al 1978). Glucose-6-phosphatase is located on the luminal surface of hepatic microsomes. Glucose-6-phosphate is transported into the microsomes by a specific translocase which is missing or inactive in GSD type Ib (Lange et al 1980). Glucose-6-phosphatase is demonstrable in GSD type Ib when microsomal membranes are disrupted by freezing or chemically, exposing the enzyme to its substrate.

Neutropenia and neutrophil dysfunction are characteristic of GSD type Ib (Beaudet et al 1980) and apparently account for the tendency for infections seen in this condition (Ambruso et al 1985), and the association with chronic inflammatory bowel disease (Roe et al 1986). Portacaval shunt procedure was reported to correct the granulocyte deficiency (Corbeel et al 1983), but this report has not been corroborated by others. One affected child has died of leukaemia. The inheritance pattern is autosomal recessive. Methods for prenatal diagnosis or carrier detection are not available.

An additional form of glycogenosis due to a microsomal transport defect for glucose-6-phosphate, inorganic pyrophosphate and carbamylphosphate has been reported in a child with insulin-dependent diabetes mellitus and designated GSD type Ic (Nordlie et al 1983).

Amylo-1,6-glucosidase (debrancher) deficiency (GSD type III, limit dextrinosis, Cori disease)

Clinical aspects The clinical manifestations can be recognized in infancy. Abdominal distension due to hepatomegaly is moderate to marked; splenomegaly is minimal or absent. Hypoglycaemia is usually mild and often accompanied by ketonuria after overnight fasting. In infancy, muscular weakness and hypotonia are common and may be the primary complaint. There is no bleeding tendency, heat intolerance, loose stools, rapid breathing or enlargement of the kidneys (helping to distinguish GSD type III from type I). These children usually survive childhood without difficulty, although growth may be slow. Hepatomegaly decreases with maturity; liver failure is rare and hepatoma has not been reported. Severe myopathy and neural involvement may begin during adolescence or early adult years (Brunberg et al 1971, DiMauro et al 1979). This has been attributed to recurring overnight depletion of amino acids in muscle, due to increased demand for gluconeogenesis in this disorder (Slonim et al 1982). Cardiac failure with mycardial glycogenosis (Olson et al 1984) and the accumulation of glycogen in sural nerve axons (Yoshikazu et al 1986) and in Schwann cells (Powell et al 1985) have been reported in GSD III.

Biochemical aspects Absence of debrancher enzyme results in glycogen accumulation in liver and in many other tissues, including leucocytes and erythrocytes. In the fasting state, blood glucose levels are sustained primarily by gluconeogenesis and by limited glycogen degradation.

Marked elevation of serum transaminase activity is common, but there is not other evidence of hepatic dysfunction. Creatinine phosphokinase activity in blood is also high and may reflect debrancher enzyme deficiency in muscle. Hyperlipidaemia may be present, but hyperuricaemia is usually absent. Blood lactate levels are normal in the fasting state and there is no rise in blood glucose or lactate values following glucagon administration. A characteristic increase in blood lactate occurs following meals and the oral administration of glucose, fructose or galactose (Fernandez et al 1969).

Histological examination of the liver shows increased fat and glycogen in hepatocytes and mild periportal fibrosis. Debrancher deficiency can be confirmed by demonstrating absence of enzyme activity in liver and in muscle. Cultured fibroblasts may be used to confirm this deficiency (van Diggelen et al 1985). Erythrocytes and leucocytes have also been used for diagnosis, but the results may be misleading (Deckelbaum et al 1972). A characteristic urinary oligosaccharide pattern has been reported in this disorder (McLaren et al 1980).

Treatment Therapy is directed towards preventing hypoglycaemia and reducing the breakdown of muscle protein for gluconeogenesis by frequent feedings and avoidance of prolonged periods of fasting. The same treatment regimens that are employed for GSD type I have been used for type III. High protein infusions, given during the night, have been advocated to treat or prevent myopathy. Limitation of fructose and galactose intake is probably not necessary, although restriction of dietary fat seems prudent. A high protein diet with particular attention to overnight protein administration can markedly improve growth.

Genetic aspects The genetics of GSD type III may be more complex than is presently understood. Amylo-1,6-

glucosidase (debrancher) and another enzyme, oligo-1,4 1,4-glucan transferase, are both associated with the same cellular protein (Brown & Illingsworth 1964). Deficiency of either or both activities might result in the same clinical picture. These two enzyme activities may be under separate genetic control. In 18 patients with GSD III, enzyme protein (CRM) could be identified immunologically in every case (Dreyfus et al 1974). Absence of debrancher activity in liver is usually associated with the same deficiency in muscle, however, limitation of this deficiency to liver has also been described. The incidence of this disease is estimated to be approximately 1:200 000 (Huijing 1973), but it is much more common in Israel (Levin et al 1967). Demonstration of debrancher enzyme deficiency in amniotic fluid cells and chorionic villi has been used for prenatal diagnosis (van Diggelen et al 1985). Detection of heterozygotes by assay of debrancher enzyme in erythrocytes has been reported (Shin et al 1984). Complexities in the assay of this enzyme have been pointed out recently (Gutman et al 1985). Successful pregnancy in a patient with GSD type III has been reported.

Hepatic phosphorylase (GSD type VI), phosphorylase kinase (GSD type IX), and phosphorylase activating system deficiencies including protein kinase deficiency (GSD type X)

Clinical aspects These disorders are less well-defined than GSD types I and III; however, their clinical appearance is similar to those disorders (de Barsy & Lederer 1980) and are usually recognizable in the first two years of life. Affected children exhibit abdominal enlargement because of hepatomegaly, mild adiposity, hypotonia and growth failure. Hypoglycaemia is either mild or absent. Lactic acidosis, bleeding tendency and loose bowel movements are not seen. Although growth is retarded in childhood, normal height and complete sexual development are eventually achieved. Abdominal distension and hepatomegaly may decrease or disappear by adolescence.

Biochemical aspects Deficiency of phosphorylase (or one of the enzymes that leads to its activation) obstructs glycogen degradation in the liver, and absence of significant fasting hypoglycaemia may be related to the fact that phosphorylase activity is usually only partially deficient and hepatic gluconeogenesis is intact.

Laboratory studies reveal a moderate elevation of serum transaminase values and hyperlipidaemia. Fasting blood glucose, lactic and uric acid levels are normal. Blood lactate values rise following meals and after glucose, galactose and fructose ingestion. Glucagon administration is reported to cause minimal glycaemic response in phosphorylase kinase deficiency (Koster et al 1973). In the authors' experience, the response to glucagon has been variable. Liver tissue obtained by biopsy shows steatosis, glycogenosis and mild periportal fibrosis. Hepatic enzyme assay reveals 75–90% reduction in phosphorylase activity in both phosphorylase and phosphorylase kinase deficiencies, but kinase activity is expected to be normal in the former disorder and decreased in the latter. Total phosphorylase activity (a plus b) is decreased in primary phosphorylase deficiency but not in phosphorylase kinase deficiency. Phosphorylase kinase deficiency appears to be the more common of these two diseases. Hepatic phosphorylase kinase deficiency may involve only liver and not muscle (X-linked type), or liver and muscle (autosomal recessive type). Deficiency of phosphorylase kinase in muscle has also been reported (Abarbanel et al 1986). Phosphorylase kinase deficiency in the X-linked form can be demonstrated with the erythrocyte enzyme assay, but not with the leucocytes (Besley 1987). Phosphorylase deficiency involves either liver alone (GSD type VI) or muscle alone (GSD type V) but not both tissues in the same patient. Protein kinase deficiency (cyclic 3'5'-AMP dependent kinase) is reported to involve both liver and muscle (Hug et al 1970).

Treatment Symptomatic hypoglycaemia is unusual, and late-onset myopathy, as seen in type III disease, does not seem to be a problem in these conditions, so that no special diet is required. The increased demand for gluconeogenesis would suggest a theoretical benefit from high protein intake. Because of liver enlargement, activities which might lead to abdominal trauma should be approached with caution.

Genetic aspects The mode of inheritance of phosphorylase kinase deficiency is complex, perhaps because the enzyme is composed of four different subunits (Cohen 1973). Both autosomal recessive (Hug et al 1969, Lederer et al 1975) and X-linked recessive inheritance (Huijing & Fernandez 1969) have been reported. Carriers of X-linked liver phosphorylase kinase deficiency can be identified by an erythrocyte assay (Besley 1987). In the autosomal form of phosphorylase kinase deficiency, decreased enzyme activity was found in liver, muscle, erythrocytes and leucocytes (Lederer et al 1980). The incidence of these disorders is estimated to be approximately 1:200 000.

Brancher deficiency (GSD type IV, amylopectinosis, Anderson disease)

Clinical aspects Brancher deficiency is one of the rarest and least studied of the glycogen storage diseases. Affected infants begin to show evidence of liver dysfunction within the first year of life, and death by 2–4 years appears to be the usual outcome. Features of hepatic failure and portal hypertension appear, including growth failure, jaundice, splenomegaly and prominent abdominal venous pattern. Hypotonia is common, and hypoglycaemia is absent (Anderson 1952).

Biochemical aspects An abnormal form of glycogen, with long chains and infrequent branch points, accumulates in many cells types, including hepatocytes, skeletal and myocardial muscle cells, fibroblasts, leucocytes and nerve cells. Hepatic cirrhosis is presumed to result from the abnormal type of glycogen which accumulates. Carbohydrate and glucagon tolerance tests are normal, providing that liver failure is not severe at the time of testing.

Deficiency of debrancher enzyme can be demonstrated in liver, in leucocytes (Brown & Brown 1966) and in cultured fibroblasts (Howell et al 1971). In histological sections of liver, staining of the abnormal glycogen with iodine produces a distinctive blue colour. This disease must be differentiated from other forms of liver failure in infancy, such as neonatal hepatitis, biliary atresia, polycystic disease of liver and kidney, Wilson disease, tyrosinosis, alpha-1-antitrypsin deficiency, etc.

Treatment No form of therapy has been successful.

Genetic aspects This disorder is inherited as an autosomal recessive defect. Heterozygotes appear to be detectable by enzyme assay of cultured skin fibroblasts. The enzyme is normally present in cultured amniotic fluid cells and prenatal diagnosis has been accomplished using cultured fibroblasts (Brown & Brown 1987).

GSD primarily involving muscle

Acid alpha-glucosidase (AAG) deficiency (GSD type II), Pompe disease, acid maltase deficiency (AMD), alpha-1,4-glucosidase deficiency

Clinical aspects AMD was first recognized in infants with hypotonia and cardiomegaly without murmur. Subsequently two, and possibly three, clinical syndromes of muscle involvement associated with AMD have been identified (Tanaka et al 1979). In the infantile form, glycogen accumulates in almost all tissues. The involvement of cardiac muscle and neural cells is the most significant for the affected infant. Manifestations usually appear within the first 6 months of life and include hypotonia and developmental delay, macroglossia, moderate hepatosplenomegaly, cardiomegaly and congestive heart failure. The condition is progressive, leading to death by 1–2 years of age. Characteristic electrocardiographic abnormalities include rapid conduction time, wide amplitude QRS complex and changes of left ventricular hypertrophy. Histological examination re-

veals glycogen accumulation in virtually every cell type. The excess glycogen is characteristically found within membrane-bound structures (lysosomes) as well as free in the cytoplasm. The late-onset forms of AMD may be manifest by gradually increasing weakness in childhood or as late as the sixth decade of life (Engel et al 1973). Skeletal muscle weakness, decreased exercise tolerance and decreased respiratory reserve are the usual features. Hepatomegaly, macroglossia, neurological involvement and cardiomegaly are absent. Death may result from complications of respiratory insufficiency.

Biochemical aspects Alpha-1,4 and alpha-1,6-glucosidase activities are associated with a single lysosomal enzyme protein (Brown et al 1970). These activities promote hydrolysis of glycogen to glucose, and absence of acid maltase results in glycogen accumulation within lysosomes. It is unclear just how this results in clinical disease.

In the infantile form, alpha-1,4-glucosidase is absent in affected tissues (skin, muscle, liver and cultured fibroblasts), assayed at both acid and neutral pH. In the late-onset forms, the enzyme activity is absent or very decreased, assayed at acid pH, but may be near normal at neutral pH (Angelini & Engel 1972). The results of enzyme assay in mixed leucocyte preparation must be interpreted with caution. Isolated lymphocytes or cultured lymphocytes, but not granulocytes are suitable for diagnosis and carrier detection (Taniguchi et al 1978). Granulocytes contain 'renal' acid maltase which is normally active in AMD patients' cells (Dreyfus & Poenaru 1980). If a mixed leucocyte preparation is used, selective removal of renal acid maltase by pH 5 precipitation is necessary for the enzyme assay to reach the diagnosis (Broadhead & Butterworth 1978). Urine acid maltase assay may also aid in laboratory diagnosis (Tanaka et al 1979). Cross reacting material (CRM) negative and CRM positive instances of the infantile form have been reported (Beratis et al 1978).

Treatment There is no specific therapy for this enzyme deficiency. The administration of purified alpha-glucosidase was not effective (Hug 1974, Tyrrell & Ryman 1976) nor was bone marrow transplantation (Watson & Goldfinch 1986). A high protein diet has produced improvement in muscle function (Slonim et al 1983).

Genetic aspects The infantile form and late-onset forms are inherited as autosomal recessive disorders. Apparently dominant inheritance of late-onset AMD has also been reported (Danon et al 1986). The carrier state can be identified in cultured fibroblasts. Prenatal diagnosis is possible using cultured amniotic fluid cells (Salafsky & Nadler 1971). The gene for alpha-glucosidase has been assigned to chromosome 17, segment q23–q25 (Halley et al 1984). Two distinct molecular abnormalities have been detected in the infantile form of AMD. These include defects in processing and production of acid alpha-glucosidase (Reuser et al 1987).

Muscle phosphorylase (MP) deficiency (GSD type V, McArdle disease)

Clinical aspects Glycogen MP deficiency usually becomes manifest in late adolescence or in the second decade of life (McArdle 1951). The principal symptoms are pain and stiffness of muscles during exercise. Strenuous activity can result in myoglobinuria. Several instances of acute renal failure due to rhabdomyolysis have been reported (Grunfeld et al 1972). Muscle groups which are stressed may become acutely swollen and tender. In later life, muscle weakness may become chronic (Engel et al 1963).

Biochemical aspects The clinical manifestations result from deficient energy production in muscle. During muscle activity, glycogen is normally broken down, providing energy for muscle contraction. Glycogen degradation is blocked in MP deficiency, and the defect in glycolysis is reflected in the absence of lactate production by muscle during ischaemic exercise. Studies using 31P nuclear magnetic resonance show a rapid exhaustion of phosphocreatinine during ischaemic exercise and indicate the importance of normal glycogen metabolism in muscle activity (Ross et al 1981). A pronounced rise in ammonia, inosine, hypoxanthine and uric acid production occurs in MP deficiency after muscular activity, apparently due to accelerated degradation of muscle purine nucleotides (ATP, ADP, AMP). These changes are also seen in GSD type III and VII (Mineo et al 1987).

Muscle biopsy for measurement of glycogen content and enzyme analysis is necessary for diagnosis of GSD type V. Muscle histology shows damaged fibres, increased glycogen content and absence of MP histochemical activity. MP activity may be present in regenerating fibres, due to the presence of a fetal-type isozyme. This isozyme has been demonstrated in cultured muscle cells from affected individuals (Meienhofer et al 1977). Phosphorylase activity in liver is normal in GSD type V.

Treatment The treatment for McArdle disease is avoidance of strenuous activity. Because the muscle symptoms result in part from lack of substrate (particularly fatty acids), the symptoms can be minimized by warming up activities which mobilize fatty acids from fat stores (Porte et al 1966). Improvement in strength was reported with a high protein diet (Slonim & Goans 1985).

Genetic aspects This rare muscle disorder is inherited as an autosomal recessive trait (Schmid & Hammaker 1961). In most cases, muscle histology shows no cross reacting material (CRM) suggesting the enzyme protein is absent. In others, CRM is detectable suggesting an inactive enzyme (Feit & Brooke 1976). Molecular heterogeneity has also been shown at the messenger RNA level with some patients lacking phosphorylase mRNA and others having reduced amounts. In four patients studied, no major deletion or rearrangement of the phosphorylase gene was detected (Gautron et al 1987). The gene for myophosphorylase has been localized to the long arm of chromosome 11 (Lebo et al 1984). Prenatal diagnosis has not yet been achieved because a gene deletion has not been shown, and because muscle tissue is needed for the enzyme assay. Furthermore, assay of fetal muscle would be expected to show the fetal isozyme, which is active in GSD V.

Muscle phosphorylase kinase deficiency

Deficiency of phosphorylase kinase limited to muscle (without liver involvement) has been reported to cause a McArdle-like disease (Abarbanel et al 1986). Heart failure in a newborn with marked glycogenosis limited to the mycocardium and phosphorylase kinase deficiency of cardiac but not skeletal muscle or liver has been reported (Yoshinobu et al 1985).

Muscle phosphofructokinase (PFK) deficiency (GSD type VII)

Clinical aspects The clinical features of PFK deficiency are very similar to those of McArdle disease (Tarui 1965). Exercise tolerance is limited by skeletal muscle cramps and pain. Symptoms usually begin during childhood and may be mild or very severe. Strenuous exercise may be followed by muscle pain, malaise, nausea and myoglobinuria (Tobin et al 1973). An infantile form of PFK deficiency, with severe muscle and neurological involvement has been described (Servidei et al 1986).

Biochemical aspects Laboratory studies show elevation of muscle enzyme values (aldolase, creatine kinase, lactate dehydrogenase and oxaloacetate transaminase) in the serum. The reticulocyte count is mildly increased, but there is no anaemia. Muscle fibres show increased glycogen content and vacuolar and degenerative changes. The activity of PFK is absent in muscle and reduced in erythrocytes. The PFK molecule is a tetramer. The muscle isozyme is composed of four identical (M) subunits, whereas erythrocyte PFK is made up of muscle and liver-type subunits. In PFK deficiency disease, the M subunit is absent and the residual PFK activity in erythrocytes reflects the presence of the liver subunit (Layzer & Rasmussen 1974).

Treatment Treatment of PFK deficiency is the same as that of MP deficiency; avoidance of strenuous exercise.

Genetic aspects PFK deficiency is rare. It appears to be inherited as an autosomal recessive disorder. The infantile form appears to be a separate entity.

Other glycogenoses

Hepatic glycogenosis with Fanconi renal tubular defect and vitamin D-resistant rickets This infrequently reported syndrome is recognized in infants on the basis of rickets, hepatomegaly and growth failure associated with increased renal clearance of glucose, amino acids, protein, phosphate and uric acid (Garty et al 1974). Affected patients have either low or normal fasting plasma glucose levels and normal fasting lactate values. After oral galactose administration there is an excessive rise in blood lactate. The glycaemic response to glucagon is variable. Histological findings show increased glycogen content in liver and muscle and steatosis of liver. Rickets is severe but improves with oral phosphate and vitamin D therapy in pharmacological doses. Pathogenesis of this disorder is unknown; no enzyme deficiency has been identified.

Hepatic glycogenosis with renal glycosuria The only patient reported thus far was a mentally retarded girl with marked hepatomegaly and renal glycosuria without other renal tubular dysfunctions. Fasting plasma glucose was normal. The glycogen content was increased in liver, muscle, erythrocytes and leucocytes. No enzyme defect was identified (Gutman et al 1965).

Glucose phosphate isomerase (GPI) deficiency The features of this disorder include severe haemolytic anaemia, hepatomegaly and muscle weakness. Liver and erythrocytes contain excessive amounts of glycogen. GPI activity is decreased in many tissues including erythrocytes and leucocytes (van Bieroliet & Staal 1977).

Glycogenosis of liver and brain with progressive neurological deterioration (GSD type VIII) In 1967, Hug et al described a child with hepatomegaly and progressive neurological deterioration. The glycogen content of liver and brain was increased, hepatic phosphorylase was in the inactive form. The phosphorylase activating system was normal. No other enzyme abnormality was identified.

Dominantly inherited cardioskeletal myopathy with lysosomal glycogen storage and normal maltase levels (Byrne et al 1986).

X–linked glycogen storage disease of liver and muscle without demonstrated enzyme defect The features include: hepatomegaly, growth retardation and hyperuricaemia (Keating et al 1985).

GLUCONEOGENIC DISORDERS ASSOCIATED WITH LACTIC ACIDOSIS

Metabolism

The maintenance of carbohydrate homeostasis in the human body is a complex process and involves the interaction of many factors. In fasting conditions blood glucose is derived mainly from glycogen breakdown (glycogenolysis) and from the conversion of lactic acid and certain amino acids to glucose (gluconeogenesis).

Gluconeogenesis takes place primarily in the liver and kidneys. The metabolic process is in part under endocrine control. During a prolonged fast, the levels of glucocorticoids may be increased. These hormones increase the synthesis of pyruvate carboxylase, glucose-6-phosphate, and aminotransferase, participants in the gluconeogenic pathway. Gluconeogenic amino acids, such as alanine, aspartic acid and glutamic acid are converted to pyruvate, oxaloacetate and α-ketoglutarate; respectively, and subsequently feed into the pathway culminating in the formation of glucose (Fig. 94.7). During fasting, epinephrine and glucagon increase, accelerating the glycogenolytic process through the activation of adenyl cyclase (as described in the section on glycogen metabolism). At the other end of the glycolytic pathway, pyruvate kinase is inactivated by a cyclic AMP protein kinase, diminishing the conversion of triose phosphate to pyruvate and lactate.

In addition to pyruvate kinase, gluconeogenesis is also tightly regulated by other key enzymes which are sensitive to allosteric control. Pyruvate carboxylase, which plays a primary role in conversion of pyruvate to oxaloacetate, is activated by acetyl CoA. When excess acetyl CoA builds up in cells, glucose synthesis is enhanced. Phosphoenolpyruvate carboxykinase is also necessary for phosphoenolpyruvate formation from oxaloacetate.

Other key enzymes in regulating the gluconeogenic pathway are fructose-1,6-diphosphatase and glucose-6-phosphatase. The former is stimulated by citrate and inhibited by AMP. Glucose-6-phosphatase and fructose-1,6-diphosphatase are known to be present in liver and intestinal tissues, whereas the pyruvate carboxylase and phosphoenolpyruvate carboxykinase have been shown to be present also in other tissues, including cultured skin fibroblasts. Genetic defects have been encountered in each of these enzymes in man. Hypoglycaemia and lactic acidosis are the most common findings. Lactic acidosis, secondary to hypoxia, shock or sepsis is not an uncommon complication in sick infants and children. For example, mitochondrial damage observed in Reye syndrome leads to lactic acidosis (Robinson et al 1977). Whatever the cause, persistent lactic acidosis usually needs prompt medical attention.

Fructose-1,6-diphosphatase deficiency

Clinical aspects

Symptoms usually begin in early infancy with hypoglycaemia, hyperlactic acidaemia and ketoacidosis (Baker &

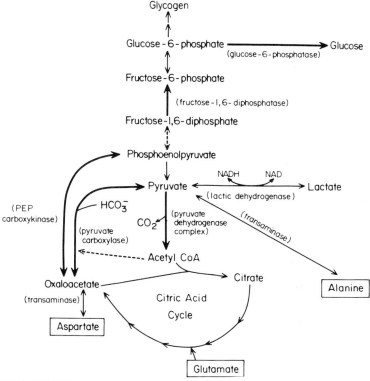

Fig. 94.7 The gluconeogenic pathway.

Winegrad 1970). The onset of symptoms often follows an infection. In some patients the onset is delayed and the clinical picture is similar to that of ketotic hypoglycaemia. The most common physical finding is hepatomegaly, resulting from fatty metamorphosis. Despite the metabolic defect, growth and intellectual development may proceed normally. Fructose-1,6-diphosphatase deficiency may be confused with glycogen storage disease type I or III, because of similarity of clinical features and of laboratory findings of hypoglycaemia and increased blood lactic acid. Confirmation of diagnosis is based upon measurement of fructose-1,6-diphosphatase activity in liver tissue.

Biochemical aspects

Prolonged fasting in the affected patient induces severe hypoglycaemia, lactic acidosis and hyperalaninaemia. The ingestion of glycerol, fructose and alanine produces hypoglycaemia, an increase in lactate and a fall in serum inorganic phosphate. Serum uric acid may also increase. The glycaemic responses to glucagon and galactose

administration have been variable. Lactate, pyruvate, β-hydroxybutyrate, alpha-ketoglutarate, and glycerol 3-phosphate accumulate in the urine (Krywawych et al 1985). The biochemical defect is a deficiency in fructose-1,6-diphosphatase activity. This enzyme is normally present in liver, kidney and intestinal tissue. It has also been found in muscle (Krebs & Woodford 1965), platelets (Karpatkin et al 1970) and lymphocytes (Fong et al 1979), however, the usefulness of these cells for diagnostic purposes has not been established.

Treatment

Treatment consists of frequent small feedings in order to prevent hypoglycaemia and limiting fructose and sorbitol intake. It has been suggested that folic acid may increase synthesis of fructose-1,6-diphosphatase (Greene et al 1972), and its use in affected children should be tested.

Genetic aspects

Fructose-1,6-diphosphatase deficiency is a rare condition inherited as an autosomal recessive trait. In parents of affected children, intermediate values of enzyme activity were found in the liver (Gitzelmann et al 1973, Saudubray et al 1973) and in cultured lymphocytes (Ito et al 1984). A family in which both the mother and a 19-month-old daughter were affected was reported (Taunton et al 1978). Fructose-1,6-diphosphatase activity in liver and intestinal mucosa were about 25% of normal. Both patients had symptomatic hypoglycaemia. The mother was unable to do her housework without having to stop several times to rest. She had unexplained episodes of crying, chilly sensations and dizziness occurring some two to five hours after meals. Biochemical studies of the liver enzyme from the mother did not reveal any difference in migration upon polyacrylamide gel electrophoresis or in K_m for fructose-1,6-diphosphate.

Pyruvate carboxylase deficiency

Clinical aspects

Clinical manifestations usually appear soon after birth. Metabolic acidosis, failure to thrive, hypotonia, anorexia, and hyporeflexia have been observed. Death within one to two months of age may occur (Saudubray et al 1976). Patients surviving the initial problems exhibit retarded growth, seizures, hypotonia and continuing metabolic acidosis. Laboratory findings include severe lactic acidosis, ketonaemia, and in some cases hyperammonaemia, citrullenaemia, hyperlysinaemia and hypoglycaemia. It has been suggested that pyruvate carboxylase deficiency is also associated with Leigh disease (Hommes et al 1968). Although the two disorders may involve the same enzyme deficiency, they now are considered to be separate entities clinically.

Biochemical aspects

The enzyme deficiency has been demonstrated in liver tissue. The assay is complicated by its dependency upon the presence of the allosteric activator, acetyl CoA. Furthermore, the enzyme is also labile. Low activities of the enzyme found in liver obtained at autopsy may reflect lability rather than a primary genetic defect. Human leucocytes and cultured skin fibroblasts also exhibit pyruvate carboxylase activity. The enzyme activity in these cells is deficient in affected patients and intermediate in known carriers (Atkin et al 1979, Atkin 1979). The enzyme is also present in cultured amniotic cells and prenatal diagnosis has been accomplished (Marsac et al 1982).

Treatment

Drastic supportive measures are usually needed. Metabolic acidosis (lactic acidosis) should be treated promptly.

Peritoneal dialysis may be helpful in reversing the clinical consequences of the metabolic defect. Biotin, thiamine and lipoic acid have been used in some patients with questionable benefit. Inclusion of glutamate and asparic acid in the diet as sources of oxaloacetate has been helpful.

Genetic aspects

Pyruvate carboxylase deficiency is inherited as an autosomal recessive disorder. The frequency of occurrence is not known. Genetic variations have been demonstrated by molecular studies. In two patients who presented with hyperammonaemia there was no CRM, while other patients had shown immuno-precipitated proteins (Robinson et al 1984).

Phosphoenolpyruvate carboxykinase deficiency

Phosphoenolpyruvate carboxykinase deficiency is rare. One patient had persistent neonatal hypoglycaemia, severe cerebral atrophy, optic nerve atrophy and fatty liver and kidneys. The enzyme defect was demonstrated in liver (Vidnes & Sovik 1976). Another patient presented at 4 months of age with failure to thrive, hepatomegaly, hypotonia, developmental delay, lactic acidaemia and fasting hypoglycaemia. Cultured skin fibroblasts showed 19% of normal activity of phosphoenolpyruvate carboxykinase (Robinson et al 1979).

Deficiencies of pyruvate dehydrogenase complex (PDHC)

Clinical aspects

The extremely variable clinical expression in this grouping suggests both clinical and biochemical heterogeneity. Patients have been described with one or more of the following findings: microcephaly, slow mental and physical development, seizures, optic atrophy of variable degree, cerebellar ataxia along with severe lactic acidosis. In some patients, post mortem examination revealed specific CNS pathology of Leigh disease (Kretzschmar et al 1987). Partial deficiency of the enzyme complex has also been observed in patients with spinocerebellar degeneration and in Friedreich ataxia (Kark & Rodriguez-Budelli 1979). Patients usually do not have hypoglycaemia, and PDHC has not been considered as a group of key enzymes in gluconeogenesis.

In patients with pyruvate dehydrogenase deficiency the levels of pyruvate, lactate and alanine are increased in blood and urine. In milder cases, random samples of blood or urine may show normal amounts of lactate. Oral glucose loads or high carbohydrate intake may induce elevations in blood lactic acid and aggravate the symptoms. In patients affected with dihydrolipoyl dehydrogenase defect branched chain amino acids may be elevated.

Biochemical aspects

PDHC comprises three principal enzymes (E_1 = pyruvate dehydrogenase or pyruvate decarboxylase; E_2 = dihydrolipoyl transacetylase; and E_3 = dihydrolipoyl dehydrogenase and five different co-enzymes (thiamine pyrophosphate, lipoic acid, coenzyme A, flavine adenine dinucleotide and nicotinamide adenine dinucleotide). In addition, a specific kinase for inactivation and a phosphatase for activation of the pyruvate dehydrogenase have been demonstrated. The sequence of the PDHC reactions is as follows (Lehninger 1975)

(1) $E_1TPP + CH_3COCOOH \rightarrow$
$$CO_2 + E_1TPP\text{-}CHOHCH_3$$
(2) $E_1TPP\text{-}CHOHCH_3 + E_2lipoic(ox) \rightarrow$
$$E_1TPP + CH_3COE_2lipoic$$
(3) $CH_3COE_2lipoic + CoASH \rightarrow$
$$CH_3COSCoA + E_2lipoic \text{ (red)}$$
(4) $E_2lipoic(red) + E_3FAD \rightarrow E_2lipoic \text{ (ox)} + E_3FADH_2$
(5) $E_3FADH_2 + NAD^+ \rightarrow E_3FAD + NADH + H^+$

Because of the complexity of this enzyme system, it is important to have available reliable methods for each enzyme assay to pinpoint the basic defect. PDHC activity is present in cultured skin fibroblasts, and therefore this tissue should be a good source for investigation. Caution is needed to avoid mycoplasma contamination because an unusually large amount of pyruvate dehydrogenase activity has been demonstrated in affected cultures (Clark et al 1978).

Treatment

Administration of thiamine and/or lipoic acid has not been helpful in most cases. Intravenous glucose administration should be done with caution because it can cause severe lactic acidosis. It is recommended that diet should be high in fats and low in carbohydrates (Cederbaum et al 1976). While this diet may be helpful in saving the patient's life, it has not prevented mental deterioration in severe cases. In patients identified as having dihydrolipoyl dehydrogenase deficiency, favourable responses to lipoic acid treatment (Matalon et al 1984) and to branched chain amino acid restriction have been observed (Sakaguchi et al 1986).

Genetic aspects

Available data suggest that deficiencies of PDHC are inherited as autosomal recessive disorders. Because of the several enzymes and cofactors involved, the specific biochemical cause should be demonstrated so as to ascertain the particular mode of inheritance. The frequency of occurrence of PDHC deficiencies may be more than now realized. Any patient who has died as a result of lactic acidosis should be considered a suspect. Prenatal diagnosis should be possible because the enzyme system is present in cultured amniotic cells. Isolation of cDNA clones for various enzyme components of the PDHC has been recently reported. This technique should be useful for diagnosis, including prenatal diagnosis.

REFERENCES

Abarbanel J M, Bashan N, Potashnik R, Osimani A, Moses S W, Herishanu Y 1986 Adult muscle phosphorylase "b" kinase deficiency. Neurology 36: 560–562

Abraham J M, Levin B, Oberholzer V G, Russell A 1967 Glucose-galactose malabsorption. Archives of Diseases in Childhood 42: 592–597

Allen J T, Gillett M, Holton J B, King G S, Pettit B R 1980 Evidence of galactosemia in utero. Lancet 1: 603

Ambruso D, McCabe E, Anderson D et al 1985 Infectious and bleeding complications in patients with glycogenosis Ib. American Journal of Diseases of Children 139: 691–697

Anderson D H 1952 Studies of glycogen disease with report of a case in which the glycogen was abnormal. In: Najjar V A (ed) Carbohydrate metabolism: a symposium on the clinical biochemical aspects of carbohydrate utilization in health and disease. Johns Hopkins Press, Baltimore, ch 1, p28

Angelini C, Engel A 1972 Comparative study of acid maltase deficiency: biochemical differences between infantile, childhood and adult types. Archives of Neurology 26: 344–349

Atkin B M 1979 Carrier detection of pyruvate carboxylase deficiency in fibroblasts and lymphocytes. Pediatric Research 13: 1101–1104

Atkin B M, Utter M F, Weinberg M B 1979 Pyruvate carboxylase and phosphoenolpyruvate carboxykinase activity in leucocytes and fibroblasts from a patient with pyruvate carboxylase deficiency. Pediatric Research 13: 38–43

Baker L, Winegrad A I 1970 Fasting hypoglycemia and metabolic acidosis associated with deficiency of hepatic fructose-1,6-diphosphatase activity. Lancet 2: 13–16

Beaudet A L, Anderson D C, Michels V V, Arion W J, Lasnge A J 1980 Neutropenia and impaired neutrophil migration in type IB glycogen storage disease. Journal of Pediatrics 97: 906–910

Beratis N G, Labadie G U, Hirschhorn K 1978 Genetic heterogeneity in acid alpha-glucosidase deficiency. American Journal of Human Genetics 30: 23A

Besley G T N 1987 Phosphorylase b kinase deficiency in glycogenosis type VIII: differentiation of different phenotypes and heterozygotes by erythrocyte enzyme assay. Journal of Inherited Metabolic Disease 10: 115–118

Beutler E, Baluda M C 1966 A simple spot screening test for

galactosemia. Journal of Laboratory and Clinical Medicine 68: 137–141

Beutler E, Baluda M C, Sturgeon P, Day R 1965 A new genetic abnormality resulting in galactose-1-phosphate uridyltransferase deficiency. Lancet 1: 353–354

Beyreiss K, Willgerodt H, Theile H 1968 Untersuchungen bei heterozygoten merkmalstagern fur fructoseintoleranz. Klinische Wochenschrift 46: 465–468

Broadhead D M, Butterworth J 1978 Pompe's disease: diagnosis in kidney and leukocytes using 4-methylumbelliferyl-a-D-glucopyranoside. Clinical Genetics 13: 504–510

Brown B I, Brown D H 1966 Lack of an alpha-1,4-glucan:alpha-1,4 glucan 6-glucosyl transferase in a case of type IV glycogenosis. Proceedings of the National Academy of Sciences (USA) 56: 725–729

Brown B I, Brown D H 1987 Prenatal screening for type IV glycogen storage disease using cultured fibroblasts. American Society Human Genetics Abstract: 795

Brown B I, Brown D H, Jeffrey P L 1970 Simultaneous absence of alpha-1,4-glucosidase and alpha 1,6-glucosidase activities (pH4) in tissue of children with type II glycogen storage disease. Biochemistry 9: 1423–1428

Brown D H, Illingsworth B 1964 The role of olio-1,4->1,4-glucantransferase and amylo-1,6-glucosidase in the debranching of glycogen. In: Whelan W J (ed) Control of glycogen metabolism, Little Brown, Boston, p139–150

Brunberg A J, McCormick W F, Schochet S S 1971 Type III glucogenosis, an adult with diffuse muscle weakness and muscle wasting. Archives of Neurology 25: 171–178

Burke V, Danks D M 1966 Monosaccharide malabsorption in young infants. Lancet 1: 1177–1180

Burman D, Holton J B, Pennock C A (eds) 1980 Inherited disorders of carbohydrate metabolism, MTP Press, Lancaster.

Byrne E, Dennett X, Crotty B et al 1986 Dominantly inherited cardioskeletal myopathy with lysosomal glycogen storage and normal acid maltase levels. Brain 109: 523–536

Cederbaum S D, Blass J P, Minkoff N, Brown W J, Cotton M E, Harris S H 1976 Sensitivity to carbohydrate in a patient with familial intermittent lactic acidosis and pyruvate dehydrogenase deficiency. Pediatric Research 10: 713–720

Chacko C M, Christian J C, Nadler H L 1971 Unstable galactose-1-phosphate uridyltransferase: a new variant of galactosemia. Journal of Pediatrics 78: 454–460

Chacko C M, Wappner R S, Brandt I K, Nadler H L 1977 The Chicago variant of clinical galactosemia. Human Genetics 37: 261–270

Chen Y-T, Cornblath M, Sidbury J B 1984 Cornstarch therapy in type I glycogen-storage disease. The New England Journal of Medicine 310: 171–175

Chen Y -T, Coleman R A, Scheinman J J, Kolbeck P C, Sidbury J B 1988 Renal disease in Type I glycogen storage disease. New England Journal of Medicine 318: 7–11

Clark A F, Farrell D F, Burke W, Scott C R 1978 The effect of mycoplasma contamination on the in vitro assay of pyruvate dehydrogenase activity in cultured fibroblasts. Clinica Chimica Acta 87: 119–124

Cohen J, Viniik A, Faller J, Fox J 1985 Hyperuricemia in glycogen storage disease Type I. Journal of Clinical Investigation 75: 251–257

Cohen P 1973 The subunit structure of rabbit-skeletal-muscle phosphorylase kinase, and the molecular basis of its activation reactions. European Journal of Biochemistry 34: 1–14

Conklin K A, Yamashiro K M, Gray G M 1975 Human intestinal sucrase-isomaltase: identification of free sucrase and isomaltase and cleavage of hybrid into active distinct subunits. Journal of Biological Chemistry 250: 5735–5741

Cook J G H, Don N A, Mann T P 1971 Hereditary galactokinase deficiency. Archives of Diseases in Childhood 46: 465–469

Corbeel L, Boogaerts M, Van den Berghe G, Everaerts M, Marchal G, Eeckels R 1983 Haematological findings in type Ib glycogen storage disease before and after portacaval shunt. European Journal of Pediatrics 140: 273–275

Danon M J, DiMauro S, Shanske S, Archer F, Miranda A 1986 Juvenile-onset acid maltase deficiency with unusual familial features. Neurology 36: 818–822

de Barsy T, Lederer B 1980 Type VI glycogenosis: identification of subgroups. In: Burman D, Holton J B, Pennock C A (eds) Inherited disorders of carbohydrate metabolism. MTP Press, Lancaster ch19, p369–380

Deckelbaum R J, Russell A, Shapira E, Cohen T, Agam G, Gutman A 1972 Type III glycogenosis: atypical enzyme activities in blood cells in two siblings. Journal of Pediatrics 81: 955–961

DiMauro S, Hartwig G, Hays A et al 1979 Debrancher deficiency: neuromuscular disorder in 5 adults. Annals of Neurology 5: 422–436

Dreyfus J C, Poenaru L 1980 White blood cells and the diagnosis of α-glucosidase deficiency. Pediatric Research 14: 342–344

Dreyfus J, Proux D, Alexander Y 1974 Molecular studies on glycogen storage diseases. Enzyme 18: 60–72

Durand P 1958 Lacttosuria idopatica in una paziente con diarrhea cronica ed acidosis Minerva Pediatrica 10: 706–711

Engel A G 1980 Acid maltase deficiency in adults: studies in four cases of a syndrome which may mimic muscular dystrophy or other myopathies. Brain 93: 599–616

Engel A G, Gomez M R Seybold M D, Lambert E H 1973 The spectrum and diagnosis of acid maltase deficiency. Neurology 23: 95–106

Engel W K, Eyerman E L, Williams H E 1963 Late onset type of skeletal muscle phosphorylase deficiency. New England Journal of Medicine 268: 135–141

Etsuro I, Yuichi S, Kyoichi K, Hirohumi M, Yoshimasa K, Hiraku Y, Yokoyama M 1987 Type Ia glycogen storage disease with hepatoblastoma in siblings. Cancer 59: 1776–1780

Feit H, Brooke M H 1976 Myophosphorylase deficiency: two different molecular etiologies. Neurology 26: 963–967

Fernandez J, Huijing F, van de Kamer J H 1969 A screening method for liver glycogen diseases. Archives of Diseases in Childhood 44: 311–317

Fernandez J, Berger R, Smit G 1984 Lactate as a cerebral metabolic fuel for glucose-6-phosphatase deficient children. Pediatric Research 18: 335–339

Fong W F, Hynic I, Lee L, McKendry J B R 1979 Increase of fructose-1,6-diphosphatase activity in cultured human peripheral lymphocytes and its suppression by phytohemagglutinin. Biochemical and Biophysical Research Communications 88: 222–228

Froesch E R 1978 Essential fructosemia and hereditary fructose intolerance. In: Stanbury J B, Wyngaarden J B, Fredrickson D S (eds) The metabolic basis of inherited diseases, 4th edn. McGraw Hill, New York, ch 6 p 121–136

Garty R, Cooper M, Tabachnik E 1974 The Fanconi syndrome associated with hepatic glycogenosis and abnormal metabolism of galactose. Journal of Pediatrics 85: 821–823

Gautron S, Daegelen D, Minnecier F, Dubocq D, Kahn A, Dreyfus J 1987 Molecular mechanisms of McArdle's disease (Muscle glycogen phosphorylase deficiency), RNA and DNA analysis. Journal of Clinical Investigation 79: 275–281

Gitzelmann R 1965 Deficiency of erythrocyte galactokinase in a patient with galactose diabetes. Lancet 2: 670–671

Gitzelmann R, Baerlock K, Prader A 1973 Hereditäre störungen in fructoseund galaktose-stoffwechsel. Monatsschrift für Kinderheilkunde 121: 174–180

Gitzelmann R, Steinmann B, Bally C, Lebherz H G 1974 Antibody activation of mutant human fructose diphosphate aldolase B in liver extracts of patients with hereditary fructose intolerance. Biochemical and Biophysical Research Communications 59: 1270–1277

Gitzelmann R, Steinmann B, Mitchell B, Haigis E 1976 Uridine diphosphate galactose 4-epimerase deficiency. IV. Report of eight cases in three families. Helvetica Paediatrica Acta 31: 441–452

Grant D B, Alexander F W, Seakins J W T 1970 Abnormal tyrosine metabolism in hereditary fructose intolerance. Acta Paediatrica Scandinavica 59: 432–434

Gray G M, Conklin K A, Townley R R W 1976 Sucrase-isomaltase deficiency. New England Journal of Medicine 294: 750–753

Greene H L, Stifel F B, Herman R H 1972 Ketotic hypoglycemia due to hepatic fructose-1,6-diphosphatase deficiency: treatment with folic acid. American Journal of Diseases of Children 124: 415–418

Greene H L, Slonim A E, O'Neil J A Jr., Burr I M 1976 Continuous nocturnal intragastric feeding for management of type I glycogen storage disease. New England Journal of Medicine. 294: 423–425

Greene H L, Slonim A E, O'Neil J A Jr., Burr I M 1979 Type I glycogen storage disease: a metabolic basis for advances in treatment. In: Barness L A (ed) Advances in Pediatrics, vol 26. Year Book Publishers, Chicago, ch 3, p 64–92

Gregori C, Besmond C, Odievre M, Kahn A, Dreyfus J C 1984 DNA analysis in patients with hereditary fructose intolerance. Annals of Human Genetics 48: 291–296

Grunfeld J, Ganeval D, Chanard J, Fardeau M, Dreyfus J 1972 Acute renal failure in McArdle's syndrome. New England Journal of Medicine 286: 1237–1242

Guthrie R 1968 Screening for inborn errors of metabolism in the newborn infant – a multiple test program. Birth Defects Original Article Series 6:92

Gutman A, Rachmilewitz E, Stein O, Eliakim M, Stein Y 1965 Glycogen storage disease, report of a case with generalized glycogenosis without demonstrable enzyme defect. Israel Journal of Medical Science 1: 14–25

Gutman A, Barash V, Schramm H, Deckelbaum T, Granot E, Acker M, Kohn G 1985 Incorporation of [^{14}C] glucose into α-1,4 bands of glycogen by leukocytes and fibroblasts of patients with type III glygcogen storage disease. Pediatric Research 19: 28–32

Halley D, Konings A, Hupkes P, Galjaard H 1984 Regional mapping of the human gene for lysosomal alpha-glucosidase by in situ hybridization. Human Genetics 67: 326–328

Henderson, M J, Holton J B, MacFall R 1983 Further observations in a case of uridine diphosphate galactose-4-epimerase deficiency with a severe clinical presentation. Journal of Inherited Metabolic Disease 6: 17–20

Henry I, Gallano P, Besmond C et al 1985 The structural gene for aldolase B (ALDB) maps to 9q13–32. Annals of Human Genetics 49: 173–180

Herman R H, Zakim D 1968 Fructose metabolism IV. Enzyme deficiencies: essential fructosuria, fructose intolerance, and glycogen storage disease. American Journal of Clinical Nutrition 21: 693–698

Hers H G 1976 The control of glycogen metabolism in the liver. In: Snell E E, Boyer P D, Meister A, Richardson C C (eds) Annual Review of Biochemistry vol 45, Annual Reviews Inc., Palo Alto, p 167–189

Holton J B, Gillett M G, MacFaul R, Young R 1981 Galactosemia: a new severe variant due to uridine diphosphate galactose-4-epimerase deficiency. Archives of Diseases in Childhood 56: 885–887

Hommes F A, Polman H A, Reerink J D 1968 Leigh's encephalomyelopathy: an inborn error of gluconeogenesis. Archives of Diseases in Childhood 43: 423–426

Howell R R, Kabach M M, Brown B I 1971 Type IV glycogen storage disease: branching enzyme deficiency in skin fibroblasts and possible heterozygote detection. Journal of Pediatrics 78: 638–642

Howell R R, Stevenson R E, Ben-Menachem Y, Phyliky R L, Berxy D H 1976 Hepatic adenomata with type I glycogen storage disease. Journal of the American Medical Association 236: 1481–1484

Hug G 1974 Enzyme therapy and prenatal diagnosis in glucogenosis type II. American Journal of Diseases of Children 128: 607–609

Hug G, Schubert W K, Chuck G, Garancis J C 1967 Liver phosphorylase: deactivation in a child with progressive brain disease, elevated hepatic glycogen and increased urinary catecholamines. American Journal of Medicine 42: 139–145

Hug G, Schubert W K, Chuck G 1969 Deficient activity of diphosphophosphorylase kinase and accumulation of glycogen in the liver. Journal of Clinical Investigation 48: 704–714

Hug G, Schubert W K, Chuck G 1970 Loss of cyclic 3'5'-AMP dependent kinase and reduction of phosphorylase kinase in skeletal muscle of a girl with deactivated phosphorylase and glucogenosis of liver and muscle. Biochemical and Biophysical Research Communications 40: 982–988

Huijung F 1973 Genetic defects of glycogen metabolism and its control. Annals of the New York Academy of Sciences 210: 290–302

Huijing F, Fernandez J 1969 X-chromosome inheritance of liver glycogenosis with phosphorylase kinase deficiency. American Journal of Human Genetics 21: 275–284

Ito M, Kurado Y, Kobashi H, Watanabe T, Takeda E, Toshima K, Miyao M 1984 Detection of heterozygotes for fructose-1,6-diphosphatase deficiency by measuring fructose-1,6-diphosphatase activity in their cultured peripheral lymphocytes. Clinica Chimica Acta 141: 27–32

Kalckar H M, Anderson E P, Isselbacher K J 1956 Galactosemia, a congenital defect in a nucleotide transferase: a preliminary report. Proceedings of the National Academy of Sciences (USA) 42: 49–51

Kark R A P, Rodriguez-Budelli M 1979 Pyruvate dehydrogenase deficiency in spino-cerebellar degeneration. Neurology 29: 126–131

Karpatkin S, Charmatz A, Langer R M 1970 Glycogenesis and gluconeogenesis in human platelets. Incorporation of glucose, pyruvate and citrate into platelet glycogen;

glycogen synthetase and fructose-1,6-diphosphatase activity. Journal of Clinical Investigation 49: 140–149

Kaufman R, Kogut M D, Donnell G N, Koch R 1979 Ovarian failure in galactosemia. Lancet 2: 737–738

Keating J, Brown B, White N, DiMauro S 1985 X-linked glycogen storage disease, a cause of hypotonia, hyperuricemia and growth retardation. American Journal of Diseases of Children 139: 609–613

Keppens S, de Wulf H 1975 The activation of liver glycogen phosphorylase by vasopressin. FEBS Letters 51: 29–32

Keppens S, de Wulf H 1976 The activation of liver glycogen phosphorylase by angiotensin II. FEBS Letters 68: 279–282

Keston A S, Meeuwisse G W, Fredrickson B 1982 Evidence for participation of mutarotase in sugar transport: absence of the enzyme in a case of glucose galactose malabsorption. Biochemical and Biophysical Research Communications 108: 1574–1580

Koster J F, Fernandez J, Slee R G, van Berkel T J C, Hulsman W C 1973 Hepatic phosphorylase deficiency: a biochemical study. Biochemical and Biophysical Research Communications 53: 282–290

Krebs H A, Woodford M 1965 Fructose-1,6-diphosphatase in striated muscle. Biochemical Journal 94: 436–445

Kretzschmar H A, DeArmond S J, Koch T K, Patel M S, Newth C J L, Schmidt K A, Packman S 1987 Pyruvate dehydrogenase complex deficiency as a cause of subacute necrotizing encephalopathy (Leigh's disease). Pediatrics 79: 370–373

Krywawych S, Wyatt S, Katz G, Lawson A M, Brenton D P 1985 Glycerol-3-phosphate excretion in fructose-1,6-diphosphatase deficiency — a new observation. Society for the Study of Inborn Errors of Metabolism. Abstract P-36

Landau B R, Marshall J S, Craig J W, Hostetler K Y, Genuth S M 1971 Quantitation of the pathways of fructose metabolism in normal and fructose intolerant subjects. Journal of Laboratory and Clinical Medicine 78: 608–618

Lang A, Groeb H, Bellkuhl B, Von Figura K 1980 A new variant of galactosemia: galactose-1-phosphate uridyl-transferase sensitive to product inhibition by glucose-1-phosphate. Pediatric Research 14: 729–734

Lange A J, Arion W J, Beaudet A L 1980 Type Ib glycogen storage disease is caused by a defect in the glucose-6-phosphate translocase of the microsomal glucose-6-phosphatase system. Journal of Biological Chemistry 255: 8381–8384

Layzer R B, Rasmussen J 1974 The molecular basis of muscle phosphofructokinase deficiency. Archives of Neurology 31: 411–417

Lebo R, Gorin F, Fletterick R, Kao F, Cheung M, Brace B, Kan Y 1984 High-resolution chromosome sorting and DNA spot-blot analyses assign McArdle's syndrome to chromosome 11. Science 225: 57–59

Lederer B, van Hoof F, van den Berghe G, Hers H 1975 Glycogen phosphorylase and its converter enzymes in hemolysate of normal human subjects and of patients with type VI glycogen-storage disease. Biochemical Journal 147: 23–35

Lederer B, van de Werve G, De Barsy T, Hers H G 1980 The autosomal form of phosphorylase kinase deficiency in man: reduced activity of the muscle enzyme. Biochemical and Biophysical Research Communications 92: 169–174

Lehninger A L 1975 Biochemistry, 2nd edn. Worth Publishers, New York, p 451

Levin S, Mosses S W, Chayoth R, Jagoda N, Steinitz K 1967 Glycogen storage disease in Israel: a clinical, biochemical and genetic study. Israel Journal of Medical Sciences 3: 397–410

Lin M S, Oizumi J, Ng W G, Alfi O S, Donnell G N 1979 Assignment of the gene for uridine diphosphate galactose-4-epimerase to human chromosome 1 by human-mouse somatic cell hybridization. Somatic Cell Genetics 5: 363–371

Lloyd M L, Olsen W A 1987 A study of the molecular pathology of sucrase-isomaltase deficiency, a defect in the intracellular processing of the enzyme. New England Journal of Medicine 316: 438–442

Lo W, Packman S, Nash S, Schmidt K, Ireland S, Diamond I, Ng W G, Donnell G N 1984 Curious neurologic sequelae in galactosemia. Pediatrics 73: 309–312

McArdle B 1951 Myopathy due to a defect in muscle glycogen breakdown. Clinical Science 10: 13–33

McLaren J, Ng W G, Roe T 1980 Abnormal urinary oligosaccharide pattern in patients with glycogen storage disease, type III. Clinical Chemistry 26: 1924–1925

McNair A, Gudmand-Hayer E, Jarnum S, Orrild L 1972 Sucrose malabsorption in Greenland. British Medical Journal 2: 19–21

Malatack J J, Iwatsuki S, Gartner J C et al 1983 Liver transplantation for type I glycogen storage disease. Lancet i: 1073–1075

Marsac C, Augereau C, Feldman G, Wolf B, Hansen T L, Berger R 1982 Prenatal diagnosis of pyruvate carboxylase deficiency. Clinica Chimica Acta 119: 121–127

Matalon R, Michals K, Justice P, Deanching M N 1977 Glucose-6-phosphatase activity in human placenta: a possible detection of heterozygote for glycogen storage disease type I. Lancet 1: 1360–1361

Matalon R, Stumpf D A, Michals K, Hart R D, Parks J K, Goodman S I 1984 Lipoamide dehydrogenase deficiency with primary lactic acidosis: Favourable response to treatment with oral lipoic acid. Journal of Pediatrics 104: 65–69

Matz D, Enzenauer J, Meune F 1975 Uber einen fall von atypischer galactosamie. Humangenetik 27: 309–313

Mayes J S, Guthrie R 1968 Detection of heterozygotes for galactokinase deficiency in a human population. Biochemical Genetics 2: 219–230

Meienhofer M C, Askanas V, Proux-Daegelen D, Dreyfus J, Engel K 1977 Muscle-type phosphorylase activity present in muscle cells cultured from three patients with myophosphorylase deficiency. Archives of Neurology 34: 779–780

Melin K, Meeuwisse G W 1969 Glucose-galactose malabsorption: a genetic study. Acta Paediatrica Scandinavica, Supplement 188: 19–24

Miller J H, Gates G F, Landing B H, Kogut M D, Roe T F 1978 Scintigraphic abnormalities in glycogen storage disease. Journal of Nuclear Medicine 19: 354–358

Mineo I, Kono N, Hara N et al 1987 Myogenic hyperuricemia, a common pathophysiologic feature of glycogenoses type III, V, and VII. New England Journal of Medicine 317: 75–80

Misuma H, Wada H, Kawakami M, Ninomiya H, Shohmori T 1981 Galactose and galactose-1-phosphate spot test for screening. Clinica Chimica Acta 111: 27–32

Mohandas T, Sparkes R S, Sparks M S, Shulkin J D 1977 Assignment of the human gene for galactose-1-phosphate uridyltransferase to chromosome 9: studies with Chinese hamster-human somatic cell hybrids. Proceedings of the National Academy of Sciences (USA) 74: 5628–5631

Moses S W, Levin S, Chayoth R, Steinitz K 1966 Enzyme induction in a case of glycogen storage disease. Pediatrics 38: 111–121

Narisawa K, Igarashi Y, Otomo H, Tada K 1978 A new variant of glycogen storage disease type I probably due to a defect in glucose-6-phosphatase transport system. Biochemical and Biophysical Research Communications 83: 1360–1364

Negishi H, Benke P J 1977 Epithelial cells and von Gierke's disease. Pediatric Research 11: 936–939

Ng W G, Donnell G N, Bergren W R 1965 Galactokinase activity in human erythrocytes of individuals at different ages. Journal of Laboratory and Clinical Medicine 66: 115–121

Ng W G, Bergren W R, Donnell G N 1973 A new variant of galactose-1-phosphate uridyltransferase in man: the Los Angeles variant. Annals of Human Genetics 37: 1–8

Ng W G, Donnell G N, Bergren W R, Alfi O, Golbus M S 1977 Prenatal diagnosis of galactosemia. Clinica Chimica Acta 74: 227–235

Ng W G, Kline F, Lin J, Koch R, Donnell G N 1978 Biochemical studies of a human low-activity galactose-1-phosphate uridyl transferase variant. Journal of Inherited Metabolic Disease 1: 145–151

Ng W G, Xu Y K, Kaufman F, Donnell G N 1987 Uridine nucleotide sugar deficiency in galactosemia: implications. Clinical Research 35: 212A

Nordlie R, Sukalski K, Munoz J, Baldwin J 1983 Type Ic, a novel glycogenosis. Journal of Biological Chemistry 258: 9739–9744

Olson L, Reeder G, Noller K, Edwards W, Howell R, Michels V 1984 Cardiac involvement in glycogen storage III. Morphologic and biochemical characterization with endomyocardial biopsy. American Journal of Cardiology 53: 980–981

Orkwiszewski K G, Tedesco T A, Croce C M 1974 Assignment of the human gene for galactokinase to chromosome 17. Nature 252: 60–62

Parker P, Burr I, Slonim A et al 1981 Regression of hepatic adenomas in type Ia glycogen storage disease with dietary therapy. Gastroenterology 81: 534–536

Peterson M L, Herber R 1967 Intestinal sucrase deficiency. Transactions of the Association of American Physicians 80: 275–283

Pickering W R, Howell R R 1972 Galactokinase deficiency: clinical and biochemical findings in a new kindred. Journal of Pediatrics 81: 50–55

Porte D, Crawford D, Jennings D B, Aber C, McIlroy M 1966 Cardiovascular and metabolic responses to exercise in McArdle's syndrome. New England Journal of Medicine 275: 406–412

Powell H, Haas R, Hall C, Wolff J, Nyhan W, Brown B 1985 Peripheral nerve in type III glycogenosis: selective involvement of unmyelinated fibre schwann cells. Muscle and Nerve 8: 667–671

Reuser A J J, Kroos M, Willemsen R, Swallow D, Tager J M, Galjaard H 1987 Clinical diversity in glycogenosis type II, Biosynthesis and in situ localization of acid α-glucosidase in mutant fibroblasts. Journal of Clinical Investigation 79: 1689–1699

Robinson B H, Gall D G, Cutz E 1977 Deficient activity of hepatic pyruvate dehydrogenase and pyruvate carboxylase in Reye's syndrome. Pediatric Research 11: 279–281

Robinson B H, Taylor J, Kahler S 1979 Mitochondrial phosphoenolpyruvate carboxykinase deficiency in a child

with lactic acidemia, hypotonia and failure to thrive. American Journal of Human Genetics 31: 60A

Robinson B H, Oei J, Sherwood W G et al 1984 The molecular basis for the two different clinical presentations of classical pyruvate carboxylase deficiency. American Journal of Human Genetics 36: 283–294

Roe T F, Kogut M D 1977 The pathogenesis of hyperuricemia in glycogen storage disease type I. Pediatric Research 11: 664–669

Roe T F, Kogut M D, Buckingham B A, Miller J, Gates G, Landing B 1979 Hepatic tumors in glycogen storage disease type I. Pediatric Research 13: 481

Roe T F, Thomas D, Gilsanz V, Isaacs H 1986 Inflammatory bowel disease in glycogen storage disease type IB. Journal of Pediatrics 109: 55–59

Ross S, Radda G, Gadian D, Rocker G, Esiri M, Falconer-Smith J 1981 Examination of a case of suspected McArdle's syndrome by ^{31}P nuclear magnetic resonance. New England Journal of Medicine 304: 1338–1342

Sadeghi-Nejad A, Presente E, Binkiewicz A, Senior B 1974 Studies of type I glycogenosis of the liver. Journal of Pediatrics 85: 49–54

Sakaguchi Y, Yoshino M, Aramaki S et al 1986 Dihydrolipoyl dehydrogenase deficiency: a therapeutic trial with branched-chain amino acid restriction. European Journal of Pediatrics 145: 271–274

Salafsky I S, Nadler H L 1971 Alpha-1,4-glucosidase activity in Pompe's disease. Journal of Pediatrics 79: 794–798

Saudubray J M, Dreyfus J C, Cepanec C, Lelo'ch H, Trung P H, Mozziconadi P 1973 Acidose lactique, hypoglycemie et hepatomegalie par deficit hereditaire en fructose-1,6-diphosphatase hepatique. Archives Francaises de Pediatrie 30: 609–632

Saudubray J M, Marsac C, Charpentier C, Cathelineau L, Besson Leaud M, Leroux J P 1976 Neonatal congenital lactic acidosis with pyruvate carboxylase deficiency in two siblings. Acta Paediatrica Scandinavica 65: 717–724

Savilahti E, Launiala K, Kuitunen P 1983 Congenital lactase deficiency, a clinical study on 16 patients. Archives of Disease in Childhood 58: 246–252

Schapira F, Kaplan J 1969 Electrophoretic abnormality of galactose-1-phosphate uridyltransferase in galactosemia. Biochemical and Biophysical Research Communications 33: 451–455

Schapira F, Schapira G, Dreyfus J C 1961/62 La lesion enzymatique de la fructosurie benigne. Enzymologia Biologica et Clinica 1: 170–175

Scherz R, Pflugshaupt R, Butler R 1976 A new genetic variant of galactose-1-phosphate uridyl transferase. Human Genetics 35: 51–55

Schmid R, Hammaker L 1961 Hereditary absence of muscle phosphorylase (McArdle's syndrome). New England Journal of Medicine 264: 223–225

Schmidt E, Schmidt F W 1979 Clinical aspects of gut enzymology. Journal of Clinical Chemistry and Clinical Biochemistry 17: 693–704

Schwenk W F, Haymond M W 1986 Optimal rate of enteral glucose administration in children with glycogen storage disease type I. The New England Journal of Medicine 314: 682–685

Scriver C R, Beaudet A L, Sly W S, Valle D (eds) 1989 The metabolic basis of inherited disease, 6th edn. McGraw Hill, New York

Segal S 1969 The Negro variant of congenital

galactosemia. In Hsia D (ed) Galactosemia. Charles C. Thomas, Springfield, Illinois, ch 23, p 176–185

Segal S, Rutman J Y, Frimpter G W 1979 Galactokinase deficiency and mental retardation. Journal of Pediatrics 95: 750–752

Service F J, Veneziale C M, Nelson R A, Ellefson R D, Go V L W 1978 Combined deficiency of glucose-6-phosphatase and fructose-1,6-diphosphatase. American Journal of Medicine 64: 696–706

Servidei S, Bonilla E, Diedrich et al 1986 Fetal infantile form of muscle phosphofructokinase deficiency. Neurology 36: 1465–1470

Shin Y, Ungar R, Rieth M, Endres W 1984 A simple assay for amylo-1,6-glucosidase to detect heterozygotes for glycogenosis type III in erythrocytes. Clinical Chemistry 30: 1717–1718

Shin Y S, Rieth M, Hayer S, Endres W 1985 Uridine diphosphogalactose, galactose-1-phosphate and galactitol concentration in patients with classical galactosemia. Society for the Study of Inborn Errors of Metabolism, Abstract p35

Simila S, Kokkonen J, Kouvalainen K 1982 Use of lactose-hydrolyzed human milk in congenital lactase deficiency. The Journal of Pediatrics 101: 584–585

Slonim A, Goans P 1985 Myopathy in McArdle's syndrome, improvement with a high-protein diet. New England Journal of Medicine 312: 355–359

Slonim A E, Weisberg C, Benke P, Evans O B, Burr I M 1982 Reversal of debrancher deficiency myopathy by the use of high-protein nutrition. Annals of Neurology 11: 420–422

Slonim A, Coleman R, McElligot M et al 1983 Improvement of muscle function in acid maltase deficiency by high-protein therapy. Neurology 33: 34–38

Soejima K, Landing B, Roe T F 1985 Pathologic studies of osteoporosis in von Gierke's disease. Pediatric Pathology 3: 307–319

Stalmans W, de Wulf H, Hers H 1971 The control of liver glycogen synthetase phosphatase by phosphorylase. European Journal of Biochemistry 18: 582–587

Stalmans W, Laloux M, Hers H 1974 The interaction of liver phosphorylase a with glucose and AMP. European Journal of Biochemistry 49: 415–427

Stamm W E, Webb D I 1975 Partial deficiency of hepatic glucose-6-phosphatase in an adult patient. Archives of Internal Medicine 135: 1107–1109

Tanaka K, Shimazu S, Oya N, Tomisawa M, Kusunoki T, Soyama K, Ono E 1979 Muscular form of glycogenosis type II (Pompe's disease). Pediatrics 63: 124–129

Taniguchi N, Kato E, Yoshida H, Iwaki S, Ohki T, Koizumi S 1978 Alpha-glucosidase activity in human leukocytes: choice of lymphocytes for the diagnosis of Pompe's disease and the carrier state. Clinica Chimica Acta 89: 293–299

Tarui S 1965 Phosphofructokinase deficiency in skeletal muscle: a new type of glycogenosis. Biochemical and Biophysical Research Communications 19: 517–523

Taunton O D, Greene H L, Stifel F B et al 1978 Fructose-1,6-diphosphatase deficiency, hypoglycemia, and response to folate therapy in a mother and her daughter. Biochemical Medicine 19: 260–276

Tedesco T A, Miller K L, Rawnsley B E, Adams M C, Markus H B, Orkwiszewski K G, Mellman W J 1977 The Philadelphia variant of galactokinase. American Journal of Human Genetics 29: 240–247

Thalhammer O, Gitzelmann R, Pantlitschko M 1968 Hypergalactosemia and galactosuria due to a galactokinase deficiency in a newborn. Pediatrics 42: 441–445

Tobin W E, Huijing F, Porro R S, Salzman R T 1973 Muscle phosphofructokinase deficiency. Archives of Neurology 28: 128–130

Tyrrell D A, Ryman B E 1976 Use of liposomes in treating type II glycogenosis. British Medical Journal 811: 88–89

van Bieroliet J-P, Staal G E 1977 Excessive hepatic glycogen storage in glucosephosphate isomerase deficiency. Acta Paediatrica Scandinavica 66: 311–315

van den Berghe G, Hue L, Hers H G 1973 Effect of the administration of fructose on the glycolytic action of glucagon, an investigation of the pathogeny of hereditary fructose intolerance. Biochemical Journal 134: 637–645

van de Werve G, Hue L, Hers H 1977 Hormonal and ionic control of the glycogenolytic cascade in rat liver. Biochemical Journal 162: 135–142

van Diggelen O P, Janse H C, Smit G P A 1985 Debranching enzyme in fibroblasts, amniotic cells and chorionic villi: pre- and postnatal diagnosis of glycogenosis type III. Clinica Chimica Acta 149: 129–134

Vidnes J, Sovik O 1976 Gluconeogenesis in infancy and childhood. III deficiencies of the extra mitochondrial form of hepatic phosphoenolpyruvate carboxykinase in a case of persistent neonatal hypoglycemia. Acta Paediatrica Scandinavica 65: 307–312

von Reuss A 1908 Zuckerausscheidung in Singlingsalter. Wiener Medizinische Wochenschrift. 58: 799–803

Waisbren S E, Norman T R, Schnell R R, Levy H L 1983 Speech and language deficits in early-treated children with galactosemia. The Journal of Pediatrics 102: 75–77

Watson J, Goldfinch M 1986 Bone marrow transplantation for glycogen storage disease type II (Pompe's disease). New England Journal of Medicine 314: 385

Wittens L A, Avruch J 1978 Insulin regulation of hepatic glycogen synthase and phosphorylase. Biochemistry 17: 406–410

Yoshikazu U, Kiyoharu I, Takemura T, Iwamasa T 1986 Accumulation of glycogen in aural nerve axons in adult-onset type III glycogenosis. Annals of Neurology 19: 294–297

Yoshinobu E, Takemura T, Sone R et al 1985 Glycogen storage disease confined to the heart with deficient activation of cardiac phosphorylase kinase: a new type of glycogen storage disease. Human Pathology 16: 193–197

Zangeneh F, Limbeck G A, Brown B I 1969 Hepatorenal glycogenosis and carcinoma of the liver. Journal of Pediatrics 74: 73–83

95. Disorders of purine and pyrimidine metabolism

J. E. Seegmiller

INTRODUCTION

In the historical introduction of scientific concepts to medicine, disorders of purine metabolism have provided a mutually fruitful meeting ground for the chemist and physician. The limited solubility of certain purine compounds leading to their precipitation as concretions of the urinary tract first brought human aberrations of purine metabolism to the attention of chemists. Thus, the Swedish chemist, Scheele, first isolated uric acid (1776) and the French chemist, Marcet, isolated xanthine (1817) from urinary calculi. In 1798 uric acid was isolated from a gouty tophus by Wollaston which he is purported to have removed from his own ear. Precipitation of uric acid on a 'huckaback' fibre, suspended in acidified serum, by the British physician, AB Garrod (1848) provided the first evidence of hyperuricaemia in gouty patients. Garrod's son, Archibald, in 1923 classified gout as an inborn error of metabolism. However, no single enzyme defect is reponsible for this disease. Instead, evidence of heterogeneity has been found with both genetic and environmental factors contributing to the hyperuricaemia responsible for development of gout. Our subsequent knowledge of more specific hereditary abnormalities in purine metabolism began less than three decades ago with the identification of the enzyme defect responsible for xanthinuria (Engelman et al 1964, Ayvazian 1964) and subsequent identification of the enzyme deficit responsible for Lesch-Nyhan disease and its variants (Seegmiller et al 1967) which in turn led to identification of other enzyme defects responsible for gouty arthritis. The past two decades has brought a burgeoning of identification of additional disorders of purine metabolism responsible for such widely different clinical conditions as immunodeficiency disease, a new type of kidney stone, haemolytic anaemia, exercise intolerance and the first enzyme defect associated with childhood autism (Fig. 95.1).

The limited solubility of certain pyrimidine compounds also provided the first indication of an abnormality of pyrimidine metabolism in a patient whose urine on cooling formed a crystalline deposit identified as orotic acid. This led to the identification of the specific enzyme defects associated with this disorder (Huguley et al 1959). More recently, a deficiency of pyrimidine 5'-nucleotidase has been found associated with a congenital primary haemolytic anaemia.

In addition, the past decade has seen assignment of additional roles for some of the products of purine metabolism. These include a modulation of free radical production by normal inflammatory cells of the body, mediated by adenosine and a possible role for uric acid as a free radical scavenger. A prime role for xanthine oxidase in production of superoxide radicals has been proposed as a potential pathological mechanism in a wide range of disorders, including reperfusion injury and development of atherosclerosis.

Defects of purine metabolism continue to provide a common meeting ground for clinicians and scientists now at the forefront of molecular genetics. Prime candidates for possible treatment by transplantation of cloned human genes are Lesch-Nyhan disease, caused by a genetic deficiency of the enzyme hypoxanthine-guanine phosphoribosyl-transferase (HPRT), and immunodeficiency diseases caused by a genetic deficiency of adenosine deaminase or purine nucleoside phosphorylase. A number of reviews have been published (Newcomb 1975, Wyngaarden & Kelley 1976, Muller et al 1977a,b, Boss & Seegmiller 1979, Seegmiller 1979a,b, Seegmiller et al 1979, Thompson & Seegmiller 1979, Mitchell & Kelley 1980, Seegmiller 1980a,b,c, Seegmiller et al 1980, Seegmiller 1985, Silverman et al 1987).

PURINE METABOLISM

Gout

Gout is a form of arthritis caused by the deposition, in and about the joints, of needle-shaped crystals of monosodium urate monohydrate from hyperuricaemic supersaturated body fluids. During the acute attacks of gouty arthritis over 95% of crystals in the joint fluid are found undergoing phagocytosis. Apparently they are being treated in the same manner as invading microorganisms, thus accounting for the intense inflammatory reaction of the attacks. The deposits of monosodium urate and the surrounding inflammatory and granulomatous response provide the characteristic pathology that differentiates gout from other forms of arthritis and from its prodromal state of hyperuricaemia.

Hyperuricaemia

The hyperuricaemia, responsible for gout, results from a heterogeneous group of environmental, physiological and genetic abnormalities and their interaction. In some

patients, the hyperuricaemia results primarily from a genetically-determined excessive synthesis of the purine precursors of uric acid. In others, the purine synthesis is normal and a diminished renal excretion of uric acid is responsible. In still others, both mechanisms contribute. The hyperuricaemia itself is entirely asymptomatic, although it may be a risk factor for development of such disorders as cardiovascular disease and diabetes mellitus (Fessel et al 1973, Fessel 1980). Patients with only a modest degree of hyperuricaemia may remain asymptomatic throughout life.

Acute gout

The degree of duration of hyperuricaemia may well be the determinants of the chance formation of the first seed

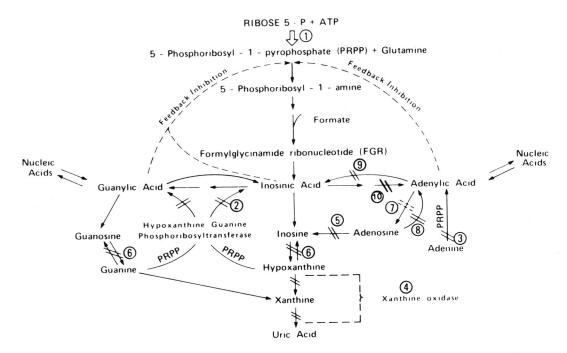

Fig. 95.1 Known enzyme defects in human purine metabolism. (1) Increased phosphoribosylpyrophosphate synthetase activity in patients with overproduction of uric acid and gout. (2) Gross deficiency of hypoxanthine guanine phosphoribosyltranferase in children with Lesch-Nyhan disease and partial deficiency of the same enzyme in patients with overproduction of uric acid and gout. (3) Adenine phosphoribosyltransferase deficiency in patients with kidney stones composed of 2-8 dioxyadenine that are often confused with uric acid stones. (4) Xanthine oxidase deficiency in patients with xanthinuria who are at increased risk for xanthine calculi of the urinary tract and, in occasional patients, myalgia from xanthine crystals in the muscle. (5) Adenosine deaminase deficiency associated with severe combined immunodeficiency disease. (6) Purine nucleoside phosphorylase deficiency associated with isolated defect in T-cells. (7) Purine 5′-nucleotidase activity is low in lymphocytes of patients with agammaglobulinaemia that may be secondary to loss of B-cells. (8) Adenosine kinase deficiency has so far been developed only in human lymphoblast cell lines. Its counterpart in patients is yet to be identified. (9) Myoadenylate deaminase deficiency is associated in some patients with development of weakness and muscle cramps after vigorous exercise and failure to show a rise in venous blood ammonia in response to muscle exercise. (10) Adenylosuccinate lyase deficiency has been found in occasional patients with childhood autism and other neurological disorders.

crystal, and thereby the age at which sufficient crystals accumulate for the first acute attack to develop. Over the years the attacks become more frequent and eventually can progress to chronic articular symptoms with permanent damage and deformity of the joint, resulting from the progressive erosion of joint surfaces by enlarging deposits of monosodium urate crystals, known as tophi. Many gouty patients also develop some evidence of renal dysfunction which, if progressive, can lead to life-threatening uraemia as the most serious complication of the disease. A portion of the renal damage can be attributed to uric acid renal lithiasis, or less commonly calcium oxalate stones. In addition, vascular changes in the kidney, hypertension and cardiovascular disease can also contribute to the overall pathology. Recent studies suggest sub-clinical lead poisoning as a major cause of renal dysfunction in patients with gout (Batuman et al 1981, Reif et al 1981).

Hyperuricaemia and gout are found in association with an ever-increasing number of other clinical disorders. Included are endocrine disorders of hypothyroidism, both hypo- and hyperparathyroidism, hypoadrenal states, myeloproliferative disorders, idiopathic hypercalciuria and psoriasis. The possibility of their being the first manifestations of one of these underlying disorders should always be considered and should lead to a complete medical evaluation to rule out these other disorders. In the present section, we will limit our discussion to the genetically-determined enzyme defects, in both carbohydrate and purine metabolism, that lead to purine overproduction as a cause of hyperuricaemia and gouty arthritis. The insight detailed studies of these disorders has given as to the normal regulatory process of purine metabolism will also be discussed.

Accompanying the increased understanding of the precise mechanisms leading to gouty athritis has been the development of rational approaches to therapeutic intervention. The result has been a dramatic improvement in the control of this disease, so that essentially all gouty patients can anticipate a life relatively unhampered by gouty arthritis, provided they follow medical advice and maintain continuous medical supervision. A number of reviews of gouty arthritis and hyperuricaemia have recently been published (Becker & Seegmiller 1974, McCarty 1974, Wyngaarden & Kelley 1976, Kelley & Weiner 1978, Boss & Seegmiller 1979, Seegmiller 1980a, Seegmiller et al 1980).

Clinical features. The presenting symptoms of acute gouty arthritis are usually sufficiently distinctive to allow its presumptive diagnosis and its differentiation from other forms of arthritis. The typical presentation consists of a monoarticular arthritis involving a peripheral joint, which shows evidence of intense inflammation, consist-ing of redness, warmth, swelling and acute tenderness, which is far greater than is seen in most other forms of arthritis. The most common presenting site is in the first metatarsophalangeal joint, which is the site of the greatest degree of physiological trauma with walking. Precipitating events may be unusual exercise, emotional upset or surgical trauma. Quite often a site of old injury determines the location for the most troublesome attacks of gout. Simkin (1977) has proposed an ingenious mechanism for concentration of urate in the first meta-tarsophalangeal joint based on the slower diffusion of urate from a traumatic effusion accumulating in this joint from excessive exercise. If untreated, the acute attack will gradually recede spontaneously over a period of one to two weeks, with complete restoration of function, but attacks will inevitably recur in the same or different joints with increasing frequency, which can eventually lead to a chronic smouldering inflammation which is usually associated with aggressive erosion of the joints, leading to permanent joint damage.

Diagnosis. The most important differential diagnosis is the distinction of gouty from septic arthritis. The latter disease can lead to substantial degrees of joint destruction within a relatively short time (Gordon et al 1986). A most direct method of distinguishing these two disorders is by the introduction of a needle into the joint space and removal of joint fluid after sterile preparation. It should be cultured, the remaining portion centrifuged and the sediment examined, with a portion stained for bacteria and the remaining portion examined under a microscope in a haemocytometer chamber. The use of cross-polarizing filters attached to an ordinary microscope will allow the ready identification of the needle-shaped crystals of monosodium urate due to their rotation of polarized light. The introduction of a red retardation filter allows the ready distinction to be made between the negatively birefringent needle-shaped crystals of monosodium urate characteristic of gouty arthritis and the positively bire-fringent trapezoidal or irregularly shaped crystals of calcium pyrophosphate which are diagnostic of chondro-calcinosis or 'pseudo gout' (McCarty 1974).

A search should also be made for gouty tophi in other parts of the body, particularly over the helix of the ears and over the points of insertion of tendons of elbows, knees or feet. If such a tophus is identified, a diagnosis of gout can quickly be made by introducing a needle and examining the contents of the needle in a drop of saline under a microscope to reveal the same needle-shaped crystals typical of gouty arthritis. The subsequent demon-stration of hyperuricaemia with a serum urate above 7.0 mg/dl provides additional confirmation of the clini-cal impression. Demonstration of crystals in fluid from the asymptomatic first metatarsophalangeal joint has proved helpful in arriving at a diagnosis (Weinberger et al 1979). Occasionally patients will be found with serum urate concentrations in the upper range of normal during the acute attack of gout. These usually return to the hyperuricaemic range when the stress of the acute attack is relieved.

Treatment. General measures for treatment include rest, elevation of the affected joint and administration of analgesics including narcotics, which is justified since this is a self-limited disease, to control the severe pain while more specific measures are being instituted. The patient should be encouraged to develop the habit of drinking at least three litres of water per day to decrease the tendency for formation of kidney stones which are commonly found in gouty patients. The acute attack responds readily to colchicine given at a dose of 0.5 mg every hour to the point of nausea, vomiting, or diarrhoea. It also responds readily to indomethacin and a wide variety of newer anti-inflammatory drugs (Boss et al 1979, Seegmiller 1980a). Phenylbutazone is no longer recommended unless other anti-inflammatory drugs have failed to control the attack.

Treatment aimed at lowering the serum urate concentration should be deferred until the acute attack of gout has been brought under control. Otherwise, experience has shown that it can lead to further exacerbation and delay in recovery from the acute attack.

Classification of gout

The period of recovery, while the patient's gout is being brought under control with prophylactic daily colchicine 0.5 mg two to three times daily as tolerated to prevent recurrences, is a convenient time to evaluate the patient's 24-hour excretion of uric acid and creatinine. Drugs such as aspirin, allopurinol or uricosuric drugs and alcoholic drinks, which are known to alter uric acid production or excretion, are stopped and the patient started on a diet virtually free of purines for a six-day period. During the last three days of the diet, the 24-hour urine is collected in a container containing 3 ml of toluene or 1/4 gram of thymol crystals, as preservative, to allow assessment of the degree of uric acid production. The urine should be stored at room temperature and analysed for both uric acid and creatinine, after care has been taken to completely dissolve, by warming and agitation, any sediment of uric acid that may be present in the bottle.

The upper range of normal excretion for an adult male is 600 mg/24 hours. Patients excreting quantities in excess of this amount are producing excessive amounts of uric acid and should be started on allopurinol after recovery from the acute attack. Allopurinol not only blocks uric acid production by inhibiting the enzyme xanthine oxidase but also diminishes excessive purine synthesis in most patients, except those with Lesch-Nyhan disease or its variants. Other indications for using allopurinol are intolerance of a uricosuric drug, recurrent calculi of the urinary tract composed of uric acid, or evidence of impaired renal function. Daily colchicine will suppress the tendency for gout patients to have an exacerbation of their disease during the first weeks to months of initiation of therapy with a drug designed to lower the serum urate concentration to the normal range. Patients should be warned of this possibility and instructed to increase the dose of colchicine at the first sign of an impending attack. Patients, with no evidence of impaired renal function, who are excreting less than 600 mg per day should be started on probenicid at a dose of 1/2 tablet (0.25 grams) daily with a gradual increase over the course of a week to a maintenance dose of 0.5 grams twice daily with additional increases in dosage as needed to maintain the serum urate concentration in the normal range (below 7.0 mg/dl). Subsequent follow-up should be done at intervals of six months for routine checks on renal function, haematology and serum urate to prevent recurrence of the disease. This approach to treatment is to maintain the serum urate in the normal range and is most gratifying to the patient who can thereby live an essentially normal life without incapacitation from gouty arthritis.

Enzyme defects associated with gout

The primary genetically-determined enzyme defects leading to gouty arthritis so far identified have all been associated with a marked overproduction of uric acid. Since an excessive production of uric acid is found in only 10–15% of gouty patients (Watts 1977), known enzyme defects probably account for less than 5% of gouty patients. The assessment of 24-hour excretion of uric acid as a routine part of the evaluation of gouty patients has the added advantage of identifying those in whom a more detailed examination for enzyme abnormalities may be appropriate.

Purine over-production and gout in glycogen storage disease type 1

A marked hyperuricaemia and modest over-production of uric acid can lead to the development of gouty arthritis in early adult life. This has been found in over 40 patients with hepatic glucose-6-phosphatase deficiency (glycogen storage disease type 1) (Alepa et al 1967, Kelley et al 1968b, Lockwood et al 1969, Seegmiller 1980a). Clinical features include hepatomegaly, retarded rate of growth and sexual development, bleeding tendencies with frequent epistaxis, early development of severe cardiovascular disease and an eating pattern in adult life of frequent small starchy meals rather than full meals. Blood shows a marked lactic acidaemia, hyperuricaemia, marked hyperlipidaemia and fasting hypoglycaemia. A number of theories have been proposed to account for the hyperuricaemia. The lactic acidaemia interferes with renal excretion of uric acid but, in addition, patients show evidence of an increased rate of purine synthesis (Alepa et al 1967, Jakovic & Sorenson 1967, Kelley et al 1968b, Roe & Kogut 1977). Greene et al (1978) provided evidence of ATP depletion and an accelerated purine nucleotide breakdown. Correction of hyperuricaemia by continuous nocturnal drip suggests a role for carbohydrate deprivation in its genesis (Benke & Gold 1977, Greene et al 1977).

Lesch-Nyhan disease

In its most severe presentation this disease is a most incapacitating neurological disorder, limited to males who present with the choreoathetosis, spasticity, mild mental retardation, 'cerebral palsy' and compulsive self-mutilation manifested by biting away lips and tongue and ends of the fingers (Lesch & Nyhan 1964). Affected children also produce markedly excessive quantities of uric acid, this forms the basis for a relatively simple screening test, in which the ratio of uric acid to creatinine in the morning urine sample is measured (Kaufman et al 1968, McInnes et al 1972). Although most patients also show an elevation of serum urate, particularly in later stages of the disease, this test cannot be used to rule out this disorder as around 5-10% show a normal serum urate.

The primary abnormality resides in a structural gene on the X chromosome coding for the synthesis of the enzyme hypoxanthine-guanine phosphoribosyltransferase, which is grossly deficient in this disorder (Seegmiller et al 1967, Seegmiller 1976). Less severe deficiencies of the same enzyme show a clinical expression with attenuation or even absence of the neurological dysfunction, but an excessive purine synthesis remains, giving rise to severe gouty arthritis with onset in early adult life and, in most cases, with the production of kidney stones composed of uric acid (Kelley et al 1967a, Kelley et al 1969, Seegmiller 1976, Seegmiller 1980c). Recurrence of the severe forms of the disease in families carrying the gene can now be prevented through monitoring of pregnancies and prenatal diagnosis (Fujimoto et al 1968, Boyle et al 1970, Van Heeswijk et al 1972, Seegmiller 1974). Several reviews have been published (Kelley et al 1969, Seegmiller 1976, Wyngaarden & Kelley 1976, Nyhan 1977, Seegmiller 1980a,b, Silverman et al 1987).

The successful cloning of the human HPRT gene (Jolly et al 1983) and the successful correction, to a substantial degree, of the HPRT-deficient human lymphoblast line cultured from an affected child by the insertion of the cloned human cDNA into a defective retroviral vector gives promise eventually of a whole new modality for possible treatment of this and other genetic diseases by gene transplantation (Willis et al 1984).

Clinical features

Although the biochemical abnormality is present prenatally, as shown by demonstration of the HPRT deficiency in amniotic cells (Fujimoto et al 1968), at birth children with this disease appear entirely normal. The first indication of the disease to many mothers is the passage of brownish to red-orange sand in the nappies, particularly noticeable when the infant becomes dehydrated. Some of the infants are very irritable with episodes of screaming, suggesting the possibility of renal colic. Most infants show normal development during the first few months of life. The first indication of impaired motor development is inability to support the head at 4-6 months of age with hypotonicity during the next year of life. Voluntary movements of both athetoid and choreoform types are present by the latter part of the first year of life, with an increase in muscle tone as the first extra-pyramidal sign. Pyramidal symptoms consisting of increased deep tendon reflexes, a sustained ankle clonus, scissoring of the lower extremities and extensor plantar responses are usually present by one year of age. An increased incidence of dislocation of the hips and club feet may in some way be related to the early hypotonicity.

Motor and physical development of affected children are grossly impaired with subnormal height and weight. Some of them show dysphagia and vomiting as prominent symptoms. An occasional patient is able to sit in a normal manner during the first year of life, which is subsequently lost with the onset of the neurological symptoms. They have a characteristic dysarthric speech, although they can usually make themselves understood to those who are caring for them. Severely affected children are never able to walk (Nyhan 1977).

Behavioural abnormalities

A compulsive aggressiveness and a self mutilation are the most variable features of the disease and are expressed in these children by biting away their lips, tongue and ends of their fingers, if given the opportunity. Biting can, in some cases, begin with the eruption of incisors. In other patients it may be delayed until early adolescence. In any given patient it can be highly variable in expression, with the patient going through periods when he shows extensive self-mutilation and other periods when this no longer is a problem. Self-mutilation tends to be correlated, at least in some cases, with emotional stress. In addition, some older children develop opisthotonic spasms which appear to be at least semivoluntary. An accompanying laryngeal spasm and stridor sometimes produces a temporary cyanosis. If the patient's head is in range of a hard object at the time of a spasm he may injure it. Children also sometimes throw themselves from the bed if left unattended or injure themselves on sharp edges of wheelchairs that are left unpadded.

Aggressive acts against others are also included in the bizarre behaviour of these children. This can take the form of biting, hitting, spitting or kicking. Physician's eye glasses are common targets for their aggression, so it is best for the examining physician to transfer them to his pocket before examining such a child. They often pinch or strike attendants in areas of sexual significance and become verbally aggressive, often with a remarkable shocking vocabulary of profanity and words that are socially unacceptable. Frequent projectile vomiting is also used by older children as one of their weapons, especially when the child becomes upset emotionally.

Even though this bizarre behaviour would be expected to alienate individuals about them, invariably these children are favourite patients of ward personnel and are charming and very responsive individuals. The children are fully aware and sensitive to their environment. They show a remarkably good sense of humour. They smile and laugh easily and appear to have far greater intelligence than their scores on intelligence tests would indicate.

Some, but not all, of the patients with less severe deficiencies of the HPRT enzyme with resulting minimal neurological dysfunction also show a compulsive behaviour. The unusual behaviour of one such patient included a compelling urge to put his hand in the cog wheels of machines which he had done on at least one occasion and lost the tip of a middle finger. He also recounted having an uncontrollable impulse to jump from a motorcycle or automobile while travelling at high speed, which had resulted in severe injuries to himself and his vehicles (Geerdink et al 1973).

Lesch-Nyhan disease and its variants are the first well-documented example of a compulsive stereotyped form of behaviour that is associated with a biochemical aberration. Since a harmless biting of lips and fingernails is a relatively common response to stress in members of the normal population, the genetic and biochemical changes could be merely producing an exaggerated response to this environmental stress.

Pathology

Autopsies reported on at least 11 patients have shown no characteristic anatomical finding in histological preparations that could be of value in characterizing the disease. Kidneys are a target for damage, leading to cardiovascular disease and death in uraemia. The most far-advanced gouty nephropathy seen at the National Institutes of Health was observed in one of Dr Nyhan's original patients who died at age 12, despite his having experienced only one acute attack of gout in the knee (Seegmiller 1968).

Biochemical features

The most extreme degree of excessive purine synthesis yet encountered in the human is found in children with Lesch-Nyhan disease. The 24-hour uric acid excretion is four to eight times that of normal individuals (Lesch & Nyhan 1964, Seegmiller et al 1967, Seegmiller 1976). The urine also contains increased amounts of the uric acid precursors 4-amino-5-imidazole carboxamide (Newcombe 1970) and hypoxanthine (Balis et al 1967). Hyperuricaemia is the eventual outcome of this overproduction but may take a number of years to develop in some patients.

Primary enzyme defect. The enzyme hypoxanthine-guanine phosphoribosyltransferase (HPRT) is normally expressed in all cells of the body with the highest specific activity found in cells of the basal ganglia and testes. The former correlates with the brain area which, if damaged, can cause analogous disorders of movement. The latter correlates with failure of sexual maturation and atrophic testes found in some patients with the most severe enzyme deficit (Watts et al 1987). A gross deficiency of the enzyme is found in all patients with Lesch-Nyhan disease (Seegmiller et al 1967, Seegmiller 1976). In patients with the most severe enzyme defect, activity is virtually absent from all cells of the body. In patients with less severe deficiencies, the HPRT activity in dialyzed erythrocyte lysates may range from less than .01 to 10 or 20% of the normal, using hypoxanthine as a substrate (Kelley et al 1967a, Kelley et al 1969, Seegmiller 1980c).

A concurrent increase in the activity of the analogous enzyme concerned with conversion of adenine to its nucleotide, adenine phosphoribosyltransferase (APRT), is a consistent finding in erythrocytes of all patients who show a severe HPRT deficiency (Seegmiller et al 1967, Seegmiller 1976), but is not found in their fibroblasts.

This increase is not found in erythrocytes of patients with a partial HPRT deficiency (Emmerson et al 1977).

HPRT activity in fibroblasts of affected children is invariably substantially higher than is found in their erythrocytes with values of around 1–3% of the activity found in normal fibroblasts (Fujimoto & Seegmiller 1970, Kelley & Meade 1971). The amount of residual activity in fibroblasts correlates inversely with the severity of clinical symptoms (Page et al 1981).

Heterozygote detection

All pedigrees have shown a pattern of inheritance consistent with X-linkage. Definitive proof came with the demonstration by radioautography of both normal and mutant phenotypes in fibroblasts grown from skin biopsies of the mothers and remains a very reliable method for heterozygote detection (Rosenbloom et al 1967a). Such a finding is entirely consistent with the single X-inactivation hypothesis proposed independently by Lyon (1961) and Beutler (1962). Demonstration of the presence of both normal and mutant cells can also be done by cloning or by selection for the mutant phenotype in the mother's fibroblasts with thioguanine or 6-azaguanine (Salzmann et al 1968, Migeon et al 1968, Felix & DeMars 1971, Fujimoto et al 1971). Heterozygotes can also be detected by assaying hair roots (Gartler et al 1971, Bakay et al 1980).

Instead of the one-third new mutations expected, examination of 47 kindreds revealed only four probands with new mutations (Francke et al 1976).

Erythrocytes of mothers of severely HPRT-deficient children invariably show an activity of HPRT in the normal range. A selective advantage of the normal stem cell over the mutant phenotype at some stage of fetal or cellular development seems to be the most satisfactory explanation. Only in heterozygotes of partial HPRT deficiency have normal and mutant erythrocytes been demonstrated (Emmerson et al 1977).

Properties of normal and mutant enzymes

HPRT has been purified up to 13 000-fold from human erythrocytes (Krenitsky et al 1969, Milman et al 1977) and to homogeneity with complete amino acid sequence (Wilson et al 1982) which agrees with the cDNA sequence (Jolly et al 1983). The magnesium and sulphhydryl groups are required for its activity and its substrates are magnesium phosphoribosylpyrophosphate (PRPP) and either hypoxanthine or guanine. It reacts with xanthine at a rate only 0.3% of that of hypoxanthine (Kelley et al 1967b). It also reacts with 6-mercaptopurine,

8-azaguanine, allopurinol and 6-thioguanine to form the respective ribonucleotides, but fails to react with adenine, uric acid, uracil, azathioprine, or oxypurinol (Krenitsky et al 1969).

The purified native enzyme is composed of two or three subunits of molecular weight 25 000. The reported molecular weights of the native enzyme range from 68 000 (Kelley & Arnold 1973) to 81 000 (Ghangas & Milman 1977). In one HPRT-deficient clone from a HeLa cell line with a missense mutation, a new protein spot was detected at the same molecular weight as the subunit, but a different position on isoelectric focusing (Milman et al 1976). Post-transcriptional alterations in the enzyme undoubtedly give rise to the three to four peaks observed on isoelectric focusing (Kelley et al 1969, Bakay & Nyhan 1971).

Considerable heterogeneity in mutations has been described. The majority of patients with the complete syndrome show no cross-reactive material (Bakay et al 1976). In some patients the mutation had produced decreased activity by reason of a decreased affinity for one of the substrates, resulting in essentially normal activity at concentrations of PRPP and guanine ten-fold greater than those generally used in the assay (Henderson et al 1976). A variety of other types of mutation in this enzyme have also been described and include differences in immunoreactive protein, electrophoretic migration, kinetic properties and amino acid sequence (Seegmiller 1980a, Silverman et al 1987).

Mechanism of purine overproduction

The excessive rates of purine synthesis observed in patients are also found in their fibroblasts (Seegmiller et al 1967, Rosenbloom et al 1968) and lymphoblasts (Lever et al 1974), providing hypoxanthine is present in the medium. If hypoxanthine is omitted from the medium, then normal cells increase their rate of purine synthesis to values quite comparable to that seen in HPRT-deficient lymphoblasts (Hershfield & Seegmiller 1977). The most reasonable explanation for the excessive rate of purine synthesis is the increased amount of phosphoribosylpyrophosphate (PRPP) accumulating as a result of the HPRT mutation. Fibroblasts cultured from affected patients show a two- to three-fold accumulation of PRPP and their erythrocytes a ten-fold accumulation over normal values (Rosebloom et al 1968, Kelley et al 1970). PRPP is a rate-limiting substrate for the presumed rate-determining reaction of purine biosynthesis catalyzed by the enzyme phosphoribosylpyrophosphate glutamine amidotransferase (Wood & Seegmiller 1973, Wood et al 1973). Further support for this concept comes from the correlation of increased intracellular PRPP in fibroblasts and excessive rates of purine synthesis as a result of a different mutation found in other families with gouty arthritis consisting of increased activity of the enzyme PRPP synthetase (see below). Both types of mutation produce an increase in intracellular PRPP in cultured fibroblasts that are associated with an excessive rate of uric acid synthesis (Rosenbloom et al 1968, Becker 1976). Recent studies of mutant fibroblasts suggest a feedback regulation of both PRPP synthetase and amido-phosphoribosyltransferase by end products with the latter reaction being more sensitive to small changes in the inhibitory activity of purine nucleotide concentrations (Becker & Kim 1987).

Molecular genetics

The normal human cDNA coding for HPRT has been cloned by Jolly et al (1983). Incorporation of this cDNA into a defective retrovirus as a vector provided a very efficient mechanism for introducing the cloned gene into a lymphoblast line cloned from a child with Lesch-Nyhan disease (Willis et al 1984). The random insertion of this gene produced clones with from 2–21% of normal HPRT activity with a substantial correction of all aberrations of purine metabolism, including the excessive rate of purine synthesis. This same vector efficiently transferred the genetic material into stem cells cultured from human bone marrow (Gruber et al 1985a). The possibility of a therapeutic benefit to the neurological dysfunction from a similar genetic correction of bone marrow stem cells of affected patients was suggested by reports of some evidence of a thymic origin for glial cells of the brain (Fujita & Kitamura 1976). Furthermore, evidence of a partial correction of mutant cell activity by close proximity to a normal cell through the mechanism of metabolic cooperation (Friedmann et al 1968) has been demonstrated with use of glial cells (Gruber et al 1985b). There is a theoretical basis for possible effectiveness of correction of bone marrow cells, which is especially attractive as a method of genetic correction of the underlying defect in the central nervous system. Furthermore, as described above, the normal HPRT activity in red cells in heterozygous females provides evidence of a selective growth advantage of normal stem cells over mutant stem cells. However, transplantation of normal bone marrow cells into a 21-year-old Lesch-Nyhan patient failed to modify the central nervous system abnormality (Nyhan et al 1986). In experimental animals the introduction of the genetically-transformed autologous stem cells back into the species of origin produce no genetically-transformed cells in the circulation. Whether or not insertion of the transformed gene into other types of cell would provide this needed therapeutic benefit remains to be demonstrated.

Treatment

General measures for treatment include avoidance of dehydration, assurance of high fluid intake and making certain that nutrition is adequate. Many of these children take a very long time to eat and in an understaffed institution may actually be malnourished. Sites of chronic irritation in the mouth from sharp edges of teeth can be eliminated by a dentist, hands can be kept away from the mouth and yet be left free for use by constructing loose fitting wrap-around fabric splints for the elbows containing wooden or plastic ribs in a fabric pocket and secured in place with the tightness desired by Velcro fasteners. These children seem to be incapable of learning from punishment, but they do respond to positive experiences and some success in behaviour modification has been achieved by simply turning away from the child when their aberrant behaviour is in evidence (Jochmus et al 1977, Nyhan 1977). Partial improvement in the self-mutilating behaviour has been reported from use of both positive and negative conditioning programmes (McGreevy & Arthur 1987).

Drugs now available are very effective in preventing the damage to kidneys produced by the excessive amounts of uric acid excreted in the urine. Allopurinol, at doses up to 10 mg/kg body weight per 24 hours, produces a striking decrease in uric acid content of both urine and serum, but fails to decrease the total purine synthesis as is seen in other types of purine overproduction. Hypoxanthine and xanthine replace the deficit in uric acid in urine. Established renal calculi composed of uric acid can thereby be substantially reduced in size. A high fluid intake of at least 50 ml/kg per day will diminish the chance of forming urinary concretions composed of xanthine that have been noted occasionally in children treated with allopurinol.

Unfortunately, no rational therapy has yet been found satisfactory for treating the neurological dysfunction. Children treated with diazepam (Valium®) are more tractable and less spastic. Hydroxytryptophan has been reported to reduce self-mutilation in children in Japan (Mizuno & Yugari 1974, 1975) but was not effective in reducing the self-mutilating behaviour in numerous other studies (Frith et al 1976, Ciaranello et al 1976, Anderson et al 1976, Nyhan 1977). A transient beneficial effect has been found with administration of combinations of the peripheral decarboxylase inhibitor carbidopa, immipramine and hydroxytryptophan (Nyhan 1977).

Prenatal diagnosis

Until a more effective therapy for the neurological aspects of this disease is developed, prevention of the disease by monitoring pregnancies is indicated. This is best done by identifying heterozygous females among the relatives of an index case (Seegmiller 1974). Index cases are readily detected by demonstrating a high ratio of uric acid to creatinine in morning urine samples (Kaufman et al 1968). Our centre has monitored 25 pregnancies at risk for carrying an affected fetus and has identified seven affected fetuses, each sufficiently early that the patients' desire to terminate the pregnancy could be met.

Increased phosphoribosyl pyrophosphate (PRPP) synthetase

The excessive production of uric acid found in 13 families with gouty arthritis has now been traced to an increased activity of phosphoribosyl pyrophosphate (PRPP) synthetase. The increased intracellular concentration of PRPP found in fibroblasts or lymphoblasts cultured from patients with this disorder provides another example, with a different mutation, of the relation of concentration of this substance with rate of purine biosynthesis de novo (Rosenbloom et al 1968, Becker 1976). This correlation provides additional evidence in support of the concept outlined above of the central role of PRPP concentrations as one important factor governing the rate of purine synthesis de novo in vivo.

Clinical presentation

In all families an excessive rate of purine synthesis was in evidence, ranging from 1.0–2.4 grams/24 hours while maintained on a diet virtually free of purines. In addition, a high incidence of renal calculi composed of uric acid was also present in these families (Seegmiller 1980a). Other clinical features in two other families include deafness (see below) (Becker et al 1980a, Becker et al 1980b).

Heterogeneity in mutations

As with patients of Lesch-Nyhan disease, considerable heterogeneity has already been detected in mutations at the PRPP synthetase locus. The patient (described by Sperling et al 1972a, Sperling et al 1972b, Zoref et al 1975) showed an enhanced rate of PRPP synthetase activity only at very low levels of inorganic phosphate added to red cell lysates. At higher phosphate concentrations the enzyme showed a normal activity. It also showed a diminished response to the feedback inhibitor, adenosine diphosphate (Zoref et al 1975). The same defect was found in two additional family members over two generations.

A different mutation in the PRPP synthetase locus was responsible for the overproduction of uric acid and gouty arthritis of two brothers described by Becker at al (1972, Becker et al 1973a,b,c, Becker & Seegmiller 1975, Becker 1976). The mutant enzyme showed a three-fold increase in enzyme activity at all concentrations of phosphate in the lysate with normal kinetics except for a three-fold increase in V_{max}. The mutant enzyme showed an increased specific activity as shown by the presence of normal amounts of cross-reacting materials on testing with antibodies to purified enzyme (Becker et al 1973c), thus delineating a most unusual type of mutation. Mutant enzyme showed a difference in electrophoretic migration from that of normal, providing evidence that it results from a mutation in a structural gene coding for the enzyme. The brothers showed an incorporation of ^{14}C-glycine into urinary uric acid that was 2½–3 times normal.

Genetics

Both the HPRT enzyme and PRPP synthetase enzyme are located in close proximity on the X chromosome. X-linkage, first suspected from pedigree studies, was later confirmed by demonstrations of normal and mutant cell populations in fibroblasts cultured from heterozygous females (Zoref et al 1977a,b, Yen et al 1978). More definitive studies mapping the adjacent locations on the X chromosome utilized the techniques of somatic cell genetics (Goss & Harris 1975, Becker et al 1979). PRPP synthetase was mapped on the long arm of the human X chromosome between the alpha galactosidase locus and the HPRT locus. This demonstration provides the first example of a gene coding for two enzymes in a metabolic sequence being found on the same chromosome of the mammalian cell.

Properties of mutant enzyme

PRPP synthetase isolated from human erythrocytes is composed of subunits of 33 200 daltons which undergo reversible association (Becker et al 1975, Meyer & Becker 1977, Becker et al 1977). The monomer or aggregates of up to eight units show only minimal if any activity. The full activity is found only in aggregates of 16 and 32 subunits and for their formation magnesium ion, inorganic orthophosphate, magnesium ATP, reaction products or nucleotide inhibitors are required.

Other defects in phosphoribosylpyrophosphate synthetase

Two different reports of a deficiency in PRPP synthetase have appeared. A severe deficiency of PRPP synthetase was first reported in a child with hypouricaemia and mental retardation who showed a remarkable and unexplained recovery of enzyme activity after treatment with adrenocorticotrophic hormone (Wada et al 1974, Iinuma et al 1975). A decrease of 30% of normal (Valentine et al 1972) was later found to be a secondary response to a three- to four-fold increase in intracellular concentration of pyrimidine-5'-nucleotides from a gross deficiency of pyrimidine-5'-nucleotidase (Valentine et al 1974) (see section below).

Hereditary xanthinuria

A gross hereditary deficiency of the enzyme xanthine oxidase results in the substitution of the precursors xanthine and hypoxanthine for uric acid as the end products of purine metabolism (Ayvazian 1964). The formation of xanthine stones of the urinary tract is the principal clinical problem of patients with xanthinuria and occurred in 40% of a series of 42 patients (Seegmiller 1980a). It was associated with a sulphite oxidase deficiency in one patient, who presented with mental retardation, seizures, nystagmus, dislocated lens, enophthalmus and developmental asymmetry of the skull (Duran et al 1979, van der Heiden et al 1979, Johnson et al 1980). Additional clinical problems observed in four patients were muscle symptoms, myalgia or arthralgia, particularly after exercise; with crystals composed of xanthine or hypoxanthine demonstrated in the muscles of three. Since the first report of xanthine urinary calculi (Marcet 1817) well over 60 additional reports of calculi have appeared. A combined deficiency of xanthine oxidase and sulphite oxidase associated with mental retardation has also been described (Herve et al 1986, Lagier et al 1986) and has been traced to a possible defect in the molybdenum-containing cofactor shared by both enzymes (Roesel et al 1986, Kramer et al 1987).

Diagnosis

The majority of patients are discovered from routine use of blood chemistry panels which reveal a serum urate that is usually less than 1.0 mg/dl in an individual who is otherwise healthy and taking none of the drugs known to lower serum urate concentrations. The diagnosis is confirmed by demonstrating the excretion of less than 100 mg of uric acid per day in the 24-hour urine, along with several hundred milligrams of hypoxanthine and xanthine, as compared to around 0.2 mg per 24 hours for the normal individual. Of these oxypurines, 50–90% is xanthine.

Heterogeneity in xanthinuria is suggested in the mutations leading to the clinical presentation of xanthinuria and is shown by the markedly variable ratios of uric acid to oxypurines that have been described indicating different degrees of severity. This procedure should also distinguish xanthinuria from other causes of hypouricaemia. In patients with a renal tubular defect, uric acid rather than oxypurines will be the major component of urine. In those with hypouricaemia from purine nucleoside phosphorylase deficiency (see below), the purine nucleosides will be present in the urine, rather than oxypurines or uric acid.

A wide variety of methods are available for the demonstration of xanthine in the urine, including paper chromatography (Dent & Philpot 1954, Thompson 1960), column chromatography (Bradford et al 1968), paper electrophoresis (Englemann et al 1964) or by enzyme assay using xanthine oxidase and uricase (Klinenberg et al 1967, Chalmers & Watts 1969). Demonstration of the enzyme defect has been done using biopsy of intestinal epithelium or liver (Ayvazian 1964, Seegmiller 1980a), but is not routinely required for the diagnosis.

Treatment

A high fluid intake and avoidance of dehydration provides the simplest and most rational approach to management. In patients with recurrent xanthine stones a restriction of the purine content of the diet should be of benefit and alkalinization of the urine may help prevent recurrence. Attempts have been made to substitute the more soluble hypoxanthine for xanthine by administration of allopurinol (Englemann et al 1964, Holmes et al 1974). Subsequent studies, however, have failed to confirm a beneficial effect (Simmonds et al 1974, Simmonds et al 1975, Salti et al 1976).

Deficiency of adenine phosphoribosyltransferase (APRT)

Four of the first six known cases of homozygous deficiency of adenine phosphoribosyltransferase (APRT) presented with calculi of the urinary tract composed of 2-8-dihydroxyadenine, a substance not previously reported in human calculi. Although the clinical presentation in each of the first four cases was in childhood, numerous subsequent cases, which now number 38, have presented with their first symptoms of urinary calculi in adult life. In most cases the stone has initially been identified as uric acid on the basis of qualitative tests. The APRT mutation seems to be far greater in the Japanese population where instances of stone formation have been found in heterozygotes (Kamitani et al 1988). In one recently described case in a black woman, renal calculi were first symptomatic at age 24 with progression in renal damage by age 42 to uraemia requiring kidney transplantation. Only after the transplanted kidney developed calculi which severely compromised its function was the correct diagnosis of APRT deficiency made. After removal of stones allopurinol treatment has prevented a recurrence and renal function has been constant for at least two years (Glicklich et al 1988). A clinical observation that could be of help to the urologist in identifying this condition is that uric acid stones are hard and tend to be yellow, whereas 2–8-dihydroxyadenine stones are friable and grey-blue on crushing. The simplest test for detection of 2–8-dihydroxyadenine is to determine the ultraviolet absorption spectrum at pH2 and compare it with that of uric acid and a known standard of 2–8-dihydroxyadenine. The latter can be produced by the prolonged action of xanthine oxidase on adenine. Confirmation of the diagnosis is found by demonstrating increased amounts of adenine in the urine and the virtual absence of APRT in dialyzed lysates of erythrocytes of the affected patient (Cartier & Hamet 1974, Debray et al 1976, Simmonds et al 1976, Van Acker et al 1977a,b, Simmonds et al 1977, Simmonds et al 1978b, Cartier et al 1980, Van Acker et al 1980). No impairment of immune function has been found (Stevens et al 1980) and both homozygotes and heterozygotes show values for uric acid in the serum and urine in the normal range. This is an example of a disease in which the heterozygous state was detected before the homozygous state was identified (Kelly et al 1968a). The reported frequency of heterozygotes is one in 233 individuals (Johnson et al 1977). Rational treatment is with allopurinol.

Immunodeficiency diseases associated with defects in purine metabolism

The discovery of specific defects in each of three sequential enzymes of purine metabolism in association with three specific types of immunodeficiency disease has added a new dimension to studies of biochemical factors regulating this complex system (Fig. 95.2). Two of these deficiencies definitely represent abnormal gene products, adenosine deaminase deficiency and purine nucleoside phosphorylase deficiency. The partial deficiency of purine-5′-nucleotidase in patients with agam-

maglobulinaemia may well be a secondary result of immaturity or loss of B cells (Thompson et al 1980, Seegmiller 1985).

Adenosine deaminase deficiency

A gross deficiency of the enzyme adenosine deaminase was reported by Giblett et al (1972) in two unrelated children with severe combined immunodeficiency disease. Since that time many more families with adenosine deaminase deficiency have been identified. All patients show a virtually complete impairment of T-cell function with varying degrees of B-cell dysfunction depending on the family or the stage of the disease (Meuwissen & Pollara 1978, Seegmiller 1980a). As a consequence, these children are vulnerable to infections of viral, bacterial and fungal origin and if untreated can succumb to overwhelming infections within the first year or so of life. About one-half of the patients with an autosomal recessive type of severe combined immunodeficiency disease are estimated to have a deficiency of adenosine deaminase (Hirschhorn 1977). Progress in our understanding of this disease has been reviewed by Tritsch and Niswander (1985) and Kredich and Hersfield (1989).

Diagnosis. Adenosine deaminase deficiency should be suspected in all patients who show recurrent infections during the first year of life. Absence of the thymus shadow on X-ray and absence of tonsils or palpable lymph nodes further supports this presumption. Many patients also show a bony abnormality of the thorax with flaring of the costochondral junction, but this has not proved to be a consistent or specific finding. Confirmation of the defect is shown by demonstrating the virtual absence of adenosine deaminase in red cells, or in fibroblasts or lymphocytes cultured from affected children. In one patient with an ADA deficiency a gross deficiency of ecto-5′-nucleotidase has also been described, which presumably was secondary to the B-cell immaturity and dysfunction (Boss et al 1981). Occasional patients have been found in whom the ADA deficiency is limited to erythrocytes and reflects an unstable enzyme. Such individuals do not have impairment of the immune system (Hirschhorn et al 1979). Diagnosis of an affected fetus during the first trimester of pregnancy was accomplished by direct analysis of ADA activity in chorionic villi in a pregnancy at risk (Dooley et al 1987).

Mechanism of pathology. One proposed mechanism of suppression of the immune system is shown in Figure 95.3. Both adenosine and deoxyadenosine are substrates for adenosine deaminase. However, adenosine kinase has a higher affinity for adenosine, thereby providing an alternative pathway for its utilization (Schnebli et al 1967). The kinase for deoxyadenosine shows a much

ENZYME DEFECT

IMMUNE SYSTEM
DEFECT

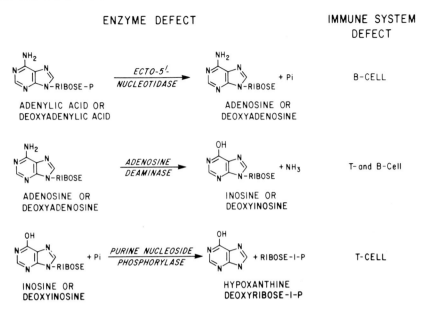

Fig. 95.2 Enzyme defects of purine nucleotide catabolism associated with various immunodeficiency diseases. Low purine-5'-nucleotidase may well be a secondary effect and reflect the paucity and immaturity of B-cells rather than being the direct product of the mutant gene.

lower affinity. Consequently, ADA-deficient children excrete, in the urine, substantial amounts of deoxyadenosine, some 6000 times that found in normal urine (Simmonds et al 1978a, Kuttesch et al 1978, Goldblum et al 1978). Erythrocytes and lymphocytes of affected children show a 10- to 20-fold increase in intracellular concentration of deoxyATP (Coleman et al 1978, Donofrio et al 1978, Cohen et al 1978a). In model systems, T-cell lines of human lymphoblasts show a greater susceptibility than B-cell lines to deoxyATP accumulation and its accompanying growth inhibition (Carson et al 1978). Impairment of growth was traced to a decreased rate of destruction of deoxyATP. This, in turn, was related to the lower activities of purine ecto-5'-nucleotidase in T-cells than in B-cells (Carson et al 1978, Thompson et al 1980).

Other workers have failed to find evidence of an increased susceptibility of normal T-cells to growth inhibition by this mechanism (Gruber et al 1985c, Gruber et al 1986, Goday et al 1986). The deoxyATP, in both the bacterial and mammalian system, is a potent allosteric inhibitor of all activities of the enzyme ribo-nucleoside diphosphate reductase which is responsible for synthesis of deoxyribonucleotide in all cells (Reichard 1972, Reichard 1978). In support of this concept is the ability of other deoxynucleosides to overcome the inhibi-

tion of mitogen-stimulated lymphocytes produced by a potent ADA inhibitor, deoxycoformycin and small amounts of deoxyadenosine (Bluestein et al 1978, Bluestein et al 1980).

Another theory for the mechanism of immunosuppression includes a permanent inhibition of the enzyme S-adenosyl-homocysteine hydrolase by deoxyadenosine that could lead to accumulation of S-adenosyl-homocysteine with a resulting inhibition of methylation reactions by S-adenosylmethionine (Hershfield 1979, Hershfield & Kredich 1979). A modest accumulation of cyclic AMP has been observed in lymphocytes of ADA-deficient patients (Schmalstieg et al 1977). The susceptibility to growth inhibition by adenosine and an ADA inhibitor of a lymphoid cell line deficient in enzymes involved in cAMP toxicity argues against this mechanism (Ullman et al 1976). The possible role of the latter two mechanisms in affected children remains to be assessed.

Treatment. Bone marrow transplantation from a histo-compatible donor has been the treatment of choice (Good & Hanson 1978). However, a transient restoration of immune function has been achieved in about half the patients by infusion at 4–6-week intervals of irradiated erythrocytes (Polmar et al 1975). Vesicles containing purified beef adenosine deaminase have produced a comparable restoration of immune function in a limited number of patients without the hazard of inducing iron accumulation that is inherent in the red cell transfusions (Hershfield et al 1987). This disease is a prime candidate for possible treatment by transplantation of the normal cDNA of the ADA gene into the patient's own bone marrow stem cells in vitro with subsequent re-population of the bone marrow with the patient's own genetically-corrected cells. Such a procedure holds promise of avoiding completely the hazard of graft versus host reaction inherent in conventional bone marrow trans-plantation.

Purine nucleoside phosphorylase deficiency

A report of a severe deficiency of the enzyme purine nucleoside phosphorylase (PNP) in a child with an isolated defect of T-cell function by Giblett et al (1975) was followed by identification of additional patients, all of whom showed evidence of gross impairment of T-cell function (Griscelli et al 1976, Wadman et al 1976, Siegenbeek et al 1976, Stoop et al 1977, Hamet et al 1977, Kredich & Hershfield 1989). Two patients have been reported who died of vaccinia infection and one with a varicella infection, pointing out the great susceptibility of these children to common viral infections. Two patients with PNP deficiencies have presented with neurological problems consisting of a tetraparesis in one case (Stoop et al 1977) and a tremor and ataxia in the other (Rich et al 1979).

Instead of excreting uric acid in the urine, these patients excrete phenomenally large amounts of the expected ribonucleoside substrates for the missing enzymes, inosine and guanosine. Totally unexpected was the presence of remarkable quantities of the correspond-ing deoxynucleosides, deoxyinosine and deoxyguanosine which constituted around one-third of the total nucleo-sides excreted (Cohen et al 1976). On a molar basis, the amount of purines excreted was comparable to the amount produced by children with Lesch-Nyhan disease (above). Since this enzyme deficit prevents these children from making hypoxanthine, a possible explanation for the excessive purine synthesis is found in the pheno-menal increase in purine synthesis produced in normal cells deprived of hypoxanthine (Hershfield & Seegmiller 1977).

One family has been described with a less severe deficiency of purine nucleoside phosphorylase associated with a clinical presentation of familial autoimmune haemolytic anaemia (Fox et al 1977, Gelfand et al 1978, Edwards et al 1978, Rich et al 1979, Rich et al 1980).

Treatment. As with patients with ADA deficiency, transfusion of irradiated erythrocytes has produced a transient return of immunological function in two

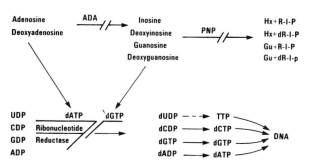

Fig. 95.3 Postulated mechanism of inhibition of lymphocyte proliferation in genetic deficiency of adenosine deaminase (ADA) or nucleoside phosphorylase (PNP).

patients with PNP deficiency (Ammann et al 1978, Zegers et al 1979, Staal et al 1980, Rich et al 1980). PNP deficiency is also a potential candidate for possible treatment by gene transplantation into the patient's bone marrow cells.

Mechanism of immunosuppression. A possible rationale for immunosuppression in this disease is very similar to that for ADA deficiency (Fig. 95.3), with the exception that deoxyguanosine leads to the deoxyGTP accumula-tion within the cells of the immune system. This nucleoside triphosphate then becomes the active inhibi-tor of the ribonucleoside diphosphate reductase leading to inhibition of production of deoxynucleosides of guan-ine, uracil and cytosine, thus preventing DNA synthesis (Cohen et al 1978a). Further evidence for this concept has been found in the resistance to deoxyguanosine toxicity of mouse T-lymphoma cells traced to a ribo-nucleoside diphosphate reductase resistant to allosteric inhibition by deoxyGTP (Gudas et al 1978, Seegmiller 1980a, Seegmiller 1985).

Significance for tumour therapy. The mechanism de-duced for the immunosuppression of either ADA or PNP deficiency points the way for possible use of inhibitors of these same enzymes, possibly with their deoxynucleo-sides, as specific therapy for conditions resulting from over-active T-cells. The most potent inhibitor known for ADA is deoxycoformycin with a Ki of 2.5×10^{-12} M (Johns & Adamson 1976, Adamson et al 1977, Agarwal et al 1979). Inhibition of ADA by the potent ADA inhibitor deoxycoformycin has been used for treatment of T-cell leukaemia with some promising results (Yu et al 1979, Smyth et al 1979, Mitchell et al 1979, Koller et al 1980, Yu et al 1980, Yu et al 1981). Although a more potent inhibitor of purine nucleoside phosphorylase than was previously available has been described (Willis et al 1980) even more potent and specific inhibitors would undoub-tedly be useful.

Decreased ecto-purine-5′-nucleotidase

A decrease in activity of the membrane-bound enzyme ecto-purine-5′-nucleotidase has been reported in lymphocytes from peripheral blood of patients with both acquired and hereditary forms of agammaglobulinaemia, and as an accompaniment of malignant lymphomas (Quagliata et al 1974, Johnson et al 1977, Edwards et al 1978). The evidence now available favours the view of the low activity reflecting immaturity and scarcity of B cells rather than a primary product of an abnormal gene. A complete absence of the enzyme activity was not found in any of the patients, and in normal controls a wide range of values was found. A possible explanation for the wide range of values in controls has been suggested by the report of Boss et al (1980) showing a decrease in the activity of this enzyme in both T and B lymphocytes with advancing age after mid-life. In normal individuals, T-cells show about one-third the activity of this enzyme found in B-cells. Some evidence has been presented that the enzyme activity may reflect a degree of B-cell immaturity (Boss et al 1979). Concurrence of low ecto-5′-nucleotidase activity in a patient with adenosine deaminase deficiency has also been found (Boss et al 1981).

X-linked agammaglobulinaemia

Affected males show a paucity of B-cells and low activities of ecto-5′-nucleotidase in peripheral blood lymphocytes. All attempts at producing long-term cultures from their peripheral blood lymphocytes have been unsuccessful. However, some of the lymphoblast lines established from peripheral blood lymphocytes of female relatives showed a low ecto-5′-nucleotidase activity during the initial phase of the cultures. However, the activity rapidly increased with prolonged culture. This observation suggested the possible identification in this manner of carriers for the gene (Thompson et al 1980). The low activity of this enzyme in T-cells may be the basis for their greater susceptibility to deoxyadenosine toxicity (see ADA deficiency above).

Myoadenylate deaminase deficiency

A gross deficiency of the enzyme adenylic acid deaminase has been found in muscle cells, but not erythrocytes or leucocytes, of five patients with exercise intolerance leading to weakness and muscle cramps as their major symptoms. They also showed decreased muscle mass, hypotonia and non-specific abnormal electromyograms. In some patients an increase in serum creatine phosphokinase was found and venous ammonia failed to rise after muscle exercise. The defects seem to be limited only to AMP deaminase generated within muscle and is not found in erythrocytes or in cultured fibroblasts or lymphoblasts (Fishbein et al 1978, Fishbein 1986). The same defect was found in six of 256 biopsies examined, but only two of the six patients had exercise related symptoms (Shumate et al 1979). In 452 muscle biopsies examined, AMP deaminase deficiency was found in 13 patients (2.9% of the specimens) but no correlation was found with exercise intolerance (Mercelis et al 1987). Furthermore, in none of the 35 biopsies from patients presenting with exercise-related muscle cramps or pains was AMP deaminase deficiency found, thus indicating that this is a relatively uncommon cause of such muscle symptoms. AMP deaminase was also found to be low in muscle tissue of patients with an early onset form of Duchenne muscular dystrophy (Kar & Pearson 1973). One patient with myoadenylate deficiency also had gouty arthritis (Dimauro et al 1980). His cultured fibroblasts showed a normal activity. An overactivity of the corresponding enzyme of liver has been proposed on theoretical grounds as a possible basis for excessive purine synthesis and gouty arthritis by Hers & Van den Berghe (1979).

Erythrocyte adenylate deaminase deficiency

In six individuals showing a complete deficiency of AMP deaminase in erythrocytes no ill health or haematological disorder was found (Ogasawara et al 1987).

Deficiency of adenylate kinase

Two sibs from consanguineous parents of an Arabian family showed a severe non-spherocytic haemolytic anaemia associated with a severe deficiency of the enzyme adenylate kinase (Szeinberg et al 1969a,b). This enzyme is normally involved in the synthesis of ADP from AMP so that its deficiency could well interfere with generation of ATP. However, the possible role in their anaemia of the glucose-6-phosphate dehydrogenase deficiency, also found in their erythrocytes, must be considered.

Ecto-nucleoside triphosphate pyrophosphohydrolase

Overactivity of the enzyme ecto-nucleoside triphosphate pyrophosphohydrolase which degrades both purine and pyrimidine nucleoside triphosphates thus liberating increased amounts of pyrophosphate, was first detected in cartilage cells of patients with chondrocalcinosis (Tennenbaum et al 1981, Howell et al 1984, Muniz et al 1984). This same enzyme was also found elevated in synovial fluid with highest values in patients with articular chondrocalcinosis and intermediate activities in synovial fluid from patients with osteoarthritis (Caswell et al 1983). The fact that an elevation of this same enzyme was found in fibroblasts cultured from sporadic cases of chondrocalcinosis (Ryan et al 1986) suggests an overproduction of pyrophosphate as the underlying mechanism. The fact that this same group were unable to find elevations of this enzyme in fibroblasts cultured from patients with familial forms of the disease seems most curious, but may well reflect the genetic heterogeneity underlying this disease.

Other abnormalities

An increase in adenosine deaminase activity was found in erythrocytes of 12 members affected with haemolytic anaemia in a family of 23, spanning three generations. They showed splenomegaly, a reticulocytosis averaging 6%, a negative Coomb's test for autoimmune haemolytic anaemia and no evidence of haemoglobinopathy (Valentine et al 1977). It was inherited in a dominant pattern and affected 5 of 10 males and 8 of 13 females. A low ATP content of the erythrocytes, as a result of this enhanced enzyme activity, seems to be the basis for the chronic haemolysis. The possibility of treatment with the very potent inhibitor of adenosine deaminase, deoxycoformycin, should be considered (Mitchell & Kelley 1980).

Other unidentified disorders of purine metabolism

Several families have been described with increased rates of purine synthesis associated with neurological dysfunction. These include a child originally thought to have autistic behaviour (Nyhan et al 1969, Becker et al 1978) but who, on repeated examinations several years later, had an increased activity of phosphoribosylpyrophosphate synthetase and deafness (Becker et al 1980a,b). An association of excessive uric acid synthesis with ataxia, weakness, deafness and renal insufficiency with varying degrees of disability have been reported in a large family (Rosenberg et al 1970) but this also was later found to be associated with overactive phosphoribosylpyrophosphate synthetase (Becker et al 1986). A girl with an encephalopathy, self-mutilation and excessive uric acid production, but no hyperuricaemia, has also been reported by Hooft et al (1968).

DISORDERS OF PYRIMIDINE METABOLISM

Hereditary orotic aciduria

A severe inherited deficiency of two enzymes of pyrimidine metabolism, orotate phosphoribosyltransferase and orotidine 5'-phosphate decarboxylase, characterizes the metabolic abnormality of hereditary orotic aciduria. The resulting interruption of the biosynthesis of pyrimidine nucleotides in affected patients results in the excretion in their urine of large amounts of orotic acid, the substrate for the first of the missing enzymes. On cooling the urine, crystalline deposits of orotic acid form along the wall of the container.

Clinical symptoms

Twelve patients have now been described, 11 of which are summarized in a review by Seegmiller (1980a). Affected patients appear normal at birth but in the first year of life develop a severe megaloblastic anaemia resistant to usual forms of treatment, with an accompanying retardation of physical and mental development (Huguley et al 1959). The original patient died from an overwhelming varicella infection at the age of two years, suggesting the possibility of T-cell dysfunction (see PNP deficiency above). In one recently-diagnosed patient evidence of immune dysfunction was found (Perignon, personal communication).

Treatment

Since these children are incapable of making pyrimidines, they are the counterpart of auxotrophic bacteria and have a new dietary requirement of pyrimidines. The administration of uridine, at a dose of 1.5 g per day, produced a dramatic decline in orotic acid excretion as a result of feed-back inhibition and produced a prompt reticulocyte response and development of a normal appearance of bone marrow within 20 days. The children resumed growth. This dietary supplement, adjusted at intervals for increases in body requirements, seems to be a fully adequate form of treatment (Becroft & Phillips 1965, Haggard & Lockhart 1967, Becroft & Phillips 1969).

Orotic aciduria associated with defects in urea synthesis

Genetically-determined human deficiencies in each of the five enzymes involved in urea synthesis have been found (Levine et al 1974). In each case hyperammonaemia was a prominent feature of the clinical disorder which also included vomiting, lethargy and coma. In the few cases that have been examined so far an orotic aciduria has been found (MacLeod et al 1972, Beaudry et al 1975). Presumably, the orotic aciduria arises from excessive carbamyl phosphate formed in the mitochondria in response to the hyperammonaemia which then leaks into the cytoplasm where it becomes a precursor for pyrimidine nucleotide synthesis.

Deficiency of pyrimidine 5'-nucleotidase in patients with non-spherocytic haemolytic anaemia

A selective autosomal recessively inherited deficiency of the enzyme pyrimidine 5'-nucleotidase limited to erythrocytes results in a non-spherocytic haemolytic anaemia. Increased concentrations of pyrimidine nucleotides are present in all erythrocytes (Valentine et al 1974, Rochant 1975, Vives-Corrons et al 1976, Ben-Bassat et al 1976, Torrance et al 1977, Miewa et al 1977). A decrease of activity of this same enzyme is seen as a very sensitive index of lead poisoning (Valentine et al 1976).

Xeroderma pigmentosum

A defect in some stage in excision and repair of thymidine dimers of DNA induced by ultraviolet light is the fundamental defect found in patients with xeroderma pigmentosum. Their clinical presentation includes abnormalities of pigmentation on exposed areas of the skin, produced by sunlight, and numerous malignancies in the same area of the skin (Cleaver 1968, Robbins et al 1974, Robbins et al 1976, Cleaver & Kraemer 1989). It is inherited in an autosomal recessive manner and heterogeneity of the genetic lesion involved is shown by correction of the defect by cell fusion of fibroblasts cultured from patients from different families. Nine complementation groups have been so identified (Cleaver & Kraemer 1989). No fully effective treatment has been devised, other than prevention of exposure to sunlight and the removal of superficial dermis with an electric dermatome to retard development of malignant tumours (Epstein et al 1972).

Additional functions of purine metabolism and intermediates

A number of most unexpected functions of purine compounds have recently emerged. In addition to being a vasodilator, adenosine serves as a modulator of free-radical production by normal inflammatory cells of the blood stream, particularly the macrophages (Cronstein et al 1985). Considerable evidence has accumulated of the effectiveness of adenosine precursors in ameliorating the ill effects of ischaemia and particularly reperfusion injury (Gruber et al 1989). A prime role for xanthine oxidase in the production of superoxide radicals was revealed by the discovery of superoxide dismutase by Fridovich and McCord (1969). In subsequent years McCord proposed that free-radical mediated damage from xanthine oxidase and other sources in vivo might play a substantial role in producing reperfusion injury (McCord 1988). Subsequent work by more recent workers has cast some doubt on the single role of xanthine oxidase in all types of reperfusion injury, particularly since certain organs have virtually no xanthine oxidase activity (Watts et al 1965, Downey et al 1987) and evidence has been provided that the xanthine oxidase inhibitors, allopurinol or oxypurinol, previously used as indicators of the role of xanthine oxidase in the process, each by itself has free-radical scavenging properties (Das et al 1987). In recent years work from Steinberg's laboratory has provided evidence of a free radical mechanism being an important factor in marking LDL particles for phagocytosis by macrophages in arterial walls in the early stages of development of atherosclerosis (Carew et al 1987) and the value of an antioxidant in preventing in part the development of atherosclerosis in the Watanabe rabbit. Although over the years uric acid has been regarded as essentially a waste product, recent investigators have pointed out that the same prosimian ancestor that lost the enzyme uricase also lost the ability to synthesize ascorbic acid and suggest that the reducing properties of uric acid might very well replace some of the reducing activity of ascorbic acid in scavenging free radicals (Ames et al 1981). Since ascorbic acid in the presence of ferrous iron is a commonly used system for generating hydroxyl radicals, failure of uric acid to produce such radicals might very well provide some advantage in reducing the exposure of human tissues to free radicals.

REFERENCES

Adamson R H, Zaharevitz D W, Johns D G 1977 Enhancement of the biological activity of adenosine analogs by the adenosine deaminase inhibitor 2'-deoxycoformycin. Pharmacology 15: 84–89

Agarwal R P, Spector T, Parks P E 1979 Tight-binding inhibitors: IV. Inhibition of adenosine deaminase by various inhibitors. Biochemical Pharmacology 26: 259–267

Alepa F P, Howell R R, Klinenberg J R, Seegmiller J E 1967 Relationships between glycogen storage disease and tophaceous gout. American Journal of Medicine 42: 58–66

Ames B N, Cathcart R, Schiviers E, Hochstein P 1981 Uric acid provides an antioxidant defense in humans against oxidant and radical caused aging and cancer: A hypothesis. Proceedings of the National Academy of Sciences (USA) 78: 6858–6862

Ammann A J, Wara D W, Allen T 1978 Immunotherapy and immunopathologic studies in a patient with nucleoside phosphorylase deficiency. Clinical Immunology and Immunopathology 10: 262–269

Anderson L T, Herrmann L, Dancis J 1976 The effect of

1-5-hydroxytryptophan on self-mutilation in Lesch-Nyhan disease: A negative report. Neuropaediatrie 7: 439–442

Ayvazian J H 1964 Xanthinuria and hemochromatosis. New England Journal of Medicine 270: 18–22

Bakay B, Nyhan W L 1971 The separation of adenine and hypoxanthineguanine phosphoribosyltransferase isoenzymes by disc gel electrophoresis. Biochemical Genetics 5: 81–90

Bakay B, Becker M A, Nyhan W L 1976 Reaction of antibody to normal human hypoxanthine phosphoribosyltransferase with products of mutant genes. Archives of Biochemistry and Biophysics 177: 415–426

Bakay B, Tucker-Pian C, Seegmiller J E 1980 Detection of Lesch-Nyhan Syndrome carriers: Analysis of hair roots for HPRT by agarose gel electrophoresis and autoradiography. Clinical Genetics 17: 1–6

Balis M E, Krakoff I H, Berman P H, Dancis J 1967 Urinary metabolites in congenital hyperuricosuria. Science 156: 1122–1123

Batuman V, Maesaka J K, Haddad B, Tepper E, Landy E, Wedeen R P 1981 The role of lead in gout nephropathy. New England Journal of Medicine 304: 520–523

Beaudry M A, Letarte J, Collu R, Leboeuf G, Ducharme J R, Melancon S B, Dallairf L 1975 Chronic hyperammonemia with orotic aciduria: Evidence of pyrimidine pathway stimulation. Diabetic Metabolism 1: 29–37

Becker M A 1976 Patterns of phosphoribosylpyrophosphate and ribose-5-phosphate concentration and generation in fibroblasts from patients with gout and purine overproduction. Journal of Clinical Investigation 57: 308–318

Becker M A, Kim M 1987 Regulation of purine synthesis de novo in human fibroblasts by purine nucleotides and phosphoribosylpyrophosphate. Journal of Biological Chemistry 262: 14531–14537

Becker M A, Seegmiller J E 1974 Genetic aspects of gout. In: Annual Review of Medicine, Annual Reviews, Inc. 25: 15–28

Becker M A, Seegmiller J E 1975 Recent advances in the identification of enzyme abnormalities underlying excessive purine synthesis in man. Arthritis and Rheumatism 18: 687–694

Becker M A, Meyer L J, Wood A W, Seegmiller J E 1972 Gout associated with increased PRPP synthetase activity. Arthritis and Rheumatism 15: 430A

Becker M A, Meyer L J, Wood A W, Seegmiller J E 1973a Purine over-production in man associated with increased phosphoribosylpyrophosphate synthetase activity. Science 179: 1123–1126

Becker M A, Kostel P J, Meyer L J, Seegmiller J E 1973b Human phosphoribosylpyrophosphate synthetase: Increased enzyme specific activity in a family with gout and excessive purine synthesis. Proceedings of the National Academy of Sciences USA 70: 2749–2752

Becker M A, Meyer L J, Wood A W, Seegmiller J E 1973c Gout with purine overproduction due to increased phosphoribosylpyrophosphate synthetase activity. American Journal of Medicine 55: 232–242

Becker M A, Kostel P J, Meyer L J 1975 Human phosphoribosylpyrophosphate synthetase: Comparison of purified normal and mutant enzymes. Journal of Biological Chemistry 250: 6822–6830

Becker M A, Meyer L J, Huisman W H, Lazar C S, Adams W B 1977 Human phosphoribosylpyrophosphate synthetase:

Relation of activity and quaternary structure. In: Muller M M, Kaiser E, Seegmiller J E (eds) Advances in Experimental Medicine and Biology, 76a. Plenum Press, New York, 71–79

Becker M A, Raivio K O, Bakay B, Adams W B, Nyhan W L 1978 Superactive phosphoribosylpyrophosphate (PRPP) synthetase with altered regulatory and catalytic functions. Abstracts of 29th Annual Meeting of the American Society of Human Genetics, p 22a

Becker M A, Yen R C K, Itkin P, Goss S J, Seegmiller J E, Bakay B 1979 Regional localization of the gene for human phosphoribosylpyrophosphate synthetase on the X-chromosome. Science 203: 1016–1019

Becker M A, Raivio K O, Bakay B, Adams W B, Nyhan W L 1980a Superactive phosphoribosylpyrophosphate synthetase with altered regulatory and catalytic properties. In: Rapado A, Watts R W E, DeBruyn C H M M (eds) Advances in Experimental Medicine and Biology. Plenum Press, New York, 122A: p 387–392

Becker M A, Raivio K O, Bakay B, Adams W B, Nyhan W L 1980b Variant human phosphoribosylpyrophosphate synthetase altered in regulatory and catalytic functions. Journal of Clinical Investigation 65: 109–120

Becker M A, Losman M J, Rosenberg A L, Mehlman I, Levinson D J, Holmes E W 1986 Phosphoribosylpyrophosphate synthetase superactivity. Arthritis and Rheumatism 29: 880–888

Becroft D M O, Phillips L I 1965 Hereditary orotic aciduria and megablastic anaemia: a second case, with response to uridine. British Medical Journal 1: 547–552

Becroft D M O, Phillips L I, Simmonds A 1969 Hereditary orotic aciduria: long-term therapy with uridine and a trial of uracil. Pediatric Pharmacology Therapy 75: 885–891

Ben-Bassat I, Brok-Simoni F, Kende G, Holtzmann F, Ramot B 1976 A family with red cell pyrimidine 5'-nucleotidase deficiency. Blood 47: 919–922

Benke P J, Gold S 1977 Purine metabolism in therapy of Von Gierke's disease. Pediatric Research 1: 837a

Beutler E 1962 Biochemical abnormalities associated with hemolytic states. In: Weinstein I M, Beutler E (eds) Mechanisms of Anaemia, McGraw-Hill, New York, p 195–236

Bluestein H G, Willis R C, Thompson L F, Matsumoto S, Seegmiller J E 1978 Accumulation of deoxyribonucleotides as a possible mediator of immunosuppression in hereditary deficiency of adenosine deaminase. Transactions of the Association of American Physicians SCI: 394–402

Bluestein H G, Thompson L F, Albert D A, Seegmiller J E 1980 Altered deoxynucleoside triphosphate levels paralleling deoxynucleoside toxicity in adenosine deaminase inhibited human lymphocytes. In: Rapado A, Watts R W E, DeBruyn C H M M (eds) Advances in Experimental Medicine and Biology. Plenum Press, New York, 122A: 427–432

Boss G R, Seegmiller J E 1979 Hyperuricemia and gout: Recent developments in classification, complications and management. New England Journal of Medicine 300: 1459–1468

Boss G R, Thompson L F, Spiegelberg H L, Waldman T A, O'Connor R D, Hamburger R N, Seegmiller J E 1979 Lymphocyte ecto-5'-nucleotidase activity as a marker of B-cell maturation. Transactions of the Association of American Physicians XCII: 309–315

Boss G R, Thompson L F, Spiegelberg H L, Pichler W J,

Seegmiller J E 1980 Age dependency of lymphocyte ecto-5'-nucleotidase activity. Journal of Immunology 125: 679–682

Boss G R, Thompson L F, O'Connor R D, Ziering R W, Seegmiller J E 1981 Ecto-5'-nucleotidase deficiency: Association with adenosine deaminase deficiency and non-association with deoxyadenosine toxicity. Clinical Immunology & Immunopathology 19: 1–7

Boyle J A, Raivio K O, Astrin K H, Schulman J D, Graf M L, Seegmiller J E, Jacobsen C B 1970 Lesch-Nyhan syndrome: Prevention control by prenatal diagnosis. Science 169: 688–689

Bradford M J, Krakoff I H, Leeper R, Balis M E 1968 Study of purine metabolism in a xanthinuric female. Journal of Clinical Investigation 47: 1325–1332

Carew T E, Schwenke D C, Steinberg D 1987 Antiatherogenic effect of probucol unrelated to its hypocholesterolemic effect: Evidence that antioxidants in vivo can selectively inhibit low density lipoprotein degradation in macrophage-rich fatty streaks and slow the progression of atherosclerosis in the Watanabe heritable hyperlipidemic rabbit. Proceedings of the National Academy of Sciences USA 84: 7725–7729

Carson D A, Kaye J, Seegmiller J E 1978 Differential sensitivity of human leukemia T cell lines and B cell lines to growth inhibition by deoxyadenosine. Journal of Immunology 121: 1726–1731

Carson D A, Kaye J, Matsumoto S, Seegmiller J E, Thompson L 1979 Biochemical basis for the enhanced toxicity of deoxyribonucleosides toward malignant human T cell lines. Proceedings of the National Academy of Sciences USA 76: 2430–2433

Cartier M P, Hamet M 1974 A new metabolic disease: The complete deficit of adenine phosphoribosyltransferase and lithiasis of 2,8-dihydroxyadenine. C R Academy of Science, Paris, 279: 883–886

Cartier P, Hamet M, Vincens A, Perignon J L 1980 Complete adenine phosphoribosyltransferase (APRT) deficiency in two siblings: Report of a new case. In: Rapado A, Watts R W E, DeBruyn C H M M (eds) Advances in Experimental Medicine and Biology. Plenum Press, New York, 122A: 343–348

Caswell A, Guilland-Cumming D F, Hearn P R, McGuire M K B, Russell R G G 1983 Pathogenesis of chondrocalcinosis and pseudogout. Metabolism of inorganic pyrophosphate and production of calcium pyrophosphate dihydrate crystals. Annals of the Rheumatic Diseases 42: 27–37

Chalmers R A, Watts R W E 1969 The separate determination of xanthine and hypoxanthine in urine and blood plasma by an enzymatic differential spectrophotometric method. Analyst 94: 226–233

Ciaranello R D, Anders T F, Barchas J D, Berger P A, Cann H M 1976 The use of 5-hydroxytryptophan in a child with Lesch-Nyhan syndrome. Child Psychiatry in Human Development 7: 127–133

Cleaver J E 1968 Defective repair replication of DNA in xeroderma pigmentosum. Nature 218: 652–656

Cleaver J E, Kraemer K H 1989 Xeroderma pigmentosa. In: Scriver C R et al (eds) The metabolic basis of inherited disease, 6th edn. McGraw Hill, New York, p 2949–2971

Cohen A, Doyle D, Martin D W, Ammann A J 1976 Abnormal purine metabolism and purine overproduction in a patient deficient in purine nucleoside phosphorylase. New England Journal of Medicine 295: 1449–1454

Cohen A, Gudas L J, Ammann A J, Staal G E J, Martin D W 1978a Deoxyguanosine triphosphate as a possible toxic metabolite in immunodeficiency associated with purine nucleoside phosphorylase deficiency. Journal of Clinical Investigation 61: 1405–1409

Cohen A, Hirschhorn R, Horowitz S D, Rubinstein A, Polmar S H, Hong R, Martin D W 1978b Deoxyadenosine triphosphate as a potentially toxic metabolite in adenosine deaminase deficiency. Proceedings of the National Academy of Sciences USA 75: 472–476

Coleman M S, Donofrio J, Hutton J J, Hahn L, Daoud A, Lampkin B, Dyminski J 1978 Identification and quantitation of adenine deoxynucleotides in erythrocytes of a patient with adenosine deaminase deficiency and severe combined immunodeficiency. Journal of Biological Chemistry 253: 1619–1626

Cronstein B N, Kramer S B, Rosenstein E D, Weissman G, Horschhorn R 1985 Adenosine modulates the generation of superoxide anion by stimulated human neutrophils via interaction with a specific cell surface receptor. Annals of the New York Academy of Sciences 451: 291–301

Das D K, Engelman R M, Clement R, Otani H, Prasad M Rm, Rao P S 1987 Role of xanthine oxidase inhibitor as free radical scavenger: a novel mechanism of action of allopurinol and oxypurinol in myocardial salvage. Biochemical and Biophysical Research Communications 148: 314–319

Debray H, Cartier P, Temstet A, Cendron J 1976 Child's urinary lithiasis revealing a complete deficit in adenine phosphoribosyltransferase. Pediatric Research 10: 762–766

Dent C E, Philpot G R 1954 Xanthinuria, an inborn error (or deviation) of metabolism. Lancet 1: 182–185

Dimauro S, Miranda A F, Hays A P, Franck W A, Hoffman G S, Schoenfeldt R S, Singh N 1980 Myoadenylate deaminase deficiency. Journal of Neurological Science 47: 191–202

Donofrio J, Coleman J S, Hutton J J, Daoud A, Lampkin B, Dyminsky J 1978 Overproduction of adenine deoxynucleosides and deoxynucleotides in adenosine deaminase deficiency with severe combined immunodeficiency disease. Journal of Clinical Investigation 62: 884–887

Dooley T, Fairbanks L D, Simmonds H A et al 1987 First trimester diagnosis of adenosine deaminase deficiency. Prenatal Diagnosis 7: 561–565

Downey J M, Miura T, Eddy L J, Chambers D E, Mellert T 1987 Xanthine oxidase is not a source of free radicals in the ischemic rabbit heart. Journal of Molecular and Cellular Cardiology 19: 1053–1060

Duran M, Korteland J, Beemer F A, van der Heiden C, de Bree P K, Brink M, Wadman S K, Lombeck I 1979 Variability of sulfituria: Combined deficiency of sulfite oxidase and xanthine oxidase. In: Hommes F A (ed) Models for the Study of Inborn Errors of Metabolism. Elsevier/North Holland, Amsterdam

Edwards N L, Magilavy D B, Cassidy J T, Fox I H 1978 Lymphocyte ecto-5'-nucleotidase deficiency in congenital agammaglobulinemia. Clinical Research 26: 513A

Emmerson B T, Johnson L A, Gordon R B 1977 HGPRT-positive and HGPRT-negative erythrocytes in heterozygotes for HGPRT deficiency. In: Muller M M, Kaiser E, Seegmiller J E (eds) Advances in Experimental Medicine and Biology. Plenum Press, New York, p 359–360

Engelmann K, Watts R W E, Klinenberg J R, Sjoerdsma A,

Seegmiller J E 1964 Clinical, physiological and biochemical studies of a patient with xanthinuria and pheochromocytoma. American Journal of Medicine 37: 839–861

Epstein E H, Burk P G, Cohen I K, Decker P 1972 Dermatome shaving in the treatment of xeroderma pigmentosum. Archives of Dermatology 105: 589–590

Felix J S, DeMars R 1971 Detection of females heterozygous for the Lesch-Nyhan syndrome by 8-azaguanine-resistant growth of cultured human fibroblasts. Journal of Laboratory and Clinical Medicine 77: 596–604

Fessel W J 1980 High uric acid as an indicator of cardiovascular disease. The American Journal of Medicine 68: 401–404

Fessel W J, Siegelaub A B, Johnson E S 1973 Correlates and consequences of asymptomatic hyperuricemia. Archives of Internal Medicine 132: 44–54

Fishbein W N 1986 Myoadenylate deaminase deficiency: primary and secondary types. Toxicology and Industrial Health 2: 105–118

Fishbein W N, Armbrustmacher V W, Griffin J L 1978 Myoadenylate deaminase deficiency: A new disease of muscle. Science 200: 545–548

Fox I H, Andres C M, Gelfand E W, Biggar D 1977 Purine nucleoside phosphorylase deficiency: Altered kinetic properties of a mutant enzyme. Science 197: 1084–1086

Franke U, Felsenstein J, Gartler S M, Migeon B R, Dancis J, Seegmiller J E, Bakay B F, Nyhan W L 1976 The occurrence of new mutants in the X-linked recessive Lesch-Nyhan disease. American Journal of Human Genetics 28: 123–137

Fridovich I, McCord J M 1969 Superoxide dismutase. An enzyme function for erythrocuprein (hemocuprein). Journal of Biological Chemistry 244: 6049–6055

Friedmann T, Seegmiller J E, Subak-Sharpe J H 1968 Metabolic cooperation between genetically marked human fibroblasts in tissue culture Nature 220: 272–274

Frith C D, Johnstone E C, Joseph M H, Powell R J, Watts R W E 1976 Double-blind clinical trial of 5-hydroxytryptophan in a case of Lesch-Nyhan syndrome. Journal of Neurology, Neurosurgery and Psychiatry 39: 656–662

Fujimoto W Y, Seegmiller J E 1970 Hypoxanthine-guanine phosphoribosyltransferase deficiency: Activity in normal, mutant, and heterozygote cultured human skin fibroblasts. Proceedings of the National Academy of Sciences USA 65: 577–584

Fujimoto W Y, Seegmiller J E, Uhlendorf B W, Jacobson C B 1968 Biochemical diagnosis of an X-linked disease in utero. Lancet 2: 511–512

Fujimoto W Y, Subak-Sharpe J H, Seegmiller J E 1971 Hypoxanthine-guanine phosphoribosyltransferase deficiency: Chemical agents selective for mutant or normal cultured fibroblasts in mixed and heterozygote cultures. Proceedings of the National Academy of Sciences USA 68: 1516–1519

Fujita S, Kitamura T 1976 Origin of brain macrophages and the nature of the microglia. In: Zimmerman M M (ed) Progress in Neuropathology, vol 111. Grune & Stratton, New York, p 1–50

Garrod A B 1848 Observations on certain pathological conditions of the blood and urine in gout, rheumatism and Bright's disease. Transactions of the Medical Society of London 31: 83–98

Garrod A E 1923 Inborn errors of metabolism. Oxford, London

Gartler S M, Scott R C, Goldstein J L, Campbell B, Sparkes R 1971 Lesch-Nyhan syndrome: Rapid detection of heterozygotes by use of hair follicles. Science 172: 572–574

Geerdink R A, DeVries W H M, Willemse J, Oei T L, DeBruyn C H M M 1973 An atypical case of hypoxanthine-guanine phosphoribosyltransferase deficiency (Lesch-Nyhan syndrome). Clinical Genetics 4: 348–352

Gelfand E W, Dosch H M, Biggar W D, Fox I H 1978 Partial purine nucleoside phosphorylase deficiency: Studies of lymphocyte function. Journal of Clinical Investigation 61: 1071–1081

Ghangas G S, Milman G 1977 Hypoxanthine phosphoribosyltransferase: Two dimensional gels from normal and Lesch-Nyhan hemolysates. Science 196: 1119–1120

Giblett E R, Anderson J E, Cohen F, Pollara B, Meuwissen H J 1972 Adenosine-deaminase deficiency in two patients with severely impaired cellular immunity. Lancet 2: 1067–1069

Giblett E R, Ammann A J, Wara D W, Sandman R, Diamond L K 1975 Nucleoside-phosphorylase deficiency in a child with severely defective T-cell immunity and normal B-cell immunity. Lancet 1: 1010–1013

Glicklich D, Gruber H E, Matas A J et al 1988 2,8-dihydroxyadenine urolithiasis: report of a case first diagnosed after renal transplant. Quarterly Journal of Medicine 69: 785–793

Goday A, Simmonds H A, Fairbanks L D, Morris G S 1986 B-lymphocytes, thymocytes and platelets accumulate high dATP levels in simulated ADA deficiency. In: Nyhan W L, Thompson L F, Watts R W E (eds) Advances in Experimental Medicine & Biology vol 195A. Plenum, New York, p 515–520

Goldblum R M, Schmalstieg F C, Nelson J A, Mills G C 1978 Adenosine deaminase (ADA) and other enzyme abnormalities in immune deficiency state. In: Summitt R L, Bergsma D (eds) Cell Surface Factors, Immune Deficiencies. Twin Studies, National Foundation of March of Dimes Birth Defects, Original Article Series, New York, XIV: 73–84

Good R A, Hansen M A 1976 Primary immunodeficiency disease. Advances in Experimental Medicine and Biology 73B: 155–178

Gordon T P, Reid C, Rozenbilds M A, Ahern M 1986 Crystal shedding in septic arthritis: case reports and in vivo evidence in an animal model. Australian and New Zealand Journal of Medicine 16: 336–340

Goss J, Harris H 1975 New method for mapping genes in human chromosomes. Nature, London 255: 680–684

Greene H L, Slonim A E, O'Neill J A, Burr I M 1977 Continuous nocturnal intragastric feeding for management of Type 1 glycogen-storage disease. New England Journal of Medicine 294: 423–425

Greene H L, Wilson F A, Hefferan P, Terry A B, Moran J R, Slonim A E, Claus T H, Burr I M 1978 ATP depletion, a possible role in hyperuricemia in glycogen storage disease Type 1. Journal of Clinical Investigation 62: 321–328

Griscelli C, Hamet M, Ballet J J 1976 Third Workshop Internal Cooperative Group for Bone Marrow Transplantation in Manhattan, New York

Gruber H E, Finley K D, Hershberg R M et al 1985a Retroviral vector-mediated gene transfer into human hematopoietic progenitor cells. Science 230: 1057–1061

Gruber H E, Koenker R, Luchtman L A, Willis R C, Seegmiller J E 1985b Glial cells metabolically cooperate: A potential requirement for gene replacement therapy. Proceedings of the National Academy of Sciences 82: 6662–6666

Gruber H, Cohen A, Redelman D, Bluestein H 1985c Levels of dATP in ADA-inhibited human peripheral blood B and T lymphocytes cultured in deoxyadenosine. Annals of the New York Academy of Sciences 451: 315–318

Gruber H E, Cohen A H, Firestein G S, Redelman D, Bluestein H G 1986 Deoxy-ATP accumulation in adenosine deaminase-inhibited human B and T lymphocytes: In: Nyhan W L, Thompson L F, Watts R W E (eds) Advances in Experimental Medicine and Biology vol 195A, Plenum, New York, p 503–507

Gruber H E, Hoffer M D, McAllister D R, Laikind P K, Lane T A, Schmid-Schoenbein G W, Engler R L 1989 Increased adenosine release from ischemic myocardium by AICA riboside: Effects on flow granulocytes and injury, (in press)

Gudas L J, Ullman B, Cohen A, Martin D W 1978 Deoxyguanosine toxicity in a mouse T lymphoma: Relationship to purine nucleoside phosphorylase-associated immune dysfunction. Cell 14: 531–538

Haggard M E, Lockhart L H 1967 Megaloblastic anemia and orotic aciduria. A hereditary disorder of pyrimidine metabolism responsive to uridine. American Journal of Disabled Children 113: 733–740

Hamet M, Griscelli C, Cartier P, Ballet J, DeBruyn C, Hosli P 1977 A second case of inosine phosphorylase deficiency with severe T-cell abnormalities. In: Muller M M, Kaiser E, Seegmiller J E (eds) Advances in Experimental Medicine and Biology 76A. Plenum Press, New York, p 477–480

Henderson J F, Dossetor J B, Dasgupta M K, Russel A S 1976 Uric acid lithiasis associated with altered kinetics of hypoxanthine-guanine phosphoribosyltransferase. Clinical Biochemistry 9: 4–8

Hers H G, Van den Berghe G 1979 Enzyme defect in primary gout. Lancet 1: 585–586

Hershfield M S 1979 Apparent suicide inactivation of human lymphoblast S-adenosylhomocysteine hydrolase by 2′-deoxyadenosine and adenine arabinoside. Journal of Biological Chemistry 254: 22–25

Hershfield M S, Kredich N M 1979 In vivo inactivation of erythrocyte S-adenosylhomocysteine hydrolase by 2′-deoxyadenosine in adenosine deaminase-deficient patients. Journal of Clinical Investigation 63: 807–811

Hershfield M S, Seegmiller J E 1977 Regulation of de novo purine synthesis in human lymphoblasts: Similar rates of de novo synthesis during growth by normal cells and mutants deficient in hypoxanthine-guanine phosphoribosyltransferase activity. Journal of Biological Chemistry 252: 6002–6010

Hershfield M S, Buckley R H, Greenberg M L et al 1987 Treatment of adenosine deaminase deficiency with polyethylene glycol-modified adenosine deaminase. New England Journal of Medicine 316:589–596

Herve F, Berger J P, Soulier J 1986 Sulfite and xanthine oxidase deficiency: a diagnosis basis on 2 simple tests. Annals of Pediatrics 33: 857

Hirschhorn R 1977 Defects of purine metabolism in immunodeficiency disease. In: Schwartz R S (ed) Progress in Clinical Immunology. Grune & Stratton, San Francisco, p 67–83

Hirschhorn R H, Roegner V, Jenkins T, Seaman C,

Piomelli S, Borkowsky W 1979 Erythrocyte adenosine deaminase deficiency without immunodeficiency: Evidence for an unstable mutant enzyme. Journal of Clinical Investigation 64: 1130–1139

Holmes E W, Mason D H, Goldstein L I, Blount R E, Kelley W N 1974 Xanthine oxidase deficiency: Studies of a previously unreported case. Clinical Chemistry 20: 1076–1079

Hooft C, Van Nevel C, DeSchaepdryver A F 1968 Hyperuricosuric encephalopathy without hyperuricemia. Archives of Disabled Children 43: 734–737

Howell D S et al 1984 NTP pyrophosphohydrolase in human chondrocalcinotic and osteoarthritic cartilage. II. Further studies on histologic and subcellular destruction. Arthritis and Rheumatism 27: 193–199

Huguley C M, Bain J A, Rivers S L, Scoggins R B 1959 Refractory megablastic anemia associated with excretion of orotic acid. Blood 14: 615–634

Iinuma K, Wada Y, Onuma A, Tanabu M 1975 Electroencephalographic study of an infant with phosphoribosylpyrophosphate synthetase deficiency. Tohoku Journal of Experimental Medicine 116: 53–55

Jakovcic S, Sorensen L B 1967 Studies of uric acid metabolism in glycogen storage disease associated with gouty arthritis. Arthritis and Rheumatism 10: 129–134

Jochmus I, Koch A, Wilhelmstroop-Meyer A 1977 Verhaltenstherapie der autoagressionen beim Lesch-Nyhan-Syndrom. Monatsschrift Kinderheilkunde 125: 839–841

Johns D G, Adamson R H 1976 Enhancement of the biological activity of cordycepin (3′-deoxyadenosine) by the adenosine deaminase inhibitor 2′-deoxycoformycin. Biochemical Pharmacology 25: 1441–1444

Johnson J L, Waud W R, Rajagopalan K V, Duran M, Beemer F A, Wadman S K 1980 Inborn errors of molybdenum metabolism: Combined deficiencies of sulfite oxidase and xanthine dehydrogenase in a patient lacking the molybdenum cofactor. Proceedings of the National Academy of Sciences USA 77: 3715–3719

Johnson L A, Gordon R B, Emmerson B T 1977 Adenine phosphoribosyltransferase: A simple spectrophotometric assay and the incidence of mutation in the normal population. Biochemical Genetics 15: 265–272

Johnson S M, Asherson G L, Watts R W E, North M E, Allsop J, Webster A B D 1977 Lymphocyte-purine 5′-nucleotidase deficiency in primary hypogammaglobulinaemia. Lancet 1: 168–170

Jolly D J, Okayama H, Berg P et al 1983 Isolation and characterization of a full length, expressible cDNA for human hypoxanthine guanine phosphoribosyltransferase. Proceedings of the National Academy of Sciences USA 80: 477–481

Kamatani N, Sonoda T, Nishioka K 1988 Distribution of patients with 2,8-dihydroxyadenine urolithiasis and adenine phosphoribosyltransferase deficiency in Japan. Journal of Urology 140 (6): 1470–1472

Kar N C, Pearson C M 1973 Muscle adenylic acid deaminase activity. Neurology 23: 478–482

Kaufman J M, Greene M L, Seegmiller J E 1968 Urine uric acid to creatinine ratio. A screening test for inherited disorders of purine metabolism. Journal of Pediatrics 73: 583–592

Kelley W N, Arnold W J 1973 Human hypoxanthine-guanine phosphoribosyltransferase: Studies on the normal and mutant forms of the enzyme. Federation

Proceedings 32: 1656-1659

Kelley W N, Meade J C 1971 Studies on hypoxanthine-guanine phosphoribosyltransferase in fibroblasts from patients with the Lesch-Nyhan syndrome: Evidence for genetic heterogeneity. Journal of Biological Chemistry 246: 2953-2958

Kelley W N, Weiner I M (eds) 1978 Uric Acid. Springer-Verlag, New York, p 639

Kelley W N, Rosenbloom F M, Henderson J F, Seegmiller J E 1967a A specific enzyme defect in gout associated with overproduction of uric acid. Proceedings of the National Academy of Sciences USA 57: 1735-1739

Kelley W N, Rosenbloom F M, Henderson J F, Seegmiller J E 1967b Xanthine phosphoribosyltransferase in man: Relationship to hypoxanthine-guanine phosphoribosyltransferase. Biochemical and Biophysical Research Communications 28: 340-345

Kelley W N, Levy R I, Rosenbloom F M, Henderson J F, Seegmiller J E 1968a Adenine phosphoribosyltransferase deficiency: A previously undescribed genetic defect in man. Journal of Clinical Investigation 47: 2281-2289

Kelley W N, Rosenbloom F M, Seegmiller J E, Howell R R 1968b Excessive production of uric acid in Type 1 glycogen storage disease. Journal of Pediatrics 72: 488-496

Kelley W N, Greene M L, Rosenbloom F M, Henderson J F, Seegmiller J E 1969 Hypoxanthine-guanine phosphoribosyltransferase deficiency in gout. A review. Annals of Internal Medicine 70: 155-206

Kelley W N, Greene M L, Fox I H, Rosenbloom F M, Levy R I, Seegmiller J E 1970 Effects of orotic acid on purine and lipoprotein metabolism in man. Metabolism 19: 1025-1035

Klinenberg J R, Goldfinger S, Bradley K H, Seegmiller J E 1967 An enzymatic spectrophotometric method for the determination of xanthine and hypoxanthine. Clinical Chemistry 13: 834-841

Koller C A, Mitchell B S, Grever M R, Mejias E, Malspeis L, Metz E N 1980 Treatment of acute lymphoblastic leukemia with 2'-deoxycoformycin: Clinical and biochemical consequences of adenosine deaminase inhibition. Cancer Treatment 64: 1949-1952

Kramer S P, Johnson J L, Ribeiro A A, Millington D S, Rajagopalan K M 1987 The structure of the molybdenum cofactor. Journal of Biological Chemistry 262: 16357-16363

Kredich N M, Hershfield M S 1989 Immunodeficiency diseases caused by adenosine deaminase deficiency and purine nucleoside phosphorylase deficiency. In: Scriver C R et al (eds) The metabolic basis of inherited disease, 6th edn. McGraw Hill, New York, p 1045-1076

Krenitsky T A, Papainnou R, Elion G B 1969 Human hypoxanthine phosphoribosyltransferase. I. Purification, properties, and specificity. Journal of Biological Chemistry 244: 1263-1270

Kuttesch J F, Schmalstieg F C, Nelson J A 1978 Analysis of adenosine and other adenine compounds in patients with immunodeficiency diseases. Journal of Liquid Chromatography 1: 97-109

Lagier P, Tessonnier J M, Collet S et al 1986 Combined sulfite and xanthine oxidase deficiency due to an anomaly in the metabolism of molybdenum cofactor. Annals of Pediatrics 33: 825-828

Lesch M, Nyhan W L 1964 A familial disorder of uric acid metabolism and central nervous system function. American Journal of Medicine 36: 561-570

Lever J E, Nuki G, Seegmiller J E 1974 Expression of purine overproduction in a series of 8-azaguanine-resistant diploid human lymphoblast lines. Proceedings of the National Academy of Sciences USA 71: 2679-2683

Levine R L, Hoogenraad N J, Kretchmer N 1974 A review: Biological and clinical aspects of pyrimidine metabolism. Pediatric Research 8: 724-734

Lockwood D H, Merimee T J, Edgar P J, Greene M L, Fujimoto W Y, Seegmiller J E, Howell R R 1969 Insulin secretion in type 1 glycogen storage disease. Journal of American Diabetes Association 18: 755-758

Lyon M F 1961 Gene action in the X-chromosome of the mouse. Nature 190: 372-373

McCarty D J 1974 Crystal deposition joint disease. Annual Review of Medicine 25: 279-288

McCord J M 1988 Free radicals and myocardial ischemia: overview and outlook. Free Radical Biology and Medicine 4: 9-14

McGreevy P, Arthur M 1987 Effective behavioral treatment of self-biting by a child with Lesch-Nyhan Syndrome. Developmental Medicine and Child Neurology 29: 529-540

McInnes R, Lamm P, Clow C L, Scriver C R 1972 A filter paper sampling method for the uric acid: Creatinine ratio in urine. Normal values in the newborn. Pediatrics 49: 80-84

MacLeod P, Mackenzie S, Scriver C R 1972 Partial ornithine carbamyl transferase deficiency: An inborn error of the urea cycle presenting as orotic aciduria in a male infant. Canadian Medical Association Journal 107: 405-408

Marcet A 1817 An essay on the chemical history and medical treatment of calculous disorders. London

Mercelis R, Martin J J, deBarsy T, Van den Berghe G 1987 Myoadenylate deaminase deficiency: absence of correlation with exercise intolerance in 452 muscle biopsies. Journal of Neurology 234: 385-389

Meuwissen H J, Pollara B 1978 Combined immunodeficiency and inborn errors of purine metabolism. Blut 37: 173-181

Meyer L J, Becker M A 1977 Human erythrocyte phosphoribosylpyrophosphate synthetase. Dependence of activity on state of subunit association. Journal of Biological Chemistry 252: 3919-3925

Miewa S, Nakashima K, Fujii H, Matsumoto M, Nomura K 1977 Three cases of hereditary hemolytic anaemia with pyrimidine 5'-nucleotidase deficiency in a Japanese family. Human Genetics 37: 361-364

Migeon B R, DerKaloustian V M, Nyhan W L, Young W J, Childs B 1968 X-linked hypoxanthine-guanine phosphoribosyltransferase deficiency: heterozygote has two clonal populations. Science 160: 425-427

Milman G, Lee E, Ghangas G S, McLaughlin J R, George M 1976 Analysis of HeLa cell hypoxanthine phosphoribosyltransferase mutants and revertants by two-dimensional polyacrylamide gel electrophoresis: Evidence for silent gene activation. Proceedings of the National Academy of Sciences USA 73: 4589-4593

Milman G, Krauss S W, Olsen A S 1977 Tryptic peptide analysis of normal and mutant form of hypoxanthine phosphoribosyltransferase from HeLa cells. Proceedings of the National Academy of Sciences USA 74: 926-930

Mitchell B S, Kelley W N 1980 Purinogenic immunodeficiency diseases: Clinical features and molecular mechanisms. Annals of Internal Medicine 92: 826-831

Mitchell B S, Koller C A, Heyn R 1979 Disappearance of

acute T cell lymphoblastic leukemia following therapy with 2'-deoxycoformycin. Blood 54: 253

Mizuno T I, Yugari Y 1974 Self-mutilation in the Lesch-Nyhan syndrome. Lancet 1: 761

Mizuno T, Yugari Y 1975 Prophylactic effect of 1-5-hydroxytryptophan on self-mutilation in the Lesch-Nyhan syndrome. Neuropaediatrie 6: 13–23

Muller M M, Kaiser E, Seegmiller J E (eds) 1977a In: Advances in Experimental Medicine and Biology, vol 76A. Plenum Press, New York, p 641

Muller M M, Kaiser E, Seegmiller J E (eds) 1977b In: Advances in Experimental Medicine and Biology, vol 76B. Plenum Press, New York, p 373

Muniz O, Pelletier J P, Pelletier J M et al 1984 NTP pyrophosphohydrolase in human chondrocalcinotic and osteoarthritic cartilage. I. Some biological characteristics. Arthritis and Rheumatism 27: 186–192

Newcombe D S 1970 The urinary excretion of aminoimidazolecarboxamide in the Lesch-Nyhan syndrome. Pediatrics 46: 508–512

Newcombe D S 1975 Inherited biochemical disorders and uric acid metabolism. University Park Press, Baltimore, p 282

Nyhan W 1977 Behavior in the Lesch-Nyhan syndrome. In: Chess S, Thomas A (eds) Annual Progress in Child Psychiatry and Child Development, 10th Annual Edition, p 175–194

Nyhan W L, James J A, Teberg A J, Sweetman L, Nelson L G 1969 A new disorder of purine metabolism with behavioral manifestations. Journal of Pediatrics 74: 20–27

Nyhan W L, Johnson H G, Kaufman I A, Jones K L 1980 Serotonergic approaches to the modification of behavior in the Lesch-Nyhan syndrome. Applied Research in Mental Retardation 1: 25–40

Nyhan W L, Page T, Gruber H E, Parkman R 1986 Bone marrow transplantation in Lesch-Nyhan disease. Birth Defects 22: 113–117

Ogasawara N, Goto H, Yamada Y, Nishigaki I 1987 Deficiency of AMP deaminase in erythrocytes. Human Genetics 75: 15–18

Page T, Bakay B, Nissinen E, Nyhan W L 1981 Hypoxanthine guanine phosphoribosyltransferase variants: Correlation of clinical phenotype with enzyme activity. Journal of Inherited Metabolic Disease 4: 203–206

Polmar S H, Wetzler E M, Stern R C, Hirschhorn R 1975 Restoration of in vitro lymphocyte responses with exogenous adenosine deaminase in a patient with severe combined immunodeficiency. Lancet 2: 743–746

Quagliata F, Faig D, Conklyn M, Silber R 1974 Studies on the lymphocyte 5'-nucleotidase in chronic lymphocytic leukemia, infectious mononucleosis, normal subpopulations, and phytohemagglutinin-stimulated cells. Cancer Research 34: 3197–3202

Reichard P 1972 Control of deoxyribonucleotide synthesis in vitro and in vivo. Advances in Enzyme Regulation 10: 3–16

Reichard P 1978 From deoxynucleotides to DNA synthesis. Federation Proceedings 37: 9–14

Reif M C, Constantiner A, Levitt M F 1981 Chronic gouty nephropathy: A vanishing syndrome? New England Journal of Medicine 304: 535–536

Rich K C, Arnold W J, Palella T, Fox I H 1979 Cellular immune deficiency with autoimmune hemolytic anemia in purine nucleoside phosphorylase deficiency. American Journal of Medicine 67: 172–176

Rich K C, Mejias E, Fox I H 1980 Purine nucleoside phosphorylase deficiency: Improved metabolic and immunologic function with erythrocyte transfusions. New England Journal of Medicine 303: 937–977

Robbins J H, Kraemer K H, Lutzner M A, Festoff B W, Coon H G 1974 Xeroderma pigmentosum: An inherited disease with sun sensitivity, multiple cutaneous neoplasms, and abnormal DNA repair. Annals of Internal Medicine 80: 221–248

Robbins J H, Kraemer K H, Andrews A D 1976 Inherited DNA repair defects in H. sapiens: Their relation to UV-associated processes in xeroderma pigmentosum. In: Yuhas J M, Tennant R W, Regan J D (eds) Biology of Radiation Carcinogenesis. Raven Press, New York

Rochant H, Dreyfus B, Rosa R, Boiron M 1975 First case of pyrimidine 5'-nucleotidase deficiency in a male. International Society of Hematology, European & African Third Meeting, London, August 24–28, Abstract 19

Roe T E, Kogut M D 1977 The pathogenesis of hyperuricemia in glycogen storage disease Type 1. Pediatric Research 11: 664–669

Roesel R A, Bowyer F, Blankenship P R, Hommes F A 1986 Combined xanthine and sulphite oxidase defect due to a deficiency of molybdenum cofactor. Journal of Inherited Metabolic Disease 9: 343–347

Rosa R, Rochant H, Dreyfus B, Valentin E, Rosa J 1977 Electrophoretic and kinetic studies of human erythrocytes deficient in pyrimidine 5'-nucleotidase. Human Genetics 38: 209–215

Rosenberg A L, Bergstrom L, Troost B T, Bartholomew B A 1970 Hyperuricemia and neurologic deficits, a family study. New England Journal of Medicine 282: 992–997

Rosenbloom F M, Kelley W N, Henderson J F, Seegmiller J E 1967a Lyon hypothesis and X-linked disease. Lancet 2: 305–306

Rosenbloom F M, Kelley W N, Miller J, Henderson J F, Seegmiller J E 1967b Inherited disorder of purine metabolism: Correlation between central nervous system dysfunction and biochemical defects. Journal of American Medical Association 202: 175–177

Rosenbloom F M, Henderson J F, Caldwell I C, Kelley W N, Seegmiller J E 1968 Biochemical bases of accelerated purine biosynthesis de novo in human fibroblasts lacking hypoxanthine-guanine phosphoribosyltransferase. Journal of Biological Chemistry 243: 1116–1173

Ryan L M, Wortmann R L, Karas B, Lynch M P, McCarty D J 1986 Pyrophosphohydrolase activity and inorganic pyrophosphate content of cultured human skin fibroblasts. Elevated levels in some patients with calcium pyrophosphate dihydrate deposition disease. Journal of Clinical Investigation 77: 1689–1693

Salti I S, Kattuah N, Alam S, Wehby V, Frayha R 1976 The effect of allopurinol on oxypurine excretion in xanthinuria. Journal of Rheumatology 3: 201–204

Salzmann J, DeMars R, Benke P 1968 Single-allele expression at an X-linked hyperuricemia locus in heterozygous human cells. Proceedings of the National Academy of Sciences USA 60: 545–552

Scheele K W 1931 Examen Chemicum Calculi Urinarn, Opuscula II, p 73, 1776. Cited from Levene P A, Bass L W 1931 Nucleic Acids, New York, Chemical Catalog Company

Schmalstieg F C, Nelson J A, Mills G C, Monahan T M, Goldman A S, Goldblum R M 1977 Increased purine nucleotides in adenosine deaminase-deficient lymphocytes. Journal of Pediatrics 91: 48–51

Schnebli H P, Hill D L, Bennett L L 1967 Purification and properties of adenosine kinase from human tumor cells of type H. Ep. No 2. Journal of Biological Chemistry 242: 1997–2004

Seegmiller J E 1968 Lesch-Nyhan syndrome – management and treatment. Federation Proceedings 27: 1097–1104

Seegmiller J E 1974 Amniotic fluid and cells in the diagnosis of genetic disorders. In: Natelson S, Scommegna A, Epstein M B (eds) Amniotic Fluid: Physiology, Biochemistry, and Clinical Chemistry. John Wiley and Sons, New York, 1: 291–316

Seegmiller J E 1976 Inherited deficiency of hypoxanthine-guanine phosphoribosyltransferase in X-linked uric aciduria (the Lesch-Nyhan syndrome and its variants). In: Harris H, Hirschhorn K (eds) Advances in Human Genetics. Plenum Press, New York, p 75–163

Seegmiller J E 1979a Abnormalities of purine metabolism in human immunodeficiency diseases. In: Baier H P, Drummond G I (eds) Physiological and Regulatory Functions of Adenosine and Adenine Nucleotides. Raven Press, New York, p 395–408

Seegmiller J E 1979b Disorders of purine and pyrimidine metabolism. In: Freinkel N (eds) Contemporary Metabolism, Plenum, New York, 1: 1–85

Seegmiller J E 1980a Diseases of purine and pyrimidine metabolism. In: Bondy P K, Rosenberg L E (eds) Metabolic Control and Disease, 8th edn. W B Saunders, Philadelphia, p 777–937

Seegmiller J E 1980b Possible mechanisms of immunodeficiency disease associated with hereditary defects in enzymes of purine degradation. In: Seligman M, Hitzig W H (eds) Primary Immunodeficiencies INSERM Symposium, Elsevier/North-Holland Biomedical Press, p 269–277

Seegmiller J E 1980c Human aberrations of purine metabolism and their significance for rheumatology. Annals of Rheumatic Diseases 39: 103–117

Seegmiller J E 1985 Overview of possible relation of defects in purine metabolism to immune deficiency. Annals of the New York Academy of Sciences 451: 9–19

Seegmiller J E, Rosenbloom F M, Kelley W N 1967 Enzyme defect associated with a sex-linked human neurological disorder and excessive purine synthesis. Science 155: 1682–1684

Seegmiller J E, Bluestein H, Thompson L, Willis R, Matsumoto S, Carson D 1979 Primary aberrations of purine metabolism associated with impairment of the immune response. In: Hommes F A (ed) Models for the Study of Inborn Errors of Metabolism. Elsevier/North-Holland Biomedical Press, p 153–168

Seegmiller J E, Thompson L, Bluestein H, Willis R, Matsumoto S, Carson D 1980 Nucleotide and nucleoside metabolism and lymphocyte function. In: Gelfand E W, Dosch H M (eds) Biological Basis of Immunodeficiency. Raven Press, New York, p 251–268

Shumate J B, Katnik R, Ruiz M, Kaiser K, Frieden C, Brooke M H, Carroll J E 1979 Myoadenylate deaminase deficiency. Muscle and Nerve 2: 213–216

Siegenbeek van Heukelom L H, Staal G E J, Stoop J W, Zegers B J M 1976 An abnormal form of purine nucleoside phosphorylase in a family with a child with severe defective T-cell and normal B-cell immunity. Clinica Chimica Acta

72: 117–124

Silverman L J, Kelley W N, Palella T D 1987 Genetic analysis of human hypoxanthine-guanine phosphoribosyltranferase deficiency. Enzyme 38: 36–44

Simkin P A 1977 The pathogenesis of podagra. Annals of Internal Medicine 86: 230–233

Simmonds H A, Levin B, Cameron J S 1974 Variations in allopurinol metabolism by xanthinuric subjects. Clinical Sciences and Molecular Medicine 47: 173–178

Simmonds H A, Levin B, Cameron J S 1975 Variations in allopurinol metabolism by xanthinuric subjects. Clinical Sciences and Molecular Medicine 49: 81–82

Simmonds H A, Van Acker K J, Cameron J S, Snedden W 1976 The identification of 2,8-dihydroxyadenine, a new component of urinary stones. Biochemical Journal 157: 485–487

Simmonds H A, Van Acker K J, Cameron J S, McBurney A 1977 Purine excretion in complete adenine phosphoribosyltransferase deficiency: Effect of diet and allopurinol therapy. In: Muller M M, Kaiser E, Seegmiller J E (eds) Advances of Experimental Medicine and Biology 76B, Series: Purine Metabolism in Man II: Physiological, Pharmacological, and Clinical Aspects. Plenum Press, New York, p 304–311

Simmonds H A, Panayi G S, Corrigall V 1978a A role for purine metabolism in the immune response: Adenosine-deaminase activity and deoxyadenosine catabolism. Lancet 1: 60–63

Simmonds H A, Rose G A, Potter C F et al 1978b Adenine phosphoribosyltransferase deficiency presenting with supposed 'uric acid' stones: pitfalls of diagnosis. Proceedings of the Royal Society of Medicine 71: 791–795

Smyth J F, Chassin M M, Harrap K R, Adamson R H, Johns D G 1979 2-deoxycoformycin (DCF): Phase 1 trial and clinical pharmacology. Proceedings of the American Society of Clinical Oncology 20: 187

Sperling O, Boer P, Persky-Brosh S, Kanarek E, DeVries A 1972a Altered kinetic property of erythrocyte phosphoribosylpyrophosphate synthetase in excessive purine production. European Journal of Clinical Biological Research 17: 703

Sperling O, Eilam G, Persky-Brosh S, DeVries A 1972b Accelerated erythrocyte 5-phosphoribosyl-1-pyrophosphate synthesis. A familial abnormality associated with excessive uric acid production and gout. Biochemical Medicine 6: 310–316

Staal G E J, Stoop J W, Zegers B J M, Siegenbeek van Heukelom L H, Van der Vlist M J M, Wadman S K, Martin D W 1980 Erythrocyte metabolism in purine nucleoside phosphorylase deficiency after enzyme replacement therapy by infusion of erythrocytes. Journal of Clinical Investigation 65: 103–108

Stevens W J, Peetermans M E, Van Acker K J 1980 Immunological evaluation of a family deficient in adenine phosphoribosyltransferase (APRT). In: Rapado A, Watts R W E, DeBruyn C H M M (eds) Purine Metabolism in Man-III. Advances in Experimental Medicine and Biology. Plenum Press, New York, 122a: 355–359

Stoop J W, Zegers B J M, Hendricks G F M et al 1977 Purine nucleoside phosphorylase deficiency associated with selective cellular immunodeficiency. New England Journal of Medicine 296: 651–655

Szeinberg A, Gavendo S, Cahane D 1969a Erythrocyte adenylate-kinase deficiency. Lancet 1: 315–316

Szeinberg A, Kahana D, Gavendo S, Zaidman J, Ben-Ezzer J 1969b Hereditary deficiency of adenylate kinase in red blood cells. Acta Haematologica 42: 111–126

Tenenbaum J et al 1981 Comparison of phosphohydrolase activities from articular cartilage in calcium pyrophosphate deposition disease and primary osteoarthritis. Arthritis and Rheumatism 24: 492–500

Thompson L F, Seegmiller J E 1979 Adenosine deaminase deficiency and severe combined immunodeficiency disease. In: Meister A (ed) Advances in Enzymology. Wiley p 167–210

Thompson L F, Boss G R, Spiegelberg H L, Bianchino A, Seegmiller J E 1980 Ecto-5'-nucleotidase activity in lymphoblastoid cell lines derived from heterozygotes for congenital X-linked agammaglobulinemia. Journal of Immunology 125: 190–193

Thompson R V 1960 Purines and pyrimidines and their derivatives. In: Chromatographic and Electrophoretic Techniques. Interscience Publishers, New York, 1: 231–235

Torrance J D, Karabus C D, Shinier M, Meltzer M, Katz J, Jenkins T 1977 Haemolytic anaemia due to erythrocyte pyrimidine 5'-nucleotidase deficiency. South African Medical Journal 52: 671–673

Tritsch G I, Niswander P W 1985 Purine catabolism as a source of superoxide in macrophages. Annals of the New York Academy of Sciences 451: 279–290

Ullman B, Cohen A, Martin D W 1976 Characterization of a cell culture model for the study of adenosine deaminase- and purine nucleoside phosphorylase-deficient immunologic disease. Cell 9: 205–211

Valentine W N, Anderson H M, Paglia D E, Jaffe E R, Konrad P N, Harris S R 1972 Studies of human erythrocyte nucleotide metabolism. II Nonspherocytic hemolytic anemia, high red cell ATP, and ribosephosphate pyrophosphokinase (RPK, E.C.2.7.6.1) deficiency. Blood 39: 674–684

Valentine W N, Fink K, Paglia D E, Harris S R, Adams W S 1974 Hereditary hemolytic anemia with human erythrocyte pyrimidine 5'-nucleotidase deficiency. Journal of Clinical Investigation 54: 866–879

Valentine W N, Paglia D E, Fink K, Madokoro G 1976 Lead poisoning: Associated with haemolytic anemia, basophilic stippling, erythrocyte pyrimidine 5'-nucleotidase deficiency, and intraerythrocytic accumulation of pyrimidine. Journal of Clinical Investigation 58: 926–932

Valentine W N, Paglia D E, Tartaglia A P, Gilsanz F 1977 Hereditary hemolytic anemia with increased red cell adenosine deaminase (45- to 70-fold) and decreased adenosine triphosphate. Science 195: 783–785

Van Acker K J, Simmonds H A, Cameron J S 1977a Complete deficiency of adenine phosphoribosyltransferase: Report of a family. In: Muller M M, Kaiser E, Seegmiller J E (eds) Advances in Experimental Medicine and Biology, 76A. Plenum Press, New York, p 295–302

Van Acker K J, Simmonds H A, Potter C, Cameron J S 1977b Complete deficiency of adenine phosphoribosyltransferase. Report of a family. New England Journal of Medicine 297: 127–132

Van Acker K J, Simmonds H A, Potter C F, Sahota A 1980 Inheritance of adenine phosphoribosyltransferase (APRT) deficiency. In: Rapado A, Watts R W E, DeBruyn C H M M (eds) Purine Metabolism in Man-III. Advances in Experimental Medicine and Biology. Plenum Press, New York, 122A: 349–353

van der Heiden C, Beemer F A, Brink W, Wadman S K, Duran M 1979 Simultaneous occurrence of xanthine oxidase and sulfite oxidase deficiency. A molybdenum dependent inborn error of metabolism? Clinical Biochemistry 12: 206–208

Van Heeswijk P J, Blank C H, Seegmiller J E, Jacobson C B 1972 Preventive control of the Lesch-Nyhan syndrome. Obstetrics and Gynecology 40: 109–113

Vives-Corrons J L, Montserrat-Costa E, Rozman C 1976 Hereditary hemolytic anemia with erythrocyte pyrimidine 5'-nucleotidase deficiency in Spain. Clinical, biological and family studies. Human Genetics 34: 285–292

Wada Y, Nishimura Y, Tanabu M, Yoshimura Y, Iinuma K, Yoshida T, Arakawa T 1974 Hypouricemic mentally retarded infant with a defect of 5-phosphoribosyl-1-pyrophosphate synthetase of erythrocytes. Tohoku Journal of Experimental Medicine 113: 149–157

Wadman S K, De Bree P K, Van Gennip A H, Stoop J W, Zwegers B J M, Staal G E J, Siegenbeek van Heukelom L H 1976 Urinary purines in a patient with a severely defective T-cell immunity and a purine nucleoside phosphorylase deficiency. Clinical Chemistry and Clinical Biochemistry 14: 326–331

Watts R W E 1977 Chairman panel discussion: Hyperuricemia as a risk factor. In: Muller M M, Kaiser E, Seegmiller J E (eds) Advances in Experimental Medicine and Biology 76A. Plenum Press, New York, p 342–364

Watts R W E, Watts J E M, Seegmiller J E 1965 Xanthine oxidase activity in human tissues and its inhibition by allopurinol (4-hydroxypyrazolo (3,4-d) pyrimidine). Journal of Laboratory and Clinical Medicine 66: 688–697

Watts R W E, Harkness R A, Spellacy E, Taylor N F 1987 Lesch-Nyhan syndrome: growth delay, testicular atrophy and a partial failure of the 11β-hydroxylation of steroids. Journal of Inherited Metabolic Disease 10: 210–223

Weinberger A, Schumacher H R, Agudelo C A 1979 Urate crystals in asymptomatic metatarsophalangeal joints. Annals of Internal Medicine 91: 56–57

Willis R C, Robbins R K, Seegmiller J E 1980 An in vivo and in vitro evaluation of 1-B-D-ribofuranosyl-1,2,4-triazole-3-carboxamidine: An inhibitor of human lymphoblast purine nucleoside phosphorylase. Molecular Pharmacology 18: 287–295

Willis R C, Jolly D J, Miller A D et al 1984 Partial phenotypic correction of human Lesch-Nyhan (HPRT-deficient) lymphoblasts with a transmissible retroviral vector. Journal of Biological Chemistry 259: 7842–7849

Wilson J W, Tarr G, Mahoney W, Kelley W 1982 Human hypoxanthine-guanine phosphoribosyltransferase: complete amino acid sequence of the erythrocyte enzyme. Journal of Biological Chemistry 257: 10978–10985

Wood A W, Seegmiller J E 1973 Properties of 5-phosphoribosyl-1-pyrophosphate amidotransferase from human lymphoblasts. Journal of Biological Chemistry 248: 138–143

Wood A W, Becker M A, Seegmiller J E 1973 Purine nucleotide synthesis in lymphoblasts cultured from normal subjects and a patient with Lesch-Nyhan syndrome. Biochemical Genetics 9: 261–274

Wyngaarden J B, Kelley W N 1976 Gout and hyperuricemia. Grune & Stratton, New York, p 55

Yen R C K, Adams B, Lazar C, Becker M A 1978 Evidence for X-linkage of human phosphoribosylpyrophosphate synthetase. Proceedings of the National Academy of

Sciences USA 75: 482–485

Yu A, Kung F, Bakay B, Nyhan W L 1979 Preliminary clinical trial of deoxycoformycin in human T-cell leukemia. Journal of Clinical Chemistry and Clinical Biochemistry 17: 451–452

Yu A L, Kung F H, Bakay B, Nyhan W L 1980 In vitro and in vivo effect of deoxycoformycin in human T-cell leukemia. In: Rapado A, Watts R W E, DeBruyn C H M M (eds) Purine Metabolism in Man-III. Plenum Press, New York, p 373–379

Yu A L, Bakay B, Kung F H, Nyhan W L 1981 The effect of 2'-deoxycoformycin on the metabolism of purines and the survival of malignant cells in a patient with T-cell leukemia. Cancer Research 41: 2677–2682

Zegers B J M, Stoop J W, Staal G E J, Wadman S K 1979 An approach to the restoration of T-cell function in a purine nucleoside phosphorylase deficient patient. Ciba

Foundation Symposium 68: 231–247

Zoref E, DeVries A, Sperling O 1975 Mutant feedback-resistant phosphoribosylpyrophosphate synthetase associated with purine overproduction and gout. Phosphoribosylpyrophosphate and purine metabolism in cultured fibroblasts. Journal of Clinical Investigation 56: 1093–1099

Zoref E, DeVries A, Sperling O 1977a Evidence for X-linkage of phosphoribosylpyrophosphate synthetase in man. Studies with cultured fibroblasts from a gouty family with mutant feedback-resistant enzyme. Human Heredity 1: 73–80

Zoref E, DeVries A, Sperling O 1977b X-linked pattern of inheritance of gout due to mutant feedback-resistant phosphoribosylpyrophosphate synthetase. In: Muller M M, Kaiser E, Seegmiller J E (eds) Advances in Experimental Medicine and Biology, 76A. Plenum Press, New York, p 287–292

96. Disorders of organic acid metabolism

S. I. Goodman

INTRODUCTION

Organic acidaemias are a group of inborn errors of (usually) amino acid metabolism in which the diagnostic accumulated compounds are acids that, because they do not contain amino group, do not react with ninhydrin. They were first reported in 1961, albeit unknowingly, when idiopathic hyperglycinaemia was described as a syndrome of mental retardation, hyperglycinaemia, and episodic ketoacidosis, neutropenia and thrombocytopenia induced by protein intake or infection (Childs et al 1961). It was realized some years later that the clinical and biochemical features of this disease, which had become known as ketotic hyperglycinaemia, were usually caused by organic acidaemias, and in particular by methylmalonic acidaemia (Rosenberg et al 1968), propionic acidaemia (Hsia et al 1971), and 2-methyl-3-hydroxybutyric acidaemia (Hillman & Keating 1974).

Isovaleric acidaemia was the first organic acidaemia to be recognized, largely because industrial chemists recognized the odour surrounding a particular patient as being due to a short-chain fatty acid (Budd et al 1967). The description of this condition led to a search for others, usually by combined gas chromatography-mass spectrometry (GC-MS), and to the rapid delineation of the remaining disorders described in this section.

The ability of GC-MS to simultaneously separate and identify the components of complex mixtures has made it the method most widely used to identify and investigate organic acidaemias. GC alone will exclude disease in most (80–90%) patients, and can be performed in any well equipped clinical laboratory. Large peaks in other samples, while usually due to drugs and food additives and not to the abnormal acids of disease, will necessitate referral to a laboratory with enough experience in organic acid analysis by GC-MS to ensure rapid and accurate diagnosis.

Clinical features vary but, in general, organic acidaemia should be suspected, and urine organic acids examined (the compounds are not effectively reabsorbed from the glomerular filtrate by the renal tubule) in the following situations:

1. Clinical features of ketotic hyperglycinaemia (see above).
2. Presence of an unusual odour.
3. Acute disease in infancy, especially when associated with metabolic acidosis, hypoglycaemia, or hyperammonaemia.
4. Chronic or recurrent metabolic acidosis, with or without an anion gap.
5. Progressive extrapyramidal disease in childhood.
6. Reye syndrome when recurrent, familial, or in infancy.
7. Neurological syndrome with alopecia and rash.

Pedigree data and/or enzyme measurements in obligate heterozygotes have shown that most organic acidaemias are inherited as autosomal recessive traits, but in a few instances, as in methylmalonic acidaemia due to the *cbl D* defect, pedigree data is too scanty and knowledge of the primary defect too uncertain to exclude X–linked inheritance. Prenatal diagnosis is relatively simple because the enzyme defects are usually expressed in cultured amniotic cells, and because the affected fetus often excretes large and easily detected amounts of abnormal organic acids into the amniotic fluid.

ISOVALERIC ACIDAEMIA

Clinical course

The clinical course of isovaleric acidaemia, first recognized in 1966 because of the distinctive 'cheesey', 'sour', or 'sweaty feet' odour of isovaleric acid (Tanaka et al 1966, Budd et al 1967), varies considerably. Some patients develop poor feeding, acidosis, seizures and the characteristic odour during the first few days of life, with coma and death following quite soon if the diagnosis is not made and appropriate treatment begun (Newman et

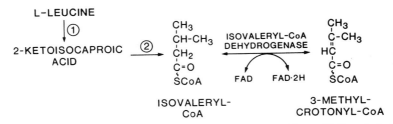

Fig. 96.1 Early steps in oxidation of L-leucine. (1) Leucine: 2-ketoglutarate transaminase. (2) Branched-chain ketoacid decarboxylase. Electrons pass from the FAD of isovaleryl-CoA dehydrogenase into the electron transport chain via an electron transfer flavoprotein (ETF).

al 1967, Budd et al 1967). Others show only episodes of vomiting, lethargy, encephalopathy, pancytopenia, and odour precipitated by infections or protein ingestion (Ando et al 1971). Developmental retardation is common. Fatty changes in the liver and kidneys are often found at autopsy. The disorder is due to deficiency of isovaleryl-CoA dehydrogenase (Rhead & Tanaka 1980), an enzyme in L-leucine metabolism which oxidizes isovaleryl-CoA to 3-methylcrotonyl-CoA (Fig. 96.1)

Pathogenesis

The primary metabolites of isovaleryl-CoA which are accumulated are isovalerylglycine (Tanaka & Isselbacher 1967), 3-hydroxyisovaleric acid (Tanaka et al 1968), and isovaleric acid. The first, produced by glycine-N-acylase catalyzed conjugation in the liver, is excreted at all times, while the latter two, which are produced by ω-oxidation and de-esterification, appear only when isovaleryl-CoA accumulation exceeds the glycine conjugating capacity of the liver, as after a protein load or during infection. The relationship of the compounds to the clinical and post-mortem findings is not well understood.

Diagnosis and differential diagnosis

Diagnosis is suggested by the clinical course and odour and confirmed by demonstrating isovalerylglycine in urine and deficiency of isovaleryl-CoA dehydrogenase in tissues. Several of the same clinical and organic acid findings may occur in glutaric acidaemia type II, but other organic acids are usually present, and the tissue activity of isovaleryl-CoA dehydrogenase is normal.

Treatment

Diets low in protein or leucine reduce the accumulation of isovaleryl-CoA and appear to decrease the number and severity of acute episodes while permitting normal intellectual development (Levy et al 1973). Oral glycine

probably increases the liver's capacity to form isovaleryl glycine, which is probably less toxic than isovaleric acid itself, and several catastrophically sick infants have been treated with it with remarkable effect (Cohn et al 1978).

Genetics

Family studies, in which males and females are affected with approximately equal frequency, suggest inheritance as an autosomal recessive trait. Prenatal diagnosis, based on decreased enzyme activity in cultured amniocytes and the presence of isovalerylglycine in amniotic fluid, has been reported (Hine et al 1986).

3-METHYLCROTONYLGLYCINAEMIA AND COMBINED CARBOXYLASE DEFICIENCY

Clinical course and heterogeneity

3-Methylcrotonylglycinaemia was first described in 1970 in a 4½ month-old girl with feeding problems, developmental delay, severe hypotonia, and an odour like that of cat's urine (Eldjarn et al 1970, Stokke et al 1972). It has since been described many times, sometimes in similar circumstances (Gompertz et al 1973, Keeton & Moosa 1976) but much more often in slightly older patients with a variety of neurological symptoms and/or acidosis, alopecia and a candida-like rash (Gompertz et al 1971, Roth et al 1976, Cowan et al 1979).

Accumulation and excretion of 3-methylcrotonylglycine and/or 3-hydroxyisovaleric acid can be due to severe biotin deficiency or to mutations of 3-methylcrotonyl-CoA carboxylase (a biotin-containing enzyme of leucine oxidation), holocarboxylase synthetase, or biotinidase (Fig. 96.2). Because defects of the latter enzymes also cause deficient carboxylation of propionyl-CoA and pyruvic acid, they are said to cause 'combined carboxylase deficiency'. Isolated deficiency of 3-methylcrotonyl-CoA carboxylase has been described in only a few patients (Gizelmann et al 1987), and combined carboxy-

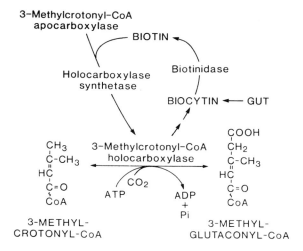

Fig. 96.2 Relation of carboxylation of 3-methylcrotonyl-CoA to the activities of biotinidase and holocarboxylase synthetase. Holocarboxylase synthetase also links biotin to apocarboxylases for propionyl-CoA, acetyl-CoA and pyruvate, and biotinidase releases biotin from proteins and enzymes which contain it.

lase deficiency is much more common, with holocarboxylase synthetase deficiency usually causing symptoms somewhat earlier than biotinidase deficiency (Wolf et al 1983a, Burri et al 1985). The syndrome of neurological abnormalities, rash, and alopecia is frequent in both forms of combined carboxylase deficiency.

Pathogenesis

Neurological symptoms in combined carboxylase deficiency are probably due to lactic and pyruvic acidaemia, resulting from deficiency of pyruvate carboxylase. The alopecia and candida-like skin rashes also occur in severe biotin deficiency (Scott 1958), but their cause is not clear.

Diagnosis

Diagnosis is suggested by finding large amounts of 3-hydroxyisovaleric acid and/or 3-methylcrotonylglycine in urine, and evaluation should then include assays of biotinidase in serum and of 3-methylcrotonyl-CoA carboxylase and holocarboxylase synthetase in cultured fibroblasts. Since similar clinical and laboratory findings may occur in severe biotin deficiency, especially during parenteral hyperalimentation (Kien et al 1981, Mock et al 1985), the adequacy of biotin intake should also be evaluated.

The frequency of biotinidase deficiency, together with the irreversibility of some neurological sequelae and the ease with which the condition can be treated with biotin, have led to its inclusion in several newborn screening programs, and several affected patients have been detected and treated successfully before the onset of symptoms (Wolf et al 1985).

Treatment

Large doses of biotin, e.g. 10 mg/24 hours, produce rapid clinical improvement and almost complete disappearance of abnormal urine organic acids in combined carboxylase deficiency (Gompertz et al 1971, 1973, Keeton & Moosa 1976, Cowan et al 1979), but are not usually effective in isolated deficiency of 3-methylcrotonyl-CoA carboxylase.

Genetics

3-Methylcrotonyl-CoA carboxylase deficiency, and both forms of combined carboxylase deficiency, are transmitted as autosomal recessive traits, but carrier detection is simple only in biotinidase deficiency, where serum biotinidase accurately distinguishes controls from heterozygous carriers (Wolf et al. 1983b). Prenatal diagnosis, while perhaps possible by demonstrating abnormal organic acids in amniotic fluid and/or deficient enzyme activity in cultured amniotic cells, has not been reported.

3-HYDROXY-3-METHYLGLUTARIC ACIDAEMIA

Clinical course

Hydroxymethylglutaric acidaemia was first described in a seven-month-old boy who developed apnoea and cyanosis, hepatomegaly, acidosis, and severe hypoglycaemia without ketonuria, shortly after an attack of diarrhoea and vomiting (Faull et al 1976), and additional patients have presented in infancy, with hypoglycaemia and acidosis (Schutgens et al 1979), and at the age of 2 years, with what appeared to be Reye syndrome (Robinson et al 1980). It is due to deficiency of hydroxymethylglutaryl-CoA lyase (Wysocki & Hähnel 1976a), an enzyme of leucine oxidation which is also involved in the synthesis of ketone bodies (Fig. 96.3).

Pathogenesis

The most prominent organic acids in this condition are 3-hydroxy-3-methylglutaric, 3-methylglutaconic and 3-hydroxyisovaleric (Wysocki et al 1976, Faull et al 1976,

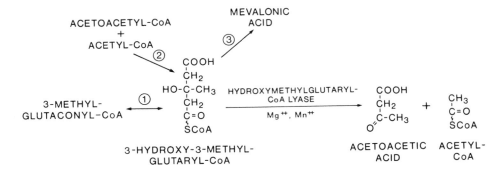

Fig. 96.3 The reaction catalyzed by hydroxymethylglutaryl-CoA lyase. (1) Methylglutaconyl-CoA hydratase. (2) Hydroxymethylglutaryl-CoA synthetase. (3) Hydroxymethylglutaryl-CoA reductase. (Reproduced with permission of Alan R. Liss, Inc.)

Duran et al 1978a, Robinson et al 1980), and especially after protein ingestion and in situations that normally favour ketone body formation. Moreover, because ketone bodies cannot be made, metabolic adjustments based on their oxidation by tissues are compromised.

Diagnosis and differential diagnosis

The diagnosis should be entertained in all patients with hypoglycaemia without ketosis in infancy and childhood, and confirmed by the organic aciduria and hydroxymethylglutaryl-CoA lyase deficiency in tissues. The observation that the same organic aciduria can occur without lyase deficiency in fibroblasts (Truscott et al 1979) makes enzyme diagnosis mandatory.

Treatment

Biochemical control might be expected from a low protein (or leucine) diet, together with measures to prevent catabolism and ketosis. One patient with the disorder had no attacks of acidosis for fourteen months after diagnosis (Wysocki & Hähnel 1978) suggesting that the approach is indeed effective.

Genetics

Hydroxymethylglutaric acidaemia is inherited as an autosomal recessive trait, and heterozygote detection is possible by demonstrating intermediate lyase activity in leucocytes (Wysocki & Hähnel 1976b). 3-Methylglutaconic acid excretion in maternal urine increased during a pregnancy with an affected fetus (Duran et al 1979), and prenatal diagnosis can probably also be made by analyzing organic acids in amniotic fluid and/or by assaying hydroxymethylglutaryl-CoA lyase in cultured amniotic cells.

2-METHYL-3-HYDROXYBUTYRIC ACIDAEMIA

Clinical course

2-Methyl-3-hydroxybutyric acidaemia was first described in a 6-year-old boy with episodes of acidosis and encephalopathy appearing after upper respiratory tract infections (Daum et al 1973), and several additional patients have now been described (e.g. Gompertz et al 1974). The disease usually presents beyond the first year of life and, without treatment, mental retardation or death during an episode of ketoacidosis is common. One patient developed hyperammonaemia and features of ketotic hyperglycinaemia in infancy (Hillman & Keating 1974), however, and another was apparently well, suffering only from intermittent headaches, at the age of 15 years (Halvorsen et al 1979).

This condition is apparently due to deficiency of the potassium-dependent acetoacetyl-CoA thiolase which catalyzes the cleavage of both 2-methylacetoacetyl-CoA and acetoacetyl-CoA (Robinson et al 1979) (Fig. 96.4).

Pathogenesis

The acids which accumulate include normal ketone bodies, e.g. 3-hydroxybutyric and acetoacetic, and 2-methyl-3-hydroxybutyric and 2-methylacetoacetic, which derive in part from metabolite backup and in part from the entry of 2-methylacetoacetyl-CoA into the hydroxymethylglutaryl-CoA cycle. Tiglyl-CoA, which is excreted as the glycine conjugate in this condition as

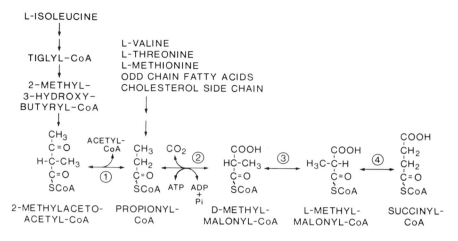

Fig. 96.4 Formation and metabolism of propionyl-CoA. (1) Acetoacetyl-CoA thiolase. (2) Propionyl-CoA carboxylase. (3) Methylmalonyl-CoA racemase. (4) Methylmalonyl-CoA mutase. Adenosylcobalamin is the specific coenzyme for methylmalonyl-CoA mutase.

well as in propionic acidaemia and methylmalonic acidaemia, may cause hyperglycinaemia by inhibiting the conversion of glycine to serine (Hillman & Otto 1974).

Diagnosis and differential diagnosis

Diagnosis is suggested by the clinical course and a consistent pattern of urine organic acids, and should be confirmed whenever possible by demonstrating tissue deficiency of acetoacetyl-CoA thiolase. Because 2-methyl-3-hydroxybutyric acid is often excreted in normal ketosis (Landaas 1975), diagnosis during acute episodes may be difficult unless tiglyglycine is present and the disorder should not be ruled out unless oral L-isoleucine loading fails to produce 2-methyl-3-hydroxybutyric aciduria.

Treatment

A low protein diet decreases the frequency and severity of episodes of acidosis and permits normal growth and development (Daum et al 1973, Hillman & Keating 1974, Gompertz et al 1974).

Genetics

Family studies, which show approximately equal numbers of males and females to be affected, unaffected parents to excrete 2-methyl-3-hydroxybutyric acid after isoleucine loads (Daum et al 1973, Gompertz et al 1974), and parental consanguinity (Daum et al 1973),

suggest inheritance as an autosomal recessive trait. Heterozygote detection and prenatal diagnosis are probably possible, but have not been reported.

PROPIONIC ACIDAEMIA

Clinical course and heterogeneity

Propionic acidaemia was first described in 1968 in an infant who died with severe metabolic acidosis and a serum propionic acid concentration of $5.4 \times 10^{-3}M$ (Hommes et al 1968), and many additional patients have been reported since that time. The disorder may present in the first week of life with feeding difficulties, lethargy, vomiting and life-threatening acidosis, hypoglycaemia, and hyperammonaemia, or the course may be chronic, with poor feeding, failure to thrive, and episodes of vomiting, ketoacidosis, hyperglycinaemia and neutropenia triggered by infection or protein ingestion (Wadlington et al 1975, Shafai et al 1978). Seizures and developmental retardation are common. Postmortem examination often shows fatty infiltration of the liver.

Propionic acidaemia fibroblasts are deficient in propionyl-CoA carboxylase (Fig. 96.4) (Hsia et al 1971), and can be divided into three main complementation groups, one of which, designated *bio*, is discussed in the section on 3-methylcrotonylglycinaemia. Two groups of cells, termed *pcc A* and *pcc C*, are deficient in propionyl-CoA carboxylase alone (Gravel et al 1977, Wolf et al 1978). Heterozygous carriers of *pcc A* mutations, but not *pcc C* mutations, show intermediate activity of propionyl-CoA carboxylase in leucocytes and fibroblasts, results which can be explained if the enzyme is composed of non-identical subunits, one of which is produced in considerable excess but both of which are needed for activity (Wolf & Rosenberg 1978).

Pathogenesis

The metabolites of propionyl-CoA most characteristic of propionic acidaemia are 3-hydroxypropionic, methylcitric, and propionic acid (Ando et al 1972a,b). The first is apparently formed by β-oxidation, the second by citrate synthetase catalyzed condensation with oxaloacetic, and the latter by simple de-esterification. The pathogenesis of the clinical phenotype is not clear. Marked hyperammonaemia probably contributes appreciably to the severe encephalopathy of patients presenting as newborns, possibly because propionyl-CoA inhibits the synthesis of N-acetylglutamate, the major allostearic activator of carbamyl phosphate synthetase (Coude et al 1979). The cause of vomiting, encephalopathy, hypoglycaemia, and the postmortem findings in patients without hyperammonaemia is more obscure. The contention that mitochondrial toxicity plays a role in pathogenesis is supported by observations that methylcitrate inhibits the citrate-malate shuttle as well as several enzymes of citrate and isocitrate metabolism (Cheema-Dhadli et al 1975), and that propionate inhibits mitochondrial oxidation of pyruvate and 2-ketoglutarate (Gregersen 1979).

Diagnosis

Diagnosis will be suggested by the clinical presentation and a consistent pattern of urine organic acids, but should be confirmed whenever possible by examining activities of propionyl-CoA, 3-methylcrotonyl-CoA, and pyruvate carboxylase in peripheral leucocytes and cultured fibroblasts.

Treatment

Acute therapy is directed to treating shock, acidosis, hypoglycaemia and hyperammonaemia with fluids, bicarbonate, glucose and even exchange transfusion and/or dialysis. Biotin should be tried in large doses, i.e. 10 mg/24 hours, but it only rarely reduces organic acidaemia in patients who do not have combined carboxylase deficiency. In biotin non-responders, i.e. the vast majority of patients, treatment involves dietary restriction of propiogenic amino acids or protein. Some patients do well on such regimen, achieving normal growth and development, albeit with ketoacidosis complicating acute infections (Brandt et al 1974), but most do not.

Genetics

All forms of propionic acidaemia are inherited as autosomal recessive traits, but only carriers of the *pcc A* mutation can be identified by intermediate tissue activity of propionyl-CoA carboxylase. Prenatal diagnosis of *pcc A* and *pcc C* disease is possible by showing propionyl-CoA carboxylase deficiency in cultured amniotic cells (Gompertz et al 1975) and/or accumulation of methylcitrate in amniotic fluid (Sweetman et al 1979).

METHYLMALONIC ACIDAEMIA

Clinical course and heterogeneity

Since almost simultaneous initial descriptions of methylmalonic acidaemia in 1967 by groups in Norway (Stokke et al 1967) and Great Britain (Oberholzer et al 1967), it has been one of the most frequently reported and extensively investigated human inborn errors of metabolism. The clinical presentation, course, and postmortem findings are virtually identical to those of propionic acidaemia (Rosenberg et al 1968). Hyperammonaemia has been observed with increasing frequency, particularly in acutely ill infants (Packman et al 1978). The course may be quite different in patients with the *cbl C* and *cbl D* defects, most of whom present during infancy with seizures, hypotonia, microcephaly or profound developmental retardation, and eventually develop megaloblastic anaemia (Levy et al 1970, Dillon et al 1974, Carmel et al 1980). Some, however, present with only mild developmental delay (Anthony & McLeay 1976, Goodman et al 1970). Thrombophlebitis and pulmonary embolism have complicated the course of one patient with the *cbl D* mutation (Goodman, unpublished).

The metabolic block in methylmalonic acidaemia is at methylmalonyl-CoA mutase, and Figure. 96.5 shows that this can be caused by defects in the mutase itself as well as by those of adenosylcobalamin biosynthesis. Five genetic complementation groups have now been defined in methylmalonic acidaemia fibroblasts. One, *mut*, contains cells with mutations in the apomutase, two, *cbl C* and *cbl D*, contain cells deficient in biosynthesis of methylcobalamin and adenosylcobalamin, and two, *cbl A* and *cbl B*, are deficient only in the synthesis of adenosylcobalamin (Gravel et al 1975, Willard et al 1978). Some *mut* lines contain no detectable mutase activity while activity can be restored to others by the addition of adenosylcobalamin (Willard & Rosenberg 1977). The only patient reported with methylmalonyl-CoA racemase deficiency (Kang et al 1972) in fact belongs to the *mut* group (Willard & Rosenberg 1979a). *Cbl B* lines are deficient in ATP:cob(I)alamin adenosyl transferase and, since only

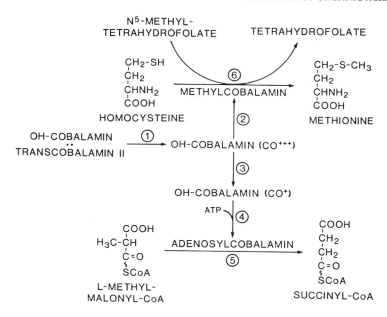

Fig. 96.5 Relationship of B_{12} metabolism to that of L-methylmalonyl-CoA and homocysteine. Details of Steps (1) and (2) are not known. Step (3) involves transport into the mitochondrion and reduction of Co^{+++} to Co^+. (4) ATP:cob(I)alamin adenosyl transferase. (5) L-methylmalonyl-CoA mutase. (6) N^5-methyltetrahydrofolate: homocysteine methyltransferase. (Reproduced with permission of Alan R. Liss, Inc.)

some of these cell lines recover mutase activity when grown in the presence of hydroxycobalamin, there is heterogeneity even within this group (Fenton & Rosenberg 1978, Willard & Rosenberg 1979b). The specific defects in the remaining groups are not known, but the *cbl A* defect probably involves the reduction of cob(III)alamin to cob(I)alamin (Fenton & Rosenberg 1978).

Pathogenesis

Methylmalonic acid, the compound most characteristic of the methylmalonic acidaemias, derives from de-esterification of the mutase substrate. Derivatives of propionyl-CoA, i.e. 3-hydroxypropionate and methylcitrate, are also accumulated, as are abnormal ketone bodies derived from the entry of propionyl-CoA into the hydroxymethylglutaryl-CoA cycle. Defective synthesis of methylcobalamin in *cbl C* and *cbl D* patients cause N^5-methyltetrahydrofolate homocysteine methyltransferase deficiency, and thus homocystinaemia and homocystinuria.

Because propionyl-CoA accumulates in this disorder, many of the points made in the discussion of propionic acidaemia also pertain to methylmalonic acidaemia.

Hypoglycaemia has been attributed to inhibition of pyruvate carboxylase by methylmalonyl-CoA (Utter et al 1974) and to inhibition of mitochondrial transport of malate, 2-ketoglutarate, and isocitrate by methylmalonic acid (Halperin et al 1971). The megaloblastosis which is often observed in patients with the *cbl C* and *cbl D* defects is probably due to the trapping of folic acid as N^5-methyltetrahydrofolate (Carmel et al 1980).

Diagnosis

Diagnosis is suggested by the clinical course and the presence of large quantities of methylmalonic acid in urine. A careful search for homocystinaemia and/or homocystinuria should always be made; when present, it is accompanied by low methionine and high cystathionine in serum and not, as in cystathionine synthetase deficiency by high methionine and low cystathionine. Whenever possible, tissue enzymes should be assayed and the defect assigned to a complementation group.

Excretion of methylmalonic acid in B_{12} deficiency is usually not as pronounced as in the inherited disorders. The only reported patient in whom this was not so was the breast-fed, 6-month-old son of a woman who had eaten no animal protein for 8 years; in addition to methylmalonic acidaemia, the child had homocystinuria, a very low serum B_{12} megaloblastic anaemia, and marked central nervous system disturbances (Higginbottom et al 1978).

Treatment

As in propionic acidaemia, treatment is directed first to treating shock, acidosis, hypoglycaemia and hyperammonaemia. Therapy with B_{12} should be tried but its effects are so apt to be confused with those of vomiting and failure to feed that responsiveness to B_{12} should also be assessed later, during a period of relatively constant protein intake.

B_{12} responsiveness has been examined rigorously in few patients, but the impression is that those with *cbl* defects usually respond and those with *mut* defects do not. In some B_{12} responders, hydroxocobalamin (1 mg/day $\times$ 2–5 days) has a greater and more sustained effect than the same dose of cyanocobalamin (Goodman et al 1972) but, since both may eventually cause toxic symptoms, it may be best to combine cobalamin therapy with moderate protein restriction. Homocystinuria in *cbl* C and *cbl* D patients does not respond to B_{12} as well as methylmalonic aciduria, and betaine hydrochloride, which promotes transmethylation of homocysteine by betaine: homocysteine methyltransferase may be useful in such cases (Goodman, unpublished).

Treatment of B_{12} nonresponders is by restriction of protein or propiogenic amino acids to amounts which just permit normal growth and development. Although striking successes with dietary treatment have been reported (Nyhan et al 1973), most patients do not do well and often die during episodes of ketoacidosis (Kaye et al 1974, Duran et al 1978b).

One woman with an affected B_{12}-responsive fetus was given large doses of cyanocobalamin during the last nine weeks of pregnancy and her methylmalonic acid excretion, which had been increasing, began to decrease. The infant was treated with B_{12} and a low-protein diet immediately after birth, apparently with a favourable outcome (Ampola et al 1975). The relevance of these observations is in question, however, as it has not yet been shown that the fetus suffers irreversible damage in utero.

Genetics

All forms of congenital methylmalonic acidaemia appear to be transmitted as autosomal recessive traits, although X–linked inheritance of the *cbl* D defect has not been excluded. Intermediate activity of methylmalonyl-CoA mutase and ATP:cob(I)alamin adenosyltransferase in fibroblasts can be used to characterize heterozygous carriers of *mut* and *cbl* B disease (Fenton & Rosenberg 1978, Willard & Rosenberg 1979a), but carriers of the other mutations cannot yet be distinguished. All forms can probably be diagnosed in utero by demonstrating defective conversion of methylmalonyl- to succinyl-CoA in cultured amniotic cells (Willard & Rosenberg 1977), but prenatal diagnosis of the *cbl* C and *cbl* D forms has not been reported to date. The amniotic fluid methylmalonic acid concentration has been elevated in several affected fetuses (Morrow et al 1970, Mahoney et al 1975, Ampola et al 1975).

GLUTARIC ACIDAEMIA

Course and heterogeneity

Glutaric acidaemia may be one of the more common organic acidaemias but its course is so different from most of these disorders that the diagnosis can easily be missed. The disorder presents after a 3-month to 2-year period of normal development either with hypotonia and loss of head control or with an acute episode of vomiting and encephalopathy following a relatively minor infection. Seizures, abnormal movements, hypoglycaemia, hepatomegaly and acidosis may be noted during the episode. Whatever the presentation, extrapyramidal symptoms e.g, dystonia, athetosis, and chorea, develop and progress (Goodman et al 1975, Kyllerman & Steen 1977, Whelan et al 1979). Death may occur during an episode of acidosis and hypoglycaemia. The course is more attenuated when the mutant enzymes have more residual activity (Gregersen et al 1977, Brandt et al 1978, Christensen & Brandt 1978). Fatty changes in the viscera and neuronal loss in the putamen and lateral aspects of the caudate have been described at autopsy (Goodman et al 1977).

This disorder is due to deficiency of glutaryl-CoA dehydrogenase (Fig. 96.6), the enzyme which oxidizes glutaryl-CoA, an intermediate of lysine, hydroxylysine and tryptophan metabolism to crotonyl-CoA (Goodman et al 1975).

Pathogenesis

The organic acids characteristic of glutaric aciduria are glutaric, 3-hydroxyglutaric and glutaconic. The first and second are usually present (Stokke et al 1975, Goodman et al 1977, Gregersen & Brandt 1979), but the third is present only occasionally, especially during ketoacidosis. Perhaps relevant to the pathogenesis of striatal degeneration is the observation that all three acids are powerful in-

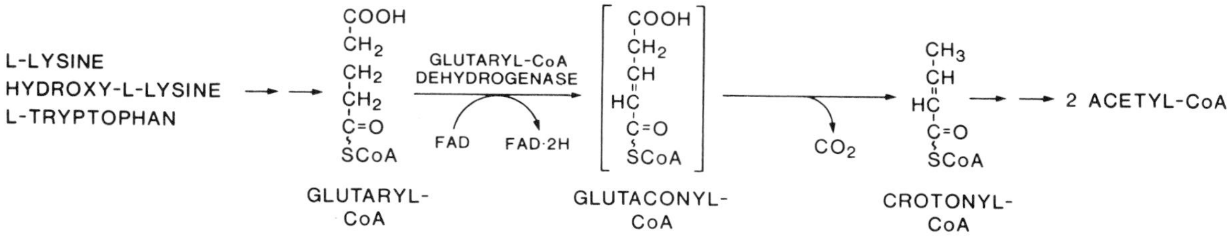

Fig. 96.6 The reaction catalyzed by glutaryl-CoA dehydrogenase, which probably dehydrogenates and decarboxylates the substrate. If glutaconyl-CoA is an intermediate, it is probably not readily dissociated from the enzyme. Electrons pass from the FAD of glutaryl-CoA dehydrogenase into the electron transport chain at coenzyme Q, probably through the electron transfer flavoprotein (ETF). (Reproduced with permission of Alan R. Liss, Inc.)

hibitors of neuronal glutamate decarboxylase (Stokke et al 1976), the enzyme responsible for the synthesis of GABA.

Diagnosis

Diagnosis should be suspected in any child with progressive dyskinesis and will be confirmed by the presence of glutaric aciduria and deficient tissue activity of glutaryl-CoA dehydrogenase. The main disorder from which the organic acid findings must be distinguished is glutaric acidaemia type II (see below), in which additional organic acids are excreted and tissue activity of glutaryl-CoA dehydrogenase is normal.

Treatment

Treatment is seldom successful, perhaps because irreversible striatal changes are already present at diagnosis. Restriction of dietary protein or glutarigenic amino acids reduce glutaric acid excretion but have little clinical effect. Riboflavin produced clinical improvement and a modest decrease in glutaric aciduria in two Danish patient observed by the author. Lioresal®, the *p*-chlorophenyl analogue of GABA, has improved some patients (Brandt et al 1979), and had no effect on others.

Genetics

Glutaric acidaemia is inherited as an autosomal recessive trait, and leucocytes of heterozygotes contain intermediate activities of glutaryl-CoA dehydrogenase (Goodman & Kohlhoff 1975). Prenatal diagnosis is possible by demonstrating enzyme deficiency in amniotic cells in culture and/or large amounts of glutaric acid in amniotic fluid (Goodman et al 1980).

MEDIUM- AND LONG-CHAIN ACYL-CoA DEHYDROGENASE DEFICIENCIES

Clinical course and heterogeneity

Deficiencies of medium- (MCAD) and long-chain acyl-CoA dehydrogenase (LCAD), two enzymes of fatty acid β-oxidation, usually cause Reye syndrome-like episodes of hypoketotic hypoglycaemia, hepatomegaly and encephalopathy or, less often, sudden death in infancy (Stanley et al 1983, Hale et al 1985, Duran et al 1986, Taubman et al 1987). The two cannot be distinguished clinically, but MCAD deficiency is by far the more common. Although Reye syndrome-like episodes may be fatal, they tend to become less frequent and severe with time, and prolonged survival is not unusual.

Pathogenesis

Limited synthesis of acetyl-CoA, and resulting decreases in pyruvate carboxylase and N-acetylglutamate synthetase activities, may cause hypoglycaemia and hyperammonaemia. The latter may contribute to the encephalopathy that characterizes the acute episode, but other possible factors are reduced circulating levels of ketone bodies and, in MCAD deficiency, high serum levels of octanoic acid (Duran et al 1985).

Cardiomyopathy may be due to decreased delivery of glucose and ketone bodies to a tissue unable to oxidize long-chain fatty acids, in LCAD deficiency because of the primary defect, and in MCAD deficiency due to carnitine deficiency secondary to loss of carnitine esters such as octanoylcarnitine in the urine (Duran et al 1985, Roe et al 1985).

Diagnosis

Diagnosis is based upon recognizing the lack of an appropriate ketone response to fasting and, in MCAD deficiency, by demonstrating octanoylcarnitine in urine when the patient is not carnitine depleted or on a diet containing medium-chain triglycerides. Assays of MCAD (and LCAD) activity in fibroblasts are probably necessary only when urine octanoylcarnitine cannot be demonstrated. Normal urine organic acids do not exclude these conditions, since excretion of dicarboxylic acids and other products of microsomal and peroxisomal oxidation of fatty acids is apt to be intermittent.

Treatment

Acute management is directed to treating hypoglycaemia, and long-term measures include providing carbohydrate snacks before bedtime and vigorous treatment of intercurrent infections. Because muscle weakness and cardiomyopathy in MCAD deficiency may result from secondary carnitine deficiency, oral carnitine may be indicated. Medium-chain triglycerides are contraindicated in MCAD deficiency, where they may cause serum octanoic acid to rise, but may be a useful energy source in LCAD deficiency.

Genetics

Both MCAD and LCAD deficiency are inherited as autosomal recessive traits, and heterozygous carriers can be distinguished from controls by enzyme assays on cultured fibroblasts (Frerman & Goodman 1985a). While theoretically possible by enzyme assays on cultured amniocytes, neither condition has been diagnosed in utero.

GLUTARIC ACIDAEMIA TYPE 11

Clinical course and heterogeneity

Glutaric acidaemia type II (multiple acyl-CoA dehydrogenation deficiency) was first described in 1976 in a baby who died at 3 days of age with profound hypoglycaemia, metabolic acidosis, the 'smell of sweaty feet,' and a complex organic aciduria dominated by glutaric, ethylmalonic, 3-hydroxyisovaleric, and C6, C8, and C10 dicarboxylic acids (Przyrembel et al 1976). Many additional patients have since been described, often with renal cysts and onset and death in early infancy, and several others with Reye-like episodes and skeletal muscle weakness beginning in childhood or even adolescence (Goodman & Frerman 1984).

Pathogenesis

In some patients the condition is due to deficiency of electron transfer flavoprotein (EFT), and in others

to deficiency of ETF:ubiquinone oxidoreductase (ETF:QO), enzymes which act sequentially to transfer electrons from a number of mitochondrial flavoenzymes of fatty- and amino acid oxidation into the respiratory chain (Frerman & Goodman 1985b).

The defect in fatty acid and β-oxidation leads to hypoketotic hypoglycaemia, and the excretion of large quantities of carnitine esters in the urine to carnitine depletion (Di Donato et al 1986), and to cardiomyopathy, which is a common cause of death.

Diagnosis

Diagnosis can be made by demonstrating the characteristic organic aciduria, and it is not usually necessary to assay ETF and ETF:QO activities.

Treatment

Treatment with carbohydrate, bicarbonate, and dietary manipulation is not usually effective, but provision of riboflavin (to augment residual activity of ETF or ETF:QO) and carnitine has shown promise in some patients (Mooy et al 1984).

Genetics

ETF and ETF:QO deficiency are both inherited as autosomal recessive traits (Frerman & Goodman 1985b, Amendt & Rhead 1986) and, while carrier detection is probably possible by enzyme assay, it cannot be done reliably or cheaply enough to justify its routine use. The infantile form of the disease can usually be diagnosed in utero by demonstrating increased amounts of glutaric acid in amniotic fluid (Mitchell et al 1983, Jakobs et al 1984). Enzyme assays on cultured amniotic cells are not usually necessary.

PYROGLUTAMIC ACIDAEMIA (5-OXOPROLINAEMIA)

Clinical course and heterogeneity

Pyroglutamic acidaemia was first described in an 18-year-old man with chronic metabolic acidosis, mental retardation ataxia, and spastic quadriplegia (Jellum et al 1970, Kluge et al 1972). Four additional patients have been described, all of whom developed severe metabolic acidosis and evidence of haemolysis, i.e. indirect hyperbilirubinaemia, anaemia and reticulocytosis, in infancy. The haemolytic anaemia tends to become compensated, but metabolic acidosis is persistent and requires treatment (Hagenfeldt et al 1974, Larsson et al 1974, Spielberg et al 1977). The condition is due to deficiency of glutathione synthetase (Wellner et al 1974).

Pathogenesis

The γ-glutamyl cycle, a series of reactions concerned with the synthesis and breakdown of glutathione, is shown in Figure 96.7. It is not clear why pyroglutamic acid is excreted in glutathione synthetase deficiency instead of γ-glutamylcysteine, but it is thought that decreased levels of glutathione may release γ-glutamylcysteine synthetase from feedback inhibition, and that γ-glutamylcysteine is then formed and converted to pyroglutamic acid faster than it can be hydrolyzed by 5-oxoprolinase (Wellner et al 1974).

One of the postulated functions of glutathione in the cell is to maintain membrane integrity, and haemolytic anaemia in pyroglutamic acidaemia may be due to glutathione deficiency. Indeed, in a form of glutathione synthetase deficiency in which the mutant enzyme is active but unstable, deficiency of glutathione is more marked in erythrocytes than in nucleated cells, and haemolytic anaemia occurs without pyroglutamic acidaemia (Mohler et al 1970, Spielberg et al 1978). The observation that amino acid transport is normal in pyroglutamic acidaemia (Larsson et al 1974, Spielberg et al 1977) does not support a major role for the γ-glutamyl cycle in carrier mediated transport of amino acids.

Diagnosis and differential diagnosis

The serum and urine concentrations of pyroglutamic acid are so high in this condition that diagnosis is fairly simple, provided that the patient is not receiving Nutramigen®, a formula which can contain as much as 6 mg pyroglutamic acid/g powder (Oberholzer et al 1975). As 5-oxoprolinase deficiency could also conceivably cause pyroglutamic acidaemia, diagnosis should be confirmed by enzyme assay whenever possible.

Treatment

Treatment of acidosis with bicarbonate is simple and appears to permit normal growth and development.

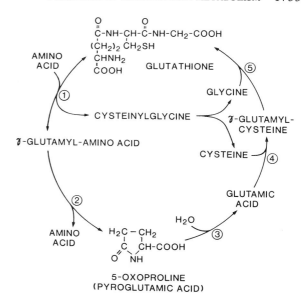

Fig. 96.7   The gamma-glutamyl cycle. (1) γ-Glutamyltranspeptidase. (2) γ-Glutamylcyclotransferase. (3) 5-Oxoprolinase. (4) β-Glutamylcysteine synthetase. (5) Glutathione synthetase. (Reproduced with permission of Alan R. Liss, Inc.)

Genetics

Pyroglutamic acidaemia is inherited as an autosomal recessive trait, with glutathione synthetase activity in tissues of heterozygous carriers being intermediate between those of patients and controls (Wellner et al 1974, Spielberg et al 1977). Prenatal diagnosis has not been reported but may be possible by demonstrating glutathione synthetase deficiency in cultured amniotic cells or increased pyroglutamic acid in amniotic fluid; amniotic fluid of one affected fetus contained about 15 times the normal concentration of pyroglutamic acid at term (Larsson et al 1974).

REFFERENCES

Amendt B A, Rhead W J 1986 The multiple acyl-coenzyme A dehydrogenation disorders, glutaric aciduria type II and ethylmalonic-adipic aciduria: Mitochondrial fatty acid oxidation, acyl-CoA dehydrogenase, and electron transfer flavoprotein activities in fibroblasts. Journal of Clinical Investigation 78: 205–213.

Ampola M G, Mahoney M J, Nakamura E, Tanaka K 1975 Prenatal therapy of a patient with vitamin B_{12}-responsive methylmalonic acidaemia. New England Journal of Medicine 293: 313–317

Ando T, Klingberg W G, Ward A N, Rasmussen K, Nyhan

W L 1971 Isovaleric acidaemia presenting with altered metabolism of glycine. Pediatric Research 5: 478–486

Ando T, Rasmussen K, Nyhan W, Hull D 1972a 3-Hydroxypropionate: Significance of β-oxidation of propionate in patients with propionic acidaemia and methylmalonic acidaemia. Proceedings of the National Academy of Sciences USA 69: 2807–2811

Ando T, Rasmussen K, Wright J M, Nyhan W L 1972b Isolation and identification of methylcitrate, a major metabolic product of propionate in patients with propionic acidaemia. Journal of Biological Chemistry 247: 2200–2204

Anthony M, McLeay A C 1976 A unique case of

derangement of vitamin B_{12} metabolism. Proceedings of the Australian Association of Neurologists 13: 61–65

Brandt I K, Hsia Y E, Clement D H, Provence S A 1974 Propionic-acidaemia (ketotic hyperglycinaemia): Dietary treatment resulting in normal growth and development. Pediatrics 53: 391–395

Brandt N J, Gregersen N, Christensen E, Grøn I H, Rasmussen K 1979 Treatment of glutaryl-CoA dehydrogenase deficiency (glutaric aciduria): Experience with diet, riboflavin and GABA analogue. Journal of Pediatrics 94: 669–673

Budd M A, Tanaka K, Holmes L B, Efron M L. Crawford J D, Isselbacher K J 1967 Isovaleric acidaemia: Clinical features of a new generic defect of leucine metabolism. New England Journal of Medicine 277: 321–327

Burri B J, Sweetman L, Nyhan W L 1985 Heterogeneity of holocarboxylase synthetase in patients with biotin-responsive multiple carboxylase deficiency. American Journal of Human Genetics 37: 320–337

Carmel R, Bedros A A, Mace J W, Goodman S I 1980 Congenital methylmalonic aciduria-homocystinuria with megaloblastic anaemia: Observations on response to hydroxyocobalamin and on the effect of homocysteine and methionine on the deoxyuridine suppression test. Blood 55: 570–579

Cheema-Dhadli S, Leznoff C C. Halperin M L 1975 Effect of 2-methylcitrate on citrate metabolism: Implications for the management of patients with propionic acidaemia and methylmalonic aciduria. Pediatric Research 9: 905–908

Childs B, Nyhan W L, Borden M A, Bard L, Cooke R E 1961 Idiopathic hyperglycinaemia and hyperglycinuria, a new disorder of amino acid metabolism. I. Pediatrics 27: 522–538

Christensen E, Brandt N J 1978 Studies on glutaryl-CoA dehydrogenase in leukocytes, fibroblasts and amniotic fluid cells. The normal enzyme and the mutant form in patients with glutaric aciduria. Clinica Chimica Acta 88: 267–276

Cohn R M, Yudkoff M, Rothman R, Segal S 1978 Isovaleric acidaemia: Use of glycine therapy in neonates. New England Journal of Medicine 299: 996–999

Coude F X, Sweetman L, Nyhan W L 1979 Inhibition by propionyl-coenzyme A of N-acetylglutamate synthetase in rat liver mitochondria. Journal of Clinical Investigation 64: 1544–1551

Cowan M J, Packman S, Wara D W, Ammann A J, Yoshino M, Sweetman L, Nyhan W 1979 Multiple biotin-dependent carboxylase deficiencies associated with defects in T-cell and B-cell immunity. Lancet 2: 115–118

Daum R S, Scriver C R, Mamer O A, Delvin E, Lamm P, Goldman H 1973 An inherited disorder of isoleucine catabolism causing accumulation of α-methylacetoacetate and α-methyl-β-hydroxybutyrate, and intermittent metabolic acidosis. Pediatric Research 7: 149–160

Di Donato S, Frerman F E, Rimoldi M, Rinaldo P, Taroni F, Wiesmann U N 1986 Systemic carnitine deficiency due to lack of electron transfer flavoprotein:ubiquinone oxidoreductase. Neurology 36: 957–963

Dillon M J, England J M, Gompertz D et al 1974 Mental retardation, megaloblastic anaemia, methylmalonic aciduria, and abnormal homocysteine metabolism due to an error in B_{12} metabolism. Clinical Science and Molecular Medicine 47: 43–61

Duran M, Ketting D, Wadman S K, Jakobs C, Schutgens R B H, Veder H A 1978a Organic acid excretion in a patient with 3-hydroxy-3-methylglutaryl-CoA lyase deficiency: facts and artefacts. Clinica Chimica Acta 90: 187–193

Duran M, Bruinvis L, Ketting D, Wadman S K 1978b Deranged isoleucine metabolism during ketotic attacks in patients with methylmalonic acidaemia. Journal of Inherited Metabolic Disease 1: 105–107

Duran M, Schutgens R B H, Ketel A, Heymans H, Berntssen M W J, Ketting D, Wadman S K 1979 3-Hydroxy-3-methylglutaryl coenzyme A lyase deficiency: Postnatal management following prenatal diagnosis by analysis of maternal urine. Journal of Pediatrics 95: 1004–1007

Duran M, Mitchell G, de Klerk J B C et al 1985 Octanoic acidaemia and octanoylcarnitine excretion with dicarboxylic aciduria due to defective oxidation of medium-chain fatty acids. Journal of Pediatrics 107: 397–404

Duran M, Hofkamp M, Rhead W J, Saudubray J–M, Wadman S K 1986 Sudden child death and 'healthy' affected family members with medium-chain acyl-coenzyme A dehydrogenase deficiency. Pediatrics 78: 1052–1057

Eldjarn L, Jellum E, Stokke O, Pande H, Waaler P E 1970 β-Hydroxyisovaleric aciduria and β-methylcrotonylglycinuria: A new inborn error of metabolism. Lancet 2: 521–522

Faull K, Bolton P, Halpern B et al 1976 Patient with defect in leucine metabolism. New England Journal of Medicine 294: 1013

Fenton W A, Rosenberg L E 1978 Genetic and biochemical analysis of human cobalamin mutants in cell culture. Annual Review of Genetics 12: 223–248

Frerman F E, Goodman S I 1985a Fluorometric assay of acyl-CoA dehydrogenases in normal and mutant human fibroblasts. Biochemical Medicine 33: 38–44

Frerman F E, Goodman S I 1985b Deficiency of electron transfer flavoprotein or electron transfer flavoprotein ubiquinone oxidoreductase in glutaric acidemia type II fibroblasts. Proceedings of the National Academy of Sciences USA 82: 4517–4520

Gitzelmann R, Steinmann B, Niederweisser A, Fanconi S, Suormala T, Baumgartner R 1987 Isolated (biotin-resistant) 3-methylcrotonyl-CoA carboxylase deficiency presenting at age 20 months with sopor, hypoglycaemia and ketoacidosis. Journal of Inherited Metabolic Disease 10 (Suppl 2): 290–292

Gompertz D, Draffan G H, Watts J L, Hull D 1971 Biotin-responsive β-methylcrotonylglycinuria. Lancet 2: 22–24

Gompertz D, Bartlett K, Blair D, Stern C M M 1973 Child with a defect in leucine metabolism associated with β-hydroxyisovaleric aciduria and β-methylcrotonylglycinuria. Archives of Disease in Childhood 48: 975–977

Gompertz D, Saudubray J M, Charpentier C, Bartlett K, Goodey P A, Draffan D H 1974 A defect in L-isoleucine metabolism associated with α-methyl-β-hydroxybutyric and α-methylacetoacetic aciduria: Quantitative *in vivo* and *in vitro* studies. Clinica Chimica Acta 57: 269–281

Gompertz D, Goodey P A, Thom H, et al 1975 Prenatal diagnosis and family studies in a case of propionic-acidaemia. Clinical Genetics 8: 244–250

Goodman S I, Frerman F E 1984 Glutaric acidaemia type II (multiple acyl-CoA dehydrogenation deficiency). Journal of Inherited Metabolic Disease 7 (Suppl 1): 33–37

Goodman S I, Kohlhoff J G 1975 Glutaric Aciduria:

Inherited deficiency of glutaryl-CoA-dehydrogenase activity. Biochemical Medicine 13: 138–140

Goodman S I, Moe P G, Hammond K B, Mudd S H, Uhlendorf B W 1970 Homocystinuria with methylmalonic aciduria: Two cases in a sibship. Biochemical Medicine 4: 500–515

Goodman S I, Keyser A J, Mudd S H, Schulman J D, Turse H, Lewy J 1972 Responsiveness of congenital methylmalonic-aciduria to derivatives of vitamin B_{12}. Pediatric Research 6: 138

Goodman S I, Markey S P, Moe P G, Miles B S, Teng C C 1975 Glutaric aciduria: A 'new' disorder of amino acid metabolism. Biochemical Medicine 12: 12–21

Goodman S I, Norenberg M D, Shikes R H, Breslich D J, Moe P G 1977 Glutaric aciduria: Biochemical and morphologic considerations. Journal of Pediatrics 90: 746–750

Goodman S I, Gallegos D A, Pullin C J et al 1980 Antenatal diagnosis of glutaric acidaemia. American Journal of Human Genetics 32: 695–699

Gravel R A, Mahoney M J, Ruddle F H, Rosenberg L E 1975 Genetic complementation in heterokaryons of human fibroblasts defective in cobalamin metabolism. Proceedings of the National Academy of Sciences USA 72: 3181–3185

Gravel R A, Lam K F, Scully K J, Hsia Y E 1977 Genetic complementation of propionyl-CoA carboxylase deficiency in cultured human fibroblasts. American Journal of Human Genetics 29: 378–388

Gregersen N 1979 Studies on the effects of saturated and unsaturated shortchain monocarboxylic acids on the energy metabolism of rat liver mitochondria. Pediatric Research 13:1227–1230

Gregersen N, Brandt N J 1979 Ketotic episodes in glutaryl-CoA dehydrogenase deficiency (glutaric aciduria). Pediatric Research 13: 977–981

Gregersen N, Brandt N J, Christensen E, Grøn I, Rasmussen K, Brandt S 1977 Glutaric aciduria: Clinical and laboratory findings in two brothers. Journal of Pediatrics 90: 740–745

Hagenfeldt L, Larsson A, Zetterström R 1974 Pyroglutamic aciduria: Studies in an infant with chronic metabolic acidosis. Acta Paediatrica Scandinavica 63: 1–8

Hale D E, Batshaw M L, Coates P M et al 1985 Long-chain acyl CoA dehydrogenase deficiency: An inherited cause of non-ketonic hypoglycemia. Pediatric Research 19: 666–671

Halperin M L, Schiller C M, Fritz I B 1971 The inhibition by methylmalonic acid of malate transport by the dicarboxylate carrier in rat liver mitochondria. Journal of Clinical Investigation 50: 2276–2282

Halvorsen S, Stokke O, Jellum E 1979 A variant form of 2-methyl-3-hydroxybutyric and 2-methylacetoacetic aciduria. Acta Paediatrica Scandinavica 68: 123–128

Higginbottom M C, Sweetman L, Nyhan W L 1978 A syndrome of methylmalonic aciduria, homocystinuria, megaloblastic anaemia and neurologic abnormalities in a vitamin B_{12}-deficient breast-fed infant of a strict vegetarian. New England Journal of Medicine 299: 317–323

Hillman R E, Keating J P 1974 Beta-ketothiolase deficiency as a cause of the 'ketotic hyperglycinaemia syndrome'. Pediatrics 53: 221–225

Hillman R E, Otto E F 1974 Inhibition of glycine-serine interconversion in cultured human fibroblasts by products of isoleucine catabolism Pediatric Research 8: 941–945

Hine D G, Hack A M, Goodman S I, Tanaka K 1986

Stable isotope dilution analysis of isovalerylglycine in amniotic fluid and urine and its application for the prenatal diagnosis of isovaleric acidemia. Pediatric Research 20: 222–226

Hommes F A, Kuipers J R G, Elema J D, Jansen J F, Jonxis J H P 1968 Propionicacidaemia, a new inborn error of metabolism Pediatric Research 2: 519–524

Hsia Y E, Scully K J, Rosenberg E 1971 Inherited propionyl-CoA carboxylase deficiency in 'ketotic hyperglycinaemia'. Journal of Clinical Investigation 50: 127–130

Jakobs C, Sweetman L, Wadman S K, Duran M, Saudubray J-M, Nyhan W L 1984 Prenatal diagnosis of glutaric aciduria type II by direct chemical analysis of dicarboxylic acids in amniotic fluid. European Journal of Pediatrics 141: 153–157

Jellum E, Kluge T, Börreson H C, Stokke O, Eldjarn L 1970 Pyroglutamic aciduria--A new inborn error of metabolism. Scandinavian Journal of Clinical and Laboratory Investigation 26: 327–335

Kang E S, Snodgrass P J, Gerald P S 1972 Methylmalonyl Coenzyme A racemase defect: Another cause of methylmalonic aciduria. Pediatric Research 6: 875–879

Kaye C I, Morrow G, Nadler H L 1974 In vitro 'responsive' methylmalonic acidaemia: A new variant. Journal of Pediatrics 85: 55–59

Keeton B R, Moosa A 1976 Organic aciduria: Treatable cause of floppy infant syndrome. Archives of Disease in Childhood 51: 636–638

Kien C L, Kohler E, Goodman S I et al 1981 Biotin-responsive in vivo carboxylase deficiency in two siblings with secretory diarrhoea receiving total parenteral nutrition. Journal of Pediatrics 99: 546–550

Kluge T, Börreson H C, Jellum E, Stokke O, Eldjarn L, Fretheim B 1972 Esophageal hiatus hernia and mental retardation: Life-threatening postoperative metabolic acidosis and potassium deficiency linked with a new inborn error of nitrogen metabolism. Surgery 71: 104–109

Kyllerman M, Steen G 1977 Intermittently progressive dyskinetic syndrome in glutaric aciduria. Neuropadiatrie 8: 397–404

Landaas S 1975 Accumulation of 3-hydroxyisobutyric acid, 2-methyl-3-hydroxybutyric acid and 3-hydroxyisovaleric acid in ketoacidosis. Clinica Chimica Acta 64: 143–154

Larsson A, Zetterström R, Hagenfeldt L, Andersson R, Dreborg S, Hörnell H 1974 Pyroglutamic aciduria (5-oxoprolinuria), an inborn error in glutathione metabolism. Pediatric Research 8: 852–856

Levy H L, Mudd S H, Schulman J D, Dreyfus P M, Abeles R H 1970 A derangement in B_{12} metabolism associated with homocystinemia, cystathioninemia, hypomethioninemia and methylmalonic aciduria. American Journal of Medicine 48: 390–397

Levy H L, Erickson A M, Lott I T, Kurtz D J 1973 Isovaleric acidaemia: Results of family study and dietary treatment. Pediatrics 52: 83–94

Mahoney M J, Rosenberg L E, Lindblad B, Waldenström J, Zetterström R 1975 Prenatal diagnosis of methylmalonic aciduria. Acta Paediatrica Scandinavica 64: 44–48

Mitchell G, Saudubray J M, Benoit Y et al 1983 Antenatal diagnosis of glutaric aciduria type II. Lancet 1: 1099

Mock D M, Baswell D L, Baker H, Holman R T, Sweetman L 1985 Biotin deficiency complicating parenteral alimentation: Diagnosis, metabolic repercussions, and treatment. Journal of Pediatrics 106: 762–769

Mohler D N, Majerus P W, Minnich V, Hess C E, Garrick

M D 1970 Glutathione synthetase deficiency as a cause of hereditary hemolytic disease. New England Journal of Medicine 283: 1253–1257

Morrow G, Schwarz R H, Hallock J A, Barness L A 1970 Prenatal detection of methylmalonic acidaemia. Journal of Pediatrics 77: 120–123

Mooy P D, Przyrembel H, Giesberts M A H, Scholte H R, Blom W, van Gelderen H H 1984 Glutaric aciduria type II: Treatment with riboflavine, carnitine and insulin. European Journal of Pediatrics 143: 92–95

Newman C G H, Wilson B D R, Callaghan P, Young L 1967 Neonatal death associated with isovalericacidaemia. Lancet 2: 439–442

Nyhan W L, Fawcett N, Ando T, Rennert O M, Julius R L 1973 Response to dietary therapy in B$_{12}$-unresponsive methylmalonic acidaemia. Pediatrics 51: 539–548

Oberholzer V G, Levin B, Burgess E A, Young W F 1967 Methylmalonic aciduria: An inborn error of metabolism leading to chronic metabolic acidosis. Archives of Disease in Childhood 42: 492–504

Oberholzer V G, Wood C B S, Palmer T, Harrison B M 1975 Increased pyroglutamic acid levels in patients on artificial diets. Clinica Chimica Acta 62: 299–304

Packman S, Mahoney M J, Tanaka K, Hsia Y E 1978 Severe hyperammonaemia in a newborn infant with methylmalonyl-CoA mutase deficiency. Journal of Pediatrics 92: 769–771

Przyrembel H, Wendel U, Becker K, Bremer H J, Bruinvis L, Ketting D, Wadman S K 1976 Glutaric aciduria type II: Report on a previously undescribed metabolic disorder. Clinica Chimica Acta 66: 227–239

Rhead W J, Tanaka K 1980 Demonstration of a specific mitochondrial isovaleryl-CoA dehydrogenase deficiency in fibroblasts from patients with isovaleric acidaemia. Proceedings of the National Academy of Sciences USA 77: 580–583

Robinson B H, Sherwood W G, Taylor J, Balfe J W, Mamer O A 1979 Acetoacetyl-CoA thiolase deficiency: A cause of severe ketoacidosis in infancy simulating salicylism. Journal of Pediatrics 95: 228–233

Robinson B H, Oei J, Sherwood G, Slyper A H, Heininger J, Mamer O A 1980 Hydroxymethylglutaryl-CoA lyase deficiency: Features resembling Reye syndrome. Neurology 30: 714–718

Roe C R, Millington D S, Maltby D A, Bohan T P, Kahler S G, Chalmers R A 1985 Diagnostic and therapeutic implications of medium-chain acylcarnitines in the medium-chain acyl-CoA dehydrogenase deficiency. Pediatric Research 19: 459–466

Rosenberg L E, Lilljeqvist A, Hsia Y E 1968 Methylmalonic aciduria: An inborn error leading to metabolic acidosis, long-chain ketonuria and intermittent hyperglycinaemia. New England Journal of Medicine 278: 1319–1322

Roth K, Cohn R, Yandrasitz J, Preti G, Dodd P, Segal S 1976 Beta-methylcrotonic aciduria associated with lactic acidosis. Journal of Pediatrics 88: 229–235

Schutgens R B H, Heymans H, Ketel A, Veder H A, Duran M, Ketting D, Wadman S K 1979 Lethal hypoglycaemia in a child with a deficiency of 3-hydroxy-3-methylglutarylcoenzyme A lyase. Journal of Pediatrics 94: 89–91

Scott D 1958 Clinical biotin deficiency (egg white injury). Acta Medica Scandinavica 162: 69–70

Shafai T, Sweetman L, Weyler W, Goodman S I,

Fennessey P V, Nyhan W L 1978 Propionic acidaemia with severe hyperammonaemia and defective glycine metabolism. Journal of Pediatrics 92: 84–86

Spielberg S P, Kramer L I, Goodman S I, Butler J, Tietze F, Quinn P, Schulman J D 1977 5-Oxoprolinuria: Biochemical observations and case report. Journal of Pediatrics 91: 237–241

Spielberg S P, Garrick M D, Corash L M, Butler J D, Tietze F, Rogers L, Schulman J D 1978 Biochemical heterogeneity in glutathione synthetase deficiency. Journal of Clinical Investigation 61: 1417–1420

Stanley C A, Hale D E, Coates P M et al 1983 Medium-chain acyl CoA dehydrogenase deficiency in children with non-ketotic hypoglycaemia and low carnitine levels. Pediatric Research 17: 877–884

Stokke O, Eldjarn L, Norum K R, Steen-Johnsen J, Halvorsen S 1967 Methylmalonic acidaemia: A new inborn error of metabolism which may cause fatal acidosis in the neonatal period. Scandinavian Journal of Clinical and Laboratory Investigation 20: 313–328

Stokke O, Eldjarn L, Jellum E, Pande H, Waaler P E 1972 Beta-methylcrotonyl-CoA carboxylase deficiency: A new metabolic error in leucine degradation. Pediatrics 49: 726–735

Stokke O, Goodman S I, Thompson J A, Miles B S 1975 Glutaric aciduria: Presence of glutaconic and β-hydroxyglutaric acids in urine. Biochemical Medicine 12: 386–391

Stokke O, Goodman S I, Moe P G 1976 Inhibition of brain glutamate decarboxylase by glutarate, glutaconate, and β-hydroxyglutarate: Explanation of the symptoms in glutaric aciduria? Clinica Chimica Acta 66: 411–415

Sweetman L, Weyler W, Shafai T, Young P E, Nyhan W L 1979 Prenatal diagnosis of propionic acidemia. Journal of the American Medical Association 242: 1048–1052

Tanaka K, Isselbacher K J 1967 The isolation and identification of N-isovalerylglycine from urine of patients with isovaleric acidaemia. Journal of Biological Chemistry 242: 2966–2972

Tanaka K, Budd M A, Efron M L, Isselbacher K J 1966 Isovaleric acidaemia: A new genetic defect of leucine metabolism. Proceedings of the National Academy of Sciences USA 56: 236–242

Tanaka K, Orr J C, Isselbacher K J 1968 Identification of β-hydroxyisovaleric acid in the urine of a patient with isovaleric acidaemia. Biochimica et Biophysica Acta 152: 638–641

Taubman B, Hale D E, Kelley R I 1987 Familial Reye-like syndrome: A presentation of medium–chain acyl-coenzyme A dehydrogenase deficiency. Pediatrics 79: 382–385

Truscott R J W, Halpern B, Wysocki S J, Hähnel R, Wilcken B 1979 Studies on a child suspected of having a deficiency in 3-hydroxy-3-methylglutaryl-CoA lyase. Clinica Chimica Acta 95:11–16

Utter M F, Keech D B, Scrutton M G A 1974 A possible role for acetyl CoA in the control of glyconeogenesis. In: Weber G (ed) Advances in Enzyme Regulation, vol 2. Pergamon, New York, p 49–68

Wadlington W B, Kilroy A, Ando T, Sweetman L, Nyhan W L 1975 Hyperglycinaemia and propionyl CoA carboxylase deficiency and episodic severe illness without consistent ketosis. Journal of Pediatrics 86: 707–712

Wellner V P, Sekura R, Meister A, Larsson A 1974 Glutathione synthetase deficiency, an inborn error of metabolism involving the γ-glutamyl cycle in patients with 5-oxoprolinuria (pyroglutamic aciduria). Proceedings of the National Academy of Sciences USA: 71:2505–2509

Whelan D T, Hill R, Ryan E D, Spate M 1979 L-Glutaric acidaemia: Investigation of a patient and his family. Pediatrics 63: 88–93

Willard H F, Rosenberg L E 1977 Inherited deficiencies of human methylmalonyl CoA mutase activity: Reduced affinity of mutant apoenzyme for adenosylcobalamin. Biochemical and Biophysical Research Communications 78: 927–934

Willard H F, Rosenberg L E 1979a Inherited deficiencies of methylmalonyl CoA mutase activity: Biochemical and genetic studies in cultured skin fibroblasts. In: Hommes F A (ed) Models for the Study of Inborn Errors of Metabolism. Elsevier, New York, p 297–310

Willard H F, Rosenberg L E 1979b Inborn errors of cobalamin metabolism: Effect of cobalamin supplementation in culture on methylmalonyl CoA mutase activity in normal and mutant human fibroblasts. Biochemical Genetics 17: 57–75

Willard H F, Ambani L M, Hart C, Mahoney M J, Rosenberg L E 1976 Rapid prenatal and postnatal detection in inborn errors of propionate, methylmalonate, and cobalamin metabolism: A sensitive assay using cultured cells. Human Genetics 32: 277–283

Willard H F, Mellman I S, Rosenberg L E 1978 Genetic complementation among inherited deficiencies of methylmalonyl-CoA mutase activity Evidence for a new class of human cobalamin mutant. American Journal of Human Genetics 30: 1–13

Wolf B, Rosenberg L E 1978 Heterozygote expression in propionylcoenzyme A carboxylase deficiency. Journal of Clinical Investigation 62: 931–936

Wolf B, Hsia Y E, Rosenberg L E 1978 Biochemical differences between mutant propionyl-CoA carboxylases from two complementation groups. American Journal of Human Genetics 30: 455–464

Wolf B, Grier R E, Allen R J et al 1983a Phenotypic variation in biotinidase deficiency. Journal of Pediatrics 103: 233–237

Wolf B, Grier R E, Allen R J, Goodman S I, Kien C L 1983b Biotinidase deficiency: The enzymatic defect in late-onset multiple carboxylase deficiency. Clinica Chimica Acta 131: 273–281

Wolf B, Heard G S, Jefferson L G, Proud V K, Nance W E, Wissbecker K A 1985 Clinical findings in four children with biotinidase deficiency detected through a statewide neonatal screening program. New England Journal of medicine 313: 16–19

Wysocki S J, Hähnel R 1976a 3 Hydroxy-3-methylglutaric aciduria : Deficiency of 3-hydroxy-3-methylglutaryl coenzyme A lyase. Clinica Chimica Acta 71:349–351

Wysocki S J, Hähnel R 1976b 3-Hydroxy-3-methylglutaric aciduria: 3-hydroxy-3-methylglutaryl-coenzyme A lyase levels in leukocytes. Clinica Chimica Acta 73: 373–375

Wysocki S J, Hähnel R 1978 3-methylcrotonylglycine excretions in 3-hydroxy-3-methylglutaric aciduria. Clinica Chimica Acta 86: 101–108

Wysocki S J. Wilkinson S P, Hähnel R, Wong C Y B, Panegyres P K 1976 3-Hydroxy-3-methylglutaric aciduria, combined with 3-methylglutaconic aciduria. Clinica Chimica Acta 70: 399–406

97. Renal tubular disorders

R. Hillman

INTRODUCTION

All small molecules not tightly bound to protein are filtered by the glomerulus. The renal tubules are the primary mechanism by which the body can reabsorb these compounds. The proximal tubules (and, for bicarbonate and water, the distal tubules and collecting ducts) are responsible for reabsorbing 80–98% of those solutes which are filtered by the glomerulus. Although a few substances are secreted by the kidney, most disorders of tubular function lead to decreased reabsorption and thus increased loss in the urine. Disorders of renal tubular function must be divided both by the segment of the tubule which is involved and by the substrate or substrates whose transport is effected. Molecules are reabsorbed by mechanisms which are both specific and saturable. In addition there is some suggestion that the entry step of substrates into the renal tubule from the brush border side of the tubule (the lumen) is under different genetic control than the exit step through the basal lateral membranes into the blood. The majority of the disorders of transport that have been described involve defects in the proximal tubule. Many of these disorders, though genetically well defined, are of little clinical significance. Sometimes, as in Hartnup disease, the renal defect seems to be less important than the corresponding defect in transport in the intestine (Hillman et al 1986).

Transport in the proximal tubule is largely energy dependent and is driven by oxidative metabolism of a variety of substrates. Experimentally it can be supported by acetate, lactate, and a variety of other organic acids. The distal tubules, and particularly the collecting ducts, are more dependent on energy derived from glycolysis. Many substrates are co-transported with sodium and much of the driving force for movement across membranes is provided by the electrochemical potential difference generated by Na^+ and H^+ movements. Thus, compounds which interfere with the energy metabolism of the kidney or with ATP'ase activity can have effects on many different transport systems in the tubule. Those disorders of generalized proximal tubular function will be discussed first.

GENERALIZED DISORDERS OF TUBULAR FUNCTION (THE FANCONI SYNDROME)

The Fanconi syndrome is a generalized tubular disorder which leads to multiple transport abnormalities. These include increased urinary loss of several organic substrates including amino acids, glucose, bicarbonate and organic acids, and the loss of inorganic ions essential for the body's homeostasis including calcium, magnesium, sodium, potassium and, perhaps most important clinically, phosphorus (Morris & Sebastian 1983). Clinically, the syndrome is usually defined by the combination of glucosuria, phosphaturia, generalized amino aciduria, and renal tubular acidosis. In addition there is usually increased renal excretion of small molecular weight proteins. The metabolic abnormalities can lead to metabolic bone disease (rickets or osteomalacia) and stunted growth, which often form the most important aspect of the disease in young children.

The Fanconi syndrome can be caused by a variety of inherited diseases and by a variety of toxins to the renal tubules (Table 97.1). In the absence of other known

Table 97.1 Inherited causes of the Fanconi syndrome

1. Familial idiopathic
2. Cystinosis
3. Disorders of phosphorylated sugar metabolism including Galactosaemia, Glycogen storage disease, and hereditary Fructose Intolerance
4. Lowe Syndrome
5. Wilson disease
6. Tyrosinaemia
7. Medullary Cystic Disease
8. Rickets with secondary hyperparathyroidism

disease, it can also exist in an isolated form that is inherited as an autosomal recessive or dominant. Probably the most common causes of hereditary Fanconi syndrome are secondary to cystinosis and galactosaemia.

The clinical presentation of the Fanconi syndrome (Harrison 1958) depends on the age of the patient and the other manifestations of the primary disease. Idiopathic Fanconi syndrome in the absence of other disease may manifest itself primarily as bone disease, as a GI problem presenting as vomiting, anorexia, constipation probably due to volume depletion, accompanied by chronic acidosis, or be picked up incidentally on a routine urine analysis. The diagnosis of idiopathic Fanconi syndrome can only be made after an exhaustive search for the other possible causes.

Families where the Fanconi syndrome has been inherited as an autosomal dominant have been reported by Ben-Ishay et al (1961) and by Hunt et al (1966). Smith et al (1976) reported a family where the syndrome appeared in four successive generations. All of these families with dominant inheritance have a relatively mild disease and are usually termed the adult Fanconi syndrome. Variation within the families has been relatively great, with some patients having only the urinary findings of the disease without overt clinical expression and others presenting with severe rickets.

Two autosomal recessive forms of the disease have been differentiated. In the severe childhood form of the recessively inherited disease the picture is much like cystinosis and some questions must be raised as to whether the early reports of this mode of inheritance (Clay et al 1953) might not represent undiagnosed secondary causes of the syndrome. The most convincing pedigree is that of Klajman and Arber (1967) who described a consanguineous Iraqi Jewish family with six affected siblings. Dent and Harris's (1956) family with adult onset Fanconi syndrome was shown by Brenton et al (1981) to have a dominant form. Thus the autosomal recessive inheritance of a distinct adult form of the disease must be questioned.

DISORDERS OF AMINO ACID TRANSPORT

Except for tryptophan (and perhaps homocysteine), which is largely bound to protein, amino acids are filtered freely by the glomerulus. Most of the amino acids are normally reabsorbed in the proximal tubule leaving only very small amounts in the resulting urine ultrafiltrate. Glycine and histidine, which are less efficiently reabsorbed than the other amino acids, account for most of the alpha amino nitrogen found in the urine. Only the very small infant, particularly the premature, excretes significant quantities of amino acids other than glycine and histidine. In these children alanine, proline, hydroxyproline, serine and threonine are commonly present in significant quantities and it is the author's impression that the more immature infants also excrete cystine.

Amino acids are reabsorbed by energy dependent mechanisms of high specificity (Hillman et al 1968). In most cases, transport is coupled to the movement of sodium ion. Essentially the transport systems for amino acids can be thought of as group specific (Table 97.2). Studies of families with inherited defects in transport have confirmed that these groups which have been best described in other animals do in fact represent the primary mechanisms for the reabsorption of amino acids in man. Transport systems are present for the neutral amino acids, the amino acids having two ammonium groups including cystine (usually called the dibasic amino acids), the acidic amino acids, and the grouping of the imino acids (proline and hyroxyproline) plus glycine. Studies in animals suggest that each of these groups may have several transport systems, with a major system of high affinity, but secondary systems with lower affinities for the same substrates (Scriver & Wilson 1967, Scriver 1968). This concept has been partially supported in man by the description of 'variant' amino acid transport disorders with different combinations of amino acids found in the urine than in classical diseases. In addition, the transport systems described in Table 97.2 apply only to the brush border side of the tubule. Transport across the basal lateral membrane is by different mechanisms. Thus far in humans a defect has only been described for the basic amino acids (lysinuric protein intolerance) in the basal lateral transport system (Rajantie et al 1981).

The genetics of transport in the human is not as straight-forward as once believed. In Hartnup disease (see below) amino acids other than those found in the neutral systems are found in the urine and stool. For several of the amino acids, transport system defects may be found in the kidney alone, in kidney plus intestine, or in the intestine alone. Thus, much must still be learned about the genetic mechanisms controlling transport of amino acids.

Table 97.2 Amino acid transport systems

1 Neutral amino acid system L (leucine preferring)
2 Neutral amino acid system A (alanine preferring)
3 Imino-glycine system
4 Acidic amino acid system
5 Dibasic amino acid system (includes cystine)

Glycine and the imino acids

Joseph et al (1958) described a child with marked increases in the urinary excretion of proline, hydroxyproline and glycine. Since then numerous other reports of similar patients have been made, and screening studies (Levy et al 1972) have reported that the incidence may be as high as 1 in 20 000 in the general population. Initially these findings were reported to be associated with a variety of neurological complications but later familial studies, as well as the population screening, suggested that this is a benign condition inherited as an autosomal recessive trait (Rosenberg et al 1968). This transport system has a much higher affinity for the imino acids than for glycine (Hillman & Rosenberg 1969). Heterozygotes for this defect may excrete only glycine in the urine and a dominantly inherited glycinuria has been reported independently in three generations (Greene et al 1973). This transport system is quite late in developing, as shown by Segal and his co-workers (Reynolds et al 1979), and these amino acids are commonly found in the urine of young infants, particularly those who are premature. Like many of the other disorders of amino-acid transport in the kidney, a defect in transport in the intestine has also been reported (Goodman et al 1967). The primary importance of this hereditary condition is that it can be mistaken for a defect in glycine metabolism, either primary or secondary to one of the organic acidaemias.

Dibasic amino acids and cystine

Classical cystinuria

Cystinuria is not only a significant clinical disease but is also important historically because it was one of the original inborn errors reported by Garrod in his famous Croonian lectures (1908). In classical cystinuria the urinary excretion of lysine, ornithine, arginine and cystine is greatly increased compared to normal (Segal & Thier 1989). Although the absolute increase in cystine is less than that of the other amino acids, because it is far less soluble than the others it forms stones. Serum amino acids are normal in this condition.

Three hereditary patterns of classical cystinuria have been described (Rosenberg et al 1966). All are inherited as autosomal recessives and the homozygotes cannot be distinguished. Heterozygotes, however, can be separated on two bases. The primary distinction is whether or not the heterozygotes excrete increased amounts of cystine and lysine in their urine. In so-called type I heterozygotes the excretion is normal. It is increased (but not to clinically significant levels) in type II and III hetero-

zygotes. Type II and III heterozygotes can be distinguished only by studying transport in the intestine. Type II heterozygotes have a transport defect in the intestine as well as the kidney but type III heterozygotes have normal or only slightly reduced transport in the intestine. The reports of patients resulting from the union of differing heterozygotes suggest that these mutations are allelic.

The incidence of clinical cystinuria is reported to vary widely in different populations. In Sweden the incidence is reported to be only 1 in 100 000 (Boström & Tottie 1959) while in Libyan Jews it is reported to be as high as 1 in 2500 (Weinberger et al 1974). Results of newborn screening suggest a high incidence in many populations (1 in 15 000 in Boston, 1 in 11 000 in Vienna, 1 in 17 000 in Sydney) but these figures must be accepted very conditionally because of the increased secretion normally noted in newborns and particularly because of the obervation by Scriver (1986) that newborn heterozygotes are difficult to distinguish from homozygotes.

Other forms of dibasic amino aciduria

Cystine excretion in the absence of other dibasic amino acids has been reported (Brodehl et al 1967). The two sibs with this condition were without stones, but were only 2 and 4 years old when reported. Dibasic amino aciduria in the absence of cystine excretion was reported in 13 members of a family (Whelan & Scriver 1968). These patients were also asymptomatic. Most importantly, the description of lysinuric protein intolerance has led to the first documentation of a basal lateral transport defect of dibasic amino acids, rather than a brush border defect (Rajantie et al 1980). This disorder leads to marked decreased protein tolerance because of hyperammonaemia and suggests that the urea cycle is not a perfect cycle but requires the intake of the dibasic amino acids. The defect can be partially overcome by giving citrulline, which is not transported by the same system and can be converted in the liver to arginine and ornithine. This disease has been reported throughout the world but has a particularly high incidence in Finland (1 in 60 000). The author is following an extended pedigree of American blacks which, along with a report from Japan, suggests that the disease is not limited to northern Europeans.

Neutral amino acids

Hartnup Disease is primarily a disease of neutral amino acid transport. However histidine, glutamine and asparagine are also increased in the urine. It can be distinguished from a generalized amino aciduria because cystine and the dibasic amino acids, the imino acids, and the dicarboxylic amino acids are not increased. The clinical manifestations of the disease are very variable (Scriver et al 1987). Clinically the patients may have any combination of cerebellar ataxia, emotional instability, delayed development and a pellagra-like rash. However, recent evidence suggests that the renal defect in the absence of an intestinal transport defect is of less significance than the combined defect, or the presence of an intestinal transport defect alone (Scriver 1987). The clinical manifestations have been believed to be due to tryptophan malabsorption leading to niacin deficiency. However, it is the author's experience that patients who have clinical manifestations other than rash (primarily developmental delay and ataxia) continue to have slow development even when receiving large amounts of niacin and a good protein intake. The presence of an intestinal transport defect is suggested by the presence of large amounts of indoles and particularly of tryptamine in the urine, resulting from the intestinal bacteria utilizing the malabsorbed tryptophan. Stool amino acids can then be measured directly.

The disease appears to be inherited as an autosomal recessive. Several reports of consanguineous cases have appeared. There seem to be three forms of the disease. The classical form of the disorder has defects in both the renal tubular and intestinal transport systems (Scriver 1965). The form of the disease usually detected on newborn screening has only urinary manifestations (Levy et al 1972). A disorder affecting only the gut transport systems was described which was associated with growth and developmental delay (Hillman et al 1986). Recently we (unpublished data) have found the same condition in a family with two affected sibs and a mild transport defect in other family members, suggesting the heterozygous state. This pedigree is strongly suggestive of autosomal recessive inheritance.

Acidic amino acids

Massive excretion of aspartic acid and glutamic acid has been reported twice in single patients (Teijema et al 1974, Melancon et al 1977). Presumably this condition is inherited as an autosomal recessive condition. The clinical manifestations in the two patients were quite different and the significance of this condition is unknown.

RENAL TUBULAR ACIDOSIS

Proximal renal tubular acidosis (Type 2 RTA)

Proximal renal tubular acidosis is caused by a change in the mechanism for bicarbonate reabsorption such that

not all the bicarbonate is reasorbed when the filtered load (the serum bicarbonate concentration) is in the normal range. The alteration is only in the proximal and not in the distal tubule so that normal acidification mechanisms in the distal tubule can still lower the urine pH and excrete an acid load. As the serum bicarbonate concentration decreases, a filtered load is reached where all the remaining bicarbonate can be reabsorbed.

Nearly all the reports of proximal renal tubular acidosis in the absence of the Fanconi syndrome have been in young children, most before 2 years of age (Morris & Sebastian 1983). The disease appears to express itself more commonly in males than females. A fairly mild expression of isolated proximal renal tubular acidosis with a dominant expression has been published (Brenes et al 1977). However, the great predominance of males (about 4 to 1, male to female) would suggest an X-linked recessive form of inheritance in other cases. This mode of inheritance cannot be considered proven, however, because no family history can be demonstrated in a majority of the cases (Scriver et al 1977).

In most cases the patients present with a failure to thrive or simply to grow normally. The only physical findings are related to the growth failure. The only laboratory finding usually is hyperchloraemic acidosis, usually of only moderate degree. The findings of the Fanconi syndrome are otherwise absent and this diagnosis is made when other signs of proximal tubular disease are excluded.

Distal renal tubular acidosis (Type 1 RTA)

This is inherited as an autosomal dominant disease. The inheritance is clearly different from the proximal tubular disease described above. Randall's (1967) follow-up of the pedigree described by himself and Targgart (1961) shows several instances of male to male transmission. This disease presents with nephrocalcinosis, fixed urinary specific gravity, a low urinary pH of about 5, low serum bicarbonate concentrations and hypocalcaemia. The bone manifestations are very variable, but may be severe.

There appears to be a second variant of this disease which is associated with perception deafness (Morris 1970). This variant is also inherited as an autosomal dominant. Carbonic anhydrase type B in red cells was reported to be unstable in this disease (Kondo et al 1978) perhaps relating its pathophysiology to the other instance of a similar defect; this is described next.

Carbonic anhydrase II deficiency

Renal tubular acidosis associated with osteopetrosis has been reported by Sly et al (1972, 1983, 1985). In this syndrome patients present in early childhood with fractures. They are later found to have cerebral calcifications of the basal ganglia. All have evidence of renal tubular acidosis and are found to have deficiency of the enzyme carbonic anhydrase II. About half of all reported cases have occurred in families of Arab descent in the Middle East or North Africa. The disease is clearly an autosomal recessive, based both on pedigree studies and on more recent enzymatic and DNA studies.

DISORDERS OF SUGAR TRANSPORT

At least two transport systems mediate the reabsorption of sugars. The most important is the system which transports glucose and galactose. Also present in the proximal tubule are systems for the transport of a variety of other sugars. Fructose is not actively transported by the tubule and the condition known as fructosuria is due to overflow rather than a reabsorption defect. As with the amino acids, defects have been described which affect the intestine as well as the kidney. Thus the genetics of sugar transport may be more complex than has thus far been described. Because heterozygotes for sugar transport defects may spill small amounts of sugar in the urine, these disorders have been described as having dominant modes of inheritance (Hjarne 1927). However, all have now been shown to be clearly inherited as autosomal recessive disorders.

Renal glycosuria

Renal glycosuria may be thought of as two disorders.

Firstly, patients may have a low threshold for glucose but a normal total capacity to reabsorb it. Thus these patients spill glucose at a serum concentration where it is normally reabsorbed. Their total daily loss of glucose in the urine is not great, however, because absorption continues to increase with increasing serum concentrations. This disorder is mainly of importance because it may be confused with diabetes mellitus and because a low renal threshold for glucose may make urine monitoring of a diabetic difficult.

Secondly, patients may have a decreased capacity to reabsorb glucose with or without a decreased threshold. These patients may spill very large amounts of glucose in a day, sometimes as much as 100 g. These two types of defect appear to be allellic. Elsas and Rosenberg (1969, 1971) showed that both types of defect can appear in the same family, and that compound heterozygotes have clinical glycosuria. Recently, Oemar et al (1987) described a family where glucose reabsorption appeared to be completely absent. Presumably, in this family there was a complete absence of the carrier protein, rather than a kinetic abnormality as seen in the other described cases. The abnormality is limited to the proximal tubule. De Marchi et al (1984) suggested that the gene is linked to HLA. Clinically these patients have few problems other than those caused by iatrogenic confusion with diabetes. Polydipsia and polyuria have been described. In the author's experience the two major problems have been nocturia in children and yeast infections of the vagina both in children and adults, presumably due to the high sugar content of the urine.

Fructosuria

Fructosuria in the absence of fructose intolerance (fructose-phosphate aldolase deficiency) is not a renal tubular disease. Instead, this benign condition is the result of a defect in hepatic fructokinase. It is inherited as an autosomal recessive trait (Laron 1961).

Pentosuria

Pentosuria was also one of the original inborn errors described in the Garrod lectures (1908). Patients excrete 1–4 g of pentose, primarily 1–xylulose each day (Khachadurian 1962). It is a benign condition which occurs primarily in Ashkenazi Jews of Polish origin, and in Lebanese. This disease, like fructosuria, is usually a disorder of metabolism rather than transport. Wang and Van Eys (1970) demonstrated that the defect is in the enzyme NADP-xylitol dehydrogenase. Heterozygotes have intermediate levels of the enzyme, confirming its autosomal recessive form of inheritance. We have seen one other patient where this enzyme is of normal activity. This suggests either that another enzyme may be involved, or that a primary renal condition (also benign) may exist. Unfortunately the patient, when told he did not have diabetes, refused further studies.

HYPOPHOSPHATAEMIC RICKETS

Hypophosphataemic rickets is discussed elsewhere in this text. It is included here because it is caused by another defect of the tubule reabsorption systems and because it is also related to the general reabsorption defects described above. Hypophosphataemic rickets behaves as an X-linked dominant trait in most families. However, Scriver et al (1977) described an autosomal dominant pedigree.

SUMMARY

The renal tubules reabsorb 80–95% of filtered small molecules by energy dependent mechanisms. Disorders, primary or secondary, which interfere with these mechanisms can cause disorders of reabsorption of sugars, amino acids, bicarbonate and phosphate, as well as of an assortment of organic acids. Specific transport systems are under genetic control. Thus, inherited disorders affecting the reabsorption of only one or a group of compounds occur in the absence of more generalized disease. With the notable exceptions of bicarbonate and phosphate, the urinary loss does not seem to produce nutritional deficiencies. Cystine transport deficiency produces problems primarily because of this compound's low solubility. In other cases, these inherited conditions are benign but it is most important to recognize them because they cause confusion with defects in metabolism where increased serum levels of a compound exceed the tubules' capacity for reabsorption.

REFERENCES

Ben-Ishay D, Dreyfuss F, Ullmann T D 1961 Fanconi syndrome with hypouricemia in an adult: a family study. American Journal of Medicine 31: 793

Boström H, Tottie K 1959 Cystinuria in Sweden. II: The incidence of homozygous cystinuria in Swedish school children. Acta Paediatria 48: 345

Brenes L G, Brenes J N, Hernandez M M 1977 Familial renal tubular acidosis: a distinct clinical entity. American Journal of Medicine 63: 244

Brenton D P, Isenberg D A, Cusworth D C et al 1981 The adult presenting idiopathic Fanconi syndrome. Journal of Inherited Metabolic Diseases 4: 211

Brodehl J, Gallissen K, Kowalewski S 1967 Isolated cystinuria (without lysine-ornithine-arginuria) in a family with hypocalcemic tetany. Klinische Wochenschrift 45: 38

Clay R D, Darmady E M, Hawkins M 1953 The nature of the renal lesion in the Fanconi syndrome. Journal of Pathology and Bacteriology 65: 551

De Marchi S, Cecchin E, Basile A et al 1984 Close genetic linkage between HLA and renal glycosuria. American Journal of Nephrology 4: 280

Dent C E, Harris H 1956 Hereditary forms of rickets and osteomalacia. Journal of Bone and Joint Surgery 38B: 204

Elsas L J, Rosenberg L E 1969 Familial renal glycosuria: a genetic reappraisal of hexose transport by kidney and intestine. Journal of Clinical Investigation 48: 1845

Elsas L J, Busse D, Rosenberg L E 1971 Autosomal recessive inheritance of renal glycosuria. Metabolism 20: 968

Garrod A E 1908 The Croonian Lectures. Lancet 2: 1,73,142,214

Goodman S I, McIntyre C A O'Brien D 1967 Impaired intestinal transport of proline in a patient with familial iminoaciduria. Journal of Pediatrics 71: 246

Greene M L, Lietman P S, Rosenberg L E, Seegmiller J E 1973 Familial Hyperglycinuria: New defect in renal tubular transport of glycine and iminoacids. American Journal of Medicine 54: 265

Harrison H E 1958 The Fanconi syndrome. Journal of Chronic Diseases 7: 346

Hillman R E, Rosenberg L E 1969 Amino acid transport by isolated mammalian renal tubules. II: Proline transport systems. Journal of Biological Chemistry 244: 4494

Hillman R E, Albrecht I, Rosenberg L E 1968 Identification and analysis of multiple glycine transport systems in isolated mammalian renal tubules. Journal of Biological Chemistry 243: 5566

Hillman R E, Stewart A, Miles J H 1986 Amino acid transport defect in intestine not affecting kidney. Pediatric Research 20: 200

Hjarne V 1927 Study of orthoglycaemic glycosuria with particular reference to its hereditability. Acta Medica Scandinavica 67: 422

Hunt D D, Stearns G, McKinley J B et al 1966 Long-term study of a family with Fanconi syndrome without cystinosis. American Journal of Medicine 40:492

Joseph R, Ribierre M, Job J-C, Girault M 1958 Maladie familiale associante des convulsions a debut tres precoce, une hyperalbuminorachie et une hyperaminoacidurie. Archives Francaises de Pediatraie 15: 374

Khachadurian A K 1962 Essential pentosuria. American Journal of Human Genetics 14: 249

Klajman A, Arber I 1967 Familial glycosuria and aminoaciduria associated with a low serum alkaline phosphatase. Israel Journal of Medical Science 3: 392

Kondo T, Taniguchi N, Taniguchi K et al 1978 Inactive form of erythrocyte carbonic anhydrase B in patients with primary renal tubular acidosis. Journal of Clinical Investigation 62: 610

Laron Z 1961 Essential benign fructosuria. Archives of Diseases of Childhood 36: 273

Levy H L, Madigan P M, Shih V E 1972 Massachusetts metabolic screening program. I: Technique and results of urine screening. Pediatrics 49: 825

Melancon S B, Dallaire L, Lemieux B et al 1977 Dicarboxylic aminoaciduria: An inborn error of amino acid metabolism. Journal of Pediatrics 91: 422

Morris R C 1970 Renal tubular acidosis. Mechanisms, classification and implications. New England Journal of Medicine 281: 1405

Morris R C, Sebastian A 1983 Renal tubular acidosis and Fanconi syndrome. In: Stanbury et al (eds) The Metabolic Basis of Inherited Disease. McGraw-Hill, New York, p 1808

Oemar B S, Byrd D J, Brodehl J 1987 Complete absence of tubular glucose reabsorption: a new type of renal glucosuria (type O). Clinical Nephrology 27: 156

Rajantie J, Simell O, Rapola J et al 1980 Lysinuric protein intolerance: a two year trial of dietary supplementation therapy with citrulline and lysine. Journal of Pediatrics 97: 927

Rajantie J, Simell O, Perheentupa J 1981 Lysinuric protein intolerance: basolateral transport effect in renal tubuli. Journal of Clinical Investigation 67: 1078

Randall R E 1967 Familial renal tubular acidosis revisited. Annals of Internal Medicine 66: 1024

Randall R E, Targgart W H 1961 Familial renal tubular acidosis. Annals of Internal Medicine 54: 1108

Reynolds R, Roth K S, Hwang S M, Segal S 1979 On the development of glycine transport systems by rat renal cortex. Biochimica et Biophysica Acta 511: 274

Rosenberg L E, Downing S E, Durant J L, Segal S 1966 Cystinuria: biochemical evidence for three genetically distinct diseases. Journal of Clinical Investigation 45: 365

Rosenberg L E, Durant J L, Elsas L J 1968 Familial iminoglycinuria: an inborn error of renal tubular transport. New England Journal of Medicine 278: 1407

Scriver C R 1965 Hartnup disease; a genetic modification of intestinal and renal transport of certain neutral alpha-amino acids. New England Journal of Medicine 273: 530

Scriver C R 1968 Renal tubular transport of proline, hydroxyproline and glycine III. Genetic basis for more than one mode of transport in human kidney. Journal of Clinical Investigation 47: 823

Scriver C R (abstract) 1986 American Society for Human Genetics

Scriver C R 1987 (personal communication)

Scriver C R, Wilson O H 1967 Amino acid transport in human kidney: Evidence for genetic control of two types. Science 155: 1428

Scriver C R, MacDonald W, Reade T M et al 1977 Hypophosphatemic non-rachitic bone disease. American Journal of Medical Genetics 1: 101

Scriver C R, Mahon B, Levy H L et al 1987 The Hartnup phenotype: mendelian transport disorder, multifactorial disease. American Journal of Human Genetics 40: 401

Segal S, Thier S 1989 Cystinurias. In: Scriver CR et al (eds) The metabolic basis of inherited disease, 6th edn. McGraw-Hill, New York, p 99

Sly W S, Lang R, Avioli L, Haddad J et al 1972 Recessive osteopetrosis: a new clinical phenotype. American Journal of Human Genetics 24: 34

Sly W S, Hewett-Emmett D, Whyte M P et al 1983 Carbonic anhydrase II deficiency identified as the primary defect in the autosomal recessive syndrome of osteopetrosis with renal tubular acidosis and cerebral calcification. Proceedings of the National Academy of Sciences 80: 2752

Sly W S, Whyte M P, Sundaram V, Tashian R E et al 1985 Carbonic anhydrase II deficiency in 12 families with the autosomal recessive syndrome of osteopetrosis with renal tubular acidosis and cerebral calcification. New England Journal of Medicine 313: 139

Smith R, Lindenbaum R H, Walton R J 1976 Hypophosphataemic osteomalacia and Fanconi syndrome of adult onset with dominant inheritance: possible relationship with diabetes mellitus. Quarterly Journal of Medicine 45: 387

Teijema H L, van Gelderen H H, Giesberta M A et al 1974 Dicarboxylic aminoaciduria: an inborn error of glutamate and aspartate transport with metabolic implications, in combination with hyperprolinemia. Metabolism 23: 115

Wang Y M, Van Eys J 1970 The enzymatic defect in essential pentosuria. New England Journal of Medicine 282: 892

Weinberger A, Sperling O, Rabinovitz M et al 1974 High frequency of cystinuria among Jews of Libyan origin. Human Heredity 24: 568

Whelan D T, Scriver C R 1968 Hyperdibasic aminoaciduria: an inherited disorder of amino acid transport. Pediatric Research 2: 525

98. The inherited porphyrias

Robert J. Desnick   Andrew G. Roberts   Karl E. Anderson

INTRODUCTION

The inherited porphyrias are a diverse group of inborn errors of metabolism, each resulting from the deficient activity of a specific enzyme in the haem biosynthetic pathway. An exception is the enzyme deficiency in porphyria cutanea tarda (PCT) which can be either inherited or acquired. Depending on the primary site of porphyrin accumulation these disorders have been classified as either 'hepatic' or 'erythropoietic'. The major clinical manifestations result from the accumulation of porphyrin precursors and/or porphyrins which cause neurological symptoms and/or cutaneous photosensitivity (Table 98.1). Neurological manifestations occur only in some hepatic porphyrias in association with excess amounts of the porphyrin precursors, δ aminolevulinic acid (ALA) and porphobilinogen (PBG). Although the pathophysiological mechanism(s) underlying the neurological involvement remain poorly understood, these symptoms can be life-threatening. Sensitivity to sunlight results from the excitation by long-wave ultraviolet light of excess tissue porphyrins leading to skin damage, scarring and deformation. The clinical exacerbation and/or severity of these disorders are determined partly by environmental and metabolic factors, such as hormones, drugs and nutrition, which increase the production of porphyrin precursors and/or porphyrins. In these 'ecogenic' disorders, environmental, physiological and genetic factors interact to cause clinical expression of the disease. The recent isolation and characterization of several of the haem biosynthetic enzymes and their genes have provided greater understanding of this essential biosynthetic pathway and have permitted the first studies of the molecular lesions which cause specific porphyrias.

THE HAEM BIOSYNTHETIC PATHWAY

The haem biosynthetic enzymes

The haem biosynthetic pathway is shown in Figure 98.1. The first and last three enzymes are functional in the mitochondrion, the other four function in the cytosol. Each of eight haem biosynthetic enzymes is encoded by a nuclear gene. To date, the full-length human cDNAs for the first five enzymes have been isolated and sequenced (Raich et al 1986, Romeo et al 1986a, Wetmur et al 1986,

Table 98.1 Classification of the human porphyrias

Type/Porphyria	Deficient enzyme	Inheritance*	McK**	Photosensitivity	Neurovisceral symptoms
Hepatic					
ALA-dehydratase deficiency	ALA-dehydratase	AR	12527	−	+
Acute intermittent porphyria (AIP)	HMB-synthase	AD	17600	−	+
Hereditary coproporphyria (HCP)	COPRO-oxidase	AD	12130	+	+
Variegate porphyria (VP)	PROTO-oxidase	AD	17620	+	+
Porphyria cutanea tarda (PCT)	URO-decarboxylase	AD	17610	+	−
Erythropoietic					
Congenital erythropoietic porphyria (CEP)	URO-synthase	AR	26370	+ + +	−
Erythropoietic protoporphyria (EPP)	Ferrochelatase	AD	17700	+	−

* AR = Autosomal Recessive, AD = Autosomal Dominant, for clinical manifestations.
** McK = Catalogue number (McKusick 1988).

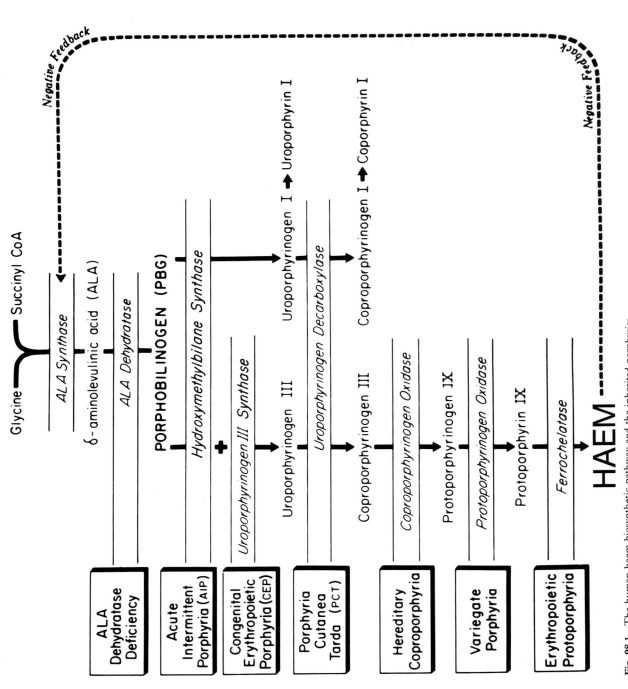

Fig. 98.1   The human haem biosynthetic pathway and the inherited porphyrias.

Bowden et al 1987, Grandchamp et al 1987, Astrin et al 1988, Tsai et al 1988). The chromosomal locations of five haem biosynthetic genes have been assigned by somatic cell or in situ hybridization techniques to four different chromosomes (Wang et al 1981, Grandchamp et al 1983, Romeo et al 1986b, Potluri et al 1987, Astrin et al 1988) (Table 98.2). Each of the enzymes in the pathway is briefly described below.

ALA-Synthase

The first enzyme in the pathway is ALA-synthase. This enzyme catalyzes the condensation of glycine, activated by pyridoxal phosphate, and succinyl coenzyme A, to form ALA. ALA-synthase is the rate-limiting enzyme for the pathway, at least in the liver, where it also is inducible by a variety of drugs, steroids and other chemicals (e.g. Granick 1966). Recently, distinct erythroid and non-erythroid (i.e. hepatic) forms of ALA-synthase, encoded by separate genes, have been identified in the chicken (Yamamoto et al 1985, Riddle et al 1989). Should future studies identify erythroid and non-erythroid forms of human ALA-synthase, this finding would provide a basis for the tissue-specific regulation of this pathway (see below). The full-length cDNA encoding human hepatic ALA-synthase has been cloned and sequenced (Astrin et al 1988, Bowden et al 1987). The human hepatic ALA-synthase gene has been assigned to the chromosomal region 3p21 by in situ hybridization techniques (Astrin et al 1988). To date, no disorder has been reported due to the deficiency of ALA-synthase activity. Presumably, a genetic lesion resulting in markedly decreased ALA-synthase activity would not be compatible with life, unless there were different genes encoding the erythroid and non-erythroid enzymes. For example, an X-linked form of sideroblastic anaemia and pyridoxine responsiveness may result from an altered form of ALA-synthase which has a decreased affinity for pyridoxine and an increased sensitivity to a mitochondrial protease (Aoki et al 1979).

ALA-Dehydratase

The second enzymatic reaction in the pathway, catalyzed by ALA-dehydratase, is the condensation of two molecules of ALA to form a cyclic compound, the pyrrole, porphobilinogen (PBG). Purified human ALA-dehydratase is composed of eight identical 31 kDa subunits and eight atoms of zinc (Anderson & Desnick 1979). The zinc atoms are required for both stability and catalytic activity (Jaffe et al 1984). Recently, the full-length cDNA encoding human ALA-dehydratase was isolated (Wetmur et al 1986). Sequence analysis revealed that the zinc atoms are bound to each subunit by a typical zinc finger domain consisting of four cysteine and two histidine residues. The zinc atoms protect essential sulph-hydryl groups of the enzyme and can be displaced by lead and other heavy metals. In fact, the measurement of erythrocyte ALA-dehydratase activity is used as a highly sensitive index of lead exposure (Morgan & Burch 1972). The gene for human ALA-dehydratase has been assigned by in situ hybridization to the chromosomal region 9q34 (Potluri et al 1987). There are two common alleles at the ALA-dehydratase locus, ALAD-1 and ALAD-2, which are responsible for the occurrence of three electrophoretically distinguishable ALA-dehydratase forms, designated 1–1, 1–2, and 2–2 (Battistuzzi et al 1981, Astrin et al 1987). The frequency of the three erythrocyte ALA-dehydratase phenotypes in Caucasian populations is 1–1, ~80%; 1–2, ~18% and 2–2, ~1%, giving gene frequencies of 0.9 and 0.1 for the ALAD-1 and ALAD-2 alleles, respectively. In Hispanics and American Blacks, the gene frequency of the ALAD-2 allele is lower (Astrin et al 1987), and in a Liberian population the ALAD-2 allele was not detected (Benkmann et al 1983). It has been hypothesized that the occurrence of this common polymorphism in the Caucasian population may be associated with a susceptibility to lead poisoning (Astrin et al 1987). A recessively inherited hepatic porphyria due to deficient ALA-dehydratase activity has been described recently (Doss et al 1980, Thunnel et al 1987).

Table 98.2 Chromosomal localization of the haem biosynthetic genes

Structural gene	Chromosomal assignment	Method*	Reference
ALA-synthase (hepatic)	3p21	cDNA	Astrin et al 1988
ALA-dehydratase	9q34	cDNA	Potluri et al 1987
HMB-synthase	11q23qter	SCH	Wang et al 1981
URO-decarboxylase	1p34	cDNA	Romeo et al 1986a
COPRO-oxidase	9	SCH	Granchamp et al 1983

* cDNA = In situ hybridization with cDNA probe; SCH = analysis of somatic cell hybrids.

Hydroxymethylbilane synthase

As shown in Figure 98.1, the formation of uroporphyrinogen III from four molecules of PBG occurs by a two-step process catalyzed by the third and fourth enzymes in the pathway, hydroxymethylbilane synthase (HMB-synthase, formerly known as PBG-deaminase or uroporphyrinogen I synthase) and uroporphyrinogen III synthase (URO-synthase). HMB-synthase catalyzes the head to tail condensation of four PBG molecules by a series of deaminations to form the linear tetrapyrrole, hydroxymethylbilane (HMB). HMB can slowly cyclize nonenzymatically to form uroporphyrinogen I. Because HMB-synthase activity is almost as low as ALA-synthase activity in most normal tissues, it may become rate-limiting when the enzyme is partially deficient or when there is an excess supply of PBG. The half-normal level of HMB-synthase is the enzymatic defect in acute intermittent porphyria (AIP) (Strand et al 1970).

HMB-synthase, purified from human erythrocytes, has been separated into multiple forms (designated A, B, C, D and E) by DEAE-cellulose chromatography or SDS-polyacrylamide gel electrophoresis (Anderson & Desnick 1980). These represent the native enzyme (A) and enzyme-substrate complexes of the mono- (B), di- (C), tri- (D), and tetrapyrrole (E) intermediates. Two tissue-specific isozymes of HMB-synthase are produced by a single gene which has been mapped to the chromosomal region 11q23→qter by the use of somatic cell hybrids (Wang et al 1981). Both forms are monomeric proteins; the erythroid-specific form is approximately 38 kDa, while the non-erythroid form is approximately 40 kDa (Grandchamp et al 1987). The human cDNAs encoding the erythroid and non-erythroid forms have been cloned and sequenced (Raich et al 1986, Grandchamp et al 1987). Subsequent characterization showed that the chromosomal gene for HMB-synthase has 15 exons and that tissue specificity for this enzyme results from alternative splicing of exons 1 and 2. In erythroid cells, the major transcript is transcribed from exons 2–15, with exon 2 containing the erythroid promoter. In non-erythroid cells, the HMB-synthase is encoded by transcript exons 1 and 3–15, with exon 1 containing the non-erythroid promoter. Only in erythroid cells are both transcripts and both enzyme forms present.

Uroporphyrinogen III synthase

Uroporphyrinogen III synthase (URO-synthase or cosynthase) catalyzes the rapid cyclization of HMB and rearranges (by inversion of) the pyrrole D ring just prior to closure of the uroporphyrinogen molecule to form the asymmetrical and physiological type III isomer (Fig. 98.1). In the absence of URO-synthase, HMB non-enzymatically cyclizes to form the uroporphyrinogen I isomer. This non-physiological compound can be metabolized to coproporphyrinogen I, but further metabolism cannot proceed since the next enzyme is stereo-specific for the III isomer. Human URO-synthase has been purified from erythrocytes and its physical and kinetic properties have been characterized (Tsai et al 1987). The enzyme is a monomer with a subunit molecular weight of 29.5 kDa. Recently, the full-length cDNA encoding this enzyme has been cloned and sequenced, and large amounts of the enzyme have been produced by expression of the cDNA in E. coli (Tsai et al 1988). To date, the chromosomal location of the URO-synthase gene has not been determined. HMB-synthase and URO-synthase are both cytosolic enzymes and may exist as an enzyme complex, possibly in association with the other two cytosolic enzymes of the pathway (Tsai et al 1988). URO-synthase activity is markedly deficient, but not absent, in congenital erythropoietic porphyria (CEP) (Romeo & Levin 1969).

Uroporphyrinogen decarboxylase

Uroporphyrinogen III is an octacarboxylate porphyrinogen, and compared to other uroporphyrinogen isomers is the preferred substrate for uroporphyrinogen decarboxylase (URO-decarboxylase), the fifth enzyme in the pathway. This cytosolic enzyme catalyzes the sequential removal of the four carboxyl groups from the acetic acid side chains of uroporphyrinogen III (clockwise, starting with ring D) to form the four methyl groups of coproporphyrinogen III, a tetracarboxylate porphyrinogen. URO-decarboxylase, purified from human erythrocytes, is a monomeric protein with a molecular weight of 42 kDa (de Verneuil et al 1983). This enzyme catalyzes all four decarboxylations. The full-length cDNA for the human enzyme has been isolated and sequenced (Romeo et al 1986a). The chromosomal gene, encoding URO-decarboxylase, which is ~3 kb in length and contains 10 exons (Romana et al 1987), has been regionally localized to chromosome 1p34 by in situ hybridization techniques (Romeo et al 1986b). Recently evidence for two isozymes in human erythrocytes has been presented (Mukerji & Pimstone 1987). Half-normal and near-total deficiencies of this enzymatic activity cause the metabolic defects in porphyria cutanea tarda (PCT) and hepatoerythropoietic porphyria (HEP), respectively (de Verneuil et al 1978, Elder et al 1981).

Coproporphyrinogen oxidase

This mitochondrial enzyme catalyzes the decarboxylation of two of the four propionic acid groups of coproporphyrinogen III (on rings A and B) to form the vinyl groups of protoporphyrinogen IX, a dicarboxylate porphyrinogen. Coproporphyrinogen oxidase (COPRO-oxidase) is functional in mitochondria between the inner and outer membranes (Elder & Evans 1978, Grandchamp et al 1978) and requires molecular oxygen for its activity. A 3-carboxylate porphyrinogen (termed harderoporphyrinogen because the corresponding porphyrin was first isolated from the rodent Harderian gland) is an intermediate in the two-step decarboxylation. Because coproporphyrinogen I, formed by decarboxylation of uroporphyrinogen I, is not a substrate for this enzyme, it is not metabolized to haem. COPRO-oxidase has not been purified from human sources, nor has the human cDNA been isolated. The purified bovine liver enzyme is a monomer with a molecular weight of 71.6 kDa (Yoshinaga & Sano 1980). The locus for the human gene encoding COPRO-oxidase has been assigned to chromosome 9 (Grandchamp et al 1983). The half-normal activity of COPRO-oxidase is the metabolic defect in hereditary coproporphyria (HCP) (Elder et al 1976). The homozygous form of HCP and harderoporphyria result from more severe deficiencies of COPRO-oxidase activity (Grandchamp et al 1977, Nordmann et al 1983).

Protoporphyrinogen oxidase

The seventh enzyme in the pathway, protoporphyrinogen oxidase (PROTO-oxidase), catalyzes the oxidation of protoporphyrinogen IX to protoporphyrin IX by the removal of six hydrogen atoms. The product of the reaction is a porphyrin (oxidized form) in contrast to the preceding several substrates which are porphyrinogens (reduced forms). This oxidation occurs readily under aerobic conditions in vitro in the absence of the enzyme. PROTO-oxidase is an integral protein of the mitochondrial inner membrane (Deybach et al 1985). The enzyme has not been purified from human sources, nor has the cDNA been isolated. The murine enzyme has been purified and shown to be a monomer of 65 kDa (Dailey & Karr 1987) whose activity is inhibited by bilirubin (Ferriera & Dailey 1988). Presumably the human enzyme also is inhibited by bilirubin, accounting for the decreased levels of PROTO-oxidase activity in Gilbert disease (McColl et al 1985a). The half-normal activity of this enzyme is the enzymatic defect in variegate porphyria (VP) (Brenner & Bloomer 1980).

Ferrochelatase

The final step in haem biosynthesis is the insertion of ferrous iron into protoporphyrin IX to form haem. This reaction is catalyzed by ferrochelatase, an enzyme also known as haem-synthetase or protohaem-ferro-lyase. Ferrochelatase is associated with the inner side of the inner mitochondrial membrane (Jones & Jones 1969, McKay et al 1969), is specific for the reduced form of iron (Fe^{2+}), but can utilize other metals (e.g. Zn^{2+} and Co^{2+}) and other 2-carboxylate porphyrins. The human enzyme has not been purified to homogeneity, nor has the cDNA been cloned. However the bovine enzyme has been shown to have a monomeric molecular weight of 40–44 kDa, which aggregates to a 240 kDa form at low salt concentrations (Dailey & Fleming 1986, Bloomer et al 1987). The bovine enzyme first binds iron, then the porphyrin. Iron binding is mediated by two vicinal sulph–hydryl groups. Ferrochelatase activity is half-normal in erythropoietic protoporphyria (EPP) (Bonkowsky et al 1975, Bottomley et al 1975) and is also sensitive to inhibition by lead (Taketani & Tokunaga 1981).

Regulation of haem biosynthesis

In the liver, the haem biosynthetic pathway is under negative feedback control. The concentration of 'free' haem regulates the synthesis and mitochondrial translocation of hepatic ALA-synthase. Haem represses the synthesis of mRNA for ALA-synthase and can also interfere with the transport of a cytosolic form of the enzyme into mitochondria (Hayashi et al 1969, Whiting 1976, Ades et al 1987). ALA-synthase is inducible by many of the same chemicals that induce cytochrome P-450, a family of haemoproteins in the endoplasmic reticulum of the liver and other tissues (Anderson et al 1982). Because most of the haem synthesized in liver is used for the synthesis of cytochrome P-450, the induction of hepatic ALA-synthase and cytochrome P-450 might be expected to occur in a coordinated fashion. When the regulatory 'free' haem pool becomes depleted, which may occur, for example, when more haem is required for synthesis of haemoproteins, the synthesis of ALA-synthase is increased (Sassa & Kappas 1983). Conversely, repression of ALA-synthase synthesis results from augmentation of the regulatory haem pool. The evidence that ALA-synthase functions as a rate-controlling enzyme, at least in the liver, includes its relatively low V_{max} (compared to most other enzymes in the pathway), its inducibility and short half-life, and its great sensitivity to repression by cellular haem (at concentrations $< 10^{-6}$M). Low affinity of the enzyme for glycine suggests that the intracellular glycine concentration also determines the rate of ALA formation.

In erythroid cells, ALA-synthase appears to be less involved in the regulation of the pathway. Studies using cultured erythroleukaemia cells and normal bone marrow cultures suggest that the more distal enzymes, such as HMB-synthase (Beru & Goldwasser 1985) and ferrochelatase, may have major rate-limiting functions during erythroid differentiation and haem formation. Haem regulates the rate of its synthesis in erythroid cells primarily by controlling the transport of iron (required for ferrochelatase) into reticulocytes (Neuwirt & Ponka 1977). The rate of haem synthesis increases during normal or stimulated erythroid differentiation; there is a coordinated increase in the activities of the haem biosynthetic enzymes during this process (Sassa 1976). In erythroid cells, an erythroid form of ALA-synthase may be synthesized by a separate erythroid gene in order to facilitate the continuous production of haem for haemoglobin. The control of haem biosynthesis in tissues other than the liver and erythroid cells has not been the subject of intensive investigation. In all cells, these enzymes make haem for cytochromes and other haemoproteins. However, it is possible that neurons may depend in part on surrounding non-neural cells for haem or haem precursors (Whetsell & Kappas 1981).

CLASSIFICATION AND DIAGNOSIS OF THE INHERITED PORPHYRIAS

Hepatic and erythropoietic porphyrias

The inherited porphyrias have been classified as hepatic or erythropoietic, based on whether the excess production of porphyrin precursors and/or porphyrins takes place primarily in the liver or in the erythron. The rapid onset of neurological symptoms, especially pain, is indicative of the acute hepatic porphyrias. During an acute attack, individuals affected by these porphyrias have markedly elevated urinary concentrations of the porphyrin precursors, ALA and PBG. In contrast, individuals affected with an erythropoietic porphyria have elevated erythrocyte porphyrins which become deposited in the skin and tissues and lead to the cutaneous manifestations (Table 98.3). This classification is useful, but is not rigid. For example, autosomal dominant hepatic porphyrias may have erythropoietic features (i.e. cutaneous manifestations) in homozygous cases.

Diagnosis

For medical management and genetic counselling, it is important to establish which inherited porphyria is present in a given patient. Because many of the symptoms of the various porphyrias are nonspecific and can mimic other more common diseases, diagnosis is often delayed. In addition, incorrect diagnoses of a porphyria in patients with symptoms due to other diseases are not uncommon. When a porphyria is suspected clinically, an initial classification can be based on the symptomatology. The next step involves determination of the levels of the

Table 98.3   The major metabolites accumulated in the human porphyrias

Type/Porphyria	Increased erythrocyte porphyrins	Porphyrin excretion	
		Urine	*Stool*
Hepatic			
ALA-dehydratase deficiency	—	ALA, Copro III	—
Acute intermittent porphyria (AIP)	—	ALA, PBG	—
Hereditary coproporphyria (HCP)	—	ALA, PBG Copro III	Copro III
Variegate porphyria (VP)	—	ALA, PBG Copro III	Copro III Proto IX
Porphyria cutanea tarda (PCT)	—	Uro III, 7-Carboxylate	Isocopro
Erythropoietic			
Congenital erythropoietic porphyria (CEP)	Uro I	Uro I	Copro I
Erythropoietic protoporphyria (EPP)	Proto IX	—	Proto IX

ALA = δ-aminolevulinic acid; PBG = porphobilinogen; Copro I = coproporphyrin I; Copro III = coproporphyrin III; Isocopro = isocoproporphyrin; Uro I = uroporphyrin I; Uro III = uroporphyrin III; Proto = protoporphyrin IX.

porphyrin precursors and porphyrins in the urine and faeces. Tests for porphyria may be difficult to interpret because abnormal porphyrin results can occur in some disorders other than true porphyrias, and minimally elevated levels of porphyrins or their precursors may have little or no diagnostic significance.

Intermediates that accumulate in excess in the porphyrias may be excreted unchanged or undergo chemical modifications prior to excretion. ALA and PBG are colourless and non-fluorescent compounds. Porphyrinogens are also colourless and non-fluorescent and are subject to autoxidation to the corresponding porphyrins outside the cell. Porphyrins are reddish in colour and fluoresce when exposed to long-wave ultraviolet light. Excess ALA, PBG, uroporphyrin I and III and 7-, 6-, and 5-carboxylate porphyrins are excreted mostly in the urine. Porphyrins with fewer carboxylate groups are progressively less water soluble. Coproporphyrins are excreted partly in urine and partly in bile, whereas harderoporphyrin and protoporphyrin are excreted almost entirely in the bile and faeces. There is evidence that coproporphyrin I is more readily excreted in bile than is coproporphyrin III, which may explain the increase in the ratio of these isomers that occurs when hepatobiliary function is impaired (Kaplowitz et al 1972).

Urinary ALA and PBG are easily quantitated by chemical methods (e.g. Mauzerall & Granick 1956) and the urinary porphyrin isomers can be separated and quantitated by high performance liquid chromatograpy (e.g. Lim & Peters 1984). Faecal porphyrins can be extracted and semi-quantitatively analyzed by thin layer chromatography. These studies, if carried out properly, especially in the presence of symptomatology, should identify a specific profile of accumulated precursors and/or porphyrins. However, the definitive diagnosis of a particular porphyria requires the demonstration of the specific enzymatic defect. Assays are available for each of the eight haem biosynthetic enzymes using erythrocytes, lymphocytes, cultured lymphoblasts or cultured fibroblasts (Bishop & Desnick 1982).

INBORN ERRORS OF HAEM BIOSYNTHESIS

ALA-Dehydratase deficient porphyria

Clinical manifestations

This hepatic porphyria is the most recently described. The disease is inherited as an autosomal recessive trait. To date, only three unrelated males in Europe have been recognized. The affected homozygotes have less than 5% of normal activity in their erythrocytes whereas their parents have about half-normal levels of activity. Two of the three reported patients were unrelated German males who had onset of symptoms during adolescence. Their major clinical manifestations resembled those of AIP, including abdominal pain and neuropathy. In contrast the third patient, a Swedish infant, had more severe disease characterized by failure to thrive. Presumably, the earlier age of onset in the Swedish patient and markedly more severe manifestations reflect a more significant deficiency of ALA-dehydratase activity.

Biochemical findings

All three affected individuals had markedly increased urinary excretion of ALA and coproporphyrin III. ALA-dehydratase activity was present, but markedly reduced in erythrocytes (< 5% of normal). The enzyme activity was not restored to normal by the in vitro addition of sulph–hydryl reagents such as dithiothreitol. Immunological studies in each of the three reported cases revealed the presence of non-functional enzyme proteins that cross-reacted with anti-ALA-dehydratase antibodies (de Verneuil et al 1985, Fujita et al 1987a). Differences in size or charge of the mutant enzymes were not detected (de Verneuil et al 1985). The presence of cross-reactive immunological material (CRIM), indicated that the mutant genes were transcribed and translated, but that the resultant CRIM-positive proteins had markedly altered catalytic properties and somewhat decreased stabilities.

It should be noted that both lead and succinylacetone (which is structurally similar to ALA and accumulates in hereditary tyrosinaemia) inhibit ALA-dehydratase, causing increased urinary excretion of ALA and ALA-mediated clinical manifestations (Anderson et al 1977, Lindblad et al 1977, Sassa & Kappas 1983). Therefore, lead intoxication and hereditary tyrosinaemia (fumarylacetoacetase deficiency) should be considered in the differential diagnosis of ALA-dehydratase deficient porphyria.

Genetics

ALA-dehydratase deficient porphyria is inherited as an autosomal recessive trait. The frequency of this recently recognized disorder is unknown. Onset and severity of the disease is variable, presumably depending on the amount of residual ALA-dehydratase activity. Heterozygotes are clinically asymptomatic, do not excrete increased levels of ALA and can be detected by demonstration of intermediate levels of erythrocyte ALA-dehydratase activity. To date, the prenatal diagnosis of this disorder has not been made, but should be possible by determination of the ALA-dehydratase activity in cultured chorionic villi or amniocytes.

Acute intermittent porphyria

AIP is an autosomal dominant ecogenetic condition resulting from half-normal levels of HMB-synthase activity. Although the enzyme deficiency can be demonstrated in most individuals who inherit a mutant allele, clinical expression of this hepatic porphyria is highly variable. Activation of the disease is clearly related to ecogenic factors which can precipitate the disease manifestations. Symptomatic patients always have increased urinary excretion of the porphyrin precursors ALA and PBG. However, the great majority of heterozygotes with HMB-synthase deficiency remain clinically asymptomatic ('latent') and may never have increased urinary excretion of ALA and PBG.

Clinical manifestations

The neurovisceral and circulatory disturbances that characterize this disease may result from the effects of ALA and/or PBG toxicity on the nervous system, although this mechanism has not been proven. Symptoms, which rarely occur before puberty, are often nonspecific and a high index of suspicion is needed to suggest the proper diagnosis. The disease can be disabling but is only occasionally fatal. Abdominal pain, the most common symptom, is usually steady and poorly localized, but may be cramping. Signs of ileus, including abdominal distention and decreased bowels sounds are common. However, increased bowel sounds and diarrhoea may occur. The abdominal manifestations are neurological rather than inflammatory, so tenderness, fever and leucocytosis are generally absent or mild. Other manifestations include nausea, vomiting, constipation, tachycardia, hypertension, mental symptoms, pain in the limbs, head, neck or chest, muscle weakness and sensory loss. Tachycardia, hypertension, restlessness, fine tremors, and excess sweating may be due to sympathetic overactivity. Dysuria and bladder dysfunction may occur and urinary retention may require catheterization.

Peripheral neuropathy in AIP is primarily motor and appears to result from axonal degeneration rather than demyelinization (Cavanagh & Mellick 1965, Sweeney et al 1970, Ridley 1975). Fortunately, significant neuropathy does not develop in all patients with acute attacks, even when abdominal symptoms are severe. Weakness most commonly begins in the proximal muscles, and more often in the arms than in the legs. The course and degree of involvement are variable. Tendon reflexes may be little affected or hyperactive in early stages, but are usually decreased or absent with advanced neuropathy. Paresis can be asymmetrical and focal. Cranial nerves, most commonly the tenth and seventh, can be affected. Rarely, involvement of the optic nerves or occipital lobes may produce blindness. There may be sensory involvement with areas of paraesthesia and loss of sensation. Muscle weakness can progress to respiratory and bulbar paralysis and death. This seldom occurs unless the porphyria is not recognized, harmful drugs not discontinued, and appropriate treatment not instituted. Sudden death, presumably due to cardiac arrhythmia, may also occur. Even advanced neuropathy is potentially reversible.

The central nervous system also may be involved. Anxiety, insomnia, depression, disorientation, hallucinations and paranoia, which can be especially severe during acute attacks, may suggest a primary mental disorder. Some patients have been mistakenly regarded as hysterical. Depression and other mental symptoms may be chronic in AIP patients. Surveys of psychiatric patients suggest that the disease is often unrecognized in such individuals (Tishler et al 1985). Seizures may occur as part of the acute neurological manifestations of AIP, as a result of hyponatraemia, or due to causes unrelated to porphyria. Treatment of seizures is problematical because virtually all anti-seizure drugs (except bromides) have at least some potential for exacerbating AIP (clonazepam may be less likely to do so than phenytoin or barbiturates). Hyponatraemia may be due to inappropriate ADH secretion, or may result from vomiting, diarrhoea and poor intake, or from excess renal sodium loss. AIP may also predispose to chronic hypertension and may be associated with impairment of renal function. An acute attack may resolve quite rapidly, with abdominal pain disappearing within a few hours, and paresis within a few days. After a severe attack, motor function and mental health may continue to improve for several years, but may leave some residual weakness.

Precipitating factors

Most of the factors known to precipitate acute porphyric attacks have the potential to induce the synthesis of hepatic ALA-synthase, thereby increasing the levels of ALA, PBG, the other haem pathway intermediates and haem. Normally the amount of HMB-synthase, particularly in the liver, is low, but sufficient to avoid any accumulation of PBG when influenced by environmental, metabolic and hormonal factors which can increase the flux of ALA, PBG and porphyrinogens through the pathway. However, AIP heterozygotes with only 50% of normal activity are functioning at a level of enzyme that is insufficient to metabolize the increased levels of PBG that result from the influence of these precipitating factors. More than one factor may contribute simultaneously to the biochemical alterations which cause the clinical expression of the disease.

Endogenous steroid hormones are probably the most important precipitating factors. This is indicated by a number of clinical features of the disease, including: (1) the rarity of symptoms and excess porphyrin precursor excretion before puberty; (2) more frequent clinical expression in women than in men; (3) premenstrual attacks of the disease in some women and their prevention by the administration of LHRH analogues (Anderson et al 1986); (4) exacerbation of AIP due to exogenous steroids including oral contraceptive preparations; and (5) the presence of more subtle abnormalities in steroid hormone metabolism, such as a deficiency of hepatic steroid 5α-reductase activity which can predispose to the excess production of steroid hormone metabolites that are inducers of ALA-synthase in the liver.

Attacks of porphyria can occur during pregnancy. However, pregnancy is usually well tolerated (Milo et al 1989). Earlier reports of worsening symptoms during pregnancy may have been due to the use of barbiturates and perhaps reduced caloric intake. Thus, clinical experience and experimental data indicate that pregnancy is not contraindicated in AIP if harmful drugs are avoided and if attention is given to proper nutrition.

Drugs are important causes of AIP attacks. Many patients with AIP do well because they avoid harmful drugs. Most porphyrinogenic drugs induce ALA-synthase and haem synthesis in the liver. Induction of ALA-synthase is closely associated with induction of cytochrome P-450, a process which increases the demand for haem synthesis in the liver. Some drugs can also increase haem turnover by promoting the destruction of cytochrome P-450, at least in experimental systems (Marks 1985). An attack following ingestion of a harmful drug in an HMB-synthase-deficient heterozygote may not be due to the drug alone. Rather, it is likely that other predisposing factors such as endogenous hormones and nutritional factors also play a role. Drugs are only rarely reported to cause acute symptoms in children with HMB-synthase deficiency. A large retrospective study of risk from anaesthetic use in AIP concluded that barbiturates or other inducing drugs are quite frequently detrimental in patients who already have porphyric symptoms but seldom exacerbate latent disease (Mustajoki & Heinonen 1980). HMB-synthase deficient heterozygotes who require long-term anticonvulsants for epilepsy do not always suffer exacerbations of porphyria. However, it is recommended that exposure to porphyrinogenic drugs be avoided in all HMB-synthase-deficient heterozygotes, including children. The major drugs known or strongly suspected by most observers to be harmful in AIP, HCP or VP, as well as drugs that are known to be safe are listed in Table 98.4. Other reviews and more extensive lists of drugs that are harmful, safe, or in intermediate categories, are available (Kappas et al 1983, Moore et al 1987). The choice of anaesthetic agents also has been studied in animal models and reviewed (Blekkenhorst et al 1980, Mustajoki & Heinonen 1980).

Clinical experience suggests that a low caloric intake, usually instituted in an effort to lose weight, is a common contributing cause of acute attacks. Caloric or carbohydrate restriction can precipitate acute symptoms of AIP and increase porphyrin precursor excretion. Therefore, even brief periods of starvation during weight reduction, postoperative periods, or with intercurrent illnesses should be avoided in patients with this disease. It has also been found that the administration of intravenous glucose (at least 300 g per 24 hours) is effective in treating acute attacks of AIP.

Attacks of porphyria can also be provoked by intercurrent infections and other illnesses, and by major surgery. The mechanisms are not understood, but may involve metabolic stress, impaired nutrition, and the increased

Table 98.4 Categories of safe and unsafe drugs in AIP, HCP and VP

Unsafe	Safe
Barbiturates	Narcotic analgesics
Sulphonamide antibiotics	Aspirin
Meprobamate	Acetaminophen
Glutethimide	Phenothiazines
Methyprylon	Penicillin and derivatives
Ethchlorvynol	Streptomycin
Mephenytoin	Glucocorticoids
Succinimides	Bromides
Carbamazepine	Insulin
Valproic Acid	Atropine
Pyrazolones	
Griseofulvin	
Ergots	
Synthetic oestrogens and progestins	
Danazol	
Alcohol	

production of steroid hormones and their ALA-synthase-inducing metabolites.

Biochemical findings

Urinary excretion of porphyrin precursors is markedly increased during acute attacks of AIP, with PBG excretion generally ranging from approximately 50–200 mg/24 h. Excretion of ALA is usually about half that of PBG. If monitored, increased ALA and PBG excretion can often be demonstrated in an AIP heterozygote for some time before an attack. It is useful to follow ALA and PBG excretion in a symptomatic patient because the concentrations of these compounds generally decrease with clinical improvement. Such decreases are particularly dramatic after haematin infusions. A normal result of a quantitative test for urinary PBG virtually excludes hepatic porphyria as a cause for the acute symptoms. After AIP has become clinically expressed, it is distinctly unusual for excretion of these precursors to decrease to normal levels, unless the disease becomes clinically latent for a prolonged period. Since ALA and PBG are colourless, the reddish urine in AIP is due to increased porphyrins. Brownish discolouration may be due to porphobilin, a degradation product of PBG, or dipyrrylmethenes. Faecal porphyrins are usually normal or minimally increased in AIP, which can help to distinguish this disorder from HCP and VP. HMB-synthase should be measured in erythrocytes to confirm a diagnosis of AIP, and family members should be tested in order to identify other AIP heterozygotes (Pierach et al 1987).

Nature of the enzymatic defect

The metabolic defect in AIP results from the half-normal activity of HMB-synthase. The nature of the defective enzymatic activity has been the focus of recent biochemical and immunological studies. Four major classes of mutation have been identified demonstrating the occurrence of genetic heterogeneity at the HMB-synthase locus (Desnick et al 1985). The majority of AIP heterozygotes had no cross-reactive immunological material (CRIM) produced by the mutant allele (designated CRIM-negative type I). The possible molecular lesions responsible for CRIM-negative mutations include complete or partial gene deletions as well as point mutations or insertions that alter the processing or stability of the mRNA, create chain terminating codons, or appreciably alter the conformation or stability of the mutant protein. The CRIM-negative type I mutations are probably heterogeneous at the molecular level. A much less common CRIM-negative mutation (designated CRIM-negative type II) results in a deficient enzyme in non-erythroid tissues, but normal enzymatic activity in erythrocytes. This variant form of AIP was first well described in Finland (Mustajoki & Tenhunen 1985). Subsequent molecular studies have shown that the molecular lesion in a CRIM-negative type II family of Dutch ancestry was a point mutation in the canonical 5' splice donor site of intron 1 which caused abnormal splicing of the HMB-synthase transcript (Grandchamp et al 1989). This tissue-specific splicing mutation provides an explanation for the deficient activity in the liver and other non-erythroid tissues and normal levels of activity in erythrocytes. Two types of CRIM-positive mutation (designated Types 1 and 2) have been characterized (Anderson et al 1981, Desnick et al 1985). In both types of mutation, the mutant alleles were expressed, but the enzyme proteins had altered kinetic and/or stability properties. Presumably the CRIM-positive mutations result from single base substitutions in the coding region of the HMB-synthase gene.

Pathophysiology

A number of hypotheses have been proposed to explain neural damage in AIP and related disorders, but none has been satisfactorily substantiated (Bonkowsky & Schady 1982, Yeung Liawah et al 1987). The possibility that ALA or PBG might be neurotoxic is favoured by the increased production of these precursors during acute porphyric attacks (Becker & Kramer 1977). ALA is taken up by most tissues more readily than is PBG, and is then further metabolized, whereas PBG appears to cross the blood-brain barrier more readily (Bonkowsky et al 1971). These intermediates may be converted in vivo to other substances which may have neurotoxic potential. AIP, HCP, VP, ALA-D deficient porphyria, plumbism and hereditary tyrosinaemia are all associated with increased ALA and similar neurological manifestations, which favours a neuropathic role for ALA. ALA is structurally analogous to gamma-aminobutyric acid (GABA) and can interact with GABA receptors. Experimental observations of these and other effects of ALA on neurological function are reviewed in more detail elsewhere (Moore et al 1977, Kappas et al 1983, Litman & Correia 1985).

Genetics

AIP is inherited as an autosomal dominant trait and is an excellent example of an ecogenic disorder since its expression is usually precipitated by hormonal, metabolic, dietary or environmental factors (see above). The disease is panethnic, but is probably most common in Scandinavia, Britain and Ireland (Wetterberg 1967). One severely affected child may have been a homozygous case of AIP (Gregor et al 1977, Kordac et al 1985). The gene encoding HMB-synthase has been localized to 11q23→qter (Wang et al 1985). Molecular cloning revealed the presence of two cDNAs for HMB-synthase, one encoding the non-erythroid form, the other erythroid specific (Raich et al 1986, Grandchamp et al 1987). The occurrence of erythroid and non-erythroid forms was suggested initially by biochemical studies (Grandchamp et al 1987). Subsequent isolation and characterization of the chromosomal gene revealed that two transcripts were encoded by a single gene, which had two promoters, one responsible for the expression of the 'housekeeping' and the other for the erythroid-specific transcript (Chretien et al 1988). The enzymatic diagnosis of family members whose HMB-synthase activity is inconclusive can be confirmed by RFLP studies in informative families using three polymorphic sites in the HMB-synthase gene (Llewellyn et al 1987, Lee et al 1988). It is likely that other informative RFLPs in or flanking the gene will be identified to permit more accurate heterozygote diagnosis. The prenatal diagnosis of an affected heterozygous fetus has been made (Sassa et al 1975).

Treatment

Acute attacks usually require hospitalization for treatment of severe pain, nausea and vomiting, and for administration of intravenous glucose, and haematin. Hospitalization also facilitates close monitoring of nutritional status, investigation of the precipitating cause or causes of an attack, and observation for neurological complications and electrolyte imbalances. Efforts should be directed to identifying and removing the inciting factors. Narcotic analgesics are usually required for abdominal pain. Nausea, vomiting, anxiety, restlessness, and other intestinal symptoms generally respond well to chlorpromazine or other phenothiazines. Large doses of phenothiazines are usually not required and may produce unpleasant side-effects in AIP patients. Chloral hydrate can be employed for insomnia and diazepam in low doses is probably safe if a minor tranquilizer is required.

Although treatment with intravenous glucose (at least 300 g per 24 hours) has been recommended for patients hospitalized with attacks of porphyria (Tschudy & Lamon 1980), a more complete nutritional regimen including intravenous vitamins, lipids, and amino acids might be beneficial, particularly if oral feeding is not possible for a prolonged period. However, the safety and efficacy of parenteral nutrition regimens in AIP patients have not been studied. Haematin given by intravenous infusion is more effective than glucose in reducing porphyrin precursor excretion (Bonkowsky et al 1971, Yeung Laiwah & McColl 1987); however, severe neurological damage and subacute or chronic symptoms are unlikely to respond (Lamon et al 1979, Bissell 1988). Although the recommended dose is 4 mg/kg body weight infused intravenously once or twice in 24 hours, lower dose regimens (e.g. 1–1.5 mg/kg once in 24 hours) may be equally effective (Bissell 1988). The pharmacokinetics of the drug and the duration of response of porphyrin precursor excretion (Petryka et al 1976) suggest that treatment once in 24 hours should be effective. Haem arginate has been reported not to produce phlebitis or an anticoagulant effect and is more stable than haematin (Tokola et al 1986). Similar advantages have been described with use of an albumin-bound lyophilized haematin preparation (Fuchs & Ippen 1987). Diagnosis is more difficult during, and for several days after, haematin administration because of the capacity of this treatment to normalize porphyrin precursor excretion. A clinical response to haematin is dependent upon the degree of neuronal damage, and may not be observed for at least 48 hours.

Administration of LHRH analogues is clearly effective for women with frequent premenstrual attacks of porphyria (Anderson et al 1986). Some improvement may occur in women with attacks only partly due to cyclical hormone changes. Continuing experience indicates that women who respond to LHRH analogue administration are unlikely to require this treatment for a major portion of their reproductive years, and after several years may no longer require ovulatory suppression.

Congenital erythropoietic porphyria

This erythropoietic porphyria, also known as Gunther disease, is due to the markedly deficient activity of URO-synthase. The accumulated uroporphyrinogen I is oxidized to uroporphyrin I, which is deposited in the tissues and fluids of individuals affected with this autosomal recessive trait.

Clinical manifestations

Severe cutaneous photosensitivity begins in early infancy and is manifested by increased friability and blistering of the epidermis on the hands and face and other sun-exposed areas. Bullae and vesicles contain serous fluid and are prone to rupture and infection. The skin may be thickened, with areas of hypo- and hyper-pigmentation. Hypertrichosis of the face and extremities is often prominent. Sunlight, other sources of ultraviolet light and minor skin trauma are the major environmental factors which increase the severity of the cutaneous manifestations. Recurrent vesicles and secondary infection can lead to cutaneous scarring and deformities, as well as loss of digits and facial features such as the eyelids, nose and ears. Corneal scarring can lead to blindness. Porphyrins deposited in the teeth produce a reddish-brown colour in natural light, termed erythrodontia. The teeth may fluoresce on exposure to long-wave ultraviolet light. Porphyrin deposition in bone also occurs. Bone demineralization has been described (Piomelli et al 1986).

Haemolysis is a feature of the disease and the more severely affected homozygotes may be transfusion dependent. Anaemia due to haemolysis can be severe, but may be minimal or absent if compensation by the bone marrow is adequate. Splenomegaly is found in most cases. Affected individuals who are not transfusion dependent typically have a milder form of the disease. Later onset adult patients have been described and represent about a third of all CEP patients. Life expectancy may be shortened by infection or haematological complications.

Haemolysis in CEP is often accompanied by anisocytosis, poikilocytosis, polychromasia, basophilic stippling, reticulocytosis, increased nucleated red cells, absent haptoglobin, increased unconjugated bilirubin, increased faecal urobilinogen and increased plasma iron turnover. Haemolysis probably results from the accumulated uroporphyrinogen I in erythrocytes and secondary splenomegaly develops in response to the increased uptake of abnormal erythrocytes from the circulation. Splenic enlargement may contribute to the anaemia and also result in leucopenia and thrombocytopenia. The latter is sometimes associated with significant bleeding (Pain et al 1975, Weston et al 1978) and splenectomy may be beneficial in such cases.

Thus a number of factors lead to the phenotypic variability in CEP. These include: (1) the amount of residual URO-synthase activity; (2) the resultant degree of haemolysis and consequent stimulation of erythropoiesis; and (3) exposure to ultraviolet light. Therefore, as in other porphyrias, an interplay of environmental factors with the deficient enzyme activity determine clinical expression of this disease.

Biochemical findings

Uroporphyrin I accumulation in the bone marrow, erythrocytes, plasma, urine and faeces, is the biochemical hallmark of the disease. Reddish coloured urine is noted shortly after birth. Urinary porphyrins are primarily uroporphyrin I and coproporphyrin I, with excess excretion of the intermediate 7-, 6-, and 5-carboxylate porphyrins as well. There is a great predominance of the type I isomers, although the type III isomers are also in excess. Urinary excretion of ALA and PBG is not increased. Faecal porphyrins are markedly increased with a predominance of coproporphyrin I. In contrast, the urine porphyrins in EPP are normal. In addition, hepatoerythropoietic porphyria (HEP), which has recently been shown to be a distinct disease from CEP and represents the homozygous form of familial PCT, is distinguishable from CEP by high levels of isocoproporphyrin in faeces and urine, and decreased URO-decarboxylase activity in erythrocytes. Very rare homozygous forms of VP and HCP may also be characterized by photosensitivity in childhood and increased erythrocyte porphyrins.

Affected homozygotes and asymptomatic heterozygotes for CEP can be detected by assaying URO-synthase in erythocytes, cultured lymphoblasts or cultured fibroblasts (Tsai et al 1987). Affected fetuses can be detected in utero by measuring porphyrins in amniotic fluid (Kaiser 1980) and the URO-synthase activity in cultured amniotic fluid cells (Deybach et al 1980). It is notable that URO-synthase activity is not totally deficient in homozygotes, since the enzyme must produce sufficient uroporphyrinogen III formation for the production of haem.

Genetics

The deficient activity of URO-synthase is the enzymatic defect in CEP (Romeo & Levin 1969, Deybach et al 1981, Tsai et al 1987). Although the chromosomal localization of the gene for human URO-synthase has not

been determined, the full length cDNA encoding the human enzyme has been cloned, sequenced and expressed in large quantities in E.coli (Tsai et al 1988). Thus efforts to identify the specific gene defects in unrelated patients with URO-synthase deficiency are now possible. Occurrence and expression of the disease is the same in males and females. To date about 100 cases have been reported.

Treatment

For homozygotes with severe manifestations, blood transfusions given in sufficient amounts to significantly suppress erythropoiesis appear to be the most effective form of treatment. For example, Piomelli et al (1986) described a case in which frequent transfusions designed to maintain the haematocrit above 32% completely suppressed the symptoms of CEP. Deferoxamine administration in conjunction with the transfusion regimen reduced iron overload to some degree, and splenectomy substantially reduced the transfusion requirements in that patient (Piomelli et al 1986). More recently, oral charcoal has been reported to be effective in depleting the accumulated uroporphyrin I (Pimstone et al 1987). This approach may be useful for patients who are not transfusion dependent and have milder disease. For all CEP homozygotes, protection of the skin from sunlight and minor trauma is highly important. Sunscreen lotions may be helpful. β-carotene may be of some value in CEP (Mathews-Roth 1979) and is unlikely to be harmful. Prompt treatment of bacterial infections which commonly complicate cutaneous blisters may help in preventing scarring and mutilation. Hospitalization for treatment of cellulitis, bacteraemia, and other severe infections with systemic antibiotics is sometimes required.

Porphyria cutanea tarda

Among the porphyrias, PCT is unique, since this cutaneous phenotype occurs in both sporadic (type I) and familial (type II) forms. In type I PCT, URO-decarboxylase activity is normal in erythrocytes, but is decreased in the liver. In type II PCT, the half-normal enzymatic activity is present systemically, consistent with its autosomal dominant transmission. The homozygous form of familial PCT is termed hepatoerythropoietic porphyria (HEP). In addition, the hepatic deficiency of this enzyme and a biochemical pattern resembling familial PCT can be produced by certain halogenated aromatic hydrocarbons. The most notable cause of environmentally-induced type I PCT was an outbreak in Turkey due to ingestion of wheat treated with the fungicide hexachlorobenzene.

Clinical manifestations

Cutaneous photosensitivity is the major clinical feature of both type I and type II PCT. Neurological manifestations are not observed. Skin lesions develop on sun-exposed areas such as the face, dorsa of the hands and feet, forearms, and legs. Fluid-filled vesicles and bullae are more common in the summer than in the winter. Sun-exposed skin becomes friable and minor trauma may precede the formation of bullae or may cause denudation of the skin. Small white plaques, termed 'milia', are also common and may precede or follow vesicle formation. Bullae and denuded areas of skin tend to heal slowly. Lesions can become infected, especially when severe and recurrent. Other cutaneous manifestations include hypertrichosis and hyperpigmentation, especially of the face, that can present in the absence of vesicles. Thickening, scarring and calcification of affected areas of skin is sometimes striking and has been termed 'pseudo-scleroderma' because it can mimic the cutaneous changes of systemic sclerosis. The skin lesions in PCT are generally indistinguishable from those in VP and HCP. The lesions of CEP are also similar but more severe.

Patients with PCT often have a history of alcohol abuse. A number of associated factors clearly contribute to the pathogenesis of PCT but do not themselves produce the disease. In addition to alcohol, liver damage, excess iron and the intake of oestrogens are the most important of these contributing factors. While liver histopathology is almost always evident, it is usually not diagnostic of alcoholic liver disease. PCT can also be induced by exposure to various chemicals. An extensive outbreak of 'PCT' occurred in eastern Turkey in 1955–1958 due to the ingestion of wheat treated with the fungicide hexachlorobenzene (Schmid 1960). Subsequently, hexachlorobenzene was shown to produce a porphyria similar to PCT and hepatic URO-decarboxylase deficiency in animals (Taljaard et al 1972). Cases of PCT in humans have been reported after exposure to other chemicals including di- and trichlorophenols and 2, 3, 7, 8-tetrachlorodibenzo-(p)-dioxin (TCDD), dioxin) (Lynch et al 1975, Doss et al 1984). Rarely, PCT is associated with chronic haemodialysis for end-stage renal disease (Praga et al 1987). Iron overload is common in haemodialysis patients and is likely to be a major contributing factor in those who develop PCT.

Patients with PCT are at risk to develop hepatocellular carcinoma. In several series, the incidence has ranged from 4–47% (Kordac 1972, Cortes et al 1980, Salata et al 1985). These tumours are apparently a complication of PCT and do not themselves contain or produce porphyrins in large amounts (Cortes et al 1980). Their cause is unknown but could relate to long-standing liver damage in PCT, haemosiderosis, exposure to halogenated chemicals that are also carcinogenic, or to the effects of porphyrin deposition in the liver.

Hepatoerythropoietic porphyria (HEP), the homozygous form of familial PCT (Elder et al 1981), is a rare condition that resembles CEP. Clinically, the disease presents with onset of blistering skin lesions, hypertrichosis, scarring and red urine in infancy or childhood. The disease is genetically heterogeneous and unusually mild cases have been described (Fujita et al 1987b, Toback et al 1987).

Biochemical findings

In patients with either type I or type II PCT, porphyrins are increased in the liver, plasma, urine and stool. Except for a slight increase in ALA in some patients, porphyrin precursor excretion is normal. Urinary porphyrins consist mostly of uroporphyrin and 7-carboxylate porphyrin, with lesser amounts of coproporphyrin, and 5- and 6-carboxylate porphyrins (Elder 1977). The excess urinary uroporphyrin in PCT is predominantly isomer I; 7- and 6-carboxylate porphyrins are mostly isomer III; 5-carboxylate porphyrin and coproporphyrin are approximately equal mixtures of isomers I and III.

The major faecal porphyrins in PCT are often of the isocoproporphyrin series. Plasma porphyrins also are increased in PCT (Moore et al 1973); the distribution pattern is similar to that in urine. Isocoproporphyrin may be present in plasma and urine (Day et al 1979). Levels of porphyrin in the skin are increased. The highest concentrations occur in areas which have not been exposed to light, suggesting that light destroys porphyrins in the skin (Malina et al 1978). Increased liver porphyrins are composed mostly of uroporphyrin and 7-carboxylate porphyrin.

The biochemical findings in HEP (homozygous familial PCT) are similar to those in PCT. In addition, the erythrocyte protoporphyrin concentration is increased.

Genetics

The deficient activity of URO-decarboxylase in type II PCT is inherited as an autosomal dominant trait. Enzymatic activity in liver, erythrocytes and cultured skin fibroblasts is approximately 50% of normal in clinically affected and latent family members (de Verneuil et al 1978). Immunoreactive enzyme is reduced by approximately 50% in familial PCT (Elder et al 1983).

Thus, most cases of familial PCT are CRIM-negative, since the mutant allele does not express detectable enzyme protein. HEP is the homozygous form of familial PCT (Elder et al 1981). In 16 reported cases of HEP, URO-decarboxylase activity has been found to be 3–28% of normal (Fujita et al 1987a). Kinetic and immunochemical studies of the enzyme from unrelated patients with HEP revealed most to have markedly reduced enzyme activity and immunoreactive enzyme protein; both reduced to below 7% of normal (de Verneuil et al 1984). In a milder case of HEP, the enzyme activity was reduced to 16% (Fujita et al 1987b). Heterozygotes for HEP may be symptomatic.

In a study of the members of several unrelated type II PCT families, no major deletions, rearrangements or RFLPs were detected at the URO-decarboxylase locus using the full-length cDNA as a probe (Hansen et al 1988a). In heterozygotes from two PCT families, northern analyses revealed normal mRNA sizes and amounts (Hansen et al 1988b). The specific molecular defect that caused HEP in two related patients from Tunisia has been determined. de Verneuil and co-workers (1986) identified a point mutation (G to A) in exon 8 at position 860 of the coding region of URO-decarboxylase. This mutation results in a glycine to glutamic acid substitution at position 281, which alters the stability of the enzyme protein. This mutation has also been found in two unrelated Spanish HEP patients, but not in two unrelated patients from Italy and Portugal, nor in 13 unrelated heterozygotes with familial PCT (de Verneuil et al 1988). Another point mutation, a G to T transversion at position 860, which results in a glycine to valine substitution, was found in an unrelated patient with PCT (Garey et al 1989).

In type I PCT, the decreased hepatic URO-decarboxylase activity is not accompanied by a decrease in the concentration of the enzyme protein (Elder et al 1985). In type I patients, URO-decarboxylase activity returns to normal following a prolonged remission. Kushner et al (1985) postulated that a genetic defect, transmitted as an autosomal recessive trait, may be the underlying cause of type I PCT and that the additional presence of hepatic siderosis is required for clinical expression. Added support for this hypothesis is the finding of four Spanish families, with at least two relatives in each, having clinically manifest PCT with decreased hepatic URO-decarboxylase activity, but normal levels in erythrocytes and other tissues (Roberts et al 1988). It is unlikely that a mutation at the URO-decarboxylase locus results in the selectively decreased activity of the enzyme in the liver, since human URO-decarboxylase is encoded by a single gene on the short arm of chromosome 1 which

transcribes the same mRNA in erythroid and non-erythroid tissues (de Verneuil et al 1986, Romeo et al 1986a). The existence of only one mRNA is consistent with the observation that the erythroid and hepatic enzymes are physically and kinetically indistinguishable (Elder & Urquhart 1984). However, these findings could be consistent with a mutation that alters URO-decarboxylase such that it is susceptible to inactivation in the liver (Kushner 1982). Such an inactivation process could result from the presence of an induced or toxic compound present in the hepatocytes of individuals with type I PCT. Kinetic data from Mukerji and Pimstone (1985) suggest that PCT may be associated with an intrinsically abnormal enzyme with altered chemical properties. The findings are also consistent with the expression of a gene at some other locus that produces a gene product in response to acquired factors, such as alcohol and hepatic siderosis, which inhibits the activity of hepatic URO-decarboxylase. Analogously, the development of chronic porphyria in certain inbred mice by selected polyhalogenated aromatic hydrocarbons is influenced by levels of hepatic iron stores and by the inherited inducibility of certain forms of cytochrome P-450 (Smith & Francis 1983). Thus, development of type I PCT may involve both acquired and genetic factors that are capable of stimulating and modulating ALA formation and cytochrome P-450 induction.

Treatment

The diagnosis of PCT should be firmly established before treatment is initiated, because VP and HCP are unresponsive to measures that are highly effective in PCT. Imaging studies are advisable to exclude complicating hepatocellular carcinoma and to serve as a baseline for follow-up. Patients should abstain from alcohol, oestrogens, iron supplements, or other exogenous agents which contribute to exacerbation of the disease. Although improvement after cessation of alcohol can be dramatic (Ramsay et al 1974), the results are generally unpredictable or slow (Topi et al 1984). Phlebotomy can produce remissions in almost all patients and remains the standard therapy for PCT (Ramsay et al 1974). The aim is to gradually reduce the excess hepatic iron which contributes to activation of PCT. About 500 ml blood can be removed at intervals of 1–2 weeks. Remission of photosensitivity due to PCT usually begins as plasma ferritin and porphyrin levels decrease. The intervals can be lengthened as evidence of iron deficiency develops. After a remission is obtained, continued phlebotomies may not be needed, even if ferritin levels later return to normal. However, it is advisable to follow porphyrin levels and reinstitute phlebotomies if porphyrin levels begin to rise. Even cutaneous scarring and pseudoscleroderma can improve with phlebotomies (Ramsay et al 1974). Abnormal liver function tests may also improve (Adjarov & Ivanov 1980). Liver histological abnormalities may not completely resolve.

Small doses of chloroquine or hydroxychloroquine have been reported to be effective in producing remissions of PCT (Tsega et al 1981). The drug complexes with the excess porphyrin, and promotes its excretion. Especially with higher doses of these drugs, the excess porphyrins accumulate in plasma prior to urinary excretion, and this can account for a transient increase in photosensitivity. A low dose chloroquine regimen is a useful alternative when repeated phlebotomies are contraindicated (Ashton et al 1984).

Hereditary coproporphyria

This disease is a hepatic porphyria which results from the deficient activity of COPRO-oxidase (Elder et al 1976). It is inherited as an autosomal dominant trait whose clinical expression is influenced by ecogenic and metabolic factors. HCP is clinically very similar to AIP, although generally somewhat milder. Photosensitivity sometimes occurs. HCP has been reported mostly in Britain, Europe and North America, and is less frequent than AIP. Two biochemically distinguishable forms of HCP have been reported in homozygous affected individuals. One form, designated harderoporphyria, is characterized by about 10% residual COPRO-oxidase activity and the accumulation of primarily harderoporphyrin, whereas the other form of homozygous HCP results from a more marked enzymatic deficiency (approximately 2% of normal) and the accumulation primarily of coproporphyrin III.

Clinical manifestations

HCP can be exacerbated by many of the same factors that cause attacks in AIP, including barbiturates and other drugs, and endogenous or exogenous steroid hormones (Brodie et al 1977). The disease is latent before puberty and symptoms are more common in adult women than men. Neurovisceral symptoms are virtually identical to those of AIP. However the disease is probably less severe than AIP, and only a few patients have been reported to expire from respiratory paralysis. Hepatitis and other causes of impaired liver function can cause increased porphyrin retention and worsen photosensitivity in HCP (Elder et al 1976).

Several cases of homozygous HCP, with cutaneous lesions beginning in early childhood, have been documented (Grandchamp et al 1977, de Verneuil et al 1983, Doss et al 1984).

Biochemical findings

Excretion of coproporphyrinogen III is markedly increased in the urine and faeces of symptomatic heterozygotes with HCP as well as in many asymptomatic (or latent) heterozygotes. Increased urinary excretion of ALA, PBG and uroporphyrin is observed during acute attacks. With resolution of symptoms, ALA and PBG levels revert to normal more readily than in AIP. Porphyrin excretion patterns in homozygous HCP resemble those observed in heterozygotes, but reflect a more profound enzymatic deficiency. Harderoporphyria is characterized by a marked increase in faecal harderoporphyrin excretion as well as coproporphyrin.

COPRO-oxidase activity is about 50% of normal in cultured fibroblasts (Elder et al 1976), circulating lymphocytes (Nordmann & Grandchamp 1978) and leucocytes (Kordac et al 1984) of HCP heterozygotes. This enzyme cannot be assayed in erythrocytes, which do not contain mitochondria. Moreover, assays for COPRO-oxidase are not readily available. For screening of family members, measurement of faecal porphyrins is advisable. However, children with the enzymatic deficiency may not excrete excess porphyrins (Grandchamp & Nordmann 1977).

Genetics

The enzyme defect is inherited as an autosomal dominant trait. Homozygous cases with a much more profound enzyme deficiency have been described (Grandchamp et al 1977, Nordmann et al 1983). Although human COPRO-oxidase has not been purified to homogeneity for characterization of its physical and genetic properties, the locus of the gene encoding COPRO-oxidase has been assigned to human chromosome 9 by somatic cell genetic techniques (Grandchamp et al 1983).

In one case of homozygous HCP, the residual COPRO-oxidase activity (approximately 2% of normal) had a normal K_m value (Grandchamp et al 1977). In contrast, three cases in a family with harderoporphyria provided evidence for a different COPRO-oxidase defect. The mutant enzyme exhibited increased thermostability and reduced affinity for both harderoporphyrinogen and coproporphyrinogen III, consistent with a structurally altered enzyme (Nordmann et al 1983). A single active site on the normal enzyme is believed to carry out both decarboxylations, and most of the harderoporphyrinogen formed from coproporphyrinogen III is not released before being further decarboxylated to protoporphyrinogen IX. The reduced affinity of the mutant enzyme for both substrates in this family may cause harderoporphyrinogen to dissociate from the enzyme more readily than normal and be excreted in faeces as harderoporphyrin. The heterozygous parents of these patients had intermediate harderoporphyrin excretion. Thus, at least two different types of mutation producing different abnormalities of COPRO-oxidase can lead to HCP and its more severe homozygous forms.

Treatment

Exacerbations of HCP are treated in the same manner as in AIP. Cholestyramine may be of some value for photosensitivity occurring with liver dysfunction (Hunter et al 1971). Phlebotomy and chloroquine are not effective.

Variegate porphyria

This disease, inherited as an autosomal dominant trait, is a hepatic porphyria and results from the deficient activity of PROTO-oxidase. The disorder is described as 'variegate' because it can present with neurological manifestations, photosensitivity, or both. 'Dual porphyria' refers to patients who have features of both VP and PCT and presumably have inherited genes for both disorders (Day 1986).

Clinical manifestations

Clinical expression of the disease before puberty is rare. The neurovisceral manifestations of VP are indistinguishable from those of AIP or HCP. Skin manifestations are very similar to those of PCT and HCP, and usually of longer duration, and occur apart from the neurovisceral symptoms. Photosensitivity is more common than in HCP. Drugs, steroids, and nutritional factors that are detrimental in AIP can also provoke exacerbations of VP (Perloth et al 1968). In a survey of 300 patients in South Africa (Eales 1980), the most common clinical features included abdominal pain, tachycardia, vomiting, constipation, hypertension, neuropathy, back pain, confusion, bulbar paralysis, psychiatric complaints, fever, urinary frequency, and dysuria. Skin manifestations were present in 85% of the patients studied. Photosensitivity may be less commonly associated with VP in more northern countries where sunlight is less intense (Muhlbauer et al 1982).

Biochemical findings

Marked increases in faecal protoporphyrin and coproporphyrin and in urinary coproporphyrin are characteristic of VP. Faecal porphyrins may remain normal until near puberty. Meso- and deuteroporphyrins are also increased and derived from the actions of gut bacteria on protoporphyrin. Urinary and faecal coproporphyrin are mostly type III. Urinary ALA, PBG, and uroporphyrin are increased during acute attacks, but may be normal or only slightly increased during remission. Plasma porphyrins, consisting in part of a dicarboxylate porphyrin tightly bound to plasma proteins, are increased in VP, particularly when photosensitivity is present (Poh-Fitzpatrick 1980). The neutral fluorescence spectrum of plasma porphyrins is characteristic and can rapidly distinguish VP from PCT, HCP and EPP. The emission maximum is at 626 nm in VP, 619 nm in PCT, CEP, HCP and AIP, and 634 nm in EPP (Poh-Fitzpatrick 1980).

PROTO-oxidase activity is approximately half-normal in cultured skin fibroblasts and lymphocytes from VP patients (Brenner & Bloomer 1980). However, the assay of PROTO-oxidase activity in cultured cells is difficult and not widely available for diagnosis and family screening. Measurement of faecal porphyrins in relatives of known VP patients is recommended to detect latent cases; levels may not be increased in all heterozygotes, especially children and elderly subjects (Eschbach et al 1987). Since it is likely that a significant number of adults with inherited PROTO-oxidase deficiency excrete normal amounts of porphyrins in urine and faeces, more of these individuals would be identified if assays for this enzyme were more readily available for family screening (Mustajoki et al 1987). The isolation of the cDNA encoding this enzyme would permit the development of molecular diagnosis.

Protoporphyrinogen IX, the substrate for this enzyme, accumulates in patients with VP and undergoes auto-oxidation to protoporphyrin IX, which is characteristically increased in VP. A close functional association between PROTO-oxidase in the inner mitochondrial membrane and COPRO-oxidase in the intermembrane space may relate to the excess excretion of both protoporphyrin and coproporphyrin in this disease (Deybach et al 1981). HMB-synthase has been reported to be somewhat decreased in some VP patients in two series. However, this enzyme is usually within the normal range in VP (Muhlbauer et al 1982). Reports that ferrochelatase activity is approximately 50% of normal in cells from VP patients have not been confirmed.

Genetics

PROTO-oxidase deficiency, which is transmitted as an autosomal dominant trait, is the underlying genetic defect in VP. Although the cDNA encoding this enzyme has not been cloned, pedigree analysis of several large South African families has established synteny of PROTO-oxidase with α_1-antitrypsin, thereby provisionally assigning the gene to chromosome 14 (Bissort et al 1988). In most countries VP is less common than AIP, with the notable exception of South Africa, where three out of every 1000 Caucasians have inherited VP (Dean 1971). Most cases can be traced to a couple who emigrated from Holland and were married in South Africa in 1688.

Several cases of homozygous VP with marked reductions in PROTO-oxidase have been documented (Kordac et al 1984, Murphy et al 1986, Mustajoki et al 1987). The heterozygous parents of the patients had approximately half-normal enzyme activity, as expected. Photosensitivity, and in some cases neurological symptoms and developmental disturbances including growth retardation, were noted in infancy or childhood. All cases had increased erythrocyte zinc protoporphyrin levels, a characteristic finding in all homozygous porphyrias so far described.

Because the porphyrias are uncommon, the coincidental presence of two inherited porphyrias in the same family would be expected to be very rare. However, kindreds with individuals having both VP and familial PCT have been described (e.g. Eales et al 1980, Martasek et al 1983). This has been termed 'dual porphyria' (Day 1986).

In a large family from Britain, some individuals had acute porphyric attacks and evidence of deficiencies of both PROTO-oxidase and HMB-synthase (McColl et al 1985b). The disease in this family has been termed 'Chester porphyria'. Photosensitivity was not observed. It is presently unclear whether the porphyria in this lineage should be considered a variant of VP or AIP.

Treatment

Treatment of acute attacks of VP with glucose, haematin, and other measures employed in AIP are usually effective. Other therapies such as propranolol, D-penicillamine, haemodialysis, alkalization of urine, and β-carotene are of little or no benefit. Repeated venesections and chloroquine are highly effective in PCT, but not in VP (Cramers & Jepsen 1980). Measures to protect the skin from sunlight with appropriate clothing including gloves and a broad-rimmed hat, as well as opaque sunscreen preparations are useful. Exposure to short-wave ultraviolet light which does not excite porphyrins, may provide some protection by increasing skin pigmentation (Day 1986).

Erythropoietic protoporphyria

This erythropoietic porphyria, due to the partially deficient activity of ferrochelatase, is inherited as an autosomal dominant trait. Excess protoporphyrin is found in erythroid cells, plasma, bile, and faeces of heterozygotes in whom EPP is clinically expressed. EPP has also been termed erythrohepatic protoporphyria and protoporphyria. EPP is the most common form of erythropoietic porphyria and after PCT is perhaps the second most common porphyria. Well over 300 cases have been reported (De Leo et al 1976). Although the disease seems most common in Caucasians, it does occur in other races, including Blacks (Poh-Fitzpatrick 1977).

Clinical manifestations

Photosensitivity of sun-exposed areas usually begins in childhood. Cutaneous symptoms are generally more troublesome in the spring and summer. Burning, itching, erythema and swelling are the most common symptoms and can occur within minutes of sun exposure (De Leo et al 1976). Oedema of the skin may be diffuse and resemble angioneurotic oedema. Burning and itching can occur without obvious skin damage. Vesicles and bullae are absent or sparse, and in one series were reported in only 10% of cases (De Leo et al 1976). Thus the cutaneous features of this disease are distinct from those of PCT and VP.

Other characteristic and more subtle skin changes have been noted. These include areas of skin lichenification, leathery pseudovesicles, labial grooving, and nail changes (Eales 1980). Some residual scarring from vesicles or severe swelling may occur, but this is rarely severe or deforming. Pigment changes, friability, and hirsutism also are not characteristic of EPP. Unlike CEP, there is no fluorescence of the teeth. It is notable that neuropathic manifestations are not found in EPP.

Pathophysiology

Porphyrins absorb light maximally at wavelengths near 400 nm (the Soret band) and enter an excited energy state that is manifested by fluorescence and, in the presence of O_2, the formation of singlet oxygen and other oxygen species that can produce tissue damage (Sandberg & Romslo 1981). This may be accompanied by lipid peroxidation (Goldstein & Harber 1972), oxidation of amino acids and cross-linking of proteins in cell membranes (De Goeij & Van Steveninch 1976). In EPP, the skin is maximally sensitive to 400 nm light. Histological changes predominantly in the upper dermis in EPP may include amorphous material deposited around blood vessels, and resemble the findings in PCT.

There is little evidence for impaired erythropoiesis or abnormal iron metabolism in this disease (Bottomley et al 1975). Liver function is usually normal in EPP, sometimes even when protoporphyrin in the liver appears to be considerably increased. A minority of patients with EPP develop chronic liver disease, which can progess rapidly and lead to death from liver failure (Bloomer 1988). However, EPP can present with advanced liver disease as the major manifestation (Singer et al 1978). Upper abdominal pain may suggest biliary obstruction, and unnecessary laparotomy to exclude this possibility can be detrimental (Bloomer 1988). The potentially life-threatening hepatic complications of EPP are incompletely understood, but are often preceded by increasing levels of erythrocyte and plasma protoporphyrin, abnormal liver function tests, marked deposition of protoporphyrin in liver cells and bile canaliculi and sometimes increased photosensitivity.

Biochemical findings

Protoporphyrin concentrations are increased in bone marrow, circulating erythrocytes, plasma, bile, and faeces of EPP patients. Other haem pathway intermediates do not accumulate. Thus, urinary porphyrin and porphyrin precursor concentrations are normal. Nucleated erythroid cells in the bone marrow in EPP display little or no fluorescence due to protoporphyrin, and bone marrow fluorescence is almost entirely found in reticulocytes which are likely to be the primary source of protoporphyrin in this condition. Erythrocyte protoporphyrin in EPP is free and not complexed with zinc as in lead poisoning and iron deficiency. Zinc protoporphyrin in the latter two conditions is bound to haemoglobin, perhaps at the haem binding site, and persists in the red cell as long as it circulates. Free protoporphyrin in EPP binds less readily to haemoglobin and diffuses more easily into plasma. Thus, erythrocyte protoporphyrin in EPP declines much more rapidly with erythrocyte age than in most other conditions in which erythrocyte protoporphyrin is increased.

A partial deficiency of ferrochelatase activity has been found in bone marrow, reticulocytes (Bottomley et al 1975), liver, cultured fibroblasts (Bonkowsky et al 1975), and leucocytes from patients with EPP (Bottomley et al 1975). A deficiency of this enzyme was also demonstrated by increased protoporphyrin accumulation after ALA

loading of cultured skin fibroblasts and mitogen stimulated lymphocytes (Sassa et al 1982). Although ferrochelatase is deficient in all cells in EPP, the deficient activity becomes rate-limiting for protoporphyrin metabolism to haem primarily in bone marrow reticulocytes.

Genetic defect

EPP is inherited as an autosomal dominant trait (Donaldson et al 1967). There is considerable variation in phenotypic expression. For example, some obligate heterozygotes have little or no increase in erythrocyte protoporphyrin. Plasma and faecal levels of protoporphyrin may be better indicators of the genetic defect in some individuals than in others. The cause of the considerable inter-individual variability in protoporphyrin levels and clinical severity among heterozygotes for this enzyme deficiency is not clear.

Ferrochelatase activity in tissue lysates of EPP patients has been reported to be only 10–25% of normal (Bonkowsky et al 1975, De Goeij et al 1975), which is lower than expected for an autosomal dominant enzymopathy. Kinetic data suggesting an inhibitor or a reduced K_m for a porphyrin substrate (Bloomer 1980) are also not readily explained. Mitochondrial structure and function have been reported to be normal in EPP (Bloomer 1980). Altered heat stability of the enzymatic activity in EPP bone marrow preparations, and the inability of EPP fibroblasts to incorporate zinc into protoporphyrin have been interpreted as indications of a structurally altered enzyme (Kramer & Viljoen 1980).

Treatment

β-carotene has been developed primarily as a drug for treating EPP, and its clinical benefits have been substantiated in large series of patients (Mathews-Roth et al 1977, Thomsen et al 1979). Tolerance to sunlight is improved in most patients, sometimes considerably. This is observed 1–3 months after treatment is begun. Doses of 120–180 mg per 24 hours in adults are usually required to maintain serum carotene levels in the recommended range of 600–800 μg/dl. Using pure preparations of β-carotene, no side-effects other than a mild and dose-related skin discolouration due to carotenaemia have been noted (Mathews-Roth et al 1977). The mechanism of action of β-carotene is not fully established but may involve quenching of singlet oxygen or free radicals. The drug appears less effective in other forms of porphyria associated with photosensitivity such as CEP and PCT.

Cholestyramine, which may interrupt the enterohepatic circulation of protoporphyrin and promote its faecal excretion, has been reported to reduce liver protoporphyrin and improve cutaneous symptoms in some EPP patients (Kniffen 1970). This and other porphyrin absorbents should be considered especially in patients with complicating hepatic dysfunction. Splenectomy may be beneficial when EPP is complicated by haemolysis and splenomegaly. Avoidance of iron deficiency, caloric restriction, and drugs or hormone preparations that impair hepatic excretory function may also be important (Bloomer 1979). Treatment of the hepatic

complications of EPP is difficult and must be individualized. Resolution may occur spontaneously, at least in part, if another reversible cause of liver dysfunction, such as viral hepatitis or alcohol, is contributing (Bonkowsky & Schned 1986). Other therapeutic options include transfusions and intravenous haematin to suppress erythroid and hepatic protoporphyrin production and, if present, the correction of iron deficiency. Some patients with EPP and liver failure have undergone liver transplantation (Morton et al 1988).

REFERENCES

Ades I Z, Stevens T M, Drew P D 1987 Biogenesis of embryonic chick liver δ-aminolevulinate synthase: regulation of the level of mRNA by hemin. Archives of Biochemistry and Biophysics 253: 297–304

Adjarov D, Ivanov E 1980 Clinical value of serum γ-glutamyl transferase estimation in porphyria cutanea tarda. British Journal of Dermatology 102: 541–545

Anderson K E, Fischbein A, Kestenbaum D, Sassa S, Alvares A P, Kappas A 1977 Plumbism from airborne lead in a firing range. An unusual exposure to a toxic heavy metal. American Journal of Medicine 63: 306–312

Anderson K E, Freddara U, Kappas A 1982 Induction of hepatic cytochrome P-450 by natural steroids: relationship to the induction of δ-aminolevulinate synthase and porphyrin accumulation in the avian embryo. Archives of Biochemistry and Biophysics 217: 597–608

Anderson K E, Spitz I M, Sassa S, Bardin C W, Kappas A 1986 Intranasal luteinizing hormone-releasing hormone agonist for prevention of cyclical attacks of acute intermittent porphyria. In: Nordmann Y (ed) Porphyrins and porphyrias. Colloque INSERM, John Libbey Eurotext 134: 225–231

Anderson P M, Desnick R J 1979 Purification and properties of δ-aminolevulinic acid dehydratase from human erythrocytes. Journal of Biological Chemistry 254: 6924–6930

Anderson P M, Desnick R J 1980 Purification and properties of uroporphyrinogen I synthase from human erythrocytes. Identification of stable enzyme-substrate intermediates. Journal of Biological Chemistry 255: 1993–1999

Anderson P M, Reddy R M, Anderson K E, Desnick R J 1981 Characterization of the PBG-deaminase deficiency in acute intermittent porphyria. I. Immunologic evidence for heterogeneity of the genetic defect. Journal of Clinical Investigation 68: 1–12

Aoki Y, Muranaka S, Nakabayashi K, Ueda Y 1979 δ-Aminolevulinic acid synthetase in erythroblasts of patients with pyridoxine-responsive anemia. Hypercatabolism caused by the increased susceptibility to the controlling protease. Journal of Clinical Investigation 64: 1196–1203

Ashton R E, Hawk J L M, Magnus I A 1984 Low-dose oral chloroquine in the treatment of porphyria cutanea tarda. British Journal of Dermatology 3: 609–613

Astrin K H, Bishop D F, Kaul B, Davidow B, Wetmer J G, Desnick R J 1987 Human δ-aminolevulinate dehydrogenase isozymes and lead toxicity. Annals of the New York Academy of Sciences 514: 23–29

Astrin K H, Desnick R J, Bishop D F 1988 Assignment of human (d)-aminolevulinate synthase (ALAS) to chromosome 3. Cytogenetics and Cell Genetics 46: 573

Battistuzzi G, Petrucci R, Silvagni L, Urbani F R, Caiola S 1981 δ-aminolevulinate dehydrase: a new genetic polymorphism in man. Annals of Human Genetics 45: 223–229

Beattie A D, Moore M R, Goldberg A, Ward R L 1973 Acute intermittent porphyria: Response of tachycardia and hypertension to propranolol. British Medical Journal 3: 257–268

Becker D M, Kramer S 1977 The neurological manifestations of porphyria: A review. Medicine 56: 411–426

Benkmann H G, Bogdanski P, Goedde W H 1983 Polymorphism of delta aminolevulinic acid dehydratase in various populations. Human Heredity: 33: 62–64

Beru N, Goldwasser E 1985 The regulation of heme biosynthesis during erythropoietin-induced erythroid differentiation. Journal of Biological Chemistry 260: 9251–9257

Bishop D F, Desnick R J 1982 Assays of the heme biosynthetic enzymes. Enzyme 28: 91–231

Bissbort S, Hitzeroth H W, du Wertzel D P 1988 Linkage between the variegate porphyria (VP) and the α-1-antitrypsin (PI) genes on human chromosome 14. Human Genetics 79: 289–290

Bissell D M 1988 Treatment of acute hepatic porphyria with hematin. Journal of Hepatology 6: 1–7

Blekkenhorst G H, Harrison G G, Cook E S, Eales L 1980 Screening of certain anaesthetic agents for their ability to elicit acute porphyric phases in susceptible patients. British Journal of Anaesthesia 52: 759–762

Bloomer J R 1979 Pathogenesis and therapy of liver disease in protoporphyria. Yale Journal of Biological Medicine 52: 39–43

Bloomer J R 1980 Characterization of deficient heme synthase activity in protoporphyria with cultured skin fibroblasts. Journal of Clinical Investigation 65: 321–327

Bloomer J R 1988 The liver in protoporphyria. Hepatology 8: 402–407

Bloomer J R, Hill H D, Morton K O, Anderson-Burnham L A, Straka J G 1987 The enzyme defect in bovine protoporphyria. Journal of Biological Chemistry 262: 7902–7905

Bonkowsky H L, Schned A R 1986 Fatal liver failure in protoporphyria: synergism between ethanol excess and the genetic defect. Gastroenterology 90: 191–201

Bonkowsky H L, Schady W 1982 Neurologic manifestations of acute porphyria. Seminars in Liver Disease 2: 108–124

Bonkowsky H L, Tschudy D P, Collins A et al 1971 Repression of the overproduction of porphyrin precursors in acute intermittent porphyria by intravenous infusions of hematin. Proceedings of the National Academy of Sciences USA 8: 2725–2731

Bonkowsky H L, Bloomer J R, Ebert P S, Mahoney M J 1975 Heme synthetase deficiency in human protoporphyria: Demonstration of the defect in liver and cultured skin fibroblasts from patients with protoporphyria. Journal of Clinical Investigation 56: 1139–1148

Bottomley S S, Tanaka M, Everett M A 1975 Diminished erythroid ferrochelatase activity in protoporphyria. Journal of Laboratory and Clinical Medicine 86: 126–131

Bowden M J, Borthwick I A, Healy H M, Morris C P, May B K, Elliott W H 1987 Sequence of human 5-aminolevulinate synthase DNA. Nucleic Acids Research 15: 8563

Brenner D A, Bloomer J R 1980 The enzymatic defect in variegate porphyria: studies with human cultured skin fibroblasts. New England Journal of Medicine 302: 765–769

Brodie M J, Thompson G G, Moore M R et al 1977 Hereditary coproporphyria. Demonstration of the abnormalities in haem biosynthesis in peripheral blood. Quarterly Journal of Medicine 46: 229–233

Cavanagh J B, Mellick R S 1965 On the nature of the peripheral nerve lesions associated with acute intermittent porphyria. Journal of Neurology, Neurosurgery and Psychiatry 28: 320–327

Chretien S, Dubart A, Beaupain D L 1988 Alternative transcription and splicing of the human porphobilinogen deaminase gene results either in tissue-specific or in housekeeping expression. Proceedings of the National Academy of Sciences USA 85: 6–10

Cortes J M, Oliva H, Paradinas F J, Hernandez-Guio C H 1980 The pathology of the liver in porphyria cutanea tarda. Histopathology 4: 471

Cramers M, Jepsen L V 1980 Porphyria variegata: Failure of chloroquin treatment. Acta Dermato Venereologica 60: 89–99

Dailey H A, Fleming J E 1986 The role of arginyl residues in porphyrin binding to ferrochelatase. Journal of Biological Chemistry 261: 7902–7905

Dailey H A, Karr S W 1987 Purification and properties of murine protoporphyrinogen oxidase. Biochemistry 26: 2697–2701

Day R S 1986 Variegate porphyria. Seminars in Dermatology 5: 138–154

Day R S, Pimstone N R, Eales L 1978 The diagnostic value of blood plasma porphyrin methyl ester profiles produced by quantitative TLC. International Journal of Biochemistry 9: 897–904

Day R S, Eales L, Pimstone N R 1979 Familial symptomatic porphyria in South Africa. South African Medical Journal 56: 909–913

Dean G 1971 The porphyrias: a study of inheritance and environment. 2nd edn. Pitman Medical, London

De Goeij A F P M, Van Steveninch J 1976 Photodynamic aspects of protoporphyrin on cholesterol and unsaturated fatty acids of erythrocyte membranes in protoporphyria and in normal red blood cells. Clinica Chimica Acta 68: 115–121

De Goeij A F P M, Christianse K, Van Steveninck J 1975 Decreased haem synthetase activity in blood cells of patients with erythropoietic protoporphyria. European Journal of Clinical Investigation 5: 397–404

De Leo V A, Poh-Fitzpatrick M, Mathews-Roth M, Harber L C 1976 Erythropoietic protoporphyria. 10 years experience. American Journal of Medicine 60: 8–20

Desnick R J, Ostasiewicz L T, Tishler P A, Mustajoki P 1985 Acute intermittent porphyria: characterization of a novel mutation in the structural gene for porphobilinogen deaminase. Journal of Clinical Investigation 76: 865–874

de Verneuil H, Aitken G, Nordmann Y 1978 Familial and sporadic porphyria cutanea tarda. Two different diseases. Human Genetics 44: 145–151

de Verneuil H, Sassa S, Kappas A 1983 Purification and properties of uroporphyrinogen decarboxylase from human erythrocytes. Journal of Biological Chemistry 258: 2454–2460

de Verneuil H, Beaumont C, Deybach J-C et al 1984 Enzymatic and immunological studies of uroporphyrinogen decarboxylase in familial porphyria cutanea tarda and hepatoerythropoietic porphyria. American Journal of Human Genetics 36: 613–622

de Verneuil H, Doss M, Brusco N, Beaumont C, Nordmann Y 1985 Hereditary hepatic porphyria with delta aminolevulinate dehydratase deficiency: immunologic characterization of the non-catalytic enzyme. Human Genetics 69: 174–177

de Verneuil H, Grandchamp B, Beaumont C et al 1986 Uroporphyrinogen decarboxylase structural mutant (Gly 282 → Glu) in a case of porphyria. Science 234: 732–734

de Verneuil H, Hansen J, Picat C et al 1988 Prevalence of the 281 (gly→glu) mutation in hepatoerythropoietic porphyria and porphyria cutanea tarda. Human Genetics 78: 101–102

Deybach J C, Grandchamp B, Grelier M et al 1980 Prenatal exclusion of congenital erythropoietic porphyria (Gunther's disease) in a fetus at risk. Human Genetics 53: 217–222

Deybach J C, de Verneuil H, Phung N et al 1981 Congenital erythropoietic porphyria (Gunther's disease): Enzymatic studies on two cases of late onset. Journal of Laboratory Clinical Medicine 97: 551–557

Deybach J C, da Silva V, Grandchamp B, Nordmann Y 1985 The mitochondrial location of protoporphyrinogen oxidase. European Journal of Biochemistry 149: 431–435

Donaldson E M, Donaldson A D, Rimington C 1967 Erythropoietic protoporphyria: A family study. British Medical Journal 1: 659–662

Doss M, Von Tiepermann R, Schneider J 1980 Acute hepatic porphyria syndrome with porphobilinogen synthase defect. International Journal of Biochemistry 12: 823–827

Doss M, Sauer H, Von Tiepermann R, Colombi A M 1984 Development of chronic hepatic porphyria (porphyria cutanea tarda) with inherited uroporphyrinogen decarboxylase deficiency under exposure to dioxin. International Journal of Biochemistry 16: 369–373

Eales L 1980 Liver involvement in erythropoietic protoporphyria (EPP). International Journal of Biochemistry 12: 915–921

Eales L, Day R S, Blekkenhorst G H 1980 The clinical and biochemical features of variegate porphyria: An analysis of 300 cases studied at Groote Schuur Hospital, Cape Town. International Journal of Biochemistry 12: 837–848

Elder G H 1977 Porphyrin metabolism in porphyria cutanea tarda. Seminars in Hematology 14: 227–245

Elder G H, Evans J O 1978 Evidence that the coproporphyrinogen oxidase activity of rat liver is situated in the intermembrane space of mitochondria. Biochemical Journal 172: 345–347

Elder G H, Urquhart A J 1984 Human uroporphyrinogen decarboxylase. Do tissue specific isoenzymes exist? Biochemical Society Transactions 12: 661–662

Elder G H, Evans J O, Thomas N et al 1976 The primary enzyme defect in hereditary coproporphyria. Lancet ii: 1217–1219

Elder G H, Smith S G, Herrero C et al 1981 Hepatoerythropoietic porphyria: A new uroporphyrinogen decarboxylase defect or homozygous porphyria cutanea tarda? Lancet i: 916–919

Elder G H, Sheppard D M, Tovey J A, Urquhart A J 1983 Immunoreactive uroporphyrinogen decarboxylase in porphyria cutanea tarda. Lancet 1: 1301–1304

Elder G H, Urquhart A J, De Salamanca R E et al 1985 Immunoreactive uroporphyrinogen decarboxylase in the liver in porphyria cutanea tarda. Lancet ii: 229–232

Eschbach J W, Egrie J C, Downing M R et al 1987 Correction of the anemia of end-stage renal disease with recombinant human erythropoietin. New England Journal of Medicine 316: 73–78

Ferriera G C, Dailey H A 1988 Mouse protoporphyrinogen oxidase: Kinetic parameters and demonstration of inhibition by bilirubin. Biochemical Journal 250: 597–603

Fowler C S, Word J M 1975 Porphyria variegata provoked by the contraceptive pill. British Medical Journal 1: 663–664

Fuchs T, Ippen H 1987 Treatment of acute intermittent porphyria with a new albumin-bound lyophilized hematin. Deutsche Medizinische Wochenschrift 112: 1302–1305

Fujita H, Sassa S, Lundgren J, Holmberg L, Thunell S, Kappas A 1987a Enzymatic defect in a child with hereditary hepatic pophyria due to homozygous δ-aminolevulinic acid dehydratase deficiency: immunochemical studies. Pediatrics 80: 880–885

Fujita H, Sassa S, Toback A C, Kappas A 1987b Immunochemical study of uroporphyrinogen decarboxylase in a patient with mild hepatoerythropoietic porphyria. Journal of Clinical Investigation 79: 1533–1537

Garey J R, Hansen J L, Lyle M 1989 A point mutation in the coding region of uroporphyrinogen decarboxylase associated with familial porphyria cutanea tarda. Blood 73:892–895

Goldstein B D, Harber L C 1972 Erythropoietic protoporphyria: Lipid peroxidation and red cell membrane damage associated with photohemolysis. Journal of Clinical Investigation 51: 892–900

Grandchamp B, Nordmann Y 1971 Decreased lymphocyte coproporphyrinogen III oxidase activity in hereditary corproporphyria. Biochemical and Biophysical Research Communications 74: 1089–1094

Grandchamp B, Phung N, Nordmann Y 1977 Homozygous case of hereditary coproporphyria. Lancet ii: 1348–1352

Grandchamp B, Phung N, Nordmann Y 1978 The mitochondrial localization of coproporphyrinogen III oxidase. Biochemical Journal 176: 97–102

Grandchamp B, Weil D, Nordmann Y et al 1983 Assigment of the human coproporphyrinogen oxidase gene to chromosome 9. Human Genetics 64: 180–183

Grandchamp B, de Verneuil H, Beaumont C, Chretien S, Walter O, Nordmann Y 1987 Tissue-specific expression of porphobilinogen deaminase, two-isoenzymes from a single gene. European Journal of Biochemistry 162: 105–110

Grandchamp B, Picat C, Mignotte J H P et al 1989 Tissue-specific splicing mutation in acute intermittent porphyria. Proceedings of the National Academy of Sciences USA 86: 661–668

Granick S 1966 The induction in vitro of the synthesis of δ-aminolevulinic acid synthetase in chemical porphyria. A response to certain drugs, sex, hormones, and foreign chemicals. Journal of Biological Chemistry 241: 1359–1375

Gregor A, Kostrzewska E, Prokurat H, Pucek Z, Torbicka E 1977 Increased protoporphyrin in erythrocytes in a child with acute intermittent porphyria. Archives of Disease in Childhood 52: 947–950

Hansen J L, O'Connell P, Romana M et al 1988a Familial porphyria cutanea tarda: hybridizaion analysis of the uroporphyrinogen decarboxylase locus. Human Heredity 38: 283–286

Hansen J L, Pryor M A, Kennedy J B et al 1988b Steady-state levels of uroporphyrinogen decarboxylase mRNA in lymphoblastoid cell lines from patients with familial porphyria cutanea tarda and their relatives. American Journal of Human Genetics 42: 847–853

Hayashi N, Yoda B, Kikuchi G 1969 Mechanism of allylisopropylacetamide-induced increase of δ-aminolevulinate synthetase in liver mitochondria. IV. Accumulation of the enzyme in the soluble fraction of rat liver. Archives of Biochemistry and Biophysics 131: 83–91

Hunter J A A, Khan S A, Hope E et al 1971 Hereditary coproporphyria. Photosensitivity, jaundice and neuropsychiatric manifestations associated with pregnancy. British Journal of Dermatology 84: 301–308

Jaffe E K, Salowe S P, Chen N T, Dehaven P A 1984 Porphobilinogen synthase modification with methylmethanethiosulfonate. A protocol for the investigation of metalloproteins. Journal of Biological Chemistry 259: 5032–5036

Jones M S, Jones O T G 1969 The structural organization of heme synthesis in rat liver mitochondria. Biochemical Journal 113: 507–514

Kaiser I H 1980 Brown amniotic fluid in congenital erythropoietic porphyria. Obstetrics and Gynecology 56: 383–385

Kaplowitz N, Javitt N, Kappas A 1972 Coproporphyrin I and III excretion in bile and urine. Journal of Clinical Investigation 51: 2895–2899

Kappas A, Sassa S, Anderson K E 1983 The porphyrias. In: Stanbury J B, Wyngaarden J B, Fredrickson D S, Goldstein J L, Brown M S (eds) The metabolic basis of inherited disease. McGraw-Hill New York, p 1301–1384

Kniffen J C 1970 Protoporphyrin removal in intrahepatic porphyrastasis. Gastroenterology 58: 1027

Kopp W 1984 Harderoporphyrin coproporphyuria. Lancet 1: 292

Kordac V 1972 The frequency of occurrence of hepatocellular carcinoma in patients with porphyria cutanea tarda in long-term follow-up. Neoplasia 19: 135–139

Kordac V, Deybach J C, Martasek P 1984 Homozygous variegate porphyria. Lancet 1: 851–854

Kordac V, Martasek P, Zeman J et al 1985 Increased erythrocyte protoporphyrin in homozygous variegate porphyria. Photodermatology 2: 257–259

Kramer S, Viljoen J D 1980 Erythropoietic protoporphyria: Evidence that it is due to a variant ferrochelatase. International Journal of Biochemistry 12: 925–931

Kushner J P 1982 The enzymatic defect in porphyria cutanea tarda. New England Journal of Medicine 306: 799–800

Kushner J P, Edwards C Q, Dadone M M, Skolnick M H 1985 Heterozygosity for HLA-linked hemochromatosis as a likely cause of the hepatic siderosis associated with sporadic porphyria cutanea tarda. Gastroenterology 88: 1232–1238

Lamon J M, Frykholm B C, Hess R A, Tschudy D P 1979 Hematin therapy for acute porphyria. Medicine 58: 252–260

Lee J S, Anvset M, Lindsten J et al 1988 DNA polymorphisms within the porphobilinogen deaminase gene in two Swedish families with acute intermittent porphyria. Human Genetics 79: 379–381

Lim C K, Peters T J 1984 Urine and faecal porphyric profiles by reversed-phase high performance liquid chromatography in the porphyrias. Clinica Chimica Acta 139: 55–63

Lim H W, Petrez H D, Goldstein I M, Gigli I 1981 Complement-derived chemotactic activity is generated in human serum containing uro-porphyrin after irradiation with 405 nm light. Journal of Clinical Investigation 67: 1072–1077

Lindblad B, Lindstedt S, Steen G 1977 On the enzymic defects in hereditary tyrosinemia. Proceedings of the National Academy of Sciences USA 74: 4641–4645

Litman D A, Correia M A 1985 Elevated brain tryptophan and enhanced 5-hydroxytryptamine turnover in acute hepatic heme deficiency: clinical implications. Journal of Pharmacology and Experimental Therapeutics 232: 337–345

Llewellyn D H, Kalsheker N A, Elder G H, Harison P, Chretier S, Goossens M 1987 A MspI polymorphism for the human porphobilinogen gene. Nucleic Acids Research 15: 1342

Lynch R E, Lee G R, Kushner J P 1975 Porphyria cutanea tarda associated with disinfectant misuse. Archives of Internal Medicine 135: 549–552

McColl K E L, Thompson G G, Moore M R, Goldberg A 1985a Abnormal haem biosynthesis in Gilbert's syndrome. Gut 26: Abstract 564

McColl K E L, Thompson G G, Moore M R et al 1985b Chester porphyria: biochemical studies of a new form of acute porphyria. Lancet 2: 796–799

McKay R, Druyan R, Getz G S, Rabinowitz M 1969 Intramitochondrial localization of δ-aminolevulate synthetase and ferrochelatase in rat liver. Biochemical Journal 114: 455–461

McKusick V A 1988 Mendelian inheritance in man, 8th edn. Johns Hopkins University Press, Baltimore

Malina L, Miller V L, Magnus I A 1978 Skin porphyrin assay in porphyria. Clinica Chimica Acta 83: 55–59

Marks G S 1985 Exposure to toxic agents: the heme biosynthetic pathway and hemoproteins as indicator. CRC Critical Reviews in Toxicology 15: 151–179

Martasek P, Kordac V, Jirsa M 1983 Variegate porphyria and porphyria cutanea tarda. Archives of Dermatology 119: 537–538

Mathews-Roth M M, Pathak M A, Fizpatrick T B et al 1977 Beta carotene therapy for erythropoietic

Mathews-Roth M M, Pathak M A, Fitzpatrick T B et al 1977 Beta carotene therapy for erythropoietic protoporphyria and other photosensitivity diseases. Archives of Dermatology 113: 1229–1234

Mauzerall D, Granick S 1956 The occurrence and determination of delta-aminolevulinic acid and porphobilinogen in urine. Journal of Biological Chemistry 219: 435–446

Milo R, Neuman M, Klein C, Caspi E, Arlazoroff A 1989 Acute intermittent porphyria in pregnancy. Obstetrics and Gynecology 73: 450–452

Moore M R 1980 International review of drugs in acute porphyria 1980. International Journal of Biochemistry 12: 1089–1097

Moore M R, Thompson G G, Allen B R et al 1973 Plasma porphyrin concentrations in porphyria cutanea tarda (short communication). Clinical Science and Molecular Medicine 45: 711–715

Moore M R, McColl K E L, Rimington C, Goldberg A 1987 Disorders of porphyrin metabolism. Plenum, New York.

Morgan J M, Burch H B 1972 Comparative tests for the diagnosis of lead poisoning. Archives of Internal Medicine 130: 335–341

Morton K O, Schneider F, Weiner M K, Straka J G, Bloomer J R 1988 Hepatic and bile porphyrins in patients with protoporphyria and liver failure. Gastroenterology 94: 1488–1492

Muhlbauer J E, Pathak M A, Tishler P V, Fitzpatrick T B 1982 Variegate porphyria in New England. Journal of the American Medical Association 247: 3095–3102

Mukerji S K, Pimstone N R 1985 Reduced substrate affinity for human erythrocyte uroporphyrinogen decarboxylase constitutes the inherent biochemical defect in porphyria cutanea tarda. Biochemistry and Biophysics Research Communications 127: 517–525

Mukerji S K, Pimstone N R 1987 Evidence for two uroporphyrinogen decarboxylase isoenzymes in human erythrocytes. Biochemical and Biophysical Research Communications 146: 1196–1203

Murphy G M, Hawk J L M, Magnus I A, Barrett D F, Elder G H, Smith S G 1986 Homozygous variegate porphyria: two similar cases in unrelated families. Journal of the Royal Society of Medicine 79: 361–364

Mustajoki P, Heinonen J 1980 General anesthesia in "inducible" porphyrias. Anesthesiology 53: 15–20

Mustajoki P, Tenhunen R 1985 Variant of acute intermittent porphyria with normal erythrocyte uroporphyrinogen-I-synthase activity. European Journal of Clinical Investigation 15: 281–284

Mustajoki P, Tenhunen R, Niemi K M, Nordmann Y, Kaariainen H, Norio R 1987 Homozygous variegate porphyria. Clinical Genetics 32: 300–305

Neuwirt J, Ponka P 1977 Regulation of haemoglobin synthesis. Martinus Nijhoff Medical Division, the Hague, Netherlands.

Nordmann Y, Grandchamp B 1978 Hereditary coproporphyria: demonstration of a genetic defect in coproporphyrinogen metabolism. Monograms in Human Genetics 10: 217–221

Nordmann Y, Grandchamp B, de Verneuil H et al 1983 Harderoporphyria: a variant hereditary coproporphyria. Journal of Clinical Investigation 72: 1139–1149

Pain R W, Welch F W, Woodruffe A J et al 1975 Erythropoietic uroporphyria of Gunther first presenting at 58 years with positive family studies. British Medical Journal 3: 621

Perlroth M G, Tschudy D P, Ratner A et al 1968 The effect of diet in variegate porphyria. Metabolism 71: 10–41

Petryka Z J, Dhar G J, Bossenmaier I 1976 Hematin clearance in porphyria. In: Doss M (ed) Porphyrins in human disease. S Karger, Basel p 259–270

Pierach C A, Weimer M K, Cardinal R A et al 1987 Red blood cell porphobilinogen deaminase in the evaluation of acute intermittent porphyria. Journal of the American Medical Association 7: 60–61

Pimstone N R, Gandhi S N, Mukerji S K 1987 Therapeutic efficacy of oral charcoal in congenital erythropoietic porphyria. New England Journal of Medicine 316: 390–393

Piomelli S, Lamola A A, Poh-Fitzpatrick M B et al 1975 Erythropoietic protoporphyria and Pb intoxication: The molecular basis for difference in cutaneous photosensitivity. I. Different rates of disappearance of protoporphyrin from the erythrocytes, both in vivo and in vitro. Journal of Clinical Investigation 56: 1519–1527

Piomelli S, Poh-Fitzpatrick M B, Seaman C et al 1986 Complete suppression of the symptoms of congenital erythropoietic porphyria by long-term treatment with high-level transfusions. New England Journal of Medicine 314: 1029–1031

Poh-Fitzpatrick M B 1977 Erthropoietic porphyrias: Current mechanistic, diagnostic, and therapeutic considerations. Seminars in Hematology 14: 211–227

Poh-Fitzpatrick M B 1980 A plasma porphyrin fluorescence marker for variegate porphyria. Archives of Dermatology 116: 543–547

Potluri V R, Astrin K H, Wetmur J G, Bishop D F, Desnick R J 1987 Chromosomal localization of the structural gene for human ALA-dehydratase to 9q34 by in situ hybridization. Human Genetics 76: 236–239

Praga M, Enriguez de Salamanca R, Andres A et al 1987 Treatment of hemodialysis-related porphyria cutanea tarda with deferoxamine. New England Journal of Medicine 316: 547–548

Raich N, Romeo P H, Dubart A, Beaupain D, Cohen-Solal M, Goossens M 1986 Molecular cloning and complete primary sequence of human erythrocyte porphobilinogen deaminase. Nucleic Acids Research 14: 5955–5968

Ramsay C A, Magnus I A, Turnbull A, Barker H 1974 The treatment of porphyria cutanea tarda by venesection. Quarterly Journal of Medicine 43: 169–172

Riddle R D, Yamamoto M, Engel J D 1989 Expression of δ-aminolevulinate synthase in avian cells: separate genes encode erythroid specific and basal isozymes. Proceedings of the National Academy of Sciences USA: 86: 792–796

Ridley A 1975 Porphyric neutropathy. In: Dyck P J, Thomas P K, Lambert E H (eds) Peripheral Neuropathy, Saunders, Philadelphia vol. 2: 942–953

Roberts A G, Elder G H, Newcombe R G et al 1988 Heterogeneity of familial porphyria cutanea tarda. Journal of Medical Genetics 25: 669–676

Romana M, Dubart A, Beaupain D, Chabret C, Goossens M, Romeo P H 1987 Structure of the gene for human uroporphyrinogen decarboxylase. Nucleic Acids Research 15: 7345–7356

Romeo G, Levin E Y 1969 Uroporphyrinogen III cosynthetase in human congenital erythropoietic porphyria. Proceedings of the National Academy of Sciences USA 63: 856–863

Romeo P H, Raich N, Dubart A 1986a Molecular cloning and nucleotide sequence of a complete human uroporphyrinogen decarboxylase cDNA. Journal of Biological Chemistry 261: 9825–9831

Romeo P H, Raich N, Dubart A, Beaupain D, Mattei M G, Goosens M 1986b Molecular cloning and tissue-specific expression analysis of human porphobilinogen deaminase and uroporphyrinogen decarboxylase. In: Nordmann Y (ed) Porphyrias and porphyrias. Colleque INSERM/John Libbey Eurotext 134: 25–34

Salata H, Cortes J M, de Salamanca R E et al 1985 Porphyria cutanea tarda and hepatocellular carcinoma. Journal of Hepatology 1: 477–487

Sandberg S, Brun A 1982 Light-induced protoporphyrin release from erythrocytes in erythropoietic protoporphyria. Journal of Clinical Investigation 70: 693–698

Sandberg S, Romslo I 1981 Porphyrin-induced photodamage at the cellular and the subcellular level as related to the solubility of the porphyrin. Clinica Chimica Acta 109: 193–197

Sassa S 1976 Sequential induction of heme pathway enzymes during erythroid differentiaton of mouse Friend leukemia virus-infected cells. Journal of Experimental Medicine 143: 305–315

Sassa S, Kappas A 1983 Hereditary tyrosinemia and the heme biosynthetic pathway. Journal of Clinical Investigation 71: 625–634

Sassa S, Solish G, Levese R D, Kappas A 1975 Studies in Porphyria IV: Expression of the gene defect of acute hepatic intermittent porphyria in cultured human skin fibroblasts and amniotic cells: prenatal diagnosis of the porphyric trait. Journal of Experimental Medicine 142: 722–731

Sassa S, Zalar G L, Poh-Fitzpatrick M B et al 1982 Studies in porphyria X. Functional evidence for a 50% deficiency of ferrochelatase activity in mitogen-stimulated lymphocytes from patients with erythropoietic protoporphyria. Journal of Clinical Investigation 69: 809–815

Schmid R 1960 Cutaneous porphyria in Turkey. New England Journal of Medicine 263: 397–398

Singer J A, Plaut A G, Kaplan M M 1978 Hepatic failure and death from erythropoietic protoporphyria. Gastroenterology 74:588

Smith A, Francis J 1983 Synergism of iron and hexachlorobenzene inhibits hepatic uroporphyrinogen decarboxylase in inbred mice. Biochemical Journal 214: 909–918

Strand L J, Felsher B F, Redeker A G, Marner H S 1970 Enzymatic abnormality in heme biosynthesis in acute intermittent porphyria: Decreased hepatic conversion of porphobilinogen to porphyrins and increased delta-aminolevulinic acid synthetase activity. Proceedings of the National Academy of Sciences USA 67: 1315–1320

Strand L J, Felsher B F, Redeker A G, Masver H S 1972 Decreased red cell protoporphyrinogen I synthetase activity in intermittent acute porphyria. Journal of Clinical Investigation 51: 2530–2536

Sweeney V P, Pathak M A, Asbury A K 1970 Acute intermittent porphyria: Increased ALA-synthetase activity during an acute attack. Brain 93: 369–380

Taketani S, Tokunaga R 1981 Rat liver ferrochelatase. Purification, properties and stimulation by fatty acids. Journal of Biological Chemistry 256: 12748–12753

Taljaard J J F, Shanley B C, Deppe W M, Joubert S M 1972 Porphyrin metabolism in experimental hepatic siderosis in the rat II. Combined effect of iron overload and hexachlorobenzene. British Journal of Haematology 23: 513–519

Thomsen K, Schmidt H, Fischer A 1979 Beta-carotene in erythropoietic protoporphyria: 5 years' experience. Dermatologica 159:82

Thunell S, Holmberg L, Lundgren J 1987 Aminolevulinate dehydrase porphyria in infancy. A clinical and biochemical study. Journal of Clinical Chemistry and Clinical Biology 25: 5–14

Tishler P V, Woodward B, O'Connor J et al 1985 High prevalence of intermittent acute porphyria in a psychiatric patient population. American Journal of Psychiatry 142: 1430–1436

Toback A C, Sassa S, Poh-Fitzpatrick M B et al 1987 Hepatoerythropoietic porphyria: clinical, biochemical, and enzymatic studies in a three-generation family lineage. New England Journal of Medicine 316: 645–650

Tokola O, Tenhunen R, Volin L, Mustajoki P 1986 Pharmacokinetics of intravenously administered haem arginate. British Journal of Clinical Pharmacology 22: 331–335

Topi G C, Amantea A, Griso D 1984 Recovery from porphyria cutanea tarda with no specific therapy other than avoidance of hepatic toxins. British Journal of Dermatology 3: 75–82

Tsai S-F, Bishop D F, Desnick R J 1987 Purification and properties of uroporphyrinogen III synthase from human erythrocytes. Journal of Biological Chemistry 262: 1268–1273

Tsai S F, Bishop D F, Desnick R J 1988 Human uroporphyrinogen III synthase: Molecular cloning, nucleotide sequence and expression of a full-length cDNA. Proceedings of the National Academy of Sciences USA 85: 7049–7053

Tschudy D P, Lamon J M 1980 Porphyrin metabolism and the porphyrias. In: Bondy P K, Rosenberg L E (eds) Duncan's diseases of metabolism, 8th edn. Saunders, Philadephia p 939

Tsega E, Besrat A, Damtew B et al 1981 Chloroquine in the treatment of porphyria cutanea tarda. Transactions of the Royal Society of Tropical Medicine and Hygiene 75: 401–404

Tu J-B, Blackwell R Q, Feng Y-S 1971 Clinical and biochemical studies of hereditary hepatic porphyria in Chinese subjects in Taiwan. Metabolism 20: 629–635

Wang A L, Arredondo-Vega F X, Giampietro P F et al 1981 Regional gene assignment of human porphobilinogen deaminase and esterase-A4 to chromosome 11q23→11qter. Proceedings of the National Academy of Sciences USA 78: 5734–5738

Weston M J, Nicholson D C, Lim C K et al 1978 Congenital erythropoietic uroporphyria (Gunther's disease) presenting in a middle aged man. International Journal of Biochemistry 9: 921–925

Wetmur J G, Bishop D F, Cantelmo S, Desnick R S 1986 Human (d)-aminolevulinate dehydratase. Nucleotide sequence of a full-length cDNA clone. Proceedings of the National Academy of Sciences USA 83: 7703–7707

Wetterberg L 1967 A neuropsychiatric and genetical investigation of acute intermittent porphyria. Svenska Bokfolaget, Norstedts: Scandinavian University Books

Whetsell W O Jr., Kappas A 1981 Protective effect of exogenous heme against lead toxicity in organotypic cultures of mouse dorsal root ganglia (DRG): Electron microscopic observations. Journal of Neuropathology and Experimental Neurology 760: Abstract 334

Whiting M J 1976 Synthesis of δ-aminolevulinate synthase by isolated liver polyribosomes. Biochemical Journal 158: 391–400

Yamamoto M, Yew N, Federspiel M, Dodgson J B, Hayashi N, Engel J D 1985 Isolation of recombinant cDNA, encoding chicken erythroid δ-aminolevulinate synthase. Proceedings of the National Academy of Sciences USA 82: 3702–3706

Yeung Laiwah A C, McColl K E L 1987 Management of attacks of acute porphyria. Drugs 34: 604–616

Yeung Laiwah A C, Moore M R, Goldberg A 1987 Pathogenesis of acute porphyria. Quarterly Journal of Medicine 241: 377–392

Yoshinaga T, Sano S 1980 Coproporphyrinogen oxidase. II. Reaction mechanism and role of tyrosine residues on the activity. Journal of Biological Chemistry 255: 4727–4731

99. Disorders of copper metabolism

D. M. Danks

GENERAL BACKGROUND

Copper is an essential micronutrient for man and animals, being a component of a number of important enzymes (Underwood 1977, Mason 1979, Danks 1980, Howell & Gawthorne 1987). Table 99.1 lists those enzymes or cellular functions for which copper has been proved essential. This list is probably not yet complete as other proteins appear to contain copper (e.g. clotting factor V). The consequences of nutritional copper deficiency observed in man and other animals correspond quite well to those which would be expected in the light of these functions (Table 99.2, Danks 1980). The precise effects differ between species, as does the order in which these effects develop on a deficient diet.

The adult human body contains 70–100 mg of copper, and the daily requirement is of the order of 1–5 mg. Absorption occurs in the upper small intestine by active processes which have not been fully defined. An equivalent amount is excreted in the bile, and very little of this biliary copper is reabsorbed. Renal losses are very small, filtered copper being reabsorbed efficiently. A moderate amount of copper is present in sweat, and in very hot climates this may become significant to the copper balance.

Copper absorbed from the intestine is transported by serum albumin bound to the amino-terminal tripeptide and is largely taken up by the liver. Histidine acts as an intermediary in the hepatic uptake process. A role for a newly recognised protein called transcuprein has been suggested. Some of the copper taken up by the liver reappears in the plasma over the next 48 hours in caeruloplasmin, a ferroxidase which may serve a role in the transport of copper to other tissues, but this process is poorly understood (Frieden 1980).

Copper must be delivered to the intra-cellular sites of synthesis of the various copper enzymes. Copper ions are very reactive and could not be tolerated free in body tissues. A very efficient system of specific transport processes must exist ensuring that copper ions are always

held complexed to larger molecules which deliver the copper to the sites where it is required. Genes must code for each of these transport molecules, and one can therefore anticipate a considerable number of genetic defects affecting copper homeostasis and availability.

To date three genetic defects are known in man. Wilson disease was discovered in 1912 and was shown to be related to copper homeostasis in 1948. Menkes syndrome was described in 1962 (Menkes et al 1962) and first shown to be related to copper metabolism in 1972 (Danks et al 1972b). The occipital horn syndrome has been related to copper deficiency more recently (Byers et al 1980, Peltonen et al 1983).

Availability of mice affected by mutations apparently homologous to those causing Menkes syndrome and the occipital horn syndrome and the use of tissue culture studies has advanced the understanding of these conditions. Neither of these advantages has been available to

Table 99.1 Copper enzymes in man

Common name	Functional role	Known or expected consequence of deficiency
Cytochrome oxidase	Electron transport chain	Uncertain
Superoxide dismutase	Free radical detoxification	Uncertain
Tyrosinase	Melanin production	Failure of pigmentation
Dopamine β hydroxylase	Catecholamine production	Neurological effects, type uncertain
Lysyl oxidase	Cross-linking of collagen and elastin	Vascular rupture
Caeruloplasmin	Ferroxidase ?other roles	Anaemia
Enzyme not known	Cross-linking of keratin (disulphide bonds)	Pili torti

Table 99.2 Effects seen in nutritional copper deficiency in man, sheep, rats, pigs, and in Menkes syndrome

Effect	Man	Sheep	Rat	Pig	Menkes syndrome
Anaemia	+ +	+ +	+ +	+ +	−
Neutropenia	+	+	+	+	−
Abnormal hair structure	±	+ +	+	+	+ +
Depigmentation	±	+	+	+	+
Arterial rupture	?	−	+	+ +	+ +
Myocardial fibrosis	?	−	+	+	−
Osteoporosis	+	±	+	+ +	+
Emphysema	?	−	+	−	+
Cerebellar ataxia	−	+ *	+ *	+ *	+
Other brain damage	−	+ *	+ *	+	+ +

*Seen only after fetal copper deficiency

those studying Wilson disease, but recent discoveries offer new possibilities, mentioned below. References throughout this chapter are to recent articles which review a particular topic. No attempt is made to cite first observations of particular findings.

WILSON DISEASE

The majority of the statements in this section can be supported and expanded by reference to a recent monograph (Scheinberg & Sternlieb 1984). Only a few facts need separate referencing.

Clinical features

Clinical presentation is generally with liver disease or with neurological disturbance. Hepatic symptoms may occur at any age, but are more frequently seen in childhood between the ages of 8 and 16 years (Odievre et al 1974, Sass-Kortsak 1975). Presentation with neurological symptoms before the age of 14 years is very unusual and is most frequent between the ages of 20 and 40 years.

Almost any symptom of liver disease may be seen, but acute presentation is surprisingly frequent for a basic process which is undoubtedly very slow and gradual in its effects. Some children are diagnosed only in the second or third episode of acute jaundice, earlier episodes being ascribed to hepatitis – a tragic situation if the final episode is fulminant and fatal. Haemolysis is often a prominent feature of the more severe acute hepatic episodes, and some patients present with haemolysis unaccompanied by other features of liver failure. However, liver disease is always found on investigation of such patients.

Dysarthria and deterioration of coordination and voluntary movement are the most frequent neurological symptoms. These are often accompanied by involuntary

movements and by disorders of posture and tone. A concomitant loss of intellectual function and/or disturbances of behaviour may or may not be seen at the onset, but always develops later. Untreated, these symptoms progress to bulbar palsy and death.

Osteoarthropathy, renal tubular acidosis, renal calculi, and cardiomyopathy are seen quite frequently and may occasionally be the presenting feature. Kayser-Fleischer rings provide the most valuable diagnostic sign of Wilson disease, but do not cause any symptoms. Golden-brown granular pigmentation is seen in the outer crescent of the iris at the limbus. Sometimes they can be observed with the naked eye, but slit lamp examination is required in many patients to detect this sign. Anaemia, cataracts, and hypoparathyroidism (Carpenter et al 1983) are occasional features.

Regardless of the mode of presentation, some degree of liver disease is always present if evidence is sought.

Laboratory and cell culture findings

Typically serum caeruloplasmin is greatly reduced, and the non-caeruloplasmin copper concentration is increased. The net effect is a moderate reduction in the total serum copper level. Urinary copper excretion is increased, and the excretion is very greatly augmented after administration of penicillamine. Liver copper concentration is greatly increased. Typical figures are quoted in Table 99.3.

The ultimate test for Wilson disease at the present time is the demonstration of a gross reduction of incorporation of copper isotope into caeruloplasmin. Total plasma radioactivity continues to fall over 48 hours after intravenous injection of ^{64}Cu in patients with Wilson disease. A secondary rise in radioactivity is seen in normal subjects from 4 hours through to 48 hours due to the appearance of labelled caeruloplasmin. Intermediate

Table 99.3 Typical copper measurements in Wilson disease

	Wilson disease	Normal (adults)
Serum caeruloplasmin		
OD units per ml	0–0.25	0.25–0.49
mg/l	0–200	200–400
Serum copper μmol/l	3–10	11–24
Urinary copper		
(μg per 24 hours)		
Untreated	100–1000	<40
On penicillamine– 250 mg 6 hourly	1500–3000	100–600

results (i.e. smaller secondary rise) are seen in some heterozygotes for Wilson disease and in patients with copper retention secondary to other forms of liver disease.

Other tests reveal the damaging effects of the disease on the various organs affected and are useful in diagnosis. Some results are relatively specific and others quite nonspecific. Any or all liver functions may be deranged; no particular pattern of derangement is characteristic. Generalised aminoaciduria, glucosuria and defective urinary acidification are frequent and similar to those found in many other diseases damaging renal tubules. Anaemia (normochromic), neutropenia, and thrombocytopenia are occasionally seen. Some microscopic findings in liver biopsies were proposed to be rather specific (e.g. marked glycogen accumulation in hepatocyte nuclei), but most authors now agree that the changes are variable and nonspecific.

Investigation of patients with neurological symptoms generally includes EEG, which only rarely gives a specific result, and CT scan, in which increased radiolucency of the basal ganglia has been described, but has not proved a constant finding.

Fibroblastic cells grown from skin biopsies have been found to accumulate abnormally high concentrations of copper (Goka et al 1976, Chan et al 1980, Camakaris et al 1980a). The change is not marked as in Menkes disease, nor entirely consistent, and has not proved useful in diagnosis, although it does offer some possibilities for research into the basic defect.

Diagnosis

Wilson disease is an important condition because it is one of the very few treatable causes of chronic liver disease and of chronic brain degeneration. Clinicians must therefore keep it in mind. It is numerically significant in both these clinical situations. Indeed, it is the most frequent single cause of cirrhosis in later childhood,

causing approximately 20% of all cases of cirrhosis which develop between the ages of 4 and 16 years (Sass-Kortsak 1975).

Paediatricians should, therefore, take the attitude that chronic liver disease presenting after 4 or 5 years of age is due to Wilson disease until proved otherwise. A similar attitude to adult patients is probably justified, but is harder to promote because the high frequency of alcoholic liver disease tends to obscure the situation. Wilson disease can cause effects indistinguishable from chronic active hepatitis, and presentation with cirrhosis is possible even in late middle age.

The classical diagnostic tests (examination for Kayser-Fleischer rings, measurement of serum copper and caeruloplasmin and the 24 hour urinary excretion of copper) will identify 95% of adult cases, but fail in approximately 15–20% of childhood cases. The copper content of a needle liver biopsy should therefore be measured in every child with chronic liver disease. A sample of about 5 mg should be analysed to avoid erroneous interpretation due to uneven distribution of copper in the liver. Copper levels above 500 μg per gram dry weight are usually diagnostic, but such levels may occur in some other forms of liver disease, and ^{64}Cu studies may be needed to finalise the diagnosis. Only by taking this aggressive attitude will the tragic failure to diagnose Wilson disease be eliminated.

Treatment

Penicillamine is a very effective drug for the treatment of Wilson disease, using 1–3 g per 24 hours in adult patients or in older children. Dosage is monitored by 24 hour urinary excretion of copper, which should be kept in the range of 1–3 mg daily. Serious complications were frequent when DL-penicillamine was used, but are uncommon with pure D-penicillamine. A nephrotic syndrome was very frequent and is still encountered occasionally. Thrombocytopenia, skin rashes, and the rare skin lesion elastosis perforans are the most common complications. A short course of prednisolone may control these effects, but they may persist and necessitate withdrawing the drug. Bone marrow aplasia can occur.

When serious complications of penicillamine therapy develop and persist, other chelating drugs may be considered (e.g. triethylene tetramine). An alternative is administration of zinc, which competes with copper for intestinal absorption. Negative copper balance sufficient for effective control of the disease can be achieved with doses of 50 mg (as sulphate or as acetate, best given on an empty stomach) three times in 24 hours (Hoogenraad et al 1983, Hill et al 1987, Milanino et al 1989).

Penicillamine has an effect on clinical features only

after several weeks (neurological features) or several months (liver disease). Consequently, it is very difficult to save patients who present in a fulminant episode of liver failure, which can be associated with the release into the circulation of as much as 30 mg of copper daily (author's experience). A method of removing copper rapidly during acute fulminant liver failure is needed. Peritoneal dialysis and plasmaphoresis are the most effective measures. Haemodialysis is a poor substitute for peritoneal dialysis for this purpose (author's experience). Albumin infusion may increase the binding of the large amount of non-caeruloplasmin copper present in these episodes; tetrathiomolybdate is able to bind this copper rapidly and strongly (author's experience), but its place in therapy is not yet clear. All too often these measures prove insufficient and liver transplantation needs to be considered early enough to be effective.

In neurological cases which are diagnosed only after considerable damage has occurred, and while awaiting a response to penicillamine, L-dopa may be useful as a symptomatic measure.

Genetics and genetic heterogeneity

Inheritance is autosomal recessive as indicated by the occurrence of the disease in sibs with the expected segregation ratio and by parental consanguinity. The incidence is not known accurately, but is in the range of 1 in 50 000 to 1 in 100 000 live births. The gene locus is closely linked to that of esterase D and that concerned in retinoblastoma at 13q14 (Bonne-Tamir et al 1986).

The range of disease effects and severity is wide, and allelic heterogeneity is almost certain. However, the most striking difference – that between hepatic and neurological presentation – does not seem to be explained by allelic variation. Many families have been described in which one sib has presented with liver manifestations and another with neurological onset. Females more often present with liver disease and males with neurological features. A particularly mild neurological form has been described in New York among Jewish immigrants from Eastern Europe (Bearn 1960).

Heterozygotes do not show any clinical manifestations. Approximately 10% have lowered levels of serum copper and caeruloplasmin. An intermediate secondary rise in plasma radioactivity after ^{64}Cu is seen in heterozygotes as a group, but cannot be used to identify individual heterozygotes.

Genetic counselling

Sibs of a patient with Wilson disease have a 1 in 4 risk of developing the disease. These sibs should be examined for liver or neurological disease, for Kayser-Fleischer rings and by measuring serum copper, serum caeroloplasmin and urinary copper, or by linkage analysis. Patients older than the index case may be assumed to be unaffected if no abnormalities are detected. Younger sibs should be investigated more fully using liver biopsy or ^{64}Cu studies if initial tests are normal.

Investigation of potential heterozygotes has little value, because available tests are not reliable and cannot be interpreted when applied to individuals with low a priori risks of being heterozygotes (e.g. spouses of aunts or uncles who may be heterozygotes). Linkage analysis may identify heterozygotes within affected families but is useless in the unrelated spouses.

The risk to offspring of affected individuals is low. Over 50 pregnancies with normal babies have been reported in patients in good clinical health on penicillamine treatment during pregnancy. Two reports have described babies with unusual connective tissue changes born to women on penicillamine therapy for cystinuria and rheumatoid arthritis respectively (Mjølnerød et al 1971, Linares et al 1979). Interference with collagen cross-linking by penicillamine itself or by reduced availability of copper was blamed. Copper accumulation in tissues is probably protective in Wilson disease. For the present, it seems reasonable to continue penicillamine during pregnancy if the maternal disease has been treated for a relatively short time. In long-treated patients, no clinical effects are seen during rests from therapy for six or nine months, and cessation during pregnancy might be preferable. On the other hand, longer-term withdrawal of treatment for periods exceeding two years has proved lethal (Walshe & Dixon 1986).

Prenatal diagnosis/presymptomatic diagnosis

Prenatal diagnosis is now possible in many families by linkage analysis using esterase D or linked anonymous DNA probes. Many may doubt the place of prenatal diagnosis in a disease of late onset for which effective treatment is available.

Mass screening of newborn babies has been suggested, and simple methods of measuring serum caeruloplasmin do exist. However, the very low levels seen in normal newborn babies make recognition at this age very difficult. Early symptomatic diagnosis of first cases in families through constant awareness should be sufficient.

Pathogenesis

The basic biochemical defect is unknown. It is not a defect in the structure of caeruloplasmin. The gene coding for caeruloplasmin is at 3q25 (Yang et al 1986) and that involved in Wilson disease is close to 13q14 (Bonne-Tamir et al 1986). Genetically determined deficiency of caeruloplasmin does not cause liver or brain disease (Edwards et al 1979). The two most fundamental defects are slow production of caeruloplasmin and severe interference with biliary excretion of copper. Presumably the defect lies in some step common to both these processes. The difficulty of studying these processes in the liver and the lack of a satisfactory animal model have hindered research. Work with cell cultures (see above), Bedlington terriers, and toxic milk mice (see below) may change this situation.

Copper accumulates progressively in Wilson disease, and the sub-cellular distribution changes during the course of the disease. Some have suggested that aggregates of copper metallothionein in lysosomes are less toxic than cytoplasmic copper-metallothionein.

The rate of accumulation and other unknown factors influence the degree of liver damage. Intercurrent virus infections may play a part in precipitating symptomatic liver disease. If liver damage is not too severe, the patient lives on and copper 'overflows' from the liver to the brain, eyes, kidney, myocardium and many other tissues. This overflow can also occur in copper accumulation secondary to other forms of liver disease. This fact and the improvement seen after liver transplantation support the idea that the extrahepatic effects are secondary to overflow from the liver.

Haemolytic crises are associated with very high levels of non-caeruloplasmin plasma copper. It is likely that some acute hepatic insult (e.g. an intercurrent virus infection) releases more copper than can be complexed in the plasma and induces acute copper poisoning with haemolysis and further liver damage.

Animal models

Attempts to mimic Wilson disease by chronic copper poisoning of laboratory animals are very artificial and unsatisfactory as models for the disease. Bedlington terriers with a recessively inherited disease involving hepatic copper accumulation (Su et al 1982a,b) and progressive liver disease may have a similar defect. The defect in toxic milk mice seems to resemble Wilson disease even more closely (Rauch 1983), and these animals could be studied more readily if they are made available in the future.

MENKES SYNDROME

A more detailed review has been published (Danks 1987) and provides more detailed documentation of original sources.

Clinical features

The full clinical syndrome comprises abnormal hair, progressive cerebral degeneration, hypopigmentation, bone changes, arterial rupture and thrombosis, ureteric and bladder diverticulae, and hypothermia (Danks et al 1972a, Danks 1987).

Premature delivery is very frequent, as is neonatal hyperbilirubinaemia. Hypothermia is common in the neonatal period and even in older babies. At this stage, the child's appearance may be normal with fine normal hair. However, some patients have trichorrhexis nodosa and monilethrix at birth, and the characteristic facies may also be apparent. Neonatal symptoms may resolve, and the baby may seem normal during the next month or two although growth may be slow. By about 2 or 3 months of age, the more flagrant symptoms of developmental delay, loss of early developmental skills, and convulsions appear. Cerebral degeneration then dominates the clinical picture with various vascular complications, particularly intracranial, and death occurs between the age of 6 months and 3 years in most cases.

The hair becomes tangled, lustreless and greyish, with a stubble of broken hairs palpable over the occiput and temporal regions where the hair rubs on sheets. Pili torti are found microscopically (Figs 99.1 and 99.2). The facies is quite characteristic with pudgy cheeks and abnormal eyebrows and is recognisable even in babies who have no hair. Skeletal X-rays show osteoporosis and widening of the flared metaphyses with spiky protrusions at the edges, which may fracture (Kozlowski & McCrossin 1979). Rib fractures are common. Wormian bones are usually seen in the skull. The combination of these bony changes with a subdural haematoma may lead to the erroneous diagnosis of child abuse. Studies to demonstrate the brain substance (CT scan or air studies) may show macroscopic patches of brain destruction. Arteriograms show elongation, tortuosity and variable calibre of major arteries throughout the brain, viscera and limbs, with areas of localised dilatation and other areas of marked narrowing (Danks et al 1972a). Emphysema, bladder or ureteric diverticulae, and retinal tears have been described. The bladder or ureteric diverticulae may rupture or become infected.

One very mildly affected patient has been described who presented at the age of 2 years with mild mental retardation and marked cerebellar ataxia (Procopis et al 1981). At 9 years, he is intellectually normal but still has some ataxia (Danks 1988). He has been treated with injections of copper histidine since diagnosis. Pili torti were present, bone changes were very mild, and arteriography showed generalised elongation and uniform dilatation of arteries. CT scan was normal. Another

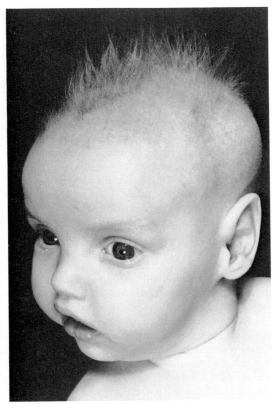

Fig. 99.1 Typical appearance of baby with Menkes syndrome aged 5 months.

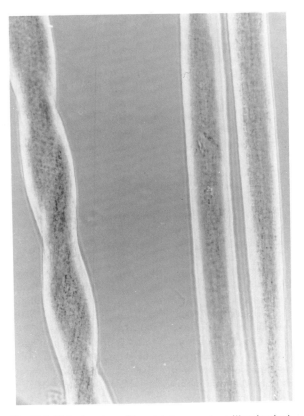

Fig. 99.2 Hair showing pili torti (phase contrast illumination).

patient aged 9 years has low normal intelligence, mild ataxia, bladder diverticulae, and loose skin and joints (Westman et al 1988). Several other patients have lived 10 years or more despite profound brain damage present from the first year. These are not truly mild affected individuals.

Laboratory and cell culture findings

Serum copper and caeruloplasmin levels are very low. Interpretation is complicated by the changing values for these measurements during the first weeks in normal babies, who are born with very little caeruloplasmin (and therefore very low serum copper levels) and achieve adult levels by about 2 years. The rise is rapid in the first weeks in normal babies. Levels in affected babies cannot be distinguished from normal until 2 weeks (Grover et al 1979).

Liver content of copper is grossly reduced, and duodenal or jejunal biopsy shows greatly increased copper content (Table 99.4). Oral ^{64}Cu is poorly absorbed; ^{64}Cu given intravenously is cleared from plasma and incorpor-

ated into caeruloplasmin quite normally (Lucky & Hsia 1979). Typical copper measurements are shown in Table 99.4.

Disturbances of copper handling in cultured cells comprise the most definitive test for the disease (Chan et al 1978, Camakaris et al 1980b, Prins & van den Hamer 1980). Cells (fibroblastic, amniotic or lymphoid) show increased copper content, increased sensitivity to killing

Table 99.4 Typical copper measurements in Menkes syndrome at usual age of diagnosis

	Menkes disease (3–12 months)	Normal (3–12 months)
Serum caeruloplasmin		
OD units per ml	<0.08	>0.25
mg/l	<50	>200
Serum copper μmol/l	<6	>12
Liver copper		
μg/g dry weight	10–20	140–70
Duodenal copper		
μg/g dry weight	50–80	7–29

Table 99.5 Findings of Menkes syndrome in cultured cells (fibroblastic or amniotic) used diagnostically in our laboratory (Camakaris et al 1980)

	Normal cells	Menkes cells
Copper content (μg per 10^6 cells)		
in normal medium	0.023 ± 0.013*	0.282 ± 0.091*
with added copper	0.113 ± 0.074*	0.770 ± 0.156*
(6 μg per ml)		
^{64}Cu content after 24 hours (μg ^{64}Cu per 10^6 cells)	0.004 ± 0.001*	0.060 ± 0.019*
^{64}Cu efflux over subsequent 24 hours in culture (% of content at 24 hours)	70–90%	0–5%

*Standard deviation

by copper added to culture medium, increased retention of ^{64}Cu added to culture medium for 24 hours, and markedly decreased release of this ^{64}Cu if cells are then grown for a further 24 hours in medium free of isotope. Typical results are shown in Table 99.5. These findings are influenced by the phase of fibroblastic cell growth at the time of testing. Use of confluent cultures which have been held in a non-dividing state by reducing the fetal calf serum in medium containing very little copper gives most reproducible results in our experience. Special care is needed in prenatal diagnosis using amniotic cells.

Reduced levels of various copper enzyme activities have been demonstrated. Light and electron microscopy show changes in elastin in the aortic wall which are consistent with defective cross–linking (Oakes et al 1976). Hair keratin analyses show defective disulphide bonding (Danks et al 1972b).

Diagnosis

Diagnosis can be made with great confidence by the clinical features. Microscopic examination of the hair is very helpful even in a mild case. Low levels of serum copper and caeruloplasmin will clinch the diagnosis. Assay of copper in gut mucosal or liver biopsies may be used, or studies of cell cultures, which comprise the ultimate test, showing marked abnormality even in the mild case (Procopis et al 1981).

Treatment

No form of treatment has yet been shown to be truly effective. Copper has been administered parenterally in a number of different forms – copper sulphate, copper chloride, copper EDTA, copper glycinate, copper histi-

dinate, and copper albumin complex. Copper nitriloacetate is the only form of copper which has proved to be absorbed from the intestine (Grover et al 1979). All these forms of treatment have corrected the hepatic copper deficiency and restored normal levels of serum copper. Some improvement in physical condition has resulted, but has not prevented fatal outcome or prevented the continuing cerebral degeneration. Restoration of normal brain copper levels has not been achieved (Grover et al 1979). Copper histidinate is the most physiological of these treatments and has definitely modified the course of the disease when started before symptoms developed in one Canadian boy (Sass-Kortsak, personal communication) and in one Swiss boy (Baerlocher et al 1983).

There may be a critical phase in brain development when copper is especially important – 7–10 days of age in brindled mice (Wenk & Suzuki 1982). It is likely that many of the effects of the disease are already established in utero and that postnatal treatment cannot be fully effective. However, the search should be continued for some chemical form of copper which can bypass the disturbance in copper transport and deliver the copper to the copper enzymes which require it, even in the brain.

Genetics and genetic heterogeneity

Numerous pedigrees show X–linked recessive inheritance which is further supported by the mosaic skin depigmentation seen in a Black heterozygous female (Volpintesta 1974) and the pili torti seen in some heterozygotes (Moore & Howell 1985). Mental retardation has been described in two girls, sisters of severely affected males (Iwakawa et al 1979, Barton et al 1983) and in a girl with an X;2 translocation (Kapur et al 1987). The fact that the breakpoint was at Xp13 suggests this as the Menkes locus, an interpretation which accords with linkage results (Horn et al 1984).

Experience in Melbourne in 1966–71 suggested an incidence of 1 in 35 000 (Danks et al 1972a), but further experience indicates a figure nearer to 1 in 100 000.

The mildly affected boys described recently (see above) presumably represent allelic variants.

Heterozygotes may show abnormalities in cultured cells similar to those seen in affected males, but X–chromosome inactivation confounds the situation quite seriously. In fact, only about half of obligate heterozygotes are identified by studies on a single skin biopsy (Camakaris et al 1980b, Horn 1980). Use of two or three biopsies from separate sites improves the diagnostic ability considerably, as does cloning of the fibroblastic cells grown from a biopsy (Horn et al 1980). Development of a test using hair roots seems desirable. At present, one can say that presence of pili torti, of mosaic skin pigmentation, or of abnormal cell culture results demonstrates heterozygosity in a female relative, but one cannot exclude heterozygosity with confidence.

Prenatal diagnosis

Any or all of the disturbances of copper metabolism in cultured cells which are described above can be used for prenatal diagnosis. Experience in Melbourne supports the idea of using all four characteristics and taking great care to standardise the cell culture conditions. ^{64}Cu retention after 24 hours has been used alone by other groups (Horn 1976), but is particularly susceptible to alteration according to the phase of cell culture and to the copper content of the medium in our experience. Release of ^{64}Cu during a subsequent 24 hours in media without isotope is least affected by culture variables, and is the most reliable single test in our laboratory. The elevated copper content of chorionic samples can be used for earlier diagnosis, but great care is needed to avoid copper contamination (Tønnesen et al 1985, 1989).

Prenatal diagnosis should probably be concentrated on in a few laboratories heavily involved with research on cellular copper metabolism.

Pathogenesis

The primary defect causes accumulation of copper in cells in a form unavailable to the sites of copper enzyme synthesis (Prins & Van den Hamer 1980, Danks & Camakaris 1983, Danks 1987). The precise fault in copper transport within the cells is not yet identified. Deficiency of a copper transport protein seems likely, allowing diversion of copper to bind to metallothionein and accumulate in this form.

Because copper transport is defective in the intestinal mucosa, profound copper deficiency develops. This is aggravated by defective reabsorption of copper from the urinary filtrate. Even that copper which is absorbed is bound to metallothionein and is poorly available in most tissues. The effective copper deficiency is much greater than the levels measured in various tissues would suggest.

Before birth, functional copper deficiency is probably less severe (Danks 1987), but is presumably still present, since symptoms are apparent at birth.

The actual clinical features can be explained by failure of the various copper enzymes listed in Table 99.1 and they match up rather closely with the effects of copper deficiency listed in Table 99.2. The absence of anaemia and neutropenia is remarkable and unexplained.

Animal models

The *mottled* mutants in the mouse exhibit disturbances of copper metabolism which are so similar to those of Menkes syndrome that homology of the loci is proposed,

especially because both loci are X-chromosomal (Hunt 1974). Of the mottled variants, presumed to be allelic, *brindled* is nearest to typical Menkes syndrome in severity. Research on these animals has advanced understanding of the human disease very greatly (Prins & Van den Hamer 1980, Danks & Camakaris 1983, Danks 1986).

OCCIPITAL HORN SYNDROME

Connective tissue abnormalities in this X-linked condition have been recognised for some years. It has been identified as a copper deficiency disease more recently (Byers et al 1980, Peltonen et al 1983). The previous names of 'X-linked cutis laxa' and 'Ehlers-Danlos syndrome type IX' have been discarded.

Clincal features

Most boys with this condition present during childhood with loose skin, loose joints, hernias, or complications of bladder diverticulae or ureteric abnormalities. The ossified horn on the occipital region may be palpable, but is more often seen only on X-rays. Abnormalities in the shape of the lateral ends of clavicles and in metaphyses of the long bones are also observed. Statements, positive or negative, about the other clinical features that might be expected in copper deficiency are lacking in most of the reports, but in individual patients one can discern abnormalities of facial appearance, hair, and arteries (Sartoris et al 1984).

Laboratory and cell culture findings

Serum copper and caeruloplasmin levels are low, but may occasionally be only just below the lower limit of normal. Lysyl oxidase activity in skin and cultured cells is greatly reduced (Kuivaniemi et al 1985). Copper studies in cultured cells show abnormalities which are indistinguishable from those seen in Menkes disease (Peltonen et al 1983). The levels of copper in liver, in intestinal mucosa, or in other relevant tissues have not been reported, nor have measurements of other copper enzymes. Diagnosis can be made by the clinical features and family history and by measurement of copper levels in serum or in cultured cells.

Treatment

There have been no reports of copper treatment in this disease.

Genetics and genetic heterogeneity

The X-linked inheritance of this condition is well documented even though only three families have been described. Prenatal diagnosis has not been described, but could presumably be performed by the methods used in Menkes disease. One would expect identical results.

Pathogenesis

This condition may be a mild allelic variant of Menkes disease. The different balance of the various features of copper deficiency in the occipital horn syndrome relative to Menkes disease is reminiscent of the differences between blotchy and brindled mice. It is possible that there is one locus involved in copper transport on the X chromosome in humans and in mice, and an array of mutations affecting its function to different degrees. Alternatively, there may be several gene loci closely linked on the X chromosome and concerned in sequential steps of intracellular copper transport. Menkes disease and the brindled mutation may be homologous to one another and the occipital horn syndrome and the blotchy mutant may be homologous lesions of another locus (Danks 1986).

OTHER POSSIBLE GENETIC DEFECTS OF COPPER METABOLISM

Since the distribution of copper throughout the body, including absorption and excretion, must involve many separate gene-controlled functions, there must be many genetic diseases of copper transport still to be discovered. These should be sought among diseases with abnormal hair, with depigmentation, with arterial degeneration, and with each of the other symptoms that are known to occur in copper deficiency (Table 99.2). Other diseases due to copper accumulation may also exist.

Liver diseases associated with hepatic copper retention

Since the majority of copper excreted from the body is put out in the bile, one might expect copper retention as a secondary effect in a number of liver diseases. This is true, but the occurrence of copper retention is not as predictable as one might expect. In particular, it should be a constant feature of diseases like extrahepatic biliary atresia which cause complete obstruction to bile flow. While some patients do show gross copper retention, others have normal levels of liver copper. The levels of

liver copper are very variable in most forms of liver disease with occasional patients showing high levels (Smallwood et al 1968, Reed et al 1972). The reason for these differences must be sought in future work which will also need to evaluate the role of copper chelation in the treatment of these patients.

Hepatic copper retention is a more consistent feature of some liver diseases and may be the basic cause of the disease. In *primary biliary cirrhosis* the copper accumulation in liver cells exceeds even that seen in Wilson disease. Penicillamine therapy has been shown to be beneficial, but not to the same degree as in Wilson disease. A rather specific secondary interference with copper excretion is most probable (Scheinberg & Sternlieb 1984), but the possibility of a primary defect in copper transport must not be dismissed. Genetic factors are not established as important in primary biliary cirrhosis.

Indian childhood cirrhosis is consistently associated with hepatic copper retention (Tanner & Portmann 1981). As yet no trials of penicillamine therapy have been reported. Copper transport in cultured cells appears normal (Camakaris, personal communication). Genetic factors are considered important in the cause of this particular form of childhood liver disease, and a primary defect in copper transport is possible.

Several patients with different forms of *neonatal cholestatic liver disease* have been shown to accumulate large amounts of copper in the liver (Evans et al 1978, Smith & Danks 1978, Kaplinsky et al 1980). The cases reported are rather heterogenous in their basic causes, and more studies will be needed to see whether any particular forms of neonatal liver disease are involved. The two forms that warrant closest attention are the recessively inherited condition of neonatal cholestatic jaundice and lymphoedema described by Aagenaes (1974) and the arterioductular hypoplasia syndrome (Alagille et al 1987). One child with the former syndrome developed extreme hepatic copper accumulation before dying of cirrhosis at the age of 5 years, and had also deposited enough copper in the basal ganglia to produce signs of lenticular degeneration very similar to those in Wilson disease (Smith & Danks 1978). More patients with this condition should be studied. In arterio-ductular hypoplasia copper retention is frequent, but is more likely to be secondary. This condition shows autosomal dominant inheritance.

REFERENCES

Aagenaes O 1974 Hereditary recurrent cholestasis with lymphoedema - Two new families. Acta Paediatrica Scandinavica 63: 465–471

Alagille D, Estrada A, Haochouel M, Gautier M, Odievre M, Dommergues J P 1987 Syndromic paucity of interlobular

bile ducts (Alagille syndrome or arteriohepatic dysplasia)-review of 80 cases. Journal of Pediatrics 110: 195–200

Baerlocher K E, Steinmann B, Rao V H, Gitzelmann R, Horn N 1983 Menkes' disease: Clinical, therapeutic and biochemical studies. Journal of Inherited Metabolic Diseases 6(Suppl 2): 87–88

Barton N W, Dambrosia J M, Barranger J A 1983 Menkes

kinky-hair syndrome: Report of a case in a female infant. Neurology 33(Suppl 2): 154.

Bearn A G 1960 Genetic analysis of Wilson's disease. Annals of Human Genetics 24: 33–43

Bonne-Tamir B, Farrer L A, Frydman M, Kanaaneh H 1986 Evidence for linkage between Wilson disease and esterase D in three kindreds: Detection of linkage for an autosomal recessive disorder by the family study method. Genetic Epidemiology 3: 201–209

Byers P H, Siegel R C, Holbrook K A, Narayanan A S, Bornstein P, Hall J G 1980 X-linked cutis laxa: Defective cross-link formation in collagen due to decreased lysyl oxidase activity. New England Journal of Medicine 303: 61–65

Camakaris J, Ackland L, Danks D M 1980a Abnormal copper metabolism in cultured cells from patients with Wilson's disease. Journal of Inherited Metabolic Diseases 3: 155–158.

Camakaris J, Danks D M, Ackland L, Cartwright E, Borger P, Cotton R G H 1980b Altered copper metabolism in cultured cells from human Menkes' syndrome and mottled mouse mutants. Biochemical Genetics 18: 117–131

Carpenter T O, Carnes D L Jr., Anast C S 1983 Hypoparathyroidism in Wilson's disease. New England Journal of Medicine 309: 873–877

Chan W Y, Garnica A D, Rennert O M 1978 Cell culture studies of Menkes' kinky hair disease. Clinica Chimica Acta 88: 495–507

Chan W Y, Cushing W, Cofeman M A, Rennert O M 1980 Genetic expression of Wilson's disease in cell culture: a diagnostic marker. Science 208: 299–300

Danks D M 1980 Copper deficiency in humans. Excerpta Medica Amsterdam (Ciba Symposium 79) 209–220

Danks D M 1986 Of mice and men, metals and mutations. Journal of Medical Genetics 23: 99–106

Danks D M 1987 Copper deficiency in infants with particular reference to Menkes' disease. In: Howell J McD, Gawthorne J M (eds) Copper in Man and Animals. C R C Press Boca Raton

Danks D M 1988 The mild form of Menkes disease: progress report on the original case. American Journal of Medical Genetics 30: 859–864

Danks D M, Camakaris J 1983 Mutations affecting trace elements. In: Harris H, Hirshhorn K (eds) Advances in Human Genetics. Plenum Press, New York, 13: 149–216

Danks D M, Campbell P E, Stevens B J, Mayne V, Cartwright E 1972a Menkes' kinky hair syndrome: an inherited defect in copper absorption with widespread effects. Pediatrics 50: 188–201

Danks D M, Stevens B J, Campbell P E, Gillespie J M, Walker-Smith J, Blomfield J, Turner B 1972b Menkes' kinky-hair syndrome. Lancet i: 1100–1103

Edwards C Q, Williams D M, Cartwright G E 1979 Hereditary hypoceruloplasminemia. Clinical Genetics 15: 311–316

Evans J, Newman S, Sherlock S 1978 Liver copper levels in intrahepatic cholestasis of childhood. Gastroenterology 75: 875–878

Frieden E 1980 Caeruloplasmin: a multifunctional metalloprotein of vertebrate plasma. Excerpta Medica Amsterdam (Ciba Symposium 79): 93–124

Goka T J, Stevenson R E, Hefferan P M, Howell R R 1976 Menkes' disease: a biochemical abnormality in cultured human fibroblasts. Proceedings of the National Academy of Sciences USA 73: 604–606

Grover W D, Johnson W C, Henkin R I 1979 Clinical and biochemical aspects of trichopoliodystrophy. Annals of Neurology 5: 65–71

Hill G M, Brewer G J, Prasad A S, Hydrick C R, Hartmann D E 1987 Treatment of Wilson's disease with zinc: I. Oral zinc therapy regimens. Hepatology 7: 522–528

Hoogenraad T U, Van den Hamer C J A 1983 Three years of continuous oral zinc therapy in 4 patients with Wilson's disease. Acta Neurologica Scandinavica 67: 356–364

Horn N 1976 Copper incorporation studies on cultured cells for prenatal diagnosis of Menkes' disease. Lancet i: 1156–1158

Horn N 1980 Menkes' X-linked disease: heterozygous phenotypic in cloned fibroblast cultures. Journal of Medical Genetics 17: 257–261

Horn N, Mooy P, McGuire V M 1980 Menkes' X-linked disease, two clonal cell populations in heterozygotes. Journal of Medical Genetics 17: 262–266

Horn N, Stene J, Mollekaer M A, Friedrich U 1984 Linkage studies in Menkes disease. The Xg blood group system and C-banding of the X chromosome. Annals of Human Genetics 48: 161–172

Howell J McC, Gawthorne J M (eds) 1987 Copper in Man and Animals. C R C Press, Boca Raton

Hunt D M 1974 Primary defect in copper transport underlies mottled mutants in the mouse. Nature 249: 852–854

Iwakawa Y, Niwa T, Tomita M et al 1979 Menkes' kinky hair syndrome: report on an autopsy case and his female sibling with similar clinical manifestations. Brain Development (Tokyo) 11: 260–266

Kaplinsky C, Sternlieb I, Javitt N, Rotem Y 1980 Familial cholestatic cirrhosis associated with Kayser-Fleischer rings. Pediatrics 65: 782–788

Kapur S, Higgins J V, Delp K, Rogers B 1987 Menkes Syndrome in a girl with X-autosome translocation. American Journal of Medical Genetics 26: 503–510

Kozlowski K, McCrossin R 1979 Early osseous abnormalities in Menkes' kinky-hair syndrome. Pediatric Radiology 8: 191–194.

Kuivaniemi H, Peltonen L, Kivirikko K I 1985 Type IX Ehlers-Danlos syndrome and Menkes syndrome: the decrease in lysyl oxidase is associated with a corresponding deficiency in the enzyme protein. American Journal of Human Genetics 37: 798–808

Linares A, Zarranz J J, Rodriguez-Alarcon J, Diaz-Perez J L 1979 Reversible cutis laxa due to maternal D-penicillamine treatment. Lancet ii: 43

Lucky A W, Hsia Y E 1979 Distribution of ingested and injected radiocopper in two patients with Menkes' kinky-hair disease. Pediatric Research 13: 1280–1284

Mason K E 1979 A conspectus of research on copper metabolism and requirements in man. Journal of Nutrition 109: 1979–2066

Menkes J H, Alter M, Steigleder G K, Weakley D R, Sung J H 1962 A sex-linked recessive disorder with retardation of growth, peculiar hair and focal cerebral and cerebellar degeneration, Pediatrics 29: 764–779

Milanino R, Marrella M, Moretti U, Velo, G P, Deganello A, Ribezzo G, Tato L 1989 Oral zinc sulphate as primary therapeutic intervention in a child with Wilson disease. European Journal of Pediatrics 148: 654–655

Mjølnerød O K, Rasmussen K, Dommerud S A, Gjeruldsen S T 1971 Congenital connective-tissue defect probably due to D-penicillamine treatment in pregnancy. Lancet i: 673–675

Moore C M, Howell R 1985 Ectodermal manifestations in Menkes disease. Clinical Genetics 28: 532–540

Oakes B W, Danks D M, Campbell P E 1976 Human copper deficiency: ultrastructural studies of the aorta and skin in a child with Menkes' syndrome. Experimental and Molecular Pathology 25: 82–98

Odievre M, Vedrenne J, Landrieu P, Alagille D 1974 Les formes hepatiques 'pures' de la maladie de Wilson chez l'enfant: à propos de dix observations. Archives Francaises de Pediatrie 31: 215–222

Peltonen L, Kuivaniemi H, Palotie A, Horn N, Kaitila I, Kivirikko K L 1983 Alterations of copper and collagen metabolism in the Menkes syndrome and a new subtype of Ehlers-Danlos Syndrome. Biochemistry 22: 6156–6162

Prins H W, Van den Hamer C J A 1980 Abnormal copper-thionein synthesis and impaired copper utilisation in mutated brindled mice: model for Menkes' disease. The Journal of Nutrition 110: 151–157

Procopis P, Camakaris J, Danks D M 1981 A mild form of Menkes' syndrome. Journal of Pediatrics 98:97–99

Rauch H 1983 Toxic milk, a new mutation affecting copper metabolism in the mouse. Journal of Heredity 74: 141–144

Reed G B, Butt E M, Landing B H 1972 Copper in childhood liver disease: A histologic, histochemical and chemical survey. Archives of Pathology 93: 249–255

Sartoris D J, Luzzatti L, Weaver D D, MacFarlane J D, Hollister D W, Parker B R 1984 Type IX Ehlers-Danlos syndrome: A new variant with pathognomonic radiographic features. Radiology 152: 665–670

Sass-Kortsak A 1975 Wilson's disease: a treatable cause of liver disease in children. Pediatric Clinics of North America 22: 963–984

Scheinberg I H, Sternlieb I 1984 Wilson's Disease. Saunders, Philadelphia

Smallwood R A, Williams H A, Rosenoer V M, Sherlock S 1968 Liver copper levels in liver disease: studies using neutron activation analysis. Lancet ii: 1310–1313

Smith A L, Danks D M 1978 Secondary copper accumulation with neurological damage in child with chronic liver disease. British Medical Journal 2: 1400–1401

Su L C, Ravanshad S, Owen C A Jr., McCall J T, Zollman P E, Hardy R M 1982a. A comparison of copper-loading disease in Bedlington terriers and Wilson's disease in humans. American Journal of Physiology 243: G226–G230

Su L C, Owen C A Jr., Zollman P E, Hardy R M 1982b. A defect of biliary excretion of copper in copper-laden Bedlington terriers. American Journal of Physiology 243: G231–G236

Tanner M S, Portmann B 1981 Indian childhood cirrhosis. Archives of Disease in Childhood 56: 4–6

Tønnesen T, Horn N, Sondergaard F, Mikkelsen M, Bouoe J, Damsgaard E, Heydorn K 1985 Measurement of copper in chorionic villi for first-trimester diagnosis of Menkes disease. Lancet 1: 1038

Tønnesen T, Gerdes A-M Damsgaard E, Miny P, Holzgreve W, Sondergaard F, Horn N 1989 First-trimester diagnosis of Menkes disease: intermediate copper values in chorionic villi from three affected male fetuses. Prenatal Diagnosis 9: 159–165

Underwood E J 1977 Trace elements in human and animal nutrition, 4th edn. Academic Press, New York

Volpintesta E J 1974 Menkes' kinky hair syndrome in a black infant. American Journal of Diseases of Children 128: 244–246

Walshe J M, Dixon A K 1986 Dangers of non-compliance in Wilson's disease. Lancet 1: 845–847

Wenk G, Suzuki K 1982 The effect of copper supplementation on the concentration of copper in the brain of the brindled mouse. Biochemical Journal 205: 485–487

Westman J A, Richardson D C, Rennert O M, Morrow G III 1988 Atypical Menkes steely hair disease. American Journal of Medical Genetics 30: 853–858

Yang F, Naylor S L, Lum J B et al 1986 Characterization, mapping, and expression of the human ceruloplasmin gene. Proceedings of the National Academy of Sciences, USA 83: 3257-3261

100. Disorders of iron metabolism and related disorders

Marcel Simon

There are many disorders of iron metabolism. Most of them – notably those associated with the haemoglobino-pathies, with certain anaemias and with the porphyrias – are dealt with in other chapters of this book. In this chapter we shall be concerned with: (1) a common disease, idiopathic haemochromatosis; (2) possible relations between the haemochromatosis allele and secondary iron overload; (3) a condition on which recent reports called interest, neonatal haemochromatosis; and (4) congenital atransferrinaemia.

CLASSIFICATION OF IRON OVERLOAD DISEASES

Idiopathic haemochromatosis is the 'prototype' of iron overload diseases. A number of variants exist, which are listed in Table 100.1.

Iron overload caused by increased intestinal absorption is mainly deposited in parenchymal tissue, leading to tissue damage. When iron overload is induced by administration of parenteral iron, including blood transfusions, the reticuloendothelial system is affected first, without marked tissue damage (Powell et al 1980); however, as iron accumulation increases, parenchymal tissue is also involved and widespread organ dysfunction occurs (Schafer et al 1981).

IDIOPATHIC HAEMOCHROMATOSIS

Definition

Idiopathic (primary, genetic or hereditary) haemochromatosis (IH), a condition involving and probably arising from an iron overload state affecting several organs, is a recessively transmitted disease controlled by a

Table 100.1 Classification of diseases with iron overload (from Simon et al 1988a, published with permission)

Diseases with iron overload	Mechanisms of iron overload				Frequency of iron overload in the disease	Degree of iron overload in the disease
	Increased intestinal absorption	*Increased iron intake*	*Parenteral administration*	*Transfusion*		
Idiopathic haemochromatosis	++				high	high
Neonatal haemochromatosis					high	high
Secondary iron overload						
a – associated with anaemia						
– aplastic anaemia				++	medium	variable
– haemolytic anaemia (spherocytosis)	?				low	variable
– ineffective erythropoiesis						
· sideroblastic anaemias	+			++	high	high
· beta-thalassaemia	+			++	high	high
· other haemoglobinopathies	+			++	low	?
b – associated with (alcoholic) liver disease	?				medium	low
c – bantou siderosis		+ (dietary)			high	variable
d – dialysed patients		+ (medicinal)	+	+	medium	variable
e – metabolic disorders						
porphyria cutanea tarda	?				high	low
atransferrinaemia	++				high	high

gene located on chromosome 6 near the A-locus of the HLA system. Fibrosis of certain organs, particularly the liver, should no longer be included in the definition of the disease, since ideally the diagnosis should be established before the onset of fibrosis. Haemochromatosis was first described by Trousseau in 1865 and given its present name following the studies of von Recklinghausen in 1889.

Clinical features of idiopathic haemochromatosis

Organic and metabolic manifestations

Skin pigmentation is pronounced, often grey but sometimes brown, is diffuse, but affects mainly exposed areas of skin. Mucosal pigmentation may be seen, with slate-grey patches in the mouth. About half the patients show cutaneous atrophy, ichthyosiform changes and flattening of the nails or true spoon nail (Chevrant-Breton et al 1977). Loss of body hair is common.

In advanced forms of the disease pronounced hepatomegaly is a constant finding. The liver is firm. Portal hypertension is rare and liver tests may be normal or show a slight elevation in serum transaminases and a fall in sulphobromophthalein excretion.

Glucose tolerance is commonly impaired and diabetes mellitus, requiring insulin administration, used to be seen in about 60% of patients (Dymock et al 1972, Simon et al 1973b). Nowadays, with early diagnosis and treatment, diabetes occurs much less often (Edwards et al 1980, Simon et al 1984). Significant pathological and functional changes include iron overload in pancreatic B cells, a reduction in their number and in their secretory granules (Rahier et al 1987), an impaired hepatic insulin extraction (Niederau et al 1984, Rumbak et al 1987) and a progressive reduction in B-cell insulin secretion (Simon et al 1984). Shared heredity between ordinary diabetes and the diabetes of haemochromatosis has been proposed (Balcerzak et al 1966, Saddi & Feingold 1974b) but this association seems in reality weak and merely due to chance (Simon et al 1984).

Hypogonadism is the main endocrine abnormality and can be attributed, on the basis of a reduced response to luteinizing hormone releasing hormone (LHRH) or the Clomiphene stimulation test, to gonadotrophin deficiency (Tourniaire et al 1974, Walsh et al 1976, Charbonnel et al 1981). Prolactin deficiency has also been described (Walton et al 1983, Kley et al 1985, Lufkin et al 1987). Cases of hypothyroidism and hyperthyroidism have been reported (Edwards et al 1983). Plasma parathyroid hormone is often slightly increased (Pawlotsky et al 1975).

Heart disease is most commonly revealed by electrocardiographic abnormalities consisting of a decrease in

QRS amplitude and T-wave flattening or inversion and by echocardiographic changes. Myocardial disease is seen clinically in 15–20% of cases and produces congestive heart failure and/or arrhythmias such as atrial fibrillation or even ventricular tachycardia or fibrillation (Mattheyses et al 1978).

Bone demineralization is common (Delbarre 1960) and one half to two thirds of patients suffer from joint disease (Schumacher 1964). This takes the form either of attacks of pseudogout, or more often a moderate chronic rheumatic disease affecting mainly the metacarpophalangeal joints of the second and third fingers and the hips. Radiography shows chondrocalcinosis, especially of the knees, and/or appearances of subchondral joint disease, particularly of the metacarpophalangeal joints. Many joints may be affected.

Other manifestations of the disease include easy fatigability, abdominal pain, increased pancreatic and/or biliary secretion in response to secretin stimulation, and vitamin A and C deficiency.

Laboratory tests and the investigation of iron overload

An increase, even a small one, in iron stores leads to an increase in serum iron and in the saturation of its carrier protein transferrin. In idiopathic haemochromatosis, serum iron levels are commonly greater than 30 μmol/l (170 μg/dl). Elevated transferrin saturation, above 0.62 (N$\approx$0.30), has been proposed as a good diagnostic criterion (Dadone et al 1982).

To evaluate the severity of iron overload, routine assay of serum ferritin (Addison et al 1972, Worwood 1979) has replaced the desferrioxamine test. Normal serum ferritin levels are less than 200 μg/l in females and 300 μg/l in males, while patients often have levels >1000 μg/l. Measurement of erythrocyte ferritin would also be of particular interest (Cazzola et al 1983, Cruickshank et al 1987).

These tests give false positive results in cases of liver disease with hepatic cell necrosis, especially alcoholic liver disease. In inflammatory diseases and malignancies, serum iron is usually decreased and serum ferritin increased.

Nuclear magnetic resonance has so far not proved useful for evaluating iron overload.

Computed tomography shows an increased liver attenuation coefficient correlated to iron overload (Howard et al 1983, Roudot-Thoraval et al 1983). While CT is useful in severe overload, its sensitivity and specificity are less satisfactory in cases of moderate and minimal overload (Guyader et al 1987).

Magnetic susceptibility techniques, based on the paramagnetic properties of ferritin and haemosiderin, may be of great value in estimating iron concentration in the liver (Brittenham et al 1982), but they are presently available in only a few laboratories.

Finally, liver needle biopsy is often necessary to confirm and quantify the iron overload. Histological examination of a liver biopsy specimen reveals marked iron deposition in hepatocytes and Kupffer cells. Evidence of fibrosis and, in advanced cases, of cirrhosis, is also seen. Hepatic iron concentration measured biochemically (Barry & Sherloch 1971) is proportional to total body iron: normally it does not exceed 36 μmol (2000 μg)/g dry weight (Brissot et al 1981) but it may reach 1000 μmol/g in patients with haemochromatosis.

HLA associations

The finding of an association with certain HLA antigens, notably HLA-A3 with or without B7 and B14, is indicative of a genetic component in idiopathic haemochromatosis (Simon et al 1975, Simon et al 1976). However, these antigens are clearly not specific and are absent in a quarter of haemochromatosis patients.

Overall picture, natural history and treatment

Major manifestations of the disease are found in 8 or 9 cases out of 10 in men, who also exhibit earlier onset of the disease – usually around the forties – than women. Mortality may ensue through heart failure or carcinoma of the liver, which may develop, once cirrhosis has set in, even after correction of iron overload (Bradbear et al 1985). Hence the need for early detection of mild cases with only skin hyperpigmentation and hepatic involvement without cirrhosis, or of still latent or subclinical cases detected by family studies. In clinically mild cases complete cure is possible; in latent cases, the disease can be prevented altogether.

Treatment consists essentially of weekly phlebotomies removing 400 to 500 ml of blood at each session until excess iron is removed. Further phlebotomy sessions are done at less frequent intervals to prevent subsequent iron build-up. A response to phlebotomy is seen in the patient's general state of health, skin changes, liver abnormalities and heart condition. Other aspects of the disease show little or no response. Survival is greatly increased (Bomford & Williams 1976, Niederau et al 1985).

Pathogenesis of idiopathic haemochromatosis

Certain aspects of the pathogenic process have been well documented. They concern notably the role of the excess iron, the mechanisms of tissue damage and the implication of non-transferrin-bound iron. Yet important questions, especially as to the cause of the iron overload, remain unresolved.

Consequences of iron overload

The degree of iron overload in an organ does not always correspond exactly to the severity of tissue damage. Nevertheless, there are sound arguments in favour of the pathogenic role of iron: (1) parenchymal iron overload states in man, whatever the cause, are associated with similar clinical features; (2) phlebotomy therapy improves the clinical picture and prolongs survival in advanced cases (Bomford & Williams 1976, Niederau et al 1985) and, as far as can be judged at present, cures or prevents the disease in mild or latent cases respectively; (3) removal of excess iron by phlebotomy totally restores to normal certain biochemically measurable abnormalities, such as excess biliary or pancreatic secretion following secretin stimulation (Simon et al 1973a) or ascorbic acid deficiency (Brissot et al 1978); (4) experimental models of iron overload, recently developed by dietary supplementation with carbonyl iron, mimic idiopathic haemochromatosis and lead to tissue damage (Bacon et al 1983).

The damaging effect of excess iron on tissues (Gordeuk et al 1987) could arise through several mechanisms (not mutally exclusive): (1) fragility of the iron-loaded lysosomes, notably due to membrane lipid peroxidation, which causes leakage of hydrolytic enzymes capable of damaging subcellular organelles (Selden et al 1980, Peters et al 1985); (2) iron-induced peroxidation (through the intermediary of free radicals) in hepatic mitochondria and microsomes, as shown in studies using rats with chronic iron overload (Bacon et al 1983), leading to functional abnormalities of these organelles (Bacon et al 1985, Bacon et al 1986); and (3) direct effect of iron on collagen synthesis (Weintraub et al 1985).

There is an increase in non-transferrin-bound iron in idiopathic haemochromatosis (Hershko & Peto 1987). This unbound iron can promote the formation of free hydroxyl radicals and stimulate the peroxidation of phospholipid liposomes (Gutteridge et al 1985). It has been shown that the myocardial uptake of low-molecular weight iron in cultured rat heart cells results in lipid peroxidation and abnormal rhythmicity and contractility (Link et al 1985).

Causes of iron overload

Iron overload in the liver (and probably in other organs) is greatly facilitated by the presence of non-transferrin-bound iron (Brissot et al 1985).

It has been well established that the only possible source of the excess iron is increased absorption, but the underlying metabolic defect remains unknown. This defect could affect many tissues, but at least two sites appear to be involved: the intestinal mucosa and the liver. Biopsy specimens of intestinal mucosa removed from haemochromatosis patients have been found to take up more iron than specimens from normal individuals (Cox & Peters 1978). Iron administered to haemochromatosis patients was found to be deposited in the liver – even after removal of excess iron and in iron deficiency states – before being used for erythropoiesis (Pollycove et al 1971, Batey et al 1978).

Many studies have been conducted to determine the role of the two principal proteins implicated in iron metabolism, transferrin and ferritin. There appears to be no reason to incriminate transferrin: its gene has been localized to chromosome 3 (Yang et al 1984); it has the same electrophoretic pattern and sialic acid content in patients with idiopathic haemochromatosis as in controls (Tsan & Shelfel 1985); for equivalent saturations, it does not affect iron turnover differently and it also links normally with tissue receptors (Cazzola et al 1985); there is no increase in transferrin receptors in haemochromatosis patients (Banerjee et al 1986). Many years ago, Crosby (1963) postulated that there was an abnormality concerning ferritin, but it has yet to be demonstrated. Recently a family of genes or pseudogenes mapping on nearly a dozen chromosomes has been demonstrated for the ferritin H sub-unit (Cragg et al 1985); one of these is localized, as is the haemochromatosis gene, to chromosome 6 near the HLA region; yet to date it has not been established whether this gene is functional and what relationship it could have with the haemochromatosis gene.

The possibility of a reticuloendothelial disorder being involved, as proposed by Astaldi et al (1966) and by Cattan et al (1967), who noted abnormally low concentrations and an abnormal distribution of iron in villous macrophages, remains open to debate.

Essentially, what is required is to identify the abnormal gene and its product and thereby the basic cause of the disorder.

Genetics

The genetics of haemochromatosis has been the subject of several recent reviews (Simon et al 1988a, Simon & Brissot 1988).

Historical background

Sheldon's inborn error of metabolism theory, postulated in 1935, was widely disputed right up to the sixties (MacDonald 1964). A number of successive observations, however, gradually lent weight to the view of the disease being an inherited trait. Iron absorption was found to be increased in certain relatives of idiopathic haemochromatosis patients, instances of familial occurrence of haemochromatosis were reported, and major disturbances in biochemical body iron parameters were seen among relatives of patients with idiopathic haemochromatosis, but not among those of patients with haemochromatosis secondary to alcoholic liver disease; the eating habits of haemochromatosis patients were found to differ little or not at all from those of control subjects.

Every conceivable mode of inheritance has been advanced. While the arguments in favour of an autosomal recessive trait have gradually gained strength, until quite recently they were far from achieving universal acceptance. Nevertheless, compilation and analysis of phenotypic data finally provided strong evidence in favour of recessive inheritance (Saddi & Feingold 1974a), as did statistical proof of major forms of the disease occurring significantly more frequently in sibs than in age matched offspring (Simon et al 1977a). What clinched the matter and finally proved the hereditary nature of the disease and its recessive mode of transmission was the discovery of an association with certain HLA antigens (Simon et al 1975, Simon et al 1977b).

Association between idiopathic haemochromatosis and the HLA complex

The association between haemochromatosis and HLA antigens A3 (Simon et al 1975), B7 (Walters et al 1975, Simon et al 1976) and B14 (Simon et al 1976) has been confirmed by more than twenty studies (review in Simon et al 1988a). All have reported an increase in A3, found in 55–100% of patients (average 73%) as compared to 19–31% in controls, and B7 in 28–86% of patients (average 47%) as compared to 9–34% in controls. B14 prevalence was increased in only half of the reported series but very significantly in some. Antigen A11 does not undergo the decrease in frequency observed in other locus A alleles due to the high frequency of A3; this means there is a relative increase in A11 (Le Mignon et al 1983). A specific linkage between A11 and the IH gene has been demonstrated (Lalouel et al 1985). A slight increase in DRw6 (31.6% in 168 patients as opposed to 18.6% in 166 controls) has been observed; however the difference was no longer significant if the large number of comparisons made was taken into account (Le Mignon 1982). A significant increase in DR2 has also been reported (Doran et al 1981). The distribution of CW, Bf and Glo loci antigens has not been found to be altered (Le Mignon 1982).

The HLA marking of the haemochromatosis allele is haplotypic. The marking haplotypes can be divided into three groups (Simon et al 1987). Group I includes haplotypes with an increased frequency and a stronger linkage disequilibrium than in controls: A3, B7 (21.1% vs 6.1%; $p < 10^{-10}$); A3, B14 (13.8% vs 1.5%; $p < 10^{-10}$); A11, B5; A11, B35. Group II is made up of haplotypes with increased frequencies but without any linkage disequilibrium (A3, B12; A3, B15). Haplotypes in group III do not have an increased frequency in haemochromatosis, but their alleles are in linkage disequilibrium in IH and in controls: A2, B12; A1, B8; A9, B7; A29, B12. Haplotypes also extend to other loci; for example A3, B7 is actually A3, B7, BfS, DR2 and A3, B14 is A3, B14, BfF, DRw6 (Simon et al 1987).

The haplotypes carrying B7 or B14 without A3 are not more frequent in haemochromatosis than in controls, but those carrying A3 without B7 or B14 show a significantly increased frequency ($p < 10^{-7}$) (Simon et al 1987). The A allele is thus the only independent marker of the haemochromatosis gene, the B alleles being secondary markers only because they themselves are linked to allele A.

Proof of recessive inheritance

A family pattern in agreement with recessive transmission is shown in Figure 100.1. It implies that in a proband's sibship only those sibs carrying the same two HLA haplotypes as the proband have haemochromatosis. Sibs that have only one haplotype in common with the proband, as presumptive heterozygotes, are either totally disease-free or may show signs of mild iron overload of no clinical consequence. Sibs that share no haplotype with the proband are presumed not to carry the gene.

The first families reported showed a clear association between HLA identity with the proband and disease state in sibs (Simon et al 1977b). This association has been confirmed by all the subsequent series involving a significant number of families (Lipinski et al 1978, Valberg et al 1980, Doran et al 1981). The frequency of this association appeared incompatible with random distribution or with a distribution resulting from dominant inheritance (Le Mignon 1982). The analysis of large pedigrees led to the same conclusions (Kravitz et al 1979, Edwards et al 1981).

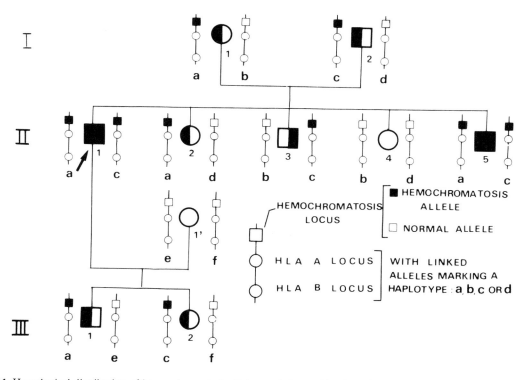

Fig. 100.1 Hypothetical distribution of haemochromatosis alleles, each in combination with a particular HLA haplotype, among relatives of a patient with idiopathic haemochromatosis (person II-I). The topographic relations between the presumed haemochromatosis locus and the HLA loci are diagrammatic approximations.
■ homozygous male; ◐ heterozygous female; ○ 'gene free' female.
(from the New England Journal of Medicine (1979) 301: 169–174, reprinted with permission.)

Exceptions to the general rule are seen, such as diseased sibs who are only half-HLA-identical to the proband or, exceptionally, HLA-different. Pseudo-dominant inheritance from one generation to the next has also been observed. Such exceptions can be explained by genetic recombination between the haemochromatosis allele and the marker HLA haplotype – a rare event because of their close linkage – and, more commonly, by homozygous-heterozygous matings (Simon et al 1979, Bassett et al 1982). Figure 100.2 illustrates such a mating: the proband (II 1) is daughter of a patient who died from haemochromatosis (I 2). She inherited a second allele, linked to the HLA-A3, B14 haplotype, from her mother, who in fact showed signs of mild iron overload. Such exceptions, once elucidated, are entirely consistent with recessive inheritance.

Studies of unrelated patients added further evidence. These studies were based on the supposition that an HLA allele, HLA-A3 as it turns out, in frequent haplotype association with the haemochromatosis allele would be distributed differently among haemochromatosis patients, depending on whether the haemochromatosis allele itself had to be present in the homozygous or heterozygous state to produce the disease. These studies very soon provided evidence of recessive inheritance (Simon et al 1977a,b), confirmed by applying the formulae proposed by Thomson and Bodmer (1977) to currently available data (Table 100.2)

Gene mapping

It is now established beyond any doubt that the haemo-chromatosis gene maps near the HLA class I genes as a whole. The cumulative results from lod score studies (Simon et al 1977b, Lipinski et al 1978, Kravitz et al 1979, Fauchet et al 1980, Doran et al 1981, Dadone et al 1982, Lalouel et al 1985) confirm close linkage with the probability error of less than 10^{-60}. The distance between the haemochromatosis locus and the HLA class I locus is probably less than one centiMorgan (Lalouel et al 1985).

The demonstration that the A3 allele is the only

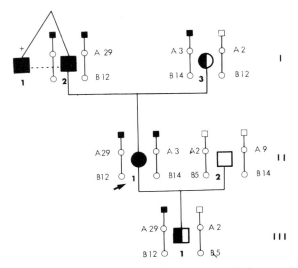

Fig. 100.2 A family with pseudo-dominant transmission. (From Simon et al 1979, Nouvelle Presse Médicale 8: 421–424, published with permission)

independent marker of the haemochromatosis gene (Simon et al 1987) makes it possible to map this gene closer to locus A than to locus B, at least in terms of genetic distance.

One point still being investigated is whether the haemochromatosis locus maps between the A locus and the B locus or beyond the A locus in relation to the B locus and the centromere. Debate over this issue has provided arguments in favour of the first possibility (Edwards et al 1986) as well as the second (David et al 1986, Simon et al 1987), yet no formal proof of either hypothesis has yet been found.

Towards gene identification

The product of the haemochromatosis gene responsible for the phenotypic expression of the disease is unknown. This handicaps the application of molecular genetic techniques. Nevertheless the gene may be unmasked

Table 100.2 Distribution of 390 unrelated patients with haemochromatosis as A3 homozygous, A3 heterozygous, or lacking A3 (from Simon et al 1988a, published with permission)

	A3 Homozygotes	A3 Heterozygotes	Non-A3 Patients
Expected numbers for dominant inheritance	42	247	101
Expected numbers for recessive inheritance	94	195	101
Observed numbers	102	187	101

Difference between expected and observed: for dominant inheritance, $X^2 = 100$, $p < 10^{-10}$; for recessive inheritance, $X^2 = 1$, N.S.

indirectly by studying restriction polymorphisms using HLA probes, and also ferritin probes since a ferritin gene (or pseudogene) has also been localized to the HLA region (Cragg et al 1985). To date, comparisons of polymorphism patterns of patients and controls have not been conclusive. A recent study with HLA probes of a particular family with two HLA-identical sibs of a heavily iron loaded proband, who were themselves disease-free, revealed that certain DNA fragments were missing in the proband's genome; these missing fragments could be related to the haemochromatosis gene (David et al 1986), but further studies are necessary for confirmation.

One or several genes

Expression varies from one patient to another. Juvenile haemochromatosis, in particular, is considered by some to be a distinct entity (Lamon et al 1979). Expression can also vary from one family to another (Muir et al 1984). The hypothesis of two functionally different HLA-linked major genes has been postulated (Bomford et al 1977). In fact, a large body of evidence to date supports the hypothesis of one HLA-linked major recessive gene (Simon et al 1980b, 1988a, Powell et al 1987). Nevertheless, the possibility of weakly expressed variants of the HLA-linked gene cannot be excluded (Simon et al 1988a), no more than that of minor gene(s) non HLA-linked which could explain the observation (Valberg et al 1980, Le Mignon et al 1983) of significantly higher iron overload biochemical parameters in non-carrier (HLA different) relatives as compared to controls.

Phenotypic expression of the haemochromatosis gene

In the heterozygous state no clinical expression is observed. Biochemical (increased serum iron and transferrin saturation and/or serum ferritin) or histological expression has been reported in one fifth to one third of cases, dependent upon the number of laboratory tests performed (Simon et al 1988a).

An absence of expression has been observed in the homozygous state, rarely in the adult male, but much more frequently in the premenopausal female and in young subjects of both sexes. Our present knowledge of gene prevalence would lead us to expect that the absence of expression, or weak expression, are greater than had been thought previously.

The search for a discriminating phenotypic test for homozygosity has been the subject of several studies. Dadone et al (1982) proposed transferrin saturation as the most reliable test, with high sensitivity and specificity for a threshold level of 62%. Borwein et al (1983) reached similar conclusions. However for patients under 35,

Bassett et al (1984) found that ferritin level predicted the homozygous state more effectively than did transferrin saturation. Finally, Bassett et al (1984) have proposed a liver iron concentration/age index as the best diagnostic criterion.

However, these tests were usually established using controls who were subjects related to patients. The predictive value of these tests is thus considerably lowered if they are applied to patients with particular diseases (such as alcoholic liver disease), who can show perturbed biochemical tests without iron overload (Brissot et al 1981), or simply when applied to the general population (for epidemiological studies) because the predictive value of a test is a function of disease prevalence (the lower the prevalence, the lower the predictive value).

What is the explanation for the HLA marking of the haemochromatosis gene?

The HLA genes do not themselves play any role in the disease. Various hypotheses have been proposed to explain the present conformation of gene marking. One supposes a selective pressure of the haemochromatosis gene on certain HLA haplotypes (Edwards et al 1981) and, conversely, another proposes a selective pressure exerted by the A3, B7 haplotype on the haemochromatosis gene (Saddi et al 1981). The hypothesis which fits best with the largest number of observed facts assumes a series of events: rare (perhaps unique) mutation(s) – chromosome recombinations – migrations (Simon et al 1980a, Ritter et al 1984, Simon et al 1987). The most ancient mutation would have placed the IH gene in an A3, B7 haplotype. The haemochromatosis, A3, B7 sequence would have been transmitted with or without modifications due to recombinations: ancient recombinations (either between A and B for A3, B14 or between haemochromatosis and A for A11 haplotypes) corresponding to the above cited group I haplotypes; recent recombinations (either between A and B for haplotypes in group II or between haemochromatosis and A for haplotypes in group III). Migrations would have produced the geographical distribution of haplotypes seen today: A3, B7 is found throughout the world; A3, B14 is not; certain regions have their particular haplotype, as, for example, central Sweden with A1, B8 (Ritter et al 1984) and northeast Italy with A3, B35 (Piperno et al 1986).

Prevalence of the haemochromatosis gene

Results of the main series reported to date are summarized in Table 100.3. Some of these studies may overestimate the global prevalence of the gene and of the

Table 100.3   Prevalence of idiopathic haemochromatosis (from Simon & Brissot 1988, published with permission)

Means of study	Country	Authors	Prevalences		
			Gene	*Heterozygotes*	*Homozygotes*
Autopsy	U S A	MacDonald 1965	0.042	0.081	0.0018
	Scotland	MacSween & Scott 1973	0.045	0.085	0.002
	Sweden (southern)	Lindmark and Erikson 1985	0.030	0.058	0.0009
Biochemical tests	Sweden (central)	Olsson et al 1983	0.070	0.132	0.005
	U S A	Expert Scientific Working Group 1985	0.038	0.073	0.0014
Biochemical tests and family studies	U S A (Utah)	Dadone et al 1982	0.069	0.128	0.005
	Australia	Bassett et al 1982	0.088	0.160	0.0077
	Canada (Ontario)	Borwein et al 1983	0.056	0.106	0.003
	France (Brittany)	Simon et al 1985b	0.064	0.120	0.004

disease for two reasons: first, they were conducted in regions where there was an a priori assumption of high prevalence; second, they were, at least partially, based on diagnostic tests whose predictive value was determined in families of haemochromatosis patients and applied to the general population without correction of this predictive value (see 'Phenotypic expression' above). The series reported by Lindmark and Eriksson (1985) and by the Expert Scientific Working Group (1985) avoid this bias and would suggest that gene frequency is hardly less than 0.03 and the homozygous state less than 0.001 in Caucasian populations, values which have been observed to be greatly exceeded in certain regions. We are working with a disease which is frequent but all too often undiagnosed.

Screening and prevention

Physicians should be aware of the early minimal signs such as melanodermia, a slightly enlarged liver, or metacarpophalangeal arthropathy, and of their value for early diagnosis. Appropriate laboratory tests and possibly liver biopsy should follow. In regions where the disease

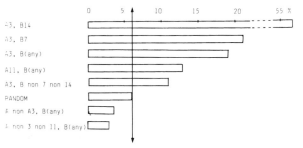

Fig. 100.3 Risk of homozygosity in a relative sharing one haplotype with the proband (obligatory heterozygote) depending on his (her) unshared haplotype (for haemochromatosis gene prevalence = 0.06) (from the Annals of the New York Academy of Sciences, 1988, 526: 11–22, reprinted with permission).

has a high prevalence, serum iron and transferrin saturation should be part of systematic check-ups during the third or fourth decade. Every diagnosis of idiopathic haemochromatosis should lead to a family screening programme with phenotypic examinations and genotypic analysis. Here, HLA typing is essential. As shown in Figure 100.1 sibs who are HLA-identical to the proband can be identified as homozygotes, while other sibs can be identified as heterozygotes (when they share one haplotype with the proband) or non carriers (when they have neither of the proband's haplotypes). Diagnosis of overt haemochromatosis in an HLA haploidentical sib reveals the presence of a supplementary haemochromatosis gene in the parental gene pool and indicates the sibship issued from a homozygote-heterozygote mating; the genetic situation of other family members should then be re-evaluated.

HLA typing should not be overlooked when tracking down a homozygous state in obligatory heterozygous individuals, especially offspring. Indeed, the risk that the other chromosome 6 also carries the gene is related to the HLA haplotype it carries. An estimation of this risk was proposed by Conte and Rotter (1984) based on antigens and association of antigens A and B in patients with haemochromatosis. Simon et al (1988b) proposed a direct method, based on haplotypes, and applicable (at least) in regions where sufficiently large family studies have been conducted: the probability of a homozygous state in an obligatory heterozygous individual is calculated from the frequency of the haplotype marking his other chromosome both in haemochromatosis and in the general population, and from the prevalence of the haemochromatosis gene; the probability for all the haplotypes is proportional to the frequency of the gene. The results for a certain number of haplotypes are given in Figure 100.3. The risk of a given haplotype carrying the haemochromatosis gene varies from less than 3% to nearly 60%. The high risk associated with the haplotype A3, B14 is illustrated in the pedigree given in Figure 100.2.

Each family member can then be counselled as to the most appropriate course of action: no need for further studies in non carriers; regular examination (every five or ten years?) for heterozygous relatives (but it may soon appear that there is no need for such periodic studies); and regular blood withdrawal for homozygous relatives if there is any phenotypic expression.

In many cases this approach should prevent a disease which is at best disabling, and at worst leads to death from heart failure or cancer of the liver.

THE IDIOPATHIC HAEMOCHROMATOSIS ALLELE AND SECONDARY IRON OVERLOAD

It has been postulated that the IH gene is involved in iron overload states formerly considered secondary. This has been discussed in a large body of publications over the last few years and has been the subject of recent reviews (Simon 1985, Simon & Brissot 1988).

Alcoholic liver disease

It has been suggested that the iron overload observed in patients with alcoholic liver disease might be related to a dependency on a heterozygous state for idiopathic haemochromatosis. This has been clearly ruled out. Actually, the prevalence of the HLA antigen A3 is identical in this condition to that observed in controls (22%) and significantly less than that observed in a heterozygous population (about 57%) (Simon et al 1977c).

Reciprocally, the iron overload in haemochromatosis is not increased further by alcohol abuse (Lesage et al 1983).

Anaemias

Family studies have shown an occasional occurrence of the haemochromatosis gene in idiopathic refractory sideroblastic anaemia, hereditary spherocytosis, beta-thalassaemia trait and haemoglobin Olympia.

Involvement of the haemochromatosis gene in idiopathic refractory sideroblastic anaemia has been proposed (Cartwright et al 1980), but this possibility is formally refuted by findings based on a large series using HLA markers (Simon et al 1985a).

In a group of individuals with the beta-thalassaemia trait Fargion et al (1985) found a significantly increased prevalence of A3 in those who showed high serum ferritin levels. But the frequency of iron overload in these patients was so great that one hesitates to attribute it to the haemochromatosis gene in all cases, especially since

the regions of high prevalence of these two diseases do not coincide.

Chronic renal failure and maintenance haemodialysis

Patients with chronic renal failure undergoing haemodialysis receive large quantities of oral and parenteral iron and present iron overload which has been suggested by numerous studies (following that by Bregman et al 1980) to result from an effect of the haemochromatosis gene and by others to be completely independent of the haemochromatosis gene. The pathophysiological mechanism proposed was a non-inhibition of intestinal absorption by parenteral iron. Unfortunately the conclusions of many of these studies must be taken with utmost caution because of erroneous methodology, the most flagrant of which is the use of A3 *and* B7 *and* B14 as 'haemochromatosis alleles', while A3 is only a truly independent marker, B7 and B14 having no significance without the presence of A3. Further studies with better methods are needed.

Porphyria cutanea tarda

Family studies (Kushner et al 1985), which are increasing in number (Edwards et al 1987), favour frequent involvement of the haemochromatosis gene in the sporadic form of porphyria cutanea tarda, at least in certain regions. On the other hand, in a large series (Beaumont et al 1987), unrelated patients were compared to controls and the frequency of the A3 antigen was found to be normal and less than that expected for a population heterozygous for the haemochromatosis gene. This would exclude any substantial involvement. Perhaps these differences result from selection bias. Sporadic porphyria cutanea tarda probably needs a complementary factor for expression. Alcohol is an important factor in certain areas and is involved much more often than any other, including the haemochromatosis gene. In other regions where alcohol intake is lower, expression of porphyria cutanea tarda could depend on other factors, including the haemochromatosis gene.

Consequently, it can be stated that the haemochromatosis gene is not involved at all, or at most only occasionally in certain secondary iron overloads, while in others the importance of its role still remains to be assessed by further studies.

NEONATAL HAEMOCHROMATOSIS

Neonatal (or perinatal) haemochromatosis was first described by Cottier in 1957. In a recent review, Knisely et al (1987) presented 25 known cases fulfilling the following requirements: (1) a rapidly progressive clinical course with death in utero or in the early neonatal period; (2) increased tissue iron deposition in multiple organs, particularly the liver, pancreas, heart and endocrine glands, with the extrahepatic reticulo-endothelial system relatively unaffected; and (3) no evidence for haemolytic disease, syndromes associated with haemosiderosis, or exogenous iron overload from transfusions. Both sexes were equally affected. The incidence of prematurity was 40%. Presenting signs were nonspecific and generally reflected multisystem failure. The main pathological findings were diffuse hepatic fibrosis or frank cirrhosis, giant-cell transformation of hepatocytes and striking deposition of haemosiderin in hepatocytes with smaller amounts in biliary epithelium and Kupffer cells. Liver iron was not only increased in terms of concentration (Knisely et al 1987) but also in absolute values (Silver et al 1987) and it has been suggested that it is directly involved in pathogenesis (Silver et al 1987). The 25 cases reported include five sib pairs, one set on three sibs and one pair of half-sibs. Laboratory tests made in certain relatives showed some cases of increased serum iron or transferrin saturation; the mother and brother of one patient had undetectable serum ferritin (Jacknow et al 1983). Knisely et al (1987) suggested codominant transmission. The mechanisms involved in the overload have not been established. At present there is no evidence which would suggest any relationship between neonatal haemochromatosis and the classical form of idiopathic haemochromatosis.

ATRANSFERRINAEMIA

Acquired transferrin deficiency, such as that due to protein-poor nutrition (Lahey et al 1958) and in which outcome is related to the degree of the deficiency, is fairly common. A number of transferrin variants, without associated disease, are known (Kirk 1968). Only a very small number of cases, however, of congenital atransferrinaemia have been reported (Heilmeyer et al 1961, Cap

et al 1968, Sakata 1969, Goya et al 1972, Loperena et al 1974).

The original case report by Heilmeyer et al (1961) outlined the clinical, biochemical and genetic features of the disease. The patient was a 7-year-old girl with a history of anaemia from the age of three months, for which numerous transfusions had been performed. The anaemia was associated with a tendency to infection, poor growth, skin hyperpigmentation, hepatomegaly and heart disease. Serum iron and serum transferrin were extremely low. Iron absorption was fairly elevated and plasma iron turnover greatly increased. Death was sudden. At autopsy, lesions were found similar to those associated with haemochromatosis, with iron deposition and fibrosis of the heart, pancreas and liver. Both parents had low serum transferrin levels and could be considered heterozygous in accordance with a recessive mode of transmission. Similar findings have been described in the few other reported cases.

In the patient described by Goya et al (1972) it was established that the congenital disorder involved the synthesis and not the breakdown of transferrin. Monthly administration of transferrin-rich plasma fractions proved effective in correcting the anaemia, and associated phlebotomies in removing excess iron stores (Dorantes-Mesa et al 1986) although desferrioxamine infusions could have been more appropriate.

ACKNOWLEDGEMENTS

The author would like to express his thanks to those whose contribution was essential in personal works about genetics of haemochromatosis, especially to M. Bourel, R. Fauchet, B. Genetet, P. Brissot, Y. Deugnier, J. Y. Le Gall, V. David, C. Beaumont, J. L. Alexandre, C. Scordia, L. Le Mignon, J. Yaouanq, J. Y. Poirier, G. Edan, J. P. Hespel, M. P. Lefoie.

Professor Simon died in 1988 after revising his chapter which was subsequently updated by his collaborator Dr Jacqueline Yaouanq.

REFERENCES

Addison G M, Beamish M R, Hales C N, Hodgkins M, Jacobs A, Llewellin P 1972 An immunoradiometric assay for ferritin in the serum of normal subjects and patients with iron deficiency and iron overload. Journal of Clinical Pathology 75: 326–329

Astaldi G, Meardi G, Lisinot T 1966 The iron content of jejunal mucosa obtained by Crosby's biopsy in hemochromatosis and hemosiderosis. Blood 28: 70–82

Bacon B R, Tavill A S, Brittenham G M, Park C H 1983 Hepatic lipid peroxidation in vivo in rats with chronic iron overload. Journal of Clinical Investigation 71: 429–439

Bacon B R, Park C H, Brittenham G M, O'Neill R, Tavill A S 1985 Hepatic mitochondrial oxidative metabolism in rats with chronic dietary iron overload. Hepatology 5: 789–797

Bacon B R, Healey H F, Brittenham G M et al 1986 Hepatic microsomal function in rats with chronic dietary iron overload. Gastroenterology 90: 1844–1853

Balcerzak S P, Westerman M P, Lee R E, Doyle A P 1966 Idiopathic hemochromatosis. A study of three families. American Journal of Medicine 40: 857–873

Banerjee D, Flanagan R P, Cluet J, Valberg L S 1986 Transferrin receptors in the human gastrointestinal tract. Relation to body iron stores. Gastroenterology

91: 861–869

Barry M, Sherlock S 1971 Measurement of liver-iron concentration in needle-biopsy specimens. Lancet 1: 100–103

Bassett M L, Doran T J, Halliday J W, Bashir H V, Powell L W 1982 Idiopathic hemochromatosis: demonstration of homozygous-heterozygous mating by HLA typing of families. Human Genetics 60: 352–356

Bassett M L, Halliday J W, Ferris R A, Powell L W 1984 Diagnosis of hemochromatosis in young subjects: predictive accuracy of biochemical screening tests. Gastroenterology 87: 628–633

Batey R G, Pettit J E, Nicholas A W, Sherlock S, Hoffbrand D M 1978 Hepatic iron clearance from serum in treated hemochromatosis. Gastroenterology 75: 856–859

Beaumont C, Fauchet R, Phung L N, de Verneuil H, Gueguen M, Nordmann Y 1987 Porphyria cutanea tarda and HLA-linked hemochromatosis. Evidence against a systematic association. Gastroenterology 92: 1833–1838

Bomford A, Williams R 1976 Long term results of venesection therapy in idiopathic hemochromatosis. Quarterly Journal of Medicine 45: 611–627

Bomford A, Eddleston A L W F, Kennedy L A, Batchelor I H, Williams R 1977 Histocompatibility antigens as markers of abnormal iron metabolism in patients with idiopathic haemochromatosis and their relatives. Lancet 1: 327–329

Borwein S T, Ghent C N, Flanagan P R, Chamberlain M J, Valberg L S 1983 Genetic and phenotypic expression of hemochromatosis in Canadians. Clinical and Investigative Medicine 6: 171–179

Bradbear R A, Bain C, Siskind V et al 1985 Cohort study of internal malignancy in genetic hemochromatosis and other chronic nonalcoholic liver diseases. Journal of the National Cancer Institute 75: 81–84

Bregman H, Gelfan M C, Winchester J F, Manz H J, Knepshield J H, Schreiner G E 1980 Iron overload associated myopathy in patients on maintenance haemodialysis: a histocompatibility linked disorder. Lancet 2: 882–885

Brissot P, Deugnier Y, Le Treut A, Regnouard F, Simon M, Bourel M 1978 Ascorbic acid status in idiopathic hemochromatosis. Digestion 17: 479–487

Brissot P, Herry D, Verger J P, Messner M, Regnouard F, Ferrand B, Simon M, Bourel M 1981 Assessment of liver iron content in 271 patients: reevaluation of direct and indirect methods. Gastroenterology 80: 557–565

Brissot P, Wright T L, Ma W L, Weisiger R A 1985 Efficient clearance of non-transferrin-bound iron by rat liver. Implications for hepatic iron loading in iron overload states. Journal of Clinical Investigation 76: 1463–1470

Brittenham G M, Farelli D E, Harris J W et al 1982 Magnetic-susceptibility measurement of human iron stores. New England Journal of Medicine 307: 1671–1675

Cap J L, Lehotska V, Mayerova A 1968 Kongenitalna atransferrinemia i 11 mesacneho dietata. Ceskoslovenska Pediatrie 23: 1020–1075

Cartwright G E, Edwards C Q, Skolnick M H, Amos D B 1980 Association of HLA-linked haemochromatosis with idiopathic refractory sideroblastic anaemia. Journal of Clinical Investigation 65: 989–992

Cattan D, Marche Cl, Jori G P, Debray C 1967 Le stock martial des villosités duodéno-jéjunales. L'absorption

martiale vue par l'histologie. Nouvelle Revue Francaise d'Hématologie 7: 259–270

Cazzola M, Dezza L, Bergamaschi G et al 1983 Biologic and clinical significance of red cell ferritin. Blood 5: 1078–1087

Cazzola M, Huebers H, Sayers M H, MacPhall A P, Eng M, Finch C A 1985 Transferrin saturation, plasma iron turnover and transferrin uptake in normal humans. Blood 66: 935–939

Charbonnel B, Chupin M, Le Grand A, Guillon J 1981 Pituitary function in idiopathic hemochromatosis: hormonal study in 36 male patients. Acta Endocrinologica 98: 178–183

Chevrant-Breton J, Simon M, Bourel M, Ferrand B 1977 Cutaneous manifestations of idiopathic haemochromatosis. Archives of Dermatology 113: 161–165

Conte W J, Rotter J I 1984 The use of association data to identify family members at high risk for marker linked diseases. American Journal of Human Genetics 36: 152–166

Cottier H 1957 Uber ein der häemochromatose. Vergleichbares krankheitsbild bei neugeborenen. Schweizerische Medizinische Wochenschrift 87: 39

Cox T M, Peters T J 1978 Uptake of iron by duodenal biopsy specimens from patients with iron-deficiency anaemia and primary haemochromatosis. Lancet 1: 123–124

Cragg S J, Drysdale J, Worwood M 1985 Genes for the 'H' subunit of human ferritin are present on a number of human chromosomes. Human Genetics 71: 108–112

Crosby W H 1963 The control of iron balance by the intestinal mucosa. Blood 22: 441–449

Cruickshank M K, Ninness J, Curtis A et al 1987 Usefulness of erythrocyte ferritin analysis in hereditary hemochromatosis. Canadian Medical Association Journal 136: 1259–1264

Dadone M M, Kushner J P, Edwards C Q, Bishop D T, Skolnick M H 1982 Hereditary haemochromatosis. Analysis of laboratory expression of the disease by genotype in 18 pedigrees. American Journal of Clinical Pathology 78: 196–207

David V, Paul P, Simon M et al 1986 DNA polymorphism related to the idiopathic hemochromatosis gene: evidence in a recombinant family. Human Genetics 74: 113–120

Delbarre D 1960 L'ostéoporose des hémochromatoses. Semaine des Hopitaux de Paris 36: 3279–3284

Doran T J, Bashir H V, Trejaut J, Bassett M L, Halliday J W, Powell L W 1981 Idiopathic haemochromatosis in the Australian population: HLA linkage and recessivity. Human Immunology 2: 191–200

Dorantes-Mesa S, Marquez J L, Valencia-Mayoral P 1986 Sobrecarga de hierro en atransferrinemia hereditaria. Boletin Medico del Hospital Infantil de Mexico 43: 99–101

Dymock I W, Cassar J, Pyke D A, Oakley W G, Williams R 1972 Observations on the pathogenesis, complications and treatment of diabetes in 115 cases of haemochromatosis. American Journal of Medicine 52: 203–210

Edwards C Q, Cartwright G E, Skolnick M H, Amos D B 1980 Homozygosity for hemochromatosis: clinical manifestations. Annals of Internal Medicine 93: 519–525

Edwards C Q, Skolnick M H, Kushner J P 1981 Hereditary hemochromatosis: contributions of genetic analyses. Progress in Hematology 12: 43–71

Edwards C Q, Kelly T M, Ellwein G, Kushner J P 1983 Thyroid disease in hemochromatosis. Increased incidence in homozygous men. Archives of Internal Medicine 143: 1890–1893

Edwards C Q, Griffen L M, Dadone M M, Skolnick M H, Kushner J P 1986 Mapping the locus for hereditary hemochromatosis: localization between HLA-B and HLA-A. American Journal of Human Genetics 38: 805–811

Edwards C Q, Griffen L M, Skolnick M H, Dadone M M, Kushner J P 1987 Evidence of an HLA-linked hemochromatosis (HC) allele in probands with sporadic porphyria cutanea tarda (S-PCT) and first degree relatives. First International Conference on Hemochromatosis. New York, April 27–29, Abst. 5

Expert Scientific Working Group 1985 Summary of a report on assessment of the iron nutritional status of the United States population. American Journal of Clinical Nutrition 42: 1318–1330

Fargion S, Piperno A, Panaiotopoulos N, Taddei M T, Fiorelli G 1985 Iron overload in subject with beta-thalassaemia trait: role of idiopathic haemochromatosis gene. British Journal of Haematology 61: 487–497

Fauchet R, Simon M, Genetet B, Bourel M 1980 Idiopathic hemochromatosis. In: Terasaki P (ed) Histocompatibility testing. Eighth International Histocompatibility Workshop, UCLA Tissue Typing Laboratory, Los Angeles, p 707–710

Gordeuk V P, Bacon B R, Brittenham G M 1987 Iron overload: causes and consequences. Annual Revue of Nutrition 7: 485–508

Goya N, Miyazake S, Kodate S Y, Uskio B 1972 A family of congenital atransferrinemia. Blood 40: 239–245

Gutteridge J M C, Rowley D A, Griffith E, Halliwell B 1985 Low-molecular-weight iron complexes and oxygen radical reactions in idiopathic haemochromatosis. Clinical Science 68: 463–467

Guyader D, Gandon Y, Deugnier Y et al 1987 Interêt de la tomodensitométrie (TDM) dans l'évaluation de la surcharge hépatique en fer de l'hémochromatose idiopathique. Association Française pour l'Etude du Foie, Paris, 1–3 Octobre

Heilmeyer L, Keller W, Vivell O et al 1961 Congenital transferrin deficiency in a seven year old girl. German Medical Monthly 6: 385

Hershko C, Peto T E A 1987 Non-transferrin plasma iron. British Journal of Haematology 66: 149–151

Howard J M, Ghent C N, Carey L S, Flanagran P R, Valberg L S 1983 Diagnostic efficacy of hepatic computed tomography in the detection of body iron overload. Gastroenterology 84: 209–215

Jacknow G, Johnson D, Freese D, Smith C, Burke B 1983 Idiopathic neonatal iron storage disease. Laboratory Investigation 48: 7P

Kirk R L 1968 The world distribution of transferrin variants and some unsolved problems. Acta Geneticas Medicae et Gemellologiae 17: 613

Kley J K, Niederau C, Stremmel W, Lax R, Strohmeyer G, Krüskemper H I 1985 Conversion of androgens to estrogens in idiopathic hemochromatosis. Journal of Clinical Endocrinology 1: 1–6

Knisely A S, Magid M S, Dische M R, Cutz E 1987 Neonatal hemochromatosis. Birth Defects 23: 75–102

Kravitz K, Skolnick M, Cannings C et al 1979 Genetic linkage between hereditary hemochromatosis and HLA. American Journal of Human Genetics 31: 601–619

Kushner J P, Edwards C Q, Dadone M M, Skolnick M H 1985 Heterozygosity for HLA-linked hemochromatosis as a likely cause of the hepatic siderosis associated with sporadic porphyria cutanea tarda. Gastroenterology 88: 1232–1238

Lahey M E, Behar M, Viteri F, Scrimshaw N S 1958 Values for copper, iron and iron-binding capacity in the serum in kwashiorkor. Pediatrics 22: 72–79

Lalouel J M, Le Mignon L, Simon M et al 1985 A combined qualitative (disease) and quantitative (serum iron) genetic analysis of idiopathic hemochromatosis. American Journal of Human Genetics 37: 700–718

Lamon J M, Marynick S P, Roseblatt R, Donelly S 1979 Idiopathic hemochromatosis in a young female. A case study and review of the syndrome in young people. Gastroenterology 76: 178–183

Le Mignon L 1982 Etude génétique de l'hémochromatose idiopathique: le point à propos de 147 enquêtes familiales comportant un groupage HLA. Thèse Med., Rennes

Le Mignon L, Simon M, Fauchet R 1983 An HLA-A11 association with the hemochromatosis allele. Clinical Genetics 24: 171–176

Lesage G D, Baldus W P, Fairbanks V F et al 1983 Hemochromatosis: genetic or alcohol-induced? Gastroenterology 84: 1471–1477

Lindmark B, Eriksson S 1985 Regional differences in the idiopathic hemochromatosis gene frequency in Sweden. Acta Medica Scandinavica 218: 299–304

Link G, Pinson A, Hershko C 1985 Heart cells in culture: a model of myocardial iron overload and chelation. Journal of Laboratory and Clinical Medicine 106: 147–153

Lipinski M, Hors J, Saleun J P 1978 Idiopathic hemochromatosis: Linkage with HLA. Tissue Antigens 11: 471–474

Loperena L, Dorantes S, Medrano E et al 1974 Atransferrinemia hereditaria. Boletin medico del Hospital Infantil Vol XXXI, n°3

Lufkin E G, Baldus W P, Bergstralh E J, Kao P C 1987 Influence of phlebotomy treatment on abnormal hypothalamic-pituitary function in genetic hemochromatosis. Mayo Clinic Proceedings 62: 473–479

MacDonald R A 1964 Hemochromatosis and hemosiderosis. Thomas Books, Springfield

MacDonald R A 1965 Hemochromatosis and cirrhosis in different geographic areas. American Journal of the Medical Sciences 249: 36–46

MacSween R N M, Scott A R 1973 Hepatic cirrhosis: a clinico-pathological review of 520 cases. Journal of Clinical Pathology 26: 936–942

Mattheyses M, Hespel J P, Brissot P et al 1978 Myocardiopathie de l'hémochromatose. Archives des maladies du coeur et des vaisseaux 71: 371–379

Muir W A, McLaren G D, Braun V, Askari A 1984 Evidence for heterogeneity in hereditary hemochromatosis. Evaluation of 174 persons in nine families. American Journal of Medicine 76: 806–814

Niederau C, Berger M, Stremmel W et al 1984 Hyperinsulinaemia in iron-cirrhotic haemochromatosis: impaired hepatic insulin degradation? Diabetologia 26: 441–444

Niederau C, Fischer R, Sonnenberg A, Stremmel W, Trampisch H J, Strohmeyer G 1985 Survival and causes of death in cirrhotic and in non cirrhotic patients with primary hemochromatosis. New England Journal of Medicine 313: 1256–1262

Olsson K S, Ritter B, Rosen U, Heedman P A, Staugard F 1983 Prevalence of iron overload in Swedish males as studied by serum ferritin. Acta Medica Scandinavica 213: 145–150

Pawlotsky Y, Simon M, Hany Y, Brissot P, Bourel M 1975 High plasma parathyroid in primary haemochromatosis. Scandinavian Journal of Rheumatology 4: suppl. 8

Peters T J, O'Connel M J, Ward R J 1985 Role of free-radical mediated lipid peroxidation in the pathogenesis of hepatic damage by lysosomal disruption. In: Poli G., Cheesemen K H, Dianzani M V, Slater T F (eds) Free Radicals in Liver Injury. IRL Press, Oxford, p 107–115

Piperno A, Fargion S, Panaiotopoulos N, Del Nino E, Taddei M T, Fiorelli G 1986 Idiopathic haemochromatosis and HLA antigens in Italy: is A3 BW35 HLA haplotype a marker for idiopathic haemochromatosis gene in north east regions? Journal of Clinical Pathology 39: 125–128

Pollycove M, Fawwaz R A, Winchell H S 1971 Transient hepatic deposition of iron in primary hemochromatosis with iron deficiency following venesection. Journal of Nuclear Medicine 12: 28–30

Powell L W, Basset M L, Halliday J W 1980 Hemochromatosis. Gastroenterology 78: 374–381

Powell L W, Ferluga J, Axelsen E, Halliday J W 1987 Is all hereditary hemochromatosis HLA related? First International Conference on Hemochromatosis, New York, April 27–29. Abst. 3

Rahier J, Loozen S, Goebbels R M, Abrahem M 1987 The haemochromatic human pancreas: a quantitative immunohistochemical and ultrastructural study. Diabetologia 30: 5–12

Ritter B, Safwenberg J, Olssonn K S 1984 HLA as a marker of the hemochromatosis gene in Sweden. Human Genetics 68: 62–66

Roudot-Thoraval F, Halphen M, Lardé D et al 1983 Evaluation of liver iron content by computed tomography: its value in the follow-up of treatment in patients with idiopathic hemochromatosis. Hepatology 3: 974–979

Rumbak M J, Joffe B I, Seftel H C, Kalk W J, Bezwoda W R 1987 Plasma C-peptide and insulin responses to intravenous glucagon stimulation in idiopathic haemochromatosis. South African Medical Journal 71: 351–353

Saddi R, Feingold J 1974a Idiopathic haemochromatosis. An autosomal recessive disease. Clinical Genetics 5: 234–241

Saddi R, Feingold J 1974b Idiopathic haemochromatosis and diabetes mellitus. Clinical Genetics 5: 242–247

Saddi R, Muller J Y, Pouliquen A, Kaplan C, Sylvestre R 1981 HLA — A3, B7 linkage disequilibrium in hemochromatotic patients with or without insulin dependent diabetes. Tissue Antigens 17: 473–479

Sakata T 1969 A case of congenital atransferrinemia. Shonika Shinnryo 32: 1523–1529

Schafer A, Cheron R, Dwyy R et al 1981 Clinical consequences of acquired transfusional iron overload in adults. New England Journal of Medicine 304: 319–324

Schumacher H R 1964 Hemochromatosis and arthritis. Archives of Rheumatology 7: 41–50

Selden C, Owen M, Hopkins J M P, Peters T J 1980 Studies on the concentration and intracellular localization of iron proteins in liver biopsy specimens from patients with iron overload with special reference to their role in lysosomal disruption. British Journal of Haematology 44: 359–603

Sheldon J H 1935 Haemochromatosis. Oxford University Press, London.

Silver M M, Beverley D W, Valberg L S, Cutz E, Phillips M J, Shakeed W A 1987 Perinatal hemochromatosis: clinical, morphologic and quantitative iron studies. American Journal of Pathology 128: 538–554

Simon M 1985 Secondary iron overload and the haemochromatosis allele. British Journal of Haematology 60: 1–5

Simon M, Brissot P 1988 The genetics of haemochromatosis. Journal of Hepatology 6: 116–124

Simon M, Gosselin M, Kerbaol M, Delanoe G, Trebaul L, Bourel M 1973a Functional study of exocrine pancreas in idiopathic haemochromatosis, untreated and treated by venesection (32 cases). Digestion 8: 485–496

Simon M, Vongsavanthong S, Hespel J P, Le Cornu M, Bourel M 1973b Diabète et hémochromatose. 1-Le diabète dans l'hémochromatose. A propos de 130 cas personnels d'hémochromatose. Semaine des Hôpitaux de Paris 49: 2125–2132

Simon M, Pawlotsky Y, Bourel M, Fauchet R, Genetet B 1975 Hémochromatose idiopathique. Maladie associée à l'antigène tissulaire HLA-A3. Nouvelle Presse Médicale 4: 1432

Simon M, Bourel M, Fauchet R, Genetet B 1976 Association of HLA-A3 and HLA-B14 antigens with idiopathic haemochromatosis. Gut 17: 332–334

Simon M, Alexandre J L, Bourel M, Le Marec B, Scordia C 1977a Heredity of idiopathic haemochromatosis: a study of 106 families. Clinical Genetics 11: 327–341

Simon M, Bourel M, Genetet B, Fauchet R 1977b Idiopathic hemochromatosis. Demonstration of recessive inheritance and early detection by family HLA typing. New England Journal of Medicine 297: 1017–1021

Simon M, Bourel M, Genetet B, Fauchet R, Edan G, Brissot P 1977c Idiopathic hemochromatosis and iron overload in alcoholic liver disease: differentiation by HLA phenotype. Gastroenterology 73: 655–658

Simon M, Hespel J P, Fauchet R et al 1979 Hérédité récessive de l'hémochromatose idiopathique: deux observations de transmission pseudo-dominante reconnue comme récessive par l'étude de la surcharge en fer et des génotypes HLA dans les familles. Nouvelle Presse Médicale 8: 421–424

Simon L, Alexandre J L, Fauchet R, Genetet B, Bourel M 1980a The genetics of hemochromatosis. In: Steinberg A G, Bearn A G, Motulsky A G, Childs B (eds) Progress in Medical Genetics. Saunders, Philadelphia, p 1356–1368

Simon M, Fauchet R, Hespel J P et al 1980b Idiopathic hemochromatosis. A study of biochemical expression in 247 heterozygous members of 63 families. Evidence for a single major HLA-linked gene. Gastroenterology 78: 703–708

Simon M, Le Mignon L, Edan G, Le Reun M, Hespel J P 1984 Diabètes d'"autres types": pancréatite chronique et hémochromatose. Journées Annuelles de Diabétologie de l'Hôtel Dieu, Flammarion, Paris, p 85–114

Simon M, Beaumont C, Briere J et al 1985a Is the HLA-linked haemochromatosis allele implicated in idiopathic refractory sideroblastic anaemia? British Journal of Haematology 60: 75–80

Simon M, Le Mignon L, Fauchet R et al 1985b Prevalence of the haemochromatosis allele in Brittany (France), as inferred from family patterns. European Iron Club Meeting, Amersfoort, Sept 18–20th. Abst

Simon M, Le Mignon L, Fauchet R et al 1987 A study of 609 haplotypes marking for the hemochromatosis gene: (1) mapping of the gene near the HLA-A locus and characters required to define a heterozygous population and (2) hypothesis concerning the underlying cause of hemochromatosis-HLA association. American Journal of Human Genetics 41: 89–105

Simon M, Fauchet R, Le Gall J Y, Brissot P, Bourel M 1988a Immunogenetics of idiopathic hemochromatosis and secondary iron overload. In: Farid N E (ed) Immunogenetics of Endocrine Disorders Alan Liss, New York, p 345–371

Simon M, Yaouanq J, Le Gall J Y, Fauchet R, Brissot P, Bourel M 1988b Genetics of hemochromatosis: HLA association and mode of inheritance. In: Weintraub L R, Edwards C Q, Krikker M (eds) Hemochromatosis, Proceedings of the first international conference. Annals of New York Academy of Sciences 526: 11–22

Thomson G, Bodmer W 1977 The genetic analysis of HLA and disease associations. In: Dausset G, Svejgeard A (eds) HLA and Disease. Munkksgaard, Williams and Wilkins, Copenhagen, Baltimore, p 84–93

Tourniaire J, Fevre M, Mazenod B, Ponsin G 1974 Effects of clomiphene citrate and synthetic LHRH on serum luteinizing hormone (LH) in men with idiopathic hemochromatosis. Journal of Clinical Endocrinology and Metabolism 38: 1122–1124

Trousseau A 1865 Clinique Médicale de l'Hôtel-Dieu de Paris. Baillère, Paris, p 663–698

Tsan M F, Sheffel V 1985 Transferrin sialic acid contents of patients with hereditary hemochromatosis. American Journal of Hematology 20: 359–363

Valberg L S, Lloyd D A, Ghent C et al 1980 Clinical and biochemical expression of the genetic abnormality in idiopathic hemochromatosis. Gastroenterology 79: 884–892

von Recklinghausen F D 1889 Uber haemochromatose Klinische Wochenschrift 26: 925

Walsh C H, Wright A D, Williams J, Holder G 1976 A study of pituitary function in patients with idiopathic hemochromatosis. Journal of Clinical Endocrinology and Metabolism 43: 866–872

Walters J M, Watt P W, Stevens F M, McCarthy C F 1975 HLA antigens in haemochromatosis. British Medical Journal 4: 520

Walton C, Kelly W F, Laing I, Bullock D E 1983 Endocrine abnormalities in idiopathic haemochromatosis. Quarterly Journal of Medicine 205: 99–100

Weintraub L R, Goral A, Grasso J, Franzblau C, Sullivan A, Sullivan S 1985 Pathogenesis of hepatic fibrosis in experimental iron overload. British Journal of Haematology 59: 321–331

Worwood M 1979 Serum ferritin. CRC Critical Reviews in Clinical Laboratory Sciences 10: 171–204

Yang S, Lum J B, McGill J R et al 1984 Human transferrin: cDNA characterization and chromosomal localization. Proceedings of the National Academy of Sciences of the United States of America 81: 2752–2756

101. The mucopolysaccharidoses

J. Spranger

The genetic mucopolysaccharidoses are hereditary, progressive disorders caused by the excessive intralysosomal accumulation of glycosaminoglycans (acid mucopolysaccharides) in various tissues. Glycosaminoglycans are long-chain complex carbohydrates consisting of a variety of uronic acids, amino sugars and neutral sugars. They are usually linked to proteins to form proteoglycans. Proteoglycans are major constituents of the ground substance of connective tissue. They are also present in mitochondria, nuclear and cell membranes (Kraemer & Smith 1974, Dietrich et al 1976).

The major glucosaminoglycans are chondroitin-4-sulphate, chondroitin-6-sulphate, heparan sulphate, dermatan sulphate, keratan sulphate and hyaluronic acid. In the organism these substances are degraded by the sequential action of lysosomal enzymes leading to a stepwise shortening of the glycosaminoglycan chain (Fig. 101.1). Absent activity of a lysosomal enzyme results in the gradual accumulation of partially degraded glycosaminoglycan molecules in lysosomes. Distended lysosomes accumulate in the cell (Fig. 101.2) and interfere with normal cell function.

Some clinical manifestations of the mucopolysaccharidoses such as coarse facial features, thick skin, corneal clouding and organomegaly can be regarded as the direct expression of glycosaminoglycan accumulation in tissue. Others, such as mental retardation, growth deficiency, skeletal dysplasia are the result of defective cell function. Joint contractures and hernias point to an interference of accumulated glycosaminoglycans with other metabolic substances such as collagen or fibronectin.

Different mucopolysaccharidoses are caused by different enzyme deficiencies leading to the accumulation of biochemically different glycosaminoglycan degradation products. As a general rule, the impaired degradation of heparan sulphate is more closely associated with mental deficiency and the impaired degradation of dermatan sulphate, chondroitin sulphates and keratan sulphate with mesenchymal abnormalities. Some of the salient features of the mucopolysaccharidoses are summarized in Table 101.1.

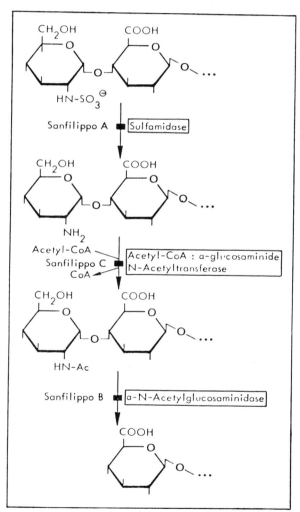

Fig. 101.1 Enzymatic degradation of N-sulphoglucosaminyl residues in heparan sulphate by the sequential action of three lysosomal enzymes. The deficiency of any of these three enzymes leads to clinically indistinguishable forms of mucopolysaccharidosis III: Sanfilippo disease A, B or C.

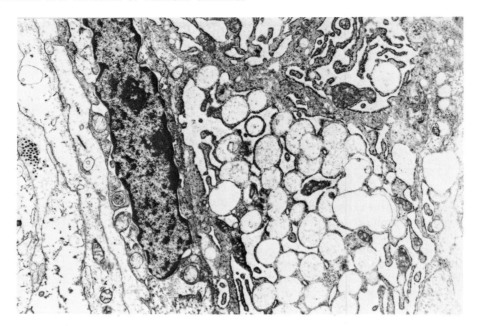

Fig. 101.2   The cytoplasm of an osteoblast from a patient with mucopolysaccharidosis II is filled with numerous membrane-bound vacuoles containing a fine granular material (buffered glutaraldehyde x 6000).

MUCOPOLYSACCHARIDOSIS I-H (HURLER DISEASE)

Hurler disease is characterized by the combinations of progressive mental degeneration with a peculiar clinical phenotype. The characteristic 'Hurler phenotype' consists of gross facial features, enlarged and deformed skull, small stature, corneal opacities, hepatosplenomegaly, valvular heart defects, thick skin, joint contractures and hernias (Fig. 101.3).

The clinical features become more apparent with age. In infancy nonspecific signs are found such as a slightly enlarged head, chronic rhinitis and hernias. A diagnosis may be suspected on the basis of broad ribs and coarse bone structure in a routine chest film. It can be confirmed by demonstrating an elevated urinary excretion of glycosaminoglycans and appropriate enzyme studies. By the end of the first year of life the Hurler phenotype becomes evident. Growth is still normal at that age but slows down thereafter. The disorder is progressive and usually leads to death before the age of 14 years. Death commonly occurs from cardiac failure due to valvular incompetence and chronic respiratory infections. The patients are severely demented but usually retain a certain degree of emotional contact. Early death during infancy has been observed following endocardial fibroelastosis (Stephan et al 1989).

Complications include chronic upper respiratory infection, large hernias, cardiac insufficiency and increased cranial pressure due to impaired spinal fluid circulation caused by thickened leptomeninges and subarachnoidal cysts. Torsion of the enlarged spleen has been observed.

X-rays show a pattern of skeletal abnormalities called 'dysostosis multiplex'. Its major features are a large skull with a deep, elongated, J-shaped sella, oar-like ribs, deformed, hook-shaped lower thoracic and upper lumbar vertebrae, pelvic dysplasia, shortened tubular bones with expanded diaphyses and dysplastic epiphyses (Fig. 101.4). The bone structure is coarse and irregular. The abnormalities become more distinct with age.

Blood smears show abnormal cytoplasmic inclusions in lymphocytes. The urinary excretion of dermatan sulphate and heparan sulphate is increased. The diagnosis is confirmed by assay in leucocytes and cultured fibroblasts of the enzyme alpha-L-iduronidase.

Mucopolysaccharidosis I-H is inherited as an autosomal recessive trait. Prenatal diagnosis is possible by measuring the iduronidase activity and the incorporation of labelled sulphate in glycosaminoglycans of cultured amniotic cells.

No causal therapy is available. Attempts at enzyme replacement using plasma transfusions have failed. Reversal of clinical features and biochemical improvement has been reported in several patients with Hurler disease after bone marrow transplantation (Hobbs et al 1986).

MUCOPOLYSACCHARIDOSIS I-S (SCHEIE DISEASE)

Scheie disease is a milder manifestation of iduronidase deficiency than Hurler disease. It is rarely diagnosed before the age of 6 years. Its major clinical features are coarse but not Hurler-like facial features, corneal clouding and joint contractures, notably of the fingers. Heart murmurs are caused by stenosis and/or regurgitation at the heart valves, mostly of the aorta. Some patients are deaf. They are of normal or almost normal height and their intelligence is unimpaired. Their life expectancy is generally good, depending on the rate of progression of cardiac disease. Complications include retinopathy, glaucoma, the carpal tunnel syndrome, pes cavus and hernias.

X–rays show minimal changes of dysostosis multiplex with broad ribs, small carpal bones with proximal convergence of the finger rays, and mild hypoplasia of the lower portions of the iliac bones of the pelvis. The urinary excretion of dermatan sulphate and heparan sulphate is increased.

Mucopolysaccharidoses I-H and I-S are probably allelic mutations involving the alpha-L-iduronidase locus. Cell fusion studies show no complementation of Hurler and Scheie cells (Galjaard 1980). The different severity of Hurler and Scheie disease may be caused by a higher residual activity of alpha-L-iduronidase towards its natural substrates in the latter.

Therapeutic measures include operative procedures for correction of the carpal tunnel syndrome, glaucoma

Table 101.1 The genetic mucopolysaccharidoses

Number	Eponym	Main clinical features	Defective enzyme	Assay in:	Genetics
MPS I-H	Pfaundler-Hurler	Severe Hurler phenotype, mental retardation, corneal clouding, death usually before age 14 years	α-L-iduronidase	L,F,Ac	AR
MPS I-S	Scheie	Stiff joints, corneal clouding, aortic valve disease, normal intelligence, survive to adulthood	α-L-iduronidase	L,F,Ac	AR
MPS I-H/S	Hurler/Scheie	Phenotype intermediate between I-H and I-S; genetic heterogeneity possible in this group, but at least some patients are Hurler-Scheie double heterozygotes	α-L-iduronidase	L,F,Ac	AR
MPS II-XR	Hunter	Severe course: similar to MPS I-H but usually clear cornea. Mild course: milder clinical phenotype, later manifestation and survival to adulthood without or with mild mental retardation. Deafness	Iduronate sulphate sulphatase	S,L, Ac? Af?	XR
MPS III-A	Sanfilippo A	Behavioural problems, aggression, progressive dementia, seizures, survival to second or third decade of life possible, considerable intrafamilial variability, mild dysmorphism, coarse hair, clear corneae, usually normal height	Heparan-S-sulphaminidase	L,F,Ac	AR
MPS III-B	Sanfilippo B		N-ac-α-D-glucosaminidase	S,F,Ac	AR
MPS III-C	Sanfilippo C		Ac-CoA-glucosaminide N-acetyltransferase	F,Ac?	AR
MPS III-D	Sanfilippo D		N-ac-glucosamine-6-sulphate sulphatase	L,F	AR
MPS-IV-A	Morquio A	Short-trunk type of dwarfism, fine corneal opacities, characteristic bone dysplasia, final height below 125 cm	Galactosamine-6-sulphate sulphatase	F,Ac?	AR
MPS IV-B	Morquio B	Same as IV-A but milder, adult height over 120 cm	β-galactosidase	L,F,Ac	AR
MPS V	No longer used	formerly Scheie disease			
MPS VI	Maroteaux-Lamy	Hurler phenotype with marked corneal clouding and normal intelligence. Mild, moderate and severe expression in different families (?allelic mutations)	N-acetyl-galactosamine α-4-sulphate sulphatase (Arylsulphatase B)	S,L,F Ac	AR
MPS VII	Sly	Highly variable. Dense inclusions in granulocytes	β-glucuronidase	S,L,F,Ac	AR

L = Leucocytes; S = Serum; F = Cultured fibroblasts; Ac = Cultured amniotic cells; Af = Amniotic fluid; AR = autosomal recessive; XR = X-chromosomal recessive and aortic disease. Corneal transplants may become necessary.

MUCOPOLYSACCHARIDOSIS I-H/S (HURLER-SCHEIE COMPOUND)

Given a gene frequency of 1 in 330 for Mucopolysaccharidosis I-H and 1 in 700 for Mucopolysaccharidosis I-S there must be patients carrying both the Hurler and the Scheie gene (McKusick et al 1972). The frequency of these double heterozygotes in the population is estimated as $2 \times (1:330) \times (1:700) = 1:115\,000$ (versus 1:100 000 for Hurler disease and 1:500 000 for Scheie disease).

The phenotype of these patients would be expected to be less severe than that for MPS I-H and more severe than that for MPS I-S. A number of such patients has been observed (Spranger et al 1974, Leisti et al 1976, Stevenson et al 1976). They are short, have corneal opacities, joint contractures, hepatomegaly, abnormal heart valves and other features of Mucopolysaccharidosis I-H. In contrast to the latter they are less severely retarded, have puckish rather than Hurler-like facial features and may survive into adulthood. Their skeletal abnormalities are less severe than in Hurler disease. Destruction of the sellar region, probably caused by arachnoid cysts, seems to be relatively common (Winters et al 1976, McKusick et al 1978).

OTHER FORMS OF α-IDURONIDASE DEFICIENCY

The genetic concept of Mucopolysaccharidosis I-H/S requires that the incidence of parental consanguinity is not increased. However in several families with alpha-L-iduronidase deficiency, and an intermediate Hurler-Scheie phenotype, parental consanguinity has been recorded. Some patients look different from the so-called I-H/S compound cases (Roubicek et al 1985). Thus there may be other forms of alpha-L-iduronidase deficiency in addition to the I-H/S compound, Hurler and Scheie disease. Fusion studies of alpha-iduronidase deficient fibroblasts from patients with severe, mild, and intermediate phenotypes suggest that they are caused by allelic mutations (Fortuin & Kleijer 1980).

MUCOPOLYSACCHARIDOSIS II (HUNTER DISEASE)

The clinical features of mucopolysaccharidosis II are similar to those of mucopolysaccharidosis I-H with the notable exception of the cornea which is generally clear. Only rarely are corneal opacities found in a child with

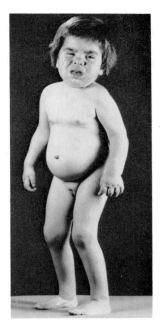

Fig. 101.3 3-year-old patient with mucopolysaccharidosis I-H. Note coarse facial features, dense hair, disproportionately short trunk, protuberant abdomen and multiple flexion contractures of the joints.

Hunter disease. Conversely, clear corneae are the exception in Hurler disease (Gardner & Hay 1974, Spranger et al 1978). Nodular skin lesions giving the skin a pebbled appearance are seen in some patients and are probably unique to mucopolysaccharidosis II.

The disease may take a rapid, an intermediate or a slow course. Patients with a *rapid course* are almost as severely affected as patients with Hurler disease, with first manifestations in late infancy, rapid physical and mental deterioration, and death in early puberty.

In its *mild form* the disease is detected later and the patients survive to adulthood. They are slightly short, of heavy build with moderately coarse facial features, hoarse voice, joint contractures notably of the fingers, median nerve entrapment, enlarged liver and spleen, and herniae. Hearing defects are almost invariably present. Atypical retinitis pigmentosa and chronic papilloedema with impairment of vision are commonly found. Heart disease due to valvular thickening, myocardial and ischaemic factors is a problem. Patients with the mild form are mentally normal. In the adult patients reported by Karpati et al (1974) multiple nerve entrapment and moderate shortness of stature were the only clinical symptoms.

X-ray studies show dysostosis multiplex in a milder

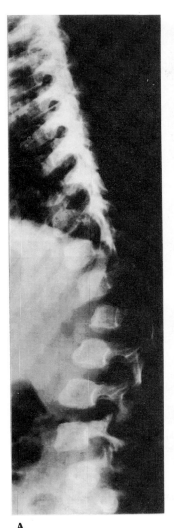

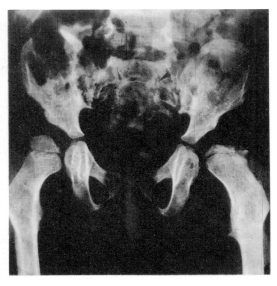

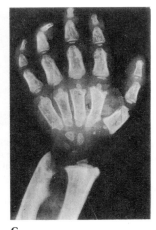

Fig. 101.4 Dysostosis multiplex. **A** 4 years. The vertebral bodies have an ovoid shape which is abnormal for this age. There is an ossification defect in the anterosuperior aspect of the bodies of L-2 to L-4. L-2 is hypoplastic and dorsally displaced. **B** 4 years. The basilar portions of the iliac bones are hypoplastic, the acetabular fossae are shallow and the iliac wings are flared. The capital femoral epiphyses are small, and the femoral necks are broad and in valgus position. **C** 8 years. The tubular bones are abnormally short, wide and deformed. The proximal and middle phalanges are bullet-shaped. The second to fifth metacarpals are narrow at their bases. The epiphyses are irregular. The carpal bones are small. The distal articular surfaces of the ulna and radius are slanted towards each other. The bone trabeculation is coarse and the cortices are thin.

A

C

and more slowly progressive form than in mucopolysaccharidosis I-H. In adult patients the only pathological findings may be small carpal bones and mild dysplasia of the pelvis and femoral heads with premature arthrosis (Grossman & Dorst 1973). The urine contains large amounts of heparan sulphate and dermatan sulphate.

Mucopolysaccharidosis II is an X-linked recessive condition caused by a deficiency of the enzyme iduronate sulphate sulphatase. The enyzme activity can be determined in serum, lymphocytes and cultured fibroblasts. Prenatal diagnosis is possible by measurement of iduronate sulphate sulphatase in amniotic fluid and by S^{35} incorporation studies in cultured amniotic cells (Liebaers & Neufeld 1975, Liebaers et al 1977) and in chorionic villi (Pannone et al 1986).

Severe and mild forms have been described in the same family (Yatziv et al 1977) and the differing severity of the manifestations is probably the expression of variability. In most families, however, the affected males are affected to a similar degree (Young et al 1982). Carrier detection is difficult but can be attempted by iduronate sulphate sulphatase determination in hair roots (Chase et al 1986), serum (Archer et al 1983) or fibroblasts (Tønnesen et al 1983).

In a single female patient with full expression of Hunter disease, deficient activity of iduronate sulphate sulphatase was caused by a partial deletion of the long arm of the X chromosome, most probably of band Xq25, and non-random inactivation (Broadhead et al 1986). Therapeutically, bone marrow transplantation has been attempted, with uncertain results (Hobbs et al 1986). Symptomatic measures are indicated as in other mucopolysaccharidoses.

MUCOPOLYSACCHARIDOSIS III (SANFILIPPPO DISEASE)

Mucopolysaccharidosis III is clinically characterized by comparatively mild dysmorphism and progressive dementia. First clinical symptoms usually appear after the second year of life. They relate to behavioural problems and include sleep disturbances, lack of concentration, short attention span and impulsiveness. Later, hyperactivity and aggressiveness occur. Psychomotor skills are gradually lost. The patients stop speaking. Convulsions occur. The most prominent clinical feature is abundant and coarse, often blond hair (Fig. 101.5). The patients are of normal height and their corneae are clear. Liver and spleen are not, or only mildly, enlarged.

The course of the disease is relentless and leads to a vegetative state. Most patients die before the age of 20 years from aspiration pneumonia. Intrafamilial variability may be considerable. Some patients are retarded from infancy, others may attend the first grades of school. Some patients die before the age of 10, others survive into middle adulthood. Patients with mucopolysaccharidosis III-A are somewhat more severely affected than those with type B, with earlier onset, more rapid progression of the disease and earlier death in the second decade of life (Van de Kamp et al 1981). Type C seems to be of intermediate severity.

There are mild skeletal changes of dysostosis multiplex with thickened calvaria, ovoid vertebral bodies and hypoplasia of the lower portions of the pelvic ilia. Peripheral lymphocytes contain conspicuous inclusions. The urinary excretion of heparan sulphate and chondroitin sulphates is elevated.

The disorder is caused by the deficiency of any of multiple lysosomal enzymes involved in the degradation of heparan sulphate (Fig. 101.1): sulphamidase (mucopolysaccharidosis III-A), alpha-N-acetyl-glucosaminidase (mucopolysaccharidosis III-B) and acetyl-CoA-alpha-glucosaminide-N-acetyl-transferase (mucopolysaccharidosis III-C). Clinically, the three enzyme deficiencies cannot be differentiated. They are inherited as autosomal recessive disorders. Mucopolysaccharidosis III-A seems to be more common than mucopolysaccharidoses III-B and III-C. Prenatal diagnosis is possible. A fourth type of Sanfilippo disease, MPS III-D, has re-

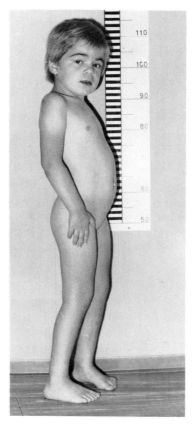

Fig. 101.5 5-year-old patient with mucopolysaccharidosis III. The hair is abundant. The facial features are slightly coarse. The patient is of normal height.

cently been described (Gatti et al 1982). It is caused by a deficiency of N-ac-glucosamine-6-sulphate sulphatase, an enzyme that acts specifically to remove sulphate from position 6 of N-ac-glucosamine in heparan sulphate (not shown in Fig. 101.1). Combined deficiency of sulphamidase and β-mannosidase has been described in a 3-year-old boy with the clinical appearance of Sanfilippo A disease (Wenger et al 1986). The relation between the two enzymatic deficiencies is presently unknown.

Therapy is symptomatic. Control of hyperactivity is difficult and may require a combination of sedatives and psychorelaxants including haloperidol. Barbiturates are frequently without effect.

MUCOPOLYSACCHARIDOSIS IV (MORQUIO DISEASE)

The main clinical features of Morquio disease are a short-trunk type of dwarfism with normal intelligence and without Hurler-like facial characteristics. Historically, the disorder has been confused with numerous spondyloepiphyseal dysplasias. It was clearly defined by Maroteaux and Lamy (1963).

The first signs appear in the second or third year of life. Thoracic deformity, kyphosis and/or genu valgum and growth retardation are noted. Other features gradually develop until finally a characteristic pattern of clinical findings has emerged with a prominent lower face, enamel hypoplasia of the teeth, short neck, protruding upper sternum, accentuated spinal curves, genu valgum, prominent and loose joints and short fingers (Fig. 101.6A). Slit-lamp examination shows fine corneal opacities and audiometry reveals hearing loss. Adult height is below 120 cm in most patients in mucopolysaccharidosis IV-A and between 120 cm and 140 cm in mucopolysaccharidosis IV-B.

The most important complication is spinal cord compression at the upper cervical level due to atlantoaxial instability. This is caused by a combination of

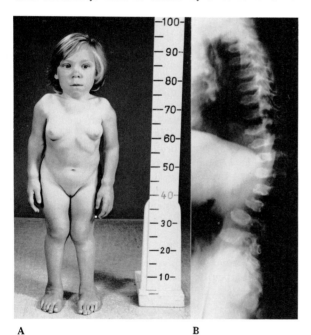

A   **B**

Fig. 101.6 A A 12-year-old girl with mucopolysaccharidosis IV, Morquio disease. The spine is disproportionately short. The lower half of the face is slightly accentuated. The joints are prominent and there are genu valga. **B** The vertebral bodies are flattened, more markedly in their dorsal than in their anterior portions. There is anterior pointing. At the lumbodorsal junction the anterior portions of the vertebral bodies are slightly hypoplastic. In some patients the hypoplasia is more marked, with a resultant kyphosis and narrowing of the spinal canal at this level.

odontoid hypoplasia and ligamentous hyperlaxity. The first symptoms of a cervical myelopathy are easy fatiguability. Later subtle neurological signs develop. If undetected, the condition may lead to quadriplegia. Spinal cord compression may also occur at the level of D-12 to L-2 where anterior hypoplasia of the vertebral bodies leads to an acute kyphosis with encroachment upon the spinal canal. Other complications are multiple arthroses, and aortic regurgitation, which develops in some patients.

X-ray studies show a characteristic spondyloepiphyseal bone dysplasia with platyspondyly, anterior hypoplasia of the vertebral bodies at the thoracolumbar junction, odontoid hypoplasia, hypoplastic basilar portions of the ilia of the pelvis, genu valga, marked epiphyseal dysplasia and shortening of the tubular bones (Fig. 101.6B). Children excrete excessive amounts of keratan sulphate in the urine. This is not the case in adults with Morquio disease. Failure to detect keratan sulphate in the urine is either caused by the older age of the patient or by improper biochemical technique: keratan sulphate is notoriously difficult to detect in the urine.

Morquio disease is heterogeneous. Type IV-A is caused by the deficiency of N-acetyl-galactosamine-6-sulphate-sulphatase (Singh et al 1976). Most patients with this defect have the classical, severe Morquio phenotype with adult height below 120 cm. Others are less severely affected, and still others have an almost normal adult height (Beck et al 1986). Type IV-B is caused by the deficiency of a β-galactosidase with specificity for keratan sulphate and chondroitin sulphates (Arbisser et al 1977). The deficiency may be caused by defects of the primary structure of the enzyme or by defects in its post-translational processing (Hoogeven et al 1984).

The disorders are inherited as autosomal recessive traits. Prenatal diagnosis should be possible by appropriate enzyme assay in cultured amniotic cells.

The most important therapeutic measure is the prevention of cervical myelopathy. Preventive fusion of the cervical spine is recommended (Kopits et al 1972, Lipson 1977). Genu valga are corrected by osteotomy. Dental care and hearing are important.

MUCOPOLYSACCHARIDOSIS VI (MAROTEAUX-LAMY DISEASE)

Patients with mucopolysaccharidosis VI have a Hurler-like phenotype with normal intelligence. There is a mild and a severe form.

The *severe form* manifests itself in early childhood with thoracic deformities, lumbodorsal kyphosis, hernias and genu valga. Coarse facial features develop. Growth is retarded and ceases at about 10 years. Macrocephaly and hydrocephaly are found in some patients and are caused by thickened meninges, possibly arachnoidal cysts leading to impaired flow and reabsorption of spinal fluid. Other complications are optic atrophy, buphthalmos, cardiac insufficiency and the carpal tunnel sequence. The patients may survive into their third decade of life. They are severely handicapped by visual loss, joint contractures and by social problems stemming from their unusual appearance. Their mental performance remains relatively normal.

The *mild form* is recognized later and the patients may live into late adulthood. In its mildest expression, stiffness of the hands, corneal opacities, hernias and body height below 160 cm with only slightly coarse facial features are the only symptoms. More commonly, adolescents and adults with the mild form have distinctly Hurler-like facial features, dense corneal clouding, short stature, joint contractures, organomegaly and cardiac involvement.

Radiographs show dysostosis multiplex, the severity of which corresponds to the degree of clinical involvement. Dense granulations are found in neutrophils of peripheral blood smears. The urine contains excessive amounts of dermatan sulphate.

The disease is caused by a deficiency of the enzyme N-acetyl-galactosamine-4-sulphate sulphatase (arylsulphatase B). It is inherited as an autosomal recessive trait. Evidence of genetic heterogeneity has been presented with the observation of biochemically different mutant enzymes (Black et al 1986). Prenatal diagnosis has been performed (Kleijer et al 1976).

Therapeutic measures include shunting procedures to relieve increased intracranial pressure, corneal grafting, operative treatment of the carpal tunnel syndrome and hip replacement in adults with severe coxarthrosis. Replacement of defective heart valves may be considered in patients with the mild form of the disease.

MUCOPOLYSACCHARIDOSIS VII

Mucopolysaccharidosis VII is caused by a deficiency of the enzyme β-glucuronidase. Up to 1985 about 20 cases had been described which were classified in a mild and a severe form (Lee et al 1985). Titration patterns resulting from an enzyme immunoassay ssupport the assumption of genetic heterogeneity (Bell et al 1977). Variability of intrafamilial expression has also been observed (Guibaud et al 1979).

In its mildest form, thoracic kyphosis and mild scoliosis are the only clinical findings (Danes & Degnan 1974, Gitzelmann et al 1978). One patient with this mild form had, in addition, fibromuscular dysplasia of the aorta and minimal coarsening of the face (Beaudet et al 1975).

Other patients have more severe manifestations. They attract medical attention in later infancy or early childhood because of slightly coarse facial features, hepatosplenomegaly, hernias, thoracic deformities and thoracolumbar kyphosis (Gehler et al 1974, Beaudet et al 1975, Pfeiffer et al 1977, Guibaud et al 1979). The patients are moderately mentally retarded. Recurrent respiratory infections are a major problem.

One patient seems to be an example of a severe form of the disease (Beaudet et al 1975). He presented with neonatal jaundice and hepatosplenomegaly. He had multiple hernias, gross corneal clouding, severely delayed psychomotor development, recurrent infections and died at 2.9 years of age.

Radiographs show minimal flattening of the vertebral bodies in mild cases and more pronounced changes of dysostosis multiplex in more severely affected patients. Dense Alder-type inclusions are found in peripheral granulocytes, and the original description of the so-called Alder anomaly may very well have been made in sibs with β-glucuronidase deficiency (Alder 1944). Increased amounts of glycosaminoglycans are found in the urine. The diagnosis is established by determination of β-glucuronidase activity in serum, leucocytes or fibroblasts.

The β-glucuronidase deficiencies are probably inherited as autosomal recessive conditions. The structural locus for β-glucuronidase has been assigned to chromosome 7 (Grzeschik 1975, Lalley et al 1975). Prenatal diagnosis has been performed (Maire et al 1979).

REFFERENCES

Alder A 1944 Über konstitutionell bedingte Granulationsveranderungen der Leukozyten. Helvetica Paediatrica Acta 11: 161–165

Arbisser A I, Donelly K A, Scott C I, DiFerrante N, Singh J, Stevenson R E, Aylesworth A S, Howell R R 1977 Morquio-like syndrome with beta galactosidase deficiency and normal hexosamine sulphatase activity: mucopolysaccharidosis IVB. American Journal of Medical Genetics 1: 195–205

Archer I M, Young I D, Rees D W et al 1983 Carrier detection in Hunter syndrome. American Journal of Medical Genetics 16: 61–69

Beaudet A L, DiFerrante N A, Ferry G D, Nichols B L, Mullins C E 1975 Variation in the phenotypic expression of β-glucuronidase deficiency. Journal of Pediatrics 86: 388–394

Beck M, Glössl J, Grubisic A, Spranger J 1986 Heterogeneity of Morquio disease. Clinical Genetics 29: 135–159

Bell C E, Sly W S, Brot F E 1977 Human β-glucuronidase

deficiency mucopolysaccharidosis. Journal of Clinical Investigations 59: 97-105

Black S H, Pelias M Z, Miller J B, Blither M G, Shapira E 1986 Maroteaux-Lamy syndrome in a large consanguineous kindred. American Journal of Medical Genetics 25: 273-279

Broadhead D M, Kirk J M, Burt A et al 1986 Full expression of Hunter's disease in a female with an X-chromosome deletion leading to non-random inactivation. Clinical Genetics 30: 392-398

Cantz M, Gehler J 1976 The mucopolysaccharidoses: inborn errors of glycosaminoglycans catabolism. Human Genetics 32: 233-235

Chase D S, Morris A H, Ballabio A et al 1986 Genetics of Hunter Syndrome: carrier detection, new mutations, segregation and linkage analysis. Annals of Human Genetics 50: 349-360

Danes B S, Degnan M 1974 Different clinical and biochemical phenotypes associated with β-glucuronidase deficiency. Birth Defects: Original Article Series 10: No 12: 251-257

Dietrich C P, Sampaio L O, Toledo O M S 1976 Characteristic distribution of sulphated mucopolysaccharides in different tissues and in their respective mitochondria. Biochemical and Biophysical Research Communications 71: 1-10

Fortuin J J H, Kleijer W J 1980 Hybridization of fibroblasts from Hurler, Scheie and Hurler/Scheie compound patients: Support of the hypothesis of allele mutations. Human Genetics 65: 155-159

Galjaard H 1980 Genetic metabolic diseases, 1st edn. Elsevier, North Holland, Amsterdam, ch 3, p 114

Gardner R J M, Hay H R 1974 Hurler's syndrome with clear corneas. Lancet II: 845

Gatti R, Borrone C, Durand P et al 1982 Sanfilippo type D disease: clinical findings in two patients with a new variant of mucopolysaccharidosis III. European Journal of Pediatrics 138: 168-171

Gehler J, Cantz M, Tolksdorf M, Spranger J, Gilbert E, Drube H 1974 Mucopolysaccharidosis VII: β-glucuronidase deficiency. Humangenetik 23: 149-158

Gitzelmann R, Wiesmann U N, Spycher M A, Herschkowitz N, Giedion A 1978 Unusually mild course of β-glucuronidase deficiency in two brothers (mucopolysaccharidosis VII), Helvetica Paediatrica Acta 33: 413-428

Grossman H, Dorst J P 1973 The mucopolysaccharidoses and mucolipidoses. Progress in Pediatric Radiology. Karger Basel, 4: 495-499

Grzeschik K H 1975 Assignment of human genes: β-glucuronidase to chromosome 7, adenylate kinase 1 to 9, a second enzyme with enolase activity to 12, and mitochondrial IDH to 15. Gene Mapping Conference. Baltimore, 3: 142-148

Guibaud P, Maire I, Goddon R, Teyssier G, Zabot M T, Mandon G 1979 Mucopolysaccharidose type VII par déficit en β-glucuronidase: Etude d'une famille. Journal de Genetique Humaine 27: 29-43

Hobbs J R, Hugh-Jones K, Chambers J D et al 1986 Lysosomal enzyme replacement therapy by displacement bone marrow transplantation with immunoprophylaxis. Advances in Clinical Enzymology 3: 184-210

Hoogeven A T, Graham-Kawashima H, D'Azzo A, Galjaard H 1984 Processing of human β-galactosidase in GM$_1$ gangliosidosis and Morquio B syndrome. Journal of Biological Chemistry 259: 1974-1977

Karpati G, Carpenter S, Eisan A A, Wolfe L S, Feindel W 1974 Multiple peripheral nerve entrapments. An unusual phenotype variant of the Hunter syndrome (mucopolysaccharidosis II) in a family. Archives of Neurology 31:418-422

Kleijer W J, Wolffers G M, Hoogeven A, Niermeijer M F 1976 Prenatal diagnosis of Maroteaux-Lamy syndrome. Lancet II: 50

Kopits S E, Perovic M N, McKusick V A, Robinson R A, Bailey J A 1972 Congenital atlantoaxial dislocations in various forms of dwarfism. Journal of Bone and Joint Surgery. 54-A: 1349-1350

Kraemer P M, Smith D A 1974 High molecular-weight heparan sulphate from the cell surface. Biochemical and Biophysical Research Communications 56: 423-429

Lalley P A, Brown J A, Eddy R L, Haley L L, Shows T B 1975 Assignment of the gene for β-glucuronidase (β-GUS) to chromosome 7 in man. Gene Mapping Conference, Baltimore, 3: 184-187

Lee J E, Falk R E, Ng W G, Donnell G N 1985 β-glucuronidase deficiency. American Journal of Diseases of Children 139: 57-59

Leisti J, Rimoin D L, Kaback M, Shapiro L J, Matalon R 1976 Allelic mutations in the mucopolysaccharidoses. Birth Defects: Original Article Series 12: 6, 81-91

Liebaers I, Neufeld E F 1975 Iduronate sulphatase deficiency in serum and lymphocytes of Hunter patients. Abstract, Annual Meeting, American Society of Human Genetics, Baltimore, October 8-11

Liebaers I, DiNatale P, Neufeld E F 1977 Iduronate sulphatase in amniotic fluid: an aid in the prenatal diagnosis of the Hunter syndrome. Journal of Pediatrics 90: 423-425

Lipson S J 1977 Dysplasia of the odontoid process in Morquio's syndrome causing quadriparesis. The Journal of Bone and Joint Surgery 59-A: 340-344

McKusick V A 1972 Heritable disorders of connective tissue, 4th edn. Mosby, Saint Louis, p 521-686

McKusick V A, Howell R R, Hussels I E, Neufeld E F, Stevenson R E 1972 Allelism, non-allelism and genetic compounds among the mucopolysaccharidoses. Lancet I: 993-996

McKusick V A, Neufeld E F, Kelly T E 1978 The mucopolysaccharide storage diseases. In: Stanbury J B, Wyngaarden J B, Frederickson D S (eds) The metabolic basis of inherited disease, 4th edn. McGraw-Hill, New York, ch 53, p 1290

Maire I, Mandon G, Zabot M T, Mathieu M 1979 β-Glucuronidase deficiency: enzyme studies in an affected family and prenatal diagnosis. Journal of Inherited Metabolic Diseases 2: 29-34

Maroteaux P, Lamy M 1963 La maladie de Morquio. Etude clinique, radiologique et biologique. Presse Médicale 71: 2091-2094

Neufeld E F 1974 The biochemical basis for mucopolysaccharidoses and mucolipidoses. Progress in Medical Genetics 10: 81-101

Nwokoro N, Neufeld E F 1979 Detection of Hunter heterozygotes by enzymatic analysis of hair roots. American Journal of Human Genetics 31:42-49

Pannone N, Gatti R, Lombardo C, Di Natale P 1986 Prenatal diagnosis of Hunter syndrome using chorionic villi. Prenatal Diagnosis 6: 207-210

Pfeiffer R A, Kresse H, Bäumer N, Sattinger E 1977 Beta-glucuronidase deficiency in a girl with unusual clinical features. European Journal of Pediatrics 126: 155–161

Rampini S U 1976 Klinik der Mukopolysaccharidosen. Enke Stuttgart

Roubicek M, Gehler J, Spranger J 1985 The clinical spectrum of alpha-iduronidase deficiency. American Journal of Medical Genetics 20: 471–481

Singh J, DiFerrante N, Niebes P. Tavella P 1976 N-acetylgalactosamine-6-sulphate sulphatase in man. Absence of the enzyme in Morquio disease. Journal of Clinical Investigation 57: 1036–1040

Spranger J 1972 The systemic mucopolysaccharidoses. Ergebnisse der Inneren Medizin und Kinderheilkunde. Springer, Berlin 32: 165–265

Spranger J, Gehler J, O'Brien J F, Cantz M 1974 Chondroitin-sulphaturia with alpha-iduronidase deficiency. Lancet II: 1082

Spranger J, Cantz M, Gehler J, Liebaers I, Theiss W 1978 Mucopolysaccharidosis II (Hunter disease) with corneal opacities. European Journal of Pediatrics 129: 11–16

Stephan M J, Stevens J L, Wenstrup R J, Greenberg C R, Gritter H L, Hodges G F, Guller B 1989 Mucopolysaccharidosis I presenting with endocardial fibroelastosis of infancy. American Journal of Diseases of Children 143: 782–784

Stevenson R E, Howell R R, McKusick V A, Suskind R, Hanson J W, Elliott D E, Neufeld E F 1976 The iduronidase-deficient mucopolysaccharidoses: clinical and roentgenographic features. Pediatrics 57: 111–122

Tønnesen T, Güttler F, Lykkelund C 1983 Reliability of the use of fructose 1-phosphate to detect Hunter cells in fibroblast-cultures of obligate carriers of the Hunter syndrome. Human Genetics 64: 371–375

Van de Kamp J J P, Niermeijer M F, von Figura K, Giesberts M A H 1981 Genetic heterogeneity and clinical variability in the Sanfilippo syndrome (A, B, and C) Clinical Genetics 20: 152–160

Wenger D A, Sujansky E, Fennessey P V, Thompson J N 1986 Human β-mannosidase deficiency. New England Journal of Medicine 315: 1201–1205

Winters P R, Harrod M J, Molenich-Heetred S A, Kirkpatrick J, Rosenberg R N 1976 Alpha-iduronidase deficiency and possible Hurler-Scheie genetic compound. Neurology 26: 1003–1007

Yatziv S, Erickson R P, Epstein C J 1977 Mild and severe Hunter syndrome (MPS II) within the same sibships. Clinical Genetics 11: 319–326

Young I D, Harper P S, Archer I M, Newcombe R G 1982 A clinical and genetic study of Hunter's syndrome. 1. Heterogeneity. Journal of Medical Genetics 10: 401–407

102. The oligosaccharidoses

J. G. Leroy

INTRODUCTION

In the first comprehensive paper (Spranger & Wiedemann 1970) on a number of hereditary disorders clinically related to both the mucopolysaccharidoses and the sphingolipidoses, the term mucolipidosis was introduced into the literature. Excessive urinary excretion of acid mucopolysaccharides (AMPS) is not observed in the mucolipidoses, but dysostosis multiplex in varying degrees is reminiscent of the mucopolysaccharidoses, while macular cherry-red spot and demyelination in peripheral nerves in some of the entities provide links with the sphingolipidoses. Although useful as a concept, mucolipidosis is a misnomer in the chemical sense because in most of the entities originally included there is no true storage of either mucopolysaccharides or lipids. The metabolism of the carbohydrate in glycoproteins and glycolipids is adversely affected in the mucolipidoses, resulting in excess presence and excretion of oligosaccharides. Therefore the term oligosaccharidosis has become the preferred substitute for the name mucolipidosis, which will not be used in this review. Table 102.1 lists the disorders which more or less fit the definition of oligosaccharidosis.

GENERAL CONSIDERATIONS ON GENETICS AND MANAGEMENT

Each one of the nosological entities among the oligosaccharidoses is inherited as an autosomal recessive trait with a recurrence risk of 1 in 4 for sibs of probands. All known primary metabolic defects involve lysosomal acid hydrolases directly or indirectly. Effective treatment is not available.

The molecular understanding of intracellular synthesis, processing and routing of endogenous lysosomal hydrolases and their receptor mediated compartmentalization has now advanced considerably (Kornfeld 1986, von Figura & Hasilik 1986). However the multiple and complex requisites for effective enzyme substitution therapy are unlikely to be met in the near future. Management of the oligosaccharidoses thus remains an object for preventive medicine. Such prevention paradoxically finds its retrospective foundation in early diagnosis in the proband, and its practical strategies in genetic counselling and prenatal diagnosis. Fetal monitoring by assay of the relevant lysosomal hydrolase in chorionic villi or in cultured amniotic fluid cells is available. Elective abortion is of increasing importance within the scheme of prevention.

Prospective preventive measures like mass screening programmes remain unrealistic. Detection of heterozygosity, though usually possible in the patients' parents, is not reliable in other relatives, because the ranges of specific enzyme activities in heterozygotes and homozygous normals overlap. This limitation of enzyme studies is likely to be circumvented soon, as direct structural information on the genes governing structure and function of lysosomal enzymes is either forthcoming or already emerging.

Supportive management of patients cannot be effective without simultaneous guidance to their parents and healthy sibs. It must include all modern clinical measures to deal with complications, and constant attention to their basic right to human happiness.

THE SIALIDOSES

Because of the primary deficiency of glycoprotein specific acid sialidase they share, and because of the intracellular accumulation and excessive urinary excretion of sialylated glycoproteins and oligosaccharides in each one of them, four clinically different disease entities have been given the common name of sialidosis (Durand et al 1977). This term should be reserved exclusively for the clinical conditions due to the isolated primary deficiency of glycoprotein sialidase.

Table 102.1 The oligosaccharidoses and allied disorders

Group designation *Type*	Primary metabolic deficiency	Secondary metabolic features*	Number in McKusick** catalogue	Chromosomal location**
– Sialidosis (S)				
· Neonatal (hydropic) sialidosis (NS)			(25655)	
· Infantile sialidosis (nephrosialidosis) (IS)			25615	
· Childhood dysmorphic sialidosis (CDS) (Spranger syndrome)	glycoprotein sialidase	–	25240	6p21.3
· Juvenile (adult) normosomatic sialidosis (JNS) (Cherry-red spot-myoclonus (CRSM) syndrome)			25655	
– Recognition marker phosphotransferase deficiency				
· I-cell disease (ICD)	glc-Nac-1 phosphotransferase	non-membrane bound lysosomal hydrolases	25250	4q21–q23
· Pseudo-Hurler polydystrophy (PHP)			25260	
– Galactosialidosis				
· Neonatal (hydropic) galactosialidosis (NGS)	32 kDa protective glycoprotein	glycoprotein sialidase and β-D-galactosidase	25654	20
· Late infantile galactosialidosis (IGS)				
· Juvenile (adult) galactosialidosis (JGS)				
– Mannosidosis	acid α-D-mannosidase	–	24850	19p13.2–q12
– [β-mannosidase deficiency]	β-mannosidase	–	–	?
– Fucosidosis	α-L-fucosidase	–	23000	1q34
– G$_{M1}$-Gangliosidosis***				
· Infantile (type 1) G$_{M1}$-gangliosidosis			23050	
· Juvenile (type 2) G$_{M1}$-gangliosidosis			23060	
· Adult (type 3) G$_{M1}$-gangliosidosis	β-D-galactosidase		23065	3p21–cen
· Morquio syndrome type B (Mucopolysaccharidosis IV B)			25301	
– Aspartylglucosaminuria (AGU)	1-aspartamido-β-N-glcNac-amino hydrolase	aspartyl-glucosamine	20840	4q21–qter
– Winchester syndrome‡	?	special trisaccharide	27795	?
Allied Disorders‡‡				
– Sialic acid storage disease (SASD)				
· Infantile type	?	free sialic acid	26992	?
· Salla disease (late infantile SASD)			26874	
– Berman syndrome	ganglioside sialidase?	ganglioside sialidase	25265	?
– Mucosulphatidosis (Multiple sulphatase deficiency) (MSD)	protective factor common to sulphatases	multiple sulphatases	27220	?

*: Beyond excessive oligosacchariduria in the true oligosaccharidoses, enzyme functions mentioned in this column are deficient; often of diagnostic importance; see text.

**: Original references in McKusick (1988); Data on the human Gene Map as of March 1, 1988.

***: Group of clinical phenotypes not discussed within this chapter; see chapter on Gangliosidoses and Mucopolysaccharidoses; molecular aspects in the various entities due to β-D-galactosidase deficiency have been treated by Hoogeveen et al 1985.

‡: Tentative and temporary classification pending improved physiopathological knowledge.

‡‡: Not true oligosaccharidoses according to strict chemical criteria.

Childhood Dysmorphic Sialidosis (CDS) (Spranger syndrome)

Initially named lipomucopolysaccharidosis when first delineated in 1968 by Spranger, and renamed mucolipidosis I (ML I) (Spranger & Wiedemann 1970), this disorder remains the prototype among the sialidoses.

Clinical manifestations

Complaints of slow psychomotor development usually arise in early childhood, when coarse facial features and thoracolumbar kyphosis are also noted. At first puffy face, depressed nasal bridge and broad maxilla are reminiscent of MPS-IH or hypothyroidism. Developmental landmarks are reached with delay. Intellectual development and physical growth are slower than normal, with height being below the third percentile between the ages of 3 and 5 years, when similarity of the facies with that in the Hurler syndrome becomes more striking. The lower median part of the nose has a bulbous shape with anteverted nostrils. Gingival hypertrophy is mild to moderate. The teeth are widely spaced, the tongue is enlarged and the maxillary part of the face prominent. The thoracic cage is barrel shaped, with pectus excavatum and thoracolumbar kyphosis. Hepatomegaly, although an early feature in some patients, is inconsistent or absent in others. Splenomegaly is rare. Hernias can be present. Sensorineural deafness is already present in early childhood. The clinical picture is only fully developed in late childhood, with the appearance of progressive ataxia, nystagmus, muscle wasting and loss of strength. By then, ophthalmological examination reveals a cherry-red macular spot, often strabismus and, inconsistently, cataract and corneal opacity. Subsequently a coarse tremor and myoclonic jerks complete the neurological syndrome. Mental deterioration is not a feature and seizures have not been observed, but sensory deficits, irregular deep tendon reflexes and decreased nerve conduction velocity are consistent indications of peripheral nerve involvement. It is of interest that limitation of large joint movements is only minimal, and that the small joints of the hands are not affected. Progression of dysmorphic sialidosis is very slow. The patients become chair-bound from adolescence. Adverse effects of the neurological deficits and pneumonia have been considered the causes of death in adolescence or early adulthood (Kelly & Graetz 1977, Spranger et al 1977, Winter et al 1980, King et al 1984).

Radiographic findings

The radiological manifestations of childhood dysmorphic sialidosis can also be summarized by the term dysostosis multiplex. They progress slowly to a moderate degree of abnormality. The skull is mildly dolichocephalic and shows progressive thickening of the calvaria and sclerosis at the base. The vertebral bodies, initially of biconvex configuration, have irregular end plates. Ossification defects in the lower thoracic and upper lumbar region result in antero-inferior beaking of a few vertebrae. Kyphosis is prominent. Moderate scoliosis is often observed, in addition to flaring of iliac wings and mildly dysplastic acetabula. Short tubular bones show osteopenia and irregularly distributed coarse trabeculation (Spranger et al 1974, Winter et al 1980).

Histopathology and chemical pathology; diagnosis

Peripheral lymphocytes contain abnormal vacuoles. In bone marrow smears histiocytic cells have a foamy cytoplasm. Histopathological changes are noticed in neurons as well as in mesenchymal and visceral cells. Hepatocytes as well as Kupffer cells are filled with cytoplasmic vacuoles and granules. Electron micrographs show enlarged membrane-bound lysosome-like organelles filled with reticulo-granular material. These vesicular structures fill major portions of the cytoplasm (Freitag et al, quoted in Spranger et al 1977).

The discovery of an increased urinary excretion of several oligosaccharides (Humbel 1975) led to the structural elucidation of these compounds as glycoprotein-derived sialyloligosaccharides in which sialic acid residues occupy the terminal non-reducing position (Strecker et al 1977 and Strecker's earlier work quoted therein). The urinary oligosaccharide pattern is rather typical in sialidosis patients (Fig. 102.1, Sewell 1980). Similar oligosaccharides are excreted in I-cell disease (ICD) and in pseudo-Hurler polydystrophy (PHP) urine, but less excessively so. A profound deficiency of a glycoprotein specific sialidase is the primary enzyme defect in CDS and in the other sialidoses (Cantz et al 1977). As a consequence, the degradation of $a2 \rightarrow 3$ and $a2 \rightarrow 6$ neuraminosyl linkages in the sialoglycan parts of glycoprotein is impaired. The normal activity in CDS brain is explained through interference by the sialidase active towards gangliosides, which in brain and in cultured fibroblasts is unaffected (Pallman et al 1980).

The demonstration in fibroblasts of a deficiency of sialidase active towards water-soluble substrates establishes the diagnosis in the sialidoses. Here this deficiency is not associated with deficient intracellular activity of several other lysosomal hydrolases. Parents of patients with dysmorphic sialidosis have intermediate sialidase activity (Cantz et al 1977). The enzyme defect in patients can also be demonstrated in leucocytes.

Storage products have not been amply studied in CDS.

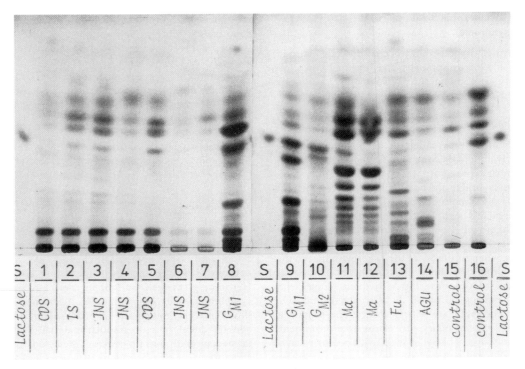

Fig. 102.1 Thin-layer chromatograms of urinary oligosaccharides (Courtesy of Dr G. Strecker, Lille, France). Silica gel (Merck) plates; development in n-butanol/acetic acid/water (2 : 1 : 1, v/v); Compounds visualized with orcinol (Humbel 1975).

S : standard
1,5 : CDS : Childhood Dysmorphic Sialidosis
2 : IS : Infantile Sialidosis (Nephrosialidosis)
3,4,6,7 : JNS : Juvenile Normosomatic Sialidosis
8,9: G_{M1} gangliosidosis type 1

10 : G_{M2} gangliosidosis ; type Sandhoff
11,12 : Mannosidosis
13 : Fucosidosis
14 : Aspartylglucosaminuria (AGU)
15,16 : Control urine

In brain there is an increase of lipid-bound and protein-bound sialic acid and of all gangliosides (Berra et al 1979). The accumulation of free and bound sialic acid in sialidosis fibroblasts matches that in I-cells (Cantz & Messer 1979).

Juvenile (adult) normosomatic sialidosis (JNS) (Cherry-red spot-myoclonus (CRSM) syndrome)

Almost simultaneously with the discovery of the primary metabolic defect in CDS a deficiency of acid sialidase was found to be the enzyme defect in the cherry-red spot-myoclonus syndrome (CRSM syndrome) (O'Brien 1977).

The designation CRSM syndrome correctly refers to the main clinical features: slowly progressive reduction of visual acuity, with onset in some patients before 10 years of age; and a crippling, often generalized action myoclonus appearing in the second decade of life. A macular cherry-red spot is almost consistently found, but the time of its first appearance cannot be determined without

prospective observations in younger sibs of probands. Seizures in these patients are not associated with loss of consciousness and probably represent repetitive bursts of generalized severe myoclonus. JNS patients consistently have nystagmus. Initially some of them complain of burning pains in the limbs. Cerebellar ataxia is also reported, but is hard to evaluate in the presence of much abnormal extrapyramidal activity. Important points in this syndrome are: absence of dysostosis multiplex even in patients with mild scoliosis; absence of psychomotor retardation and mental deficiency except for terminal deterioration; absence of corneal clouding even in slit-lamp examination; absence of facial coarsening. For a review of the original literature see Lowden and O'Brien (1979). Patients with JNS were also reported by Rapin et al (1978), Thomas et al (1978, 1979). Patients with visual disturbance and cherry-red spot only, and thus without any extrapyramidal sign (Durand et al 1977), probably do not represent a separate entity because in some patients a long time-lag is observed between the onset of reduced vision and that of myoclonus (Tsvetkova et al 1987). As the enzyme diagnosis in patients with JNS is sometimes delayed until adulthood, oligosacchariduria may no longer be detectable. Even in the presence of severe neurological disease, the ocular fundus may be unremarkable (Harzer et al 1986). Peripheral neuropathy has been documented in JNS, thus linking this entity to CDS pathologically too (Steinman et al 1980). The residual activity of sialidase is higher in fibroblasts from JNS than in those from CDS patients (O'Brien & Warner 1980). The parents of patients have intermediate levels of sialidase activity (Thomas et al 1978). Somatic cell hybrids between CDS- and JNS-fibroblast strains do not show enzymatic complementation, providing evidence of functional allelism of the mutant genes (Hoogeveen et al 1980a).

Infantile sialidosis (IS) (Nephrosialidosis)

The disorder described originally in two sibs with early appearing and severe clinical features of CDS with an identical isolated deficiency of acid sialidase (Den Tandt & Leroy 1980) may be called infantile sialidosis (IS). It has subsequently been observed by Aylsworth et al (1980). Because glomerular nephropathy is considered an essential component and was fatal in one of the original patients, this disorder has also been termed nephrosialidosis (Maroteaux et al 1978).

Neonatal (Hydropic) sialidosis (NS)

Glycoprotein sialidase deficiency can apparently result in fetal and/or neonatal non-immune hydrops, ascites and hepatosplenomegaly. The findings of excessive excretion of urinary oligosaccharides and of glycoprotein sialidase deficiency establish the diagnosis in these very sick infants. In bone marrow cells, and in liver biopsy specimens, foamy hepatocytes, Küppfer cells and endothelial cells containing large empty-appearing vacuoles are readily apparent. In one patient only glycoprotein sialidase was totally deficient (Beck et al 1984) but in another an additional deficiency of β-D-galactosidase was not ruled out (Laver et al 1983).

DISORDERS DUE TO DEFECTIVE RECOGNITION MARKER(S) ON LYSOSOMAL HYDROLASES

I-cell disease (ICD)

Clinical manifestations

I-cell disease (ICD) is a slowly progressive disorder with clinical onset at birth and fatal outcome in childhood.

The neonate with ICD has a low birth weight. His facies is plump and swollen, his skin thick and particularly stiff about the ears. Congenital hernias are consistently present in males. One or more orthopaedic abnormalities are common: clubfoot; dislocation of the hip(s); thoracic deformity or kyphosis. Despite generalized hypotonia, the range of movement in the shoulders is already limited.

Unlike Hurler syndrome (MPS-IH) there is no temporary acceleration of skeletal growth around one year of age. Instead, growth decelerates within 6 months from birth and often ceases before 15 months. Growth failure is always severe and a final height of 80 cm is rarely exceeded. Head size is proportional to stature. Stiffening of all joints occurs from the first year of life. Psychomotor retardation is extreme in some patients but rather mild in others. Upper respiratory infection and otitis recur frequently. Breathing is noisy. The facies resembles that of patients with MPS-IH but shows consistent differences: small orbits and hypoplastic supraorbital ridges; prominent eyes; tortuous pattern of prominent periorbital veins; telangiectatic capillaries over midface and cheeks; impressive gingival swelling and prominent mouth. Hepatosplenomegaly is moderate or absent. The corneae are clear but haziness is found on slit lamp examination (Leroy et al 1971). In the longer-surviving patients, coarsening of facial features, broadening of hands and wrists and cardiac murmurs are common. The abdomen is protuberant with an umbilical hernia often being present (Fig. 102.2). Bronchopneumonia and congestive heart failure are the usual causes of death.

Within the clinical phenotype of ICD there exists more variation than is usually encountered in biochemically well defined autosomal recessive disorders. However, affected sibs have more similar clinical features, indicating genetic heterogeneity between families.

Radiographic features

The radiological abnormalities in MPS-IH and in G_{MI}-gangliosidosis type 1 are qualitatively indistinguishable from those in ICD. Excessive periosteal new bone formation along the long tubular bones before one year of age is a feature shared with the patient who has infantile G_{MI}-gangliosidosis. In ICD 'dysostosis multiplex', a term introduced to summarize the general radiographic findings in these and related disorders, is quantitatively most severe at any given time in the clinical course. Excellent radiographic descriptions are available (Spranger et al 1974, Maroteaux 1982). The radiographs most informative in making a diagnosis include lateral skull, lateral spine, anteroposterior thorax and pelvis, humerus and hands with wrists.

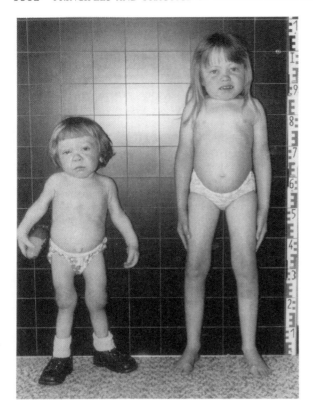

Fig. 102.2 3½-year-old patient with I-cell disease (left of figure) and a 10-year-old girl with pseudo-Hurler polydystrophy.

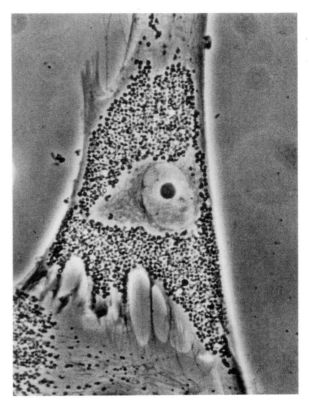

Fig. 102.3 Living inclusion cell (I-cell) as observed by phase contrast microscopy. A juxtanuclear zone, including the Golgi apparatus, is free of granular inclusions.

Laboratory findings; 'The I-cell phenomenon'; diagnosis

The name 'I-cell' disease originated from the observation in the phase contrast microscope of a large number of cytoplasmic granular inclusions in the patients' skin fibroblasts cultured in vitro (Fig. 102.3). These cells were called 'Inclusion cells' or 'I-cells' and the corresponding disorder I-cell disease (Leroy & DeMars 1967). The cytoplasmic inclusions are swollen lysosomes with pleomorphic contents (DeMars & Leroy 1967, Hanai et al 1971, Tondeur et al 1971). The original definition of the I-cell phenomenon was a morphological one. It was soon extended by several biochemical findings, some of which are also apparent in vivo. In 'I-cells' the activity of a large number of lysosomal acid hydrolases is considerably decreased or absent (Leroy & Spranger 1970, Leroy et al 1972). These include the glycoprotein and ganglioside sialidases (Cantz & Messer 1979, Pallman et al 1980). The activity of the same acid hydrolases is greatly increased in the culture media of I-cells and also in the patients' extracellular fluids (Wiesmann et al 1971a, 1971b). In postmortem tissues the specific activity of β-D-galactosidase and of acid sialidase is reduced, but that of other acid hydrolases is within normal limits (Leroy et al 1972, Cantz & Messer 1979, Eto et al 1979, Pallman et al 1980). Findings in leucocytes are inconsistent but probably similar. The 'I-cell' phenomenon is specific except for its presence also in pseudo-Hurler polydystrophy (see below). As a secondary effect of the genetic defect, it remains of considerable diagnostic significance in both disease. Its presence also in cultured amniocytes as well as in chorionic villi has been used successfully in prenatal diagnosis of ICD (Aula et al 1975, Matsuda 1975, Gehler et al 1976, Poenaru et al 1984).

The secondarily impaired degradation of glycoproteins is sufficiently extensive in vivo to result in excessive urinary excretion of several sialyloligosaccharides (Humbel 1975, Strecker et al 1977, Sewell 1980). However the excretion pattern in the sialidoses is qualitatively similar (Fig. 102.1).

Histopathology and chemical pathology

The single most characteristic pathological feature is the presence of a large number of cytoplasmic, unit membrane-bound vacuoles in connective tissue cells, irrespective of the organ in which they are located. Such abnormal cells are particularly abundant in skin, gingiva, heart valves and the zones of endochondral and membranous bone formation. Pericytes of capillaries, adventitial cells and Schwann and perineural cells are affected. In the renal glomeruli there is foamy transformation only in the visceral and not in the parietal cells of Bowman's capsule. Changes in neurons and glial cells are minimal, inconsistent and possibly of a secondary nature. The heterogeneous osmiophilic bodies in hepatocytes are considered of questionable significance. Kupffer cells do not contain such dense bodies and appear normal (Martin et al 1975, 1984). In ICD, connective tissue cells are primarily affected. Whereas in cultured fibroblasts the cytoplasmic granules are filled with pleomorphic material, the corresponding in vivo inclusions in mesenchymal cells are either empty or contain only sparse granulofibrillar material.

On the one hand there is neither histochemical nor biochemical evidence of significant storage of lipids, mucopolysaccharides or lipid- and protein-bound sialic acid in brain and visceral organs in ICD (Leroy et al 1972, Dacremont et al 1974, Martin et al 1975, Berra et al 1979, Eto et al 1979). On the other hand I-cells accumulate 'SO$_4$-containing compounds including mucopolysaccharides' (Schmickel et al 1975) and lipids (Leroy et al 1972) in addition to free and bound sialic acid (Thomas et al 1976). Apparently the multiple secondary enzyme deficiencies in I-cells, isolated in vitro from other tissues, result in storage of metabolites.

The I-cell phenomenon is not apparent in postmortem viscera although the primary enzyme deficiency (see below) is expressed in these parenchymatous tissues (Waheed et al 1982).

The primary metabolic defect

In cell lines derived from the patients' parents a small number of I-cells is consistently observed (DeMars & Leroy 1967). In the serum of these obligate heterozygotes there is a slight but definite increase of several acid hydrolases (Van Elsen & Leroy 1973, Van Elsen et al 1976). By receptor-mediated pinocytosis, I-cells can take up extracellular bovine β-D-glucuronidase and human a-L-iduronidase (Hickman & Neufeld 1972). Once captured, the exogenous enzymes are maintained in I-cells and display a normal turnover rate. However, a-L-iduronidase and β-D-glucuronidase obtained from I-cell culture medium are not taken up by indicator MPS-IH or MPS VII fibroblasts respectively, nor is ICD N-acetyl-β-D-hexosaminidase (hex) pinocytosed by a G_{M2}-gangliosidosis Sandhoff type cell line. Thus the ICD primary metabolic defect is responsible for the lack in lysosomal hydrolases of a common recognition marker essential for their adsorption to specific receptors and subsequent intracellular routing. The carbohydrate nature of the common recognition marker was first shown by Hickman et al (1974). Subsequently mannose-6-phosphate and phosphorylated mannans were found to be effective inhibitors of adsorptive pinocytosis of hydrolases, and pretreatment with alkaline phosphatase abolished receptor-mediated pinocytosis of hydrolases and underscored the role of phosphate in the recognition marker (Kaplan et al 1977). Direct chemical analysis has also demonstrated the presence of mannose-6-phosphate in high mannose-type oligosaccharides specifically released from urinary a-N-acetyl-glucosaminidase (von Figura & Klein 1979), bovine testicular β-D-galactosidase (Distler et al 1979) and human splenic β-glucuronidase (Natowicz et al 1979). In I-cells phosphorylation and processing of the newly synthesized precursor proteins, which are of larger molecular size than the mature intracellular hydrolases, do not occur. The enzymes encountered in ICD culture media are unphosphorylated. They have no phosphate containing recognition marker (Hasilik & Neufeld, 1980a,b) which is needed to gain access to the lysosomal compartment. In control fibroblasts, intralysosomal enzymes are fully processed and only small amounts of phosphorylated precursors are found extracellularly (Bach et al 1979a).

A major portion of the $^{32}P_i$ groups in newly phosphorylated high mannose-type oligosaccharides in biosynthetic intermediates of lysosomal enzymes is blocked by N-acetylglucosamine which renders the mannose-6-phosphate containing carbohydrate chains insensitive to alkaline phosphatase (Hasilik et al 1980, Tabas & Kornfeld 1980). The mere finding of the phosphodiesters suggested their formation by enzymatic transfer of N-acetyl-glucosamine-1-phosphate onto C_6 of mannose. Glycopeptide of thyroglobulin and β-hexosaminidase dephosphorylated by acid hydrolysis, acting as acceptors, can be phosphorylated by an enzyme in microsomes from rat liver, human placenta, postmortem organs and normal human fibroblasts, in the presence of UDP-N-acetylglucosamine acting as the donor molecule. This specific reaction is deficient in fibroblasts and parenchymatous organs from patients with I-cell disease or pseudo-Hurler polydystrophy. Thus the primary defect in these disorders is a deficiency in UDP-N-acetylglucosamine: lysosomal hydrolase N-acetylglucosamine-1-phosphotransferase (Hasilik et al 1981, Reitman et al

1981, Waheed et al 1982) for which the term GlcNac-phosphotransferase is adopted here as a trivial name. A microsomal N-acetylglucosamine 1-phosphodiester α-N-acetyl-glucosaminidase, immunologically and catalytically distinct from the lysosomal α-N-acetylglucosaminidase, hydrolyses as a glycosidase the blocking N-acetylglucosamine residues, and thereby exposes the mannose 6-phosphate recognition marker (Varki & Kornfeld 1980, Waheed et al 1981). This 'deblocking' enzyme is normal in I-cells. Because of the basic metabolic defect in ICD the mannose 6-phosphate (M6P) marker is lacking in lysosomal enzymes, resulting in the secretion of at least those precursor hydrolases which depend on the M6P recognition pathway for their correct subcellular distribution. The two distinct M6P receptors recently purified, and structurally characterized by cloning of the corresponding cDNAs (Dahms et al 1987, Lobel et al 1987, Pohlmann et al 1987, Stein et al 1987), are most probably normal in ICD. The discovery of the enzyme defect in ICD has increased knowledge of the biosynthesis and processing of lysosomal enzymes, their mannose 6-phosphate dependent in vivo transport, and the specific plasma membrane receptors involved. The relative role of this mechanism in intracellular routing and distribution of glycoproteins is gradually emerging. These matters have recently been adequately reviewed (Kornfeld 1986, von Figura & Hasilik 1986, Dahms et al 1989, Tong et al 1989).

Pseudo-Hurler polydystrophy (PHP)

This disorder has been delineated and named pseudo-Hurler polydystrophy (PHP) by Maroteaux (Maroteaux & Lamy 1966). It was called mucolipidosis III (Spranger & Wiedemann 1970) before its biochemical alignment with ICD was known.

Clinical manifestations

Complaints of physical slowness, joint stiffness and slow mental development about the age of 3 years mark the clinical onset. The patient's facies is plump, and the range of movement in shoulders and hips already reduced. Growth rate is slower than normal and head circumference remains proportional to stature, which is below normal in adults. The corneae are clear by inspection but show opacities on slit lamp examination. Liver and spleen are usually not enlarged (Kelly et al 1975, Leroy & Van Elsen 1975). Mental deficiency in PHP patients is mild and non-progressive. The course of the disease is very slow and characterized by increasing joint stiffness. PHP patients of advanced age have been reported (Langer, quoted in Kelly et al 1975) but insufficient data on life expectancy are available (see Fig. 102.2).

There is generalized osteoporosis. Bone age is considerably delayed. Dysostosis multiplex, though variable between patients, is generally mild, except for the severe and progressive lesions in the hips, (Spranger et al 1974, Kelly et al 1975) where secondary arthritic changes are a considerable problem. Stiffness in the shoulders is of soft tissue origin. Urinary excretion of AMPS is normal. That of sialyl-oligosaccharides is excessive, complex and indistinguishable from that found in ICD urine (Humbel 1975, Strecker et al 1977, Sewell 1980). This finding is nevertheless of some help in diagnosis (Fig. 102.1).

Diagnosis; the relationship between PHP and ICD

The I-cell phenomenon is apparent in PHP fibroblasts as in ICD cultures. Thus PHP derived cells are also I-cells. The activity of many acid hydrolases is considerably reduced in the cells and elevated in the conditioned culture media (Thomas et al 1973, Berman et al 1974a). The residual activity of β-D-galactosidase (Leroy & O'Brien 1976) and of sialidase (Den Tandt & Leroy 1980) is higher in I-cells from PHP patients than in those from ICD donors. Contrary to findings in ICD, in oligosaccharides isolated from PHP acid hydrolases, a small amount of phosphorylation is encountered (Hasilik & Neufeld 1980b). It is tempting to correlate these findings with the milder clinical phenotype in PHP. Of direct diagnostic importance is the fact that in serum of patients there is also a greatly increased activity of many acid hydrolases.

The dividing line between PHP patients and ICD patients with mild mental handicap and protracted course may not be clear, but differences in growth rate, final height and degree of dysostosis multiplex form the strongest grounds for distinguishing between the two disorders.

The presence of the I-cell phenomenon in both disorders points towards a closely related pathogenesis, as has been proved by the finding of the same enzyme defect (Reitman et al 1981).

In vitro complementation studies reveal no less than three complementation groups among patients with deficient GlcNac-phosphotransferase. Apparently all patients with ICD tested so far, and some with PHP, belong to a single complementation group A (Mueller et al 1985). The complementation groups B and C comprise only cell lines from clinical PHP donors. Recent claims are that at least the catalytic subunit in the mutant GlcNac-phosphotransferase is smaller than normal in the A group cells and larger than normal in the B complementation group (Ben-Yoseph et al 1986). The exceptional C group I-cells have a normal GlcNac-phosphotransferase activity when tested with the exogenous α-methylmannoside as a phosphate acceptor, but a significantly reduced one when endogenous glycoproteins isolated from placenta serve as GlcNac-phosphate acceptors (Varki et al 1981, Mueller et al 1985, Little et al 1986). Thus GlcNac-phosphotransferase appears to be an oligomeric protein with at least one subunit for enzymatic catalysis and one for recognition of acceptor and/or substrate. At least a few structural and possibly regulatory genes are involved in controlling GlcNac-phosphotransferase activity. Unfortunately, prospective and controlled studies on the correlation between clinical phenotype and complementation group have not yet been undertaken.

THE GALACTOSIALIDOSES

Deficiency of β-D-galactosidase in skin and conjunctival tissues was found by Goldberg et al (1971) in a proband with 'a new syndrome which combines clinical features of several storage diseases, but which is nonetheless unique'. In similar patients glycoprotein sialidase is also markedly reduced (Wenger et al 1978). Meanwhile, three clinical phenotypes have been discerned among patients with a combined deficiency of acid sialidase and β-D-galactosidase, and with typical, excessive urinary excretion of sialyloligosaccharides (Table 102.1). The designation galactosialidosis proposed by Andria et al (1981) applies to all three entities because of their clinical and metabolic relationship with G_{M1}-generalized gangliosidosis and with sialidosis, from each of which they are genetically distinct. Most frequent among patients is the juvenile (adult) type of galactosialidosis. In addition, late infantile galactosialidosis, or the Goldberg-Wenger syndrome, and a neonatal hydropic type have been delineated. Somatic cell hybridization has demonstrated that the defects in the various types of galactosialidosis do not mutually complement and thus are caused by allelic mutations (Hoogeveen et al 1980a). The responsible molecular defect is the lack of a nonenzymic 32-kDa glycoprotein required for the aggregation of the 64-kDa β-galactosidase monomers and their protection against intralysosomal proteolytic degradation and for the activation of acid sialidase (Hoogeveen et al 1980b, D'Azzo et al 1982, Verheyen et al 1985). Contrary to findings in patients with G_{M1}-gangliosidosis the deficiency of β-D-galactosidase is not found in all tissues or in plasma. It is also less complete than in patients with isolated primary β-galactosidase deficiency. In obligate heterozygotes β-D-galactosidase is normal but sialidase activity is intermediate. Patients with any of the galactosialidoses have vacuolated peripheral lymphocytes, aligning them with all storage disorders due to a lysosomal hydrolase deficiency.

Juvenile (Adult) galactosialidosis (JGS) (Goldberg-Wenger syndrome)

Although variable, the clinical onset of the most frequent galactosialidosis occurs from late childhood till early adult life (Goldberg et al 1971, Miyatake et al 1979, Okada et al 1979, Suzuki et al 1983). More patients are reported from Japan than from anywhere else. Intrafamily variation between patients is smaller than interfamily differences. The composite clinical picture of the fully developed Goldberg-Wenger syndrome consists of the following signs and symptoms: (1) slowly progressive cerebellar ataxia, tremor and action myoclonus, pyramidal but no extrapyradmidal signs and no nystagmus; (2) decreasing visual acuity and cherry-red spot in the macula; (3) mild dysostosis multiplex, mild coarsening of facial features and moderately short stature; (4) moderate intellectual impairment, which is unusual in the initial stages of the disease. In addition, angiokeratoma is frequently observed. Most patients show corneal opacities on slit-lamp examination. Hearing loss is occasionally present.

Late infantile galactosialidosis (IGS)

A few patients with clinical onset of the disorder during or before the second year of life have been reported. In them, coarse facial features, hepatosplenomegaly, anterior-inferior beaking of lumbar vertebral bodies with kyphosis, dysostosis multiplex and developmental delay are noted (Andria et al 1978, Strisciuglio et al 1984) without ophthalmological or neurological signs. It is likely that these abnormalities will develop as the patients become older. Unfortunately no follow-up reports are available. In these patients the normally formed immature 52-kDa precursor appears to be altered structurally and thus is poorly converted into the active 32-kDa protective glycoprotein, whereas in JGS patients the complete lack of the glycoproteinous protector of β-D-galactosidase and acid sialidase is associated with insufficient synthesis of its 52-kDa precursor. In the neonatal or early infantile hydropic type galactosialidosis (next section) the total lack of 32-kDa non-enzymic protector is due to a still more marked reduction of 52-kDa precursor (Palmeri et al 1986).

Neonatal (Hydropic) galactosialidosis (NGS)

Three unrelated neonates presenting with a condition clinically almost indistinguishable from G_{M1}-gangliosidosis type 1, but with extensive oedema and ascites, have been diagnosed as having a combined deficiency of glycoprotein sialidase and β-galactosidase. One patient died as a newborn, the two others at 6 and 8 months of age respectively. They had a plump facies, depressed nasal bridge, cloudy corneae, macular cherry-red spot and conjunctival telangiectasia with similar lesions over the lower abdomen. In the longer surviving patients respiratory infection recurred frequently and both congestive heart failure and renal failure were the compounding causes of death, in addition to anaemia and thrombocytopenia. Radiographically the skeletal changes were identical to those in G_{M1}-gangliosidosis and ICD (Gravel et al 1979, Lowden et al 1981). At present it remains difficult to classify the Japanese infant reported by Okada et al (1983), because she was clinically and metabolically intermediate between NGS and IGS. In addition, this patient had features in common with nephrosialidosis or IS patients.

MANNOSIDOSIS

The nosological delineation of mannosidosis almost coincided with the discovery of the responsible metabolic defect by Öckerman (1967a, b).

Clinical and radiographic features

The neonatal period is uneventful in mannosidosis, but even during the patients' first year of life recurrent respiratory infections and otitis require hospital admissions. Psychomotor progress slows in the second year and walking is achieved with delay or, in some instances, not at all, as in the first recorded patient. Belated onset of speech and psychomotor retardation are the usual reasons for clinical evaluation. In childhood, signs and symptoms are: normal stature, macrocephaly, prominent forehead, plump facies, clear corneae, persistent epicanthic folds, low nasal bridge, noisy breathing, thick lips and prominent jaw and mouth. Joint mobility is minimally impaired. The abdomen is protuberant with an umbilical hernia as a rule. In boys inguinal hernias or hydroceles are common. Hepatosplenomegaly is mild to moderate in young patients, but disappears in adolescence. Mild kyphosis is common. Hearing loss of both the conductive and the sensorineural type, clumsy broadbased gait and deficiency of motor skills are almost always present from later childhood on. Although hypotonia is common, deep tendon reflexes are usually increased in the lower limbs. Occasionally hypertonia is found. Speech and language remain at an elementary level. The patients' disposition is usually agreeable, but sudden episodes of anger or aggressiveness and periods of sleep disturbance are regularly reported. Ophthalmological examination does not reveal any retinal changes but regularly detects cataract.

In most instances the clinical course is rather mild and barely progressive, with slowly coarsening facial and body features. Data on life expectancy are scarce. Apparently most patients survive well into adulthood and are found among the mentally retarded with normal stature and hearing defects (Loeb et al 1969a, Autio et al 1973, Farriaux et al 1975, Booth et al 1976, Kistler et al 1977). Some patients are more severely affected (Aylsworth et al 1976) and have a fatal course in childhood due to complications such as refractory viral infection, as in one patient with associated cellular immunodeficiency (Desnick et al 1976). In sibs reported from Israel (Bach et al 1978) corneal clouding was apparent. These patients, possibly examples of a variant mannosidosis, also showed marked limitation of joint mobility. In general the number of case reports is still too limited to fully assess clinical heterogeneity.

Radiographic findings can be summarized as mild and slowly progressive dysostosis multiplex. Thickening and sclerosis of the calvaria and macrocephaly are the most consistent findings. Long tubular bones including clavicles and ribs, are undermodelled. The lumbar gibbus is associated with antero-inferior beaking of some lumbar vertebrae. The metacarpals and phalanges show slightly widened diaphyses, proximal pointing and coarse trabeculation. There is mild iliac flaring and coxa valga.

Deficiency of acid α-D-mannosidase; formal diagnosis

The diagnosis of mannosidosis is based on the demonstration in tissue or body fluids of a severe deficiency of lysosomal α-D-mannosidase with optimal activity near pH 4.5. In postmortem tissues of the original patient the large residual activity was mainly due to isozymes active at more neutral pH (Carroll et al 1972, Poenaru & Dreyfus 1973). Precautions against other α-mannosidases which may interfere with the enzyme assay are particularly relevant when the artificial p-nitrophenyl- or 4-methylumbelliferyl-mannoside substrates are used.

The activity of α-D-mannosidase can be determined most easily in total homogenates of leucocytes and/or cultured fibroblasts, where at pH 4.2 interference of neutral isozymes is negligible and the specific activity of lysosomal α-D-mannosidosis is only a small proportion of that in controls.

Similar results in cultured amniotic fluid cells and postmortem organs respectively establish prenatal diagnosis or confirmation of mannosidosis. By DEAE-cellulose chromatography normal tissue acid α-D-mannosidase is resolved into two components called A and B (Phillips et al 1974a). Both are activated by Zn^{2+} and inhibited by Co^{2+} and EDTA. Both are deficient in mannosidosis, where the corresponding mutant enzyme is activated by Co^{2+} (Desnick et al 1976, Halley et al 1980). The neutral enzyme peak C is eluted at slightly higher salt concentration. This cytosolic enzyme is unaffected in mannosidosis and activated by Co^{2+}. There is no immunological cross-reaction between the C form and antibodies raised against the acidic forms of a-D-mannosidase (Phillips et al 1975).

In human plasma or serum, the 'intermediate' form of a-D-mannosidase is predominant and the lysosomal enzyme much less abundant. The former is thermolabile at 56° C and most active at pH 5.5–6.0 (Hirani et al 1977), but the latter is thermostable. Serum or plasma lysosomal mannosidase can be measured most reliably at its pH optimum of 4.6 only after thermoinactivation (56°C) of the samples dialysed against phosphate buffered saline (Hirani & Winchester 1980, Van Elsen & Leroy 1981). In some instances, an apparent increase in the K_m value of the mutant a-D-mannosidase has been found (Beaudet & Nichols 1976, Desnick et al 1976, Halley et al 1980). The correlation between differences in enzyme substrate affinity and clinical heterogeneity has been studied insufficiently.

A neurodegenerative disorder with autosomal recessive inheritance, also known as mannosidosis, exists in Angus cattle (Phillips et al 1974b) and has been detected in cats (Burditt el al 1980). Deficiency of the lysosomal a-D-mannosidase is the responsible metabolic defect in both animal models. The structural gene governing acidic lysosomal a-D-mannosidase in humans is located on chromosome 19 (Champion & Shows 1977).

Histopathology and chemical pathology

Vacuolization in peripheral lymphocytes is very prominent in all patients reported. In liver tissue numerous clear vacuoles are seen in hepatocytes, and in Kupffer cells. The cellular inclusions also exist in histiocytes of bone marrow, in endothelial cells of sinusoid vessels and in lymphocytes of spleen and lymph nodes (Kjellman et al 1969, Loeb et al 1969a, Autio et al 1973, Desnick et al 1976, Kistler et al 1977). Throughout the central nervous system the cytoplasm of neurons is distended, packed with an abundance of single membrane-bound vacuoles with remarkably clear, sparsely dispersed reticulogranular material (Desnick et al 1976). The severe morphological changes in hepatocytes and neurons are not due to storage of large macromolecules but to the accumulation of abnormal amounts of mannose-containing oligosaccharides derived from improperly degraded carbohydrate chains in glycoproteins (Öckerman 1969). That mannosidosis must be considered an oligosaccharidosis is shown by the demonstration of excessive urinary excretion of mannose containing-oligosaccharides (Fig. 102.1) by

simple screening tests of silica gel thin layer chromatography (Humbel 1975, Sewell 1980). With more refined methods of analytical chemistry the structure of the oligosaccharides excreted has been worked out in detail (Strecker 1977, Yamashita et al 1980) thus relating the mannose-rich metabolites to the lysosomal enzyme defect.

β-mannosidase deficiency

Originally described in goats (Jones & Dawson 1981) total deficiency of β-mannosidase has now also been detected in a young boy (Wenger et al 1986) and in two adult mentally retarded sibs (Cooper et al 1986). From the age of 18 months the boy showed slowly coarsening features, cessation of speech development, hyperactivity, mental deficiency and mild skeletal abnormalities. In addition to β-mannosidase, heparine sulphamidase (see Sanfilippo A disease) also had a low activity in leucocytes and skin fibroblasts. His urine contained excessive amounts of glycosaminoglycans and oligosaccharides. The adults were studied because of mental retardation without associated neurological signs. In these latter patients no physical abnormalities were observed and heparine sulphamidase was not studied.

FUCOSIDOSIS

This disorder was originally recognized as an atypical mucopolysaccharidosis (Durand et al 1966, 1968) with normal urinary excretion of AMPS. With the demonstration that the vacuoles in peripheral lymphocytes and liver are abnormally swollen lysosomes, a search among the lysosomal hydrolases for the responsible metabolic defect led to the finding of a profound deficiency of a-L-fucosidase in tissues and body fluids (Van Hoof & Hers 1968).

Clinical and radiographic findings

An initial symptom-free interval of 6–12 months is followed by frequent upper respiratory infections at the time when delay in psychomotor development becomes overt. Physical examination at this stage reveals slightly coarse facies, thickened lips and tongue, thick skin and generalized hypotonia with depressed deep tendon reflexes. Some patients never learn to walk alone. Abundant sweating with increased salinity of the sweat has been noticed in young patients. Slowing of linear growth occurs from about the age of 2 years (Durand et al 1969, Loeb et al 1969b, Patel et al 1972). Mild hepatosplenomegaly, inconsistently observed in early childhood, is absent in older patients. Mild thoracolumbar kyphosis and cardiomegaly are more often radiographic than clinical findings. The corneae are clear and the ophthalmological findings normal except for some tortuosity and irregularity of calibre in the retinal vessels (Libert et al 1977). Before 3 years of age, and earlier in some patients, the clinical course is characterized by progressive loss of motor skills, apathy, hypertonia and spasticity with hyper-reflexia, sometimes seizures, increasing mental deterioration and finally dementia and decerebrate rigidity. Patients with this natural course extending over only a few years (Durand et al 1969) or a slightly longer period (Loeb et al 1969b) succumb to complications of their neurodegenerative disease and have been considered examples of fucosidosis type 1 (Tondeur 1977).

The observation of several patients with severe mental deficiency, an almost non-progressive disease, mild radiographic abnormalities, angiokeratoma and telangiectasia, reported when in their teens or twenties (Patel et al 1972, Gatti et al 1973, Kousseff et al 1973, Borrone et al 1974, MacPhee et al 1975) prompted the suggestion of a second phenotype, fucosidosis type 2. These patients, surviving beyond adolescence and into early adulthood, probably represent the majority of cases. Late in their disease they have recurrent attacks of dehydration due to inability to control body temperature (Patel et al 1972).

As more information on the natural course and the extent of the clinical spectrum of fucosidosis becomes available, the hypothesis of two distinct clinical phenotypes can hardly be maintained. Vascular markings and skin lesions are not seen only in older patients with slow evolution. Even in early childhood extensive subcutaneous telangiectasia may be found, especially on the thenar and hypothenar eminences, on the lateral aspect of the sole and also over the thorax. Pinhead-sized skin lesions similar to angiokeratomas in Fabry disease may also develop on many regions of the body even during childhood (Patel et al 1972, Gatti et al 1973, Kousseff et al 1973). Patients with either type of disease have been observed in one large pedigree (Durand et al 1976) or in a single sibship (Christomanou & Beyer 1983). In somatic cell hybridization experiments with fibroblast cultures derived from the two types of patient, no mutual complementation is observed (Beratis et al 1976). Advances in molecular biology are soon likely to confirm that a large number of different point mutations and molecular deletions within or about the structural gene locus, known to be located on chromosome 1 (McKusick 1988) will offer a more solid basis for explaining differences between patients and correlating clinical phenotype and course (Fukushima et al 1985).

Radiographic changes are either absent or mild in young patients. Skeletal age lags behind the patients' chronological age. Lumbar vertebrae are either slightly hypoplastic or normal in the presence of dorsolumbar kyphosis. Thus true dysostosis multiplex is not encountered in fucosidosis. Instead, mild spondyloepiphyseal dysplasia is often found in longer surviving subjects.

α-L-Fucosidase deficiency; formal diagnosis

Assay of α-L-fucosidase in leucocytes using the fluorescent 4-methylumbelliferyl-α-L-fucopyranoside as a substrate is at present the method of choice for establishing or excluding the diagnosis of fucosidosis (Robinson & Thorpe 1974). The profound deficiency of α-L-fucosidase found in tissues (Patel el al 1972, Matsuda et al 1973, Borrone et al 1974, MacPhee et al 1975) is similar in both patients with rapidly advancing disease and those with the more protracted course.

α-L-fucosidase deficiency has been shown in liver, brain, kidney and other visceral organs (Van Hoof & Hers 1968, Loeb et al 1969b, Robinson & Thorpe 1974) and in cultured fibroblasts (Zielke et al 1972, Matsuda et al 1973).

Determination of α-L-fucosidase activity in serum is of no value in the diagnosis of fucosidosis, because in about 12% of normal individuals the average serum enzyme activity is only about 5% of that in the rest of the population (Ng et al 1976, Van Elsen et al 1983). In these normal individuals with variant α-L-fucosidase in serum, the enzyme in leucocytes has normal activity.

Pathological findings

Weakly PAS positive vacuoles are found in peripheral lymphocytes. In hepatocytes studied with the electron microscope two types of unit-membrane bound cytoplasmic vacuoles are seen: one type has very light, loosely structured contents; the other type is filled with rounded osmiophilic lamellar structures. The Küpffer cells contain similar vacuole-like bodies. Also histiocytes, glomerular endothelium, epithelial and other cell types in conjunctiva and skin (irrespective of the presence of angiokeratoma) as well as bronchial and rectal mucosa endothelial cells are swollen by similar lysosome-like structures (Libert et al 1977). In brain, neuronal and myelin loss is considerable. In the small proportion of neurons left, large unit-membrane bound vacuoles are consistently observed.

Fucose-containing oligosaccharides are excreted excessively in the urine (Strecker 1977). Simple screening by thin layer chromatography can distinguish the pattern of oligosaccharide excretion in fucosidosis from that in other oligosaccharidoses, provided the appropriate known samples are included in the study (Humbel 1975, Fig. 102.1). In brain and liver, fucose containing glycosylceramide is considerably increased (Dawson 1972). In fucosidosis, increased antigenicity of the fucose containing blood group substances would be expected, and has in fact been observed (Staal et al 1977).

The complexity of the products stored is part of the reason why enzyme study is the most important means of establishing the diagnosis, although urinary screening for oligosaccharides and electron microscopic study of skin or conjunctiva biopsy specimens are important in directing the efforts of the biochemistry laboratory. The latter point is illustrated well by the recent report on a Black proband with a rapid clinical course of fucosidosis and a markedly decreased thermostability of the high residual activity of the mutant acidic a-L-fucosidase (Blitzer et al 1985).

ASPARTYLGLUCOSAMINURIA (AGU)

The excessive urinary excretion of aspartylglucosamine, first detected by Jenner and Pollitt (1967) in mentally retarded adults with coarse facies reminiscent of that in some of the mucopolysaccharidoses, is the biochemical marker which linked AGU to the oligosaccharidoses and pointed to the deficiency of the lysosomal enzyme 1 - aspartamido - β - N - acetylglucosamine -aminohydrolase (Pollitt et al 1968). AGU occurs at relatively high frequency in Finland (Autio et al 1973) but has also been observed in other countries (Hreidarsson et al 1983). The disorder becomes apparent from early childhood with progressive mental deficiency, coarsening features and speech and language impairment. In younger patients hepatosplenomegaly may be found.

Cardiac valve thickening is observed in a minority of cases. Uncontrolled behaviour is a regular problem in the management of patients. Lymphocytic vacuolization and radiographic abnormalities are consistent but nonspecific findings. Thin-layer chromatography of urinary oligosaccharides will detect the disorder (Fig. 102.1).

THE WINCHESTER SYNDROME

An abnormal oligosaccharide containing one fucose and two galactose residues is excreted excessively in the urine of patients with short stature, progressive joint stiffness simulating severe rheumatoid arthritis and, radiologically, destructive skeletal changes and osteoporosis, mainly about the joints.

This syndrome was first described by Winchester et al (1969). More recently other examples of this disorder with a still unknown metabolic defect but morphological indications of excessive collagen turnover have been reported (Dunger et al 1987). Similar patients were probably reported earlier by Hollister et al (1974) and by Landing and Nadorra (1986). There is no evidence of either lysosomal storage or involvement in this disorder, which is probably heterogeneous, as several features are not shared by all patients reported.

ALLIED DISORDERS

A number of nosological entities have traditionally been considered members of the group of oligosaccharidoses. However, by strictly chemical criteria they are not. Nevertheless, the clinical phenotypes warrant their discussion within a chapter on the oligosaccharidoses.

Sialic acid storage diseases (SASD)

The metabolic hallmark in these patients is the excessive urinary excretion and intracellular accumulation of free sialic acid. The primary metabolic error remains unknown but is probably related to defective transport of sialic acid about the lysosomes. Clear membrane bound and swollen lysosomal inclusions are found in peripheral lymphocytes, as well as in many parenchymal and connective tissue cells.

According to the strictly chemical definitions of the terms, patients with SASD neither have an oligosaccharidosis nor a sialidosis. At least two clinical phenotypes have been discerned: the more severe infantile form with fatal outcome already in early childhood; and the late infantile onset type with slowly progressive disease of the central nervous system but without significant interference with life expectancy. The latter disorder has been observed most frequently in northern Scandinavia (Renlund 1984). At present no data on in vitro complementation are available to answer formally the question of functional allelism of the mutant genes in these clinical conditions. The likely direct correlation between degree of derangement of sialic acid metabolism and severity of the clinical features has so far been insufficiently documented.

Infantile SASD

The early infantile form of SASD is characterized by deficient psychomotor and somatic development, axial hypotonia with hypertonia of the limbs, hypopigmentation, coarse facial features, loose stools, hepatosplenomegaly, inguinal hernias, recurrent infections and hypochromic anaemia. Inconsistently mild dysostosis multiplex, punctate calcifications, laryngomalacia and cardiomegaly are recorded (Tondeur et al 1982, Stevenson et al 1983, Paschke et al 1986). Intercurrent respiratory infection in infancy or early childhood is the usual cause of death in these bedridden, nearly immobile, profoundly retarded patients. It is of interest that in some of the patients with infantile SASD, congenital or neonatal ascites and non-immune hydrops are the presenting clinical signs (Hancock et al 1982, Gillan et al 1984) prompting a differential diagnosis with the neonatal hydropic type sialidosis (NS), neonatal galactosialidosis (NGS) and infantile G_{M1}-gangliosidosis.

Salla disease (Late Infantile SASD)

Because of its relatively frequent occurrence in northern Finland, Salla disease is a convenient eponym for the milder type of SASD with onset in later infancy or early childhood and with chronic clinical course. Other main features are moderate to severe psychomotor retardation, with ambulation usually achieved, but minimal speech development, ataxia, nystagmus, rigidity, pyramidal spasticity with hyperactive tendon reflexes, particularly in the lower limbs, and convulsions. In most patients hepatosplenomegaly is equivocal or absent, although exceptions are known (Wilcken et al 1987). There is neither general nor facial dysmorphia and there are no detectable radiographic changes of the skeleton. Motor nerve conduction velocities have been consistently normal.

Some patients may have a milder phenotype (Fontaine et al 1968, Palo et al 1985) yet their clinical evolution falls well within the spectrum of clinical variability expected for Salla disease, which has also been observed outside Finland (Baumkötter et al 1985, Wolburg-Buchholz et al 1985, Echenne et al 1986).

Prior to the elucidation of the primary metabolic defect, and without the results of in vitro complementation tests, it is impossible to resolve the question of whether the original patient of Fontaine et al (1968) and the one recently described from Australia (Wilcken et al 1987), who likewise shows ultrastructural changes of mitochondria instead of abnormalities of lysosomes, are in fact genetically different from patients with Salla disease.

Berman syndrome

From the time of the first clinical observation by Berman et al (1974a) this disorder has been aligned with the mucolipidoses and subsequently called mucolipidosis IV (ML IV) (Merin et al 1975), because of some clinical features shared with the mucopolysaccharidoses and the lipidoses. Anatomo- and chemicopathological findings indicate that this by now clinically well delineated disorder, which occurs mainly, but not exclusively, in Ashkenazi Jewish children (Amir et al 1987), is in fact a true lipidosis with only minor storage of gangliosides but with significant accumulation in brain and liver of various phospholipids. The urinary excretion of the latter is also increased (Tellez-Nagel et al 1976, Crandall et al 1982). Storage of phospholipids also occurs in cultured fibroblasts, in addition to the accumulation of glycosaminoglycans, but that of gangliosides is equivocal (Bach et al 1979b). However, internalized exogenous gangliosides are poorly metabolized in the patients' fibroblasts (Zeigler & Bach 1986). That the reduced activity of solubilized ganglioside sialidase is the primary defect in the Berman syndrome has not been rigorously proved. Oligosaccharide excretion in the urine is normal, a finding which supports the contention that the syndrome is not really a type of oligosaccharidosis.

Slowing psychomotor development in the first year of life and corneal opacities with signs of visual deficiency, either from birth or from early childhood, are the presenting signs. Independent walking and effective oral language are never achieved. A stable level of mental defect and of low grade social contact is soon reached without further deterioration even into early adulthood which already has been reached by the oldest known patients. Although physical development and growth are deficient, at no time is there any radiological abnormality of the skeleton. The patients remain hypotonic but with brisk deep tendon reflexes. There is neither facial coarsening nor macrocephaly. Organomegaly is not observed (Amir et al 1987).

In conjunctival or skin biopsy specimens, but also in cultured fibroblasts and amniocytes as well as in parenchymal organs, grossly swollen lysosomal bodies filled with membraneous lamellar inclusions are observed with the electron microscope. This ultrastructural finding appears to be sufficiently typical to be used effectively as a marker of cellular pathology in prenatal diagnosis (Kohn et al 1982).

Mucosulphatidosis: Multiple sulphatase deficiency (MSD)

The first patients with this rare disorder were described by Austin, who subsequently found a deficiency of several sulphatases (Austin et al 1965). The clinical and pathological phenotypes, succinctly reviewed by Eto et al (1983), are composites of features encountered in some of the mucopolysaccharidoses and in metachromatic leucodystrophy. Consequently the disorder was originally incorporated into the group of mucolipidoses.

Clinically, the disorder manifests itself late in the first year of life with psychomotor retardation, moderate hepatosplenomegaly, recurrent respiratory infections, inguinal hernias in males, radiographic features of dysostosis multiplex, and increased urinary excretion of AMPS. The skin can show scaling. Neurodegenerative symptoms are apparent before 2 years of age, with loss of acquired skills, progressive quadriplegia, ataxia, nystagmus, convulsions, decrease and loss of vision and hearing. The corneae are clear.

Ophthalmological examination shows loss of retinal pigment, grey maculae and atrophy of the optic nerve discs. The disorder ends fatally before adolescence and sometimes in early childhood. Reports of this disorder remain scarce but lend support to the phenotype described (Nevsimalova et al 1984). Not surprisingly, clinical variants are also observed, such as the neonatal form of MSD with more rapid course and fatal outcome described by Vamos et al (1981) and a late onset variant (MSD$_v$) with slow clinical progression. The latter muta-tion does not show in vitro complementation in hybrids derived from MSD$_v$ and MSD fibroblasts (Tanaka et al 1987). The apparently allelic mutations affect a gene, the product of which renders a common stability to the multiplicity of known sulphatases (Waheed et al 1982). The diagnosis can be made formally by demonstrating deficiencies of lysosomal arylsulphatases A and B, and of microsomal arylsulphatase C. Several other sulphatases have also been found deficient. For the data on chemical pathology, histopathology and molecular aspects of the sulphatases involved, the reader is referred to well documented reviews (Austin 1973, Eto et al 1983, Kolodny & Moser 1983).

REFERENCES

Amir N, Ziotogora J, Bach G 1987 Mucolipidosis type IV: clinical spectrum and natural history. Pediatrics 79: 953–959

Andria G, Del Giudice E, Reuser A J J 1978 Atypical expression of β-galactosidase deficiency in a child with Hurler-like features but without neurological abnormalities. Clinical Genetics 14: 16–23

Andria G, Strisciuglio P, Pontarelli G, Sly W S, Dodson W E 1981 Infantile neuraminidase and β-galactosidase deficiencies (galactosialidosis) with mild clinical courses. In: Perspectives in inherited metabolic diseases vol 4. Ermes, Milan p 379–395

Aula P, Rapola J, Autio S, Raivio K, Karjalainen O 1975 Prenatal diagnosis and fetal pathology of I-cell disease (mucolipidosis type II). Journal of Pediatrics 87: 221–226

Austin J H 1973 Studies in metachromatic leukodystrophy. XII. Multiple sulfatase deficiency. Archives of Neurology 28: 258–264

Austin J, Armstrong D, Shearer L 1965 Metachromatic form of diffuse cerebral sclerosis. V. The nature and significance of low sulfatase activity: a controlled study of brain, liver and kidney in four patients with MLD. Archives of Neurology 13: 593–614

Autio S, Norden N E, Ockerman P A, Riekkinen P, Rapola J, Louhimo T 1973a Mannosidosis: clinical, fine-structural and biochemical findings in three cases. Acta Paediatrica Scandinavica 62: 555–565

Autio S, Visakorpi J K, Jarvinen H 1973b Aspartylglycosaminuria (AGU). Further aspects of its clinical picture, mode of inheritance and epidemiology, based on a series of 57 patients. Annals of Clinical Research 5: 149–155

Aylsworth A S, Taylor H A, Stuart C M, Thomas G H 1976 Mannosidosis: phenotype of a severely affected child and characterization of α-mannosidase activity in cultured fibroblasts from the patient and his parents. Journal of Pediatrics 88: 814–818

Aylsworth A S, Thomas G H, Hood J L, Libert J 1980 A severe infantile sialidosis: clinical biochemical and microscopic features. Journal of Pediatrics 96: 662–668

Bach G, Kohn G, Lasch E E, Massri M E, Ornoy A, Sekeles E, Legum C, Cohen M M 1978 A new variant of mannosidosis with increased enzymatic activity and mild clinical manifestation. Pediatric Research 12: 1010–1015

Bach G, Bargal R, Cantz M 1979a I-cell disease: deficiency of extracellular hydrolase phosphorylation. Biochemical and Biophysical Research Communications 91: 976–981

Bach G, Zeigler M, Schaap T, Kohn G 1979b Mucolipidosis type IV: ganglioside sialidase deficiency. Biochemical and Biophysical Research Communications 90: 1341–1347

Baumkötter J, Cantz M, Mendla K, Baumann W, Friebolin H, Gehler J, Spranger J 1985 N-acetylneuraminic acid storage disease. Human Genetics 71: 155–159

Beaudet A L, Nichols B L 1976 Residual altered α-mannosidase in human mannosidosis. Biochemical and Biophysical Research Communications 68: 292–297

Beck M, Bender S W, Reiter H L, Otto W, Bässler R, Dancygier H, Gehler J 1984 Neuraminidase deficiency presenting a non-immune hydrops fetalis. European Journal of Pediatrics 143: 135–139

Ben-Yoseph Y, Potice M, Michell D A, Pack B A, Melancon S B, Nadler H C 1986 Altered molecular size of N-acetyl-glucosaminylphosphotransferase in I-cell disease and pseudo-Hurler polydystrophy. 7th International Congress in Human Genetics, Berlin, Abstract, 22–26 September 1986

Beratis N G, Turner B M, Hirschhorn K 1976 Reply: on genetic variants in fucosidosis. Journal of Pediatrics 89: 690

Berman E R, Kohn G, Yatziv S, Stein H 1974a Acid hydrolase deficiencies and abnormal glycoproteins in Mucolipidosis III. Clinica Chimica Acta 52: 115–124

Berman E R, Livni H, Shapira E, Merin S, Levij S I 1974b Congenital corneal clouding with abnormal systemic storage bodies : a new variant of mucolipidosis. Journal of Pediatrics 84: 519–526

Berra B, Di Palma S, Lindi C, Sandhoff K 1979 Content of gangliosides and protein-bound sialic acid in post-mortem brain of patients with mucolipidosis I and II (ML I and ML II). Cell and Molecular Biology 25: 281–284

Blitzer M G, Sutton M, Miller J B, Shapiro E 1985 A thermolabile variant of α-L-fucosidase — clinical and laboratory findings. American Journal of Medical Genetics 20: 535–539

Booth C W, Chen K K, Nadler H L 1976 Mannosidosis: clinical and biochemical studies in a family of affected adolescents and adults. Journal of Pediatrics 88: 821–824

Borrone G, Gatti R, Trias X, Durand P 1974 Fucosidosis: clinical biochemical, immunologic and genetic studies in two new cases. Journal of Pediatrics 84: 727–730

Burditt L J, Chotai K, Hirani S, Nugent P G, Winchester B

G 1980 Biochemical studies on a case of feline mannosidosis. Biochemical Journal 189: 467–473

Cantz M, Messer H 1979 Oligosaccharide and ganglioside neuraminidase activities of mucolipidosis I (sialidosis) and mucolipidosis II (I-cell disease) fibroblasts. European Journal of Biochemistry 79: 113–118

Cantz M, Gheler J, Spranger J 1977 Mucolipidosis I: increased sialic acid content and deficiency of an α-N-acetyl-neuraminidase in cultured fibroblasts. Biochemical and Biophysical Research Communications 74: 732–738

Carroll N, Dance N, Masson P K, Robinson D, Winchester B G 1972 Human mannosidosis. The enzymic defect. Biochemical and Biophysical Research Communications 49: 579–583

Champion M J, Shows T B 1977 Mannosidosis: assignment of the lysosomal α-mannosidase B gene to chromosome 19 in man. Proceedings of the National Academy of Sciences USA 74: 2968–2972

Christomanou H, Beyer D 1983 Absence of α-fucosidase activity in two sisters showing a different phenotype. European Journal of Pediatrics 140: 27–29

Cooper A, Sardharwalla I B, Roberts M M 1986 Human β-mannosidase deficiency. New England Journal of Medicine 315: 1231

Crandall B F, Philippart M, Brown M J, Bluestone D A 1982 Review article: mucolipidosis IV. American Journal of Medical Genetics 12: 301–308

Dacremont G, Kint J A, Cocquyt G 1974 Brain sphingolipids in I-cell disease (mucolipidosis II). Journal of Neurochemistry 22: 599–602

Dahms N M, Lobel P, Breitmeyer J, Chirgwin J M, Kornfeld S 1987 46 kD mannose 6-phosphate receptor: cloning, expression and homology to the 215 kD mannose 6-phosphate receptor. Cell 50: 181–192

Dahms N M, Lobel P, Kornfeld S 1989 Mannose 6-phosphate receptors and lysosomal enzyme targeting. Journal of Biological Chemistry 264: 12115–12118

Dawson G 1972 Glycosphingolipid abnormalities in liver from patients with glycosphingolipid and mucopolysaccharide storage diseases. In: Volk B W, Aronson S M (eds) Sphingolipids, Sphingolipidoses and Allied Disorders Plenum Press, New York, p 395–413

d'Azzo A, Hoogeveen A T, Reuser A J J, Robinson D, Galjaard H 1982 Molecular defect in combined β-galactosidase and neuraminidase deficiency in man. Proceedings of the National Academy of Sciences USA 79: 4532–4539

DeMars R I, Leroy J G 1967 The remarkable cells cultured from a human with Hurler's syndrome: An approach to visual selection for in vitro genetic studies. In Vitro 2: 107–118

Den Tandt W R, Leroy J G 1980 Deficiency of neuraminidase in the sialidoses and the mucolipidoses. Human Genetics 53: 383–388

Desnick R J, Sharp H L, Grabowski G A, Brunning R D, Quie P G, Sung J H, Gorlin R J, Ikonne J U 1976 Mannosidosis: clinical, morphologic, immunologic and biochemical studies. Pediatric Research 10: 985–996

Distler J, Hieber V, Sahagian G, Schmickel R, Jourdian G W 1979 Identification of mannose-6-phosphate in glycoproteins that inhibit the assimilation of β-galactosidase by fibroblasts. Proceedings of the National Academy of Sciences USA 76: 4235–4239

Dunger D B, Dicks-Mireaux C, O'Driscoll P, Lake B, Eroser R, Show D G, Grant D B 1987 Two cases of Winchester syndrome: with increased urinary oligosaccharide excretion. European Journal of Pediatrics 146: 615–619

Durand P, Borrone C, Della Cella G 1966 A new mucopolysaccharide lipid storage disease. Lancet ii: 1313

Durand P, Borrone C, Della Cella G, Philippart M 1968 Fucosidosis. Lancet i: 1198

Durand P, Borrone C, Della Cella G 1969 Fucosidosis. Journal of Pediatrics 75: 665–674

Durand P, Borrone C, Gatti R 1976 On genetic variants in fucosidosis. Journal of Pediatrics 89: 688–690

Durand P, Gatti R, Cavalieri S, Borrone C, Tondeur M, Michalski J C, Strecker G 1977 Sialidosis (Mucolipidosis I). Helvetica Paediatrica Acta 32: 391–400

Echenne B, Vidal M, Maire I, Michalski J C, Baldet P, Astruc J 1986 Salla disease in one non-Finnish patient. European Journal of Pediatrics 145: 320–322

Eto Y, Owada M, Katagawa T, Kokubun Y, Rennert O W 1979 Neurochemical abnormality in I-cell disease: chemical analysis and a possible importance of β-galactosidase deficiency. Journal of Neurochemistry 32: 397–405

Eto Y, Kureha Y, Tada Y, Toshiharu T, Kihei M 1983 MSD multiple sulfatase deficient disorder. A review of clinical, pathological, biochemical and pathogenic findings. Acta Paediatrica Japan 25: 17–21

Farriaux J P, Legouis I, Humbel R et al 1975 La Mannosidose. A propos de 5 observations. La Nouvelle Presse Medicale 4: 1867–1870

Fontaine G, Biserte G, Montreuil J, Dupont A, Farriaux J P 1968: La sialurie: un trouble metabolique original. Helvetica Paediatrica Acta 23 (suppl. XVII) 1–32

Fukushima H, De Wet J R, O'Brien J S 1985 Molecular cloning of a cDNA for human α-L-fucosidase. Proceedings of the National Academy of Sciences USA 82: 1262–1265

Gatti R, Borrone C, Trias X, Durand P 1973 Genetic heterogeneity in fucosidosis. Lancet ii: 1024

Gehler J, Cantz M, Stoeckenius M, Spranger J 1976 Prenatal diagnosis of mucolipidosis II (I-cell disease). European Journal of Pediatrics 122: 201–206

Gillan J E, Lowden J A, Gaskin K, Cutz E 1984 Congenital ascites as a presenting sign of lysosomal storage disease. Journal of Pediatrics 104: 225–231

Goldberg M, Cotlier E, Fichenscher L G, Kenyon K, Enat R, Borowsky S A 1971 Macular cherry-red spot, corneal clouding and β-galactosidase deficiency. Archives of Internal Medicine 128: 387–398

Gravel R A, Lowden J A, Callahan J W, Wolfe L S, Ng Yin Kin N M K 1979 Infantile sialidosis: a phenocopy of type 1 G_{M1} gangliosidosis distinguished by genetic complementation and urinary oligosaccharides. American Journal of Human Genetics 31: 669–679

Halley D J J, Winchester B G, Burditt L J, d'Azzo A, Robinson D, Galjaard H 1980 Comparison of the α-mannosidases in fibroblast cultures from patients with mannosidosis and mucolipidosis II and from controls. Biochemical Journal 187: 541–543

Hanai J, Leroy J G, O'Brien J S 1971 Ultrastructure of cultured fibroblasts in I-cell disease. American Journal of Diseases of Children 122: 34–38

Hancock L W, Thaler N M, Howitz A L, Dawson G 1982 Generalized N-acetylneuraminic acid storage disease: quantitation and identification of the monosaccharide accumulating in brain and other tissues. Journal of Neurochemistry 38: 803–809

Harzer K, Cantz M, Sewell A C et al 1986 Normomorphic sialidosis in two female adults with severe neurologic disease and without sialyl oligosacchariduria. Human Genetics 74: 209–214

Hasilik A, Neufeld E F 1980a Biosynthesis of lysosomal enzymes in fibroblasts. Synthesis as precursors of higher molecular weight. Journal of Biological Chemistry 255: 4937–4945

Hasilik A, Neufeld E F 1980b Biosynthesis of lysosomal enzymes in fibroblasts. Phosphorylation of mannose residues. Journal of Biological Chemistry 255: 4946–4950

Hasilik A, Klein U, Waheed A, Strecker G, von Figura K 1980 Phosphorylated oligosaccharides in lysosomal enzymes: identification of p-N-acetylglucosamine (1) - phospho (6) mannose diester groups. Proceedings of the National Academy of Sciences USA 77: 7074–7078

Hasilik A, Waheed A, von Figura K 1981 Enzymatic phosphorylation of lysosomal enzymes in the presence of UDP-N-acetylglucosamine. Absence of the activity in I-cell fibroblasts. Biochemical and Biophysical Research Communications 98: 761–767

Hickman S, Neufeld E F 1972 A hypothesis for I-cell disease: defective hydrolases that do not enter lysosomes. Biochemical and Biophysical Research Communications 49: 992–999

Hickman S, Shapiro L J, Neufeld E F 1974 A recognition marker required for uptake of a lysosomal enzyme by cultured fibroblasts. Biochemical and Biophysical Research Communications 57: 55–61

Hirani S, Winchester B G 1980 Plasma α-D-mannosidase in mucolipidosis II and mucolipidosis III. Clinica Chimica Acta 101: 251–256

Hirani S, Winchester B G, Patrick A D 1977 Measurement of the α-mannosidase activities in human plasma by a differential assay. Clinica Chimica Acta 81: 135–144

Hollister D W, Rimoin D L, Lachman R S, Cohen A H, Reed W B, Wilbur Westin G 1974 The Winchester syndrome: a non-lysosomal connective tissue disease. Journal of Pediatrics 84: 701–709

Hoogeveen A T, Verheyen F W, d'Azzo A, Galjaard H 1980a Genetic heterogeneity in human neuraminidase deficiency. Nature 285: 500–502

Hoogeveen A T, Verheyen F W, Galjaard H 1980b The relation between human lysosomal β-galactosidase and its protective protein. Journal of Biological Chemistry 255: 4937–4945

Hoogeveen A T, Graham-Kawashima H, d'Azzo A, Galjaard H 1985 Processing of human β-galactosidase in G$_{M1}$-gangliosidosis and Morquio B syndrome. Journal of Biological Chemistry 259: 1974–1977

Hreidarsson S, Thomas G H, Valle D L, Stevenson R E, Taylor H, McCarty J, Coker S B, Green W R 1983 Aspartylglucosaminuria in the United States. Clinical Genetics 23: 427–435

Humbel R 1975 Biochemical screening for mucopolysaccharidosis, mucolipidosis and oligosaccharidosis. Helvetica Paediatrica Acta 30: 191–200

Jenner F A, Pollitt R J 1967 Large quantities of 2-acetamido-1- (β-L-aspartamido)-1, 2-dideoxyglucose in the urine of mentally retarded siblings. Biochemical Journal 103: 48–49

Jones M Z, Dawson G 1981 Caprine β-mannosidosis: inherited deficiency of β-D-mannosidase. Journal of Biochemical Chemistry 256: 5185-5188

Kaplan A, Fischer D, Achard D, Sly W 1977 Phosphohexosyl recognition is a general characteristic of pinocytosis of lysosomal glycosidases by human fibroblasts. Journal of Clinical Investigation 60: 1088–1093

Kelly T E, Graetz G 1977 Isolated acid neuraminidase deficiency: a distinct lysosomal storage disease. American Journal of Medical Genetics 1: 3–46

Kelly T E, Thomas G H, Taylor H A et al 1975 Mucolipidosis III (pseudo-Hurler polydystrophy): clinical and laboratory studies in a series of 12 patients. Johns Hopkins Medical Journal 137: 156–175

King M, Cockburn F, MacPhee G B, Logan R W 1984 Infantile type 2 sialidosis in a Pakistani family — a clinical and biochemical study. Journal of Inherited Metabolic Disease 7: 91–96

Kistler J P, Lott I T, Kolodny E H et al 1977 Mannosidosis: new clinical presentation, enzyme studies and carbohydrate analysis. Archives of Neurology 34: 45–51

Kjellman B, Gamstorp I, Brun A, Ockerman P A, Palmgren B 1969 Mannosidosis: A clinical and histopathologic study. The Journal of Pediatrics 75: 366–373

Kohn G, Sekeles E, Arnon J, Ornay A 1982 Mucolipidosis IV: prenatal diagnosis by electron microscopy. Prenatal Diagnosis 2: 301-307

Kolodny E H, Moser H W 1983 Sulfatide lipidosis: metachromatic leucodystrophy. In: Stanbury J B et al (eds) The Metabolic Basis of Inherited Disease, 5th edn. McGraw-Hill, New York, p 881–905

Kornfeld S 1986 Trafficking of lysosomal enzymes in normal and disease states. Journal of Clinical Investigation 77: 1–6

Koster J F, Niermeyer M F, Loonen M C B, Galjaard H 1976 β-galactosidase deficiency in an adult: a biochemical and somatic cell genetic study on a variant of G$_{M1}$-gangliosidosis. Clinical Genetics 9: 427–432

Kousseff B G, Beratis N G, Danesino C, Hirschhorn K 1973 Genetic heterogeneity in fucosidosis. Lancet ii: 1387–1388

Landing B H, Nadorra R 1986 Infantile systemic hyalinosis. Pediatric Pathology 6: 55–79

Laver J, Fried K, Beer S I, Iancu T C, Heyman E, Bach G, Zeigler M 1983 Infantile lethal neuraminidase deficiency (Sialidosis). Clinical Genetics 23: 97–101

Leroy J G, DeMars R I 1967 Mutant enzymatic and cytological phenotypes in cultured human fibroblasts. Science 157: 805–806

Leroy J G, O'Brien J S 1976 Mucolipidosis II and III: different residual activity of beta-galactosidase in cultured fibroblasts. Clinical Genetics 9: 533–539

Leroy J G, Spranger J W 1970 I-cell disease (cont.) New England Journal of Medicine 283: 598–599

Leroy J F, Van Elsen A F 1975 Natural history of a mucolipidosis. Twin girls discordant for ML III. Birth Defects: Original Article Series XI(6): 325–334

Leroy J G, Spranger J W, Feingold M, Opitz J M, Crocker A C 1971 I-cell disease: a clinical picture. Journal of Pediatrics 79: 360–365

Leroy J G, Ho M W, MacBrinn M C, Zielke K, Jacob J, O'Brien J S 1972 I-cell disease: biochemical studies. Pediatric Research 6: 752–759

Libert J, Tondeur M, Martin J J 1977 La fucosidose: aspects anatomopathologiques et microscopie electronique. In: Farriaux J P (ed) Les oligosaccharidoses Crouan & Roques, Lille, p 51–58

Little L E, Mueller O T, Honey N K, Shows T B, Miller A L 1986: Heterogeneity of N-acetylglucosamine-1-phosphotransferase within mucolipidosis III. Journal of Biological Chemistry 261: 733–738

Lobel P, Dahms N M, Breitmeyer J, Chirgwin J M, Kornfeld S 1987 Cloning of the bovine 215-kDa cation-independent mannose 6-phosphate receptor. Proceedings of the National Academy of Sciences USA 84: 2233–2237

Loeb H, Tondeur M, Toppet M, Cremer N 1969a Clinical, biochemical and ultrastructural studies of an atypical form of mucopolysaccharidosis. Acta Paediatrica Scandinavica 58: 220–228

Loeb H, Tondeur M, Jonniaux G, Mockel-Pohl S, Vamos-Hurwitz 1969b Biochemical and ultrastructural studies in a case of mucopolysaccharidosis 'F' (Fucosidosis). Helvetica Paediatrica Acta 24: 519–537

Lowden J A, O'Brien J S 1979 Sialidosis: a review of human neuraminidase deficiency. American Journal of Human Genetics 31: 1–18

Lowden J A, Cutz E, Skomorowski M A 1981 Infantile type 2 sialidosis with β-galactosidase deficiency. In: Tettamanti G, Durand P, Di Donato S (eds) Sialidases and Sialidoses Edi. Ermes, Milan, p 261–280

McKusick V A 1988 Mendelian Inheritance in Man, 8th edn. The Johns Hopkins University Press, Baltimore

MacPhee G B, Logan R W, Primrose D A A 1975 Fucosidosis: how many cases undetected? Lancet ii: 462–463

Maroteaux P 1982 Maladies osseuses de l'enfant, 2nd edn. Flammarion, Paris

Maroteaux P, Lamy M 1966 La pseudopolydystrophie de Hurler. Presse Medicale 71: 2889–2892

Maroteaux P, Humbel R, Strecker G, Michalski J C, Maude R 1978 Un nouveau type de sialidose avec atteinte renale: la nephrosialidose. Archives Francaises de Pediatrie 35: 819–829

Martin J J, Leroy J G, Farriaux J-P, Fontaine G, Desnick R J, Cabello A 1975 I-cell disease (mucolipidosis II). A report on its pathology. Acta Neuropathologica (Berlin) 33: 285–305

Martin J J, Leroy J G, Van Eygen M, Ceuterick C 1984: I-cell disease: a further report on its pathology. Acta Neuropathologica (Berlin) 64: 234–242

Matsuda I U 1975 Prenatal diagnosis of I-cell disease. Humangenetik 30: 69–73

Matsuda I, Arashima S, Anakura M, Ege A, Hayata I 1973 Fucosidosis. Tohuku Journal of Experimental Medicine 109: 41–48

Merin S, Levni N, Berman E R, Yatziv T 1975 Mucolipidosis IV. Ocular, systemic and ultrastructural findings. Investigative Ophthalmology 14: 437–448

Miyatake T, Atsumi Y, Obayaski T, Mizuno Y, Ando S, Ariga T, Matsui-Nakamura K, Yamada T 1979 Adult type neuronal storage disease with neuraminidase deficiency. Annals of Neurology 6: 232–244

Mueller O T, Little L E, Miller A L, Lozzio C B, Shows B 1985 I-cell disease and pseudo-Hurler polydystrophy: heterozygote detection and characteristics of the altered N-acetyl-glucosamine-phosphotransferase in genetic variants. Clinica Chimica Acta 150: 175–183

Natowicz M R, Chi M M-Y, Lowry O H, Sly W S 1979 Enzymatic identification of mannose-6-phosphate on the recognition marker for receptor-mediated pinocytosis of β-glucuronidase by human fibroblasts. Proceedings of the National Academy of Sciences USA 76: 4322–4326

Nevsimalova S, Elleder M, Smid P, Zemankova M 1984 Multiple sulfatase deficiency in homozygous twins. Journal of Inherited Metabolic Diseases 7: 38–40

Ng W G, Donnell G N, Koch R, Bergren W R 1976 Biochemical and genetic studies of plasma and leucocyte α-L-fucosidase. American Journal of Human Genetics 28: 42–50

O'Brien J S 1977 Neuraminidase deficiency in the cherry red spot-myoclonus syndrome. Biochemical and Biophysical Research Communications 79: 1136–1141

O'Brien J S, Warner T G 1980 Sialidosis: delineation of subtypes by neuraminidase assay. Clinical Genetics 17: 35–38

O'Brien J S, Gugler E, Giedeon A, Wiesmann U, Herschkowitz N, Meier C, Leroy J 1976 Spondyloepiphyseal dysplasia, corneal clouding, normal intelligence and acid β-galactosidase deficiency. Clinical Genetics 9: 495–504

Öckerman P A 1967a A generalized storage disorder resembling Hurler's syndrome. Lancet ii: 239–241

Öckerman P A 1967b Deficiency of beta-galactosidase and alpha-mannosidase: primary enzyme defects in gargoylism and a new generalized disease. Acta Paediatrica Scandinavica 177: 35–36

Öckerman P A 1969 Mannosidosis: isolation of oligosaccharide storage material from brain. Journal of Pediatrics 75: 360–365

Okada S, Yutaka T, Kato T, Ikehara C, Yabuuchi H, Okawa M, Inui M, Chiyo H 1979 A case of neuraminidase deficiency associated with a partial β-galactosidase defect. European Journal of Pediatrics 130: 239–249

Okada S, Sugino H, Kato T, Yukata T, Koike M, Dezawa T, Yamano T, Yabuuchi H 1983 A severe infantile sialidosis (β-galactosidase-α-neuraminidase deficiency) mimicking G_{M1}-gangliosidosis type 1. European Journal of Pediatrics 140: 295–298

Pallman B, Sandhoff K, Berra B, Miyatake T 1980 Sialidase in brain and fibroblasts in three patients with different types of sialidosis. In: Svennerholm L, Mandel P, Dreyfus H, Urban P F (eds) Structure and function of gangliosides Plenum Press, New York, p 401–414

Palmeri S, Hoogeveen A T, Verheyen F W, Galjaard H 1986 Galactosialidosis: molecular heterogeneity among distinct clinical phenotypes. American Journal of Human Genetics 38: 137–148

Palo J, Rauvala H, Finne J, Haltia M, Palmgren K 1985 Hyperexcretion of free N-acetylneuraminic acid — a novel type of sialuria. Clinica Chimica Acta 145: 237–242

Paschke E, Trinkl G, Erwa W, Pavelka M, Mutz I, Roscher A 1986 Infantile type of sialic acid storage disease with sialuria. Clinical Genetics 29: 417–424

Patel V, Watanabe I, Zeman W 1972 Deficiency of α-L-fucosidase. Science 176: 426–427

Phillips N C, Robinson D, Winchester B G 1974a Human liver α-D-mannosidase activity. Clinica Chimica Acta 55: 11–19

Phillips N C, Robinson D, Winchester B G, Jolly R D 1974b Mannosidosis in Angus Cattle. Biochemical Journal 137: 363–371

Phillips N, Robinson D, Winchester B 1975 Immunological characterization of human liver α-D-mannosidase. Biochemical Journal 151: 469–475

Poenaru L, Dreyfus J C 1973 Electrophoretic heterogeneity of human α-mannosidase. Biochimica et Biophysica Acta 303: 171–174

Poenaru L, Castelman L, Dumez Y, Thepot F 1984 First trimester prenatal diagnosis of mucolipidosis II (I-cell disease) by chorionic biopsy. American Journal of

Human Genetics 36: 1379–1385

Pohlmann R, Nagel G, Schmidt B et al 1987 Cloning of a cDNA encoding human cation-dependent mannose 6-phosphate specific receptor. Proceedings of the National Academy of Sciences USA 84 : 5575–5579

Pollitt R J, Jenner F A, Merskey H 1968 Aspartylglucosaminuria: an inborn error of metabolism associated with mental defect. Lancet 2: 253–255

Rapin I, Goldfischer S, Katzman R, Engel J, O'Brien J S 1978 The cherry-red spot-myoclonus syndrome. Annals of Neurology 3: 234–242

Reitman M L, Varki A, Kornfeld S 1981 Fibroblasts from patients with I-cell disease and pseudo-Hurler polydystrophy are deficient in uridine 5'-diphosphate N-acetylglucosamine: glycoprotein N-acetylglucosaminylphospho-transferase activity. Journal of Clinical Investigation 67: 1574–1579

Renlund M 1984 Clinical and laboratory diagnosis of Salla disease in infancy and childhood. Journal of Pediatrics 104: 232–236

Robinson D, Thorpe R 1974 Fluorescent assay of α-L-fucosidase. Clinica Chimica Acta 55: 65–69

Sando G N, Neufeld E F 1977 Recognition and receptor mediated uptake of a lysosomal enzyme α-L-iduronidase by cultured human fibroblasts. Cell 12: 619–627

Schmickel R D, Distel J, Jourdian G W 1975 Accumulation of sulfate containing acid mucopolysaccharides in I-cell fibroblasts. Journal of Laboratory and Clinical Medicine 86: 672–682

Sewell A C 1980 Urinary oligosaccharide excretion in disorders of glycolipid, glycoprotein and glycogen metabolism. European Journal of Pediatrics 134: 183–194

Spranger J W, Wiedemann H R 1970 The genetic mucolipidoses. Humangenetik 9: 113–139

Spranger J, Langer L O, Wiedemann H R 1974 Bone dysplasias Fisher, Stuttgart

Spranger J, Gehler J, Cantz M 1977 Mucolipidosis I — a sialidosis. American Journal of Medical Genetics 1: 21–29

Staal G E J, Van Der Heyden McM, Troost J, Moes M, Borst-Eilers E 1977 Fucosidosis and Lewis substances. Clinica Chimica Acta 76: 155–157

Stein M, Zijderhand-Bleekemolen J E, Geuze H, Hasilik A, von Figura K 1987 Mr 46,000 mannose 6-phosphate specific receptor: its role in targeting of lysosomal enzymes. The Embo Journal 6: 2677–2681

Steinman L, Tharp B R, Dorfman L J, Forno L S, Sogg R L, Kelts K A, O'Brien J S 1980 Peripheral neuropathy in the cherry-red spot-myoclonus syndrome (sialidosis type I). Annals of Neurology 7: 450–456

Stevenson R E, Lubinsky M, Taylor H A, Wenger D A, Schroer R J, Olmstead P M 1983 Sialic acid storage disease with sialuria: clinical and biochemical features in the severe infantile type. Pediatrics 72: 441–449

Strecker G 1977 Glycoproteines et glycoproteinoses. In: Farriaux J P (ed) Les Oligosaccharidoses. Crouan & Roques, Lille, p 13–30

Strecker G, Peers M C, Michalski J C et al 1977 Structure of nine sialyloligosaccharides accumulated in urine of eleven patients with three different types of sialidosis. European Journal of Biochemistry 75: 391–403

Strisciuglio P, Creek K E, Sly W S 1984 Complementation, cross correction and drug correction studies of combined β-galactosidase neuraminidase deficiency in human fibroblasts. Pediatric Research 18: 167–171

Suzuki Y, Sakubarz H, Yamanaka T, Ko Y M, Okamura Y

1983 Galactosialidosis (β-galactosidase-neuraminidase deficiency) : a new hereditary metabolic disease with abnormal degradation of enzyme molecules. Acta Paediatrica Japonica 25: 31–37

Tabas I, Kornfeld S 1980 Biosynthetic intermediates of β-glucuronidase contain high mannose oligosaccharides with blocked phosphate residues. Journal of Biological Chemistry 255: 6633–6639

Tanaka A, Hirabayashi M, Ishii M, Yamaoka S, Kawamura M, Nishida M, Isshiki G 1987 Complementation studies with clinical and biochemical characterizations of a new variant of multiple sulfatase deficiency. Journal of Inherited Metabolic Diseases 10 : 103–110

Tellez-Nagel I, Rapin I, Iwamoto T, Johnson A B, Norton W T, Nitowsky H 1976 Mucolipidosis IV. Clinical, ultrastructural, histochemical and chemical studies of a case including a brain biopsy. Archives of Neurology 33: 828–835

Thomas G H, Taylor H A, Reynolds L W, Miller C S 1973 Mucolipidosis III (pseudo-Hurler polydystrophy) Multiple lysosomal enzyme abnormalities in serum and cultured fibroblast cells. Pediatric Research 7: 751–756

Thomas G H, Tiller G E, Reynolds L W, Miller C S, Bace J W 1976 Increased levels of sialic acid associated with a sialidase deficiency in I-cell disease (Mucolipidosis II) fibroblasts. Biochemical and Biophysical Research Communications 71: 188–195

Thomas G H, Tipton R E, Ch'ien L T, Reynolds L W, Miller C S 1978 Sialidase (α-N-acetyl-neuraminidase) deficiency: the enzyme defect in an adult with macular cherry-red spots and myoclonus without dementia. Clinical Genetics 13: 369–379

Thomas P K, Abrams J D, Swallow D, Stewart G 1979 Sialidosis type 1: cherry red spot-myoclonus syndrome with sialidase deficiency and altered electrophoretic mobilities of some enzymes known to be glycoproteins. Journal of Neurology, Neurosurgery and Psychiatry 42: 873–880

Tondeur M 1977 La fucosidose. In Farriaux J P (ed) Les Oligosaccharidoses Crouan & Roques, Lille, p 43–49

Tondeur M, Vamos-Hurwitz E, Mockel-Pohl S, Dereume J P, Cremer N, Loeb H 1971 Clinical, biochemical and ultrastructural studies in a case of chondrodystropy presenting the I-cell phenotype in tissue culture. Journal of Pediatrics 79: 366–378

Tondeur M, Libert J, Vamos E, Van Hoof F, Thomas G H, Strecker G 1982 Infantile form of sialic acid storage disorder: clinical ultrastructural and biochemical studies in two siblings. European Journal of Pediatrics 139: 142–147

Tong P Y, Gregory W, Kornfeld S 1989 Ligand interactions of the cation-independent mannose 6-phosphate receptor. The stoichiometry of mannose 6-phosphate binding. Journal of Biological Chemistry 264: 7962–7969

Tsvetkova I V, Petushkova N A, Zolotuchina T V, Kucharenko V I, Rosenfeld E L 1987 Biochemical study of sialidosis type 1 in a Russian family. Journal of Inherited Metabolic Disease 10: 18–23

Ullrich K, Mersmann G, Weber E, von Figura K 1978 Evidence for lysosomal enzyme recognition by human fibroblasts via a phosphorylated carbohydrate moiety. Biochemical Journal 170: 643–650

Vamos E, Liebaers I, Bousard N, Libert J, Perlrutter N 1981 Multiple sulfatase deficiency with early onset. Journal of Inherited Metabolic Disease 4: 103–104

Van Elsen A F, Leroy J G 1973 I-cell disease (mucolipidosis II). Serum hydrolases in obligate heterozygotes. Humangenetik 20: 119–123

Van Elsen A F, Leroy J G 1981 a-D-Mannosidases in serum of patients with I-cell disease (ICD). Clinica Chimica Acta 112: 159–165

Van Elsen A F, Leroy J G, Vanneuville F J, Vercruyssen A L 1976 Isoenzymes of serum N-acetyl-beta-D-glucosaminidase in the I-cell disease heterozygote. Human Genetics 31: 75–81

Van Elsen A F, Leroy J G, Wauters J G, Willems P J, Buytaert C, Verheyen K 1983 In vitro expression of alpha-L-fucosidase activity polymorphism observed in plasma. Human Genetics 64: 235–239

Van Hoof F, Hers H G 1968 Mucopolysaccharidosis by absence of a-fucosidase. Lancet 1: 1198

Varki A, Kornfeld S 1980 Identification of a rat liver a-N-acetylglucosaminyl phosphodiesterase capable of removing "Blocking" a-N-acetylglucosamine residues from phosphorylated high mannose oligosaccharides of lysosomal enzymes. Journal of Biological Chemistry 255: 8398–8401

Varki A, Reitman M L, Kornfeld S 1981 Identification of a variant of mucolipidosis III (pseudo-Hurler polydystrophy); a catalytically active N-acetylglucosaminylphosphotransferase that fails to phosphorylate lysosomal enzymes. Proceedings of the National Academy of Sciences USA 78: 7773–7777

Verheyen F W, Palmeri S, Hoogeveen A T, Galjaard H 1985 Human placental neuraminidase: activation, stabilization and association with β-galactosidase and its "protective" protein. European Journal of Biochemistry 149: 315–321

von Figura K, Hasilik A 1986 Lysosomal enzymes and their receptors. Annual Review of Biochemistry 55: 167–193

von Figura K, Klein U 1979 Isolation and characterization of phosphorylated oligosaccharides from a-N-acetylglucosaminidase that are recognized by cell-surface receptors. European Journal of Biochemistry 94: 347–354

von Figura K, Voss B 1979 Cell-surface-associated lysosomal enzymes in cultured human skin fibroblasts. Experimental Cell Research 121: 267–276

Waheed A, Pohlman R, Hasilik A, von Figura K 1981 Subcellular location of two enzymes involved in the synthesis of phosphorylated recognition markers in lysosomal enzymes. Journal of Biological Chemistry 256: 4150–4152

Waheed A, Pohlman R, Hasilik A, von Figura K, van Elsen A, Leroy J 1982 Deficiency of UDP-N-acetylglucosamine: lysosomal enzyme N-acetylglucosamine-1-phosphotransferase in organs of I-cell patients. Biochemical and Biophysical Research Communications 105: 1052–1058

Wenger D A, Tarby T J, Wharton C 1978 Macular cherry-red spot and myoclonus with dementia: coexistent neuraminidase and β-galatosidase deficiencies. Biochemical and Biophysical Research Communications 82: 589–595

Wenger D A, Sujansky E, Fennessey P V, Thompson J N 1986 Human β-mannosidase deficiency. New England Journal of Medicine 315: 1201–1205

Wiesmann U N, Lightbody J, Vassella F, Herschkowitz N N 1971a Multiple lysosomal enzyme deficiency due to enzyme leakage? New England Journal of Medicine 284: 109–110

Wiesmann U N, Vassella D, Herschkowitz N N 1971b I-cell disease: leakage of lysosomal enzymes into extracellular fluids. New England Journal of Medicine 285: 1090–1091

Wilcken B, Don N, Greenaway R, Hammond J, Sosula L 1987 Sialuria: a second case. Journal of Inherited Metabolic Disease 10: 97–102

Winchester P, Grossman H, Wan Ngo Lim, Shannon Danes B 1969 A new mucopolysaccharidosis with skeletal deformities simulating rheumatoid arthritis. American Journal of Roentgenology 106: 121–128

Winter R M, Swallow D M, Baraitser M, Purkiss P 1980 Sialidosis type 2 (acid neuraminidase deficiency): clinical and biochemical features of a further case. Clinical Genetics 18: 203–210

Wolburg-Buchholz K, Schlote W, Baumkotter J, Cantz M, Holder H, Harzer K 1985 Familial lysosomal storage disease with generalized vacuolization and sialic aciduria. Sporadic Salla disease. Neuropediatrics 16: 67–75

Yamashita K, Tachibana Y, Mihara K, Okada S, Yabuuchi H, Kobata A 1980 Urinary oligosaccharides of mannosidosis. Journal of Biological Chemistry 255: 5126–5133

Zeigler M, Bach G 1986 Internalization of exogenous gangliosides in cultured skin fibroblasts for the diagnosis of mucolipidosis IV. Clinica Chimica Acta 157: 183–190

Zielke K, Veath M L, O'Brien J S 1972 Fucosidosis: deficiency of a-L-fucosidase in cultured skin fibroblasts. Journal of Experimental Medicine 136: 197–199

103. Gangliosidoses and related lipid storage diseases

Alan K. Percy

INTRODUCTION

Recent clinical and biochemical advances have dramatically expanded our understanding of the gangliosidoses and related disorders. As a group, these disorders share the following common features: (1) they are genetic; (2) they are characterized, with notable exceptions, by degenerative processes affecting the central and/or peripheral nervous system; (3) they involve the tissue storage in abnormal concentration of a normal lipid or glycolipid and in some cases a glycoprotein or mucopolysaccharide as well; and (4) the molecular defect in many of them is the deficiency of a lysosomal acid hydrolase. The gangliosides and related sphingolipids have been implicated in a group of lipid storage diseases call the sphingolipidoses. The sphingolipidoses will be described in the context of the accumulated sphingolipid and the relevant biochemical defect (Svennerholm 1969, Pilz et al 1979, Sandhoff & Christomanou 1979, Herschkowitz & Schulte 1984, Lake 1984, Moser 1985). A separate group of CNS storage diseases, the neuronal ceroid lipofuscinoses, is less well understood in terms of a specific biochemical abnormality (Percy 1987). Four clinically distinct entities will be discussed. Finally, four other disorders of lipid metabolism involving tissue storage will be outlined (Percy et al 1979, Fishman & Percy 1984).

HISTORICAL ASPECTS

The gangliosidoses and related sphingolipidoses represent the summation of clinical and laboratory observations extending back 100 years. Clinical and pathological descriptions for each of these disorders have been available for many years. Our understanding of their molecular basis, however, has only developed in the last quarter of a century. One of these disorders, Tay-Sachs disease, provides a perspective. With his description, in 1881, of a child with generalized weakness and cherry-red macular degeneration, Waren Tay (1881) signalled a century of activity involving many biomedical disciplines and culminating in our present understanding of the sphingolipidoses.

Following the identification and characterization of the stored lipid utilizing improved techniques in lipid chemistry (Svennerholm & Zettergren 1957, Svennerholm 1962), the biochemical lesion could then be defined (Okada & O'Brien 1969). This biochemical definition, however, did not represent the end of the story. Rather, the need for interdisciplinary collaboration has expanded with the application of molecular genetic techniques, with the awareness of heterogeneity within many of these disorders, and with the clinical implications relative to accurate clinical diagnosis, genetic counselling and prenatal detection.

CLINICAL CONSIDERATIONS

Pathogenetic correlations

The disorders of lipid storage share a common biochemical pathogenesis. The storage or accumulation of a specific compound might represent excess synthesis and/or deficient degradation of the accumulated material. In each of these disorders with a defined biochemical lesion, lipid storage is the result of deficient activity of a specific degradative enzyme. In particular, the sphingolipidoses represent the deficiency of a specific lysosomal (degradative) enzyme with the resultant intracellular (lysosomal and cytoplasmic) and interstitial accumulation of sphingolipid or other lipid material.

Lipids are important constituents of all biological membranes participating critically in cell structure and function. Individual lipid constituents exhibit considerable variability from tissue to tissue, particularly among the specialized membranes of the nervous system. As might be anticipated, the lipid storage diseases, especially the sphingolipidoses, reflect the tissue distribution of the disease-related lipid.

In general, the sphingolipidoses involving the central nervous system may be divided into two groups, one group predominantly affecting the white matter or myelin-containing portion of the nervous system, and thus called *leucodystrophies*, the second impinging on neuronal or grey matter processes. Storage of sphingolipids which predominate in the white matter, namely galactosylceramide (and galactosylsphingosine) and sulphatide, is representative of diseases in the former group. Since the leucodystrophies generally have their onset during infancy and early childhood, the principal initial manifestations of these white matter disorders are delayed or decline in motor development and abnormalities of gait along with upper motor neuron or long tract findings. Disorders of the second group are represented by the gangliosidoses and are accompanied by early symptoms including seizures, intellectual difficulties, and visual abnormalities. This clinical formulation of entities involving grey or white matter pertains only during first stages of the disease. As the process advances, dysfunction of the nervous system disseminates and specificity of white or grey matter involvement is lost. The concept, however, may focus the diagnostic process during the initial clinical assessment (Freeman & McKhann 1969).

Biochemical basis

The stored materials in most of the disorders considered in this chapter belong to a class of compounds known as sphingolipids. A preliminary understanding of the structure of these compounds is necessary for an appreciation of the clinical-biochemical correlations.

Definition and tissue localization

The sphingolipids are a group of compounds sharing a common basic component called ceramide (Fig. 103.1). Ceramide is a long chain amino alcohol to which is attached a fatty acid covalently linked to the amino group. The individual sphingolipids are formed by the addition of specific groups to the terminal alcohol position of ceramide. The unique physicochemical characteristics of each sphingolipid derive from this particular side chain and from the fatty acid. With the single exception of sphingomyelin, one or more of the hexose units, glucose, galactose or N-acetylgalactosamine, is added to the alcohol group. Several of the sphingolipids are uncharged at physiological pH, but three types, the sulphatides, the sphingomyelins, and the gangliosides have a charged group(s) under physiological conditions. The fatty acid chain length may vary from 14 to 26 carbon units, particularly in neural tissue where longer chain fatty acids are found predominantly. In addition, the fatty acids may demonstrate variable unsaturation with one or more double bonds.

The gangliosides, a sub-group of the sphingolipids, are characterized by N-acetyl-neuraminic acid (NANA, sialic acid) linked covalently to the hexose units. Gangliosides vary in two respects: (1) length of sugar side chain may vary from two to four hexose groups; and (2) the number of NANA groups per molecule may vary from one to four. At least 15 chemically-distinct gangliosides have been identified in neural tissue, although four major gangliosides constitute more than 80% of the total (Molin et al 1987).

The sphingolipids are ubiquitous in human tissues (Mårtensson 1969), principally as components of cellular membranes. The concentration of the individual sphingolipids varies greatly from tissue to tissue. For example, the neutral sphingolipid glucosylceramide is a common constituent of liver and spleen, yet is not present in significant quantity in neural tissue (Svennerholm & Svennerholm 1963). Hence, the principal clinical manifestations of glucosylceramidosis (Gaucher disease) involve the liver and spleen. Conversely, galactosylceramide and sulphatide are prominent constituents of the nervous system, particularly of myelin, and, to a lesser extent, of kidney. Disorders involving these lipids affect the nervous system predominantly. Globoside is the major glycosphingolipid in kidney and erythrocytes. Sphingomyelin is prominent in all human membranes.

Gangliosides with four hexose units attached to the ceramide and one or more NANA derivatives are major components of neurons and neuronal membranes and may be integrally involved in synaptic transmission. The smallest ganglioside, GM3, predominates in non-neural tissues, where it may comprise more than 70% of the total ganglioside fraction (Svennerholm 1970).

Metabolic interrelations

As one might suspect from the common chemical backbone, the sphingolipids are closely related in terms of their metabolism. Biosynthesis reflects enzyme-mediated addition of the various relevant substituents to ceramide in sequential fashion, utilizing appropriate uridyl or cytidyl nucleotides. Sphingolipid degradation is also stepwise, involving specific hydrolases acting at the free terminal, non-reducing end of the sugar chain. Should any one hydrolase be missing, or be present in rate-limiting amounts, degradation cannot proceed. Total degradation of a glycosphingolipid thus requires the action, sequentially and in concert, of a series of enzymes each having a very high degree of specificity for the terminal sugar and for the anomeric configuration of the glycosidic bond (Fig. 103.1).

Beginning in 1964, a deficiency in the activity of each of these degradative enzymes has been associated with a

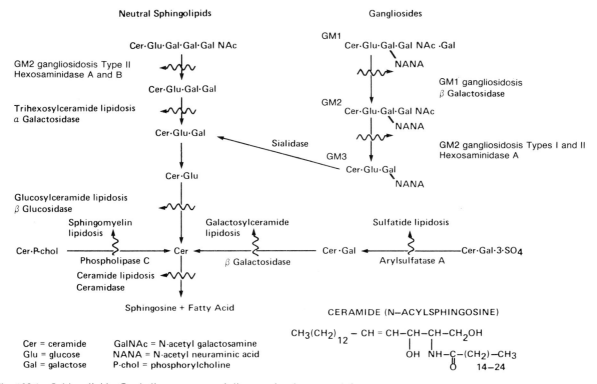

Fig. 103.1 Sphingolipids. Catabolic sequence and disease-related enzyme defects.

human genetic disorder. A specific catabolic enzyme deficiency interrupts the metabolic sequence and the sphingolipid preceding the defective enzyme accumulates. In general, this accumulation occurs in the tissue(s) where the relevant sphingolipid or one of its precursors is a prominent constituent. That is, storage of neural sphingolipids invariably results in neural dysfunction, whereas deposition of predominantly extraneural sphingolipids manifests visceral involvement and may even spare the central nervous system. Regardless, the sphingolipid accumulation within the cell occurs, at least in part, within the *lysosomes*, the subcellular site of the degradative (hydrolytic) enzymes.

Lysosomes are important intracellular organelles containing enzymes which perform vital housekeeping chores within the cell by degrading or hydrolyzing complex compounds to small molecules which can then be recycled or eliminated. Lysosomes, identified by de Duve and co-workers (1955), are membrane-bound and contain a repertoire of hydrolytic enzymes optimally-active at acid pH. These enzymes are primarily involved in the degradation of intralysosomal macromolecules which represent either the turnover of normal cellular constituents or are molecules imbibed by pinocytosis.

Having postulated that some human diseases might be due to the deficient activity of a lysosomal hydrolase resulting in intralysosomal accumulation of various molecules, Hers (1963) demonstrated the deficiency of an acid glucosidase in type II glycogen storage disease. Similar deficiencies were soon described for the sphingolipid storage diseases. Austin et al (1965) reported deficiency of arylsulphatase A in metachromatic leucodystrophy, and Brady and co-workers (1965) found a reduced level of glucocerebrosidase activity in Gaucher disease. Since that time, hydrolase deficiencies in most of the other 'lipid storage' diseases have been established.

THE SPHINGOLIPIDOSES

The storage of each major sphingolipid (Fig. 103.1) has now been associated with a clinical disorder. Dysfunction of the central nervous system is a prominent feature in each disorder with the exception of Fabry disease, and variant forms of Gaucher and Niemann-Pick disease.

Presently, there are eight distinct diseases representing accumulation of a specific sphingolipid. An additional disorder has been associated with the ganglioside

GM3, but remains to be established as a clinical entity. One or more variant forms differing in age at onset, in clinical presentation as reflected in the tissues involved, and in clinical course have been identified for several of these disorders. Differences in enzyme-substrate specificity, enzyme stability, tissue distribution, or residual activity may account for the observed variability in these disorders (von Figura et al 1987).

Present nomenclature is based on the disease-related lipid and the known metabolic inter-relationship of the sphingolipids. While the familiar eponyms are included, the biochemical classification better describes this family of disorders.

Gangliosidoses

GMI-gangliosidoses

GM1 gangliosidoses are characterized by the accumulation of the ganglioside GM1 (Fig. 103.1). Presently, three forms of GM1-gangliosidosis have been recognized (Landing et al 1964, O'Brien et al 1972, Wenger et al 1980a) (Table 103.1).

Type 1 GM1-gangliosidosis (generalized gangliosidosis) is a devastating disease which appears in infancy, with death usually resulting before the second birthday. The disease is marked by severe bony abnormalities resembling the appearance of the child with Hurler syndrome, hepatosplenomegaly and profound motor and mental retardation. Initial complaints consist of feeding difficulties or failure to thrive. The infants are hypoactive or hypotonic, appear to have both facial and peripheral oedema, frontal bossing, and a depressed nasal bridge with hypertelorism. The gums are commonly hypertrophied and the tongue enlarged. Pigmentary changes of the macula resembling the cherry-red spot of Tay-Sachs disease occur in about half the cases described. There is an exaggerated startle response to noise. Mental and motor development is severely retarded from birth, the infants showing little interest in their environment. Initially, bony changes are mainly observed in the long bones of the extremities as periosteal new bone formation, but with progression of the disease, involvement of the vertebral bodies becomes prominent. There is also widening of the long bones reflecting enlargement of the marrow space secondary to cellular lipid storage. In addition, as the disease progresses, flexion contractures of the joints appear, especially involving the fingers, knees, and elbows. Characteristically, the hands appear very broad with short stubby fingers. Macrocephaly may develop later on, although not nearly as severe or impressive as is seen in Tay-Sachs disease. The pathology of Type I GM1-gangliosidosis includes vacuolation of the peripheral lymphocytes, the accumulation of histiocytes in the visceral organs, mainly the liver and spleen, and the accumulation of intracytoplasmic material in cells of bone marrow. The most devastating lipid accumulation occurs in neurons throughout the nervous system and may, indeed, be seen in the ganglion cells of the rectum. Viewed by electron microscopy this stored material is noted within the lysosomes resembling the membranous cytoplasmic bodies first described in Tay-Sachs disease.

Type II GM1-gangliosidosis differs from Type I in

Table 103.1   GM1-Gangliosidosis

	Type I Generalized Gangliosidosis	Type II Juvenile	Type III Adult
Age at onset	Infancy	6–12 months	Adolescence to adulthood
Prognosis	Death by age 2	Death by age 3–10	Prolonged survival
Mode of inheritance	AR	AR	AR
Neurological signs	Psychomotor deterioration Cherry-red maculae Seizures	Psychomotor deterioration Ataxia Seizures	Dystonia Bradykinesia Gait difficulty Variable dementia
Systemic signs	Hurler-like features Hepatosplenomegaly	No dysmorphism Mild or no hepatomegaly	No dysmorphism
Stored material	GM1-ganglioside Asialo-GM1-ganglioside Keratan sulphate	GM1-ganglioside Asialo-GM1-ganglioside Keratan sulphate	GM1-ganglioside Asialo-GM1-ganglioside Keratan sulphate
Enzyme defect	Ganglioside β-galactosidase	Ganglioside β-galactosidase	Ganglioside β-galactosidase
Prenatal diagnosis feasible	Yes	Yes	Yes

AR = Autosomal recessive

that the symptoms and signs do not appear until late infancy, and death may not result until the end of the first decade. Bony involvement is mild and in the usual case, mental and motor development may appear normal through the first year of life. Initially, gait disturbance, or ataxia, occurs followed by the loss of attempts at speech. No organomegaly or evidence of macular degeneration is noted. Progressive weakness and hypotonia follow, with the eventual development of seizures. By the end of the second year interest in the environment is usually lost and deterioration to a vegetative state after this point is fairly rapid. Pathological findings in Type II GM1-gangliosidosis are very similar to those described for Type I, although usually less extensive. Despite the absence of organomegaly, there is evidence of histiocyte accumulation in the liver.

Type III GM1-gangliosidosis is a relatively recently described variant whose onset is usually in adolescence or early adulthood. Several of the reported cases involved Japanese individuals (Ushiyama et al 1985, Mutoh et al 1986a). Initial involvement of pyramidal and extrapyramidal systems includes gait disturbances and dystonia. Speech is slurred and intellectual involvement is variable and mild. Visceromegaly and cherry-red maculae are absent, and mild vertebral abnormalities have been noted. Progression is slow. The principal neural pathology is confined to intraneuronal storage in the basal ganglia (Goldman et al 1981).

Biochemical Defect The chemical abnormalities described for GM1-gangliosidosis are similar for each type; namely, GM1-ganglioside and its asialo-form (from the action of the lysosomal enzyme, α-sialidase) is stored in the central nervous system (Fig. 103.1). In addition, mucopolysaccharide (a keratan sulphate-like compound) can be found in the visceral organs in both Type I and Type II patients (Suzuki 1968). The GM1-ganglioside has been isolated from the visceral organs of Type I patients, but similar isolations have not been made for Type II. The biochemical defect is the failure to cleave the terminal galactose from the GM1-ganglioside molecule (Fig. 103.1) and the keratan sulphate-like compound. In each disorder there is a profound deficiency in the activity of the enzyme β-galactosidase, which is responsible for removing this terminal galactose (Okada & O'Brien 1968, O'Brien et al 1972). Observations from liver and cultured fibroblasts suggest that the deficiency is less profound in Type II disease, although the level of deficiency is similar in brain for the two types. The β-galactosidase activity represents a family of enzymes (isoenzymes) and separation of these isoenzymes reveals at least three distinct zones of activity. There is general agreement that two of these isoenzymes are absent in

GM1-gangliosidosis whereas the third, isoenzyme A, may or may not be present. While isoenzyme A is detectable in Type I disease, in Type II disease it is, in fact, increased. The existing isoenzyme A activity may be sufficient to confine the major pathophysiological changes to the nervous system in Type II disease. At the present time, this remains the only explanation for these two different types of GM1-gangliosidosis (Singer & Schafer 1972, O'Brien 1975).

Hybridization studies with Type I and Type III cells failed to produce complementation, suggesting that the mutations are allelic. In addition, Morquio B syndrome appears to belong to the same complementation group (Mutoh et al 1986b). In Type I and Type III fibroblasts, defective β-galactosidase protein is formed, preventing compartmentation in lysosomes (Hoogeveen et al 1986).

GM2-gangliosidoses

Type I GM2-gangliosidosis (Tay-Sachs disease) is, perhaps, the most familiar sphingolipidosis affecting the nervous system (Table 103.2). This disorder occurs commonly in Jewish families, particularly those from eastern Europe (Ashkenazi) and in French Canadians from eastern Quebec. The carrier frequency for this autosomal recessive gene is approximately 3% of Jewish individuals descended from European regions, and is similarly increased in the French Canadian group. About 1/3600 infants of Ashkenazi (Eastern European) Jewish ancestry has Tay-Sachs disease and about 1/30 individuals in this group is a carrier of the mutant gene. Tay-Sachs disease is not restricted to the Jewish or French Canadian populations, however, having been reported in virtually every ethnic and racial group. It is a particularly devastating disease which presents in the period of infancy, often around the fifth or sixth month of life, and is usually fatal within five years. These infants may appear normal initially, but within six months are characterized by apathy, hypotonia, and delayed psychomotor development. As in GM1-gangliosidosis these infants exhibit an exaggerated startle response to noise. This feature is commonly the indication for seeking medical attention. Physical examination includes cherry-red spots in the macular areas of the retinae (Fig. 103.2). This represents lipid storage in the ganglion cells of the retina obscuring the choroidal vessels lying behind (Fig. 103.3). In the foveal region of the retina where the ganglion cells are sparse the vascularity of the underlying choroid then projects as the cherry-red spot. The cherry-red appearance disappears over time, so that its absence in an advanced stage of neurological impairment should not exclude the diagnosis (Kivlin et al 1985). This disease progresses fairly rapidly, with early psychomotor retarda-

Table 103.2   GM2-Gangliosidosis

	Type I Late Infantile Tay-Sachs	Type II Sandhoff	Type III Juvenile Type I
Age at onset	4–12 months	4–12 months	2–5 years
Prognosis	Death by age 5	Death by age 5	Death by age 15
Mode of inheritance	AR	AR	AR
Neurological signs	Psychomotor deterioration Cherry-red maculae Exaggerated startle Seizures Irritability	Psychomotor deterioration Cherry-red maculae Exaggerated startle Seizures Irritability	Psychomotor deterioration Seizures Gait difficulty Ataxia
Systemic signs	—	Hepatosplenomegaly	—
Stored material	GM2-ganglioside Asialo GM2-ganglioside Lyso GM2-ganglioside	GM2-ganglioside Asialo GM2-ganglioside Globoside Lyso GM2-ganglioside	GM2-ganglioside Asialo GM2-ganglioside GM2-ganglioside
Enzyme defect	Hexosaminidase A	Hexosaminidase A and B	Hexosaminidase A
Prenatal diagnosis feasible	Yes	Yes	Yes

AR = Autosomal recessive

tion, blindness usually by 12–18 months, and the appearance of seizures. There is no hepatosplenomegaly. Macrocephaly, a common feature of this disease, particularly in children who survive past the first year of life, is a reflection of glial proliferation, and is not a representation of lipid storage per se. Pathological features of this disorder are principally those of swollen, stuffed neurons (Fig. 103.4) and secondary gliosis. Despite a lack of clinical evidence of extraneural involvement, there are lipid-laden cells identifiable in liver, spleen and lung. Electron microscopy reveals membranous cytoplasmic bodies composed of concentric layers of dense membranes located throughout the cytoplasm of the involved neurons representing lipid-laden lysosomes.

A juvenile form of GM2-gangliosidosis, sometimes called the juvenile form of Tay-Sachs disease, is more aptly denoted as GM2-gangliosidosis Type III (Brett et al 1973). This form appears between the ages of 2 and 5 as a progressive deterioration of psychomotor behaviour and an insidious disturbance of gait. Death usually occurs within 15 years. No predilection for Jewish individuals is evident. Physical examination is similar to that in Type I GM2-gangliosidosis, with the notable absence of macrocephaly and cherry-red maculae. Optic atrophy or retinitis pigmentosa may be seen instead. Pathological examination reveals similar, although generally less extensive, neuronal storage of lipid than in Type I.

Biochemical Defect   Types I and III GM2-gangliosidosis are characterized by storage of the GM2-ganglioside (Fig. 103.1). Normally a very minor ganglioside component, in this disease the GM2-ganglioside is increased enormously, representing approximately 90% of the

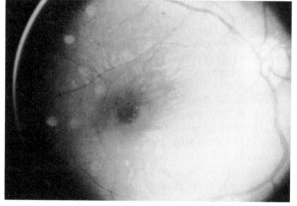

Fig. 103.2   Cherry-red macula.

ganglioside fraction in neural tissue. GM2-ganglioside is also increased in liver and spleen when compared to normal tissue. In addition, the *asialo* form of the GM2-ganglioside, i.e. GM2-ganglioside minus the NANA group (Fig. 103.1), is also present in excess, and may represent up to 5% of the total glycolipid fraction in brain. Recently, lyso-GM2 (GM2-ganglioside minus the fatty acid) has been isolated from brains of Type I and II individuals, a finding analogous to those in Krabbe and Gaucher diseases and metachromatic leucodystrophy (Rosengren et al 1987). Lyso-compounds are regarded as cytotoxic and probably important in the pathogenesis of the central nervous system dysfunction.

The enzymatic defect in GM2-gangliosidosis is characterized by failure to hydrolyze the terminal amino sugar

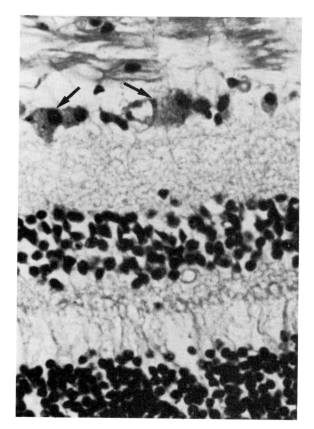

Fig. 103.3 Lipid-laden retinal ganglion cells. Haematoxylin and eosin.

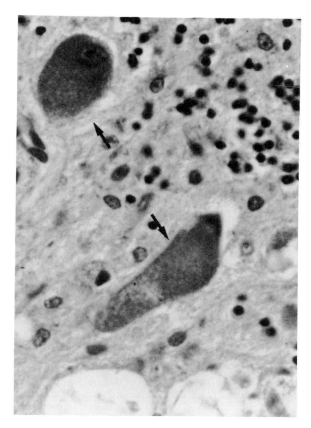

Fig. 103.4 Lipid-laden neurons from brain of patient with GM2-gangliosidosis. Luxol fast blue-haematoxylin and eosin.

from the GM2-ganglioside (Fig. 103.1). This enzyme is known as hexosaminidase and occurs as two major forms, or isoenzymes, designated A and B. Total hexosaminidase activity, representing the hydrolytic action of both hexosaminidase A and B, may be elevated in tissues from children with Type I and III GM2-gangliosidosis. Hexosaminidase A is virtually absent, however, with a compensatory increase in hexosaminidase B accounting for the normal or elevated levels of total hexosaminidase activity (Okada & O'Brien 1969). In the juvenile form of type III there is partial deficiency of the hexosaminidase A isoenzyme, perhaps accounting for the delayed onset and longer course of this form.

Hexosaminidase A is a thermolabile protein composed of alpha and beta subunits ($\alpha\beta_A\beta_B$); hexosaminidase B is heat stable and contains only β subunits $2(\beta_A\beta_B)$ (Mahuran et al 1985). The α subunit appears to map to chromosome 15, while the β subunit is associated with chromosome 5 (Gilbert et al 1975).

Significant advances in the molecular genetics of GM2-gangliosidosis have emerged recently (Neufeld 1989). Classical (Type I) GM2-gangliosidosis is marked by the absence of cross-reacting material for the α-subunit of hexosaminidase A, indicating a failure of protein synthesis (Proia & Neufeld 1982). Using a cDNA clone coding for the α subunit, Myerowitz and Proia (1984) noted failure of fibroblasts from Ashkenazi Tay-Sachs individuals to synthesize the mRNA for the α subunit, whereas cells from a variant form of GM2-gangliosidosis produced mRNA. These data were extended to discriminate the French-Canadian and Ashkenazi forms indicating that the α subunit gene of the French-Canadian form contained a 5–8 kilobase deletion, whereas the Ashkenazi α subunit gene was intact (Myerowitz & Hogikyan 1987). Additional mutations have been identified recently within the Ashkenazi population (Arpaia et al 1988, Paw et al 1989).

Type II GM2-gangliosidosis

Type II GM2-gangliosidosis (Sandhoff disease) is considered separately from Types I and III because the clinical and biochemical findings differ (Sandhoff et al 1968). Age at onset and progression of disease resemble Type I (Table 103.2). This disease is not seen predominantly in Jewish individuals, but is accompanied by psychomotor retardation, blindness with cherry-red maculae, and exaggerated startle response to noise. Enlargement of the liver and spleen is prominent and represents the principal clinical difference from Type I.

Biochemical Defect   Type II manifests the striking accumulation, particularly in neural tissue, of GM2-ganglioside as well as the lyso- and the asialo-form of GM2 (Fig. 103.1.) This asialo-form may represent as much as one-third of the total glycolipid fraction of the brain. In addition to GM2 storage, globoside, the common neutral glycolipid of red blood cells and kidney (Fig. 103.1), accumulates in the abdominal organs, the liver, kidney and spleen. Globoside has the same terminal amino sugar as GM2-ganglioside. The biochemical abnormality of Type II GM2-gangliosidosis is total deficiency of hexosaminidase activity. Both isoenzyme A and B activities are absent in tissues of individuals with the disorder, whereas hexosaminidase S, a minor isoenzyme, is increased (Sandhoff et al 1971).

GM2-variants

Additional types of GM2-gangliosidosis have been described (Table 103.3). One, termed the AB variant, is characterized by the onset of dementia, gait difficulties, and seizures in a 6-year-old child without macular or visual abnormalities. Neuronal membranous cytoplasmic bodies typical of Tay-Sachs disease were seen at postmortem examination. The enzymatic lesion is particularly interesting. Total hexosaminidase activity using artificial substrate was normal or increased, and activity of the A isoenzyme with the same substrate was about 50% of control values, but hexosaminidase activity was absent with the natural substrate, GM2-ganglioside. The enzymatic defect involves the absence of an *activating* substance essential for the binding of GM2 to the hexosaminidase molecule (Conzelmann & Sandhoff 1978). O'Neill et al (1978) described an adult AB variant presenting with seizures, dementia, and normal pressure hydrocephalus. Hexosaminidase A and B were normal using artificial substrate.

Another reported variant featuring cherry-red maculae and cerebellar ataxia, without seizures or dementia,

Table 103.3   GM2-Gangliosidosis

Heterogeneity of hexosaminidase deficiency diseases

Type		Clinical features	Biochemical abnormality	Subunit notation*
I.	Late Infantile (Tay-Sachs)	Blindness, seizures, psychomotor deterioration	Hex A deficiency, B increased	$\alpha_O \beta_A \beta_B$ $2(\beta_A \beta_B)$
II.	Sandhoff	Similar to Type I, visceromegaly	Hex A and B deficiency	$\alpha \beta_O$ $2(\beta_O)$
III.	Juvenile Type I	Ataxia, spasticity, seizures, psychomotor deterioration, anterior horn cell disease	Hex A and B deficiency	$\alpha_D \beta_A \beta_B$ $2(\beta_A \beta_B)$
IV.	Juvenile Sandhoff Type II	Cerebellar ataxia, cherry red maculae, intact mentation	Hex A and B deficiency	$\alpha \beta_D$ $2(\beta_D)$
V.	AB Variant	Similar to Type I	Deficiency of Hex A activator protein	$\alpha \beta_A \beta_B$ $2(\beta_A \beta_B)$
VI.	Motor neuron variant	ALS-like syndrome	Hex A deficiency	$\alpha_D \beta_A \beta_B$ $2(\beta_A \beta_B)$
VII.	Chronic	Spinocerebellar degeneration distal muscle wasting, dystonia, intact mentation	Hex A deficiency	$\alpha_D \beta_A \beta_B$ $2(\beta_A \beta_B)$
VIII.	Spinal muscle variant	Spinal muscular atrophy, fasciculations, intact mentation and bulbar muscles	Hex A deficiency	$\alpha_D \beta_A \beta_B$ $2(\beta_A \beta_B)$
IX.	Late infantile (Tay-Sachs) variant	Blindness, seizures, psychomotor deterioration	Hex A deficiency versus natural substrate or sulphated artificial substrate	$\alpha_D \beta_A \beta_B$ $2(\beta_A \beta_B)$

* Hexosaminidase subunit representation

Isoenzyme	*Subunit Structure*	
Hexosaminidase A	$\alpha \beta_A \beta_B$	α_O = absent α-subunit; β_O = absent β-subunit
Hexosaminidase B	$2(\beta_A \beta_B)$	$\alpha_\triangle$ = defective α-subunit; $\beta_\triangle$ = defective β-subunit
Hexosaminidase S	2α	

appears to be an adult form of Type II (Oonk et al 1979). Hexosaminidase B activity is absent and hexosaminidase A is severely deficient. A third variant (chronic form) with slow progression of cerebellar ataxia and distal muscle wasting and without seizures, dementia or macular changes, revealed normal total hexosaminidase activity and profoundly reduced hexosaminidase A activity in serum (Johnson et al 1977). In leucocytes, hexosaminidase activity was about 50% of control values.

A variant, clinically identical with Type I GM2-gangliosidosis, has been distinguished from Type I by the presence of α subunit cross-reacting material and by the recognition of altered substrate-enzyme binding (Bayleran et al 1987). Hybridization failed to demonstrate complementation with Type I cells, indicating an α subunit mutation (Sonderfeld et al 1985) and a cDNA clone derived from mRNA revealed a single base substitution to account for the altered enzyme activity (Ohno & Suzuki 1988). A clinically-similar variant represented an abnormal, short α-chain which was not processed further and failed to associate with β-chain to form mature hexosaminidase A (Zokaeem et al 1987). Also, in some variants of hexosaminidase α-chain deficiency, altered or abnormal α- and β-subunit association was noted (d'Azzo et al 1984).

Yet another variant (adult) was identified in the course of a Tay-Sachs screening programme. A young adult, in good health, was noted to have a profound deficiency in serum and fibroblast hexosaminidase A activity. Subsequently he has developed typical features of amyotrophic lateral sclerosis, including muscle weakness, wasting and fasciculations. Rectal biopsy revealed neuronal inclusions similar to those noted in classical Tay-Sachs disease (Yaffe et al 1979). Additional examples have been described more recently (Mitsumoto et al 1985).

At least nine forms of GM2-gangliosidosis (Table 103.3) have been described. Types I, III, VI, VII, VIII and IX may be caused by mutations at the α subunit locus, and Types II and IV by mutations at the β subunit locus. Type V appears to represent a mutation at a separate locus distinct from the α and β loci. This formulation results from the assignment of genes for hexosaminidase (Hex) A and B to separate chromosomes (Gilbert et al 1975) and subunit structure representation (Mahuran et al 1985) in which the Hex A is denoted by $\alpha\beta_A\beta_B$, Hex B by $2(\beta_A\beta_B)$.

GM3-gangliosidosis

GM3-gangliosidosis is a disorder described in two males within a single family (Max et al 1974). Respiratory difficulty and seizures began within the first days of life.

Lethargy, poor feeding, macroglossia and gingival hyperplasia were noted. The infant was hypotonic, developed little and had frequent generalized seizures. Death occurred at 3 months of age. The brain from one child contained large amounts of GM3-ganglioside and virtually no GM2 or GM1 ganglioside. A novel biosynthetic defect in ganglioside production was noted. Activity of UDP-GalNAc: GM3 N-acetylgalactosaminyltransferase which converts GM3 to GM2 ganglioside was severely diminished in his brain and liver. The genetics of this disorder is unclear, but X–linked recessive transmission is possible.

Other sphingolipidoses

Sphingomyelin lipidoses (Niemann-Pick disease)

This group of disorders is characterized by an abnormal accumulation of sphingomyelin (Fig. 103.1). Four clinical forms have been described (Table 103.4) but deficient enzyme activity has been noted in only two (Brady et al 1966).

The infantile or acute form (Type I), representing about 80% of sphingomyelin lipidosis cases, appears in early infancy, with failure to thrive and hepatomegaly. Psychomotor deterioration is prominent, leaving the child devastated by 12 months of age. Death results by age 4. As with Tay-Sachs disease, this form is especially common in eastern European Jews (Ashkenazi). A characteristic, although not diagnostic finding, is the appearance of foam cells in the bone marrow. Approximately half the patients have cherry-red maculae. Pathological findings are generalized, with foam cells appearing throughout the reticuloendothelial system. Neuropathological findings include marked neuronal storage, numerous foam cells representing lipid storage in glial cells, and glial proliferation. Electron microscopy of the foam cells reveals multi-laminated concentric cytoplasmic inclusions.

Type II has been called the chronic form because of the absence of neurological involvement and because of an apparently prolonged survival. Enlargement of liver and spleen is evident in early childhood. The earliest diagnosed patients are now in their 30s and 40s without neurological impairment.

Types III and IV are clinically similar, and there is no compelling pathological or biochemical reason to separate them. Type IV signifies a cluster of cases in Nova Scotia, all traced to a single mutation in ancestors of French Acadians (Winsor & Welch 1978). Both types appear in early childhood (age 1–6) with death by adolescence. Hepatosplenomegaly is the prominent finding initially, but evidence of neurological involvement soon appears,

Table 103.4 Sphingomyelin Lipidosis

Niemann-Pick disease

	Type I Infantile (85%)	Type II Adult	Type III Late Infantile	Type IV Nova Scotia
Age at onset	Infancy	Childhood	1–6 years	1–6 years
Prognosis	Death by age 4	Prolonged survival	Death in teens	Death in teens
Mode of inheritance	AR	AR	AR	AR
Neurological signs	Severe psychomotor deterioration	Usually spared	Psychomotor deterioration Ataxia Vertical gaze deficit	Psychomotor deterioration Ataxia Vertical gaze deficit
Systemic signs	Failure to thrive Hepatosplenomegaly Recurrent respiratory infections	Hepatosplenomegaly Cirrhosis Hypersplenism Respiratory infections	Hepatosplenomegaly initial feature	Hepatosplenomegaly initial feature
Stored material	Sphingomyelin	Sphingomyelin	Cholesterol Neutral lipids	Cholesterol Neutral lipids
Enzyme defect	Sphingomyelinase (phospholipase C)	Sphingomyelinase	Cholesterol compart- mentation and esterification	Cholesterol compart- mentation and esterification
Prenatal diagnosis feasible	Yes	Yes	No	No

AR = Autosomal recessive

manifested as gait disturbance, vertical gaze problems, and gradual intellectual deterioration. Recent studies indicate a broader spectrum of clinical findings (Fink et al 1989).

Biochemical defect Types I and II sphingomyelin lipidosis are marked by the abnormal accumulation of sphingomyelin in most tissues. In Type I, the accumulation is so extensive that sphingomyelin may represent 2–5% of the body weight (Kamoshita et al 1969). Because of its clinical course, Type II has not yet been examined thoroughly. Nonetheless, sphingomyelin content of liver and spleen is several-fold greater than in controls. Sphingomyelin accumulation in Types III and IV is less significant (Philippart et al 1969), and recent observations indicate no specific sphingolipid increase in Type III (Vanier 1983). There is a 3–4 fold increase in spleen; in the liver, sphingomyelin content may be normal. Activity of the enzyme, sphingomyelinase, is deficient in Types I and II. The different clinical courses of these two types is not explained by any quantitative difference in sphingomyelinase deficiencies, each form having similar residual activities (Gal et al 1980). Sphingomyelinase activity in Types III and IV is normal to mildly reduced. Christomanou (1980) reported deficient sphingomyelinase and glucocerebrosidase activating factor (heat-stable and non enzymic) in Type III tissues and concluded that previous in vitro analyses utilizing exogenous detergents had masked this deficiency. However, Fujibayashi and Wenger (1985) demonstrated normal activator protein using specific antibodies in cells from the variant forms. Inclusion of Types III and IV as disorders of sphingo-

myelin storage is probably unwarranted. Correction of the sphingomyelinase deficiency has been demonstrated in fibroblasts from Type III using lipoprotein-free culture conditions (Thomas et al 1989). Indeed, abnormal uptake and processing of exogenous cholesterol has been noted in Types III and IV fibroblasts (Butler et al 1987, Pentchev et al 1987). Further, differential esterification of exogenous and endogenous cholesterol supports the notion of a fundamental abnormality in compartmentation of cholesterol as the basis for these variant forms of Niemann-Pick disease (Mazière et al 1987).

Prenatal diagnosis of Type III was aided by the reduction of sphingomyelinase activity in fetal tissues to 20–50% of control levels, whereas postnatal tissues yielded control level activities (Harzer et al 1978, Wenger 1985).

Sulphatide lipidoses (Metachromatic leucodystrophy – MLD)

This disorder is represented by four clinical forms, three of which differ in age at onset, rate of progression and clinical findings, but share a quantitatively similar deficiency of the lysosomal hydrolase, arylsulphatase A (Table 103.5). The fourth is a separate entity, clinically and biochemically. The late infantile form (Type I), the most common of the four, usually presents from 12–24 months. Progressive loss of motor milestones with gait difficulty and hypotonia are first noted and, subsequently, a decline in speech and mentation. Cherry-red maculae have been described. Death usually occurs by

Table 103.5   Sulphatide Lipidosis

Metachromatic Leucodystrophy

	Late infantile	Juvenile	Adult	Mucosulphatidosis
Age at onset	6–24 months	4–8 years	15 years or older	6–18 months
Prognosis-year	Death in 5–6 years	Death in 10–15 years	Slow progression	Death by age 10–12
Mode of inheritance	AR	AR	AR	AR
Neurological signs	Gait difficulty	Gait difficulty	Dementia	Gait difficulty
	Hypotonia	Ataxia	Depression	Hypotonia
	Ataxia	Intellectual decline	Psychosis	Ataxia
	Rapid deterioration		Motor difficulty	Rapid deterioration
Systemic signs	–	–	–	Coarse features
				Hepatosplenomegaly
				Skeletal deformity
				Ichthyosis
Stored material	Sulphatide	Sulphatide	Sulphatide	Sulphatide
	Lyso-sulphatide	Lyso-sulphatide	Lyso-sulphatide	Cholesterol sulphate
				Mucopolysaccharide
Enzyme defect	Sulphatide sulphatase	Sulphatide sulphatase	Sulphatide sulphatase	Multiple sulphatases
	(Arylsulphatase A)	(Arylsulphatase A)	(Arylsulphatase A)	
Prenatal diagnosis feasible	Yes	Yes	Yes	Yes

AR = Autosomal recessive

age 6. Diagnosis may be aided by finding an increase in CSF protein and a decrease in nerve conduction velocity (Hagberg et al 1960).

A juvenile form (Type II) occurs at 4–8 years with cerebellar ataxia and gait dysfunction progressing to death in the second decade (Haberland et al 1973, Haltia et al 1980). Juvenile metachromatic leucodystrophy may actually represent two patterns of disease (McKhann 1984). Alternatively, juvenile metachromatic leucodystrophy will present at 6–16 years of age, with personality and behaviour changes and declining school performance. Seizures are common and motor dysfunction eventually ensues. Progression of this form is slower, and survival is possible into late adolescence or early adulthood. An adult form (Type III) appears in the late teens or later, with a psychosis or dementia and evidence of long tract involvement. Survival may be prolonged well into adult life (Percy et al 1977).

Pathological studies are abundant for the late infantile form, but are less extensive for the two delayed forms. The late infantile and juvenile forms manifest involvement predominantly of white matter, nerve tracts, and peripheral nerves. Loss of myelin, glial proliferation and the appearance of metachromatically-staining material is characteristic (Fig. 103.5). In addition, metachromatic material may be identified in peripheral nerve, liver, gall bladder, spleen, kidney, pancreas, lung and lymph nodes. While the cerebral cortex is relatively spared in the late infantile and juvenile forms, significant neuronal storage of metachromatic material is seen in adult cases. Segmental demyelination is invariably present in peripheral nerve. Electron microscopy of brain and nerve reveals granular cytoplasmic inclusions which are multi-laminated (Fig. 103.6). Stored material is present in cellular components in addition to lysosomes (Inui et al 1987).

Biochemical defect   The metachromatic material stored in this disorder is the sulphated derivative of galactosylceramide called sulphatide (Fig. 103.1). Sulphatide accumulates in both neural and non-neural tissues in this disorder, due to a deficiency in the activity of the lysosomal enzyme, sulphatide sulphatase (Mehl & Jatzkewitz 1963). This enzyme appears identical with one of the arylsulphatase isoenzymes, arylsulphatase A (Austin et al 1963). The reduction of arylsulphatase A activity in each form is profound and quantitatively similar whether employing the natural or artificial substrate (Percy & Kaback 1971). While the clinical-biochemical discrepancy is not resolved by in vitro enzyme analyses, tissue culture studies reveal differences which could explain the clinical variations noted. When cultured skin fibroblasts are incubated in the presence of sulphatide, cells from patients with sulphatidosis Type I have little ability to remove the sulphatide; cells from patients with Type II disease are somewhat better, and those from Type III patients are better still (Porter et al 1971). von Figura et al (1986) described instability of the arylsulphatase A synthesized in juvenile and adult MLD cells as a possible explanation for the metabolic abnormality in these variants.

The fourth form of metachromatic leucodystrophy is termed multiple sulphatase deficiency disease. This condition is genetically and biochemically perplexing. These patients have significant defects in the activity of a

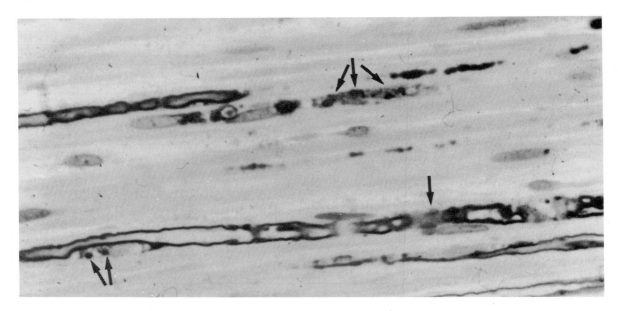

Fig. 103.5 Metachromatic (reddish-brown) material in longitudinal section of peripheral nerve from patient with sulphatide lipidosis.

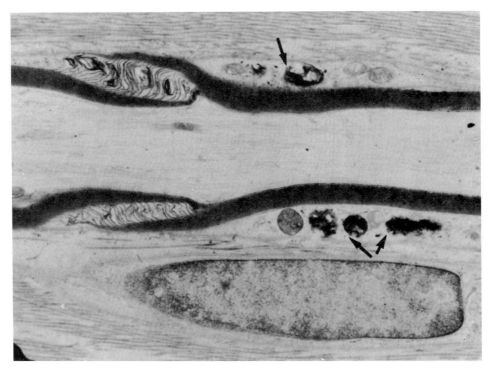

Fig. 103.6 Densely-staining storage material in Schwann cell cytoplasm adjacent to myelin sheath. Electron micrograph of peripheral nerve from a patient with sulphatide lipidosis.

variety of sulphatases. Arylsulphatase A, arylsulphatase B, iduronate sulphatase and heparan-N-sulphatase, all lysosomal enzymes involved in glycolipid or mucopolysaccharide catabolism, are reduced in these patients, as is the microsomal enzyme steroid sulphatase (Murphy et al 1971). Since distinct autosomal and X-chromosomal genes are involved in the coding for these enzyme proteins, the precise location of the genetic lesion is unclear. Clinically, these children are similar to juvenile or late infantile MLD patients, but in addition have hepatosplenomegaly and increased urinary mucopolysaccharide excretion. Many of these patients then show features both of a lipidosis and a mucopolysaccharidosis. A neonatal form has also been described. Under suitable conditions, cultured skin fibroblasts from such patients reveal significant activities of arylsulphatase A, suggesting that in the intact cell the enzyme is synthesized but, for as yet unknown reasons, may not be accessible to its substrate (Fluharty et al 1978). More recently, Eto et al (1987) demonstrated instability of arylsulphatase A in cultured fibroblasts, suggesting premature degradation of the respective sulphatases.

A further variant was recently described in which arylsulphatase A activity was about 50% of control levels (or in the heterozygote range) using both natural and artificial substrates (Shapiro et al 1979). The patient developed symptoms at age 4 with seizures, mental deterioration, and initial hypotonia and hyporeflexia progressing to spasticity. Cultured skin fibroblasts were unable to hydrolyze exogenous sulphatide whereas cells from the mother behaved as control preparations. Deficiency of 'activating factor' for sulphatide degradation could explain these findings (Stevens et al 1981). Indeed, Fujibayashi and Wenger (1986) and Wenger et al (1989) demonstrated failure of these fibroblasts to produce activator protein. Molecular genetic techniques will certainly define the error in gene coding.

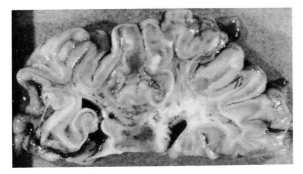

Fig. 103.7 Virtual absence of white matter in brain from patient with galactosylceramide lipidosis.

Galactosylceramide lipidosis (Krabbe disease)

The appearance of multinucleated or globoid cells in brain characterizes this disorder. Hence, the term globoid cell leucodystrophy has been synonymous with Krabbe disease (Table 103.6). Onset is in the first six months and progression is relentless, leading to death by age 2. Feeding difficulty, irritability and failure of psychomotor development are noted clinically, resulting in spasticity, cortical blindness, optic atrophy and deafness. The peripheral nerves are also involved, as indicated by decreased nerve conduction velocity. Cerebrospinal fluid protein is almost always elevated. Pathological findings are confined to the nervous system. The brain is small and of rubbery consistency. Grey matter is relatively spared; white matter is almost devoid of myelin (Fig. 103.7). Glial cell proliferation (gliosis) is profound and numerous macrophages and multinucleated globoid cells are noted (Fig. 103.8). Peripheral nerves are marked by segmental demyelination without evidence of globoid cells.

Electron microscopy of the globoid cells reveals cytoplasmic inclusions which have a hollow tubular appearance similar to, but distinct from, those seen in glucosylceramide lipidosis. Typical globoid cells have been produced experimentally by intracerebral injection of galactosylceramide or by culturing retinal cells in the presence of galactosyl- or glucosylceramide (Austin 1963, Sourander et al 1966).

Biochemical defect Galactosylceramide lipidosis is a unique disorder of sphingolipid catabolism. Instead of lipid storage there is an absolute deficiency of galactosylceramide as well as the other sphingolipids. However, when the globoid cells are isolated, chemical analysis reveals a relative accumulation of galactosylceramide. This observation, and the previously described experiments inducing globoid cells, prompted the analyses which revealed deficient galactosylceramide β-galactosidase activity (Fig. 103.1). This β-galactosidase enzyme is distinct from the enzyme involved in Gm_1-gangliosidosis (Suzuki & Suzuki 1970). Recently, Svennerholm et al (1980) reported a 100-fold accumulation of galactosylsphingosine (psychosine), the deacylated galactosylceramide, in white matter from affected infants. The cytopathic effect of galactosylsphingosine on oligodendroglia could explain the absolute deficiency of galactosylceramide.

A variant form of galactosylceramide lipidosis has been described with onset in childhood from age 4 to 8. The principal findings are gait disturbance and progressive psychomotor deterioration. Pathological findings are similar to the infantile form and the deficiency of galactosylceramide β-galactosidase activity is quantitatively similar. The clinical course is somewhat longer,

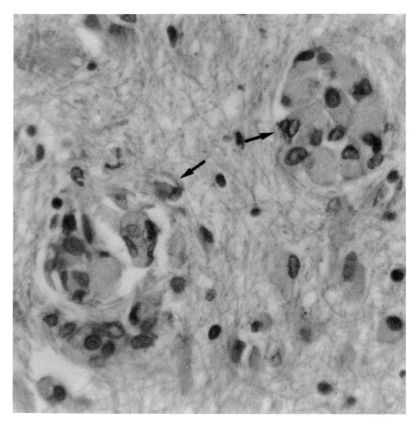

Fig. 103.8   Typical multinucleated 'globoid' cells in brain from patient with galactosylceramide lipidosis. Haematoxylin and eosin.

however, with death in the second decade. In contrast to the infantile form, peripheral nerve function as measured by nerve conduction velocity was normal in this juvenile variant (Young et al 1972).

A further variant was described by Dunn et al (1976). This child had the early onset of signs and symptoms, a prolonged course, and typical enzymatic abnormalities, but lacked globoid cells on histological examination.

Trihexosylceramide lipidosis (Fabry disease)

This disorder is the only sphingolipid disorder which generally spares the central nervous system from direct involvement, and is the only sphingolipidosis inherited as an X–linked recessive (Table 103.7). Fabry disease has its onset in childhood or adolescence and may run a variable course. Death usually occurs in middle adulthood, or at least by the end of the fifth decade. Pathological manifestations of this disease are predominantly noted in the skin, kidneys and cornea. The disease may appear as episodes of burning pain, particularly in the distal extremities, often associated with fever and elevation of

the erythrocyte sedimentation rate. Cutaneous vascular lesions called *angiokeratoma corporis diffusum* may also represent the initial manifestations. These lesions are usually symmetrical, occurring over the abdomen, lower back, the buttocks, hips and thighs, as well as the genitalia. Lesions have also been noted in the mouth and conjunctivae. The skin lesions are actually dilated vessels or angiectases with diffuse lipid infiltration of vascular endothelium. Similar lesions have been noted in individuals with fucosidosis and sialidosis and thus are not specific for Fabry disease. Exceptional patients may have central nervous system involvement presenting with manifestations of cerebrovascular insufficiency (Lou & Reske-Nielsen 1971). Peripheral oedema is often present without tangible explanation. Recently, reduced motor nerve conduction velocities were noted in 8 of 12 affected males and one-third of obligate carriers (Sheth & Swick 1979). The peripheral neuropathy is painful and often disabling but may respond to treatment with carbamazepine or phenytoin. Signs of renal dysfunction do not usually appear until adulthood, but ultimately the complications of chronic renal failure ensue. Death

Table 103.6 Galactosylceramide Lipidosis
Krabbe disease or globoid cell leucodystrophy

	Infantile	Late infantile
Age at onset	Infancy	1–4 years
Prognosis	Death by age 2	Death by age 10–12
Mode of inheritance	AR	AR
Neurological signs	Irritability	Ataxia
	Extensor rigidity	Gait difficulty
	Optic atrophy	Visual loss
	Cortical blindness	Psychomotor decline
	Rapid deterioration	
Stored material	Galactosylceramide	Galactosylceramide
	Galactosylsphingosine (psychosine)	Galactosylsphingosine (psychosine)
Enzyme defect	Galactosylceramide β-galactosidase	Galactosylceramide β-galactosidase
Prenatal diagnosis feasible	Yes	Yes

AR = Autosomal recessive

usually results either from renal failure itself, or from the cardiac and/or cerebral complications of hypertension or vascular disease. Many female carriers, by Lyonization, show some involvement, although in an attenuated form, most commonly manifested as hazy clouding of the cornea (Bird & Lagunoff 1978). Survival of female carriers may be normal, although they often succumb to the same complications as the hemizygous males (Burda & Winder 1967).

Pathological examinations reveal a generalized involvement of the endothelial lining of the blood vessels and reticuloendothelial systems, of epithelial tissues of cornea, kidney and skin and of the ganglion cells of the autonomic nervous system and the Schwann cells of the peripheral nervous system (Sima & Robertson 1978). The vaso-occlusive events reflect the vascular endothelial cell

Table 103.7 Trihexosylceramide Lipidosis
Fabry disease or angiokeratoma corporis diffusum

Age at onset	Adolescence to early adulthood
Prognosis	Prolonged survival
Mode of inheritance	XLR
Neurological signs	Painful dysaesthesia (hands and feet)
	Cerebrovascular occlusion
Systemic signs	Renal failure
	Cardiac failure
	Cutaneous angiectasia (genitalia, buttocks, thighs, lower abdomen)
Stored material	Trihexosylceramide
Enzyme defect	Trihexosylceramide α-galactosidase
Prenatal diagnosis feasible	Yes

XLR = X-linked recessive

storage of sphingolipid. Motor neurons themselves are ordinarily spared. Electron microscopy (EM) reveals cytoplasmic inclusions in lysosomes with a laminated structure and regular periodicity distinct from the inclusions seen in the other sphingolipidoses. CNS neuronal inclusions have been noted in the amygdala by EM (Grunnet & Spilsbury 1973).

Biochemical defect Fabry disease is marked by the accumulation of trihexosylceramide (Fig. 103.1) and digalactosylceramide in most tissues of the body. Both compounds accumulated have, as the terminal disaccharide, two galactose units linked in an alpha configuration. This is pertinent in that the enzymatic defect consists of markedly reduced α-galactosidase activity (Brady et al 1967). Digalactosylceramide is present in human tissues in very small amounts under normal circumstances, and only in this disorder does it increase abnormally. Careful analysis of α-galactosidase synthesis and post-translational processing in fibroblasts from Fabry patients has demonstrated various defects in synthesis, processing and intralysosomal stability. Thus, as with the other disorders of lysosomal hydrolases, remarkable heterogeneity exists among the individuals with Fabry disease (Lemansky et al 1987, Bernstein et al 1989). In addition, a full length cDNA clone coding for human α-galactosidase has been isolated (Calhoun et al 1985) and utilized for accurate diagnosis of this disorder but, more importantly, the accurate assessment of potential carriers, heterozygous females (Desnick et al 1987). Carrier detection by enzyme assay fails to identify all carriers because of the variability in X–inactivation.

Renal transplantation has been employed as a rational mode of intervention (Clarke et al 1972). Results of chronic dialysis or renal transplantation have been promising with regard to improved renal function. Other aspects of the disease have not improved substantially, however.

Glucosylceramide lipidoses (Gaucher disease)

Glucosylceramide lipidosis occurs in three clinically-distinct forms (Table 103.8), each involving the accumulation of glucosylceramide: Type I – Adult or chronic form (CNS spared), Type II – infantile form (early CNS involvement) and Type III – Juvenile form (late CNS involvement).

The adult or chronic form (Type I) represents about 80% of the total cases. This form is, like Tay-Sachs and Niemann-Pick disease, associated with eastern European Jews (Ashkenazi). Symptoms often occur in childhood, and usually by adolescence, with progressive splenomegaly and evidence of hypersplenism (pancytopenia). Affected individuals usually reach adulthood, and those with later onset may have normal life expectancy. The chronicity of the disease is denoted by massive hepatosplenomegaly and by bony lesions. These bony lesions consist of expansion of the bone marrow space and pathological fractures. CNS pathology consists of perivascular storage with intense glio-mesodermal fibrillary reaction and typical Gaucher cells, but with no neuronal storage (Soffer et al 1980). The infantile form, Type II (about 15% of reported cases), is a fulminant disease, appearing in infancy, usually with failure to thrive, laryngospasm, recurrent pulmonary infections and hepatosplenomegaly. Neurological signs occur early in infancy and progress rapidly, resulting in spasticity, strabismus and persistent extension of head and neck (extensor rigidity). Seizures may also appear, while cherry-red maculae are generally absent. Death occurs usually by age 2. The characteristic pathological finding is the appearance of Gaucher cells throughout the reticuloendothelial system, especially in bone marrow and visceral organs. These are reticuloendothelial cells containing cytoplasmic fibrillary tangles simulating wrinkled tissue paper. Perivascular Gaucher cells are visible in brain along with evidence of neuronal storage and degeneration. Electron microscopy of Gaucher cells reveals numerous inclusions which resemble hollow tubules.

The juvenile form (Type III) is represented mainly by a cluster of cases from Sweden. Splenomegaly may be noted during the first year of life, but development may be normal until intellectual deterioration becomes manifest from age 4 to 8. Death usually comes by age 15. Pathological findings generally resemble those of Type II.

Biochemical defect Glucosylceramide lipidosis is marked by the accumulation of glucosylceramide. Glucosylceramide is stored in extra-neural organs in each form of Gaucher disease, but only in Type II and Type III does the sphingolipid accumulate in brain. In addition, deacylated (lyso) glucosylceramide or glucosylsphingosine, analogous to the lyso-sphingolipids noted previously in GM2-gangliosidosis, Krabbe disease and MLD, accumulates and represents an important cytotoxic component of the pathogenesis in this disorder.

Glucosylceramide (Fig. 103.1) occupies a strategic position in the degradation pathway of globoside and gangliosides. Brady and co-workers (1965) found glucosylceramide β-glucosidase activity to be deficient in glucosylceramide lipidosis. This observation was particularly significant. It clearly defined for the first

Table 103.8 Glucosylceramide Lipidosis

	Gaucher disease		
	Type I Adult (80%)	Type II Infantile (15%)	Type III Norrbotten (Sweden)
Age at onset	By adolescence	Infancy	4–8 years
Prognosis	Prolonged survival	Death by age 2	Death by age 10–15
Mode of inheritance	AR	AR	AR
Neurological signs	Spared	Psychomotor deterioration Extensor posturing	Motor difficulties Seizures Progressive dementia
Systemic signs	Hepatosplenomegaly Hypersplenism Pathological fractures Arthritis	Failure to thrive Hepatosplenomegaly Laryngospasm and stridor	Initially hepatosplenomegaly
Stored material	Glucosylceramide Glucosylsphingosine	Glucosylceramide Glucosylsphingosine	Glucosylceramide Glucosylsphingosine
Enzyme defect	Glucosylceramide β-glucosidase	Glucosylceramide β-glucosidase	Glucosylceramide β-glucosidase
Prenatal diagnosis feasible	Yes	Yes	Yes

AR = Autosomal recessive

time a sphingolipid hydrolase deficiency and prompted the intense investigative interest which has resolved the primary enzymatic deficiency in each sphingolipid storage disease.

Types I and II have residual enzyme activity (glucosylceramide β-glucosidase) which is inversely proportional to the rate of progression of the disorder. The infantile form has little detectable activity, while the adult or chronic form has from 5–15% of control levels (Brady 1966). Reduced enzyme activity has been described in Type III patients representing about 15–20% of control levels (Hultberg et al 1973, Hultberg 1978, Nishimura & Barranger 1980). Accurate correlation of clinical involvement with leucocyte residual enzyme activity appears imprecise, although Svennerholm et al (1986) demonstrated discrimination of Types II and III brain enzyme activity using the natural substrate, glucosylceramide. Recently, the severity of Type I disease has been related to specific mutations within the β-glucosidase genome (Zimran et al 1989).

Substantial data are available regarding synthesis and post-translational processing of glucosylceramide β-glucosidase (Aerts et al 1987, Jonsson et al 1987, Sorge et al 1987). Multiple different mutations in the β-glucosidase gene appear to account for the variable clinical expression of Gaucher disease (Beutler et al 1984, Sorge et al 1985, Fabbro et al 1987, Bergmann et al 1989, Theophilus et al 1989). Even Type I disease among the Ashkenazi involves more than one mutation. Molecular genetic techniques utilizing cDNA coding for native enzyme should provide assistance in resolving this variability. Indeed, mutant enzyme from one Type II patient represented a single base substitution, resulting in the amino acid change from leucine to proline. Comparison of restriction fragments derived from other patients indicated a correlation of this mutation with neurological involvement (Tsuji et al 1987). Extension of these observations to additional patients is essential.

Ceramide lipidosis – lipogranulomatosis (Farber disease)

Lipogranulomatosis (Table 103.9) is a very unusual and devastating disorder of early infancy, recently added to the sphingolipidosis category (Crocker et al 1967). Irritability, a weak, hoarse cry, lymphadenopathy, joint swelling, multiple subcutaneous nodules, and severe psychomotor retardation characterize this disorder. Cherry-red maculae have been noted. The clinical course is relentlessly progressive with recurrent fever and pulmonary infiltrates. Death usually occurs by age 2. Pathological changes are generalized. Diffuse extraneural granulomas involve skin, lung, liver, spleen and joint capsules. The granulomas typically contain lipid-

Table 103.9 Ceramide Lipidosis
Farber disease or lipogranulomatosis

Age at onset	Infancy
Prognosis	Death by age 2
Mode of inheritance	AR
Neurological signs	Psychomotor deterioration
Systemic signs	Subcutaneous granulomas
	Pulmonary infiltrates
	Skeletal deformities
	Dermatitis
	Hoarseness
Stored material	Ceramide
Enzyme defect	Ceramidase
Prenatal diagnosis feasible	Yes

AR = Autosomal recessive

laden cells (histiocytes). Neuropathological findings include neuronal storage, glial proliferation, and foci of myelin loss. Retinal ganglion cells accumulate lipid material as well.

Biochemical defect Two types of sphingolipid accumulate in lipogranulomatosis. There is a mild elevation of ganglioside, mainly GM3, or haematoside (Fig. 103.1) in *visceral* organs. Brain ganglioside levels appear normal. The major sphingolipid stored is ceramide (Fig. 103.1) which is increased 10-fold in kidney and 60-fold in liver. Ceramide levels in grey matter appear normal while a 5-fold increase is noted in white matter. In cultured fibroblasts, exogenous ceramide accumulates in lysosomes, producing lamellar and curvilinear membranous inclusions (Chen & Decker 1982). The postulated defect in ceramide catabolism (Fig. 103.1) has been confirmed by delineation of ceramidase deficiency in kidney, liver and cultured fibroblasts (Sugita et al 1972, Dulaney et al 1976).

NEURONAL CEROID LIPOFUSCINOSES

The neuronal ceroid lipofuscinoses (NCL), a clinically well described but pathophysiologically poorly understood group of neurodegenerative diseases (Fig. 103.9), are similar to the sphingolipidoses in many respects. Yet the chemical nature of the 'stored' material is not known, nor is the specific enzyme deficiency. There are four recognized clinical disorders with an autosomal recessive inheritance pattern (Table 103.10). As a group, they are often referred to as Batten disease (Lake 1984).

Type I is an infantile form of neuronal ceroid lipofuscinosis described extensively in the Finnish population. Profound mental and motor deterioration and blindness appear at age 1–2 years. The electroretinogram (ERG) is reduced or absent and the visual evoked response (VER) is absent. Progression is relentless, with

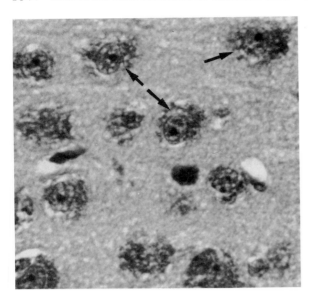

Fig. 103.9 Neuronal cytoplasmic accumulation of lipofuscin in neuronal ceroid lipofuscinosis. Luxol fast blue-haematoxylin and eosin.

death in the first decade. Pathologically, severe microcephaly with brain atrophy and an absence of cerebral cortical neurons is noted (Hagberg et al 1974). Brain lipids are dramatically reduced (Svennerholm et al 1975, Bourre et al 1979). Svennerholm et al (1987) recently reported a dramatic increase in the neutral oligoglycosphingolipids, while confirming the drastic reduction in neural sphingolipids and in phosphoglyceride polyunsaturated fatty acids.

Type II, Jansky-Bielschowsky disease, usually begins at age 2-4 with seizures. Death occurs by age 10. Dementia, blindness with optic atrophy, retinitis pigmentosa and macular degeneration are commonly seen. The ERG is decreased or absent, whereas the VER displays an exaggerated response. Diffuse cortical atrophy was noted by computed tomography (Valavanis et al 1980). Type III, Batten-Spielmeyer-Sjögren-Vogt disease, usually appears later in childhood and has a somewhat more indolent course. Visual symptoms are particularly common in this disease, blindness being a relatively early finding. The ERG and VER are decreased to absent. Macular degeneration with 'salt and pepper' pigmentary retinal changes are characteristic. Peripheral blood lymphocytes frequently show vacuolization, a finding occasionally observed in Jansky-Bielschowsky patients. Progressive dementia over ten years or more precedes death in the second decade. The fourth type of neuronal ceroid lipofuscinosis, Kufs disease, starts as a slowly progressive dementia at age 15-20. Seizures are occasion-

ally seen, but visual or retinal changes are rare. Interestingly, instances of Kufs disease have been found in families in which Jansky-Bielschowsky or Spielmeyer-Sjögren-Vogt disease has occurred. The precise genetic mechanism accounting for these three clinical syndromes (Types II-IV) is therefore uncertain and clarification awaits further biochemical advances. Pathologically, the four disorders are characterized by autofluorescent lipopigments in a number of viscera and in the brain (Fig. 103.10). By electron microscopy this pigment is found within neurons appearing in a characteristic granular, curvilinear or fingerprint pattern (Aquas et al 1980). Granular inclusions predominate in the infantile form, curvilinear inclusions in the late infantile form (Jansky-Bielschowsky) and fingerprint in the juvenile form (Spielmeyer-Sjögren-Vogt). Definitive diagnosis of NCL is made at present by brain biopsy or at autopsy. Alternatively, autofluorescent material may be identified in buffy coat preparations and characteristic inclusions can be detected by electron microscopy applied to peripheral blood lymphocytes or skin, conjunctiva or rectal myenteric plexus biopsies. MacLeod et al (1985) have successfully diagnosed the late infantile form in uncultured amniotic fluid cells at 16 weeks' gestation. This technique should be applicable to other forms of NCL.

The molecular defect in these disorders remains elusive. The origin of the autofluorescent lipofuscin is thought to represent peroxidation of tissue lipids with polymerization of the resulting products. A deficiency of leucocyte peroxidase activity was described previously in patients with the Batten variant (Armstrong et al 1974). Subsequent studies from different centres contradicted these initial findings. Since a reduction in cellular peroxidase activity might explain the lipopigment accumulation interest in this area has been rekindled, with later reports of glutathione peroxidase deficiencies in erythrocytes from patients with the Type I (Finnish) and Type III (Batten) forms (Westermarck & Sandholm 1977, Jensen et al 1978). Alternatively, the autofluorescent material was shown to contain retinoyl complexes and peroxidized polyunsaturated fatty acids (Wolfe et al 1977).

More recently, the pigments were linked to the dolichols, polyisoprenoid alcohols important in the glycosylation of glycoproteins. Elevated levels of urinary dolichols were noted in some NCL patients and suggested as a diagnostic marker (Wolfe et al 1983). However, subsequent studies have failed to reveal consistent abnormalities in dolichol levels or in dolichol-related metabolic events (Paton & Poulos 1984, Bennett et al 1985, Paton & Poulos 1987). Using a sheep model of NCL, Palmer et al (1986a,b) concluded that this model did not represent a lipidosis or storage of lipid

Table 103.10 Neuronal ceroid lipofusinosis

	Type I Infantile [Santavuori]	Type II Late infantile [Jansky-Bielschowsky]	Type III Juvenile [Spielmeyer- Sjögren-Vogt]	Type IV Adult [Kufs]
Age at onset	1–2 years	2–4 years	5–10 years	Adolescence to adulthood
Prognosis	Death by age 10	Death by age 10	Death by age 20	Prolonged survival
Mode of inheritance	AR	AR	AR	AR
Neurological signs	Psychomotor deterioration Microcephaly Myoclonus, seizures Retinal atrophy Blindness	Seizures Dementia Ataxia Retinitis pigmentosa Macular degeneration	Visual loss Dementia Retinitis pigmentosa Ataxia Seizures	Slowly progressive dementia Seizures Vision spared
Systemic signs	–	–	–	–
Stored material	Autofluorescent lipopigment	Autofluorescent lipopigment	Autofluorescent lipopigment	Autofluorescent lipopigment
Enzyme defect	Unknown	Unknown	Unknown	Unknown
Prenatal diagnosis feasible	Uncertain	Yes	Yes	Uncertain

AR = Autosomal recessive

breakdown products. Rather, the stored material was mainly composed of protein (70% by weight). The major protein component had a molecular weight of 3500. These authors postulated a defect in lysosomal protein catabolism.

OTHER LIPIDOSES

Four disorders of lipid metabolism involving tissue storage will be described briefly (Table 103.11). These are phytanic acid lipidosis (Refsum disease), Wolman disease and cholesterol ester lipidosis, which appear to share a common enzymatic deficiency, and cholestanol lipidosis (cerebrotendinous xanthomatosis).

Phytanic acid lipidosis (Refsum disease)

Phytanic acid lipidosis, a clinically-complex, potentially-treatable disorder transmitted as an autosomal recessive, often appears in childhood and usually by age 20 (Table 103.11). It was originally called *heredopathia atactica polyneuritiformis* because of the prominent cerebellar ataxia and peripheral neuropathy (Refsum 1960). The mode of onset is variable and may involve extremity weakness, unsteadiness of gait, failing vision particularly at night, or anosmia. The complete clinical syndrome includes cerebellar ataxia, retinitis pigmentosa, symmetrical motor and sensory peripheral neuropathy, epiphyseal dysplasia, manifested in a shortened fourth metatarsal bone, syndactyly, hammer toes, cartilage degeneration and pes cavus. Clinical investigations reveal elevated CSF protein, decreased nerve conduction velo-

city, and conduction defects in the EKG. Remissions and exacerbations, the latter often as a result of intercurrent febrile illness, surgical procedures or pregnancy, are typical, with an overall pattern of progressive disability. Pathological findings include hypertrophic interstitial peripheral neuropathy with demyelination, retinal degeneration, and glial proliferation in brain.

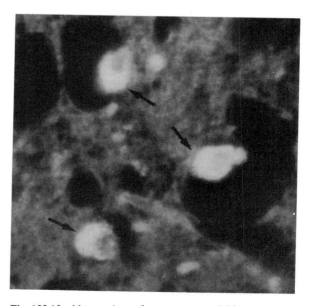

Fig. 103.10 Neuronal autofluorescent material in neuronal ceroid lipofuscinosis.

Table 103.11 Other Lipidoses

	Phytanic acid lipidosis [Refsum]	Triglyceride and cholesterol ester lipidosis [Wolman]	Cholesterol ester lipidosis	Cholestanol lipidosis [Cerebrotendinous xanthomatosis]
Age at onset	Adolescence	Infancy	Childhood	Late childhood to early adolescence
Prognosis	Prolonged survival	Death by 3 months	Normal life expectancy	Prolonged survival
Mode of inheritance	AR	AR	AR	AR
Neurological signs	Ataxia Deafness Polyneuropathy Retinitis pigmentosa Visual decline	Spared clinically	Spared	Xanthomas of brain Ataxia Dementia
Systemic signs	Ichthyosis	Adrenal calcification Hepatosplenomegaly Failure to thrive (marasmus)	Hepatomegaly Short stature Anaemia Diarrhoea	Xanthomas over extensor tendons Cataracts
Stored material	Phytanic acid	Triglycerides Cholesterol esters	Cholesterol esters	Cholestanol Cholesterol
Enzyme defect	Phytanic acid oxidase	Acid lipase	Acid lipase	Cholesterol 24-hydroxylase
Prenatal diagnosis feasible	Yes	Yes	Yes	Uncertain

AR = Autosomal recessive

Biochemical defect

Plasma phytanic acid (normally present only in trace amounts) may represent 5–30% of the total fatty acid fraction and tissue phytanic acid may account for 50% of total fatty acids. Phytanic acid levels in peripheral nerves usually exceed those in the central nervous system (MacBrinn & O'Brien 1968).

Phytanic acid is a natural product, the major source being chlorophyll-containing foods and foods derived from ruminant animals, namely cows. Hence, phytanic acid lipidosis is unique among the lipid storage disorders in that the accumulating material is derived from exogenous sources and does not represent accretion of a normal membrane constituent. Metabolism of phytanic acid by the usual fatty acid β-oxidation pathway is precluded by the methyl side-group, thus, an initial α-oxidation step is required. A defect in this α-oxidation step was noted in patients with phytanic acid lipidosis and intermediate levels were found in obligate heterozygotes (Stokke et al 1961, Steinberg & Hutton 1972).

Phytanic acid oxidation is now associated with the subcellular organelle, the peroxisome (Skjeldal et al 1986). The important role of the peroxisome in cellular metabolism has been recognized recently and has helped clarify the biochemical abnormalities of several disorders, including adrenoleucodystrophy and phytanic acid lipi-dosis (Refsum disease). In addition, clarity has also developed in relationship to Zellweger syndrome, neonatal adrenoleucodystrophy, and neonatal phytanic acid lipidosis (Percy & Fishman 1987).

Since phytanic acid is obtained from dietary sources, a diet low in phytanic acid offers a potential mode of therapy. Improvement of affected patients has been noted in terms of reduced plasma phytanic acid levels and amelioration of the peripheral neuropathy. No improvement was noted in cerebellar or cranial nerve function. Early institution of dietary restriction might delay or even prevent disease onset (Refsum 1984). Plasma phytanic acid levels may be lowered acutely by plasmapheresis (Lundberg et al 1972, Gibberd et al 1979).

Triglyceride and cholesterol ester lipidosis

Two clinical entities, one with limited survival, the other with normal life expectancy, are associated with the accumulation of cholesterol esters and triglycerides (Table 103.11).

The first disorder, Wolman disease (Abramov et al 1956, Crocker et al 1965), is a devastating autosomal recessive disorder of early infancy with death by 12–18 months. Failure to thrive, with poor feeding and malabsorption, hepatosplenomegaly, and adrenal enlargement with calcifications are noted at onset. Primary central nervous system involvement is unusual. Lipid-laden histiocytes are seen in the bone marrow and in most organs including occasional histiocytic collections in brain. The second disorder, cholesterol ester lipidosis, has been described in only half a dozen families. Moderate hepatomegaly (liver function normal) occurs in childhood and foam cells are found in the bone marrow, liver and intestine. Disability is minimal and life expectancy appears normal. In addition, three affected sibs have been described with a clinical picture intermediate between Wolman disease and cholesterol ester lipidosis (Beaudet et al 1977).

Biochemical defect These disorders are characterized by tissue accumulation of cholesterol esters and triglycerides, the latter being less prominent in cholesterol ester lipidosis. In liver, the magnitude of increase is similar in each disorder. Brain lipid analyses from patients with Wolman disease reveal no consistent abnormality. Plasma cholesterol and triglyceride levels have usually been normal in Wolman disease and increased (mainly cholesterol esters) along with low density lipoproteins in cholesterol ester lipidosis, representing a major risk factor for the occurrence of occlusive vascular disease in the latter.

Acid phosphatase (a lysosomal hydrolase) activity in the limiting membrane of stored lipid material suggested defective lysosomal function in Wolman disease. Deficient activity of an acid lipase or esterase has been noted histochemically in liver and peripheral blood smears (Lake 1971), and biochemically in liver, spleen, leucocytes and fibroblasts (Patrick & Lake 1969). Wolman patients exhibited no evidence of acid lipase activity. In contrast, the patients designated as cholesterol ester lipidosis had about 15-20% control activity (Beaudet et al 1974, Hoeg et al 1984). Heterozygote detection has been established in leucocytes and fibroblasts.

Using cultured fibroblasts from individuals with Wolman disease, Salvayre et al (1987) noted that the stored cholesterol and triglycerol esters in lysosomes appeared to result from exogenous lipids, whereas triglycerides synthesized within the cell remained in non-lysosomal cytoplasmic granules. In addition to defective catabolism of lipid esters, Wolman cells may be unable to regulate lipoprotein receptors and thus demonstrate excessive lipoprotein uptake as well. In this regard, the cholesterol ester lipidoses appear to resemble the Types III and IV Niemann-Pick disease (sphingomyelin lipidosis).

In summary, these observations suggest that Wolman disease and cholesterol ester lipidosis represent phenotypic variants of a similar, although quantitatively differ-ent, biochemical defect in acid lipase activity, as reflected in cholesterol ester and triglyceride storage.

Cholestanol lipidosis (cerebrotendinous xanthomatosis)

Cholestanol lipidosis is an extremely unusual disorder (50-60 cases) involving the clinical constellation of dementia, xanthomas, cataracts and progressive neurological dysfunction (Menkes et al 1968). Onset is usually in late childhood or adolescence in the form of a dementia, followed by the appearance of cataracts and xanthomas. Progressive neurological dysfunction, including ataxia and gait difficulty, leads to death usually by age 30-40. Xanthomas are most commonly found on the Achilles tendon but may also be found on triceps tendons, tibial tuberosity, or extensor tendons of the fingers. With advanced disease, pain and vibratory sensation may be lost, and distal muscular atrophy is evident. Sural nerve biopsies demonstrate typical segmental demyelination (Argov et al 1986).

Pathological changes in the brain include glial proliferation, myelin loss and foam cells in perivascular spaces. Cerebral grey matter is spared, while the white matter is devastated. Granulomas virtually replace cerebellar white matter. Xanthomas consist of birefringent crystals with multinucleated giant cells and mononuclear cells.

Biochemical defect Cholestanol levels are markedly increased in all tissues. While the usual plasma lipids are normal, plasma cholestanol may be increased several-fold. Interestingly, the tendon xanthomas reveal cholesterol storage predominantly with mild elevation of cholestanol. Cholesterol levels in brain are increased only slightly. Cholestanol (dihydrocholesterol) is itself derived from a minor pathway of cholesterol catabolism. Recent reports indicate that one of the final steps in the conversion of cholesterol to bile acids is impaired in this disorder. Inability to oxidize the cholesterol side-chain results in defective synthesis of the bile acids, cholic acid and chenodeoxycholic acid, and excretion of precursors in bile and urine. Increased levels of cholestanol would arise in response to shunting cholesterol from its usual bile acid pathway to the cholestanol pathway.

Delineation of the enzymatic defect has been difficult, due partly to methodological problems involving the sterol intermediates in bile acid synthesis. Cholesterol biosynthesis is high, but bile acid synthesis is reduced, suggesting a defect in the conversion of cholesterol to bile acids. Salen et al (1979) noted a reduction of liver microsomal 24-hydroxylase activity to 25% of control levels. Together with the pattern of bile intermediates formed, the enzymatic data support the primary defect as one of abnormal 24-hydroxylation. Subsequently, Oftebro et al (1980) reported a lack of cholesterol 26-hydroxylation in liver of one affected individual. However, the absence of this enzyme in normal liver makes interpretation difficult. Carrier detection is also problematic. Recently Koopman et al (1986) utilized cholestyramine-stimulation of bile acid synthesis as a provocative test and were able to discriminate carriers from non-affected individuals.

Treatment of cholestanol lipidosis is based on the premise that provision of adequate cholic or cheno-deoxycholic acid would suppress endogenous sterol biosynthesis by a feedback mechanism. Using cheno-deoxycholic acid, Berginer et al (1982) noted an improved EEG pattern in nine patients. In addition to reducing plasma cholestanol levels to normal, no further progression or some improvement was also noted in neurological function (Berginer et al 1984) and in visual and brainstem auditory evoked responses (Pedley et al 1985). Alternatively, cholic acid has been similarly effective and is devoid of significant side-effects (diarrhoea, nausea, pruritus, altered liver function tests) as well as being less expensive (Koopman et al 1985).

Lewis et al (1983) described the beneficial effects of an inhibitor of cholesterol biosynthesis, mevinolin, with regard to plasma cholestanol and hepatomegaly. No change in neurological status was noted after five months of therapy.

GENETICS

Each of the sphingolipidoses, with the exception of trihexosylceramide lipidosis (Fabry disease), is transmitted as an autosomal recessive trait which requires that each parent must be a carrier or obligate heterozygote for the disease-related recessive gene. Fabry disease, on the other hand, is inherited as an X–linked recessive, and as a result the female heterozygote may, by Lyonization (Lyon 1962), manifest signs and symptoms as in the affected male.

With the advent of appropriate enzyme assays for each of these disorders, it is now possible to screen high-risk individuals for heterozygosity; i.e. determination of the disease-related enzyme activity in potential carriers for a given disorder should yield values which are intermediate between the affected level and the normal control range. In general, activity of the disease-related enzyme in the heterozygote is 30–60% of normal control values, while affected individuals manifest less than 10% of the disease-related enzyme activity. By this method, it has been possible to provide some measure of genetic counselling for each of these disorders. The ramifications of this genetic counselling will be discussed below.

PATIENT EVALUATION

A thorough history and physical assessment are essential in evaluating the patient with an inherited lipid storage disorder. Significant historical data may be derived from a detailed family history such as evidence of consanguinity or previous children with similar difficulties.

One should ask specifically about untimely childhood deaths from unknown or ill-defined causes in this or previous generations. Occasionally, the parents will describe a previous child who was given the diagnosis of 'progressive cerebral palsy' or 'progressing encephalitis'. Since cerebral palsy is non-progressive, such a description should alert the clinician.

In many instances the lipid storage disorders profoundly affect psychomotor development. When acquired skills are lost, or expected milestones are never achieved, little doubt exists about the progressive nature of the disease process. However, it is often difficult to decide whether a plateau in development represents normal variation or evidence of psychomotor delay. As a rule, the pattern of development in the child with a non-progressive central nervous system disorder resulting, for example, from the impact of neonatal hypoxia or asphyxia, will be continuous but at a slower rate than normal. The child with a lipid storage disorder affecting the central nervous system may appear to exhibit a similar pattern at first glance but, as the disease process progresses, serial assessments will show that the actual rate of development is slowing.

The physical examination may also provide important clues. The presence of organomegaly suggests a storage disease. Bony abnormalities or dysmorphic facial features are encountered in patients with the mucolipidoses and with the sphingolipidosis, GM1-gangliosidosis. Ophthalmological findings include corneal changes (trihexosylceramide lipidosis), cherry-red maculae (GM1-gangliosidosis, GM2-gangliosidosis-Tay-Sachs disease, sphingomyelin lipidosis-type I, sialidosis Type I, ceramide lipidosis (Farber disease) and, rarely, sulphatide lipidosis), optic atrophy (sphingolipidoses), and retinal pigmentary changes (neuronal ceroid lipofuscinoses, phytanic acid lipidosis-Refsum disease). Since the peripheral nerves may also be involved, one may see the interesting, if not confusing, combination of hypotonia and hyporeflexia and Babinski signs. Cerebellar ataxia and nystagmus may be prominent features of sulphatide lipidosis, the infantile forms of neuronal ceroid lipofuscinoses, or phytanic acid lipidosis.

Definitive diagnosis of those diseases for which the biochemical lesion is known can be accomplished by demonstrating deficient activity of the disease-related enzyme in appropriate tissues such as leucocytes or cultured skin fibroblasts. Enzyme assays are now available for the rapid and accurate diagnosis of the sphingolipidoses, phytanic acid lipidosis (Refsum disease), the cholesterol ester lipidoses, and cholestanol lipidosis. When a definitive diagnosis is established, it is crucial that other family members (parents and sibs) be tested.

Prior to the development of definitive biochemical methodologies, diagnosis depended on tissue biopsy and appropriate histological examination. Using peripheral nerve, rectal myenteric plexus, or brain, characteristic inclusions were identified, along with other neuropathological findings. For those diseases which can be established in leucocytes or cultured skin fibroblasts by relevant enzyme testing, nerve or brain biopsy is no longer acceptable. Skin biopsies should be employed when a diagnosis cannot be established clinically or biochemically, and then only under carefully controlled conditions where professional expertise will guarantee proper handling of the tissue (Martin & Jacobs 1973, O'Brien et al 1975, Farrell & Sumi 1977).

Brain biopsy demands even more stringent controls requiring the multidisciplinary approach which will ensure skilled histology, electron microscopy, neurochemistry, and neurobiochemistry. Brain biopsy should not be conducted in hospitals lacking such a multidisciplinary capability. The goal of brain biopsy in otherwise ill-defined neurodegenerative diseases must be to provide a diagnosis, if possible, and to guide the physician in counselling the family relative to prognosis and to possible genetic implications. The family needs to understand that the procedure is unlikely to benefit the child directly, but may provide important information regarding the disease process itself and, thereby, enhance future approaches to patients with these problems.

PREVENTION

Where an identifiable at-risk population can be defined, as in Tay-Sachs disease, and carriers identified with easily available tissue, population screening is a rational undertaking and provides important information on gene frequency (Cantor et al 1987). Programmes currently in force have screened in excess of 700 000 individuals (Kaback, personal communication) and monitored more than 600 at risk pregnancies for Tay-Sachs disease (Kaback et al 1977). For the other disorders of sphingolipid metabolism, we are presently dependent on the detection of index cases. Unless there is previous evidence of one of these disorders, an affected individual must be identified and the diagnosis established before the other members of that family can receive the benefits of genetic counselling. Recent recognition of pseudo-deficiency (low enzyme activity in clinically normal individuals) for lysosomal hydrolases (e.g. MLD, Krabbe

disease) has created difficulty in establishing heterozygosity. Pseudo-arylsulphatase A deficiency has been linked to an altered enzyme protein which has reduced stability (Ameen & Chang 1987). Resolution of the pseudo-deficiency state can be achieved in cultured fibroblasts by examining the degradation of exogenous natural substrate (Fluharty et al 1978). Similar pseudo-deficiency has been noted in families of Krabbe disease patients.

PRENATAL DIAGNOSIS

In the last few years each of the sphingolipidoses has been detected in trophoblasts or amniocytes and the diagnosis has been confirmed in aborted tissues (Wenger 1985). Since the probability of the fetus being affected for these disorders is one in four and since the abortion procedure is without major difficulty, the monitoring of pregnancies of at-risk couples has become an integral part of genetic counselling. In instances where the family desires additional, phenotypically-normal children, the physician can now ensure the realization of this possibility. Attention must be given to possible pseudo-deficiency status as noted above.

THERAPY

Effective and satisfactory treatment in terms of reversing the molecular defect is currently unavailable for the sphingolipidoses. This can be stated unequivocally in relation to those disorders which affect the nervous system. Individuals with trihexosylceramide lipidosis (Fabry disease) have been treated with renal transplantation (Clarke et al 1972). Since the life-threatening aspects of this disorder involve chronic renal insufficiency, renal transplantation or chronic dialysis is a potentially favourable mode of therapy. The observed lowering of blood sphingolipid levels may be due to graft-produced enzyme, but may also be due in part to improved glomerular filtration and the effects of immunosuppressive therapy. However, despite improved renal function, disease progression has not been altered consistently. Fetal liver cells were transplanted into three adults with Fabry disease (Touraine et al 1982). Despite a lack of increased α-galactosidase activity in leucocytes, clinical improvement or stabilization was noted in terms of dysaesthesias, renal function and cutaneous lesions, and no neurological abnormalities occurred over follow-up periods from 28 to 77 months. Similar, although less extensive, studies have been performed with splenic transplantation in Gaucher patients (Groth et al 1972) and hepatic transplantation in Niemann-Pick disease (Delvin et al 1974).

Specific enzyme replacement therapy has not yet been achieved for any of the lysosomal storage diseases. Enthusiasm for this modality arose following the demonstration that defective mucopolysaccharide metabolism could be normalized in cell culture systems by exposure to appropriate 'corrective factors' or enzymes. Numerous theoretical and practical difficulties exist, including large-scale isolation of the relevant lysosomal enzymes, potential immunological complications after repeated injection and, in the case of those disorders with prominent central nervous system involvement, the physical-chemical blood brain barrier. In an attempt to circumvent these problems laboratory models have been developed to explore chemical alteration of the blood brain barrier, enabling brain uptake of the lysosomal hydrolases (Barranger et al 1977) and a variety of alternative delivery systems involving entrapment of the enzymes in liposomes (Reynolds et al 1978) or autologous erythrocyte membranes (Ihler et al 1973). The latter manoeuvres are directed at reducing antigenicity and, for patients with lysosomal storage diseases sparing the CNS may represent an effective alternative.

In recent years bone marrow transplantation following pharmacological removal of recipient marrow has been employed with some measure of success (Hobbs 1987). Delivery of the relevant enzyme to the central nervous system in cells has been demonstrated (Hoogerbrugge et al 1988). Whether this is sufficient to reverse neurological dysfunction remains to be established. In the case of Type I GM1-gangliosidosis, bone marrow transplantation was ineffective (Shaw et al 1986). Conversely, individuals with Gaucher disease (glucosylceramide lipidosis) Type III have benefited from bone marrow transplantation, particularly if preceded by splenectomy (Hobbs et al 1987). Progressive neurological changes have not been noted, although reversal of existing abnormalities has not occurred. The presence of hepatic fibrosis is a negative indicator. Sphingomyelin lipidosis Type II (Vellodi et al 1987) and Wolman disease (Hobbs et al 1986) were successfully engrafted and improvement resulted, although the latter child succumbed to sepsis. Despite presence of the relevant enzyme in brain in the murine model of Krabbe disease (galactosylceramide lipidosis), disease progression was slowed, but not halted (Ichioka et al 1987). In a patient with juvenile metachromatic leucodystrophy (sulphatide lipidosis) progression of clinical neurological changes was slowed, but nerve conduction velocities continued to deteriorate (Lipton et al 1985, Krivit et al 1987).

In summary, bone marrow transplantation appears to be unsatisfactory at present for the treatment of the storage diseases in which progressive neurological dysfunction is prominent. In particular, reversibility of neurological changes has not been demonstrated. With regard to structural pathology, alterations in central nervous system both by light and electron microscopy (Fig. 103.11) have been noted in affected fetuses (GM1- and GM2-gangliosidosis) aborted at 20 weeks' gestation (Percy et al 1973). Unless these changes are found to be reversible, appropriate therapy may have to commence during intrauterine life. One should weigh the risks and benefits of bone marrow transplantation carefully in children whose disease process involves the nervous system. At present, the potential benefit seems insufficient.

Attention is being directed to molecular genetic strategies for treatment (Anderson 1984). Significant groundwork remains to be accomplished. The availability of a number of animal models of lysosomal storage diseases provides the opportunity to evaluate these critical questions, and it seems likely that progress will be made in this area in the future (Baker et al 1979, Pritchard et al 1980, Wenger et al 1980b).

ACKNOWLEDGEMENTS

Dawna Armstrong M D, Department of Pathology, Baylor College of Medicine, Houston, Texas, kindly assisted with the illustrative reproductions. Nancy Ivy provided secretarial assistance. Texas Children's Hospital, through funds to the Section of Pediatric Neurology, supported the preparation of this chapter.

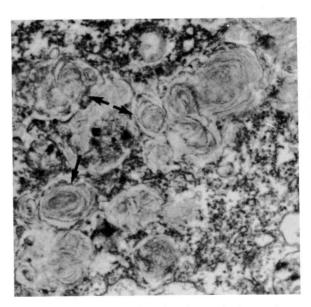

Fig. 103.11 Membranous inclusions in anterior horn cell from fetus (20 weeks' gestation) with GM2-gangliosidosis. Reproduced from Percy et al (1973).

REFERENCES

Detailed information regarding the disorders discussed above may be found in following review articles: Scriver C R, Beaudet A L, Sly W S, Valle D (eds) 1989 The metabolic basis of inherited disease, 6th edn, McGraw Hill, New York, ch 51, 57–59, 64–72

Abramov A, Schorr S, Wolman M 1956 Generalized xanthomatosis with calcified adrenals. American Journal of Diseases of Children 91: 282–286

Aerts J M F G, Donker-Koopman W E, van Laar C et al 1987 Relationship between the two immunologically distinguishable forms of glucocerebrosidase in tissue extracts. European Journal of Biochemistry 163:583–589

Ameen M, Chang P L 1987 Pseudo arylsulfatase A deficiency. Biosynthesis of an abnormal arylsulfatase A. FEBS Letters 219: 130–134

Anderson W F 1984 Prospects for human gene therapy. Science 226: 401–409

Aquas A P, Moura Nunes J F, Hasse Ferreira A D, Vital J P 1980 Neuronal ceroid lipofuscinosis: ultrastructural study of lymphocytic dense bodies. Neurology 30: 976–980

Argov Z, Soffer D, Eisenberg S, Zimmerman Y 1986 Chronic demyelinating peripheral neuropathy in cerebrotendinous xanthomatosis. Annals of Neurology 20: 89–91

Armstrong D, Dimmitt S, Van Vormer D E 1974 Studies in Batten's disease I: Peroxidase deficiency in granulocytes. Archives of Neurology 30: 144–152.

Arpaia E, Dumbrille-Ross A, Maler T et al 1988 Identification of an altered splice site in Ashkenazi Tay-Sachs disease. Nature 333: 85–86

Austin J 1963 Studies in globoid (Krabbe) leukodystrophy. Archives of Neurology 9: 207–231.

Austin J H, Balasubramanian A S, Pattabiraman T N, Saraswathi S, Basu D K, Bachhawat B K 1963 A controlled study of enzymic activities in three human disorders of glycolipid metabolism. Journal of Neurochemistry 10: 805–816

Austin J, Armstrong D, Shearer L 1965 Metachromatic form of diffuse cerebral sclerosis V. The nature and significance of low sulfatase activity. Archives of Neurology 13: 593–614

Baker H J, Reynolds G D, Walkley S U, Cox N R, Baker G H 1979 The gangliosidoses: comparative features and research applications. Veterinary Pathology 16: 635–649

Barranger J A, Pentchev P G, Rapoport S I, Brady R O 1977 Augmentation of brain lysosomal enzyme activity following enzyme infusion with concomitant alteration of the blood-brain barrier. Annals of Neurology 1: 496

Bayleran J, Hechtman P, Kolodny E, Kaback M 1987 Tay-Sachs disease with hexosaminidase A: Characterization of the defective enzyme in two patients. American Journal of Human Genetics 41: 532–548

Beaudet A L, Lipson M H, Ferry G D, Nichols, B L Jr. 1974 Acid lipase in cultured fibroblasts: cholesterol ester storage disease. Journal of Laboratory and Clinical Medicine 84: 54–61

Beaudet A L, Ferry G D, Nichols B L Jr. Rosenberg H S 1977 Cholesterol ester storage disease: Clinical, biochemical, and pathological studies. Journal of Pediatrics 90: 910–914

Bennett M J, Mathers N J, Hemming F W, Zweije-Hofman I, Hosking G P 1985 Urinary sediment dolichol excretion in patients with Batten disease and other neurodegenerative and storage disorders. Pediatric Research 19: 213–216

Berginer V M, Radwan H, Korczyn A D, Kott E, Salen G, Shefer S 1982 EEG in cerebrotendous xanthomatosis (CTX). Clinical Electroencephalography 13: 89–96

Berginer V M, Salen G, Shefer S 1984 Long-term treatment of cerebrotendinous xanthomatosis with chenodeoxycholic acid. New England Journal of Medicine 311: 1649–1652

Bergmann J E, Grabowski G A 1989 Posttranslational processing of human lysosomal acid β-glucosidase: A continuum of defects in Gaucher disease Type I and Type II fibroblasts. American Journal of Human Genetics 44: 741–750

Bernstein H S, Bishop D F, Astrin K H et al 1989 Fabry disease: six gene rearrangements and an exonic point mutation in the α-galactosidase gene. Journal of Clinical Investigation 83: 1390–1399

Beutler E, Kuhl W, Sorge J 1984 Cross-reacting material in Gaucher disease fibroblasts. Proceedings of the National Academy of Sciences USA 81: 6506–6510

Bird T D, Lagunoff D 1978 Neurologic manifestations of Fabry disease in female carriers. Annals of Neurology 4: 537–540

Bourre J M, Haltia M, Daudu O, Monge M, Baumann N 1979 Infantile form of so-called neuronal ceroid lipofuscinosis: Lipid biochemical studies, fatty acid analysis of cerebroside sulfatides and sphingomyelin, myelin density profile and lipid composition. European Neurology 18: 312–321.

Brady R O 1966 The sphingolipidoses. New England Journal of Medicine 275: 312–318

Brady R O, Kanfer J N, Shapiro D 1965 Metabolism of glucocerebrosides. II evidence of an enzymatic deficiency in Gaucher's disease. Biochemical and Biophysical Research Communications 18: 221–225

Brady R O, Kanfer J N, Mock M, Frederickson D S 1966 The metabolism of sphingomyelin II: evidence of an enzymatic deficiency in Niemann-Pick disease. Proceedings of the National Academy of Sciences USA 55: 366–369

Brady R O, Gal A E, Bradley R M, Mårtensson E, Warshaw A L, Laster L 1967 Enzymatic defect in Fabry's disease, ceramidetrihexosidase deficiency. New England Journal of Medicine 276: 1163–1167

Brett E M, Ellis R B, Haas L, Ikonne J U, Lake B D, Patrick A D, Stephens R 1973 Late onset GM2-gangliosidosis. Archives of Disease in Childhood 48: 775–785

Burda C D, Winder P R 1967 Angiokeratoma corporis diffusum universale (Fabry's disease) in female subjects. American Journal of Medicine 42: 293–301

Butler J D, Comly M E, Kruth H S et al 1987 Niemann-Pick variant disorders: Comparison of errors of cellular cholesterol homeostasis in group D and group C fibroblasts. Proceedings of the National Academy of Sciences USA 84: 556–560

Calhoun D H, Bishop D F, Bernstein H S, Quinn M, Hantzopoulos P, Desnick R J 1985 Fabry disease: Isolation of a cDNA clone encoding human α-galactosidase A. Proceedings of the National Academy of Sciences USA 82: 7364–7368

Cantor R M, Roy C, Lim J S T, Kaback M M 1987 Sandhoff disease heterozygote detection: A component of population screening for Tay-Sachs disease carriers. II. Sandhoff disease gene frequencies in American Jewish and Non-Jewish populations. American Journal of Human Genetics 41: 16–26

Chen W W, Decker G L 1982 Abnormalities of lysosomes in human diploid fibroblasts from patients with Farber's disease. Biochimica et Biophysica Acta 718: 185–192

Christomanou H 1980 Niemann-Pick disease, Type C: Evidence for the deficiency of an activating factor stimulating sphingomyelin and glucocerebroside degradation. Hoppe-Seyler's Zeitschrift fur Physiologische Chemie 361: 1489–1502

Clarke J T R, Guttman R D, Wolfe L S, Beaudoin J G, Morehouse D D 1972 Enzyme replacement therapy by renal allotransplantation in Fabry's disease. New England Journal of Medicine 287: 1215–1218

Conzelmann E, Sandhoff K 1978 AB variant of infantile Gm$_2$-gangliosidosis: deficiency of a factor necessary for stimulation of hexosaminidase A-catalyzed degradation of ganglioside Gm$_2$ and glycolipid Ga$_2$. Proceedings of the National Academy of Sciences USA 75: 3979–3983

Crocker A C, Vawter G F, Neuhauser E B D, Rosowsky A 1965 Wolman's disease: three patients with a recently described lipidosis. Pediatrics 35: 627–640.

Crocker A C, Cohen J, Farber S 1967 The 'Lipogranulomatosis' syndrome; review with report of patient showing milder involvement. In: Aronson S M, Volk B W (eds) Inborn Disorders of Sphingolipid Metabolism. Pergammon Press, Oxford, p 485–503.

d'Azzo A, Proia R L, Kolodny E H, Kaback M M, Neufeld E F 1984 Faulty association of α- and β-subunits in some forms of β-hexosaminidase A deficiency. Journal of Biological Chemistry 259: 11070–11074

de Duve C, Pressman B C, Gianetto R, Wattiaux R, Appelmans F 1955 Tissue fractionation studies. Intracellular distribution patterns of enzymes in rat-liver tissue. Biochemical Journal 60: 604–617

Delvin E, Glorieux F, Daloze P, Gorman J, Block P 1974 Niemann-Pick type A: enzyme replacement by liver transplantation. American Journal of Human Genetics 26: 25A

Desnick R J, Bernstein H S, Astrin K H, Bishop D F 1987 Fabry disease: Molecular diagnosis of hemizygotes and heterozygotes. Enzyme 38: 54–64

Dulaney J T, Milunsky A, Sidbury J R, Hobolth N, Moser H W 1976 Diagnosis of lipogranulomatosis (Farber's disease) by use of cultured fibroblasts. Journal of Pediatrics 89: 59–61

Dunn H G, Dolman C L, Farrell D F, Tischler B, Hasinoff C, Woolf L I 1976 Krabbe's leukodystrophy without globoid cells. Neurology 26: 1035–1041.

Eto Y, Gomibuchi I, Umezawa F, Tsuda T 1987 Pathochemistry, pathogenesis and enzyme replacement in multiple-sulfatase deficiency. Enzyme 38: 273–279

Fabbro D, Desnick R J, Grabowski G A 1987 Gaucher disease: genetic heterogeneity within and among the subtypes detected by immunoblotting. American Journal of Human Genetics 40: 15–31

Farrell D F, Sumi S M 1977 Skin punch biopsy in the diagnosis of juvenile neuronal ceroid-lipofuscinosis. Archives of Neurology 34: 39–44

Fink J K, Filling-Katz M R, Sokol J et al 1989 Clinical spectrum of Niemann-Pick disease type C. Neurology 39: 1040–1049

Fishman M A, Percy A K 1984 Update on febrile seizures and inherited lipid storage diseases. In: Appel S H (ed) Current Neurology, vol 5. John Wiley, New York p 117–162

Fluharty A L, Stevens R L, Davis L L, Shapiro L J, Kihara H 1978 Presence of arylsulfatase A (ARS A) in multiple sulfatase deficiency disorder fibroblasts. American Journal of Human Genetics 30: 249–255.

Freeman J M, McKhann G M 1969 Degenerative diseases of the central nervous system. Advances in Pediatrics 16: 121–175

Fujibayashi S, Wenger D A 1985 Studies on a sphingolipid activator protein (SAP-2) in fibroblasts from patients with lysosomal storage diseases, including Niemann-Pick disease Type C. Clinica Chimica Acta 146: 147–156

Fujibayashi S, Wenger D A 1986 Biosynthesis of the sulfatide/Gm$_1$ activator protein (SAP-1) in control and mutant cultured skin fibroblasts. Biochimica et Biophysica Acta 875: 554–562

Gal A E, Brady R O, Barranger J A, Pentchev P G 1980 The diagnosis of type A and type B Niemann-Pick disease and detection of carriers using leucocytes and a chromogenic analogue of sphingomyelin. Clinica Chimica Acta 104: 129–132

Gibberd F B, Page N G R, Billimoria J D, Retsas S 1979 Heredopathia atactica polyneuritiformis (Refsum's disease) treated by diet and plasma exchange. Lancet 1: 575–578

Gilbert F, Kucherlapati R, Creagan R P, Murnane M J, Darlington G J, Ruddle F H 1975 Tay-Sachs' and Sandhoff's diseases: the assignment of genes for hexosaminidase A and B to individual human chromosomes. Proceedings of the National Academy of Sciences USA 72: 263–267

Goldman J E, Katz D, Rapin I, Purpura D P, Suzuki K 1981 Chronic Gm$_1$ gangliosidosis presenting as dystonia: I. Clinical and pathological features. Annals of Neurology 9: 465–475

Groth C G, Blomstrand R, Hagenfeldt L, Ockerman P A, Samuelsson K, Svennerholm L 1972 Metabolic changes following splenic transplantation in a case of Gaucher's Disease. In: Volk B W, Aronson S M (eds) Sphingolipids, Sphingolipidoses, and Allied Disorders. Plenum Press, New York, p 633–639

Grunnet M L, Spilsbury P R 1973 The central nervous system in Fabry's disease. Archives of Neurology 28: 231–234.

Haberland C, Brunngraber E, Witting L, Daniels A 1973 Juvenile metachromatic leucodystrophy. Acta Neuropathologica 26: 93–106

Hagberg B, Sourander P, Svennerholm L, Voss H 1960 Late infantile metachromatic leukodystrophy of the genetic type. Acta Paediatrica Scandinavica 49: 135–153

Hagberg B, Haltia M, Sourander P, Svennerhom L, Eeg-Olofsson O 1974 Polyunsaturated fatty acid lipidosis - infantile form of so-called neuronal ceroid lipofuscinosis I: Clinical and morphological aspects. Acta Paediatrica Scandinavica 63: 752–763

Haltia T, Palo J, Haltia M, Icén A 1980 Juvenile metachromatic leukodystrophy. Archives of Neurology 37: 42–46

Harzer K, Schlote W, Peiffer J, Benz H U, Anzil A P 1978 Neurovisicidosis lipidosis compatible with Niemann-Pick disease type C. Acta Neuropathologica 43: 97–104

Hers H G 1963 α-Glucosidase deficiency in generalized

glycogen storage disease (Pompe's disease). Biochemical Journal 86: 11–16

Herschkowitz N, Schulte F J 1984 Gangliosidoses and leukodystrophies: A correlative approach in neurobiology. Neuropediatrics 15(Suppl): 1–112

Hobbs J R 1987 Experience with bone marrow transplantation for inborn errors of metabolism. Enzyme 38: 194–206

Hobbs J R, Hugh-Jones K, Shaw P J et al 1986 Wolman's disease corrected by displacement bone marrow transplantation with immunoprophylaxis. Bone Marrow Transplantation 1 (Suppl 1): 347

Hobbs J R, Hugh-Jones K, Shaw P J, Lindsay I, Hancock M 1987 Beneficial effects of pre-transplant splenectomy on displacement bone marrow transplantation for Gaucher's syndrome. Lancet 1: 1111–1115.

Hoeg J M, Demosky S J Jr. Pescovitz O H, Brewer H B Jr 1984 Cholesteryl ester storage disease and Wolman disease: Phenotypic variants of lysosomal acid cholesteryl ester hydrolase deficiency. American Journal of Human Genetics 36: 1190–1203

Hoogerbrugge P M, Suzuki K, Suzuki K, Poorthuis B J H M, Kobayashi T, Wagemaker G, van Bekkum D W 1988 Donor-derived cells in the central nervous system of twitcher mice after bone marrow transplantation. Science 239: 1035–1038

Hoogeveen A T, Reuser A J J, Kroos M, Galjaard H 1986 GM1-gangliosidosis: Defective recognition site on β-galactosidase precursor. Journal of Biological Chemistry 261: 5702–5704

Hultberg B 1978 β-glucosidase activities in the Norrbotten type of juvenile Gaucher's disease. Acta Neurologica Scandinavica 58: 89–94

Hultberg B, Sjoblad S, Ockerman P A 1973 4-methylum-belliferyl-β-glucosidase in cultured human fibroblasts from controls and patients with Gaucher's disease. Clinica Chimica Acta 49: 93–97

Ichioka T, Kishimoto Y, Brennan S, Santos G W, Yeager A M 1987 Hematopoietic cell transplantation in murine globoid cell leukodystrophy (the twitcher mouse): Effects on levels of galactosylceramidase, psychosine, and galactocerebrosides. Proceedings of the National Academy of Sciences USA 84: 4259–4263

Ihler G, Glew R H, Schnure F W 1973 Enzyme loading of erythrocytes. Proceedings of the National Academy of Sciences USA 70: 2663–2666

Inui K, Furukawa M, Nishimoto J et al 1987 Metabolism of cerebroside sulphate and subcellular distribution of its metabolites in cultured skin fibroblasts derived from controls, metachromatic leukodystrophy, globoid cell leukodystrophy and Farber disease. Journal of Inherited Metabolic Disease 10: 293–296

Jensen G E, Shukla V K S, Gissel-Nielsen G, Clausen J 1978 Biochemical abnormalities in Batten's syndrome. Scandinavian Journal of Clinical and Laboratory Investigation 38: 309–318

Johnson W G, Chutorian A, Miranda A 1977 A new juvenile hexosaminidase deficiency disease presenting as cerebellar ataxia. Neurology 27: 1012–1018

Jonsson L M V, Murray G J, Sorrell S H et al 1987 Biosynthesis and maturation of glucocerebrosidase in Gaucher fibroblasts. European Journal of Biochemistry 164: 171–179

Kaback M M, Nathan T J, Greenwald S 1977 Tay-Sachs disease: heterozygote screening and prenatal diagnosis – US experience and world perspective. In: Kaback M (ed) Progress in clinical and biological research in Tay-Sachs: screening and prevention. Alan Liss, New York, p 13–36

Kamoshita S, Aron A, Suzuki K, Suzuki K 1969 Infantile Niemann-Pick disease, a chemical study. American Journal of Diseases of Children 117: 379–394

Kivlin J D, Sanborn G E, Myers G G 1985 The cherry-red spot in Tay-Sachs and other storage diseases. Annals of Neurology 17: 356–360

Koopman B J, Wolthers B G, van der Molen J C, Waterreus R J 1985 Bile acid therapies applied to patients suffering from cerebrotendinous xanthomatosis. Clinica Chimica Acta 152: 115–122

Koopman B J, Waterreus R J, Van Den Brekel H W C, Wolthers B G 1986 Detection of carriers of cerebrotendinous xanthomatosis. Clinica Chimica Acta 158: 179–186

Krivit W, Lipton M E, Lockman L A et al 1987 Prevention of deterioration in metachromatic leukodystrophy by bone marrow transplantation. American Journal of Medical Sciences 294: 80–85.

Lake B D 1971 Histochemical detection of the enzyme deficiency in blood films in Wolman's disease. Journal of Clinical Pathology 24: 617–620

Lake B D 1984 Lysosomal enzyme deficiencies. In: Adams J H, Corsellis J A N, Duchen L W (eds) Greenfield's Neuropathology, 4th edn. John Wiley, New York, 491–572.

Landing B H, Silverman F N, Craig J M, Jacoby M D, Lahey M E, Chadwick D L 1964 Familial neurovisceral lipidosis. American Journal of Diseases of Children 108: 503–522

Lemansky P, Bishop D F, Desnick R J, Hasilik A, von Figura K 1987 Synthesis and processing of α-galactosidase A in human fibroblasts: Evidence for different mutations in Fabry disease. Journal of Biological Chemistry 262: 2062–2065

Lewis B, Mitchell W D, Marenah C B, Cortese C, Reynolds E H, Shakir R 1983 Cerebrotendinous xanthomatosis: biochemical response to inhibition of cholesterol synthesis. British Medical Journal 287: 21–22

Lipton M E, Lockman L A, Jacobson R I, Krivit W 1985 Bone marrow transplant for metachromatic leukodystrophy. Annals of Neurology 18: 399

Lou H O C, Reske-Nielsen E 1971 The central nervous system in Fabry's disease. Archives of Neurology 25: 351–359

Lundberg A, Lilja L G, Lundberg P O, Try K 1972 Heredopathia atactica polyneuritiformis (Refsum's disease). European Neurology 8: 309–324

Lyon M F 1962 Sex chromatin and gene action in the mammalian X-chromosome. American Journal of Human Genetics 14: 135–148

MacBrinn M C, O'Brien J S 1968 Lipid composition of the nervous system in Refsum's disease. Journal of Lipid Research 9: 552–561

McKhann G M 1984 Metachromatic leukodystrophy: Clinical and enzymatic parameters. Neuropediatrics 15(Supplement): 4–10

MacLeod P M, Dolman C L, Nickel R E, Chang E, Nag S, Zonana J, Silvey K 1985 Prenatal diagnosis of neuronal ceroid-lipofuscinosis. American Journal of Medical Genetics 22: 781–789

Mahuran D, Novak A, Lowden J A 1985 The lysosomal hexosaminidase isozymes. In: Rattazzi M C, Scandalios J G, Whitt G S (eds) Isozymes, vol 12. Alan Liss, New York, p 229–288

Mårtensson E 1969 Glycosphingolipids of animal tissue. Progress in the Chemistry of Fats and Other Lipids 10: 367–407

Martin J J, Jacobs K 1973 Skin biopsy as a contribution to diagnosis in late infantile amaurotic idiocy with curvilinear bodies. European Neurology 10: 281–291

Max S R et al 1974 Gm$_3$ (hematoside) sphingolipody-strophy. New England Journal of Medicine 291: 929–931

Mazière C, Mazière J C, Mora L, Lageron A, Polonovski C, Polonovski J 1987 Alterations in cholesterol metabolism in cultured fibroblasts from patients with Niemann-Pick disease type C. Journal of Inherited Metabolic Disease 10: 339–346

Mehl E, Jatzkewitz H 1963 Uber ein Cerebrosid-schwefelsaureester spaltendes Enzym aus Schweineniere. Hoppe-Seyler's Zeitschrift fur Physiologiche Chemie 331: 292–294

Menkes J H, Schimschock J R, Swanson P D 1968 Cerebrotendinous xanthomatosis: The storage of cholestanol within the nervous system. Archives of Neurology 19: 47–53

Mitsumoto H, Sliman R J, Schafer I A, Sternick C S, Kaufman B, Wilbourn A, Horwitz S J 1985 Motor neuron disease and adult hexosaminidase A deficiency in two families: Evidence for multisystem degeneration. Annals of Neurology 17: 378–385

Molin K, Månsson J-E, Fredman P, Svennerholm L 1987 Sialosyllactotetraosylceramide, 3'-isoLM1, a ganglioside of the lactotetraose series isolated from normal human infant brain. Journal of Neurochemistry 49: 216–219.

Moser H W 1985 Leukoencephalopathies caused by metabolic disorders. In: Koetsier J C (ed) Handbook of Clinical Neurology, vol 47, Elsevier Science Publishers, Amsterdam, p 583–604

Murphy J V, Wolfe H J, Balazs E A, Moser H W 1971 A patient with deficiency of arylsulfatases A, B, C and steroid sulfatase associated with storage of sulfatide, cholesterol sulfate and glycosaminoglycans In: Bernsohn J, Grossman H (eds) Lipid Storage Diseases: Enzymatic Defects and Clinical Implications. Academic Press, New York p 67–110

Mutoh T, Sobue I, Nasi M, Matsuoka Y, Kiuchi K, Sugimura K 1986a A family with β-galactosidase deficiency: Three adults with atypical clinical patterns. Neurology 36: 54–59

Mutoh T, Naoi M, Takahashi A, Hoshino M, Nagai Y, Nagatsu T 1986b A typical adult Gm$_1$-gangliosidosis: Biochemical comparison with other forms of primary β-galactosidase deficiency. Neurology 36: 1237–1241

Myerowitz R, Hogikyan N D 1987 A deletion involving Alu sequences in the β-hexosaminidase α-chain gene of French Canadians with Tay-Sachs disease. Journal of Biological Chemistry 262: 15396–15399

Myerowitz R, Proia R L 1984 cDNA clone for the α-chain of human β-hexosaminidase: Deficiency of α-chain mRNA in Ashkenazi Tay-Sachs fibroblasts. Proceedings of the National Academy of Sciences USA 81: 5394–5398

Neufeld E F 1989 Natural history and inherited disorders of a lysosomal enzyme, β-hexosaminidase. Journal of Biological Chemistry 264: 10927–10930

Nishimura R N, Barranger J A 1980 Neurologic complications of Gaucher's disease type 3. Archives of Neurology 37: 92–93

O'Brien J S 1975 Molecular genetics of Gm$_1$ β-galactosidase. Clinical Genetics 8: 303–313

O'Brien J S, Ho M W, Veath M L et al 1972 Juvenile Gm$_1$ gangliosidoses: clinical, pathological, chemical, and enzymatic studies. Clinical Genetics 3: 411–434

O'Brien J S, Bernett J, Veath M L, Paa D 1975 Lysosomal storage disorders: diagnosis by ultrastructural examination of skin biopsy specimens. Archives of Neurology 32: 592–599

Oftebro H, Björkhem I, Skrede S, Schreiner A, Pedersen J I 1980 Cerebrotendinous xanthomatosis: a defect in mitochondrial 26-hydroxylation required for normal biosynthesis of cholic acid. Journal of Clinical Investigation 65: 1418–1430

Ohno K, Suzuki K 1988 Mutation in Gm$_2$-gangliosidosis B1 variant. Journal of Neurochemistry 50: 316–318

Okada S, O'Brien J S 1968 Generalized gangliosidosis: beta-galactosidase deficiency. Science 160: 1002–1004

Okada S, O'Brien J S 1969 Tay-Sachs disease: generalized absence of a beta-D-N-acetylhexosaminidase component. Science 165: 698–700

O'Neill B, Butler A B, Young E, Falk P M, Bass N H 1978 Adult-onset Gm$_2$-gangliosidosis. Neurology 28: 1117–1123

Oonk J G W, Van der Helm H J, Martin J J 1979 Spinocerebellar degeneration: hexosaminidase A and B deficiency in two adult sisters. Neurology 29: 380–384

Palmer D N, Husbands D R, Winter P J, Blunt J W, Jolly R D 1986a Ceroid lipofuscinosis in sheep I. Bis (monoacylglycero) phosphate, dolichol, ubiquinone, phospholipids, fatty acids and fluorescence in liver lipopigment lipids. Journal of Biological Chemistry 261: 1766–1772

Palmer D N, Barns G, Husbands D R, Jolly R D 1986b Ceroid lipofuscinosis in sheep II. The major component of the lipopigment in liver, kidney, pancreas and brain is low molecular weight protein. Journal of Biological Chemistry 261: 1773–1777

Paton B C, Poulos A 1984 Dolichol metabolism in cultured skin fibroblasts from patients with 'neuronal' lipofuscinosis (Batten's disease). Journal of Inherited Metabolic Disease 7: 112–116

Paton B C, Poulos A 1987 Normal dolichol concentration in urine sediments from four patients with neuronal ceroid lipofuscinosis (Batten's disease). Journal of Inherited Metabolic Disease 10: 28–32

Patrick A D, Lake B D 1969 Deficiency of an acid lipase in Wolman's disease. Nature 222: 1067–1068

Paw B H, Kaback M M, Neufeld E F 1989 Molecular basis of adult-onset and chronic GM2 gangliosides in patients of Ashkenazi Jewish origin: Substitution of serine for glycine at position 269 of the α-subunit of β-hexosaminidase. Proceedings of the National Academy of Sciences USA 86: 2413–2417

Pedley T A, Emerson R G, Warner C L, Rowland L P, Salen G 1985 Treatment of cerebrotendinous xanthomatosis with chenodeoxycholic acid. Annals of Neurology 18: 517–518

Pentchev P G, Comly M E, Kruth H S et al 1987 Group C Niemann-Pick disease: faulty regulation of low-density lipoprotein uptake and cholesterol storage in cultured fibroblasts. FASEB Journal 1: 40–45

Percy A K 1987 The inherited neurodegenerative disorders of childhood: Clinical assessment. Journal of Child Neurology 2: 82–97

Percy A K, Fishman M A 1987 Peroxisomal disorders. In: Appel S H (ed) Current Neurology, vol 7. Year Book Medical Publishers, Chicago, p 295–318

Percy A K, Kaback M M 1971 Infantile and adult-onset metachromatic leukodystrophy, biochemical comparisons and predictive diagnosis. New England Journal of Medicine 285: 785–787

Percy A K, McCormick U M, Kaback M M, Herndon R M 1973 Ultrastructure manifestations of Gm_1 and Gm_2-gangliosidosis in fetal tissues. Archives of Neurology 28: 417–419

Percy A K, Kaback M M, Herndon R M 1977 Metachromatic leukodystrophy: comparison of early- and late-onset forms. Neurology 27: 933–941

Percy A K, Shapiro L J, Kaback M M 1979 Inherited lipid storage diseases of the central nervous system In: Gluck L (ed) Current Problems in Pediatrics, vol 9(11). Yearbook Medical Publishers, Chicago, p 1–51

Philippart M, Martin L, Martin J J, Menkes J H 1969 Niemann-Pick disease, morphological and biochemical studies in the visceral form with late central nervous system involvement (Crocker's group C). Archives of Neurology 20: 227–238

Pilz H, Heipertz R, Seidel D 1979 Basic findings and current developments in sphingolipidoses. Human Genetics 47: 113–134

Porter M T, Fluharty A L, Trammell G, Kihara H 1971 A correlation of intracellular cerebroside sulfatase activity in fibroblasts with latency in metachromatic leuko-dystrophy. Biochemical and Biophysical Research Communications 44: 660–666

Pritchard D H, Napthine D V, Sinclair A J 1980 Globoid cell leukodystrophy in polled Dorset sheep. Veterinary Pathology 17: 399–405

Proia R L, Neufeld E F 1982 Synthesis of β-hexosamini-dase in cell-free translations and in intact fibroblasts: An insoluble precursor α-chain in a rare form of Tay-Sachs disease. Proceedings of the National Academy of Sciences USA 79: 6360–6364

Refsum S 1960 Heredopathia atactica polyneuritiformis reconsideration. World Neurology 1: 334–337

Refsum S 1984 Heredopathia atactica polyneuritiformis (Refsum's disease): Clinical and genetic aspects of Refsum's disease. In: Dyck P J, Thomas P K, Lambert E G (eds) Peripheral Neuropathy, vol II. Saunders, Philadelphia p 868–890

Reynolds G D, Baker H J, Reynolds R H 1978 Enzyme replacement using liposome carriers in feline Gm_1-gangliosidosis fibroblasts. Nature 275: 754–755

Rosengren B, Månsson J-E, Svennerholm L 1987 Composition of gangliosides and neutral glycosphingolipids of brain in classical Tay-Sachs and Sandhoff disease: More lyso-Gm_2 in Sandhoff disease? Journal Neurochemistry 49: 834–840

Sachs B 1887 On arrested cerebral development with special reference to its cortical pathology. Journal of Nervous and Mental Diseases 14: 541–553

Salen G, Shefer S, Cheng F W, Dayal B, Batta A K, Tint G S 1979 Cholic acid biosynthesis: the enzymatic defect in cerebrotendinous xanthomatosis. Journal of Clinical Investigation 63: 38–44

Salvayre R, Negre A, Maret A, Radom J, Douste-Blazy L 1987 Extracellular origin of the lipid lysosomal storage in cultured fibroblasts from Wolman's disease. European Journal of Biochemistry 170: 453–458

Sandhoff K, Christomanou H 1979 Biochemistry and genetics of gangliosidoses. Human Genetics 50: 107–143

Sandhoff K, Andreae U, Jatzkewitz H 1968 Deficient hexosaminidase activity in an exceptional case of Tay-Sachs disease with additional storage of kidney globoside in visceral organs. Pathologia Europaea 3: 278–285

Sandhoff K, Harzer K, Wässle W, Jatzkewitz H 1971 Enzyme alterations and lipid storage in three variants of Tay-Sachs disease. Journal of Neurochemistry 18:2469–2489

Shapiro L J et al 1979 Metachromatic leukodystrophy without arylsulfatase A deficiency. Pediatric Research 13: 1179–1181

Shaw P J, Hugh-Jones K, Hobbs J R, Cooper A, Lealman G T 1986 Gm_1-gangliosidosis: failure to halt neurological regression by bone marrow transplantation. Bone Marrow Transplantation 1 (Suppl 1): 339

Sheth K J, Swick H M 1979 Peripheral nerve conduction in Fabry disease. Annals of Neurology 7: 319–323

Sima A A F, Robertson D M 1978 Involvement of peripheral nerve and muscle in Fabry's disease. Archives of Neurology 35: 291–301

Singer H S, Schafer I A 1972 Clinical and enzymatic variations in Gm_1-generalized gangliosidosis. American Journal of Human Genetics 24: 454–463

Skjeldal O H, Stokke O, Norseth J, Lie S O 1986 Phytanic acid oxidase activity in cultured skin fibroblasts. Diagnostic usefulness and limitations. Scandinavian Journal of Clinical and Laboratory Investigation 46: 283–287

Soffer D, Yamanaka T, Wenger D A, Suzuki K, Suzuki K 1980 Central nervous system involvement in adult-onset Gaucher's disease. Acta Neuropathologica 49: 1–6

Sonderfeld S, Brendler S, Sandhoff K, Galjaard H, Hoogeveen A T 1985 Genetic complementation in somatic cell hybrids of four variants of infantile Gm_2 gangliosidosis. Human Genetics 71: 196–200

Sorge J, Gelbart T, West C, Westwood B, Beutler E 1985 Heterogeneity in type I Gaucher disease demonstrated by restriction mapping of the gene. Proceedings of the National Academy of Sciences USA 82: 5442–5445

Sorge J A, West C, Kuhl W, Treger L, Beutler E 1987 The human glucocerebrosidase gene has two functional ATG initiator codons. American Journal of Human Genetics 41: 1016–1024

Sourander P, Hansson H A, Olsson Y, Svennerholm L 1966 Experimental studies on the pathogenesis of leukodystrophies. II: the effect of sphingolipids on various cell types in cultures from the nervous system. Acta Neuropathologica 6: 231–242

Steinberg D, Hutton D 1972 Phytanic acid storage disease. In: Volk B W, Aronson S M (eds) Sphingolipids, sphingolipidoses and allied disorders. Plenum Press, New York, p 515–532

Stevens R L, Fluharty A L, Kihara H et al 1981 Cerebroside sulfatase activator deficiency induced metachromatic leukodystrophy. American Journal of Human Genetics 33: 900–906

Stokke O, Try K, Eldjarn L 1961 α-Oxidation as an alternative pathway for the degradation of branched chain fatty acids in man, and its failure in patients with

Refsum's disease. Biochimica et Biophysica Acta 144: 271–284

Sugita M, Dulaney J T, Moser H W 1972 Ceramidase deficiency in Farber's disease (lipogranulomatosis). Science 178: 1100–1102

Suzuki K 1968 Cerebral Gm$_1$-gangliosidosis: chemical pathology of visceral organs. Science 159: 1471–1472

Suzuki K, Suzuki Y 1970 Globoid cell leukodystrophy (Krabbe's disease): deficiency of galactocerebroside β-galactosidase. Proceedings of the National Academy of Sciences USA 66: 302–309

Svennerholm E, Svennerholm L 1963 Neutral glycolipids of human blood serum, spleen, and liver. Nature 198: 688–689

Svennerholm L 1962 The chemical structure of normal human brain and Tay-Sachs ganglioside. Biochemical and Biophysical Research Communications 9: 436–446

Svennerholm L 1969 New principles for the classification of glycolipidoses. Metabolism 5: 60–70

Svennerholm L 1970 Ganglioside metabolism. In: Florkin M, Stotz E H (eds) Comprehensive Biochemistry, vol 18. Elsevier Amsterdam, ch IV

Svennerholm L, Zettergren L 1957 Infantile amaurotic idiocy. Acta Pathologica et Microbiologica Scandinavica 41: 127–134

Svennerholm L, Hagberg B, Haltia M, Sourander P. Vanier M T 1975 Polyunsaturated fatty acid lipidosis, II lipid biochemical studies Acta Paediatrica Scandinavica 64: 489–496

Svennerholm L, Vanier M T, Månsson J-E 1980 Krabbe Disease: a galactosylsphingosine (psychosine) lipidosis. Journal of Lipid Research 21: 53–64

Svennerholm L, Månsson J-E, Rosengren B 1986 Cerebroside β-glucosidase activity in Gaucher brain. Clinical Genetics 30: 131–135

Svennerholm L, Fredman P, Jungbjer B et al 1987 Large alterations in ganglioside and neutral glycosphingolipid patterns in brains from cases with infantile neuronal ceroid lipofuscinosis/polyunsaturated fatty acid lipidosis Journal of Neurochemistry 49: 1772–1783

Tay W 1881 Symmetrical changes in the region of the yellow spot in each eye of an infant. Transactions of the Ophthalmological Societies of the United Kingdom 1: 55–57

Theophilus B, Latham T, Grabowski G A et al 1989 Gaucher disease: molecular heterogeneity and phenotype-genotype correlations. American Journal of Human Genetics 45: 212–225

Thomas G H, Tuck-Muller C M, Miller C S et al 1989 Correction of sphingomyelinase deficiency in Niemann-Pick Type C fibroblasts by removal of lipoprotein fraction from culture media. Journal of Inherited Metabolic Disease 12: 139–151

Touraine J L, Malik M C, Maire I, Veyron P, Zabot M T, Rolland M O, Mathieu M 1982 Fetal liver transplantation in congenital enzyme deficiencies in man. Experimental Hematology 10 (Suppl 10); 46–47

Tsuji S, Choudary P V, Martin B M, Stubblefield B K, Mayor J A, Barranger J A, Ginns E I 1987 A mutation in the human glucocerebrosidase gene in neuronopathic Gaucher disease. New England Journal of Medicine 316: 570–575

Ushiyama M, Ikeda S, Nakayama J, Yanagisawa N, Hanyu N, Katsuyama T 1985 Type III (chronic) Gm$_1$-

gangliosidosis: Histochemical and ultrastructural studies of rectal biopsy. Journal of the Neurological Sciences 71: 209–223

Valavanis A, Friede R L, Schubiger O, Hayek J 1980 Computed tomography in neuronal ceroid lipofuscinosis. Neuroradiology 19: 35–38

Vanier M T 1983 Biochemical studies in Niemann-Pick disease I. Major sphingolipids of liver and spleen. Biochimica et Biophysica Acta 750: 178–184

Vellodi A, Hobbs J R, O'Donnell N M, Coulter B S, Hugh-Jones K 1987 Treatment of Niemann-Pick disease type B by allogeneic bone marrow transplantation. British Medical Journal 295: 1375–1376

von Figura K, Steckel F, Conary J, Hasilik A, Shaw E 1986 Heterogeneity in late-onset metachromatic leukodystrophy. Effects of inhibitors of cysteine proteinases. American Journal of Human Genetics 39: 371–382

von Figura K, Hasilik A, Pohlmann R, Braulke T, Lemansky P, Stein M 1987 Mutations affecting transport and stability of lysosomal enzymes. Enzyme 38: 144–153.

Wenger D A, DeGala G, Williams C et al 1989 Clinical, pathological, and biochemical studies on an infantile case of sulfatide/GM1 activator protein deficiency. American Journal of Medical Genetics 33: 255–265

Wenger D A 1985 Disorders of lipid metabolism. In: Milunsky A (ed) Genetic Disorders and the Fetus, 2nd edn. Plenum, New York, p 205–255

Wenger D A, Sattler M, Mueller O T, Myers G G, Schneiman R S, Nixon G W 1980a Adult Gm$_1$-gangliosidosis: clinical and biochemical studies on two patients and comparison to other patients called variant or adult Gm$_1$-gangliosidosis Clinical Genetics 17: 323–334

Wenger D A, Sattler M, Kudoh T, Snyder S P, Kingston R S 1980b Niemann-Pick disease: a genetic model in Siamese cats. Science 208: 1471–1473

Westermarck T, Sandholm M 1977 Decreased erythrocyte glutathione peroxidase activity in neuronal ceroid lipofuscinosis (NCL) corrected with selenium supplementation. Acta Pharmacologica et Toxicologica 40: 70–74

Winsor E J T, Welch J P 1978 Genetic demographic aspects of Nova Scotia Niemann-Pick disease (type D). American Journal of Human Genetics 30: 530–538

Wolfe L S, Ng Ying Kin N M K, Baker R R, Carpenter S, Anderman F 1977 Identification of retinoyl complexes as the autofluorescent component of the neuronal storage material in Batten disease. Science 195: 1360–1362

Wolfe L S, Ng Ying Kin N M K, Palo J, Haltia M 1983 Dolichols in brain and urinary sediment in neuronal ceroid lipofuscinosis. Neurology 33: 103–106

Yaffe M G et al 1979 An amyotrophic lateral sclerosis-like syndrome with hexosaminidase A deficiency: a new type of Gm$_2$-gangliosidosis. Neurology 29: 611

Young E, Wilson J, Patrick A D, Crome L 1972 Galactocerebrosidase deficiency in globoid cell leukodystrophy of late onset. Archives of Disease in Childhood 47: 449–450

Zimran A, Gross E, West C et al 1989 Prediction of severity of Gaucher's disease by identification of mutations at DNA level. Lancet ii: 349–352

Zokaeem G, Bayleran J, Kaplan P, Hechtman P, Neufeld E F 1987 A shortened β-hexosaminidase α-chain in an Italian patient with infantile Tay-Sachs disease. American Journal of Human Genetics 40: 537–547.

104. The peroxisomal disorders

R. B. H. Schutgens   H. S. A. Heymans   R. J. A. Wanders

INTRODUCTION

Considerable progress has been achieved in recent years in our understanding of the important role of peroxisomes in essential metabolic functions in human cells. It also has become clear that dysfunction of peroxisomes can have serious clinical consequences.

Since 1983 it has been found in a growing number of genetic disorders that there is a relation between disease and peroxisomal dysfunction.

The term 'peroxisomal disorders' was introduced by Goldfischer and Reddy (1984) to describe this newly recognized group of genetic diseases resulting from either a general or a more limited impairment of peroxisomal functions. In this chapter we will first summarize present knowledge about the role of peroxisomes in human cellular metabolism; subsequently the clinical and biochemical characteristics of the different peroxisomal disorders, the biochemical procedures used in prenatal and postnatal diagnosis, the outcome of studies on the genetic relationship between the different peroxisomal diseases and perspectives for treatment will be described in more detail.

PEROXISOMES

Peroxisomes (microbodies) are subcellular organelles bounded by a single lipid trilayer membrane surrounding a granular matrix of soluble proteins. First described by Rhodin (1954) in a morphological study of the mouse kidney, peroxisomes were later found to be widely distributed in eukaryotic organisms and appear to be ubiquitous both in plant and mammalian cells, including cultured skin fibroblasts and nervous tissue (Tolbert & Yamazaki 1969, Hruban et al 1972, Novikoff et al 1973, Böck et al 1980, Holtzmann 1982, Arias et al 1985). The number and size of peroxisomes in mammalian tissues vary considerably, being plentiful in gluconeogenic cells (liver and kidney), steroid secreting cells (adrenal cortex), sebaceous cells, myelin-forming cells and many cells of the digestive tract, and relatively rare in smooth muscle and fibroblasts. The use of alkaline 3,3'-diamino-benzidine (DAB) makes it possible to stain peroxisomes for light and electron microscopy (Fahimi 1968, Novikoff & Goldfischer 1969). Besides this cytochemical procedure, peroxisomes can also be identified by immuno-cytochemical procedures which utilize either the peroxidase-labelled Fab fragments of the antibodies raised against peroxisomal enzymes (Reddy et al 1981, Yokota et al 1987) or the protein A-gold method (Bendayan & Reddy 1982). Normally new peroxisomes appear to form by division of pre-existing peroxisomes. This has been visualised most clearly in methanol-grown yeast (Osumi et al 1975). Sometimes mammalian peroxisomes are interconnected in a peroxisome reticulum (Lazarow & Moser 1989). An extreme example of this is demonstrated in the mouse preputial gland by Gorgas (1984) who found that all the peroxisomes within a cell are interconnected. In these cells, new peroxisomes appear to form by budding from the pre-existing peroxisome. No information about this aspect is available for human cells.

Metabolic role of peroxisomes

Treatment of rodents with hypolipidaemic drugs like clofibrate, thyroid hormone, or certain plasticizers leads to a marked proliferation of peroxisomes and induction of certain peroxisomal enzymes (Lazarow 1977, Moody & Reddy 1977, Fringes & Reith 1980, Reddy et al 1987).

Biochemically, peroxisomes were initially characterized by de Duve and Baudhuin (1966) who demonstrated that organelles enriched in urate oxidase, D-aminoacid oxidase and catalase could be isolated from rat liver. These organelles, for which the term peroxisomes was introduced, were subsequently found to contain many other flavin oxidases, accepting L-a-hydroxyacids, D- and L-aminoacids, fatty acyl-CoA esters, polyamines (Höltta 1977), glutaryl-CoA and oxalate as substrates (RH2) and producing hydrogen peroxide as a reaction product. The hydrogen peroxide produced is sub-

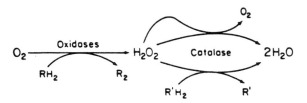

Fig. 104.1 Peroxisomal respiratory pathway (from De Duve & Baudhuin 1966).

sequently reduced by catalase to water by either a peroxidatic or catalitic mechanism depending upon the availability of substrates (R′H2) like alcohol, formate, nitrite and quinones (Fig. 104.1). These reactions of peroxisomal respiration may be responsible for as much as 20% of the oxygen consumption of the liver. Energy originating from these oxidative peroxisomal processes is not conserved as ATP but contributes to thermogenesis (De Duve & Baudhuin 1966). Peroxisomes of brown adipose tissue are strikingly induced during cold adaptation (Nedergaard et al 1980). More recently discovered biochemical functions in mammalian peroxisomes are in the β-oxidation of (very) long chain fatty acids (Lazarow & de Duve 1976) including the very long chain saturated fatty acids lignoceric acid (C24:0) and hexacosanoic acid (C26:0) (Singh et al 1984, Wanders et al 1987a,b), the biosynthesis of ether linked glycerolipids (Hajra & Bishop 1982), biosynthesis of bile acids (see Schutgens et al 1986), purine catabolism (Lazarow 1982), ethanol detoxification (Thurman & McKenna 1974), glyoxylate metabolism (Noguchi & Takada 1979), the conversion of gluconeogenic amino-acids to their corresponding keto acids, catabolism of dicarboxylic acids (Mortensen et al 1983), L-pipecolic acid (Read 1987, Trijbels et al 1987), dolichol metabolism (Appelkvist & Dallner 1987), oxidation of prostaglandins (Diczfalusy et al 1987) and most probably in phytanic acid oxidation. Krisans et al (1987) found that in rat liver 3-hydroxy-3-methylglutaryl-CoA reductase, a key regulatory enzyme in cholesterol biosynthesis, is not only an enzyme located in the endoplasmic reticulum (Brown & Goldstein 1980), but also in peroxisomes. The role of this cholestyramine inducable peroxisomal activity remains to be elucidated. Several excellent reviews have provided a more detailed account of the enzymic composition and the general properties of peroxisomes in different cell types (Böck et al 1980, Tolbert 1981, Lazarow 1982, De Duve 1983, Fahimi & Sies 1987).

CLINICAL CHARACTERISTICS

The absence of peroxisomes in hepatocytes and renal proximal tubules in cerebro-hepato-renal (Zellweger) syndrome (ZS), first described by Goldfischer et al (1973) formed the beginning of an extensive study of clinical and biochemical characteristics of genetic diseases that were recognised as peroxisomal disorders. A tentative classification scheme for this group of diseases is presented in Table 104.1

Group 1: Disorders with a general impairment of peroxisomal functions with severely reduced number of peroxisomes

Zellweger syndrome (McKusick 21410)

This is usually a lethal disease with severe clinical, pathological and biochemical abnormalities, including a typical craniofacial dysmorphism and neuronal migration disturbances present at birth. From these phenomena we can conclude that the deterioration in this autosomal recessive disease starts prenatally, an important consideration with respect to treatment (see later). The 'classic' type of ZS is characterized by the association of: (1) dysmorphogenesis (Fig. 104.2); (2) severe neurological dysfunction; (3) neurosensory defects; (4) regressive changes; (5) renal cysts and calcific stippling; (6) failure to thrive and early death; and (7) absence of recognizable liver peroxisomes (see Kelly 1983, Schutgens et al 1986, 1987, Monnens & Heymans 1987, Lazarow & Moser 1989) (Table 104.2).

At least 150 patients with a worldwide distribution have been described. Danks et al (1975) postulated that the incidence is about 1 in 100 000 live births. However, before specific biochemical diagnostic procedures were available, many patients probably died in early life without proper diagnosis. From our own experience during recent years we conclude that in the Netherlands the incidence is at least 1 in 40 000 live births.

Next to this 'classic' type of ZS a growing number of ZS patients with a milder phenotype of the disease are recognized (Barth et al 1985, 1987, Bleeker-Wagemakers et al 1986, Holmes et al 1987). The main clinical features in these patients, ranging in age from 3–16 years, are moderate to severe pyschomotor retardation, tapetoretinal degeneration, sensorineural deafness, hepatomegaly and absence of recognizable peroxisomes in liver. Biochemically these patients show a generalized peroxisomal dysfunction and cannot be differentiated from classic ZS.

Infantile Refsum Disease (IRD)

Patients with this disease share many clinical features with ZS, but they differ from the classic type of ZS with respect to age of onset, initial symptoms, degree of dysfunction and survival (Poll-Thé et al 1987a,b). Only about 10 patients have been described so far.

Table 104.1   Classification of peroxisomal disorders

Group 1. General impairment of peroxisomal functions with severely reduced number of peroxisomes in all cell types.
    a. Zellweger (cerebro-hepato-renal) syndrome (classic type, milder type)
    b. Infantile Refsum disease
    c. Neonatal adrenoleucodystrophy
    d. Hyperpipecolic acidaemia
Group 2. Activities of multiple peroxisomal enzymes are deficient with variable number of peroxisomes in liver.
    a. Rhizomelic chondrodysplasia punctata
    b. Zellweger-like syndrome
Group 3. Deficiency of only a single peroxisomal enzyme and normal number of peroxisomes in all cell types.
    a. (i) X–linked adrenoleucodystrophy
       (ii) X–linked adrenomyeloneuropathy
    b. Adult-type Refsum (phytanic acid storage) disease
    c. Primary hyperoxaluria type I
    d. Zellweger variants
       (i) Peroxisomal acyl-CoA oxidase deficiency (= pseudo neonatal adrenoleucodystrophy)
       (ii) Bifunctional enzyme deficiency
       (iii) Peroxisomal thiolase deficiency (= pseudo Zellweger syndrome)
       (iv) Others
    e. Acatalasia

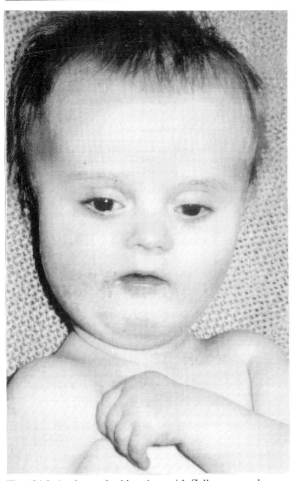

Fig. 104.2 An 8-month-old patient with Zellweger syndrome.

Initially this disorder was placed in relation to the adult form of Refsum (phytanic acid storage) disease (Scotto et al 1982) because both disorders show an accumulation of phytanic acid in serum and in mesenchymal and parenchymal liver cells due to a deficiency of phytanic acid α-oxidation. However, later studies have shown that IRD patients lack liver peroxisomes and show the same panel of peroxisomal enzyme defects as Zellweger and neonatal adrenoleucodystrophy patients, thus differing fundamentally from adult Refsum disease both in clinical and biochemical features (Table 104.2). Complementation analyses with cultured fibroblasts from IRD and ZS patients support the hypothesis that IRD and mild ZS are both clinically and biochemically indistinguishable (Tager et al 1987).

Neonatal adrenoleucodystrophy (NALD, McKusick 20237)

This is an autosomal recessive disease with many points of resemblance to ZS (Table 104.2, Kelly et al 1986). In general, patients with NALD are clinically slightly less profoundly affected than ZS patients. They live longer, dysmorphic features are milder and occasionally absent, and they do not have renal cortical cysts and calcific stippling of the bones. Complementation studies with cultured fibroblasts from NALD and ZS patients have demonstrated mutual correction of the defect in plasmalogen synthesis (Tager et al 1987) and in other biochemical phenomena like catalase latency (Brul et al 1988).

Hyperpipecolic acidaemia (HPA, MuKusick 23940)

This has been reported in only seven patients; in three

hyperpipecolic acidaemia was associated with Joubert syndrome (Poll-Thé et al 1987a). In some patients the disease is characterized by minor dysmorphic features, hypotonia, neurological dysfunction, neurosensory deficit and hepatomegaly. Studies of plasma, cultured fibroblasts or postmortem tissue have demonstrated the same morphological and biochemical defects as in ZS and NALD. Complementation studies with cultured fibroblasts from an HPA patient, described by Thomas et al (1975), and ZS patients have revealed that they do not mutually correct the peroxisomal defects; it is therefore questionable whether HPA is distinct from ZS.

Group 2: Disorders with a deficiency of multiple peroxisomal enzymes and variable number of peroxisomes

Several distinct forms of genetically caused chondrodysplasia punctata have been described. In 1971, Spranger and co-workers described two major types: the rhizomelic type with an autosomal recessive mode of inheritance (McKusick 21510) and the Conradi-Hünermann type (McKusick 11865) with autosomal dominant inheritance. Clinical characteristics of the rhizomelic type are dwarfism, severe symmetrical shortening of the proximal extremities, flat face, congenital cataracts, bone changes, multiple joint contractures, and severe psychomotor retardation (Table 104.2). The epiphyseal and extra-epiphyseal calcifications are symmetrical and usually severe. Other radiological findings are the marked metaphyseal changes and coronal cleft of the vertebral bodies. It is described that most patients die before the age of 2 years; in our experience with 14 rhizomelic chondrodysplasia punctata (RCDP) patients survival is much longer, as only two patients died in the first year of life, while the others vary in age from 11 months to 18 years (average 6 years 10 months).

A third form of chondrodysplasia punctata has been described exclusively in female patients with presumed lethality in the affected male fetus (Happle 1979). This suggests an X–linked dominant mode of inheritance.

Finally, a fourth type has been recognized in which chondrodysplasia occurred in a pattern consistent with an X-linked recessive mode of inheritance (Curry et al 1984).

So far peroxisomal abnormalities have only been found in the rhizomelic type of chondrodysplasia punctata (RCDP).

Electron microscopic studies of needle biopsy material of liver from two RCDP patients revealed a variable number of irregularly shaped peroxisomes (Heymans et al 1986).

Zellweger-like syndrome is another disorder belonging to this group (Suzuki et al 1988).

Group 3: Deficiency of only a single peroxisomal enzyme with normal number of peroxisomes.

X–linked adrenoleucodystrophy (X-ALD, McKusick 30010)

This should be considered in any prepubertal boy who displays changes in behaviour and progressive deterioration of intellectual functions, vision and gait. This will be followed by central deafness, spastic quadraparesis or hemiplegia evolving to a variable degree of decorticate posturing and usually death during adolescence (Table 104.2). The main pathological feature is a demyelinating process that resembles multiple sclerosis. Axons may be involved in the advanced stage of the disease. The phenotype of X-ALD is varied, ranging from the severe childhood form described above to a milder adult variant, referred to as adrenomyeloneuropathy (AMN). Some persons with the biochemical defect seem to remain asymptomatic (Moser & Moser 1989). Most females heterozygous for X-ALD are asymptomatic, but some present with a chronic nonprogressive spinal cord syndrome, suggesting that the diagnosis of symptomatic ALD carrier status should be considered in women with evidence of white matter disease (Noetzel et al 1987).

Adult Refsum (phytanic acid storage) disease (McKusick 26650)

This is a rare autosomal recessive disorder affecting adults. In most patients this disease is clinically characterized by peripheral neuropathy, ataxia, retinitis pigmentosa and nerve deafness (Table 104.2, Steinberg 1989). Whether adult Refsum disease can be classified as a peroxisomal disorder is still controversial as it is not yet clear whether phytanic acid α-oxidation activity, the deficient metabolic activity in this disease, is a peroxisomal or a mitochondrial activity in human liver. However, phytanic acid oxidase is deficient in all peroxisomal disorders listed in groups 1 and 2.

Primary hyperoxaluria type 1 (McKusick 25990)

This is a rare genetic disorder of glyoxylate metabolism. Patients usually present during the first decade of life with recurrent calcium oxalate nephrolithiasis and nephrocalcinosis. Considerable heterogeneity is noticed within the disorder, with some patients presenting with only minimal renal damage and others showing an acute neonatal form with rapid progression and early death (Williams & Smith 1983).

Zellweger variants

This is the name used to cover a growing number of patients with many clinical features similar to ZS, but with abundant liver peroxisomes. Detailed studies in a limited number of patients revealed defects at different levels in peroxisomal β-oxidation of (very) long chain fatty acids and/or bile acids. In the patient described by Goldfischer et al (1986) as pseudo-ZS with a clinical presentation very similar to 'classic' ZS, the defect was found to be limited to the level of peroxisomal 3-ketoacyl-CoA thiolase only, while the activities of the other peroxisomal fatty acid oxidation enzymes and the peroxisomal enzymes of plasmalogen metabolism were normal (Schram et al 1987). In another patient, described as pseudo-NALD, the defect was identified at the level of a deficient peroxisomal acyl-CoA oxidase (Poll-Thé et al 1988). The latter patient displayed no dysmorphia and showed a clinical presentation similar to that observed in NALD. Recently a patient with peroxisomal bifunctional enzyme deficiency has been described (Watkins et al 1989). Much can be learned from these patients about the pathophysiology in ZS and NALD respectively. Other patients belonging to this group were described by Clayton et al (1987); at least ten others are known (Schutgens et al 1988a).

Acatalasia (McKusick 11550)

This is described in different patients with varying degrees of catalase deficiency. No pathological lesions except for gangrenous oral lesions have been reported in human acatalasia. Peroxisomes or the peroxisomal localization of the residual catalase activity have not been examined specifically in acatalatic subjects.

Table 104.2 Clinical and morphological characteristics of main peroxisomal disorders

	Zellweger syndrome		Neonatal ALD	RCDP	X-linked ALD	Adult Refsum
	at birth	*after 6 months*				
Craniofacial features						
High forehead	+++	+	++	++	−	−
Wide open fontanels/sutures	+++	+	++	−	−	−
Epicanthus	+++	++	++	+++	−	−
External ear deformities	+++	+++	++	−	−	−
High arched palate	+++	+++	++	−	−	−
Neurological manifestations						
Psychomotor retardation	++	+++	+	+++	progressive	−
Hypotonia	+++	+++	+++	++	−	−
Hypo-/areflexia	+++	+	++		−	++
Seizures/abnormal EEG	+	++	+++		++	−
Hearing impairment	+++	+++	+++	++	+	++
Neurological deterioration	−	−	++		+++	++
Neuronal migration defects	+++	+++	++		−	−
White matter degeneration	++	++	+++		+++	−
Ocular abnormalities						
Cataract	++	++	+	+++	−	++
Chorioretinopathy	+++	+++	+++	++	−	+++
Optic nerve dysplasia	+++	+++	+++	++	++	+
Liver abnormalities						
Hepatomegaly	+	++	++	−	−	−
Fibrosis/cirrhosis	+	++	++	−	−	−
Peroxisomal absence/decrease	+++	+++	+++	−	−	−
Lamellar inclusions	++	+++	+++		−	−
Other manifestations						
Renal cysts	+++	+++	−	−	−	−
Adrenal atrophy	+	++	+++	−	+++	−
Cryptorchidism/Clitoromegaly	++	++	++	−	−	−
Chondrodysplasia calcificans	+	+	−	+++	−	−
Synacthen test abnormal	++	++	++		+++	−

+++ very frequently present; ++ frequently present; + sometimes present; − absent.
EEG = electroencephalogram; ALD = adrenoleucodystrophy; RCDP = rhizomelic chondrodysplasia punctata.

BIOCHEMICAL OBSERVATIONS

Diagnostic procedures

Patients with a generalized peroxisomal disorder show absence of recognizable peroxisomes in the liver (Goldfischer et al 1973, Roels et al 1986, Kelly et al 1986). In addition, catalase activity in liver biopsy samples or in cultured skin fibroblasts is found in the cytosol rather than in subcellular organelles (Wanders et al 1984). This represents a way of demonstrating the absence of integral peroxisomal structure and is also of value as a diagnostic assay. Moreover, patients with a generalised peroxisomal disorder (group 1) show a set of biochemical abnormalities which are presumed to be secondary to the defective peroxisome structure. These include impairment of the metabolism of very long chain fatty acids (VLCFA), pipecolic acid, intermediates of bile acid biosynthesis, phytanic acid and defects in the biosynthesis of plasmalogens, resulting in specific abnormalities in plasma, tissues and or cultured fibroblasts (see Schutgens et al 1986, Moser & Moser 1989) (Table 104.3). Amniocytes or chorionic villus samples can be used for prenatal diagnosis (Moser et al 1984, Poll-Thé et al 1987c, Schutgens et al 1989).

Diagnostic tests include measurement of acyl CoA: dihydroxyacetone phosphate acyltransferase (DHAP-AT) activity in blood platelets, and fibroblasts (Schutgens et al 1984, 1989), of the de novo plasmalogen biosynthesis in skin fibroblasts, amniocytes or chorionic villus

fibroblasts, intracellular localization of catalase in fibroblasts or amniocytes, detection of the phytanic acid, tri(di)hydroxycoprostanoic acid and/or VLCFA levels in plasma and of peroxisomal β-oxidation activity with lignoceric acid (C24:0) or hexacosanoic acid (C26:0) as a substrate in fibroblasts or amniocytes. Limited screening tests in blood(cells) can be done in as little as 2 ml of EDTA-blood; subsequently a more detailed biochemical study can be done in fibroblasts. Urine can be analyzed for elevated pipecolic acid levels and for abnormal bile acids.

Heterozygote detection is not possible, probably reflecting the fact that these biochemical changes are secondary to an as yet unidentified primary biochemical defect or defects at the level of the biogenesis of peroxisomes (see below).

Rhizomelic chondrodysplasia

This is biochemically characterized by a deficiency of the peroxisomal key enzymes in plasmalogen biosynthesis, DHAP-AT and alkyl DHAP synthase, phytanic acid α-oxidation activity (Heymans et al 1986, Schutgens et al 1988b, Table 104.3) and by a lack of maturation of peroxisomal thiolase enzyme protein (Hoefler et al 1988, Heikoop et al 1990). The peroxisomal β-oxidation system is undisturbed. Diagnostic tests for RCDP include measurement of DHAP-AT activity in blood platelets, fibro-

Table 104.3   Biochemical characteristics of the main peroxisomal disorders

Parameter	Zellweger syndrome	Refsum disease		ALD		RCDP
		infantile	adult	neonatal	X-linked	
Metabolites in plasma						
Very long-chain fatty acids (C_{26}/C_{22} ratio)	↑↑	↑	n	↑↑	↑	n
Pipecolic acid	↑↑/↑	↑	n	↑	n	n
Intermediates of bile acid biosynthesis (THCA/DHCA)	↑	↑	n	↑	n	n
Phytanic acid	↑/↑↑	↑	↑↑	↑	n	↑↑
Enzyme activities (tissue/fibroblasts)						
DHAP-AT	↓↓	↓	n	↓	n	↓
Alkyl DHAP synthase	↓	↓	n	↓	n	↓
Catalase						
total	n	n	n	n	n	n
% particulate	<5	<5	n	<5	n	n
Plasmalogens (tissues/fibroblasts)						
Content	↓	↓	n	↓	n	↓
De novo biosynthesis	↓↓	↓	n	↓	n	↓↓
Peroxisomal β-oxidation activity						
Palmitic ($C_{16:0}$) acid	↓	↓	n	↓	n	n
Hexacosanoic ($C_{26:0}$) acid	↓	↓	n	↓	↓	n

↑↑ = severely elevated; ↑ = elevated; ↓ = decreased; ↓↓ = severely decreased; n = normal.

blasts, amniocytes or chorionic villus samples, analysis of the de novo plasmalogen biosynthesis in fibroblasts, measurement of the plasma phytanic acid level and the detection of the decreased plasmalogen level in erythrocytes, amniocytes or chorionic villus samples.

Heterozygotes for RCDP cannot be recognized biochemically.

X-ALD/AMN

This can be diagnosed postnatally and prenatally by demonstrating increased VLCFA levels in plasma (Moser et al 1984a), cultured skin fibroblasts or amniocytes (Moser et al 1982, Singh et al 1984b), or by demonstrating the impaired hexacosanoic acid (C26:0) β-oxidation in liver, cultured skin fibroblasts or chorionic villus fibroblasts from patients (Table 104.3, Wanders et al 1987c).

The ALD gene has been localized to the q28 segment of the X chromosome (Migeon et al 1981). Linkage has been established between ALD and a cloned DNA probe (St14) providing the possibility of first trimester prenatal diagnosis of X-ALD by linkage analysis (Boué et al 1985).

Most, but not all female heterozygotes for X-ALD can be recognised biochemically by determination of elevated VLCFA levels in plasma or cultured skin fibroblasts (Moser et al 1983, Moser & Moser 1989).

Adult Refsum disease

This can be recognized biochemically by detecting severely decreased phytanic acid oxidase activity in cultured fibroblasts or more easily, by detecting elevated phytanic acid levels in plasma from affected individuals (Steinberg 1989).

Hyperoxaluria type I

Patients with this disease can be identified by elevated urinary excretion of oxalate and glycolate (see Williams & Smith 1983). A more specific diagnostic test is the detection of deficient activity of the peroxisomal enzyme alanine: glyoxylate aminotransferase, in liver samples from patients (Danpure & Jennings 1986, Wanders et al 1987d). Unfortunately this enzyme activity is not expressed in cultured fibroblasts or amniocytes, preventing the use of these cells in the prenatal diagnosis of the severe neonatal type of the disease.

Primary biochemical defect

Immunoblot studies have shown that livers, kidneys and fibroblasts from ZS patients lack the immunoreactive proteins of peroxisomal acyl-CoA oxidase, bifunctional protein and 3-ketoacyl-CoA oxidase (Tager et al 1985, Suzuki et al 1986a). The deficiency of these enzymes accounts for the accumulation of VLCFA in the generalized peroxisomal disorders (Table 104.3), since this peroxisomal oxidation is required for VLCFA oxidation. Pulse-labelling studies in fibroblasts from ZS and IRD patients have shown that precursors of acyl-CoA oxidase and peroxisomal thiolase enzyme proteins are formed normally on free ribosomes in the cytoplasm, but their maturation is impaired, resulting in rapid degradation (Schram et al 1986, Suzuki et al 1986b). Indirect evidence indicates that this also includes the first two enzymes in the biosynthesis of plasmalogens, DHAP-AT and alkyl-DHAP synthase. However, biosynthesis and stability of catalase is normal in ZS fibroblasts. It is assumed that the primary biochemical lesion in the genetic disorders of group 1 (ZS, IRD, NALD, HPA) is at the level of a not yet defined essential peroxisomal membrane protein, or of a protein essential for the transfer of newly synthesized peroxisomal enzymes from the cytoplasm into the peroxisomes. Absence of peroxisomal structure, or a defect in the machinery for importing matrix proteins into the peroxisomal membrane, results in abnormally rapid degradation of some, but not all, peroxisomal enzyme proteins. This accounts for the multiple enzyme defects in the generalized peroxisomal disorders. All biochemical abnormalities observed in these diseases must therefore be considered to be secondary to this phenomenon; it is also clear that heterozygotes do not exhibit these biochemical abnormalities as stable peroxisomes are present in their cells. Progress has been made recently in studies on the biogenesis of peroxisomes (Lazarow 1987, Santos et al 1988), but the exact nature of the biochemical defect in ZS and related disorders has not yet been clarified.

In RCDP, liver immunoblotting experiments have shown that the different peroxisomal β-oxidation enzyme proteins are normally present with the exception of the peroxisomal thiolase protein which is only present in its 44 kDa precursor form.

Presumably this phenomenon has no effect on the overall in vivo peroxisomal β-oxidation capacity since there is no accumulation of very long chain fatty acids in RCDP patients. In contrast, severe abnormalities were found in the activities of DHAP-AT and alkyl DHAP synthase and in phytanic acid metabolism. The observation that there is a normal intracellular localization of catalase in RCDP fibroblasts indicates that at least in this type of cell peroxisomes are normally present. The finding of multiple biochemical abnormalities in RCDP, and the normal results in the obligate heterozygotes, suggest that these abnormalities are secondary phenomena resulting from an underlying defect which remains to be elucidated. We can only speculate that this primary lesion can be at the level of a specific receptor at the peroxisomal membrane or of a protein that is normally active in the intracellular transport or the import of a specific group of newly synthesized peroxisomal enzymes.

The primary defect in X-ALD/AMN has recently been identified. Following a suggestion by Hashmi et al (1986), Wanders et al (1987b) obtained direct evidence that the defect in X-ALD is at the level of a deficient peroxisomal very long chain fatty acyl-CoA synthetase activity. This explains the accumulation of VLCFA in patients, and the earlier finding that X-ALD fibroblasts are not able to metabolize VLCFA, whereas the CoA-esters are degraded normally.

The primary defect in adult type Refsum disease has been located at the level of a deficient α-oxidative pathway for phytanic acid, involving an initial α-hydroxylation followed by decarboxylation to generate the 19-carbon homologue, pristanic acid (Steinberg 1989).

Primary hyperoxaluria type I results from a deficiency of peroxisomal alanine: glyoxylate aminotransferase (Danpure & Jennings 1986, Wanders et al 1987d). Recently we found that immunoreactive alanine:glyoxylate aminotransferase protein is absent in the liver of a patient with the severe neonatal type of the disorder (Wanders 1988).

Genetic relationship

Complementation analysis after somatic fusion of fibroblasts was used to investigate the genetic relationship between the various diseases in which there is a simultaneous impairment of several peroxisomal functions (groups 1 and 2). So far six different complementation groups have been found; one for RCDP; one for cell lines from ZS, IRD and HPA; one for another ZS cell line; two for NALD; and finally one for yet another ZS cell line (Roscher et al 1986, Brul et al 1988). It was concluded that substantial genetic heterogeneity exists within the group of peroxisomal disorders characterized by a generalized impairment of peroxisomal functions, even within the clinically relatively homogeneous ZS, and that mutations in different genes can lead to the same clinical and biochemical phenotype. Moreover, at least six genes are required for the assembly of a functional peroxisome.

TREATMENT

No effective treatment for the generalized peroxisomal disorders has been found. This is not surprising, bearing in mind that dysmorphogenesis, especially of the CNS, begins prenatally. Treatment of two ZS patients with the peroxisome proliferator clofibrate was ineffective as assessed biochemically, morphologically and clinically (Lazarow et al 1985). Dietary supplementation with 1-alkylglycerols was tried in two other ZS patients, both with a milder phenotype. It was observed that erythrocyte phosphoethanolamine plasmalogen composition returned to control levels, but clinical improvement seemed only limited (Holmes et al 1987).

In RCDP no effective treatment has been described. Theoretically, treatment by dietary supplementation with 1-alkylglycerols and restriction of phytanic acid intake is indicated.

Interest in testing a dietary approach to X-ALD stemmed from awareness of the clinical benefit produced in patients with adult Refsum disease when their phytanic acid intake was reduced (Steinberg 1989). This restriction of phytanic acid brings about normalization of plasma phytanic acid levels, improvement in peripheral nerve function, and stabilization of the retinal lesion and deficits resulting from central nervous system involvement. As Kishimoto et al (1980) demonstrated that a substantial percentage of the accumulated C26:0 in postmortem ALD brain was derived from food, a diet restricted in VLCFA and especially C26:0 was developed, but failed to reduce plasma C26:0 levels or cause clinical improvement (Moser et al 1987). Probably the explanation for this phenomenon is the fact that the C26:0 which accumulates in X-ALD is both of dietary and endogenous origin (Tsuji et al 1984). Subsequently Rizzo et al (1987) found that oleic acid (C18:1), and especially erucic acid (C22:1), reduced the rate of C26:0 synthesis in cultured skin fibroblasts from control subjects. This has led to dietary therapy in which dietary restriction of C26:0 is combined with measures aimed at lowering endogenous C26:0 synthesis by administration of C18:1 or C22:1 (Rizzo et al 1989). A substantial reduction of the plasma C26:0 levels in X-ALD patients was obtained with this regimen, but whether any clinical improvement can be obtained is still under investigation.

Theoretically the same approach can be followed in patients affected by ZS variants resulting from a defect in the peroxisomal β-oxidation system.

Treatment of hyperoxaluria type I is directed towards decreasing oxalate excretion by inhibition of oxalate synthesis, and towards increasing calcium oxalate solubility at a given urinary concentration of oxalate. Pyridoxine in large doses has been successful in reducing oxalate synthesis in some patients (see Williams & Smith 1983).

ACKNOWLEDGEMENTS

The authors' studies referred to in this paper were supported by grants from the Netherlands Organization for Pure Scientific Research (ZWO) under the auspices of the Netherlands Foundation for Medical and Health Research (MEDIGON) and the Princess Beatrix Fund (The Hague, The Netherlands). All studies were performed in close collaboration with Drs P.G. Barth, H. van den Bosch, A.W. Schram, J.M. Tager and Mrs G. Schrakamp.

REFERENCES

Appelkvist E L, Dallner G 1987 Dolichol metabolism and peroxisomes. In: Fahimi H D, Sies H (eds) Peroxisomes in biology and medicine. Springer, Berlin, p 53–66

Arias J A, Moser A B, Goldfischer S 1985 Ultrastructural and cytochemical demonstration of peroxisomes in cultured fibroblasts from patients with peroxisomal deficiency disorders. Journal of Cell Biology 100: 1789–1792

Barth P G, Schutgens R B H, Bakkeren J A J M, Dingemans K P, Heymans H S A, Douwes A C, van der Klei-van Moorsel J M 1985 A milder variant of Zellweger syndrome. European Journal of Pediatrics 144: 338–342

Barth P G, Schutgens R B H, Wanders R J A et al 1987 A sibship with a mild variant of Zellweger syndrome. Journal of Inherited Metabolic Disease 10: 253–259

Bendayan M, Reddy J K 1982 Immunocytochemical localization of catalase and heat-labile enoyl-CoA hydratase in the livers of normal and peroxisome proliferator-treated rats. Laboratory Investigations 47: 364–369

Bleeker-Wagemakers E M, Oorthuys J W E, Wanders R J A, Schutgens R B H 1986 Long term survival of a patient with the cerebro-hepato-renal (Zellweger) syndrome. Clinical Genetics 29: 160–164

Böck P, Kramar R, Pavelka R 1980 Peroxisomes and related particles in animal tissues. Cell Biology Monographs 71. Springer, Wien

Boue J, Oberle I, Heilig R et al 1985 First trimester prenatal diagnosis of adrenoleukodystrophy by determination of very long chain fatty acid levels and by linkage analysis to a DNA probe. Human Genetics 69: 272–274

Brown M S, Goldstein J L 1980 Multivalent feedback regulation of HMG-CoA reductase, a control mechanism coordinating isoprenoid synthesis and cell growth. Journal of Lipid Research 21: 505–517

Brul S, Westerveld A, Strijland A et al 1988 Genetic heterogeneity in the cerebro-hepato-renal (Zellweger) syndrome and other inherited disorders with a generalized impairment of peroxisomal functions: a study using complementation analysis. Journal of Clinical Investigation 81: 1710–1715

Clayton P T, Lake B D, Hjelm M et al 1987 Bile acid analyses in "pseudo-Zellweger" syndrome – clues to the defect in peroxisomal β-oxidation. Abstract of the 25th SSIEM annual symposium, Sheffield Abstract 0-4

Curry C J R, Magenis E, Brown M 1984 Inherited chondrodysplasia punctata due to a deletion of the terminal short arm of an X-chromosome. New England Journal of Medicine 311: 1010–1015

Danks D M, Tippett P, Adams C, Cambell O 1975 Cerebro-hepato-renal syndrome of Zellweger. A report of eight cases with comments upon the incidence, the liver lesion, and a fault in pipecolic acid metabolism. Journal of Pediatrics 86: 382–387

Danpure C J, Jennings P R 1986 Peroxisomal alanine: glyoxylate aminotransferase deficiency in primary hyperoxaluria type I. Federation of European Biochemical Societies Letters 201: 20–24

De Duve C 1983 Microbodies in the living cell. Scientific American, May Issue: 52–62

De Duve C, Baudhuin P 1966 Peroxisome (microbodies and related particles). Physiological Reviews 46: 323–357

Diczfalusy U, Alexon S E H, Pedersen J I 1987 Chain shortening of prostaglandin F2a by rat liver peroxisomes. Biochemical and Biophysical Research Communications 144: 1206–1213

Fahimi H D 1968 Cytochemical localization of peroxidase activity in rat hepatic microbodies (peroxisomes). Journal of Histochemistry and Cytochemistry 16: 547–550

Fahimi H D, Sies H (eds) 1987 Peroxisomes in biology and medicine. Springer, Berlin

Fringes B, Reith A 1980 The formation of microbodies (Mb) under triiodothyronine (T3) influence in rat liver. A serological study by electron microscopy. European Journal of Cell Biology 22: 166 Abstract M493

Goldfischer S, Reddy J K 1984 Peroxisomes (Microbodies) in Cell Pathology. International Review of Experimental Pathology 26: 45–84

Goldfischer S, Moore C L, Johnson A B et al 1973 Peroxisomal and mitochondrial defects in the cerebro-hepato-renal syndrome. Science 183: 62–64

Goldfischer S, Collins J, Rapin I et al 1986 Pseudo-Zellweger syndrome: deficiencies in several peroxisomal oxidative activities. Journal of Pediatrics 108: 25–32

Gorgas K 1984 Peroxisomes in sebaceous glands. V. Complex peroxisomes in the mouse preputial gland. Serial sectioning and three-dimensional reconstruction studies. Anatomical Embryology 169: 261–270

Hajra A K, Bishop J E 1982 Glycerolipid biosynthesis in peroxisomes via the acyl dihydroxy-acetone phosphate pathway. Annals of the New York Academy of Sciences 386: 170–182

Happle R 1979 X-linked dominant chondrodysplasia punctata: a review of literature and report of a case. Human Genetics 53: 65–73

Hashmi M, Stanley W, Singh I 1986 Lignoceroyl-CoASH ligase: enzyme defect in fatty acid β-oxidation in X-linked adrenoleukodystrophy. Federation of European Biochemical Societies Letters 196: 247–250

Heikoop J C, Just W W, van Roermund C W T et al 1990 Deficiency in peroxisomes and impaired processing of 3-oxoacyl-CoA thiolase in rhizomelic chondrodysplasia punctata. Journal of Clinical Investigation (in press)

Heymans H S A, Oorthuys J W E, Nelck G, Wanders R J A, Dingemans K P, Schutgens R B H 1986 Peroxisomal abnormalities in rhizomelic chondrodysplasia punctata. Journal of Inherited Metabolic Disease 9 (suppl 2): 329–331

Hoefler G, Hoefler S, Watkins P A et al 1988 Biochemical abnormalities in rhizomelic chondrodysplasia punctata. Journal of Pediatrics 112: 726–733

Holmes R D, Wilson G, Hajra A 1987 Oral ether lipid therapy in patients with peroxisomal disorders. Journal of Inherited Metabolic Disease 10 (suppl 2): 239–241

Höltta E 1977 Oxidation of spermidine and spermine in rat liver: purification and properties of polyamine oxidase. Biochemistry 16: 91–100

Holtzmann E 1982 Peroxisomes in nervous tissue. Annals of the New York Academy of Sciences. 386: 523–525

Hruban Z, Vigil E L, Slsers A, Hopkins E 1972 Microbodies: constituent organelles of animal cells. Laboratory Investigation 27: 184–191

Kelly R I 1983 Review: the cerebro-hepato-renal syndrome of Zellweger, morphologic and metabolic aspects. American Journal of Medical Genetics 16: 503–517

Kelly R I, Datta N S, Dobyns W B 1986 Neonatal adrenoleukodystrophy: new cases, biochemical studies, and differentiation from Zellweger and related peroxisomal polydystrophy syndromes. American Journal of Medical Genetics 23: 869–901

Kishimoto Y, Moser H W, Kawamura N et al 1980 Adrenoleukodystrophy: evidence that abnormal very long chain fatty acids of brain cholestrol esters are of exogenous origin. Biochemical and Biophysical Research Communications 96: 69–76

Krisans S K, Pazirandeh M, Keller G A 1987 Localisation of 3-hydroxy-3-methyl-glutaryl-coenzyme A reductase in rat liver peroxisomes. In: Fahimi H D, Sies H (eds) Peroxisomes in biology and medicine. Springer, Berlin, p 40–52

Lazarow P B 1977 Three hypolipidemic drugs increase hepatic palmityol-coenzyme A oxidation in the rat. Science 197: 580–581

Lazarow P B 1982 Peroxisomes. In: Arias I, Popper H, Schachter D, Shafitz D A (eds) Liver: biology and pathology. Raven Press, New York, p 27–39

Lazarow P B 1987 The role of peroxisomes in mammalian cellular metabolism. Journal of Inherited Metabolic Disease 10 (Suppl 1): 11–22

Lazarow P B, de Duve C 1976 A fatty acyl-CoA oxidizing system in rat liver peroxisomes: enhancement by clofibrate, a hypolipidemic drug. Proceedings of the National Academy of Sciences USA 73: 2043–2046

Lazarow P B, Moser H W 1989 Disorders of peroxisome biogenesis. In: Scriver C R, Beaudet A L, Sly W S, Valle D (eds) The metabolic basis of inherited disease, 6th edn. McGraw-Hill, New York, p 1479–1509

Lazarow P B, Black V, Shio H et al 1985 Zellweger syndrome: biochemical and morphological studies on two patients treated with clofibrate. Pediatric Research 19: 1356–1364

McKusick V A 1988 Mendelian inheritance in man, 8th edn. Johns Hopkins University Press, Baltimore

Migeon B R, Moser H W, Moser A B, Axelman J, Sillence D, Norum R A 1981 Adreno-leukodystrophy: evidence for X-linkage in activation and selection favoring the mutant allele in heterozygous cells. Proceedings of the National Academy of Sciences USA 72: 5066–5070

Monnens L, Heymans H S A 1987 Peroxisomal disorders: clinical characterization. Journal of Inherited Metabolic Disease 10 (Suppl 1): 23–32

Moody D E, Reddy J K 1977 Hepatic peroxisomes (microbody) proliferation in rats fed plasticizers and related compounds. Toxicological Applied Pharmacology 45: 497–505

Mortensen P B, Gregersen N, Rasmussen K 1983 The β-oxidation of dicarboxylic acids in isolated mitochondria and peroxisomes. Journal of Inherited Metabolic Disease 6 (Suppl 2): 123–124

Moser H W 1986 Peroxisomal disorders. Journal of Pediatrics 108: 89–91

Moser H W, Moser A B 1989 Adrenoleucodystrophy (X-linked). In: Scriver C R, Beaudet A L, Sly W S, Valle D (eds) The metabolic basis of inherited disease, 6th edn. McGraw-Hill, New York, p 1511–1532

Moser H W, Moser A B, Powers J M, Nitowski H M, Schaumburg H H, Norum R A, Migeon B R 1982 The prenatal diagnosis of adrenoleukodystrophy. Demonstration of increased hexacosanoic acid levels in cultured amniocytes and fetal adrenal gland. Pediatric Research 16: 172–175

Moser H W, Moser A E, Trojak J E et al 1983 Identification of female carriers of adrenoleukodystrophy. Journal of Pediatrics 103: 54–59

Moser H W, Moser A R, Singh I, O'Neill B P 1984a Adrenoleukodystrophy: survey of 303 cases: biochemistry, diagnosis and therapy. Annals of Neurology 16: 628–641

Moser A E, Singh I, Brown F R III, Solish G I, Kelley R I, Benke P J, Moser H W 1984b The cerebro-hepato-renal (Zellweger) syndrome. Increased levels and impaired degradation of very long chain fatty acids and their use in prenatal diagnosis. The New England Journal of Medicine 310: 1141–1146

Moser A B, Borel J B, Odone A et al 1987 A new dietary therapy for adrenoleukodystrophy: biochemical and preliminary clinical results in 36 patients. Annals of Neurology 21: 240–249

Nedergaard J, Alexson S, Cannon B 1980 Cold adaptation in the rat: increased brown fat peroxisomal β-oxidation relative to maximal mitochondrial oxidative capacity. American Journal of Physiology 239: C208–C216

Noetzel M J, Landau W M, Moser H W 1987 Adrenoleukodystrophy carrier state presenting as a chronic non-progressive spinal cord disorder. Archives of Neurology 44: 566–567

Noguchi T, Takada Y 1979 Peroxisomal localization of alanine: glyoxylate aminotransferase in human liver. Archives of Biochemistry and Biophysics 196: 645–647

Novikoff A B, Goldfischer S 1969 Visualisation of peroxisomes (microbodes) and mitochrondria with diaminobenzidine. Journal of Histochemistry and Cytochemistry 17: 675–680

Novikoff A B, Novikoff P M, Davis C, Quintana J 1973 Are microperoxisomes ubiquitous in mammalian cells? Journal of Histochemistry and Cytochemistry 21: 737–755

Osumi M, Fuuzumi F, Terasshi Y, Tamaka A, Fukui S 1975 Development of microbodies in Candida tropicalis during incubation in a n-alkane medium. Archives of Microbiology 103: 1–11

Poll-Thé B T, Saudubray J M, Ogier H, Lombes A, Munnich A, Frézal J 1987a Clinical approach to inherited peroxisomal disorders. In: Vogel F, Sperling K (eds) Human Genetics, Proceedings of the 7th International Congress Berlin Springer, Berlin, p 345–351

Poll-Thé B T, Saudubray H M, Ogier H A M et al 1987b Infantile Refsum's disease: an inherited peroxisomal disorder; comparison with Zellweger syndrome and neonatal adrenoleukodystrophy. European Journal of Pediatrics 146: 477–483

Poll-Thé B T, Saudubray J M, Rocchiccioli F et al 1987c Prenatal diagnosis and confirmation of infantile Refsum's disease. Journal of Inherited Metabolic Disease 10 (Suppl 2): 229–232

Poll-Thé B T, Roels F, Ogier H et al 1988 A new peroxisomal disorder with enlarged peroxisomes and a specific deficiency of acyl-CoA oxidase (pseudo neonatal adrenoleukodystrophy). American Journal of Human Genetics 42: 422–434

Read W 1987 Personal communication

Reddy J K, Rao M S, Lalwani N D, Reddy M K, Nemali M R, Alvares K 1987 Induction of hepatic peroxisome proliferation by Xenobiotics. In: Fahimi H D, Sies H (eds) Peroxisomes in biology and medicine. Springer, Berlin, p 255–263

Reddy M K, Qureshi S A, Hollenberg P F, Reddy J 1981 Immunochemical identity of peroxisomal enoyl-CoA hydratase with the peroxisome-proliferation-associated 80 000 mol wt polypeptide in rat liver. Journal of Cell Biology 89: 406–417

Rhodin J 1954 Correlation of ultrastructural organisation and function in normal and experimentally changed proximal tubule cells of the mouse kidney. Doctoral thesis, Karolinska Institute, Stockholm, Aktiebolaget Godvil p 76

Rizzo W B, Phillips M W, Dammann A L et al 1987 Adrenoleukodystrophy: dietary oleic acid lowers hexacosanoate levels. Annals of Neurology 21: 232–239

Rizzo W B, Leshner R T, Odone R et al 1989 Dietary erucic acid therapy for X-linked adrenoleucodystrophy. Neurology 39: 1415–1422

Roels F, Cornelis A, Poll-Thé B T, Aubourg P, Ogier H, Scotto J, Saudubray J M 1986 Hepatic peroxisomes are deficient in infantile Resum disease: A cytochemical study of 4 cases. American Journal of Medical Genetics 25: 257–271

Roscher A, Höfler S, Höfler G, Paschke E, Paltanf F 1986 Neonatal adrenoleukodystrophy (NALD) and cerebro hepato renal syndrome (CHRS): Genetic complementation analysis of impaired peroxisomal plasmalogen biosynthesis. Abstracts 24th Annual SSIEM Meeting, Amersfoort, Abstract 03

Santos M J, Imanaka T, Shio H, Small G M, Lazarow P B 1988 Peroxisomal membrane ghosts in Zellweger syndrome-aberrant organelle assembly. Science 239: 1536–1538

Schram A W, Strijland A, Hashimoto T, Wanders R J A, Schutgens R B H, van den Bosch H, Tager J M 1986 Biosynthesis and maturation of peroxisomal β-oxidation enzymes in fibroblasts in relation to the Zellweger syndrome and infantile Refsum disease. Proceeding of the National Academy of Sciences USA 83: 6156–6158

Schram A W, Goldfischer S, van Roermund C W T et al 1987 Human peroxisomal 3-oxoacyl-coenzyme A thiolase deficiency. Proceedings of the National Academy of Sciences USA 84: 2494–2496

Schutgens R B H, Romeijn G J, Wanders R J A, van den Bosch H, Schrakamp G, Heymans H S A 1984 Deficiency of acyl-CoA: dihydroxy-acetone phosphate acyltransferase in patients with Zellweger (cerebro-hepato-renal) syndrome. Biochemical and Biophysical Research Communications 120: 179–184

Schutgens R B H, Heymans H S A, Wanders R J A, van den Bosch H, Tager J M 1986 Peroxisomal disorders: A newly recognised group of genetic diseases. European Journal of Pediatrics 144: 430–440

Schutgens R B H, Wanders R J A, Nijenhuis A et al 1987 Genetic diseases caused by peroxisomal dysfunction: New findings in clinical and biochemical studies. Enzyme 38: 161–176

Schutgens R B H, Wanders R J A, Tager J M, van den

Bosch H 1988a Unpublished observations

Schutgens R B H, Heymans H S A, Wanders R J A et al 1988b Multiple peroxisomal enzyme deficiencies in rhizomelic chondrodysplasia punctata. Comparison with Zellweger syndrome, Conradi-Hünermann syndrome and the X-linked dominant type of chondrodysplasia punctata. Advances in Clinical Enzymology 6: 57–65

Schutgens R B H, Schrakamp G, Wanders R J A et al 1989 Prenatal and perinatal diagnosis of peroxisomal disorders. Journal of Inherited Metabolic Disease 12 (Suppl. 1): 118–134

Scotto J M, Hadchouel M, Odievre M et al 1982 Infantile phytanic acid storage disease, a possible variant of Refsum's disease: three cases including ultrastructural studies of the liver. Journal of Inherited Metabolic Disease 5: 83–90

Singh I, Moser A E, Goldfischer S, Moser H W 1984a Lignoceric acid is oxidized in the peroxisome: implications for the Zellweger cerebrohepatorenal syndrome and adrenoleukodystrophy: Proceedings of the National Academy of Sciences USA 81: 4203–4207

Singh I, Moser A E, Moser H W, Kishimoto Y 1984b Adrenoleukodystrophy: Impaired oxidation of very long chain fatty acids in white blood cells, cultured skin fibroblasts, and amniocytes. Pediatric Research 18: 286–290

Spranger J W, Opitz J M, Bidder U 1971 Heterogeneity of chondrodysplasia punctata. Humangenetik 11: 190–212

Steinberg D 1989 Refsum disease. In: Scriver C R, Beaudet A L, Sly W S, Valle D (eds) The metabolic basis of inherited disease, 6th edn. McGraw-Hill, New York, p 1533–1550

Suzuki Y, Orii T, Mori M, Tatibana M, Hashimoto T 1986a Deficient activities and proteins of peroxisomal β-oxidation enzymes in infants with Zellweger syndrome. Clinica Chimica Acta 156: 191–196

Suzuki Y, Orii T, Hashimoto T 1986b Biosynthesis of peroxisomal β-oxidation enzymes in infants with Zellweger syndrome. Journal of Inherited Metabolic Disease 9: 292–296

Suzuki Y, Shimozawa N, Orii T et al 1988 Molecular analysis of peroxisomal β-oxidation enzymes in infants with Zellweger syndrome and Zellweger-like syndrome. Clinica Chimica Acta 172: 65–76

Tager J M, Westerveld R, Strijland H, Schram A W, Schutgens R B H, van den Bosch H, Wanders R J A 1987 Complementation analysis of peroxisomal disease by somatic cell fusion. In: Fahimi H D, Sies H (eds) Peroxisomes in biology and medicine. Springer, Berlin, p 353–357

Thomas G H, Haslam H A, Gatschaw M O, Capute A J, Neidengoud L, Ranson J L 1975 Hyperpipecolic acidemia associated with hepatomegaly, mental retardation, optic nerve dysplasia and progressive neurological disease. Clinical Genetics 8: 370–382

Thurman R G, McKenna W 1974 Activation of ethanol utilisation in perfused liver from normal and ethanol pretreated rats. The effect of hydrogen peroxide generating substrates. Hoppe Seylers Zeitschrift zur Physiologische Chemie 355: 336–340

Tolbert N E, Yamazaki R K 1969 Leaf peroxisomes and their relation to photorespiration and photosynthesis. Annals of the New York Academy of Sciences 168: 325–341

Tolbert N E 1981 Metabolic pathways in peroxisomes and glyoxysomes. Annual Review of Biochemistry 50: 133–157

Trijbels J M F, Monnens L A H, Melis G, van den Broek-van Essen M, Bruckwilder M 1987 Localisation of pipecolic acid metabolism in rat liver peroxisomes: probable explanation for hyperpipecolataemia in Zellweger syndrome. Journal of Inherited Metabolic Disease 10: 128–135

Tsuji S, Ohno T, Miyatake T et al 1984 Fatty acid elongation activity in fibroblasts from patients with adrenoleukodystrophy (ALD). Journal of Biochemistry 96: 1241–1247

Wanders R J A 1988 Unpublished observations

Wanders R J A, Kos M, Roest B et al 1984 Activity of peroxisomal enzymes and intracellular distribution of catalase in Zellweger syndrome. Biochemical and Biophysical Research Communications 123: 1054–1061

Wanders R J A, Schutgens R B H, Heymans H S A et al 1987a Biochemical analysis in peroxisomal disorders. In: Fahimi H D, Sies H (eds) Peroxisomes in biology and medicine. Springer, Berlin, p 341–352

Wanders R J A, van Roermund C W T, van Wijland M J A et al 1987b X-linked adrenoleukodystrophy: defective peroxisomal oxidation of very long chain fatty acids but not of very long chain fatty acyl-CoA esters. Clinica Chimica Acta 165: 312–329

Wanders R J A, van Roermund C W T, van Wijland M J A et al 1987c Peroxisomal fatty acid β-oxidation in relation to the accumulation of very long chain fatty acids in cultured skin fibroblasts from patients with Zellweger syndrome and other peroxisomal disorders. The Journal of Clinical Investigation 80: 1778–1783

Wanders R J A, van Roermund C W T, Westra R et al 1987d Alanine glyoxylate aminotransferase and the urinary excretion of oxalate and glycollate in hyperoxaluria type I and the Zellweger syndrome. Clinica Chimica Acta 165: 311–319

Watkins P A, Chen W W, Harris C J et al 1989 Peroxisomal bifunctional enzyme deficiency. Journal of Clinical Investigation 83: 771–777

Williams H E, Smith L H 1983 Primary hyperoxaluria. In: Stanbury J B, Wijngaarden J B, Fredrickson D S, Goldstein J L, Brown M S (eds) The Metabolic Basis of Inherited Disease, 5th edn. McGraw-Hill, New York, p 204–228

Yokota S, Völkl P, Hashimoto T, Fahimi H D 1987 Immunoelectron microscopy of peroxisomal enzymes; their substructural association and compartmentalization in rat kidney peroxisomes. In: Fahimi H D, Sies H (eds) Peroxisomes in biology and medicine. Springer, Berlin, p 115–127

105. Pharmacogenetics

David A. Price Evans

INTRODUCTION

In this chapter we shall not deal primarily with metabolic disorders which give rise to spontaneous disease but rather with how the genetic constitution of patients determines to a considerable degree what happens when they receive drug medications. Two main classes of polymorphism will be discussed, those affecting drug metabolism and those influencing pharmacologic effect. HLA associated abnormal drug reactions and interethnic variability in drug response will also be considered.

SINGLE GENE PHENOMENA

Drug metabolism

All phenotypes common

Acetylation This polymorphism was found as a result of studying the fate of isoniazid in tuberculous patients. Some patients were found to have a relatively high plasma concentration at a standard time following a standard dose, whilst other patients had a relatively low plasma concentration under the same circumstances. An individual fell into the same class on repeated testing. Family studies disclosed the property to be controlled by two alleles at one autosomal locus (Evans et al 1960), a conclusion more recently confirmed by segregation analysis (Iselius & Evans 1983) (Fig. 105.1).

It was suspected that these alleles might work by governing the acetylation of isoniazid. This suspicion was proved correct in two ways: (1) sulphadimidine (sulphamethazine) which only undergoes one important biotransformation, namely acetylation, was shown to have this enzymic conjugation controlled by the same alleles; (2) the degree of acetylation of isoniazid in vitro by liver tissue corresponded with the in vivo phenotype of the individual from whom the tissue was derived.

The enzyme governed by the alleles is N-acetyltransferase, present in liver and intestinal mucosa. It is not known whether the alleles control enzyme structure

or rate of synthesis (Weber 1986). In the rabbit N-acetyltransferase polymorphism, which is very similar to the human polymorphism, the slow acetylator phenotype is due to a gene deletion (Blum et al 1989).

Drug compounds which are polymorphically acetylated include: isoniazid, sulphadimidine, sulphapyridine (especially as derived from salicylazo-sulphapyridine), hydralazine, dapsone, procaine amide, aminoglutethimide, prizidilol and amrinone; also nitrazepam and clonazepam (following reduction of the nitro group to give an amine). Polymorphic acetylation of phenelzine has been put forward as an idea on the basis of its possessing a hydrazino-moiety the same as isoniazid and hydralazine. Recent metabolic studies do not support this idea.

It has been found that in the metabolism of caffeine, polymorphic N-acetyltransferase is responsible for the production of 5-acetylamino-6-formylamino-3-methyl uracil (AFMU). Consequently phenotyping can now be carried out by measuring the ratio of AFMU (or its more stable deformylated product AAMU) to 1-methyl xanthine in the urine after a subject has ingested a cup of coffee (Grant et al 1984).

The importance of the acetylation polymorphism in practical therapeutics is shown in Table 105.1.

The ethnic distribution of the alleles controlling the acetylator polymorphism shows one interesting and unexplained fact. Along the Eastern littoral of Asia and associated islands is a cline. The Eskimos are almost all rapid acetylators, as are 90% of the Japanese. This percentage falls steadily towards the equator. No clear pattern has emerged regarding allele frequencies in other geographic locations (Karim et al 1981). Since hydralazine-induced systemic lupus erythematosus (SLE) is almost always a disorder of slow acetylators, surveys have been made of spontaneous SLE. It would appear, however, that patients with this disorder have a normal distribution of the alleles controlling the acetylation polymorphism.

There is a statistical association between slow acetylation and bladder cancer. The acetylation of aniline and the carcinogen benzidine is polymorphic. It is clear

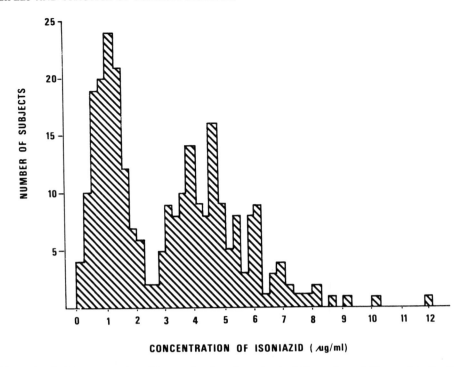

Fig. 105.1 Plasma isoniazid concentrations 6 hours after drug ingestion in 267 members of 53 complete family units. All received approximately 9.8 mg of isoniazid per Kg body weight (from Evans et al 1960).

Table 105.1 Acetylator phenotypes in therapeutics

Drug (i.e. environmental factor)	Phenotype	Effect observed
Isoniazid	Slow	More prone to develop peripheral neuropathy on therapy with conventional doses
	Slow	More prone to adverse effects of phenytoin when simultaneously treated for tuberculosis with INH
	Slow	More prone to hepatotoxicity when treated for tuberculosis with rifampicin and INH
	Rapid	Less favourable results of treating open pulmonary tuberculosis with a once-weekly isoniazid dosage regime
Hydralazine	Slow	Develop antinuclear antibodies and systemic lupus erythematosus-like syndrome
	Rapid	Require higher doses to control hypertension
Salicyl-azo-sulphapyridine	Slow	Increased incidence of various adverse reactions in healthy subjects and when drug used to treat ulcerative and Crohn's colitis. Better response in rheumatoid arthritis
Dapsone	Rapid	Higher doses needed to control dermatitis herpetiformis (disputed)
	Slow	More adverse haematological effects
Prizidilol	Slow	Greater antihypertensive effects.

Genetic polymorphism of acetylation has been described for sulphadimidine, sulphapyridine, amrinone and the amine metabolites of nitrazepam and clonazepam produced in the body as a result of reduction, and for these drugs no firm association of a clinical event with either phenotype has been defined. Procaine amide has been shown to be polymorphically acetylated; and the correlation of clinical effects with plasma concentration makes it likely that the acetylator phenotype is relevant in clinical practice.

therefore that slow acetylators are more prone than rapid acetylators to develop the cancer, because they cannot inactivate and excrete the carcinogenic compounds. Other associations are summarised by Evans (1989).

Oxidation of debrisoquine and sparteine. Debrisoquine has been in clinical use for some years as a post-ganglionic sympathetic blocker type of antihypertensive. Studies of its metabolic fate revealed oxidation at a number of sites, by far the most important of which was on the carbon atom at the 4 position on the heterocyclic ring. The parent compound and the main metabolite can be simultaneously measured in urine in one gas chromatographic procedure.

Examination of the urine for debrisoquine and 4-hydroxydebrisoquine following a single small oral dose of the compound was performed in a population of healthy persons. Three out of 93 were shown to be in a category of their own, excreting only a very small amount of the metabolite (and much more of the unchanged drug) as compared to the other 90 persons. These three persons were termed 'poor metabolisers (PM)' and the remainder 'extensive metabolisers (EM)'. This polymorphism has been confirmed by studying large numbers of subjects (Fig. 105.2).

An otherwise drug-free individual on re-testing falls in the same phenotype class. The response is quantified as $\log_{10}$ metabolic ratio:

$$\log_{10}\left\{\frac{\text{conc. debrisoquine}}{\text{conc. 4-hydroxydebrisoquine}}\right\}$$

Family studies have shown poor metabolisers to be homozygous for the allele controlling the recessive phenotype.

Sparteine is an alkaloid formerly in clinical use as an anti-arrhythmic and oxytocic drug. In view of what follows, it is interesting to note that it was abandoned because of 'the unpredictability of its effects'. It has proved possible to measure sparteine and two of its metabolites (dehydrosparteines) in the urine by a single gas chromatographic assay following a single small oral dose.

This procedure has been carried out in a standardized manner on a population of 360 subjects and it has been found that 5% form a separate phenotype lacking the ability to produce the metabolites (Eichelbaum et al 1979).

Correlation studies in random individuals and within families have proved that the same alleles control both the debrisoquine and sparteine polymorphisms. These alleles are located on chromosome 22 linked to P1 (22q11.2-qter).

Results from various in vivo and in vitro correlation studies suggest that the oxidation of a large range of therapeutic compounds is controlled by the 'debrisoquine/sparteine' alleles. These drugs include propranolol, metoprolol, timolol, bufuralol and other β-adrenergic blockers, guanoxan, phenacetin, metiamide, 4-methoxyamphetamine, methoxyphenamine, dextromethorphan, encainide, imipramine, clomipramine and other tricyclic antidepressants. The oxidation of carbamazepine, phenytoin tolbutamide and quinidine is not controlled by the 'debrisoquine' alleles.

Sparteine oxidation in vitro is inhibited by debrisoquine and tricyclic antidepressants. In vivo it is practically abolished in quinidine-treated patients.

The same enzymes which oxidize debrisoquine and sparteine also oxidize bufuralol, and have been shown to be of two types, P 450 bufI and P 450 bufII. These enzymes are respectively governed by the alleles controlling extensive and poor metabolism. Bufuralol like many drugs is enantiomeric. Enzyme I has a marked selectivity for the (+) enantiomer ($\frac{-}{+}= 0.15$) whereas enzyme II is non-stereoselective ($\frac{-}{+}=1.03$). The values for K_m and K_i (quinine) are also very different for the two forms of the enzyme (Gut et al 1986).

Hypotension has long been known to be an adverse effect of debrisoquine (the same as for many antihypertensives). An explanation for some of the cases of hypotension is afforded by the observation that PM subjects are more prone to hypotension than are EM subjects following a single therapeutic dose.

It may be speculated (but there is no proof) that persons prone to adverse reactions following the therapeutic

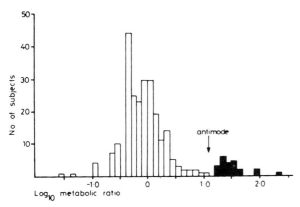

Fig. 105.2   The frequency distribution of

$$\log_{10}\left\{\frac{\text{concentration of urinary debrisoquine}}{\text{concentration of urinary 4 hydroxydebrisoquine}}\right\}$$

(from Evans et al 1980).

administration of sparteine in the past may well have been non-metabolizers.

The case of perhexiline, whose oxidation is polymorphically controlled by the sparteine/debrisoquine alleles, is of particular interest. The parent compound stays in the body for much longer in the PM phenotype after a single dose than in the EM, and this difference is magnified by repeated dosing. Perhexiline (used to treat angina pectoris) causes adverse reactions including liver toxicity and peripheral neuropathy. Amongst 20 patients with angina and perhexiline neuropathy 10 were PM, whereas no PM was found amongst 14 patients treated with perhexiline who had not developed neuropathy; among 38 anginal patients who had never received perhexiline three were PM. Patients with perhexiline liver damage have also been studied. Amongst four of them there were three PM, whereas amongst 70 patients with liver damage due to various other causes there were six PM. This evidence suggests that the PM phenotype is very much more prone to develop the adverse effects of this compound. Poor metabolizers of debrisoquine are at much greater risk than extensive metabolizers of developing adverse reactions on tricyclic antidepressants and β-adrenergic blockers.

The 'typed panel' approach has shown that poor hydroxylators of debrisoquine are also poor hydroxylators of phenformin. A family study has demonstrated genetic polymorphism for hydroxylation of the latter drug, with allele frequencies not significantly different from those of debrisoquine and sparteine. Plasma lactate concentrations were elevated to a greater extent after phenformin in poor hydroxylators than in extensive hydroxylators. Lactic acidosis (often fatal) occurred in some patients being treated with phenformin for their diabetes. Some patients were investigated with debrisoquine after recovery and were shown to be poor hydroxylators.

Some interactions could be of clinical significance. For example, rifampicin causes a 30% increase of the metabolic clearance of sparteine in EM, whereas in PM subjects no effect on the overall elimination of the drug was seen. With regard to associations of spontaneous disorders with the polymorphism, it has been reported that there are statistically significant associations of PM with Parkinsonism and with systemic lupus erythematosus, and of EM with various cancers (Caporaso et al 1989). There is no association between the PM phenotype and alcoholic liver cirrhosis.

Molecular genetics Preliminary results indicate that the PM phenotype is due to 'splicing errors' producing defective mRNA from the P450 db1 (P450 C2D1) gene (Gonzales et al 1988a) which is localized on chromosome 22 (Gonzales et al 1988b). It seems that there are three linked genes, one 'normal' and two containing various abnormalities at this locus (Kimura et al 1989).

Mephenytoin In studies to investigate the kinetic consequences of stereoselective 5-mephenytoin hydroxylation during long-term racemic mephenytoin dosing in normal subjects, Kupfer and colleagues (1984) detected one person with a very low ability to perform aromatic hydroxylation of the compound. The recovery of 4-hydroxy-mephenytoin after a single oral dose of the compound was much lower (3%) as compared with other people (41%). Both parents and three brothers of this anomalous subject were studied and two brothers were found to have the same poor capacity for mephenytoin hydroxylation (PM_M). The proband had normal mephenytoin demethylation ability and, when tested with debrisoquine, was found to be an extensive metabolizer of that compound (EM_M). The suggestion from those original observations that PM_M is an autosomal recessive phenotype has been substantiated by further family studies.

It has been found that the demethylated metabolite of S-mephenytoin, 5-phenyl 5-ethyl hydantoin (S-nirvanol), is also polymorphically 4-hydroxylated and this polymorphism is under the control of the same alleles as the oxidation of mephenytoin itself. There is an advantage in using nirvanol as a test drug because both parent drug and metabolite are excreted in the urine. This circumvents a major difficulty with using mephenytoin itself where there is very little excretion of the parent compound and the phenotyping test result is expressed as the fraction of the dose excreted as 4-hydroxymephenytoin in a given time. Such an index could be influenced by factors such as intestinal absorption and completeness of urinary collection.

Mephobarbital oxidation has been shown to be co-regulated by the mephenytoin alleles.

The possibility that the mephenytoin/nirvanol polymorphism is regulated by the same alleles as the debrisoquine/sparteine polymorphism has been investigated (Kupfer & Preisig 1984). A total of 221 unrelated, normal, European, volunteer subjects were tested with both debrisoquine and mephenytoin and showed the following distribution of phenotypes: $EM_D EM_M 189$, $PM_D EM_M 20$, $EM_D PM_M 9$, $PM_D PM_M 3$. In another survey, 83 Caucasians tested with sparteine and mephenytoin showed: $EM_S EM_M 75$, $EM_S PM_M 2$, $PM_S EM_M 6$. These results indicate that the two polymorphisms are genetically independent.

A detailed enzyme analysis was carried out using liver microsomal preparations from both extensive and poor metabolizers (PM) of mephenytoin (Meier et al 1985).

The 4-hydroxylation reaction in PM showed an increased K_m, a decreased rate of S-mephenytoin hydroxylation, and loss of stereoselectivity for the hydroxylation of R- and S-enantiomers as compared with the EM phenotype. The formation of 4-hydroxymephenytoin from the R-enantiomer and the demethylation reaction remained unaffected. These results indicate that the mephenytoin polymorphism is caused by a partial or complete absence or inactivity of a cytochrome P450 isozyme with high activity for S-mephenytoin.

Surveys in different ethnic groups have revealed that the frequency of PM_M in Chinese populations is not significantly different to that in Europeans. In randomly selected Japanese, however, 7 out of 31 were PM_M, which indicates a significantly higher frequency in this ethnic group (Wilkinson et al 1989).

Gene localisation By examining rat-human hybrid cell chromosomes, Meehan et al (1988) showed that the mephenytoin P450 gene occurs in the region 10q24.1 to 10q24.3.

Ethanol It is a common observation that individuals differ markedly in their responses to ethanol. Recent studies have shed some light on the basis for this variability. Of particular interest is the inter-ethnic difference in the pharmacological effects of ethanol. Both Wolff (1972) and Ewing et al (1974) showed that flushing after alcohol ingestion was more common in Orientals than in Caucasians. Ewing et al (1974) suggested that this phenomenon might have as its basis a greater production of acetaldehyde in Orientals, controlled by genetic factors. Reed et al (1976) and Hanna (1978) showed that ethanol metabolism was more rapid in Orientals than in Caucasians and the latter research group also showed a higher acetaldehyde production in Orientals.

A great deal of attention has been focused on liver alcohol dehydrogenase variants in different ethnic groups, but despite some elegant biochemical genetics these studies have not hitherto shed light on the basis of phenotypic differences in response to ethanol.

In the last few years the focus of attention has moved to acetaldehyde dehydrogenase (ALDH) (the liver cytosolic form is controlled by genes located on 9q). This enzyme also exhibits polymorphism in vitro. Harada et al (1980b) demonstrated the existence of four isozymes in human liver. These have different K_m values as well as showing differences on isoelectric focusing; evidence favouring the view that they have different molecular structures. Absence of the highly active band I isozyme was found in 52% of 40 Japanese – a phenomenon not observed in 68 Germans (Harada et al 1980a).

An important step forward in the investigation of the epidemiological significance of ALDH was the discovery that individuals could be phenotyped for absence of ALDH I by examination of hair roots. The symptoms of alcohol sensitivity such as dysphoria, facial flushing, elevation of skin temperature, abdominal discomfort, muscle weakness, dizziness, and increased heart rate vary between different populations and correlate with the frequency of ALDH I deficiency, both b;eing more common in Pacific Asiatics. Likewise, the blood acetaldehyde concentration after ethanol is raised in ALDH I deficiency. Japanese alcoholics have been found to have a lower frequency of ALDH I deficiency than the general population which suggests the possibility that this phenotype is protective against the disorder (Goedde et al 1983).

Thiopurine methyltransferase Thiopurine methyltransferase (TPMT) catalyses the S-methylation of a variety of potentially toxic thiopurine drugs such as 6-mercaptopurine, 6-thioguanine and azathioprine. Not only is S-methylation an important catabolic pathway for these drugs but S-methylated ribonucleotides of thiopurines are 'active' metabolites capable of inhibiting purine biosynthesis. Erythrocyte TPMT activity is trimodal, with the least activity mode contributing one person in 298. Population studies and segregation analysis of family data indicate that TPMT activity is controlled by two alleles at an autosomal locus.

By making use of healthy kidney tissue from subjects requiring nephrectomy, and obtaining red cells from the same individuals, a correlation between TPMT activity in the two tissues was observed. This finding indicates that the same alleles control the TPMT enzyme activity in red cells and kidney (Woodson et al 1982).

Azathioprine and 6-mercaptopurine (6MP) are widely used as cytotoxins and immunosuppressives. Azathioprine is rapidly cleared in the body to yield 6MP which is believed to exert its cytotoxic effect by being incorporated into DNA to form 6-thioguanine nucleotides (6TGN). High concentrations of 6TGN have been found in the red cells of patients treated with 6MP who have developed myelosuppression. Lennard et al (1987) found that there was a negative correlation between red cell TPMT activity and red cell 6TGN concentrations in children with 6MP. These results strongly suggest that a genetically determined low red cell TPMT activity is a significant risk factor for the development of myelosuppression on 6MP therapy.

Some phenotypes rare

Pseudocholinesterase When succinyl choline (suxamethonium) was introduced into clinical practice as a short-term muscle relaxant, occasional patients were found who suffered from prolonged apnoea. Plasma pseudocholinesterase was known to hydrolyse the drug and so terminate its action. Therefore, the activity of this enzyme was investigated and the persons who suffered from the prolonged apnoea were found to have relatively low activities. In some individuals it became apparent that the low plasma activity was produced by a pathological process, e.g. liver disease, poisoning by organophosphorous compounds, malnutrition, severe anaemia, hyperpyrexia, infectious diseases, cardiac failure, uraemia, catatonia and malignancy (Lehmann & Liddell 1961). However in many individuals such an explanation was not tenable, and so the possibility arose that the low plasma enzyme activity was an inherited trait. Family studies of subjects with prolonged apnoea revealed healthy relatives who also had low plasma pseudocholinesterase activities (Lehmann & Simmons 1958).

The study of the enzyme by means of the inhibitors dibucaine and fluoride revealed the presence of isozymes controlled by four autosomal alleles designated E_1^u (usual), E_1^a (atypical, detected by dibucaine), E_1^f (detected by fluoride) and E_1^s (silent). The locus is at 3q25.2.

Genotypes which do not possess E_1^u have increased sensitivity to succinyl choline and are at risk of developing prolonged apnoea with customary doses. However, some individuals who develop prolonged apnoea do not have any pathological lesion which could be held responsible, and type $E_1^u E_1^u$ on the above tests.

The practical question that is frequently asked is 'When in clinical practice should individuals have their plasma examined for pseudocholinesterase variants?'. The answer is that plasmas should be examined (in laboratories used to doing the tests) in individuals who have a history of unexplained prolonged apnoea following previous operations, and also in relatives of such persons.

Acatalasia Formerly catalase was considered to be essential to the functioning of mammalian cells. In 1946 however, a clinical observation by Professor Takahara showed that this presumption was not correct (see Takahara 1952). A girl aged 11 years had been much afflicted by gangrene around the teeth, of which she had lost several. Thereafter, caries involving the maxilla was followed by the development of an inflammatory mass in the maxillary sinus. After excising the inflammatory mass, Professor Takahara poured hydrogen peroxide on the raw surface as was his custom. Instead of frothing bright red, the wound became brownish-black. From this simple but startling observation, he deduced that the blood and tissues of this patient did not contain catalase. Subsequent biochemical investigations showed his deduction to have been correct. Subsequently further similar patients with oral gangrene were discovered in Japan and Korea.

An investigation of the genetics of the condition revealed that patients with the oral gangrene syndrome were homozygotes. Heterozygotes could be identified in Japanese pedigrees as a distinctly separate mode in a frequency distribution of blood catalase values.

Electrophoretic studies of catalase in normal homozygotes, heterozygotes and acatalasics have shown that the 'abnormal' catalase has a different electrophoretic activity from normal. Both forms are demonstrable in heterozygotes. The abnormal form has greater heat lability at 55°C in Swiss (but not in Japanese) acatalasics. On the other hand, in Japanese acatalasics the 'abnormal' catalase can be distinguished from the normal form by immunological techniques.

There thus appears to be definite evidence of the existence of different types of acatalasia. The chromosomal location for catalase genes is 11p1305–1306.

Diphenylhydantoin (Phenytoin) This compound is metabolised by para-oxidation of one phenyl ring in the endoplasmic reticulum of the human liver cell. Three families have been described by Kutt (1971) in which the mother and one or more offspring seemed to have a relative inability to carry out this metabolic biotransformation. Other similar families have been described subsequently. These individuals appear to be in quite a separate class from ordinary subjects, suggesting that they are expressing a distinct Mendelian character. The practical result is a high plasma steady state drug concentration and a long half-life. The high steady state concentration on conventional doses renders the subject unusually prone to the toxic effects of the drug, i.e. ataxia, nystagmus, slurred speech, inattention, etc.

Rare reactions to phenytoin are known to occur, characterized by fever, skin rash, hepatotoxicity, lymphadenopathy and various blood dyscrasias. These reactions occur some weeks after the initiation of treatment. Light has been shed on their mechanism of production by some novel research (Spielberg et al 1981). The lymphocytes of persons who had experienced such reactions were exposed to phenytoin metabolites generated by a murine hepatic microsomal system, and their subsequent viability assessed by trypan blue exclusion. Dose-dependent toxicity was demonstrated, a response which was not found in control lymphocytes. Phenytoin itself did not induce the toxicity. The lymphocytes of control subjects were made liable to toxicity by the inhibition of epoxide hydrolase. The parents of affected individuals showed intermediate responses, whilst sibs were either normal or resembled the probands. Detoxification of non-arene oxide metabolites (e.g. of acetaminophen) was normal in the patients' cells. It was concluded therefore that a heritable response to arene oxides may predispose some patients to hepatotoxicity.

This information has been applied to the study of

phenytoin-associated birth defects. Twenty-four children exposed to phenytoin throughout gestation had their lymphocytes studied by the technique described above and 14 were found to possess the abnormality. These 14 had more of the major birth defects (congenital heart disease, cleft lip/palate, microcephaly and major genitourinary, eye and limb defects) than the other 10, but minor birth defects were equally distributed through both groups. These findings suggest that incapacity to detoxify arene oxide increases the risk of a phenytoin-exposed embryo to develop major birth defects (Strickler et al 1985).

Phenacetin A remarkable pedigree was described by Shahidi (1968) in which two individuals had a relative inability to de-ethylate phenacetin. Since this major pathway accepted less substrate, more of the drug was converted to minor metabolites, such as phenetidine, than is normally the case. These metabolites have a methaemoglobin-producing propensity, and it was in fact the clinical observation of methaemoglobinaemia which caused this family to be studied so intensively.

Bishydroxycoumarin (Dicoumarol) A single pedigree has been described (Vessell 1975) in which individuals have a relative inability to hydroxylate the compound. The consequence is a greater sensitivity than normal to the anticoagulant effect produced by ordinary dosages.

Pharmacological effects

All phenotypes common

Glucose-6-phosphate dehydrogenase deficiency This is the commonest pharmacogenetic trait. The enzyme polymorphism first came to light as a result of studying persons who had developed haemolysis as an adverse reaction to treatment of their malaria with pamaquine and primaquine.

Very soon it was realised that the deficiency was in the enzyme glucose-6-phosphate dehydrogenase (G6PD) and assays of the activity of this enzyme superseded the glutathione stability test as a phenotyping procedure.

A large number of other drugs in addition to primaquine are known to precipitate haemolysis in G6PD-deficient subjects. The ingestion of the bean *Vicia faba* can also produce the same effect and this is the basis of favism–an affliction described in antiquity.

Clinical observation revealed that Mediterranean G6PD-deficient individuals were more severely affected than Black G6PD-deficient subjects after primaquine ingestion. When the purified enzyme was subjected to a number of biochemical procedures, e.g. electrophoresis, pH optimum, temperature stability, Michaelis constant with various substrates, etc., it was found that there are, in various populations, a large number of different structural variants. The type responsible for G6PD-deficiency in Blacks (termed A-) is caused by a single amino acid substitution compared with the normal form, with asparagine being replaced by aspartic acid (Yoshida 1967). In the Black form of deficiency, leucocyte G6PD activity is normal. In the Mediterranean and Chinese forms of the deficiency leucocyte G6PD activity is reduced.

The locus controlling G6PD is situated on the X chromosome at Xq22 quite close to the locus for deuteranopia (estimated recombination fraction 5%).

The geographic distribution of G6PD-deficiency is similar to that of malaria – a fact which gave rise to the speculation that it might have a protective role. Support for this idea was derived from a finding in malarious heterozygotes. Due to Lyonisation, heterozygotes have some erythrocytes which are normal and some which are G6PD-deficient. It has been found that the latter type of cell is less frequently parasitized than the former (Beutler 1978). A large number of G6PD variants have been identified all over the world by means of various laboratory techniques, and molecular genetic techniques are providing precise identifications of different mutants (Beutler & Yoshida 1988, Beutler 1989).

Black and Mediterranean G6PD-deficient subjects are quite healthy, provided their red cells are not subjected to chemical stresses. The situation is different in the rare Northern European kindred where a chronic non-spherocytic anaemia may have G6PD-deficiency as its basis (e.g. McCann et al 1980).

Some phenotypes rare

Malignant hyperthermia This is a fatal condition which supervenes unexpectedly in an otherwise fit subject during anaesthesia – usually with halothane and or succinyl choline chloride (Britt & Kalow 1968). Soon after induction of anaesthesia the muscles go into massive spasm and the body temperature quickly rises to a high level. The patient becomes acidotic and it is probably the cardiac effects of the acidosis which often cause sudden death.

Related individuals have suffered from this catastrophe and the disposition of these individuals within pedigrees suggests that it is inherited as a rare Mendelian dominant character.

In vitro studies performed with voluntary muscle strips obtained at biopsy from susceptible individuals have shown an abnormal contraction in response to halothane, succinyl chlorine or caffeine (Moulds & Denborough 1974a). The contraction was prevented by procaine. In a calcium-free bath, muscle tissue from an affected person gave an initial sustained contraction when exposed to caffeine or halothane, but re-exposure to these agents when the muscle had relaxed following a change of bath liquid did not produce a second contracture. A second contracture could be produced, however, if the bath liquid contained calcium. The suggestion has therefore been made that in malignant hyperthermia the calcium-storing sarcolemma and sarcoplasmic reticulum release abnormally large amounts of calcium in response to the action of the precipitating drug.

The investigation of muscle biopsies along the above lines has been proposed as a preoperative screening test for relatives of subjects known to have suffered from malignant hyperthermia (Ørding 1988).

Some predictive value may also be obtained by a careful physical examination, since clinically evident myopathy of a minor degree may be present, and a serum creatine kinase, since this is raised in some susceptible subjects (Moulds & Denborough 1974b).

During anaesthesia, signs of onset of the condition are a rise in temperature, muscular rigidity and a rise in end-tidal carbon dioxide concentration. Appropriate general measures and specific therapy with dantrolene must be put into effect immediately (Ellis 1984).

Resistance to oral anticoagulants This rare Mendelian dominant character was discovered as a result of a clinical observation. A man who had sustained a myocardial infarction failed to show a lowering of his plasma prothrombin concentration following conventional doses of warfarin (O'Reilly et al 1964). It transpired that the desired effect of the drug did occur when dosage was increased to a high level. His dose-response curve was grossly displaced to the right, compared with ordinary patients. Otherwise he had no unusual features. Other persons with the same phenotype were discovered in his pedigree. Later a second, independent and much larger pedigree was described in which persons with the same phenotype occurred (O'Reilly 1970). More recently still, a third family has been described (Alving et al 1985). This 'warfarin-resistance' is an autosomal dominant trait and is accompanied by resistance to other oral anticoagulants, e.g. dicoumarol (but not, of course, heparin). The pharmacokinetics of warfarin are normal in resistant subjects.

It is clear that there is some mechanism in the liver producing 'anticoagulant resistant' individuals which is not affected to the same extent by a given concentration as in ordinary individuals. The precise nature of the biochemical mechanism controlled by this rare allele remains unknown.

Warfarin resistance in wild rats, which has been described from more than one focus in the UK and from the USA and Denmark, is also inherited as an autosomal dominant character. It would seem to be exactly analogous to the rare disorder in man and it has as its basis a variant type of vitamin K epoxide reductase, in the liver

endoplasmic reticulum, with a lower V_{max} and K_m for vitamin K epoxide than that found in the warfarin-sensitive phenotype (Hildebrandt et al 1984).

Haemoglobin Zurich This unstable haemoglobin was originally discovered because a young girl and her father had suffered severe haemolysis following treatment with conventional doses of different sulphonamides (Frick et al 1962).

The cause of the haemolysis was found to be within the red cells which showed inclusion bodies during the acute stage. Electrophoretic studies showed that the two patients possessed haemoglobin A and also an abnormal haemoglobin, named 'Zurich', which had a mobility intermediate between A and S. Structural studies showed that histidine, which usually occupies position 63 of the β chain, is replaced by arginine (Bachmann & Marti 1962).

Subsequently ferrokinetic and ^{51}Cr tagged red cell survival studies showed that red blood cells from the original patients had a shorter life span than normal. Affected individuals also suffer from mild anaemia and episodic mild jaundice (when they have not been on drugs).

It appears, therefore, that haemoglobin Zurich is normally unstable. But when the patient has ingested sulphonamides the precipitation of the haemoglobin is greatly speeded up and a massive haemolysis results.

Some individuals with haemoglobin Zurich have not suffered from this low-grade uninduced haemolysis. On closer scrutiny these individuals turned out to be smokers. Haemoglobin Zurich has twice as much affinity for carbon monoxide as haemoglobin A, and it appears to be stabilised in smokers, so protecting them from haemolysis (Virshup et al 1983).

Similar clinical manifestations would be expected with other unstable haemoglobins. An example is haemoglobin H (formed of four β chains and no α chains) which has been described by Rigas and Koler (1961).

HLA AND ADVERSE REACTIONS

Many adverse reactions to drugs have an allergic or hypersensitivity basis. Their occurrence seems entirely unpredictable. Yet probably even the most common of these, penicillin hypersensitivity, has a much higher concordance amongst monozygous than dizygous twins, suggesting the possibility of a genetic basis (Lader et al 1974).

However, three examples have been published which seem to form the basis of a new branch of pharmacogenetics in that they indicate a role for the HLA system (or some closely related genetic entity) in the predisposition to adverse reactions to drugs.

Firstly, 14 out of 15 individuals who developed proteinuria after auriothiomalate ('gold') therapy for rheumatoid arthritis were found to be of HLA type DRw3, which has a frequency of only about 8% in the Caucasian population (Wooley et al 1980).

Secondly, patients with hydralazine-SLE, who have long been known to be almost always slow acetylators, have now been found to be predominantly (75%) possessors of antigen DRw4, which only occurs in about 25% of the general Caucasian population (Batchelor et al 1980).

INTER-ETHNIC VARIABILITY

The subject of inter-ethnic variability of drug metabolism and effect is recognised to be of growing importance. A recent volume (Kalow et al 1986) summarizes much of the existing knowledge.

This topic is obviously an important one because it has practical implications in therapeutics. The same phenomena may have importance in occupational health (e.g. acetylator status of industrial workers handling aromatic amines, and the paroxonase activity of agricultural workers).

WHICH SCREENING TESTS ARE WORTH DOING?

The answer to this question has recently been discussed (Evans 1986) and depends on a number of clinical variables:

1. The severity of a possible adverse reaction;
2. The strength of the association which has been demonstrated between:
   a. efficacy and susceptible phenotype;
   b. adverse reaction and susceptible phenotype;
3. The chance of finding a patient with a susceptible phenotype;
4. The availability of alternative drugs.

In practice, certain combinations of possibilities do not occur. For example, if there were a drug which caused a severe adverse reaction whenever it was given to an individual of susceptible phenotype, and such individuals were common in the population, then such a drug would soon be banned!

On the other hand if a drug only caused an occasional mild adverse reaction it would not be worth mounting expensive screening tests to guard against the event.

The availability of equally efficacious drugs, equally acceptable to the patient, and no more expensive, usually means that drugs causing severe adverse reactions, even

only in occasional subjects, will drop out of usage (e.g. perhexilene).

So reflection indicates that screening for susceptible phenotypes has only a limited applicability.

In populations where the susceptible phenotype is common and the adverse reaction severe (e.g. porphyria variegata in South Africa), then routine screening is clearly essential.

It is certainly worth screening for G6PD deficiency and many blood banks carry out this precaution.

Where there is a family history of a serious adverse reaction occurring in a rare phenotype (e.g. apnoea after succinylcholine, or malignant hyperpyrexia) then it is worth screening the family members.

CONCLUSIONS

Known pharmacogenetic alleles may well represent only a fraction of those which exist but are, as yet, undiscovered. It is therefore clearly sensible to think of the possibility of a genetic explanation when an unusual adverse reaction is observed.

The family history may reveal the presence of a clinically important dominant character. In such a situation the patient may be at risk, e.g. from malignant hyperpyrexia or porphyria following anaesthesia. If such a suspicion is generated, then it is wise to carry out appropriate investigations not only on the patient but also on available relatives.

A novel adverse reaction may reveal a new allele. Knowledge of new alleles is in itself of value for a variety of subsequent genetic investigations. It must be emphasised that the key to making such advances lies in studying the relatives of the proband.

Clinical trials should be designed so that the groups to be compared contain representative numbers of the different phenotypes in a polymorphism.

When a drug is released for use in a new population, then a new type of adverse reaction may be observed, or there may be a different incidence of known reactions.

The monitoring of plasma concentrations of drugs has been in existence for a long time (e.g. salicylates and sulphonamides) but is now feasible for a great variety of compounds; and modern techiques, especially HPLC, allow metabolites to be assayed along with the original drug molecules. In the interpretation of data obtained in this way there are a number of pharmacological considerations of importance. One of the aims of the procedure, however, is to obtain an estimate of the inter-individual variability whose basis is to a considerable extent determined by heredity.

On a broader biological basis the taking of a drug represents an environmental change. The phenotypes within a genetic polymorphism may respond to this environmental factor in different ways, e.g. some phenotypes may be more prone to adverse reactions, whereas others may benefit.

Statistical associations between pharmacogenetic phenotypes and 'spontaneous' disorders (i.e. not drug-induced) may shed new light on aetiological mechanisms.

REFERENCES

Alving B M, Strickler M P, Knight R D, Barr C F, Berenberg J L 1985 Hereditary warfarin resistance. Investigation of a rare phenomenon. Archives of Internal Medicine 145: 499–501

Bachman F, Marti H R 1962 Hemoglobin Zurich II. Physiochemical properties of the abnormal hemoglobins. Blood 20: 272–286

Batchelor J R, Welsh K I, Tinoco R M et al 1980 Hydralazine-induced systemic lupus erythematosus: Influence of HLA-DR and sex on susceptibility. Lancet 1: 1107–1109

Beutler E 1978 Glucose-6-phosphate dehydrogenase deficiency. In: Stanbury J B, Wyngaarden J B, Fredrickson D S (eds) Metabolic Basis of Inherited Disease, 4th edn. McGraw-Hill, New York, ch 60, p 1430–1451

Beutler E 1989 Glucose-6-phosphate dehydrogenase: New perspectives. Blood 73: 1397–1401

Beutler E, Yoshida A 1988 Genetic variation of glucose-6-phosphate de-hydrogenase. A catalog and future prospects. Medicine (Baltimore) 67: 311–334

Blum M, Grant D M, Demierre A, Meyer U A 1989 N-acetylation pharmacogenetics: A gene deletion causes absence of arylamine N-acetylation in liver of slow acetylator rabbits. Proceedings of the National Academy of Sciences, USA 86: 9554–9558

Britt B A, Kalow W 1968 Hyper-rigidity and hyperthermia associated with anaesthesia. Annals of the New York Academy of Sciences 151: 947–958

Caporaso N, Hayes R B, Dosemeci M et al 1989 Lung cancer risk, occupational exposure and the debrisoquine metabolic phenotype. Cancer Research 49: 3675–3679

Eichelbaum M, Spannbrucker N, Steincke B, Dengler H J 1979 Defective N-oxidation of sparteine in Man: A new pharmacogenetic defect. European Journal of Clinical Pharmacology 16: 183–187

Ellis F R 1984 Malignant hyperpyrexia. Archives of Disease in Childhood 59: 1013–1015

Evans D A P 1986 Therapy. In: Kalow W, Goedde H W, Agarwal D P (eds) Ethnic differences in reactions to drugs and xenobiotics. Alan Liss, New York, p 491–526

Evans D A P 1989 N-Acetyltransferase. Pharmacology and Therapeutics 42: 157–234

Evans D A P, Manley K A, McKusick V A 1960 Genetic control of isoniazid metabolism in man. British Medical Journal 2: 485–491

Evans D A P, Mahgoub A, Sloan T P, Idle J R, Smith R L 1980 A family and population study of the genetic polymorphism of debrisoquine oxidation in a white British population. Journal of Medical Genetics 17: 102–105

Ewing J A, Rouse B A, Pellizzari E D 1974 Alcohol sensitivty and ethnic background. American Journal of Psychiatry 131: 206–210

Frick P G, Hitzig W H, Betke K 1962 Hemoglobin Zurich I. A new hemoglobin anomaly associated with acute hemolytic episodes with inclusion bodies after sulphonamide therapy. Blood 20: 261–271

Goedde H W, Agarwal D P, Harada S 1983 The role of alcohol dehydrogenase and aldehyde dehydrogenase isozymes in alcohol metabolism, alcohol sensitivity and alcoholism. In: Rattazzi M C (ed) Isozymes: current topics in biological and medical research, vol 8, Cellular localization metabolism and physiology. Alan Liss, New York, p 175–193

Gonzales F J, Skoda R C, Kimura S et al 1988a Characterization of the common genetic defect in humans deficient in debrisoquine metabolism. Nature 331: 442–446

Gonzales F J, Vilbois F, Harduzck J P et al 1988b Human debrisoquine 4-hydroxylase (P450 II D1); cDNA and deduced amino-acid sequence and assignment of the CYP2D locus to chromosome 22. Genomics 2: 174–179

Grant D M, Tang B K, Kalow W 1984. A simple test for acetylator phenotype using caffeine. British Journal of Clinical Pharmacology 17: 459–464

Gut J, Catin T, Dayer P, Kronbach T, Zanger U, Meyer U A 1986 Debrisoquine/sparteine-type polymorphism of drug oxidation. Journal of Biological Chemistry 261: 11734–11743

Hanna J M 1978 Metabolic responses of Chinese, Japanese and Europeans to alcohol. Alcoholism: Clinical and Experimental Research 2: 89–92

Harada S, Misawa S, Agarwal D P, Goedde H W 1980a Liver alcohol dehydrogenase and aldehyde dehydrogenase in the Japanese: Isozyme variation and its possible role in alcohol intoxication. American Journal of Human Genetics 32: 8–15

Harada S, Agarwal D P, Goedde H W 1980b Electrophoretic and biochemical studies of human aldehyde dehydrogenase isozymes in various tissues. Life Sciences 26: 1773–1780

Hildebrandt E F, Preusch P C, Patterson J L, Suttie J W 1984 Solubilization and characterization of vitamin K epoxide reductase from normal and warfarin-resistant rat liver microsomes. Archives of Biochemistry and Biophysics 228: 480–492

Iselius L, Evans D A P 1983 Formal genetics of isoniazid metabolism in man. Clinical Pharmacokinetics 8: 541–544

Jurima M, Inaba T, Kadar D, Kalow W 1985 Genetic polymorphism of mephenytoin p(4')-hydroxylation: difference between Orientals and Caucasians. British Journal of Clinical Pharmacology 19: 483–487

Kalow W, Goedde H W, Agarwal D P (eds) 1986 Ethnic differences in reactions to drugs and xenobiotics. Progress in Clinical and Biological Reseach Alan Liss, New York, 214: 1–583

Karim A K M B, Elfellah M S, Evans D A P 1981 Human acetylator polymorphism: Estimate of allele frequency in Libya and details of global distribution. Journal of Medical Genetics 18: 325–330

Kimura S, Umeno M, Skoda R C, Meyer U A, Gonzales F J 1989 The human debrisoquine 4-hydroxylase (CYP2D) locus: sequence and identification of the polymorphic CYP2D gene, a related gene and a pseudogene. American Journal of Human Genetics 45: 889–904

Kupfer A, Preisig R 1984 Pharmacogenetics of mephenytoin: A new drug hydroxylation polymorphism in man. European Journal of Clinical Pharmacology 26: 753–759

Kupfer A, Desmond P, Patwardhan R, Schenker S, Branch R A 1984 Mephenytoin hydroxylation deficiency: Kinetics after repeated doses. Clinical Pharmacology and Therapeutics 35: 33–39

Kutt H 1971 Biochemical and genetic factors regulating dilantin metabolism in Man. Annals of the New York Academy of Sciences 179: 704–722

Lader M, Kendell R, Kasriel J 1974 The genetic contribution to unwanted drug effects. Clinical Pharmacology and Therapeutics 16: 343–347

Lehmann H, Liddell J 1961 The cholinesterases. In: Evans F T, Gray T C (eds) Modern Trends in Anaesthesia 2. Butterworth, London, ch 8, p 164–205

Lehmann H, Simmons P H 1958 Sensitivity to suxamethonium. Lancet 2: 981–982

Lennard L, VanLoon J A, Lilleyman J S, Weinshilboum R M 1987 Thiopurine pharmacogenetics in leukaemia: Correlation of erythrocyte thiopurine methyltransferase activity and 6–thioguanine nucleotide concentrations. Clinical Pharmacology and Therapeutics 41: 18–25

McCann S R, Smithwick A M, Temperley I J, Tipton K 1980 G6PD (Dublin): Chronic non-spherocytic haemolytic anaemia resulting from glucose-6-phosphate dehydrogenase deficiency in an Irish kindred. Journal of Medical Genetics 17: 191–193

Meehan R R, Gosden J R, Rout D et al 1988 Human cytochrome P-450 PB-1: A multigene family involved in mephenytoin and steroid oxidations that maps to chromosome 10. American Journal of Human Genetics 42: 26–37

Meier U T, Dayer P, Male P-J, Kronbach T, Meyer U A 1985 Mephenytoin hydroxylation polymorphism: Characterization of the enzymatic deficiency in liver microsomes of poor metabolizers phenotyped in vivo. Clinical Pharmacology and Therapeutics 38: 488–494

Moulds R F W, Denborough M A 1974a Biochemical basis of malignant hyperpyrexia. British Medical Journal 2: 241–244

Moulds R F W, Denborough M A 1974b Identification of susceptibility to malignant hyperpyrexia. British Medical Journal 2: 245–247

Ørding H 1988 Diagnosis of susceptibility to malignant hyperthermia in man. British Journal of Anaesthesia 60: 287–302

O'Reilly R A 1970 The second reported kindred with hereditary resistance to oral anticoagulant drugs. New England Journal of Medicine 282: 1448–1451

O'Reilly R A, Aggeler P M, Hoag M S, Leong L S,

Kropatkin M L 1964 Hereditary transmission of exceptional resistance to coumarin anticoagulant drugs - the first reported kindred. New England Journal of Medicine 271: 809–815

Reed T E, Kalant H, Gibbins R J, Kapur B M, Rankin J G 1976 Alcohol and acetaldehyde metabolism in Caucasians, Chinese and Amerinds. Canadian Medical Association Journal 115: 851–852

Rigas D A, Koler R D 1961 Decreased erthrocyte survival in hemoglobin H disease as a result of the abnormal properties of hemoglobin H. The benefit of splenectomy. Journal of Hematology 18: 1–17

Shahidi N T 1968 Acetophenetidin-induced methaemoglobinaemia. Annals of the New York Academy of Sciences 151: 822–832

Spielberg S P, Gordon G B, Blake D A, Goldstein D A, Herlong F 1981 Predisposition to phenytoin hepatotoxicity assessed in vitro. New England Journal of Medicine 305: 722–727

Strickler S M, Miller M A, Andermann E, Dansky L V, Seni M-H, Spielberg S P 1985 Genetic predisposition of phenytoin-induced birth defects. Lancet 2: 746–749

Takahara S 1952 Progressive oral gangrene probably due to lack of catalase in the blood (acatalasaemia) Lancet 2: 1101–1104

Vesell E S 1975 Pharmacogenetics - the individual factor in drug response. Triangle 14: 125–130

Virshup D M, Zinkham W H, Sirota R L, Caughey W S 1983 Unique sensitivity of Hb Zürich to oxidative injury by phenazopyridine: Reversal of the effects by elevating carboxyhaemoglobin levels *in vivo* and *in vitro*. American Journal of Hematology 14: 315–324

Weber W W 1986 Commentary: The molecular basis of hereditary acetylation polymorphism. Drug Metabolism and Disposition 14: 377–381

Wilkinson G R, Guengerich F P, Branch R A 1989 Genetic polymorphism of 5-mephenytoin hydroxylation. Clinical Pharmacology and Therapeutics 43: 53–76

Wolff P H 1972 Ethnic differences in alcohol sensitivity. Science 175: 449–450

Woodson L C, Dunnette J H, Weinshilboum R M 1982 Pharmacogenetics of human thiopurine methyltransferase: Kidney-erythrocyte correlation and immunotitration studies. Journal of Pharmacology and Therapeutics 222: 174–181

Wooley P H, Griffin J, Panayi G S, Batchelor J R, Welsh K I, Gibson T J 1980 HLA-DR antigens and toxicity to sodium auriothiomalate and D-penicillamine in rheumatoid arthritis. New England Journal of Medicine 303: 300–302

Yoshida A 1967 A single amino acid substitution (asparagine to aspartic acid) between normal (B+) and the common Negro variant (A+) of human glucose-6-phosphate dehydrogenase. Proceedings of the National Academy of Sciences (Biochemistry) 57: 835–840

Yoshida A, Beutler E 1983 G-6-PD variants: Another update. Annals of Human Genetics 47: 25–38

106. Cancer genetics

R. Neil Schimke

INTRODUCTION

Cancer research has largely focused on the identification of environmental carcinogens. Indeed, scarcely a day passes without a pronouncement of some new agent (or some old agent newly studied) that has been causally implicated in human carcinogenesis, usually on the basis of studies in experimental animals. Until recently, very little attention was paid to the possibility that man's genotype, or at least the genes in some men, might be the initiating factor and thereby provide fertile substrate for an environmental carcinogen. For obvious reasons, geneticists have concentrated on those unifactorial disorders in which malignancy is a regular enough occurrence to be noteworthy, having left consideration of common cancers to epidemiologists. It has been shown quite clearly that familial aggregation does exist even for common neoplasms and that this aggregation cannot be totally accounted for by the environment (Schneider & Chaganti 1986). Hence, there has been a recent quickening of interest in cancer genetics in man. The topic has been reviewed in some detail in a series of publications, and the interested reader should consult these for general background as well as more specific information on the diseases considered in this chapter (Lynch 1976, Mulvihill et al 1977a, Schimke 1978, Chaganti & German 1985, Knudson 1986).

THE GENETIC AETIOLOGY OF CANCER

It is now quite clear that a variety of aneuploid states, single gene disorders and even polygenic conditions may predispose to malignancy, although the precise molecular mechanisms are not always clear. In conditions such as Bloom syndrome, where the gene mutation results in deficient DNA ligase I activity and hence defective DNA repair, it is easy to visualize a cause and effect relationship (Willis & Lindahl 1987). It is more difficult to account for the hereditary component of breast or colon cancer, since these are internal, site specific malignancies occurring in older individuals. For this reason, initial attention was focused on early onset tumours such as retinoblastomas, where treatment was generally effective and careful follow-up was possible. The hereditary fraction of all retinoblastomas may be in excess of 25%. When inherited, the predisposition to retinoblastoma behaves as an autosomal dominant trait with penetrance in excess of 90% (Vogel 1979). After evaluation of the available data, Knudson and his colleagues (1986) theorized that development of an embryonal malignancy such as retinoblastoma requires two mutational events. With heritable tumours, the first mutation would be germinal, the second somatic. The consequences of this reasoning would be that inherited tumours would tend to be multifocal (or bilateral when appropriate) and have an earlier age of onset. Decreased penetrance and less than complete monozygotic twin concordance could be explained by the absence of a somatic event, even in a genetically susceptible individual. Nonfamilial tumours would tend to be unifocal and later in onset, since two somatic events would be required. For tumours such as retinoblastoma, the theory has been established in fact. As discussed in more detail elsewhere in this text susceptible individuals in retinoblastoma families have been found by DNA analysis to have constitutional heterozygosity for a small region on chromosome 13 (13q14.11) (Cavanee et al 1986). The tumours themselves have lost this constitutional heterozygosity via a number of different mechanisms. In other words, loss or mutation of both alleles at the putative retinoblastoma (Rb) locus appears in some fashion to initiate malignancy. Similar findings have been noted for other neoplasms, not all of which are recognizably genetic (Table 106.1).

Whether this 'two-hit' model is generally applicable remains to be established. Nonetheless, it seems likely that the normal allele in some fashion regulates retinal differentiation, such that total loss of regulatory control results in malignancy; i.e. the normal allele is a tumour suppressing gene (Sager 1989).

Table 106.1 Tumours in which alterations in both respective homologous chromosomes have been seen

Tumour	Chromosome
Retinoblastoma	13q
Osteogenic sarcoma	13q
Wilms tumour	11p
Hepatoblastoma	11p
Rhabdomyosarcoma	11p
Bladder carcinoma	11p
Acoustic neuroma	22q
Meningioma	22q
Colorectal carcinoma	5q
Small cell lung carcinoma	3p
Renal cell carcinoma	3p

Considerable interest has also been generated by the study of oncogenes and their action (Druker et al 1989). While there is no firm evidence that oncogenes per se cause cancer in man, especially heritable cancer, they do seem to promote the malignant phenotype, especially when they are modified by rearrangement and translocation (Duesberg 1987). Careful cytogenetic study, initially of leukaemia and lymphoma, and later of solid tumours, has led to the inescapable conclusion that chromosome alterations are not random (Sandberg & Turc-Carel 1987). Moreover, the majority of cellular oncogenes can be precisely localized to breakpoints involved in tumour-specific chromosome rearrangements (Heim & Mitelman 1987). It is the general feeling that oncogene activation may be exceedingly important in determining the grade or severity of malignancy, even to the point of inducing the metastatic phenotype (Egan et al 1987).

CANCER FAMILIES

Most of the tumours to be discussed in this chapter are site specific; e.g. hereditary retinoblastoma, familial phaeochromocytoma, etc. In addition to this, a number of families have been described in which there is a pattern of malignancies within the family, but not every individual necessarily has the same neoplasm. In general, the tumours in such families are the common malignancies seen in man, but there are some unusual features. First of all, the tumour tends to occur at an earlier average age; e.g. colon carcinoma in the third or fourth decade, versus the usual onset in the 60s or 70s. Secondly, it is not uncommon for an individual to have more than one primary tumour; e.g. both colon and endometrial carcinoma. Third, the tumours may be multicentric. Fourth, in these families usually more than 25% of the individuals in direct lineal descent from the proband are affected, the exact percentage obviously depending upon

the age of these individuals. Fifth, for practical purposes, the cancer predisposition in these families behaves as an autosomal dominant trait with about 60% penetrance. Two cancer family syndromes have been tentatively identified, and it is quite likely that others exist (Table 106.2). The more common of the two is also appropriately called hereditary adenocarcinomatosis to indicate that the great bulk of affected individuals suffer from adenocarcinoma at various but rather predictable sites (Lynch et al 1977). The other syndrome is less clearly delineated, since there is a broad array of tumours represented, the chief ones of which are breast carcinoma and sarcomas in adults and embryonal neoplasms in children (Li & Fraumeni 1982, Lynch et al 1985).

This is not to say that other types of cancer families do not exist. For example, it appears that some members of families in which the proband has hereditary immunodeficiency have an increased incidence of malignancy, particularly of the lymphoreticular system (Conley et al 1980). Other families may have unique cancer-predisposing genes analogous to the so-called 'private' blood groups (Anderson 1978). In still other instances, heterozygotes for certain rare recessive disorders, which in themselves predispose to cancer, may represent a population at increased risk for cancer. As will be seen, the majority of man's cancer predisposition seems to be inherited by an autosomal dominant mechanism. Yet there are a few diseases, all autosomal recessive, in which the incidence of malignancy is quite high (Table 106.3). Virtually all of these have been found to have abnormalities in DNA repair after a variety of different insults. It is logical to assume that heterozygotes for these disorders might display partial defects in the same mechanisms to such an extent that they too would be at increased risk for the development of a tumour, although the number of families studied is small and the issue is controversial (Swift et al 1980). For example, Swift et al (1987) have calculated that more than 8% of patients with breast cancer in the USA are heterozygotes for ataxia-telangiec-

Table 106.2 Cancer types seen in two probable varieties of cancer family syndrome

Type I	Type II
Endometrium	Breast
Ovary	Sarcoma
Breast	Embryonal
Prostate	Brain
Colon	Leukaemia
Stomach	Lymphoma
Pancreas	Adrenal
Skin	Thyroid
Melanoma	Bladder

Table 106.3 Neoplasms in some autosomal recessive disorders

Fanconi anaemia
Leukaemia
Oesophageal carcinoma
Skin carcinoma
Hepatoma
Ataxia-telangiectasia
Leukaemia
Lymphoma
Ovarian cancer
Gastric cancer
Brain tumours
Colon cancer
Bloom syndrome
Leukaemia
Carcinoma of tongue
Oesophageal carcinoma
Colon carcinoma
Wilms tumour
Xeroderma pigmentosum
Skin cancer
Melanoma
Leukaemia
Cancer of oropharynx
Werner syndrome
Sarcoma
Hepatoma
Breast carcinoma
Thyroid carcinoma
Leukaemia

tasia. Whether these calculations are accurate or not remains to be proved; nonetheless, it does appear that persons harbouring certain recessive genes in the heterozygous state are at increased risk for cancer and therefore constitute a special type of cancer family syndrome.

EMBRYONAL TUMOURS

There are a number of tumours best considered as embryonal since they are often congenital and must thus originate in utero. Study of the molecular genetics of these tumours has proved to be most rewarding, as illustrated by retinoblastoma.

Retinoblastoma

The genetic specifics of this tumour and the molecular mechanisms that underlie its pathogenesis are discussed in detail elsewhere in this text. Of considerable interest has been the observation that survivors of retinoblastoma develop second tumours, notably osteosarcomas. The osteosarcomas show the same loss of constitutional heterozygosity of chromosome 13 as do the retinoblastomas (Hansen et al 1985). This finding indicates that a

single pleiotropic germinal mutation may predispose to a variety of tissue specific tumours, depending upon the tissue in which the somatic event occurred.

The range of potential tumours may well be restricted, perhaps in part by age. In other words, retinoblastoma is rare beyond age 5, such that the effect of the loss of heterozygosity at the Rb locus in retinal cells would no longer lead to malignancy. The bones may harbour no such age restriction, although reported osteosarcomas tend to develop at the usual time; i.e. in adolescence and early adult life. Additional data collected on retinoblastoma families suggest that other cancers more typical of older individuals, such as lung and bladder cancer, may occur later in life (Strong et al 1984, Tarkkanen & Karjalainen 1984). Molecular studies of these tumours should prove most rewarding. Pinealoma appears unusually frequent with bilateral retinoblastoma, an observation that, recognizing the vestigial photoreceptor function of the pineal, has given rise to the whimsical application of the term 'trilateral retinoblastoma' (Bader et al 1982). The *N-myc* oncogene may be amplified and overexpressed in retinoblastoma as in neuroblastoma, when this is found it usually portends a poorer prognosis (Lee et al 1984).

Wilms tumour

Wilms tumour comprises about 15% of all childhood neoplasms with half the tumours developing before age 3. It has been estimated that 1/3 of all cases may be hereditary, although a substantially smaller proportion was uncovered in a US tumour registry (Breslow & Beckwith 1982). When inherited, Wilms tumour is transmitted as an autosomal dominant trait with roughly 60% penetrance (Knudson & Strong 1972). Monozygotic twin concordance is about 50%. Most gene carriers probably have unilateral disease with as many as 1/3 of supposedly sporadic unilateral tumours being heritable. Unlike most heritable tumours, the age of onset is not appreciably younger than sporadic cases. Bove & McAdams (1976) found coexistent anomalous metanephric differentiation in all bilateral, and in 14 of 60 unilateral cases of Wilms tumour. Gallo (1978) reported similar findings in 12 of 61 cases, and of these 12, four subsequently developed tumours in the opposite kidney. These findings argue in favour of a basic heritable defect in differentiation of the metanephric blastema analogous to that previously postulated for retinoblastoma. The parallel is apt since some patients with heritable Wilms tumour have also been found to suffer from loss of constitutional heterozygosity for a DNA segment contained in the 11p13 chromosome region (Dao et al 1987). Other patients with Wilms tumour, usually with a visible deletion of 11p13, have other anomalies including aniridia, ambiguous genitalia in males and varying degrees of retardation (Drash syndrome) (Eddy & Mauer 1985). The frequently cryptorchid testes carry a 20-30% risk of malignancy. It is likely that the complex of anomalies is, in reality, a contiguous gene syndrome, with symptoms dependent upon the extent of the deleted 11p13 segment (Schmickel 1986).

Second tumours in survivors of Wilms tumour are not common, but it is only recently that mortality statistics have substantially improved. These tumours generally develop in the irradiated tumour bed or after treatment of metastases. Soft tissue sarcomas, hepatoblastomas, thyroid carcinoma, acute leukaemia and colon carcinoma have been reported (Meadows et al 1977). Unfortunately, in none of these reports of second tumours is information provided about family history. Except in a patient with Wilms tumour and the Beckwith-Wiedemann syndrome, no cytogenetic or molecular studies have been done on second tumours (see below). It may well be that the patient with the familial form of Wilms tumour is at greater risk for a second neoplasm. If this reasoning is correct, then patients with hereditary diseases should be treated as far as possible with surgery alone.

Patients with hemihypertrophy seem to have a greater incidence of embryonal malignancy (Müller et al 1978). About 3% of patients with Wilms tumour have hemihypertrophy but data on the converse are not available. Hemihypertrophy is usually an isolated finding, but dominant pedigrees are known, and minor degrees probably go unnoticed. A family has been reported in which a woman with hemihypertrophy had three children with Wilms tumour (one bilateral, two unilateral) and another with a renal malformation (Meadows et al 1974). The latter also has been found with increased frequency in conjunction with Wilms tumour (Bove & McAdams 1976).

Wilms tumour has been reported in Sotos syndrome, Klippel-Trenaunay syndrome, Beckwith-Wiedemann syndrome, and von Recklinghausen disease, conditions which feature growth disturbances of one form or another. The Beckwith-Wiedemann syndrome is probably an incompletely penetrant autosomal dominant trait with a high incidence of embryonal malignancy, particularly Wilms tumour, adrenal cortical carcinoma and hepatoblastoma (Sotelo-Avila et al 1980). Molecular study of three disparate tumours in a patient with Beckwith-Wiedemann syndrome (Wilms tumour, hepatoblastoma, rhabdomyosarcoma) showed loss of constitutional heterozygosity for DNA in the 11p13 region in all three tumours (Koufos et al 1985). These findings support the previously offered contention that a single primary mutational event may underlie different malignancies as is seen in patients with retinoblastoma and osteosarcoma. The available evidence suggest that regulatory control of the potential for malignancy is dominant, since insertion of a normal human 11p chromosome into a Wilms tumour cell line suppresses the ability of the cells to induce tumours when transplanted into nude mice (Weissman et al 1987). However, genes located in the 11p15.5 region may also be of considerable importance, since loss of alleles in this region have been found in Wilms tumour and adrenocortical carcinoma (Henry et al 1989).

Neuroblastoma

The neuroblastoma tumour cell is derived from the neural crest, a ubiquitous tissue that gives rise to a number of structures including the adrenal medulla and the autonomic ganglia (Schimke 1979). While the adrenal is a favoured site, more than half the tumours are located outside these glands. Adequate genetic studies of neuroblastoma are lacking for two conflicting reasons. On the one hand, survival is poor, but paradoxically some tumours, especially in females, mature to ganglioneuroma or ganglioneurofibroma and as such may never be detected except serendipitously (Wilson & Draper 1974). In situ neuroblastomas are present in as many as 1/200 children at autopsy, an incidence far less than the 1/10 000 of frank tumours (Bolande 1977). Comparatively few familial cases of neuroblastoma have been reported, although the tumour has been described in twins, in sibs and in two generations (Schimke 1979). Autosomal dominant inheritance of the familial tumour would seem to be the most likely interpretation of the data. The gene defect could on occasion present as heterochromia iridis or as aganglionic megacolon (Knudson & Meadows 1976).

The proportion of heritable cases of neuroblastoma is unknown but, like the other embryonal neoplasms, the genetic form is more likely to be multifocal and become evident earlier. More than one tumour may be present at birth and the question arises as to whether the disease is already disseminated or represents multifocal, primary, and hence by definition, genetic disease. For example, a special group of children has been defined who present with small, commonly bilateral adrenal lesions, along with additional nodules in liver, skin and bone marrow, but who frequently show spontaneous regression of their tumours (Evans et al 1980). The neuroblastoma nodules in this setting, termed stage IV-S, are not truly malignant but probably represent collections of neural crest tissue bearing only a germinal mutation (a single 'hit') that has interfered with their normal development (Knudson & Meadows 1980).

Second tumours in neuroblastoma survivors include thyroid, renal and basal cell carcinoma, glioma and osteogenic sarcoma, virtually all of which arose in previously irradiated areas (Li 1977, Meadows et al 1977). One patient has been reported with congenital neuroblastoma, later multiple phaeochromocytomas and eventually multifocal renal cell carcinoma (Fairchild et al 1979).

Cytogenetic studies in neuroblastoma patients have not been rewarding as in the other embryonal neoplasms. Deletion of the short arm of chromosome 1 tends to be the most common finding. Excess numbers of small, paired chromatin bodies known as double minutes are also regularly seen. A single child with neuroblastoma and trisomy 13 has been reported (Feingold et al 1971). Neuroblastoma has been seen in the fetal hydantoin syndrome (Seeler et al 1979). It is conceivable that this substance is both teratogenic and oncogenic in certain susceptible individuals, since Wilms tumour has also been described in an infant exposed in utero (Taylor et al 1980). Genomic amplification of the *N-myc* oncogene tends to be associated with more aggressive tumour behaviour (Seeger et al 1985).

Hepatoblastoma and hepatoma

Hepatoblastoma is a rare tumour almost invariably developing before age 2. There is very little evidence for genetic aetiology, save for two reports of affected infant sibs (Fraumeni et al 1969, Napoli & Campbell 1977). The tumour has been reported with 'overgrowth' syndromes such as congenital hemihypertrophy, cerebral gigantism, and the Beckwith-Wiedemann syndrome (Müller et al 1978, Sotelo-Avila et al 1980). In these situations, the genetics is that of the primary syndrome. It has also been seen in two Japanese sibs with type Ia glycogen storage disease (Ito et al 1987). Hepatoblastoma has also been reported in families with polyposis coli (Li et al 1987). It is not known whether all hepatoblastomas show changes in the 11p13 chromosome region, as was seen in the Beckwith-Wiedemann syndrome.

Hepatocellular carcinoma or hepatoma is also uncommonly familial, and when it occurs in relatives is almost invariably related to some prior hepatotoxic insult such as neonatal hepatitis, biliary atresia or cirrhosis of virtually any cause. Genetic syndromes in which hepatoma has been reported are listed in Table 106.4. It must be emphasized that hepatoma is an uncommon accompaniment of these conditions. A deletion of the 11p13–11p14 region was found in one chromosome in a hepatocellular carcinoma associated with hepatitis B virus (Rogler et al 1985). The presumption was that the deletion was generated by integration of the virus into the host

Table 106.4 Genetic syndromes in which hepatoma may occur

Haemochromatosis
Fanconi anaemia
Ataxia-telangiectasia
Osler-Rendu-Weber syndrome
Tyrosinaemia
Alpha-1 antitrypsin deficiency
Familial cirrhosis
Byler disease
Werner syndrome

genome. Similar events with different viruses could be responsible for somatic mutations in both hereditary and sporadic tumours.

Teratomas

The majority of congenital teratomas develop in the sacrococcygeal area and a few of them are malignant. In later childhood they are generally gonadal in origin, apparently arising by parthenogenesis from a single germ cell. The sacrococcygeal tumours may be discovered only incidentally (Ashcraft et al 1975, Yates et al 1983). Teratoma-free individuals who transmit the autosomal dominant tendency may have radiographically detectable sacral defects, anterior sacral meningocele, anorectal abnormalities, or recurrent perianal abscesses, illustrating the extreme degree of variability of the gene defect. Hereditary teratomas may be more common than generally recognized, since many of them may be asymptomatic.

Sarcomas

The relationship between sarcomas and other childhood neoplasms, particularly retinoblastoma, has been noted earlier. There is significant sib-sib correlation between osteogenic sarcoma, rhabdomyosarcoma, hamartomas and other unusual sarcomas (Miller 1968). The earliest to appear is the rhabdomyosarcoma, but the tumour accounts for only about 2% of all deaths from cancer below age 15. It is rarely familial except as a facet of the Li-Fraumeni or type II cancer family syndrome.

The same is true in general with osteogenic sarcoma. For example, a man who had osteogenic sarcoma of the tibia at age 15 developed another such tumour of the mandible at age 40 (Epstein et al 1970). He has two children with tumours, one an osteogenic sarcoma, the other an adreno-cortical carcinoma. In another family two sibs and their grandfather had sarcoma and a maternal aunt had leukaemia and breast cancer (Bottomly et al 1971). The aunt had two children with acute leukaemia and another with an adrenal carcinoma. There are a few examples of familial osteogenic sarcoma occurring as isolated tumours, but not in sufficient quantity to construct a genetic hypothesis (Colyer 1979). The tumours generally are not multiple and they develop during the adolescent growth spurt at the usual sites where rapid bone growth is taking place. The reports are mostly of sibs, but two generation occurrence has been noted (Parry et al 1979). In such families it is probably worthwhile to look for evidence of heritable conditions known to be associated with sarcomas, such as neurofibromatosis, multiple exostoses, enchondromatosis, osteogenesis imperfecta, fibrous dysplasia and, in older individuals, Paget disease. Mulvihill et al (1977b) described an American Indian family in which multiple sibs had varying combinations of limb anomalies, erythrocyte macrocytosis and childhood osteogenic sarcoma. The father had the limb deformities and macrocytosis. An abnormality in regulation of bone formation was postulated.

Loss of constitutional heterozygosity of chromosome 13 has been found in sporadic osteosarcoma patients without retinoblastoma or a family history of such (Dryja et al 1986). Moreover, female sibs with osteosarcoma have been reported who had a heritable constitutional 13;14 chromosomal rearrangement (Gilman et al 1985). The tumours were not studied cytogenetically. Other non-osteogenic sarcomas have not shown specific alterations in chromosome 13 (Hansen et al 1985). Ewing sarcoma has been described in sibs who had constitutional cytogenetic alterations (Joyce et al 1984). Chromosome studies on eight sporadic Ewing tumour cell lines have shown a consistent reciprocal translocation between chromosomes 11 and 12, most likely t(11;12)(q24q12) (Aurias et al 1983, Turc-Carel et al 1983). It is quite possible that deletions in one of those two chromosomes act to initiate this particular sarcoma.

HAMARTOMA SYNDROMES

Neurofibromatosis

Neurofibromatosis is the prototype of the hamartoma syndromes, with an incidence of about 1/3000 births. The clinical features and the diagnostic criteria for this autosomal dominant trait have been well-described (Riccardi & Eichner 1986). A variety of tumours may complicate neurofibromatosis (Table 106.5) but the overall incidence of NF-related malignancy is unlikely to exceed a few percent. The most common tumours are those sarcomas that develop as a degenerative complication of the neurofibromas. Central nervous system tumours are next most frequent, the whole array of

Table 106.5 Some tumours described in patients with neurofibromatosis

Neurinoma	Phaeochromocytoma
Glioma	Paraganglioma
Ganglioneuroma	MEN syndromes
Schwannoma	Carcinoid
Meningioma	Leukaemia
Neuroblastoma	Nephroblastoma
Fibroma	Rhabdomyosarcoma
Sarcoma	Hepatoma

gliomas having been reported (Horton 1976). In children, the CNS lesions may provide a clue to the diagnosis, since the characteristic skin changes are often not present in early life. In one reported series of meningiomas in children it was concluded that nearly a quarter were the direct result of neurofibromatosis (Merten et al 1974). The neurofibromatosis gene has been localized to chromosome 17 (Barker et al 1987, Seizinger et al 1987a). The application of molecular probes to this chromosome may provide considerable insight, not only into neurofibromatosis, but also the malignant facet of the condition as well. However, since the neurofibromas per se are not clonal in origin, the development of malignant degeneration may have a more complex aetiology (Fialkow 1977).

It is now clear that at least two forms of neurofibromatosis exist, since the gene for a separate central form comprising acoustic neuromas, gliomas, meningiomas and spinal neurofibromas has been mapped to chromosome 22 (Seizinger et al 1987b). Loss of genes on this chromosome appears to be responsible for malignancy in all these lesions (Seizinger et al 1986).

Congenital fibromatosis is a disorder in children that may simulate neurofibromatosis (Baird & Worth 1976). Affected individuals have fibrous, leiomyomatous tumour masses throughout the body that spontaneously regress, providing vital visceral function is not disturbed by their presence. It is inherited as an autosomal recessive trait.

Von Hippel-Lindau syndrome

The diagnostic hallmarks of this condition are haemangioblastomas of the retina and cerebellum, although these vascular tumours can develop anywhere in the brain or spinal cord (Horton et al 1976). Cysts have been reported in a variety of organs, including the liver, kidney, pancreas and epididymus and these are often the only sign of the disease (Levine et al 1982). Hypernephroma, often bilateral, may occur in 20% or more of the patients (Malek et al 1987). In some families the renal cell carcinoma may be the only sign of the disease (Richard et al 1973). Phaeochromocytomas also occur, but much less commonly. Some patients with the syndrome have had nonfunctional pancreatic islet cell tumours, a topic discussed in detail later. Whether the patients with adrenal medullary and pancreatic tumours represent a distinct subgroup is not clear at present, although the parallel with the multiple endocrine neoplasia syndromes, particularly types IIa and IIb, is obvious. Autosomal dominant inheritance is the accepted mode of genetic transmission for the von Hippel-Lindau syndrome.

Tuberous sclerosis

A wide variety of hamartomas characterize this disorder, notably in the brain, skin, retina, kidney and heart, although such tumours may be found in any organ. Malignant degeneration, usually sarcomatous in type, can occur, but probably in no more than a few percent of cases, and metastatic spread is rare. Even the characteristic brain tumours are histologically benign, although they often interfere with neurological function either by direct encroachment on vital structures or through obstructive hydrocephalus. More invasive brain tumours have been described, particularly in younger individuals, including glioblastomas and ependymomas (Horton 1976). Optic gliomas may cause considerable visual disability. The kidney tumour is a mixed neoplasm, generally referred to as an angiomyolipoma, that only rarely becomes truly malignant, although cystic degeneration and stone formation are common. Wilms tumour has been noted, but it was almost certainly coincidental (Grether et al 1987). The diagnostic skin lesions and the more rare cardiac rhabdomyomas are virtually never malignant. The trait is an autosomal dominant with considerable variation in expressivity. The gene has tentatively been mapped to chromosome 9.

Basal cell nevus syndrome

The chief feature of this disorder is the skin tumour, but other developmental abnormalities in the skeleton may be diagnostically useful, since the basal cell nevi are not present in children (Gorlin & Sedano 1972). Medulloblastomas are also seen. Interestingly, when children with the brain tumours are irradiated, basal cell carcinomas develop in an accelerated fashion in the irradiated scalp, neck and shoulder areas, whereas in non-irradiated affected adults, the nevi are more common in sun-exposed areas. Other tumours reported include meningioma, astrocytoma, rhabdomyosarcoma, fibrosarcoma, melanoma, ovarian fibroma and carcinoma, hamartoma-tous gastric polyps and mesenteric cysts (Southwick & Schwartz 1979). It is inherited as a quite variable autosomal dominant. Apart from the medulloblastomas and ovarian tumours, the other tumours may be coincidental.

Blue rubber bleb nevus syndrome

The name of this autosomal dominant syndrome is most descriptive, as affected patients have blister-like vascular nevi not only on the body surface, but potentially in the viscera as well (Gorlin 1976). The nevi may be painful, and tend to bleed, but are not malignant. Associated cancers have been described, but not with sufficient specificity or frequency for any firm conclusions to be made about the total neoplastic potential of the syndrome (Lichtig 1971). A similar, but independent condition is familial angiolipomatosis, an autosomal recessive disorder in which affected sibs have multiple subcutaneous tumours, particularly in the neighbourhood of joints (Hapnes et al 1980). There is no known malignant predisposition.

Cowden syndrome (Multiple hamartoma syndrome)

Patients with this disorder are often quite striking in their physical appearance, in that they have multiple papillomas of the oral cavity, hair follicle hamartomas, and angiomas, lipomas and cysts almost anywhere in the body (Gentry et al 1975). Affected females have developed breast and uterine cancer, and both sexes have had colon and thyroid cancer. This disorder is a rare autosomal dominant. Patients without the typical facies may not be correctly diagnosed, so the overall incidence of malignancy is unknown.

Other hamartoma syndromes

The Sturge-Weber syndrome is generally placed in this category, but it appears not to confer an increased risk of malignancy. Another neurocutaneous syndrome, the linear sebaceous nevus syndrome, has a high incidence of malignancy, as attested by one study of 25 patients (Andriola 1976). The tumours have developed in diverse locations such as brain, skin, salivary glands, heart, oesophagus and jaw. Both these conditions are sporadic. Two other non-heritable hamartoma syndromes should be mentioned; the Klippel-Trenaunay-Weber (angio-osteohypertrophy) and the Maffucci syndromes. Bilateral Wilms tumour has been reported in the former (Ehrich et al 1978) and while the association may have been coincidental, it has been mentioned that embryonal tumours tend to occur in syndromes involving aberrant growth patterns. Chondrosarcomas and angiosarcomas can develop in the Maffucci syndrome (enchondromas and haemangiomas) and, curiously, there seems to be an increased incidence of pituitary and perhaps other endocrine tumours as well (Schnall & Genuth 1976, Lowell & Mathog 1979). Other conditions that could easily be classified as hamartomatous include the Gardner, Peutz-Jegher, and Turcot syndromes but, as all feature intestinal polyposis, they are discussed elsewhere in this book.

ENDOCRINE GLAND NEOPLASMS

Secretory tumours of any of the endocrine glands obviously have extensive physiological implications, whether they are malignant or not. From a diagnostic point of view confusion frequently reigns due to the predilection of malignant endocrine tumours to produce ectopic hormones as well. There are three well-defined multiple endocrine neoplasia syndromes (MENS), two of which share certain features (Schimke 1984).

MEN I (Werner syndrome)

This condition consists of tumours or hyperplasia of, in order of decreasing frequency of involvement, parathyroids, pancreatic islet cells, and pituitary (Yamaguchi et al 1980). The clinical presentation is variable, depending upon the function status of the various glands at the time of diagnosis. In some instances the affected individual is totally asymptomatic, the presence of the syndrome being detected only by systematic screening. More than 90% of the patients present with hypercalcaemia or symptoms referable to a pituitary tumour; e.g. headaches, visual disability or galactorrhoea-amenorrhoea. Less commonly they develop signs of acromegaly, Cushing syndrome, or thyroid dysfunction. Tumours of the latter organ are unusual and are not medullary in type, this neoplasm being characteristic of the other two MENS. About 60% of affected family members have two glands involved, and 20% eventually have three or more. Generally speaking, the only consistent truly malignant part of the syndrome involves the islet cells, where the presentation may be that of insulinoma, the Zollinger-Ellison syndrome, the glucagonoma syndrome or pancreatic cholera. Other tumours described in MEN I include lipomas, Schwannomas, thymomas and cutaneous leiomyomas.

Symptoms of the syndrome may develop at any age, but the condition is uncommon in childhood and rarely presents initially after age 60. As with the other MEN syndromes, MEN I is an autosomal dominant disorder probably with complete penetrance, but with considerable variability in expression. Identical twins have been

described who were concordant for the presence of the syndrome, but discordant at the time of presentation for specific gland involvement (Bahn et al 1986). The basic genetic lesion is unknown and involvement of the various glands cannot be totally accounted for (Schimke 1986). Once the diagnosis is made, periodic screening studies must be undertaken in all first-degree family members (Marx et al 1986). The MEN I gene has been mapped to the long arm of chromosome 11 (Nakamura et al 1989).

MEN IIa (Sipple syndrome)

Medullary thyroid carcinoma, phaeochromocytoma and parathyroid hyperplasia constitute the triad of findings characteristic of this syndrome. The thyroid tumour is actually derived from the parafollicular cells whose prime secretory product is calcitonin, the excessive secretion of which, while causing no symptoms, is extraordinarily useful in diagnosis. Parafollicular or C-cell hyperplasia probably always precedes frank malignancy by months or even years. The thyroid tumours once they develop are multifocal, and this is also true of the adrenal medullary neoplasms, although with the latter tumours, it is not uncommon for years to elapse between the detection of one tumour and the development of another. The phaeochromocytomas may be extra-adrenal and are also preceded by premonitory adrenal medullary hyperplasia (Carney et al 1975). The parathyroid glands are generally diffusely hyperplastic. As with islet cells, the medullary thyroid tumour may secrete a variety of substances besides calcitonin; e.g. ACTH, serotonin, vasoactive intestinal polypeptide, and so forth, again generating diagnostic confusion. Other tumours reported in MEN II include brain tumours, breast carcinoma, leukaemia and cancer of the pyriform sinus, but in no case is the association strong enough to be considered more than coincidental.

The thyroid tumour is ultimately malignant, although even with frank lymph node involvement prolonged survival is common. The incidence of true malignancy of the adrenal medullary tumours is probably higher than with sporadic phaeochromocytomas. Oddly enough, they often do not respond to the usual provocative tests, and may actually be detected only incidentally, a factor that may account in part for the higher malignant potential.

MEN IIa is an autosomal dominant disorder with nearly complete penetrance by age 50. Baylin et al (1978), using tissue from patients with MEN IIa who were also heterozygous for two electrophoretically distinguishable G6PD variants, have established that the syndrome results from a clonal event, in that each separate tumour focus has either the A or the B phenotype. This finding is in keeping with the 'two-hit' hypothesis, in that a second somatic event would be necessary before a given cell would undergo malignant transformation and clonal growth. Further support for this hypothesis is derived from study of monozygotic twins who were concordant for thyroid carcinoma but discordant for phaeochromocytoma (Pohl et al 1977).

Provocative testing with either or both calcium and pentagastrin has been used in individuals at risk for MEN IIa. These substances stimulate secretion of large amounts of calcitonin by the C-cells even during their preneoplastic stages, thereby allowing for curative thyroidectomy. Once basal serum calcitonin levels are elevated, the tumour is beyond the confines of the thyroid capsule. The MEN IIa gene has now been mapped to chromosomes 10 (Simpson et al 1987) and it is likely that molecular probes will prove more useful than calcitonin measurements for early diagnosis. The prevailing opinion is that thyroidectomy should be carried out as soon as the gene carrier is identified (Telander et al 1986).

MEN IIb (Mucosal neuroma syndrome)

MEN IIb also includes medullary thyroid carcinoma and phaeochromocytoma, but in addition affected individuals have a rather striking habitus, including the virtually pathognomonic feature of mucosal neuromas, not only in the oropharynx but literally throughout the gastrointestinal tract (Schimke 1973, Carney & Hayles 1978). Other features that distinguish MEN IIb from MEN IIa include the lack of parathyroid involvement in the former disorder and the poorer prognosis, the mean survival being substantially less.

MEN IIb is also an autosomal dominant disorder, but calculations of penetrance are not yet possible, since no systematic study of enough families has been undertaken to see whether mucosal neuromas could be present without the more malignant aspects of the syndrome. When the typical facies are present, it is important to remove the thyroid totally as soon as possible, since thyroid malignancy may be present by age 2, and no therapy save surgery is consistently effective (Moyes & Alexander 1977). The behaviour of the phaeochromocytoma in MEN IIb is similar to that in MEN IIa.

Possible MEN syndromes

There are a host of reports of patients with two or more endocrine tumours, often of a type that suggests overlap of the recognized MEN syndromes. Virtually all of the cases are sporadic, and it is not clear that they are distinct syndromes.

One endocrine tumour association may be unique; i.e. that of phaeochromocytoma with pancreatic islet cell tumours, a combination of neoplasms that may be familial or occur sporadically. The phaeochromocytomas tend to be multiple and have an early age of onset. The islet cell tumours, which may be benign or malignant, are generally not secretory, at least not for any known hormones, a situation unlike that seen with MEN I where more than 75% of such lesions are functional (Carney et al 1980). In one affected family, the proband had multiple islet cell tumours and multicentric phaeochromocytomas, her daughter had a unilateral phaeochromocytoma, and her mother had bilateral phaeochromocytoma and a pituitary tumour (Janson et al 1978). While it is tempting to consider this complex as MEN III, it is interesting that about half the reported patients either had the von Hippel-Lindau syndrome, or had first-degree relatives with this condition (Hull et al 1979). In the family just noted, the proband also had benign adenomas in both kidneys, findings reminiscent of the von Hippel-Lindau syndrome. Pancreatic adenomas, functional status unknown, have also been described in this condition (Horton et al 1976). Conceivably, the von Hippel-Lindau syndrome may be more clinically variable than previously thought or, alternatively, it may be genetically heterogenous.

Other familial endocrine tumours

Familial examples of pituitary adenomas exclusive of MEN I are rare. Levin et al (1974) recorded brothers with acromegaly, and a mother-daughter pair have had the galactorrhoea-amenorrhoea syndrome (Linquette et al 1967). The latter complex is commonplace in endocrine clinics and has been related by some clinicians to the extensive contemporary use of oral contraceptives; hence, no genetic interpretation of familial aggregation is possible.

There are numerous reports in the literature of familial hyperparathyroidism such that autosomal dominant inheritance seems assured (Marx et al 1977). What is less clear is what proportion of these families actually has one of the MEN syndromes, the other facets not having become evident at the time the family is recorded. A reasonable estimate might be about one third. Hyperparathyroidism has been reported in patients with papillary thyroid carcinoma on a nonfamilial basis. While external ionizing radiation has been implicated as a potential cause of both lesions, the evidence is far from convincing (LiVolsi & Feind 1976).

A few families have been recorded with multiple individuals affected with papillary or follicular carcinomas (Stoffer et al 1986), but no firm genetic hypothesis can be constructed. Recognized predisposing factors include long-standing goitre, particularly if associated with certain inborn errors of thyrosine biosynthesis (Cooper et al 1981) and external irradiation. Papillary thyroid cancer has been reported in the Gardner, Cowden and Werner syndromes. Both papillary and follicular neoplasms have also been reported in the cancer family syndrome.

Pancreatic islet cell tumours, no matter what their secretory capacity, are only rarely familial, except when part of MEN I or the aforementioned phaeochromocytoma-islet cell tumour complex. A father and daughter with insulinomas have been reported (Tragl & Mayr 1977). In another family, one member had a glucagonoma and other individuals had elevated plasma levels of high molecular weight glucagon in a pattern consistent with autosomal dominant inheritance, but whether these family members actually had islet cell tumours is unknown (Boden & Owen 1977). A familial form of nesidioblastosis has been recorded in sibs (Schwartz et al 1979). Pathologically this abnormality is characterized by a diffuse and disorganized formation of new islet cells. Neonatal hypoglycaemia is the presenting feature and the clinical course may be relentless unless early subtotal pancreatectomy is performed, and even this may not be entirely effective. Autosomal recessive inheritance of this peculiar entity is likely, but it is not strictly speaking a cancer syndrome.

Only about 10% of adult patients with adrenal cortical hyperfunction have primary adrenal disease. In children, however, adrenal carcinoma is much more likely, with the presenting features either of the Cushing syndrome or, more commonly, of virilization (Gilbert & Cleveland 1970). Earlier reports of familial occurrence of adrenal cortical tumours may well have represented untreated sibs with the mild, non-salt losing forms of the adrenogenital syndrome, conditions in which the pathological anatomy of the adrenal glands is often quite bizarre, due to the continued stimulation by ACTH. True malignancy in this setting is quite rare, as metastatic disease from such a source has not been successfully documented. Other instances of familial adrenal cortical carcinoma seem to be part of the cancer family syndrome (Schimke 1978). One rather interesting autosomal dominant syndrome comprises adrenocortical micronodular dysplasia (with Cushing syndrome), cardiac myxomas, multiple lentigines and spindle cell skin tumours (Danoff et al 1987). Adrenal cortical tumours may complicate the Gardner and Beckwith-Wiedemann syndromes.

Embryonic tumours of the adrenal medulla have been discussed earlier. Phaeochromocytoma may be part of MEN IIa and IIb, of von Recklinghausen disease and the von Hippel-Lindau syndrome, all autosomal dominant disorders. In addition, the tumour has a separate hereditary basis in some instances, although also as an autoso-

mal dominant trait. About 10% of all cases are hereditary with the hereditary form showing the expected features of frequent bilateral and/or extra-adrenal location. The various paraganglia are embryonically related to the adrenal medulla, and it is not surprising to find tumours of structures such as the glomus jugulare or the carotid bodies in patients with familial phaeochromocytoma (Pollack 1973). However, paragangliomas, or as some would prefer, chemodectomas, may occur on a familial basis in the absence of recognized phaeochromocytomas (Kahn 1977).

Carcinoid tumours are considered by some to be a form of endocrine neoplasia, predominantly because the tumours are secretory, but also because they occur as a component of MEN I and, in sporadic instances, with phaeochromocytoma. In these settings, the tumours are almost invariably foregut in location. Familial carcinoids independent of these other neoplasms are largely confined to the lower gastrointestinal tract, and are quite rare.

REPRODUCTIVE SYSTEM

Testicular tumours

Testicular tumours are diagnosed in less than 1/50 000 males. Most are of germ cell origin, except in children where teratomas and stromal tumours predominate. Gonadal teratomas usually develop parthenogenetically, especially in females. Nongonadal teratomas arise mitotically and these have the same karyotype as the host, although a tetraploid XXXY mediastinal lesion has been described (Kaplan et al 1979). While familial examples of testicular teratomas are rare, bilateral lesions have been described in sibs, one pair of which had the Klinefelter syndrome (Gustavson et al 1975, Shinohara et al 1980). Interestingly enough, mediastinal choriocarcinomas occur more often than expected in the Klinefelter syndrome (Schimke et al 1983). Seminoma has also been noted in a patient with Klinefelter syndrome (Isurugi et al 1977), but in this instance the gonad was cryptorchid, and it is well known that the incidence of malignancy in cryptorchid testes is increased at least 10-fold (Verp & Simpson 1987).

Familial aggregation of testicular tumours independent of the above and of the intersex states have been reported, albeit infrequently. Less than 70 such families have been noted, with the disease appearing in twins, sibs and, less commonly, two generations (Fuller & Plenk 1986). There is a greater tendency for the tumours to be bilateral in these families, and monozygotic twin concordance is high, bespeaking simply inherited tendency for neoplasia in some families. Also supporting a prime genetic role is the documented ethnic difference between

African Blacks and white Englishmen (30-fold higher in the latter), a difference that persists even after migration of the Blacks from Africa. At the present time, however, no clearly defined mode of inheritance for testicular tumours has been established, although it is quite likely that bilateral tumours have a greater tendency to be heritable, perhaps as a sex-limited autosomal dominant trait.

Ovary

Ovarian cancer is about five times more common than testicular cancer. About 90% of the tumours are derived from germinal epithelium and they tend to occur in older women. No definitive environmental risk factors have been identified (Annegars et al 1979). In contrast, a number of papers have documented multigeneration transmission of ovarian cancer (Simpson & Photopoulos 1976), but oddly enough the tumours are uncommonly bilateral and the age of onset is usually similar to the non-familial cases.

In children, ovarian teratomas predominate and they do tend to be bilateral, frequently also undergoing torsion (Brown 1979). A number of familial instances of teratomas have been described. Arrhenoblastomas and dysgerminomas have also been reported in females over two generations (Jensen et al 1974). Ovarian fibromas have been recorded in four generations of a family (Dumont-Herskowitz et al 1978). Perhaps 5–10% of ovarian tumours are due to simply inherited predisposing factors, behaving either as a sex-limited autosomal or an X–linked dominant trait. Table 106.6 summarizes some disorders in which gonadal tumours, either testicular or ovarian, may occur.

Gonadal tumours in intersex states

Gonadal tumours probably never occur in individuals with intersex states unless the gonad contains a Y-chromosome cell line (Verp & Simpson 1987). The risk is

Table 106.6 Disorders in which gonadal tumours appear

XO/XY mosaicism
True hermaphroditism
XY pure gonadal dysgenesis
Testicular feminization
Cryptorchidism
Cancer family syndrome
Peutz-Jegher syndrome
Gardner syndrome
Basal cell nevus syndrome
Ataxia-telangiectasia
Stein-Leventhal syndrome

variable, however, ranging from zero in XX males who are H-Y antigen positive to 20–30% in patients with XO/XY mosaicism or with H-Y positive, XY pure gonadal dysgenesis. Gonadal malignancy has been documented in true hermaphroditism, but it is rare. The risk for patients with the complete form of testicular feminization syndrome is less than 5% but those with the incomplete varieties, of which there are many, have not yet developed gonadal neoplasms. Inborn errors of steroid metabolism leading to sexual ambiguity do not seem to predispose to true malignancy in either sex. Testicular tumours in males with virilizing forms of the adrenogenital syndrome have been reported, but these disappear after cortisol therapy and are generally considered to be hypertrophied adrenal rest tissue.

Genital cancer

Cancer of the genitalia, exclusive of the uterus, is rare, and genetic factors are of no aetiological significance. There is no firm evidence that cancer of the cervix is at all genetic, except when it develops as a complication of the hereditary diseases dyskeratosis congenita and ectodermal dysplasia. Of greater interest to epidemiologists has been the association between maternal ingestion of diethylstilbestrol and vaginal cancer in female offspring. A large co-operative study of such individuals revealed that 34% had vaginal changes, often referred to as vaginal adenosis, but the actual cancer incidence was low, being about 1/1000 women exposed (Robboy et al 1979). The risk is age-related, in that the vast majority develop lesions prior to age 20.

Endometrial cancer has a more prominent genetic component, 16 of 154 patients in one series having an affected first-degree relative (Lynch et al 1967). Evaluation of the pedigrees revealed that about 10% of the multiply affected families contained members with other adenocarcinomas, a finding suggestive of the cancer family syndrome. Oestrogen use has been correlated with endometrial cancer, although the various studies are not in complete agreement (Hulka et al 1980). It has been suggested that the use of both oestrogens and progesterone confers a protective effect. To what extent the use of unopposed oestrogen might interact with heritable factors is not known, but would be worthy of further study. Endometrial carcinoma has been reported in the Turner syndrome, but virtually all patients had received unopposed oestrogens. As mentioned earlier, those with XO/XY and Turner phenotype are at substantial risk for gonadal neoplasms, but they should properly be considered as having mixed gonadal dysgenesis rather than the Turner syndrome. There is some evidence that individuals with the Turner syndrome may be unduly prone to tumours of neural crest derivatives (Wertelecki et al 1970).

Uterine sarcomas have been reported in the Werner syndrome, and both endometrial and breast cancer have been seen in sclerotylosis. Uterine leiomyomas (fibroids) are so common that no good genetic studies have been performed.

Prostate

In situ prostate carcinoma may occur in 10-15% of males over the age of 50 (Lynch et al 1966). Since cancer is, in general, a disease of older individuals, prostate tumours could easily occur in families by chance alone, hence no firm evidence for genetic factors has emerged. A statistical relationship between prostate cancer and breast, ovarian and endometrial cancer in female relatives was established in one study (Thiessen 1974). All these tumours are part of the cancer family syndrome, so that men with this kind of history may be at greater risk of having second tumours and of having offspring with similar afflictions. It seems unlikely that such men constitute more than 1–2% of the entire prostate cancer population.

Breast cancer

In the United States, the average lifetime probability of a woman developing breast cancer is about 7%. The tumour accounts for more than 20% of all female neoplasms and is the main cause of death in women (Anderson 1977). The incidence rates have risen in Western countries since the turn of the century, for unknown reasons. A host of adverse and protective circumstances have been associated with breast cancer, all of which are statistically interesting but of little value in defining a high risk population, much less an individual. Ethnic differences have been noted which appear to be related to environmental factors since they increase with migration from a low to a high incidence area (MacMahon et al 1975).

The first familial report of breast cancer was by Broca in 1886 who noted the disease in 10 of 24 female relatives. Other families with equally impressive numbers have been described. Lynch et al (1984) found that 5% of 225 consecutively ascertained breast cancer patients had a family history consistent with a breast cancer syndrome. More extensive family histories may more than double this incidence (Lynch & Lynch 1986). Other estimates of the heritable fraction of breast cancer range from 8% (based on the incidence of bilaterality) to a theoretical prediction of three- to four-fold higher. Within this genetically predisposed group there is evidence of heterogeneity, in that only about half of patients have had relatives with breast cancer alone, the remainder having a positive family history of breast carcinoma and/or other tumours; e.g. ovary, endometrium, colon and soft tissue sarcomas (Go et al 1983). Not surprisingly, the disease in families tends to appear earlier, even premenopausally and is often, if not initially, eventually bilateral (Anderson & Badzioch 1985a). The lifetime probability of developing breast cancer in the female progeny of a woman with premenopausal, bilateral disease is high enough to be consistent with autosomal dominant inheritance of a mammary tumour susceptibility gene (Anderson & Badzioch 1985b). In favour of this interpretation is a report suggesting linkage of such a gene with the glutamate-pyruvate transaminase locus (King et al 1983). In other families, notably those containing members with other tumours, no such linkage has been found.

Anderson (1974) noted that 8 of 234 (3.4%) pedigrees of breast cancer patients showed an associated adenocarcinoma at other sites, especially ovary, endometrium and colon, and an additional 14 (6%) showed aggregation of breast cancer with sarcomas, embryonal tumours and leukaemia. The data of Lynch et al (1978a) suggest that about 30% of familial breast cancer occurs in families in which these other tumours appear as well. In general, these latter families conform to the two general types of cancer family syndrome mentioned earlier. It is also quite possible that other breast cancer syndromes exist, but these are not yet well delineated.

Definition of that fraction of women with a genetic predisposition becomes exceedingly important, since environmental risk factors are so poorly defined, save for those individuals with a previous history of therapeutic chest irradiation (Li et al 1983). It is the genetically predisposed group that should be screened more vigorously. Fibrocystic disease is probably a high-risk indicator (Hutchinson et al 1980). Interestingly, in breast cancer families the increased risk extends to, and may be transmitted by, males (La Raja et al 1985). Outside the confines of such families male breast cancer is uncommon and heritability is low in otherwise normal men (Schwartz et al 1980). Males with the Klinefelter syndrome have a 20-fold increased risk of mammary cancer, and the tumour has also been noted in true hermaphrodites, perhaps in both instances on the basis of abnormal oestrogen levels and/or metabolism, although such has not been shown to be significant in women with breast carcinoma.

Breast carcinoma is a feature of the Cowden and Torre-Muir syndromes and it has also been reported in genetically determined immune deficiency states.

GASTROINTESTINAL CANCER

Gastrointestinal tumours, particularly of the colorectum, are among the most common neoplasms in man. In the past, much emphasis has been placed on those environmental factors that might predispose to malignancy. While such clearly exist, it is evident that heredity must also play a role, even in common cancers, although the genetic input varies with tumour site.

Oropharynx

While anatomical purists might quibble, the oropharynx, along with the rectum, could be considered as the squamous cell extremes of the gastrointestinal tract. The heritable disorders that predispose to neoplasia in these structures are few, and in general are associated with high cell turnover and/or abnormal DNA repair (Schimke 1980). For example, in X-linked dyskeratosis congenita, leukoplakia of the oral and rectal mucosa may give rise to squamous cell carcinoma. The same tumour type has been reported in dominantly inherited ectodermal dysplasia, in both dominant and recessive epidermolysis bullosa, and in xeroderma pigmentosum and the Bloom syndrome. These latter two conditions are discussed in greater detail elsewhere in this text.

Oesophagus

The bulk of oesophageal carcinoma is felt to develop because of nutritional deficiency and/or dietary peculiarities, largely because of the unusual geographic distribution of the disease, being more prevalent in central Africa and the Middle East. For example, in the Caspian littoral of Iran, the highest incidence rates in the world are found, perhaps as high as 400 per 100 000 population (Ghadirian 1985). Hence, families with multiple affected individuals in these areas provide no insight into any potential genetic mechanisms. Ashley (1969), studying oesophageal cancer in Wales, concluded that the greater the Welsh ancestry, the more likely the risk of developing the disease with an average two-fold risk over non-Welsh individuals living in Wales. The absolute risk in Wales is clearly low, given the population incidence of the disease.

Oesophageal cancer may complicate some rare genetic disorders, such as the previously mentioned dyskeratosis congenita and epidermolysis bullosa, and also the autosomal recessive Fanconi syndrome, another disorder in which DNA repair mechanisms are abnormal. Cancer of the oesophagus along with other GI cancers has been reported in common variable immunodeficiency for reasons which are not totally clear, although decreased immune surveillance is a plausible hypothesis (Spector et ,

al 1978). A similar rationale could be invoked for the increased incidence of oesophageal cancer in coeliac disease and in the more benign variant of scleroderma termed the CREST syndrome. In the latter condition, recurrent acid reflux may be of greater aetiological significance, and in the former, nutritional deficiency may play a prominent role. Both coeliac disease and the CREST syndrome are reportedly autoimmune disorders and, like the other autoimmune diseases, the genetics are quite complex with very little evidence for any major inherited component.

The most noteworthy genetic disease with oesophageal cancer is the late-onset form of tylosis. Virtually all patients with this rare, autosomal dominant disorder develop oesophageal malignancy by the seventh decade (Harper et al 1970). Another autosomal dominant form of tylosis appears in infancy and does not predispose to any known malignancy. Sclerotylosis can be distinguished from either of the above conditions by additional atrophic skin changes beyond the palmar-plantar areas (Hariez et al 1968). Oesophageal tumours have not been described in this condition, but cancer of the tongue, tonsil, breast and uterus have been reported.

Stomach

There is some disagreement concerning the role of genetics in the development of gastric cancer (Anderson 1978, Lehtola 1978). While pedigrees purportedly showing autosomal dominant inheritance have been published, the data are equally compatible with a polygenic hypothesis. Specific environmental carcinogens have not been identified in man, although substances like ethanol and certain nitroso compounds have been implicated. Histology may be significant, since heritability is greater with the diffuse rather than either the intestinal or undifferentiated cell types (Lehtola 1978). Ethnic factors seem to be important, as does the simultaneous presence of blood group A and pernicious anaemia, the latter usually accompanied by atrophic gastritis. Pernicious anaemia is generally associated with anti-parietal cell antibodies, and patients not uncommonly have other evidence of autoimmune disease. Individuals with immune deficiency states, such as adult-onset common variable immunodeficiency and ataxia-telangiectasia seem to be predisposed to gastric cancer to such an extent as to perhaps constitute a subpopulation of individuals at increased risk for this neoplasm (Spector et al 1978).

Gastric malignancy also appears to be more frequent in heterozygotes for the various autosomal recessive disorders with defective DNA repair. Gastric tumours may complicate some of the colon polyposis syndromes which are generally dominantly inherited. One apparently unique family has been described, in which 10 members over three generations suffered only gastric polyposis with a high frequency of associated stomach cancers (Santos & Magalhaes 1980). There were no recognized intestinal polyps. Familial aggregation of gastric carcinoma, melanoma and basal cell carcinoma has been reported in a pattern consistent with autosomal dominant inheritance (Weston et al 1986). Gastric cancer has also been reported in the cancer family syndrome. However, in the absence of any of these aforementioned risk factors, the absolute risk of a relative of a gastric cancer patient developing the same tumours is really quite low.

Benign stomach tumours have been noted in the basal cell nevus and Cowden syndromes (Schimke 1980).

Small intestine

Tumours of the small bowel are rare, and when they occur are more likely to be one facet of more complex disorders such as the Gardner, Peutz-Jeghers, colon polyposis syndromes, or cancer family syndromes (Love 1985). In fact, the risk of small intestinal malignancy, particularly in the periampullary structures, is increased in the Gardner syndrome 100- to 200-fold (Pauli et al 1980). Islet cell tumours and carcinoid tumours have been found in the duodenum in multiple endocrine neoplasia type I. Small bowel lymphomas have been described in multiple members of some families, but since most of these are male, the opinion has been advanced that these individuals have the Duncan syndrome, an X-linked selective immunodeficiency to Epstein-Barr virus (see later).

Gallbladder

The most significant predisposing agent to gallbladder cancer is felt to be stones; yet the latter are so common and the former so rare that other factors must be of importance. Indians in the southwestern United States have a higher incidence of gallstones and a six-fold increased incidence of gallbladder cancer when compared to the non-Indian population. While shared environment; i.e. reservation living and a high fat, high carbohydrate diet must be of significance, families have been reported in which detribalized individuals have developed the disease (Devor & Buechley 1979). This might indicate that the Indian heritage adds to the risk conferred by environment.

Liver

In nutritionally deprived areas of the world, both cirrhosis and hepatocellular carcinoma are not uncommon. Elsewhere, if exposure to environmental hepatotoxins can be excluded, familial aggregation of liver cancer is rare (Hagstrom & Baker 1968). There are a number of heritable diseases involving the liver where carcinoma has developed (Table 106.4). Hepatitis B antigen may conceivably be transmitted from one generation to the next via the placenta, giving rise to apparent dominant hepatoma (Ohbayashi et al 1972). An unusual family has been described in which the affected individuals had various combinations of liver cell adenomas or carcinomas and diabetes mellitus (Foster et al 1978). Two younger female members also had sclerocystic ovaries, along with hepatic adenomas and mild diabetes mellitus. Neither had been on oral contraceptives. Save for these few exceptions, the heritability of hepatic carcinoma should be considered as being quite low.

Pancreas

The incidence of adenocarcinoma of the pancreas appears to be increasing at about 15% per decade in the Western world. Suspected inciting agents are multiple, but alcohol, tobacco and certain industrial carcinogens have been most often incriminated. Calcific pancreatitis, either acquired or heritable, seems to predispose. Pancreatic cancer has been reported in ataxia-telangiectasia and in the cancer family syndrome. Islet cell carcinomas are an integral feature of multiple endocrine neoplasia and may develop in the von Hippel-Lindau syndrome. Familial aggregation of pancreatic cancer is otherwise virtually non existent (Ehrenthal et al 1987).

Colorectum

Cancer of the colorectum is second only to lung cancer as a cause of morbidity and mortality in the Western world. Exclusive of the heritable polyposis syndromes, which account for less than 5% of all colon cancer, most cases are sporadic, with a negative family history. However, that genetic factors are operational to some extent is indicated by the results of one series where 26% of patients had a positive family history (Lovett 1976) and surveys which suggest that the relatives of an index case have a three- to four-fold increased risk of developing colorectal cancer during their lifetime; i.e. if the lifetime probability of large bowel cancer is 5% an affected first-degree relative would increase the probability to at least 15% (Anderson 1980). However, these figures may be both an underestimate and an oversimplification. For example, pedigree studies of non-polyposis colorectal cancer have revealed some other markers that may indicate a greater liability to cancer in some families; e.g. earlier average age of onset in the index case, multiple tumours, simultaneous or independent presence of endometrial carcinoma in a first-degree female relative or gastric cancer in relatives of either sex, and a predominant right-sided location. It has been suggested that within the colorectal cancer patient category there are subgroups in whom the cancer liability behaves as an autosomal dominant trait with moderately high penetrance (Lynch et al 1985). These reputed entities are the cancer family syndrome or hereditary adenocarcinomatosis, hereditary gastrocolonic cancer, hereditary isolated colon cancer and the Torre-Muir syndrome, the latter clearly an autosomal dominant condition featuring sebaceous cysts, adenocarcinomas of the large and small bowel and uterus, squamous cell carcinoma of the mucous membranes, and transitional cell carcinoma of the urinary system (Fahmy et al 1982). Whether the former non syndromic colorectal cancer families represent one or a series of entities is not clear, but there is evidence that in these families the tumour develops in or prior to the fifth decade, the lesions are more likely to be right-sided (2/3 versus about 1/4 of sporadic cases) and they tend to be multiple about 20% of the time. Prolonged survival also seems to characterize this group of patients, perhaps because of the more vigorous use of early detection procedures (Lynch et al 1978b). Whether one disease or many, it is possible that these families may well represent the bulk of patients at increased risk of colorectal cancer, the families of the remaining patients having essentially no greater risk than the general population. In other words, the population-based studies showing increased risk to relatives may represent a composite figure for a heterogeneous disease consisting of some patients with high risk and others with low risk. Clearly, detailed histories and prospective studies are indicated to evaluate this possibility, since in the aggregate these individuals could conceivably comprise 5–10% of colon cancer patients. Marker studies, while perhaps not useful on a population basis, may provide clues to cancer susceptibility within families (Kopelovich 1980, Fearon et al 1990).

Multiple polyposis syndromes

These conditions are of considerable interest to the geneticist because they are heritable, with the exception of the Cronkhite-Canada syndrome, a rather enigmatic disorder in which the adenomatous gastrointestinal polyps are generally considered to be inflammatory (Daniel et al 1982). Some of the syndromes with polyposis are complex and have extracolonic features that facilitate diagnosis, such as the Gardner and Peutz-Jegher syndromes.

Gardner syndrome

The Gardner syndrome consists of the triad of colon polyps, sebaceous cysts and osteomas, but the gene has

Table 106.7 Tumours reported in the Gardner syndrome

Colon polyps and adenocarcinoma
Carcinoma of duodenum
Carcinoma of ampulla of Vater
Osteoma and osteosarcoma
Papillary thyroid carcinoma
Adrenal carcinoma
Bladder carcinoma
Fibroma and fibrosarcoma
Lipoma
Leiomyoma
Epidermoid cyst
Ovarian fibroma and carcinoma
Brain tumour
Melanoma
Parotid fibroma

multiple pleiotropic effects and tumours of a host of organs have been described (Table 106.7). It is inherited as a quite variable autosomal dominant disorder with complete penetrance (Naylor & Gardner 1977). The probability of malignant degeneration of the colon polyps is essentially 100% by age 40. While the diagnosis may be difficult to make in childhood, almost all patients have some extracolonic manifestation of the gene by the third decade. The presence of clumped, pigmented ocular fundus lesions may be particularly valuable in early detection of a gene carrier (Traboulsi et al 1987). Danes (1978) has found increased tetraploidy in epithelial cell cultures taken from tissues known to undergo malignant change in the Gardner syndrome. Cells from benign tumours such as lipomas, cysts and fibromas and skin fibroblasts did not show this phenomenon. The significance of this finding is not at the moment clear. The polyps have been shown to be multiclonal in origin (Hsu et al 1983). The gene maps to chromosome 5q at a site identical with, or at least close to, the gene for polyposis coli (Nakamura et al 1988). It is possible that both the Gardner syndrome and familial polyposis coli are due to a single gene mutation with considerable phenotypic variability. Alternatively they may be allelic.

Some families have been described whose features are in part compatible with the Gardner syndrome but in which other clinical findings are sufficiently different for the authors to feel that they were dealing with a distinct entity (Binder et al 1978). Alternatively, occasional patients with familial polyposis coli have had skin lesions of one sort or another, or osteomas, prompting the suggestion that the two syndromes are in reality one (McConnell 1980). These seem unlikely in view of Gardner's elaborate analysis (Naylor & Gardner 1977) but it illustrates the complexity of adequate nosology when overlapping clinical features are present and the basic genetic lesion is unknown.

Familial polyposis coli

This is the classic autosomal dominant polyposis syndrome in which the colon contains few to literally thousands of adenomatous polyps (Kussin et al 1979). Gastric polyps also occur but less commonly. Colon polyps have been detected in the first year of life or as late as the eighth decade, but the average age of onset is in the mid-twenties. Patients are generally managed by early colectomy with ileoprotoctomy, remaining rectal polyps having been found to regress in some instances. More recent data suggest that the incidence of recurrent rectal cancer is high if rectal polyps are present and low if not, so that the former group must be watched carefully if a conservative surgical approach is adopted (Bess et al 1980). The gene has been localized to chromosome 5 (5q21–22) (Bodmer et al 1987). Loss of constitutional heterozygosity appears to be an important mechanism for transformation of polyps to carcinoma in this syndrome, a situation analogous to that seen in retinoblastoma and Wilms tumour (Solomon et al 1987).

Peutz-Jegher syndrome

The buccal and labial pigmentation should alert the clinician to the diagnosis of this condition in which the gastrointestinal polyps are hamartomas and are generally considered benign, although they may cause bleeding or obstruction. Malignant degeneration does occur, however, especially if the polyps are in the stomach and duodenum, although the magnitude of this risk is probably no greater than 5%. Of considerable interest is the fact that affected females have an increased risk of sex-cord ovarian tumours, and Sertoli cell tumours of both ovary and testis have been seen (Giardiello et al 1987). Breast and endometrial carcinomas have also been described.

Juvenile polyposis

In this autosomal dominant condition the polyps appear in childhood, histologically are usually cystic hamartomas and are benign. Simultaneous adenomatous polyps have also been reported, however, and these may be malignant (Goodman et al 1979). In some families adenomatous polyps have been found in adults and juvenile polyps in children, raising the spectre of age-related, environmentally-induced degenerative changes. Treatment is generally conservative, with caution dictating that more aggressively appearing lesions should be removed under fibroscopic visualization.

Turcot syndrome

This is the only polyposis syndrome known to be inherited as an autosomal recessive (Itoh & Ohsato 1985).

Proposed dominant forms are less clearly delineated and may actually represent the Gardner syndrome (Lewis et al 1983). The extracolonic feature is a glioma. The condition is quite rare, only a few cases having been reported.

Other syndromes with polyps

Benign colon polyps occur in the Cowden syndrome. In neurofibromatosis and the mucosal neuroma syndrome, gangliomas of the colon may stimulate polyps, but they are virtually never malignant. Colon carcinoma has also been reported in some of the heritable immunodeficiency states, particularly those with absent IgA (Spector et al 1978).

URINARY TRACT MALIGNANCY

Hypernephroma in families is rare, with fewer than 50 instances having been documented in the literature (Lyons et al 1977, Li et al 1982). In some of these families, the affected individuals may have had the von Hippel-Lindau syndrome, a condition in which the incidence of renal cell carcinoma may exceed 20%, and one in which the renal tumour may precede the other more diagnostic features (Richard et al 1973). Associations of familial renal cell carcinoma with various HLA types have been sought and found, notably with Bw17, A2, B12, Bw21 and Aw30/31, but none of these are convincing, nor have they been established as very useful for predicting which relatives will likewise be affected (Pilepich et al 1978). One family has been described in which 10 individuals over three generations had either uni- or bilateral hypernephroma (Cohen et al 1979). Also segregating in this family was a balanced translocation between chromosomes 3 and 8. Five hypernephroma patients carried the translocation and three others must have had it according to pedigree analysis. The c-myc gene is apparently involved in the translocation (Drabkin et al 1985). Other workers have found that loss of alleles on the short arm of chromosome 3 seem to be rather consistent findings in sporadic renal cell carcinoma (Zbar et al 1987). Alleles in the same region are also lost in small cell lung tumours (see later), but whether they are alleles at the same locus is not yet known. In general, the heritability of hypernephroma should be considered low.

Familial examples of cancer of the renal pelvis, ureter and bladder are even more scarce and most workers feel these tumours are more directly related to environmental exposure to aromatic hydrocarbons. Only one family with ureteral cancer has been described, a mother and son being affected (Burkland & Juzek 1966). Transitional cell carcinoma of the renal pelvis has been noted in the cancer family syndrome (Frischer et al 1985). Genetic factors may play some role in the aetiology of bladder cancer in some families, although the data in these families are perhaps more suggestive of the cancer family syndrome in which the genitourinary malignancy could be considered just one component (Lynch et al 1979). These lesions are usually transitional cell carcinomas. A study of 101 unrelated patients with this tumour suggested a statistically significant association with blood group A and HLA types B5 and Cw4 (Herring et al 1979). Bladder cancer seems to be unusually frequent in elderly relatives of patients with familial retinoblastoma. In view of scarcity of familial reports, there would seem to be very little risk for lower urinary tract cancer in first-degree relatives of an affected individual, unless the family history is striking, or a common environmental carcinogen can be identified. Bladder carcinomas tend to lose genes on the short arm of chromosome 11, but this is not invariably true, perhaps indicative of aetiological heterogeneity (Fearon et al 1985).

CANCER OF THE RESPIRATORY TRACT

There is little doubt that cigarette smoking is of prime aetiological importance in bronchogenic carcinoma. Small cell or squamous cell lung tumours are virtually non-existent in non-smokers, save for those exposed to whole body irradiation, to chlormethyl ethyl ether or to uranium ore (Greco & Oldham 1979). Tokuhata & Lilienfeld (1963) showed more lung cancer in families of lung cancer probands even when there was no smoking history. Ooi et al (1986) found that even after control of the confounding environmental elements, there was a 2.4-fold greater risk of lung cancer among relatives of probands. There is evidence that smoking may act synergistically with other factors which may have at least partial genetic control, such as a tendency to develop chronic obstructive pulmonary disease (Cohen et al 1977). Alpha-1-antitrypsin phenotypes MZ or ZZ account for some, but not all, differences in tendency towards COPD (Kueppers et al 1977). The value of aryl hydrocarbon hydroxylase inducibility as a potential marker for lung cancer susceptibility remains in question. Loss of constitutional heterozygosity of 3p alleles appears to be a consistent finding in small cell lung tumours (Brauch et al 1987, Naylor et al 1987) and an occasional finding in non-small cell tumours. It is quite conceivable that some component of tobacco induces the allele loss that seems to be important in initiation of lung carcinoma.

In view of the fact that lung cancer is so common in the Western world, the lack of familial aggregation on purely environmental grounds is surprising, and perhaps under-reported (Mulvihill 1976). Carcinoma of the larynx should probably be considered together with bronchogenic carcinoma, both on anatomical and epidemiological grounds, since it essentially never appears in non-smokers.

Pulmonary fibrosis, whether idiopathic, caused by chronic infection, or associated with scleroderma, seems to predispose to adenocarcinoma of the lung. This tumour may be a facet of the cancer family syndrome, particularly that variety with the breast cancer-sarcoma complex. Bronchial carcinoid is an irregular feature of MEN I, and mucosal neuromas of the bronchi and larynx may complicate MEN IIb.

Nasopharyngeal carcinoma is a peculiar small cell tumour of ill-defined origin that occurs predominantly in Chinese and Alaskan natives. Because of this ethnic predilection, genetic factors must be of some importance and must account for some of the recognized familial aggregation (Lanier et al 1979). That this is not the whole story is supported by the finding that affected individuals have high antibody titres to EB virus, the same virus incriminated in tumour formation in non-genetic Burkitt lymphoma and in X–linked selective immunodeficiency syndrome. These findings suggest that not only tumour induction but tumour type and even site may depend in part on selective immune deficiency to EB virus, perhaps inherited by a Mendelian mechanism (Schimke et al 1987).

TUMOURS OF THE CENTRAL NERVOUS SYSTEM

The world-wide incidence of CNS tumours is about 1/10 000, about 90% of which occur in the brain. The mortality is age-dependent with children doing less well, brain tumours being second only to leukaemia as a cause of death in children under age 15. The implication is that adult lesions are less virulent, more effectively treated, or that the patients die of other causes. Most neurologists feel that heredity is not of major importance in the pathogenesis of brain tumours. However, relatives of glioma patients have been estimated to have a four- to ten-fold increased risk of the same tumour (von Metz et al 1977) and for children the frequency of sib pairs with brain tumours is nine times greater than that expected by chance (Miller 1968). That the genetic predisposition is not limited to the CNS is attested by the occurrence in sibs of tumours such as adrenocortical carcinoma, osteogenic sarcoma and leukaemia at a rate much higher than expected (Draper et al 1977, Meadows et al 1977). In adults, extraneural primaries are most common in meningioma patients, one series of 76 such individuals harbouring 20 additional malignancies, 12 of which were in the gastrointestinal tract or the lung (Bellur et al 1979). Another series associated meningiomas with breast carcinoma (Schoenberg 1975). Some of the patients may be members of cancer families, but pertinent detailed family history is not sufficient to draw conclusions in this regard.

Save for a few select families with the cancer family syndrome or with recognized conditions in which CNS tumours occur with unusual frequency, the heritability of brain tumours is likely to be low. Single gene inheritance may be operating in some instances where familial aggregation is particularly striking, but even here multi-factorial causation cannot be excluded (Delleman et al 1978, Challa et al 1983).

Autosomal recessive conditions in which brain tumours have been reported include the Werner and Turcot syndromes and ataxia-telangiectasia. Heterozygotes for the latter disorder may also be at increased risk for brain tumours (Swift 1976). Acoustic neuromas, along with gliomas and meningiomas occur in families as a facet of central neurofibromatosis. As mentioned earlier, this gene is located on chromosome 22.

SKIN

Cancer of the integument is common along light-skinned races. The usual cell types are basal or squamous cell, with melanomas being less frequent. Heritable non-syndromic varieties of basal and squamous cell tumours probably exist, but the lesions are relatively common, are for the most part age-dependent and may be aetiologically related to a host of environmental carcinogens. No systematic genetic survey has been undertaken.

Melanoma has been more extensively studied from a genetic point of view. It has been estimated that 5–10% of all melanomas are heritable (Greene et al 1985). Despite this the genetics remain unclear, especially since affected children are about twice as likely to have an affected mother than father, implicating possible cytoplastic or even intrauterine effects. A rather interesting lesion, an inherited nevus variously called the B-K mole syndrome, the familial atypical mole malignant melanoma (FAMMM) syndrome, or the dysplastic nevus syndrome, seems to be inordinately susceptible to malignant transformation, and could account for some, but certainly not all instances of familial melanoma (Kopf et al 1986). There is suggestive evidence that the gene for familial cutaneous melanoma may be linked to the Rh locus on chromosome 1 (Greene et al 1983).

There are a number of genetic disorders in which skin cancer can occur; some of these are listed in Table 106.8.

LEUKAEMIA AND LYMPHOMA

Leukaemia is usually considered to be either lymphocytic or non-lymphocytic in type, and either variety may be acute or chronic. Leukaemia may occur at any age, and this factor along with the absence of any detailed prospective family studies have hampered genetic investigation. The proportion of cases with a heritable component has been variously estimated as 0–25%. Monozygotic twin concordance is about 25%, but this must be accepted with reservation, since concordance beyond age 5 is rare and the twins tend to be affected within weeks to months of each other, suggesting the possibility of cross-transfusion of a single malignant clone through the common placental circulation. Identical cytogenetic alterations have been found in the leukaemia cell lines in twin pairs studied in detail, and this lends support to the common circulation hypothesis (Chaganti et al 1979). Risks to sibs in childhood leukaemia are two to four times higher than the population incidence, but the absolute risk under these circumstances is low (Gunz et al 1975). The risk to adult relatives of these children is unknown. It is possible that the risk will also vary depending on the type of leukaemia.

Acute leukaemia

Acute leukaemia tends to be more a disease of childhood, with the lymphocytic form (ALL) predominant in the first five years, and nonlymphocytic leukaemia (ANLL) becoming evident later. In some instances the cell type is so primitive that accurate classification is impossible. A number of impressive pedigrees, some multigenerational, have been published (Davidson et al 1978, Gunz et al 1978, Luddy et al 1978). Consanguinity is generally not impressive, save for one study in Japan (Kurita et al 1974) and another in a religious and cultural isolate (Feldman et al 1976). In one instance, X-linked inheritance was suggested, although male-limited autosomal dominant inheritance could not be excluded (Li et al 1979). T-cell leukaemia can be familial, but not necessarily genetic,

Table 106.8 Genetic syndromes with basal, squamous cell carcinoma or melanoma

Basal cell nevus syndrome
Dyskeratosis congenita
Hidrotic ectodermal dysplasia
Multiple cylindromas of Brooke
Multiple keratoacanthoma
Flegel disease
Porokeratosis of Mibelli
Albinism
Epidermodysplasia verruciformis
Epidermolysis bullosa dystrophica
Fanconi panmyelopathy
Rothmund-Thompson syndrome
Xeroderma pigmentosum
Neurocutaneous melanosis
B-K mole syndrome
Familial melanoma
Cancer family syndrome

because of common infection with human immunodeficiency virus (HIV) (Miyamoto et al 1985). Some families have had markers suggested as being predictors of an ultimate leukaemia state. While these putative markers may be useful within a family, they are likely to be of little reliability in a population survey. HLA identity has been reported in one sib pair with ALL (Blattner et al 1978), in sibs with myeloproliferative disease (Cervantes et al 1984), and in sibs with hairy cell leukaemia (Wylin et al 1982). Restricted genetic heterogeneity at the HLA loci has been reported in patients with ALL, suggesting that there may be subpopulations at greater than average risk (MacSween et al 1980), such as black American children (Budowle et al 1985). Studies of ALL in G6PD heterozygotes has suggested that the disease is both clonal in origin and that it may be heterogeneous in terms of whether it is expressed in stem cells or becomes evident in a more differentiated cell line (Fialkow et al 1979).

A reasonable interpretation of the available data suggests that perhaps 5% of all cases of acute leukaemia result from an autosomal dominant predisposition, although polygenic inheritance cannot be excluded with certainty. If there is no one else affected in the family the risk to any first-degree relative is small. An important caveat is to be certain that the proband does not suffer from a simply inherited genetic disease in which acute leukaemia has been reported (Table 106.9). Others may exist, as exemplified by the sibs reported by Greenberg et al (1981) who had both polyposis coli and acute myelocytic leukaemia.

Cytogenetic alterations are found in the majority of malignant cell lines in acute leukaemia (LeBeau & Rowley 1986). Although there is considerable variability,

Table 106.9 Syndromes in which acute leukaemia has been reported

Neurofibromatosis
Ataxia-telangiectasia
Glutathione reductase deficiency
Incotinentia pigmenti
Immune deficiency diseases
Rubenstein-Taybi syndrome
Kostmann syndrome
Fanconi anaemia
Bloom syndrome
WT syndrome
Schwachman syndrome
Klinefelter syndrome
Poland anomaly
Trisomy 21
Trisomy 13
Trisomy 8
Cancer family syndrome

the changes are not random. Generally, the more complex the cytogenetic alteration, the poorer the prognosis, whether in children or adults. In children, the cytogenetic changes are less consistent, but the basic patterns tend to be similar.

Chronic leukaemia

There is no firm evidence for a genetic aetiology of chronic myelogenous leukaemia (CML), only a small number of families having been reported in which more than one member was affected. More than 80% of patients with CML have the Philadelphia (Ph[1]) chromosome, the cells harbouring this anomaly all having been derived from a single clone (Fialkow 1977). In families where more than one individual had CML, the Ph[1] chromosome is generally present (Svarch & de la Torre 1977). CML in children is uncommon, and about half the cases are Ph[1] negative. The absence of this chromosome generally portends a poorer prognosis. When Ph[1] positive CML enters an acute phase, a variety of cytogenetic aberrations supervene as with ANLL, a double Ph[1] chromosome configuration being quite common. The cytogenetic alteration involves translocation of the Abelson (c-abl) oncogene from chromosome 9 to chromosome 22. The breakpoint regions in chromosome 9 appear to be variable, whereas those in chromosome 22 consistently appear in the breakpoint cluster region (bcr) (Shtivelman et al 1985).

The data in regard to genetic factors in chronic lymphocytic leukaemia (CLL) are more substantial. It tends to be more common in elderly individuals and long-term survival is not unusual. About 90% of the time the involved lymphocyte is B-cell in type, only a few percent being T-cells and the remainder non-T, non-B or null cells (Nowell et al 1980). Familial occurrence of CLL occurs more frequently than expected by chance. Impressive sibship aggregation and apparent two-generation transmission have been seen often enough to implicate genetic factors. In one of the earliest reports, 56-year-old identical twin brothers were affected within three months of one another (Dameshek et al 1929). A follow-up report 28 years later documents the disease in a 53-year-old son of one of the twins (Gunz & Dameshek 1957).

Exactly what might be inherited is unknown. Immunological abnormalities have been detected in both affected and unaffected family members, but they are not always consistent (Cohen et al 1979). Some family members with CLL may have virtually identical clinical courses with the same morphological and functional characteristics, and the same surface markers (Blattner et al 1976, Branda et al 1978) whereas in other families, not only is the immune defect discordant, but the disease may assume a different form; e.g. lymphosarcoma, reticulum cell sarcoma, hairy cell leukaemia or acute leukaemia (Cohen et al 1979). Some relatives have even had CML. Non-leukaemic malignancies occur commonly in patients with CLL or lymphocytic lymphosarcoma, showing an overall incidence of 34.4% (Hyman 1969). Roughly 40% of these patients developed the other neoplasm before the CLL, the remainder being about equally divided between those whose onset of combined neoplasia was within three months and those whose non-leukaemic tumour developed later. In another retrospective series of 102 patients it was concluded that the overall risk of subsequent malignancy was increased three-fold (Manusow & Weinerman 1975). It is interesting that the families of most patients with CLL contain relatives with non-leukaemic malignancy as well.

The basic genetic lesion would appear to reside in some defective immune function, perhaps in immune surveillance, in suppressor cell function, or in some subtle alteration that allows for the persistence of an oncogenic antigen. Based on a review of the available pedigrees, it seems reasonable to postulate that 10–15% of patients with CLL have their disease on the basis of a heritable predisposition that behaves in a manner consistent with autosomal dominance. However, in view of the variable clinical presentation in some families, it is also possible that the disease is heterogeneous, comprising both dominant and polygenic forms.

Chromosome studies in CLL most commonly reveal t(8;14), t(11;14) or t(14;18) translocations. The disease seems to be clinically heterogeneous, ranging from pure CLL to hairy cell leukaemia, Sezary syndrome and so forth.

Lymphoma

Most authorities classify lymphoma as being Hodgkin (HD) or non-Hodgkin in type. The latter not uncommonly occurs in families of patients with CLL, and unfortunately both types of lymphoma may develop in a given family, such that the genetic issue is confused (Buehler et al 1975). Moreover, examination of such families frequently reveals not only the expected immunological abnormalities in affected relatives, but also nonlymphomatous tumours in some (Clark et al 1987). Whether this simply reflects a more general loss of immune surveillance capability or denotes a type of cancer family syndrome is not clear.

Family studies of HD are fairly extensive (Grufferman et al 1977). The usual aggregation is that of sibs, but parent-child and affected cousins have been reported. In fact, HD has been described in colleagues at work, in

teacher-student pairs, in drug addicts, in neighbours, in relatives working in the same environment and, rarely, even in spouses (Nagel et al 1978). In one extensive study of sib pairs, Grufferman et al (1977) found, from personal experience and literature review, 46 sib pairs under age 45, 30 of whom were concordant for sex. They concluded that both genetic and common environmental factors were important in aetiology. The risk of a relative developing HD has been estimated to be three- to seven-fold higher than the basic age-adjusted population risk (Robertson et al 1987). HLA studies by and large have not shown an impressive association between HD and any particular allele or haplotype. In 13 families prone to HD, the probands showed an excess of Bw35 (Greene et al 1979). In general, affected sibs tend to be HLA concordant, a finding that suggests to some authors that susceptibility to HD is recessive (Hors et al 1980). The discovery of multiple affected individuals in consanguineous families would tend to support this hypothesis. However, the numbers studied are small and no firm conclusion can be drawn at present, An occupational exposure to wood and wood products has been suggested to be of importance in some families, presumably genetically predisposed, as evidenced by multiple affected members (Greene et al 1978).

Lymphomas commonly complicate the heritable immunodeficiency disease. A peculiar form of lymphoma may be seen in the autosomal recessive Chediak-Higashi syndrome. Cytogenetic rearrangements involving chromosome 14 are among the most common alterations seen in lymphomas. The t(14;18) translocation results in placement of a candidate proto-oncogene bcl-2 (B-cell leukaemia-lymphoma) on chromosome 18 near or within the immunoglobulin heavy chain region on chromosome 14 (Weiss et al 1987). The rearrangement is particularly common in follicular lymphoma.

Multiple myeloma

Multiple myeloma and the related condition, Waldenstrom macroglobulinaemia, are diseases of old age. Familial instances of these conditions are relatively few and two generation occurrence, while uncommon, has been reported (Grosbois et al 1986). Interestingly, in some unaffected family members benign monoclonal gammopathy has been discovered. A series of twenty asymptomatic monoclonal gammopathy patients has been described, in which individuals were followed for up to 14 years (Fine et al 1979). Four cases evolved into malignant disease, two into macroglobulinaemia and two into myeloma, indicating that the appellation 'benign' is not always appropriate. As with many other lymphoreticular malignancies, immunoglobulin abnormalities have also been recorded in unaffected family members. As association of multiple myeloma in American blacks with HLA–Cw5 has been suggested (Leech et al 1983). Undoubtedly both elements, i.e. the presence of paraproteins and immune markers, must relate to the basic pathogenetic mechanism, but it is not at all clear that these are primarily genetic. The heritability of myeloma appears to be low, with relatives having no more than a five-fold risk of developing malignant lymphoreticular disease at some time of their life.

Familial histocytosis

This condition has a number of alternative names including familial reticuloendotheliosis, familial Letterer-Siwe disease and erythrophagocytic lymphohistocytosis, the latter being particularly descriptive of the typical heavy, largely perivascular infiltrate found at autopsy. The disease in adults, also termed histiocytic medullary reticulosis, is not known to have a genetic component whereas the childhood form is not only heritable but heterogeneous, both autosomal and X–linked recessive forms having been described (Janka 1983). In the autosomal recessive form affected infants fail to thrive, develop anaemia and neutropenia, occasionally with paradoxical eosinophilia, diarrhoea, hepatosplenomegaly, occasional rash and hyperlipidaemia, and histocytic infiltration of virtually every organ, including the central nervous system. The condition is usually rapidly progressive. There is some question of whether the disorder is truly a malignancy or is a basic immunodeficiency disease with secondary histocytic proliferation. Defects in both T- and B–cell function have been identified, but it is not clear whether these are primary or secondary. Some affected children have responded, albeit transiently, to immunosuppressive therapy, a seemingly unlikely phenomenon if the disorder is actually a primary immunodeficiency state (Lilleyman 1980).

The X–linked form is more clearly an immunodeficiency disease, and apparently a selective one, in that affected males respond inappropriately to EB virus (Harrington et al 1987). For reasons as yet unknown, the disease has a number of phenotypes ranging from fatal infectious mononucleosis, through non-Hodgkin and/or Burkitt lymphoma or a dysgammaglobulinaemia. Earlier reports of familial intestinal lymphoma and sibs with fatal infectious mononucleosis probably represented this entity. However, not all forms of increased susceptibility to EB virus need be necessarily X–linked (Schimke et al 1987). Gut lymphoma has been described in male and female sibs, one aged 51 and the other 54, both of whom had high EB virus titres (Freedlander et al 1978). Joncas et al (1976) have noted a family in which sibs and first cousins were variously affected with nasopharyngeal carcinoma (one with EB virus titre greater than 640), Burkitt lymphoma and myeloma. Polyclonal B–cell lymphoma occurred during the course of EB virus infection in a female child whose parents were first cousins (Robinson et al 1980). Thus it is conceivable that a number of different genetic types of lymphohistocytosis may exist, the primary lesion most likely being related to altered immunity to EB virus in some cases and to unknown agents in other instances.

IMMUNE DEFICIENCY STATES

It has long been known that patients who have deficient immunity, either on the basis of a genetic defect or because of immunosuppressive and/or cytotoxic therapy, have an increased incidence of malignancy. In both types of patients, lymphoma and leukaemia are among the predominant lesions, but tumours in a variety of other sites have been described as well (Penn 1978). A survey of 267 individuals with genetically determined immunodeficiency disease (GDID) and malignancy revealed the following: (1) the tumour type in a child with GDID is generally a non-Hodgkin lymphoma; in an adult, lymphoma and carcinoma occur in about equal proportions; (2) the lymphomas are mostly lymphoreticular or histocytic, with the former being either B- or T–cell more commonly than null type; (3) gastric carcinomas are much more common than expected, especially in adolescence and early adult life; (4) in some instances, there are cell patterns that are unique, such as the excess of epithelial malignancies in girls with ataxia-telangiectasia and the association of myelogenous leukaemia in boys with the X–linked Wiscott-Aldrich syndrome (Spector et al 1978). The incidence of malignancy varies with the GDID, being highest with Wiscott-Aldrich syndrome (15.4%), followed by ataxia-telangiectasia (11.7%), selective IgM deficiency (10%) and common variable immunodeficiency, all ages combined (4.3%). A much larger series of patients with Wiscott-Aldrich syndrome confirmed the high incidence of cancer in those males, with 36 of 301 individuals (12%) being affected, 30% of whom had either lymphoreticular malignancies or leukaemia (Perry et al 1980). In view of the suggested increased incidence of malignancies in heterozygotes with ataxia-telangiectasia, it would be of interest to examine the first-degree female relatives of boys with Wiscott-Aldrich syndrome to see if any consistent pattern emerged. No increase was noted in families of patients with severe combined immunodeficiency syndrome (Morrell et al 1987).

REFERENCES

Anderson D E 1974 Genetic study of breast cancer: identification of high risk group. Cancer 34: 1090–1097

Anderson D E 1977 Breast cancer in females. Cancer 40(4 Suppl): 1855–1860

Anderson D E 1978 Familial cancer and cancer families. Seminars in Oncology 5: 11–16

Anderson D E 1980 Risk in families of patients with colon cancer. In: Winawer S, Schottenfeld D, Sherlock P (eds) Colorectal cancer: prevention, epidemiology and screening. Raven Press, New York, p 109–115

Anderson D E, Badzioch M D 1985a Bilaterality in familial breast cancer patients. Cancer 56: 2092–2098

Anderson D E, Badzioch M D 1985b Risk of familial breast cancer. Cancer 56: 383–387

Andriola M 1976 Nevus unius lateralis and brain tumors. American Journal of Diseases of Children 130: 1259–1261

Annegers J F, Strom H, Decker D G, Dockerty M B, O'Fallon W M 1979 Ovarian cancer. Cancer 43: 723–729

Ashcraft K, Holder T M, Harris D J 1975 Familial presacral teratomas. Birth Defects 11: 143–146

Ashley D J 1969 Oesophageal cancer in Wales. Journal of Medical Genetics 6:70–75

Aurias A, Rimbaut C, Buffe D, Dubousset J, Mazabrand A 1983 Chromosome translocations in Ewing's sarcoma. New England Journal of Medicine 309: 496–497

Bader J L, Meadows A T, Zimmerman L E, Rorke L B, Voute P A, Champion L A A, Miller R W 1982 Bilateral retinoblastoma with ectopic intracranial retinoblastoma: trilateral retinoblastoma. Lancet 2: 582–583

Bahn R S, Scherthauer B W, van Heerden J A, Laws E R Jr., Harvath E, Gharib H 1986 Nonidentical expression of multiple endocrine neoplasia type I in identical twins. Mayo Clinic Proceedings 61: 689–696

Baird P A, Worth A J 1976 Congenital generalized fibromatosis: an autosomal recessive condition. Clinical Genetics 9: 488–494

Barker D, Wright E, Nguyen K, et al 1987 Gene for von Recklinghausen neurofibromatosis in the pericentric region of chromosome 17. Science 236: 1100–1102

Baylin S B, Hsu S H, Gann D S, Smallridge R C, Wells S A Jr. 1978 Inherited medullary thyroid carcinoma: a final monoclonal mutation in one of multiple clones of susceptible cells. Science 199: 429–431

Bellur S N, Chandra V, McDonald L W 1979 Association of meningiomas with extra neural primary malignancy. Neurology 29: 1165–1168

Bess M A, Adson M A, Elveback L R, Moertel C G 1980 Rectal cancer following colectomy for polyposis. Archives of Surgery 115: 460–467

Binder M K, Zablen M A, Fleischer D E, Sue D Y, Dwyer R M, Hanelin L 1978 Colon polyps, sebaceous cysts, gastric polyps, and malignant brain tumor in a family. American Journal of Digestive Diseases 23: 460–466

Bishop J M 1987 The molecular genetics of cancer. Science 235: 305–316

Blattner W A, Strober W, Muchmore A V, Blaese R M, Broder S, Fraumeni J F Jr. 1976 Familial chronic lymphocytic leukemia. Annals of Internal Medicine 84: 554–557

Blattner W A, Naiman J L, Mann D L, Wimer R S, Dean J S, Fraumeni J F Jr. 1978 Immunogenetic determinants of familial acute lymphocytic leukemia. Annals of Internal Medicine 89: 173–176

Boden G, Owen O E 1977 Familial glucagonemia – an autosomal dominant disorder. New England Journal of Medicine 296: 534–538

Bodmer W F, Bailey C J, Bodmer J et al 1987 Localization of the gene for familial adenomatous polyposis on chromosome 5. Nature 328: 614–616

Bolande R P 1977 Childhood tumors and their relationship to birth defects. In: Mulvihill J J, Miller R W, Fraumeni J F Jr. (eds) Genetics of human cancer. Raven Press, New York, p 43–75

Bottomly R H, Trainer A L, Condet P T 1971 Chromosome studies in a "cancer family". Cancer 28: 519–528

Bove K E, McAdams A J 1976 The nephroblastomatosis complex and its relationship to Wilms' tumor: a clinocopathologic study. Perspectives in Pediatric Pathology 3: 185–223

Branda R F, Ackerman S K, Handwerger B S, Howe R B, Douglas S D 1978 Lymphocyte studies in familial chronic lymphatic leukemia. American Journal of Medicine 64: 508–514

Brauch H, Johnson B, Hovis J et al 1987 Molecular analysis of the short arm of chromosome 3 in small cell and non-small-cell carcinoma of the lung. New England Journal of Medicine 317: 1109–1113

Breslow N E, Beckwith J B 1972 Epidemiological features of Wilms' tumor: results of the national Wilms' tumor study. Journal of the National Cancer Institute 68: 429–436

Brocca P P 1866–1869 Traité des Tumeurs, vols 1 & 2 E. Asselin, Paris

Brown E H 1979 Identical twins with twisted benign cystic teratoma of the ovary. American Journal of Obstetrics and Gynecology 134: 879–880

Budowle B, Dearth J, Bowman P et al 1985 Genetic predisposition to acute lymphocytic leukemia in American blacks. Cancer 55: 2880–2882

Buehler S K, Firme F, Fodor G, Fraser G R, Marshall W H, Vaze P 1975 Common variable immunodeficiency, Hogdkin's disease and other malignancies in a Newfoundland family. Lancet 1: 195–197

Burkland C E, Juzek R H 1966 Familial occurrence of carcinoma of the ureter. Journal of Urology 96: 697–701

Carney A, Sizemore G W, Tyce G M 1975 Bilateral adrenal medullary hyperplasia in multiple endocrine neoplasia, type 2. Mayo Clinic Proceedings 50: 3–10

Carney J A, Hayles A B 1978 Alimentary tract manifestations of multiple endocrine neoplasia, type 2b. Mayo Clinic Proceedings 52: 543–548

Carney J A, Go V L W, Gordon H, Northcutt R C, Pease A G E, Sheps S G 1980 Familial pheochromocytoma and islet cell tumor of the pancreas. American Journal of Medicine 68: 515–521

Cavenee W K, Murphee A L, Shull M M, Benedict W F, Sparkes R S, Kock E, Nordenskjold M 1986 Prediction of familial predisposition to retinoblastoma. New England Journal of Medicine 314: 1201–1207

Cervantes F, Ribera J-M, Sanchez-Bisano J, Bruges R, Rosman C 1984 Myeloproliferative disease in two young siblings. Cancer 54: 899–902

Chaganti R S K, German J L (eds) 1985 Genetics in Clinical Oncology. Oxford, New York

Chaganti R S K, Miller D R, Meyers P A, German J 1979 Cytogenetic evidence of the intrauterine origin of acute leukemia in monozygotic twins. New England Journal of Medicine 300: 1032–1034

Challa V R, Goodman H O, Davis C H Jr. 1983 Familial

brain tumors: studies of two families and review of recent literature. Neurosurgery 12: 18–23

Clark J W, Tucker M A, Greene M H 1987 Clinical and laboratory observations in a lymphoma-prone family. Cancer 60: 864–869

Cohen A J, Li F P, Berg S, Marchetto J, Tsai S, Jacobs S C, Brown R S 1979 Hereditary renal cell carcinoma associated with a chromosomal translocation. New England Journal of Medicine 301: 592–595

Cohen B H, Diamond E L, Graves C G et al 1977 A common familial component in lung cancer and chronic obstructive pulmonary disease. Lancet 2: 523–526

Cohen H J, Shimm D, Paris S A, Buckley C E III, Kremer W B 1979 Hairy cell leukemia-associated familial lymphoproliferative disorder: immunologic abnormalities in unaffected family members. Annals of Internal Medicine 90: 174–179

Colyer R A 1979 Osteogenic sarcoma in siblings. Johns Hopkins Medical Journal 145: 131–135

Conley C L, Misiti J, Laster A J 1980 Genetic factors predisposing to chronic lymphocytic leukemia and to autoimmune disease. Medicine 59: 323–334

Cooper D S, Axelrod A, DeGroot L J, Vickery A L Jr., Maloof F 1981 Congenital goiter and development of metastatic follicular carcinoma with evidence for a leak of non-hormonal iodide: clinical pathological, kinetic and biochemical studies and a review of the literature. Journal of Clinical Endocrinology and Metabolism 52: 294–306

Dameshek W, Savitz H A, Arbor B 1929 Chronic lymphatic leukemia in twin brothers, age 56. JAMA 92: 1343–1349

Danes B S 1978 Increased in vitro tetraploidy: tissue specific in the heritable colorectal cancer syndromes with polyposis coli. Cancer 41: 2330–2334

Daniel E S, Ludurg S L, Lewin J, Ruprecht R M, Rajacich G M, Schwabe A D 1982 The Cronkhite-Canada syndrome. Medicine 61: 293–309

Danoff A, Jormark S, Lorber D, Fleisher N 1987 Adrenocortical micronodular dysplasia, cardiac myxomas, lentigines, and spindle cell tumors. Archives of Internal Medicine 147: 443–448

Dao D D, Schroeder W T, Chao L-Y et al 1987 Genetic mechanisms of tumor-specific loss of 11p DNA sequences in Wilms' tumor. American Journal of Human Genetics 41: 202–217

Davidson R J L, Walker W, Watt J L, Page B M 1978 Familial erythroleukemia: a cytogenetic and hematologic study. Scandinavian Journal of Haematology 20: 351–359

Delleman J W, DeJong J G Y, Bleeker G M 1978 Meningiomas in five members of a family over two generations, in one member simultaneously with acoustic neurinomas. Neurology 28: 567–570

Devor E J, Buechley R W 1979 Gallbladder cancer in Hispanic New Mexicans. Cancer Genetics and Cytogenetics 1:139–145

Drabkin H A, Bradley C, Hart I, Bleskau J, Li F P, Patterson D 1985 Translocation of c-myc in the hereditary renal cell carcinoma associated with a t(3;8)(p14.2;q24.13) chromosome translocation. Proceedings of the National Academy of Sciences (USA) 82: 6980–6984

Draper G J, Heaf M M, Wilson L M K 1977 Occurrence of childhood cancer among sibs and estimation of familial risks. Journal of Medical Genetics 14: 81–95

Druker B J, Mamon H J, Roberts T M 1989 Oncogenes and growth factors and signal transduction. New England Journal of Medicine 321: 1383–1391

Dryja T P, Rapaport J M, Epstein J, Goorin A M, Weichselbaum R, Koufos A, Cavenee W K 1986 Chromosome 13 homozygosity in osteosarcoma without retinoblastoma. American Journal of Human Genetics 38: 59–66

Duesberg P H 1987 Cancer genes: rare recombinants instead of activated oncogenes (A Review). Proceedings of the National Academy of Sciences (USA) 84: 2117–2124

Dumont-Herskowitz R E, Safari H S, Senior B 1978 Ovarian fibroma in four successive generations. Journal of Pediatrics 94: 621–624

Eddy A A, Mauer S M 1985 Pseudohermaphroditism, glomerulopathy, and Wilms' tumor (Drash syndrome): frequency in end-stage renal failure. Journal of Pediatrics 106: 584–587

Egan S E, Wright J A, Jarolim L, Yanugihara K, Bassin R H, Greenberg A H 1987 Transformation by oncogenes encoding protein kinases induces the metastatic phenotype. Science 238: 202–205

Ehrenthal D, Haeger L, Griffen T, Compton C 1987 Familial pancreatic adenocarcinoma in three generations. Cancer 59: 1661–1664

Ehrich J H H, Ostertag J, Flatz S, Kamran D 1978 Bilateral Wilms' tumor in Klippel-Trenaunay syndrome. Archives of Disease in Childhood 54: 405

Epstein L I, Bixler D, Bennett J E 1970 An incident of familial cancer including 3 cases of osteogenic sarcoma. Cancer 25: 889–891

Evans A E, Chatten J, D'Angio G J, Gerson J M, Robinson J, Schnaufer L 1980 A review of 17 IV-S neuroblastoma patients at the children's hospital of Philadelphia. Cancer 45: 833–839

Fahmy A, Burgdorf W H C, Schosser R H, Pitha J 1982 Muir-Torre syndrome. Cancer 49: 1898–1903

Fairchild R S, Kyner J L, Hermreck A, Schimke R N 1979 Neuroblastoma, pheochromocytoma, and renal cell carcinoma: occurrence in a single patient. JAMA 242: 2210–2211

Fearon E R, Feinberg A P, Hamilton S H, Vogelstein B 1985 Loss of genes on the short arm of chromosome 11 in bladder cancer. Nature: 318:377–380

Fearon E R, Joe K R, Nigro J M et al 1990 Identification of a chromosome 18q gene that is altered in colorectal cancers. Science 247: 49–56

Feingold M, Gheraodi G, Simons C 1971 Familial neuroblastoma and trisomy 13. American Journal of Diseases of Children 121: 451–452

Feldman J G, Lee S L, Seligman B 1976 Occurrence of acute leukemia in females in a genetically isolated population. Cancer 38: 2548–2550

Fialkow P J 1977 Clonal original stem cell evolution of human tumors. In: Mulvihill J J, Miller R W, Fraumeni J F Jr. (eds) Genetics of human cancer. Raven Press, New York, p 439–453

Fialkow P J, Singer J W, Adamson J W, Berkow R L, Friedman J M, Jacobson R J, Moohr J W 1979 Acute nonlymphocytic leukemia. New England Journal of Medicine 301: 1–5

Fine J M, Laubin P, Muller J Y 1979 The evolution of asymptomatic monoclonal gammopathies. Acta Medica Scandinavica 205: 339–341

Foster J H, Donohue T A, Berman M M 1978 Familial liver-cell adenomas and diabetes mellitus. New England Journal of Medicine 299: 239–241

Fraumeni J F Jr., Rosen P J, Hull E W, Barton R F, Shapiro

S R, O'Connor J F 1969 Hepatoblastoma in infant sisters. Cancer 24: 1086–1090

Freedlander E, Kissen L H, McVee J G 1978 Gut lymphoma presenting simultaneously in two siblings. British Medical Journal 1: 80–81

Frischer Z, Waltzer W C, Gonder M J 1985 Bilateral transitional cell carcinomas of the renal pelvis in the cancer family syndrome. Journal of Urology 134: 1197–1198

Fuller D B, Plenk H P 1986 Malignant testicular germ cell tumors in a father and two sons. Cancer 58: 955–958

Gallo G E 1978 Pathology of "uninvolved" renal parenchyma in nephroblastoma. Pediatric Research 12: 1030

Gentry W C Jr., Reed W B, Siegel J M 1975 Cowden disease. Birth Defects 11: 137–141

Ghadirian P 1985 Family history of esophageal cancer. Cancer 56: 2112–2116.

Giardiello F M, Welsh S B, Hamilton S R et al 1987 Increased risk of cancer in the Peutz-Jeghers syndrome. New England Journal of Medicine 316: 1511–1514

Gilbert G, Cleveland W W 1970 Cushing's syndrome in infancy. Pediatrics 46: 217–222

Gilman P A, Wang N, Fan S-F, Reede J, Khan A, Leventhal B G 1985 Familial osteosarcoma associated with 13;14 chromosomal rearrangement. Cancer Genetics and Cytogenetics 7: 123–132

Go RCP, King M-C, Bailey-Wilson J, Elston R C, Lynch H T 1983 Genetic epidemiology of breast cancer and associated cancers in high risk families. I. Segregation analysis. Journal of the National Cancer Institute 71: 455–461

Goodman Z D, Yardley J H, Milligan F D 1979 Pathogenesis of colonic polyps in multiple juvenile polyposis. Cancer 43: 1906–1913

Gorlin R J 1976 Some soft tissue heritable tumors. Birth Defects 12: 7–14

Gorlin R J, Sedano H O 1972 The multiple nevoid basal cell carcinoma syndrome. Birth Defects 7: 140–148

Greco F A, Oldham R K 1979 Current concepts in cancer: small cell lung cancer. New England Journal of Medicine 301: 355–358

Greenberg M S, Anderson K C, Marchetto D J, Li F P 1981 Acute myelocytic leukemia in two brothers with polyposis coli and carcinoma of the colon. Annals of Internal Medicine 95: 702–703

Greene M H, Brinton L A, Fraumeni J F Jr., D'Amico R 1978 Familial sporadic Hodgkin's disease associated with occupational wood exposure. Lancet 2: 626–627

Greene M H, McKeen E A, Li F P, Blattner W A, Fraumeni J F Jr. 1979 HLA antigens in familial Hodgkin's disease. International Journal of Cancer 23: 777–780

Greene M H, Goldin L R, Clark W H Jr. et al 1983 Familial cutaneous malignant melanoma: autosomal dominant trait possibly linked to the Rh locus. Proceedings of the National Academy of Sciences (USA) 80: 6071–6075

Greene M H, Clark W H Jr., Tucker M A et al 1985 Acquired precursors of cutaneous malignant melanoma: the familial dysplastic nevus syndrome. New England Journal of Medicine 312: 91–97

Grether P, Carnevale A, Pasquel P 1987 Wilms' tumor in an infant with tuberous sclerosis. Annales de Genetiques 30: 183–185

Grosbois B, Gueguen M, Fauchet R et al 1986 Multiple myeloma in two brothers. Cancer 58: 2417–2421

Grufferman S, Cole P, Smith P G, Lukes R J 1977 Hodgkin's disease in siblings New England Journal of Medicine 296: 248–250

Gunz F, Dameshek W 1957 Chronic lymphocytic leukemia in a family, including twin brothers and a son. JAMA 164: 1323–1324

Gunz F W, Gunz J P, Veale A M O, Chapman C J, Houston I B 1975 Familial leukemia: a study of 909 families. Scandinavian Journal of Haematology 15: 117–131

Gunz F W, Gunz J P, Vincent P C, Bergin M, Johnson F L, Bashir H, Kirk R L 1978 Thirteen cases of leukemia in a family. Journal of the National Cancer Institute 60: 1243–1250

Gustavson H, Gamstorp I, Meruling S 1975 Bilateral teratoma of the testes in two brothers with 47, XXY Klinefelter's syndrome. Clinical Genetics 8: 5–10

Hagstrom R M, Baker T D 1968 Primary hepatocellular carcinoma in three siblings. Cancer 22: 142–150

Hansen M F, Koufos A, Gallie B L et al 1985 Osteosarcoma and retinoblastoma: a shared chromosomal mechanism revealing recessive predisposition. Proceedings of the National Academy of Sciences (USA) 82: 6216–6220

Hapnes S A, Boman H, Skeie S O 1980 Familial angiolipomatosis. Clinical Genetics 17: 202–208

Hariez C, Deminatti M, Agache P, Mennecier M 1968 Une genodysplasie non encore individualise: la genodermatose sclero-atrophiante et keratodermique des extremities frequemment degenerative. Semaine des hopitaux de Paris 44: 481–488

Harper P S, Harper R M J, Howel-Evans A 1970 Carcinoma of the esophagous with tylosis. Quarterly Journal of Medicine 39: 317–333

Harrington D S, Weisenburger D D, Purtilo D T 1987 Malignant lymphoma in the X-linked lymphoproliferative syndrome. Cancer 59: 1419–1429

Heim S, Mitelman F 1987 Nineteen of 26 cellular oncogenes precisely localized in the human genome map to one of the 83 bands involved in primary cancer-specific rearrangements. Human Genetics 75: 70–72

Henry I, Grandjovan S, Barichard F et al 1989 Tumor-specific loss of 11p15.5 alleles in del 11p13 Wilms tumor and in familial adrenocortical carcinoma. Proceedings of the National Academy of Sciences (USA) 86: 3247–3251

Herring D W, Cartwright R A, Williams D R 1979 Genetic associations of transitional cell carcinoma. British Journal of Medicine 51: 73–77

Hors J, Steinberg G, Andrieu J M et al 1980 HLA genotypes in familial Hodgkin's disease: excess of HLA identical sibs. European Journal of Cancer 16: 809–815

Horton W A 1976 Genetics of central nervous system tumors. Birth Defects 12: 91–97

Horton W A, Wong V, Eldridge R 1976 von Hippel-Lindau disease. Archives of Internal Medicine 136: 769–777

Hsu S H, Luk G D, Krush A J, Hamilton S R, Hoover H H Jr. 1983 Multiclonal origin of polyps in Gardner syndrome. Science 221: 951–953

Hulka B S, Fowler W C, Kaufman D G et al 1980 Estrogen and endometrial cancer: cases and two control groups from North Carolina. American Journal of Obstetrics and Gynecology 137: 92–101

Hull M T, Warfel K A, Muller J, Higgins J T 1979 Familial islet cell tumors in von Hippel-Lindau's disease. Cancer 44: 1523a–1526

Hutchinson W B, Thomas D B, Hamlin W B, Roth G J, Peterson A V, Williams B 1980 Risk of breast cancer in women with benign breast disease. Journal of the National Cancer Institute 65: 13–20

Hyman G A 1969 Increased incidence of neoplasia in

association with chronic lymphocytic leukemia. Scandinavian Journal of Haematology 6: 99–104

Isurugi K, Imao S, Hirose K, Aoki H 1977 Seminoma in Klinefelter's syndrome with 47, XXY, 15+ karyotype. Cancer 39: 2041–2047

Ito E, Sato Y, Kawauchi K, Munakata H, Kamata Y, Yoduno H, Yokoyama M 1987 Type Ia glycogen storage disease with hepatoblastoma in siblings. Cancer 59: 1776–1780

Itoh H, Ohsato K 1985 Turcot syndrome and its characteristic colonic manifestations. Diseases of the Colon and Rectum 28: 399–402

Janka G E 1983 Familial hemophagocytic lymphohistiocytosis. European Journal of Pediatrics 140: 221–230

Janson K L, Roberts J A, Varela M 1978 Multiple endocrine adenomatous: in support of the common origin theories. Journal of Urology 119: 161–165

Jenson R D, Norris H J, Fraumeni J H Jr. 1974 Familial arrhenoblastoma and thyroid adenoma. Cancer 33: 218–223

Joncas J H, Rioux E, Robitaille R, Wastriaux J P 1976 Multiple cases of lymphoma in a Canadian family. Bibliotheca Hematologica 43: 224–276

Joyce M J, Harmon D C, Mankin H J, Suit H D, Schuller A L, Truman J T 1984 Ewing's sarcoma in female siblings. Cancer 53: 1959–1962

Kahn L B 1977 Vagal body tumor (nonchromaffin paraganglioma, chemodectoma and carotid body-like tumor) with cervical node metastases and familial association. Cancer 39: 2367–2377

Kaplan C G, Askin F B, Benirschke K 1979 Cytogenetics of extragonadal tumors. Teratology 19: 261–266

King M-C, Go R C P, Lynch H T et al 1983 Genetic epidemiology of breast cancers in high-risk families. II. Linkage analysis. Journal of the National Cancer Institute 71: 463–467

Knudson A G Jr. 1986 Genetics of human cancer. Annual Review of Genetics 20: 231–252

Knudson A G Jr., Meadows A T 1976 Developmental genetics of neuroblastoma. Journal of the National Cancer Institute 57: 675–682

Knudson A G Jr., Meadows A T 1980 Regression of neuroblastoma IV- S: a genetic hypothesis. New England Journal of Medicine 302: 1254–1256

Knudson A G Jr., Strong L C 1972 Mutations and cancer: a model for Wilms' tumor of the kidney. Journal of the National Cancer Institute 48: 313–324

Kopelovich L 1980 Hereditary adenomatosis of the colon and rectum: recent studies on the nature of cancer promotion and cancer prognosis in vitro. In: Winawer S J, Schottenfeld D, Sherlock P (eds) Colorectal cancer: prevention, epidemiology and screening. Raven Press, New York, p97–108

Kopf A W, Hellman L J, Rogers G S et al 1986 Familial malignant melanoma. JAMA 256: 1915–1919

Koufos A, Hansen M F, Copeland N G, Jenkins N A, Lampkin B C, Cavenee W K 1985 Loss of heterozygosity in three embryonal tumors suggests a common pathogenetic mechanism. Nature 316: 330–334

Kueppers F, Miller R D, Gordon H, Hepper N G, Offord K 1977 Familial prevalence of chronic obstructive pulmonary disease in a matched pair study. American Journal of Medicine 63: 336–342

Kurita S, Kamei Y, Ota K 1974 Genetic studies on familial leukemia. Cancer 34: 1098–1101

Kussin S Z, Lipkin M, Winawer S J 1979 Inherited colon

cancer: clinical implications. American Journal of Gastroenterology 72: 448–457

Lanier A P, Bender T R, Tschopp C F, Dohan P 1979 Nasopharyngeal carcinoma in an Alaskan Eskimo family: report of three cases. Journal of the National Cancer Institute 62: 1121–1124

LaRaja R D, Pagnozz J A, Rothenberg R E, Georgiou J, Sabatini M T, Hirschman R J 1985 Carcinoma of the breast in three siblings. Cancer 55: 2709–2711

LeBeau M M, Rowley J D 1986 Chromosomal abnormalities in leukemia and lymphoma: clinical and biological significance. Advances in Human Genetics 15: 1–54

Lee W H, Murphee A L, Benedict W F 1984 Expression and amplification of the N-myc gene in primary retinoblastoma. Nature 309: 458–460

Leech S H, Bryan C F, Elston R C, Rainey J, Bickers J N, Pelias M Z 1983 Genetic studies multiple myeloma. Cancer 51: 1408–1411

Lehtola J 1978 Family study of gastric carcinoma with special reference to histologic types. Scandinavian Journal of Gastroenterology 13 (Suppl 5): 3–54

Levin S R, Hofeldt F D, Becker N, Wilson C B, Seymour R, Forsham P H 1974 Hypersomatotropism and acanthosis nigricans in two brothers. Archives of Internal Medicine 134: 365–367

Levine E, Collins D L, Horton W H, Schimke R N 1982 CT screening of the abdomen in von Hippel-Lindau disease. American Journal of Roentgenology 139: 505–510

Lewis J H, Ginsburg A L, Toomey K E 1983 Turcot's syndrome. Cancer 51: 524–528

Li F P 1977 Second malignant tumors after cancer in childhood. Cancer 40: 1899–1902

Li F P, Fraumeni J F Jr. 1982 Prospective study of a family cancer syndrome JAMA 247: 2692–2694

Li F P, Marchetto D J, Vawter G F 1979 Acute leukemia and preleukemia in eight males in a family: an X-linked disorder? American Journal of Hematology 6:61–69

Li F P, Marchetto D J, Brown R S 1982 Familial renal carcinoma. Cancer Genetics and Cytogenetics 7: 271–275

Li F P, Corkery J, Vawter G, Fine W, Sallan S E 1983 Breast carcinoma after cancer therapy in childhood. Cancer 51: 521–523

Li F P, Thurber W A, Seddon J, Homes G E 1987 Hepatoblastoma in families with polyposis coli. JAMA 257: 2475–2477

Lichtig C 1971 Multiple skin and gastrointestinal hemangiomas (blue rubber-bleb nevus). Dermatologica 142: 356–362

Lilleyman J S 1980 The treatment of familial erythrophagocytic lymphohistiocytosis. Cancer 46: 468–470

Linquette M, Herlaut M, Laine E, Fossati P, DuPont-LeCompte J 1967 Adenome a prolactie chez une jeune fille dont la niere etait porteuse d'un adenoma hypophysaire avec amenorrhee-galactorrhee. Annales d'endocrinologie 28: 773–776

LiVolsi V A, Feind C R 1976 Parathyroid adenoma and nonmedullary thyroid carcinoma. Cancer 38: 1391–1393

Love R R 1985 Small bowel cancers, B-cell lymphatic leukemia, and six primary cancers with metastases and prolonged survival in the cancer family syndrome of Lynch. Cancer 55: 499–502

Lovett H E 1976 Family studies in cancer of the colon and rectum. British Journal of Surgery 63: 13–18

Lowell S H, Mathog R H 1979 Head and neck manifestations of Mafucci's syndrome. Archives of Otolaryngology 105: 427–430

Luddy R E, Champion L A A, Schwartz A D 1978 A fatal myeloproliferative syndrome in a family with thrombocytopenia and platelet dysfunction. Cancer 41: 1959–1963

Lynch H T (ed) 1976 Cancer Genetics. Thomas, Springfield, Il

Lynch H T, Larsen A L, Magnuson C W, Krush A J 1966 Prostate carcinoma and multiple primary malignancies. Cancer 19: 1891–1897

Lynch H T, Krush A J, Larsen A L 1967 Heredity and endometrial carcinoma. Southern Medical Journal 60: 231–235

Lynch H T, Harris R E, Lynch P M, Guirgis H A, Lynch J F, Bardawill W A 1977 Role of heredity in multiple primary cancer. Cancer 40: 1849–1854

Lynch H T, Harris R E, Guirgis H A, Maloney K, Carmody L L, Lynch J F 1978a Familial association of breast/ovarian carcinoma. Cancer 41: 1543–1549

Lynch H T, Bardawill W A, Harris R E, Lynch P M, Guirgis H A, Lynch J F 1978b Multiple primary cancers and prolonged survival. Diseases of the Colon and Rectum 21: 165–168

Lynch H T, Walzak M P, Fried R, Domina A H, Lynch J F 1979 Familial factors in bladder carcinoma. Journal of Urology 122: 458–461

Lynch H T, Albano W A, Danes B S et al 1984 Genetic predisposition to breast cancer. Cancer 53: 612–622

Lynch H T, Katz D A, Bogard P J, Lynch J F 1985a The sarcoma, breast cancer, lung cancer, and adrenocortical carcinoma syndrome revisited. Childhood Cancer. American Journal of Diseases of Children 139: 134–136

Lynch H T, Kimberling W, Albano W A et al 1985b Hereditary nonpolyposis colorectal cancer (Lynch syndromes I and II). Cancer 56: 934–938

Lynch H T, Lynch J F 1986 Breast cancer genetics in an oncology clinic: 328 consecutive patients. Cancer Genetics and Cytogenetics 22: 369–371

Lyons A R, Logan H, Johnston G W 1977 Hypernephroma in two brothers. British Medical Journal 1: 816–817

McConnell R B 1980 Genetics of family polyposis. In: Winawer P, Schottenfeld D, Sherlock P (eds) Colorectal cancer: prevention epidemiology and screening. Raven Press, New York, p 69–71

MacMahon B, Cole P, Brown J B 1975 Factors that influence mammary carcinogenesis. New England Journal of Medicine 292: 974–975

MacSween J M, Fernandez L A, Eastwood S L, Pyesmany A F 1980 Restricted growth heterogeneity in families of patients with acute lymphocytic leukemia. Tissue Antigens 16: 70–72

Malek R S, Omess P J, Benson R C Jr., Zinke H 1987 Renal cell carcinoma in von Hippel-Lindau syndrome. American Journal of Medicine 82: 236–238

Manusow D, Weinerman B H 1975 Subsequent neoplasia in chronic lymphocytic leukemia. JAMA 232: 267–269

Marx S J, Spiegel A M, Brown F M, Aurbach G O 1977 Family studies in patients with primary parathyroid hyperplasia. American Journal of Medicine 62: 698–706

Marx S J, Vinik A I, Santen R J, Floyd J C Jr., Mills J L, Green J III 1986 Multiple endocrine neoplasia type I: assessment of laboratory tests to screen for the gene in a large kindred. Medicine 65: 226–241

Meadows A T, Lichtenfeld J L, Koop C E 1974 Wilms' tumor in three children of a woman with congenital hemihypertrophy. New England Journal of Medicine 291: 23–24

Meadows A T, D'Angio G J, Mike V, Banfi A, Harris C, Jenkins R D T, Schwartz A 1977 Patterns of second malignant neoplasms in children. Cancer 40: 1901–1911

Merten D F, Gooding C A, Newton T H, Malamud N 1974 Meningiomas of childhood and adolescence. Journal of Pediatrics 84: 696–750

Miller R W 1968 Deaths from childhood cancer in sibs. New England Journal of Medicine 279: 122–126

Miyamoto Y, Yamaguchi K, Nishimura H et al 1985 Familial adult T-cell leukemia. Cancer 55: 181–185

Morrell D, Chase C L, Surf M 1987 Cancer in families with severe combined immune deficiency. Journal of the National Cancer Institute 78: 455–458

Moyes C D, Alexander F W 1977 Mucosal neuroma syndrome presenting in a neonate. Developmental Medicine and Child Neurology 19: 518–534

Müller S, Gadner H, Weber B, Vogel M, Riekm H 1978 Wilms' tumor and adrenocortical carcinoma with hemihypertrophy. European Journal of Pediatrics 127:219–226

Mulvihill J J 1976 Host factors in human lung tumors: an example of ecogenetics in oncology. Journal of the National Cancer Institute 57: 3–7

Mulvihill J J, Miller R W, Fraumeni J F Jr. (eds) 1977a Genetics of Human Cancer. Raven Press, New York

Mulvihill J J, Gralnick H R, Whang-Peng J, Leventhal B E 1977b Multiple childhood osteosarcomas in an American Indian family with erythroid macrocytosis and skeletal anomalies. Cancer 40: 3115–3122

Nagel G A, Nagel-Studer E, Seiler W, Hofer H O 1978 Malignant lymphoma in 4 of 5 siblings. International Journal of Cancer 22: 675–679

Nakamura Y, Lathrop M, Lappert M et al 1988 Localization of the genetic defect in familial adenomatous polyposis within a small region of chromosome 5. American Journal of Human Genetics 43: 638–644

Nakamura Y, Larsson C, Julier C et al 1989 Localization of the genetic defect in multiple endocrine neoplasia type I within a small region of chromosome 11. American Journal of Human Genetics 44: 751–755

Napoli V M, Campbell W C 1977 Hepatoblastoma in infant sisters and brothers. Cancer 39: 2647a–2650

Naylor E W, Gardner E J 1977 Penetrance and expressivity of the gene responsible for the Gardner syndrome. Clinical Genetics 11: 381–393

Naylor S L, Johnson B E, Minna J P, Sakaguchi A Y 1987 Loss of heterozygosity of chromosome 3p markers in small cell lung cancer. Nature 329: 451–454

Nowell P, Daniele R, Rowland D Jr., Finan J 1980 Cytogenetics of chronic B-cell and T-cell leukemia. Cancer Genetics and Cytogenetics 1: 273–280

Ohbayashi A, Okochi K, Mayumi M 1972 Familial clustering of a symptomatic carrier of Australian antigen and patients with chronic liver disease or primary liver cancer. Gastroenterology 62: 617–625

Ooi W L, Elston R C, Chen V W, Bailey-Wilson J, Rothschild H 1986 Increased familial risk for lung cancer. Journal of the National Cancer Institute 76: 217–222

Parry D M, Mulvihill J J, Miller R W 1979 Sarcomas in a child and her father. American Journal of Diseases of Children 133: 130–132

Pauli R M, Pauli M E, Hale J G 1980 Gardner syndrome and periampillary malignancy. American Journal of Medical Genetics 6: 205–219

Penn I 1978 Malignancies associated with immunosuppressive or cytotoxic therapy. Surgery 83: 492–502

Perry S III, Spector B D, Schuman L M et al 1980 The Wiscott-Aldrich syndrome in the United States and Canada (1972–1979). Journal of Pediatrics 92: 72–78

Pilepich M V, Berkman E M, Goodchild N T 1978 HLA typing in familial renal carcinoma. Tissue Antigens 11: 487–488

Pohl G, Boeckl O, Galvan G, Salis-Samaden R, Steiner H, Thurner J 1977 Konkordantes medullares Schilddrusenkarzinom bei einigen Zwillingen mit diskordantem Phaochromozytom (Sipple syndrom). Wiener Klinische Wochenschrift 89: 481–484

Pollack R S 1973 Carotid body tumors – idiosyncracies. Oncology 27: 81–91

Riccardi V M, Eichner J E 1986 Neurofibromatosis. Phenotype, Natural History and Pathogenesis. Johns Hopkins University Press, Baltimore

Richard R D, Mebust W K, Schimke R B 1973 A prospective study in von Hippel-Lindau disease. Journal of Urology 110: 27–30

Robboy S J, Kaufman R H, Prat J et al 1979 Pathologic findings in young women enrolled in the National Cooperative Diethylstilbestrol Adenosis (DESAD) project. Obstetrics and Gynecology 53: 309–317

Robertson S J, Lowman J T, Grufferman S et al 1987 Familial Hodgkin's disease. Cancer 59: 1314–1319

Robinson J E, Brown N B, Andiman et al 1980 Diffuse polyclonal B-cell lymphoma during primary infection with Epstein-Barr virus. New England Journal of Medicine 302: 1293–1297

Rogler C E, Sherman M, Su C Y et al 1985 Deletion on chromosome 11p associated with a hepatitis B integrator site in hepatocellular carcinoma. Science 230: 319–322

Sager R 1989 Tumor suppressor genes, the puzzle and the promise. Science 236: 1406–1412

Sandberg A A, Turc-Carel C 1987 The cytogenetics of solid tumors. Cancer 59: 387–395

Santos J G, Magalhaes J 1980 Familial gastric polyposis. Journal of Human Genetics 28: 293–297

Schimke R N 1973 Phenotype of malignancy: the mucosal neuroma syndrome. Pediatrics 52: 283–285

Schimke R N 1978 Genetics and cancer in man. Churchill Livingstone, Edinburgh

Schimke R N 1979 The neurocristopathy concept: fact or fiction. In: Advances in neuroblastoma research. Raven Press, New York, p13–24

Schimke R N 1980 Genetic syndromes with gastrointestinal cancer. In: Genetics and heterogeneity in common gastrointestinal disease. Academic Press, New York, p 377–389

Schimke R N 1984 Genetic aspects of multiple endocrine neoplasia. Annual Review of Medicine 35: 25–31

Schimke R N 1986 Multiple endocrine neoplasia: search for the oncogenic trigger. New England Journal of Medicine 314: 1315–1316

Schimke R N, Madigan C M, Silver B J, Fabian C J, Stephens R L 1983 Choriocarcinoma, thyrotoxicosis and the Klinefelter syndrome. Cancer Genetics and Cytogenetics 9: 1–7

Schimke R N, Collins D L, Cross D 1987 Nasopharyngeal carcinoma, aplastic anemia, and various malignancies in a family: possible role of Epstein-Barr virus. American Journal of Medical Genetics 27: 195–202

Schmickel R D 1986 Contiguous gene syndromes: a component of recognizable syndromes. Journal of Pediatrics 109: 231–241

Schnall A M, Genuth S M 1976 Multiple endocrine adenomas in a patient with the Maffucci syndrome. American Journal of Medicine 61: 952–956

Schneider N R, Chaganti R S K 1986 Genetic epidemiology of familial aggregation of cancer. Advances in Cancer Research 47: 1–36

Schoenberg B S 1975 Nervous system neoplasms and primary malignancies at other sites. Neurology 25: 702–712

Schwartz R M, Newell R B, Hauch J F, Fairweather W H 1980 A study of familial breast carcinoma and a second report. Cancer 46: 2697–2701

Schwartz S S, Rich B H, Lucky A W et al 1979 Familial nesidioblastosis: severe neonatal hypoglycemia in two families. Journal of Pediatrics 95: 44–53

Seeger R C, Brodeur G M, Sather H, Dalton A, Siegel S E, Wong K Y, Hammond D 1985 Association of multiple copies of the N-myc oncogene with rapid progression of neuroblastoma. New England Journal of Medicine 313: 1111–1116

Seeler R A, Israel J N, Royal J E, Kaye C I, Rao S, Abulabam M 1979 Ganglioneuroblastoma and fetal hydantoin-alcohol syndrome. Pediatrics 63: 524–527

Seizinger R B, Martuza R L, Gusella J F 1986 Loss of genes on chromosome 22 in tumorigenesis of human acoustic neuroma. Nature 322: 644–647

Seizinger B R, Rouleau G A, Ozeluis L J 1987a Genetic linkage of von Recklinghausen neurofibromatosis to the nerve growth factor receptor gene. Cell 49: 589–594

Seizinger B R, Rouleau G A, Ozeluis L J et al 1987b Common pathogenic mechanism for three tumor types in bilateral acoustic neurofibromatosis. Science 236: 317–319

Shinohara M, Komatsu H, Kawamura T, Yokoyama M 1980 Familial testicular teratoma in 2 children: familial report and review of the literature. Journal of Urology 123: 552–555

Shtivelman E, Lifshitz B, Gale R P, Canaani E 1985 Fused transcript of abl and bcr genes in chronic myelogenous leukemia. Nature 315: 550–554

Simpson J L, Photopoulos G 1976 Hereditary aspects of ovarian and testicular neoplasia. Birth Defects 12: 51–60

Simpson N E, Kidd K K, Goodfellow P J et al 1987 Assignment of multiple endocrine neoplasia 2A to chromosome 10 by linkage. Nature 328: 528–530

Solomon E, Voss R, Hall V et al 1987 Chromosome 5 allele loss in human colorectal carcinomas. Nature 328: 616–618

Sotelo-Avila C, Gonzalez-Crussi F, Fowler J W 1980 Complete and incomplete forms of the Beckwith-Wiedeman syndrome: their oncogenic potential. Journal of Pediatrics 86: 47–50

Southwick G J, Schwartz R A 1979 The basal cell nevus syndrome. Cancer 44: 2294–2305

Spector B D, Perry G S III, Kersey J H 1978 Genetically determined immunodeficiency disease (GDID) and malignancy: report from the immunodeficiency-cancer registry. Clinical Immunology and Immunopathology 11: 12–29

Stoffer S S, Van Dyke D L, Bacj J V, Szpunar W, Weiss L 1986 Familial papillary carcinoma of the thyroid. American Journal of Medical Genetics 25: 775–782

Strong L C, Herson J, Haas C, Elder K, Chakraboty R, Weiss K M, Majunder P 1984 Cancer mortality in relatives of retinoblastoma patients. Journal of the National Cancer Institute 73: 303–311

Svarch E, de la Torre E 1977 Myelomonocytic leukemia with a preleukemic syndrome and a Ph[1] chromosome in monozygotic twins. Archives of Disease in Childhood 52: 72–74

Swift M, Sholman L, Perry M, Chase C 1976 Malignant neoplasms in the families of patients with ataxia telangiectasia. Cancer Research 36: 209–215

Swift M, Caldwell R J, Chase C 1980 Reassessment of cancer predisposition of Fanconi anemia heterozygotes. Journal of the National Cancer Institute 65: 863–867

Swift M, Reitnauer P J, Morrell D, Chase C L 1987 Breast and other cancers in families with ataxia-telangiectasia. New England Journal of Medicine 316: 1289–1294

Tarkkanen A, Karjalainen K 1984 Excess of cancer deaths in close relatives of patients with bilateral retinoblastoma. Ophthalmologica 189: 143–146

Taylor W F, Myers M, Taylor W R 1980 Extrarenal Wilms' tumor in an infant exposed to intrauterine phenytoin. Lancet 2: 481–482

Telander R L, Zimmerman D, van Heerden J A, Sizemore G W 1986 Results of early thyroidectomy for medullary thyroid carcinoma in children with multiple endocrine neoplasia type 2. Journal of Pediatric Surgery 21: 1190–1194

Thiessen E J 1974 Concerning a familial association between breast cancer and both prostatic and uterine malignancies. Cancer 34: 1102–1107

Tokuhata G K, Lilienfeld A M 1963 Familial aggregation of lung cancer in humans. Journal of the National Cancer Institute 30: 289–312

Traboulsi E I, Krush A J, Gardner E J et al 1987 Prevalence and importance of pigmented ocular fundus lesions in Gardner's syndrome. New England Journal of Medicine 316: 661–667

Tragl K H, Mayr W R 1977 Familial islet-cell adenomatosis. Lancet 2: 426–428

Turc-Carel C, Philip I, Berger M–P, Philip T, Lenoir G M 1983 Chromosome translocation in Ewing's sarcoma. New England Journal of Medicine 309: 497–498

Verp M S, Simpson J L 1987 Abnormal sexual differentiation and neoplasia. Cancer Genetics and Cytogenetics 25: 191–218

Vogel F 1979 Genetics of retinoblastoma. Human Genetics 52: 1–54

Von Metz I P, Bots G T, Enotz L J 1977 Astrocytoma in three sisters. Neurology 27: 1038–1041

Weiss L M, Warnke R A, Sklar J, Cleary M L 1987 Molecular analysis of the t(14;18) chromosome translocation in malignant lymphomas. New England Journal of Medicine 317: 1185–1189

Weissman B E, Saxon P J, Pasquale S R, Jones G R, Geiser A G, Stanbridge E J 1987 Introduction of a normal human chromosome 11 into a Wilms' tumor cell line controls its tumorigenic potential. Science 236: 175–180

Wertelecki W, Fraumeni J F Jr., Mulvihill J J 1970 Nongonadal neoplasia in Turner's syndrome. Cancer 26: 485–488

Weston B, Grufferman S, Kostyu D, Barton C S, Grant J 1986 Familial aggregation of melanoma, basal cell carcinoma and gastric adenocarcinoma. Cancer 57: 2230–2234

Willis A E, Lindahl H 1987 DNA ligase I deficiency in Bloom's syndrome. Nature 325: 355–357

Wilson L M, Draper G J 1974 Neuroblastoma, its natural history and prognosis: a study of 487 cases. British Medical Journal 3: 301–307

Wylin R F, Greene M H, Palutke M, Khilanani P, Tabaczka P, Swiderski G 1982 Hairy cell leukemia in three siblings. Cancer 49: 538–542

Yamaguchi K, Kameya T, Abe K 1980 Multiple endocrine neoplasia type I. Clinics in Endocrinology and Metabolism 9: 261–284

Yates V D, Wilroy R S, Whitington G L, Simmons J C H 1983 Anterior sacral defects: an autosomal dominantly inherited condition. Journal of Pediatrics 102: 239–242

Zbar B, Brauch H, Talmadge C, Linehan M 1987 Loss of alleles of loci on the short arm of chromosome 3 in renal cell carcinoma. Nature 327: 721–724

107. Oncogenes

James V. Watson   Karol Sikora

INTRODUCTION

Oncogenes are a family of unique sequences of DNA whose abnormal expression is associated with the development of malignant cell behaviour. They were first demonstrated in rapidly transforming RNA viruses. Their significance lies in the discovery that they are not viral in origin but are derived from normal cellular DNA and appear in retroviruses as a consequence of recombinant events between the virus and the host's genetic information. The presence of a retrovirus acquired oncogene leads to uncontrolled proliferation, differentiation arrest and possibly metastasis, the hallmarks of malignancy. The exact mechanisms by which transformation is achieved remain unclear, but sequence homology with growth factors and their receptors, together with functional characteristics pointing to a role in cell cycle control, provide intriguing leads in the study of the signalling mechanisms that regulate cell growth. The exact relationship between viral oncogenes and their normal cellular parents, the proto-oncogenes, remains controversial. It is likely, however, that proto-oncogenes do have malignant potential and, when activated by the process of amplification, mutation, translocation and deletion, can promote tumour formation. Recent techniques in oligopeptide immunisation have been used to develop sets of monoclonal antibodies against oncogene products. These novel reagents have been used to investigate oncogene function in normal and neoplastic tissue and have already demonstrated their potential as tumour markers with prognostic capability. Furthermore, by purifying and analysing oncoproteins, their function can be explored and this may possibly open new avenues for therapy.

There are three conventional approaches to the treatment of cancer, surgery, radiotherapy and chemotherapy. The first two are effective in dealing with local disease in a wide variety of malignancies. Despite its widespread use, chemotherapy is only effective in prolonging survival of certain relatively rare tumour types. For common cancers such as lung, colon and breast it has little efficacy in prolonging life. The problem in devising strategies for selective tumour cell destruction is the similarity of the cancer cell to its normal counterpart.

Observations on the mutagenicity of carcinogens, the presence of damaged and translocated chromosomes in malignant cells, and the recognition of families with an inherited predisposition to the development of cancer led to the belief that the key to understanding the differences between normal and malignant cells lay in the study of the genome. It was predicted that the genetic changes took place in the small discrete sequences of DNA termed 'oncogenes'. The problem lies in the complexity of the human genome. With 50 000 functional genes buried within thousands of kilobases of non-coding sequences, where should the search begin?

TUMOUR VIRUSES

A genetic basis for cancer can be traced to the experiments of Peyton Rous who observed that cell free filterable tumour extracts could transmit sarcomas in chickens (Rous 1911). Apart from this observation little of significance took place in the first half of this century. However, in 1951 it was reported that a virus-induced murine leukaemia could be transmitted vertically from one generation to the next (Gross 1951). In 1958 It was shown that mouse parotid tumours cultivated in vitro resulted in propagation of an oncogenic virus (Stewart et al 1958). This was subsequently shown to induce tumours in rats, mice, hamsters, rabbits and guinea pigs and was called 'polyoma' in recognition of its cross species oncogenic potential. Furthermore, purified DNA from polyoma was found to be oncogenic, and Friend (1965) showed that this virus could transform cells in vitro. Infection and subsequent transformation of cells with polyoma is associated with the expression of three viral proteins, large-, middle- and small-T antigens (Smith & Ely 1983). Large-T of polyoma confers indefinite growth and a reduced requirement for growth factors (Rassoulzadegan et al 1982, 1983). Middle-T expression gives rise to anchorage independence, but the function of polyoma small-t is not known.

Further experiments which helped to establish a genetic basis for oncogenesis were reported by Martin in 1970. He subjected Rous sarcoma virus to an alkylating agent. On subsequent infection temperature sensitive mutants were produced. At permissive temperatures the cells were transformed, but reverted to their normal non-transformed phenotype at high temperatures (Martin 1970).

Many of the oncogenic viruses are made of RNA, a discovery which had profound consequences for the whole of biology. The reaction DNA→RNA→protein is thermodynamically driven towards protein and the back reaction DNA← RNA was initially thought to be impossible. However, the very existence of RNA viruses containing no DNA signalled that there had to be a mechanism for converting the message in the RNA sequence back into DNA. The enzyme responsible for this conversion, reverse transcriptase, was isolated from Rous sarcoma virus in 1970 by Baltimore and by Temin & Mizutani. This work ushered in the era of recombinant DNA technology.

The genome of the non-oncogenic RNA viruses is small, with only three genes. These are gag, pol and env, respectively encoding core protein, reverse transcriptase and envelope. When infection takes place the cell recognises the injected RNA as its own messenger which is then translated to protein. The protein product of the pol gene is reverse transcriptase. This constructs a DNA copy complementary to the RNA of the virus which is back-spliced into the host cell genome. The term retrovirus derives from this ability to perform the retroconversion of RNA into DNA, and hence replication using the DNA synthesis mechanisms of the cell. Duesberg & Vogt (1970), using ribonuclease-induced partial deletions, showed that the Rous sarcoma virus contains an extra gene. This was called src, an acronym derived from sarcoma. The genomes of most of the oncogenic retroviruses also contain an extra gene, which may be one of many. Each is named after the tumour with which that particular oncogene is associated. The gene associated with chicken myelocytomatosis is called myc; myb derives from chicken myeloblastosis; and ras from rat sarcoma. There are two major ras gene families named after the discoverers of the transmitting agents, Harvey (Ha- or H-ras) and Kirsten (Ki- or K-ras).

CELLULAR ONCOGENES

A surprising observation was made by Stehlin et al in 1976 when the v-src gene was cloned and shown to have a homologue in perfectly normal cells. By 1982 it had been shown that many oncogenes in RNA viruses have cellular homologues (Bishop & Varmus 1982). This had given rise to a nomenclature problem which was resolved by the simple expedient of adding a 'v-' prefix to the viral gene identifier and a 'c-' prefix to the cellular counterpart (Coffin et al 1981). It now transpires that oncogenes of RNA viruses have been derived from cellular genes. The evidence for this comes firstly from a comparison of the genetic structure in RNA viruses and eukaryotes. A typical gene of, for example, 1000 bases in eukaryotic cells may in fact span 20–30 kilobases within the genome and is divided into regions called introns and exons. The whole of the gene is transcribed to RNA. The introns are excised and the exons are spliced end-to-end to form the messenger RNA which is then translated to protein. The genetic code of RNA viruses does not contain introns. Furthermore, the RNA is constructed by a cell and must originally have been derived from the DNA of a cell. Initial confirmation of this was obtained by Hanafusa et al (1977). Rous sarcoma virus mutants deficient in segments of the v-src oncogene were used to infect chickens but the characteristic sarcomas were not observed. However, when virus was recovered and used to reinfect different animals the tumours were induced. The partially deleted v-src gene had been reconstituted in the virus particles after one passage through animals. It could only have been reconstructed from the cellular homologue.

Many cellular oncogenes, including that encoding the transformation associated protein p53 ('p' for protein, 53 for relative molecular weight in kilodaltons) do not have viral homologues. This protein was discovered in cells infected with the SV40 DNA virus which express two antigens called large-T and small-t (Rigby & Lane 1983). Under some conditions p53 is bound to large-T to form stable complexes (Lane & Crawford 1979, Linzer & Levine 1979, McCormick & Harlow 1980, Oren et al 1981). SV40 large-T is associated with indefinite growth and anchorage independence (Kriegler et al 1984) and some evidence suggests that small-t of SV40 has an effect on the cytoskeleton (Graessman et al 1980).

TRANSFECTION

Absolute confirmation of a genetic basis of cancer was obtained by transfection, which is the process whereby DNA foreign to the cell is incorporated into its genome. Although the frequency of transfectants was low, it was shown that DNA from human bladder and lung cancer could give rise to transformation of 3T3 mouse fibroblasts (Weinberg 1981). The genes responsible for the malignant change were found to belong to the ras family (Der et al 1982).

ONCOGENE FUNCTION

The final connection between oncogenes and proliferation control was made in 1983 when c-*sis* was shown to encode a subunit of platelet derived growth factor, PDGF, (Doolittle et al 1983, Waterfield et al 1983). This association was consolidated in the succeeding two years when the v-*erb* B and c-*fms* genes respectively were shown to encode the intracellular domain of the receptor for epidermal growth factor, EGF, (Downward et al 1984) and a transmembrane receptor for macrophage colony stimulating factor, CSF 1 (Roussel et al 1984, Scherr et al 1985). However, disordered proliferation control is only one aspect of cancer, the second major characteristic is the propensity for metastasis. Further discoveries have potentially linked this phenomenon with disordered functioning of oncogenes encoding cytoskeleton elements. The v-*fgr* gene encodes a hybrid protein containing a portion of the actin molecule (Naharro et al 1984) and *onc*-D codes for a non-muscle tropomyocin (Martin-Zanca et al 1986).

MOLECULAR PATHOLOGY IN ONCOGENESIS

A number of chromosome abnormalities are associated with cancer (Gilbert 1983). Some are gross, with the duplication of one, or more, or all chromosomes. Others are more subtle. A number of molecular mechanisms including gene amplification, mutation, promotor insertion, translocation and rearrangements are now known to be implicated in cancer (Green 1989).

The 'Philadelphia' chromosome (Rowley 1973) is a consistent finding in the chronic myeloid leukaemia (CML) and results from a 9:22 translocation. The c-*abl* oncogene is located at the breakpoint (de Klein et al 1982). The c-*mos* gene is associated with the 8:21 translocation in acute myeloid leukaemia (Neel et al 1982). The c-*myc* gene is translocated from chromosome 8 to 14 (most commonly) or to chromosomes 2 or 22 in Burkitt lymphoma. The 8:14 translocation joins c-*myc* to the immunoglobulin γ_1 genes (Hamlyn & Rabbitts 1983) possibly removing c-*myc* from its normal control region giving rise to activation. c-Ki-*ras* is amplified, over-expressed and associated with karyotypic abnormalities in mouse adrenocortical tumour cells (Schwab et al 1983a). The association of cellular homologues of viral oncogenes with translocation breakpoints has given rise to searches for oncogenes at other known breakpoints. This approach is beginning to yield dividends and is revealing a new generation of oncogenes which do not appear to have viral homologues (Bishop 1984, Varmus 1984).

Any chromosome abnormality which is visible by existing banding patterns represents massive genomic rearrangements in molecular terms. However, very subtle changes, not apparent by banding, may have profound consequences. The avian leukosis virus (ALV), unlike most retroviruses, does not contain an extra gene (Cooper & Neiman 1980). The new DNA in the infected cells which is complementary to the viral RNA was found close to the c-*myc* gene. This gave rise to a 50-fold increase in the number of c-*myc* mRNA copies (copy number) with concomitant malignant transformation (Hayward et al 1981). Apart from the specific genes the retroviruses contain flanking long terminal repeats (LTR). These genomic segments are thought to be involved in the insertion process and in 'promoting' activation of the genes after insertion. Complementary ALV DNA close to the c-*myc* gene may, therefore, activate the latter by alteration of normal promotor function or by insertion of the viral promotor.

Gene amplification has been found in a myelocytic cell line and in the primary from which the cell line was derived (Favera et al 1982). In one patient with chronic myelocytic leukaemia the c-*myc* gene was amplified 16-fold and rearranged within the genome during episodes of transformation (McCarthy et al 1984). Amplification of the c-*myc* gene has also been reported in cell lines derived from a very poor prognosis group of patients with small cell lung cancer (Little et al 1983).The N-*myc* gene which bears some homology with c-*myc* is amplified up to 100-fold in both neuroblastoma (Schwab et al 1983b) and retinoblastoma (Lee et al 1984). As yet we have very little idea of how these lesions are produced in humans. However, a variety of carcinogens can each induce reliable mutation of specific cellular genes which are associated with their specific tumours in experimental animals. These include a methylbenzanthracine-induced mouse papilloma and c-Ha-*ras* (Balmain et al 1984); γ-radiation with thymic lymphoma and c-Ki-*ras* in the mouse (Guerrero et al 1984a) and a number of nitroso-urea compounds associated with mouse breast carcinoma and c-Ha-*ras* (Sukumar et al 1983); mouse thymic lymphoma and N-*ras* (Guerrero et al 1984b); and rat neuroblastoma with c-*neu* (Schechter et al 1984).

ONCOPROTEIN FUNCTION

Although specific biochemical functions have been assigned to some of the oncoproteins (Bishop 1985) we do not as yet know how those functions, or the derangement of those functions, are integrated to produce the neoplastic phenotype. Duesberg (1985), playing devil's advocate, has pointed out that the only 'true' oncogenes are those found in retroviruses. These genes have the capacity not only to induce, but also to maintain malignant transformation, apparently in a single step, by either insertion of a gene, a long terminal repeat, or both. The protein products of *sis*, *erb* and *fms* are undoubtedly concerned with growth control. The *neu* protein probably also comes into this category as it is serologically related to EGF receptor (Schechter et al 1984). Apart from that, our detailed knowledge of oncoprotein function and the physiology which underlies transformation is as scanty as the preceding statements. Furthermore, the oncogenes found in retroviruses are not identical to their cellular homologues, the proto-oncogenes (Hunter 1984). As a result of the molecular pathology induced by carcinogenesis, either the coding or control regions of the proto-oncogenes are modified (Krontiris 1983, Cooper & Lane 1984). These changes can subvert the normal growth control processes by increased, or inappropriate, production of normal oncogene products, or by expression of aberrant proteins (Der & Cooper 1983, Stewart et al 1984a). However, although our lack of physiological understanding is enormous, there are some very interesting observations which will eventually gel into a coherent whole (Zeillinger et al 1989).

The v-*sis* protein can transform appropriate cells but PDGF cannot. However, v-*sis* encodes only the β2 subunit of the growth factor. The product of either v-*sis* or its cellular homologue may not have to be secreted from the cell to produce transformation (Betsholtz et al 1984). Hence, inappropriately increased production of the β2 subunit may 'short-circuit' one of the normal proliferation control mechanisms within the cell. The normal c-*fos* protein does not induce transformation, but modification of the carboxy terminus by manipulation of the gene can give rise to transformation (Miller et al 1984). There is also a difference between the carboxy termini of pp60^{v-src} and pp60^{c-src} which may be related to the transforming capacity of the former (Takeya & Hanafusa 1983).

Many of these proteins, including those encoded by *erb*-B, *fms*, *yes*, *src*, *ras*, *mos* and *fes* for example, have protein kinase activity (Hunter & Cooper 1985). pp60^{v-src} phosphorylates tyrosine (Hunter & Sefton 1980) and is found in adhesion plaques of infected cells (Rohrschneider 1980). These findings aroused interest as tyrosine is one of the more unusual amino acids to undergo phosphorylation and the cytoskeleton protein vinculin is abundant in adhesion plaques. It anchors actin microfilaments to the plasma membrane, which is part of the mechanism resposible for adherence of cells to the substratum. The tyrosine residues of vinculin are specifically hyperphosphorylated by a factor of about eight in Rous sarcoma virus infected cells, compared with those that are not infected (Sefton et al 1981). This modifies the protein's normal function. Cells infected with heat sensitive Rous sarcoma virus mutants (Martin 1970)

exhibit dramatic cytoskeleton changes at pp60^{v-src} permissive temperatures. Within 15–20 minutes of a temperature decrease 'flowers', observed by fluorescence, appeared on the upper surface of infected cells. These 'flowers' were composed of myosin, tropomyacin, α-actin and actin (Boschek et al 1981). The authors postulated that '. . . the microfilament-anchorage protein, as yet unidentified, might serve as a direct target for pp60^{v-src}'. It seems inconceivable that the 'as yet unidentified' microfilament-anchorage protein could have been anything other than vinculin.

Regulatory signal transducing G-proteins have been shown to have homology with *ras* proteins (Hurley et al 1984). The product of the N-*ras* gene, p21^{N-ras}, seems to link the effects of growth factor stimulation of receptors with inositol phospholipid metabolism (Wakelman et al 1986) which is increased in cells stimulated into the division cycle. Increased phosphoinositole turnover is mediated via a guanine nucleotide regulatory G-protein which may, therefore, be p21^{N-ras} or closely related.

p53 has been implicated not only in transformation (Crawford 1983, Eliyahu et al 1984) but also in cell proliferation (Milner & McCormick 1980, Milner & Milner 1981, Sarnow et al 1981, Mercer et al 1982). Elevated levels are found in cells transformed by radiation and chemicals as well as with viral agents (Deleo et al 1979, Lane & Crawford 1979, Linzer & Levine 1979, Rotter et al 1981, Rotter 1983). It may play a part in regulation of DNA synthesis, as microinjection of an anti-p53 monoclonal antibody inhibits growth factor induced DNA synthesis in 3T3 cells (Mercer et al 1982). However, p53 is a normal protein functioning in proliferation control (Milner & McCormick 1980, Mercer et al 1982, Reich & Levine 1984). We can surmise that expression of p53 must be under extremely strict regulation in normal cells in order to contain its oncogenic potential. This control can operate at several levels including transcription (Milner & Milner 1981), mRNA transcript copy number (Reich et al 1983) and protein turnover (Oren et al 1981, Reich et al 1983). It also appears to exist in two distinct forms. A number of antibodies have been raised to this protein and Milner (1984) has shown that one antibody recognises a p53 epitope in quiescent cells which is occluded after stimulation. A second antibody recognises an epitope after stimulation which is not exposed before stimulation. Both antibodies immunoprecipitate at 53 kDa. These results suggest that there may be a conformation change in the protein after stimulation which is related to the different functional states of quiescent and stimulated cells.

At least three cellular oncogenes with viral homologues (*fos*, *myb* and *myc*) encode proteins which are nuclear associated. The functions of these proteins are not yet known, though increasing evidence suggests that the c-*myc* product is involved in cell proliferation regulation (Kelly et al 1983, 1984, Makino et al 1984, Greenberg & Ziff 1984, Rabbitts et al 1985, Dang et al 1989). It may also play a part in differentiation as mRNA copy number shows a peak at 4-5 weeks in developing placenta (Pfeiffer-Ohlsson et al 1984) and a peak during spermatogenesis with stem cells and mature sperm showing very low levels (Stewart et al 1984b). This protein has a molecular weight of 62 kDa, $p62^{c-myc}$, and is one of a discrete set of non-histone and non-matrix nuclear proteins which elute from the nucleus at salt concentrations below 200mM (Evan & Hancock 1985). This suggests a DNA function which can be modulated rapidly by ionic changes within the physiological range. The turnover of both the protein and its mRNA is rapid, with half-lives in the order of 20–30 minutes in exponentially growing cells (Hann et al 1985, Rabbitts et al 1985). c-*myc* mRNA exhibited an increase within two hours of serum stimulation in serum deprived cells, but did not thereafter show a cyclical variation correlating with cell cycle phase, nor did it decrease in density arrested cells maintained in the presence of growth factors (Thompson et al 1985). The most recent evidence suggests that $p62^{c-myc}$ is intimately involved in the replicon complex of proteins responsible for initiation and maintenance of DNA synthesis (Studzinski et al 1986, Karn et al 1989).

Although our exact knowledge is still sparse, it is quite obvious that the oncogenes code for proteins which are intimately involved in the basic contol mechanisms of one of the most fundamental of all cellular functions, the drive to proliferate. Normally, growth is tightly regulated with considerable precision by a well integrated molecular chain carrying signals from the exterior to the nucleus. The available evidence suggests that there will be a number of sub-categories, at least five, under the heading of proliferation. These include genes encoding extracellular signal transmitters (c-*sis*); signal receivers on the external membrane (c-*fms*); signal transducers at the plasma membrane (v-*erb* B amd c-*fms*); intracellular transmitters (N-*ras*); and signal receivers plus transducers in the nucleus. Likely possibilities for the last category include oestrogen receptor, which has recently been shown to have extensive homology with the steroid receptor encoded by v-*erb*-A (Green et al 1986), and the proteins encoded by c-*myc*, c-*fos* and c-*myb*. There is some evidence already that $p62^{c-myc}$ is concerned with triggering and/or maintaining stimulated cells in the division cycle. p53 is also a candidate for this group, with a possible role in the initiation and/or control of DNA synthesis.

It would seem possible that growth factors such as EGF and possibly also transferrin, the interleukins and insulin, together with their receptors, will be found to be encoded by 'oncogenes'. It is becoming increasingly obvious that these genes are not exclusive to cancer, it is just that they first became apparent in cancer through the virus connection and their involvement in proliferation. All diseases in which proliferation or differentiation are disordered or required including, for example, both rheumatoid and osteo-arthritis, granulomatous processes, proliferative vasculitis, bone marrow response to anaemia or infection and wound healing are likely to be attended by alterations in 'oncogene' expression.

Some aspects of the cancer jig-saw which relate to proliferation are beginning to fall into place. However, we have hardly begun to address the most important aspect of human cancer in practical terms, that of metastasis. The majority of unsuccessfully treated cancer patients die from metastatic disease, as local disease is generally curable. The inappropriate cell proliferation of cancer is most likely to be due to failure of negative servo control mechanisms which normally regulate growth to within extraordinarily narrow limits. By the same token, the metastasis phenomenon is also likely to be due to a failure of control mechanisms which would normally constrain cells to recognise their correct 'geographical' location. All cells possess the potential capacity for mobility. Metastatic cancer cells exhibit inappropriate mobility. Mobility is associated with motility. The proteins of the cytoskeleton confer motility. It would seem to be highly significant that two oncogenes, v-*fgr* and *onc*-D, encode cytoskeleton elements both coupled with tyrosine kinase activity (Naharro et al 1984, Martin-Zanca et al 1986). Thus, we have a second major category of 'oncogenes', those concerned with sub-cellular architecture and hence possibly with metastatic potential, to complement those involved with proliferation. These two categories, namely disordered proliferation and metastasis, constitute the fundamental pathological diad of cancer.

RELEVANCE OF ONCOGENES TO HUMAN CANCER

Clinical observation does not support a single step to the malignant phenotype as observed with retroviruses in animals. Hyperkeratotic lesions of the hands and face of Caucasians exposed to tropical sun may, or may not, progress to frankly invasive squamous cell carcinoma. Few would doubt that the lesions are premalignant. Villous adenomata of the colon are recognised as being premalignant, but the final transformation to the fully malignant invasive phenotype may take years. Another good example is transitional cell papillomata of the bladder which may take 20 years before invasion takes place. Also, the bladder lining may undergo metaplastic change to a squamous epithelium in response to the chronic irritation of vesicolithiasis before development of squamous cancer. Carcinoma in situ of the uterine cervix may considerably antedate invasion of the basement membrane, as may comparable ductal epithelial changes in the breast. A 'loose' parallel has been found in model systems. Land et al (1983) have shown that full transformation to a neoplastic phenotype may require the 'co-operation' of two or more genes. A *ras* gene point mutation did not transform, but a combined co-transfection with v-*myc* gave rise to full transformation. A similar phenomenon was also found with p53 and *ras* (Parada et al 1984).

Apart from oncogene amplification which has been documented in a number of human tumours (Favera et al 1982, Little et al 1983, Lee et al 1984, Schwab et al 1983b, McCarthy et al 1984), there seems little doubt that oncogenes are significantly involved in human malignancy at the level of transcription. The c-*myc* oncogene is expressed in tumour material from patients with haemopoetic neoplasia (Rothberg et al 1984) and genes of the *ras* family appear to be over-expressed in a number of tumours. K-*ras* and H-*ras* mRNA has been found elevated in colonic carcinoma, colonic polyps (Spandidos & Kerr 1984) and breast cancer (Spandidos & Agnantis 1984). In 54 patients, covering 20 different malignancies, it was shown that more than one cellular oncogene was transcriptionally active (Slamon et al 1984, Lemoine et al 1989). Furthermore, in the majority of 14 patients in which it was possible to study both normal and malignant tissue from the same organ, there was increased transcriptional activity of oncogenes in the malignant tissue.

The vast majority of studies carried out to date in both tissue culture and human cancer have relied upon hybridization techniques using radioactive probes for either DNA (Southern 1975) or mRNA (Thomas 1980). These methods, particularly the latter, require fresh tissue which is not always obtainable in sufficient quantities from cancer patients. Also, it may take a considerable time to accumulate sufficient material and information to make meaningful clinical correlates with fresh tissue. This applies particularly to the rare tumours. Pathology departments are notorious for hoarding their archival material, which contains a huge store of information, locked up in wax awaiting release. Moreover, neither the gene nor its message is the effector molecule; this is the province of the protein. Herein lie the possibilities for extending clinical applications using monoclonal antibodies (Kohler & Milstein 1975) directed to specific oncoproteins, for example p53 (Harlow et al 1981), $p21^{c-ras}$ (Furth et al 1982) and $p62^{c-myc}$ (Evan et al

1985). Antibodies can now be raised to hydrophilic synthetic peptides predicted from the base sequence of cloned genes (Niman et al 1983) and as many oncogenes have now been completely sequenced we will soon have panels of such antibodies available for routine use in diagnosis, screening, monitoring, prognosis and possibly therapy.

FUTURE APPLICATIONS

Anti-oncoprotein antibodies have now been used for localization in tissue sections and for quantitation of levels in serum, urine and in populations of single cells.

Diagnosis, screening, prognosis and monitoring

Immunocytochemical localization with antibodies has been used to define differential *ras* expression in benign and malignant colonic disease (Thor et al 1984). Studies with an anti–$p62^{c-myc}$ monoclonal antibody, MYC 1-6E10 (Evan et al 1985), have shown that normal colonic mucosa exhibited maximal expression in the maturation zones of the crypts of Lieberkuhn where there was mixed nuclear and cytoplasmic staining (Stewart et al 1986). However, $p62^{c-myc}$ is known to be nuclear associated (Evan & Hancock 1985) and in further more extensive studies it has been shown that this protein is redistributed from a nuclear to a cytoplasmic location with increasing maturation of the normal colonic mucosa (Sundaresan et al 1987). This has also been shown in mucosa freshly fixed within seconds of biopsy (Forgacs et al 1986) and active exclusion of the protein from the nucleus may be part of the normal control mechanism for regulating proliferation and differentiation. In familial polyposis coli, which inexorably progresses to the malignant invasive phenotype, nuclear staining persisted to the surface of the crypts and in carcinomas the staining was predominantly nuclear (Sundaresan et al 1987). Quantitative studies comparing normal with dysplastic mucosa and carcinomas developing in patients with ulcerative colitis have shown that the nuclear $p62^{c-myc}$ content increased with the transition from 'mild' to 'severe' dysplasia (Forgacs et al 1986) and that the protein content is raised in carcinomas (Watson et al 1987). Furthermore, the protein content was also raised in morphologically normal colonic mucosa derived from malignant, compared with non-malignant, specimens (Watson et al 1990). These studies used flow cytometric techniques (Watson 1980, 1981, 1987) to quantitate the oncoprotein content with total DNA simultaneously in individual nuclei extracted from tissue sections (Watson et al 1985) using an adaptation of the method of Hedley et al (1983). The results from archival material using fluorescence techniques complemented those obtained with Northern and Western blotting using fresh tissue (Sikora et al 1987).

Studies have also been carried out in testicular cancer biopsies. p62^{c-myc} was expressed in only small amounts in the normal testis. Seminomas exhibited increased nuclear and cytoplasmic staining. Undifferentiated teratomas showed barely detectable staining, whereas well differentiated epithelial structures and yolk-sac elements exhibited intense staining (Sikora et al 1985). Parallel flow cytometric quantitation was carried out, which enabled significance limits to be assigned to the qualitative results obtained by immunocytochemistry. Low p62^{c-myc} levels were found in normal testicular tissue and significantly elevated levels were found in both teratoma ($p < 0.001$) and seminoma ($p < 0.001$). However, the oncoprotein level increased significantly with increasing differentiation in teratoma ($p < 0.01$). Patients with intermediate and undifferentiated tumours who developed recurrence had lower levels than those who were disease free since their initial treatment, $p < 0.05$ (Watson et al 1986), hence prognostic information is potentially forthcoming. Sainsbury et al (1985) have also obtained prognostic information in breast cancer patients by assaying EGF receptor (v-erb-B) and oestrogen receptor (v-erb-A).

Flow technology has been used in uterine cervix neoplasia to assay for p62^{c-myc} in archival specimens (Hendy-Ibbs et al 1987). Normal biopsies exhibited higher p62^{c-myc} levels than carcinomas, $p < 0.00001$. There was a progressive decrease in oncoprotein level with progression from cervical intraepithelial neoplasia, stage I (CIN I) to CIN III, $p < 0.05$. Furthermore, the maximum fluorescence signal in the normal tissues occurred at a lower antibody concentration compared with tumour tissue, $p < 0.00001$. There was no correlation with histological grade, stage, age or prognosis in patients with invasion. These techniques have now been adapted for tissue sampled from colposcopy clinics, with a view to automated prescreening of cervical smears in an attempt to exploit the obvious diagnostic potential of the simultaneous DNA/p62^{c-myc} assay (Elias-Jones et al, 1986, Sowani et al 1989).

The findings in colonic neoplasia and seminoma were partially anticipated, but those in both the histological breakdown of teratoma and in cervical carcinoma were completely contrary to expectation. The latter finding was particularly controversial as Riou et al (1985) have reported amplification of both the c-myc and H-ras oncogenes in carcinoma of the cervix associated with papilloma virus infection (Durst et al 1983). However, an increase in either the gene or mRNA copy number (or both), which would give rise to an increased protein production rate, need not necessarily be reflected in a marked increase in the total protein content, for two main reasons. Firstly, inappropriately increased message may result in rate limitation at the protein synthesis level.

Secondly, an increase in protein degradation may offset an increased production rate. The latter is most likely to occur with a protein which has a short half-life and, clearly, this is a distinct possibility for p62^{c-myc} with a half-life of 20–30 minutes in rapidly cycling and stimulated cells (Greenberg & Ziff 1984, Rabbitts et al 1985). Hence, the lower absolute levels in carcinoma of the cervix compared with normal, and in undifferentiated compared with the better differentiated teratomas, may reflect an increased protein turnover and an increased cell production rate in both cases. Further possibilities include post-translational protein modification in the more malignant teratomas and in cervical carcinoma, giving rise to an alteration or partial occlusion of the epitope recognised by the antibody and a possible increase in the susceptibility of the protein to proteolysis in neoplastic cells in the preparation for the assay. There is a small shred of evidence that post-translational protein modification may occur in cervical carcinoma. Maximum binding was observed at different antibody concentrations in the normal and malignant cells, which might indicate a change in binding constant.

These various findings suggest the potential for the oncoproteins to become a new generation of tumour markers, and they have also been detected in serum and urine. Crawford et al (1982) have detected antibodies against the cellular protein p53 in sera from patients with breast cancer. Anti-peptide antibodies have detected and compared oncogene-related proteins in urine in normal subjects, pregnancy and cancer patients (Niman et al 1985). Similar studies have been conducted using an antibody to the c-myc protein. A 40 000 Dalton breakdown product of p62^{c-myc}, or a related protein, was detected in cancer patients and in pregnancy (Chan et al 1987) and the p40 serum levels decreased after hemicolectomy for carcinoma, raising the possibility of monitoring for recurrence with regular sampling. Diagnostic scanning is another possibility as a radiolabelled anti-p62^{c-myc} antibody has been used to localize lung cancer (Chan et al 1986).

Therapy

The scope for developing diagnostic, screening, prognostic and monitoring assays using probes for the oncogenes and their products is enormous. Although it is obvious how these assays will relate to overall management, it is not so obvious how a knowledge of oncogenes and their products will relate directly to therapy. Nevertheless, possibilities do exist (Steel 1989). Tamoxifen has been used for breast cancer patients for almost two decades, yet it is only recently that oestrogen receptor has been shown to be homologous with the protein encoded by v-erb-A (Green et al 1986). Moreover, many of the oncoproteins involved in the pathology are slightly abnormal; examples from experimental systems include those encoded by *fos* and *src*. The v-*erb*-B oncogene encodes the intracellular and transmembrane domains, plus a truncated portion of the external domain of the EGF receptor in some human cancers. If this truncated extracellular domain is *unique* to the tumour cells in which it is found it may be possible to use targeted monoclonal antibody-mediated killing with coupled toxins or radioisotopes. Complement mediated killing is another possibility. It is probably unlikely that all oncoproteins will be found to be abnormal in human systems. However, if any intracellular oncoproteins are found to be abnormal they could be blocked by small synthetic peptides without blocking the normal counterpart. These possibilities are mere speculation at present and it seems highly unlikely that a universal 'magic oncogene-related bullet' will be forthcoming for all cancer, and full therapeutic possibilities will have to await elucidation and understanding of oncogene physiology. However, a real start has been made and we believe that we are just at the very beginning of a renaissance in cancer treatment which will be based on an understanding of the fundamental biochemical differences between normal and malignant cells. That understanding will come from objective measurements made at the molecular level, and the differences will be exploited for the benefit of the cancer patient.

REFERENCES

Balmain A, Ramsden M, Bowden G T, Smith J 1984 Activation of the mouse Harvey-*ras* gene in chemically induced benign skin papillomas. Nature 307:658–660

Baltimore D 1970 RNA-dependent DNA polymerase in virons of RNA tumour viruses. Nature 226: 1209–1211

Betsholtz C, Wetermark B, Ek B, Heidin C H 1984 Coexpression of a PDGF-like growth factor and PDGF receptors in a human osteosarcoma cell line: implications for autocrine receptor activation. Cell 39: 447–457

Bishop J M 1984 Trends in oncogenes. Trends in Genetics 1: 245–249

Bishop J M 1985 Viral oncogenes. Cell 32: 23–36

Bishop J M, Varmus H 1982 Functions and origins of retroviral transforming genes. In: Weiss R, Teich N, Varmus H, Coffin J (eds) Molecular Biology of Tumour Viruses, Part III, RNA Tumour Viruses. Cold Spring Harbor Press, New York p999–1108

Boschek C B, Jockusch B M, Friis R R, Back R, Grundmann E, Bauer H 1981 Early changes in the distribution and organization of microfilament proteins during cell transformation. Cell 24: 175–184

Chan S Y T, Evan G I, Ritson A, Watson J V, Wraight P, Sikora K 1986 Localization of lung cancer by a radiolabelled monoclonal antibody against the c-*myc* oncogene product. British Journal of Cancer. 54: 761–769

Chan S Y T, Gabra H, Hill F, Evan G, Sikora K 1987 A novel tumour marker related to the c-*myc* oncogene product. Molecular and Cellular Probes 1: 73–82

Coffin J H, Varmus H E, Bishop J M et al 1981 Proposal for naming host cell derived inserts in retrovirus genomes. Journal of Virology 40: 953–957

Cooper G M, Lane M A 1984 Cellular transforming genes and oncogenesis. Biochimica et Biophysica Acta 738: 9–20

Cooper G M, Neiman E 1980 Transforming genes of neoplasms induced by avian leukosis virus. Nature 287: 656–659

Crawford L 1983 The 53000 dalton cellular protein and its role in transformation. International Review of Experimental Pathology 25: 1–50

Crawford L V, Pim D C, Bulbrook R D 1982 Detection of antibodies against the cellular protein p53 in sera from patients with breast cancer. International Journal of Cancer 30: 403–408

Dang C V, McGuire M, Buckmire M, Lee W M 1989 Involvement of the 'leucine zipper' region in the oligomerization and transforming activity of human c-*myc* protein. Nature 337: 664–666

de Klein A, Kessel A G, Grosveld G, Botram C R, Hagemeijer A, Groffen J, Stephenson J R 1982 A cellular oncogene is translocated to the Philadelphia chromosome in chronic myelocytic leukaemia. Nature 300: 765–767

Deleo A B, Jay G, Appella E, Dubois G C, Law L W, Old J 1979 Detection of a transformation-related antigen in chemically induced sarcomas and other transformed cells in the mouse. Proceedings of the National Academy of Sciences 76: 2420–2424

Der C J, Cooper G M 1983 Altered gene products are associated with activation of cellular *ras*^{K} genes in human lung and colon carcinomas. Cell 32: 201–208

Der C J, Krontiris T G, Cooper G M 1982 Transforming genes of human bladder and lung carcinoma cell lines are homologous to the *ras* gene of Harvey and Kirsten sarcoma viruses. Proceedings of the National Academy of Sciences USA 79: 3637–3640

Doolittle R F, Hunkerpiller M W, Hood L E, Devare S G, Robbins K C, Aaronson S A, Antoniades H W 1983 Simian sarcoma virus *onc* gene, v-*sis*, is derived from the gene (or genes) encoding a platelet derived growth factor. Science 211: 275–276

Downward J, Yardem Y, Mayes E et al 1984 Close similarities of epidermal growth factor receptor and v-*erb* B oncogene protein sequences. Nature 307: 521–527

Duesberg P H 1985 Activated proto-onc genes: Sufficient or necessary for cancer? Science 228: 660–677

Duesberg P H, Vogt P K 1970 Differences between the ribonucleic acids of transforming and non-transforming avian tumour viruses. Proceedings of the National Academy of Sciences 67: 1673–1680

Durst M, Gissman L, Ikenberg H, zur Hausen H 1983 A papilloma-virus DNA from a cervical carcinoma and its prevalence in cancer biopsy samples from different geographic regions. Proceedings of the National Academy of Sciences 80: 3812–3815

Elias-Jones J, Hendy-Ibbs P, Cox H, Evan G I, Watson J V 1986 Cervical brush biopsy specimens suitable for DNA and oncoprotein analysis using flow cytometry. Journal of Clinical Pathology 39: 577–581

Eliyahu D, Raz A, Gruss P, Gival D, Oren M 1984 Participation of p53 cellular tumour antigen in transformation of normal embryonal cells. Nature 312: 646–649

Evan G I, Hancock D C 1985 Studies on the interaction of the human c-*myc* protein with cell nuclei: p62[c-myc] as a member of a discrete subset of nuclear proteins. Cell 43: 253–261

Evan G I, Lewis G K, Ramsay G, Bishop J M 1985 Isolation of monoclonal antibodies specific for human and mouse proto-oncogene products. Molecular and Cellular Biology 5: 3610–3616

Favera D R, Wong-Staal F, Gallo R 1982 Onc gene amplification in promyelocytic leukaemia cell line (HL-60) and in the primary from the same patient. Nature 299: 61–63

Forgacs I C, Sunderesan V, Evan G, Wight D G D, Neale G, Hunter J O, Watson J V 1986 Abnormal expression of c-*myc* oncogene product in dysplasia and neoplasia associated with ulcerative colitis. Gut 7: A1285

Friend M 1965 Cell transformation ability of a temperature sensitive mutant of polyoma virus. Proceedings of the National Academy of Sciences 53: 486–491

Furth M E, Davis L J, Fleurdelys B, Scolnick E 1982 Monoclonal antibodies to the p21 product of the transforming gene of Harvey murine sarcoma virus and of the cellular ras gene family. Journal of Virology 43: 294–304

Gilbert F 1983 Chromosome aberrations and oncogenes. Nature 303: 475

Graessman A, Graessman M, Tjian R, Topp W C 1980 Simian virus 40 small-t protein is required for loss of actin cable network in rat cells. Journal of Virology 33: 1182–1191

Green M R 1989 When the products of oncogenes and antioncogenes meet. Cell 56: 1–3

Green S, Walter P, Kurman V, Krust A, Bornert J-M, Argos P, Chambon P 1986 Human oestrogen receptor cDNA: sequence, expression and homology to v-*erb*-A. Nature 320: 134–139

Greenberg M E, Ziff E B 1984 Stimulation of 3T3 cells induces transcription of the c-*fos* proto-oncogene. Nature 311:433–438

Gross L 1951 Spontaneous leukaemia developing in C3H mice following inoculation, in infancy, with AK-leukaemia extracts, or AK-embryos. Proceedings of the Society for Experimental Biology and Medicine 76: 27–32

Guerrero I, Villasante A, Corces V, Pellicer A 1984a Activation of a c-K-ras oncogene by somatic mutation in mouse lymphomas induced by γ-radiation. Science 225: 1159–1162

Guerrero I, Villasante A, D'Eustachio P, Pellicer A 1984b Isolation, characterization, and chromosome assignment of mouse N-ras gene from carcinogen-induced thymic lymphoma. Science 225: 1041–1043

Hamlyn P H, Rabbitts T H 1983 Translocation joins the c-*myc* and the immunoglobulin γ₁ genes in Burkitt's lymphoma revealing a third exon in the c-*myc* oncogene. Nature 304: 135–139

Hanafusa H, Haplern C C, Buckhagen D L, Kawai S 1977 Recovery of avian sarcoma viruses from tumours induced by transformation-defective mutants. Journal of Experimental Medicine 146: 1735–1747

Hann S R, Thompson C B, Eisenman R N 1985 c-*myc* oncogene protein is independent of the cell cycle in human and avian cells. Nature 314: 366–369

Harlow E, Crawford L V, Pim P C, Williamson N M 1981 Monoclonal antibodies specific for simian virus 40 tumour antigens. Journal of Virology 39: 861–869

Hayward W S, Neel B G, Ashin S M 1981 Activation of a cellular onc gene by promotor insertion in ALV-induced lymphoid leukaemias. Nature 290: 475–479

Hedley D W, Friedlander M I, Taylor I W, Rugg C A, Musgrove E A 1983 Method for analysis of cellular DNA content of paraffin-embedded pathological material using flow cytometry. Journal of Histochemistry and Cytochemistry 31: 1333–1335

Hendy-Ibbs P, Cox H, Evan G I, Watson J V 1987 Flow cytometric quantitation of DNA and c-*myc* oncoprotein in archival biopsies of uterine cervix neoplasia. British Journal of Cancer 55: 275–282

Hunter T 1984 Oncogenes and proto-oncogenes: How do they differ? Journal of the National Cancer Institute 73: 773–785

Hunter T, Cooper J A 1985 Protein-tyrosine kinases. Annual Review of Biochemistry 54: 897–930

Hunter T, Sefton B M 1980 Transforming gene product of Rous sarcoma virus phosphorylates tyrosine. Proceedings of the National Academy of Sciences 77: 1311–1315

Hurley J B, Simon M I, Teplow D B, Robinshaw J D, Gilman A G 1984 Homologies between signal transducing G proteins and ras gene products. Science 226: 860–863

Karn J, Watson J V, Lowe A D, Green S M, Vedeckis W 1989 Regulation of cell cycle duration by c-*myc* levels. Oncogene 4: 773–787

Kelly K, Cochran B H, Stiles C D, Leder P 1983 Cell specific regulation of the c-*myc* gene by lymphocyte mitogens and platelet derived growth factor. Cell 35: 603–610

Kelly K, Cochran B H, Stiles C D, Leder P 1984 The regulation of c-*myc* by growth signals. Current Topics in Microbiology and Immunology 113: 117–126

Kohler G, Milstein C 1975 Continuous cultures of fused cells secreting antibody of predefined specificity. Nature 256: 495–496

Kriegler M, Perez C F, Hardy C, Botchan M 1984 Transformation mediated by the SV40 T-antigens; separation of the overlapping SV40 early genes with a retroviral vector. Cell 38: 483–491

Krontiris T G 1983 The emerging genetics of human cancer. New England Journal of Medicine 309: 404–409

Land H, Parada L F, Weinberg R A 1983 Tumorigenic conversion of primary embryo fibroblasts requires at least two cooperating oncogenes. Nature 304: 596–602

Lane D P, Crawford L V 1979 T-antigen is bound to a host protein in SV40-transformed cells. Nature 278: 261–263

Lee W W Murphee A L, Benedict W F 1984 Expression and amplification of the N-*myc* gene in primary retinoblastoma. Nature 309: 458–460

Lemoine N R, Mayall E, Wyllie F et al 1989 High frequency of *ras* oncogene activation in all stages of human thyroid tumorigenesis. Oncogene 4: 159–164

Linzer D I H, Levine A J 1979 Characterization of a 54K Dalton cellular SV40 tumour antigen present in SV40-transformed cells and uninfected embryonal carcinoma cells. Cell 17: 43–52

Little C D, Nau M M, Carney D N, Gazdar A F, Minna J D 1983 Amplification and expression of the c-*myc* oncogene in human lung cancer cell lines. Nature 306: 194–196

McCarthy D M, Rassool F V, Goldman J M, Graham S V, Binnie G D 1984 Genomic alterations involving the c-*myc* proto-oncogene locus during the evolution of a case of chronic granulocytic leukaemia. Lancet 2: 1362–1365

McCormick F, Harlow E 1980 Association of a murine 53,000 Dalton phosphoprotein with simian virus 40 large-T antigen in transformed cells. Journal of Virology 34: 213–224

Makino R, Hayashi K A, Sugimura T 1984 c-*myc* is induced in rat liver at a very early stage of regeneration or by cycloheximide treatment. Nature 310: 697–698

Martin G S 1970 Rous sarcoma virus; a function required for the maintenance of the transformed state. Nature 227: 1021–1023

Martin-Zanca D, Hughes S H, Barbacid M 1986 A human oncogene formed by the fusion of truncated tropomysin and protein tyrosine kinase sequences. Nature 319: 743–748

Mercer W E, Nelson D, Deleo A B, Old L J, Baserga R 1982 Microinjection of monoclonal antibody to protein p53 inhibits serum-induced DNA synthesis in 3T3 cells. Proceedings of the National Academy of Sciences 79: 6309–6312

Miller A D, Curran T, Verma I M 1984 c-*fos* protein can induce cellular transformation: A novel mechanism for activation of a cellular oncogene. Cell 36: 51–60

Milner J 1984 Different forms of p53 detected by monoclonal antibodies in non-dividing and dividing lymphocytes. Nature 310: 143–145

Milner J, McCormick F 1980 Lymphocyte stimulation: concanavalin A induces the expression of a 53K protein. Cell Biology International Reports 4: 663–667

Milner J, Milner S 1981 SV40–53K antigen: A possible role for 53K in normal cells. Virology 112: 785–788

Naharro G, Robins K, Reddy E P 1984 Gene product of v-*fgr* onc: hybrid protein contains a portion of actin and a tyrosine-specific protein kinase. Science 223: 63–66

Neel B G, Jhan War S C, Chaganti R S K, Hayward W S 1982 Two human c-*onc* genes are located on the long arm of chromosome 8. Proceedings of the National Academy of Sciences, USA 79: 7842–7846

Niman H L, Houghten R A, Walker L E, Reisfeld R A, Wilson I A, Hogle J M, Lerner R A 1983 Generation of protein-reactive antibodies by short peptides in an event of high frequency: Implications for the structural basis of immune recognition. Proceedings of the National Academy of Sciences 80: 4949–4953

Niman H L, Thompson A M H, Yu A et al 1985 Anti-peptide antibodies detect oncogene-related proteins in urine. Proceedings of the National Academy of Sciences 82: 7924–7928

Oren M, Malzman W, Levine A J 1981 Post-translational regulation of the 54K cellular tumour antigen in normal and transformed cells. Molecular and Cellular Biology 1: 101–110

Parada L F, Land H, Weinberg R A, Wolf D, Rotter V 1984 Co-operation between gene encoding p53 tumour antigen and *ras* in cellular transformaton. Nature 312: 649–651

Pfeiffer-Ohlsson S, Goustin A S, Rydnert J, Wahlstrom T, Bjersing L, Stehelin D, Ohlsson R 1984 Spatial and temporal pattern of cellular *myc* oncogene expression in developing human placenta; Implications for embryonic cell proliferation. Cell 38: 585–596

Rabbitts P H, Watson J V, Lamond A et al 1985

Metabolism of c-*myc* gene products: c-*myc* mRNA and protein expression in the cell cycle. EMBO Journal 4: 2009–2015

Rassoulzadegan M, Cowie A, Carr A, Glaichenhous N, Karmen R 1982 The role of individual polyoma virus early proteins in oncogenic transformation. Nature 300: 713–718

Rassoulzadegan M, Naghashfar Z, Cowie A, Carr A, Grisoni M, Kamen R, Cuzin F 1983 Expression of the large-T protein of polyoma virus promotes the establishment in culture of 'normal' rodent fibroblast cell lines. Proceedings of the National Academy of Sciences 80: 4354–4358

Reich N C Levine A J 1984 Growth regulation of a cellular tumour antigen, p53, in non-transformed cells. Nature 308: 199–201

Reich N C Oren M, Levine A J 1983 Two distinct mechanisms regulate the level of a cellular tumour antigen, p53. Molecular and Cellular Biology 3: 2143–2150

Rigby P W, Lane D P 1983 Structure and function of Simian virus 40 large-T antigen. In: Klein G (ed) Advances in Viral Oncology, vol. 3. Raven Press, New York, p31–58

Riou G, Barrois M, Tordjman I, Dutronquay V, Orth G 1985 Presence de genomes de papillomavirus et amplification des oncogenes c-*myc* et c-Ha-*ras* dans des cancers envahissants du col de l'uterus. Compte Rendu de l'Académie des Sciences, Paris 299: 575–580

Rohrschneider L R 1980 Adhesion plaques of Rous sarcoma virus transformed cells contain the *src* gene product. Proceedings of the National Academy of Sciences 77: 3514–3518

Rothberg P G, Erisman M D, Diehl R E, Roviatti U G, Astrin S M 1984 Structure and expression of the oncogene c-*myc* in fresh tumour material from patients with haemopoetic malignancies. Molecular and Cellular Biology 4: 1096–1103

Rotter V 1983 p53, a transformation-related cellular-encoded protein, can be used as a biochemical marker for the detection of primary mouse tumour cells. Proceedings of the National Academy of Sciences 80: 2613–2617

Rotter V, Boss M A, Baltimore D J 1981 Increased concentration of an apparently identical cellular protein in cells transformed by either Ableson murine leukaemia or other transforming agents. Journal of Virology 38: 336–346

Rous P 1911 Transmission of a malignant new growth by means of a cell-free filtrate. Journal of the American Medical Association (Chicago) 6: 198–202

Roussel M F, Rettenmier C W, Look A T, Scherr C J 1984 Cell surface expression of v-*fms*-coded glycoproteins is required for transformation. Molecular and Cellular Biology 4: 1999–2009

Rowley J D 1973 A new consistent chromosomal abnormality in chronic myelogenous leukaemia identified by quinacrine fluorescence and Giemsa staining. Nature 243: 290–293

Sainsbury J R C, Farndon J R, Sherbet G V, Harris A L 1985 Epidermal growth factor receptors and oestrogen receptors in human breast cancer. Lancet i: 364

Sarnow P, Ho Y S, Williams J, Levine A J 1981 Adenovirus Elb-58K tumour antigen and SV40 large tumour antigen are physically associated with the same 54kd cellular protein in transformed cells. Cell 28: 387–394

Schechter A L, Stern D F, Vaidyanathan L, Decker S J, Drebin J A, Green M I, Weinberg R A 1984 The *neu* oncogene: an *erb*-B-related gene encoding a 185 000-M$_r$ tumour antigen. Nature 312: 513–517

Scherr C J, Rettenmier C W, Sacca R, Rousel M F, Look A T, Stanley E R 1985 The c-*fms* proto-oncogene product is related to the receptor for the mononuclear phagocytic growth factor, CSF 1. Cell 41: 665–676

Schwab M, Alitalo K, Varmus H E, Bishop J M, George D 1983a A cellular oncogene c-Ki-*ras* is amplified, overexpressed and located with karyotypic abnormalities in mouse adrenocortical tumour cells. Nature 303: 497–501

Schwab M, Alitalo K, Klempenauer K H et al 1983b Amplified N-*myc* with limited homology to *myc* cellular oncogene is shared by human neuroblastoma cell lines and a neuroblastoma tumour. Nature 305: 245–248

Sefton B M, Hunter T, Ball E H, Singer S J 1981 Vinculin: a cytoskeletal target for the transforming protein of Rous sarcoma virus. Cell 24: 165–174

Sikora K, Evan G, Stewart J, Watson J V 1985 Detection of the c-*myc* oncogene product in testicular cancer. British Journal of Cancer 52: 171–176

Sikora K, Chan S Y T, Evan G I, Markham N, Stewart J, Watson J V 1987 c-*myc* expression in colorectal cancer. Cancer 59: 1289–1295

Slamon D J, Dekernion J B, Verma I M, Cline M J 1984 Expression of cellular oncogenes in human malignancies. Science 224: 256–262

Smith A E, Ely B K 1983 The biochemical basis of transformation by polyoma virus. In: Klein G (ed) Advances in Viral Oncology, vol 3 Raven Press, New York, p 3–30

Southern E M 1975 Detection of specific sequences among DNA fragments by gel electrophoresis. Journal of Molecular Biology 98: 503–517

Sowani A, Ong G, Dische S et al 1989 c-*myc* oncogene expression and clinical outcome in carcinoma of the cervix. Molecular and Cellular Probes 3: 117–123.

Spandidos D A, Agnantis N J 1984 Human malignant tumours of the breast, as compared to their respective normal tissue, have elevated expression of the Harvey *ras* oncogene. Anticancer Research 4: 269–272

Spandidos D A, Kerr I B 1984 Elevated expression of the human *ras* oncogene family in premalignant tumours of the colorectum. British Journal of Cancer 49: 681–688

Steel C M 1989 Peptide regulatory factors and malignancy. Lancet ii: 30–34

Stehlin D, Varmus H E, Bishop J M, Vogt P K 1976 DNA related to transforming genes of avian sarcoma virus is present in normal avian DNA. Nature 260: 170–173

Stewart J, Evan G I, Watson J V, Sikora K E 1986 Detection of the c-*myc* oncogene product in colonic polyps and carcinomas. British Journal of Cancer 53: 1–6

Stewart S E, Eddy B E, Borgese N G 1958 Neoplasms in mice inoculated with a tumour agent carried in tissue culture. Journal of the National Cancer Institute 20: 1223–1243

Stewart T A, Pattengale P K, Leder P 1984a Spontaneous mammary adenocarcinomas in transgenic mice carry and express MTV/myc fusion genes. Cell 38: 627–637

Stewart T A, Bellve A R, Leder P 1984b Transcription and promoter usage of the c-*myc* gene in normal somatic and spermatogenic cells. Science 226: 707–710

Studzinski G P, Brelvi Z S, Feldman S C, Watt R A 1986 Participation of c-*myc* in DNA synthesis of human cells. Science 234: 467–470

Sukumar S, Notorio V, Martin-Zanca D, Barbacid M 1983 Induction of mammary carcinomas in rats by nitros-methylurea involves malignant activation of H-*ras*-1 locus by single point mutation. Nature 306: 658–661

Sundaresan V, Forgacs I, Wight D, Evan G I, Watson J V 1987 Abnormal distribution of the c-*myc* oncogene product in familial polyposis coli. Journal of Clinical Pathology 40: 1274–1281

Takeya T, Hanafusa H 1983 Structure and sequence of the cellular gene homologous to the RSV *src* gene and the mechanism for generating the transforming virus. Cell 32: 881–890

Temin H, Mizutani S 1970 RNA- dependent DNA polymerase in virons of Rous sarcoma virus. Nature 226: 1211–1213

Thomas P S 1980 Hybridization of denatured RNA and small DNA fragments transferred to nitrocellulose. Proceedings of the National Academy of Sciences, USA 77: 5201–5205

Thompson C B, Challoner P B, Neiman P E, Groudine M 1985 Levels of c-*myc* oncogene mRNA are invariate throughout the cell cycle. Nature 314; 363–366

Thor A, Horan Hand P, Wunderlich D, Caruso A, Muraro R, Schlom J 1984 Monoclonal antibodies define differential *ras* gene expression in malignant and benign colonic disease. Nature 311: 562–564

Varmus H E 1984 The molecular genetics of cellular oncogenes. Annual Review of Genetics 18: 553–612

Wakelman M J O, Davies S A, Houslay M D, McKay I, Marshall C J, Hall A 1986 Normal p21^{N-ras} couples bombesin and other growth-factors to inositole phosphate production. Nature 323: 173–176

Waterfield M D, Scrace G T, Whittle N et al 1983 Platelet derived growth factor is structurally related to the putative transforming protein p28^{sis} of simian sarcoma virus. Nature 304: 35–39

Watson J V 1980 Enzyme kinetic studies in cell populations using fluorogenic substrates and flow cytometric techniques. Cytometry 1: 143–151

Watson J V 1981 Dual laser beam focussing for flow cytometry through a single crossed cylindrical lens pair. Cytometry 2: 14–19

Watson J V 1987 Flow cytometry in Biomedical Science. Nature 325: 741–742

Watson J V, Sikora K E, Evan G I 1985 A simultaneous flow cytometric assay for c-*myc* oncoprotein and cellular DNA in nuclei from paraffin embedded material. Journal of Immunological Methods 83: 179–192

Watson J V, Stewart J, Evan G I, Ritson A, Sikora K 1986 The clinical significance of flow cytometric c-*myc* oncoprotein quantitation in testicular cancer. British Journal of Cancer 53: 331–337

Watson J V, Stewart J, Cox H, Sikora K E, Evan G I 1987 Flow cytometric quantitation of the c-*myc* oncoprotein in archival neoplastic biopsies of the colon. Molecular and Cellular Probes 1: 151–157

Watson J V, Stewart J, Cox H, Sikora K E, Evan G I 1990 c-*myc* oncoprotein levels are raised in morphologically normal colonic mucosa derived from malignant compared with non-malignant specimens. (In submission)

Weinberg R A 1981 Use of transfection to analyse genetic information and malignant transformation. Biochimica et Biophysica Acta 651: 25–35

Zeillinger R, Kury F, Czerwenka K et al 1989 HER-2 amplification, steroid receptors and epidermal growth factor receptor in primary breast cancer. Oncogene 4: 109–114

Applied Genetics

108. Genetic counselling

R. Skinner

The last few decades have seen a dramatic decrease in the importance of environmental causes of ill-health in developed countries. As a result there has been a sharp increase in the relative importance of genetic and partially genetic disorders as causes of present day morbidity and mortality, particularly amongst children. Many studies in recent years have shown that roughly 30% of admissions to, and between 40 and 50% of deaths occurring in, paediatric hospitals are accounted for by children with genetic disorders or congenital malformations. Genetic diseases are almost always serious, are not curable, and relatively few are amenable to satisfactory modes of treatment. Thus, in the current situation the prevention of this group of diseases remains of paramount importance. At the present time the most effective means of preventing genetic diseases remains the provision of genetic counselling for individuals at risk of having a child with a serious genetic disorder, coupled with prenatal diagnosis where possible.

One of the prime requirements of an effective genetic counselling programme is the comprehensive ascertainment of those individuals in the population who are at risk of having an affected child so that they can be offered genetic advice. There are a number of ways in which such individuals can be ascertained, but these fall mainly in two categories. Population screening is one obvious way of ascertaining people at risk, but such methods are accompanied by many problems, both practical and ethical. The main way in which ascertainment is achieved, therefore, is as a result of routine diagnosis when an individual is found to have a disorder known to be genetic. The families of such individuals can then be screened and advice offered to those at risk of having affected children. This approach can of course be greatly facilitated by the use of a genetic register system designed for this purpose. The intricacies and usage of both population screening and genetic registers for the ascertainment of individuals in need of genetic counselling have been reviewed elsewhere in this text and will therefore not be discussed further here.

Traditionally, genetic counselling has been viewed as the process by which individuals seeking advice are provided with all the information that is required to enable them to make a wholly informed decision on what their future reproductive plans will be. Therefore, this has mainly taken the form of what has been termed 'factually-oriented' counselling. The last decade however, has seen increasing recognition of the importance of the many psychological aspects of such counselling. Awareness of the variety of problems which may lessen the degree of communication between counsellor and counsellee, of the feelings of guilt often attendant on the birth of a handicapped child, and of the dynamics of the coping and decision-making processes themselves, have led to the trend by most genetic counsellors to move away from traditional approaches towards what Kessler (1979) has described as more 'person-oriented' counselling and to be more aware of the need to ensure comprehensive support and follow-up for those receiving counselling. This aspect of genetic counselling will be explored towards the end of the chapter when the more basic, factual aspects of the problem have been considered.

BASIC INFORMATION NEEDED FOR GENETIC COUNSELLING

Before a counsellor can embark upon giving definitive genetic advice he must have available to him certain basic, essential information. He must at least have a precise and fully confirmed diagnosis in the index patient, an accurate pedigree of the family, and know the mode of inheritance of the disorder at hand so that the precise risk of occurrence or recurrence can be estimated. The person responsible for gathering this information together after the referral of a family to a genetic advisory centre will vary from centre to centre. Although a medically qualified geneticist will certainly be required to evaluate the accuracy of a diagnosis, whether by personal examination of the proband or from scrutiny of the relevant documentation, the family details and pedigree can well be coordinated by another suitably trained member of the team, a nurse, social worker or genetic associate.

A precise diagnosis of the disease in the proband is essential if accurate genetic advice is to be given. This is largely because of the problem of genetic heterogeneity which will be discussed below. Knowing the mode of inheritance of the disease within the family is of course mandatory so that the genetic implications can be assessed and explained. The mode of inheritance may be obvious once the diagnosis is established, if dealing with a well known genetic disorder. If not, it may have to be assessed on the basis of the individual family's pedigree – hence the need for accurate recording of the family data.

When in possession of an established diagnosis and when the mode of inheritance is known, then the counsellor is able to estimate the recurrence risks involved either from first principles in the case of unifactorial disorders (with or without modification by carrier detection tests), or from empirical data in the case of chromosome or multifactorial disorders. These risks can then be explained and explored with those seeking advice.

DIAGNOSTIC PROBLEMS IN GENETIC COUNSELLING

Genetic heterogeneity

One of the major problems for genetic counsellors is the occurrence of *genetic heterogeneity*, which often complicates the establishment of a precise diagnosis. Genetic heterogeneity is the phenomenon whereby certain disorders, though superficially resembling one another at the clinical level, may result from quite different genetic defects. Thus, similar disorders may be caused by different mutations at the same locus or by mutations at different loci and may therefore have quite different modes of inheritance. Congenital methaemoglobinaemia is a good example. Here a very similar clinical appearance can result either from autosomal recessive mutations leading to a reduction in erythrocyte methaemoglobin reductase (the enzyme itself being polymorphic) or from dominant mutations at either the α or β chain loci resulting in a number of different haemoglobinopathies. Other excellent examples of well defined genetic disorders which exhibit marked heterogeneity at both the clinical and genetic levels are the Ehlers-Danlos syndrome, the mucopolysaccharidoses and the various muscular dystrophies. Needless to say, if faced with a child with a mucopolysaccharidosis one's genetic advice to the parents would be quite different if the child proved to have X-linked Hunter syndrome rather than any of the other autosomal recessive forms.

Phenocopies

Another important reason for having an accurate diagnosis is to ensure that the disease in question is genetic in origin. The occurrence of *phenocopies* can give rise to considerable difficulty in genetic counselling. Such conditions, although they mimic genetic disorders, are caused by environmental factors and are therefore unlikely to recur. A frequent example of this problem is microcephaly. Although this congenital malformation may be inherited as an autosomal recessive trait, it may also result from intrauterine exposure of the fetus to teratogens such as rubella, toxoplasmosis or maternal radiation. In addition to intrauterine infections and radiation, a variety of other influences including maternal disease, drug ingestion and mechanical factors in the uterus such as amniotic bands, may also give rise to phenocopies.

The sporadic case

The occurrence of an isolated or *sporadic case* within a family poses a problem familiar to all who are regularly involved in genetic counselling. The small size of modern families makes this a common problem. Here the pedigree information is of no value and the counsellor is entirely dependent on a clinical or laboratory diagnosis to establish the mode of inheritance concerned and the risks to various family members. Many different situations may lead to the occurrence of a sporadic case and all of these must be considered:

1. The disorder may prove to be non-genetic (or only partially genetic) and therefore have little risk of recurring.
2. The disorder may be due to a chromosome anomaly which, if neither parent is a healthy carrier, will have only a low risk of recurring.
3. The disorder may have a multifactorial or polygenic aetiology with a definite, but again usually low or moderate risk of recurrence, the actual risk depending on the condition in question.
4. The disorder may represent a new dominant mutation within the family with very little risk of recurrence in sibs. Before reassurance is given great care must be taken, however, to ensure that neither parent is in fact affected, even only slightly.
5. The individual may have an autosomal recessive condition and be the first affected child born to healthy, unsuspecting heterozygous parents. The recurrence risk would then be 1 in 4.
6. If the affected individual is a male then the disorder may be an X-linked recessive one. This may either

represent a new mutation (more common if it is a lethal disease) or the mother may prove to be a carrier with high risks to further children.

Clearly, accurate genetic advice can only be given if a precise diagnosis is established and the mode of inheritance of the disease is well defined. Only then can true risks of recurrence, either empiric or theoretical, be estimated. Needless to say situations do occur, especially when dealing with complex, multiple malformation syndromes, where a diagnosis cannot be reached and hence genetic advice cannot be given. All genetic counsellors must be prepared on occasion to admit that they cannot give an accurate assessment of the genetic implications for a particular, atypical family; they are not clairvoyant!

Illegitimacy

Anyone drawing up a family's pedigree must be aware of the possibility that illegitimacy may be present in the family and could drastically alter the implications of the situation for the person seeking advice. Often such information is given freely by the mother or implied by a family member. Frequently however this vital fact is not volunteered and can only be suspected in a puzzling situation. Illegitimacy itself does not of course present any difficulty, it is clear knowledge of the true father of a child which is important. Recent studies have indicated that as many as 15% of children in Edinburgh are not the offspring of their putative fathers. Presumably in a more liberal environment an even higher figure could apply.

The problems associated with disputes about the true paternity of a child, and methods of resolving them, are comprehensively discussed elsewhere in this text.

GENETIC COUNSELLING IN CHROMOSOME DISORDERS

The pooled data from several series in which chromosome studies have been done, comprising 47 000 consecutive live-born children, have shown that roughly 1 in 150 babies (5.81/1000) has a recognizable chromosomal abnormality (Nielsen 1975). Of these, 3.75/1000 had an autosomal anomaly, and 2.06/1000 had a sex chromosome anomaly. Thus chromosome anomalies are relatively common and are therefore conditions frequently encountered by most genetic centres.

The vast majority of chromosomal disorders show only a very low risk of recurring within the family, except when a family member is found to be a balanced translocation carrier or when maternal age complicates the issue. In spite of the usual low risks of recurrence

involved it is important that every effort be made to identify high risk situations since chromosomal abnormalities are so easily and accurately detected during pregnancy by fetal chromosome studies.

Trisomy 21

The single most common and most important chromosomal disorder from the counselling point of view is Down syndrome. This abnormality occurs in roughly 1 in 700 live-births and is mainly accounted for (95%) by trisomy 21. Its increased frequency amongst the offspring of older mothers is well recognised and must be considered carefully when giving genetic counselling. The now well documented increased risk associated with increased paternal age (when maternal age is kept constant) is of much lesser magnitude. Two main problems associated with trisomy 21 present themselves to the genetic counsellor: the risk to the older mother and the risk to the mother of a previously affected child with trisomy 21.

Table 108.1 lists the maternal age related incidence and risk figures for Down syndrome. From these it can be seen that the risk of having a child with trisomy 21 has already risen above the overall population level by a maternal age of 35 years, increasing gradually up to 40 years and thereafter more rapidly. Data from amniocentesis results suggest a slightly higher risk than that derived from live-birth studies (Table 108.1).

After the birth of one child with trisomy 21, the risk of another such child being born to the couple is higher than the normal risk. This increased risk is more marked in mothers of both low and high extremes of maternal age than in mothers with maternal ages of 25–35 years. Combined amniocentesis data (Mikkelsen 1979) show the overall risk to be about 0.5% specifically for another child with Down syndrome. After the age of 35 years a woman with a previous affected child would seem to run about twice the normal age-specific risk of having a further child with Down syndrome.

Maternal age

It is important to remember that Down syndrome is not the only chromosome anomaly related to maternal age. Trisomies of certain other autosomes (which occur in live-borns) occur more frequently in the offspring of older mothers, as do the XXY and XXX sex chromosome anomalies. The XYY and XO syndromes are however not related to maternal age. At any particular maternal age the risk of having a child with any form of chromosomal aneuploidy is roughly twice the age related risk of having a child with Down syndrome.

Table 108.1 Age-specific rates of Down syndrome in live-births and at amniocentesis

Maternal age in years	No. cases per 1000 live-births*	Risk at birth*	Risk of DS at amniocentesis+	Risk of any aneuploidy at amniocentesis+
35	3.09	1/324	1/222	1/133
36	1.96	1/510	1/204	1/102
37	2.94	1/340	1/130	1/75
38	3.10	1/322	1/110	1/68
39	7.57	1/132	1/76	1/54
40	10.50	1/95	1/83	1/43
41	14.50	1/69	1/43	1/33
42	12.59	1/80	1/30	1/16
43	15.72	1/64	1/56	1/25
44	36.91	1/27	1/18	1/13
45	33.64	1/30	1/30	1/20
46	28.11	1/36	1/12	1/7

*Data from Trimble and Baird 1978
+Data from Ferguson-Smith 1979

Autosomal abnormalities other than trisomy 21

Available data on the recurrence risks for any of these anomalies are scanty. Nevertheless, recurrence seems to be rare except where a familial translocation is involved. Maternal age can however be a complicating factor and should be borne in mind.

Sex chromosome anomalies

Recurrence of any of the sex chromosome anomalies within families is extremely rare and reassurance can be given. The relationship between maternal age and the XXY or XXX syndrome should however be borne in mind.

A common reason for sex chromosome abnormalities to be brought to a genetic counsellor, apart from diagnostic situations and the birth of an affected child, is the detection of a sex chromosome abnormality in a live-birth screening programme or in the products of a spontaneous abortion. In the former situation, the parents are usually anxious to discuss the prognosis of the condition discovered unexpectedly in their apparently healthy offspring. In the latter situation, information is usually wanted about the risk of such an abnormality occurring in any future live-born child.

Chromosomal translocations

The most common translocations encountered by the genetic counsellor are those involving chromosome 21 and D/D group translocations. No matter what the translocation involved, the recurrence risk is small unless one of the parents is a balanced carrier of the translocation. Since such individuals may have a relatively high risk of abnormality in their offspring, it is essential to test all close relatives of a patient with an unbalanced translocation in order to identify unsuspected balanced carriers, so that they can be offered prenatal diagnosis if appropriate.

Some 4% of all patients with Down syndrome prove to have unbalanced translocations and in about half of them this is familial. Most commonly chromosome 21 is translocated to a D group chromosome, usually chromosome 14 (less commonly 13 or 15). Alternatively it may be translocated to another G group chromosome which may be chromosome 22, or the two 21 chromosomes are translocated onto each other. Table 108.2 shows the risk of live-born chromosomally abnormal children amongst the offspring of balanced carriers of translocations involving chromosome 21.

Table 108.2 Recurrence risk of Down syndrome due to various chromosome aberrations (From Emery & Mueller (1988), with permission)

Karyotypes Patient	Father	Mother	Chance of recurrence %
Translocation			
D/G	N	C	10-15
	C	N	5
21/22	N	C	10-15
	C	N	5
21/21	C	N	100
	N	C	100
Trisomy 21	N	N	1
Translocation or mosaic	N	N	small

C = carrier; N = normal

Balanced D/D group translocations are not uncommon and are usually not associated with unbalanced chromosome defects in live-born offspring (de Grouchy 1976).

Recurrent spontaneous abortion

Repeated studies of the chromosomes of early spontaneous abortions consistently show a very high rate of chromosome abnormality. This is especially so in those occurring before 12 weeks of gestation when some 60% show abnormalities (Boué & Boué 1975). Many of the chromosome abnormalities commonly found in abortions do not occur in live-births. Since chromosome anomalies are such a common cause of abortion, there have been several studies of the chromosomes of couples who have had repeated spontaneous abortions. In more than 10% of such couples one partner is found to have a balanced chromosome anomaly (Kaosaar & Mikelsaar 1973, Kim et al 1975). It is therefore valuable to do chromosome studies on all couples when no adequate gynaecological reason can be found to account for repeated spontaneous abortions, so that prenatal chromosome studies can be considered if appropriate. Certain couples are at increased risk for either repeated chromosomally abnormal abortions or chromosomally normal abortions (Hassold 1980). Where there is no apparent cause for recurrent abortion, an immunological basis has been postulated (Mowbray et al 1985).

GENETIC COUNSELLING IN MULTIFACTORIAL DISORDERS

A multifactorial disorder is presumed to result largely from the additive effect of a number of factors, some undoubtedly genetic and others environmental. Since the genetic component in the aetiology of such conditions is not simple, but results from a combination of many genes, estimation of recurrence risks from first principles is not possible. Nevertheless it is still possible to give reasonably accurate genetic advice by resorting to the use of *empiric risks* of recurrence (see below). Diseases thought to be inherited in this way include most of the commoner birth defects as well as most of the important chronic diseases of later adulthood and thus are frequent problems for the genetic counsellor. It is fortunate, in view of the frequency of these disorders, that the recurrence risks within the family are almost always low.

Empiric risks of recurrence

These are risks of recurrence estimated directly from family data. Thus they provide statistical estimates of

recurrence which may be of great value in counselling families with a multifactorial disorder. Empiric risks are available now for many multifactorial conditions, and some of these can be seen in Table 108.3.

The accuracy and usefulness of empiric risk data have been comprehensively reviewed by Carter (1977). He concluded that such data can be extremely accurate and valuable, providing careful attention is paid to several sources of error in its collection and application. Sources of error include the precision of the diagnosis in the proband, accurate collection of family data, random sampling of probands, adequate size of the study group, and appropriateness of the population studied (as risks may vary considerably between populations).

Factors modifying the risks for the individual family

After finding a satisfactory empiric risk estimate for the disorder in question, the genetic counsellor's next move should be to consider whether or not the risk needs to be modified for the particular patient or family seeking advice. Factors which need consideration include the severity of the disorder in the affected individual, the sex of the patient, the presence or not of other affected individuals in the family, parental consanguinity, and any relevant predisposing environmental factors.

The degree of severity with which the patient is affected is important as the recurrence risk is likely to increase with increasing severity. Thus the recurrence risk in sibs if the proband has a unilateral cleft lip is about 4% but is 6% if a bilateral cleft lip is present.

Where the sex ratio of the condition differs significantly from unity, the recurrence risk is likely to be higher when the patient is of the sex less often affected. Thus the risk to sibs of a male proband with congenital pyloric stenosis is 3% whereas to the sibs of an affected female it is 8%, the malformation being five times more common in males than in females.

The occurrence of other affected individuals in the family in addition to the proband may significantly increase the risk, especially if a first-degree relative is involved. The risk to the sibs of an isolated child with club feet is only 3%, but if one parent is also affected the risk to subsequent children is about 10%.

Lastly, the presence of consanguinity between the parents should be recorded. However, this has little effect on the risk for multifactorial disorders, only increasing it by 1–2%.

GENETIC COUNSELLING IN UNIFACTORIAL DISORDERS

These disorders segregate within affected families according to Mendel's laws and therefore risk figures for

Table 108.3 Empiric risks for some common disorders (in per cent) (from Emery & Mueller 1988, with permission)

Disorder	Incidence	Sex ratio M:F	Normal parents having a second affected child	Affected parent having an affected child	Affected parent having a second affected child
Anencephaly	0.20	1:2	5*	–	–
Cleft palate only	0.04	2:3	2	7	15
Cleft lip ± cleft palate	0.10	3:2	4	4	10
Club foot	0.10	2:1	3	3	10
Cong. heart disease (all types)	0.50	1:1	1–4	1–4	10
Diabetes mellitus (juvenile, insulin-dependent)	0.20	1:1	6	1–2	–
Dislocation of hip	0.07	1:6	6	12	36
Epilepsy ('idiopathic')	0.50	1:1	5	5	10
Hirschsprung disease	0.02	4:1			
short segment			3	2	–
long segment			12	–	–
Hypospadias (in males)	0.20	–	10	10	–
Manic-depressive psychoses	0.40	2:3	10–15	10–15	–
Mental retardation ('idiopathic')	0.30–0.50	1:1	3–5	10	20
Profound childhood deafness	0.10	1:1	10	8	–
Pyloric stenosis	0.30	5:1			
male proband			2	4	13
female proband			10	17	38
Renal agenesis (bilat.)	0.01	3:1			
male proband			3	–	–
female proband			7	–	–
Schizophrenia	1–2	1:1	10	16	–
Scoliosis (idiopathic, adolescent)	0.22	1:6	7	5	–
Spina bifida	0.30	2:3	5*	4*	–
Tracheo-oesophageal fistula	0.03	1:1	1	1	–

*Anencephaly or spina bifida

various family members can be readily and accurately estimated in most situations. Thus genetic counselling is usually straightforward, provided an accurate diagnosis can be established. The actual risks calculated from pedigree data alone may be modified and made more accurate in a variety of situations. Thus, taking into account the ages of family members may drastically alter the basic risks when dealing with an autosomal dominant disorder of variable or late onset. Similarly, appropriate biochemical or DNA investigations may be very valuable in estimating the probable carrier status of an individual, particularly a woman in a family in which an X–linked recessive disorder is segregating (see below).

Mendelian inheritance can be established in a variety of ways, but most commonly this results from knowing the diagnosis, a characteristic pedigree pattern being found even if the diagnosis remains in doubt, or a combination of the diagnosis of a known Mendelian disorder and a compatible pedigree pattern. The recent tendency towards smaller family size may not allow the develop-ment of a typical pedigree pattern and therefore isolated cases are frequently encountered.

Autosomal dominant disorders

In families with an autosomal dominant disorder, risks of recurrence can be easily calculated from first principles. Therefore genetic counselling in such disorders should be relatively simple. However, in practice many factors associated with dominant inheritance may cause great problems in the genetic counselling situation. If an individual is definitely heterozygous for an autosomal dominant gene then there is a 50% risk of transmitting the gene to any offspring, regardless of the sex of the child or the severity of the condition. Problems arise in counselling when the condition has variable or late onset, or when variable expressivity or incomplete penetrance can make it difficult to be sure whether an apparently unaffected member of the family is either truly normal or a heterozygote with minimal or no manifestations of the gene.

When giving genetic counselling in late onset autosomal dominant disorders there is no problem in risk estimation for clearly affected family members, but one of the major problems arising is at what age one can assume an apparently unaffected person to be genetically normal and therefore not about to develop the disease. When data are available on age related occurrence rates, such as those for Huntington chorea, then substantial modification of the basic a priori risk for an individual can often be made, particularly if the individual or an apparently unaffected parent is well into middle-age. The other major problem associated with counselling in late onset dominant disorders is that individuals found to be affected may already have families before genetic advice is found to be necessary. Not only does this mean additional individuals at risk, but it is also a situation which proves emotionally very traumatic. Also traumatic are occasions when the counsellor has to indicate that a counsellee is himself at high risk. This may have to be done so that the counsellee can appreciate the risk of a dominant disorder in his children.

The problems associated with variable expressivity and incomplete penetrance have been discussed elsewhere in this text. It remains merely to emphasize the importance of ensuring that great caution be exercised before full reassurance is given to apparently unaffected family members when variable expressivity or incomplete penetrance is suspected.

The same problem arises in the case of apparently new mutations, great care being required to ensure that neither supposedly normal parent is minimally affected. The lower the fitness of affected individuals the higher is the likelihood that an isolated case has been caused by a new mutation.

Autosomal recessive disorders

The major difficulty in dealing with autosomal recessive disorders is being confident that this is in fact the mode of inheritance in question. So frequently the counsellor is faced (because of small family size) with an isolated case or perhaps two affected sibs, who by chance may both be male and hence raise the possibility of X-linkage. Usually autosomal recessive inheritance is established by confirmation of the diagnosis of a recongnized genetic disorder and perhaps further supported by consanguinity of the parents if it is a rare disease.

Once this mode of inheritance is firmly established counselling is usually straightforward, since recessive conditions seldom show many of the problems of dominant conditions such as variable expression. Certainly

heterogeneity may occur, but this is often defined at the biochemical level (often as enzyme kinetic variations) and each different form of the disorder 'runs true' within families, the mode of inheritance remaining unaltered. A frequent query from the parents of children with recessive disorders concerns the genetic implications for both the affected child himself and any normal sibs. In both cases of course the risk to offspring is small provided their partner does not have the same recessive gene – hence the need to warn against marrying within the family in such situations.

X–linked recessive disorders

As X–linked dominant disorders are few and rare, in practice most of the X–linked disease met by genetic counsellors is X–linked recessive in aetiology.

As in the other unifactorial situations, counselling in X–linked recessive disorders is relatively straightforward, and a priori risks can easily be estimated using first principles. However, these disorders do present some interesting counselling problems. The most important is in trying to differentiate between normal women in the family (who are at low risk of having affected children) and healthy heterozygous carriers (whose offspring are at very high risk). It is in these disorders most of all that a priori risks can be modified considerably by conditional information (either clinical or from biochemical or DNA studies) which can thus drastically alter the risks given at genetic counselling, and hence perhaps the whole orientation of the problem for a family. Females heterozygous for X–linked genes show a much greater degree of phenotypic variation than is seen with autosomal recessive disorders, which is thought to arise because of Lyonisation.

The carrier state can be demonstrated to different degrees in many situations, either in terms of clinical or biochemical manifestations of the gene, or by the use of recombinant DNA techniques. Developments in recombinant DNA technology have revolutionised the approach to carrier detection in the last few years through the availability of gene probes or linked RFLPs in many situations. Discussion of this aspect of carrier detection and examples of how carrier detection tests are applied can be found in chapters devoted to the individual disorders. Such tests are particularly useful for the detection of carriers of Duchenne muscular dystrophy.

THE PRACTICAL ASPECTS AND EFFECTIVENESS OF GENETIC COUNSELLING

The process of genetic counselling can reasonably be divided into four consecutive phases: an initial phase in which all necessary information is gathered and the diagnosis in the proband established; a phase during which facts about the disease, the genetic implications and the possible options are imparted to and discussed with the counsellee; a phase during which the counsellee evaluates, assimilates and learns to cope with the information given; and finally a phase during which decisions are reached about eventual reproductive choices and adjustment is made to the changed milieu created by genetic counselling.

Essential prelude to genetic counselling

Either at the initial visit or before the prospective counsellee even comes to the genetic centre, a certain amount of essential groundwork needs to be done in preparation for the definitive genetic counselling session or sessions. Primarily, this is required to provide the basic core of information which enables assessment of the prognostic information and recurrence risks to be explained to the counsellee. It can also be used to assimilate valuable indications of the emotional status of the counsellees and their expectations and possible reactions to the counselling situation, which can have such marked influences on the counselling session.

This phase of counselling includes the gathering of information and the diagnostic work-up required to establish and confirm the diagnosis of the condition in question and its mode of inheritance within the family. Usually, therefore, a fairly routine series of events takes place in most counselling clinics. These include drawing up an accurate pedigree of both sides of the family, clinical examination of the proband (if alive) and any family members at risk, and performing any appropriate laboratory investigations. If the proband is no longer alive then the appropriate hospital records will have to be found and carefully inspected. Once a diagnosis is established, and any necessary tests done then the actual risks for various family members can be estimated.

A prior, sensitive appraisal of the psychological status of the prospective counsellees, and knowledge of any socio-economic or religious factors which may influence their attitude to the situation, can help to make the actual genetic counselling session much more successful. Here also prior warning of the counsellee's expectations from the session can be very helpful. For example, lengthy and detailed explanation of probability estimates for further children are not very relevant if the counsellee has been sterilized already and is concerned about the genetic implications for the children already born in the family.

The type of person who gathers such important precounselling information will vary from clinic to clinic. This need not be a physician genetic counsellor, but can just as well be a social worker, health visitor, nurse, psychologist or genetic assistant. Confirmation of the diagnosis in question should however always be the ultimate responsibility of the physician.

The factual content of genetic counselling

Although for most genetic counsellors the emphasis in the counselling situation is shifting very much away from primary concern with the basic facts of the situation to evaluation of the patient's problems and worries in a much wider context, the factual content of the counselling process remains a very important aspect. After all, it is concern about this that has usually motivated the counsellee to seek advice in the first instance. Thus great care must be taken in the evaluation of the facts and their communication to the counsellee. The way in which these facts are presented to the counsellee is determined largely by whether the counselling is to be 'directive' or 'non-directive' in approach. Certainly most counsellors now opt for the latter course in most situations.

Many people involved in genetic counselling would agree that there is a certain amount of basic information that must be included in the counselling process in order for it to be a complete and meaningful experience for the counsellee. Certainly, there should be full discussion of at least the diagnosis and prognosis of the condition in question, the genetic risks involved for that particular individual and the options or courses of action available.

The importance of establishing the correct diagnosis has already been discussed. Of equal importance is the need to divulge and explain this diagnosis to the counsellee and to discuss fully the prognosis of the condition and the nature and availability of treatment. There is much evidence to show that parents are just as much influenced in their decision making by the implications of what has been termed the 'burden' of the disease as they are by the actual genetic risks involved.

Most counsellees come expecting to hear about the genetic risks involved in their particular situation. Thus care must be taken in assessing these risks accurately and in communicating them as clearly as possible. Evidence from many follow-up studies shows that most subjects do remember the level of risk they were told at counselling, although not always in numerical form, but rather whether it was a high or low risk of recurrence. In practical terms therefore great refinement of risk estimation is not relevant (Carter et al 1971, Emery et al 1972, Leonard et al 1972, Emery et al 1979). The mode in which this type of information is explained to counsellees is also of the utmost importance. Many individuals seen for counselling have little or no concept of probability theory (Pearn 1973, Lippmann-Hand & Fraser 1979a) and thus the skill of a good counsellor is shown by his ability to judge prospective clients and tailor the information and mode of delivery to their particular needs. In this area too, more than any other, the mode of presentation of the information can greatly influence the interpretation of the facts. Although most counsellors would certainly claim to be non-directive in their approach, few would deny that in some situations they do deliver the risk figures in such a way that their clients are left in little doubt about their gravity!

Discussion of the options open to a couple makes the counselling process more comprehensive and relevant, for this is one of the aspects of the problem which will have a profound influence on their decision making. If the occurrence or recurrence risk involved is low then the major decision for a couple is whether it is acceptably low to them in the context of their own circumstances. If, however, the risk is a high one then other factors become more important, such as the availability and limitations of prenatal diagnosis, or of adoption, or perhaps of artificial insemination. For those couples who finally decide that in their circumstances they do not wish to have a child, or further children, then good contraceptive advice is of paramount importance, not only as a means of reducing one of the possible sources of marital disharmony which can follow counselling, but also to prevent unplanned, high risk pregnancies occurring, as shown in some of the earlier follow-up studies (Carter et al 1971, Leonard et al 1972).

Psychological aspects of counselling

Many so-called 'counselling failures' result from a lack of true communication between counsellor and counsellee. Thus, great thought must be given to the process of communication and the factors affecting it. Poor communication can result from a variety of problems associated with the counsellees. Lack of motivation on their behalf, or overt anxiety or even hostility, can seriously disrupt the counselling relationship. Perhaps the factor most commonly found by counsellors to cause difficulties in effective communication is the educational background of their client, and in particular the client's knowledge of biology (Antley & Seidenfeld 1978, Emery et al 1979). The environment in which the counselling takes place can also greatly influence the process, no young person for instance will be as much at ease or as receptive in their own home, overheard by insensitive family members, as in a more detached hospital setting. On the other hand, a particularly independent couple may be more at ease in the privacy of their own home. In relation to communication it must be remembered that not all situations viewed by counsellors to be failures

may necessarily be true failures, but may rather represent the counsellee's genuinely felt difference of interpretation of the situation. The prospect of having a blind child may certainly be perceived very differently by a blind counsellee who copes well with life, than by a fully sighted counsellor.

The psychological needs and the issues associated with the genetic counselling process are many and complicated. As well as having to cope and come to terms with emotionally traumatic information, clients need to make decisions on future reproductive plans and may also need to make fundamental alterations to their feelings about themselves and about interpersonal relationships. A knowledge of these various psychological aspects is important for genetic counselling if it is to be of value to the majority of clients. These factors have been reviewed in depth in various publications including McCollum and Silverberg (1979), Lippmann-Hand and Fraser (1979b) and Emery and Pullen (1984).

Much has now been written about the psychodynamics of the coping process, and this has been well reviewed by Falek (1977). Realization that this standard, sequential process occurs in response to genetic counselling, in the same way that it may follow any other major stressful event such as bereavement, has added greatly to our understanding of many patients' responses at various stages of the counselling process. Thus for counsellees to achieve the goal of psychological homeostasis, and be in a position then to make the important decisions that are necessary, they must have experienced the four phases of the coping process known to follow exposure to stressful situations. These four phases are initial shock and denial, anger and/or guilt, anxiety, and depression, all familiar situations to those involved in counselling. Awareness that these phases are the natural course of events, and identification of the phases reached by individual counsellees, can help the counsellor to plan his approach more successfully. It will also allow the astute counsellor to recognize the occasional need for more specialist psychiatric help for a particular client to resolve coping problems before a suitable stage of psychological adjustment to allow decision making can be reached.

When the stage of decision making comes, then too it is important to remember that this is a dynamic process and one which may need skilled guidance from the counsellor. The many factors involved in this area are comprehensively reviewed by Pearn (1979) and Lippmann-Hand and Fraser (1979b) as are their practical relevance in the genetic counselling situation. The fundamental force at play is the counsellee's basic reproductive drive, but this is subject to modification by a variety of factors, depending on individual circumstances and attitudes.

Lastly, with respect to the psychological aspects of counselling, mention must be made of the importance of adequate support and follow-up facilities. Two main areas are important here. Firstly, adequate follow-up and support by personnel trained in psychosocial counselling can help to lessen the emotional trauma involved, not only in receiving genetic counselling, but also in subsequent readjustments within the family and between the family and the rest of society. Secondly, evidence from many studies indicates that reinforcement of the genetic advice is helpful and necessary in many situations if the counselling process is to be of maximum benefit. There is evidence which suggests that reinforcement of the facts may be particularly indicated in certain situations such as chromosomal disorders and X-linked recessive disorders (Emery et al 1979).

Effectiveness of genetic counselling

When attention was first focused on the success or effectiveness of genetic counselling rather than its ethical problems, it led to many retrospective studies of individuals who had received genetic counselling (Carter et al 1971, Leonard et al 1972, Emery et al 1972, 1973, 1979, Reynolds et al 1974). Such studies concentrated largely on the reproductive decisions made after counselling and the accuracy with which counsellees remembered the genetic advice given, as these were relatively simple parameters to quantify. Almost uniformly these studies showed that retention of genetic advice was reasonably good (if not always perfectly accurate in strict numerical terms) and that on the whole the higher the genetic risk, the lower the proportion of counsellees deciding to plan pregnancies. They also highlighted for the first time the importance of the so-called 'burden' of the disorder (emotional as well as financial) in influencing reproductive decisions. Thus, much useful information resulted from such studies, much of which significantly altered the approach of many genetic counsellors.

However, many criticisms have been levelled at such studies. They were said to be biased, since follow-up was often done by the counsellors themselves, not to reflect adequately the changing attitudes during the period of the study, and also to show little of how such information affected individual couples and their decision making. A review of the published studies and their findings is given by Evers-Kiebooms and van den Berghe (1979). The obvious shortcomings of such retrospective studies, as well as increased awareness of the various additional dimensions of the genetic counselling process have stimulated new approaches to evaluating the effectiveness and achievements of counselling. Most studies undertaken now are prospective in design and involve in-depth analysis of the psychological aspects of the problem. Many new and excellent books dealing with the theory and practice of genetic counselling explore this area in detail.

REFFERENCES

Antley R M, Seidenfeld M J 1978 A detailed description of mother's knowledge before genetic counselling for Down syndrome. American Journal of Medical Genetics 2: 357–364

Boué A, Boué J 1975 Chromosome abnormalities and abortions. In: Coutinho B E M, Fuchs F (eds) Physiology and Genetics of Reproduction. Plenum, New York

Carter C O 1977 Risk data: How good is empiric information. In: Lubs H A, de la Cruz F (eds) Genetic Counselling. Raven Press, New York, ch 5, p407

Carter C O, Fraser Roberts J A, Evans K A, Buck A R 1971 Genetic clinic: a follow-up. Lancet i: 281–285

de Grouchy J 1976 Human chromosomes and their anomalies. In: Barltrop D (ed) Aspects of Genetics in Paediatrics. Fellowship of Postgraduate Medicine, London, ch 1, p5

Emery A E H, Mueller R F 1988 Elements of Medical Genetics, 7th edn. Churchill Livingstone, Edinburgh

Emery A E H, Pullen I (eds) 1984 Psychological aspects of genetic counselling. Academic Press, London

Emery A E H, Watt M S, Clack E R 1972 The effects of genetic counselling in Duchenne muscular dystrophy. Clinical Genetics 3: 147–150

Emery A E H, Watt M S, Clack E R 1973 Social effects of genetic counselling. British Medical Journal 1: 724–726

Emery A E H, Raeburn J A, Skinner R, Holloway S, Lewis P 1979 Prospective study of genetic counselling. British Medical Journal 1: 1253–1256

Evers-Kiebooms G, van den Berghe H 1979 Impact of genetic counselling: a review of published follow-up studies. Clinical Genetics 15: 465–474

Falek A 1977 Use of the coping process to achieve psychological homeostasis in genetic counselling. In: Lubs H A, de la Cruz F (eds) Genetic Counselling. Raven Press, New York, ch2, p179

Ferguson-Smith M A 1979 Maternal age specific incidence of chromosome aberrations at amniocentesis. In: Murken J D, Stengel-Rutkowski S, Schwinger E (eds) Prenatal Diagnosis. Enke, Stuttgart, ch1, p1

Hassold T J 1980 A cytogenetic study of repeated spontaneous abortions. American Journal of Human Genetics 32: 723–730

Kaosaar M E, Mikelsaar A-V N 1973 Chromosome investigation in married couples with repeated spontaneous abortions. Humangenetik 17: 277–283

Kessler S 1979 The genetic counsellor as psychotherapist. In: Lappe M, Twiss S B, Capron A, Murray R, Powledge T (eds) Genetic Counselling: facts, values and norms. Plenum Press, Miami

Kim H J et al 1975 Cytogenetics of fetal wastage. New England Journal of Medicine 293: 844–847

Leonard C O, Chase G A, Childs B 1972 Genetic

counselling: a consumer's view. New England Journal of Medicine 287: 433–439

Lippmann-Hand A, Clarke Fraser F 1979a Genetic counselling: provision and reception of information. American Journal of Medical Genetics 3: 113–127

Lippmann-Hand A, Clarke Fraser F 1979b Genetic counselling – the post-counselling period: 11. Making reproductive choices. American Journal of Medical Genetics 4: 73–87

McCollum A T, Silverberg R L 1979 Psychosocial advocacy. In: Hsia Y E, Hirschhorn K, Silverberg R L, Godmilow L (eds) Counselling in Genetics. Alan Liss, New York, ch 11, p 239

Mikkelsen M 1979 Previous child with Down syndrome and other chromosome aberration. In: Murken J D, Stengel-Rutkowski S, Schwinger E (eds) Prenatal Diagnosis. Enke, Stuttgart, ch 2, p 22

Mowbray J F, Gibbings C, Liddell H et al 1985 Controlled trial of treatment of recurrent spontaneous abortion by immunisation with paternal cells. Lancet i: 941–943

Nielsen J 1975 Chromosome examination of newborn children. Purpose and ethical aspects. Humangenetik 26: 215

Pearn J H 1973 Patients' subjective interpretation of risks offered in genetic counselling. Journal of Medical Genetics 10: 129–134

Pearn J H 1979 Decision-making and reproductive choice. In: Hsia Y E, Hirschhorn K, Silverberg R L, Godmilow L (eds) Counselling in Genetics, Alan Liss, New York, ch 10, p 223

Reynolds B DeV, Puck M H, Robinson A 1974 Genetic counselling: an appraisal. Clinical Genetics 5: 177–187

Trimble B K, Baird P A 1978 Maternal age and Down syndrome: age specific incidence rates by single year intervals. American Journal of Medical Genetics 2: 1–5

109. Newborn genetic screening

R. W. Erbe G. R. Boss

INTRODUCTION

Genetic screening is a search in a population for persons that possess genotypes which: (1) are associated with disease or predispose to disease; (2) may lead to disease in their descendants; or (3) produce other variations not known to be associated with disease (Committee for the Study of Inborn Errors of Metabolism 1975). Genetic screening thus serves several objectives. First, screening can lead to therapy. Newborn screening aims at the earliest possible recognition of disorders in order to intervene. Sometimes this intervention includes effective treatment to prevent the most serious consequences of the disorder, although such therapy is presently available for only a small proportion of the several thousand known genetic disorders. Second, screening can identify those individuals and couples whose pregnancies are at increased risk for producing offspring with serious genetic abnormalities. With effective therapy so limited the current approach in many instances is towards preventing the birth of affected individuals through genetic counselling including prenatal genetic diagnosis and selective abortion. Such screening is usually directed at reproductive-age persons either prior to or during pregnancy. This approach recognizes the fact that an overwhelming proportion of the genes for lethal, recessively inherited disorders are present in asymptomatic carriers who will continue to give birth to affected offspring unless they are identified prospectively and made aware of their risks and reproductive alternatives. Third, genetic screening can be a source of epidemiological data regarding birth defects.

The primary focus of this chapter is newborn genetic screening for inborn errors of metabolism as is presently performed in the relatively comprehensive programme of the Commonwealth of Massachusetts. The nature and number of newborn screening tests vary widely in different localities and may include some or all of the following: (1) prenatal (maternal) blood; (2) cord blood; (3) newborn nursery blood; (4) newborn follow-up blood; and/or (5) newborn follow-up urine. In addition to tests for classical inborn errors of metabolism newborn genetic screening may include tests for some or all of the following disorders: congenital hypothyroidism, haemoglobinopathies, α_1-antitrypsin deficiency, cystic fibrosis, Duchenne muscular dystrophy, hyperlipidaemia, adenosine deaminase deficiency and congenital adrenal hyperplasia.

HISTORICAL ASPECTS

Genetic screening as we know it dates from the 1960s. However, as early as 1908 Sir Archibald Garrod stated that inborn errors of metabolism could be recognized '...by some strikingly unusual appearance of surface tissues or of excreta, by the excretion of some substance which responds to a test habitually applied in the routine of clinical work, or by giving rise to obvious morbid symptoms' (Harris 1963). These principles were first applied on a population-wide basis to phenylketonuria (PKU). In 1934 Folling described the association of phenylketonuria with mental retardation (Folling 1934), the possibility that diets low in phenylalanine might prevent the associated mental retardation was suggested subsequently (Scriver et al 1989). Although testing for amino acid disorders initially relied on urine (Dent 1946), it soon became clear that the analysis of blood provided a more effective means for detecting PKU in newborns. In 1962 Guthrie described a bacterial growth inhibition assay for measuring blood phenylalanine concentration that required only a few drops of blood spotted on filter paper and dried (Levy 1973). After a successful field trial in Massachusetts (MacCready & Hussey 1964) screening for PKU by the Guthrie assay expanded widely in the United States and abroad at a time when important gaps still existed in knowledge regarding diagnosis and management of PKU (Committee for the Study of Inborn Errors of Metabolism 1975). Guthrie subsequently introduced microbiological assays to screen for maple syrup urine disease, histidinaemia and galactosaemia (Guthrie 1964). At about the same time, paper chromatographic methods for urinary amino acid analysis were introduced in several screening programmes (Berry et al 1959, Efron et al 1964, Scriver et al 1964).

Since the mid-1970s, newborn genetic screening for PKU and often other inborn errors has continued on a wide scale in the US and elsewhere, mainly using dried blood. Although nearly all states in the US screen for PKU, the programmes in different localities vary rather widely, and it is essential that persons concerned with genetics determine what genetic screening tests are being performed in a particular area. The radioimmunoassay for congenital hypothyroidism developed in 1974 by Dussault has been added to many newborn programmes. Moreover, new tests are still being proposed and introduced.

Screening for genetic disorders other than inborn errors of metabolism was initiated early in the 1970s. Much early experience in carrier screening and counselling was gained from programmes focusing on Tay-Sachs disease. This disorder is almost ideally suited to genetic screening because of its uniformly fatal course, the lack of effective therapy, the potential for accurate carrier state diagnosis, and the availability of valid in utero detection. The programme begun in the Baltimore-Washington area by Kaback (see chapter elsewhere in this text) provided an early model. Screening was generally preceded by educational programmes which enlisted voluntary community participation and were directed at reproductive-age adults. A number of large-scale programmes began to screen for sickle-cell trait and sickle-cell anaemia in older children and adults, and several programmes screened newborns for chromosome disorders. In contrast haemoglobinopathy screening programmes were very heterogeneous and many problems arose. Many of the programmes were too small or had little guidance from physicians. Laws that mandated testing and specified the activities of the programmes were passed in several states beginning in 1971. These laws generally made no provision for prior education, informed consent, diagnostic accuracy, or genetic counselling during screening. Although some individuals and groups had spoken out earlier in opposition to PKU screening laws, the public and professional controversies that erupted in response to haemoglobinopathy screening were even more vocal and widespread. Two milestones in the analysis of issues in genetic screening were a short report by the Research Group on Ethical, Social and Legal Issues in Genetic Counselling and Genetic Engineering (1972) and the detailed report by the Committee for the Study of Inborn Errors of Metabolism, National Research Council, National Academy of Sciences (1975). Although the controversies over issues are presently less apparent, some programmes continue to operate with flawed designs and in violation of important principles discussed in these two reports.

NEWBORN METABOLIC SCREENING

Collection of specimens

Many screening programmes in the US and other countries test only newborn blood specimens. Most larger programmes in the US test newborns for disorders in addition to PKU. Only a few laboratories screen via urine specimens or prenatal blood specimens.

The specimens and tests used in the programmes in Massachusetts are shown in Table 109.1. Newborn whole-blood specimens are collected on filter paper after heel stick when the infant has begun to ingest protein and prior to discharge from the nursery, usually days 3 to 5.

Table 109.1 Newborn metabolic screening in Massachusetts (modified from Levy 1973)

Specimen	Age obtained	Test	Primary disorder
Dried blood (newborn)	3–5 days	BIA (Phe)	PKU
		BIA (Leu)	MSUD
		BIA (Met)	Homocystinuria
		Bacterial assay (Paigen test)	Galactosaemia
		Radioimmunoassay (T₄)	Congenital hypothyroidism
		Enzyme assay	Biotinidase deficiency
		Immunoassay	Congenital toxoplasmosis
Dried urine	3–4 weeks	Efron unidimensional paper chromatography	Aminoacidurias and organic acid disorders

BIA = bacterial inhibition assay of Guthrie

Newborn urine specimens from the diaper are collected by the parents on filter paper when the infant is 3–4 weeks old using a kit given to them at the time the newborn leaves the hospital. Due to the differences in processing and tests performed, analyses of blood and urine are described separately in the following sections.

Blood

Analysis of blood specimens

In the laboratory small discs are punched out of the blood-impregnated filter paper. For the Guthrie-type bacterial inhibition tests, the discs are placed on agar gels that contain a test strain of bacteria. The principle of the test is that the inhibition of bacterial growth by a toxic compound can be reversed in a competitive manner by the presence of a structurally similar physiological compound. The Guthrie PKU test uses a strain of *B. subtilis* sensitive to beta-2-thienylalanine. The growth inhibition produced by this compound can be reversed by phenylalanine, phenylpyruvic acid or phenyllactic acid. The bacteria are mixed with agar and the toxic compound and poured into a plate. The disc containing the blood (or urine) to be tested is placed on the agar with as many as 100 such discs per plate (Fig. 109.1). The amount of bacterial growth is directly proportional to the amounts of phenylalanine, phenylpyruvic acid or phenyllactic acid present in the blood or other physiological fluid, with the actual concentrations estimated by comparison with a series of standards in the centre of the plate. Similar bacterial inhibition assays developed by Guthrie are used in screening programmes to measure the concentrations of leucine for maple syrup urine disease, of histidine for histidinaemia, of methionine for one of the three aetiologies of homocystinuria and of tyrosine for tyrosinaemia (Table 109.2). A bacterial inhibition assay for lysine to detect hyperlysinaemia has not been used in screening. In general the tests devised by Guthrie are sensitive, reliable and, when performed appropriately, not subject to interference by other compounds, not even antibiotics.

Increased concentrations of galactose in physiological fluids can be detected by means of a direct inhibition assay developed by Guthrie in which a galactose-1-phosphate uridyltransferase-deficient strain of *E. coli* is killed when galactose or galactose-1-phosphate or both are present in the specimen being tested. In contrast to the Guthrie bacterial inhibition assays noted above, a

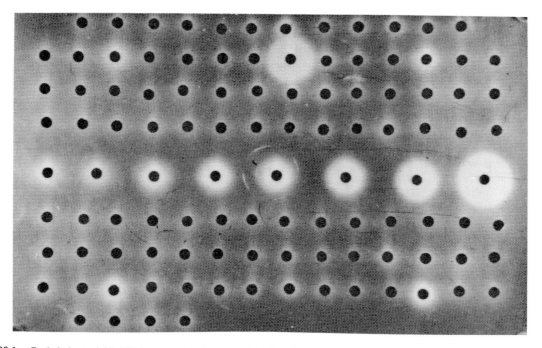

Fig. 109.1 Guthrie bacterial inhibition test plate for phenylalanine. Dried blood disc towards top centre is from an infant with phenylketonuria. The bacterial growth surrounding this disc is in response to a phenylalanine concentration greater than 20 mg/dl. The centre row of discs consists of standard specimens containing concentrations of phenylalanine ranging from 2 mg/dl on the far left to 50 mg/dl on the far right. (Reprinted from Levy (1973) with permission.)

Table 109.2 Guthrie bacterial inhibition assays

Compound detected	Disorder
Phenylalanine	Phenylketonuria
	Hyperphenylalaninaemic states
Leucine	Maple syrup urine disease
Histidine	Histidinaemia
Galactose	Galactosaemia
Methionine	Homocystinuria (one type, due to cystathionine synthase deficiency)
	Liver disease
Tyrosine	Tyrosinaemia
	Liver disease

positive result in the Guthrie test for galactosaemia consists of the absence of bacterial growth around the specimen. A disadvantage of this test is the tendency of the transferase-deficient strain of *E. coli* on which it depends to lose its sensitivity to galactose (Levy & Hammersen 1978). In contrast, the assay introduced by Paigen et al (1982) uses a strain of *E. coli* blocked in the galactose pathway at uridine diphosphogalactose-4-epimerase. These mutant bacteria cannot resist lysis by a particular bacteriophage except in the presence of galactose. Like the Guthrie assay, discs of dried blood on the Paigen test are surrounded on the plate by bacterial growth in direct proportion to the blood galactose concentration. Since it measures both galactose and, when alkaline phosphatase is added, galactose-1-phosphate, this test detects galactosaemia due to transferase deficiency, kinase deficiency or epimerase deficiency and the procedure is technically simple. On the other hand, false positives may occur due to nongalactosaemic liver disease or other causes.

Another useful test employs blood eluted from a dried specimen to measure the activity of the enzyme, galactose-1-phosphate uridyltransferase, the enzyme deficient in classical galactosaemia (Beutler & Baluda 1966). Similar tests were subsequently devised for other enzymes, notably glucose-6-phosphate dehydrogenase, pyruvate kinase and glutathione reductase. These assays require that the enzymes remain active for several days after the blood has been applied to the filter paper and that enough enzyme activity is present in a drop of blood to permit accurate measurement. The blood is eluted from the filter paper strip and the transferase or other activity measured by means of the fluorescence of NADPH. False positive results are quite frequent in the transferase assay and are often due to inactivation by heat and humidity, a greater problem in warm environments. In view of the relative strengths and weaknesses, it is probably best to combine initial screening by means of a galactose metabolic assay with follow up using the Beutler transferase assay.

Biotinidase activity is also measured using blood-impregnated filter paper. In the semiquantitative assay used in screening (Wolf et al 1987), biotinidase releases p-aminobenzoate from the artificial substrate, biotinyl-p-aminobenzoate. Colour developing reagents added subsequently cause samples with biotinidase activity to become purple, while samples lacking biotinidase activity remain clear or straw-coloured. A quantitative colorimetric assay for biotinidase activity in serum is used to confirm positive screening tests and to identify heterozygotes. The frequency of false-positive results is relatively low, about 1:1000. Biotinidase activity is low in some premature infants due to functional immaturity of the liver.

Confirmatory tests

It must be emphasized that a single abnormal screening test result does not establish a specific diagnosis. Screening tests usually differ from diagnostic tests in regard to sensitivity, specificity and other important characteristics. The abnormality reflected by the positive screening test result may have more than one possible genetic or nongenetic cause, and the aetiology in each particular case must be ascertained. Moreover, transient abnormalities and artifacts must be distinguished.

Confirmation of PKU, galactosaemia and other inborn errors of metabolism requires additional blood specimens as well as urine testing. If these further tests yield abnormal results, specific diagnostic evaluation must be carried out before an appropriate plan of management can be formulated.

Disorders and conditions detected by newborn blood screening

The estimated frequencies of metabolic disorders or conditions detectable by newborn blood screening are listed in Table 109.3. Although detailed description of these disorders is beyond the scope of this chapter, aspects especially pertinent to screening are considered below.

PKU and hyperphenylalaninaemias

As in many inherited disorders, the detection of a primary abnormality, hyperphenylalaninaemia, requires the consideration of a spectrum of genetic heterogeneity before proper diagnosis and management are possible. The failure to appreciate that several disorders as well as

Table 109.3 Frequencies of some metabolic disorders and conditions detected by screening newborn blood.

Disorder or condition	Frequency
Hyperphenylalaninaemias	
PKU	1: 13 000
Other hyperphenylalaninaemia	1: 20 000
Galactosaemia	1: 50 000
Biotinidase deficiency	1: 72 000
Maple syrup urine disease	1: 170 000
Hypermethioninaemia	
(homocystinuria)	1: 200 000
Hereditary tyrosinaemia	Very low

benign metabolic conditions can cause hyperphenylalaninaemia was a serious early problem in newborn metabolic screening (Committee for the Study of Inborn Errors of Metabolism 1975, Erbe 1981).

Upon detection of hyperphenylalaninaemia, the several aetiologies that must be distinguished include: (1) transient hyperphenylalaninaemia; (2) persistent non-PKU hyperphenylalaninaemia; (3) classical PKU; and (4) a defect in pterin synthesis or metabolism. The phenylalanine concentration in newborn blood is normally less than 2 mg/dl. The Guthrie bacterial inhibition test is positive when the phenylalanine concentration exceeds 2 mg/dl. The diagnosis of classical PKU is generally assigned when: (a) blood phenylalanine concentrations are 20 mg/dl or greater in follow-up specimens while the infant is ingesting a diet normal for age; and (b) tyrosine concentration in blood is no greater than 5 mg/dl. Urinary concentrations of phenylalanine and its metabolites, such as orthohydroxyphenylacetic acid, may also be elevated in these infants. When these criteria are met a low-phenylalanine diet should be instituted promptly in order to prevent the mental retardation seen in untreated PKU. The rationale for confirming this diagnosis by a phenylalanine challenge as well as a protocol for that purpose have been recommended for all patients three months after initial diagnosis (O'Flynn et al 1980).

Classical PKU is due to deficiency of hepatic phenylalanine hydroxylase and must be distinguished from another type of block in the phenylalanine hydroxylating system in which tetrahydrobiopterin (BH_4), the phenylalanine hydroxylating cofactor, is deficient. This group of disorders is characterized by hyperphenylalaninaemia with progressive neurological deterioration despite a low phenylalanine diet (Smith et al 1986). In one of these, dihydropteridine reductase (DHPR) deficiency, the regeneration of tetrahydrobiopterin is disrupted, thereby interfering with the conversion of phenylalanine to

tyrosine. Since tyrosine and tryptophan hydroxylases also require BH_4, the conversion of tyrosine to DOPA and tryptophan to 5-hydroxytryptophan (and to serotonin) is also impaired, thus disrupting neurotransmitter synthesis as one important consequence. Similarly, at least two inherited deficiencies of enzymes in the pathway of biopterin synthesis also cause deficient hydroxylation of these three aromatic amino acids. Since the degrees of hyperphenylalaninaemia and the usual clinical manifestations of classical PKU, dihydropteridine reductase deficiency and the biopterin synthesis deficiencies are similar during the newborn period, accurate diagnosis requires a combination of in vivo and in vitro tests. Although phenylalanine hydroxylase activity can be assayed only in the liver, dihydropteridine reductase can be assayed in white blood cells and in cultured skin fibroblasts and amniotic fluid cells (Scriver et al 1989).

Hyperphenylalaninaemias not due to PKU or tetrahydrobiopterin deficiency are generally associated with less elevation of the plasma phenylalanine concentration, are transient, disappear in the first months of life, and require no specific therapy (O'Flynn et al 1980). In most instances the hyperphenylalaninaemia is accompanied by transient hypertyrosinaemia.

It has been emphasized that all hyperphenylalaninaemic subjects identified in newborn screening programmes must be appropriately studied to distinguish those with malignant phenotypes due to blocks in tetrahydrobiopterin generation from the 97–99% of subjects who will either respond to low-phenylalanine diets or who need no treatment (Scriver et al 1989).

Although most newborns with PKU have plasma phenylalanine concentrations above 6 mg/dl when first tested, occasional phenylketonuric newborns have much milder elevations on initial testing, especially if prior protein intake is low or the infant is discharged early from the nursery. Accordingly, concerns about possible false negative initial PKU tests have been raised and arrangements for routine retesting recommended. Sepe et al (1979) surveyed by questionnaire the results of routine follow-up blood screening of infants for PKU in the 13 states that conduct such studies. Some 2 382 300 routine follow-up blood specimens were obtained from infants aged 2–6 weeks, and 11 of these infants, or 1:217 000, were found to have persistent hyperphenylalaninaemia not detected by the initial newborn screening. Seven of these infants had milder forms of hyperphenylalaninaemia that did not require treatment, while four had PKU. This analysis of follow-up blood specimens showed that additional cases of PKU were detected at a frequency of 1:596 000 which increased the cost for each PKU case found to $263 000 or 30 times the $8700 cost of identifying a PKU infant by routine screening. The survey clearly indicated that incomplete testing poses a problem. Based on the observed compliance rate of 80% for initial testing, it was estimated that some 640 000 infants each year in the US are not tested and 54 of these would have PKU.

As another approach to evaluate the effectiveness of newborn PKU screening, subsequently-born sibs of children with PKU or mild hyperphenylalaninaemia were followed prospectively (Meryash et al 1981). Each of the 16 infants with PKU and one of two with mild hyperphenylalaninaemia had an elevated blood phenylalanine concentration detectable by the Guthrie assay within the first one to two days after birth. This early detection was possible despite the fact that three of the 16 infants had been breast fed and three had not received protein feedings. It seems likely from these and other studies that the instances of unrecognized cases of PKU result mainly from failure to be screened and from human error.

Maternal PKU can be detected by cord blood or prenatal testing. The importance of this condition stems from the occurrence of mental retardation in the non-phenylketonuric offspring of mothers with PKU. Lenke and Levy (1980) collected data on 524 pregnancies in 155 women having PKU or other forms of hyperphenylalaninaemia. A higher rate of spontaneous abortion was found and, moreover, the 423 live-born offspring showed a marked increase in the frequencies of mental retardation, microcephaly and congenital heart disease. Indeed, of mothers having blood phenylalanine concentrations of 20 mg/dl or greater, one or more of their children was mentally retarded in 95% of instances. It seems that prenatal dietary therapy might prevent or at least lessen fetal damage but this has not yet been proven (Ghavami et al 1986).

Galactosaemia

At least three disorders of galactose metabolism are detectable in newborn screening. They are appropriate targets for newborn screening because of the need for early intervention. The most frequent of these disorders is classical galactosaemia due to deficiency of galactose-1-phosphate uridyl transferase which is normally present in most tissues including liver, skin fibroblasts and red blood cells (Segal 1989). In this disorder transferase activity is undetectable and the untreated clinical course is characterized by failure to thrive, jaundice, hepatomegaly and often death in infancy, especially due to E. coli sepsis (Levy et al 1977). Untreated infants who survive develop mental retardation, cirrhosis and cataracts. Early diagnosis can lead to effective treatment and hence

screening is needed. Moreover, even when the infant is obviously ill, the correct diagnosis of this rare inborn error of metabolism is made infrequently by the primary physicians so that identification by screening is essential.

Several variant forms of transferase deficiency have been described (Segal 1989). In the so-called Negro variant, low but detectable levels of transferase activity are present in liver and intestinal mucosa but not erythrocytes, and the clinical course is milder. Variants such as Rennes and Indiana may be associated with some or all of the serious clinical abnormalities, while the Duarte variant is characterized by diminished erythrocyte transferase activity and altered electrophoretic mobility of the transferase without clinical abnormalities.

The other galactose metabolic disorders are galactokinase deficiency and uridine diphosphate galactose-4-epimerase deficiency. These are much less frequent than transferase deficiency galactosaemia. Galactokinase deficiency leads to cataract formation in older untreated patients without other evidence of galactose toxicity, while epimerase deficiency is usually unassociated with any clinical abnormalities. Treatment of galactosaemia due to either transferase deficiency or galactokinase deficiency aims at rigorous exclusion of galactose from the diet and if instituted early is effective in preventing most or all of the serious clinical abnormalities (Segal 1989).

Cystathionine β-synthase deficiency

The screening of nearly 20 million newborns by the Guthrie bacterial inhibition assay for methionine has led to the detection of approximately 100 infants with cystathionine synthase deficient homocystinuria. This form of homocystinuria results from an autosomal recessively inherited deficiency of cystathionine β-synthase which condenses L-homocysteine and L-serine to cystathionine, using pyridoxal-5'-phosphate as a cofactor. Deficiency of this enzyme may result in clinical abnormalities that include mental retardation, ectopia lentis, vascular obstruction and musculoskeletal abnormalities. Treatment includes a low-methionine diet and pharmacological doses of pyridoxine (Mudd et al 1989).

Some cases of cystathionine synthase deficiency have escaped detection by newborn screening and this has raised concerns about possible slow rises in blood methionine (Levy 1973). The blood methionine concentration may not exceed normal (1 mg/dl) until after the first week of life in cystathionine synthase deficient infants, whereas elevations of 4 mg/dl or greater detected at 1–2 months of age are usually transient and related to a high-protein diet in healthy infants (Levy 1973). Other causes of hypermethionianemia include liver disease, tyrosinaemia (see below) and, very rarely, methionine adenosyl-transferase deficiency (Mudd et al 1989). The frequency of transient hypermethioninaemia may be decreasing now that more neonates are breast fed or otherwise have lower protein intakes than previously (Whiteman et al 1979). Other important causes of homocystinuria and homocystinaemia are due to defects in the metabolism and use of folates and cobalamins that block the trans-methylation of homocysteine to methionine (Erbe 1986). Thus, although the concentrations of homocystine and related compounds are increased in blood and urine, the concentration of methionine is low or normal, so that transmethylation disorders escape detection by assays that detect hypermethioninaemia.

Maple syrup urine disease

Use of the Guthrie bacterial inhibition assay for leucine has allowed detection of some instances of maple syrup urine disease (MSUD). This disorder results from defi-cient activity of one or more enzymes involved in the oxidative decarboxylation of the a-keto acid derivatives of leucine, isoleucine and valine (Danner & Elsas 1989). Although apparently healthy at birth, the newborn begins to feed poorly by the end of the first week. This is followed by vomiting, lethargy, muscular hypertonicity, seizures, coma and death. A distinctive urinary odour resembling maple syrup accompanies the clinical abnor-malities. With dramatic severity, the clinical illness can lead to death before the true nature of the disorder is recognized. Levy (1973) has suggested that MSUD may be underdiagnosed because the acute episode may lead to retention in the hospital and a fatal delay in submission of the appropriate specimens for screening. Attempts at treatment have involved complicated diets which have been partially successful (Danner & Elsas 1989). Several variants of MSUD with milder clinical and biochemical abnormalities have been described (Danner & Elsas 1989). A transient elevation (6 mg/dl or greater) of the blood leucine concentration occurs in 0.1–0.2% of new-borns screened.

Hereditary tyrosinaemia

In at least 1–2% of infants the blood tyrosine concentra-tion exceeds 5 mg/dl at some time during the first three months of life and the frequency is even higher in prematures (Levy 1973). Such transient tyrosinaemia usually disappears spontaneously within a few weeks, although its disappearance can sometimes be promoted by administering vitamin C or with a low-protein diet (Goldsmith & Laberge 1989).

Persistent tyrosinaemia can be caused by at least two inherited disorders. First, hereditary tyrosinaemia (tyro-sinaemia I) is an autosomal recessively inherited disorder in which the primary enzyme defect is fumarylacetoace-tate hydrolase deficiency (Goldsmith & Laberge 1989). This disorder has been recognized most frequently in the Quebec province of Canada. It is characterized by a complex set of clinical and laboratory abnormalities including hepatosplenomegaly, nodular hepatic cirrhosis, often with hepatoma formation, disturbed tyrosine and methionine metabolism with marked p-hydroxypheny-llactic aciduria (termed tyrosyluria) and renal tubular defects resulting in hyperphosphaturia, rickets, melli-turia, proteinuria and a generalized aminoaciduria of a distinct type (Goldsmith & Laberge 1989). Dietary treat-ment has been attempted with limited success.

The second hereditary disorder is termed tyrosinaemia II (Richner-Hanhart syndrome) and has been diagnosed in only a few patients (Buist et al 1985, Goldsmith & Laberge 1989). Blood tyrosine concentrations are 20–50 mg/dl on an unrestricted diet. Mental retardation is present in all cases, but hepatic and renal disease are absent. Over 1.7 million newborns in six countries were screened without finding a single instance of this dis-order. Thus either the frequency is extremely low or the rise in the blood tyrosine concentration is delayed (Levy 1973).

Other inherited disorders, particularly transferase defi-ciency galactosaemia and fructosaemia, also called here-ditary fructose intolerance, due to deficient fructose-1-phosphate aldolase, may lead to an elevation of the blood tyrosine concentration when the infant is ill. Both of these disorders elevate blood tyrosine concentration by deleterious effects on hepatic metabolism. Indeed, liver disease of any aetiology can elevate the blood tyrosine concentration and thus either tyrosinaemia or hyper-methioninaemia may signal liver disease.

Biotinidase deficiency

Biotinidase deficiency can be detected in newborns who, if treated with pharmacological doses of biotin, do not develop the otherwise serious or even fatal abnormalities seen in untreated patients. Biotin is a vitamin that is essential for the activity of four carboxylases required for the catabolism of several branched-chain amino acids, the first step of gluconeogenesis and the synthesis of fatty acids (Wolf et al 1987). These carboxylases are normally activated by the covalent enzymic attachment of biotin. One product of the eventual proteolytic degradation of these carboxylases is biocytin. Normally biotinidase hy-drolytically releases biotin from biocytin, making the biotin available for reutilization.

Biotinidase deficient persons may become biotin deficient during infancy or early childhood (Wolf et al 1985). Signs and symptoms are mainly neurological and cutaneous, and include seizures, ataxia, hearing loss, hypotonia, developmental delay, skin rash and alopecia. They also usually manifest metabolic acidosis and organic aciduria. Metabolic decompensation can terminate in coma and death. Biotinidase deficiency shows a wide range of phenotypic severity, the basis for this variation being unknown. Some affected children have neurological abnormalities without cutaneous findings or organic aciduria. Symptomatic children with biotinidase deficiency have consistently responded to treatment with biotin.

Biotinidase deficiency is inherited in an autosomal recessive pattern (Wolf et al 1985) and may be heterogeneous. The frequency of the deficiency in newborns has varied between studies but is estimated to be 1:72 000, with 95% confidence limits of 1:27 000 to 1:277 000 (Wolf et al 1987).

Urine

Analysis of urine specimens

Filter paper urine specimens can be analyzed either by unidimensional paper chromatography (Efron et al 1964, Levy et al 1980) as in Massachusetts and formerly in New South Wales, Australia, or by unidimensional thin-layer chromatography as in Quebec, Canada (Lemieux et al 1988). In the Massachusetts programme two $\frac{1}{4}$ inch diameter discs are punched out of each filter paper, one of these being analyzed for amino acids by overnight descending chromatography and ninhydrin stain while the other is analyzed for methylmalonic acid by six hour ascending chromatography developed with o-dianisidine reagent (Levy et al 1980). Each sheet of chromatography paper accommodates 25 specimens plus appropriate reference standards. The identification, analysis and interpretation of suspected abnormalities have been described in detail (Levy et al 1980), as have the procedures for follow-up and management.

Confirmatory tests

A variety of confirmatory tests are available depending on the specific disorder or condition suspected. These include spot tests of urine for specific compounds, two-dimensional chromatography, electrophoresis and gas chromatography-mass spectrometry. Tests of blood and specific enzyme assays of fluids or cells may also be appropriate.

Disorders and conditions detected by newborn urine specimens

Parents are requested to submit a filter paper urine sample at age 3–4 weeks in the Massachusetts programme and at age 2 weeks in the Quebec programme (Levy et al 1980). A major goal in screening urine at a later age than that at which newborn blood is collected is to diminish the frequency of false positives due to transient amino acid disturbances. Several transient amino acid abnormalities remain at 3–4 weeks, especially iminoglycinuria and cystinuria/lysinuria, but these usually disappear by age 3 months. In the Massachusetts programme the compliance rate averages 75%. About 1% of the specimens are inadequate for testing because, for example, they contain insufficient urine or are contaminated with diaper cream or faeces. Detailed analysis of urine screening of 108 353 newborns in the Massachusetts programme during 1976–1977 showed that: (1) 20% had been reanalyzed by unidimensional chromatography; (2) 27% had been further analyzed by some special chromatography procedure; (3) 4% were reanalyzed for methylmalonic acid; (4) 3% were analyzed by two-dimensional sequential paper chromatography; and (5) in 2% a repeat sample was sought, half because of specimen inadequacy and half because of a suspected abnormality. Importantly, this expensive reanalysis and retesting failed to detect a single infant with a clinically significant disorder not already strongly suspected from the testing of the original filter paper urine specimen. Indeed, although newborn urine screening provides important epidemiological and medical information, the failure of the programme as now conducted to identify treatable disorders had led to a question of its worth as a service (Levy et al 1980). Analysis of the programme in Australia led to similar conclusions (Wilcken et al 1980) and has been discontinued.

The frequencies of some metabolic disorders and conditions detected by screening newborn urine are listed in Table 109.4. In several cases, including disorders listed in the table, newborn urinary screening yields abnormal results but incomplete information is available about the natural history, possible medical significance and management of the disorder. Examples of such findings of uncertain significance include cystathioninaemia, hyperlysinaemia and sarcosinaemia. Several conditions detected are probably benign, including iminoglycinuria, Hartnup aminoaciduria and hyperprolinaemia. Treatable disorders detected by newborn urine screening include argininosuccinic acidaemia, methylmalonic aciduria and the Fanconi syndrome. Three of the disorders or conditions in Table 109.4 involve defects in renal transport rather than inborn errors of metabolism, viz,

Table 109.4 Frequencies of some metabolic disorders and conditions detected by screening newborn urine

Disorder or condition	Frequency
Cystinuria	1: 8 000
Iminoglycinuria	1: 12 000
Histidinaemia	1: 20 000
Hartnup disease	1: 25 000
Methylmalonic aciduria	1: 50 000
Cystathioninuria	1: 70 000
Argininosuccinic aciduria	1: 90 000
Hyperglycaemia, nonketotic	1: 180 000
Hyperprolinaemia	1: 200 000

cystinuria, iminoglycinuria and Hartnup aminoaciduria. In most other disorders involving aminoaciduria an extrarenal metabolic disturbance leads to accumulation in plasma of one or more amino acids which are filtered in amounts that exceed the reabsorption capacity of the nephron.

Certain features of specific conditions and disorders are described briefly in the following sections.

Cystinuria

Cystinuria is the most prevalent of the urinary amino acid abnormalities with a frequency of 1:8000 newborns. Cystinuria is a genetically heterogeneous, autosomal recessively inherited disorder involving defective transport of cystine, lysine, arginine and ornithine by the epithelial cells of the renal tubule and the gastrointestinal tract. These amino acids, along with cysteine-homocysteine mixed disulphide, are excreted in excessive amounts in urine. Blood amino acid concentrations are not increased. Cystine, the least soluble of all the amino acids, precipitates in urine leading to formation of renal calculi with possible obstruction, infection and loss of renal function. Most cystine renal calculi become clinically apparent during the second and third decades, although earlier or later initial presentations occur. Therapeutic approaches aim to prevent renal stone formation and include dietary alterations, alkalinization of urine, high volume fluid intake and the administration of penicillamine (Segal & Their 1989).

Three genetically distinct types of cystinuria were defined by Rosenberg et al (1966). Heterozygotes for the Type I defect can be detected only by studies of intestinal absorption where they lack active transport of cystine, lysine and arginine. In contrast, urine from heterozygotes for the Type II or Type III defects contains increased amounts of the dibasic amino acids. These heterozygotes differ from each other and from Type I heterozygotes in certain other characteristics as well (Scriver & Rosenberg

1973). While homozygotes excrete the largest quantities of cystine and dibasic amino acids, detection by screening of the quantitative pattern compatible with cystinuria in the much more numerous Type II or Type III heterozygotes leads to additional testing of a substantial number of newborns who are probably not at increased risk for urinary stones later in life (Levy et al 1980).

Iminoglycinuria

Familial iminoglycinuria is an inborn error of membrane transport with persistent and marked urinary excretion of the imino acids, proline and hydroxyproline, and of glycine without other aminoaciduria or altered blood amino acid concentrations. Genetic heterogeneity is suggested, since some families with iminoglycinuria also show defective intestinal transport of these amino acids. Adult heterozygotes have no iminoaciduria, and may or may not have hyperglycinuria. The characteristic amino acid pattern in urine is not accompanied by any consistent clinical abnormalities, thus suggesting that familial iminoglycinuria is a benign trait (Scriver 1989).

False positives for the iminoglycinuric pattern are frequent in newborns. During the first few months of life newborns and infants frequently excrete imino acids and glycine in easily measurable amounts. This transient iminoglycinuria usually disappears by 4–6 months of age. False positives for this urinary pattern are also frequent in infants who are ill with a variety of unrelated disorders. Heterozygotes for iminoglycinuria may exhibit the iminoglycinuric pattern during the first year of life, with later disappearance of the imino acids from the urine but persistence of the hyperglycinuria. Thus accurate identification of iminoglycinuria homozygotes requires testing of urine beyond the first year of life.

Histidinaemia

Elevations of the blood histidine concentration in newborns reflect: (1) transient elevations; (2) histidinaemia due to autosomal recessively inherited deficiency of L-histidine ammonia lyase (histidase); or (3) as described in one family, variant or atypical histidinaemia. Transient elevation of the histidine concentration in whole blood to 6 mg/dl or greater occurs once per 200–500 infants tested and, since this is nearly as high as the 8–20 mg/dl seen in infants with histidinaemia, false positive Guthrie screening tests may result. Since increased urinary excretion of histidine and its metabolites is more pronounced than the elevated blood histidine concentration in histidinaemia, urinary screening yields a far lower false-positive rate (Levy 1973).

The major presently unresolved question regarding

histidinaemia is whether this is a benign condition or a serious disorder. Except under unusual conditions, such as some instances of perinatal hypoxia, it seems that histidinaemia is benign (Scriver & Levy 1983).

Hartnup disease

Hartnup disease, named for the family in which the condition was first described, is a renal aminoaciduria involving monoamino-, monocarboxylic-amino acids with neutral or aromatic side chains. This characteristic aminoaciduria is the only consistent feature. Renal clearances are increased 5- to 10-fold for alanine, histidine, isoleucine, leucine, phenylalanine, serine, threonine, tryptophan and tyrosine. Asparagine and glutamine are also excreted in large quantities. The faeces usually contain increased amounts of the same amino acids. Blood amino acid levels are not increased. The urine also contains increased amounts of tryptophan metabolites produced by intestinal bacteria from unabsorbed tryptophan.

In contrast to the consistent urinary pattern of amino acids, clinical features are intermittent and variable. Indeed, individuals detected by screening are often asymptomatic, whereas skin lesions, neurological deficits and psychological changes were described earlier in some patients (Scriver et al 1987). Skin lesions resemble those of dietary pellagra and involve the face and extremities. Cerebellar signs may be present but are variable and completely reversible. Symptomatic attacks can be precipitated by sunlight, fever, emotional stress or exposure to sulphonamide drugs and are more likely to occur when the nutritional status is poor. Clinical manifestations tend to become less frequent and milder with increasing age. Attempts at therapy include an adequate diet and supplementation with nicotinic acid. The prognosis for persons with Hartnup disease appears to be good (Levy 1989b).

Hartnup disease is detected at a frequency of 1:25 000 by screening newborn urine. Transient hyperaminoacidurias of the Hartnup pattern are rare (Levy 1973). Inheritance of Hartnup disease follows an autosomal recessive pattern and parental consanguinity is increased.

Methylmalonic aciduria

Methylmalonic aciduria is one of the most frequent of the inborn errors of organic acid metabolism and is detected in 1:50 000 newborns (Levy et al 1980, Coulombe et al 1981). A special stain is used on the chromatogram of urine to detect methylmalonic acid and other organic acids (Coulombe et al 1981). Normal metabolism of methylmalonate requires the integrity of a series of apoenzymes, and the absorption and metabolic interconversion of the cobalamin derivatives required by one of these apoenzymes. At least five distinct biochemical bases for methylmalonic aciduria have been identified by means of metabolic and cell complementation studies (Rosenberg & Fenton 1989). These include methylmalonyl CoA mutase apoenzyme deficiency, two discrete defects in the synthesis of adenosylcobalamin and defective synthesis of both adenosylcobalamin and methylcobalamin.

The chemical abnormalities associated with the first four of these defects are similar and include life-threatening or fatal ketoacidosis and hyperammonaemia appearing during the first month of life. Continued episodes of ketoacidosis are associated with failure to thrive, neurological abnormalities including mental retardation, recurrent bacterial and viral infections, osteoporosis, neutropenia, thrombocytopenia and other abnormalities. Clinical abnormalities in patients with defective synthesis of both adenosylcobalamin and methylcobalamin are distinctly different, reflecting the disturbances of both methylmalonate and sulphur amino acid metabolism (Rosenberg & Fenton 1989). Metabolic studies in patients and in their cultured cells are useful in identifying the existence and nature of these various defects. Pedigree studies suggest an autosomal recessive inheritance, but methods for detecting heterozygotes are lacking. Therapy with supplementary cobalamin, including prenatally, was effective in some families (Rosenberg & Fenton 1989). A low protein diet and a synthetic formula deficient in methylmalonate and propionate precursors may also be used.

The eight Massachusetts infants detected either prenatally or as neonates illustrate the heterogeneity of observed clinical courses (Coulombe et al 1981). Two died in the newborn period, two showed a poor clinical and biochemical response to therapy, two responded to treatment and were clinically normal, and two were clinically normal without treatment, despite persistence of the methylmalonic aciduria. The last two individuals had clinically normal sibs who also had methylmalonic aciduria and were presumed to have the benign forms (Ledley et al 1984) similar to the one described by Giorgio et al (1976).

An occasional newborn is found to excrete methylmalonic acid transiently. Such methylmalonic aciduria is mild, not acompanied by clinical abnormalities and is found almost exclusively in breast-fed infants (Coulombe et al 1981). Methylmalonic aciduria was also described with cobalamin deficiency (Higginbottom et al 1978). Methylmalonic aciduria accompanied by hyperglycinuria constitutes one form of ketotic hyperglycinaemia (see below).

Cystathioninuria

Cystathioninuria was detected by means of newborn urine screening at a frequency of 1:70 000 in the Massachusetts programme (Levy 1973) but at over twice that frequency in Australia where a more sensitive method is used (Mudd et al 1989). If appropriate preservation measures are not taken, cystathionine in urine may be converted by bacterial contaminants to homocyst(e)ine, thus obscuring the diagnosis. Cystathioninuria, usually of mild degree, can occur transiently in newborns but generally resolves by 3 months of age. Cystathioninuria also has environmental causes and associations including vitamin B_6 deficiency, liver disorders of several kinds including hepatoblastoma and tumours of neural crest origin.

When cystathioninuria persists and acquired causes are ruled out, an autosomal recessively inherited deficiency of γ-cystathionase should be suspected. This hepatic enzyme uses pyridoxal-5′-phosphate as a cofactor and converts cystathionine to cysteine generating one molecule of α-ketobutyrate. Most individuals with γ-cystathionianase deficiency decrease their urinary excretion of cystathionine markedly in response to pharmacological doses of vitamin B_6. These biochemical characteristics are accompanied by no consistent clinical features (Mudd et al 1989). Since cystathioninuria is probably a benign metabolic trait, treatment appears not to be indicated.

Argininosuccinic aciduria

Deficiency of argininosuccinase leads to argininosuccinic aciduria, an autosomal recessively inherited disorder that occurs with a frequency of about 1:90 000 newborns. Although normally not detectable, argininosuccinate in this disorder appears in large amounts in urine, blood and cerebrospinal fluid, and the blood citrulline concentration is often 2–3 times normal. The increased concentration of argininosuccinate is generally directly related to protein intake but remains elevated even in the absence of symptoms. The argininosuccinate spot detected by chromatography or electrophoresis of urine is usually accompanied by two additional spots which are the anhydrides of the compound.

As part of the urea cycle, argininosuccinase normally cleaves argininosuccinate to arginine and fumarate. The activity is widely distributed and can be assayed in liver, erythrocytes, and cultured skin fibroblasts and amniotic fluid cells. The accumulation of argininosuccinate and the hyperammonaemia associated with this and other urea cycle disorders appears to be especially injurious to the immature brain (Brusilow & Horwich 1989). Additional methods have been tested to screen for other urea cycle disorders (Naylor 1981).

Based on age of presentation and natural history, three forms of argininosuccinic aciduria can be distinguished. The late-onset type occurs most frequently, with neurological abnormalities being the main feature. Feeding difficulties and vomiting may appear in infancy, followed later by seizures, intermittent ataxia and frank mental retardation. The two other clinical types exhibit a more rapid and severe course. In the neonatal type feeding problems and lethargy appear soon after birth, followed by seizures, respiratory distress, coma and death within the first 10 days of life. Onset in the subacute type is during infancy with failure to thrive, seizures and hepatomegaly.

Over one-third of the reported patients were detected by routine newborn screening. Possible treatments include a low protein diet, arginine supplementation and administration of sodium benzoate (Batshaw et al 1981). Arginine supplementation seems to be especially beneficial and may be sufficient therapy alone (Brusilow & Horwich 1989). On the other hand, the practice of obtaining newborn urine at 3–4 weeks of age for analysis may preclude effective treatment of patients with the neonatal type who become acutely ill and die at an earlier age (Levy 1973).

Hyperglycinaemia

Several pathological forms of hyperglycinuria and hyperglycinaemia must be distinguished from each other and from the hyperglycinuria without hyperglycinaemia, a frequent finding in normal newborns. Infants with both hyperglycinuria and hyperglycinaemia should be evaluated for a group of disorders of organic acid metabolism that give rise to the ketotic hyperglycinaemia syndrome. Athough the exact mechanism is unknown, organic acid intermediates that accumulate because of an inborn error of organic acid metabolism apparently produce a secondary block in glycine catabolism, perhaps cleavage of the glycine cleavage enzyme, that leads to accumulation of glycine from dietary sources and endogenous synthesis. Ketotic hyperglycinaemia presents clinically as an acute, severe illness of infancy with recurrent episodes of ketosis and acidosis often precipitated by protein intake or infection. Infants who survive may show neutropenia, thrombocytopenia, seizures and mental retardation. The most common cause of ketotic hyperglycinaemia syndrome is propionic acidaemia due to propionyl-CoA carboxylase deficiency. The syndrome can also occur with methylmalonic acidaemia, isovaleric acidaemia and a defect in isoleucine metabolism termed β-ketothiolase deficiency. A search for these disorders of organic acid metabolism is essential in any infant with hyperglycinaemia both for diagnostic accuracy and because treatment by dietary alteration is often successful.

Nonketotic hyperglycinaemia may be as frequent as ketotic hyperglycinaemia and differs from the latter in several important respects. Although it, too, often presents as an overwhelming illness early in life, ketosis and acidosis are absent, as are organic acid intermediates from blood or urine. The glycine concentration is increased 5- or more fold in plasma, 10- to 20-fold in urine, and as much as 100-fold in cerebrospinal fluid, while all other amino acids are normal. As in ketotic hyperglycinaemia, conversion of the C1 of glycine to CO_2 is blocked in vivo but, in contrast to the ketotic forms, conversion of the C2 of glycine to the C3 of serine may also be blocked (Nyhan 1989). Some patients die in infancy while many of those who survive show severe neurological abnormalities including mental retardation, seizures, opisthotonos, myoclonus and spasticity. Attempts at therapy by several approaches have reduced the plasma glycine concentration but do not cause sustained clinical improvement. In contrast, several infants with hyperglycinaemia but without evident abnormality in organic acid metabolism developed quite normally on unrestricted diets, despite having elevated plasma glycine concentrations (Levy 1973). Individuals with these other forms of hyperglycinaemia have normal concentrations of glycine in cerebrospinal fluid and brain despite the fact that their plasma glycine concentration may be as high as the patients with nonketotic hyperglycinaemia. Thus, measurement of glycine concentration in cerebrospinal fluid is an effective means of determining whether or not a hyperglycinaemic patient with neurological abnormalities has glycine encephalopathy (Perry et al 1975).

Detection by screening is more difficult in hyperglycinuric patients whose acute illness in the neonatal period leads to reduced protein intake and therefore decreased glycine excretion. Under these circumstances the glycinuria may be much less striking and resemble the amounts frequently seen in normal newborns.

Hyperprolinaemia

Hyperprolinaemia is detected by urine screening at a frequency of approximately 1:200 000 and occurs in two forms. Type I hyperprolinaemia due to a deficiency of pyrroline-5-carboxylate reductase or proline oxidase activity is probably an innocent metabolic trait despite suggestions that it is associated with hereditary nephropathy (Phang & Scriver 1989). Type II hyperprolinaemia due to δ-1-pyrroline-5-carboxylate dehydrogenase deficiency leads to more pronounced hyperprolinuria and is probably benign, although an association with neurological disease had been suggested (Phang & Scriver 1989).

Despite the specificity of the inherited block for proline metabolism, hyperprolinaemia results in iminoglycinuria, not to be confused with familial iminoglycinuria described earlier. The increased plasma concentration of proline leads to saturation by proline of the renal transport system shared by the imino acids and glycine so that, in addition to proline, hydroxyproline and glycine also appear in elevated amounts in the urine (Scriver & Rosenberg 1973).

OTHER NEWBORN SCREENING

Congenital hypothyroidism screening began in 1974 with the introduction by Dussault (Dussault et al 1975) of a radioimmunoassay procedure applicable to newborn filter paper blood specimens. Congenital hypothyroidism screening is now part of many programmes and has had the interesting effect of promoting regionalization of screening since the radioimmunoassays used for hypothyroidism are technically more complicated than the tests used for inborn error screening. In this procedure the initial test involves measurement of the newborn blood thyroxine (T_4) concentration. A filter paper disc of dried blood is incubated with radiolabelled T_4 and anti-T_4 antibodies and an inhibitor of thyroxine binding globulin. A low blood T_4 concentration leads to greater radioactive T_4 binding by the anti-T_4 antibody and reduced amounts of unbound radioactive T_4. Following separation of the bound and unbound fractions, the measurement of radioactivity in each fraction allows estimation of the blood T_4 concentration. The procedure can be automated and the data analysis completed by computer. Commonly the detection of a T_4 value two standard deviations or more below the mean is followed by measurement of the concentration of thyroid stimulating hormone (TSH) by radioimmunoassay using another disc from the blood sample. When both a low T_4 and an elevated TSH concentration are detected, the newborn's parents and physician are advised regarding the need for additional testing and possible treatment. This approach requires TSH testing in 3% of newborns and identifies congenital hypothyroidism in approximately 1:3600–5000 newborns (Rovet et al 1987). Although commonly combined with newborn screening for principally genetic disorders, only a few of the aetiologies of congenital hypothyroidism are Mendelian (Dumont et al 1989).

Screening newborns for haemoglobinopathy by newborn blood haemoglobin electrophoresis has been conducted extensively in several programmes. The early identification of infants with one of the sickling haemoglobinopathies coupled with aggressive follow-up has been shown to result in a significant reduction of mortality during the early years when the risks are especially great (Vichinsky et al 1988). Moreover, the investigators in the multicentre oral penicillin prophylaxis trial achieved an 84% reduction in the incidence of pneumococcal disease, a major cause of early morbidity and mortality in the sickling disorders, by means of inexpensive and safe treatment with penicillin (Gaston et al 1986). In addition to the treatment of affected newborns and genetic counselling of their parents, some programmes attempt to follow up the parents of carrier newborns in order to identify and counsel those couples in which both are carriers. Prenatal diagnosis of these disorders can now be offered earlier in pregnancy by means of chorionic villus sampling, and with great speed and accuracy using the polymerase chain reaction (Saiki et al 1988). Only a small percentage of those couples whose offspring are at risk for a serious globin disorder have chosen to use prenatal diagnosis. Screening programmes outside major metropolitan areas face the issue of whether to screen all newborns, accepting the additional costs and problems that accompany increasing programme size, or to attempt to identify and screen only those newborns considered to be at risk, based on racial or other criteria.

The technical feasibility of screening newborns for cystic fibrosis by measuring the serum immunoreactive trypsin in dried blood has been established (Hammond et al 1987). Moreover, accurate methods have been developed for the prenatal diagnosis of cystic fibrosis and the identification of carriers among close relatives of cystic fibrosis patients by means of closely linked DNA markers (Spence et al 1987).

The cloning of the cystic fibrosis gene (Rommens et al 1989) and the identification of a three base deletion removing phenylalanine at position 508 of the protein as the mutant allele present in the majority of cases (Kerem et al 1989, Riordan et al 1989) have made possible the direct detection of this mutant cystic fibrosis allele prenatally and postnatally in a substantial proportion of affected individuals and heterozygotes. This three base deletion, designated ΔF508, is the mutant allele found in approximately 75% of the cystic fibrosis chromosomes from patients of northern European ancestry (Lemna et al 1990), and is present in smaller proportions of cystic fibrosis chromosomes from patients from other populations. Thus approximately half of cystic fibrosis patients of northern European ancestry can be expected to be homozygous for the ΔF508 allele. Several dozen additional mutant alleles have been identified, but all of these have occurred at low frequency, essentially being confined to the families in which they were first identified. Genotyping of affected homozygotes and compound heterozygotes, and ascertainment of heterozygotes will remain incomplete until additional mutant alleles are identified.

Newborn cystic fibrosis screening has been initiated in several countries (Hammond et al 1987). Although both short- and long-term benefits have been claimed, the most convincing evidence of a short-term benefit was the demonstration by Wilcken and Brown, who screened 400 000 newborns in Australia, that the numbers of hospital days during the first two years of life was lower for the screened patients than in unscreened historical controls (Wilcken & Brown 1987). In other respects it is not yet established that early diagnosis and treatment will significantly improve the morbidity and mortality of cystic fibrosis. The suggested benefits are currently being assessed in a randomized controlled trial of newborn screening in Wisconsin.

Other programmes considered or begun are screening for a_1-antitrypsin deficiency (Sveger 1978), Duchenne muscular dystrophy (Lemieux 1987), adenosine deaminase deficiency (Moore & Meuwissen 1974), hyperlipidaemia (Wilcken 1987) and congenital adrenal hyperplasia (Thuline 1987). Their ultimate place in newborn screening programmes remains to be established.

ISSUES AND CONCERNS IN SCREENING

Most screening tests are designed to be sensitive in order to minimize false-negative results, but these tests may not be specific and they are seldom diagnostic. Accurate and definitive diagnosis requires additional testing in nearly all instances. Since false negative results do occur with every screening procedure, a negative result from screening should not preclude an appropriate evaluation for a disorder suspected clinically.

Screening programmes and procedures should meet a variety of criteria both before they are implemented and continually during their operation (Committee for the Study of Inborn Errors of Metabolism 1975). These criteria include technical, educational and organizational aspects. A high signal-to-noise ratio is needed to maximize effectiveness and minimize adverse effects. The noise in the system includes the true biological variation of the character being measured in the screened population and the variation within the testing procedure itself. As noted earlier, positive results in a screening test necessitate repeat testing with follow up and additional testing, possibly over a period of weeks or months. These can be expensive in terms of personnel, materials and parental anxiety and inconvenience. The rarer the trait being sought by screening, the higher will be the proportion of false positives.

In addition to normal biological variation and transient abnormalities, confusing artifacts are produced by contamination of blood and urine specimens with microorganisms, drugs used systemically or locally, diaper powder, food supplements and the like. Disentangling these sources of confusion and delay requires great expertise.

Finally, screening programmes should be organized and administered in such a way that they are constantly updated to incorporate the latest technical and medical advances. They must also be responsive to changes in society. The present trends towards the earlier discharge of mother and child from the hospital and the increased numbers of home births provide poignant examples of changes having major potential impact on newborn screening.

REFERENCES

Batshaw M L, Thomas G H, Brusilow S W 1981 New approaches to the diagnosis and treatment of inborn errors of urea synthesis. Pediatrics 68: 290–297

Berry H K 1959 Procedures for testing urine specimens dried on filter paper. Clinical Chemistry 5: 603–608

Beutler E, Baluda M C 1966 A simple spot screening test for galactosemia. Journal of Laboratory and Clinical Medicine 68: 137–141

Brusilow S W, Batshaw M L 1979 Arginine therapy for argininosuccinase deficiency. Lancet 1: 134–136

Brusilow S W, Horwich A L 1989 Urea cycle enzymes. In: Scriver C R, Beaudet A L, Sly W S, Valle D (eds) The Metabolic Basis of Inherited Disease, 6th edn. McGraw-Hill, New York, ch 20, p 629–663

Buist N R M, Kennaway N G, Fellman J H 1985 Tyrosinemia type II: Hepatic cytosol tyrosine aminotransferase deficiency (the "Richner-Hanhart syndrome"). In: Bickel H, Wachtel U (eds) Inherited Diseases of Amino Acid Metabolism. Georg Thieme, Stuttgart, p 203

Committee for the Study of Inborn Errors of Metabolism 1975 Genetic Screening: Programs, Principles and Research. National Academy of Sciences, Washington, D. C.

Coulombe J T, Shih V E, Levy H L 1981 Massachusetts metabolic disorders screening program. II. Methylmalonic aciduria. Pediatrics 67: 26–31

Danner D J, Elsas L J II 1989 Abnormalities of branched-chain amino acid and ketoacid metabolism. In: Scriver C R, Beaudet A L, Sly W S, Valle D (eds) The Metabolic Basis of Inherited Disease, 6th edn. McGraw-Hill, New York, ch 22, p 671–692

Dent C E 1946 Detection of amino acids in urine and other fluids. Lancet 2: 637–639

Dumont J E, Vassart G, Refetoff S 1989 Thyroid disorders. In: Scriver C R, Beaudet A L, Sly W S, Valle D (eds) The Metabolic Basis of Inherited Disease, 6th edn. McGraw-Hill, New York, ch 73, p 1843–1879

Dussault J H, Coulombe P, Laberge C, Letarte J, Guyda H, Khoury K 1975 Preliminary report on a mass screening program for neonatal hypothyroidism. Journal of Pediatrics 86: 670–674

Efron M L, Young D, Moser H W, MacCready R A 1964 A simple chromatographic screening test for the detection of disorders of amino acid metabolism. New England Journal of Medicine 270: 1378–1383

Erbe R W 1981 Issues in newborn screening. In: Bloom A D, James L S (eds) The Fetus and the Newborn (Birth Defects Original Article Series, vol 17). Alan Liss, New York, p 167

Erbe R W 1986 Inborn errors of folate metabolism. In: Blakley R L, Whitehead V M (eds) Folates and Pterins: Volume 3 - Nutritional, Pharmacological and Physiological Aspects. John Wiley, New York, p 413

Folling A 1934 Uber Ausscheidung von Phenylbrenztraubensaure in den Harn als Stoffwechselanomalie in Verbindung mit Imbezillitat. Hoppe Seyler Zeitschrift Physiologische Chemie 227: 169–176

Gahl W A, Renlund M, Thoene J G 1989 Lysosomal transport disorders - cystinosis and sialic acid storage disorders. In: Scriver C R, Beaudet A L, Sly W S, Valle D (eds) The Metabolic Basis of Inherited Disease, 6th edn. McGraw-Hill, New York, ch 107, p 2619–2647

Garrick M, Pass K, Sarjeant G 1987 Summary of the workshop on hemoglobinopathies. In: Therell B L Jr. (ed) Advances in Neonatal Screening. Excerpta Medica, Amsterdam, p 397–399

Gaston M, Verter J I, Woods G et al 1986 Prophylaxis with oral penicillin in children with sickle cell anemia: A randomized trial. New England Journal of Medicine 314: 1594–1599

Ghavami M, Levy H L, Erbe R W 1986 Prevention of fetal damage through dietary control of maternal hyperphenylalaninemia. Clinical Obstetrics and Gynecology 29: 580–585

Giorgio A J, Trowbridge M, Boone A W, Patten R S 1976 Methylmalonic aciduria without vitamin B_{12} deficiency in an adult sibship. New England Journal of Medicine 295: 310–313

Goldsmith L A, Laberge C 1989 Tyrosinemia and related disorders. In: Scriver C R, Beaudet A L, Sly W S, Valle D (eds) The Metabolic Basis of Inherited Disease, 6th edn. McGraw-Hill, New York, ch 16, p 547–562

Guthrie R 1964 Routine screening for inborn errors in the newborn: "inhibition assays," "instant bacteria" and multiple tests. International Copenhagen Congress on the Scientific Study of Mental Retardation, Denmark, August 7–14

Guthrie R, Susi A 1963 A simple phenylalanine method for detecting phenylketonuria in large populations of newborn infants. Pediatrics 32: 338–343

Hammond K, Naylor E, Wilcken B 1987 Screening for cystic fibrosis. In: Therell B L Jr. (ed) Advances in Neonatal Screening. Excerpta Medica, Amsterdam, p 377–382

Harris H 1963 Garrod's Inborn Errors of Metabolism. Oxford University Press, London

Heard G S, Wolf B, Jefferson L G et al 1986 Neonatal screening for biotinidase deficiency: Results of a 1-year pilot study. Journal of Pediatrics 108: 40–46

Higginbottom M C, Sweetman L, Nyhan W L 1978 A syndrome of methylmalonic aciduria, homocystinuria, megaloblastic anemia and neurologic abnormalities in a vitamin B_{12}-deficient breast-fed infant of a strict vegetarian. New England Journal of Medicine 299: 317–323

Kerem B-S, Rommens J M, Buchanan J A et al 1989 Identification of the cystic fibrosis gene: genetic analysis. Science 245: 1073–1080

Lemna W K, Feldman G L, Kerem B-S et al 1990 Mutation analysis for heterozygote detection and the prenatal diagnosis of cystic fibrosis. New England Journal of Medicine 322: 291–296

Ledley F D, Levy H L, Shih V E, Benjamin R, Mahoney M J 1984 Benign methylmalonic aciduria. New England Journal of Medicine 311: 1015–1018

Lemieux B 1987 Recommendations regarding neonatal screening for muscular dystrophy. In: Therell B L Jr. (ed) Advances in Neonatal Screening. Excerpta Medica, Amsterdam, p 349

Lemieux B, Auray-Blais C, Giguere R, Shapcott D, Scriver C R 1988 Newborn urine screening experience with over one million infants in the Quebec network of genetic medicine. Journal of Inherited Metabolic Disease 11: 45–55

Lenke R R, Levy H L 1980 Maternal phenylketonuria and hyperphenylalaninemia: an international survey of the outcome of untreated pregnancies. New England Journal of Medicine 303: 1202–1208

Levy H L 1973 Genetic screening. In: Harris H, Hirschhorn K (eds) Advances in Human Genetics. Plenum, New York, vol 4, p 1

Levy H L 1977 Screening for genetic disorders in the newborn. In: Altman P L, Katz D D (eds) Human Health and Disease. Federation of American Societies for Experimental Biology, Bethesda, p 107

Levy H L 1989a Disorders of histidine metabolism. In: Scriver C R, Beaudet A L, Sly W S, Valle D (eds) The Metabolic Basis of Inherited Disease, 6th edn. McGraw-Hill, New York, ch 17, p 563–576

Levy H L 1989b Hartnup disorder. In: Scriver C R, Beaudet A L, Sly W S, Valle D (eds) The Metabolic Basis of Inherited Disease, 6th edn. McGraw-Hill, New York, ch 101, p 2515–2527

Levy H L, Hammersen G 1978 Newborn screening for galactosemia and other galactose metabolic defects. Journal of Pediatrics 92: 871–877

Levy H L, Sepe S J, Shih V E, Vawter G F, Klein J O 1977 Sepsis due to Escherichia coli in neonates with galactosemia. New England Journal of Medicine 297: 823–825

Levy H L, Coulombe J T, Shih V E 1980 Newborn urine screening. In: Bickel H, Guthrie R, Hammersen G (eds) Neonatal screening for inborn errors of metabolism. Springer-Verlag, Heidelberg, p 89

MacCready R A, Hussey M G 1964 Newborn phenylketonuria detection program in Massachusetts. American Journal of Public Health 54: 2075–2081

Meryash D L, Levy H L, Guthrie R, Warner R, Bloom S,

Carr J R 1981 Prospective study of early neonatal screening for phenylketonuria. New England Journal of Medicine 304: 294–296

Moore E C, Meuwissen H J 1974 Screening for ADA deficiency. Journal of Pediatrics 85: 802–804

Mudd S H, Levy H L, Skovby F 1989 Disorders of transsulfuration. In: Scriver C R, Beaudet A L, Sly W S, Valle D (eds) The Metabolic Basis of Inherited Disease, 6th edn. McGraw-Hill, New York, ch 23, p 693–734

Naylor E W 1981 Newborn screening for urea cycle disorders. Pediatrics 68: 453–457

Nyhan W L 1989 Nonketotic hyperglycinemia. In: Scriver C R, Beaudet A L, Sly W S, Valle D (eds) The Metabolic Basis of Inherited Disease, 6th edn. McGraw-Hill, New York, ch 25, 743–753

O'Flynn M E, Holtzman N A, Blaskovics M, Azen C, Williamson M L 1980 The diagnosis of phenylketonuria. A report from the collaborative study of children treated for phenylketonuria. American Journal of Diseases of Children 134: 769–774

Paigen K, Pacholee S, Levy H L 1982 A new method of screening neonates for galactosemia and other galactose metabolic defects. Journal of Laboratory and Clinical Investigation 99: 895–907

Pass K A 1987 Newborn screening for sickle cell disease in New York. In: Therell B L Jr. (ed) Advances in Neonatal Screening. Excerpta Medica, Amsterdam, p 409–414

Perry T L, Urquhart N, MacLean J et al 1975 Nonketotic hyperglycinemia. Glycine accumulation due to absence of glycine cleavage in brain. New England Journal of Medicine 292: 1269–1273

Phang J M, Scriver C R 1989 Disorders of proline and hydroxyproline metabolism. In: Scriver C R, Beaudet A L, Sly W S, Valle D (eds) The Metabolic Basis of Inherited Disease, 6th edn. McGraw-Hill, New York, ch 18, p 577–597

Research Group on Ethical, Social and Legal Issues in Genetic Counseling and Genetic Engineering 1972 Ethical and social issues in screening for genetic disease. New England Journal of Medicine 286: 1129–1132

Riordan J R, Rommens J M, Kerem B-S et al 1989 Identification of the cystic fibrosis gene: cloning and characterization of complementary DNA. Science 245: 1066–1073

Rommens J M, Iannuzzi M C, Kerem B-S et al 1989 Identification of the cystic fibrosis gene: chromosome walking and jumping. Science 245: 1059–1065

Rosenberg L E, Fenton W A 1989 Disorders of propionate and methylmalonate metabolism. In: Scriver C R, Beaudet A L, Sly W S, Valle D (eds) The Metabolic Basis of Inherited Disease, 6th edn. McGraw-Hill, New York, ch 29, p 821–844

Rosenberg L E, Downing S E, Durant J L, Segal S 1966 Cystinuria: biochemical evidence for three genetically distinct diseases. Journal of Clinical Investigation 45: 365–371

Rovet J, Glorieux J, Heyerdahl S 1987 Summary of presentations and discussion on the psychological follow-up of CH children identified by newborn screening. In: Therell B L Jr. (ed) Advances in Neonatal Screening. Excerpta Medica, Amsterdam, p 71–77

Saiki R K, Chang C-A, Levenson C H et al 1988 Diagnosis of sickle cell anemia and β-thalassemia with enzymatically amplified DNA and nonradioactive allele-specific oligonucleotide probes. New England Journal of Medicine. 319: 537–541

Scriver C R 1989 Familial renal iminoglycinuria. In: Scriver C R, Beaudet A L, Sly W S, Valle D (eds) The Metabolic Basis of Inherited Disease, 6th edn. McGraw-Hill, New York, ch 102, p 2529–2538

Scriver C R, Levy H L 1983 Histidinaemia. Part I: Reconciling retrospective and prospective findings. Journal of Inherited Metabolic Disease 6: 51–53

Scriver C R, Rosenberg L E 1973 Amino acid metabolism and its disorders. Saunders, New York

Scriver C R, Davies E, Cullen A M 1964 Application of a simple micromethod to the screening of plasma for a variety of aminoacidopathies. Lancet 2: 230–232

Scriver C R, Mahon B, Levy H L et al 1987 The Hartnup phenotype: Mendelian transport disorder, multifactorial disease. American Journal of Human Genetics 40: 401–412

Scriver C R, Kaufman S, Woo S L 1989 The hyperphenylalaninemias. In: Scriver C R, Beaudet A L, Sly W S, Valle D (eds) The Metabolic Basis of Inherited Disease, 6th edn. McGraw-Hill, New York, ch 15, p 495–546

Segal S 1989 Disorders of galactose metabolism. In: Scriver C R, Beaudet A L, Sly W S, Valle D (eds) The Metabolic Basis of Inherited Disease, 6th edn. McGraw-Hill, New York, ch 13, p 453–480

Segal S, Their S O 1989 Cystinurias. In: Scriver C R, Beaudet A L, Sly W S, Valle D (eds) The Metabolic Basis of Inherited Disease, 6th edn. McGraw-Hill, New York, ch 99, p 2479–2496

Sepe S J, Levy H L, Mount F W 1979 An evaluation of routine follow-up blood screening of infants for phenylketonuria. New England Journal of Medicine 300: 606–609

Smith I, Howells D W, Hyland K 1986 Pteridines and mono-amines: relevance to neurological damage. Postgraduate Medical Journal 62: 113–123

Spence J E, Buffone G J, Rosenbloom C L et al 1987 Prenatal diagnosis of cystic fibrosis using linked DNA markers and microvillar enzyme analysis. Human Genetics 76: 5–10

Sveger T 1978 a_1-Antitrypsin deficiency in early childhood. Pediatrics 62: 22–25

Thuline H C 1987 Newborn screening for congenital adrenal hyperplasia (CAH). In: Therell B L Jr. (ed) Advances in Neonatal Screening. Excerpta Medica, Amsterdam, p 301–302

Vichinsky E, Hurst D, Earles A, Kleman K, Lubin B 1988 Newborn screening for sickle cell disease: Effect on mortality. Pediatrics 81: 749–755

Whiteman P D, Clayton B E, Ersser R S, Lilly P, Seakins J W T 1979 Changing incidence of neonatal hypermethioninaemia: Implications for the detection of homocystinuria. Archives of Disease in Childhood 54: 593–598

Wilcken D E L 1987 Summary of the workshop on hyperlipidemias. In: Therell B L Jr. (ed) Advances in Neonatal Screening. Excerpta Medica, Amsterdam, p 325–327

Wilcken B, Brown A R D 1987 Screening for cystic fibrosis in New South Wales, Australia: Evaluation of the results of screening 400,000 babies. In: Therell B L Jr. (ed) Advances in Neonatal Screening. Excerpta Medica, Amsterdam p 385–390

Wilcken B, Chalmers G 1985 Reduced mortality in patients with cystic fibrosis detected by neonatal screening. Lancet 2: 1319–1321

Wilcken B, Smith A, Brown D A 1980 Urine screening for aminoacidopathies: Is it beneficial? Journal of Pediatrics 97: 492–497

Wolf B, Heard G S, Jefferson L G, Proud V K, Nance W E, Weissbecker K A 1985 Clinical findings in four children with biotinidase deficiency detected through a statewide neonatal screening program. New England Journal of Medicine 313: 16–19

Wolf B, Heard G S, Jefferson L G, Mitchell P L, Bennett G, Lambert F W, Linyear A S 1987 Neonatal screening of biotinidase deficiency. In: Therell B L Jr. (ed) Advances in Neonatal Screening. Excerpta Medica, Amsterdam, p 311–315

110. Heterozygote screening

M. M. Kaback

INTRODUCTION

The specific biochemical abnormality in each of more than 200 inborn errors of metabolism in man has now been determined (McKusick 1988, Scriver et al 1989). Nearly all are inherited either as autosomal or X-linked recessive disorders. The capability to identify such conditions in relatively easily available tissues from affected individuals permits the rapid and accurate diagnosis of such disorders, minimizing the necessity for complicated and, at times, risk-associated diagnostic procedures. Many of these methods have also been applied to the prenatal detection of such conditions in the fetus during early gestation. This approach has provided a vital new option in genetic counselling for many families. In addition, in some instances, the delineation of the underlying metabolic defect has enabled investigators to develop rational and effective therapies for certain of these disorders (Desnick 1981).

In addition to the diagnostic and possible therapeutic implications of such discoveries, comparable methodologies have been employed for the detection of heterozygous carriers of many of the recessive traits involved. Accordingly, not only is a striking deficiency of enzymatic activity or metabolic dysfunction evident in the diagnosis of the homozygous or hemizygous state (the affected male with an X-linked recessive disorder), but a distinct quantitative decrease of the same function can be demonstrated in the otherwise normal individual carrying the recessive allele. In some instances variant protein products of the mutant gene can be directly demonstrated by immunological or electrophoretic methods (Harris & Hopkinson 1978). This capability to quantify gene dosage, and thereby to identify carriers of recessive traits, has been reported for many, but not all, of the inborn errors of metabolism where the primary defect is known.

In recent years, dramatic advances in the applications of molecular genetic techniques have made it possible to identify (either directly or indirectly) heterozygous carriers of an increasing number of mutant alleles. In some instances this may involve direct detection of the mutation site (e.g. sickle-cell anaemia, haemophilia-A, some types of β-thalassaemia, etc.). In other conditions where the gene has eluded isolation thus far, carrier identification has been achieved by the demonstration of polymorphic genetic markers (restriction fragment length polymorphisms – RFLPs) segregating in specific families very closely linked to the disease-associated mutant gene (e.g. Huntington chorea, cystic fibrosis). In the latter approach, carrier detection through RFLP analysis allows for a statistical probability of carrier (or disease) status to be ascertained. This method requires however, that comparable linkage determinations be (or have been) carried out on DNA from affected members of the same family. In some families, such RFLP linkage studies may be totally uninformative or only partially informative for carrier identification purposes. Clearly, as more and more gene loci are isolated and their nucleotide sequences defined, the applications of these and other sensitive and accurate molecular methods for mutant gene identification will increase accordingly.

At present however, the specific gene loci or closely linked RFLPs for the majority of inborn errors of metabolism have not yet been characterized. Accordingly, for these conditions biochemical, immunological, or other phenotype-specific methods are still employed for disease diagnosis and heterozygote detection. In certain disorders, such methods for carrier identification may be complex, tedious and at times difficult to interpret. Either significant overlap with homozygous normal individuals is evident with the method(s) employed; the procedures are associated with significant complexity and possible morbidity; or sufficient numbers of obligate heterozygotes (parents of affected children) and normal homozygotes have not as yet been studied to establish the statistical validity of the carrier identification method. These issues will be addressed in detail in subsequent parts of this chapter.

It is not the intent of this article to review all known metabolic disorders as to their current status regarding carrier detection. Rather, specific disorders will be cited solely as examples of the issues being discussed. Other chapters in this volume provide a detailed elaboration of the fundamental inborn errors associated with such conditions.

CARRIER SCREENING IN CLINICAL PRACTICE

When a patient is identified with an inborn error of metabolism or the family history reveals such a disorder in a close blood relative, the question of whether to test that individual and other family members for heterozygosity should be considered. In many instances where such tests are available and accurate, this can serve to *reduce expressed or hidden anxieties in other family members*. Since most of these disorders are individually rare, it is relatively unlikely that other family members need be too fearful of producing affected offspring. For example, taking a maximum risk situation, an American Black individual whose brother or sister is a patient with sickle-cell anaemia may be concerned about having children with this disease. Assuming they reproduce with another black person with *no known* sickle-cell anaemia in his or her family – what are the actual risks? The unaffected sib of a person with sickle-cell anaemia has two chances in three of having sickle trait (if born of the same parents as the patient with sickle-cell anaemia). The approximate overall sickle trait frequency in American blacks is about one in ten. Therefore, the likelihood that the person will be at risk for sickle-cell anaemia in his or her offspring is: $2/3 \times 1/10 = 1/15$. The likelihood that any given pregnancy will result in a child with sickle-cell anaemia is 1/4 of that risk, or 1 in 60. Although these statistics alone can be somewhat comforting, simple carrier detection studies in the appropriate persons can put this question out of the realm of 'calculation', and establish definitively whether either or both individuals are carriers. If both prospective parents are found to be carriers, then comprehensive genetic counselling with a complete discussion of all available options can be initiated. Where at-risk couples are identified, this can lead to *prevention of subsequent intrafamilial cases of disease* – a second major reason to consider carrier testing in such families.

A third rationale relates to *marital counselling*, particularly where consanguinity between prospective parents may exist. In certain situations, because of religious, moral, or other concerns, individuals might utilize such information about their carrier status in their decision regarding mate selection. This is the practice in certain Hassidic Jewish communities where strong religious proscriptions against abortion exist. Since marriages are 'arranged' (often in childhood) and require rabbinical approval, some rabbis have opted for Tay-Sachs disease (TSD) carrier testing among the children of their community. Approval for marriage is withheld by the rabbi (to whom solely the results of carrier testing are conveyed) if two carriers are 'matched'. Alternative 'arrangements' are then made without specifying the reason, thus avoiding family or individual stigmatization.

Another important consideration for carrier screening is where *artificial insemination* is being considered as an alternative for a couple who have previously had a child with autosomal recessive disorder. Potential sperm or ovum donors should be evaluated (where feasible and practical) by appropriate carrier screening tests to avoid what could otherwise be a most unfortunate tragedy. The author is aware of two children with TSD, conceived by artificial insemination, born to two unrelated families who were attempting to have an unaffected child after they had had a previous child with this fatal condition. In another instance, screening three medical students as potential sperm donors for a woman who had been previously identified as a TSD heterozygote, showed one of the three to be a TSD carrier also. Of course, he was excluded as a potential donor. Such screening, in addition to a thorough family history on all potential sperm donors for other relevant issues, can help to avert tragedy.

CARRIER SCREENING IN INDIVIDUALS OF DEFINED SUBPOPULATION GROUPS

In Table 110.1, a list of relatively 'common' autosomal recessive disorders seen in defined subpopulations in the USA is presented with data indicating the respective carrier frequencies and newborn disease incidence in those ethnic groups. Gene frequencies and incidence of the disorder may vary considerably in the same ethnic groups in other parts of the world. The fact that selected genetic diseases occur predominantly in certain ethnic, religious, or racial groups should not be surprising when one considers the relatively high degree of inbreeding seen in defined subpopulations (McKusick 1988, Ramot 1974). In addition to inbreeding, in some situations, selective environmental factors may have existed at some point in history which provided a biological (reproductive) advantage to carriers of the recessive gene (e.g. relative resistance to malaria in individuals who are heterozygous for sickle haemoglobin, β-thalassaemia or G6PD deficiency). Because of this selective effect, the gene becomes 'enriched' from one generation to the next in that population.

Because of these population distributions and the availability of relatively simple, accurate, and inexpensive carrier detection methods for the respective traits, it is possible to screen individuals in these groups and identify persons (and, more critically, couples) at risk for homozygous disease in their offspring before affected children have been born to them. With comprehensive genetic counselling, and the important new options which prenatal diagnosis can provide, many 'at-risk' families, identified through screening such subpopulations, might choose to have only children unaffected with the disorder for which they are found to be at risk.

Perhaps the most effective effort of this nature has been the experience with TSD carrier screening and prenatal diagnosis in western countries (Kaback 1981). From 1970 (when serum carrier detection methods were first described) to 1987, community-based TSD education-screening-counselling programmes have been initiated in Jewish communities throughout North America, as well as in Israel, South Africa, Europe and South America. More than 640 000 Jewish adults have been screened voluntarily and over 24 000 heterozygotes detected. Most critically, 729 couples – none of whom had had affected children previously – have been identified as being at risk for this fatal disorder in their offspring. Over 1800 pregnancies at risk for TSD have been monitored by amniocentesis, and the births of 325 infants destined to die with this disorder have been prevented. Recent data indicate that these efforts have contributed to a 60–85% decrease in the incidence of this disorder in Jewish infants throughout North America (Kaback 1982).

Most recently, similar efforts directed at the prevention of β-thalassaemia, through carrier screening and prenatal diagnosis, have been initiated in several European countries and certain areas of North America. Such programmes have had a definite effect in reducing the newborn incidence of β-thalassaemia in several Mediterranean countries as well as in the Cypriot community in Britain (Modell & Mouzouras 1982, Cao et al 1984).

Screening for sickle trait has been initiated in several parts of the world (including the USA). Although the capability to diagnose homozygous sickle-cell anaemia in early fetal life is well established – through either amniocentesis or chorionic villus sampling – this alternative has not been widely adopted. This may reflect (at least in the USA) some of the complex socio-ethical issues associated with genetic testing in minority populations (Whitten 1973, Rutkow & Lipton 1974, Fletcher et al 1985).

Recent discoveries involving the use of polymorphic markers closely linked to the gene for cystic fibrosis predict a capability for mass carrier screening for this deleterious allele in the near future. Such methods can already be applied to heterozygote identification among relatives where DNA from family members with CF is available. With the isolation of the CF gene itself, and assuming little if any heterogeneity in the mutation(s) causing CF, wide-scale screening should become a reality. This, coupled with genetic counselling and prenatal diagnosis for CF, may have a major impact in reducing the incidence of this serious disease.

It is important to remember that for these relatively 'common' autosomal disorders occurring in defined ethnic groups, there is *usually no known prior history of the disease in either side of the family*. Such a positive family history may be present in only about 20% of instances where a child with such a disorder is diagnosed. For this reason, clinicians should consider carrier screening for all individuals in these subpopulation groups where heterozygote detection is readily available. Certainly, such testing and its implications should be discussed thoroughly with the patients – or they can be referred to appropriate regional agencies for such services.

Table 110.1 Frequency and incidence estimates for selected autosomal recessive disorders in defined ethnic groups in the USA

Disease	Ethnic group	Gene frequency	Carrier frequency	'At risk' couple 'frequency'*	Disease incidence in newborns
Sickle-cell anaemia	Blacks	0.040	0.080	1 in 150	1 in 600
Tay-Sachs disease	Ashkenazi Jews	0.016	0.032	1 in 900	1 in 3600
β-Thalassaemia	Greeks, Italians	0.016	0.032	1 in 900	1 in 3600
α-Thalassaemia	S.E.Asians and Chinese	0.020	0.040	1 in 625	1 in 2500
Cystic fibrosis	N. Europeans	0.020	0.040	1 in 625	1 in 2500
Phenylketonuria	Europeans	0.008	0.016	1 in 4000	1 in 16 000

*Likelihood that both members of a couple are heterozygous for the same recessive allele (assuming nonconsanguinity and that both are of the same ethnic group).

Not only is this considered optimal preventive medicine, but considerable concern has arisen recently regarding the medicolegal implications of failing to do so (President's Commission 1983).

THERAPEUTIC IMPLICATIONS FOR HETEROZYGOTES

Although in most instances heterozygosity for a recessive trait is of no known health consequence to the individual, there are certain conditions in which the heterozygous state may impart certain health hazards.

Accordingly, in heterozygotes for certain conditions, the individual's knowledge of their carrier status may have certain therapeutic or preventive health implications for them. For example, persons with AS haemoglobin (sickle-cell trait) should be aware of possible hazards they might incur if exposed to reduced ambient oxygen concentrations, e.g. mountain climbing at high altitude, flying in an unpressurized aircraft above 8000 feet, etc. Also, alerting the anaesthetist of the AS trait of their patient prior to gaseous anaesthesia, could avert inadvertent hypoxia which might be particularly hazardous to such an individual. Heterozygous individuals for Type II hypercholesterolaemia may be predisposed to premature atherosclerotic degeneration and coronary artery insufficiency. It is believed that appropriate therapy (diet, weight control and/or specific medication) may substantially obviate the increased risk for early myocardial infarction in individuals carrying this dominantly-expressed disorder. In a similar context, persons heterozygous for α-1-antitrypsin deficiency (MZ) clearly may be predisposed to chronic obstructive pulmonary disease in early adulthood. Avoidance of tobacco smoke and other noxious inhalants may greatly reduce this risk. Having identified an individual as heterozygous for this genetic mutation, it might be of great practical value for this person to be so counselled and to be guided into appropriate job selection and/or environmentally safe areas, as well as informed of the particular importance of not smoking.

METHODS AND TISSUES USED IN CARRIER IDENTIFICATION

Depending upon the genetic nature of the condition, its expression in different organ systems, and the availability of appropriate material for examination, a variety of approaches have been employed for the purpose of heterozygote identification. Table 110.2 lists a series of approaches, ranging from physiological studies to direct mutation analysis which are utilized in carrier detection for different disorders. The disorders listed are representative only of the different categories of methods used. In some instances, combined techniques are involved for optimal ascertainment of the carrier state. For example, in Duchenne muscular dystrophy, use of biochemical (CPK) and Bayesian methods in combination has provided the best estimation of possible carrier status in certain women. Combined coagulation studies (physiological) with immunoquantitation of Factor VIII has been the optimal method for carrier identification in haemophilia A. Somatic cell methods assessing the enzymatic (HPRTase) or physiological (^{3}H-hypoxanthine incor-

Table 110.2 Methods employed for carrier detection in representative autosomal and X-linked recessive disorders

Approach	Method*	Disorder*
Physiological	Loading test kinetics	PKU,OTC
Biochemical	Quant. enzyme activity	TSD,MLD
Functional	NBT dye reduction	Chron.gran.dis.
Structural	Hb electrophoresis	Haemoglobinopathies
Somatic cell	Clonal mosaicism	Lesch-Nyhan
Immunological	Quant. immunochem.	Haemophilias
Statistical	Bayesian pedigree analysis	DMD
Genetic linkage (classical)	Xg family study	XR-MR
Genetic linkage (molecular)	RFLP analysis	CF, β-Thal.
Direct mutation analysis	Restriction site alteration, synthetic oligonucleotide probes	SSA, β-Thal, haemophilia

*NBT = Nitro-blue tetrazolium; Xg = X chromosome linked blood group;
PKU = phenylketonuria; OTC = Ornithine transcarbamylase deficiency;
TSD = Tay-Sachs disease; MLD = Metachromatic leucodystrophy;
DMD = Duchenne muscular dystrophy; XR-MR = X-linked recessive mental retardation
CF = cystic fibrosis; β-Thal = β-Thalassaemias
SSA = sickle cell anaemia

Table 110.3 Tissue used for carrier detection in representative recessive disorders

Tissue	Methods	Disorders*
Serum, plasma	Enzyme assay, immunoquantitation functional assay	TSD, haemophilias
Erythrocytes	Enzyme assay, electrophoresis	G6PD deficiency, haemoglobinopathies
Leucocytes	Enzyme assay, histology, functional tests	Gaucher, Batten, CGD
Cultivated skin fibroblasts	Enzyme assay, cloning	MLD, Hunter
Hair follicles	Enzyme assay/ratio	Lesch-Nyhan, Fabry disease
Tears	Enzyme assay	TSD
Teeth	Vertical banding	Amelogenesis imperfecta-XR
Eyes	Fundoscopy	XR-fundal dystrophies, RP
Liver, muscle biopsy	Enzyme assay, cellular histology	OTC, DMD
DNA from any somatic cells	RFLP or direct mutation site analysis	Haemoglobinopathies

*TSD = Tay-Sachs disease; CGD = Chronic granulomatous disease;
MLD = Metachromatic leucodystrophy; XR = X-linked recessive;
RP = Retinitis pigmentosa; OTC = Ornithine transcarbamylase deficiency;
DMD = Duchenne muscular dystrophy

poration) properties of clones of skin fibroblast cells have been applied effectively to carrier detection in Lesch-Nyhan syndrome. In each of the above examples, however, as well as with other disorders, advanced molecular genetic techniques (RFLP linkage, direct mutation site analysis, etc.) have either replaced the above approaches to carrier testing or are now used in conjunction with them in order to identify definitively the heterozygous individual (Ostrer & Hejtmancik 1988).

In Table 110.3, a compilation is presented of various tissues used for heterozygote detection in representative recessive disorders. In considering carrier screening in any individual (or subpopulation, for that matter) the accessibility of appropriate tissue or material for testing very much influences the feasibility and cost of such procedures. In some instances, accurate heterozygote identification can be achieved with such readily available tissues as serum, erythrocytes, or even tears. In other examples cited, optimal carrier detection may require cultured skin fibroblasts or even biopsied liver or muscle tissue. Clearly, whether to conduct such studies in individuals related to an affected person, or more generally, will be strongly influenced by such considerations.

The application of molecular techniques, involving DNA analysis, in the detection of mutant genes has had great impact on this issue. Since adequate DNA samples are readily obtained from leukocytes separated from a routine blood sample, the aforementioned reservations are in large part obviated if 'DNA methods' can be employed. In some instances, DNA from buccal cells rinsed from the mouth (or even that amount extracted from a single somatic cell) in conjunction with gene amplification techniques, such as the polymerase chain reaction, can provide sufficient material for carrier testing purposes. Accordingly, ease of testing as well as ultimate cost (particularly since such methods are readily automated) should allow for greatly expanded genetic testing for these disorders.

PROBLEMS IN HETEROZYGOTE DETECTION

Statistical constraints

The great majority of the inborn errors of metabolism alluded to in this chapter are relatively rare conditions. Although in the aggregate it is estimated that perhaps 1% of all live born infants will, at some time in life, manifest such a single-gene disorder, there are more than 2000 such disorders now recognized. This poses certain critical problems for carrier identification. The only individuals who are obligatory carriers of an autosomal recessive genetic trait are the biological parents of an affected individual (discounting the 10^{-5} to 10^{-6} possibility of new mutation). Therefore, in the establishment of a carrier identification method, it is critical that a 'significant number' of such obligatory heterozygotes be studied (and control individuals as well) before a statistical validity can be assigned to the testing method. In this regard one must be careful in interpreting many of the research publications in which only small numbers of obligate heterozygotes have been tested and where results suggest that the methods are applicable to carrier detection. Obviously, the larger the samples of obligate carriers and controls studied, and the greater the separation observed in the test results between the two groups, the greater the likelihood for significant application of the method to heterozygote identification.

It is a very different matter to study persons who the investigator knows *must be* carriers for a particular trait than individuals who are complete unknowns. Since all experiences in this context show a *distribution of test results*, both for carriers and controls, the narrowness of each distribution and the degree of separation of one from the other become critical considerations in assigning a statistical probability that any given person's test result falls into one or the other distribution.

With molecular methods, these constraints may be obviated in large part. Certainly where the specific mutation site is identifiable (either with specific cDNA probes or synthetic oligonucleotides), and where sequence information is available allowing for the amplification of relevant sequences (through polymerase chain reaction methods), direct ascertainment of mutation(s) is possible without the need for massive numbers in control studies or expansive statistical determinations. With the use of RFLPs, however, the proximity of the polymorphic marker to the disease locus is critical to interpretation since possible meiotic crossovers can confound apparent conclusions drawn by the linkage test. Here, again, substantial population studies may be necessary before the 'RFLP test' can be applied to carrier detection.

Why variability ?

One would expect that individuals who are heterozygotes for an autosomal recessive mutation would reflect 50% of the value (whatever the measurement happens to be) of that found in homozygous normal persons. This is clearly not the case. Not only is there variability of test values in heterozygotes, but considerable variation may also be evident in data derived from normals. This may reflect the limitations of the methods employed and/or the inherent *biological variability* of such functions. Assuredly, other genetic and environmental factors may influence any given biological parameter such that a definite range of results is seen in both carriers and noncarriers. In some instances where, for example, an enzymatic activity measurement is the test employed, there may be levels of activity in heterozygotes distinctly less than 50% of normal. Where the relevant enzyme is comprised of multiple subunits – only one of which is under control of the gene in question – random aggregation of normal and abnormal subunits can result in a wide range of activities in the multimeric enzyme. Other mutations may result in only partial reduction in activity of the respective polypeptide. In this instance, the heterozygote may have near normal activity, or activity of the enzyme in question which overlaps considerably with the range of measurements found in non-carriers.

With X–linked conditions, the carrier female, quite characteristically, reflects a broad range of test results extending from clearly normal levels to those seen in affected males. This is predominately a manifestation of the well-known Lyonization effect with X chromosome linked genes. This biological phenomenon makes carrier determination for such X-linked genes particularly difficult. In fact, heterozygous females who carry X-linked recessive genes are mosaic in the expression of most of the genes in question, with a certain proportion of their somatic cells expressing the normal gene and the remainder reflecting the mutant state. The reader is referred to other chapters in this volume concerning X–linked disorders for further discussion of carrier-state identification.

Other factors influencing the carrier test

In addition to the consideration that other genes in an individual's constitution might influence the expression of a distant specific gene locus, other biological factors may influence gene expression as well. Factors such as age, pregnancy and certain illnesses might influence the parameter in question, thereby altering the ability to distinguish carriers from non-carriers. Such issues need to be addressed before wide-scale application of a carrier detection method is made.

Genetic heterogeneity is another important consideration in this regard. This means that more than one genetic locus may cause a similar alteration in the test used or in the phenotype observed. If standard haemoglobin electrophoresis is the only parameter used for sickle trait identification, then persons carrying the mutation for haemoglobin-D will be incorrectly identified as AS, since S and D haemoglobin electrophorese similarly under standard conditions. In this instance, of course, the adjunct use of other methods such as haemoglobin solubility studies or sickling on deoxygenation will clarify this possible discrepancy.

In some instances, certain environmental factors such as drugs, diet, or other agents could affect biological functions and thereby influence their applicability to carrier detection. Iron deficiency can cause haematological changes which mimic the findings of those seen in heterozygotes for β-thalassaemia. Birth control medications have been shown to reduce the *relative* amount of serum hexosaminidase A, making some women taking 'the pill' appear as carriers for Tay-Sachs disease (Kaback 1977). These are only two examples where such determinations can be influenced by external factors, resulting in inaccurate carrier identification studies. Other examples may exist as well.

SENSITIVITY AND SPECIFICITY

With all of the above considerations in mind, and having assessed reasonable numbers of obligate heterozygotes and controls with the method(s) recommended, significant overlap in the distribution of carriers and non-carriers may still remain. Capabilities of any one laboratory may not be comparable with those of others reflecting, perhaps, differences in preferred methodologies or other inherent variables. Thus the ability to identify all true carriers (*sensitivity*) is reflected in the *false negative* frequency with the test employed. The identification of only true carriers (*specificity*), and not other persons with a *false positive* test, is also of paramount importance. The greater the overlap in distributions between carrier and non-carrier, the greater the likelihood for either or both types of misidentification.

In certain instances, even where a defined level of overlap is known to exist, carrier detection studies may still be appropriate. In this context, a test result clearly in the carrier range may indicate, with great likelihood, that the person is heterozygous, whereas a result in the overlap area would be less definitive and leave the possibility of carrier status indeterminate. Similarly, a result at the upper levels of the non-carrier distribution might make the probability of heterozygosity exceedingly small.

Where such difficulties exist, carrier screening is (most definitely) best restricted to use only in high risk individuals (close relatives of probands) rather than in more general or subpopulation screening. Only those approaches in which prior studies have proven the statistical reliability and accuracy of the method and its relative ease of applicability should be candidates for more general use.

COST AND FEASIBILITY

Where significant morbidity or cost would be involved in performing carrier detection studies (even where the accuracy is optimal), these issues should be considered and discussed with the individual before proceeding. Performing a skin biopsy for cultivation of fibroblast cells may have minimal morbidity, but is quite an expensive endeavour to undertake. For this reason, carrier screening using this approach should only be applicable to the highest risk individuals. Liver or muscle biopsy for such determinations obviously cannot be undertaken lightly. Again, perhaps only brothers and sisters or aunts and uncles would be at sufficient risk to warrant considering such studies. On the other hand, molecular-based DNA methods, where feasible, can be employed easily with DNA extracted from readily available somatic cells (leucocytes, skin cells, etc.) and at a reasonable cost.

AGE FOR CARRIER TESTING

As mentioned previously, for most recessive traits heterozygosity has little if any health consequences for the individual. It is only a matter relevant to reproduction. For this reason, it is the author's opinion that carrier testing is best instituted at a time just prior to, or during, the reproductive age. This has added benefits in that the person's ability to comprehend the meaning of such information is much more likely to be adequate at such an age. For this reason, carrier testing among children or young teenagers should not be undertaken routinely and should be considered only under very special circumstances. One's level of maturity and background education may be important factors in obviating any possible stigmatization which carrier identification could potentially entail. A parental request to determine the possible carrier status of their child(ren) need not be a sufficient basis to proceed. Rather, a full discussion with the parents as to the lack of health implications and possible psychosocial hazards of testing youngsters may lead to deferral of such studies until a more appropriate time.

CONCLUDING REMARKS

From its very outset a number of complex and important social and ethical issues have been identified with genetic screening (Hastings Center 1972, Bergsma 1974). Such issues as the possible personal, familial, or even more general stigmatization of the identified carrier – maintenance of utmost confidentiality of test results – rigorous protection of the individual's privacy – the informed consent of the tested individual – are but a few of the more important concerns raised. Clearly, the physician must consider all of these matters in his patient interaction where possible genetic testing is being anticipated. These issues notwithstanding, it is the author's opinion that heterozygote testing is likely to increase substantially in the future for many of the reasons cited earlier. With appropriate technical, medical and communicative expertise, the expanded utilization of these new approaches may serve to reduce the individual, familial, and societal burdens associated with many severe, currently untreatable, hereditary disorders.

ACKNOWLEDGEMENTS

This work was supported in part by a contract from the Genetic Disease section, Maternal and Child Health Branch, State of California Department of Health, and by a grant from the National Tay-Sachs and Allied Disorders Association, Incorporated.

REFERENCES

Bergsma D (ed) 1974 Ethical Social and Legal Dimensions of Screening for Human Genetic Disease, Birth Defects: Original Article Series, Vol. X, March of Dimes Birth Defects Foundation

Cao A, Pintus L, Lecca U et al 1984 Control of homozygous β-thalassemia by carrier screening and antenatal diagnosis in Sardinia. Clinical Genetics 26:2

Desnick R J 1981 Treatment of Inherited Metabolic Diseases: An Overview. In: Kaback M (ed) Genetic Issues in Pediatric and Obstetrical Practice. Year-Book Medical Publishers, New York

Fletcher J C, Berg K, Tranoy K E 1985 Ethical aspects of medical genetics: A proposal for guidelines in genetic counseling, prenatal diagnosis and screening. Clinical Genetics 27: 199

Harris H, Hopkinson D A 1978 Handbook of Enzyme Electrophoresis in Human Genetics. North-Holland, Amsterdam

Hastings Center 1972 Ethical and social issues in screening for genetic disease. New England Journal of Medicine 286: 1129

Kaback M (ed) 1977 Tay-Sachs Disease: Screening and Prevention. A R Liss, New York

Kaback M M 1981 Heterozygote Screening and Prenatal Diagnosis in Tay-Sachs Disease: A Worldwide Update. In: Callahan J W, Alexander Lowden J (eds) Lysosomes and Lysosomal Storage Diseases. Raven Press, New York

Kaback M M 1982 The control of genetic disease by carrier screening and antenatal diagnosis. Birth Defects 18: 243

McKusick V A 1988 Mendelian inheritance in man, 8th edn Johns Hopkins Press, Baltimore

Modell B, Mouzouras M 1982 Social consequences of introducing antenatal diagnosis for thalassemia. Birth Defects 18: 285

Ostrer H, Hejtmancik J F 1988 Prenatal diagnosis and carrier detection of genetic diseases by analysis of DNA. Journal of Pediatrics. 112: 679

President's Commission for the Study of Ethical Problems in Medicine and Biomedical Research 1983 Screening and Counseling for Genetics Conditions. U.S. Government. Print Office, Washington D.C.

Ramot B (ed) 1974 Genetic Polymorphisms and Diseases in Man. Academic Press, New York

Rutkow I M, Lipton J M 1974 Some negative aspects of the state health departments' policies related to screening for sickle cell anemia. American Journal of Public Health 64: 217

Scriver C R, Beaudet A L, Sly W S, Valle D 1989 The metabolic basis of inherited disease, 6th edn. McGraw-Hill, New York

Whitten J C 1973 Sickle cell programming: An imperiled promise. New England Journal of Medicine 288: 318

111. Prenatal diagnosis and therapy

Joel Charrow   *Henry L. Nadler*   *Mark I. Evans*

INTRODUCTION

In the last decade our understanding of gene structure and the mechanisms of gene expression have increased dramatically. Research in molecular genetics has made it possible to literally 'read' long stretches of the human genome and to grasp the causes of many inherited disorders on a molecular level. While these developments have had little impact on the treatment of these conditions, they have significantly enhanced our ability to diagnose genetic diseases prenatally. Prenatal diagnosis offers couples an opportunity to prevent congenital disorders and to plan their families with greater assurance. It is also essential if prenatal therapy is to be achieved, and is a prerequisite for optimal obstetric and neonatal care.

In this chapter we will review the indications for prenatal diagnosis, the evaluation of risks, the specific procedures available for studying the fetus and for analyzing fetal tissues. In addition, we will review the current status of fetal therapy.

GENERAL INDICATIONS FOR PRENATAL DIAGNOSIS

It is frequently assumed that prenatal diagnosis is offered only: (1) to couples who are known to be at high risk for producing a child with a congenital disorder; (2) when the disorder is associated with high morbidity, mortality, or significant functional impairment; and (3) when the couple is willing to terminate the pregnancy if the fetus is found to have the disorder. However, there are many situations in which all of these conditions are not fulfilled, and in which prenatal diagnosis is still highly desirable. A small number of disorders may be treated prenatally; the development and application of effective therapies is entirely dependent on accurate, early diagnosis. Some specific examples of prenatal therapy will be discussed later in this chapter. Foreknowledge of some birth defects, such as meningomyelocele, will affect the management of labour and delivery; caesarean section is

probably indicated to reduce the risk of trauma to the exposed spinal cord. There are many additional diagnoses which dictate delivery of the infant at an institution with the resources and expertise to provide optimal obstetric and neonatal care. There are also many conditions for which specific early neonatal therapy is desirable, and more easily achieved if the diagnosis is known prior to birth. For example, the metabolic disturbances which develop in a large number of inborn errors of metabolism (e.g. maple syrup urine disease) may be prevented if appropriate treatment is instituted at birth.

Even when there are no specific therapeutic implications, there is little doubt that parental anxiety is substantially reduced when there is time to learn about the child's diagnosis, mobilize support systems, and prepare for the special needs of a handicapped infant. It is important to emphasize, however, that more often than not the information derived from prenatal diagnosis is of a positive nature; the parents may be reassured and may look forward to a normal pregnancy and the birth of a healthy child. In either event it is well known that parents often act differently than they expected to, when confronted with the reality of a specific diagnosis. Although it is important that the option of termination be discussed, it is pointless and inappropriate to expect parents to have reached a decision before the diagnosis is known.

It is clear that termination of pregnancy is not the only reason for performing prenatal diagnosis. Nonetheless, it is still desirable to complete prenatal diagnostic studies early enough so that this option is not precluded. This generally means no later than 24 weeks' gestation, although closer to 20 weeks is preferable. In some countries termination may only be performed earlier in pregnancy, and in others it may be performed later.

One of the principal objections to prenatal diagnosis has been that it is nothing more than a 'search and destroy mission'. It is true that in the vast majority of instances in which a serious malformation is diagnosed, and termination is legally possible, this option will be chosen by the parents. However, it is also true that a great many more babies have been born because of prenatal diagnosis than have been aborted after prenatal diagnosis. Untold thousands of couples who otherwise would not have contemplated another pregnancy have been able to have more children precisely because it is possible to determine the well-being of the fetus early in pregnancy through prenatal diagnostic procedures.

Identifying couples 'at risk'

Who then are the subjects of prenatal diagnosis? Women over the age of 35, who are at increased risk for children with chromosome abnormalities, comprise the largest group seeking prenatal diagnosis. For most disorders, however, it is only after the birth of an affected child that prenatal diagnosis can be attempted in subsequent pregnancies. When there is no family history of a genetic disorder prenatal diagnosis may be feasible only if: (1) a population at risk can be identified; (2) the at risk population can be safely screened for unaffected carriers or for affected pregnancies; and (3) the pregnancies at risk may be monitored and the condition diagnosed with a high degree of reliability prior to 24 weeks' gestation. These criteria are unfortunately fulfilled by very few conditions: Tay-Sachs disease in Ashkenazi Jews (Kaback 1977); sickle-cell disease in Blacks (Alter et al 1976); beta-thalassaemia in Mediterranean peoples (Kan et al 1977, Fairweather et al 1978) and alpha- and beta-thalassaemia in Orientals. Because the frequency of the respective mutant allele is sufficiently high in these populations, and the means of carrier detection reliable and relatively simple, population screening for carriers can be performed and couples at risk identified.

There are a few disorders which are so common that the entire population may be considered to be at risk. For example, screening for Rhesus incompatibility, and Rh isoimmunization in women at risk, is routine. The entire population may be screened for acquired disorders as well as inherited disorders. Congenital rubella and syphilis are two such conditions for which screening of all pregnancies has been recommended for many years. Because of their high incidence, the entire population can also be considered to be at risk for neural tube defects (NTDs). These can be screened for during the 15th–20th week of pregnancy by measuring the maternal serum level of alpha-fetoprotein (see below). Unfortunately, population screening for many common genetic disorders is not yet possible.

Evaluating risks

Identifying couples who are at increased risk for having a child with a congenital disorder is the first step towards prenatal diagnosis. Such couples may be identified on the basis of their family histories or through a variety of screening methods. Determining which of these couples are candidates for prenatal diagnosis involves two further considerations: defining their numerical risk for producing a child with a congenital disorder, and evaluating the magnitude and significance of that risk to them. While the physician or genetic counsellor can determine the probability that a couple will have a child with a congenital disorder, only the parents can decide if this risk is 'too high' or 'high enough' to warrant prenatal diagnosis. All couples face a 3–4% risk of having a child with some type of birth defect. A 35-year-old woman, because of her age, faces an additional 0.6% risk of having a child with a chromosome abnormality. Whether this increase in risk appears large or small will be determined in large part by the parents' past experience, and the importance of the pregnancy to them. A childless couple who had difficulty conceiving may find the added risk associated with advanced maternal age trivial, but a woman of the same age who already has three children may find the same risk unacceptably high. Evaluating the risks of the prenatal diagnostic procedure itself is equally complex. A 0.3–0.5% chance of miscarriage resulting from amniocentesis may appear insignificant when one realizes that the risk of mid-trimester spontaneous abortion without any procedure may be as high as 3%. Furthermore, a couple who has had a child with a devastating illness may be willing to accept an even higher risk of fetal loss (such as might occur with fetoscopy), in order to prevent the recurrence of the disorder.

Performing the test

The identification of a pregnancy at high risk for a congenital disorder is the essential first step in prenatal diagnosis. Also important is the reliability of the technique used to monitor the pregnancy, and the skill and experience of those performing the procedures and the laboratory analyses. Experience in this area implies more than technical competence; an appreciation of the full range of normal, and an ability to tailor the procedure to the question being asked, are both necessary. It is also essential that the diagnosis be verified after birth of the child or termination of the pregnancy so that the analytical methods can be continually evaluated and improved. Prenatal diagnosis is not simply a laboratory exercise, it is a process which requires identification of pregnancies at risk, genetic counselling, parental education about genetics, procedures, and their risks, and emotional support at a time when difficult and sensitive issues are being decided. In addition, follow-up, both for verification of the diagnosis, and continued interaction with the parents, who are frequently guilt-ridden and uncertain of the wisdom of their decisions, cannot be neglected. Support services beyond those of the genetic counselling facility may be required, including social service, clergy, and dieticians. Good communication between the geneticist and the referring physician is essential. Lastly, the parents must feel confident that their needs, be they emotional or medical, will be met by a team with expertise in this area.

PROCEDURES FOR PRENATAL DIAGNOSIS

There are two basic approaches to identifying fetal defects: visualization and analysis of fetal tissues (Table 111.1). Which approach is taken depends on the specific information being sought.

Visualization of the fetus or fetal parts provides structural information, and may reveal anatomical abnormalities. Visualization is also frequently needed for the performances of other invasive procedures used to obtain fetal tissues for analysis.

Analysis of fetal tissue may provide a wealth of information about the genetic endowment of the fetus (Table 111.2). However, fetal tissue is obtained and analyzed only for the specific condition for which the fetus is at risk. The particular disorder which prompts the prenatal diagnostic effort usually determines the type of analysis to be done, the specific tissue which needs to be obtained for that analysis, and the optimal and safest technique for obtaining it. For example, although most biochemical analyses are performed on cells obtained by amniocentesis or chorionic villus sampling, several urea cycle enzymes are not normally expressed in these cells; prenatal diagnosis for these disorders cannot therefore be achieved by enzyme analysis of amniotic fluid (AF) cells. Prenatal diagnosis of these disorders may be achieved,

Table 111.1 Methods used for prenatal diagnosis

Visualization of the fetus
　Noninvasive:
　　Ultrasonography
　　Radiography
　Invasive:
　　Fetoscopy
　　Fetography
　　Amniography

Analysis of fetal tissues
　Amniocentesis
　Chorionic villi sampling
　Fetoscopy:
　　Fetal blood sampling
　　Fetal skin biopsy
　　Fetal liver biopsy
　Percutaneous umbilical blood sampling

Table 111.2 Types of studies performed on fetal tissues

Cytogenetic studies
Biochemical analysis:
　Quantitation of metabolites
　Quantitation of specific proteins
　Enzyme assay
DNA hybridization studies
Gene linkage analysis based on any of the above
Tissue histology

however, either by enzyme analysis of a different tissue (fetal liver), or by a different type of analysis (e.g. restriction endonuclease analysis of the DNA in amniocytes or chorionic villi).

In the following sections the specific procedures used for prenatal diagnosis will be reviewed, along with their indications and risks. Although prenatal diagnostic procedures may be performed throughout gestation, this discussion will be limited to those studies that may be completed prior to 24 weeks' gestational age.

Ultrasonography

The application of ultrasonographic methods to the study of human anatomy has had a tremendous impact on all areas of medicine. The development of high resolution real-time scanners has made it possible to visualize essentially any part of the fetus' anatomy in exquisite detail (Hobbins et al 1979, Sabbagha & Shkolnik 1980, Hill et al 1983).

Until recently only a limited amount of information could be obtained during the first trimester. However, the gestational sac can be visualized as early as 5½–6 weeks' menstrual age and cardiac activity is detectable at 7–8 weeks with generally available equipment. With the use of vaginal transducers operating at higher frequencies it is now possible to identify the embedded embryo within days of the missed period (Timor-Tritsch et al 1988) and cardiac activity can be seen by 5–6 weeks. With the progress of this technology, the gestational age at which fetal anomalies may be diagnosed is ever decreasing. First trimester ultrasound for the diagnosis of fetal anomalies may well become a routine procedure in the future. It will undoubtedly continue to play an important role in the verification of a viable embryo and for guiding the passage of instruments for invasive procedures.

Second trimester ultrasound examination may be used as the primary diagnostic modality for a large and ever growing number of anomalies, or in conjunction with invasive diagnostic and therapeutic techniques such as amniocentesis, fetoscopy, percutaneous fetal blood sampling and transfusion, and in utero shunt placement and drainage for hydronephrosis. With current equipment, examinations for fetal anomalies are best performed between 16 and 20 weeks' gestational age. At this age the fetal structures are large enough to be identified, and, if needed, the examination can still be repeated in time to allow the woman the option of termination of pregnancy.

Mid-trimester ultrasound examinations have become commonplace (performed in 30–50% of all pregnancies in the USA) and are frequently performed in the obstetrician's office. However, such studies are frequently limited in scope and detail, providing information about gestational age (based on the biparietal diameter), verification of fetal life, and the identification of multiple gestations and the placental location.

More detailed examinations ('Level II and III' studies) are best performed by ultrasonographers with special interest and expertise in fetal anatomy, pathology and physiology. Prenatal diagnosis may be most successful when a particular defect is specifically sought. A thorough examination includes a variety of measurements to assess intrauterine growth, gestational age, and identify skeletal disproportions. In addition, each part of the fetal anatomy (face, head, chest, heart, abdomen, genitourinary system, and extremities) is examined individually in detail.

A variety of relatively nonspecific ultrasound findings may provide important information about fetal well-being and may indicate the need for more detailed examination of specific structures:

Estimation of fetal size Estimation of fetal size is possible by measurement of biparietal diameter, femur length, abdominal circumference and other measurements, but the prediction of fetal weight and diagnosis of intrauterine growth retardation is still often problematic. Estimation of gestational age is also based on fetal measurements, and is a common indication for ultrasound examination.

Oligo- and polyhydramnios Although estimation of amniotic fluid volume based on measurements of uterine and fetal dimensions is possible, recognition of oligohydramnios is most often based on the subjective impression of crowding of the intrauterine contents. The finding of oligohydramnios is very ominous. If the membranes have not ruptured its presence strongly suggests impairment of renal function, and careful examination of the kidneys and collecting system is mandatory.

Polyhydramnios is associated with fetal anomalies in 20% of cases. Many of these (anencephaly, spina bifida, gastrointestinal tract obstruction, intra-thoracic cysts, diaphragmatic hernia) can be diagnosed by visualization of the involved organ.

Ascites Fetal ascites is an ominous finding associated with Rh isoimmunization, chylous ascites, urinary tract obstruction, prune belly syndrome, and a variety of multiple anomaly syndromes, many of which can be more specifically diagnosed ultrasonographically.

Hydrops fetalis The ultrasonographic finding of the generalized oedema of hydrops carries a very grave prognosis. Several conditions known to cause this condition (Rh isoimmunization, thalassaemia, chromosome abnormalities, cardiac arrhythmias) may be specifically diagnosed by other means. However, many cases are idiopathic.

Abnormal fetal anatomy

There are six general ways in which specific fetal malformations may be visualized with ultrasound (Chervenak & Isaacson 1989): (1) absence of a normally present structure; (2) presence of additional structures which distort the normal fetal contour; (3) dilation of a structure behind an obstruction; (4) herniation through a structural defect; (5) abnormal size of the fetus or specific fetal structures; and (6) absent or abnormal fetal motion.

Absence of a normally present structure The most dramatic example of this type of anomaly is anencephaly, in which the echogenic bones of the skull are absent, and the normally well defined cerebral structures are replaced by a heterogeneous mass of cystic tissue (Fig. 111.1). Anencephaly can be diagnosed with essentially 100% accuracy. Alobar holoprosencephaly, in which there is absence of the midline cerebral structures, is also readily diagnosed. Renal agenesis has also been diagnosed, although errors have occurred. This may be attributable in part to inadequate visualization in the absence of adequate amounts of amniotic fluid. In some instances it may be appropriate to inject normal saline into the amniotic cavity, or to administer furosemide to the mother, thus stimulating fetal urine production to facilitate definition of the fetal bladder.

Presence of additional structures distorting normal contour Fetal teratomas may produce distortions of the fetal contour, most frequently in the sacrococcygeal region (Fig. 111.2). They are the most common fetal neoplasm. Cystic hygromas, arising from abnormal development of the lymphatic system, produce fluid filled protrusions about the fetal neck.

Dilation of a structure behind an obstruction Dilation can be caused by an obstruction to the normal flow of body fluids or secretions, including urine, amniotic fluid, and cerebrospinal fluid. Hydrocephalus is the most common anomaly in this category and is characterized by a relative enlargement of the ventricular system and fetal head. Small bowel obstruction can cause dilation proximal to the obstruction. For example, in duodenal atresia there is a characteristic 'double bubble' resulting from enlargement of the duodenum and stomach, with narrowing of the pylorus and duodenum (Fig. 111.3).

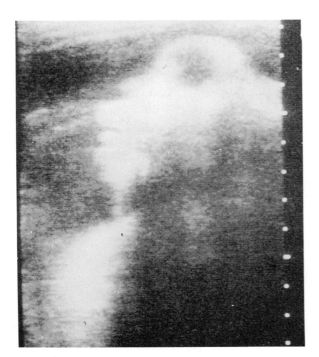

Fig. 111.1 Ultrasound of anencephalic fetus, approximately 20 weeks, showing facial profile. The remainder of the cranial vault is missing.

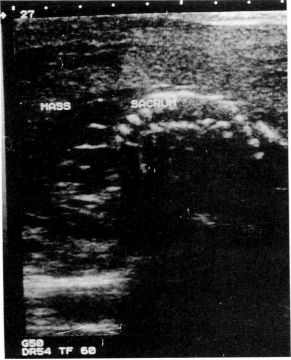

Fig. 111.2 Ultrasound of sacrococcygeal teratoma. The mass projects to the left, extending out of the sacrum.

This finding is a very important one, since as many as one third of fetuses with duodenal atresia have Down syndrome.

Urinary tract obstruction may also produce dilation of the proximal ureter or bladder, and can lead to megacystis, hydroureter, hydronephrosis and renal destruction. In some cases these findings may be indications for insertion of a suprapubic catheter in utero, to shunt the obstructed urine (see below).

Herniation through a structural defect Incomplete fusion of normal fetal structures can lead to defects through which otherwise contained structures may herniate. Defects in the development of the skull from the mesoderm which surrounds the rostral end of the neural tube may permit the formation of encephaloceles, herniations of meninges and, often, brain through the defect. Omphalocele, resulting from failure of the midgut to return to the abdomen after protruding into the umbilical cord, is another example of this type of anomaly. The protrusion of the abdominal contents can be seen sonographically. Diaphragmatic hernia, in which the abdominal organs may be present in the chest, is also readily diagnosable.

Abnormal size of the fetus or specific fetal structures Nomograms for the development of numerous fetal structures as a function of gestational age are now available (Zador et al 1988). Many fetal anomalies are best diagnosed by identifying an abnormality of the size of a structure, without there being abnormal shape or consistency. Microcephaly can be detected when the brain appears normal except for its small size. Assessments are frequently made by comparing the fetal biparietal diameter with other indices of fetal size, such as femur length. Similarly, a large number of skeletal dysplasias can be diagnosed by using fetal measurements, and ultrasonography has essentially supplanted radiographic methods for the initial prenatal diagnosis of these conditions (Grannum & Hobbins 1983, Donnenfeld & Mennuti 1987). Normative data on the lengths of the femur, tibia, humerus and ulna are available, and have made it possible to objectively assess fetal skeletal growth and proportion. Knowledge of the natural history of the disorder being sought, and sequential measurement of fetal limb lengths are critical for the diagnosis of some dysplasias (Donnenfeld & Mennuti 1987). For example, in heterozygous achondroplasia femur length is normal at 18 weeks, but growth is impaired thereafter. By 22 weeks femur length has fallen below the first percentile. Attempts to exclude the diagnosis prior to this age are obviously subject to error. Radiographic standards for normal and dysplastic fetuses are now available for corroboration of the diagnosis in utero (Ornoy et al 1988).

Absent or abnormal fetal motion The fetal heart is the most dynamic part of the fetus, and a variety of

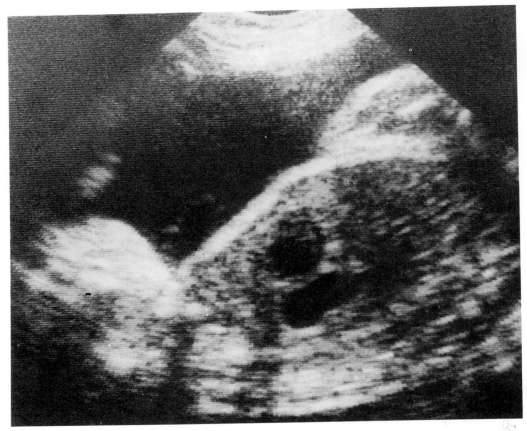

Fig. 111.3 Ultrasound of fetal abdomen at 30 weeks, showing the characteristic double-bubble of duodenal atresia. This fetus had Down syndrome.

structural defects can now be diagnosed with a combination of real-time and M-mode echocardiography (Allan et al 1984). Although false negative results still occur, their frequency has decreased dramatically. A variety of dysrhythmias and conduction disturbances have been recognized by examining and measuring cardiac valvular motion and rhythm. Structural defects which have been successfully diagnosed prior to 22 weeks include atrial septal defect, hypoplastic aortic arch, coarctation of the aorta, endocardial cushion defect, hypertrophic cardiomyopathy, mitral atresia with double outlet right ventricle, tricuspid atresia, hypoplastic left heart, and cardiac rhabdomyoma. Extra-cardiac anomalies may be found in more than 60% of cases and should be carefully looked for.

A partial listing of abnormalities which can be diagnosed in the second trimester is presented in Table 111.3 and discussed in several excellent reviews (Hobbins et al 1979, Sabbagha & Shkolnik 1980, Grannum &

Hobbins 1983, Hill et al 1983, Donnenfeld & Mennuti 1987, Vintzileos et al 1987).

There is no convincing evidence of any adverse effects of ultrasound exposure, even when repeated examinations have been performed. However, the possibility remains that unrecognized effects may occur, and further study is required (NIH Consensus Panel 1984).

In view of the apparent safety of prenatal ultrasound examinations, and the potential for the prenatal diagnosis of medically significant conditions, substantial consideration has been given to the routine examination of all pregnancies for the detection of birth defects. Indeed, this practice has been implemented in Scotland, West Germany, Belgium and Sweden, and evidence for its effectiveness presented (Persson & Kullander 1983). However, after review of the available data, the NIH Consensus Panel (1984) concluded that although routine screening can improve the detection of twins and congenital malformations, there was still insufficient

Table 111.3 Disorders diagnosable by ultrasonography in the second trimester

Hydrops	*Renal/GU*
Oligohydramnios	Cystic kidneys
Polyhydramnios	Renal agenesis
	Hydronephrosis
Face and Neck	
Branchial cleft cyst	*Skeletal anomalies*
Cleft lip/palate	Adactyly
Cystic hygroma	Ectrodactyly
Hypotelorism	Polydactyly
Micrognathia	Fractures
	Limb reduction deformities
Central Nervous System	
Anencephaly	*Skeletal dysplasias*
Encephalocele	Achondrogenesis IA,
Holoprosencephaly	IB and II
Hydranencephaly	Achondroplasia (late)
Hydrocephalus	Asphyxiating thoracic
Lipomeningocele	dysplasia
Meningomyelocele	Atelosteogenesis
Microcephaly	Campomelic dysplasia
	Chondroectodermal
Chest	dysplasia
Congenital heart disease	Diastrophic dysplasia
Cystic adenomatoid	Dyssegmental dysplasia
malformation of the lung	Hypophosphatasia,
Diaphragmatic hernia	infantile type
Pleural effusion	Kyphomelic dysplasia
Pulmonary hypoplasia	Melnick-Needles syndrome
Small thoracic cavity	Osteogenesis imperfecta
	Roberts syndrome
Abdomen/GI	Schneckenbecken dysplasia
Duodenal atresia	Short-rib polydactyly, type I
Oesophageal atresia	(Saldino-Noonan)
Gastroschisis	Short-rib polydactyly,
Omphalocele	type II (Majewski)
	Spondyloepiphyseal
	dysplasia congenita
	Thanatophoric dysplasia
	Thrombocytopenia-absent-
	radius

evidence of improved outcome or benefit to the mother or fetus to warrant routine screening at this time. Nonetheless, we believe that high quality ultrasound examinations for fetal assessment should be offered to all pregnant women.

Radiographic methods

Although mineralization of the fetal skeleton is adequate to permit radiographic examination, early experience with this modality was disappointing, and ultrasonography has essentially replaced radiographic methods for the initial diagnosis of skeletal anomalies. Fetal X-rays may be useful in defining the exact diagnosis in certain instances. Fetography and amniography have been largely supplanted by ultrasonography. In amniography, a water-soluble dye was injected into the amniotic cavity and permitted visualization of the fetal contour by contrast. In addition, some of the contrast material was swallowed by the fetus and outlined the gastrointestinal tract. In fetography, an oil-soluble contrast material was used and adhered to the fetal vernix, permitting visualization of the fetal contour.

Fetoscopy

Fetoscopy was developed as a method for direct visualization of the fetus and has been employed for cannulation of umbilical vessels for blood sampling and transfusion, fetal skin biopsy and fetal liver biopsy (Elias 1980, 1987, Rodeck et al 1982, Rodeck & Nicolaides 1983, 1986, Nicolaides & Rodeck 1984). The most widely used instruments are rigid endoscopes with an outer diameter of 1.7 mm. They contain a fibre-optic light source and self-focusing lens. The depth of focus is approximately 2 cm, and the viewing angle is 55 or 70 degrees (depending on the model). There is a variable magnification factor, depending on the viewing distance. The endoscope is inserted through an oval shaped cannula, 2.7–3.0 mm in the greater diameter. Some models have a separate channel for instruments for fetal blood sampling, transfusion or biopsy.

The procedure is best performed between the 17th and 20th weeks of gestation. Ultrasound is peformed prior to the procedure for location of the placenta and umbilical cord insertion, determination of the fetal position and selection of an insertion site, as well as for the confirmation of fetal viability, gestational age, and detection of multiple gestations. In addition, real-time ultrasonography is useful for directing and orienting the fetoscope during the procedure.

Light sedation (e.g. with diazepam) is often desirable to reduce fetal and maternal motion. Under strict aseptic conditions, the trochar and cannula are inserted through a stab incision under local anaesthesia. The trochar and cannula are advanced into the amniotic cavity, the trochar removed, and the fetoscope inserted through the cannula. Because of the short viewing distance and limited viewing angle, the area seen is usually only 2–4 cm^2. Positioning the fetoscope near the fetal part of interest is facilitated by ultrasonography. Fetal blood samples (of approximately 1 ml) can be obtained through a 25- or 27-gauge flexible needle from an umbilical vessel near the insertion of the cord in the placenta. If a biopsy is to be obtained, the cannula is positioned at the desired site (e.g. back, scalp, thorax) and if a fetoscope without a biopsy channel is being used, the fetoscope is removed, the biopsy forceps or needle inserted, and the sample

Table 111.4 Disorders which have been diagnosed by fetal skin biopsy

Disorder	Inheritance
Epidermolysis bullosa letalis	AR
Epidermolysis bullosa, recessive dystrophic	AR
Epidermolysis bullosa, recessive atrophicans inversa	AR
Epidermolytic hyperkeratosis	AD
Harlequin ichthyosis	AR
Lamellar ichthyosis	AR
Oculocutaneous albinism	AR
Sjögren Larsson syndrome	AR

Table 111.5 Conditions diagnosable by fetal blood sampling

Disorder	Inheritance
Coagulation disorders	
Congenital amegakaryocytic thrombocytopenia	AR
Haemophilia A and B	X-linked
Thrombocytopenia-absent radius	AR
Von Willebrand disease (homozygous)	
Fetal infection	
Haemoglobinopathies	AR
Immunological disorders	
Chédiak-Higashi syndrome	AR
Chronic granulomatous disease	X-linked
Severe combined immune deficiency	AR, X-linked
Wiskott-Aldrich syndrome	X-linked
Metabolic disorders	
Alpha-1-antitrypsin deficiency	AR
Galactosaemia	AR
Homocystinuria	AR
Mucopolysaccharidosis	AR
Metachromatic leucodystrophy	AR
Tay-Sachs disease	AR
Chromosome abnormalities	
Fragile-X syndrome	X-linked

taken. With some models of fetoscope the biopsy forceps may be inserted through a separate channel and the specimen taken under direct vision.

Fetoscopy has enjoyed a limited but important role in prenatal diagnosis. Because of the small viewing angle, its utility for direct visualization of the fetus is limited. It has been useful for blood sampling and intravascular transfusion, but these procedures can now be performed percutaneously under ultrasonographic guidance (see below) with smaller instruments and less risk to the pregnancy. It is quite likely that skin biopsy could also be performed percutaneously with ultrasonographic guidance. Fetal liver biopsy, which has been performed with fetoscopic guidance for the diagnosis of ornithine transcarbamylase deficiency (Rodeck et al 1982), is also amenable to this more direct approach (Holzgreve & Golbus 1981).

The major risk of fetoscopy is spontaneous abortion, which occurs after as many as 5–10% of all procedures (Rodeck & Nicolaides 1986, Elias 1987), although rates as low as 2% have been reported (Rodeck & Nicolaides 1986). Premature labour occurs in an additional 10% of patients, but this is probably only slightly higher than the expected rate. Amnionitis occurs in 0.3–0.5% of patients (Rodeck & Nicolaides 1986). Leakage of amniotic fluid per vagina occurs in 4–5% of patients. Rh isoimmunization may occur, and Rh immune globulin is generally given to Rh negative women at risk. There is little evidence for non-fatal fetal injury, although scarring at the site of a skin biopsy has been observed (Elias 1987).

Some of the genodermatoses which have been diagnosed by fetal skin biopsy are listed in Table 111.4. The analysis of fetal blood samples will be discussed below.

Placentocentesis and percutaneous umbilical blood sampling

Placentocentesis, usually performed at 18 weeks' gestation, is a method for obtaining fetal blood samples. As a result of improved ultrasound equipment, it has been replaced by direct umbilical vessel sampling, and is mentioned here because of its historical importance. The procedure was performed by direct insertion of a spinal needle into the placenta under ultrasonographic guidance (Kan et al 1974, Golbus et al 1976). The blood samples obtained were frequently contaminated with amniotic fluid or maternal blood, and the complications of the procedure included a relatively high fetal loss rate (5%), the risk of trauma to a major vessel with potentially disastrous consequences, and the danger of fetal maternal transfusion and the resultant possibility of Rh isoimmunization.

Percutaneous umbilical blood sampling (PUBS, cordocentesis) was first reported in 1983 by Daffos et al. They performed the procedure with local anaesthesia and real-time ultrasonographic guidance in pregnancies from 17–38 weeks' gestation. Using aseptic technique, a 10 cm 20-, 22- or 25-gauge spinal needle attached to a 2 ml syringe is introduced in the plane of the ultrasound and guided to the insertion of the umbilical cord at the placenta. If the cord insertion is anterior, the needle is guided through the placenta and never enters the amniotic cavity; if the insertion is posterior, the needle passes through the amniotic cavity and avoids the placenta. The cord is then penetrated 1–2 cm from its placental insertion, the stylet removed, and 1–3 ml of blood aspirated from the umbilical vessel. After removal of the needle the site is observed until bleeding ceases, usually only a few seconds (Ludomirski et al 1987). The entire procedure usually takes less than 10 minutes. Dilution of the samples with amniotic fluid may occur, but contamination with maternal blood does not appear to be a problem. Daffos et al (1985) reported a fetal loss rate (intrauterine deaths and spontaneous abortions) of 1.9% in pregnancies followed to completion. In six of the seven losses, there were other conditions identified which may have contributed to the pregnancy loss. Premature delivery (prior to 37 weeks) occurred in 5% of continuing pregnancies, which is probably no more than the expected rate.

PUBS has several advantages over fetoscopically guided blood sampling. Most importantly, the needle used is considerably smaller than a fetoscope, which probably accounts for the substantially lower risk of fetal loss. Like fetoscopy, it may be used for transfusion or partial exchange transfusion of blood directly into a fetal vessel (Grannum et al 1986).

Fetal blood sampling is indicated for the diagnosis of diseases which are manifest in the plasma or cellular components of the blood, and which cannot be diagnosed by less invasive procedures (Table 111.5). Specific examples of these, and the methods for their diagnosis are discussed in a subsequent section. In addition to these indications, there are occasions when time constraints do not permit amniocentesis and cell culture to be performed, and for this reason chromosomal or metabolic analyses may be performed on fetal blood samples. Rarely, prenatal blood sampling may be indicated because the results of chromosomal studies on cultured cells are ambiguous or inconclusive. This may occur with the prenatal diagnosis of the fragile-X syndrome, when chromosomal mosaicism has been detected, and when it is difficult to distinguish true mosaicism from pseudomosaicism (Watson et al 1984, Gosden et al 1988). Lastly, fetal blood sampling may be very useful for evaluating non-immune hydrops fetalis (Hsieh et al 1987), and for determining if fetal infection with toxoplasmosis (Desmonts et al 1985) or rubella (Daffos et al 1984) has occurred when there are signs of maternal infection with these organisms.

Amniocentesis

Transabdominal amniocentesis in combination with ultrasonography is undoubtedly the most widely used invasive technique for prenatal diagnosis because of the wealth of information that can be derived by studying material of fetal origin, namely the amniotic fluid cells and the fluid itself. Amniocentesis was first applied to the

prenatal determination of fetal sex by Barr body identification in the 1950s (Serr et al 1955, Fuchs & Riis 1956). Within 10 years, it was demonstrated that chromosome analyses could be performed on amniotic fluid cells (Steele & Breg 1966) and the first prenatal diagnosis of a chromosomal abnormality was reported (Jacobson & Barter 1967). A year later Nadler (1968) demonstrated the applicability of the technique to the diagnosis of the inborn errors of metabolism.

The amniotic fluid is probably derived from many sources: transudation of maternal serum across the placental membranes, fetal urine and tracheobronchial secretions, and secretion by the amniotic epithelium. The circulation of the fluid and origin of many of its components are still poorly understood. The volume of amniotic fluid increases during gestation to a maximum of approximately 1 litre at 38 weeks and gradually decreases thereafter (Elliot & Inman 1961). At 15–16 weeks' gestation approximately 180–200 ml is present (Wagner & Fuchs 1962) and the uterus has risen above the pelvic brim and is therefore accessible to a transabdominal approach (Gerbie & Elias 1980).

Prior to amniocentesis ultrasonography is used to: (1) verify fetal life; (2) determine gestational age; (3) diagnose multiple gestations; (4) determine placental and fetal positions; (5) detect fetal malformations or a hydatid mole; and (6) detect uterine malformations. If estimation of gestational age by measurement of biparietal diameter (BPD) is at variance with that calculated from the last menstrual period, the BPD is used for timing the amniocentesis and for the interpretation of the derived information.

Amniocentesis should be performed by an obstetrician skilled in the technique. It is commonly performed with real-time ultrasonographic guidance (Jeanty et al 1983), although certainly many thousands of procedures have been performed without the benefit of concurrent ultrasound. Immediately prior to the procedure, the woman is instructed to void. A local anaesthetic may be injected into the needle insertion site. Under strict aseptic conditions, a 3½ inch, 20- or 22-gauge spinal needle is then inserted and the stylet removed. A few drops of fluid are discarded to minimize the risk of contaminating the sample with maternal cells; if blood is present in the first drop and subsequently clears, the bloody aliquot is discarded and 20–30 ml of yellow-tinged fluid is gently aspirated, transferred to sterile tubes, and transported at room temperature to the laboratory as quickly as possible. A few drops of fluid may be observed for 'ferning' to ensure that the sample is not urine (Elias et al 1978). In diamniotic twin gestations a water soluble dye (e.g. indigo carmine) may be injected after withdrawal of the fluid. The needle is then removed and insertion in the second

Table 111.6 Indications for amniocentesis and chorionic villus sampling

Advanced maternal age
Previous child with a cytogenetic abnormality
Parental balanced translocation
First-degree relative with a neural tube defect
At risk for a diagnosable Mendelian disorder
At risk for an X-linked disorder

sac attempted. If colourless fluid is then aspirated it is probable that the first sac has not been re-entered. In many cases the fetal membranes and relationships can be clearly discerned with ultrasound, and injection of dye is unnecessary. After the procedure the woman may return to normal activity and is told to report any cramping or leakage of fluid from the puncture site or vagina.

In skilled hands an adequate sample is obtained on the first attempt in over 99% of cases, and successful amniotic fluid cell cultures are established in 98% of these. The samples can be sent to the laboratory by mail, although this increases the risk of unsuccessful culture.

The indications for amniocentesis are summarized in Table 111.6. Advanced maternal age is the most common indication and accounts for more than 90% of all prenatal diagnostic procedures (Simpson 1980). Although it is now widely appreciated that the risk of having a child with Down syndrome (trisomy 21) increases with increasing maternal age (Hook & Chambers 1977), it is perhaps less well known that the incidence of other chromosome anomalies increases as well (Table 111.7) (Hook & Chambers 1977, Hook 1981). Although it is established practice to inform women over the age of 35 of the availability of amniocentesis, the choice of 35 years as the cutoff is entirely arbitrary. In fact, the risk of a child with a chromosome abnormality begins to increase prior to age 30 and then continues to rise at an accelerated rate. We prefer to review the risks with prospective parents and let them decide at what age the risk is 'too high'.

Couples who have had a child with Down syndrome face a recurrence risk of 1% or more in each subsequent pregnancy; they are therefore considered candidates for prenatal diagnosis regardless of age. Although the recurrence risks for trisomy 18, trisomy 13, and Turner syndrome are less well established, prenatal diagnosis is often desirable for alleviation of parental anxiety.

A known cytogenetic abnormality (i.e. a balanced translocation) in one of the parents is a less frequent, but important indication for prenatal diagnosis. Such balanced translocations typically come to light after the birth of a child with an 'unbalanced' chromosomal rearrangement. Parental balanced translocations may

also be uncovered as part of the diagnostic evaluation of multiple spontaneous first trimester abortions.

A previous child or first-degree relative with a neural tube defect is another indication for amniocentesis. Although these defects are not inherited in a Mendelian fashion, a couple who has had a child with anencephaly or meningomyelocele faces approximately a 3% risk of having a second affected child. At least 90% of open defects (those in which there is communication between the subarachnoid space and the amniotic cavity) can be detected by measurement of alpha-fetoprotein in the amniotic fluid (Brock & Sutcliffe 1972, Milunsky & Alpert 1974, Crandall et al 1978, Second report of the UK collaborative study on alpha-fetoprotein in relation to neural tube defects 1979). Amniotic fluid acetylcholinesterase is also elevated in the presence of these defects and has proven to be a very useful diagnostic adjunct (Smith et al 1979, Zeisel et al 1980, Wald & Cuckle 1981, Milunsky & Sapirstein 1982).

Women who have had elevated serum alpha-fetoprotein levels on two occasions during pregnancy, and whose gestational timing has been confirmed by ultrasound examination, are at markedly increased risk of having a child with a neural tube defect and are candidates for amniocentesis for definitive diagnosis.

Many inborn errors of metabolism and lysosomal storage diseases can be diagnosed by measurement of the relevant enzyme in amniotic fluid cells grown in tissue culture. Enzyme activities can also be determined in the cell-free amniotic fluid itself, but measurement in the latter has generally been less reliable than assays performed with cultivated cells. This type of analysis is usually possible only after a couple has had one child with the disease, as it is essential that the diagnosis in the index case be firmly established before the prenatal diagnosis is attempted. In instances where carrier detection is available (such as Tay-Sachs disease) it is possible to identify pregnancies at risk prior to the birth of an affected child and to perform appropriate biochemical studies.

A growing list of inherited conditions can now be diagnosed by the analysis of fetal cells for specific genes, or segments of DNA linked to specific genes. Perhaps most notable among these diseases are the haemoglobinopathies, and other diseases in which the genetic defect is not expressed in amniotic fluid cells.

Couples who are at risk of having a child with an X-linked recessive disorder are also candidates for amniocentesis for prenatal sex determination. Such couples may be identified after the birth of an affected son or, occasionally, from review of the family history. If specific diagnosis is not possible, one can at least offer these couples the opportunity to terminate the pregnancy if the

Table 111.7 Estimated incidence of chromosome abnormalities by 1-year maternal age intervals*

Maternal age	Down Syndrome		All chromosome anomalies[†]	
	Rate/thousand live births	Fractional rate	Rate/thousand live births	Fractional rate
30	1.13	1/885	2.6	1/385
31	1.21	1/826	2.6	1/385
32	1.38	1/725	3.1	1/323
33	1.69	1/592	3.5	1/286
34	2.15	1/465	4.1	1/244
35	2.74	1/365	5.6	1/179
36	3.49	1/287	6.7	1/149
37	4.45	1/225	8.1	1/123
38	5.66	1/177	9.5	1/105
39	7.21	1/139	12.4	1/81
40	9.19	1/109	15.8	1/63
41	11.71	1/85	20.5	1/49
42	14.91	1/67	25.5	1/39
43	19.00	1/53	32.6	1/31
44	24.20	1/41	41.8	1/24
45	30.84	1/32	53.7	1/18
46	39.28	1/25	68.9	1/15
47	50.04	1/20	89.1	1/11
48	63.75	1/16	115.0	1/9
49	81.21	1/12	149.3	1/7

*Hook & Chambers 1977, Hook 1981
[†] Excludes 47,XXX

fetus is male. In this way they may at least be certain of having an unaffected daughter.

The major risk of amniocentesis is fetal loss. In the NICHD study (1976) the rate of loss (spontaneous abortions, fetal deaths in utero and stillbirths) was 3.5% in the subjects and 3.2% in the controls; after adjustment for maternal age the rates were 3.3% and 3.4%, respectively. No difference in the distribution of fetal loss at various gestational ages was observed. The rate was not increased in women requiring more than one needle insertion and was not related to the volume of fluid withdrawn. If discoloured fluid (greenish-brown) is obtained, the fetal loss rate may be increased (Hanson et al 1985). Based on these and other data (O'Brien 1984, Hanson et al 1985) the increase in risk is generally taken to be less than 0.5%.

Although in the NICHD study and others (Golbus et al 1979) ultrasonographic localization of the placenta prior to the amniocentesis did not alter the outcome, subsequent studies have suggested that the use of real-time ultrasound during the procedure reduces the rate of fetal loss (Chandra et al 1979, Crandon & Peel 1979). In addition, the use of ultrasound reduces the frequency of dry and bloody taps, and the number of needle insertions required (Romero et al 1985).

Amnionitis occurs after amniocentesis with a frequency of less than 0.1% (Murken et al 1979). Rhesus isoimmunization may occur and is of particular concern if the amniotic fluid is bloody. Examination of a Kleihauer-Betke preparation of the maternal blood smear after amniocentesis has been advocated to detect entry of fetal blood cells into the maternal circulation, but this method is not sensitive enough to detect small but significant transfusions. Rh immune globulin (Rhogam) is therefore usually given after the procedure to all Rh negative women.

Despite much concern about possible injury from fetal puncture at the time of amniocentesis, no evidence for this occurrence was found in the NICHD study. Skin scarring and dimpling have been reported, however (Karp & Hayden 1977).

Amniotic fluid leakage and vaginal bleeding occur in less than 1% of women and are usually of no significance. Premature labour pains occurred very infrequently (0.2%) in the NICHD study.

Processing of the specimen should begin immediately on its arrival in the laboratory. Usually a portion of the fluid is analyzed for alpha-fetoprotein and the remainder introduced into tissue culture for subsequent cytogenetic analysis. Other studies are performed as indicated and are

Table 111.8 Disorders of amino acid and organic acid metabolism which may be diagnosable through amniocentesis or CVS

Disorder	Inheritance	Basis of diagnosis
Argininosuccinic aciduria	AR	Enzyme assay
Citrullinaemia	AR	Enzyme assay
Cystathioninuria	AR	Enzyme assay
Dihydropteridine reductase deficiency	AR	Enzyme assay
Gamma-glutamyl synthetase deficiency	AR	Enzyme assay
Glutaric aciduria	AR	Enzyme assay
Histidinaemia	AR	Enzyme assay
Homocystinuria	AR	Enzyme assay
3-Hydroxy-3-methylglutaryl CoA lyase deficiency	AR	Enzyme assay
Hypervalinaemia	AR	Enzyme assay
Hyperglycinaemia, non-ketotic form	AR	Amniotic fluid glycine: serine
Isovaleric acidaemia	AR	Enzyme assay
Beta-Ketothiolase deficiency	AR	Enzyme assay
Maple syrup urine disease	AR	Enzyme assay
Beta-Methylcrotonic aciduria	AR	Enzyme assay
Methylene tetrahydrofolate reductase deficiency	AR	Enzyme assay
Methylmalonic acidaemia	AR	Enzyme assay
Methyltetrahydrofolate homocysteine: methyltransferase deficiency	AR	Enzyme assay
Multiple carboxylase deficiency	AR	Enzyme assay
Ornithine transcarbamylase deficiency	X-linked	DNA
Ornithinaemia	AR	Enzyme assay
5-Oxoprolinuria	AR	Enzyme assay
Phenylketonuria	AR	DNA
Prolidase deficiency	AR	Enzyme assay
Propionic acidaemia	AR	Enzyme assay
Pyruvate carboxylase deficiency	AR	Enzyme assay
Pyruvate decarboxylase deficiency	AR	Enzyme assay
Pyruvate dehydrogenase deficiency	AR	Enzyme assay
Saccharopinuria	AR	Enzyme assay
Tyrosinaemia	AR	Enzyme assay

Table 111.9 Disorders of carbohydrate metabolism which may be diagnosable through amniocentesis or CVS

Disorder	Inheritance	Basis of diagnosis
Galactokinase deficiency	AR	Enzyme assay
Galactosaemia	AR	Enzyme assay
Glucose-6-phosphate dehydrogenase deficiency	X-linked	Enzyme assay
Glycogen storage diseases		
Type II – Pompe disease	AR	Enzyme assay
Type III – Debrancher deficiency	AR	Enzyme assay
Type IV – Brancher deficiency	AR	Enzyme assay
Type VIII – Phosphorylase kinase deficiency	X-linked	Enzyme assay
Phosphohexose isomerase deficiency	AR	Enzyme assay

discussed in detail below. Tables 111.8–111.12 list the various disorders which may be diagnosed. Because the number of disorders which may be diagnosed is always increasing, these lists should not be considered complete.

Early amniocentesis

With increasing experience and confidence of needle placement under ultrasound guidance it has become possible to perform amniocentesis earlier and earlier (Evans et al 1988). Motivated by the desirability of completing prenatal diagnostic studies as early as possible, and by the limited availability of chorionic villus sampling in many areas, several prenatal diagnosis programmes have begun offering amniocentesis as early as 10–14 weeks' gestation. Limited experience in the last few years suggests that the safety of the procedure is probably comparable to traditional amniocentesis, but long-term outcome studies are not yet available.

Early amniocentesis still does not enable chromosome analysis or biochemical analyses to be performed as quickly as they can be after chorionic villus sampling (CVS). However, it may be useful in some twin pregnancies (in which sampling both fetuses may not be possible by CVS) or other circumstances in which CVS is contraindicated (see below). Early amniocentesis may also be very useful for neural tube defect detection, since this cannot be done through CVS (Evans et al 1988).

Chorionic villus sampling

Although amniocentesis has proven to be very safe and highly reliable, the desirability of a procedure which could provide information prior to 18 or 20 weeks' gestation is obvious. Although the decision to terminate a pregnancy is rarely (if ever) easy, it is perhaps more easily made earlier in pregnancy. Early attempts to use trophoblast tissue for prenatal diagnosis during the first trimester suffered from technical difficulties in obtaining the tissue, and problems culturing the cells (Kullander & Sandahl 1973, Hahnemann 1974). The first promising report of successful first trimester prenatal diagnosis by chorionic villus sampling came from the Tietung Hospital of the Anshan Iron and Steel Company in China (1975). The technique of transcervical villus aspiration was performed without ultrasonographic guidance for the prenatal determination of fetal sex. Despite the report of a high success rate and relatively low abortion rate (5%) the procedure was abandoned because of the extreme sex selection bias that occurred. The next report came from the Soviet Union (Kazy et al 1982) where, with ultrasound guidance, the technique was used in pregnancies at risk for X-linked disorders and metabolic

diseases. The method was applied soon after to the diagnosis of haemoglobinopathies using DNA hybridization techniques on uncultured trophoblast tissue (Old et al 1982) and a detailed description of the technique followed (Ward et al 1983). A method for chorion biopsy under direct vision was also described (Gosden et al 1982). It remained only for Simoni et al (1983) to adapt cytogenetic techniques to yield satisfactory karyotypes from the trophoblast tissue to establish CVS as a promising new approach to first trimester prenatal diagnosis.

The chorion frondosum consists of an outer layer of trophoblast cells and an inner layer of mesoderm. The chorion forms an arbor-like network of villi which completely surrounds the embryo. The villi which face the uterine cavity (i.e. in the decidua capsularis) eventually degenerate (chorion laeve). The villi in the decidua basalis ultimately form the placenta. At 8 weeks' gestation the chorion projects into the uterine cavity. It is 3–6 mm thick, while the overlying decidua is only 2 mm thick. CVS is usually not attempted prior to this time because of difficulty identifying the chorion before 8 weeks, and the very thin area into which the catheter would have to be manoeuvred to obtain a sample. Transcervical sampling before 8 weeks', or after 12 weeks' gestation, appears to increase the risk of fetal loss (Hogge et al 1986).

Several methods for transcervical CVS have been described (Lilford 1986). Prior to the procedure the vagina and cervix are cleaned with a povidone iodine solution, and a tenaculum may be placed on the cervix to permit manipulation to ease passage of the instruments.

One of the earlier techniques for chorion biopsy employed direct endoscopic visualization of the chorion and villi, with or without ultrasonographic guidance of the endoscope. This technique is now rarely used (Ghirardini et al 1986, Holzgreve et al 1986, Mencaglia et al 1986).

The more commonly employed technique relies entirely on ultrasound guidance, without benefit of direct vision (Fig. 111.4). A metal sound is introduced through the internal cervical os to chart the path for the catheter on the ultrasound, and to determine the degree of curvature between the cervical canal and the placenta. A malleable catheter (usually plastic with an aluminium obturator) 1–2 mm in diameter is then bent to permit easy passage through the cervix and manoeuvring to the implantation site. A flexible biopsy forceps may be used instead of a catheter (Kazy et al 1982, Goossens et al 1983). The tip of the instrument is advanced through as much of the placenta as is possible. The metal obturator is removed, a 20 cc syringe is attached to the catheter, and suction is applied. The catheter is then slowly pulled back, with some rotation, to increase tissue aspiration. The villi which are torn from the chorion are taken up in

Table 111.10 Disorders of lysosomal enzymes which may be diagnosable through amniocentesis or CVS

Disorder	Inheritance	Basis of diagnosis
Acid phosphatase deficiency	AR	Enzyme assay
Aspartylglucosaminuria	AR	Enzyme assay
Cholesterol ester storage disease	AR	Enzyme assay
Fabry disease	X-linked	Enzyme assay
Farber disease	AR	Enzyme assay
Fucosidosis	AR	Enzyme assay
Gaucher disease, Types I, II, III	AR	Enzyme assay
GM1 gangliosidosis (all types)	AR	Enzyme assay
GM2 gangliosidosis		
Tay Sachs disease	AR	Enzyme assay
Sandhoff disease	AR	Enzyme assay
Krabbe disease (Globoid cell leucodystrophy)	AR	Enzyme assay
Mannosidosis	AR	Enzyme assay
Metachromatic leucodystrophy	AR	Enzyme assay
Mucolipidosis		
Type I	AR	Enzyme assay
Type II	AR	Enzyme assay
Type III	AR	Enzyme assay
Type IV	AR	Intracellular inclusions
Mucopolysaccharidosis		
Type I H Hurler syndrome	AR	Enzyme assay
Type I S Scheie syndrome	AR	Enzyme assay
Type I H/S Hurler/Scheie	AR	Enzyme assay
Type II Hunter syndrome	X-linked	Enzyme assay
Type III A Sanfilippo A	AR	Enzyme assay
Type III B Sanfilippo B	AR	Enzyme assay
Type III C Sanfilippo C	AR	Enzyme assay
Type III D Sanfilippo D	AR	Enzyme assay
Type IV Morquio syndrome	AR	Enzyme assay
Type VI Maroteaux-Lamy	AR	Enzyme assay
Type VII Beta-glucuronidase deficiency	AR	Enzyme assay
Multiple sulphatase deficiency	AR	Enzyme assay
Niemann-Pick disease, types A, B, C	AR	Enzyme assay
Sialidosis	AR	Enzyme assay
Wolman disease	AR	Enzyme assay

Table 111.11 Other enzyme deficiencies which may be diagnosable through amniocentesis or CVS

Disorder	Inheritance	Basis of diagnosis
Acatalasia	AR	Enzyme assay
Acyl CoA dehydrogenase deficiency (short, medium, long chain)	AR	Enzyme assay
Adenosine deaminase deficiency	AR	Enzyme assay
Congenital adrenal hyperplasia (21-hydroxylase deficiency)	AR	Linkage analysis
Ehlers-Danlos syndrome		
Type VI	AR	Enzyme assay
Type VII	AR	Enzyme assay
Familial hypercholesterolaemia	AD	Enzyme assay
Hypophosphatasia	AR	Enzyme assay
Ichthyosis (steroid sulphatase)	X-linked	Enzyme assay
Lesch-Nyhan syndrome	X-linked	Enzyme assay; DNA
Nucleoside phosphorylase deficiency	AR	Enzyme assay
Orotic aciduria	AR	Enzyme assay
Porphyria		
Acute intermittent porphyria	AD	Enzyme assay
Congenital erythropoietic porphyria	AR	Enzyme assay
Coproporphyria	AD	Enzyme assay
Protoporphyria	AD	Enzyme assay
Variegate porphyria	AD	Enzyme assay
Refsum disease	AR	Enzyme assay
Sulphite oxidase deficiency	AR	Enzyme assay

Table 111.12 Miscellaneous disorders which may be diagnosable through amniocentesis or CVS

Disorder	Inheritance	Basis of diagnosis
Adrenoleucodystrophy	X-linked	Very long chain fatty acids
Alpha-1-antitrypsin deficiency	AR	DNA
Antithrombin III deficiency	AD	DNA
Chédiak-Higashi disease	AR	Amniotic fluid cell inclusions
Chromosomal abnormalities	—	Karyotype
Chromosome instability syndromes		
Ataxia telangiectasia	AR	Bleomycin induced chromosome breaks
Bloom syndrome	AR	Sister chromatid exchange
Fanconi anaemia	AR	DEB induced breaks
Xeroderma pigmentosum	AR	DNA repair synthesis
Cockayne syndrome	AR	Colony forming ability; recovery of RNA synthesis
Congenital nephrosis (Finnish type)	AR	Amniotic fluid AFP
Cystic fibrosis	AR	Amniotic fluid microvillar enzymes; DNA
Cystinosis	AR	Intracellular cystine
Duchenne/Becker muscular dystrophy	X-linked	DNA
Ehlers-Danlos syndrome, type IV	AD	DNA
Haemoglobinopathies/thalassaemias	AR	DNA
Haemophilia A and B	X-linked	DNA
Huntington chorea	AD	DNA
Menke kinky hair	X-linked	Copper accumulation
Myotonic dystrophy	AD	Linkage to secretor gene; DNA
Neural tube defects	—	Amniotic fluid AFP
Norrie disease	X-linked	DNA
Osteogenesis imperfecta		
Type I	AD	DNA
Type II, III	AD, AR	Collagen secretion, DNA
Type IV	AD	DNA
Polycystic kidney disease (adult type)	AD	DNA
Primary pituitary dysgenesis	AR	Amniotic fluid prolactin
Retinoblastoma	AD	DNA
Tangier disease	AR	Amniotic fluid apoA-I
Tuberous sclerosis	AD	DNA
Zellweger syndrome	AR	Peroxisomal enzyme assay, very long chain fatty acids

tissue culture medium and examined under the dissecting microscope to determine the adequacy of the sample. If decidua or other debris is present, this material is removed prior to any further processing of the tissue. Sample sizes vary, but usually weigh 5–20 mg. An adequate sample is successfully obtained on the first attempt by an experienced operator in 85% of cases, and after two attempts in 98% of cases. Most workers will not attempt more than two passes in a single session, because the risk of infection and spontaneous abortion may be increased.

Transcervical CVS is contraindicated in cases of vaginitis, vaginismus, active bleeding, inaccessible cervical canal, multiple gestations, and previous Rh isoimmunization (Brambati et al 1987b,c). A long and/or narrow cervical canal, or pronounced angle of the sampling route, may make a transcervical approach difficult, but are not absolute contraindications.

CVS may also be performed using a transabdominal approach. The theoretical advantages of this approach include the possibility of a lower risk of infection, and easier access to fundal placentas. It may be performed throughout pregnancy, while transcervical sampling cannot be carried out after 12 weeks. The transabdominal approach may also be easier to learn than the transcervical approach (Carpenter et al 1987) and may be suitable when the transcervical approach is contraindicated, difficult because of the pelvic anatomy, or when the transcervical approach has failed to produce satisfactory samples (Brambati et al 1987c, Carpenter et al 1987). In addition, the spinal needles used for performing transabdominal CVS are readily available. In contrast, transcervical catheters are regulated in the USA by the Federal Drug Administration as 'investigational devices', and their distribution is therefore limited.

The patient is prepared for transabdominal CVS in the

same fashion as for amniocentesis. Using ultrasonographic guidance, an 18-gauge needle is inserted through the abdominal and uterine walls to the edge of the placenta (Maxwell et al 1986). A 20-gauge needle is then passed through this, to a point in the chorion between the edge of the developing placenta and the cord insertion, and suction applied (Fig. 111.5). Alternatively, a 20-gauge needle may be passed alone, without prior insertion of the canula (Brambati et al 1987c). In experienced hands, an adequate specimen is obtained on the first attempt in 95% of cases.

The choice of approach (transcervical or transabdominal) depends on placental location and the experience of the operator. Both approaches will undoubtedly play important roles in prenatal diagnosis in the future.

As with amniocentesis there has been great concern about the risk of spontaneous abortion or fetal injury as a result of CVS. The first major problem in determining the loss rate, however, is differentiating the true procedure-related losses from the spontaneous losses. The fetal loss rate after a normal ultrasound at 8–10 weeks is estimated to be 1.4–2.7% (Gilmore & McNay 1985,

Wilson et al 1986, Liu et al 1987). However, the spontaneous abortion rate increases with maternal age (and other factors such as tobacco and alcohol consumption). Since 80–90% of CVS are performed in women over the age of 35, the spontaneous abortion rate at this age (4.0–4.3%) is more relevant (Gilmore & McNay 1985, Wilson et al 1986).

In two large published series of transcervical CVS (Hogge et al 1986, Brambati et al 1987b), the fetal loss rates in pregnancies sampled between 9 and 12 weeks ranged from 3.8% to 4.1%. This is comparable to the data from the World Health Organization registry (Jackson 1987), which now includes over 50 000 procedures worldwide. The average fetal loss rate, for all approaches (i.e. transcervical and transabdominal) since the inception of the registry was 3.7% in November 1987.

The fetal loss rate appears to increase when the procedure is performed prior to 9 weeks or after 12 weeks (Hogge et al 1986), if there are more than two catheter insertions (Brambati et al 1987b), and when the experience of the operator is limited (Hunter et al 1986). The data from the World Health Organization registry do

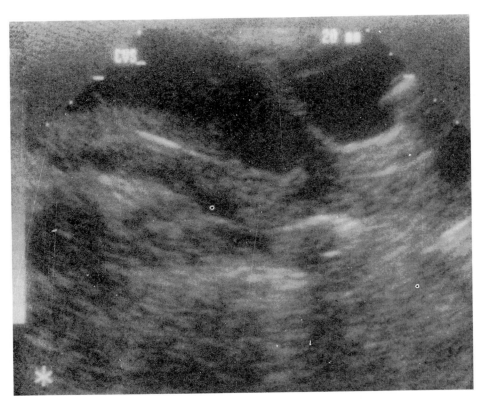

Fig. 111.4 Ultrasound of transcervical chorionic villus sampling procedure. The catheter is seen as a long white line passing through the cervix on the right, and continuing into the posterior placenta.

not indicate a difference in loss rates between the transabdominal approach and the transcervical approach, but do suggest that the use of biopsy forceps may be associated with a higher loss rate.

The reported fetal loss rates are very similar to the spontaneous abortion rates noted above, but the data are not strictly comparable. CVS permits the diagnosis of chromosome abnormalities early in gestation. If untreated, many of these pregnancies would terminate spontaneously, but instead are terminated electively when the abnormality is identified. If elective abortions for chromosome abnormalities were not performed after CVS, the rate of spontaneous abortion following the procedure would be higher than has actually been observed.

Large multicentre studies in the United States and Canada have compared the safety and efficacy of CVS with amniocentesis (Canadian Collaborative CVS-Amniocentesis Clinical Trial Group 1989, Rhoads et al 1989). These studies together examined more than 3000 women who underwent CVS, and 1990 who underwent amniocentesis. The fetal loss rate after CVS was 0.6–0.8% higher than the loss rate after amniocentesis, with a 95% upper confidence limit of 2.2–2.5%.

It appears likely that there is indeed a procedure-related increase in fetal loss rate associated with CVS. However, when CVS is performed by an experienced operator, the increased risk is probably no greater than 1% (Jackson 1986, Wilson et al 1987).

The other potential complications of CVS are of less significance, and to some degree preventable, if the procedure is performed by an experienced operator with strict adherence to aseptic technique. Uterine infection or chorioamnionitis has occurred after 0.2–0.6% of transcervical procedures, and was usually followed by loss of the pregnancy (Hogge et al 1986, Brambati et al 1987b). It has been suggested that unrecognized infection is in fact responsible for a significant percentage of spontaneous abortions which occur after the procedure (Wilson et al 1987). The occurrence of infection is not surprising in view of the normal colonization of the vagina and the observation that 30–50% of the catheters are contaminated after CVS, and 15% of the villi samples are also contaminated (Brambati et al 1987a, Perry et al 1987). Serious infections have occurred, but only rarely (Jackson 1985, Barela et al 1986, Lilford 1986).

Vaginal bleeding occurs in as many as 12% of patients in the 2-3 days following the procedure, and may last a few hours or a few days. It is usually benign, however. Intrauterine haematomas have been noted in 4% of women; these resolve prior to 16 weeks (Brambati et al 1987b). Perforation of the fetal membranes occurs very rarely in experienced centres, but despite this, oligohydramnios has been noted in 0.5% of cases, and is frequently associated with pregnancy loss (Hogge et al 1986). The rates of premature labour and non-chromosomal congenital defects do not appear to be increased, although one case of amniotic bands following CVS has been recorded (Planteydt et al 1986).

The risk of Rh isoimmunization has already been noted. That fetal-maternal transfusion can occur after CVS is evidenced by a rise in maternal serum alpha-fetoprotein after the procedure. This increase is greater after multiple catheter insertions (Blakemore et al 1986). However, the rise is transient, and does not affect the results of maternal serum alpha-fetoprotein screening for neural tube defects at 15-16 weeks.

ANALYSIS OF FETAL TISSUES

Maternal blood

The identification of Y chromosome containing cells in maternal blood samples has demonstrated that fetal cells may enter the maternal circulation as early as 15 weeks' gestation. This observation has suggested the possibility of fetal karyotyping using these cells. With the development of cell sorting methodology, it has become possible to sort leucocytes obtained from maternal blood and to prepare a fraction which is relatively 'enriched' in fetal cells (Herzenberg et al 1979). However, maternal cells still predominate, and the results of efforts to prepare fetal karyotypes from these preparations have not been encouraging. Furthermore, it is possible that fetal cells from previous gestations may persist and confuse the analysis. Multiple gestations would pose similar prob-

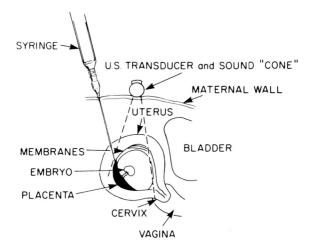

Fig. 111.5 Schematic illustration of transabdominal CVS. A spinal needle is inserted through the abdominal wall into the placenta.

lems. While there has been a great deal of excitement and interest in this approach, at the present time the technical obstacles seem overwhelming.

Maternal serum alpha-fetoprotein screening. Neural tube defects (anencephaly and meningomyelocele), which occur with a frequency of 1-2/1000 in the USA and 2-3/1000 in the UK, are among the most common of birth defects. Although most of these defects can be detected by measurement of amniotic fluid alpha-fetoprotein and/or ultrasound examination, more than 95% of all children with NTDs are born to women who have no specific indication for prenatal diagnosis. In 1973 Brock et al demonstrated that fetal AFP could be detected in maternal serum and used for the mid-trimester diagnosis of neural tube defects. By the mid 1970s maternal serum AFP (MSAFP) screening was routinely performed in the United Kingdom. Concern about the relatively high frequency of false positive results, and the difficulties in providing prompt results, counselling, and repeat testing for the large percentage of women expected to have 'positive' results, delayed the development and implementation of similar programmes in the United States until the mid 1980s.

Most programmes now recommend that MSAFP be measured at 15-16 weeks' gestation. 3-4% of women tested will have levels 2.5 times the median (Burton et al 1983). If the level is extremely elevated immediate ultrasound examination is appropriate. Otherwise, analysis of a second sample is recommended, and is normal in half of the cases. When both MSAFP levels are elevated (2% of the population) ultrasound examination is performed, and provides an explanation for the elevation in half of the cases. Most often the elevation is the result of inaccurate gestational dating, since MSAFP increases sharply in the second trimester (Fig. 111.6, bottom). Multiple gestations account for many of the remaining false positives. If the ultrasound establishes a singleton pregnancy and correct gestational age (1% of the population), amniocentesis for amniotic fluid AFP and acetylcholinesterase is recommended. However, only 10% of the women who have amniocentesis (approximately 0.1% of the population) are found to be carrying a fetus with an NTD.

MSAFP screening is subject to many difficulties and is best performed by centralized laboratories that are able to ensure the highest standards of quality control for this sensitive assay (Macri et al 1987, Simkowski 1987), and are able to accumulate sufficient data to establish reliable normative data on the levels of MSAFP in the population being screened (Evans et al 1987a). Furthermore, MSAFP screening requires prompt and conscientious follow-up, and the availability of competent and informed personnel to counsel those women whose first level is elevated (97% of whom are carrying healthy fetuses). Nonetheless, through MSAFP screening programmes it is possible to detect 90% of fetuses with NTDs.

A serendipitous use of MSAFP screening was suggested by Merkatz et al (1984), when they noted abnormally low mid-trimester MSAFP levels when the fetus was aneuploid. The statistical manipulations of such data have been refined, and have suggested a new approach to maternal age counselling for chromosome abnormalities. Instead of basing the risk of aneuploidy only on the mother's age, an adjusted risk can be established, based on the prior risk (maternal age) and how low the MSAFP is. In the clinical programme at Hutzel Hospital/Wayne State University, threshold levels for low MSAFP have been established for different maternal ages, so that a woman's risk of having an aneuploid infant (based on her age and MSAFP) is equivalent to the risk in a 35-year-old mother (i.e. approximately 1 in 200). Since the prior risk of aneuploidy for a 20-year-old woman is lower than the prior risk for a 30-year-old woman, the MSAFP level would have to be lower for the 20-year-old to fall below the threshold. In this programme, approximately 7% of women have had levels below the threshold, and an abnormal karyotype has been found in approximately 1/90 who have undergone amniocentesis. Approximately 40% of the abnormalities have been trisomy 21, 20% have been other trisomies, and the remaining patients have had a variety of different chromosomal disorders.

The protocol for the evaluation of low MSAFP is somewhat different from the NTD protocol (Evans et al 1987b). Low MSAFP values at 15 weeks (the earliest that most laboratories can interpret the data) are *not* repeated. There is some evidence that MSAFP levels in abnormal fetuses regress towards the mean with advancing gestational age; performing a repeat analysis on a sample obtained later in the pregnancy may therefore be futile (Haddow et al 1986). Furthermore, if amniocentesis and chromosome analysis are to be performed, with the results available early enough to permit termination of the pregnancy, time is of the essence.

Although the risk of chromosome abnormalities is higher in older women, most aneuploid children are born to mothers younger than 35 years. This simply reflects the higher birth rate in younger women. If cytogenetic prenatal diagnosis is offered only to women over the age of 35, only 15% of all aneuploid fetuses would be detected. By employing MSAFP screening as outlined above, as many as 40% of chromosomally abnormal fetuses could be detected (Evans et al 1987b). While not perfect by any means, the ability to place low risk patients (based on their age) into a high risk group (based on their MSAFP) has major implications for prenatal diagnosis.

Amniotic fluid

Because the amniotic fluid contains secretions of the fetal respiratory epithelium, amniotic epithelium, and fetal urine, it is rich in fetal hormones and metabolic products (Nadler & Gerbie 1969). However, the volume and composition of the fluid change throughout gestation, making it difficult to establish appropriate denominators

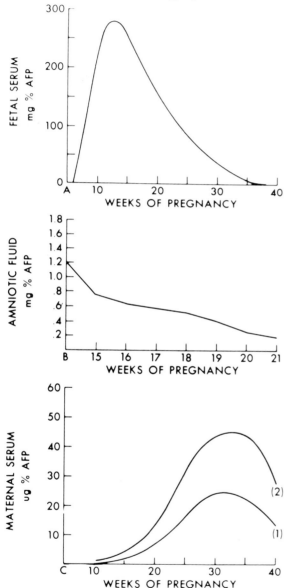

Fig. 111.6 Changes in alpha-fetoprotein concentrations during gestation. Top, fetal serum (from Gitlin & Boesman 1966; middle, amniotic fluid (from Crandall et al 1978); bottom, maternal serum (from Leighton et al 1975).

for expressing the concentrations of these products; normal ranges for most constituents are wide. For this reason analysis of amniotic fluid is infrequently used for prenatal diagnosis; analysis of cells in the amniotic fluid is preferable in a great many instances. There are, however, some important exceptions to this principle which will be discussed here.

Alpha-fetoprotein and the detection of neural tube defects. Neural tube defects are among the most common of congenital malformations. While surgical interventions have greatly improved morbidity and mortality in these disorders, primary prevention through prenatal diagnosis and termination has been possible since 1972 by the measurement of mid-trimester amniotic fluid alpha-fetoprotein levels (Brock & Sutcliffe 1972). Several excellent reviews have been written (Crandall et al 1978, Main & Mennuti 1986).

AFP is first detectable in fetal serum 30 days after conception. Early in gestation it is produced in the yolk sac, but hepatic synthesis increases steadily, and by the end of the first trimester the liver is the major site of production. The function of this albumin-like glycoprotein is unknown. Its concentration in fetal serum (Fig. 111.6, top) rises until 10–13 weeks and then declines steadily until adult levels are reached at 1 month of postnatal age. The decline in serum levels from 10–13 weeks is attributed to the increase in fetal size, since the total amount of circulating AFP remains fairly constant (Gitlin & Boesman 1966). Some of the protein is secreted in the urine and thereby enters the amniotic fluid where its concentration is 1/100 that of the fetal serum at 14 weeks. Amniotic fluid levels decline from about 2 mg/dl at 12–13 weeks to less than 0.5 mg/dl at 20 weeks (Fig. 111.6, middle) and an accurate assessment of gestational age is therefore critical for interpretation of levels (Seppälä & Ruoslahti 1972, Milunsky & Alpert 1974, Seller 1974).

The exact mechanism by which AFP levels are increased in NTDs is still unclear, but the reliability of AFP in the detection of open defects has been well established. Amniotic fluid AFP is elevated in 98% of pregnancies in which the fetus is anencephalic or has an open meningomyelocele (Second Report of the UK Collaborative Study on Alpha-fetoprotein in relation to neural tube defects 1979). Closed defects, which account for 10% of NTDs, often do not have elevated levels and may therefore escape detection. Some of these cases may be diagnosed by ultrasonography. Overall, more than 90% of all NTDs can be detected with the use of amniotic fluid and maternal serum AFP levels and ultrasonography.

Neural tube defects are not the only disorders associated with elevated amniotic fluid AFP levels. In congenital nephrosis of the Finnish type, missed abortion, severe Rh isoimmunization, oesophageal atresia, duodenal atresia, omphalocele, Turner syndrome with cystic hygromas and several chromosome abnormalities, increased AFP levels have been found (Guiband et al 1973, Seppälä 1973, Seppälä & Ruoslahti 1973a,b, Whyley et al 1974, De Bruijn & Huisjes 1975).

False positive elevations of amniotic fluid AFP may also occur. In the UK Collaborative Study, the rate of elevated AFPs without a neural tube defect was 0.8%. One third of these pregnancies subsequently ended in a spontaneous abortion. Half of the remaining fluids were blood tinged, and the presence of fetal blood in the specimens may have caused the increased level of AFP. In 1/3 of the remaining pregnancies (with clear amniotic fluid) severe congenital anomalies and other disorders associated with elevated amniotic fluid AFP were observed, so that the resulting 'practical' false positive rate was only 0.27%. This rate is approximately the same as the incidence of NTDs. This implies that an elevated amniotic fluid AFP is as likely to be a false positive as it is to be indicative of an NTD, since most amniocenteses are performed for cytogenetic indications (i.e. where there is no increased risk for an NTD). Therefore, when the amniotic fluid AFP is elevated, two complementary tests should be performed for specific diagnosis of an NTD or other defect: high quality ultrasonography, and measurement of amniotic fluid acetylcholinesterases.

Several cholinesterase isozymes are detectable in amniotic fluid (Smith et al 1979). The amniotic fluid level of acetylcholinesterase (AChE), which is synthesized in the central nervous system, is markedly elevated when there is an open NTD. AChE can be distinguished from the other isozymes by electrophoresis or with the use of specific inhibitors (Elejalde et al 1986). Elevations of AChE appear to be more specific for NTDs than are elevations of AFP (Milunsky & Sapirstein 1982). Therefore, it is routinely assayed when there is a high risk for an NTD, or for confirmation when the AFP is elevated.

Cystic fibrosis. A variety of approaches to the prenatal diagnosis of cystic fibrosis (CF) have been explored, largely without success. However, in 1983 reduced levels of several intestinal microvillar enzymes (peptidase, disaccharidases, and alkaline phosphatase) were reported in amniotic fluid samples from affected pregnancies (Brock 1983, Carbarns et al 1983, van Diggelen et al 1983). The lowered activity of these enzymes is presumed to result from a functional ileus, since reductions have also been observed in imperforate anus, duodenal atresia and other intestinal atresias (Morin et al 1987). Several cautions about the application of these observations to the prenatal diagnosis of CF must be noted, however. The

timing of the amniocentesis appears to be quite critical to the interpretation of the enzyme assays, with 17–18 weeks being optimal. More importantly, one must recognize the limited sensitivity and specificity of this approach, and the constraints they imply. When the risk of CF is 1 in 4 (i.e. in a couple with a previously affected child), the false positive rate is 1–4%, and the false negative rate is 6–8% (Brock et al 1985, Boué et al 1986). However, in a pregnancy not at increased risk for CF, an abnormal result is 30–60 times more likely to represent a false positive result than it is CF (Beaudet & Buffone 1987). For this reason, amniotic fluid microvillar enzyme analysis for prenatal diagnosis is applicable only when the risk of CF is considerably higher than the general population risk. Fortunately, the identification of probes to the short arm of chromosome 7, for nucleotide sequences which are linked to the CF gene, has permitted an alternative and more widely applicable approach based on DNA hybridization studies and linkage analysis (Farrall et al 1986, Spence et al 1987). At least 90% of families have 'informative' restriction fragment length polymorphisms (RFLPs) in this region (Beaudet & Buffone 1987). The recent cloning and sequencing of the CF gene (Rommens et al 1989) makes it possible to directly detect mutations which cause CF. Since 70% of the mutations in CF patients involve deletion of the same 3 base pairs (resulting in loss of a phenylalanine residue at position 508) (Kerem et al 1989), direct DNA based detection of the majority of cases will be possible. Furthermore, population based carrier testing based on detection of this deletion should also be possible.

Other disorders. The measurement of the abnormal metabolite succinyl acetone may be used for the prenatal diagnosis of hereditary tyrosinaemia (Gagne et al 1982). However confirmation by measurement of fumarylacetoacetase activity in amniotic fluid cells is probably indicated. The diagnosis may also be made by measurement of the enzyme activity in chorionic villi.

Although methylmalonic acidaemia (Morrow et al 1970), argininosuccinic aciduria (Fleisher et al 1977), multiple carboxylase deficiency, and propionic acidaemia may be recognized by accumulation of their respective metabolites in amniotic fluid, not all inborn errors are associated with metabolite accumulation in utero. In general, inborn errors of metabolism are most reliably diagnosed either by direct measurement of cellular enzyme activity, or by DNA hybridization methods.

The measurement of several hormone levels has been used for prenatal diagnosis of endocrinopathies. Primary pituitary dysgenesis, a rare autosomal recessive disorder, has been successfully diagnosed by means of amniotic fluid prolactin measurements (Stoll et al 1978). Determinations of pregnanetriol and 17-ketosteroid levels have been used for the diagnosis of congenital adrenal hyperplasia (CAH), but these analyses are unreliable in mid-trimester (Merkatz et al 1969). Levels of 17-alpha-hydroxyprogesterone are more consistently elevated in this disorder (Milunsky & Tulchinsky 1977) and are now used in conjunction with HLA typing of amniotic fluid cells for prenatal diagnosis of CAH.

Uncultivated amniotic fluid cells

The first application of amniocentesis to prenatal diagnosis was sex determination by examination for Barr bodies in uncultivated amniotic fluid cells. These fetal cells derive from the amnion itself, desquamation from the fetal skin, and mucosal surfaces (buccal and vaginal) and from the urine. Contamination of the fluid with maternal blood may, however, result in the presence of leucocytes. Although some of the cells possess some enzymatic activity (Nadler & Gerbie 1969), many are non-viable and serve only to render interpretation of results more difficult. At present there are no reliable enzymatic assays based on uncultivated amniotic fluid cells. DNA hybridization studies can be performed on uncultivated cells, but the use of cultivated cells is preferred.

Cultivated amniotic fluid cells

Four types of study are commonly performed using amniotic fluid cells: cytogenetic analyses, enzyme assays, linkage analyses, and DNA hybridization studies. In each case, the amniotic fluid cells are inoculated into several flasks containing tissue culture medium prior to analysis. After 2–3 weeks sufficient growth has occurred to permit harvesting of the cultures and analysis.

Cytogenetic studies

Approximately 90% of all amniocenteses are performed for cytogenetic analysis. The data presented in Table 111.7, demonstrating the increasing risk of Down syndrome and other chromosome abnormalities with advancing maternal age, form the basis for the recommendation that women over the age of 35 consider amniocentesis. Other cytogenetic indications will be discussed later. The fibroblast-like cells obtained at amniocentesis can be cultured in a variety of tissue culture media enriched with fetal calf serum, and after 1–3 weeks sufficient cells have grown to permit karyotyping. A minimum of 15 cells is examined and the modal chromosome number established. A smaller number of cells is then examined after Q- or G-banding to detect minor structural rearrangements. The original

fluid specimen should be seeded into at least two culture flasks, and samples from each studied.

Sex determination and abnormalities of chromosome number and structure can be determined with accuracy in excess of 99% (NICHD 1976, Golbus et al 1979). There are, however, a number of potential pitfalls in the interpretation of cytogenetic studies. Polyploidy has frequently been observed in amniotic fluid cell cultures and may comprise 4–100% of the cells studied (Kohn & Robinson 1970, Milunsky et al 1970, 1971). In most of the reported cases, pregnancy has not been terminated and the infants born at term have had normal karyotypes. However, liveborn infants with triploidy have been reported. Mosaicism for trisomy 20 has also been observed in AF cell cultures, and is probably of little clinical significance. Hsu et al (1987) reported their experience with this abnormality, and found no congenital defects in 85% of the infants, and only rather non-specific abnormalities, which did not conform to any pattern, in the remaining 15%. The trisomic cells were thought to be confined to specific fetal organs or extraembryonic tissues, since the abnormality was not confirmed on blood cultures.

Although true mosaicism occurs in only 0.2–0.4% of pregnancies, pseudomosaicism, resulting from the de novo appearance of a trisomic clone, occurs in as many as 2–3% of AF cell cultures (Peakman et al 1978, 1979, Hsu & Perlis 1984, Benn et al 1984). Multiple chromosomes may be involved in 0.5–1% of cultures. Chromosomes 2, 7, X, 9, 17 and 20 are most commonly involved (Hsu & Perlis 1984). Although pseudomosaicism is typically found in only one flask of cells (or in one colony if the chromosomes are examined in situ in flaskettes) it is occasionally necessary to repeat the amniocentesis or obtain fetal blood by PUBS for confirmation. Benn et al (1984) have cautioned that even with the examination of 25 cells from each of two flasks, as many as 4.5% of true mosaics may go undetected, and as many as 7% may be misdiagnosed as pseudomosaic.

Marker chromosomes are seen in approximately 0.1% of AF cell cultures, and although they are not usually associated with phenotypic abnormalities, they pose a counselling dilemma (Benn & Hsu 1984). Mosaicism is found in more than half of these cases. Since marker chromosomes may be inherited, it is imperative that chromosome analyses be performed on the parents if a marker is found.

Lastly, the normal variation in chromosome length, satellite size, or the position of specific bands may occasionally be problematic (e.g. if an inversion or translocation is present). Karyotype analysis of the parents may be the only means of interpreting unusual findings.

Fragile-X syndrome

A 'fragile site' can be demonstrated at band q27 on the long arm of the X chromosome in many mentally retarded boys, and is discussed elsewhere in this text. The linkage of the fragile site to the gene(s) causing the mental retardation render the cytogenetic abnormality useful for diagnosis, family studies, and prenatal diagnosis of hemizygous males and heterozygous females. The fragile site is most frequently evident when the cells are cultured in folate- and thymidine-deficient medium, or in the presence of fluorodeoxyuridine or methotrexate (Hecht et al 1982). The expression of the fragile site appears to depend on depletion of deoxythymidylate pools, but the precise mechanism is unknown. The fragile site can be induced in fibroblasts and amniotic fluid cells, at very low frequency, and prenatal diagnosis has been successfully performed (Jenkins et al 1981, 1984, Shapiro et al 1982). However, the laboratory procedures for achieving this are technically very demanding (Jenkins et al 1986, Shapiro & Wilmot 1986, Tommerup et al 1986) and both false negative and false positive results have occurred. The use of DNA probes and RFLPs in the region of q27 may simplify the diagnosis in the future (Buchanan et al 1987). However, at the time of writing, the analysis of fetal blood samples is probably the most reliable means of achieving prenatal diagnosis, because the frequency of the fragile site in lymphocytes is substantially higher than that observed in cultured AF cells (Webb et al 1987).

Chromosomal instability syndromes

Several of the chromosomal instability syndromes may be amenable to prenatal diagnosis by amniocentesis. For example, in Bloom syndrome an increased frequency of sister chromatid exchanges is observed in cultured lymphocytes and fibroblasts, and can be sought in cultured AF cells for prenatal diagnosis (German et al 1979). In patients with Fanconi anaemia (FA) lymphocytes and fibroblasts show spontaneous chromosomal breaks with specific sensitivity to the mutagen diepoxybutane (DEB). A number of pregnancies at risk for FA have been monitored with this technique and the outcome predicted correctly (Auerbach et al 1979, 1981). In ataxia telangiectasia (AT), spontaneous chromosomal breakage is frequently observed. AT cells may be uniquely sensitive to bleomycin, responding with decreased cell viability and increased chromosomal damage, a 'stress' test which may be applicable to prenatal diagnosis (Cohen & Simpson 1980, Schwartz et al 1985). Xeroderma pigmentosum has been diagnosed in utero by demonstration of decreased radioactive thymidine incorporation ('repair synthesis') after exposure of cultured cells to ultraviolet light (Ramsay et al 1974, Halley et al 1979). Cultured cells from children with Cockayne syndrome are hypersensitive to ultraviolet light, expressed as defective colony-forming ability, recovery of DNA synthesis, and recovery of RNA synthesis. These phenomena have been used for prenatal diagnosis in at risk pregnancies, with correct prediction of the outcome (Sugita et al 1982, Lehmann et al 1985).

Enzyme assays

There are a large number of autosomal recessive and X-linked disorders that result either in impaired production or impaired functioning of an enzyme or other type of protein. The result in either type of defect is the same: reduced functional activity of the protein. Both types of defect can be diagnosed prenatally by measurement of enzyme activity or protein function in cultured amniotic fluid cells.

Prior to attempting prenatal diagnosis by enzyme assay, there are many important considerations to be evaluated. First and foremost, it is essential that the diagnosis be confirmed in the index case, in order to establish that the pregnancy is truly at risk. Second, the enzyme in question must be expressed in amniotic fluid cells. The enzymes that are deficient in many inborn errors of metabolism (e.g. phenylketonuria, most urea cycle defects, type I glycogen storage disease) are normally expressed only in liver and prenatal diagnosis cannot be performed by assay of amniotic fluid cells. Third, it is frequently desirable to assay the enzyme in cells from the parents, prior to the attempted prenatal diagnosis, to ensure that they have detectable enzyme activity. Several examples of 'pseudodeficiency' have been described, in which heterozygotes for a specific disease *appear* to be entirely deficient in the specific enzyme (Baldinger et al 1987). This situation can arise in an individual who has one of the disease (truly deficient) alleles, and whose other allele is inactive under the laboratory assay conditions, but is active in vivo. Lastly, the laboratory performing the assay should be experienced in the specific procedure used, and should assay cells from several normal controls and affected controls at the same time as the patient's amniotic fluid cells. It is advisable that an unrelated enzyme also be assayed at the same time, to ensure that any observed deficiency of activity is not the result of cell injury or other laboratory artifact, but represents an isolated and specific defect.

Numerous autosomal recessive and X-linked enzyme deficiencies may be diagnosed prenatally by assaying amniotic fluid cell (or chorionic villi) enzyme activity, and are listed in Tables 111.8–111.12. For some of the disorders listed, prenatal diagnosis has not yet been accomplished, although there is evidence that it is possible for all of them. There will undoubtedly be other disorders, not listed, which will be amenable to this approach.

Linkage analysis

Linkage analysis is an important and now frequently used method for prenatal diagnosis of diseases in which the defective gene is not expressed in amniotic fluid cells. When two genes are linked, it is often possible to determine the nature of the linkage relations (i.e. coupling or repulsion) within a given family. When this linkage relationship is established, one can infer the presence (or absence) of one gene from the presence (or absence) of the other. Therefore, when a gene that is not expressed in amniotic fluid cells is linked to a gene that is, linkage analysis may be useful for prenatal diagnosis.

Only a few clinically useful linkage relationships were known prior to the study of restriction fragment length polymorphisms. One application of linkage analysis is the determination of fetal sex in pregnancies at risk for X-linked disorders, followed by the selective abortion of all male fetuses. Half of the aborted males, however, will not be affected. In some cases, a specific diagnosis can be reached by linkage analysis, e.g. the diagnosis of X-linked mental retardation by its linkage to the fragile site on the X chromosome.

Prenatal diagnosis of congenital adrenal hyperplasia (21-hydroxylase deficiency) is also possible by linkage analysis (Pollack et al 1979, Mornet et al 1986). The enzyme which is deficient in this disorder is normally expressed only in adrenal cortical cells, and not in amniotic fluid cells. However, the gene encoding the enzyme is closely linked to the HLA-B locus in the major histocompatibility complex on the short arm of chromosome 6. Since the HLA antigens are expressed in amniotic fluid cells, HLA typing of these cells and linkage analysis can be used for prenatal diagnosis. By determining which HLA alleles in the mother are linked to her copy of the defective 21-hydroxylase gene, and which HLA alleles in the father are linked to his copy of the defective gene, HLA typing of the fetus can be used to determine if it has inherited both defective copies and is affected with CAH. It is important to note that the linkage relationship between the HLA alleles and the 21-hydroxylase gene cannot be assumed, since different HLA haplotypes will be linked to the abnormal gene in different families.

Linkage analysis is a very powerful method for prenatal diagnosis. However, because linkage disequilibrium cannot be assumed (and is frequently not present), it is imperative that the linkage relationship be determined in the specific family under study, or the results of the prenatal studies will be uninterpretable. It is also important to recognize that linkage analysis can fail if recombination occurs between the linked genes, and recombination is therefore a potential source of error. The use of multiple linked genes, which flank the disease gene on both sides, is highly desirable, because it is then easier to recognize recombinations when they occur.

DNA hybridization studies

Although all nucleated cells contain a complete copy of the genome, many genes are expressed only in selected tissues. Diagnosis based on the analysis of a gene product is only possible if the gene is expressed in an accessible tissue. Advances in molecular biology have made it possible to diagnose genetic disorders by direct examination of the DNA present in any nucleated cell without relying on the expression of the gene in that cell type. This may well make it possible to diagnose *any* inherited disorder by analysis of amniotic fluid cells or chorionic villi.

Direct examination of genes is usually dependent on hybridization of a DNA 'probe' to the complementary sequence in the patient's DNA. This technique has provided a new means of identifying fetal sex (Gosden et al 1982, Page et al 1982). Because the Y chromosome is found only in male cells, DNA probes directed at unique Y chromosome base sequences will hybridize only with DNA from male cells.

A variety of methods have been used for identifying abnormalities in *specific* genes. When the sequence of the gene and the location of the abnormality are known (e.g. sickle-cell disease) a single base substitution may be recognized because it alters a restriction endonuclease cleavage site, or because it prevents hybridization of a specific oligonucleotide probe to that region. Complete or partial gene deletions can be recognized by their effects on the size of the DNA fragments produced by digestion with restriction endonucleases.

There are many disorders for which the precise location and sequence of the abnormal gene are unknown, or in which different mutations in the gene in different families have produced clinically identical diseases (e.g. the thalassaemias). These conditions can frequently be identified by combining DNA hybridization methods (i.e. analysis of RFLPs) with linkage analysis. This technology has made it possible to diagnose disorders for which the basic defects (abnormal proteins) have not been identified. Any genetic disorder should be diagnosable by these means. Lastly, it has recently become possible to prepare relatively large amounts of highly purified DNA from specific regions of the genome, i.e. to isolate single genes in large quantities, using a technique known as the polymerase chain reaction (Saiki et al 1985, Kogan et al 1987). Specific stretches of DNA isolated from amniotic fluid cells or chorionic villi can now be directly analyzed by a variety of hybridization methods, and may in fact be directly sequenced for prenatal diagnostic purposes.

Further description of these methods is beyond the scope of this chapter, and is provided elsewhere in this text. These methods have already permitted the prenatal diagnosis of sickle-cell disease (Kan & Dozy 1978, Chang & Kan 1982, Orkin et al 1982), alpha- and beta-thalassaemia (Orkin et al 1978, Antonarakis et al 1982, 1985b, Old et al 1986), haemophilia A (Antonarakis et al 1985a, Gitschier et al 1985) and B (Giannelli et al 1984, Peake et al 1984), Duchenne muscular dystrophy (Kunkel 1986), autosomal dominant polycystic kidney disease (Reeders et al 1986), cystic fibrosis, and a list of other disorders (Cooper & Schmidtke 1987) that is growing in length at an unprecedented rate.

Chorionic villi

It appears that any analysis that can be performed on cultured amniotic fluid cells can also be performed on chorionic villi. Because the Langhans cells of the cytotrophoblast are rapidly dividing, it is possible to perform 'direct' chromosome analyses on these cells, immediately after sampling, or after 24 hours' incubation in tissue culture medium. Alternatively, the mesenchymal cells in the core of the villi can be established in tissue culture after mechanical maceration of the villi or partial digestion with trypsin and/or collagenase. Direct analysis has the great advantage of permitting fetal chromosomal analysis to be completed within 24–48 hours. Because the analysis is not dependent on cell division in culture, direct chromosome preparations are not likely to be affected by contamination with maternal decidua cells, in which mitoses are infrequently observed. In their series of 1000 direct chromosome preparations, Simoni et al (1986b) observed a 46,XX karyotype in only two of the male fetuses. Both cases were mosaic (46,XX/46,XY) and the maternal origin of the 46,XX cells was demonstrated on the basis of banding polymorphisms.

Unfortunately, the quality of the banding in direct chromosome preparations is usually inferior to that which is typical of cultured cells, and small chromosomal rearrangements can be missed if only the direct preparations are examined (Czepulkowski et al 1986). In addition, a variety of chromosome abnormalities have been observed in direct preparations, but have not been confirmed in cultured cells, by amniocentesis, or by examination of fetal tissues (Simoni et al 1986a). The chromosome abnormalities observed in some cases involved abnormalities not seen in liveborn children (e.g. trisomy 16), but in many other cases were entirely plausible (e.g. 47,XXY or 45,X). The abnormalities have included marker chromosomes (Dalprà et al 1986, Lilford et al 1987), mosaicism (Martin et al 1986b, Cheung et al 1987), and trisomies (Bartels et al 1986, Dalprà et al 1986). In many instances these abnormalities reflect true mosaicism in placental tissue, which is not uncommon (Verjaal et al 1987), and which does not reflect the true fetal chromosomal constitution. Tragically, in some of the early cases the pregnancy was terminated and it was only upon examination of the fetal tissues that the discrepancy was uncovered.

Normal chromosome complements have been seen occasionally in direct preparations from fetuses which have subsequently proved to be abnormal, either by analysis of cultured cells or by amniocentesis (Linton & Lilford 1986, Lilford et al 1987). The missed abnormalities have included true mosaicism (Eichenbaum et al 1986) and trisomy 18 (Martin et al 1986a).

Although the quality of the banding on samples which have been cultured for six or seven days is superior to direct preparations, these analyses are more subject to difficulties from contamination with maternal cells, which may also become established in the cultures (Martin et al 1986b, Schulze & Miller 1986, Williams et al 1987). This problem has been reported in as many as 8–13% of cultures (Cooke et al 1986, Williams et al 1987), but the frequency varies with the duration of cell culture, and the care with which the villi are cleaned prior to inoculation in culture. In addition to this problem, pseudomosaicism has also been observed in cultured cells (Martin et al 1986b, Schulze & Miller 1986, Lilford et al 1987).

The frequency of ambiguous chromosome results in chorionic villi samples has varied, but even in experienced laboratories problems with interpretation may occur in 1–3% of cases (Dalprà et al 1986, Martin et al 1986b, Simoni et al 1986a, Cheung et al 1987). It is therefore recommended that chromosome analysis be performed on both direct and cultured samples in every case, and that neither be relied on alone. An algorithm for resolving discrepancies between direct and cultured results has been described by Martin et al (1986b). In most instances, the interpretation of the results is entirely uncomplicated and reliable. However, just as with amniocentesis, in rare problematic cases it may still be necessary to perform additional testing, such as amniocentesis or fetal blood sampling.

A long and rapidly growing list of inherited disorders

have been diagnosed by analysis of chorionic villi. Studies employing DNA hybridization methods can be performed directly on villi, without prior culture. In many instances, studies which are based on enzyme assays may also be performed directly on the villi. However, the level of enzyme activity expressed in chorionic villi cells is not necessarily similar to that expressed in cultured amniotic fluid cells; for some enzymes activity is lower in chorionic villi, while for others it is higher (Evans et al 1986, Kleijer 1986). The contribution of different isozymes to the measured activity of an enzyme may also be different from that in cultured amniotic fluid cells. For example, the prenatal diagnosis of metachromatic leucodystrophy using synthetic substrates for the assay of arylsulphatase A has been complicated by the activity of other arylsulphatases in trophoblasts (Sanguinetti et al 1986, Poenaru 1987).

Several enzymes are now known to express higher levels of activity in cultured villus cells than in uncultured cells (Ben-Yoseph et al 1986), and in these instances the diagnosis of the associated disorders (e.g. mucolipidosis I, II, and III, Hurler syndrome) is best achieved using cultured cells (Kleijer 1986, Poenaru 1987). On the other hand, there is some evidence that Pompe disease (acid alpha-glucosidase deficiency) may be more reliably diagnosed using uncultured cells (Grubisic et al 1986, Poenaru 1987). There is also evidence that some assay methods may be better suited to one sample type or the other. For example, in the prenatal diagnosis of a fetus affected with argininosuccinic aciduria, argininosuccinic acid lyase activity was reported as normal in uncultured cells and deficient in cultured cells (Czepulkowski et al 1986). However, in another patient the deficiency was correctly identified in intact villi, using a different assay method (Kleijer 1986). As with the cytogenetic studies, many workers have noted problems from maternal cell contamination in cultured specimens.

It is clear that enzyme assay of chorionic villi for prenatal diagnosis should only be attempted by laboratories experienced both with the biochemical methods and with chorionic villi. It is imperative that normal chorionic villi be studied simultaneously, and in many cases it is advisable to examine both uncultured and cultured material. When the results indicate that the fetus is not affected amniocentesis may be offered for confirmation, until the reliability of the specific assay conditions for chorionic villi is well established.

Fetal blood

Because the results of the analysis of a fetal blood sample can be very significantly altered if the sample is con-taminated with maternal blood, the first part of any analysis involves verification of the purity of the sample. Advantage may be taken of the fact that the fetal red blood cells are considerably larger ($120-160$ um^3) than in the adult ($80-95$ um^3). After a blood sample is obtained, it may be immediately analyzed in a particle size distribution analyzer (e.g. Coulter counter). If the distribution of cells is primarily in the smaller range, additional blood samples may be obtained. When an adequate specimen is obtained, the precise proportion of fetal cells can be determined by preparing a blood smear and counting the percentage of cells remaining after acid elution (Kleihauer-Betke technique), or by serologically determining the proportion of cells which express the fetal red cell surface antigen I (Habibi et al 1986).

Until recently, analysis of fetal blood samples provided the only means for prenatally diagnosing the haemoglobinopathies (Leonard & Kazazian 1978). Although fetal reticulocytes synthesize very small amounts of adult haemoglobins, this synthesis is sufficient for diagnosis. It may be studied by incubating the fetal reticulocytes in a medium containing radiolabelled leucine, which is incorporated into the newly synthesized proteins (primarily globins) (Alter 1979). The radiolabelled globin chains (alpha, beta and gamma) are then separated by ion exchange chromatography. The radioactivity in each type of chain is measured, and reflects the rate of synthesis of that chain type. Abnormal beta-globins are detected by their early or late elution from the ion exchange column.

As noted previously, the haemoglobinopathies may frequently be diagnosed by DNA hybridization methods, using either amniotic fluid cells or chorionic villi. This has largely replaced fetal blood sampling for the diagnosis of these conditions.

A variety of other disorders have been diagnosed by analysis of fetal blood samples (Table 111.5) (Hoyer et al 1979, Jeppsson et al 1979, Newburger et al 1979, Webb et al 1983). Prenatal diagnosis of classical haemophilia A is complicated by the presence of tissue thromboplastins in amniotic fluid which may contaminate the samples. This problem may be circumvented in some cases by measuring the ratio of factor VIII coagulant activity to factor VIII-related antigen (Firschein et al 1979). An immunoradiometric assay of factor IX has similarly been used for the diagnosis of haemophilia B (Holmberg et al 1980, Ljung & Holmberg 1982). However, both of these disorders have also been diagnosed using DNA hybridization methods (Giannelli et al 1984, Peake et al 1984, Antonarakis et al 1985a, Gitschier et al 1985, Kogan et al 1987).

Immune defects and other disorders that alter the number, morphology, or surface markers of the blood cells may also be diagnosed through fetal blood sampling (Durandy et al 1982). Chronic granulomatous disease (CGD) may be diagnosed by demonstrating lack of superoxide generation and reduction of the dye nitroblue tetrazolium in stimulated fetal leucocytes (Newburger et al 1979). CGD, which is X-linked, may now be diagnosable by linkage analysis using DNA probes flanking the CGD locus on the X chromosome. It is, of course, important to determine the fetal sex (by CVS, amniocentesis, or ultrasound) before pursuing the prenatal diagnosis of CGD (or any other X-linked condition). Several other of the conditions listed in Table 111.5 can also be diagnosed by other means. Alpha-1-antitrypsin deficiency can be diagnosed by DNA hybridization with an oligonucleotide probe. Metabolic and cytogenetic disorders can be diagnosed by analysis of amniotic fluid cells or chorionic villi, and fetal blood sampling for these studies should be reserved for those instances in which there is insufficient time for cell culture or when the results of the analysis have been ambiguous. As noted earlier, this may occur with the prenatal diagnosis of the Fragile-X syndrome, when chromosomal mosaicism has been detected, and when it is difficult to distinguish true mosaicism from pseudomosaicism (Watson et al 1984).

Fetal liver

A variety of enzymes of intermediary metabolism are expressed only in liver. The prenatal diagnosis of disorders associated with abnormalities of these enzymes cannot be accomplished by enzyme assay of amniotic fluid cells or chorionic villi. Successful needle biopsy of fetal liver at 18–20 weeks has been achieved by aspiration of tissue under ultrasonographic (Holzgreve & Golbus 1981) or fetoscopic (Rodeck et al 1982) guidance. Ornithine transcarbamylase deficiency was correctly diagnosed and excluded by analysis of fetal liver so obtained. Type I glycogen storage disease (glucose-6-phosphatase deficiency) has also been correctly diagnosed by this technique (Holzgreve & Golbus 1981). When these types of studies are undertaken, it is important that at least one additional enzyme (which is specific for liver) be assayed, to ensure that an adequate and viable sample of liver has been obtained and that absence of activity does not simply reflect an inadequate sample. It is also important to verify that the protein being assayed is normally expressed at the gestational age at which the sample is taken.

Skin biopsies

If a genetic disorder results in histological or histochemical alterations in an accessible tissue, such as skin, diagnosis can be achieved even when the biochemical basis of the disorder is not known. This approach requires biopsy of the affected tissue, followed by preparation and examination by light and/or electron microscopy. To date, this approach has been applied only to disorders in which the skin is involved, several of which are listed in Table 111.4. Definitive diagnosis requires that the histological appearance of the skin be pathognomonic for the disorder at 20 weeks' gestation.

PRENATAL THERAPY

The possibility of prenatal diagnosis of anatomical and metabolic abnormalities has raised the possibility of prenatal therapy for these conditions. In a very limited number of instances it may be possible to correct or ameliorate the fetal abnormality. Forays into prenatal therapy can be divided into three major areas: surgical, medical, and genetic.

Surgical therapies

The history of fetal surgery really begins more than 20 years ago, with the pioneering work of Liley on fetal intraperitoneal transfusions for haemolytic disease. Today both intraperitoneal and direct intravascular transfusions are relatively routine procedures, and have saved countless babies. In experienced hands, these procedures carry only a 1–2% risk.

In the late 1970s and early 1980s there was much enthusiasm for relieving excess intracranial pressure in fetuses with hydrocephalus (or more correctly, ventriculomegaly). The shunting of ventriculomegaly was performed with the hope of reducing intracranial pressure, and thereby preventing or reducing damage to the brain (Clewell et al 1982). Unfortunately, the experience gained from these efforts indicates that in more than 50% of patients with ventriculomegaly, the ventriculomegaly is not an isolated defect, and the results of shunting have been generally dismal (Manning et al 1986). In fact, in several instances shunting did not result in the hoped-for improvement of a baby from impaired to normal, but probably created a severely impaired infant from one who would have otherwise died. As a result of the poor outcomes observed, a de facto moratorium on the use of such shunts was instituted. However, recent data have suggested that this action may have been premature (Drugan et al 1988). It is now clear that there are two patient populations which must be distinguished. Patients with isolated ventriculomegaly, without other physical abnormalities, and whose ventriculomegaly worsens as the pregnancy progresses, may have a positive response to shunting. Fetuses with multiple congenital abnormalities fare less well, and probably should not be treated. In this latter group the ventriculomegaly is only one manifestation of pre-existing central nervous system damage.

Obstruction of the fetal bladder is a relatively common event which can result in destruction of the fetal kidneys and death. In male fetuses, obstructive uropathy is most commonly a consequence of posterior urethral valves. The inability to excrete urine results in distension of the bladder, and later the ureters, and finally creates hydronephrosis, destruction of the kidneys, and in some instances the prune belly syndrome. Unlike the case with ventriculomegaly, most obstructive uropathies are isolated defects, the repair of which should allow otherwise normal development.

The placement of a suprapubic, transabdominal, vesicoamniotic shunt (Fig. 111.7) is simpler than the placement of an intracranial shunt, and has been successful in over 100 cases. Data from the Fetal Surgery Registry of the International Fetal Medicine and Surgery Society indicate that, as with the intracranial shunts, the outcome of shunting is much better when the obstructive uropathy is an isolated defect, than when it is associated with other anomalies. It is essential that all possible information about the state of the fetus be obtained prior to shunting (including karyotyping), and that the procedure be reserved for fetuses with isolated defects. Histopathological studies suggest that the earlier the shunt is placed, the less likely it is that permanent renal damage has occurred (Adzick et al 1985). Most shunts have been placed between 18 and 26 weeks, with the earliest at 14 weeks.

Open fetal surgery A congenital diaphragmatic hernia with extravasation of gut into the chest cavity inhibits lung development and results in pulmonary hypoplasia and high neonatal mortality. Diaphragmatic hernia can easily be diagnosed with ultrasound, although the diagnosis is usually serendipitous. There have been a small number of cases in which maternal laparotomies have been performed, with incision of the uterus, removal of the fetus, repair of the diaphragmatic defect, and return of the fetus and amniotic fluid into the uterus to continue an intrauterine gestation. While the first several cases have formed a learning curve, it seems reasonable to expect that this type of approach may improve fetal morbidity and mortality in the future.

An interesting finding from these experiences has been that the fetal incisions have healed without scars. If fetal surgery can be shown to be safe, surgery for a variety of inherited dysmorphic syndromes might be considered prenatally, to allow more normal craniofacial development, and more extensive surgery without scarring.

Medical therapies

Fetal cardiac arrhythmias have been documented in over 700 cases in the Fetal Therapy Registry. Approximately 14% of patients with arrhythmias have an underlying structural defect and approximately 10% are chromosomally abnormal. Those cardiac arrhythmias which may lead to congestive heart failure in adult patients, lead to hydrops, and often death, in the fetus. In appropriately selected cases, cardioversion of arrhythmias has been accomplished with great success, and with obvious clinical implications.

Congenital adrenal hyperplasia (CAH) resulting from 21-hydroxylase deficiency is the most common cause of ambiguous genitalia in genetic females. The enzyme deficiency results in inadequate cortisol production, accumulation of 17-alpha-hydroxyprogesterone and, consequently, overproduction of androgens which masculinize the external genitalia. Evans et al (1985) have demonstrated that oral administration of dexamethasone to the mother, beginning at 10 weeks' gestation, suppresses the synthesis of 17-alpha-hydroxyprogesterone by the fetal adrenal gland. This effectively prevents androgen overproduction and the consequent masculinization.

In pregnancies at risk for CAH fetal sex determination can be performed at 9 weeks' gestation by chorionic villus sampling, and CAH can be diagnosed definitively by linkage analysis. If a female fetus is affected, therapy can be instituted immediately.

Several other biochemical disorders, such as B_{12} responsive methylmalonic acidaemia and multiple carboxylase deficiency, may be treated by prenatal administration to the mother of pharmacological doses of vitamins B_{12} and biotin, respectively (Ampola et al 1975, Packman et al 1982, Roth et al 1982). Although it is clear that accumulation of the abnormal metabolites may be reduced by prenatal vitamin administration in these disorders, it is not clear if this has any clinically important effect.

Prenatal treatment of congenital infections may also be achieved. Desmonts et al (1985) have successfully diagnosed congenital toxoplasmosis by fetal blood sampling. They have also shown that antibiotic treatment begun in the second trimester can very significantly ameliorate the sequelae of the disorder. The implications of their findings are considerable, but unfortunately are not immediately applicable to viral infections such as herpes or cytomegalovirus.

Gene therapy

Relatively recent advances in molecular biology have raised the possibility of a truly unique method for treating

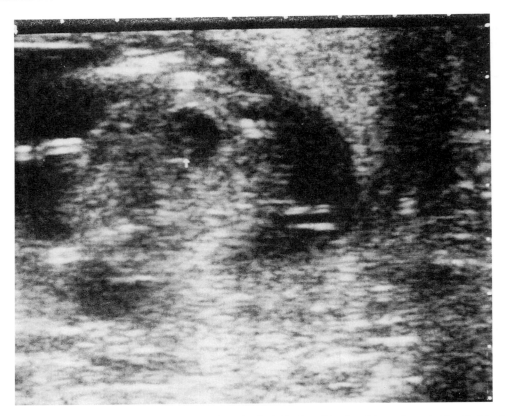

Fig. 111.7 Ultrasound showing placement of catheter into the fetal bladder. The tip of the catheter is identified by the arrow in the bladder. The shunt passes from the bladder to the left.

disease: giving the organism the ability to make its own missing (or defective) gene product. A variety of experiments have demonstrated that it is possible to introduce genes into intact cells and organisms, to have them stably integrated into the genome, and passed on from generation to generation (Anderson 1986). The development of this field has been slow and painstaking; the problem of regulating the expression of newly introduced genes is still onerous. Thus the first candidates for experimental 'gene therapy' will likely be children with lethal or very severely debilitating disorders, and ones in which finely-tuned rejuvenation of gene productivity is not critical (Anderson 1986).

Attempts are underway to introduce the genes for beta-globin and adenosine deaminase into haematopoietic stem cells, and to re-introduce those stem cells into the host bone marrow to create chimaeras in which the newly introduced gene is expressed. Adenosine deaminase deficiency will probably be the first human disease for which this type of gene therapy will be attempted. While it seems likely that the first attempts will be made during childhood, it is logical to attempt this type of therapy as early in pregnancy as possible, to allow the introduction of the new gene into the tissues before they are fully developed. Attempts to inject haematopoietic stem cells in the second trimester (via PUBS) for the treatment of haemoglobinopathies have been reported, although they have been unsuccessful to this point (Linch et al 1987). It seems likely, though, that prenatal genetic correction in the second trimester of pregnancy, or even in the preimplantation stage (in conjunction with in vitro fertilization) will be included in the therapeutic armamentarium of the future.

CONCLUSION

Tremendous progress has been made in our ability to diagnose fetal abnormalities during pregnancy. Little more than 20 years have elapsed since the first amniocentesis for chromosome analysis was reported. Since that bold step, we have seen the perfection of ultrasound technology to a point which allows us to 'see' the fetus with exquisite anatomical detail. In the last five years we have witnessed the advent of first trimester prenatal diagnosis and the application of DNA hybridization methods to the diagnosis of diseases for which the basic defect remains unknown. Ironically, it is at the intersection of the new 'molecular' technology and the classical methods of family study and linkage analysis that the greatest potential for prenatal diagnosis lies. In the years to come we can look forward to the development of libraries of DNA probes spanning the entire human genome, with each probe mapped to a specific chromosomal location. With these libraries may come the potential for easily locating the gene for *any* heritable disorder.

REFERENCES

Adzick N S, Harrison M R, Glick P L, Flake A W 1985 Fetal urinary tract obstruction: experimental pathophysiology. Seminars in Perinatology 9: 79–90

Allan L D, Crawford D C, Anderson R H, Tynan M J 1984 Echocardiographic and anatomical correlations in fetal congenital heart disease. British Heart Journal 52: 542–548

Alter B P 1979 Prenatal diagnosis of hemoglobinopathies and other hematologic diseases. Journal of Pediatrics 95: 501–513

Alter B P, Modell C B, Fairweather D et al 1976 Prenatal diagnosis of hemoglobinopathies. New England Journal of Medicine 295: 1437–1443

Ampola M G, Mahoney M J, Nakamura E, Tanaka K 1975 Prenatal therapy of a patient with vitamin B_{12}-responsive methylmalonic acidemia. New England Journal of Medicine 293: 313–317

Anderson W F 1986 Prospects for human gene therapy in the born and unborn patient. Clinical Obstetrics and Gynecology 29: 586–594

Antonarakis S E, Phillips J A III, Kazazian H H 1982 Genetic diseases: Diagnosis by restriction endonuclease analysis. Journal of Pediatrics 100: 845–856

Antonarakis S E, Copeland K L, Carpenter R J, Carta C A, Hoyer L, Caskey C T, Toole J, Kazazian H H Jr. 1985a Prenatal diagnosis of haemophilia A by factor VIII gene analysis. Lancet 1: 1407–1409

Antonarakis S E, Kazazian H H, Orkin S H 1985b DNA polymorphism and molecular pathology of the human globin gene clusters. Human Genetics 69: 1–14

Auerbach A D, Warburton D, Bloom A D, Chaganti R S K 1979 Prenatal detection of the Fanconi anemia gene by cytogenetic methods. American Journal of Human Genetics 31: 77–81

Auerbach A D, Adler B, Chaganti R S K 1981 Prenatal and postnatal diagnosis and carrier detection of Fanconi anemia by a cytogenetic method. Pediatrics 67: 128–135

Baldinger S, Pierpont M E, Wenger D A 1987 Pseudodeficiency of arylsulfatase A: A counselling dilemma. Clinical Genetics 31: 70–76

Barela A I, Kleinman G E, Golditch I M, Menke D J, Hogge W A, Golbus M S 1986 Septic shock with renal failure after chorionic villus sampling. American Journal of Obstetrics and Gynecology 154: 1100–1102

Bartels I, Rauskolb R, Hansmann I 1986 Chromosomal mosaicism of trisomy 7 restricted to chorionic villi. American Journal of Medical Genetics 25: 161–162

Beaudet A L, Buffone G J 1987 Prenatal diagnosis of cystic fibrosis. The Journal of Pediatrics 111: 630–633

Benn P A, Hsu L Y 1984 Incidence and significance of supernumerary marker chromosomes in prenatal diagnosis. American Journal of Human Genetics 36: 1092–1102

Benn P, Hsu L Y, Perlis T, Schonhaut A 1984 Prenatal diagnosis of chromosome mosaicism. Prenatal Diagnosis 4: 1–9

Ben Yoseph Y, Evans M I, Bottoms S F, Pack B A, Mitchell D A, Koppitch F C III, Nadler H L 1986 Lysosomal enzyme activities in fresh and frozen chorionic villi and in cultured trophoblasts. Clinica Chimica Acta 161: 307–313

Blakemore K J, Baumgarten A, Schoenfeld-Dimaio M, Hobbins J C, Mason E A, Mahoney M J 1986 Rise in maternal serum alpha-fetoprotein concentration after chorionic villus sampling and the possibility of isoimmunization. American Journal of Obstetrics and Gynecology 155: 988–993

Boué A, Muller F, Nezelof C et al 1986 Prenatal diagnosis in 200 pregnancies with a 1-in-4 risk of cystic fibrosis. Human Genetics 74: 288–297

Brambati B, Matarreli M, Varotto F 1987a Septic complications after chorionic villus sampling. Lancet 1: 1212–1213

Brambati B, Oldrini A, Ferrazzi E, Lanzani A 1987b Chorionic villus sampling: An analysis of the obstetric experience of 1,000 cases. Prenatal Diagnosis 7: 157–169

Brambati B, Oldrini A, Lanzani A 1987c Transabdominal chorionic villus sampling: a freehand ultrasound-guided technique. American Journal of Obstetrics and Gynecology 157: 134–137

Brock D J 1983 Amniotic fluid alkaline phosphatase isoenzymes in early prenatal diagnosis of cystic fibrosis. Lancet 2: 941–943

Brock D J H, Sutcliffe R G 1972 Alpha-fetoprotein in the antenatal diagnosis of anencephaly and spina bifida. Lancet 2: 197–199

Brock D J H, Bolton A E, Monaghan J M 1973 Prenatal diagnosis of anencephaly through maternal serum-alpha-fetoprotein measurement. Lancet 2: 923–924

Brock D J, Bedgood D, Barron L, Hayward C 1985 Prospective prenatal diagnosis of cystic fibrosis. Lancet 1: 1175–1178

Buchanan J A, Buckton K E, Gosden C M, Newton M S, Clayton J F, Christie S, Hastie N 1987 Ten families with fragile X syndrome: linkage relationships with four DNA probes from distal Xq. Human Genetics 76: 165–172

Burton B K, Sowers S G, Nelson L H 1983 Maternal serum

alpha-fetoprotein screening in North Carolina: Experience with more than twelve thousand pregnancies. American Journal of Obstetrics and Gynecology 146: 439

Canadian Collaborative CVS-Amniocentesis Clinical Trial Group 1989 Multicentre randomised clinical trial of chorion villus sampling and amniocentesis. Lancet 1: 1–6

Carbarns N J, Gosden C, Brock D J 1983 Microvillar peptidase activity in amniotic fluid: possible use in the prenatal diagnosis of cystic fibrosis. Lancet 1: 329–331

Carpenter R J, Moise K, Copeland K L, Ledbetter D H 1987 Comparison of the transabdominal and transcervical methods of chorion villus sampling. American Journal of Human Genetics 41 (Supplement): A269 Abstract 800

Chandra P, Nitowsky H M, Marion R 1979 Experience with sonography as an adjunct to amniocentesis for prenatal diagnosis of fetal genetic disorders. American Journal of Obstetrics and Gynecology 133: 519–524

Chang J C, Kan Y W 1982 A sensitive new prenatal test for sickle-cell anaemia. New England Journal of Medicine 307: 30–32

Chervenak F A, Isaacson G L 1989 Ultrasound detection of anomalies. In: Evans M I, Fletcher J C, Dixler A O et al (eds) Fetal Diagnosis and Therapy: Science, Ethics and the Law. Lippincott Harper, Philadelphia

Cheung S W, Crane J P, Kyine M, Cui M Y 1987 Direct chromosome preparations from chorionic villi: A method for obtaining extended chromosomes and recognizing mosaicism confined to the placenta. Cytogenetics and Cell Genetics 45: 118–120

Clewell W H, Johnson M L, Meier P R et al 1982 A surgical approach to the treatment of fetal hydrocephalus. New England Journal of Medicine 306: 1320–1325

Cohen M M, Simpson S J 1980 Bleomycin induced chromosome damage in ataxia telangiectasia lymphoblastoid cells. American Journal of Human Genetics 32 (Supplement): 66A Abstract 200

Cooke H M, Penketh R J, Delhanty J D 1986 An evaluation of maternal cell contamination in cultures of chorionic villi for the prenatal diagnosis of chromosome abnormalities. Clinical Genetics 30: 485–493

Cooper D N, Schmidtke J 1987 Diagnosis of genetic disease using recombinant DNA. Supplement. Human Genetics 77: 66–75

Crandall B F, Lebherz T B, Freihube R 1978 Neural tube defects. Maternal serum screening and prenatal diagnosis. Pediatric Clinics of North America 25: 619–629

Crandon A J, Peel K R 1979 Amniocentesis with and without ultrasound guidance. British Journal of Obstetrics and Gynaecology 86: 1–3

Czepulkowski B H, Heaton D E, Kearney L U, Rodeck C H, Coleman D V 1986 Chorionic villus culture for first trimester diagnosis of chromosome defects: Evaluation by two London centres. Prenatal Diagnosis 6: 271–282

Daffos F, Capella-Pavlovsky M, Forestier F 1983 A new procedure for fetal blood sampling in utero: preliminary results of 53 cases. American Journal of Obstetrics and Gynecology 146: 985–987

Daffos F, Grangeot Keros L, Lebon P, Forestier F, Capella-Pavlovsky M, Chartier M, Pillot J 1984 Prenatal diagnosis of congenital rubella. Lancet 2: 1–3

Daffos F, Capella-Pavlovsky M, Forestier F 1985 Fetal blood sampling during pregnancy with use of a needle guided by ultrasound: A study of 606 consecutive cases. American Journal of Obstetrics and Gynecology 153: 655–660

Dalprà J, Nocera G, Tibiletti M G, Gramellini F, Agosti S, Oldrini A 1986 Technical aspects and diagnostic problems of direct chromosome analysis using chorionic villus sampling in the first trimester. Human Reproduction 1: 103–106

De Bruijn H W A, Huisjes H J 1975 Omphalocele and raised alpha-fetoprotein in amniotic fluid. Lancet 1: 525–526

Desmonts G, Forestier F, Thulliez P H, Daffos F, Capella-Pavlovsky M, Chartier M 1985 Prenatal diagnosis of congenital toxoplasmosis. Lancet 1: 500–503

Donnenfeld A E, Mennuti M T 1987 Second trimester diagnosis of fetal skeletal dysplasias. Obstetrical and Gynecological Survey 42: 199–217

Drugan A, Krauss B, Zador I E et al 1988 End the moratorium on in utero ventricular shunts. Society of Perinatology and Obstetrics #248, Las Vegas, Nevada

Durandy A, Dumez Y, Guy-Grand D, Henrior R, Griscelli C 1982 Prenatal diagnosis of severe combined immunodeficiency. Journal of Pediatrics 101: 995–997

Eichenbaum S Z, Krumins E J, Fortune D W, Duke J 1986 False-negative finding on chorionic villus sampling. Lancet 2: 391–392

Elejalde B R, Peck G, de Elejalde M M 1986 Determination of cholinesterase and acetylcholinesterase in amniotic fluid. Uses in prenatal diagnosis and quality control. Clinical Genetics 29: 196–203

Elias S 1980 Fetoscopy in prenatal diagnosis. Seminars in Perinatology 4: 199–205

Elias S 1987 Use of fetoscopy for the prenatal diagnosis of hereditary skin disorders. Current Problems in Dermatology 16: 1–13

Elias S, Martin A O, Patel V A, Gerbie A B, Simpson J L 1978 Analysis for amniotic fluid crystallization in second trimester amniocentesis. American Journal of Obstetrics and Gynecology 133: 401–404

Elliot P M, Inman W H 1961 Volume of liquor amnii in normal and abnormal pregnancy. Lancet 2: 835–840

Evans M I, Chrousos G P, Mann D W et al 1985 Pharmacologic suppression of the fetal adrenal gland in utero. Attempted prevention of abnormal external genital masculinzation in suspected congenital adrenal hyperplasia. Journal of the American Medical Association 253: 1015–1020

Evans M I, Moore C, Kolodny E H et al 1986 Lysosomal enzymes in chorionic villi, cultured amniocytes, and cultured skin fibroblasts. Clinica Chimica Acta 157: 109–113

Evans M I, Belsky R L, Clementino N A et al 1987a Establishment of a collaborative university-commercial maternal serum alpha-fetoprotein screening program: a model for tertiary center outreach. American Journal of Obstetrics and Gynecology 156: 1441–1449

Evans M I, Belsky R L, Greb A, Mariona F 1987b Maternal serum alpha-fetoprotein screening. Journal of Clinical Immunoassay 10: 210–216

Evans M I, Koppich F C, Nemitz B, Quigg M H, Zador I E 1988 Early genetic amniocentesis and chorionic villus sampling: Expanding the opportunities for early prenatal diagnosis. Journal of Reproductive Medicine 33: 450–452

Fairweather D V I, Modell B, Berdoukas V et al 1978 Antenatal diagnosis of thalassemia major. British Medical Journal 1: 350–353

Farrall M, Rodeck C H, Stanier P et al 1986 First-trimester prenatal diagnosis of cystic fibrosis with linked DNA probes. Lancet 1: 1402–1405

Firschein S I, Hoyer L W, Lazarchik J et al 1979 Prenatal diagnosis of classic hemophilia. New England Journal of Medicine 300: 937–941

Fleisher L D, Rassin D K, Rogers P, Desnick R J, Gaull G E 1977 Argininosuccinic aciduria – prenatal diagnosis and studies of an affected fetus. Pediatric Research 11: 455

Fuchs F, Riis P 1956 Antenatal sex determination. Nature 177: 330

Gagne R, Lescault A, Grenier A, Laberge C, Melancon S B, Dallaire L 1982 Prenatal diagnosis of hereditary tyrosinemia: Measurement of succinyl acetone in amniotic fluid. Prenatal Diagnosis 2: 185–188

Gerbie A B, Elias S 1980 Technique for midtrimester amniocentesis for prenatal diagnosis. Seminars in Perinatology 4: 159–163

German J, Bloom D, Passarge E 1979 Bloom's syndrome. VII. Progress report for 1978. Clinical Genetics 15: 361–367

Ghirardini G, Gualerzi C, Fochi F, Spreafico L, Agnelli P, Diazzi M 1986 Chorionscopy and chorionic villi sampling. Acta Europaea Fertilitatis 17: 495–499

Giannelli F, Choo K H, Winship P R et al 1984 Characterisation and use of an intragenic polymorphic marker for detection of carriers of haemophilia B (factor IX deficiency). Lancet 1: 239–241

Gilmore D H, McNay M B 1985 Spontaneous fetal loss rate in early pregnancy. Lancet 1: 107

Gitlin D, Boesman M 1966 Serum alpha-fetoprotein, albumin and gamma-G-globulin in the human conceptus. Journal of Clinical Investigation 45: 1826–1838

Gitschier J, Lawn R M, Rotblat F, Goldman E, Tuddenham E G D 1985 Antenatal diagnosis and carrier detection of haemophilia A using a factor VIII gene probe. Lancet 1: 1093–1094

Golbus M S, Kan Y W, Naglich-Craig M 1976 Fetal blood sampling in midtrimester pregnancies. American Journal of Obstetrics and Gynecology 124: 653–655

Golbus M S, Loughman W D, Epstein C J, Halbasch G, Stephens J D, Hall B D 1979 Prenatal genetic diagnosis in 3000 amniocenteses. New England Journal of Medicine 300: 157–163

Goossens M, Dumez Y, Kaplan L, Lupker M, Chabret C, Henrior R, Rosa J 1983 Prenatal diagnosis of sickle-cell anemia in the first trimester of pregnancy. New England Journal of Medicine 309: 831–833

Gosden J R, Mitchell A R, Gosden C M, Rodeck C H, Morsman J M 1982 Direct vision chorion biopsy and chromosome specific DNA probes for determination of fetal sex in first trimester prenatal diagnosis. Lancet 2: 1416–1419

Gosden C, Nicolaides K H, Rodeck C H 1988 Fetal blood sampling in investigation of chromosome mosaicism in amniotic fluid cell culture. Lancet 1: 613–617

Grannum P A, Hobbins J C 1983 Prenatal diagnosis of fetal skeletal dysplasias. Seminars in Perinatology 7: 125–137

Grannum P A, Copel J A, Plaxe S C, Scioscia A L, Hobbins J C 1986 In utero exchange transfusion by direct intravascular injection in severe erythroblastosis fetalis. New England Journal of Medicine 314: 1431–1434

Grubisic A, Shin Y S, Meyer W, Endres W, Becker U, Wischerath H 1986 First trimester diagnosis of Pompe's disease (glycogenosis type II) with normal outcome: Assay of acid alpha-glucosidase in chorionic villus biopsy using antibodies. Clinical Genetics 30: 298–301

Guiband S, Bonnet M, Thoulon J M, Dumont M 1973 Alpha-fetoprotein in amniotic fluid. Lancet 1: 1261

Habibi B, Bretagne M, Bretagne Y, Forestier F, Daffos F 1986 Blood group antigens on fetal red cells obtained by umbilical vein puncture under ultrasound guidance: a rapid hemagglutination test to check for contamination with maternal blood. Pediatric Research 20: 1082–1084

Haddow J E, Palomaki G E, Wald N J, Cuckle H S 1986 Maternal serum alpha-fetoprotein screening for Down syndrome and repeat testing. Lancet 2: 1460

Hahnemann N 1974 Early prenatal diagnosis: A study of biopsy techniques and cell culturing from extraembryonic membranes. Clinical Genetics 6: 294–306

Halley D J J, Keijzer W, Jaspers N G J et al 1979 Prenatal diagnosis of xeroderma pigmentosum (group C) using assays of unscheduled DNA synthesis and post replication repair. Clinical Genetics 16: 137–146

Hanson F W, Tennant F R, Zorn E M, Samuels S 1985 Analysis of 2136 genetic amniocenteses: experience of a single physician. American Journal of Obstetrics and Gynecology 152: 436–443

Hecht F, Jacky P B, Sutherland G R 1982 The fragile X chromosome: current methods. American Journal of Medical Genetics 11: 489–495

Herzenberg L A, Bianchi D W, Schröder J, Cann H M, Iverson G M 1979 Fetal cells in the blood of pregnant women: Detection and enrichment by fluorescence activated cell sorting. Proceedings of the National Academy of Sciences USA 76: 1453–1455

Hill L M, Breckle R, Gehrking W C 1983 The prenatal detection of congenital malformations by ultrasonography. Mayo Clinic Proceedings 58: 805–826

Hobbins J C, Grannum P A T, Berkowitz R L, Silverman R, Mahoney M J 1979 Ultrasound in the diagnosis of congenital anomalies. American Journal of Obstetrics and Gynecology 134: 331–345

Hogge W A, Schonberg S A, Golbus M S 1986 Chorionic villus sampling: experience of the first 1000 cases. American Journal of Obstetrics and Gynecology 154: 1249–1252

Holmberg L, Gustavii B, Cordesius E et al 1980 Prenatal diagnosis of hemophilia B by an immunoradiometric assay of factor IX. Blood 56: 397–401

Holzgreve W, Golbus M S 1981 Prenatal diagnosis of ornithine transcarbamylase deficiency utilizing fetal liver biopsy. American Journal of Human Genetics 36: 320–328

Holzgreve W, Miny P, Stening C, Vancaille T, Beller F K 1986 Experiences with different techniques of chorionic villi sampling for first trimester diagnosis. Acta Europaea Fertilitatis 17: 485–490

Hook E B 1981 Rates of chromosome abnormalities at different maternal ages. Obstetrics and Gynecology 58: 282–285

Hook E B, Chambers G M 1977 Estimated rates of Down syndrome in live births by one year maternal age intervals for mothers aged 20–49 in a New York state study – Implications of the risk figures for genetic counselling and cost-benefit analysis of prenatal diagnosis programs. Birth Defects 13: 123–141

Hoyer L W, Lindsten J, Blomback M, Hagenfeldt L, Cordesius E, Strömberg P, Gustavii B 1979 Prenatal evaluation of fetus at risk for severe von Willebrand's disease. Lancet 2: 191–192

Hsieh F J, Chang F M, Ko T M, Chen H Y 1987

Percutaneous ultrasound-guided fetal blood sampling in the management of non-immune hydrops fetalis. American Journal of Obstetrics and Gynecology 157: 44–49

Hsu L Y, Perlis T E 1984 United States survey on chromosome mosaicism and pseudomosaicism in prenatal diagnosis. Prenatal Diagnosis 4: Spec No. 97–130

Hsu L Y, Kaffe S, Perlis T E 1987 Trisomy 20 mosaicism in prenatal diagnosis – a review and update. Prenatal Diagnosis 7: 581–596

Hunter A G, Muggah H, Ivey B, Cox D M 1986 Assessment of the early risks of chorionic villus sampling. Canadian Medical Association Journal 134: 753–756

Jackson L 1985 The CVS Newsletter August 28

Jackson L 1986 The CVS Newsletter September 12

Jackson L 1987 The CVS Newsletter November 24

Jacobson C B, Barter R H 1967 Intrauterine diagnosis and management of genetic defects. American Journal of Obstetrics and Gynecology 99: 795–805

Jeanty P, Rodesch F, Romero R, Venus I, Hobbins J C 1983 How to improve your amniocentesis technique. American Journal of Obstetrics and Gynecology 146: 593–596

Jenkins E C, Brown W T, Duncan C J, Brooks J, Yishay M B, Giordano F M, Nitowsky H M 1981 Feasibility of fragile X chromosome prenatal diagnosis demonstrated. Lancet 2: 1292

Jenkins E C, Brown W T, Brooks J, Duncan C J, Rudelli R D, Wisniewski H M 1984 Experience with prenatal fragile X detection. American Journal of Medical Genetics 17: 215–239

Jenkins E C, Brown W T, Wilson M G et al 1986 The prenatal detection of the fragile X chromosome: review of recent experience. American Journal of Medical Genetics 23: 297–311

Jeppsson J O, Franzen B, Sveger T, Cordesius E, Strömberg P, Gustavii B 1979 Prenatal exclusion of alpha-$_1$-antitrypsin deficiency in a high risk fetus. New England Journal of Medicine 300: 1441–1442

Kaback M M 1977 Tay-Sachs disease: Prenatal diagnosis and heterozygote screening 1969–1976. Pediatric Research 11: 458

Kan Y W, Dozy A M 1978 Antenatal diagnosis of sickle-cell anemia by DNA analysis of amniotic fluid cells. Lancet 2: 910–912

Kan Y W, Valenti C, Carnazza V, Guidotti R, Rieder R F 1974 Fetal blood sampling in utero. Lancet 1: 79–80

Kan Y W, Golbus M S, Trecartin R F et al 1977 Prenatal diagnosis of beta-thalassemia and sickle-cell anemia – experience with 24 cases. Lancet 1: 269–271

Karp L E, Hayden P W 1977 Fetal puncture during mid trimester amniocentesis. Obstetrics and Gynecology 49: 115–117

Kazy Z, Rozovsky I S, Bakharev V A 1982 Chorion biopsy in early pregnancy: A method of early prenatal diagnosis for inherited disorders. Prenatal Diagnosis 2: 39–45

Kerem B-S, Rommens J M, Buchanan J A et al 1989 Identification of the cystic fibrosis gene: Genetic analysis. Science 245: 1073–1080

Kleijer W J 1986 First-trimester diagnosis of genetic metabolic disorders. Contributions to Gynecology and Obstetrics 15: 80–89

Kogan S C, Doherty M, Gitschier J 1987 An improved method for prenatal diagnosis of genetic diseases by analysis of amplified DNA sequences: Application to hemophilia A. New England Journal of Medicine 317: 985–990

Kohn G. Robinson A 1970 Tetraploidy in cells cultured from amniotic fluid. Lancet 2: 778–779

Kullander S, Sandahl B 1973 Fetal chromosome analysis after transcervical placental biopsies during early pregnancy. Acta Obstetrica et Gynecologica Scandinavica 52: 355–359

Kunkel L M 1986 Analysis of deletions in DNA from patients with Becker and Duchenne muscular dystrophy. Nature 322: 73–77

Lehmann A R, Francis A J, Giannelli F 1985 Prenatal diagnosis of Cockayne's syndrome. Lancet 1: 486–488

Leighton P C, Gordon Y B, Kitau M J, Leek A E, Chard T 1975 Levels of alpha-fetoprotein in maternal blood as a screening test for fetal neural tube defect. Lancet 2: 1012–1015

Leonard C O, Kazazian H H Jr. 1978 Prenatal diagnosis of hemoglobinopathies. Pediatric Clinics of North America 25: 631–642

Lilford R J 1986 Chorion villus biopsy. Clinics in Obstetrics and Gynaecology 13: 611–632

Lilford R J, Irving H C, Linton G, Mason M K 1987 Transabdominal chorion villus biopsy: 100 consecutive cases. Lancet 1: 1415–1417

Linch D C, Rodeck C H, Nicolaides K, Jones H M, Brent L 1986 Attempted bone-marrow transplantation in a 17-week fetus. Lancet 2: 1453

Linton G, Lilford R J 1986 False-negative finding on chorionic villus sampling. Lancet 2: 630

Liu D T, Jeavons B, Preston C, Pearson D 1987 A prospective study of spontaneous miscarriage in ultrasonically normal pregnancies and relevance to chorion villus sampling. Prenatal Diagnosis 7: 223–227

Ljung R, Holmberg L 1982 Genetic variants of haemophilia A detected by immunoradiometric assay: Implications for prenatal diagnosis. Pediatric Research 16: 256–258

Ludomirski A, Nemiroff R, Johnson A, Ashmead G G, Weiner S, Bolognese R J 1987 Percutaneous umbilical blood sampling. A new technique for prenatal diagnosis. Journal of Reproductive Medicine 32: 276–279

Macri J N, Kasturi R V, Krantz D A, Hu M G 1987 Maternal serum alpha-fetoprotein screening. II. Pitfalls in low-volume decentralized laboratory performance. American Journal of Obstetrics and Gynecology 156: 533–535

Main D M, Mennuti M T 1986 Neural tube defects: Issues in prenatal diagnosis and counselling. Obstetrics and Gynecology 67: 1–16

Manning F A, Harrison M R, Rodeck C 1986 Catheter shunts for fetal hydronephrosis and hydrocephalus. Report of the International Fetal Surgery Registry. New England Journal of Medicine 315: 336–340

Martin A O, Elias S, Rosinsky B, Bombard A T, Simpson J L 1986a False negative finding on chorionic villus sampling. Lancet 2: 391–392

Martin A O, Simpson J L, Rosinsky B J, Elias S 1986b Chorionic villus sampling in continuing pregnancies. II. Cytogenetic reliability. American Journal of Obstetrics and Gynecology 154: 1353–1362

Maxwell D, Czepulkowski B, Lilford R, Heaton D, Coleman D 1986 Transabdominal chorionic villus sampling. Lancet 1: 123–126

Mencaglia L, Ricci G, Perino A, Cittadini E, Catinella E 1986 Hysteroscopic chorionic villi sampling: a new approach. Acta Europaea Fertilitatis 17: 491–494

Merkatz I R, New M I, Peterson R E, Seaman M P 1969 Prenatal diagnosis of adrenogenital syndrome by amniocentesis. Journal of Pediatrics 75: 977–982

Merkatz I R, Nitowsky H M, Macri J N, Johnson W E 1984 An association between low maternal serum alpha-fetoprotein and fetal chromosomal abnormalities. American Journal of Obstetrics and Gynecology 148: 886–894

Milunksy A, Alpert E 1974 The value of alpha-fetoprotein in the prenatal diagnosis of neural tube defects. Journal of Pediatrics 84: 889–893

Milunsky A, Sapirstein V S 1982 Prenatal diagnosis of open neural tube defects using the amniotic fluid acetylcholinesterase assay. Obstetrics and Gynecology 59: 1–5

Milunksy A, Tulchinsky D 1977 Prenatal diagnosis of congenital adrenal hyperplasia due to 21-hydroxylase deficiency. Pediatrics 59: 768–773

Milunsky A, Littlefield J W, Atkins L 1970 Tetraploidy in amniotic fluid cells. Lancet 2: 979

Milunsky A, Atkins L, Littlefield J W 1971 Polyploidy in prenatal genetic diagnosis. Journal of Pediatrics 79: 303–305

Morin P R, Melancon S B, Dallaire L, Potier M 1987 Prenatal detection of intestinal obstructions, aneuploidy syndromes, and cystic fibrosis by microvillar enzyme assays (disaccharidases, alkaline phosphatase, and glutamyltransferase) in amniotic fluid. American Journal of Medical Genetics 26: 405–415

Mornet E, Boué J, Raux Demay M et al 1986 First trimester prenatal diagnosis of 21-hydroxylase deficiency by linkage analysis to HLA-DNA probes and by 17-hydroxyprogesterone determination. Human Genetics 73: 358–364

Morrow G, Schwarz R H, Hallock J A, Barness L A 1970 Prenatal detection of methylmalonic acidemia. Journal of Pediatrics 77: 120–123

Murken J A, Stengel-Rutkowski S, Schwinger E 1979 Prenatal Diagnosis. Proceedings of the 3rd European conference on prenatal diagnosis of genetic disorders. Ferdinand Enke, Stuttgart

Nadler H L 1968 Antenatal detection of hereditary disorders. Pediatrics 42: 912–918

Nadler H L, Gerbie A B 1969 Enzymes in non-cultured amniotic fluid cells. American Journal of Obstetrics and Gynecology 103: 710–712

Newburger P E, Cohen H J, Rothchild S B, Hobbins J C, Malawista S E, Mahoney M J 1979 Prenatal diagnosis of chronic granulomatous disease. New England Journal of Medicine 300: 178–181

NICHD National Registry for amniocentesis study group 1976 Mid trimester amniocentesis for prenatal diagnosis: Safety and accuracy. Journal of the American Medical Association 236: 1471–1476

Nicolaides K, Rodeck C H 1984 Prenatal diagnosis. Fetoscopy. British Journal of Hospital Medicine 31: 396–405

NIH Consensus Panel 1984 Diagnostic ultrasound imaging in pregnancy. Report of a consensus conference sponsored by the National Institute of Child Health and Human Development, the Office of Medical Applications of Research, and the Food and Drug Administration, February 6–8, 1984. NIH Publication 84–667, Baltimore

O'Brien W F 1984 Midtrimester genetic amniocentesis: A review of the fetal risks. Journal of Reproductive Medicine 29: 59–63

Old J M, Ward R H T, Petrou M, Karagözlu F, Modell B,

Weatherall D J 1982 First-trimester fetal diagnosis for haemoglobinopathies: Three cases. Lancet 2: 1413–1416

Old J M, Fitches A, Heath C et al 1986 First-trimester fetal diagnosis for haemoglobinopathies: Report on 200 cases. Lancet 2: 763–767

Orkin S H, Alter B P, Altay C, Mahoney M J, Lazarus H, Hobbins J C, Nathan D G 1978 Application of endonuclease mapping to the analysis and prenatal diagnosis of thalassemias caused by globin gene deletion. New England Journal of Medicine 299: 166–172

Orkin S H, Little P F R, Kazazian H H, Boehm C D 1982 Improved detection of the sickle mutation by DNA analysis: Application to prenatal diagnosis. New England Journal of Medicine 307: 32–36

Ornoy A, Borochowitz Z, Lachman R, Rimoin D 1988 Atlas of Fetal Skeletal Radiology. Yearbook Medical Publishers, Chicago

Packman S, Golbus M S, Cowan M J et al 1982 Prenatal treatment of biotin-responsive multiple carboxylase deficiency. Lancet 1: 1435–1438

Page D, Martinville B D, Barker D, Wyman A, White R, Francke U, Botstein D 1982 Single-copy sequence hybridizes to polymorphic and homologous loci on human X and Y chromosomes. Proceedings of the National Academy of Sciences USA 79: 5352–5356

Peake I R, Furlong B L, Bloom A L 1984 Carrier detection by direct gene analysis in a family with haemophilia B (Factor IX deficiency). Lancet 1: 242–243

Peakman D C, Moreton M F, Corn B J, Robinson A 1978 Chromosomal mosaicism in amniotic fluid cell cultures. Pediatric Research 12: 455

Peakman D C, Moreton M F, Corn B J, Robinson A 1979 Chromosomal mosaicism in amniotic fluid cultures. American Journal of Human Genetics 31: 149–155

Perry T B, Vekemans M J, Lippman A, Hamilton E F, Fournier P J 1987 Early prenatal diagnosis by chorionic villi sampling. Current Problems in Dermatology 16: 14–22

Persson P H, Kullander S 1983 Long-term experience of general ultrasound screening in pregnancy. American Journal of Obstetrics and Gynecology 146: 942–947

Planteydt H T, van de Vooren M J, Verweij H 1986 Amniotic bands and malformations in a child born after pregnancy screened by chorionic villus biopsy. Lancet 2: 756–757

Poenaru L 1987 First trimester prenatal diagnosis of metabolic diseases: a survey in countries from the European community. Prenatal Diagnosis 7: 333–341

Pollack M S, Maurer D, Levine L S et al 1979 Prenatal diagnosis of congenital adrenal hyperplasia (21-hydroxylase deficiency) by HLA typing. Lancet 1: 1107–1108

Ramsay C A, Coltart T M, Blunt S, Pawsey S A, Giannelli F 1974 Prenatal diagnosis of xeroderma pigmentosum. Report of the first successful case. Lancet 2: 1109–1112

Reeders S T, Zerres K, Gal A et al 1986 Prenatal diagnosis of autosomal dominant polycystic kidney disease with a DNA probe. Lancet 2: 6–8

Rhoads G G, Jackson L G, Schlesselman S E et al 1989 The safety and efficacy of chorionic villus sampling for early prenatal diagnosis of cytogenetic abnormalities. New England Journal of Medicine 320: 609–617

Rodeck C H, Nicolaides K H 1983 The use of fetoscopy for prenatal diagnosis and treatment. Seminars in Perinatology 7: 118–124

Rodeck C H, Nicolaides K H 1986 Fetoscopy. British Medical

Bulletin 42: 296–300

Rodeck C H, Pembrey M E, Patrick A D, Tzannatos C, Whitfield A E 1982 Fetal liver biopsy for prenatal diagnosis of ornithine carbamyl transferase deficiency. Lancet 2: 297–300

Romero R, Jeanty P, Reece E A, Grannum P, Bracken M, Berkowitz R, Hobbins J C 1985 Sonographically monitored amniocentesis to decrease intraoperative complications. Obstetrics and Gynecology 65: 426–430

Rommens J M, Iannuzzi M C, Kerem B-S et al 1989 Identification of the cystic fibrosis gene: Chromosome walking and jumping. Science 245: 1059–1065

Roth K S, Yang W, Allan L, Saunders M, Gravel R A, Dakshinamurti K 1982 Prenatal administration of biotin in biotin responsive multiple carboxylase deficiency. Pediatric Research 16: 126–129

Sabbagha R E, Shkolnik A 1980 Ultrasound diagnosis of fetal abnormalities. Seminars in Perinatology 4: 213–227

Saiki R K, Scharf S, Faloona F, Mullis K B, Horn G T, Erlich H A, Arnheim N 1985 Enzymatic amplification of beta-globin genomic sequences and restriction site analysis for diagnosis of sickle cell anemia. Science 230: 1350–1354

Sanguinetti N, Marsh J, Jackson M, Fensom A H, Warren R C, Rodeck C H 1986 The arylsulphatases of chorionic villi: Potential problems in the first-trimester diagnosis of metachromatic leucodystrophy and Maroteaux-Lamy disease. Clinical Genetics 30: 302–308

Schulze B, Miller K 1986 Chromosomal mosaicism and maternal cell contamination in chorionic villi cultures. Clinical Genetics 30: 239–240

Schwartz S, Flannery D B, Cohen M M 1985 Tests appropriate for the prenatal diagnosis of ataxia telangiectasia. Prenatal Diagnosis 5: 9–14

Second report of the U.K. collaborative study on alpha-fetoprotein in relation to neural tube defects 1979 Amniotic fluid alpha-fetoprotein measurement in antenatal diagnosis of anencephaly and open spina bifida in early pregnancy. Lancet 2: 651–661

Seller M J 1974 Alpha-fetoprotein and the prenatal diagnosis of neural tube defects. Developmental Medicine and Child Neurology 16: 369–381

Seppälä M 1973 Increased alpha-fetoprotein in amniotic fluid associated with a congenital esophageal atresia of the fetus. Obstetrics and Gynecology 42: 613–614

Seppälä M, Ruoslahti E 1972 Alpha-fetoprotein in amniotic fluid: An index of gestational age. American Journal of Obstetrics and Gynecology 114: 595–598

Seppälä M, Ruoslahti E 1973a Alpha-fetoprotein in antenatal diagnosis. Lancet 1: 155

Seppälä M, Ruoslahti E 1973b Alpha-fetoprotein in Rh negative immunized pregnancies. Obstetrics and Gynecology 42: 701–706

Serr D M, Sachs L, Danon M 1955 Diagnosis of sex before birth using cells from the amniotic fluid. Bulletin of the Research Council of Israel 5B: 137

Shapiro L R, Wilmot P L 1986 Prenatal diagnosis of the fra(X) syndrome. American Journal of Medical Genetics 23: 325–340

Shapiro L R, Wilmot P L, Brenholz P et al 1982 Prenatal diagnosis of fragile X chromosome. Lancet 1: 99–100

Simkowski K W 1987 Laboratory considerations in maternal serum alpha-fetoprotein testing. Journal of Clinical Immunoassay 10: 217–221

Simoni G, Brambati B, Danesino C, Rossella F, Terzoli G L,

Ferrari M, Fraccaro M 1983 Efficient direct chromosome analyses and enzyme determinations from chorionic villi samples in the first trimester of pregnancy. Human Genetics 63: 349–357

Simoni G, Gimelli G, Cuoco C et al 1986a First trimester fetal karyotyping: one thousand diagnoses. Human Genetics 72: 203–209

Simoni G, Rossella F, Lalatta F, Fraccaro M 1986b Maternal metaphases on direct preparation from chorionic villi and in cultures of villi cells. Human Genetics 72: 104

Simpson J L 1980 Antenatal diagnosis of cytogenetic abnormalities. Seminars in Perinatology 4: 165–178

Smith A D, Wald N J, Cuckle H S, Stirrat G M, Bobrow M, Lagercrantz H 1979 Amniotic fluid acetylcholinesterase as a possible diagnostic test for neural tube defects in early pregnancy. Lancet 1: 685–690

Spence J E, Buffone G J, Rosenbloom C L et al 1987 Prenatal diagnosis of cystic fibrosis using linked DNA markers and microvillar intestinal enzyme analysis. Human Genetics 76: 5–10

Steele M W, Breg W R Jr. 1966 Chromosome analysis of human amniotic fluid cells. Lancet 1: 383–385

Stoll C, Willard D, Czernichow P, Boué J 1978 Prenatal diagnosis of primary pituitary dysgenesis. Lancet 1: 932

Sugita T, Ikenaga M, Suehara N, Furuyama J I, Yabuuchi H 1982 Prenatal diagnosis of Cockayne syndrome using assay of colony forming ability in ultraviolet light irradiated cells. Clinical Genetics 22: 137–142

Tietung Hospital of Anshan Iron and Steel Company 1975 Fetal sex prediction by sex chromatin of chorionic villi cells during early pregnancy. Chinese Medical Journal 2: 117–126

Timor-Tritsch I E, Bar Yam Y, Elgali S, Rottem S 1988 The technique of transvaginal sonography with the use of a 6.5 MHz probe. American Journal of Obstetrics and Gynecology 158: 1019–1024

Tommerup N, Aula P, Gustavii B et al 1986 Second trimester prenatal diagnosis of the fragile X. American Journal of Medical Genetics 23: 313–324

van Diggelen O P, Janse H C, Kleijer W J 1983 Disaccharidases in amniotic fluid as possible prenatal marker for cystic fibrosis. Lancet 1: 817

Verjaal M, Leschot N J, Wolf H, Treffers P E 1987 Karyotypic differences between cells from placenta and other fetal tissues. Prenatal Diagnosis 7: 343–348

Vintzileos A M, Campbell W A, Nochimson D J, Weinbaum P J 1987 Antenatal evaluation and management of ultrasonically detected fetal anomalies. Obstetrics and Gynecology 69: 640–660

Wagner G, Fuchs F 1962 Volume of amniotic fluid in the first half of human pregnancy. Journal of Obstetrics and Gynaecology of the British Commonwealth 69: 131–136

Wald N J, Cuckle H S 1981 Amniotic fluid acetylcholinesterase electrophoresis as a secondary test in the diagnosis of anencephaly and open spina bifida in early pregnancy. Report of the collaborative acetylcholinesterase study. Lancet 2: 321–324

Ward R H T, Modell B, Petrou M, Karagözlu F, Douratsos E 1983 Method of sampling chorionic villi in first trimester of pregnancy under guidance of real time ultrasound. British Medical Journal 286: 1542–1544

Watson M S, Breg W R, Hobbins J C, Mahoney M J 1984 Cytogenetic diagnosis using midtrimester fetal blood samples: Application to suspected mosaicism and other diagnostic problems. American Journal of Medical Genetics 19: 805–813

Webb T, Gosden C M, Rodeck C H, Hamill M A, Eason P E 1983 Prenatal diagnosis of X-linked mental retardation with fragile (X) using fetoscopy and fetal blood sampling. Prenatal Diagnosis 3: 131–137

Webb T P, Rodeck C H, Nicolaides K H, Gosden C M 1987 Prenatal diagnosis of the fragile X syndrome using fetal blood and amniotic fluid. Prenatal Diagnosis 7: 203–214

Whyley G A, Ward H, Hardy N R 1974 Alpha-fetoprotein levels in amniotic fluids in pregnancies complicated by Rhesus isoimmunization. Journal of Obstetrics and Gynaecology of the British Commonwealth 81: 459–465

Williams J III, Medearis A L, Chu W H, Kovacs G D, Kaback M M 1987 Maternal cell contamination in cultured chorionic villi: Comparison of chromosome Q-polymorphisms derived from villi, fetal skin, and

maternal lymphocytes. Prenatal Diagnosis 7: 315–322

Wilson R D, Kendrick V, Wittmann B K, McGillivray B 1986 Spontaneous abortion and pregnancy outcome after normal first-trimester ultrasound examination. Obstetrics and Gynecology 67: 352–355

Wilson R D, Hogge W A, Golbus M S 1987 Analysis of chromosomally normal spontaneous abortions after chorionic villus sampling. Journal of Reproductive Medicine 32: 25–27

Zador I E, Bottoms S F, Tse G M, Brindley B A, Sokol R J 1988 Nomograms for ultrasound visualization of fetal organs. Journal of Ultrasound in Medicine 7: 197–201

Zeisel S H, Milunsky A, Blusztajn J K 1980 Prenatal diagnosis of neural tube defects. V. The value of amniotic fluid cholinesterase studies. American Journal of Obstetrics and Gynecology 137: 481–485

112. Genetic registers

Andrew P. Read

The simplest register is no more than a list of interesting cases compiled for a specific purpose, and in this sense every geneticist keeps innumerable registers. Here, however, we are concerned with the use of relatively large and permanent registers to organize the delivery of genetic services. Such patient-care registers may guide research projects or provide epidemiological information, but in principle their purpose is different.

THE PURPOSE OF A GENETIC REGISTER

In 1972 a World Health Organization Scientific Group recommended that medical genetics centres should establish registers of genetically determined disorders so that genetic counselling could be offered to all who would benefit from it (WHO 1972). This remains one prime purpose of a register, but the development of DNA technology has provided another. At present few diseases can be diagnosed directly by examining the DNA of an isolated individual, but many can be tracked through pedigrees using DNA restriction fragment length polymorphisms (RFLPs) (Weatherall 1985). Gene tracking using RFLPs often requires extended pedigrees and long-term DNA storage. Prenatal diagnosis using RFLPs is inefficient if the first contact with the family happens when a pregnancy is already under way. Thus the efficient application of DNA technology requires long-term contact with extended families; this is the hallmark of a genetic register.

A register as described here does not have aims separate from the rest of the genetic service: it is a tool for dealing efficiently with some central aspects of the service. It may overlap epidemiological research registers or systems for computerised clinic notes, but its specific functions are:

1. to extend counselling from the proband to the whole family.
2. to maintain long-term contact with the family.
3. to recall children at risk at the appropriate time for any tests or counselling.
4. to ensure that appropriate DNA and other samples are stored against future needs.
5. to avoid emergency laboratory work and unnecessary prenatal interventions.
6. to avoid emergency counselling in inappropriate circumstances.

If a register fulfils these functions adequately, it will be effective at preventing genetic disease by identifying people at risk before they have an affected child and offering them counselling and diagnostic tests. Its systematic long-term follow-up will facilitate monitoring of the effect of genetic services. Depending on ascertainment policy, the register may also be a source of epidemiological and other research data.

Total ascertainment is desirable so that all families at risk are identified and offered counselling. Nevertheless, overemphasis on ascertainment brings the risk of reducing the register to little more than a list of interesting names. Insofar as the register is a tool for delivering a service, ascertainment should be a function of the resources available to carry the service workload. One way of managing with inadequate resources is to attempt complete ascertainment of a limited set of diseases, and not register other diseases at all. This has the attraction of administrative clarity, and leaves the way open to seek funding for other diseases later.

WHAT DISEASES SHOULD BE REGISTERED?

Some genetics departments register all referrals, but the critical diseases are those where the risk extends significantly beyond the nuclear family, and those where gene tracking by RFLPs is possible, or likely to become possible. In practice these include:

1. serious autosomal dominant diseases where affected people often have children, including:

   Huntington chorea
   von Recklinghausen neurofibromatosis
   Myotonic dystrophy

Familial hypercholesterolaemia
Adult polycystic kidney disease
Dominant familial cancers

2. serious X-linked diseases including:

Duchenne and Becker muscular dystrophy
Fragile-X mental retardation
Haemophilia A and B
Retinitis pigmentosa

3. balanced chromosomal translocations

4. autosomal recessive diseases where prenatal diagnosis depends on gene tracking by RFLPs, including:

Haemoglobinopathies
Cystic fibrosis
Phenylketonuria.

THE REGISTER AND THE DNA LABORATORY

Most diagnostic DNA laboratories have set out to build up banks of DNA (or cell lines) from people who may not be alive when their DNA is needed. Examples are patients with Huntington chorea and their unaffected relatives who are old enough for us to be confident they do not carry the disease gene, and boys affected with Duchenne muscular dystrophy. Their DNA is needed either to establish phase with future linked markers or to enable the nature of the mutation in that family to be defined once the gene is isolated. Deciding what categories of DNA to bank involves guesswork about future developments, but the importance of DNA banking is now widely recognised.

DNA banks require catalogues. The catalogue may not be identical to the genetic register (it will include far more diseases) but they overlap to such a degree that some functional relationship is needed. On the most simple basis the register record will include the reference numbers of any banked DNA samples, and there will be an extra category of register records for people whose only involvement with the register is through the DNA bank.

A database of families is also important in the shorter term for a DNA laboratory offering prenatal diagnosis. With many diseases – Duchenne muscular dystrophy is an outstanding example – DNA studies of the family are necessary to decide whether a woman is a carrier. If a woman is first ascertained when already pregnant, the tests cannot be done in time to decide whether or not to perform a chorion biopsy. Instead, the biopsy is sent to the laboratory, along with blood from the woman and her family, and often the test results show the biopsy was

unnecessary. Such a system puts the pregnancy at risk as well as wasting obstetric and laboratory time.

Even where the genetic status is not in doubt, unnecessary tests will be done if the family is not studied before the pregnancy. In cystic fibrosis one can safely assume that both parents of an affected child are carriers, but current methods for prenatal diagnosis require that they should be informative for gene tracking. With the present range of probes a few couples are uninformative and chorion biopsy would not help them.

Apart from avoiding unnecessary biopsies, investigating the family before a pregnancy is efficient for the laboratory. As long as the laboratory procedure is based on Southern blotting and hybridisation with radio-labelled probes, the biggest single determinant of workload is the number of probes to be used. It costs little more time or money to test ten samples with a probe than to test one. Efficient working therefore depends on batching samples, which is only possible with non-urgent requests. If a family has not been investigated beforehand, the samples must be tested urgently with all possible probes to find one for which they are informative. A laboratory working with a genetic register can screen family members sequentially with each probe, putting in the samples when there is a full batch ready for that probe; then when the chorion biopsy arrives, the urgent test needs only the probe(s) for which the couple are known to be informative. Table 112.1 shows the recent Manchester protocols for prenatal diagnosis of cystic fibrosis, and demonstrates the reduction in workload in registered families.

Both knowledge and technology are advancing so rapidly in molecular genetics that all statements on this

Table 112.1 Protocols for prenatal diagnosis of cystic fibrosis, showing the advantages of referral before pregnancy

Samples: both parents
fetus
affected child

Urgent tests: Family studied beforehand		New pregnant referral	
Digest	Probe	Digest	Probe
		TaqI	Met-D
(as determined by			Met-H
previous investigation)			XV.2c
		PstI	KM.19
		MspI	pJ3.11
		BanI	Met-D
		HhaI	CS.7
1 or 2	1 or 2	5	6

subject must be regarded as provisional. The adoption of stable non-radiolabelled probes would make it less important to handle samples in batches, and direct detection of the disease gene will remove the need for family studies in some diseases. On the other hand, increasing automation may impose its own requirement for large batches of samples, and it seems likely that family studies will continue to be necessary for diseases which are maintained by recurrent mutation rather than by selection or drift, and probably also for many biochemically ill-defined diseases. In short, for the forseeable future DNA diagnostic services will continue to need DNA banks and family databases.

GEOGRAPHICAL SCOPE

Should the register be national, regional or local? The choice is constrained by a number of factors. A more mobile population needs a register with a wider geographical base. Diseases which are treated in specialised centres will probably best be registered by the centre. Where epidemiological registers already exist, as with national cancer registers in the UK, the patient care register needs to relate to these, most simply by having the same geographical base. Any existing DNA banks will also partly determine the coverage of a register. In general, however, if the register is a tool for organizing a genetic counselling service, it should have the same geographical scope as the counselling service. In the UK this would normally be a Health Service Region, with a population of 2–5 million.

Difficulties then arise when families cross boundaries. Since one of the main criteria for inclusion in the register is that risk should extend beyond the nuclear family, these problems will be common. Despite this, local registers are preferable to national ones. One must work on the assumption that no remotely accessible computer is secure against skilled and determined hackers. Information that someone is at risk of Huntington chorea is valuable (to employers, insurers etc.), and the best way of protecting it is to disperse it onto microcomputers not connected to a telephone line. On a more mundane level, the register is most likely to be successful if the people running it are the ones who suffer when it doesn't work.

In our experience the problems of families which straddle boundaries are best contained by ensuring that in each area there is one clearly identified person who is the contact for enquiries about that disease. Even with a national register such a definition of responsibilities would be essential to avoid families suffering multiple and maybe contradictory approaches.

COMPUTERISATION

A genetic register should clearly be manipulated on a computer rather than in manual form. Developments since the first edition of this book mean that a standard desk-top microcomputer running a standard database package is entirely suitable. A stand-alone microcomputer offers good security, and using a standard database package ensures portability when the computer is replaced by a newer, more powerful, and cheaper model.

No general prescription can be offered about what data should be stored; this depends on local requirements and arrangements. As a minimum, the following functions should be available:

1. the ability to recall a patient given a reference number or name.
2. the ability to recall data on a whole family given the name or reference number of any member.
3. the ability to count or list patients by age, sex, disease, risk category, geographical area.
4. the ability to generate worklists for recall or review.
5. the ability to flag people for various actions (e.g. bleeding for DNA).
6. the ability to link individuals to a pedigree – important when spouses or unaffected relatives are bled for DNA studies, but are not otherwise included in the register.
7. the ability to check rapidly the state of progress, with any family, in counselling and in laboratory testing.

It is useful if the computer is able to update various risk calculations automatically. This requires that the records contain the pedigree structure (typically, a family number, an individual number and the number of the father and mother).

In the UK such a computer data bank would require registration under the terms of the Data Protection Act.

THE MANCHESTER GENETIC REGISTER

Genetic registers are maintained in several UK genetic centres. One of the first was the RAPID system in Edinburgh (Emery et al 1974). The North West Regional genetic register in Manchester was started in 1980 following the recommendations of a report from a working party of the Clinical Genetics Society (Emery et al 1978). Because of limited resources coverage is restricted to Duchenne and Becker muscular dystrophy, Huntington chorea and adult polycystic kidney disease.

People are eligible for registration if they are affected or at 10% or greater risk of developing (Huntington chorea, polycystic kidney disease) or carrying (Duchenne and Becker muscular dystrophy) the disease. We began by including all families referred to the Regional genetic counselling service, both retrospectively and prospectively. We then sought further families through the consultants running specialist clinics and the handicap registers maintained by the community medical service. The eventual aim is complete ascertainment of these diseases within the North West Region (population 4 million). There is a formal system of consenting to registration, which people may refuse, and this reduces the potential uses of the register as an epidemiological tool.

At the time the register was set up there were no markers for any of the diseases included; now, of course, gene tracking is available for all these diseases and the register works very closely with the molecular genetics laboratory. The work with the Duchenne muscular dystrophy families has been described elsewhere (Read et al 1986). The present status is shown in Table 112.2.

Protocols

The Manchester genetic register works to the following protocols:

1. The diagnosis is established, usually jointly by the consultant clinical geneticist and the appropriate medical specialist.
2. The proband is counselled.
3. If the proband consents he (and where appropriate his children) is registered and asked to agree that other family members be approached. He is encouraged to initiate this contact himself.
4. The family doctor of each relative at risk is informed that his patient 'might be at risk of an inherited disease', and is asked whether there is any reason why the relative should not be approached for counselling.
5. The relative is approached, again without specifying the disease or degree of risk, so that he retains a genuine option not to know.
6. If the relative agrees he is counselled and any necessary diagnostic investigations arranged. If he

consents he is then included on the register in his own right.
7. If the relative consents, but only if he consents, his family doctor is given details of the consultation and tests.
8. Everybody on the register is contacted once a year, to update the address and enquire about any changes in the family to be noted on the pedigree. They are offered an appointment if there is new information to be communicated or if they feel the need.

ETHICAL PROBLEMS

The main ethical issues concern confidentiality and the propriety of offering unsuspecting people the unsolicited information that they are at risk of an untreatable disease.

Confidentiality is a particularly difficult problem. Naturally the register will take suitable precautions to prevent unauthorised access to its data. However, with late-onset diseases like Huntington chorea there is a conflict between the desire of the relative to keep his risk secret and the interests of potential employers, insurers etc. The family doctor is the focus of this conflict. Good medical practice requires that he be fully informed, not least so that he can judge whether it would be appropriate to approach his patient for counselling. But it is the family doctor who will have to answer questions from employers, insurers etc. However legitimate these enquiries are, the register operation would collapse if its first effect were to make all members of Huntington chorea families unemployable and uninsurable. This is the reason for the carefully chosen vague wording of the letter to the relative's doctor. It is also another reason for preferring the first approach to be made by the proband rather than the register. The geneticist must bear in mind that it is not always in somebody's best interest to discover, say, that he is at risk of polycystic kidney disease if he has not yet arranged life insurance. The priorities must be set by the needs of patients and not by the desire for a tidy register.

In contrast, the ethical problems of unsolicited approaches to relatives are not severe. Our experience suggests that relatives are rarely totally unaware of their risk. Often they overestimate their personal risk, and counselling brings relief. Even when this is not true, it is not self-evidently ethical to withold from someone information without which he cannot realistically plan his life. Some have suggested that not giving the information is unethical (Fletcher et al 1985).

The risks of offering unsolicited information are minimised by careful adherence to the protocol above. This however raises another problem: what happens if the proband or the family doctor unreasonably refuse to

Table 112.2 The Manchester genetic register – status in September 1989

Disease	Families	Individuals Affected	At risk
Huntington chorea	210	295	2072
Muscular dystrophy:			
Duchenne	180	246	813
Becker	18	63	78
Polycystic kidney disease	129	265	441

agree to a relative being approached? Note that the protocol seeks the agreement, not the permission, of these people. They have no authority to forbid an approach, though the proband can forbid disclosure of his own condition. Contacts initiated through the proband can circumvent obstruction by the family doctor. If the proband witholds his agreement it is prudent to wait and try again later, hoping that meanwhile he will come to feel he has benefited from his own contacts with the register, through counselling, support, prenatal diagnosis etc. Experience has shown that patience usually yields results.

A LOOK AHEAD

A register is a long-term commitment, and some attempt must be made to foresee needs and technical possibilities ten years ahead. Counselling needs are unlikely to change radically, but the technical possibilities certainly will. Forseeing the unforseeable is difficult: one has only to think of the changes produced in the past three years by PCR (polymerase chain reaction) technology. PCR affects not only laboratory practice but also schemes for DNA banking, since it is now possible to genotype dead people from Guthrie cards or fixed tissues.

It seems certain that every common serious Mendelian disease will very soon become amenable to gene tracking. A disease should not be left off the register just because it has not yet been mapped – by next year it probably will be. On the other hand, the technology will move on. At present gene tracking is difficult, requires a good understanding of genetics, and clearly belongs in a large genetic centre. In a few years this may change. What would happen if easily used kits are sold which detect common disease genes directly, without the need for family studies?

Some diseases seem inherently complicated, genetically and at the molecular level. I believe that Duchenne muscular dystrophy and fragile-X mental retardation will always need to be handled by counsellors with a deep knowledge of genetics and by laboratories capable of more than just using kits. Other diseases seem simple – cystic fibrosis for example. If kits for direct diagnosis of the CF mutation become available, the case for keeping CF within the genetic register is not overwhelming. Many diseases – Huntington chorea is a likely candidate – will become simple at the laboratory level, but will continue to require the counselling skills and long-term contact which the genetic register is designed to provide.

As genetic knowledge increases, attention may move away from the simple Mendelian and chromosomal disorders and focus more on genetic susceptibility to common diseases. Were it to become possible to screen individuals for genetic susceptibility to cancer, heart disease, etc, and to counsel them about drugs or changes in lifestyle which could substantially lower their risk, then the genetic register would be the natural vehicle for handling such an operation. Opinions may reasonably differ on whether this is either likely or desirable.

ACKNOWLEDGEMENTS

I am deeply indebted to Lauren Kerzin-Storrar for many helpful discussions and comments, and to Rodney Harris for his encouragement.

REFERENCES

Emery A E H, Elliott D, Moores M, Smith C 1974 A genetic register system (RAPID). Journal of Medical Genetics 11: 145–151

Emery A E H, Brough C, Crawfurd M, Harper P, Harris R, Oakshott G 1978 A report on genetic registers. Journal of Medical Genetics 15: 435–442

Fletcher J C, Berg K, Tranøy K E 1985 Ethical aspects of medical genetics: a proposal for guidelines in genetic counselling, prenatal diagnosis and screening. Clinical Genetics 27: 199–205

Read A P, Kerzin-Storrar L, Mountford R C, Elles R G, Harris R 1986 A register-based system for gene tracking in Duchenne muscular dystrophy. Journal of Medical Genetics 23: 581–586

Weatherall D J 1985 The new genetics and clinical practice, 2nd edn. Oxford University Press

WHO 1972 Genetic disorders: prevention, treatment and rehabilitation. Technical report series no 497, WHO, Geneva.

113. Treatment of inherited metabolic diseases

Robert J. Desnick

INTRODUCTION

Major advances have been made in the elucidation of the molecular pathologies of inherited metabolic diseases during the past two decades. The clinical and pathophysiological manifestations have been delineated and the metabolic derangements have been characterized in an ever-increasing number of these disorders. Sophisticated chemical and enzymatic techniques as well as in vitro tissue culture systems have been developed to identify the specific enzymatic defects in more than 200 of the over 400 catalogued, recessively inherited, inborn errors of metabolism (McKusick 1988). Implementation of these techniques in major centres has made the diagnosis of these disorders a reality. Indeed, the demonstration of the specific enzyme deficiency has provided for the accurate diagnosis of affected homozygotes or hemizygotes, detection of heterozygous carriers, and the capability to diagnose prenatally and prevent the birth of affected fetuses. However, in spite of these major diagnostic achievements, patients and their families have become increasingly disappointed by the absence of specific therapies for most of these debilitating disorders.

Common pathophysiology of inherited metabolic diseases

In each of these disorders, the defective enzymatic activity results in a metabolic block (Fig. 113.1). Typically, the enzyme's substrate accumulates and there is a severe deficiency of the metabolic product. In some disorders the disease pathology results from the abnormal accumulation of the substrate, (e.g. phenylketonuria, mucopolysaccharidoses) while in others the pathological manifestations are caused by lack of the critical metabolic product (e.g. growth hormone deficiency, adrenogenital syndrome). In certain disorders, a critical cofactor for the enzyme (e.g. vitamin, trace metal) may not be available in

an active form to catalyze the reaction. For example, in classical phenylketonuria (PKU), the deficient activity of phenylalanine hydroxylase results in the accumulation of phenylalanine; the metabolic block also leads to lack of tyrosine, but the deficiency of this amino acid does not appear to be pathological. The high concentration of phenylalanine leads to the accumulation of toxic derivatives, including phenylpyruvic acid, phenylacetic acid and other phenylalanine metabolites. Pathophysiologically, the massive accumulation of a particular substrate (or the lack of a crucial metabolic product) can lead to dysfunction of a cell type, which may then impair organ function and result in the clinical manifestations of the disease.

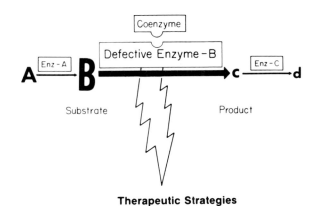

Therapeutic Strategies

Fig. 113.1 Metabolic block in an inborn error of metabolism. A mutation in the gene encoding enzyme B renders it defective (i.e. non-functional). Substrate B accumulates and product C is deficient. Some enzymes require a coenzyme (or cofactor) for catalytic function. Certain cofactor-dependent enzyme defects can be corrected by supplementation with the appropriate vitamin, trace metal, etc.

Approaches for the treatment of inherited metabolic diseases

During the past decade, considerable attention has been focused on the development of strategies to treat patients with inherited metabolic diseases (Table 113.1). Early therapeutic endeavours primarily involved attempts to alter the disease course by various metabolic manipulations. Investigators have attempted to decrease the concentrations of an accumulated substrate (or of precursors to a metabolic block) by dietary restriction, chelation, or administration of appropriate metabolic inhibitors; or, in disorders resulting from the lack of a crucial product, to replace the normal product. Following early recognition and appropriate intervention in certain of these disorders, chemical and clinical successes have been documented. Therapeutic trials at the level of the biochemical defect have involved direct administration of the appropriate gene product, the specific active enzyme or deficient cofactor, or the transplantation of allografts capable of producing the normal gene product. The limitations, as well as the encouraging successes, of these strategies for the treatment of genetic diseases have been the subject of many symposia and reviews (Matas et al 1978, Desnick & Grabowski 1981, Desnick 1983, 1987, Shapiro 1983).

Current research efforts to treat these diseases are directed towards the improvement of metabolic manipulation techniques, further development of enzyme replacement and enzyme manipulation strategies, and the evaluation of bone marrow transplantation for the correction of selected disorders. Recent attention has also focused on the potential therapeutic application of recombinant DNA (rDNA) technology. Theoretically, the ideal cure for these inherited diseases would be the insertion of the normal segment of DNA coding for the synthesis of a functional gene product. Rapid developments in rDNA technology and gene transfer methodology have provided the means to assess the potential of therapeutic endeavours at the level of the primary defect, or 'gene therapy'. This review will discuss the present status and future prospects for the treatment of inherited metabolic disorders using rDNA techniques.

APPLICATION OF rDNA TO THE TREATMENT OF INHERITED METABOLIC DISEASES

Production of biologically active substances

rDNA technology has provided the ability to synthesise human biochemical products of therapeutic importance. It is first necessary to isolate the full-length cDNA encoding the therapeutic protein. Then the cDNA can be inserted into an expression vector for the production of large amounts of the protein. A variety of expression vectors have been elegantly constructed for the production of proteins in E. coli, yeast, baculovirus-infected insect cells and mammalian cells (Mulligan & Berg 1980, Sarver et al 1981, Old & Primrose 1985, Miller et al 1986). These expression vectors are designed to facilitate insertion of the cDNA into a position behind a promotor, a powerful DNA sequence which is responsible for the initiation of transcription of the inserted cDNA sequence.

The two major types of expression systems currently in use employ prokaryotic (i.e. E. coli) and eukaryotic (i.e. yeast, baculovirus, mammalian) vector constructs. The prokaryotic systems can produce very large amounts of protein, but the bacteria lack the post-translational modification machinery to glycosylate or proteolytically cleave certain proteins for proper folding and/or stability. Proteins that are functionally active in E. coli can be produced in very large quantities at relatively low cost. However, since many human proteins are not functionally active when produced in E. coli, efforts have focused on the development and evaluation of eukaryotic expression systems.

Attractive eukaryotic systems have been used to express a variety of human proteins (Table 113.2). Notable among these are those being produced commercially, including human insulin, growth hormone, interleukin-2, somatomedins, tissue plasminogen activator and erythropoietin. Clearly, this technology should permit the production of any human protein. Efforts are

Table 113.1 Strategies for the treatment of inherited metabolic diseases

Metabolic manipulation
   Dietary restriction
   Substrate depletion techniques
      Chelation enhanced excretion
      Plasmapheresis/affinity binding
   Surgical bypass procedures
   Metabolic inhibition
   Product replacement

Gene product therapy
   Cofactor supplementation
   Enzyme induction
   Allotransplantation
   Enzyme replacement therpay

Gene therapy
   Production of human gene products
   Gene replacement

Preventive therapy
   Heterozygote screening
   Genetic counselling
   Prenatal diagnosis

Table 113.2 Examples of expressed recombinant human proteins

Protein	Expression system	Vector
Insulin	E. coli; mammalian cell culture	SV40-derived plasmid
Growth hormone	Mammalian cell culture	SV40-derived plasmid; Bovine papilloma virus
α-Interferon	Mammalian cell culture; insect cell culture	Herpes simplex-derived plasmid; Baculovirus
β-Interferon	Mammalian cell culture; insect cell culture	SV40-derived plasmid; Baculovirus
Interleukin 2	Mammalian cell culture; insect cell culture	SV40-derived plasmid; Baculovirus
Tissue plasminogen activator	E. coli; mammalian cell culture	SV40-derived plasmid
α_1-Antitrypsin	E. coli; yeast	
Erythropoietin	Mammalian cell culture	SV40-derived plasmid
Granulocyte-Macrophage Colony Stimulating Factor (GM-CSF)	Mammalian cell culture	SV40-derived plasmid
Choriogonadotropin	Mammalian cell culture	SV40-derived plasmid
β-glucosidase	insect cell culture	Baculovirus
α-galactosidase	Mammalian cell culture; insect cell culture	SV40-derived plasmid; Baculovirus

currently underway to express human Factor VIII for the treatment of haemophilia A (without the risk of infection by HIV or non-A, non-B hepatitis virus), as well as a variety of enzymes for the evaluation of enzyme replacement therapy in selected disorders (e.g. Gaucher and Fabry diseases), using adequate amounts of enzyme, made available for the first time by rDNA techniques. Thus, the ability to produce large quantities of biologically active proteins will not only have a major impact on genetic diseases, but will also be useful in a variety of areas including industry, agriculture and animal husbandry.

Germ-line gene therapy

The goal of germ-line gene therapy is the insertion of a gene or genes into the germ cells (i.e. oogonia, spermatogonia) in such a way that it will be corrective and transmitted in a Mendelian fashion from generation to generation. Experimental germ-line gene therapy in humans has been prohibited in concept, philosophy and fact by the 'Guidelines' of the NIH Recombinant DNA Advisory Committee on Human Gene Therapy. However, such experiments have been permitted in mice and serve to demonstrate the feasibility of inserting functional genes into the germ-line with subsequent cure of the murine disease.

Feasibility of germ-line gene therapy: transgenic mice

The technique for insertion of a foreign gene or DNA segment into the mouse germ line is shown in Figure 113.2. One-celled mouse embryos are removed immediately following fertilization. The male pronucleus is visible at this stage and foreign DNA can be inserted into it by microinjection. When about 100 embryos have been injected these are placed into the uterus of a pseudopregnant female mouse. Only a few will successfully undergo fetal development. After birth of the pups, the presence of the foreign gene in each is determined by Southern hybridization analyses using DNA isolated from tail biopsies.

Mice which have the foreign gene integrated into their genomes (one to several hundred copies) will transmit the gene in a Mendelian fashion. Moreover, the integrated genes tend to be expresssed with the appropriate tissue-specificity. For example, the human β-globin gene, which is normally expressed only in erthrocytes, was expressed only in these cells after transfer into the mouse germ-line (Costantini et al 1986). Because these mice can express the foreign genes, they are called 'transgenic' mice.

Using mice with specific genetic defects as the test systems, normal, foreign genes have been injected, and their incorporation into the mouse genome has effectively and dramatically cured the murine disease (Table

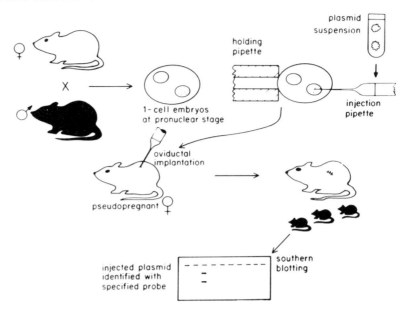

Fig. 113.2 Introducing a foreign gene into the germ-line of mice (i.e. production of transgenic mice). Immature albino females are superovulated and mated to males homozygous for the wild-type allele at the albino locus. One-celled embryos at the pronuclear stage of development (day 1 of gestation) are removed from the oviducts, after which one of the pronuclei is microinjected with the recombinant-plasmid DNA. Embryos are then reimplanted into the oviducts of albino females which have been rendered pseudopregnant by mating to vasectomized albino males. The pigmentation markers are employed to identify any offspring arising from oocytes fertilized by spermatozoa from inadequately vasectomized males. In this scheme, such embryos would be of the albino phenotype. After normal delivery, pigmented mice are evaluated by Southern hybridization for retention of microinjected DNA (Gordon et al 1980).

113.3.). For example, transfer of the rat growth hormone gene into growth hormone deficient 'Dwarf Little' mice resulted in the cure of the growth hormone deficiency and the generation of larger-than-normal mice (Hammer et al 1984). Similarly, transfer of the human β-globin gene into mice with β-thalassaemia (due to a gene deletion in the murine β-globin gene) resulted in the regulated expression of β-globin molecules in these mice, association of the murine β-globin chains with the human β-globin chains, and correction of the haematological disease (Costantini et al 1986). Such examples illustrate the fact that gene therapy is feasible and, at least in the mouse, can effectively cure a genetic disease.

However, it should also be noted that insertion of the foreign gene is random and that it is possible to cause damage by inserting the foreign gene into a chromosomal gene, thereby rendering it inactive. Although such events occur infrequently, 'insertional mutagenesis' has provided the basis for studies in developmental biology. Thus, the random integration of injected exogenous genes can be harmful as well as helpful. Future efforts must be directed to target the injected gene to a specific region within the genome (see below).

Somatic gene therapy

The insertion of genes into somatic cells, particularly those with primary disease pathology, is the goal of somatic gene therapy. As shown in Figure 113.3, the foreign genes must gain access to the cell nucleus for stable integration into the host chromosome and for the (regulated) expression of the desired gene product. In this approach, exogenous genes are not transmitted through the germ-line and therapy is limited to the diseased individual.

Retroviral vectors for gene transfer

The 'Trojan Horse' of somatic gene therapy is the retrovirus. This RNA virus can infect human cells and

Table 113.3 Correction of genetic defects in transgenic mice

Murine disease	Defective gene	Microinjected gene	Reference
Growth hormone deficiency (Dwarf Little mouse, *lit*)	Growth hormone	Rat growth hormone	Hammer et al 1984
β-Thalassaemia (*Hbb*[th−1] mouse)	β-Globin (deletion)	Human β-globin	Costantini et al 1986
Hypogonadism (hypogonadal mouse, *Hpg*)	GnRH-GAP* (3′ deletion)	Murine GnRH-GAP	Mason et al 1986
Shiverer mouse (*shi*) (defective MBP)	MBP** (3′ deletion)	Murine MBP	Readhead et al 1987

* GnRH-GAP = Gonadotropin-Releasing Hormone and GnRH-Associated Peptide
** MBP = Myelin Basic Protein

insert a DNA copy of its viral RNA genome into the host chromosome. The life cycle of the retrovirus is shown in Figure 113.4. The virus binds to the cell membrane, injects its RNA, and reverse transcriptase (Pol) converts the single-stranded viral RNA genome into a double-stranded DNA copy that can be integrated (by recombination using a virally-encoded integrase) into the host genome as a 'provirus'. The provirus is able to use the host cell machinery to transcribe and translate the viral genome and produce copies of the RNA genome as well as the essential viral proteins. The viral particle can then be assembled within the cytoplasm and infectious virus particles can cross the host cell membrane by budding and infect other cells.

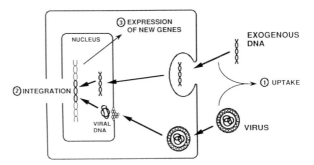

Fig. 113.3 Genetic modification of a mammallian cell. The added exogenous genetic information may be integrated into the chromosome of the recipient cell and become expressed as a new gene product.

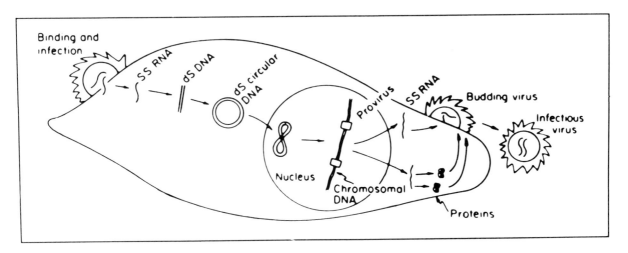

Fig. 113.4 The retroviral life cycle. After adsorption and uptake (i.e. binding and infection) of the viral genome, the single-stranded (ss) RNA is converted to double-stranded (ds) DNA by reverse transcriptase. After uptake into the nucleus, the DNA integrates randomly into a chromosome to form the provirus. The provirus serves as a template both for mRNAs to yield viral proteins and for new, full length genomic RNA. Two copies of the genomic RNA and viral proteins assemble and, by budding, release a new infectious virus to repeat the cycle (Bernstein et al 1985).

The retroviral genome and constructs for gene transfer

The structure of the retroviral genome is shown in Figure 113.5. At each end is a sequence called the long terminal repeat (LTR). This sequence contains both the promoter, and elements needed for translation of the three major viral genes, *gag*, *pol* and *env*. In addition, there is a sequence near the 5′ LTR known as the ψ (psi) site which is essential if the viral RNA transcript is to be packaged into a viral particle. If the ψ sequence is altered (i.e. ψ^-) then that RNA cannot be encapsulated in the viral particle.

Investigators have taken advantage of the ψ sequence to develop a method to package a foreign DNA sequence into a defective retroviral particle for gene therapy (Fig. 113.5). For example, the retroviral *gag*, *pol* and *env* genes can be replaced by a cDNA which encodes a therapeutic protein; this recombinant sequence would have an intact ψ region permitting the sequence to be packaged. A second 'helper' retroviral sequence which is ψ^- can be used to infect the host cells in order to produce the viral core, polymerase and envelope glycoproteins necessary for packaging. The 'helper cells' infected with the ψ^- virus are called ψ_2 packaging cells. When the ψ_2 cells are infected with a ψ^+ recombinant construct containing the foreign cDNA sequence, a defective viral particle is assembled which only contains the recombinant cDNA sequence. This viral particle is defective since it does not contain the viral genes necessary to produce the viral proteins required to assemble a normally infectious virus

particle. However, this recombinant virus can be used to introduce foreign DNA into somatic cells (i.e. bone marrow stem cells, hepatocytes or various cultured cell types) without subsequent production of infectious viral particles (Fig. 113.6).

The development of retroviral vectors for use in gene transfer experiments is an active area of investigation. Although beyond the scope of this discussion, virologists are experimenting with a variety of retroviral constructs designed for more efficient expression of foreign genes and for the production of higher titres of recombinant viral particles. Some vectors have inactivated viral promoters (by deleting a segment of the LTR) and have inserted strong promoters (i.e. TK, SV40) in front of the foreign gene or have mini-gene constructs with the foreign gene's 5′ promoter sequence next to the cDNA. For selection of infected cells, the *neo* gene has been placed in the vector (Fig. 113.7). This gene confers resistance to the antibiotic G418, permitting the positive selection of infected cells containing the retroviral construct.

Retrovirus-mediated somatic gene therapy in cultured cells and animals

Experience with retroviral systems for gene transfer has demonstrated their ability to insert and express foreign genes in mammalian cells including cultured bone marrow, fibroblasts and hepatocytes (Gilboa et al 1986, Hock & Miller 1986, Kantoff et al 1986, Williams et al

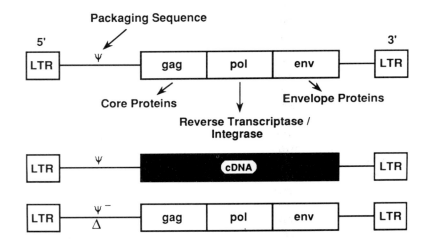

Fig. 113.5 Modification of the retroviral genome for gene transfer experiments. Schematic representation of the retroviral genome (top). Retroviral gene construct with a human cDNA replacing the *gag*, *pol*, and *env* genes (middle), and retroviral genome with a deletion of the ψ sequence which is normally for packaging the retroviral genome (bottom).

Retroviral Gene Transfer

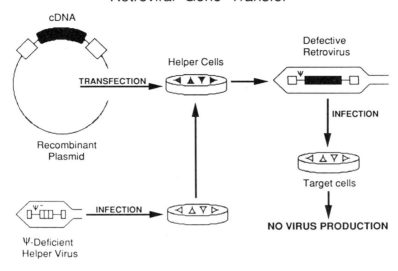

Fig. 113.6 Retrovirus-mediated somatic gene transfer. The psi-deficient (ψ^-) helper virus produces all the normal viral proteins, but cannot package its own RNA because it lacks the appropriate packaging signal. Helper cells are made by inserting the helper provirus into the genome of the helper cell. This is accomplished by infection of the cells with helper virus. Recombinant vector DNA, including a human cDNA sequence, is inserted into helper cells by transfection with a plasmid containing the human cDNA flanked by retroviral LTR sequences. Because the recombinant vector contains the ψ sequence, the vector RNA genome is automatically encapsulated by viral proteins produced by the helper provirus DNA in the helper (ψ_2) packaging cells. The resulting viral particles are released by budding from the helper cell membrane. The vector virus is capable of only one infection because it lacks the information needed to make viral proteins. Targets cells (such as human bone marrow cells) are then infected with the virus. Once the vector construct is integrated into the target cell DNA, as a provirus, the foreign gene sequence can be expressed. However, no viral particles will be produced by the transfected target cells, since the genes for the viral proteins have been deleted from the recombinant viral construct.

Retroviral Vector With Internal Promoter

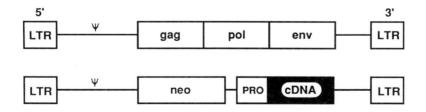

Fig. 113.7 Retroviral constructs with a selectable marker gene and foreign gene with an internal promoter. Recombinant DNA techniques are used to replace the *gag*, *pol* and *env* genes with one or more foreign genes. The foreign genes can be inserted in several different patterns. In this example, a selectable marker gene, *neo*, which confers neomycin-resistance, replaces the viral *gag* and *pol* genes and a human gene replaces the *env* gene. The *neo* gene is transcribed from the LTR promoter, while the heterologous human sequence is transcribed from a separate promoter, PRO, e.g. SV40 or metallothionein promoters.

1986, Ledley et al 1987a, Morgan et al 1987).

Investigators have consequently attempted somatic gene transfer into intact mice in order to determine if the foreign genes are expressed in vivo. These efforts have focused on the transfer of genes into bone marrow cells in short-term culture followed by transplantation of the infected cells into an irradiated host, as illustrated in Figure 113.8. In this protocol, bone marrow cells are removed from a normal mouse, placed in culture and then infected with the retroviral vector containing the foreign gene. The infection can be accomplished either by mixing the target cells with helper cells (ψ_2 packaging cells) which are producing the recombinant vector carrying the foreign gene, or they can be incubated with the medium from the helper cell culture which contains the defective recombinant viral particles. If the retroviral gene construct also contains a selectable gene, e.g. *neo*, then cells containing the foreign gene could be selected by treatment of the bone marrow culture with the antibiotic, G418. This would allow only cells containing the neomycin-resistance gene (*neo*) to survive. Thus, by selection, only bone marrow cells containing the retroviral gene construct would be infused intravenously into a mouse whose bone marrow had previously been destroyed by a lethal dose of radiation. Since the mice are inbred, the bone marrow transplant will not be subject to rejection complications. Once the stem cells have repopulated the bone marrow, the haematopoietic system would be reconstituted with cells containing the foreign gene.

Although the presence of the transferred genes has been demonstrated in mouse recipients by DNA analysis, the expression of these genes was initially disappointing. In many experiments, expression was not detectable, while in others expression was low and transient. Only recently has the expression of the foreign gene been shown in murine peripheral blood cells for prolonged periods (i.e. several months) (Lim et al 1987, Belmont et al 1988, Bender et al 1989).

A variety of strategies are being pursued to overcome the difficulty of obtaining sufficient expression of foreign genes for therapeutic purposes. Efforts are focused on designing vectors with stronger promoters so that more gene product is produced in infected cells. In addition, investigators are attempting to identify and isolate the pluripotent bone marrow stem cells so that infection can be targeted to these cells specifically. It is anticipated that future advances in gene transfer for the treatment of genetic disease will occur in the area of retrovirology and in our greater understanding of haematopoiesis.

Evaluation in animal models of human diseases

Following the successful demonstration of gene transfer in mice, it will be necessary to determine if this approach

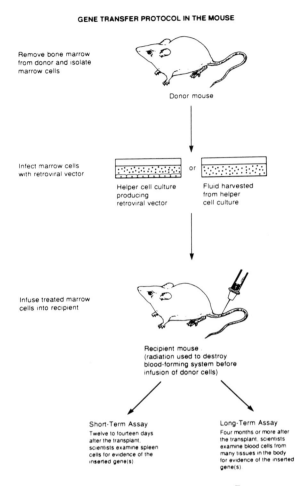

GENE TRANSFER PROTOCOL IN THE MOUSE

Remove bone marrow from donor and isolate marrow cells

Donor mouse

Infect marrow cells with retroviral vector

Helper cell culture producing retroviral vector   or   Fluid harvested from helper cell culture

Infuse treated marrow cells into recipient

Recipient mouse (radiation used to destroy blood-forming system before infusion of donor cells)

Short-Term Assay
Twelve to fourteen days after the transplant, scientists examine spleen cells for evidence of the inserted gene(s)

Long-Term Assay
Four months or more after the transplant, scientists examine blood cells from many tissues in the body for evidence of the inserted gene(s)

Fig. 113.8 Somatic gene transfer in the mouse. Bone marrow cells are removed from a normal animal or from an animal treated with drugs known to increase the proportion of stem cells in the body. A retroviral vector is used to insert foreign genes into the bone marrow cells. The cells are infected with the vector in one of two ways: they are mixed with helper cells producing the vector, or they are bathed in fluid harvested from the helper cell culture. After infection, the treated cells are infused into a mouse whose blood-forming system has been destroyed by radiation. (In mice, the donor and the recipient are usually different, but genetically identical, animals; in large animals, the treated cells would be injected back into the donor.) Long-term survival of the recipient animal depends on the introduction of enough bone marrow cells to repopulate the blood-forming system (Nichols 1988).

can be accomplished in larger animals, like dogs, cats and monkeys. The availability of well-characterized animal models of human inherited metabolic disease will greatly facilitate these studies (Desnick et at 1982, Kuehn et al 1987). For example, canine and feline analogues of human mucopolysaccharidoses (MPS) have been identified including Plott hounds and domestic cats with MPS I (α-L-iduronidase deficiency), Siamese cats with MPS VI (arylsulphatase B deficiency), and mixed breed dogs with MPS VII (β-glucuronidase deficiency). Such animals may be ideal candidates for gene therapy trials since heterologous bone marrow transplantation has been shown to have a clinically beneficial effect on the course of the disease in the recipient. The ability to obtain serial blood and biopsy specimens as well as to monitor the clinical course of the disease in treated animals and untreated affected littermates will permit a thorough evaluation of the biochemical and clinical effectiveness of gene transfer endeavours.

Disease candidates for somatic gene therapy

At present, the diseases which are considered potential candidates for somatic gene therapy are those in which bone marrow transplantation has proved to be therapeutic. In such disorders, the gene defect is manifested primarily by the deficient function or lack of a bone marrow-derived gene product (i.e. thalassaemias, haemoglobinopathies, immunodeficiencies, leucocyte and platelet defects, etc.). Successful bone marrow transplantation results in cellular replacement of normal blood elements which can produce the normal form of the defective gene product and correct the metabolic disease. A candidate of particular note is severe combined immunodeficiency disease (SCID). This disorder results from totally deficient adenosine deaminase (ADA) activity. The treatment of choice for this lethal disease is bone marrow transplantation from an enzymatically normal, HLA-identical sib. However, most patients do not have such a sib and would be candidates for other therapeutic endeavours including enzyme replacement,

bone marrow transplantation from a parent or, in the future, autologous transplantation of bone marrow cells that have been infected with a retroviral construct containing the human ADA gene. Studies in several laboratories have demonstrated that retroviral-ADA gene constructs can express the enzyme in cultured cells, including T and B cells (Kantoff et al 1986). However, attempts to transplant bone marrow containing the ADA gene into normal Rhesus monkeys and obtain sufficient and prolonged expression in peripheral cells have not been successful to date (Kantoff et al 1987).

Future prospects for somatic gene therapy: correction of the molecular lesion by homologous recombination

As has already been discussed, retrovirus-mediated gene transfer results in the random insertion of a foreign gene, which may cause damage to other genes. In order to avoid such insertional mutagenesis, experimental efforts have focused on the targeting of a specific DNA sequence to replace a defective copy of this sequence in the genome. This would allow for the correction of a genetic lesion by its replacement with the normal sequence via a recombination process. Promising results have already been obtained in tissue culture systems (Thomas & Capecchi 1986, Thomas et al 1986, Nandi et al 1988). Thus, in the future it may be possible to correct a given gene defect in somatic cells without random integration of a complete copy of the normal sequence which could inactivate a normal chromosomal gene. Instead, it may be feasible to 'surgically' remove the specific genetic lesion and insert the required sequence at the same site, resulting in the production of a normal gene product.

REFERENCES

Anderson W F 1984 Prospects for human gene therapy. Science 226: 401–409

Anderson W F, Fletcher J C 1980 Gene therapy in human beings: when is it ethical to begin. New England Journal of Medicine 303: 1293–1297

Belmont J H, MacGregor G R, Wagner-Smith K et al 1988 Expression of human adenosine deaminase in murine hematopoietic cells. Molecular and Cellular Biology 8: 5116–5125

Bender M, Gelinas R, Miller A 1989 A majority of mice show long term expression of a human β-globin gene after retrovirus transfer into hematopoietic cells. Molecular and Cellular Biology 9: 1426–1432

Bernstein A, Berger S, Huszar D, Dick J 1985 Gene transfer with retroviral vectors. In: Setlow J K, Hollaender A (eds) Genetic engineering: principles and methods, vol. 7. Plenum, New York, p 235–262

Constantini F, Chada K, Magram J 1986 Correction of

murine β-thalassemia by gene transfer into the germ line. Science 233: 1192–1194

Desnick R J 1981 Treatment of inherited metabolic diseases. An overview. In: Kaback M M (ed) Genetic issues in pediatric and obstetric practice. Year Book Medical Publishers, Chicago, p 525–566

Desnick R J 1983 Treatment of inherited metabolic diseases: current status and prospects. In: Dietz A A (ed) Genetic diseases: diagnosis and treatment. American Association of Clinical Chemistry, Washington D.C., p 183–259

Desnick R J 1987 Bone marrow transplantation in genetic diseases: a status report. In: Kaback M M, Shapiro L J (eds) Frontiers in genetic medicine. Report of the 92nd Ross conference on pediatric research, Columbus, Ohio, June 1986. p 71–83

Desnick R J, Grabowski G A 1981 Advances in the treatment of inherited metabolic diseases. In: Harris H, Hirschhorn K (eds) Advances in human genetics, vol. 11. Plenum, New York, p 281–369

Desnick R J, Patterson D F, Scarpelli D G (eds) 1982 Animal

models of inherited metabolic disease. Liss, New York

Dick J E, Magli M C, Phillips R A, Bernstein A 1986 Genetic manipulation of hematopoietic stem cells with retrovirus vectors. Trends in Genetics 2: 165–170

Eglitis M A, Kantoff P W, Gilboa E, Anderson W F 1985 Gene expression in mice after high efficiency retroviral-mediated gene transfer. Science 230: 1395–1398

Gilboa E 1987 Retrovirus vectors and their uses in molecular biology. BioEssays 5: 252–257

Gilboa E, Eglitis M A, Kantoff P W, Anderson W F 1986 Transfer and expression of cloned genes using retroviral vectors. BioTechniques 4(6): 504–512

Gordon J W, Scangos G A, Plotkin D J, Barbosa J A, Ruddle F H 1980 Genetic transformation of mouse embryos by microinjection of purified DNA. Proceedings of the National Academy of Sciences, USA 77: 7380–7384

Hammer R E, Palmiter R D, Brinster R L 1984 Partial correction of a murine hereditary growth disorder by germ-line incorporation of a new gene. Nature 311: 65–67

Hock R A, Miller A D 1986 Retrovirus-mediated transfer and expression of drug resistance genes in human haematopoietic progenitor cells. Nature 320: 275–277

Kantoff P W, Kohn D B, Mitsuya H et al 1986 Correction of adenosine deaminase deficiency in cultured human T and B cells by retrovirus-mediated gene transfer. Proceedings of the National Academy of Sciences, USA 83: 6563–6567

Kantoff P W, Gillio A, McLachlin J R et al 1987 Expression of human adenosine deaminase in non-human primates after retroviral-mediated gene transfer. Journal of Experimental Medicine 166: 219–234

Karlsson S, Papayannopoulou T, Schweiger S G, Stamatoyannopoulos G, Nienhuis A W 1987 Retroviral-mediated transfer of genomic globin genes leads to regulated production of RNA and protein. Proceedings of the National Academy of Sciences, USA 84: 2411–2415

Kuehn M R, Bradley A, Robertson E J, Evans M J 1987 A potential animal model for Lesch-Nyhan syndrome through introduction of HPRT mutations into mice. Nature 326: 295–298

Kwok W W, Schuening F, Stead R B, Miller A D 1986 Retroviral transfer of genes into canine hemopoietic progenitor cells in culture. A model for human gene therapy. Proceedings of the National Academy of Sciences, USA 83: 4552–4555

Ledley F D, Darlington G J, Hahn T, Woo S L 1987a Retroviral gene transfer into primary hepatocytes: implications for genetic therapy of liver-specific functions. Proceedings of the National Academy of Sciences, USA 84: 5335–5339

Ledley F D, Grenett H E, Bartos D P, Woo S L 1987b Retroviral mediated transfer and expression of human α-1-antitrypsin in cultured cells. Gene 61: 113–118

Ledley F D, Grenett H E, Woo S L 1987c Biochemical characterization of recombinant human phenylalanine hydroxylase produced in Escherichia coli. Journal of Biological Chemistry 162: 2228–2233

Lim B, Williams D, Orkin S 1987 Retrovirus mediated gene transfer of human ADA: expression of functional enzyme in murine hematopoietic stem cells in vivo. Molecular and Cellular Biology 7: 3459–3465

McKusick V A 1988 Mendelian inheritance in man, 8th edn. Johns Hopkins University Press, Baltimore

Mann R, Mulligan R C, Baltimore D 1983 Construction of retrovirus packaging mutant and its use to produce helper-free defective retrovirus. Cell 33: 153–159

Marx J L 1987 Probing gene action during development: the good news – and the bad – about gene therapy prospects. Science 236: 29–30

Mason A J, Pitts S L, Nikolics K, Azonyi E, Wilcox J N, Seeburg P H, Stewart T A 1986 The hypogonadal mouse: reproductive functions restored by gene therapy. Science 234: 1372–1378

Matas A J, Simmons R L, Desnick R J 1978 Clinical and experimental transplantation in enzymatic deficiency disease. Surgery, Gynecology and Obstetrics 146: 975–982

Merz B 1986 Stumbling blocks pave path to clinical trials for gene therapy. Journal of the American Medical Association 255(14): 1825–1827, 1832

Miller A D, Eckner R J, Jolly D J, Friedmann T, Verma I M 1984 Expression of a retrovirus encoding human HPRT in mice. Science 225: 630–632

Miller D W, Safer P, Miller L K 1986 An insect baculovirus host-vector system for high-level expression of foreign genes. In: Setlow J K, Hollaender A (eds) Genetic engineering, vol. 8. Plenum, New York, p 277–298

Morgan J R, Barrandon Y, Green H, Mulligan R C 1987 Expression of an exogenous growth hormone gene by transplantable human epidermal cells. Science 237: 1476–1479

Mulligan R C, Berg P 1980 Expression of a bacterial gene in mammalian cells. Science 209: 1422–1423

Nandi A, Roginski R S, Gregg R G, Smithies O, Skoultchi A I 1988 Regulated expression of genes inserted at the human chromosomal β-globin locus by homologous recombination. Proccedings of the National Academy of Sciences, USA 85: 3845–3849

Nichols E K 1988 Human gene therapy, Institute of Medicine – National Academy of Sciences. Harvard, Cambridge

Old R W, Primrose S B 1985 Cloning in yeast and other microbial eukaryotes. In: Old R W, Primrose S B (eds) Principles of gene manipulation. Blackwell, Oxford, p 195–200

Readhead C, Popko B, Takahashi N, Shine H D, Saavedra R A, Sidman R L, Hood L 1987 Expression of a myelin basic protein gene in transgenic shiverer mice: correction of the dysmyelinating phenotype. Cell 48: 703–712

Sarver N, Gruss P, Law M-F, Khoury G, Howley P M 1981 Bovine papilloma virus deoxyribonucleic acid: a novel encaryotic cloning vector. Molecular and Cellular Biology 1: 486–496

Shapiro L J 1983 Treatment of genetic diseases. In: Emery A E H, Rimoin D L (eds) Principles and practice of medical genetics, 1st edn. Churchill Livingstone, Edinburgh, p 1488–1496

Thomas K R, Capecchi M R 1986 Introduction of homologous DNA sequences into mammalian cells induces mutations in the cognate gene. Nature 324: 34–38

Thomas K R, Folger K R, Capecchi M R 1986 High frequency targeting of genes to specific sites in the mammalian genome. Cell 44: 419–428

Williams D A, Lemischka I R, Nathan D G, Mulligan R C 1984 Introduction of new genetic material into pluripotent haematopoietic stem cells of the mouse. Nature 310: 476–480

Williams D A, Orkin S H, Mulligan R C 1986 Retrovirus-mediated transfer of human adenosine deaminase gene sequences into cells in culture and into murine hematopoietic cells in vivo. Proceedings of the National Academy of Sciences, USA 83: 2566–2570

114. Paternity testing

Robert S. Sparkes *Susan E. Hodge*

INTRODUCTION

Paternity testing refers to attempts to determine whether a given man, often called the 'putative father' or under certain circumstances the 'accused man,' is in fact the father of a given child. The mother is usually assumed to be known. However, similar testing could be applied in cases where the identity of the mother is disputed, caused by the rare and regrettable cases of confusion between babies in maternity units. Originally, this testing was based primarily on just a few major blood groups, but in recent years the list of available and accepted genetic markers has expanded greatly.

Accurate determination of paternity in disputed cases is extremely important. The most common situation occurs when the mother (or alternatively the state) sues a man for paternity. It is equally critical, on the one hand, that the man be acquitted (excluded) if he is not the father and, on the other, that he be positively identified if he is. One can easily imagine other scenarios as well, for example, where a married rape victim wishes to determine whether the fetus she carries was fathered by her husband or by the rapist.

The principles of paternity testing are simple and relate to the use of polymorphic genetic traits with known and established inheritance patterns. Initially a search is made for an exclusion in which the child has one or more characteristics that could not have come from the putative father. If no exclusion is found, a calculation is made as to the likelihood of paternity.

Compared to several European countries, the use of paternity testing has been accepted relatively slowly by courts in the United States. This is probably partly due to the fact that each state establishes its own acceptance criteria for paternity testing. In the United States, this process has been accelerated by the passage of PL-93647, which requires that each state develop an appropriate plan for the determination of paternity.

For many years, the ABO, Rh, and MNSs blood types were the mainstays of paternity determination. With the increasing availability of other polymorphic genetic traits this list has been greatly expanded and accepted in many states. However, there continue to be differences as to how paternity testing is handled in each of the states.

Initially, paternity testing was directed towards finding an exclusion. More recently there has been a rather subtle shift in emphasis. Very often the objective now is to identify the father of a child positively, so that the responsibility for that child can be shifted from the state to the biological father.

In recent years, paternity questions which may reflect changes in our society have occurred more frequently. As noted in the above paragraph, there has been a tendency to shift the responsibility for the care of the child from the state (often through welfare systems) to the biological father. Second, there appears to have been an increasing tendency for children to be born out of wedlock. These, and probably other factors, have contributed to the increasing frequency with which the question of paternity has been raised.

Initially, paternity testing was done by blood typing laboratories. With the increasing use of other markers, such as HLA, isoenzymes and serum protein markers, there has been a shift to other laboratories, often associated with universities or medical centres. More recently, there has been a further shift in which commercial laboratories have become more involved.

The premise upon which paternity testing is based is that individuals can be identified through genetic testing. This in turn is based upon the study of those traits which show genetic polymorphism. Because of relative ease of sampling, most of these tests are done on blood samples. Most often, the tests have been developed for other purposes, such as genetic linkage analysis. In many instances, the results of these tests offer a relatively objective evaluation of the question of paternity, which might otherwise be based upon only legal and social considerations. As with many genetic studies, the trend appears to be moving to the use of DNA markers which can be used to establish a 'genetic fingerprint' of an individual. With some of the newer tests described below, it appears that the possibility of confirming the identity of the father of a given child may become very high indeed. It has been satisfying to many workers in the field to see the application of scientific knowledge to an increasingly important social problem.

GENETIC MARKERS FOR PATERNITY TESTING

Most of the current paternity testing still depends upon the use of polymorphic markers. The initial use of the ABO, Rh and MNSs antigen systems has been supplemented by further polymorphic red cell antigen systems (e.g. Duffy, Kell, Kidd and P). The use of red cell antigens was supplemented, and even to a large extent replaced, by the use of HLA typing. A very high degree of polymorphism for the HLA types was recognized in the early 1970s as having utility for individual identification and, therefore, application to paternity testing. With the further development of other genetic polymorphic testing systems, red blood cell isoenzymes and serum protein markers have been added to the list of genetic traits which can be used in paternity evaluation. DNA polymorphisms are now also being introduced for paternity testing.

The genetic traits used in paternity evaluation meet the requirements for individual identification. These traits show significant polymorphism in the population, the frequencies of the different types are known in the racial and ethnic groups being studied, and they have a known and consistent inheritance pattern. Moreover the tests are relatively inexpensive to carry out, they require blood samples which are easily obtained, and they are reproducible in experienced laboratories.

In addition to the above markers, chromosome polymorphisms have been used on a more limited scale, perhaps because of their cost and the somewhat subjective nature of their interpretation.

Although the HLA system has become very popular, it does have limitations. First, a complete set of typing reagents tends to be available only on a limited basis and many are not commercially available. Every laboratory may not have a broad base of testing reagents, so the testing becomes less definitive in part because of the problem of not being able to establish with certainty the haplotypes of the individuals involved.

DNA MARKERS

The initial approach using DNA markers was to consider restriction fragment length polymorphisms (RFLPs) for

analysis. However, it seemed that even though these tests had high biological potential, the cost might limit their use. This concern has been reduced by the development of other DNA polymorphic traits as first demonstrated by the 'minisatellites' developed by Jeffreys and his colleagues (1985a,b). Testing is based upon the occurrence of a family of DNA sequences that are tandemly repeated and dispersed in the human genome. Jeffreys and his colleagues first identified a minisatellite probe during the characterization of a human myoglobin gene. This is a 33 base pair subunit and was soon found to be part of, or close to, other genes. When one carries out Southern blotting of DNA from an individual using the minisatellite probes, each individual appears to have a unique, or almost unique, pattern of multiple bands. Because of this, the technique has sometimes been called 'DNA fingerprinting.' It has been estimated that as many as 20 genetic loci can be examined simultaneously. It also appears that there is great heterozygosity at each of these loci, which makes them very informative for identification purposes. Because of these factors the cost of the analysis should be relatively low, compared with other DNA studies. As discussed by Gill et al (1985), using a single probe the probability that another unrelated individual would have the same pattern is 3×10^{-11}. With a second probe, the probability becomes 5×10^{-19}, a very small probability indeed. Because of these considerations, it is likely that the standard calculation for the likelihood of paternity (see below) may eventually no longer be required. Gill et al (1985) further discussed the application of these probes to forensic problems.

NEW DEVELOPMENTS

More recently, two additional similar situations have been described. First, Vassart et al (1987) found that, under appropriate hybridizing conditions, a sequence of the M13 phage detects hypervariable minisatellites in human and other animal DNA. This was based upon finding two clusters of 15 base pair repeats within the protein III gene for the bacteriophage. The authors noted that the pattern they observed was different from that obtained with Jeffreys' probes.

Nakamura et al (1987) described the development of a 'variable number of tandem repeat' (VNTR) markers. These investigators developed these probes primarily for human gene mapping, but obviously they have application for paternity testing as well. The authors constructed a number of oligonucleotides which corresponded to consensus sequences of tandem repeats of the insulin gene, the pseudogene of zeta-globin, the myoglobin gene, and part of the core sequence of a plasmid PYNZ22.

Heterozygosity can be detected by this approach so it has the potential for application to paternity studies.

Although the systems described above are very powerful, another new development may have implications for paternity testing in the future. This is the ability to detect human DNA polymorphisms related to a single base change. While this in some ways is similar to the use of the standard RFLPs, which is based upon the presence or absence of specific DNA sequences, this technique uses a denaturing gradient gel electrophoresis (Noll & Collins 1987). With this latter technique, one does not have to depend upon having a specific restriction endonuclease to identify the DNA alteration. The denaturing of gradient gel electrophoresis permits detection of single base changes that occur within stretches of DNA forming early melting domains. It has been estimated that up to 50–70% of all base pair substitutions should be detectable with this technique. With further development in this area, it is conceivable that this technique could have application to paternity evaluation as well.

EXCLUSIONS

The following considerations are particularly important in those instances where exclusions have been demonstrated. There are two types of exclusion which can be considered. The first is a direct or first-degree exclusion in which the child has a phenotype which could not have been inherited from either the mother or the putative father. The second is an indirect or second-degree exclusion in which the child should have received a given genetic trait if the putative father is homozygous for that trait. In these situations one must always be aware of possible confounding issues; for example, one needs to be aware that in many systems there may be null alleles, or there may be a situation in which the gene is present but may not be expressed, such as the Bombay factor with the ABO red blood cell antigen. Uncommon mutations may also occur. Furthermore, in some of the complex systems such as HLA, recombination may occur, and this can confound the interpretation of the inheritance pattern in a family. If two or more systems exclude the putative father, we may have more confidence in the exclusion than when it is based on a single system.

ATTRIBUTION OF PATERNITY

Clearly, genetic markers cannot prove that a given man is the father in the same way that they can exclude him. For example, if the child is blood type O and the man is AB then, barring laboratory error, new mutation, the rare cis AB allele or the Bombay phenotype, it is simply impossible for that man to be the father of that child. In contrast, if the man is type A, and the mother is type B, and the child is AB, then the man is not excluded; but neither does it prove that he *is* the father.

On the other hand, if the man fails to be excluded at not one but many loci, and if at some of these loci the man and the child share antigens which are not very frequent in the population, then it is intuitively reasonable to interpret these facts as evidence in favour of paternity. This kind of reasoning underlies the 'paternity index'.

The paternity index (PI) was first formulated by Essen–Moeller (1938). It is first computed separately for each locus or system; then the results are combined over all tested loci. For an individual locus the PI embodies both the likelihood that the man under investigation *is* the father, and the likelihood that he *is not* the father. More specifically, consider the actual phenotype observed in the particular man. The first likelihood (x) is proportional to the probability that a man would have this phenotype if he is the father; the second (y) is proportional to the probability that the man would have this phenotype if he is not the father. The ratio of the first to the second likelihood (x/y) is the PI for that locus; it can be interpreted as the relative odds in favour of this man being the father.

For example, consider the configuration shown in Figure 114.1. The mother is homozygous 1–1 at the codominant adenosine deaminase (ADA) locus, whereas the child and the man share the relatively rare 2 allele (population frequency = 0.066). (Note that gene (allele) frequencies may vary in different racial/ethnic groups and, therefore, gene frequencies need to be known for the biological ancestry of the man being tested.) The probability of a man who is not the father having genotype 1–2 is the same as the frequency of that genotype in the

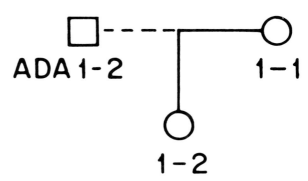

Fig. 114.1 An example in which the child and the accused man share a rare allele.

general population. Assuming Hardy–Weinberg equilibrium, $y = 2(0.066)(1-0.066) = 0.124$. The only other possible genotype for the father would be 2–2, so x will give the probability that the true father is 1–2 as opposed to 2–2. The calculation is based on Hardy–Weinberg equilibrium and Mendel's first law and also takes into account the genotypes of the mother and the child.

$$x = \frac{(0.124)(0.5)}{(0.124)(0.5) + (0.004)(1)} = 0.939.$$

Thus the relative odds, x/y, becomes $0.939/0.124 = 7.57$; this represents the PI. In other words, the man is 7.57 times more likely to be the real father than not.

A PI greater than unity tends to support paternity; a value less than 1 tends to argue against it. For an example of how the PI can be less than unity, consider Figure 114.2. Here the mother clearly contributed the rarer allele 2 to the child. The quantity y is still 0.124. However x is now smaller than y, since the true father is much more likely to have been 1–1 than 1–2.

$$x = \frac{(0.124)(0.5)}{(0.124)(0.5) + (0.872)(1)} = 0.066.$$

Here the PI is $0.066/0.124 = 0.535$, which represents odds of 1.87 to 1 against that man being the father.

The PI values for the different loci or marker systems are all mutliplied together. For example, if the PI is 7.57 for ADA, 3.1 for ABO, and 5.6 for MNSs, then these three loci alone yield a total PI of 131.4, which is considered to represent very strong odds in favour of paternity.

A somewhat more controversial quantity is the 'probability of paternity.' This probability is calculated as $PI/(1 + PI)$ and is sometimes denoted by W. Thus, a PI value of 7.57 corresponds to a probability of paternity $W = 88.3\%$; a PI of 131.4 gives rise to $W = 99.2\%$. The controversy arises because this formula assumes that the prior probability that the particular man is in fact the true father is 50%. The 50% is supposed to represent our prior ignorance, and it may not always be acceptable to all parties involved. However, it is easily shown that when the PI is high, then the value one assumes for the prior probability makes very little difference to the probability of paternity W. (For example, for $PI = 100$ the probability of paternity W is 99.0%; if instead of 0.5 we

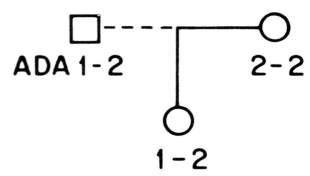

Fig. 114.2 An example yielding a paternity index less than unity.

assumed a prior probability of 0.25 the probability of paternity would drop to 97.1%, or with a prior probability of 0.75 it would rise to 99.7%.) Since most courts of law accept only fairly high values of the PI as being relevant, the debate about an appropriate choice of prior probability is more theoretical than practical.

LEGAL-SOCIAL ASPECTS

As the increased utility of genetic typing becomes known, it seems very likely that these tests will be increasingly used in paternity testing. Because of this, it is probable that certain specific laboratories will be established to do such testing, or that there will be some type of laboratory certification. Indeed, efforts are already under way by the Association of American Blood Banks to establish a certifying procedure. With each state having its own laws regarding paternity testing, it may be some time before there is a nationwide standard for paternity testing. However, this may be moved along more quickly by the increasing involvement of commercial laboratories involved in paternity testing.

The California Evidence Code (Sec. 895.5) now recognizes a PI value of 100 (corresponds to $W = 99.0\%$) as a legal criterion. For PI values below 100, the burden of proof remains on the plaintiff to demonstrate that the man is the father, whereas over 100, the burden shifts to the man to prove that he is not the father. Many other States in the USA use a less stringent criterion; requiring a W value of 98% (corresponds to $PI = 50$) is common.

REFERENCES

Essen-Moeller E 1938 Die Beweiskraft der Aehnlichkeit im Vaterschaftsnachweis. Theoretische Grundlagen. Mitt. Anthropologische Gesellschaft (Wien) 68: 9–53

Gill P, Jeffreys A J, Werrett D J 1985 Forensic application of DNA 'fingerprints.' Nature 318: 577–579
Jeffreys A J, Wilson V, Thein S L 1985a Hypervariable

minisatellite regions in human DNA. Nature 314: 67–73

Jeffreys A J, Wilson V, Thein S L 1985b Individual specific fingerprints of human DNA. Nature 316: 76–79

Nakamura Y, Leppert M, O'Connell P et al 1987 Variable number of tandem repeat (VNTR) markers for human gene mapping. Science 235: 1616–1622.

Noll W W, Collins M 1987 Detection of human DNA polymorphisms with a simplified gradient gel electrophoresis technique. Proceedings of the National Academy of Sciences, USA 84: 3339–3343

Vassart G, Georges M, Monsieur R, Brocas H, Lequarre A S, Christophe D 1987 A sequence in M13 phage detects hypervariable minisatellites in human and animal DNA. Science 235: 683–684

115. Legal considerations in the delivery of genetic care

Margery W. Shaw

INTRODUCTION

In the horse and buggy era of medicine, the doctor did not have to have a great store of medical knowledge, for the simple reason that very little was known. Too often, the only thing that could be offered a seriously ill or dying patient was condolence or reassurance. Medicine of that time is exemplified by the famous painting of the doctor sitting helplessly by the bed of a dying child while the grieving parents look on. Such medical care, for all its deficiencies, made for a solid relationship of trust between the doctor and the community.

But now there is much more. As the practice of medicine has become more scientific and specialized, the doctor-patient relationship has been transformed. Sophisticated diagnostic instruments, computers, laboratory tests, and therapeutic procedures have been interposed between the doctor and the patient. Some have said that the 'art' of medicine has been replaced by the 'science' of medicine. The complex genetic principles elucidated in this textbook attest to this kind of change. In many cases, patients and their families have benefited by these technological advances, but this explosion of scientific knowledge has also widened the gap between doctors and patients and led to poorer communication between them. Patients have higher expectations for miracle drugs and cures. When they are disappointed, some have tended to blame their doctor for complications, suffering and misfortune.

This chapter will address some of the legal problems that have arisen in clinical practice that are of particular interest to medical geneticists. These issues are divided into five topics: (1) the doctor-patient contract; (2) privacy and confidentiality, particularly as they relate to procreation, genetic counselling and genetic records; (3) the legal standard of medical care in the genetic context; (4) the duties of the physician in obtaining informed consent and providing genetic counselling; and (5) the role of the physician in promoting genetic health.

The discussion which follows is based on common law, statutory law, and constitutional laws in the United States. It is therefore not directly applicable to the laws of other countries. It is aimed at helping the physician and medical student to understand broad legal principles. It should not be construed as legal advice. Every practising physician should have an attorney-counsellor to call upon for advice in specific situations.

THE DOCTOR-PATIENT CONTRACT

A legal contract is usually an *express contract* in the sense that when two parties enter into a legal relationship there is a *written* or *oral* expression of agreement between them. In the medical setting an *implied contract* exists which is not expressed, but which is recognized in the law as binding. In other words, the doctor and the patient may not be aware that they have entered a legal contract but their actions towards each other imply that there is an agreement between them. The patient comes for advice and/or treatment; the physician agrees to try to make a diagnosis through history, physical examination and special tests as indicated, and to provide medical advice or treatment, and usually expects the payment of a fee in return for the services provided.

A legal contract ordinarily arises after arms-length bargaining between two parties who are presumed by the law to be equally capable of protecting their self-interests. But in the doctor-patient contract, the physician is at an advantage vis-a-vis the patient because of superior knowledge, training and skills. The law recognizes this inequality between the parties and considers the relationship to be a *fiduciary contract*, where the patient puts trust in the physician. In an attempt to equalize this unequal bargaining position, the law places certain *duties* on the physician and grants certain *rights* to the patient. For example, the patient has the right to refuse treatment, or to fail to keep appointments at any time, for any reason. Of course, the physician is not devoid of rights: patients may be accepted or rejected, and a physician treating a patient may terminate the contract by referring the patient to another doctor or by giving adequate notice that services will no longer be provided.

The concept of a legal contract between physician and patient is important because if the court finds that no contract exists then no legal duties of the physician arise. It is also important to note that the law recognizes the existence of uncertainties in medical diagnosis and treatment and does not impose upon the physician a duty to guarantee a cure or improvement of the medical condition. Physicians should reassure their patients, but they should not make promises which could later be construed as a breach of contract. An example, which has arisen in many legal cases, is the situation in which a physician warrants a sterilization operation and the patient later bears or begets a child. Since sterilization is sometimes desired by the patient for genetic reasons, a prudent geneticist-physician would not guarantee permanent sterility. Instead, the patient should be told that, although vasectomy and tubal ligation are nearly always effective, there is a small possibility of failure (i.e. recanalization). Likewise, the physician should never promise a patient that a sterilization procedure is reversible, thus causing the patient to rely on the possibility of future fertility.

Physicians should not fear the legal implications of a doctor-patient contract. Instead, the contract should be viewed as a legal recognition of a relationship between two people that is based on trust. The physician should regard it as an opportunity to develop an understanding of the patient's needs and a respect for the patient's self-determination in medical matters which will lead to further trust and co-operation by the patient. Distrust arises when there is little or no meaningful communication between the doctor and the patient or when the doctor, even with the best of intentions, assumes the parental role, and deceives the patient or proffers false hopes.

PRIVACY AND CONFIDENTIALITY

The historical basis of confidentiality

Whenever a doctor and a patient enter into a professional relationship there is an expectation by the patient that any personal information which is divulged will be treated as confidential. This is a cornerstone of the patient's trust in the physician. This expectation is not unrealistic; in fact it is rooted in ancient ethical concepts. The fundamental statement on medical confidentiality is found in the Hippocratic Oath (1967):

What I may see or hear in the course of treatment or even outside of the treatment in regard to the life of man, which on no account one must spread abroad, I will keep to myself, holding such things shameful to be spoken about.

This rule, taken literally, provides for no exception to absolute confidentiality. However, there are times when in the interest of the patient, or in the interest of society, exceptions are necessary. Thus, a lack of absolutism is found in the 1981 Principles of Medical Ethics of the American Medical Association (AMA 1981):

A physician shall . . . . safeguard patient confidences within the constraints of the law.

The constitutional right of privacy in reproductive decisions

The decision whether or not to bear or beget a child is a very private one, yet until 1965 there was no legally recognized right of privacy in reproductive decisions. In that year the US Supreme Court held that a Connecticut statute which prohibited married couples from using contraceptives was unconstitutional (Griswold v. Connecticut 1965). The court based its decision on a constitutional right of privacy, emanating from the rights enumerated in the First, Third, Fourth, Fifth, Ninth and Fourteenth Amendments of the US Constitution. Seven years later the US Supreme Court extended the right of privacy in the use of contraceptives to unmarried people (Eisenstadt v. Baird 1972). Then, in 1973, the landmark abortion decision (Roe v. Wade 1973) proclaimed that a zone of privacy encompassed the decision of a pregnant woman, in consultation with her physician, to choose to abort an unwanted fetus. This right cannot be invaded by the state during the first trimester. After the first trimester and until the period of viability of the fetus (i.e. the capacity of the fetus to live if separated from the womb) the state can only impose regulations on abortion to protect maternal health. When fetal viability is reached, the state may proscribe abortions except to preserve the mother's life or health.

These three decisions from the highest court firmly established the principle of reproductive privacy. In medical genetics practice, the reproductive options were widened and the physician now has considerable discretion to provide alternatives to any couple who wish to avoid the birth of a genetically defective child.

Artificial insemination by donor (AID) and in vitro fertilization (IVF) using an egg donor are two other ways to circumvent genetic catastrophes. In autosomal dominant diseases AID or IVF may be chosen, depending on whether the gene is in the paternal or maternal kindred. Either AID or IVF could avert autosomal recessive conditions, but AID will usually be the preferred alternative because it is easier, cheaper, and non-invasive. In X-linked recessive conditions AID is of no value in preventing the birth of affected sons if the mother is a carrier, but it would eliminate the possibility of carrier daughters if the father is affected. IVF with a donor egg is the only way to prevent conception of affected males (Shaw 1980a).*

Breach of confidentiality in family settings

In genetic counselling, the counsellor may face a decision as to whether or not there is a legal right to breach the time-honoured medical confidentiality rule in order to contact relatives to further delineate the disorder in question, or to warn them of their possible genetic risks. This problem can be addressed prospectively by explaining to the counsellee before the family history is taken that a situation may arise when spouses or relatives need to be informed about a particular inherited condition. By raising the issue and seeking an understanding in advance, the counsellee would have no reason to claim reliance on confidentiality. A spouse or relative may be at risk of incurring economic and emotional burdens if not informed of the possibility of a defective child and may claim that a right to know was denied if no warning was given and an affected child is born.

Although courts recognize the need to protect medical confidentiality in order to promote trust in the doctor-patient relationship and jealously guard the patient's interests in non-disclosure of medical facts, they have also recognized that there may be, at times, a compelling societal need to exercise or even encourage breaches of confidentiality in order to avert a risk of serious harm to others. For example, a psychotherapist was charged with a legal duty to warn an identifiable victim when his patient threatened violence and the therapist perceived a real danger (Tarasoff v. University in California 1976). Similarly, in order to prevent the spread of a highly infectious disease, a physician was held to a duty to warn individuals who came into contact with the patient (Simonsen v. Swenson 1920).

Thus, a physician may have a right to disclose to relatives of patients with a chromosome translocation or with a dominant or X-linked gene that they have a risk of bearing a child with a burdensome chromosomal or genetic disorder. In light of the precedents set in the

* Footnote: Since this chapter was written, a landmark decision has been announced by the U.S. Supreme Court. Although not directly overturning Roe v. Wade, the majority opinion expands each state's power to regulate and restrict abortion which may impact the woman's right to privacy. Further developments may materially affect the geneticist's freedom to advise patients regarding abortion.

psychiatric and infectious disease cases there may even be a duty to do so, although no genetic cases addressing this issue have reached appellate courts.

Confidentiality of genetic records

The clinical geneticist maintains detailed information about many individuals other than the counsellee when pedigrees are assembled or family testing is done. Because people may perceive, with some justification, that disclosure of their genetic make-up may be stigmatizing, there is a duty to prevent unconsented disclosures to third parties such as school officials, employers, or insurance companies. On the other hand, the legitimate need for access to genetic data banks for reseach studies is patently clear. Special attention should be given to protecting anonymity in stored records by the use of codes, and information on the proband or the kindred should not be released without consent of the parties involved. Epidemiologists can often analyze demographic, statistical and medical information without the need to know the identity of the individuals, and linkage studies can be analyzed anonymously. But if a need arises to collect cases of rare inherited diseases for clinical or laboratory studies then the individuals involved should give voluntary informed consent for participation. The Federal Privacy Act of 1974 provides guidelines for disclosure of medical records (Privacy Act 1974) and most states have statutes regarding confidentiality of medical data.

GENERAL PRINCIPLES OF NEGLIGENCE IN MEDICAL MALPRACTICE

Medical malpractice law is one branch of tort (non-criminal) law called negligence. Negligence is a non-intentional tort, in contrast to battery which is an intentional tort. Liability for negligence in genetic counselling does not differ from liability in other medical consultation situations. Liability in prenatal diagnosis does not differ in theory from liability in postnatal diagnosis. It is the facts in each particular situation which distinguish it from other cases; the legal reasoning is similar. Therefore, if you have a specific legal question try to analyze it as lawyers do, in the framework outlined below.

Negligence does *not* mean neglect. It is much broader than that. The most common suits brought to court because of negligence are traffic accidents. Anyone can be sued for negligence; it is not limited to medical personnel. To prove a case of negligence, the court looks to the following five criteria (all of which must be met):

1. *Standard of care* What is the acceptable behaviour

of a reasonable person under the cirumstances? The standard of reasonableness is set by comparison to one's peers. Obviously, the standard of care in driving a car is violated by drunk driving, running a red light, or speeding, since these are standards established by statutes. But speed is a good example of a fluctuating standard of behaviour based on circumstances. Even though a sign is posted on a street which indicates that 30 miles an hour is the speed limit, it would not be reasonable to drive at this speed in fog, on icy streets, in a school zone, in a parade, or in other shifting circumstances. In medical situations, a physician must meet a higher standard than a physician's assistant and a specialist must meet a higher standard than a generalist; therefore, a certified clinical geneticist would be held to a higher standard in genetic diagnosis and counselling than other physicians.

In all professions there is a *duty* to act reasonably, based on skill, education, expertise and experience. There is a duty to 'keep up' with advances in the field. Failure to keep abreast of new knowledge may be negligence. One court succinctly stated this principle (Fortner v. Koch 1935):

It is the duty of a physician in diagnosing a case to use due diligence in ascertaining all available facts and collecting data essential to a proper diagnosis.

2. *Breach of duty*   A breach of duty to meet the standard of care must be proven by a preponderance of the evidence in civil suits. 'Proof' in law does not mean the same thing as it does in science. It means that a judge or jury is convinced, by the preponderance of the evidence, that the explanation offered by the winning party is more likely than that offered by the losing party. Indisputable conclusions can seldom, if ever, be obtained. The court's decision (whether judge or a jury) is essentially a judgement call, much like an umpire's decision in baseball. It is based on the best facts available and the parties must either abide by the decision (even if they still think it is wrong) or appeal to a higher court.

3. *Injury*   The patient complaining of medical negligence must have been injured or harmed. This may be physical injury, economic loss, or emotional pain and suffering. In the context of amniocentesis, a physician could not be sued for failing to offer prenatal diagnosis in a high-risk pregancy, if the birth results in a normal infant, because there would be no legal injury.

4. *Proximate cause*   There must be a demonstrable, causal relation between the alleged negligent act and the injury, but it need not be the *sole* cause. An act may be one of omission as well as one of commission. For example, if fetoscopy has been negligently performed and there is some physical damage to the fetus, proximate cause could

be held. If, on the the other hand, the child is born with an atrioventricular septal defect, proximate cause could not be established to be related to the fetoscopy procedure. Failure to provide information on genetic risks and reproductive alternatives, when these would be relevant to a patient's decision, would only be negligence if the risk in question actually materialized. A woman who was not offered amniocentesis, even though it was indicated because of her age, could not show proximate cause if her infant had a genetic disorder that was unrelated to increased maternal age.

5. *Foreseeability*   There must be reason to believe that, at the time the breach of duty occurred, the negligent act could result in the harm complained about. Thus, the thalidomide and DES cases do not usually involve negligence because the outcomes could not have been reasonably predicted when the drugs were first prescribed. Instead, they fall under another area of the law called product liability, which does not require that the elements of negligence be present. This is a different legal issue which need not concern us here. Today, however, with the information available on the possible harmful side-effects of these drugs, a reasonable and prudent physician would not prescribe them to a pregnant woman because foreseeability of possible harm could be demonstrated.

These comments on negligence represent only the author's opinion based upon the legal principles followed by most jurisdictions. If a case is settled in a lower court it does not bind other courts unless it is appealed. Only when a legal issue is decided by the State's highest court does it become the common law of that state. If a pronouncement is made by the US Supreme Court then it is binding on all state and federal courts.

Specific legal cases involving genetic conditions

With the advances in heterozygote testing, prenatal diagnosis, and increased sophistication in predicting genetic risks, a number of cases have been heard in the courts alleging that physicians were negligent because they failed to offer diagnostic tests or failed to provide information which might be material to a decision to conceive or to continue a pregnancy. A summary of 45 cases has been published (Shaw 1986). These do not represent all cases because most trial court cases and all out-of-court settlements are not published in the legal literature.

These 45 cases include chromosomal defects, autosomal dominant, autosomal recessive and X-linked disorders, Rh-incompatibility, rubella cases, multiple congenital defects, and environmental teratogens. Thus the courts frequently recognize negligence, wrongful birth and wrongful life cases involving genetic conditions. Courts are more likely to recognize claims by the parents that they have suffered financial injury or emotional pain and suffering than to recognize the child's claim for physical pain and suffering for a genetic disease. One of the reasons that the courts give for this distinction is that as far as the child is concerned it is impossible to compare life with defects against no life at all. They argue that a logical and legal quandary exists because the child would not be here to complain if no wrong had been committed and the child thus lacks standing to sue. Some courts have warned that if the child has a legal cause of action against the physician then it would also be able to complain against its parents for allowing it to be born to suffer if the parents had been forewarned of its defects and had decided against abortion.

Several legal commentators have argued that a child should be given the right to complain that it has been born in a defective condition due to the negligence of another (Shaw 1977, 1980b, Robertson 1978, Capron 1979). In a 1960 decision by the Supreme Court of New Jersey involving a fetus that had been injured in an automobile accident and was later born alive the negligent driver was held liable. The court noted (Smith v. Brennan 1960):

Justice requires that the principle be recognized that a child has a legal right to begin life with a sound mind and body.

This concept was expanded in a comment made in a decision by an appellate court in California involving a Tay-Sachs child (Curlender v. Bioscience Laboratories 1980):

If a case arose where ... parents made a conscious choice to proceed with a pregnancy, with full knowledge that a seriously impaired infant would be born ... we see no sound public policy which should protect those parents from being answerable for the pain, suffering, and misery which they have wrought upon their offspring.

The impact of this holding caused an immediate reaction in the California legislature. A statute (California Civil Code 1982) was passed, stating in part:

(a) No cause of action arises against a parent of a child based upon the claim that the child should not have been conceived or, if conceived, should not have been allowed to have been born alive.
(b) The failure or refusal of a parent to prevent the livebirth of his or her child shall not be a defense in any action against a third party, nor shall the failure or refusal be considered in awarding damages in any such action.

Thus it is clear that the law imposes a duty on physicians to warn potential parents of high-risk pregnancies, but it imposes no corollary duty on parents to prevent the birth of defective offspring. This is in keeping with the parents' rights of reproductive privacy: when to have children, how many children to have, and the quality of life of their children. However, if one traces the history of child abuse and fetal abuse and the statutory parental duties to provide medical care for their children, it is possible that the law will evolve to prevent egregious decisions by parents that allow known defective children to be born if those children endured severe physical pain and suffering, and shortened life spans that could have been avoided.

THE DOCTRINE OF INFORMED CONSENT

The cornerstone of the informed consent doctrine was enunciated in a New York case (Schloendorff v. Society of New York Hospitals 1914):

Every human being of adult years and sound mind has a right to determine what shall be done with his own body.

In order for a genetic counsellee to make a rational and informed decision about procreation certain information must be disclosed by the counsellor. For example, the burden of the genetic disease should be discussed, the genetic risks must be revealed, and enough statistical information must be imparted so that the individual can understand and interpret the risks. Alternative courses of action must also be outlined for the counsellee. This may include carrier testing, contraception, sterilization, prenatal diagnosis, abortion, sex selection, adoption, artificial insemination, in vitro fertilization, or taking the risks of having defective children. All of the appropriate options should be discussed.

An understanding of Mendelian inheritance is often difficult to communicate to the average adult who has little knowledge of reproductive biology and the concepts of probability. With patients who are minors, who are mentally defective, or who do not speak the language of the counsellor, the problem of comprehension may be insurmountable. In these cases, an adult relative, a guardian, a translator, or an ombudsman may be needed for proxy consent or for help in relaying the message.

There are many new procedures being developed in medical genetics that require human experimentation. New approaches to prenatal diagnosis are being tested. Fetoscopy, fetal biopsies, and fetal blood sampling have met with success. Some genetic diseases are being investigated to determine whether enzyme replacement or gene replacement is feasible. Research on fetuses and fetal tissues pose a special problem. Whenever research is involved the physician-investigator must obtain permission from an institutional review board before proceeding. Special attention is given to the informed consent forms by these review committees and the subject of the experiment must be told of the potential risks and benefits that the experiment entails. The subject should also know that refusal to participate in research projects will not compromise his or her right to quality medical care.

One of the issues in informed consent that has not yet been adequately addressed by the courts is whether the physician has a duty to determine that the patient actually comprehends the consent form which is to be signed. So far, the courts have merely held physicians to the duty to make disclosures, but not to a duty to determine whether the patient understood the information imparted. The courts have, however, stated that *all* information material to a decision must be disclosed so that an informed decision can be made (Canterbury v. Spence 1972, Cobbs v. Grant 1972, Wilkinson v. Vesey 1972). It is this writer's opinion that the patient should be free to choose any course of action among the alternatives available, including refusal to accept the physician's recommendations, *except* when the choice would be harmful to another person, including a person yet unconceived or unborn. The judicial trend is towards a 'reasonable patient' standard of disclosure and away from a 'reasonable physician' standard. This means that the doctor may not pick and choose those options which other doctors disclose but must give the information that a reasonable person would want to know.

THE PHYSICIAN'S ROLE IN PROMOTING GENETIC HEALTH

The physician is in a unique position to effect changes in attitudes and behaviour towards responsible parenthood by educating and counselling his or her patients about reproduction and genetic disease. This process should begin in early childhood and continue throughout life.

Children should be helped to understand bodily functions and should learn to take responsibility for health promotion and the prevention of illness. Appointments for physical check-ups and inoculations afford the physician an opportunity to initiate meaningful dialogue with the child about the mysteries of the body, including sexual reproduction. Children are naturally curious and quite receptive to new information about themselves.

The physician should discuss the family pedigree and provide sex education to the teenager. Most states have statutes that protect the privacy of the physician-patient relationship in counselling adolescents about the use of contraceptives. The United States Supreme Court has ruled that a Massachusetts statute requiring the approval of the parents or a judge before a minor can obtain an abortion was unconstitutional as an invasion of privacy and violative of due process (Bellotti v. Baird 1979). However, a Utah statute which requires parental notification, but not parental consent, before a minor can obtain an abortion has been upheld by the US Supreme Court (H.L. v. Matheson 1981). Although state statutes require physicians to report sexually transmissible diseases, most states allow venereal disease treatment of minors without parental notification. Clow and Scriver (1977) have shown that genetic counselling and heterozygote screening of adolescents by a medical geneticist in a high school setting can be quite effective.

The physician has a continuing duty to take adequate family histories, offer diagnostic tests, and provide information about increased genetic risks to couples during their reproductive years. Opportunities for these discussions are presented by premarital examinations, prenatal visits and postnatal follow-up. It is also legally incumbent on physicians to refer patients to specialists for diagnosis and counselling or treatment if, in the exercise of due care, problems arise that are beyond the competence of the generalists (Manion v. Tweedy 1959). With the advent of board certification in clinical genetics, other physicians should recognize the need for referral for genetic testing, in-depth counselling of complex probabilities and risks, and specialized treatments for genetic disease. It will soon become possible to predict the risk or certainty for *all* inherited conditions by linkage of abnormal alleles with restriction endonuclease polymorphisms (Botstein et al 1980) or by direct gene sequencing. This will further necessitate referral to genetic specialists. Gene therapy and gene replacement will likely become commonplace in the not too distant future.

CONCLUSION

The physician who keeps abreast of new developments in medical genetics and who provides good genetic counselling and testing need have little fear of medical malpractice in genetic conditions. But it is incumbent on clinicians who deal with prospective parents to pursue continuing education courses in genetics, take careful family histories, offer genetic tests, and disclose alternative reproductive choices. All physicians should know about the availability of specialized genetic clinics if they are unable or unwilling to provide these services themselves.

REFERENCES

American Medical Association 1981 Principles of Medical Ethics, Section 4

Bellotti v. Baird, 433 U.S. 622 (1979)

Botstein D, White R L, Skolnick M, Davis R W 1980 Construction of a genetic linkage map in man using restriction fragment length polymorphisms. American Journal of Human Genetics 32: 314

California Civil Code 1982 §43.6 West

Canterbury v. Spence, 464 F.2d 772 (D.C. Cir.), *cert. denied*, 409 U.S. 1064 (1972)

Capron A M 1979 Tort liability in genetic counselling. Columbia Law Review 79: 618

Clow C L, Scriver C R 1977 Knowledge about and attitudes among high school students: the Tay-Sachs experience. Pediatrics 59: 86

Cobbs v. Grant, 8 Cal. 3d 229, 502 P.2d 1, 104 Cal. Rptr. 505 (1972)

Curlender v. Bioscience Laboratories, 106 Cal. App. 3d 811, 165 Cal. Rptr. 477 (1980)

Eisenstadt v. Baird, 405 U.S. 438 (1972)

Fortner v. Koch, 261 N.W. 762 (Mich. 1935)

Griswold v. Connecticut, 381 U.S. 479 (1965)

H.L. v. Matheson, 450 U.S. 398 (1981)

Hippocratic Oath 1967 Ancient Medicine: Selected Papers of Ludwig Edelstein. Temkin & Temkin (eds), Johns Hopkins University Press, Baltimore, p6

Manion v. Tweedy, 257 Minn. 59, 100 N.W.2d 124 (1959)

Privacy Act of 1974, 5 U.S.C. §552 (1974)

Robertson H B 1978 Toward rational boundaries of tort liability for injury to the unborn: Prenatal injuries, preconception injuries and wrongful life. Duke Law Journal 1978: 1401

Roe v. Wade, 410 U.S. 113 (1973)

Schloendorff v. Society of New York Hospitals, 105 N.E. 92 (1914)

Shaw M W 1977 Genetically defective children: Emerging legal considerations. American Journal of Law and Medicine 3: 333

Shaw M W 1980a In vitro fertilization: For infertile married couples only? Hastings Center Report 10: 4

Shaw M W 1980b The potential plaintiff: Preconception and prenatal torts. In: Milunsky A, Annas G (eds) Genetics and the Law II. Plenum Publishing, p 225–232

Shaw M W 1986 Medicolegal aspects of prenatal diagnosis. In: Milunsky A (ed) Genetic Disorders and the Fetus. Plenum Publishing, p 799–817

Simonsen v. Swenson, 104 Neb. 224, 177 N.W. 831 (1920) (per curiam)

Smith v. Brennan, 157 A.2d 497 (N.J. 1960)

Tarasoff v. Regents of the University of California, 17 Cal.3d 425, 551 P.2d 334, 131 Cal. Rptr. 14 (1976)

Wilkinson v. Vesey, 110 R.I. 606, 295 A.2d 676 (1972)

Legal cases are cited in these references according to *A Uniform System of Citation* 1972 12th edn. published by the Harvard Law Review Association, Cambridge, Massachusetts.

116. Challenges for the future

H. Galjaard

INTRODUCTION

Articles in scientific journals usually deal with new data, methodologies and concepts. Chapters in books usually review accumulated information about specific topics and, in a comprehensive multiauthor book like 'Principles and Practice of Medical Genetics', the reader may even acquire knowledge about the state of the art in a whole discipline. Not surprisingly, most authors write about all advances that have been made in the elucidation of the aetiology of congenital disease and about the new perspectives for early diagnosis, treatment, genetic counselling and prevention.

In this last chapter of the book I will try to focus on basic facts that are not yet understood, and on economic, social, psychological and ethical or religious factors which limit the application of existing methodology and may also be important in the utilization of new technologies.

The main reason for writing such a chapter is the hope that it will be a challenge for the future, especially for the younger generation interested in medical genetics.

As can be seen from the previous chapters, impressive advances have been made in various areas of human genetics. Still, many problems are unresolved at the level of the genes, proteins, molecular interactions and metabolic functions, as well as in the areas of cell differentiation, cell-cell interaction and the relationships between genetic and environmental factors.

The molecular aetiology of only a very small proportion of congenital malformations and single gene disorders is understood. As a consequence the possibilities of early laboratory diagnosis, carrier detection and prenatal diagnosis are still limited. This in turn restricts the options of a couple at risk.

However, exciting new methodologies are appearing on the horizon and their application will undoubtedly provide new insights in molecular and cellular biology.

Gradually, the importance of clinical genetics will extend from paediatric disorders to malignancies, cardiovascular diseases, psychiatric and neurological abnormalities in (late) adulthood. New diagnostic methods will become available which may offer new perspectives for treatment and prevention; they may also create new problems, both for the individual and for society.

While most experts will be excited by new methods and discoveries, the majority of the world's population has no idea about what is going on in medical genetics. According to UNESCO (1986) 40 000 young children die every day in the developing world. Of those surviving malnutrition, a considerable percentage will develop mental retardation and a marked deficit in work capacity.

Yet over the last four decades infant and child death rates in the developing world have almost halved, and the average life expectancy has increased by 40%. Also, the proportion of children entering school has increased from 30% to more than 80%. Although vast problems still have to be solved in the developing world, interest in medical genetics is no longer restricted to Western industrialized countries where congenital disorders are the major cause of infant mortality and morbidity. Several developing countries are starting to pay attention to medical genetics as well. The reasons for this include declining infant mortality and a consequent relative increase in the incidence of congenital disorders; specific problems related to a government population policy, as is the case in China; a high rate of consanguineous marriages based on social traditions, as in some Middle Eastern countries and Asian populations.

One of the challenges for the future is the transfer of knowledge to those in need of it, and in such a way that different (groups of) people may use this knowledge according to their own cultural, traditional, social and religious backgrounds. Another challenge is the creation of sufficient clinical, laboratory and teaching facilities so that people at risk for a genetic disorder will be able to use the existing methodologies for early diagnosis, treatment, genetic counselling and prevention.

The elucidation of the various complex factors responsible for the underutilization of genetic services will not only contribute to the future prevention of physical and mental handicap, but it will also help to improve the way in which we deal with the incorporation of new technologies and approaches to various health care systems.

MOLECULES AND CELLS

DNA

During the last two decades impressive progress has been made in understanding the molecular basis of hereditary disease. This can be seen from a comparison of the contents of some chapters in the first and second editions of this book, published at an interval of 7 years. A similar comparison for other chapters, however, would show that many aspects of congenital malformations, genetic diseases and multifactorial disorders are still not understood. Answers to these unresolved questions at the molecular and cellular level form a major challenge for the future.

Currently some 1800 expressed genes and more than 2500 additional RFLP and other markers have now been mapped on the human genome (see Friedmann 1990). These numbers are impressive but they also imply that 97–98% of coding human genes have not yet been identified.

The same reasoning holds for Mendelian disorders: according to McKusick's last catalogue (1988) the responsible (enzyme) protein defect has been elucidated in about 400 disorders. Again, this represents a vast amount of clinical, pathological and biochemical work, but nevertheless the molecular aetiology of more than 90% of the 4000 diseases known or believed to be due to a single-gene mutation are still not understood. Knowledge of the exact nature of the gene mutation or the protein defect often provides new perspectives for the early diagnosis of index patients, carrier detection, genetic counselling, and prenatal testing, and it also forms a necessary basis for attempts at treatment.

Many researchers who previously worked on biochemical aspects of genetic disease have moved into the area of DNA analysis. Indeed, the problems to be solved, as well as the potential to do so, are enormous. The whole human genome is believed to consist of 3×10^9 base pairs of which 1–2% are mRNA coding sequences. Some experts envisage mapping the whole human genome within one or two decades. Others have challenged the need for a centralized effort and instead propose data banks where information from many different groups, each working on their particular gene(s) of interest, can be ordered and stored.

Whatever the outcome, new methodologies for gene mapping and the analysis of DNA sequences are becoming available at a rapid rate. The use of rare cutting restriction enzymes, new methods of cosmid cloning, jumping libraries and pulsed-field or field inversion gel electrophoresis already contribute to filling the gap between the resolution of chromosome banding (down to 1000 kb) and that of restriction mapping (dozens – 100 kb). New methods using fluorescent chain-terminating dideoxynucleotides and a laser detection system already enable the sequencing of 100 bases per hour per lane, i.e. 5000 bases per day with multiple samples run simultaneously. In a Japanese project the development of a fully automated high-speed DNA sequencing machine with a capacity of 10^6 bases a day is foreseen!

Another important aspect of present and future genetic work is the theoretical basis of human genetic linkage and the development and use of computer programs for the simultaneous analysis of many loci. It seems that more geneticists with expertise in this field are needed, especially since linkage with restriction fragment length polymorphisms is being used more and more in the (prenatal) diagnosis of hereditary disease.

According to a recent survey of worldwide experience with first-trimester fetal diagnosis, some two dozen different Mendelian disorders have been diagnosed by direct or indirect demonstration of the gene mutation using DNA technology. This number will undoubtedly increase significantly in the future and will also include disorders of multifactorial aetiology if linkages with specific DNA sequences become established.

At present only a few gene mutations can be demonstrated directly by endonuclease mapping or the use of synthetic oligonucleotide probes. In the future the scope will certainly widen, as new methods become available to detect single-base substitutions. An important step forward in the practice of DNA diagnosis is the enhanced sensitivity that can be achieved by specific enzyme amplification of DNA in vitro. A major challenge for the future is a further simplification of these analytical methods to allow their wider application at relatively low costs and with readily available chemicals. In the latter context it is of great importance, especially for developing countries, that radiolabelled probes be replaced by fluorogenic ones with similar sensitivity. Only when these requirements are fulfilled will carrier detection on a large scale become feasible, and thereby prevention of the birth of first affected children in families. The recent discovery of the gene defect responsible for cystic fibrosis undoubtedly is the first step in a series of such actions that will lead to a marked decrease in the incidence of this most frequent disease among Caucasians.

Proteins

Of the 1500 Mendelian disorders inherited as autosomal recessive traits, in 20% the responsible protein defect, usually an enzyme deficiency, has been identified. Of the 2500 dominant phenotypes presently known, in only 60 cases has a non-enzymic protein defect been found (2.2%); and of the 300 X-linked disorders the responsible protein defect has been found in about 6%. From these data it can be concluded that there is still much work to do in the search for specific biochemical defects in patients with this category of congenital disorders, which also comprises 22% of those with localized malformations and 3% with multiple malformations.

To identify the molecular aetiology of a disease, accurate clinical examination and attention to unusual pathological features remain an important basis. Sometimes the search for specific abnormalities of metabolites in blood, urine or other body fluids will provide a clue to the basic protein defect. Several new analytical techniques, such as gas-chromatography-mass spectrometry, high performance liquid chromatography, and nuclear magnetic resonance have become available. In other instances careful pathological examination of cells and tissues, including the application of modern imaging techniques, may reveal specific abnormalities which ultimately point the way to a specific protein defect. During the last decades these approaches have regularly led to the discovery of 'new defects' and they will undoubtedly continue to do so. Recent examples of this include the identification of the LDL receptor defect, the discovery of peroxisomal disorders and new lysosomal storage diseases, including membrane transport defects. Advances have also been made in the elucidation of protein defects in inherited disorders of connective tissue and of the role of mitochondrial abnormalities in neuromuscular diseases.

In future, parallel to studies at the DNA level, the search for the basic protein defect in diseases like cystic fibrosis, various muscular dystrophies, skeletal disorders, hereditary cancers and psychiatric diseases will remain of great importance. Also, a better understanding at the protein level of the associations between HLA types and disorders like ankylosing spondylitis, juvenile diabetes, myasthenia gravis, multiple sclerosis and coeliac disease may contribute to the elucidation of the molecular aetiology of these diseases. The work on the genetic basis of insulin-dependent diabetes marks an important first step in this context.

Even when the basic protein defect of a Mendelian disorder has been defined several questions remain to be answered. It has become more and more clear that 'the same' protein defect may be associated with very different clinical and pathological manifestations. During the last decade the study of normal and mutant cells has yielded much information about the various steps in the post-translational modification of proteins and about the molecular mechanisms involved in the targeting of proteins to specific subcellular organelles. Different mutations affecting different steps in the processing of a protein may all result in a functional deficiency of this protein. However, the extent to which the function is affected may depend on the exact molecular nature of the defect. Despite all advances in the delineation of different mutations within one gene and of different genes involved in the processing and targeting of one protein, in most instances the cause of clinical heterogeneity within a syndrome is not yet understood.

So far, most studies on the genetic and molecular aspects of a protein defect have been performed on easily accessible cell material such as placenta, blood cells or cultured skin fibroblasts. For a proper understanding of pathogenesis and the clinical heterogeneity of genetic diseases it seems of great importance that new systems are being developed. The use of transgenic animals may be of great help in studying pathogenetic mechanisms.

More information about the targeting of proteins, mechanisms involved in recognition, uptake and intracellular transport of molecules and membrane passage is also essential for progress in the field of therapy. Difficulties in this field are illustrated by the disappointing results of (enzyme) protein replacement therapy, despite many years of work. The experimental work on models for gene therapy is also more complex than many have anticipated. The use of viral vectors and the possibility of gene targeting and gene replacement, however, mean a step forward.

Chromosomes

Because of the relatively simple instrumentation and preparation procedures involved, chromosome analysis is probably the most widely used laboratory method in the diagnosis of congenital disorders. Improvement of the staining techniques has enabled a more accurate delineation of minor structural rearrangements and deletions, and high resolution banding resolves the human genome into segments with an average size of 1000–2000 kb. In recent years some exciting new challenges in cytogenetics have appeared and new methods provide the potential to answer old questions.

Dual-laser flow sorting has enabled the isolation of relatively large amounts of single human chromosomes. DNA libraries have been prepared and more and more probes are becoming available for the detailed analysis of regions of specific chromosomes and of single genes located in specific parts of a region. Gradually, the boundaries between chromosomal abnormalities detectable with microscopic techniques and anomalies diagnosed by DNA technology will become less distinct.

Molecular methods will contribute increasingly to cytogenetics and, hopefully, will also help in the diagnosis of a large proportion of severely handicapped people who have so far remained undiagnosed.

Already the combination of conventional chromosome studies and DNA technology has enabled the identification of microdeletions, some in the order of 10^3 kb, involving several unrelated structural gene loci. Future studies on patients with complex phenotypes and symptoms associated with more than one Mendelian disorder will certainly reveal other chromosomal abnormalities at a resolution level between hundreds and thousands of kb. In this context pulsed field gel electrophoresis and other analytical methods allowing the identification of large DNA fragments may be of great help.

The use of probes for specific genes may also be useful in the identification of very small chromosome fragments and in the study of translocations, inversions or duplications. An interesting example is the finding of an exchange between small fragments of Yp and Xp, explaining the male phenotype in people with a 46,XX karyotype. Chromosome specific probes may enable (prenatal) diagnosis in interphase cells.

Apart from diagnostic applications, the use of molecular methods will be of great interest in fundamental studies on homologies between the sex chromosomes, the order of genes on chromosomes and chromosomal evolution.

Another major challenge for the future is to obtain a better understanding of the aetiology and pathogenesis of chromosomal aberrations. As far as pathogenesis is concerned, it will be virtually impossible to relate a trisomy or a monosomy of a whole chromosome, involving hundreds to a thousand coding genes, to specific metabolic disturbances and impaired cellular functions.

Syndromes with an abnormality of very small fragments of a chromosome, that may also be supernumerary or deleted as a whole, have therefore been studied. Delineation of the genes involved in the various syndromes, their exact mapping and their relationship with specific biochemical, pathological and clinical manifestations may ultimately lead to better insight into the pathogenesis of gross chromosomal anomalies.

In addition to the studies mentioned above, one of the major focuses of interest in future cytogenetics will probably be the study of chromosomal and molecular abnormalities in cancer cells.

One of the breakthroughs in tumour cytogenetics was the finding that the chromosome translocations that typify Burkitt's lymphoma and chronic myeloid leukaemia affect a known proto-oncogene. In the former c-myc is translocated into the immunoglobulin heavy chain gene cluster and it may or may not be mutated. In chronic myeloid leukaemia molecular analyses have shown that the translocation of c-abl into the bcr gene results in the expression of a fused transcript and the production of a chimaeric protein.

Recently, another fusion protein has been found in Ph$^+$ cells from patients with acute lymphocytic leukaemia. In the future other chromosomal rearrangements, as defined by molecular methods, may be found in other human malignancies. The next step will be clarification of the exact role of the mutated or chimaeric protein in causing the cellular dysregulation characteristic of each type of malignancy (see also next section).

Another important model for future research in cancer (cyto)genetics is that reported for retinoblastoma. The predisposition to this tumour is inherited as an autosomal dominant trait which can now be identified by DNA studies. A deletion of a chromosome 13q14 fragment may also be associated with retinoblastoma. Most interesting, however, is the finding that the retinoblastoma gene, although dominant in the individual, is recessive at the cellular level. A necessary step in tumorigenesis is the development of homozygosity or hemizygosity for the mutant allele. This may occur by various chromosomal mechanisms in somatic cells, such as loss of the normal allele, reduplication of the mutant allele, mitotic recombination, gene conversion or point mutation. It is also intriguing to note that surviving patients with the hereditary form of retinoblastoma have a high probability of developing other cancers such as osteosarcomas and fibrosarcomas.

A few other tumours, including Wilms tumour, have also been shown to be caused by a two step process as described above. In Wilms tumour evidence has been presented that mitotic recombination is the mechanism leading to homozygosity of a mutant gene in 11p13. It has been postulated that for this type of tumour a pair of regulatory genes that normally suppress the expression of a transforming gene is lost. Recently, the loss of an allele in 5q21-22 has been related to the development of colorectal adenocarcinomas in some patients. Other examples are the loss of a gene on 3p in lung carcinoma and a gene on 22q in meningioma.

These examples illustrate that new areas of research have opened up for the clinician, epidemiologist, cytogeneticist and molecular biologist. Challenges for the future are the discovery of new associations between specific genetic abnormalities and certain cancers, and of course the 'translation' of genetic abnormalities into a better understanding of the (abnormal) protein(s) involved. This should ultimately lead to the elucidation of the mechanisms responsible for the abnormal cell functions in various cancers.

Cells

In the previous sections on DNA, proteins and chromosomes, the necessity of understanding abnormalities at the level of cellular structures and functions has already been mentioned several times. The study of (sub)cellular structures and functions is of importance for virtually all congenital disorders, but in the near future cell biology is likely to play an especially significant role in the fields of carcinogenesis and developmental biology.

Since the pioneering work on Rous sarcoma virus, some 50 viral and cellular (proto)oncogenes have been identified. They encode a wide variety of proteins whose functions are also very diverse. The products encoded by some oncogenes act in the nucleus, others in the cytoplasm, and still others are located at the plasma membrane.

One of the actions of nuclear oncogenes is the power to immortalize cells in culture, which might be related to activation of transcription from other genes and by (dys) regulation of DNA replication.

Cytoplasmic products of proto-oncogenes usually seem to be in a resting state awaiting a stimulus to rise to an excited state for a short period of time. It is thought that the cytoplasmic products such as protein-tyrosine kinases or protein-serine/threonine kinases play a role in the phosphorylation of proteins and lipids, induction of the secretion of growth factors, and signal transduction. Oncogene mutations affecting the structure or level of the encoded proteins may create constitutive excitation and thereby dysregulation.

A large number of oncogenes code for proteins associated with or located in the plasma membrane. The best known examples are transmembrane receptor molecules for growth factors exerting protein-tyrosine kinase activity and a regulator of adenylate cyclase.

The complexity of this field is still enormous. In mammalian cells alone over 100 different protein kinases are known. The proliferation of cells is probably regulated by an elaborate circuitry of processes extending from the cell surface to the nucleus. One of the challenges for the future is the discovery of additional parts of the mechanisms involved in the regulation of normal cell proliferation. Maybe then it will become clear in which ways tumour cells arise and which exogenous and genetic factors play a role.

In this context it is worth mentioning that it has been demonstrated that some oncogenes are the direct targets of chemical carcinogens. Also, the role of growth factors and the induction of their target genes will be major foci of interest.

Another exciting new area of research is the role of oncogenes and their products in early *embryonic development*. Several important homologies have been found between genes involved in the early development of *Drosophila* and a cellular proto-oncogene. The *Drosophila* gene *dorsal* is a maternal effect locus essential for the dorsal-ventral polarity in the developing embryo 2–3 hours after fertilization. The protein encoded by this gene turned out to be almost 50% identical over an extensive region to the protein encoded by the avian oncogene v-*rel* and its cellular homologue c-*rel*. In another study homology was shown between the mouse mammary oncogene *int*-1 and the *Drosophila* gene *wingless*. The latter gene codes for a protein which probably functions in morphogenesis as a signal in cell-cell communication. In this context it should be mentioned that the *Drosophila* gene *sevenless* codes for a transmembrane tyrosine kinase receptor which plays a role in reading or interpreting positional information during the development of the compound eye. In the future it is likely that further studies along these lines will provide more insight into the regulatory mechanisms involved in embryogenesis.

At the DNA level an important step forward has been made by the finding of so-called dominant control regions (DCR). In transgenic mice the introduction of DCR sequences enhanced the expression of the human β-globin gene to endogenous levels. This effect is independent of the place of integration of the DCR in the genome.

During recent years much progress has been made in the areas of genetic markers and techniques to introduce (mutant) genes into fertilized eggs. Homozygous uniparental mouse embryos have been produced by microsurgical removal of the male pronucleus from fertilized eggs, diploidization and addition of blastomeres from normal mouse embryos to produce a chimaera. In addition, the various ways of producing transgenic animals are a promising tool.

At the molecular and cellular levels techniques are becoming available which allow the induction of specific gene mutations. The exploitation of these various techniques will enable further studies on the effect of well defined (mutant) genes during intrauterine development.

Studies on chimaeras have already shown that, in addition to the genetic information, the spatial position and immediate environment of a cell determine its fate. Therefore, processes of cell movement and cell-cell interactions are also of great importance in developmental biology. In this connection cytoskeletal structures, the apparatus of cell motion and the constituents of the cell membrane are of primary interest. During the last decade a variety of gene products have been identified which play a role in cell-cell contact, such as cell adhesion molecules, substrate adhesion molecules and cell junctional molecules. In addition to the biosynthesis and function of such (glyco)proteins attention should be paid to other components, including the functioning of growth factor receptors, (glyco)lipids and ions such as calcium.

The extracellular matrix also deserves attention; although synthesized by the cell, matrix molecules, once deposited may affect important processes like cell proliferation, migration, adhesion and differentiation.

One of the great challenges for the future is to bridge the gaps still existing between the various approaches summarized here in order to find new clues to the complex processes involved in early embryonic development and, hopefully, a better understanding of congenital malformations of unexplained aetiology. A better understanding of the interactions between genetic and environmental factors will also be of great help in studying major diseases in adulthood like cancers, cardiovascular disorders, rheumatoid arthritis and various neurological and psychiatric disorders which are thought to be multifactorial in origin.

Finally, a minority of the congenital malformations are due to environmental factors alone, as many clinical geneticists have unfortunately experienced in pregnancies where thalidomide, alcohol, abused drugs, valproic acid or other teratogens had been used. The harmfulness of these substances, as well as of certain intrauterine infections, has sometimes been discovered by the attentiveness of individual doctors. In other instances associations have been revealed by birth-defect monitoring programmes and international collaboration.

Studies of teratogens at the cellular and molecular levels may provide new insight into critical stages of embryonic development and (genetic) variability as far as drug metabolism and sensitivity of specific cell types is concerned.

PEOPLE AND SOCIETIES

Individuals

The loss of a child or confrontation with a congenital handicap causes grief in families all over the world. The ways individuals cope with it may, however, vary according to differences in individual attitudes and life situations, socioeconomic circumstances, cultural and religious backgrounds and differences among societies. Also, the possibilities of early diagnosis, counselling, prevention and treatment of congenital handicaps, as well as the means to support the handicapped child and his or her family, vary between countries and ethnic groups (see next section).

In countries where undernutrition and infectious diseases are prevented, congenital disorders have become the major cause of infant mortality. In some industrialized Western countries the proportion of deaths due to congenital disorders during the first year of life is as high as 35%.

Furthermore, studies in Great Britain have shown that at age seven 5.2% of all children have a psychomotor retardation or another physical or mental handicap and that 85% of these impairments are of congenital origin. It is therefore not surprising that couples at reproductive age show a great interest in new means of early diagnosis, carrier detection, genetic counselling and prenatal monitoring.

This increasing interest is not only due to public information about new technologies but is also associated with the marked decline of the birth rate in many countries, socioeconomic changes, the general attitude towards handicap and disease and the increasingly important role that is attributed to the health care system in solving the problems of the individual.

Many young couples in wealthy countries focus on the fulfilment of their own ideals and ambitions and will adapt their (reproductive) behaviour accordingly. In most instances both spouses have a job and would consider the birth of a handicapped baby as a (too) heavy burden on their own lives and that of any future child. Also, families are becoming more and more isolated, which implies fewer opportunities for psychological and practical support in the immediate neighbourhood. Finally, teaching of modern biology and medical genetics in schools and the flow of information about risk factors and new methods of (genetic) diagnosis have increased public awareness of the present and future possibilities for early diagnosis, treatment, and prevention of handicaps and disease.

In general, the individual at risk of affected offspring is primarily interested in what can be done about this problem now, or in the foreseeable future. The direct confrontation with an affected child or sib is of course the strongest motivation to seek help and advice about the future. Often, however, it is not easy to provide information and genetic counselling at the right moment. In societies where more than 98% of children survive into adulthood, parents who are unexpectedly confronted with the loss of a child or with a congenital handicap often feel isolated in their grief. Many young adults in Western countries have never been confronted with death and react initially with aggression and disappointment about the role of medical experts ('why did this happen to us . . . ', 'if they had acted otherwise, then . . . '). Also, most doctors involved in clinical care have focused on diagnosis and treatment and usually do not spend time providing information about the genetic background of a disorder, the (recurrence) risk and the possibilities of prevention.

One or two decades ago the majority of people asking for genetic counselling were parents who had already given birth to one or more affected children. Now, an increasing proportion of counsellees (30–50%) do not yet have any children and want advice because one or more relatives have a congenital disorder or unexplained mental or physical handicap. Genetic counselling in this category is, of course, most effective in terms of prevention. It requires, however, sufficient openness within the family which, unfortunately, is often hampered by feelings of shame, guilt, bad relationships or overprotection (to hide bad news from the children). One major task for the future is to improve information about medical genetics in such a way that new generations will understand that openness is one of the foundations in genetic counselling and hence in the prevention of disease in future pregnancies of close relatives.

Another basis for genetic counselling is an accurate diagnosis of the index patient. Again, in the case of familial disorders, cooperation of relatives is required. Every country where congenital disorders are a major cause of infant mortality and morbidity should create sufficient facilities for clinical, cytogenetic and molecular diagnosis. It is also important to have one or more cell repositories, not only for research purposes and the storage of cell material required for prenatal diagnosis in future pregnancies, but also to enable a diagnosis in situations where patients with a possible genetic disease have remained undiagnosed initially. Even for couples who have lost a child a retrospective diagnosis, when new methodologies allow this, means at least some comfort, and has the additional advantage of providing accurate information about the recurrence risk and preventive measures in the future. In view of recent advances in the elucidation of various types of congenital disorder and the accumulation of linkage data, the possibility of retrospective studies on a patient's cell material seems of increasing importance.

In the future, genetic counselling clinics will become more and more involved in questions about the risks of environmental factors and about genetic aspects of diseases manifesting in adulthood, such as certain cardio-vascular diseases and malignancies, and various neurological and psychiatric disorders. Since many clinicians and other health workers may be involved in the care of patients with such diseases the patient and his family often feel lost amid the many experts. It is therefore of great importance to integrate the various activities, including those of the clinical geneticist.

At present, the options for a couple at increased risk of having affected offspring are still quite limited. They may accept the risk or decide not to have any (further) children; they may choose artificial insemination using donor gametes or ask for prenatal monitoring with the possibility of terminating their pregnancy if there is an affected fetus. The choices are difficult and will be determined by a combination of factors, such as previous experience with an affected child or relative, the severity of the disorder and possibilities of adequate treatment, the presence of one or more healthy children, socio-economic factors, the age of the counsellees, the appraisal of the genetic risk, and the psychological strength of the couple. Other basic values are also involved; these are determined mainly by education, social background, tradition, ethical values and religion. Here, the direct environment and society play a decisive role (see next section).

In view of rapid technological advances in medical genetics and recent changes in many societies, new problems can be anticipated, in addition to the many questions that already need answers.

Which risks are considered as 'acceptable by everybody': 'low', 'moderate', 'high' or 'unacceptable'? Will counsellees be allowed to decide for themselves which risk is acceptable or not? Which criteria are being used to define whether a fetal abnormality, a handicap in childhood or a disease in adulthood is severe enough to warrant avoidance by abortion? Given financial constraints in health care, will society set limits to the magnitude of a risk and the severity of a handicap warranting further action? Do individuals have the right to refuse investigations when they fall within such limits and can they utilize diagnostic, therapeutic or preventive approaches at their own cost when they are not formally eligible? If so, how can equality of access to health care facilities still be guaranteed?

Up to now genetic counselling and neonatal screening and diagnosis have dealt mainly with information to parents about their child. In the (near) future genetics will be more and more concerned with providing information to adults about carrier status and risks of manifesting a disease in later life. Will people have the right not to know? 'Of course', everybody will answer, but the reality is less simple. Interviews with possible carriers of the gene causing Huntington chorea show that some people want to use modern DNA diagnosis but others do not want to know. If a young person at risk decides to ask for a DNA test, because for example, he does not want to transmit the mutant gene to his progeny, the diagnostic result may also imply carriership and hence future clinical deterioration, in one of his parents, who may not want to know. In the future there will be more situations where decisions by young adults may result in undesired information to their parents and other relatives.

Another problem to be solved is the restriction of information. If a person asks for genetic counselling the results of the examination may point to certain risks to the counsellee's health. If so, he or she may well be forced to provide this information to a future employer, mortgage bank, life insurance company or health insurance organization, and this may affect various aspects of the counsellee's life. Such problems will arise on a larger scale if, as predicted by some experts, new techniques enable the analysis of a larger number of genes known to be involved in major disorders. As yet, we have very little idea of how early knowledge of risks or certainties about manifesting a disease will influence people's relationships, behaviour and intrinsic feelings.

The clinical geneticist will only be able to participate fruitfully in future discussions about such complex issues if more data become available on the psychosocial aspects of reproduction, infertility, carrier status and early knowledge of incurable diseases.

Fortunately there is still time for this because the period between a breakthrough in research and large-scale application in health care is usually much longer than that anticipated by the expert and hoped for by the individual at risk.

Societies

Throughout almost the whole history of mankind individual couples needed 6-8 children if one son were to survive his father. The average life expectancy at birth was 20 years among (pre)agricultural men, and increased to 30-40 years during the (pre)industrial period. Most people were confronted daily with the fight for survival, anxiety, suffering and the loss of people in their own family or direct neighbourhood. Most people had no expectations of any real improvement in their situation, let alone the ability to exert any influence themselves.

It is only during the last century that dramatic changes in reproduction, (child) mortality, and the possibilities of preventing disease have occurred. Unfortunately, most of the improvements have remained restricted to the wealthy industrialized countries, although impressive progress is also being made in some parts of the developing world.

In most industrialized countries social security is such that a couple no longer needs children to ensure adequate financial support when they reach an advanced age or if they lose employment earlier. A combination of socio-economic factors and the availability of reliable contraceptives has led to a marked decline of the birth rate in many of these countries. Unfortunately in several other countries, i.e. most Central and East European countries, but also in Japan and the Third World, many unwanted pregnancies still occur and are terminated. Secondary infertility often results from these recurrent abortions.

In many countries of the world the average life expectancy at birth has increased during the last 50 years. In some Western European and Scandinavian countries and Japan it has become as high as 80 years for women and 72-74 years for men. This is mainly due to a marked decrease of infant mortality (6-10 per 1000) which has been accompanied by a very low birth rate of 10-13 per 1000. In other countries with a low or moderate child mortality, such as the Central and Eastern European countries, USSR, Canada, USA, Australia, New Zealand, Cuba, Costa Rica, Hong Kong, Singapore and the P.R. China, the birth rate is somewhat higher (16-19 per 1000), but still low compared with the rest of the world.

The previous section discussed how congenital disorders have become the major cause of infant mortality and morbidity in the (30) countries with a low infant mortality (< 25 per 1000). Socioeconomic reasons for couples in industrialized countries to utilize more frequently methods of early diagnosis and prevention of congenital handicaps have also been discussed. One other major reason for the increasing interest in clinical genetics from the point of view of politicians, health authorities and insurance companies in the wealthy countries is the high cost of medical and psychosocial care of the chronically handicapped. A favourable cost-benefit analysis has been used repeatedly by clinical geneticists to acquire support for new methods in prenatal and postnatal diagnosis.

Most scientific and technical advances in medical genetics have been accomplished in Western countries. Experts from these countries sometimes calculate the overall burden of genetic disease in the world and extrapolate the measures to be taken from experience in their own country or even in their own region. In doing so it should be realized that in large parts of the developing world a situation such as that described at the beginning of this section still exists. In some 40 countries, such as India, Pakistan, Bangladesh and many African countries, involving a total of 1.5 billion people, the infant mortality still varies from 100-200 per 1000, and the average life expectancy at birth is 45 years. In another 35 countries, including Indonesia, Brazil, Mexico and various countries in the Middle East, Central America and Africa, involving one billion people, the infant mortality is still 50–100 per 1000.

This implies that at least half the world population is still mainly concerned with its daily survival. In the poorest countries, those with a gross national product per capita (GNP) from less than $100 to $2500 per year, most couples have 6–8 children and lose several of them because of undernutrition and infectious diseases. Between 53% and 84% of the adult females in the 75 poorest countries are still illiterate. This implies that they cannot easily be reached with information about the use of modern contraceptives, let alone carrier detection for haemoglobinopathies or prenatal monitoring.

Generalisations about 'developed' and 'developing' countries are, however, not always justified. The P.R. China for instance, with a total population of about 1100 million people, a GNP of about $300 per capita per year, and 80–85% of its labour force in agriculture, considers itself as a developing country. Yet it has succeeded in reducing the overall mortality from 25 per 1000 in 1960 to 6–7 per 1000 in 1984, and the average life expectancy at birth has increased to nearly 70 years for women and 67 years for men. A strong governmental population policy, including a very efficient network of public information and motivation, has led to a marked reduction of the birth rate which dropped from 43 per 1000 in 1963 to about 17 per 1000 in 1984. In 1981 60% of couples already had a 'one-child certificate' indicating that they were limiting their family size to this number. The use of intrauterine devices and sterilization (usually of females) accounts for 85% of contraception. In the context of the restrictive population policy, the relatively low infant mortality, and the regional high incidence of certain congenital malformations, it is not surprising that this developing country pays increasing attention to the creation of facilities for laboratory diagnosis of genetic disease, genetic counselling and fetal diagnosis.

Other examples of countries with a relatively low income which nevertheless have succeeded in achieving a low infant mortality are Costa Rica, Jamaica and Cuba. The latter country spends much of its income on education and health care and, in spite of limited resources, has a good functioning system of clinical genetics services, including maternal serum AFP screening, neonatal screening for PKU and congenital hypothyroidism, carrier screening for haemoglobinopathies, and prenatal cytogenetics and biochemistry.

On the other hand there are countries like Libya, Oman and Saudi Arabia with a (very) high national income (up to $20 000 GNP per capita) and an infant mortality which is still too high. In some of the Arab countries the epidemiology and planning of necessary facilities for diagnosing genetic disorders are complicated by the high proportion (up to 66%) of temporary immigrants from a wide variety of countries and ethnic origins. The proportion of consanguineous marriages among the local inhabitants is not known exactly, but some have mentioned 20–40%, others even 50–80%. In a major hospital in Abu Dhabi (U.A.E.) the overall incidence of major congenital abnormalities detectable at birth (1.2%) was, however, no higher than elsewhere.

Since the incidence of certain haemoglobinopathies is relatively high in some Arab countries in the Middle East, attention has been given to the acceptability of various clinical genetics services. Again, generalization about the attitude of Islam towards genetics is not justified, since there are many different opinions, just as in other major religions. According to some religious leaders consulted in the United Arab Emirates, the Koran discourages consanguineous marriage, couples may refrain from pregnancy if they are at high risk of having affected offspring, and certain methods of birth control are acceptable if this contributes to the quality of the family. Prenatal diagnosis as such is acceptable, but termination of a pregnancy would be forbidden ('harran') after 120 days; it is permitted before 40 days ('hallal'), and in the period between 40–120 days it is allowed but not liked ('marrouh'). The latter would imply that chorionic villus analysis would in principle be feasible in certain Islamic populations. Discussions with leading obstetricians in some of the Arab countries suggest, however, that there may be large discrepancies between what is officially allowed by religious leaders and what is or is not done in practice based on traditions over centuries.

The more one travels and learns about different political systems, religions, traditions and a variety of socioeconomic factors, the more one realizes how different the role of medical genetics must be in different societies. Unfortunately most of us will judge the behaviour and activities in other societies from the point of view of our own background and moral values. The government of the USA has stopped its financial support of the United Nations Fund for Population Activities because it opposes family planning programmes as pursued, for instance, in the P.R. China. Yet visitors will not see malnourished children in this enormous country which has nearly 20 million births annually. This accomplishment becomes even more evident when one is confronted with the impressive malnutrition, suffering and loss of life in neighbouring Asian countries where family planning programmes are not so successful.

Another sensitive issue is the use of prenatal diagnosis to determine fetal sex, followed by selective termination if the fetus is female, in some countries like India. Again, most Western geneticists will find it difficult or impossible to accept such measures as being justified by the long history of preference for male progeny, which for a long time also prevailed in the Chinese culture.

It will be equally difficult for many to understand why in Japan, a country with the lowest infant mortality in the world (6 per 1000) and a high scientific and technical level, prenatal diagnosis has not really developed. The explanation provided by leading Japanese colleagues is that termination of a pregnancy on the basis of inequality is not culturally acceptable. This is in contrast to the reality of a very high number of abortions of unwanted pregnancies. 'This is completely acceptable here because these abortions are done for socioeconomic reasons and not on the basis of a judgement about the value of a fetus' was the remark of a Japanese representative at the International Conference on Bioethics in Paris, in 1985.

These examples are only a limited illustration of the enormous differences between societies. Within Western societies there are also major differences in the organization of health care, access to clinical genetics services and attitudes towards reproduction, genetic testing, fetal diagnosis and abortion. In most European countries health care, including facilities for clinical genetics, is supported by the government or national health (insurance) organizations and there is equal access for all people. In the USA the same is true for some basic facilities, but the emphasis on commercialization of diagnostic services, including those of genetic diagnosis, is much stronger. As a consequence the utilization rates among different groups of people may be very different. Also, the presence of many different ethnic groups in the USA complicates generalizations about the utilization of certain health care facilities. It is expected that by the year 2000 one third of all school children in the United States will be 'minorities'.

Experience with carrier screening for Tay-Sachs disease among Ashkenazi Jews, for sickle-cell anaemia among the Black population in the USA and for β-thalassaemia among Mediterranean populations has shown that a variety of requirements must be fulfilled to achieve sufficient participation. Among these, optimal information on the population concerned, a well prepared organization, and the collaboration of local health authorities and community and religious leaders are essential. The success of some programmes and the failure of others are another indication of the complex problems of integrating a medical technology with the many social and moral aspects of a population. A thorough analysis of the various factors leading to (non) acceptance of diagnostic, therapeutic and preventive methods in medical genetics is also of great importance for adequate planning of the utilization of future technologies.

Such studies have already shown that people at risk of having affected offspring who have different ethnic, cultural and religious backgrounds may react very differently towards similar options of avoiding the birth of a handicapped child. The decision not to reproduce is unacceptable in some societies and for some couples, and will be easier to accept in societies where voluntary childlessness has become generally accepted. The decision to terminate a pregnancy is legally unacceptable in large parts of the world, including Latin America, involving more than 360 million people, several states of the USA and countries of the Middle East.

In other societies, i.e. nearly all European countries, termination of a pregnancy before 20–24 weeks has been legalized during the last decade or two, and an increasing proportion of couples at risk choose this option as a means of preventing the birth of a handicapped child. Yet even in these countries it has taken some 15 years after the introduction of prenatal diagnosis for a significant utilization rate to be achieved.

Follow-up studies on women at risk who decided not to use facilities for prenatal diagnosis indicate that moral objections, insufficient information, fear of the procedure or loss of the pregnancy, and simply the idea 'that everything would be all right' were the main reasons for not asking for prenatal monitoring.

It is to be hoped that in the future medical genetics will play an increasing role in countries which now have to focus on fighting poverty, undernutrition and infectious diseases.

Another challenge is to create a situation where new generations of people will have sufficient knowledge about their own risks and the various alternatives to avoid having handicapped offspring. People should have the freedom to decide about their own lives and that of their children, and to make choices that fit best with their personal circumstances, religion, traditional and ethical backgrounds, and their socioeconomic and psychological strengths. It must be possible to provide optimal medical and psychosocial care to those who are handicapped and at the same time to stimulate prevention.

The challenges for the future will be different according to the interest of the reader, his or her background, training and position, the facilities available and the society to which he or she belongs. Whatever choice is made: work on DNA, proteins, chromosomes or cells, participation in clinical genetics, the organization of health care, or even changing some aspects of society, there is still much, and interesting, work for everybody to do.

ACKNOWLEDGEMENTS

The help of Dr G C Grosveld, Dr A W M van der Kamp, Prof M F Niermeyer and Dr D J J Halley is greatly appreciated.

FURTHER READING

Bender W, Peifer M 1987 Oncogenes take wing. Cell 50: 519–520

Bishop J M 1985 Viral oncogenes. Cell 42: 23–28

Bloch M, Fahy M, Fox S, Hayden M R 1989 Predictive testing for Huntington disease. American Journal of Medical Genetics 32: 217–224

Brambati B, Simoni G, Fabro S (eds) 1986 Chorionic villus sampling; fetal diagnosis of genetic diseases in the first trimester. Marcel Dekker, New York

Cao A 1987 Results of programmes for antenatal detection of thalassaemia in reducing the incidence of the disorder. Blood Reviews 1: 169–176

Cold Spring Harbor Symposia on quantitative biology 1986 vol LI Molecular Biology of Homo Sapiens. Cold Spring Harbor Lab, New York

Das R C, Robbins P W (eds) 1987 Protein transfer and organelle biogenesis. Academic Press, New York

Edelman G M, Thiery J P (eds) 1985 The cell in contact, adhesions and junctions as morphogenetic determinants. John Wiley, New York

Evers-Kieboom G, van den Berghe H 1979 Impact of genetic counselling: a review of published follow-up studies. Clinical Genetics 15: 465–474

Friedmann T 1990 The human genome project — some implications of extensive 'reverse genetic' medicine. American Journal of Human Genetics 46: 407–414

Grosveld F, Blom van Assendelft G, Greaves D, Kollias G 1987 Position-independent high level expression of the human β-globin gene in transgenic mice. Cell 51: 975–985

Grouchy J de, Turleau C 1987 Mendelian disorders and autosomal structural rearrangements. In: Sandberg A (ed) Progress and topics in cytogenetics. Liss, New York

Gusella J F 1986 Recombinant DNA techniques in the diagnosis of inherited disorders. Journal of Clinical Investigation 77: 1723–1726

Hunter T 1987 A thousand and one protein kinases. Review Cell 50: 823–829

Kaback M M (ed) 1977 Tay-Sachs disease: screening and prevention. Liss, New York

Kerem B, Rommens J M, Buchanan J A et al 1989 Identification of the cystic fibrosis gene: genetic analysis. Science 245: 1073–1079

Kogan S C, Doherty M, Gitschier J 1987 An improved method for prenatal diagnosis of genetic diseases by analysis of amplified DNA sequences. Science 317: 985–990

Kornfeld S 1986 Trafficking of lysosomal enzymes in normal and disease states. Journal of Clinical Investigation 77: 1–6

Kuliev A, Modell B, Galjaard H (eds) 1985 Perspectives in fetal diagnosis of congenital disorders. WHO/Serono report, Ares-Serono Symp, Rome

Kunkel T A, Roberts J D, Zakon R A 1987 and efficient site-specific mutagenesis without phenotypic selection. Methods in Enzymology 154: 367–382

Le Douarin N, McLaren A (eds) 1984 Chimeras in developmental biology. Academic Press, New York

McKusick V A 1988 Mendelian Inheritance in Man, 8th edn. Johns Hopkins University Press, Baltimore

Murphy D, Hanson J 1987 The production of transgenic mice by the microinjection of cloned DNA into fertilized one-cell eggs. In: Glover D M (ed) DNA — cloning, a practical approach, vol. 3. IRL Press, Oxford, p 213–248

Ott J 1985 Analysis of human genetic linkage. University Press, Baltimore

Rothman J E 1987 Protein sorting by selective retention in the endoplasmic reticulum and Golgi Stack. Cell 50: 521–522

Spranger J, Benirschke R, Hall J G et al 1982 Errors of Morphogenesis: concepts and terms. Recommendations of an International Working Group. Journal of Pediatrics 100: 160–165

Todd J A, Bell J I, McDevitt H O 1987 HLA-DQβ gene contributes to susceptibility and resistance to insulin-dependent diabetes. Nature 329: 599–604

UNESCO report 1986 The State of World's Children. Oxford University Press

Vogel F, Sperling K (eds) 1987 Human Genetics, Proceedings of the 7th International Congress, Berlin 1986. Springer, Heidelberg

Weinberg R A 1985 The action of oncogenes in the cytoplasm and nucleus. Science 230: 770–776

Wertz D C, Fletscher J C 1989 Ethical problems in prenatal diagnosis: a cross-cultural survey of medical geneticists in 12 nations. Prenatal Diagnosis 9: 145–157

INDEX

Index

Volumes 1 and 2